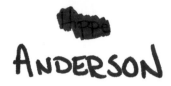

ANDERSON

D1307725

Current Veterinary Therapy 4

Food Animal Practice

Current Veterinary Therapy 4

Food Animal Practice

JIMMY L. HOWARD, D.V.M., M.S.
Diplomate, A.B.V.P. (Food Animal Practice)
Amarillo, Texas

Associate Editor
ROBERT A. SMITH, D.V.M., M.S.
Diplomate, A.B.V.P.
McCasland Chair in Beef Health and Production
Oklahoma State University
College of Veterinary Medicine
Stillwater, Oklahoma

W.B. SAUNDERS COMPANY
A Division of Harcourt Brace & Company
Philadelphia   London   Toronto   Montreal   Sydney   Tokyo

W.B. SAUNDERS COMPANY
A Division of Harcourt Brace & Company

The Curtis Center
Independence Square West
Philadelphia, Pennsylvania 19106

Library of Congress Cataloging-in-Publication Data

Main entry under title:

Current veterinary therapy.

Includes index.

ISBN 0–7216–7654–5

1. Veterinary medicine.   I. Howard, Jimmy L.   II. Title: Food animal practice 4

SF745.C784 1999   636.089′55   85-2006

CURRENT VETERINARY THERAPY 4: Food Animal Practice   ISBN 0–7216–7654–5

Printed in the United States of America.

Last digit is the print number: 9   8   7   6   5   4   3   2   1

I would like to dedicate this fourth edition of *Current Veterinary Therapy: Food Animal Practice* to a very dear friend and colleague, Dr. H. W. Leipold, who died suddenly in the interim since the last edition was published. Horst was a very special friend while I was at Kansas State University and had remained so until his death. He had contributed to all three of the previous editions of this book.

Horst was one of the most well-known pathologists in the world, with a specialty in congenital diseases. He was loved by his students, both graduate and undergraduate, and by the members of the faculty with whom he worked.

At the time of his death he was a well-respected professor of pathology at Kansas State University.

The profession has again lost a very fine member, and he will certainly be missed by all who knew him.

So this edition is in your memory, Horst.

J.L.H.

Contributors

David E. Anderson, D.V.M., M.S., Diplomate, A.C.V.S.
Assistant Professor, Food Animal Section, Department of Veterinary Clinical Sciences, College of Veterinary Medicine, The Ohio State University, Columbus, Ohio.
Abomasal Impactions of Cattle; Intestinal Volvulus in Cattle; Intraluminal Intestinal Obstruction: Trichobezoars, Phytobezoars, and Enteroliths; Intussusception; Intraluminal-Intramural Hemorrhage of the Small Intestine in Cattle; Fractures; Tendon Injuries in Cattle

Mike Apley, D.V.M., Ph.D., Diplomate, A.C.V.C.P.
Assistant Professor, Beef Production Medicine, College of Veterinary Medicine, Iowa State University, Ames, Iowa.
Bovine Respiratory Disease; Respiratory Disease Therapeutics; Section 10: Respiratory Diseases

Louis F. Archbald, D.V.M., M.S., Ph.D., M.R.C.V.S., Diplomate, A.C.T.
Professor, College of Veterinary Medicine, University of Florida, Gainesville, Florida.
Pyometra in Cattle; Dairy Herd Reproductive Efficiency; Section 13: Reproductive Diseases

Robert G. Arther, Ph.D.
Project Manager, Clinical Development, Bayer Corporation, Agriculture Division, Animal Health, Shawnee, Kansas.
External Parasiticides

Thomas L. Bailey, D.V.M., M.S., A.C.T.
Assistant Professor, Virginia-Maryland Regional College of Veterinary Medicine, Virginia Polytechnic Institute and State University, Blacksburg, Virginia.
Dairy Heifer Development and Monitoring

Aubrey N. Baird, D.V.M., M.S.
Associate Professor of Large Animal Surgery, Auburn University, Auburn, Alabama.
Interdigital Phlegmon (Interdigital Necrobacillosis); Fescue Foot

E. Lee Belden, Ph.D.
Department of Veterinary Science, College of Agriculture, University of Wyoming, Laramie, Wyoming.
Selenium Toxicosis

Dennis J. Blodgett, D.V.M., Ph.D.
Associate Professor, Virginia-Maryland Regional College of Veterinary Medicine, Virginia Polytechnic Institute and State University, Blacksburg, Virginia.
Renal Toxicants

Carole A. Bolin, D.V.M., Ph.D.
Research Leader, Zoonotic Diseases Research Unit, U.S. Department of Agriculture, National Animal Disease Center, Ames, Iowa.
Leptospirosis

Dawn M. Boothe, D.V.M., Ph.D.
Associate Professor, Department of Veterinary Physiology and Pharmacology, College of Veterinary Medicine, Texas A&M University, College Station, Texas.
Adverse Drug Reactions

Robert T. Brandt, Jr., Ph.D., M.S.
Adjunct Professor, Kansas State University, Manhattan, Kansas; Senior Professional Services Specialist, Hoechst Roussel Vet, Overland Park, Kansas.
Growth-Promoting Implants and Feed Additives in Beef Cattle Production

Deborah J. Briggs, Ph.D.
Director, Rabies Laboratory, College of Veterinary Medicine, Kansas State University, Manhattan, Kansas.
Rabies in Food Animals

Gordon W. Brumbaugh, D.V.M., Ph.D.
Associate Professor, Department of Veterinary Physiology and Pharmacology, College of Veterinary Medicine, Texas A&M University, College Station, Texas.
Adverse Drug Reactions

Marie S. Bulgin, D.V.M., M.B.A.
Professor and Clinician, Department of Animal and Veterinary Science, Caine Veterinary Teaching Center, University of Idaho, Caldwell, Idaho.
Ovine Production Medicine

R. L. Carson, D.V.M., M.S., Diplomate, A.C.T.
Associate Professor, Department of Large Animal Surgery and Medicine, College of Veterinary Medicine, Auburn University, Auburn, Alabama.
Diseases of the Penis and Prepuce; Diseases of the Male Internal Genitalia

Thomas L. Carson, D.V.M., Ph.D.
Veterinary Toxicologist and Professor, Veterinary Diagnostic Laboratory, College of Veterinary Medicine, Iowa State University, Ames, Iowa.
Investigating Feed Problems; Toxic Gases; Ergotism

Stan W. Casteel, D.V.M., Ph.D., Diplomate, A.B.V.T.
Associate Professor, Veterinary Toxicology, College of Veterinary Medicine, University of Missouri, Columbia, Missouri.
Lead Poisoning; Principal Toxic Plants of the Midwestern and Eastern States; Hepatotoxic Plants

Christopher K. Cebra, V.M.D., M.A., M.S., Diplomate, A.C.V.I.M.
Assistant Professor, Large Animal Internal Medicine, College of Veterinary Medicine, Oregon State University, Corvallis, Oregon.
Dermatologic Disorders of Sheep

Christopher C. L. Chase, D.V.M., M.S., Ph.D.
Associate Professor, Department of Veterinary Science, South
Dakota State University, Brookings, South Dakota; Associate
Veterinarian, Flandreau Veterinary Clinic, Flandreau, South
Dakota.
Porcine Reproductive and Respiratory Syndrome

M. M. Chengappa, D.V.M., Ph.D.
Department of Diagnostic Medicine/Pathobiology, College of
Veterinary Medicine, Kansas State University, Manhattan,
Kansas.
Anthrax; Section 8: Bacterial Diseases

Norbert K. Chirase, M.S., Ph.D.
Professor of Animal Science, West Texas A&M University,
Canyon, Texas; Research Animal Scientist, Texas Agricultural
Experiment Station, Amarillo, Texas.
Mineral Supplementation of Beef Cattle: Rangeland and Feedlot

Bruce L. Clark, D.V.M., Diplomate, A.C.T.
Associate Professor, College of Veterinary Medicine,
Mississippi State University, Mississippi State, Mississippi.
Dairy Production Medicine

Cyril R. Clarke, B.V.Sc., Ph.D., Diplomate, A.C.V.C.P.
Professor of Pharmacology, Department of Anatomy,
Pathology, and Pharmacology, College of Veterinary Medicine,
Oklahoma State University, Stillwater, Oklahoma.
Pasteurellosis in Cattle

Bill C. Clymer, Ph.D.
Adjunct Professor, West Texas A&M University, Amarillo,
Texas; Livestock Parasitologist, Fort Dodge Animal Health,
Fort Dodge, Iowa.
Ticks and Mites

Carmen M. H. Colitz, D.V.M., Ph.D.
Resident in Veterinary Ophthalmology, Veterinary Teaching
Hospital, North Carolina State University, Raleigh, North
Carolina.
Food Animal Ocular Neoplasia

Michael T. Collins, D.V.M., Ph.D.
Professor of Microbiology, School of Veterinary Medicine,
University of Wisconsin, Madison, Wisconsin.
Paratuberculosis (Johne's Disease)

Anthony W. Confer, D.V.M., Ph.D., Diplomate, A.C.V.P.
Endowed Chair for Food Animal Research, Professor of
Pathology, Department Head, Department of Anatomy,
Pathology and Pharmacology, College of Veterinary Medicine,
Oklahoma State University, Stillwater, Oklahoma.
Pasteurellosis in Cattle

Peter D. Constable, B.V.Sc., M.S., Ph.D.
Section Head, Food Animal Medicine and Surgery,
Department of Veterinary Clinical Medicine, University of
Illinois, Urbana, Illinois.
*Therapeutic Management of Cardiovascular Diseases; The
Ruminant Forestomach; Cecocolic Dilation and Volvulus; Atresia
Coli*

Victor S. Cortese, D.V.M., Diplomate, A.B.V.P.
Managing Veterinarian, Cattle Technical Services, Pfizer
Animal Health, Exton, Pennsylvania.
*Neonatal Immunology; Bovine Virus Diarrhea Virus and Mucosal
Disease*

Robert M. Corwin, D.V.M., Ph.D.
Professor, Parasitology-Veterinary, Department of Veterinary
Pathobiology, College of Veterinary Medicine, University of
Missouri, Columbia, Missouri.
Anthelmintic Therapy

Glenn H. Coulter, Ph.D., P.Ag.
Assistant Director, Agriculture and Agri-Food Canada,
Lethbridge Research Centre, Lethbridge, Alberta, Canada.
Management Programs for Developing Beef Bulls

Victor S. Cox, D.V.M., Ph.D.
Associate Professor, Department of Veterinary Pathobiology,
College of Veterinary Medicine, University of Minnesota, St.
Paul, Minnesota.
Downer Cow Syndrome

Timothy B. Crawford, D.V.M., Ph.D.
Associate Professor of Virology and Pathology, Department of
Veterinary Microbiology and Pathology, Washington State
University, Pullman, Washington.
Malignant Catarrhal Fever

Scott Dee, D.V.M., M.S., Ph.D.
Adjunct Professor, Department of Clinical and Population
Sciences, University of Minnesota College of Veterinary
Medicine, St. Paul, Minnesota; Swine Practitioner, Swine
Health Center, Morris, Minnesota.
Actinomyces suis *Infection*

Stanley M. Dennis, B.V.Sc., Ph.D., F.R.C.V.S., F.R.C.Path.
Professor of Pathology, College of Veterinary Medicine,
Kansas State University, Manhattan, Kansas.
Listeriosis (Circling Disease, Silage Sickness)

Linda A. Detwiler, D.V.M.
Senior Staff Veterinarian, Emergency Programs Staff, U.S.
Department of Agriculture, Animal and Plant Health
Inspection Service, Veterinary Services, Robbinsville, New
Jersey.
Bovine Spongiform Encephalopathy

**Thomas J. Divers, D.V.M., Diplomate, A.C.V.I.M,
A.C.V.E.C.C.**
Professor of Medicine, Cornell University, Ithaca, New York.
Diseases of the Nervous System; Section 16: Neurologic Diseases

John C. Doyle II, M.S., D.V.M., Ph.D.
Consultant, IAP Pty. Ltd., Toowoomba, Queensland, Australia.
Mineral Supplementation of Beef Cattle: Rangeland and Feedlot

J. P. Dubey, M.V.Sc., Ph.D.
Microbiologist, Parasite Biology and Epidemiology Laboratory,
Livestock and Poultry Sciences Institute, U.S. Department of
Agriculture, Beltsville, Maryland.
Toxoplasmosis; Sarcocystosis

Oliver Duran, D.V.M., Ph.D.
Assistant Professor, College of Veterinary Medicine, Michigan
State University, East Lansing, Michigan.
Causal Factors in Swine Pneumonia

Neil Dyer, D.V.M., M.S., A.C.V.P.
Assistant Professor, Diagnostic Pathologist, North Dakota
State University, Department of Veterinary and Micro
Sciences, Fargo, North Dakota.
Bovine Respiratory Syncytial Virus

Terry J. Engelken, D.V.M., M.S.
Assistant Professor, Diagnostic and Field Service Program, College of Veterinary Medicine, Mississippi State University, Mississippi State, Mississippi.
Breeding Season Evaluation of Beef Herds; Section 3: Herd Health Management

James England, D.V.M., Ph.D.
Director and Professor, Animal and Veterinary Science Department, Caine Veterinary Teaching and Research Center, Caldwell, Idaho.
Section 7: Viral Diseases

E. Denis Erickson, D.V.M., Ph.D.
Professor, Department of Veterinary Science, University of Nebraska, Lincoln, Nebraska.
Streptococcal Disease

Melvyn L. Fahning, M.S., D.V.M., Ph.D.
Professor and Head, Division of Theriogenology, Clinical and Population Science Department, College of Veterinary Medicine, University of Minnesota, St. Paul, Minnesota.
Retained Fetal Membranes

John M. Fairbrother, B.V.Sc., Ph.D.
Professor, Department of Pathology and Microbiology, Faculté de Médecine Vétérinaire, Université de Montréal, St. Hyacinthe, Québec, Canada.
Escherichia coli *Infections in Farm Animals*

Darrell Farmer, D.V.M.
Animal Medical Clinic, Tucumcari, New Mexico.
Practical Immunology

Gilles Fecteau, D.M.V., Diplomate, A.C.V.I.M.
Associate Professor, University of Montreal, St. Hyacinthe, Québec, Canada.
Abomasal Physiology, and Dilation, Displacement, and Volvulus

Brad Fenwick, D.V.M., M.S., Ph.D., Diplomate, A.C.V.I.M.
Department of Diagnostic Medicine/Pathobiology, College of Veterinary Medicine, Kansas State University, Manhattan, Kansas.
Actinobacillus suis *Infection; Porcine Contagious Pleuropneumonia*

Melissa R. Finley, D.V.M., Diplomate, A.C.V.I.M.
Assistant Professor, Section of Agricultural Practices, Kansas State University, Manhattan, Kansas.
Listeriosis (Circling Disease, Silage Sickness)

Sherrill Fleming, D.V.M., Diplomate, A.C.V.I.M. and A.B.V.P. (Food Animal)
Associate Professor, Food Animal Medicine, Diagnostic Laboratory and Field Services Department, College of Veterinary Medicine, Mississippi State University, Mississippi State, Mississippi.
Ovine and Caprine Respiratory Disease: Infectious Agents, Management Factors, and Preventive Strategies

James G. Floyd, Jr., D.V.M., M.S.
Extension Veterinarian and Professor, Department of Animal and Dairy Sciences, Auburn University, Auburn, Alabama.
Urolithiasis in Food Animals (Urinary Calculi, Waterbelly, Calculosis)

Deborah S. Friedman, D.V.M., Diplomate, A.C.V.O.
Clinical Ophthalmologist, Animal Emergency Center, Milwaukee, Wisconsin.
Ophthalmology of South American Camelids: Llamas, Alpacas, Guanacos, and Vicuñas

Francis D. Galey, D.V.M., Ph.D., Diplomate, A.B.V.T.
Associate Professor of Clinical Diagnostic Veterinary Toxicology, California Veterinary Diagnostic Laboratory System—Toxicology, Davis, California.
Tremorgenic Mycotoxins; Oleander (Nerium oleander) *Toxicosis*

Dale R. Gardner, Ph.D.
Research Chemist, U.S. Department of Agriculture, Animal Research Service, Poisonous Plant Research Laboratory, Logan, Utah.
Principal Poisonous Plants of the Western United States

Tam Garland, D.V.M., Ph.D.
Research Veterinarian, Department of Veterinary Physiology and Pharmacology, College of Veterinary Medicine, Texas A&M University, College Station, Texas.
Principal Toxic Plants of the Southwestern United States

Franklyn B. Garry, D.V.M., M.S., Diplomate, A.C.V.I.M.
Associate Professor, Food Animal Medicine and Surgery, Colorado State University, Fort Collins, Colorado.
Rumen Putrefaction (Esophageal Groove Dysfunction, Rumen Drinkers)

H. Allen Garverick, Ph.D.
Professor, University of Missouri, Columbia, Missouri.
Ovarian Follicular Dynamics and Endocrine Profiles in Cows With Ovarian Follicular Cysts

Brian J. Gerloff, D.V.M., Ph.D.
Owner, Seneca Bovine Services, Marengo, Illinois.
Ketosis; Fatty Liver in Dairy Cattle

Brian G. Gilger, D.V.M., M.S., Diplomate, A.C.V.O.
Associate Professor, Ophthalmology, Department of Companion Animal and Special Species Medicine, College of Veterinary Medicine, North Carolina State University, Raleigh, North Carolina.
Food Animal Ocular Neoplasia

Donald R. Gill, M.S., Ph.D.
Extension Animal Nutritionist, Oklahoma State University, Stillwater, Oklahoma.
Backgrounding and Stocker Calf Management

Juliet Rathbone Gionfriddo, D.V.M., M.S., Diplomate, A.C.V.O.
Assistant Professor of Comparative Ophthalmology, Purdue University, West Lafayette, Indiana.
Ophthalmology of South American Camelids: Llamas, Alpacas, Guanacos, and Vicuñas

M. Daniel Givens, D.V.M.
Theriogenology Resident, College of Veterinary Medicine, Auburn University, Auburn, Alabama.
Potential of Embryo Transfer for Infectious Disease Control

Robert D. Glock, D.V.M., Ph.D.
Director, Arizona Veterinary Diagnostic Laboratory, University of Arizona, Tucson, Arizona.
Swine Dysentery

Jesse P. Goff, D.V.M., Ph.D.
Veterinary Medical Officer, Metabolic Diseases and Immunology Unit, National Animal Disease Center, U.S. Department of Agriculture, Agricultural Research Service, Ames, Iowa.
Milk Fever (Parturient Paresis) in Cows, Ewes, and Doe Goats; Phosphorus Deficiency; Ruminant Hypomagnesemic Tetanies

Daniel H. Gould, D.V.M., Ph.D. Diplomate, AB. V.T.
Professor of Pathology, Department of Pathology, College of
Veterinary Medicine and Biomedical Sciences, Colorado State
University, Fort Collins, Colorado.
Toxic Syndromes Associated With Sulfur

Dee Griffin, D.V.M., M.S.
Great Plains Veterinary Educational Center, University of
Nebraska, Clay Center, Nebraska.
Section 4: Dietary Management

Charles Guard, Ph.D., D.V.M.
Associate Professor of Medicine, Ambulatory and Production
Medicine Clinic, Cornell University, Ithaca, New York.
Super Foot Rot; Digital Dermatitis

John C. Haliburton, D.V.M., Ph.D.
Head, Diagnostic Toxicology, Texas Veterinary Medical
Diagnostic Laboratory, Amarillo, Texas.
*Nonprotein Nitrogen–Induced Ammonia Toxicosis in Ruminants;
Nitrate Poisoning Associated With the Consumption of Forages or Hay*

Mark R. Hall, Ph.D.
Professor, School of Veterinary Medicine, College of
Agriculture, Professor, Department of Microbiology, School of
Veterinary Medicine and School of Medicine, University of
Nevada, Reno, Nevada.
Bovine Trichomoniasis

Ralph F. Hall, D.V.M.
Professor Emeritus, Large Animal Clinical Sciences, College of
Veterinary Medicine, University of Tennessee, Knoxville,
Tennessee.
Nonparasitic Skin Diseases of Swine

Edward D. Hamilton, D.V.M., M.Agr.
Associate Professor, Veterinary Science, South Dakota State
University, Brookings, South Dakota.
Standardized Performance Analysis

Donald R. Hanks, D.V.M.
Professor and Department Chair, School of Veterinary
Medicine, University of Nevada, Reno, Nevada.
Bovine Trichomoniasis

Donald E. Hansen, D.V.M., M.P.V.M.
Extension Veterinarian, College of Veterinary Medicine,
Oregon State University, Corvallis, Oregon.
The Bovine Practitioner's Role in Beef Quality Assurance

Roger B. Harvey, D.V.M., M.S.
Veterinary Medical Officer (Toxicology), U.S. Department of
Agriculture, Agricultural Research Service, Food Animal
Protection Research Laboratory, College Station, Texas.
Aflatoxins; Trichothecenes

Steve Henry, D.V.M.
Abilene Animal Hospital, Abilene, Kansas.
Porcine Contagious Pleuropneumonia

R. P. Herd, M.V.Sc., Ph.D.
Emeritus Professor, College of Veterinary Medicine, The Ohio
State University, Columbus, Ohio.
Helminth Parasites of the Gastrointestinal Tract

**Thomas H. Herdt, D.V.M., M.S., Diplomate, A.C.V.N. and
A.C.V.I.M.**
Professor, Department of Large Animal Clinical Sciences and
Animal Health Diagnostic Laboratory, Michigan State
University, East Lansing, Michigan.
Ketosis; Fatty Liver in Dairy Cattle; Section 5: Metabolic Diseases

Sharon K. Hietala, Ph.D.
University of California, Davis, California Veterinary
Diagnostic Laboratory System, Associate Professor of Clinical
Diagnostic Immunology, University of California, Davis,
Davis, California.
Neosporum caninum Infection and Abortion in Cattle

F. C. Hinds, M.S., Ph.D.
Professor Emeritus, Ruminant Nutrition, Department of
Animal Science, University of Wyoming, Laramie, Wyoming.
Dietary Management in Sheep

R. T. Hinnant, M.S.
Research Associate, Department of Rangeland Ecology and
Management, Texas Agricultural Experiment Station, Texas
A&M University, College Station, Texas.
*Nutritional Management of Livestock Grazing Range and Pasture
Lands*

Kent Hoblet, D.V.M., M.S.
Professor and Chairman, Department of Veterinary Preventive
Medicine, Extension Veterinarian, Dairy Cattle, The Ohio
State University, Columbus, Ohio.
Aseptic Laminitis of Cattle

Bruce W. Hoffman, D.V.M.
Veterinary Research and Consulting Services, Greeley,
Colorado.
Feedlot Production Medicine Programs

Lorraine J. Hoffman, Ph.D.
Professor and Section Leader in Bacteriology, Department of
Veterinary Diagnostic and Production Animal Medicine,
Veterinary Diagnostic Laboratory, College of Veterinary
Medicine, Iowa State University, Ames, Iowa.
Pasteurellosis in Swine

Larry D. Holler, D.V.M., Ph.D.
South Dakota State University, Animal Disease Research and
Diagnostic Laboratory, South Dakota State University,
Brookings, South Dakota.
Abortion Diagnosis in Food Animals

**Jimmy L. Howard, D.V.M., M.S., Diplomate, A.B.V.P.
(Food Animal Practice)**
Amarillo, Texas.
Section 1: Special Therapy; Section 18: Dermatologic Diseases

Bruce L. Hull, D.V.M., M.S.
Professor and Head, Department of Food Animal Medicine
and Surgery, The Ohio State University, Columbus, Ohio.
*Sole Abscesses; Vertical Wall Cracks; Horizontal Wall Cracks;
Rusterholz Ulcer; Spondylitis; Section 17: Musculoskeletal Diseases*

Elaine Hunt, D.V.M., Diplomate, A.C.V.I.M.
Associate Professor, Department of Food Animal Medicine,
College of Veterinary Medicine, North Carolina State
University, Raleigh, North Carolina.
*Diarrheal Diseases of Neonatal Calves; Section 2: Neonatal Disease
and Disease Management*

J. E. Huston, Ph.D.
Professor of Animal Science, Texas Agricultural Experiment
Station, Texas A&M University System, San Angelo, Texas.
Mineral Supplementation of Beef Cattle: Rangeland and Feedlot

Thomas J. Inzana, Ph.D.
Director, Professor of Clinical Microbiology, Virginia-Maryland Regional College of Veterinary Medicine Teaching Hospital, Virginia Polytechnic Institute and State University, Blacksburg, Virginia.
The Haemophilus somnus *Complex*

Cynthia A. Jackson, D.V.M., Diplomate, A.C.V.I.M.
Post-Doctoral Fellow, Michigan State University, East Lansing, Michigan.
Cerebellar Disease in Cattle

Lynn F. James, Ph.D.
Research Leader, U.S. Department of Agriculture Agricultural Research Service, Poisonous Plant Research Laboratory, Logan, Utah.
Principal Poisonous Plants of the Western United States

Reginald Johnson, D.V.M., M.S., Ph.D.
Research Consultant, Veterinary Research Consultants, Inc., Fort Collins, Colorado.
Bovine Leukemia Virus

Thomas R. Kasari, D.V.M., M.V.Sc., Diplomate, A.C.V.I.M.
Associate Professor of Large Animal Medicine, College of Veterinary Medicine, Texas A&M University, College Station, Texas.
Omphalitis and Its Sequelae in Ruminants

John P. Kastelic, D.V.M., Ph.D.
Research Scientist, Agriculture and Agri-Food Canada, Lethbridge Research Centre, Lethbridge, Alberta, Canada.
Management Programs for Developing Beef Bulls

William P. Kautz, D.V.M., Ph.D.
Pioneer Hybrid International, Madison, Wisconsin.
Toxicologic and Quality Evaluation of Forages and Silages

William J. Kelch, D.V.M., Ph.D.
University of Tennessee, Knoxville, Tennessee.
Fescue Toxicosis

George A. Kennedy, D.V.M., Ph.D.
Professor, Department of Diagnostic Medicine and Pathobiology, Assistant Director, Kansas Veterinary Diagnostic Laboratory, College of Veterinary Medicine, Kansas State University, Manhattan, Kansas.
Salmonellosis

Larry A. Kerr, D.V.M., M.S.
Associate Professor, College of Veterinary Medicine, University of Tennessee, Knoxville, Tennessee.
Fescue Toxicosis

Karl W. Kersting, D.V.M., M.S.
Associate Professor, Food Animal Section, College of Veterinary Medicine, Iowa State University, Ames, Iowa.
Actinobacillosis (Wooden Tongue, Woody Tongue, Big Head); Actinomycosis (Lumpy Jaw); Necrotic Stomatitis and Laryngitis (Oropharyngeal Necrobacillosis, Calf Diphtheria); Lactic Acidosis (Rumen Overload, Rumen Acidosis, Grain Overload, Engorgement Toxemia, Rumenitis)

Donald P. Knowles, Jr., D.V.M., Ph.D.
Research Leader, Animal Disease Research Unit, U.S. Department of Agriculture, Agricultural Research Service, Washington State University, Pullman, Washington.
Caprine Arthritis-Encephalitis Virus

M. M. Kothmann, M.S., Ph.D.
Professor, Department of Rangeland Ecology and Management, Texas A&M University, College Station, Texas.
Nutritional Management of Livestock Grazing Range and Pasture Lands

Jerry P. Kunesh, D.V.M., M.S., Ph.D.
Professor of Veterinary Clinical Sciences, Department of Veterinary Clinical Sciences, College of Veterinary Medicine, Iowa State University, Ames, Iowa.
Swine Erysipelas

William G. Kvasnicka, D.V.M.
Extension Veterinarian, College of Agriculture, University of Nevada, Reno, Nevada.
Bovine Trichomoniasis

Vernon C. Langston, D.V.M., Ph.D., Diplomate, A.C.V.C.P.
Associate Professor, College of Veterinary Medicine, Mississippi State University, Mississippi State, Mississippi.
Therapeutic Management of Inflammation; Antimicrobial Use in Food Animals; Therapeutic Management of Urinary Diseases

Gordon H. K. Lawson, B.V.M.&S., B.Sc., Ph.D.
Honorary Fellow, Royal (Dick) School of Veterinary Studies, Summerhall, Edinburgh, Scotland, United Kingdom.
Proliferative Enteropathy of Pigs

Hong Li, D.V.M., Ph.D.
Research Microbiologist, Animal Disease Research Unit, U.S. Department of Agriculture, Agricultural Research Service, Washington State University, Pullman, Washington.
Malignant Catarrhal Fever

D. H. Lloyd, B.Vet.Med., Ph.D., F.R.C.V.S., Diplomate, E.C.V.D.
Reader in Veterinary Dermatology, Royal Veterinary College, Hawkshead Campus, University of London, North Mymms, Hertfordshire, England, United Kingdom.
Dermatophilosis

John E. Lloyd, Ph.D.
Professor of Entomology, University of Wyoming, Laramie, Wyoming.
Flies, Lice, and Grubs

John A. Lynch, D.V.M., M.Sc., D.V.Sc., Diplomate, A.C.V.M.
Manager, Research Coordination Unit, Laboratory Services Division, University of Guelph, Guelph, Ontario, Canada.
Nocardioses

John Maas, D.V.M., M.S., Diplomate, A.C.V.N. and A.C.V.I.M.
Extension Veterinarian, School of Veterinary Medicine, University of California, Davis, Davis, California.
Analyzing Milk Diets for Calves

Bill Mahanna, M.S., Ph.D.
Senior Ruminant Nutritionist, Nutritional Team Leader, Nutritional Services, Pioneer Hi-Bred International, Inc., Johnston, Iowa.
Dairy Cow Nutritional Guidelines

Roger Marshall, B.V.Sc., Ph.D., M.S.
Formerly Associate Professor, Department of Veterinary Pathology and Public Health, Faculty of Veterinary Science, Massey University, Palmerston North, New Zealand.
Nonvenereal Campylobacteriosis

Guy-Pierre Martineau, D.V.M.
Professor, Université de Montréal, Faculté de Médecine Vétérinaire, St. Hyacinthe, Québec, Canada.
Solving Neonatal Pig Problems

Milton M. McAllister, D.V.M., Ph.D., Diplomate, A.C.V.P.
Associate Professor, University of Wyoming, College of Agriculture, Department of Veterinary Sciences, Laramie, Wyoming.
Toxic Syndromes Associated With Sulfur

Charles McCauley, D.V.M.
Resident, Food Animal Medicine and Surgery, Oklahoma State University, Stillwater, Oklahoma.
Circulatory Shock

C. Pat McCoy, D.V.M., M.S., Diplomate, A.B.V.T.
Professor, Veterinary Toxicology, College of Veterinary Medicine, Mississippi State University, Mississippi State, Mississippi.
Ionophore Toxicoses

Steve McOrist, B.V.Sc., M.V.Sc., Ph.D.
Veterinary Pathology Services, Glenside, South Australia, Australia.
Proliferative Enteropathy of Pigs

William L. Mengeling, D.V.M., M.S., Ph.D., Diplomate, A.C.V.M.
Professor and Collaborator, Department of Microbiology, Immunology, and Preventive Medicine, College of Veterinary Medicine, Iowa State University; Research Leader, Virology Swine Research Unit, National Animal Disease Center, Ames, Iowa.
Porcine Parvovirus

Delbert G. Miles, D.V.M., M.S.
Veterinary Rsearch and Consulting Service, Greeley, Colorado.
Feedlot Production Medicine Programs

Paul E. Miller, D.V.M., Diplomate, A.C.V.O.
Clinical Associate Professor of Ophthalmology, Department of Surgical Sciences, School of Veterinary Medicine, University of Wisconsin—Madison, Madison, Wisconsin.
Neurogenic Vision Loss

Todd Milton, Ph.D.
Assistant Professor, Extension Feedlot Specialist, University of Nebraska, Lincoln, Nebraska.
Protein Supplementation in Beef Cattle Diets

Dragan Momcilovic, D.V.M., Ph.D.
College of Veterinary Medicine, Department of Large Animal Clinical Sciences, University of Florida, Gainesville, Florida.
Elective Termination of Pregnancy

Larry F. Moore, D.V.M.
Consultant, Broken Arrow, Oklahoma.
External Parasiticides

Sandra E. Morgan, D.V.M., M.S.
Associate Professor, Department of Medicine and Surgery, Boren Veterinary Teaching Hospital, College of Veterinary Medicine, Oklahoma State University, Stillwater, Oklahoma.
Gossypol

Karen Moriello, D.V.M., Diplomate, A.C.V.D.
Clinical Associate Professor of Dermatology, Veterinary Medical Teaching Hospital, University of Wisconsin—Madison, Madison, Wisconsin.
Dermatophytosis (Ringworm)

Peter R. Morresey, B.V.Sc., M.A.C.V.Sc.
Resident, Theriogenology, College of Veterinary Medicine, University of Florida, Gainesville, Florida.
Bovine Mastitis

Derek A. Mosier, D.V.M., Ph.D.
Department of Diagnostic Medicine/Pathobiology, College of Veterinary Medicine, Kansas State University, Manhattan, Kansas.
Anthrax; Section 8: Bacterial Diseases

Julia M. Murphy, D.V.M.
Resident in Production Medicine, Virginia-Maryland Regional College of Veterinary Medicine, Virginia Polytechnic Institute and State University, Blacksburg, Virginia.
Dairy Heifer Development and Monitoring

T. G. Nagaraja, M.V.Sc., Ph.D.
Professor, Department of Animal Sciences, Kansas State University, Manhattan, Kansas.
Necrobacillosis Associated With Fusobacterium necrophorum

Dale R. Nelson, D.V.M., M.S.
Professor, Food Animal Medicine and Surgery, Department of Veterinary Clinical Medicine, University of Illinois, Urbana, Illinois.
Stifle Injuries

Paul Nicoletti, D.V.M., M.S.
Professor, College of Veterinary Medicine, University of Florida, Gainesville, Florida.
Brucellosis

Jerome C. Nietfeld, D.V.M., Ph.D.
Assistant Professor, Department of Diagnostic Medicine, Kansas State Veterinary Diagnostic Laboratory, Kansas State University, Manhattan, Kansas.
Salmonellosis

Daniel O'Brien, D.V.M.
Post-Doctoral Fellow, Population Medicine Center, College of Veterinary Medicine, Michigan State University, East Lansing, Michigan.
Toxic Properties of Animal Wastes and Sewage Sludge Applied to Agricultural Lands

Garrett R. Oetzel, D.V.M., M.S.
Associate Professor, Food Animal Production Medicine Section, School of Veterinary Medicine, University of Wisconsin—Madison, Madison, Wisconsin.
Milk Fever (Parturient Paresis) in Cows, Ewes, and Doe Goats

Bruce M. Olcott, D.V.M., M.S., M.B.A.
Associate Professor, Department of Veterinary Clinical Science, School of Veterinary Medicine, Louisiana State University, Baton Rouge, Louisiana.
Production Medicine and Health Problems in Goats

Olimpo Oliver, D.V.M., M.Sc., D.V.Sc.
Professor of Large Animal Medicine, Department of Animal Health, Facultad de Medicina Veterinaria, Universidad Nacional; Head of Large Animal Clinic, Universidad Nacional, Bogota, Colombia.
Tetanus, Botulism, and Blackleg; Bacillary Hemoglobinuria, Braxy, and Black Disease

Fernando A. Osorio, M.V., M.S., Ph.D., Diplomate, A.C.V.M.
Professor, Department of Veterinary and Biomedical Sciences, University of Nebraska, Lincoln, Nebraska.
Infectious Bovine Rhinotracheitis and Other Clinical Syndromes Caused by Bovine Herpesvirus Types 1 and 5

Gary D. Osweiler, D.V.M., M.S., Ph.D., Diplomate, A.B.V.T.
Professor, Veterinary Diagnostic and Production Animal Medicine; Director, Veterinary Diagnostic Laboratory, College of Veterinary Medicine, Iowa State University, Ames, Iowa.
Using Diagnostic Resources for Toxicology; Zearalenone; Fumonisins; Section 6: Physical and Chemical Diseases

Donal O'Toole, M.V.B., Ph.D., F.R.C.Path.
Department of Veterinary Sciences, University of Wyoming, Laramie, Wyoming.
Selenium Toxicosis; Malignant Catarrhal Fever

Randall S. Ott, D.V.M., M.S.
Professor and Head, Production Medicine/Theriogenology, College of Veterinary Medicine, University of Illinois, Urbana, Illinois.
Management of Reproduction of Sheep and Goats

Dale Paccamonti, D.V.M., M.S.
Associate Professor of Theriogenology, Louisiana State University, Baton Rouge, Louisiana.
Problems Associated With Artificial Insemination in Cattle

Kip E. Panter, Ph.D.
Research Scientist, U.S. Department of Agriculture, Agricultural Research Service, Poisonous Plant Research Laboratory, Logan, Utah.
Principal Poisonous Plants of the Western United States

Prem S. Paul, B.V.Sc., Ph.D., Diplomate, A.C.V.M.
Professor of Virology and Associate Dean for Research and Graduate Studies, College of Veterinary Medicine, Iowa State University, Ames, Iowa.
Porcine Parvovirus

Janet B. Payeur, D.V.M., M.P.H., Ph.D.
Head, Mycobacteria and Brucella Laboratory, Diagnostic Bacteriology Laboratory, National Veterinary Services Laboratories, Animal and Plant Inspection Services, U.S. Department of Agriculture, Ames, Iowa.
Bovine Tuberculosis

Simon Peek, B.V.Sc., M.R.C.V.S., Diplomate, A.C.V.I.M.
Assistant Professor of Large Animal Medicine, Theriogenology and Infectious Disease Management, Department of Medical Sciences, School of Veterinary Medicine, University of Wisconsin, Madison, Wisconsin.
Diseases of the Peripheral Nervous System

Louis J. Perino, D.V.M., Ph.D.
Professor of Immunology, Health, and Management, Division of Agriculture, West Texas A&M University, Canyon, Texas.
Bovine Respiratory Disease

James A. Pfister, M.S., Ph.D.
Rangeland Scientist, U.S. Department of Agriculture, Agricultural Research Services, Poisonous Plant Laboratory, Logan, Utah.
Principal Poisonous Plants of the Western United States

J. Phillip Pickett, D.V.M., Diplomate, A.C.V.O.
Associate Professor of Ophthalmology, Department of Small Animal Clinical Sciences, Virginia-Maryland Regional College of Veterinary Medicine, Virginia Polytechnic Institute and State University, Blacksburg, Virginia.
Ophthalmic Examination Techniques for Food Animals; Selected Eye Diseases of Food and Fiber-Producing Animals; Section 15: Eye Diseases

Robert H. Poppenga, D.V.M., Ph.D., Diplomate, A.B.V.T.
Associate Professor of Veterinary Toxicology, School of Veterinary Medicine, University of Pennsylvania, Kennett Square, Pennsylvania.
Toxic Properties of Animal Wastes and Sewage Sludge Applied to Agricultural Lands

Maria E. Prado, M.V.
Medicine Resident, Department of Medicine and Surgery, College of Veterinary Medicine, Oklahoma State University, Stillwater, Oklahoma.
Bloat, or Rumen Tympany

John F. Prescott, M.A., Vet.M.B., Ph.D.
Professor, Department of Pathobiology, University of Guelph, Guelph, Ontario, Canada.
Systemic Mycoses; Leptospirosis

Robbi H. Pritchard, Ph.D.
Ruminant Nutrition, Department of Animal and Range Sciences, South Dakota State University, Brookings, South Dakota.
Ration Management in Feedlot Cattle

D. Owen Rae, D.V.M., M.P.V.M.
Associate Professor, Rural Animal Medicine Service, Large Animal Clinical Sciences, College of Veterinary Medicine, University of Florida, Gainesville, Florida.
Evaluation of Beef Cattle Reproductive Performance

Merl F. Raisbeck, D.V.M., M.S., Ph.D., Diplomate, A.B.V.T.
Professor of Veterinary Toxicology, University of Wyoming, Laramie, Wyoming.
Selenium Toxicosis; Toxic Syndromes Associated With Sulfur

Richard F. Randle, D.V.M., M.S.
Veterinary Medical Extension and Continuing Education, College of Veterinary Medicine, University of Missouri, Columbia, Missouri.
Urinary Disorders Associated With the Neonate; Infectious Pyelonephritis in Cattle; Section 14: Urinary Diseases

David T. Ramsey, D.V.M., Diplomate, A.C.V.O.
Assistant Professor, Department of Small Animal Clinical Sciences, Veterinary Medical Center, Michigan State University, East Lansing, Michigan.
Ophthalmic Therapeutics; Surface Ocular Microbiology in Food and Fiber-Producing Animals

Lawrence E. Rice, D.V.M., M.S.
Professor Emeritus, Department of Medicine and Surgery, Oklahoma State University, Stillwater, Oklahoma.
Development of Replacement Heifers

Gavin F. Richardson, D.V.M., M.V.Sc., Diplomate, A.C.T.
Professor of Theriogenology, Department of Health Management, Atlantic Veterinary College; Service Chief,

Theriogenology, University of Prince Edward Island, Charlottetown, Prince Edward Island, Canada.
Metritis and Endometritis; Bovine Vaginitis

E. J. Richey, D.V.M.
Professor, Large Animal Clinical Sciences, College of Veterinary Medicine, University of Florida, Gainesville, Florida.
Bovine Anaplasmosis

Robert K. Ridley, D.V.M., Ph.D.
Professor, Veterinary Parasitology, College of Veterinary Medicine, Kansas State University, Manhattan, Kansas.
Parasites of the Respiratory System

D. Michael Rings, D.V.M., M.S., Diplomate, A.C.V.I.M.
Professor, Food Animal Medicine, Surgery, and Theriogenology, Veterinary Clinical Sciences, College of Veterinary Medicine, Ohio State University Veterinary Teaching Hospital, The Ohio State University, Columbus, Ohio.
Esophageal Obstruction (Choke); Pharyngeal Lacerations and Retropharyngeal Lacerations and Retropharyngeal Abscesses in Cattle; Abomasal Physiology, and Dilation, Displacement, and Volvulus; Abomasal Emptying Defect in Sheep; Atresia Coli; Ovine Contagious Foot Rot; Section 12: Digestive Diseases

Marylou B. Rings, D.V.M.
Veterinary Clinical Associate, Ohio State College Veterinary Medicine, Marysville Ambulatory, Marysville, Ohio.
Rectal Prolapse in Food Animals

Carlos A. Risco, D.V.M., Diplomate, A.C.T.
Associate Professor, College of Veterinary Medicine, University of Florida, Gainesville, Florida.
Dairy Herd Reproductive Efficiency

Farrel R. Robinson, D.V.M., Ph.D.
Professor Emeritus of Toxicology and Pathology, Purdue University, West Lafayette, Indiana.
Forensic and Legal Aspects of Food Animal Toxicoses

Joe D. Roder, D.V.M., Ph.D., Diplomate, A.B.V.T.
Adjunct Professor, College of Veterinary Medicine, Mississippi State University, Mississippi State, Mississippi; Laboratory Manager, CAVL, Amarillo, Texas.
Ionophore Toxicoses

Karen C. Rogers, D.V.M., M.S.
Veterinary Consultant, Greeley, Colorado.
Feedlot Production Medicine Programs

Joseph S. Rook, D.V.M.
Associate Professor, Department of Large Animal Clinical Sciences, College of Veterinary Medicine, Michigan State University, East Lansing, Michigan.
Pregnancy Toxemia of Ewes

Kurt D. Rossow, D.V.M., Ph.D.
Assistant Professor, South Dakota State University, Brookings, South Dakota.
Porcine Reproductive and Respiratory Syndrome

Allen J. Roussel, Jr., D.V.M., M.S., Diplomate, A.C.V.I.M.
Associate Professor and Associate Department Head, Department of Large Animal Medicine and Surgery, College of Veterinary Medicine, Texas A&M University, College Station, Texas.
Fluid Therapy, Transfusion, and Shock; Colostrum and Passive Immunity; Omphalitis and Its Sequelae in Ruminants

Richard Rubenstein, Ph.D.
Adjunct Professor, College of Staten Island; Laboratory Head, Molecular and Biochemical Neurology, New York State Institute for Basic Research in Developmental Disabilities, Staten Island, New York.
Bovine Spongiform Encephalopathy

Nicolas Sattler, D.M.V.
Large Animal Internal Medicine Resident, University of Montreal, St. Hyacinthe, Québec, Canada.
Abomasal Physiology, and Dilation, Displacement, and Volvulus

Beverly Schmitt, D.V.M., M.S.
Chief, Diagnostic Virology Laboratory, National Veterinary Services Laboratories, Ames, Iowa.
Vesicular Stomatitis Virus in Swine and Cattle

Danny W. Scott, D.V.M., Diplomate, A.C.V.D.
Professor of Medicine, College of Veterinary Medicine, Cornell University, Ithaca, New York.
Viral Skin Diseases; Protozoal Skin Diseases; Immunologic Skin Diseases; Environmental Skin Diseases; Disorders of Pigmentation and Epidermal Appendages; Neoplastic Skin Diseases; Miscellaneous Skin Diseases

Brad Seguin, D.V.M., Ph.D.
Professor, Theriogenology Division, Department of Clinical and Population Sciences, College of Veterinary Medicine, University of Minnesota, St. Paul, Minnesota.
Estrus Synchronization

Susan D. Semrad, V.M.D., Ph.D., Diplomate, A.C.V.I.M.
Associate Professor, University of Wisconsin—Madison, Madison, Wisconsin.
Dermatophytosis (Ringworm)

James A. Shmidl, D.V.M., M.S.
Manager, Toxicology and Regulatory Affairs (Retired), Bayer Corporation, Agriculture Division, Animal Health, Shawnee, Kansas.
External Parasiticides

Nonie L. Smart, D.V.M., Ms.C., Ph.D.
Veterinary Microbiologist, Animal Health Laboratory, University of Guelph, Guelph, Ontario, Canada.
Haemophilus parasuis *Infection (Glasser's Disease)*

Billy I. Smith, D.V.M., M.S.
Courtesy Assistant Professor, College of Veterinary Medicine, University of Florida, Gainesville, Florida.
Lactation Failure in Swine

Craig A. Smith, D.V.M., Ph.D., Diplomate, A.C.T.
Assistant Editor, American Veterinary Medical Association, Schaumburg, Illinois.
Management of Reproductive Problems in Swine Herds

Herb Smith, D.V.M., Ph.D.
Professor, Department of Veterinary and Microbiological Sciences, North Dakota State University, Fargo, North Dakota.
Bovine Respiratory Syncytial Virus

Robert A. Smith, D.V.M., M.S., Diplomate, A.B.V.P.
McCasland Chair in Beef Health and Production, College of Veterinary Medicine, Oklahoma State University, Stillwater, Oklahoma.
Backgrounding and Stocker Calf Management; Section 9: Protozoal Diseases

J. Glenn Songer, Ph.D.
Professor, Department of Veterinary Science and
Microbiology, University of Arizona, Tucson, Arizona.
Swine Mycobacterial Disease; Corynebacterium *Species Infections;*
Clostridial Enterotoxemia (Clostridium perfringens)

Steven D. Sorden, D.V.M., Ph.D.
Assistant Professor of Veterinary Pathology, Department of
Veterinary Diagnostic and Production Animal Medicine,
College of Veterinary Medicine, Iowa State University, Ames,
Iowa.
Diagnostic Methods for Respiratory Disease

C. A. Speer, B.Sc., M.Sc., Ph.D.
Professor of Veterinary Molecular Biology, College of
Agriculture, Montana State University, Bozeman, Montana.
Coccidiosis

**Henry Staempfli, D.V.M., Diplomate, A.C.V.I.M. (Large
Animals)**
Associate Professor, Large Animal Medicine, Department of
Clinical Studies, Ontario Veterinary College, University of
Guelph, Guelph, Ontario, Canada.
*Tetanus, Botulism, and Blackleg; Bacillary Hemoglobinuria, Braxy,
and Black Disease*

Bryan L. Stegelmeier, D.V.M., Ph.D., Diplomate, A.C.V.P.
Veterinary Pathology, U.S. Department of Agriculture,
Agricultural Research Service, Poisonous Plant Research
Laboratory, Logan, Utah.
Principal Poisonous Plants of the Western United States;
Pyrrolizidine Alkaloid Toxicosis

George C. Stewart, Ph.D.
Associate Professor of Diagnostic Medicine/Pathobiology,
College of Veterinary Medicine, Kansas State University,
Manhattan, Kansas.
Staphylococcal Disease

Guy St. Jean, D.M.V., M.S., Diplomate, A.C.V.S.
Professor of Surgery and Head, Department of Clinical
Sciences, School of Veterinary Medicine, Ross University,
Basseterre, St. Kitts, West Indies.
Abomasal Impactions of Cattle; Intestinal Volvulus in Cattle;
Intraluminal Intestinal Obstruction: Trichobezoars, Phytobezoars,
and Enteroliths; Intussusception; Intraluminal-Intramural
Hemorrhage of the Small Intestine in Cattle; Septic Arthritis

**Johannes Storz, D.V.M., Ph.D., Dr.H.C., Diplomate,
A.C.V.M.**
Professor and Head, Department of Veterinary Microbiology
and Parasitology, School of Veterinary Medicine, Louisiana
State University, Baton Rouge, Louisiana.
Respiratory Disease of Cattle Associated With Coronavirus Infections

Barbara Straw, D.V.M., Ph.D.
Professor, College of Veterinary Medicine, Michigan State
University, East Lansing, Michigan.
Causal Factors in Swine Pneumonia

Robert N. Streeter, D.V.M., M.S., Diplomate, A.C.V.I.M.
Assistant Professor, Department of Medicine and Surgery,
Oklahoma State University, Stillwater, Oklahoma.
Circulatory Shock; Bloat, or Rumen Tympany; Traumatic
Reticuloperitonitis and Its Sequelae; Section 11: Circulatory Diseases

David A. Stringfellow, D.V.M., M.S.
Associate Professor, Department of Pathobiology, College of
Veterinary Medicine, Auburn University, Auburn, Alabama.
Potential of Embryo Transfer for Infectious Disease Control

Raymond W. Sweeney, V.M.D.
Associate Professor of Medicine, University of Pennsylvania
School of Veterinary Medicine, Kennett Square, Pennsylvania.
Hypokalemia Syndrome in Dairy Cows; Spinal Cord Diseases

Robert C. Thaler, M.S., Ph.D.
Animal Nutrition, Swine Production, South Dakota State
University, Brookings, South Dakota.
Dietary Management in Pigs

James R. Thompson, D.V.M., M.S.
Associate Professor, Food Animal Section, College of
Veterinary Medicine, Iowa State University, Ames, Iowa.
Actinobacillosis (Wooden Tongue, Woody Tongue, Big Head);
Actinomycosis (Lumpy Jaw); Necrotic Stomatitis and Laryngitis
(Oropharyngeal Necrobacillosis, Calf Diphtheria); Lactic Acidosis
(Rumen Overload, Rumen Acidosis, Grain Overload, Engorgement
Toxemia, Rumenitis)

Mark C. Thurmond, D.V.M., Ph.D.
Professor of Clinical Epidemiology, School of Veterinary
Medicine, University of California, Davis, Davis, California.
Neosporum caninum *Infection and Abortion in Cattle*

**John F. Timoney, B.Sc., M.S., Ph.D., D.Sc., M.V.B.,
M.R.C.V.S.**
Keeneland Professor of Infectious Diseases, University of
Kentucky, Lexington, Kentucky.
Streptococcal Disease

Alfonso Torres, D.V.M., M.S., Ph.D.
Adjunct Professor (Courtesy Appointment), College of
Veterinary Medicine, Cornell University, Ithaca, New York;
Director, Plum Island Animal Disease Center, U.S.
Department of Agriculture, Agricultural Research Service,
Greenport, New York.
Foot-and-Mouth Disease

Vincent Traffas, D.V.M.
Traffas Veterinary Services, P.A., Smith Center, Kansas.
Breeding Season Evaluation of Beef Herds

Roderick C. Tubbs, D.V.M., M.S., M.B.A.
Swine Veterinarian, Green River Swine Consultation, Bowling
Green, Kentucky.
Cystitis, Pyelonephritis, and Miscellaneous Diseases of Swine

Eric Tulleners, D.V.M., Diplomate, A.C.V.S.
Lawrence Baker Sheppard Associate Professor of Surgery,
Chief, Section of Surgery, University of Pennsylvania, Kennett
Square, Pennsylvania.
Coxofemoral Luxations

Jean-Pierre Vaillancourt, D.V.M., M.Sc., Ph.D.
Associate Professor, College of Veterinary Medicine, North
Carolina State University, Raleigh, North Carolina.
Solving Neonatal Pig Problems

Richard L. Walker, D.V.M., Ph.D., M.P.V.M.
Associate Professor of Clinical Microbiology, California
Veterinary Diagnostic Laboratory System, School of Veterinary
Medicine, University of California, Davis, Davis, California.
Bovine Venereal Campylobacteriosis

Robert D. Walker, M.S., Ph.D.
Professor of Microbiology, Section Chief, Bacteriology/
Mycology, College of Veterinary Medicine, Michigan State
University, East Lansing, Michigan.
Actinobacillosis; Actinomycosis

Bimbo Welker, D.V.M., M.S.
Clinical Associate Professor and Director, Ambulatory
Services, Ohio State University, Marysville, Ohio.
*Diagnostic Methods in Food Animal Cardiology; Acquired Diseases
of the Heart; Interdigital Hyperplasia (Interdigital Fibroma, Corn);
Osteomyelitis*

Cecelia A. Whetstone, Ph.D.
Formerly Research Leader, U.S. Department of Agriculture,
Agricultural Research Service, Plum Island Animal Disease
Center, Greenport, New York.
Foot-and-Mouth Disease

Stephen D. White, D.V.M., Diplomate, A.C.V.D.
Associate Professor, College of Veterinary Medicine and
Biomedical Sciences, Colorado State University, Fort Collins,
Colorado.
Bacterial Skin Diseases

**Robert H. Whitlock, D.V.M., Ph.D., Diplomate,
A.C.V.I.M.**
Associate Professor of Medicine, University of Pennsylvania,
New Bolton Center, Kennett Square, Pennsylvania.
Vagal Indigestion; Abomasal Ulcers; Brain Stem Diseases of Cattle

Marlyn S. Whitney, D.V.M., Ph.D.
Clinical Pathologist, Texas Veterinary Medical Diagnostic
Laboratory, Amarillo, Texas.
Hematology of Food Animals

Dwight F. Wolfe, D.V.M., M.S.
Professor and Head, Department of Large Animal Surgery and
Medicine, College of Veterinary Medicine, Auburn University,
Auburn, Alabama.
*Management of the Repeat Breeder Female; Diseases of the Testes
and Epididymis*

**Phillip R. Woods, D.V.M., Ph.D., M.R.C.V.S., Diplomate,
A.C.V.I.M.**
Assistant Professor of Medicine and Surgery, College of
Veterinary Medicine, Oklahoma State University, Stillwater,
Oklahoma.
Colostrum and Passive Immunity

A. M. Zajac, D.V.M., Ph.D.
Associate Professor, Virginia-Maryland Regional College of
Veterinary Medicine, Blacksburg, Virginia.
Helminth Parasites of the Gastrointestinal Tract

Preface to the Fourth Edition

Current Veterinary Therapy 4: Food Animal Practice is a timely, updated edition in the field of food animal practice. The material is, as the name implies, current. Some of the material is less than 6 months old. For this edition we have a new associate editor, Dr. Robert A. Smith, 12 new consulting editors, and more than 200 different authors. Most of the authors are also new, giving a fresh approach in many areas. Of course, we have some of the tried-and-true authors who have been with us since the beginning. Dr. Smith has done an excellent job in putting together a large portion of this edition. We have some exciting new additions to this volume as well as updates of all other material.

This edition continues to have the same purpose as the original edition, that is, to provide a quick, concise resource book containing material on the prevention, therapy, management, and review of food animal diseases. Again, it is not encyclopedic in scope, but some of the sections are miniature books within a book. Some of the extra special sections include the chapters on herd health management, dietary management, physical and chemical disorders, bacterial and fungal diseases, diseases of the digestive system, and diseases of the musculoskeletal system. These chapters need a thorough examination.

The responsibility for the scientific material contained in each article is solely that of the article's author. The consulting editors, Dr. Smith, and I have attempted to standardize the manuscript form without altering the scientific content. The authors have presented outstanding, up-to-date material in excellently prepared manuscripts. Most of the authors are world known authorities in their special fields. Many of the authors have published books of their own. We consider our main strength to be that we have always had the best authors in the field of veterinary medicine.

Again, it is impossible to thank everyone who had a part in producing this edition. I will thank God for allowing me to remain around for these almost 20 years since we started this series. Also thanks to my wonderful wife who has assisted me and supported me for almost 50 years. Thanks also go out to all the editors and authors of past editions who have contributed so much in the past, and now to this wonderful crew who have put the edition together. One of the consulting editors needs special thanks: Dr. Bruce L. Hull of Ohio State University has been a consulting editor for all four editions and, as usual, has done an outstanding job. I would like to mention all of the authors who have written in all four editions, but we do not have space, and I'm afraid I would leave someone out. A special thanks is due to the outstanding staff of W.B. Saunders Company for their excellent work in editing, proofreading, organizing, and keeping things moving in an orderly fashion.

I hope you will find this book a worthwhile addition to your library, and I recommend you use it often.

JIMMY L. HOWARD

Contents

SECTION **7**
Viral Diseases 283
Consulting Editor:
James England, D.V.M., Ph.D.

SECTION 8
Bacterial Diseases 319
Consulting Editors:
  M. M. Chengappa, D.V.M., Ph.D.
  Derek A. Mosier, D.V.M., Ph.D.

Special Therapy

Consulting Editor

Jimmy L. Howard, D.V.M., M.S., Diplomate, A.B.V.P. (Food Animal Practice)

Water and salt, known for centuries to be elements essential to life, are as critical to survival today as ever. Because of the extreme importance of water and electrolytes to biologic processes, many organ systems are involved in their regulation and balance. The gastrointestinal tract, kidneys, skin, and several endocrine glands function to maintain body water and electrolyte concentration in delicate balance despite large changes in intake and loss. However, life-threatening imbalances can occur rapidly when these homeostatic mechanisms are overwhelmed.

■ Fluid Therapy, Transfusion, and Shock Therapy

Allen J. Roussel, Jr., D.V.M., M.S., Diplomate, A.C.V.I.M.

WATER AND ELECTROLYTE BALANCE

Total body water constitutes approximately 60% of the mass of the adult ruminant and pig. Total body water is inversely related to body fat; therefore, fattened livestock have relatively less body water. On the other hand, neonates have relatively more body water, as much as 86% of body mass. Total body water is divided into two major physiologic compartments that have imperfect anatomic corollaries. The largest compartment is the intracellular fluid compartment (ICF), which accounts for about two thirds of total body water. The extracellular fluid compartment (ECF) makes up the balance. Extracellular water can further be divided into the intravascular fluid compartment and the interstitial fluid compartment. Intravascular fluid or plasma volume makes up about 5% of total body mass. Water and certain molecules, such as urea, move freely from one compartment to the next, but the movement of certain ions and molecules is restricted or controlled by membrane channels and pumps. The osmolality of body fluids is relatively constant in healthy animals, about 300 mOsm/kg. Sodium, the most important extracellular cation, constitutes about 95% of the total cation pool. Major ECF anions include chloride and bicarbonate. The most important intracellular cation is potassium. The inverse relation of sodium and potassium inside and outside the cells is maintained by the Na^+, K^+-ATPase pump found in almost all mammalian cell membranes. Phosphate, proteins, and other anions balance the charge of K^+ and the other cations inside the cells.

When dehydration occurs, all fluid compartments are affected, but not uniformly. Rapid dehydration causes disproportionate reduction in the intravascular compartment, followed by contraction of the interstitial compartment, and finally by contraction of the ICF. In time equilibration occurs, and all compartments become dehydrated.

Depletion of body water and electrolytes usually occurs simultaneously, but the relative amount of water and electrolytes lost is not constant. If excess free water is lost owing to evaporative loss or water deprivation, electrolyte *content* of the ECF will not increase, but electrolyte *concentration* will increase. This can be most easily measured by analyzing plasma sodium, which will rise above normal concentration. If body water and electrolytes are lost in the same relative proportions as they are found in the ECF, volume contraction or dehydration will be isotonic. Measuring plasma electrolytes will reveal a normal sodium concentration. In some situations, sodium loss may exceed water loss, which results in hypotonic or at least hyponatremic dehydration. This is seen in ruminants with ruptured bladder when Na^+ moves into the peritoneal cavity, and in some calves with diarrhea when sodium is lost in the feces. Most clinically dehydrated ruminants and swine have isotonic or nearly isotonic fluid losses. Therefore it is essential to supply electrolytes, particularly sodium, in addition to water for rehydration and volume replacement. Failure to do so will result in relative water excess, which will be quickly corrected by the kidneys, subsequently returning the animal to a volume-depleted state again.

FLUID AND ELECTROLYTE REPLACEMENT THERAPY

Fluid therapy in food animals is both challenging and rewarding. Although it is often technically difficult, labor-intensive, and inconvenient, this basic therapeutic modality produces clinical results that no sophisticated surgical technique or expensive miracle drug can duplicate.

The principles of therapy are relatively simple; the physical, logistic, and economic constraints can be (and are) overcome by creative, resourceful practitioners. Administration of effective and economical fluid and electrolyte replacement therapy is achievable by every large animal practitioner.

Many of the principles of fluid therapy are the same for all classes of livestock. However, there are enough differences between neonatal and mature ruminants in terms of the abnormalities frequently encountered and solutions subsequently required to correct them to warrant separate discussions. Most of the research and clinical experience has been derived from cattle, but the same principles apply to other ruminants as well.

Fluid Therapy for Calves

The most frequent indication for fluid therapy for calves is neonatal calf diarrhea. Regardless of the etiologic organism, the metabolic changes resulting from diarrhea in calves are similar. They include (1) dehydration, (2) acidosis, (3) electrolyte abnormalities, and (4) negative energy balance or hypoglycemia, or both.

The major cause of dehydration in these calves is fecal fluid loss, which can be as much as 13% of body weight in 24 hours. Compounding this problem is decreased intake from either anorexia or withdrawal of milk by the owner.

Acidosis results from bicarbonate and strong cation loss in the stool, lactic acid accumulation in tissues, decreased renal excretion of acid, and increased production of organic acid in the colon in malabsorptive diarrheas. Along with water and bicarbonate, sodium, chloride, and potassium are lost in the feces, which results in a total body deficit of these ions.

Negative energy balance can occur in diarrheal calves owing to decreased milk intake, decreased digestion or absorption of nutrients, or replacement of milk with low-energy oral rehydration solutions. In some calves with malabsorptive disease, acute hypoglycemia may occur. Increased energy demand, such as that resulting from cold weather or fever, exacerbates these problems.

Patient Assessment

Dehydration. Acute dehydration can most accurately be quantified by monitoring body weight. This is seldom possible except during rehydration because accurate baseline weights are not usually available. Serial measurements of packed cell volume (PCV) and total plasma protein (TPP) provide assessment of the relative state of hydration, but without baseline data these measurements can be misleading. The range of PCV in healthy neonatal calves is 22% to 43%, much too variable to provide quantitative information of hydration status, at least with a single sampling. The TPP is even more variable, depending greatly on the degree of colostral immunoglobulin absorption that occurred, as well as hydration. The PCV aids in assessment of rehydration efforts and can be used to help prevent overhydration, but TPP may be less useful. Proteins are contained in other fluid compartments, which makes the volume of distribution of plasma proteins larger than the plasma volume. Therefore, PCV is a more reliable indicator of changes in blood volume than is TPP.

Without a reliable quantitative measure for hydration status, we must rely on estimates based on clinical signs. Table 1 provides a rough guideline for estimating the degree of dehydration in cattle. However, this table, like many others, is based on clinical experience and response to therapy, not on scientific evidence. Naylor found that calves assessed to be 8% to 10% dehydrated by a clinical scoring system, and rehydrated accordingly, gained only about 5.2% of their body weight in 24 hours, even though they were no longer clinically dehydrated. Perhaps the ICF compartment had not equilibrated; thus restoration of total body water was not accomplished, or perhaps our method of assessment overestimates dehydration. Regardless, rehydration based on estimated degree of dehydration is clinically successful. Rather than become overly concerned with pinpointing the exact degree of dehydration, veterinarians should be concerned whether intravenous therapy is needed, or whether voluntary or forced oral supplementation will suffice. Rather than defining an exact long-term fixed plan for rehydration, we should begin with a reasonable plan and adjust it as needed. In other words, *guess and reassess*.

Empirically, 8% dehydration is the severity beyond which it is considered that oral fluid therapy will not suffice. Clinical signs associated with severe dehydration include marked enophthalmos, prolonged skin tenting, dry mucous membranes, and moderate to severe depression. Calves displaying these signs will benefit the most from intravenous therapy. In general, calves that readily suckle quantities of rehydration solution sufficient to meet their replacement, maintenance, and ongoing loss needs will respond to oral solutions. Many of the more severely dehydrated calves will respond to forced oral solutions as well, but intravenous replacement is preferred.

Acidosis. Acidemia can quickly and accurately be assessed when a blood gas analyzer is available. These units are becoming more affordable, but access to such a unit is still not common in private large animal practice. It may be beneficial for practitioners to have several samples analyzed occasionally as a means of evaluating how effective their empirical treatment regimens are. Blood samples submerged in ice water can be held up to 24 hours before analysis of pH and blood gases. Therefore practitioners could have the samples analyzed after the fact as a self-education experience for help in future cases. Samples should be collected anaerobically into a heparinized syringe, and the needle should be capped with a rubber stopper immediately. Consult your laboratory for details.

Measurement and assessment of total carbon dioxide (TCO_2) will provide essentially equivalent clinical data in assessment of nonrespiratory acidosis or alkalosis, which is the type of acid-base disturbance most frequently encountered in conscious animals. TCO_2 measurement is available with many units that measure electrolytes. Blood tubes should be filled to capacity if TCO_2 is to be measured, to avoid falsely low values. In most cases in practice, the degree of acidosis will be estimated. Although some authors have published tables that suggest base deficit may be estimated based on the same criteria as dehydration, these estimates have not been evaluated experimentally. An attempt has been made to develop a depression score that would estimate acidosis by evaluating a battery of clinical signs of diarrheal, acidotic calves. Unfortunately, the scoring system was inaccurate at predicting the degree of acidosis in calves. They also described several calves with moderate to severe metabolic acidosis without diarrhea or dehydration, demonstrating the fallacy of predicting acid-base status strictly on the basis of hydration. It was also determined that dehydrated calves greater than 1 week of age had more severe acidosis (mean base deficit of 19.5 mEq/L) than did those less than 1 week of age (mean deficit of 14.4 mEq/L). As a rule of thumb, severely diarrheal calves less than 1 week of age can be assumed to have a base deficit of 10 to 15 mEq/L, whereas those greater than 1 week of age can be assumed to have a base deficit of 15 to 20 mEq/L.

Electrolyte Imbalance. Laboratory analysis of serum or plasma electrolytes is of limited benefit in evaluating the replacement needs of diarrheal calves and, if misinterpreted, could

Table 1 **GUIDE TO ESTIMATION OF FLUID REPLACEMENT REQUIREMENT**	
% of Body Weight Needed	**Clinical Signs**
6–7	Slight enophthalmos, skin turgor slightly increased, mucous membranes moist
8–9	Eyes obviously sunken, skin turgor obviously increased, mucous membranes tacky
10–12	Eyes deeply sunken in orbits, skin tents and does not return, mucous membranes dry, depression evident

lead to inappropriate therapy. Plasma represents a very small portion of total body water, and the concentration of electrolytes in a blood sample must be interpreted in light of that fact. If sodium and chloride are within normal limits and a calf has lost 20% of ECF volume, then the calf has a total body sodium and chloride deficit of nearly 20%. Because sodium and chloride concentrations are often within or below the reference range in diarrheal calves, it is extremely important to provide these electrolytes in replacement solutions. Failure to do so will result in dilution of the already deficient ions.

A potentially more misleading laboratory value than plasma sodium and chloride is plasma potassium. Many dehydrated, acidemic calves are hyperkalemic, yet they have a total body potassium deficit. This paradox is the result of a shift of potassium out of the ICF compartment into the ECF compartment during acidemia. The ECF, which normally contains only about 5% of the body's total exchangeable potassium, has a greater than normal concentration of potassium. Because of the fecal and urinary losses, however, ICF potassium concentration and total body potassium content are decreased.

Blood Glucose. Blood glucose determination can be made by a serum analyzer or by a rapid method using a hand-held meter. Hypoglycemia in calves results in weakness, lethargy, coma, convulsions, and opisthotonos. Negative energy balance is not easily quantified because it can result from inadequate intake, malabsorption-maldigestion, or increased metabolic demand due to fever or low ambient temperature. If milk is withheld for more than 48 hours, especially in cold weather, a serious energy deficit can occur. Weak or recumbent calves that do not appear to be dehydrated, but are emaciated, are usually suffering from malabsorption or malnutrition. Sometimes these calves respond, at least temporarily, to intravenous dextrose infusion.

Estimating Fluid and Electrolyte Replacement Requirements

The first priority in treatment of a dehydrated calf should be restoration of ECF volume. When estimating the volume of fluid needed by a patient, the veterinarian should consider not only the deficit but also maintenance requirements and compensation for continuing loss. Daily maintenance fluid requirement for the neonatal calf is 50 to 100 mL/kg, whereas ongoing fluid loss can range from minimal amounts to as much as 4 L in 24 hours. One must avoid overemphasizing the estimate of the degree of dehydration and the calculation of volume *replacement* needed, while neglecting to include maintenance and ongoing loss into the calculations. In many cases, the actual deficit is less than half of the total 24-hour volume requirement.

Second in priority to correcting ECF volume depletion is correcting acidosis. It has been suggested that the restoration of ECF volume alone would allow the kidneys to eliminate acid in sufficient quantity to restore normal acid-base balance. This has been disproved in calves with moderate to severe acidemia. Neither intravenously nor orally administered solutions without alkalinizing agents resolved acidosis expeditiously even though ECF volume was restored.

Acidosis can be corrected by the administration of HCO_3^- or so-called bicarbonate precursors, salts of weak organic acids. Alternatives to bicarbonate include lactate, acetate, gluconate, propionate, and citrate. Studies in calves have demonstrated the superior alkalinizing efficiency of bicarbonate, compared with L-lactate and acetate.

Sodium bicarbonate is the most economical and readily available alkalinizing agent; however, it cannot be heat-sterilized. It also should not be used in solutions containing calcium because an insoluble compound will form.

Alternative alkalinizing agents offer both advantages and disadvantages as well. Lactate is a widely used alkalinizing agent in veterinary medicine, although it has several shortcomings. Hepatic perfusion and function are necessary for its metabolism, and endogenous lactate (lactic acid) that accumulates during hypovolemia and shock can reduce its metabolism. Also, commercial preparations of lactated Ringer's solution contain racemic mixtures of D- and L-lactate. Only the L-isomer is metabolized efficiently, whereas most of the D-isomer is excreted in the urine unchanged. Therefore, the alkalinizing potential of the racemic mixture is only about half of the alkalinizing potential of an equimolar amount of the L-isomer. Acetate has the advantage of being metabolized by peripheral tissues and of having no significant endogenous source and no unmetabolized isomer. Citrate can be used in oral rehydration solutions, but its calcium-chelating properties preclude its inclusion in solutions for intravenous administration. Gluconate, an alkalinizing agent used in combination with acetate in some commercially prepared solutions for intravenous administration to human beings, dogs, and horses, has been shown to be ineffective as an alkalinizing agent in calves when administered intravenously, but it is effective when administered orally.

Rate of administration of alkalinizing agents, especially sodium bicarbonate, is a controversial subject. Some concern is warranted because rapid intravenous administration of 8.3% sodium bicarbonate can cause serious side effects. Rapid injection of this solution can cause hypernatremia and hyperosmolality as well as rapid alkalinizing. Another complication reported to be associated with the use of sodium bicarbonate for alkalinization is cerebrospinal fluid (CSF) acidosis. This condition was reported in 1967 in two human patients who received sodium bicarbonate infusions; however, whereas numerous warnings about CSF acidosis can be found in the veterinary literature, I am not aware of a documented clinical case of CSF acidosis in domestic animals and therefore do not hesitate to replace the total calculated deficit of bicarbonate in the initial deficit replacement solution.

When blood gas analysis is available, the value for the base deficit (BD) can be used to calculate total base requirement by use of the formula

$$0.6 \times BD \times \text{body weight} = \text{base requirement in mEq.}$$

We have found 0.6 to be an accurate estimate of the bicarbonate space in young calves, while 0.3 is recommended for mature cattle. When the value for TCO_2 or bicarbonate is known, it can be subtracted from 25, and the difference can be used in place of BD in the formula. When it is not possible to quantify acid-base status, an estimate of 10 to 20 mEq/L may be used to formulate fluids for intravenous use for diarrheal calves. Remember that calves greater than 1 week of age tend to become more severely acidotic.

The addition of glucose to rehydration solutions has three benefits. In orally administered solutions, glucose enhances sodium absorption in the small intestine via a transmembrane cotransport system. Once absorbed or injected, glucose also stimulates the release of insulin, which in turn enhances the movement of potassium from the ECF to the ICF. Last, glucose provides readily available energy. Glucose concentrations of 1% to 2% in intravenously administered solutions have produced favorable clinical results and usually do not result in significant glucosuria or osmotic diuresis. Additional glucose may be provided in oral solutions. In selected cases, total or partial parenteral nutrition may be beneficial to calves with severe prolonged malabsorptive diarrhea. In one study, calves receiving parenteral nutrition gained more weight but did not have better survivability than those receiving traditional therapy.

The importance of replacing sodium and chloride should not

be overlooked. Remember that total body sodium and chloride are deficient in dehydrated calves, even when plasma concentrations are normal.

The administration of potassium to a hyperkalemic patient seems absurd at first, but the objective is to replace the total body potassium deficit that exists despite hyperkalemia. Administration of potassium to hyperkalemic acidemic calves can be accomplished safely if bicarbonate and dextrose are administered concurrently. As previously mentioned, dextrose and bicarbonate enhance the movement of potassium from the ECF to the ICF. Ideally, the initial liter or so of intravenously administered rehydration solution should contain less potassium than subsequent volumes. However, practicality often dictates the use of a single solution for rehydration. There seems to be little danger in including up to 20 mEq of potassium per liter if bicarbonate and dextrose are included in the solution.

Formulating a Solution for Intravenous Administration

There are as many "correct" ways to formulate solutions for intravenous administration in calves as one can imagine. The following is a list of suggested criteria for intravenously administered solutions:

1. Osmolality between 300 and 450 mOsm/L.
2. Sodium and chloride concentrations near or slightly less than normal plasma concentrations.
3. Potassium concentration 10 to 20 mEq/L. (Because 1 g of potassium chloride contains 14 mEq potassium, inclusion of 1 g of potassium chloride per liter fulfills this criterion.)
4. Dextrose at 10 to 20 g/L of solution (1% to 2%).
5. Sodium bicarbonate or a suitable metabolizable base calculated to meet the measured deficit (or an estimated base deficit of 10 to 20 mEq/L if laboratory values are not available).

Of course, commercial solutions like lactated Ringer's can be used. In most cases, sodium bicarbonate will be required in addition to correct acidosis. Dextrose and additional potassium should also be added. Remember that bicarbonate should not be mixed in the same container with calcium-containing solutions, such as lactated Ringer's.

Whereas it may be ideal to rehydrate a patient over 24 to 48 hours, bovine practitioners must often use the maximal safe infusion rate rather than the ideal. Overhydration and hypertension can be detected when central venous pressure is monitored, but this luxury is seldom available to the practitioner. A maximum of 80 mL/kg/hour has been suggested as a "safe" flow rate. A more conservative rate of 50 mL/kg/hour is probably a reasonable, relatively safe maximal infusion rate. With use of this infusion rate, most calves can be rehydrated in 2 to 3 hours. During rapid intravenous administration of fluids, the veterinarian or attendant should periodically monitor heart rate, respiratory rate and character, and attitude, adjusting the flow rate if necessary. Extra caution should be exercised when administering intravenous fluids to hypothermic calves.

When possible, it is desirable to administer approximately 1 L of the solution rapidly to reverse hypovolemic shock, and then administer the balance over a period of hours. This will maximize the benefit of the therapy by minimizing the diuresis that is sometimes induced by rapid fluid administration. If it is impractical or impossible to administer the total 24-hour requirement, or even the total deficit by intravenous infusion, 1 or 2 L of fluid administered intravenously may be enough to improve the circulatory status of a calf so that the balance of the calf's requirement may be provided by the oral route. In other words, a relatively small volume of fluids administered intravenously may convert a calf from the "intravenous fluid required" to the "oral fluid satisfactory" category. Fluids for maintenance and continued loss may be administered orally or by slow intravenous infusion. Alternatively, intravenously administered hypertonic saline solution combined with intraruminally administered electrolyte solution may be administered.

Hypertonic Saline Solution (HSS). The sheer size of mature cattle and the great quantity of fluid required to resuscitate and rehydrate them has prevented many veterinarians from taking full advantage of intravenous fluid therapy. HSS (7.2% NaCl) offers the advantages of low cost and rapid administration, as well as efficacy, for treatment of shock and dehydration. HSS is commercially available, or it can be made by adding 72 g of NaCl to a liter of sterile distilled water. It should be administered at a dose of 4 mL/kg over 3 to 10 minutes. Rapid administration is essential because it works by transiently creating intravascular hyperosmolality. Intravascular volume increases by 3 to 4 mL per milliliter administered. The water is recruited from the interstitial and intracellular compartments. The effect of HSS is transient and must be supplemented by additional volume replacement. Colloids such as dextran and hetastarch enhance the efficacy of HSS by prolonging its effect. They add, however, substantially to its cost. If HSS is administered to dehydrated cattle it *must be accompanied by intraruminal water or followed by isotonic crystalloid solutions.* The volume of intraruminal water that should accompany HSS administration to dehydrated cattle should be approximately 10 times the volume of the HSS. Acidosis, hypokalemia, and hypocalcemia, if present, must be addressed separately by oral, intraruminal, or parenteral administration.

Oral Rehydration Therapy for Calves

The popularity of oral rehydration solution (ORS) for calves is an accurate reflection of the success of this therapeutic modality. Veterinarians and stockmen alike have witnessed the results of oral rehydration and have promoted its use. There are many products commercially produced, each with its advantages and shortcomings. The following discussion should help veterinarians make informed decisions concerning the use of these products.

Advantages of ORS. There are several obvious advantages of oral fluid therapy over intravenous fluid therapy. Economy of materials, time, and equipment is the major advantage in treating food animals. The ORS can be carried and stored in dry form, mixed with tap water, administered by nursing bottle or by stomach tube, and administered as infrequently as every 12 hours. Whereas suckling delivers the solution more directly to the abomasum by inducing reticular groove closure, intubation is also an accepted means of delivery in neonatal calves. A slight delay in absorption may occur after intubation, which could be beneficial if a depot effect is desired rather than an immediate effect. Finally, the gradual absorption of the ORS allows more flexibility in the formulation of these solutions than of those for intravenous use. Greater concentrations of potassium, glucose, and total osmoles can be supplied in ORS than in intravenous solutions.

Characteristics of ORS. Several types and numerous individual formulations of ORS are available commercially. Although a significant difference in constituents exists, all of these solutions can be used successfully. Included in all ORS formulations are substantial amounts of sodium, chloride, potassium, and glucose. Most contain bicarbonate or another alkalinizing agent. Many contain glycine, acetate, or citrate to enhance sodium and water absorption. Calcium, magnesium, and phosphorus are present in some. Additives such as psyllium are now included as antidiarrheal agents.

The major differences between formulations occur in the

following constituents: glucose, alkalinizing agents, and total osmolality. The variety of combinations of constituents in to-day's commercial ORS market allows the veterinarian to choose the type of solution that will perform best in a given situation. High-energy solutions approach the maintenance needs of the calf and reduce weight loss, compared with low-energy solutions. However, if a significant amount of glucose reaches the colon, it may exacerbate diarrhea. If milk intake is withdrawn or reduced for more than 24 hours, moderate- to high-energy solutions should probably be used.

Whenever acidosis is moderate to severe, ORS with alkalinizing agents must be used to restore normal acid-base status in a timely manner. According to Naylor's work, alkalinizing solutions are more likely to be needed for older calves. Nonalkalinizing solutions are indicated for clients who monitor calves closely and institute fluid therapy early in the course of disease before dehydration or acidosis becomes severe. Alkalinizing potential and alkalinity of solutions do not necessarily parallel each other. Solutions containing sodium bicarbonate as an alkalinizing agent are alkaline, whereas some solutions containing a metabolizable base are actually acidic when consumed. Bicarbonate-containing solutions are therefore more likely to alkalinize the abomasum and allow the proliferation of bacteria and possibly the passage of pathogens to the intestines. The clinical significance of this is unproven, but experimentally it is easier to produce colibacillosis in calves if sodium bicarbonate is administered before bacterial challenge. The high-energy solutions mentioned must also be hyperosmolar, because the energy source is glucose. Reasonable arguments can be made for both isosmolar and hyperosmolar solutions. Intuitively, it seems reasonable that consumption of hyperosmolar solutions would result in movement of free water into the gastrointestinal lumen along the osmotic gradient. Such a shift in water would exacerbate the preexisting dehydration. There is evidence that a slight transient shift occurs, but no adverse effects have been shown. On the other hand, a villus countercurrent mechanism causes the interstitium of the villus tip to become hyperosmolar during absorption, which makes a hyperosmolar solution "isosmotic" relative to the interstitial fluid in closest proximity. However, the merit of creating a luminal osmolality equal to the interstitium is questionable, because one of the theories explaining the purpose of the countercurrent mechanism and resulting villus hyperosmolality is that the gradient established between the lumen and interstitium enhances water absorption from the lumen. If this gradient is reduced or negated by hypertonic solutions, water absorption could theoretically be reduced.

There is probably not one "ideal" ORS for all situations. In addition to the medical and physiologic considerations, other factors (such as cost, convenience, and palatability) must be considered when an ORS is chosen.

Using ORS for Optimal Results. In order to maximize the benefit of ORS, there are certain practices to adopt and others to avoid. The controversy over whether ORS should be used as a supplement to milk feeding or as a replacement is still unsettled, but a consensus is forming on a few points. There is evidence in people that removing all food from the diet results in rapid loss of digestive and absorptive capability of the intestines. In calves, weight loss is accelerated by withdrawing milk and replacing it with ORS, especially the lower-energy solutions. Therefore it is desirable to maintain calves on milk if the intestinal damage is not so great that a severe malabsorptive osmotic diarrhea results. However, recent studies show that consumption of bicarbonate-containing solutions interspersed between milk feedings results in decreased weight gain, possibly due to poor digestibility of the milk. Also, when ORS was mixed 1:1 with milk and fed to healthy calves, diarrhea was noted. From these studies, it can be concluded that ORS should not be mixed with milk or milk replacer and that nonbicarbonate-containing solutions may be preferred if calves are not taken off milk during the time that fluids are being administered. If milk is completely withdrawn from the diet, it should probably be reintroduced after 24 hours or less to avoid excessive weight loss. Reduction of daily intake is preferable to complete withdrawal.

FLUID THERAPY IN MATURE RUMINANTS

Although some of the principles of fluid therapy of mature ruminants are similar to those of calves and other species, many important exceptions exist. When assessing hydration status, one must remember that body weight and rumen fill can be misleading. Cattle with carbohydrate engorgement may not lose weight and may actually look full, but much of the fill is intraruminal water, which is unavailable to the animal. Also, skin tent and enophthalmos must be evaluated in light of the body condition. Emaciated cows may have sunken eyes and skin that tents, regardless of their hydration status. When deciding on route of administration, one should consider not only hydration status but cardiovascular status as well. For example, cattle with strangulating-obstructing gastrointestinal disease, especially those soon to undergo standing surgery, will benefit from intravenous fluid therapy even if they are not severely dehydrated because they may be in or near shock and cardiovascular collapse.

The volume required for complete rehydration of a large cow or bull is substantial and may dissuade practitioners from using this mode of therapy. It should be remembered that 10 to 20 L of fluid administered rather rapidly may be lifesaving, even though it represents less than half of the total fluid deficit. By use of at least some intravenous fluid (isotonic or hypertonic), intravascular volume can be restored, an underlying problem can be remedied by surgical or medical means, and oral fluids can be supplied to replace the rest of the deficit. To reduce the cost of administering intravenous fluids, practitioners may consider formulating their own solutions. Dry ingredients can be preweighed and packaged and mixed with sterile distilled water immediately before administration. Another disadvantage of commercially available solutions, besides the expense, is that relatively few are appropriate for most cattle.

Unlike neonates, adult ruminants do not usually require alkalinizing fluids when they are dehydrated. A few conditions (such as choke, carbohydrate engorgement, and diabetes mellitus) are consistently associated with acidosis. Renal failure, fatty liver, ketosis, severe diarrhea, pneumonia, and pregnancy toxemia are often associated with acidosis. Abomasal volvulus, displacement and impaction, intussusception, and cecal torsion are causes of moderate to severe alkalosis. In a study of mature dehydrated cattle, only about 22% had metabolic acidosis. Therefore, nonalkalinizing solutions will be the fluid of choice for most dehydrated mature ruminants. Usually accompanying alkalosis is hypochloridemia. Sequestration of chloride in the proximal small intestine, abomasum, and rumen results in hypochloridemic alkalosis. Alkalosis and anorexia contribute to hypokalemia in many sick cattle. Lactating dairy cattle are often hypocalcemic as well. To address these metabolic problems, we have used the following formulation at our hospital:

140 g of NaCl
30 g of KCl
10 g of CaCl$_2$ or Ca Borogluconate
q.s. to 20 L ± Dextrose ≤ 50% soln

This solution may be administered intraruminally via tube or intravenously. If it is administered intravenously, one bottle of commercially prepared calcium borogluconate solution may be substituted for the calcium chloride, and up to a liter of 50% dextrose may be added if ketosis is a concurrent problem.

When administering solutions intraruminally, I prefer to pass a medium-sized nasogastric tube through the nasal cavity instead of using a Frick mouth speculum. The procedure is less stressful to the patient and allows the veterinarian to administer fluids unassisted. Be aware that on a relative weight basis, the nasal cavity of the cow is smaller than that of the horse, so a relatively smaller tube must be used. If nutritional supplementation is needed, pelleted feed (with no large pieces of grain) can be soaked in warm water, made into a slurry, and pumped by use of a marine bilge pump or a commercially available cattle pump system.

Intravenous administration of fluids may be accomplished through a jugular catheter. A 10- to 14-gauge catheter is sufficient to permit rapid fluid administration. Cyanocrylic glue is effective for affixing the catheter to the skin. I prefer to use a 30-in. extension set connected to the catheter and held in place by elastic tape wrapped around the cow's neck. The extension set may be taped so that the end is positioned at the dorsum of the cow's neck to allow easy access for attachment to the intravenous administration set or for injections. An alternative to the jugular is the auricular vein. It is easily accessible and is more convenient to use if cattle must be restrained in a head-catch during fluid administration. A 14- to 18-gauge 1- or 2-in. catheter is placed in the vein, glued, and taped in place, with or without an extension set (Fig. 1). Because of the smaller size of the vein, speed of fluid administration is limited; however, the rate of administration is great enough to rehydrate even a severely dehydrated cow in a reasonable amount of time. An auricular vein catheter can also be used as an access for repeated intravenous infusions. One must be aware that an auricular

artery courses down the dorsum of the pinna. It should be identified by palpation of a pulse and avoided. Use of a rubber band as a tourniquet at the base of the ear usually collapses the artery and distends the veins.

USE OF BLOOD AND PLASMA

Whole Blood. Whole blood is indicated when the red blood cell mass is below that necessary to carry an adequate amount of oxygen to the tissues. The point at which transfusion is necessary is determined in large part by the time course over which the red blood cells were lost or destroyed. The slower the process, the more tolerant the animal is to a low PCV. Cattle that become anemic gradually can tolerate a PCV as low as 8% if they are not stressed, and I have seen parasitized goats with a PCV of 5% survive without transfusion. Transfusion has been recommended at a PCV of 12% to 15% if the anemia develops acutely. However, the most important indicator for determining if transfusion is indicated is the overall condition of the animal determined by respiratory rate and character, heart rate, and neurologic status. Another important fact to consider before deciding to transfuse is whether the stress of transfusion itself is likely to result in death.

Although plasma is more desirable, whole blood transfusion can be used to provide immunoglobulins to calves with failure of passive transfer. Achieving an adequate plasma immunoglobulin concentration in a calf with complete failure of passive transfer with the use of whole blood is difficult because the volume required may result in volume overload, polycythemia, or hemolytic icterus. Therefore, whole blood is most useful in calves

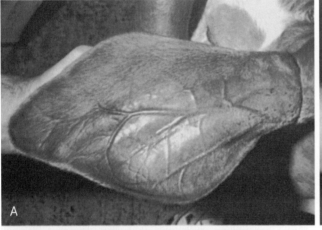

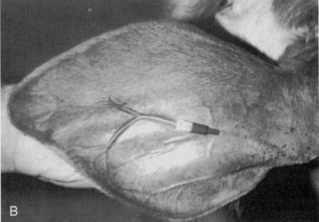

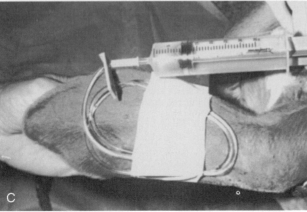

Figure 1

Ear vein catheterization. *A,* A rubber band is used as a tourniquet at the base of the ear. The veins are easily visible when distended. *B,* The catheter is inserted in the vein, capped with an injection cap, flushed with heparinized saline, and glued to the ear with cyanoacrylate. *C,* A simple tape bandage is applied to protect and secure the catheter.

Table 2
DRUG REFERENCE LIST

Name of Drug	Company	Species	Dose
Dexamethasone	Many	Bovine	0.5 mg/kg for shock
Flunixin meglumine (Banamine)	Schering-Plough Animal Health, Kenilworth, N.J.	Bovine	2.2 mg/kg
Ketoprofen (Ketofen)	Fort Dodge Laboratories, Fort Dodge, Iowa	Bovine	3 mg/kg
Prednisolone sodium succinate (Solu-Delta Cortef)	The Upjohn Company, Kalamazoo, Mich.	Bovine	1.1 mg/kg

with partial failure of passive transfer. Up to 2 L of whole blood can be safely administered to a 45-kg calf.

Transfusion reactions are extremely rare in cattle that have not been transfused previously. A practical means of determining compatibility is to infuse a small quantity of blood, about 0.5 mL/kg body weight, and wait 10 minutes before proceeding with the transfusion. Blood should be administered slowly (10 mL/kg/hour or less) through a blood administration set with an appropriate filter. Usually, 10 to 15 mL/kg are administered. Reported signs of transfusion reaction include hiccupping, dyspnea, muscle tremor, salivation, lacrimation, and fever. Epinephrine hydrochloride 1:1000 should be administered (at 4 to 5 mL intramuscularly to an adult cow) if signs of anaphylaxis occur.

Although many diseases are transmissible by transfusion, bovine leukosis and anaplasmosis are two of the most important. If a known uninfected donor is unavailable, the donor should probably be a herdmate of the recipient. This will at least prevent inadvertent introduction of a new pathogen into the herd.

It is safe to remove 10 to 15 mL/kg of blood from a healthy donor. Remember, however, that if this same dose is given to a recipient, the rise in PCV will be small (3% to 4%) and the duration short because exogenous red blood cells are rapidly destroyed by the recipient. Only 25% remain after the fourth day.

When blood is collected for immediate use, sodium citrate is an effective and inexpensive anticoagulant. It should be purchased or formulated to a 2.5% to 4.0% solution and added as one part solution to nine parts of blood. If blood is to be stored for more than a few hours, acid citrate dextrose solution should be used.

Plasma. Plasma is indicated in cases of hypoproteinemia and failure of passive transfer. Because ruminant red blood cells do not settle by gravity, centrifugation is required. The large volumes required to raise the recipient's plasma protein concentration significantly make plasma transfusion a relatively uncommon practice. In attempting to provide an acceptable immunoglobulin concentration to a calf with complete failure of passive transfer, 2 L of plasma should be administered. Commercially prepared plasma is currently available for purchase.

SHOCK

Shock in its broadest sense is a condition in which there is decreased tissue perfusion, cellular hypoxia, and ultimately cell death.

There are three major types of shock: hypovolemic, cardiogenic, and vasculogenic. The type of shock most commonly encountered in cattle is vasculogenic, specifically endotoxic or septic shock. Endotoxin is a constituent of the cell wall of gram-negative bacteria. It is released when bacterial cells die. Causes of endotoxic shock in cattle include colisepticemia, coliform mastitis, septic metritis, and pasteurellosis.

Endotoxic shock is characterized by dyspnea, depression, congested mucous membranes, recumbency, and death. Cardiovascular effects include decreased mean arterial blood pressure and cardiac output, and increased pulmonary arterial pressure. The traditional treatment for shock in food animals is rapid intravenous infusion of crystalloid solutions. The rate of administration should be rapid, especially initially. In most cattle, 75 mL/kg/hour is probably safe for infusion of isosmotic solutions for at least 30 to 60 minutes. HSS has been used successfully to treat shock.

In endotoxic shock, corticosteroids, flunixin meglumine, and ketoprofen have been shown to be effective in reducing the cardiopulmonary effects. The "shock" dose of corticosteroids used in research protocols for cattle has been 2 mg/kg for dexamethasone and 1.1 mg/kg for prednisolone sodium succinate, although many veterinarians use smaller doses. Flunixin meglumine and ketoprofen are approved for use in cattle in Europe at a daily dose of 2 mg/kg and 3 mg/kg, respectively (Table 2). More frequent dosing may be needed in endotoxemia. These drugs must be used in an appropriate extralabel fashion.

BIBLIOGRAPHY

Naylor JM: Severity and nature of acidosis in diarrheic calves over and under one week of age. Can Vet J 28:168–173, 1987.

Roussel AJ: Fluid and electrolyte therapy. Vet Clin North Am Food Anim Pract 6:1, 1990.

St Jean G, Constable PD, Yvorchuck K: The clinical use of hypertonic saline solution in food animals with hemorrhagic and endotoxic shock. Agri Pract 14:6–11, 1993.

■ Therapeutic Management of Inflammation

Vernon C. Langston, D.V.M., Ph.D., Diplomate, A.C.V.C.P.

That many disease names have the suffix -itis (e.g., peritonitis, pleuritis, etc.) implies that inflammation plays a prominent role in many afflictions. Indeed, the inflammatory process is a part of the normal defense mechanism which first localizes and then aids in the repair of damaged tissue. This is true most notably in the acute phases. However, widespread or chronic inflammation may become detrimental. In these cases therapeutic interruption of the inflammatory process is required to avoid inadequate tissue perfusion, tissue fibrosis, and loss of function. Because pharmacologic intervention is usually performed at the inflammatory mediator level, a brief review of the inflammatory process is in order.

Following an insult to tissue a variety of mediators derived from cells, plasma, or tissues are released. Those mediators manipulated pharmacologically in the food animal clinical setting include histamine and the eicosanoid mediators (prostaglandins, leukotrienes, and thromboxanes).

Histamine is found in mast cells and basophils. Following release it causes prominent vasodilation and edema which result in the well-known signs of inflammation: redness (erythema), warmth, swelling, pain, and loss of function. Histamine is the prominent mediator, however, for only the first 30 to 60 minutes post injury.

While histamine is of obvious importance in such acute conditions as anaphylactoid shock, in most other instances it plays a secondary role to the eicosanoid mediators. As Figure 1 illustrates, following tissue injury phospholipases convert the fatty acids of cell membranes (e.g., arachidonic acid) into intermediaries which are subsequently acted upon by lipoxygenases or cyclo-oxygenases which produce leukotrienes or prostaglandins, respectively.

The leukotrienes are responsible for a variety of actions on vascular and airway smooth muscle, including pronounced bronchoconstriction. Additionally, many of them are strongly chemotactic to white blood cells (WBCs) which move into an area to remove the offending organism or agent. If the WBCs are overwhelmed and die in significant numbers, their lysosomal enzymes containing large amounts of free radicals will be released into the tissues, thereby aggravating the inflammation. (Free radicals may also be generated by other processes.) At present there are no clinically available drugs that can selectively inhibit the lipoxygenase pathway.

Prostaglandins are a group of autocoids with tremendously diverse and often opposite actions. The exact role of the prostaglandins (and related thromboxanes) in inflammation and disease is not totally understood. It is, however, well accepted that these agents are capable of sensitizing pain receptors, causing fever and altering blood flow. Since prostaglandins regulate a number of normal body mechanisms, including gastrointestinal mucus production and renal blood flow, it is not surprising that drugs which interfere with cyclo-oxygenase activity cause gastrointestinal ulceration and renal papillary necrosis as common side effects.

Table 1 lists some common anti-inflammatory drugs and their dosages.

ANTIHISTAMINES

Antihistamines act by binding to the H_1 cellular receptors of histamine, thereby serving as a competitive antagonist to histamine. Although they have been suggested for treatment of a variety of illnesses, including laminitis, mastitis, and pneumonia, their use in food animals has remained empirical. They are of doubtful efficacy in most food animal diseases with the exception of allergies. When used, the following points should be kept in mind:

1. Antihistamines do not reverse the effects of histamine; they only prevent its binding. In an acute allergic reaction (i.e., anaphylaxis) primary emphasis must be placed on physiologically reversing life-threatening hypotension, laryngeal edema, etc. In such situations epinephrine and fluid support are usually the preferred treatment with antihistamines used as ancillary agents to minimize the effects of subsequent histamine release.

2. Antihistamines commonly have anticholinergic properties and cause a drying effect on epithelial surfaces. This is of special importance as regards the respiratory tract where secretions may become thick and tenacious. Although they might be useful when an allergic component is suspected, their use in most respiratory diseases is probably best avoided. If used, patient hydration should be well maintained.

3. All of the antihistamines used in veterinary medicine cross the blood-brain barrier and may cause sedation. Paradoxically, sudden high concentrations, as seen with rapid intravenous (IV) administration, may cause central nervous system (CNS) stimulation. Therefore, intramuscular (IM), subcutaneous (SC) or slow IV administration is mandatory.

CYCLO-OXYGENASE INHIBITORS (NONSTEROIDAL ANTI-INFLAMMATORY DRUGS)

The cyclo-oxygenase–inhibiting drugs, also known as nonsteroidal anti-inflammatory drugs (NSAIDs), are one of the most commonly used classes of drugs in veterinary practice.

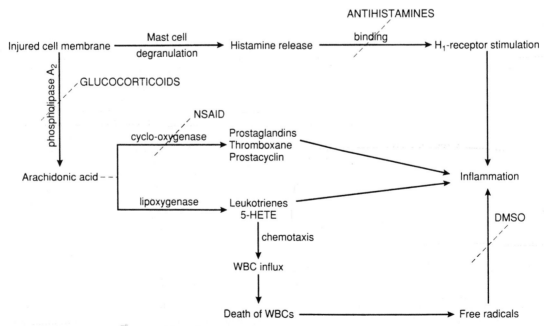

Figure 1
Site of action of common anti-inflammatory agents.

Table 1
COMMON ANTI-INFLAMMATORY DRUGS AND THEIR DOSAGES

Generic Name	Trade Name*	Source	Species	Dosage
Antihistaminic Drugs				
Diphenhydramine	Benadryl	Parke-Davis, Morris Plains, N.J.	Cattle	0.5–1.0 mg/kg IM or IV q.6–8h.
Tripelennamine	Re-Covr injection†	Solvay Animal Health, Mendota Heights, Minn.	Cattle	1 mg/kg IM or IV q.6–12h.
			Swine	1 mg/kg IM or IV q.6–12h.
Nonsteroidal Anti-Inflammatory Drugs				
Aspirin	Aspirin 60 grain†	W.A. Butler, Dublin, Ohio	Cattle	100 mg/kg PO q.12h.
			Swine	10 mg/kg PO q.6h.
Flunixin	Banamine solution	Schering-Plough Animal Health, Kenilworth, N.J.	Cattle, swine	1.1–2.2 mg/kg IV, IM, PO§
Ketoprofen	Ketofen	Fort Dodge Animal Health, Fort Dodge, Iowa	Cattle	2–4 mg/kg IV, IM, q.24h.
Phenylbutazone	Butaject	Vetus Animal Health, c/o Burns Veterinary Supply, Farmers Branch, Tex.	Cattle	10 mg/kg IV or PO priming dose 5 mg/kg IV or PO q.48h.
			Swine	4 mg/kg IV or PO q.24h.
Glucocorticoids‖				
Dexamethasone				
Sodium phosphate	Dexaject SP	Vetus Animal Health, c/o Burns Veterinary Supply, Farmers Branch, Tex.	Cattle, swine	Shock: 0.5–1.0 mg/kg IV Inflammation: 0.15 mg/kg IV or IM q.24–48h.
Solution¶	Azium‡	Schering-Plough Animal Health, Kenilworth, N.J.	Cattle, swine	Same as sodium phosphate form
Isoflupredone acetate	Predef 2X†	Pharmacia & Upjohn, Kalamazoo, Mich.	Cattle	Ketosis: 0.04 mg/kg IM
Prednisolone sodium succinate	Solu-Delta-Cortef	Pharmacia & Upjohn, Kalamazoo, Mich.	Cattle, swine	Shock: 10–30 mg/kg IV Inflammation: 1 mg/kg IM s.i.d.
Prednisone suspension	Meticorten	Schering-Plough Animal Health, Kenilworth, N.J.	Cattle, swine	Inflammation: 1 mg/kg IM s.i.d.
Dimethyl Sulfoxide				
DMSO solution	Domoso	Fort Dodge Animal Health, Fort Dodge, Iowa	Cattle, swine	CNS inflammation: 1 g/kg IV as a 10% solution once daily

IM, intramuscular; IV, intravenous; SC, subcutaneous; PO, orally; DMSO, dimethyl sulfoxide.
*No footnote symbol indicates use in the United States is extralabel.
†Labeled for use in the United States in cattle at the stated dose.
‡Labeled for use in the United States in cattle, but dose quoted is higher than label recommendation (withdrawal times may be longer).
§Repeat flunixin as needed based on clinical response but not more often than q.8–12h. in cattle or q.12–24h. in pigs.
‖Adjust to lowest effective dose if therapy exceeds 3–5 days.
¶Product is in a solution with propylene glycol and alcohol. Although it may be given slowly IV, the sodium phosphate form is preferred for this route because of its quicker onset and minimal cardiovascular depression.

Members of this family typically have a triad of effects, namely, anti-inflammatory, analgesic, and antipyretic. These agents have occasionally been referred to as "antiprostaglandins"; however, this nomenclature would seem to imply that the drugs work by binding prostaglandins or blocking their effects. In actuality they do neither, but rather work by inhibiting the cyclo-oxygenase (i.e., prostaglandin synthetase) pathway, thereby reducing prostaglandin and thromboxane production.

Although classified as anti-inflammatory drugs, they are probably used more in veterinary medicine for their analgesic and antipyretic effects, the first action occurring by virtue of decreasing the synthesis of prostaglandins which sensitize pain receptors (peripheral and central mechanisms may exist) and the latter by resetting the temperature regulatory center of the hypothalamus toward normal. The NSAIDs possess rather limited anti-inflammatory capabilities by comparison with glucocorticoids; however, they are occasionally used for this purpose because of the high incidence of side effects associated with glucocorticoid therapy. Typically, a higher dose is required for the purpose of combating inflammation as opposed to controlling fever and pain. There is evidence that these agents are helpful in combating endotoxic shock.

As a group the NSAIDs tend to behave as weak acids, often highly bound to plasma proteins. They are metabolized extensively by the liver and removed by the kidneys. As with most drugs that undergo extensive hepatic metabolism, interspecies pharmacokinetic variation is high and extrapolation of doses among species is not recommended.

If all NSAIDs worked by the same mechanism it might be presumed that they would all have the same clinical uses. This is not the case, as there is tremendous variation among drugs, particularly when used as analgesics.

Aspirin

The first NSAID to be used in modern medicine was aspirin (acetylsalicylic acid). Aspirin is only given orally, and following its absorption is quickly converted to salicylic acid which serves as the active metabolite. Other salicylates exist but are seldom used in clinical medicine. Aspirin is unique among the NSAIDs in that it irreversibly binds to platelet cyclo-oxygenase producing a mild anticoagulant effect in all common domestic animals except cattle.[1] This irreversibility is not seen with the other salicylates or NSAIDs and occurs at a dose much lower than that required for other effects. Cattle and horses rapidly excrete the drug and therefore require large doses to maintain therapeutic plasma concentrations. It is effective as an antipyretic and for the control of mild to moderate somatic pain (skin, muscle, etc.). Aspirin has little effect on visceral pain. Though labeled for use in cattle in the United States, it has never undergone formal approval in this species.

Phenylbutazone

The best known NSAID in veterinary medicine is phenylbutazone. It has the ability to block mild to moderate somatic and visceral pain. As with salicylates, phenylbutazone has large species differences in metabolism, with an elimination half-life of

36 hours in the cow[2] vs. 5 hours in the horse.[3] This long half-life makes it particularly attractive in treating fractious cattle as dosing can be done at 48-hour intervals rather than the 12-hour intervals needed with most other NSAIDs. While veterinarians should realize that the use of all NSAIDs in food animals falls under the guidelines applicable to the Animal Medicinal Drug Use Clarification Act (AMDUCA), the long half-life of phenylbutazone coupled with its potential to cause aplastic anemia in man warrants judicious use in animals destined for slaughter. Because of its extensive protein binding and long half-life in cattle, a loading dose of 1.5 to 2.0 times the maintenance dose is usually employed.

Dipyrone

Dipyrone is closely related to phenylbutazone but has less anti-inflammatory action. It is an antipyretic and can also control mild to moderate somatic and visceral pain. Because dipyrone has the potential to cause aplastic anemia in humans and its pharmacokinetics and residue profile are unknown, the Food and Drug Administration (FDA) strongly discourages the use of dipyrone in food animals.

Flunixin

Flunixin meglumine is an NSAID approved for use in the horse, but it is commonly used in the cow and pig. The drug has excellent analgesic activity, especially for control of severe visceral pain. It also performs well as an antipyretic and anti-inflammatory agent. It has been shown to be effective in reducing signs and lesions associated with parainfluenza virus type 3 pneumonia in cattle.[4] Flunixin may be one of the few drugs beneficial in the treatment of 3-methylindole toxicity (atypical bovine pulmonary emphysema).[5] It is reputed to be useful in the management of endotoxemia such as that associated with coliform mastitis and *Pasteurella* pneumonia in cattle and agalactia and hypogalactia in swine. As it is relatively nonirritating, SC or IM injections can be given. It has also been shown to be absorbed orally in cattle.

RX
Fog
Fever

Ketoprofen

Ketoprofen is an NSAID approved for use in horses as an injectable formulation but is finding increasing extralabel use in cattle for a variety of indications. Though touted to be a dual cyclo-oxygenase and lipoxygenase inhibitor, the magnitude of the lipoxygenase inhibition is small enough to make this attribute of questionable clinical significance. Ketoprofen was found equally effective to flunixin as an analgesic in the treatment of mild to moderate equine colic; however, some clinicians feel flunixin may be the better agent for more severe pain.[6] Though a variety of NSAIDs have been shown to be of benefit in endotoxemia disease models, ketoprofen is one of the few such drugs to undergo a clinical trial where its benefit was proved. More specifically, in a study involving naturally occurring coliform mastitis, ketoprofen-treated animals had a more rapid return toward normal milk production than did cows not receiving ketoprofen.[7] In the horse, the drug may be less ulcerogenic and nephrotoxic than other common NSAIDs.[8]

Contraindications and Side Effects

By far the most common side effect of the NSAIDs is gastrointestinal ulceration with associated bleeding, which also represents the major contraindication to the use of these drugs. The reason is not totally known but appears to be due to an alteration of the normal mucus which protects the gastrointestinal system (prostaglandin E_1 [PGE_1] and E_2 [PGE_2] and prostaglandin A [PGA] are involved in normal mucus production). While there may be some variation in the propensity of different drugs to induce gastrointestinal ulceration (perhaps due to differing affinities for Cox 1 vs. Cox 2 enzyme subtypes),[9] it is seen with all drugs in this category.

Nephrotoxicity is occasionally reported. Most commonly a renal papillary necrosis is observed. As PGE_2 is necessary for normal renal blood flow, blocking its production with resultant impaired circulation may be the underlying pathophysiologic mechanism of nephrotoxicity.

Thromboxane production by platelets is a major contributing factor in normal coagulation. Cyclo-oxygenase inhibition thus results in some degree of impaired platelet adhesion and may cause a tendency toward increased bleeding. This is normally a reversible process except where aspirin is used.

Other side effects sometimes seen include hypersensitivities, and in humans bronchoconstriction and delayed parturition have been reported. Because of their ability to displace other highly protein-bound drugs, adverse drug interactions involving anesthetics or coumarin anticoagulants have been observed. Bone marrow suppression has been reported as a rare but serious complication of NSAID therapy. This occurs most commonly with the pyrazolone derivatives phenylbutazone and dipyrone.

GLUCOCORTICOIDS

Of all the anti-inflammatory agents there is no doubt that the glucocorticoids are the most effective. A variety of mechanisms have been proposed to explain their actions, including stabilization of lysosomal membranes and decreased influx of WBCs. It is now well accepted that their major anti-inflammatory effects occur by inhibition of phospholipase. As seen in Figure 1, this early interruption of the arachidonic acid cascade leads to decreased production of all the eicosanoids.

Although the glucocorticoids have many common physiologic effects, there are differences which make certain agents preferable in a given situation. Table 2 lists the common glucocorticoids, their potency, mineralocorticoid activity, and duration of hypothalamic-pituitary suppression (biologic half-life). Several points deserve mention here. First, regarding potency, note that this term is intended for comparison between agents to achieve a stated effect, not whether one agent is capable of achieving an effect that another cannot. For example, normal cortisol secretion is approximately 1 mg/kg/day. To have an anti-inflammatory effect, a good rule of thumb is that five times that amount is required. Thus a dose of 5 mg/kg/day of cortisol approximates 1 mg/kg/day prednisolone or 0.15 mg/kg/day dexamethasone. In selecting a glucocorticoid, potency is not an important concern as long as proper dosage adjustments are made. Primarily one should consider:

1. How rapid an onset is desired
2. The desired duration of effects
3. The desirability of mineralocorticoid activity
4. Whether abortifacient activity is an issue

In selecting an agent for administration, it is important, as regards onset and duration, to realize that both the drug and its formulation must be considered. If a rapid onset is desired, it could be argued that prednisolone achieves intracellular penetration earlier than does dexamethasone, making it more desirable in acute situations. However, in large animal medicine the longer biologic half-life (allowing for less frequent dosing) and lower cost make dexamethasone a preferred glucocorticoid.

Table 2
CHARACTERISTICS OF SOME COMMON GLUCOCORTICOIDS

Glucocorticoid	Anti-Inflammatory Potency*	Mineralocorticoid Potency*	Biologic Half-Life	Abortifacient Potential
Hydrocortisone	1	1.0	8–12 hr (short)	+
Prednisolone	4	0.8	12–36 hr (intermediate)	+
Triamcinolone	5	0.0	12–36 hr (intermediate)	+
Isoflupredone	17	0.0†	—	+
Dexamethasone	29	0.0	36–54 hr (long)	+ + +
Betamethasone	30	0.0	36–54 hr (long)	+ + +
Flumethasone	30	0.0	36–54 hr (long)	+ + +

*Potency is relative to hydrocortisone.
†Isoflupredone has some mineralocorticoid activity in dogs. Evidence suggests that repeated high doses of isoflupredone may contribute to hypokalemia in cattle.

While these characteristics of the parent drug are of obvious importance, formulation of the glucocorticoid preparation is often more relevant. When an immediate effect is desired, the water-soluble form of the steroid is preferred (i.e., sodium phosphate or sodium succinate salts), whereas if a long duration is desired, the water-insoluble (repository) form would be used (i.e., acetate, acetonide, or dipropionate salts). For example, in treating endotoxic shock with its rapid onset, the sodium phosphate form is preferable over the conventional dexamethasone base (in propylene glycol and water). Dexamethasone acetate would be inappropriate here because of its delayed onset.

Differences also exist in the mineralocorticoid activity of the glucocorticoids. Usually this tendency toward sodium retention and potassium excretion is of limited clinical significance. A rare exception is cardiac disease where sodium (and hence fluid) retention may further decompensate the patient. Of greater significance is the observation that glucocorticoid treatment with repeated doses of isoflupredone (9-fluoroprednisolone) has resulted in hypokalemia in some cattle prone toward anorexia or ketosis.[10] Because this syndrome was only recently recognized, it has been hypothesized that changes in dairy management may be cofactors in the precipitation of the hypokalemia. Large extralabel doses of the steroid, recent calving, diet (anionic or high potassium rations), and administration of oral propionate compounds have been considered as contributing causes to the condition, but at present this remains speculative. Whether the hypokalemia encountered in this situation is related to an unrecognized mineralocorticoid effect from isoflupredone (single doses have minimal mineralocorticoid activity in the cow, but some activity is reported in the dog) or to another, unknown, mechanism remains to be determined, as does the incidence of this side effect. Isoflupredone remains a valuable glucocorticoid for use in cattle; however, until this matter is resolved label instructions should be followed with repeated large doses of isoflupredone avoided unless careful monitoring is available. This syndrome has not been associated with steroids largely devoid of mineralocorticoid activity such as dexamethasone (see Table 2).

Of particular importance to food animal veterinarians is the abortifacient activity of the different agents. Although all glucocorticoids have the potential to induce abortion, this phenomenon is seen most often in ruminants in the last half of gestation following administration of C^{16}-methylated agents such as dexamethasone. Steroid-induced abortion usually results in placental retention. When glucocorticoids must be administered to the pregnant animal, the nonmethylated compounds such as prednisolone or isoflupredone will lower the risk of abortion.[11] In other species glucocorticoids are considered potential teratogens if given during the first trimester of pregnancy.

Clinical Uses

The glucocorticoids have been used in a number of specific clinical conditions, including shock, CNS edema, and ketosis. The benefit of glucocorticoids in shock has remained controversial; although seldom contraindicated, it now appears that they are of limited benefit in most forms of shock. An exception to this is in endotoxic (septic) shock where early high doses of glucocorticoids may stabilize the condition of the animal, allowing for correction of the underlying infection. (There is evidence from human clinical trials that steroids do not change the eventual mortality rate in septic shock; that is, the patient improves only to die later.)

Methylprednisolone and perhaps dexamethasone have the ability to limit damage following CNS trauma provided high doses are given shortly after the injury. They are also effective in reducing cerebral edema associated with certain CNS neoplasms. Because of their immunosuppressive properties, care should be taken to rule out the presence of CNS infection before proceeding with glucocorticoid therapy.

The glucocorticoids are also used to treat bovine ketosis. Although these agents decrease the peripheral utilization of glucose, the gluconeogenic properties produce higher blood glucose concentrations, thereby ameliorating CNS signs. Many of the beneficial effects seen in lactating dairy cattle may come from the ability of glucocorticoids to decrease milk production, thereby decreasing energy demands. It is probably wise to warn the dairyman of this side effect when treating lactating dairy cattle. As mentioned earlier, repetitive use of steroids having significant mineralocorticoid activity should be avoided in these patients.

Dexamethasone, betamethasone, and flumethasone have been shown to increase surfactant production in the fetus. In those instances where completion of the full term of pregnancy is unlikely, treatment of the dam with low doses (i.e., 0.02 mg/kg IM) 24 to 48 hours prior to induction or cesarean section may reduce the incidence of neonatal respiratory distress syndrome.

The following rules of thumb apply to the clinical uses of glucocorticoids in the general treatment of inflammatory disease:

1. A single large dose of a glucocorticoid seldom causes harm.
2. If used in bacterial infections, bactericidal antimicrobials may be preferred to bacteriostatic agents because of glucocorticoid-induced dysfunction of phagocytes. Animals suffering from infectious diseases controlled primarily by cell-mediated immunity (i.e., systemic mycoses, mycobacterial infections) should not receive glucocorticoids (unless clinical judgment deems them absolutely necessary and if appropriate antifungal and antimycobacterial therapy is instituted).

3. If chronic therapy is required, the lowest possible dose which achieves the desired effect should be sought. Alternate-day therapy with a nonrepository intermediate-acting agent further decreases the incidence of adrenal insufficiency and immunosuppression. As iatrogenic hypoadrenocorticism is a rare but serious consequence of chronic steroid administration, doses should be gradually rather than abruptly reduced.

4. Remember that glucocorticoids are primarily palliative therapy. Diagnosis and treatment of the underlying disease should be instituted.

Contraindications and Side Effects

Few drugs affect such a wide variety of tissues as do the glucocorticoids. Of the myriad effects that can occur following their use, the contraindications to administration of a glucocorticoid include gastrointestinal ulceration, systemic mycoses, and mycobacterial infections. Corneal ulceration prohibits ophthalmic use. All of the drugs in this class tend to delay healing and promote infection; therefore, their use in animals with bone fractures or following abdominal surgery is discouraged. If they must be used in any of these conditions, an intermediate-acting water-soluble product such as prednisolone sodium succinate is preferred so that the duration of activity is minimized. If sepsis is suspected, bactericidal antimicrobials are preferred over bacteriostatic agents, as phagocyte activity is inhibited by glucocorticoids. Conditions in small animals which may be exacerbated by glucocorticoid administration include diabetes mellitus (owing to the anti-insulin effect), pancreatitis, osteoporosis (owing to increased calcium excretion), and renal disease (owing to catabolic effects). In addition to their abortifacient activity these agents are teratogenic in the first trimester, making their use in pregnant animals undesirable. Prednisone (inactive prodrug) should not be used in patients with hepatic failure, as a functioning liver is required for transformation to active prednisolone.

DIMETHYL SULFOXIDE (DMSO)

DMSO has many characteristics which make it a useful agent in the treatment of inflammation. Although most of the anti-inflammatory effects have been attributed to its ability to scavenge free radicals, it also may potentiate endogenous glucocorticoid effects, decrease the influx of WBCs into an area, and limit fibrous tissue formation following injury. Its ability to act as a percutaneous carrier for other drugs with molecular weights of less than 3000 has also attracted a great deal of interest.

Topically (its approved route in the dog and horse) DMSO can be used to treat a variety of musculoskeletal conditions such as tendonitis or desmitis. It is also used in an extralabel manner IV to treat CNS edema or trauma or pneumonia.

When used to treat CNS edema or trauma, a dose of 0.5 to 1.0 g/kg is usually given IV once daily as a 10% solution. Higher concentrations (which can cause hemolysis) or rapid administration may cause nonspecific histamine release resulting in collapse. Even the 10% solution is still quite hypertonic and a marked diuresis is common.

Surprisingly, no scientific data exist to document the efficacy of DMSO as an adjunct treatment in bovine pneumonia. It has been used empirically at IV doses of 0.02 to 1.0 g/kg.

In addition to the hemolysis and histamine release mentioned above, DMSO is a potential teratogen and ideally, should be avoided in pregnant animals. DMSO may potentiate the effects of cholinesterase-inhibiting agents such as organophosphate insecticides or phenothiazine tranquilizers. Although chronic high-dose administration has been reported to cause cataract formation in the dog, this is of doubtful clinical significance.

REFERENCES

1. Gentry PA, Tremblay RRM, Ross ML: Failure of aspirin to impair bovine platelet function. Am J Vet Res 50(6):919–922, 1989.
2. Lees P, Ayliffe T, Maitho TE: Pharmacokinetics, metabolism and excretion of phenylbutazone in cattle following intravenous, intramuscular and oral administration. Res in Vet Sci 44:57–67, 1988.
3. US Pharmacopeia Drug Information. Vol 1: Drug Information for the Health Care Professional. September 1995 Update. Rockville, Md, US Pharmacopeia Convention, 1996, p 702.
4. Selman IE, Allan EM, Gibbs HA, et al: Effect on anti-prostaglandin therapy in experimental parainfluenza type 3 pneumonia in weaned, conventional calves. Vet Rec 115:101–105, 1984.
5. Selman IE, Allan EM, Gibbs HA, et al: The effect of anti-prostaglandin therapy in an acute respiratory distress syndrome induced in experimental cattle by the oral administration of 3-methylindole. Bovine Pract 20:124–126, 1985.
6. Betley M, Sutherland SF, Gregorick MJ, et al: The analgesic effect of ketoprofen for use in treating equine colic as compared to flunixin meglumine. Equine Pract 13:11–16, 1981.
7. Shpigel NY, Chen R, Winkler M, et al: Anti-inflammatory ketoprofen in the treatment of field cases of bovine mastitis. Res Vet Sci 56:62–68, 1994.
8. MacAllister CG, Morgan SJ, Borne AT, et al: Comparison of adverse effects of phenylbutazone, flunixin meglumine, and ketoprofen in horses. J Am Vet Med Assoc 202:71–77, 1993.
9. Spangler RS: Cyclooxygenase 1 and 2 in rheumatic diseases: Implications for nonsteroidal anti-inflammatory drug therapy. Semin Arthritis Rheum 26:435–446, 1996.
10. Sielman ES, Sweeney RW, Whitlock RH, et al: Hypokalemia syndrome in dairy cows: 10 cases (1992–1996). J Am Vet Med Assoc 210:240–243, 1997.
11. Lauderdale JW: Effect of corticoid administration on bovine pregnancy. J Am Vet Med Assoc 160:867–871, 1972.

BIBLIOGRAPHY

Booth NH, McDonald LE (eds): Veterinary Pharmacology and Therapeutics, ed 6. Ames, Iowa State University Press, 1988.
Calvert CA, Cornelius LM: Symposium on the use and misuse of steroids (peer reviewed). Vet Med August 85:810–865, 1990.
Ellis C (ed): International Symposium on Nonsteroidal Anti-inflammatory Agents. Orlando, Fla, Veterinary Learning Systems, 1986.
Upson DW: Upson's Handbook of Veterinary Pharmacology, ed 2. Lenexa, Kan, VM Publishing, 1985.

■ Adverse Drug Reactions

Gordon W. Brumbaugh, D.V.M., Ph.D.
Dawn M. Boothe, D.V.M., Ph.D.

Adverse drug reactions (ADRs) are defined as any unintended and undesirable response to a drug and can be categorized as either type A or type B. Type B (idiosyncratic or "bizarre") ADRs are unpredictable responses to a drug. Although they affect only a small percent of the animal population, they occur regardless of the dose of drug administered. Hypersensitivity reactions and genetic idiosyncrasies are examples of type B reactions. Because of the rarity of these reactions, many animals must receive a particular drug before this type of ADR is recognized and can be declared as an inherent risk of using the medication in animals. In contrast, type A (idiopathic or "augmented") ADRs are usually concentration- or dose-dependent and are more likely to occur when an improper dosing regimen is used that results in concentrations of drug outside the therapeutic range. Type A ADR may be manifested as an exaggerated pharmacologic response, as a toxic response (e.g., tissue damage) if the concentration is above the therapeutic range, or as therapeutic failure if the concentration lies below the therapeutic range.

The dosing regimen and the disposition of the drug in the body are important determinants of systemic concentrations of a drug. Events that determine disposition of a drug include the rate and extent of drug *absorption* from the site of administration, *distribution* of the drug from the circulation into tissues, and clearance of the drug by *metabolism* or *excretion* or both. The chemistry of the drug largely determines the role each of these events has in the drug's disposition. However, these events can be altered in a patient by a variety of factors, thus increasing the potential of type A adverse drug reactions. These factors can be described as physiologic, pharmacologic, or pathologic.

PHYSIOLOGIC FACTORS

Many type A adverse reactions occur because a dosing regimen in one species has been inappropriately extrapolated to another. Generally, species that are physiologically similar tend to have the same pattern of disposition of a drug. Thus, while a similar dosing regimen might be used for ruminants, a different one is often needed for monogastric animals (e.g., pigs). Species differences affect all phases of disposition of a drug.

Major determinants of gastrointestinal *absorption* of a drug include gastrointestinal pH, surface area, motility, and blood flow. Each of these determinants may vary among species, resulting in differences in the rate and extent of absorption among species. For example, the gastrointestinal pH of pigs varies from 1 to 7. Although ruminal pH is less variable (5.5 to 6.5), it can be markedly affected by ration or diet. Ruminants present another unique challenge for orally administered drugs. Ruminal contents might dilute or destroy the drug, or be destroyed by the drug before the drug reaches the site of absorption. The site of parenteral administration may also lead to a different rate and extent of absorption of a drug. For example, studies with calves have shown that the most consistent absorption of ampicillin occurs if the drug is administered either intramuscularly in the middle gluteal muscles or subcutaneously over the ribs.

Major determinants of *distribution* of drugs include the extent of binding to proteins in plasma and other extracellular fluids (particularly albumin), the fat-to-lean distribution of body weight, and the size of body compartments to which the drug might be distributed. The concentration of a drug in plasma varies inversely with the amount of tissue to which the drug is distributed. Administration of a lipid-soluble drug to animals with a greater proportion of body fat, such as pigs, finished steers, and lambs, may decrease the amount of drug available to target tissues, resulting in therapeutic failure because of inadequate concentrations of drug in plasma. Alternatively, if the drug does not distribute into fat, but an animal with a high proportion of fat is dosed on the basis of total body weight, concentrations of the drug in plasma may be higher than those produced in lean animals (e.g., unfinished animals, steers, goats, and cows) receiving a similar dose. An exaggerated response may occur in such animals. Distribution of drugs into the gastrointestinal tract of ruminants and the mammary glands of dairy cattle depends on the drug's chemistry, degree of ionization in the tissue, and lipid-solubility of the drug. If the pH is appropriate, a drug can accumulate in tissues by ion trapping. Two potential problems can occur: (1) less drug is available for distribution to target organs; and (2) drugs may be trapped in edible tissues, where it serves as a source of exposure to suckling calves or human consumers of milk products. In the latter case, violative milk residues become a major concern.

Species differences in the *metabolism* of drugs can be profound and clinically significant. Metabolism of drugs occurs primarily in the liver in two phases. Phase I metabolism chemically changes the drug so that it is more amenable to phase II metabolism. Phase II reactions are synthetic: a large molecule (e.g., glucuronic acid or sulfate) is added to the drug or its phase I metabolite. With rare exceptions, phase II reactions inactivate the drug and increase its water-solubility so that excretion is facilitated. Few differences in metabolism have been documented among food animals. The elimination half-life of phenylbutazone is at least 36 hours in cattle, but much less (9 hours) in several other species. Metabolism of drugs by microbes in the gastrointestinal tract can result in type A reactions, particularly therapeutic failure. Species differences in the *excretion* of drugs are also likely to exist among food animals, although their role in the advent of type A adverse drug reactions has not been established.

Age-related differences in the disposition of drugs can play a significant role in the advent of ADRs, although usually these differences are not as marked in cattle. Briefly, the *pediatric* patient is predisposed to changes in disposition of drugs for the following reasons: (1) Its gastrointestinal tract is more permeable, particularly for the first 24 hours following birth. More drug is absorbed than in adult animals and this might result in violative residues. (2) The drug is distributed to a larger volume of tissue. Total body water is greater and the concentration of serum albumin is less in pediatric patients than in adults. (3) Metabolism of drugs is generally less, particularly in neonates, because drug-metabolizing enzymes mature at different rates during the first 3 months of life. (4) Finally, renal elimination of drugs is less in neonates for the first few days of life than it is in adults. Age-related changes in disposition of drugs in the *geriatric* patient can be more dramatic than those in the pediatric patient, but geriatric bovine patients are particularly rare.

Sex differences in drug disposition have not been documented in food animals. In those species in which such differences have been identified, the sequelae are usually minor and clinically insignificant; however, the female of all species is predisposed to selected type A ADRs because of her reproductive activity. Drugs may cause embryocidal or teratogenic effects, abortion, changes in parturition, or altered lactation. Occasionally, the male reproductive tract is selectively susceptible to some type A ADRs.

Type A ADRs may reflect interspecies or intraspecies variations in the ratio of body mass to body weight. Although body surface area is the best estimate of body mass, drugs are usually dosed on a per-unit body weight (i.e., pounds or kilograms). Unfortunately, charts with conversion of weight to body surface area that have been validated for large animals are not available to the practitioner. Differences between body weight and "true lean body weight" can be important contributors to adverse reactions in selected populations of animals: obese versus starved animals; animals with edema or ascites; dehydrated animals; animals with large tumors; and animals with filled gastrointestinal compartments.

An often overlooked factor that can lead to type A adverse reactions is environmental temperature. Flow of blood at sites of parenteral administration can be altered by ambient temperature, which will change absorption. For example, hypothermia can cause peripheral vasoconstriction, decreased metabolic processes, and reduced intestinal motility. The newborn animal is particularly susceptible to the effects of hypothermia.

PHARMACOLOGIC FACTORS

Pharmacologic factors, or drug interactions, occur whenever the action or disposition of one drug is modified by another, concurrently administered drug. The incidence of drug interactions increases as the number of drugs administered increases, as the duration of drug therapy increases, and in the presence of disease. Drug interactions can be pharmaceutical, pharmaco-

---

Table 1
EXAMPLES OF PHARMACEUTICAL DRUG INTERACTIONS

Drug	Interactions
	In Vitro
Atropine sulfate and barbiturates	Diazepam
Gentamicin sulfate	Carbenicillin, cephalosporins, heparin sodium
Tetracyclines	Divalent and trivalent cations (calcium, aluminum, magnesium), cephalosporins, tylosin, chloramphenicol sodium succinate, hydrocortisone sodium succinate, sodium bicarbonate
Meperidine and barbiturates	Sodium bicarbonate, heparin sodium, methylprednisolone sodium succinate
Calcium gluconate and carbonate	Phosphate, sulfate salts, tetracyclines
Semisynthetic penicillins	Aminoglycosides, barbiturates, diazepam, phenothiazine neuroleptics, vitamin B complexes
	In Vivo
Aminoglycosides	Penicillins
Tetracyclines	Divalent or trivalent cations
Protamine	Heparin
Calcium gluconate and sodium sulfonamide	Can form gels in veins
Kaolin	Rifampin, lincomycin, and other drugs following oral administration

---

Table 3
EXAMPLES OF INTERACTIONS OF DRUGS AND DIETARY CONSTITUENTS

Drug or Dietary Nutrient	Effect
Sulfafurazole	Impaired absorption
Ampicillin and other semisynthetic penicillins (except amoxicillin)	Impaired absorption
Cephalexin	Impaired absorption
Tetracyclines	Impaired absorption
Lincomycin	Impaired absorption
Rifampin	Impaired absorption
Griseofulvin	Enhanced absorption in presence of fat

---

kinetic, or pharmacodynamic, depending on the phase of drug action in which they occur.

Pharmaceutical drug interactions occur when two or more chemically incompatible drugs are combined (Tables 1 and 2). This may occur prior to (in vitro) or following (in vivo) administration. Interactions in vitro can occur among drugs and additives (e.g., base or salt forms, solubilizers, stabilizers). Pharmaceutical drug interactions are often accompanied by a change in the physical or chemical nature of the drug. These changes usually alter dissolution, diffusion, absorption and distribution of the drug. In some instances, one or more drugs are inactivated. The most common pharmaceutical interactions are those that occur when drugs intended for injection are mixed with fluids (see Table 2) or with one another for convenience prior to administration. Pharmaceutical incompatibilities can occur in the gastrointestinal tract after oral administration but prior to absorption. Occasionally, interactions between a drug and dietary constituent lead to adverse drug reactions (Table 3).

Pharmacokinetic drug interactions occur in vivo when one drug alters any phase of disposition of a second, concurrently administered drug. These interactions can be profound and occasionally are life-threatening. Pharmacokinetic drug interactions that alter *absorption* of drugs usually follow oral administration. The effect of changes in gastric motility depends on the site of absorption of the drug (Table 4). Because most drugs are absorbed from the small intestine, drugs that slow ruminal or abomasal motility tend to delay emptying and the rate of absorption. Although the total amount of drug absorbed might not be affected, the peak plasma concentration of the drug may be decreased. Drugs that increase motility may have the opposite effect. Drugs that alter small intestinal motility frequently do not change the absorption of an orally administered drug because the surface area of the intestines is too large. However, drugs that increase or decrease blood flow in the gastrointestinal tract may cause parallel changes in the absorption of some drugs. Finally, some drugs can cause malabsorption of other drugs or nutrients due to their toxic effects on the gastrointestinal tract.

Absorption from intramuscular and subcutaneous sites can be decreased by drugs that decrease regional blood flow. Some topical preparations contain drugs that are included to increase the permeability of the skin (e.g., dimethyl sulfoxide [DMSO]) and, thus, drug absorption.

Most clinically important pharmacokinetic interactions that alter *distribution* result from competition of protein-bound drugs for protein binding sites. Examples of highly protein-bound (>85%) drugs include most nonsteroidal anti-inflammatory drugs and some sulfonamides. Because protein binding is reversible and competitive, the drug with the highest affinity for protein (usually albumin) will displace a drug with less affinity.

Table 2
EXAMPLES OF PHARMACEUTICAL DRUG-FLUID INTERACTIONS

Drug	Fluid
Ampicillin	Glucose and dextran fluids
Oxytetracycline	Ca^{2+} or Mg^{2+}, glucose fluids
Gentamicin sulfate	Any (>1 g/L)
Diazepam	Any
Methylprednisolone	Sodium succinate and sodium lactate solutions
Sodium bicarbonate	Sodium lactate, Ringer's, any solution with Ca^{2+}

Table 4
DRUGS THAT INDUCE OR INHIBIT DRUG METABOLISM ENZYMES

Inducers
  Chlorinated hydrocarbons
  Griseofulvin
  Phenobarbital (and other barbiturates)
  Phenylbutazone
  Phenytoin
  Theophylline
Inhibitors
  Chloramphenicol
  Cimetidine, ranitidine
  Prednisolone
  Phenylbutazone
  Quinidine

Table 5
EXAMPLES OF PHARMACODYNAMIC DRUG INTERACTIONS THAT INCREASE DRUG ADVERSITY

Drug 1	Adversity	Drug 2
Aminoglycosides	Otoxicity and nephrotoxicosis	Furosemide
Aminoglycosides	Neuromuscular and cardiac blockade	Most general anesthetics*
Pancuronium gallamine	Enhanced neuromuscular blockade	Lincomycin Clindamycin Polymixins
Tetracyclines	Neuromuscular blockage	General anesthetics (or during hypocalcemia)
Halothane and methoxyflurane	Sensitized myocardium to arrhythmogenic effects of catecholamines	Thiobarbiturates potentiate the effect†
Diamidine antiprotozoals	Anticholinesterase inhibitors	Organophosphates
Succinylcholine	Prolonged flaccid paralysis	Cholinesterase inhibitors
Methoxyflurane	Renal failure	Tetracyclines

*Reversed with Ca^{2+} and anticholinesterase antagonist.
†Premedication with acepromazine, lidocaine, or propranolol reduces this effect.

Because the free (unbound) form of the drug is pharmacologically active, the potential for adverse reactions is increased. Competition for protein binding can also occur in tissues. Distribution to organs also may be changed by drugs that alter regional blood flow.

Changes in *metabolism* of drugs, induced by pharmacokinetic drug interactions, can be profound and clinically significant. Phase I hepatic drug–metabolizing enzymes are susceptible to induction or inhibition by other compounds. Many drugs have been identified as potential inducers or inhibitors (Table 5); some drugs (e.g., phenylbutazone) are capable of either effect, depending on the enzyme involved. If *induction* of enzymes occurs, metabolism increases. Clearance of concurrently administered drugs that are also metabolized by the liver will increase, and therapeutic failure may follow. A toxic or a pharmacologic response may also occur, however, if production of a toxic phase I metabolite or a pharmacologically active drug is increased. Drugs vary in their ability to induce enzymes, and several days to weeks of administration may be required for enzyme induction to occur. A similar period may be necessary for resolution of induction after the inducing drug has been discontinued.

Drugs can also *inhibit* metabolizing enzymes, although these effects are probably not as clinically significant as are those resulting from induction. Clearance of a concurrently administered drug that is metabolized by the liver is usually decreased. As the drug accumulates, the potential for a toxic or an exaggerated pharmacologic response increases. Generally, inhibition does not require long-term administration of the drug, and the effects of inhibition may resolve faster than those of induction. Drug metabolism may also be decreased by drugs that decrease hepatic blood flow (e.g., theophylline and cimetidine); however, this interaction is significant only for drugs characterized by extensive and rapid hepatic clearance (e.g., propranolol, lidocaine). In such instances, the clearance of a drug will decline in concert with decreased hepatic blood flow.

Pharmacokinetic drug interactions may alter the *excretion* of some drugs, although these changes are probably not as clinically important as those that affect drug metabolism. Changes in biliary elimination are rare and usually result from competition for excretory proteins. Pharmacokinetic drug interactions during renal excretion often reflect drug-induced changes in renal blood flow and glomerular filtration. In addition, drugs, and particularly weak acids, compete for active tubular secretion. Finally, renal excretion of a drug may be changed by drugs that alter urinary pH. As the drug becomes more ionized, less is resorbed from the tubules and more is excreted. If the pH increases the amount of un-ionized drug, more drug is resorbed from the tubules into the plasma. Clearance of the drug would then be decreased.

Pharmacodynamic drug interactions occur when one drug directly alters the physiologic response to another drug (Table 6). They can either enhance the response to a drug (*agonistic*) or they can inhibit the response (*antagonistic*). Agonistic interactions can be additive or synergistic. This may occur either at the same receptor or at different sites but with the same physiologic reaction. Many drug combinations result in agonistic effects. Examples include the combination of selected antimicrobials. Antagonistic interactions decrease the response to a drug, owing to competition at the same receptor site (e.g., atropine and anticholinesterases) or at distant but physiologically related sites. Although antagonistic pharmacodynamic interactions often produce an undesirable side effect, they may also be of therapeutic benefit. Examples of some therapeutically beneficial antagonistic interactions include the combination of chemicals for restraint or anesthesia and the reversal of the action of narcotics.

PATHOLOGIC FACTORS

Dosage regimens recommended for a pharmaceutical preparation generally are based on controlled studies with normal, healthy animals. The patient, however, is usually diseased. Pathophysiologic changes that accompany disease can profoundly alter disposition of drugs, which predisposes the diseased patient to type A ADRs. Diseases of the liver and kidneys are probably most important because these organs are responsible for most clearance of drugs.

Effects of renal disease on disposition of drugs have been well documented in selected species. Disease-induced decreases in glomerular filtration and tubular secretion will markedly decrease renal clearance of drugs and metabolites. In general, clearance of drugs eliminated by glomerular filtration will decline in proportion to decreased renal blood flow. These changes become important if the drug is toxic, and particularly if the drug is nephrotoxic (e.g., aminoglycosides). The effects of renal disease on drug clearance can be estimated based on changes in

Table 6
DRUGS THAT HAVE BEEN SUBJECTS OF REPORTS OF ADVERSE REACTIONS IN CATTLE

Antimicrobial
Tranquilizer
Ionophores
Vitamin/mineral
Endocrine/hormone
Antihistamine
Antiparasitic
Dextrose, multiple electrolytes
Nonsteroid anti-inflammatory
Antibloat

Data from Tjálve H: Adverse reactions to veterinary drugs reported in Sweden during 1991–1995. J Vet Pharmacol Ther 20:105, 1997.

the patient's clearance of creatinine. Likewise, dosing regimens of drugs that are excreted by glomerular filtration can be individualized to the patient, based on the patient's creatinine clearance (*pt CrCl*) or its serum creatine concentrations, according to the formula:

$$\text{New dose} = \text{normal dose} \quad \times \frac{\text{pt CrCl}}{\text{normal CrCl}}$$

$$\text{New interval} = \text{normal interval} \times \frac{\text{normal CrCl}}{\text{Clpt CrCl}}$$

Physiologic changes that accompany renal disease may alter other determinants of disposition of drugs. Examples include changes in serum protein binding (because of protein loss through the glomerulus or competition with accumulated endogenous substrates) and fluid, electrolyte, and acid-base imbalances.

The effects of hepatic disease on drug disposition are very complex. Both hepatic blood flow and metabolic enzyme activity decline with progressing hepatic disease. Hepatic clearance of drugs proportionately decreases. Changes in protein binding also occur owing to decreased synthesis of albumin or increased formation of globulins. These will affect the rate of hepatic clearance, because unbound drugs are generally cleared faster by the liver than are protein-bound drugs. Changes in hepatic clearance are particularly important for orally administered drugs that undergo hepatic first-pass metabolism (i.e., most of the drug is removed from the blood by the liver the first time the drug passes through the liver). The bioavailability of such drugs increases as hepatic blood flow decreases. Plasma drug concentrations may develop in the toxic range if the normal oral dose is administered. Changes in protein concentration can also alter drug distribution, as can changes in fluid, electrolyte, and acid/base balance. The effects of hepatic disease on drug disposition depend on the drug, its degree of protein binding, how rapidly the drug is removed by the liver, the type of hepatic disease, and the species to which the drug is being administered. Unfortunately, the complexity of hepatic disease precludes making general recommendations regarding the alteration of dosing regimens in the patient with hepatic disease. Caution should be exercised when administering toxic drugs, and particularly drugs that are hepatotoxic.

Because cardiac output is important to the normal function of all body organs, cardiovascular disease can affect all determinants of drug disposition. These effects can be profound in an animal suffering from hypotensive or endotoxic shock. In general, regional blood flow to body organs decreases in the presence of cardiac disease. Both oral and parenteral absorption can decrease. Regional distribution of drugs to target organs declines. Because blood flow to the heart and brain is maintained, these organs may receive a greater proportion of drug and are susceptible to drug-induced toxicity. Blood flow to organs of excretion (i.e., kidney and liver) parallels cardiac output; consequently, excretion of drugs decreases.

Diseases of other body systems can also dramatically alter drug disposition. For example, gastrointestinal disease may alter drug absorption because of changes in the gastrointestinal pH, epithelial permeability, or motility. Malnutrition can alter drug disposition because of hypoproteinemia and altered metabolism. Endocrinologic disorders can alter body metabolism as well as homeostasis of fluid and electrolytes. Finally, diseases of any organ will affect the response of that organ to a drug. If the organ is the target of drug therapy, therapeutic failure may occur owing to changes in receptors, intracellular messengers, or subcellular physiology. Alternatively, diseased organs are not as capable of repair following insult or toxicity as healthy organs

are. As the pathologic effects of disease are reversed, disposition is likely to change again, which may predispose the patient to ADRs.

TYPE B ADVERSE DRUG REACTIONS

Type B ADRs are bizarre reactions that are unrelated to the dose or the anticipated pharmacologic effect of the drug. Because type B adverse reactions are unpredictable and occur in a very small percent of the population, they are nearly unavoidable and are an inherent part of veterinary medicine. Type B reactions have been attributed to genetic or idiosyncratic factors or hypersensitivities (allergic reactions). Some species differences reflecting different receptor sensitivity may be considered type B. For example, cattle, and particularly Brahman or Brahman-crossed cattle, are more sensitive to the depressant effects of xylazine, whereas sheep tend to react adversely to haloxon. Cattle react to morphine by exhibiting excitation rather than depression.

The most common type B ADR is probably hypersensitivity. The incidence of drug hypersensitivities is not great. Most drugs are too small to induce an immune response. Rather they (or their metabolites) must covalently bond with a larger macromolecule to induce an allergic response. The drug molecule is referred to as a *hapten* (as opposed to *antigen*), and the allergic reaction can be manifested against the drug, the macromolecule, or both. Drugs can cause any type of immune-mediated response (i.e., types I through IV) and any component of a drug's formulation can cause the allergic reaction. For example, carriers and solubilizers may result in the sudden release or activation of autacoids such as histamine, serotonin, kinins, prostaglandins, leukotrienes, and platelet-activating factors. Signs indicative of an anaphylactic response may result. Microbiologic (contaminating) products may also stimulate an immune reaction. Cross-reactivity between closely related compounds (e.g., β-lactam antibiotics such as penicillins and cephalosporins, or any of the chemically related sulfonamides) may result in a similar response. Drugs of different pharmacologic classification may incite anaphylaxis as well. An example is allergic reaction to furosemide by an animal that is allergic to sulfonamides. This is because the sulfonamide grouping induces the reaction and is present on both drugs.

Drug allergies are characterized by the following conditions: (1) the patient was previously exposed to the drug or a drug with chemical similarity; (2) the reaction occurs every time the drug (and in some cases, similar drugs) is administered; (3) the reaction is not correlated to the amount of drug administered; and (4) the response occurs or worsens regardless of the dose.

AVOIDANCE OF ADVERSE DRUG REACTIONS

The incidence of type A ADRs can be decreased by the following means: (1) limiting the clinic's pharmacy to selected, representative drugs; (2) becoming thoroughly familiar with these drugs; (3) being thoroughly informed of the clinical status of the patient, particularly of factors that may predispose the patient to adverse reactions; (4) collecting appropriate baseline data prior to initiating drug therapy, with emphasis on drug history and on organs of drug elimination and organs that are targets for drug-induced toxicity; (5) altering the dosage regimen (dose or interval) if indicated, based on clinical assessment, clinical laboratory tests, or therapeutic drug monitoring; (6) selecting the least toxic drug; (7) avoiding concurrent administration of drugs to reduce the incidence of drug interactions; (8) alternating the times at which drug is administered; (9)

following, when possible, the recommended dosage regimen for each species without modifying the drug's preparations; and (10) monitoring the patient for response and discontinuing the drug if indicated by therapeutic success, failure, or toxicity.

Anaphylactoid reactions are not immunologic, not related to pharmacologic action of the drug, and are partly predictable. They result from drug-induced release of chemical mediators (particularly histamine), which causes pathophysiologic responses typical of anaphylaxis. However, unlike anaphylaxis, prior exposure of the drug is not necessary. Cationic drugs such as radiocontrast dyes and amphotericin B are capable of causing direct mast cell degranulation and thus an anaphylactoid response. Anaphylactoid reactions are partly dose-dependent.

Clinical signs, biochemical monitoring, and therapeutic drug monitoring are important tools that can be used to guide drug therapy in the patient predisposed to toxic responses. Signs of drug toxic effects can be difficult to discern from signs of the patient's illness, however. Although biochemical tests are more specific, some drugs alter the results of those tests but are not necessarily indicative of drug-induced organ pathology. Practitioners must be informed regarding the potential of a drug to alter the results of tests before an assumption of drug-induced toxicity is made. Therapeutic drug monitoring is the most specific means of guiding drug therapy. It is particularly applicable to therapy with selected antimicrobials (i.e., aminoglycosides), antiarrhythmics, and anticonvulsants. Measurement of concentrations of drugs in plasma is important for drugs that are toxic, when therapeutic success is critical (i.e., when an organ or life is threatened), or when therapeutic response is difficult to assess (e.g., with antimicrobials). Several laboratories throughout the United States offer therapeutic drug monitoring services. Clinical pharmacology consultation is offered at these and other locations to support the efforts of practitioners in reducing the incidence of adverse drug reactions.

REFERENCES

1. Riviere JE: Veterinary clinical pharmacokinetics: Part I. Fundamental concepts. Compend Contin Educ Small Anim Pract 10:24–30, 1988.
2. Pond SM: Pharmacokinetic drug interactions. In Benet LZ, Massoud N, Grunbertoglio JU (eds): Pharmacokinetic Basis for Drug Treatment. New York, Raven Press, 1985, pp 195–220.
3. Baggott J: Principles of Drug Disposition in Domestic Animals: The Basis of Veterinary Clinical Pharmacology. Philadelphia, WB Saunders, 1979, pp 73–112.
4. Green TP, Mirkin BL: Clinical Pharmacokinetics: Pediatric Considerations. Philadelphia, Lea & Febiger, 1976, pp 269–282.
5. Massoud N: Pharmacokinetic considerations in geriatric patients. Philadelphia, Lea & Febiger, 1976, pp 283–310.
6. Wilkinson GR, Branch RA: Effects of hepatic disease on clinical pharmacokinetics. In Benet LZ, Massoud N, Grunbertoglio JU (eds): Pharmacokinetic Basis for Drug Treatment. New York, Raven Press, 1985, pp 49–62.
7. Brater DC, Chennavasin P: Effects of renal disease: Altered pharmacokinetics. In Benet LZ, Massoud N, Grunbertoglio JU (eds): Pharmacokinetic Basis for Drug Treatment. New York, Raven Press, 1985, pp 149–172.
8. Tjälve H: Adverse reactions to veterinary drugs reported in Sweden during 1991–1995. J Vet Pharmacol Ther 20:105–110, 1997.

■ Antimicrobial Use in Food Animals

Vernon C. Langston, D.V.M., Ph.D., Diplomate, A.C.V.C.P.

Antimicrobials are the most widely used class of pharmaceutical in veterinary medicine. Many practitioners become accustomed to using specific antimicrobials for specific diseases in a relatively routine manner. While this approach is sufficient in most instances, the interactions between host, drug, and pathogen can be quite complex and therefore this review is offered to better address unusual or difficult cases as well as provide background information on antibiotic families and individual drugs as they relate to food animals. This topic is particularly relevant given the increasing incidence of bacterial resistance to antimicrobials and the role that indiscriminate antibiotic use has played in its development.

Antimicrobial therapy as discussed in this chapter addresses those infections associated with bacterial, rickettsial, spirochetal, and mycoplasmal organisms. (For simplicity the terms *gram-positive* and *gram-negative* will refer to aerobic and facultative anaerobic bacteria. *Anaerobes* will refer to obligate anaerobic bacteria, both gram-positive and gram-negative unless otherwise defined.) It is axiomatic that infections due to fungal or viral elements will be unresponsive and certainly the indiscriminate use of antimicrobials merely promotes the development of bacterial resistance.

SELECTION CRITERIA*

The following questions must be considered in the selection of an antimicrobial drug regimen:

1. Does the diagnosis warrant antibiotic therapy?
2. What organisms are involved?
3. What is the in vitro antibiotic susceptibility of the organism?
4. In what region of the body and in what cell is the organism located? Will the antibiotic penetrate to the organism? If the organism is intracellular, does it leave the host cell often enough to be susceptible to extracellular antibiotics?
5. Is the antibiotic likely to be active in the local environment of the organism?
6. What drug formulation and dosage regimen will maintain the appropriate antimicrobial concentration for a long enough period of time?
7. What side effects might be expected during treatment? What potential for toxicity does the drug have? Do the benefits outweigh the risks?
8. Will the chosen drug pose a potential residue problem?
9. Is this the most cost-effective therapy?

Identification of Causative Agent

A presumptive diagnosis must be established before any sound decisions regarding therapeutic approaches can be made. That the diagnosis should be the basis for all treatment decisions is often ignored.

It is not always necessary to culture samples from all patients with infectious diseases to identify the organism involved. Often,

---

*Significant portions of this section are reproduced with permission from Langston VC, Davis LE: Factors to consider in the selection of antimicrobial drugs for therapy. Compendium Continuing Educ Pract Vet 11:355–364, 1989.

the practitioner can base a diagnosis on clinical experience of related or similar cases. The signs of some infectious diseases are so clear-cut that the need for further microbiologic identification is minimal, but for infectious diseases of unknown cause or for those attributable to organisms with irregular antibiotic sensitivity patterns, there is no substitute for identifying the causative agent.

Isolation and identification of the causative agent are applicable to treatment of an individual animal and can be applicable to herd management. Culturing of samples obtained from representative animals can help confirm the clinical diagnosis and provide required information should initial antimicrobial treatment prove ineffective. In addition, portions of the samples can be stained and examined immediately; such analysis, which may reveal the shape of the organism and whether the organism is gram-positive or gram-negative, can be useful to the practitioner in the immediate selection of a drug for therapy while other diagnostic tests are being performed.[1]

Sensitivity Testing

Once the causative organism is identified, a decision regarding the need for antimicrobial sensitivity testing can be made. In some cases, no further testing is required. For example, clostridial organisms are all sensitive to high doses of penicillin G, while sensitivity testing of aerobic gram-negative enteric organisms is beneficial because most of them have highly erratic sensitivity patterns. Table 1 indicates those organisms with reasonably predictable sensitivity patterns. For treating cases in which sensitivity testing is not practical, various references are available that list the relative frequency of resistance encountered in different organisms.[2–6] Some variation in resistance in various geographic areas should be expected, and clinical judgment therefore must be used.

The Kirby-Bauer sensitivity test is the most commonly used in vitro sensitivity test. It is easy to perform and, if standardized, provides useful information at a relatively low cost. In an attempt to more precisely define the concentration of drug needed to inhibit growth, many laboratories have adopted a microtiter minimum inhibitory concentration (MIC) method of testing. The MIC method of antibiotic susceptibility testing offers advantages over the Kirby-Bauer method in that it provides a quantitation of how sensitive the organism is rather than a mere qualitative categorization. To properly use this additional information from an MIC it is necessary, however, to know the likely concentration of drug reaching the organism, that is, plasma or tissue drug distribution profiles. In either method the test organism is usually classified as sensitive, intermediate, or resistant to selected antimicrobial agents. The interpretation is based on normally achieved plasma drug concentrations; however, drug concentrations may vary from tissue to tissue (e.g., brain vs. blood) as well as within the dose schedule (peak vs. trough).

In general, an organism resistant to an antibiotic in vitro can be considered to be resistant in vivo; however, an organism that is sensitive in vitro may be clinically ineffective in vivo. Numerous host-drug-parasite interactions must be considered before even limited trust can be placed in the performance of a drug against an organism that is sensitive in vitro. Nevertheless, sensitivity testing remains the best source of objective data for rationally choosing an antibiotic drug for therapy. For a more detailed discussion on proper use of susceptibility tests, see Respiratory Disease Therapeutics in Section 10.

Penetration

Once the cause of the infectious process and its antimicrobial sensitivity pattern are known, the question of drug penetration to the infectious organism must be considered. Drug penetration to the organism depends on the location of the organism and the ability of the drug to penetrate to that site. Whether the organisms are likely to be intracellular or extracellular and whether they are protected by natural (e.g., blood-brain and blood-milk) or pathologic (e.g., thrombus) tissue barriers must be considered.

The ability of an antimicrobial drug to cross biologic membranes depends on various factors, including lipid solubility, pK of the drug relative to environmental pH, protein binding, molecular size, and in certain instances specific cellular transport mechanisms.[7] If the organism is extracellular and not protected by a tissue barrier, water-soluble antimicrobial agents may be acceptable. Such drugs are also effective against infections by facultative intracellular parasites with high turnover rates (e.g., coccidiosis) in which host-cell lysis releases the organism into fluids that contain the antimicrobial agent. For organisms that spend most of their time within host cells or behind tissue barriers, however, greater lipid solubility can be a distinct advantage for an antimicrobial drug.[8] Table 2 shows the ratios for the concentration of various antibiotics in milk to that in plasma; such ratios reflect the principles of drug penetration. In general, a higher ratio indicates a better ability to cross membranes (with ratios greater than 1 usually attributable to ion trapping). The exception may be the blood-brain barrier where endothelial tight junctions limit passive diffusion. Also, in certain instances transport mechanisms exist to move drug out of the central nervous system (CNS). The ability of a drug to cross the blood-brain barrier is most attributable to low protein binding and inherent lipid-solubility characteristics. Accordingly, drugs that are likely to adequately penetrate the CNS without relying on inflammation would include the human-labeled third-generation cephalosporins (such as cefotaxime), potentiated sulfonamides, rifampin, and perhaps florfenicol and the fluoroquinolones. At the time of this writing, only florfenicol is approved in the United States for use in a food animal.

Inflammation may enhance the penetration of antimicrobial drugs into tissues that they would normally enter in restricted amounts. For instance, penicillin G rarely reaches therapeutic concentrations in the CNS of a healthy animal, but in cases of bovine listeriosis early use of this agent can be efficacious.[9] For many drugs, however, the effect of inflammation on penetration is unknown or not reproducible.

Local Activity

A drug must maintain its activity while in contact with the organism. In most cases, drug activity is maintained in the local environment. Notable exceptions include such drugs as the aminoglycosides and sulfonamides. Aminoglycosides have maximum activity in an aerobic environment with a slightly alkaline pH[10, 11]; because staphylococcus-induced abscesses are neither aerobic nor alkaline, therapeutic failure is often encountered despite in vitro sensitivity. Although not bound extensively by plasma proteins, the aminoglycosides are bound to a high degree by intracellular constituents. Such binding usually is not a problem because the drug does not penetrate most cell membranes (except in the kidney where it undergoes pinocytosis), but purulent fluids may contain cellular debris that is rich in intracellular particles that may bind aminoglycosides, thus reducing their efficacy.[12] Sulfonamides also lose much of their activity in purulent debris as this material contains large amounts of protein and para-aminobenzoic acid (PABA), substances that bind and antagonize sulfonamides, respectively.[13] In some diseases, the early use of sulfonamides may be beneficial, whereas the drug may be largely inactivated later in the course of the illness.

Table 1
SUSCEPTIBILITY PATTERNS OF BACTERIA

Bacteria	Organism Location	Stain Affinity	Oxygen Requirements	Shape (if Applicable)	Probable Susceptibility
Actinobacillus	Extracellular	Gram-negative	Facultative anaerobic	Rod	Variable
Anaplasma	Obligate intracellular	NA	NA		Tetracycline
Bacteroides	Extracellular	Gram-negative	Anaerobic	Rod	Penicillin (except B. fragilis), lincomycin
Bordetella	Extracellular	Gram-negative	Aerobic	Rod	Variable
Campylobacter	Extracellular	Gram-negative	Aerobic	Rod	Variable
Chlamydia	Obligate intracellular	NA	NA		Tetracycline
Clostridium	Extracellular	Gram-positive	Anaerobic	Rod	Penicillin
Corynebacterium	Facultative intracellular	Gram-positive	Facultative anaerobic	Rod	Penicillin,* erythromycin
Escherichia coli	Extracellular	Gram-negative	Facultative anaerobic	Rod	Variable
Enterobacter	Extracellular	Gram-negative	Facultative anaerobic	Rod	Variable
Eperythrozoon	Attached to host cell membrane	NA	NA		Tetracycline, arsenicals
Erysipelothrix	Extracellular	Gram-positive	Facultative anaerobic	Rod	Variable
Fusobacterium	Extracellular	Gram-negative	Anaerobic	Rod	Penicillin, macrolide
Haemophilus	Extracellular	Gram-negative	Facultative anaerobic	Rod	Variable
Klebsiella	Extracellular	Gram-negative	Facultative anaerobic	Rod	Variable
Leptospira	Extracellular	Weakly gram-negative	Aerobic	Spirochete	Tetracycline, penicillin G
Listeria	Facultative intracellular	Gram-positive	Aerobic	Rod	Variable
Mycobacterium	Facultative intracellular	Acid-fast	Aerobic	Rod	Variable
Mycoplasma	Attached to host cell membrane	NA	NA		Tylosin, erythromycin, tilmicosin, enrofloxacin, tetracycline, lincomycin
Nocardia	Facultative intracellular	Variable	Aerobic		Variable
Pasteurella	Extracellular	Gram-negative	Facultative anaerobic	Rod	Variable
Proteus	Extracellular	Gram-negative	Facultative anaerobic	Rod	Variable
Pseudomonas	Extracellular	Gram-negative	Aerobic	Rod	Variable
Salmonella	Facultative intracellular or extracellular	Gram-negative	Facultative anaerobic	Rod	Variable
Staphylococcus	Facultative intracellular or extracellular	Gram-positive	Facultative anaerobic	Coccus	Variable
Streptococcus	Extracellular	Gram-positive	Facultative anaerobic	Coccus	Penicillin (β-hemolytic streptococci)
Treponema	Extracellular	Weakly gram-negative	Anaerobic or microaerophilic	Spirochete	Variable

NA, not applicable.
*Organism often resistant in vivo.
Adapted from Burrows GE: Systemic antibacterial drug selection and dosage. Bovine Pract 15:103–110, 1980.

While not as severely affected, activity of the β-lactam antibiotics may be diminished in purulent debris. Though they cause a break in the cell wall, this injury in itself is not necessarily fatal to the bacteria. Rather, osmotic gradients across the now unprotected bacterial cell membrane cause the cell to swell and eventually rupture. The loss of this osmotic gradient has been hypothesized to be the reason that β-lactam antibiotics may be less effective in diseases involving abscesses and excessive purulent debris, particularly if drainage is not employed.

Dosage and Formulation

The selected antimicrobial drug must contact the organism in a concentration high enough and for a period long enough to have its effect. The dose, route of administration, and drug formulation affect the concentration of the drug over time. Different formulations of ampicillin (e.g., sodium ampicillin and ampicillin trihydrate) do not provide identical concentrations in tissue; therefore, for infections with organisms that require high MICs of ampicillin, sodium ampicillin may be effective in cases in which ampicillin trihydrate is not. As a rule, the more slowly a drug is absorbed, the lower the peak plasma concentration will be. As Figure 1 shows, benzathine penicillin G provides penicillin in the body for a long period but at extremely low concentrations.[6] Its efficacy is thus questionable in most veterinary diseases. Such repository formulations usually have zero-order or mixed absorption kinetics; that is, increasing the dose results in longer duration of drug in the body (residue) but does not result in a proportional increase in plasma concentrations.

Though much remains to be determined, some strides have been made in understanding the relationship between drug concentration curves (pharmacokinetics) and bacterial killing (pharmacodynamics). The antibiotics are now often divided into three basic dynamics of bacterial killing. The β-lactam antibiotics (penicillins and cephalosporins) have time-dependent killing. That is, better effects are seen when the concentrations of drug continuously meet or exceed the MIC (or some multiple thereof), especially for gram-negative infections. This implies that in critically ill patients frequent dosing intervals may be preferred. Most bacteriostatic antibiotics are also thought to have time-dependent dynamics.

The aminoglycosides have concentration-dependent killing. For this type of bacterial killing the outcome correlates with maximum exposure to high pulse concentrations of the drug. Plasma concentration may then be allowed to drop well below the MIC of the organism throughout much of the dosing interval without adversely affecting the outcome. Accordingly, once-daily administration of the total daily dose of aminoglycoside has been shown experimentally and in human medicine to maintain

Table 2
MILK-TO-PLASMA ULTRAFILTRATE RATIOS*†

Drug	Range‡
Sulfacetamide[50]	0.08–0.11
Sulfadimethoxine[51]	0.13–0.24
Penicillin[52]	0.13–0.26
Sulfadiazine[50]	0.16–0.19
Gentamicin[53]	0.20–0.50
Cephaloridine[52]	0.24–0.28
Ampicillin[52]	0.24–0.30
Spectinomycin[54]	0.37–1.12
Sulfathiazole[50]	0.37 (mean)
Sulfadimidine[50]	0.59–0.62
Kanamycin[53]	0.60–0.80
Sulfanilamide[50]	0.97–1.04
Tylosin[54]	1.00–5.35
Tetracycline[55]	1.22–1.91§
Lincomycin[56]	2.50–6.25
Trimethoprim[57]	3.00–4.90
Erythromycin[58]	6.00–7.30

*Milk-to-plasma ultrafiltrate ratios are not available for florfenicol or the fluoroquinolones, though both are known to distribute well into milk. Based on distribution studies and the characteristics of these drugs, it is probable that free drug concentrations would be approximately equivalent between milk and plasma, that is, a ratio of approximately 1.
†A higher ratio indicates a better ability to cross membranes.
‡Results often varied with pH of milk.
§Sequestration by calcium may have raised milk concentrations.

similar cure rates to the total daily dose divided evenly and given at 8-hour intervals.[14] Though veterinary clinical studies are lacking, this protocol is in common use, particularly in equine medicine, although some advise caution in using once-daily treatment protocols for severely immunocompromised patients.

The third recognized dynamic of bacterial killing is the area under the inhibitory curve (AUIC). The AUIC is the total drug exposure over 24 hours (as determined by area under the curve measurements) divided by the MIC of the offending pathogen. For the fluoroquinolone ciprofloxacin, AUIC scores of 125 or greater for life-threatening gram-negative pneumonia are best associated with a successful outcome.[15] Because AUIC values are independent of the dosing interval, it is believed that long dosing intervals (e.g., once daily) may be as effective as frequent intervals (e.g., twice daily) assuming the same total daily dose of drug is administered.

Combination Therapy

In general, combinations of antibiotics are best avoided although the reasons for using combination therapy may be well grounded in certain instances (e.g., mixed infections not susceptible to a single agent). At other times, combination therapy to gain a wide spectrum is substituted in lieu of more aggressive diagnostic procedures. Regardless of the reason for combination therapy, the guidelines discussed in this section may be useful.

Such antibiotic combinations as trimethoprim-sulfadiazine and penicillin-aminoglycoside have demonstrated synergism and are sound choices. Others, such as penicillin-tetracycline, have demonstrated antagonism.[16] In the past, it was believed that in general only antibiotics with similar activity should be combined (e.g., bactericidal with bactericidal). This dogma was based primarily on human clinical trials where the combination of penicillin G–chlortetracycline or ampicillin-chloramphenicol-streptomycin had a much higher mortality in treating meningitis than did the use of single-drug therapy; hence the view that bactericidal and bacteriostatic drugs are antagonistic.[17, 18] Conversely, the combination of streptomycin and oxytetracycline, bactericidal and bacteriostatic drugs, respectively, has proved more efficacious in treating brucellosis than oxytetracycline alone.[19] Also, whether an agent is bactericidal or bacteriostatic often depends on the dose, and, frequently, antagonistic/synergistic relationships are very genus-, species-, and even isolate-specific. Thus, while it is probably wise to avoid the β-lactam–tetracycline combination, whether combining other bactericidal and bacteriostatic antibiotics affects clinical outcome remains to be seen. If the rationale behind the assertion is true (i.e., a bactericidal drug must have rapidly dividing bacteria in order to be effective), the need to use antimicrobials of similar activity would probably be of most importance in treating immunocompromised patients or when a rapid bactericidal action is necessary (e.g., meningitis).

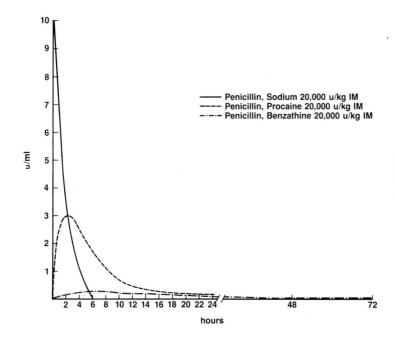

Figure 1
Plasma concentrations of penicillin in the cow. (Adapted from Burrows GE: Systemic antibacterial drug selection and dosage. Bovine Pract 15:103–110, 1980.)

The mechanism of action of the antimicrobial drugs should also be considered in combination therapy. The agents should act at different sites to avoid competing for the same enzymes and substrates.[20] Table 3 indicates the site of action of common antimicrobial drugs. For example, a combination of erythromycin and lincomycin would be undesirable because both drugs act at the 50S ribosome level; a more logical combination might include lincomycin, which acts at the 50S subunit, with spectinomycin, which acts at the 30S subunit.

All other considerations being equal, the antimicrobial with the narrowest spectrum should be chosen, whether for sole use or in combination with another antimicrobial. Choosing a drug with a narrow spectrum reduces selection pressure for resistance to the broad-spectrum agents.

Prophylactic Antimicrobials

The practitioner is sometimes confronted with situations where antimicrobials may be appropriate to prevent rather than treat disease. Such use may range from prevention of a specific organism (e.g., anaplasmosis, leptospirosis) to situations requiring broad-spectrum coverage such as protection of immunocompromised patients or surgical patients (particularly in field situations where aseptic technique may be jeopardized). The following are suggestions for proper prophylactic antimicrobial use:

- When a specific organism is being targeted, use a drug with the narrowest spectrum that will prevent the disease. This avoids exposure of incidental bacteria to broader-spectrum antimicrobials and hence decreases pressure toward bacterial resistance.
- Prophylactic antimicrobial treatment can be effective in preventing certain highly susceptible organisms for reasonably long periods of time (e.g., use of tetracyclines to prevent anaplasmosis). Long-term prophylaxis against "infection" (e.g., protection of immunocompromised patients) is not possible because invasion of resistant bacteria almost always occurs.
- For surgical prophylaxis the greatest efficacy will occur if the antibiotics are given prior to surgery so that the drugs are incorporated into clots, fibrin, and so on, as they are formed. This also allows the antimicrobial to encounter relatively low numbers of bacteria when fewer inactivating enzymes and purulent debris are likely to be present. Studies have indicated that treatment beyond 2 days postoperatively is unlikely to improve the outcome and will only add to bacterial resistance problems. A good rule of thumb for surgical prophylaxis is the 2×2 rule: 2 hours before and 2 days after surgery.[21]

Extra-label Drug Use

New antibiotics have improved the food animal veterinarian's armamentarium of antimicrobials substantially in the last decade, particularly for the treatment of respiratory disease in beef cattle. It should be remembered, however, that use of a drug in a nonapproved species; for indications not listed in the labeling; at altered dosage, frequencies, or routes of administration other than those stated in the labeling constitutes extra-label drug use.

In most instances, extra-label use seldom results in problems for the practitioner. In those few instances in which a practitioner's use of pharmaceuticals is questioned, the strongest defense often lies in the rationale for the drug selection. The concepts discussed here can help the practitioner justify extra-label use, especially if culture and sensitivity results document

that it is unlikely that approved doses of any other drugs would have been successful. Because extra-label use is subject to the Animal Medicinal Drug Use Clarification Act of 1994 (AMDUCA) and its regulations,[22] the following synopsis of those regulations is offered.

Pertinent Points of the Animal Medicinal Drug Use Clarification Act

Definition

Extra-label use means use of a drug in an animal in a manner that is not in accordance with the approved labeling. This includes, but is not limited to, use in species not listed in the labeling, use for indications (disease or other conditions) not listed in the labeling, use at dosage levels, frequencies, or routes of administration other than those stated in the labeling, and deviation from the labeled withdrawal time based on these different uses. Such use is limited to treatment modalities when the health of an animal is threatened or suffering or death may result from failure to treat.

Conditions for Use

The following conditions must be met for extra-label use of animal and human drugs in food-producing animals:

1. When there is no approved animal drug that contains the same active ingredient in the required dosage form and concentration that is labeled for such use, or all approved animal drugs are clinically ineffective for its intended use.

2. The use must occur within the context of a valid veterinarian-client-patient relationship. A valid veterinarian-client-patient relationship is one in which:

- A veterinarian has assumed the responsibility for making medical judgments regarding the health of the animal(s) and the need for medical treatment, and the client (the owner of the animal or other caretaker) has agreed to follow the instructions of the veterinarian
- There is sufficient knowledge of the animal(s) by the veterinarian to initiate at least a general or preliminary diagnosis.
- The practicing veterinarian is readily available for follow-up in case of adverse reactions or failure of the therapy regimen. Such a relationship can exist only when the veterinarian has recently seen and is personally acquainted with the keeping and care of the animal(s) by virtue of examination of the animal(s), or by medically appropriate and timely visits to the premises where the animal(s) is kept.

3. Prior to prescribing or dispensing an approved animal or human drug for an extra-label use in food animals, the veterinarian must:

- Make a careful diagnosis and evaluation of the conditions for which the drug is to be used.
- Establish a substantially extended withdrawal period supported by appropriate scientific information, if applicable.
- Institute procedures to ensure that the identity of the treated animal(s) is carefully maintained.
- Take appropriate measures to assure that assigned withdrawal times are met and no illegal drug residues occur.
- Ensure that such use is in accordance with an appropriate medical rationale.

4. Any drug prescribed and dispensed for extra-label use shall bear or be accompanied by labeling information adequate to assure the safe and proper use of the product. Such information shall include the following:

Table 3
COMMON ANTIMICROBIAL DRUG CHARACTERISTICS

Drug	Action	Site of Action	Mechanism of Action	Gram-Positive	Gram-Negative	Anaerobes Clostridium	Anaerobes Other	Mycoplasma	Leptospira	Rickettsia	Elimination Renal	Elimination Liver
Aminoglycosides	Bactericidal	30S ribosome subunit	Protein synthesis; misreading of genetic code	Sensitive*	Sensitive	Resistant	Resistant		Sensitive		Primary	
Cephalosporins	Bactericidal	Cell wall	Inhibits cross-linkage	Sensitive	1st-generation: varies; 3rd generation: sensitive	Sensitive‡,§	Sensitive‡,§				Primary	
Florfenicol	Bacteriostatic	50S ribosome subunit	Protein synthesis; inhibits translocation	Sensitive	Sensitive	Sensitive‡,§	Sensitive‡,§				Primary	Secondary
Fluoroquinolones	Bactericidal	Enzyme	Inhibits DNA gyrase	Sensitive*	Sensitive	Resistant	Resistant	Sensitive		Variable	Primary	Secondary
Lincomycin	Bacteriostatic	50S ribosome subunit	Protein synthesis; inhibits initiation	Sensitive	Resistant	Sensitive	Sensitive	Sensitive	Sensitive†		Secondary	Primary
Macrolides	Bacteriostatic	50S ribosome subunit	Protein synthesis; inhibits translocation	Sensitive	Resistant (*Pasteurella* may be sensitive)	Erythromycin: sensitive‡,§	Varies	Sensitive	Erythromycin: sensitive‡,§		Secondary	Primary
Penicillins	Bactericidal	Cell wall	Inhibits cross-linkage	Sensitive	Narrow: resistant; broad: varies; extended: sensitive	Sensitive	Sensitive†		Sensitive		Primary	
Potentiated sulfonamide	Bactericidal	Enzyme	Sulfonamide competes with PABA; trimethoprim competes for dihydrofolic acid reductase	Sensitive	Sensitive	Sensitive‡,§	Sensitive‡,§				Primary	
Spectinomycin	Bacteriostatic	30S ribosome subunit	Protein synthesis; inhibits translocation	Resistant	Sensitive		Resistant	Sensitive‡,§			Primary	
Sulfonamides	Bacteriostatic	Enzyme	Inhibits folate synthesis by competing with PABA	Sensitive	Sensitive						Primary	
Tetracyclines	Bacteriostatic	30S ribosome subunit	Protein synthesis; inhibits attachment of transfer RNA	Sensitive	Sensitive	Sensitive§	Varies	Sensitive	Sensitive	Sensitive	Primary	Secondary

*Many streptococci are resistant.
†Except *B. fragilis.*
‡In vivo efficacy not well established.
§Other agents usually preferred.

- The name and address of the prescribing veterinarian. If the drug is dispensed by a pharmacy, the labeling shall include the name of the prescribing veterinarian and the name and address of the dispensing pharmacy, and may include the address of the prescribing veterinarian.
- The established name of the drug or, if formulated from more than one active ingredient, the established name of each ingredient.
- Any directions for use, including the class or species or identification of the animal or herd, flock, pen, lot, or other group of animals being treated, in which the drug is intended to be used; the dosage, frequency, and route of administration; and the duration of therapy.
- Any cautionary statements.
- The veterinarian's specified withdrawal time.

5. If scientific information on the human food safety aspect of the use of the drug in food-producing animals is not available, the veterinarian must take appropriate measures to assure that the animal and its food products will not enter the human food supply.

6. Extra-label use of an approved human drug in a food-producing animal is not permitted if an animal drug approved for use in food-producing animals can be used in an extra-label manner for the particular use.

Banned Drugs

The following drugs are prohibited for extra-label use in food-producing animals:

- Chloramphenicol
- Clenbuterol
- Diethylstilbestrol (DES)
- Dimetridazole
- Ipronidazole
- Other nitroimidazoles such as metronidazole
- Furazolidone (except for approved topical use)
- Nitrofurazone (except for approved topical use)
- Sulfonamide drugs in lactating dairy cattle (except approved use of sulfadimethoxine, sulfabromomethazine, and sulfaethoxypyridazine)
- Fluoroquinolones
- Glycopeptides (such as vancomycin)

Banned Uses

The following specific extra-label uses are not permitted:

- Use by a layperson (except when under the supervision of a licensed veterinarian)
- Extra-label use in or on an animal feed
- Extra-label use resulting in any residue which may present a risk to the public health or is above an established safe concentration or tolerance

Compounding

Extra-label use from compounding of approved animal or human drugs is permitted if:

1. All relevant portions of AMDUCA have been complied with.

2. There is no approved animal or human drug that, when used as labeled or in conformity with criteria established by AMDUCA, will, in the available dosage form and concentration, appropriately treat the condition diagnosed.

3. Compounding from a human drug for use in food-producing animals will not be permitted if an approved animal drug can be used for the compounding.

4. The compounding is performed by a licensed pharmacist or veterinarian within the scope of a professional practice.

5. Adequate procedures are followed that ensure the safety and effectiveness of the compounded product.

6. The scale of the compounding operation is commensurate with the established need (e.g., similar to that of comparable practices).

7. All relevant state laws relating to the compounding of drugs for use in animals are followed.

Record Requirements

Veterinarians shall maintain the following records of extra-label uses. Such records shall be legible, documented in an accurate and timely manner, and be readily accessible to permit prompt retrieval of information if requested by the Food and Drug Administration (FDA). Such records shall include the identification of the animals and shall be maintained either as individual records or, in food animal practices, on a group, herd, flock, or per-client basis. Records shall be adequate to provide the following information:

- The established name of the drug and its active ingredient, or if formulated from more than one ingredient, the established name of each ingredient
- The condition treated
- The species of the treated animal(s)
- The dosage administered
- The duration of treatment
- The number of animals treated
- The specified withdrawal, withholding, or discard time(s), if applicable, for meat, milk, eggs, or any food which might be derived from any food animals treated

A veterinarian shall keep all required records for 2 years or as otherwise required by federal or state law, whichever is greater.

Withdrawal Times

With the increase in extra-label drug use has come the problem of estimating withdrawal times for antibiotics. In most instances, withdrawal recommendations published in the package insert for approved products may not apply to the larger doses often used. Two resources that the veterinarian can use for help in estimating withdrawal times are the Food Animal Residue Avoidance Database (FARAD) and the veterinary monographs within the U. S. Pharmacopeia Drug Information (USPDI). FARAD is a superb resource for estimating withdrawal times for animal exposure to a variety of compounds. At the time of this writing, however, funding for FARAD is in jeopardy. The USPDI is a collection of expert panel–reviewed drug monographs detailing accepted usage of those drugs. Withdrawal time recommendations for extra-label use of veterinary drugs in food animals have recently been implemented. Though the recommendations are in reference only to the USPDI suggested dosage, it is one of the few proactive sources of food animal withdrawal time information. The continuation of the Veterinary USPDI is, however, being studied.

One should remember that withdrawal time recommendations for extra-label use are estimates only. The best advice is to be conservative in recommending withdrawal times. When a more definitive answer is needed, the in vitro antibiotic screening tests may be of use in avoiding residues. These tests (e.g., Delvotest P, G. B. Fermentation Industries) can be particularly useful in testing milk for antimicrobial residues. Many milk cooperatives now offer such testing services to their members. The tests used to check urine for antimicrobial activity (e.g., L.A.S.T., Granite Diagnostics) are also useful when one considers that the kidney swab assay is the most commonly used regulatory test. Some antibiotics (e.g., erythromycin) have primary routes of elimination other than the kidney; for such drugs, negative tests of urine may have limitations in predicting nondetectable residues.

Kinetic modeling may offer some help in predicting residue patterns, particularly if no depot or preferential tissue binding occurs. When such binding does occur, kinetic modeling can still be useful if the parameters for the tissue in question are determined.[23]

Bacterial Resistance

The introduction of modern antimicrobials in this century no doubt led many to believe such drugs would greatly diminish if not eliminate bacterial diseases as a cause of suffering and death. All too quickly it became evident that sooner or later bacteria develop resistance to virtually any antimicrobial agent. Accordingly, the veterinarian can encounter a great deal of antimicrobial resistance, particularly to the older antimicrobials such as penicillin G, tetracyclines, and sulfonamides. While antimicrobial resistance of veterinary pathogens has been of concern to the profession for some time, the issue of antimicrobial use in animals is gaining increasing scrutiny because of real or perceived threats to human health. Increased bacterial resistance of pathogens affecting humans can occur as zoonotic pathogens such as *Salmonella* or via transmission of R factor plasmids from veterinary pathogens or saprophytic flora to human pathogens.[24-26]

Bacterial resistance mechanisms can be divided into three broad categories. The first is by enzymatic degradation or inactivation of the drug such as with penicillinase production by *Staphylococcus* spp. A second method is alteration of the binding site of the drug. Examples of this mechanism would include altered penicillin binding proteins preventing a β-lactam from integrating into the bacterial cell wall, or altered bacterial DNA gyrase preventing a fluoroquinolone antibiotic from binding and inactivating the enzyme. Lastly, the bacteria can produce changes in membrane permeability preventing sufficient accumulation of drug within the bacterial cell. Bacteria resistant to tetracyclines contain active transport mechanisms that can pump the drug out faster than it can diffuse into the cell.

Of greater clinical consequence than how resistance occurs is how it is spread. Resistance mechanisms can be carried on the bacterial chromosome or on genetic material carried in plasmids. Chromosomal mutations imparting resistance can only be passed to subsequent generations of that organism, a process termed *vertical transmission*. Resistance due to plasmids or transposons can, however, be passed by transference of that genetic material from one to another species or even another genus. It is this horizontal transmission (R factor transmission) that has the greatest ability to disseminate drug resistance and thus has a much larger impact on bacterial populations. Table 4 identifies the resistance mechanisms used by various bacteria and how they are transmitted.

In the end it is selection pressure from exposure to an antimicrobial that promotes bacterial resistance. Though the impact of an individual practitioner in development of resistance may seem small, it is imperative that the veterinarian understand the importance of appropriate antimicrobial usage from a broader perspective. The following suggestions are made to minimize resistance development:

1. Make sure that the diagnosis warrants antimicrobial therapy. For example, nonsepticemic collibacillosis in calves and coliform mastitis in cows often respond to supportive measures without antibiotic therapy.

2. Avoid broad-spectrum antimicrobials when a narrow-spectrum drug will suffice. There is little reason to use anything beyond penicillin G in most streptococcal infections.

3. When possible use culture and sensitivity data to direct therapy. When empirical choices must be made, take into account the isolates likely in a given disease and their probable

---

Table 4
MECHANISMS AND TRANSMISSION OF RESISTANCE TO COMMON ANTIMICROBIALS

Antimicrobial	Mechanism of Resistance	Transmission	Examples
Aminoglycosides	Enzymatic degradation or inactivation of drug; altered binding site (ribosomal); change in membrane permeability	Plasmid	*Staphylococcus*, Enterobacteriaceae, *Klebsiella*, Serratia, Enterococcus Enterococcus Pseudomonas
Chloramphenicol	Enzymatic degradation or inactivation of drug (chloramphenicol acetyltransferase)	Plasmid	Enterobacteriaceae, *Haemophilus*, *Streptococcus*
Fluoroquinolones	Altered binding site (altered DNA gyrase); change in membrane permeability	Chromosomal Chromosomal	Enterobacteriaceae Enterobacteriaceae, *Pseudomonas*, *Staphylococcus*
Macrolides and lincosamides	Altered binding site (methylated ribosomal RNA)	Plasmid and transposon	*Staphylococcus*, *Streptococcus*
Penicillins and cephalosporins	Enzymatic degradation or inactivation of drug (β-lactamase); altered binding site (penicillin-binding proteins); change in membrane permeability	Plasmid, chromosomal, or transposon Chromosomal Chromosomal?	*Bacteroides*, *Campylobacter*, *Haemophilus*, *Moraxella*, *Pseudomonas*, *Staphylococcus*, *Streptococcus* *Staphylococcus*, *Enterococcus*, *Haemophilus* Enterobacteriaceae, *Klebsiella*, *Pseudomonas*
Sulfonamides	Altered binding site (altered dihydropteroate synthetase)	Plasmid	*Staphylococcus*, *Streptococcus*, *Enterococcus*, Enterobacteriaceae, *Pseudomonas*
	Change in membrane permeability	Plasmid	
Tetracyclines	Change in membrane permeability (increased efflux)	Plasmid and chromosomal	*Bacteroides*, Enterobacteriaceae, *Enterococcus*, *Haemophilus*, *Moraxella*, *Pseudomonas*, *Staphylococcus*, *Streptococcus*
Trimethoprim	Altered binding site (altered dihydrofolate reductase)	Plasmid	*Staphylococcus*, Enterobacteriaceae, *Pseudomonas*
Vancomycin	Altered binding site	Plasmid	*Enterococcus*

Data from references 59–62.

susceptibility profiles. While ideally this information is derived from first-hand experience, regional diagnostic laboratories can sometimes be of help in this regard.

4. Use appropriate dosages. When combination therapy is warranted, use full doses of each antimicrobial. Table 5 lists common antimicrobial dosages.

5. Treat well past resolution of the disease.

6. Avoid overuse of newer agents when an older drug is likely to be effective.

7. Use topical agents to which development of resistance is uncommon.

8. Use prophylactic antibiotics at full dosages. (See Prophylactic Antimicrobials for suggestions on proper use.)

INDIVIDUAL FAMILIES OF ANTIBIOTICS

β-Lactams

The β-lactam antibiotics include the penicillins and cephalosporins. They are bactericidal antibiotics that cause a break in the cell wall of susceptible bacteria. The cell wall injury in itself is not fatal to the bacteria but autolysins are activated that weaken the cell membrane allowing osmotic gradients across the membrane to cause the cell to swell and eventually lyse. It has been hypothesized that a decrease in this osmotic gradient may be the reason that β-lactam antibiotics may be less effective in diseases involving abscesses and excessive purulent debris, particularly if drainage is not employed. The bactericidal properties are thought to be time-dependent in nature, implying that it is preferred that concentrations above the MIC (or some multiple thereof) be maintained throughout the dosing interval, particularly for gram-negative infections. Thus, in the severely ill animal, frequent dosing intervals may be preferred for this family of antibiotics.

The β-lactams as a family are relatively lipid insoluble and tend to be restricted primarily to extracellular fluid spaces. Though they achieve adequate concentrations in most tissues, penetration across many physiologic barriers is limited. Inflammation may allow adequate penetration into the CNS, and β-lactams can be effective if the organism is highly sensitive (e.g., listeriosis). Although some hepatic elimination may occur with certain β-lactams, they are removed predominantly by renal active transport mechanisms. Hypersensitivities are the primary adverse reactions associated with the β-lactams.

Penicillins

Narrow-Spectrum Penicillins

The penicillins are divided into narrow, broad, and extended (anti-*Pseudomonas*) classifications. Penicillin G (benzyl penicillin), a narrow-spectrum penicillin, was the first true antibiotic discovered and remains a mainstay for antibiotic treatment in many species. Penicillin G is effective against many gram-positive bacteria, including most streptococcal infections (except enterococci); however, many staphylococcal isolates are resistant due to penicillinase production. It is the drug of choice for most clostridial infections and is highly effective in other obligate anaerobic infections. One anaerobe, *Bacteroides fragilis* (often isolated in infections associated with fecal contamination), is, however, almost always resistant to penicillin G, and other agents should be used if this organism is suspected. Spirochetes are generally sensitive, though the drug may not clear the carrier state in leptospirosis. The majority of gram-negative organisms are resistant.

Penicillin G is available in three formulations: crystalline, penicillin G procaine, and benzathine penicillin G. The crystalline forms, sodium or potassium penicillin, can be given intravenously (IV) as well as intramuscularly (IM; peak concentrations occur within 30 minutes of injection). Penicillin G potassium should be administered slowly when given IV to avoid cardiac arrhythmias. Crystalline penicillin use is often employed when an immediate onset is desired, as may occur in unexpected contamination of a surgical field or peracute life-threatening clostridial diseases (e.g., blackleg) where death may be imminent if the animal is not treated rapidly. The drug has a short elimination half-life and requires administration at least four times daily. Though such intense therapy is appropriate in severe infections it is often impractical in most food animal settings; hence, in severe field cases crystalline penicillin G may be given to produce rapid high concentrations while concomitantly an IM dose of penicillin G procaine is administered. Therapy would then be continued at high-dose penicillin G procaine twice daily.

By linking the penicillin molecule to a procaine molecule, a repository formulation is produced in penicillin G procaine. Though the peak concentrations (C_{max}) are smaller and the time of the peak concentrations (T_{max}) is delayed, the duration of the concentration is extended. Dosing intervals of every 12 hours are preferred for extremely ill animals although once-daily dosing in field situations may be appropriate. Though the drug may be given subcutaneously (SC), this route has been associated with extensive hemorrhage at the injection site when using the large extra-label doses needed against most pathogens, and hence IM administration is recommended.

Benzathine penicillin is an extremely long-acting penicillin G preparation that unfortunately fails to produce therapeutic concentrations against nearly any bacteria of veterinary significance and has little place in veterinary medicine. In those preparations combining procaine and benzathine penicillin G, it is most probably the procaine formulation that is providing a benefit.

Penicillin V is an oral narrow-spectrum penicillin that could be given to preruminant calves (e.g., 1 to 2 weeks of age) or swine. The drug is, however, seldom employed for this use.

Dicloxacillin is of importance as an intramammary infusion, particularly for staphylococcal mastitis, because of its resistance to penicillinase. If an in vitro susceptibility test does not include dicloxacillin, the results associated with oxacillin may be extrapolated.

Broad-Spectrum Penicillins

The broad-spectrum penicillins include ampicillin and amoxicillin. Although these drugs may be slightly less effective against gram-positive pathogens than penicillin G, as the categorization implies they can treat more of the gram-negative bacteria, including many *Pasteurella* spp. Resistance to these drugs is, however, common (e.g., 41% to 77% resistance for *Pasteurella haemolytica* and 68% resistance for *Escherichia coli*).[27, 28] Moderately susceptible organisms can be treated, but only at high doses. In these cases, ampicillin sodium given at least three times daily is required due to the fact that the trihydrate forms (ampicillin trihydrate and amoxicillin trihydrate) will produce subtherapeutic concentrations.

The spectra of ampicillin and amoxicillin are similar and susceptibility profiles can usually be extrapolated. As such, the drugs are largely interchangeable when given by injection. Amoxicillin is approximately twice as well absorbed when given orally to monogastric animals and is the preferred oral form of the two drugs in swine and preruminant calves. Amoxicillin is well absorbed when given orally to calves at 2 weeks of age but undetectable in serum when given at 6 weeks of age. Hetacillin

Table 5
COMMON ANTIMICROBIAL DOSAGES*

Generic Name	Trade Name	Source	Dosage†
Amoxicillin			
Trihydrate injection	Amoxi-Inject	Pfizer Animal Health, Exton, Pa.	Cattle: 6.6–22 mg/kg IM q.8, 12, or 24h. Swine: same
Oral	Amoxi-Tabs		Preruminant calves: 10–22 mg/kg PO q.12–24h. Swine: same
Ampicillin			
Sodium injection	Amp-Equine	Pfizer Animal Health	Cattle: 10–20 mg/kg IV q.6–8h. Swine: same
Trihydrate injection	Polyflex	Fort Dodge Laboratories, Fort Dodge, Iowa	Cattle: 4.4–22 mg/kg IM q.8, 12, or 24h. Swine: same
Ceftiofur			
Sodium	Naxcel	Pharmacia & Upjohn, Kalamazoo, Mich.	Cattle: 1.1–2.2 mg/kg IM q.24h.
Sterile suspension	Excenel		Swine: 3–5 mg/kg IM q.24h.
Erythromycin injection	Erythro-200	Rhone Merieux, Athens, Ga.	Cattle: 2.2–8.8 mg/kg IM q.24h.; for pneumonic pasteurellosis, some authors suggest 15 mg/kg IM q.12h.
Florfenicol	Nuflor	Schering-Plough Animal Health, Kenilworth, N.J.	20 mg/kg IM q.48h.‡
Lincomycin hydrochloride			
Injection	Lincomix	Pharmacia & Upjohn	Cattle: 5–10 mg/kg IM q.12–24h. Swine: 11 mg/kg IM q.24h.
Oral powder	Lincomix		Cattle: contraindicated Swine: 8.4 mg/kg PO q.24h. in water
Oxytetracycline			
Injection	Liquamycin 100	Pfizer Animal Health	Cattle: 6.6–11 mg/kg IM or IV q.12–24h. Swine: 6.6–11 mg/kg IM or IV q.24h.
Long-acting injection	Liquamycin LA-200		Cattle: 20 mg/kg IM q.72h.‡ Swine: 20 mg/kg IM
Penicillin G			
Potassium or sodium	Pfizerpen	Pfizer Animal Health	Cattle: 20,000 units/kg IV or IM q.6h. Swine: same
Procaine	Pfi-pen G		Cattle: 20,000–60,000 units/kg IM q.24h. Swine: same
Potentiated sulfonamide (sulfadiazine and trimethoprim)	Tribrissen	Coopers Animal Health, Mundelein, Ill.	Preruminant calves: 30 mg/kg (25 mg/kg sulfadiazine and 5 mg/kg trimethoprim) PO q.12–24h. Swine: 30 mg/kg (25 mg/kg sulfadiazine and 5 mg/kg trimethoprim) PO q.24h.
Spectinomycin	Spectam injectable	Rhone Merieux	Cattle: 20 mg/kg IV or IM q.12–24h. Swine: 6.6–22 mg/kg IM q.24h. Piglets: 15–20 mg/kg PO q.12h.
Sulfachlorpyridazine			
Bolus or powder	Vetisulid	Solvay Animal Health, Mendota Heights, Minn.	Calves: 33–49.5 mg/kg PO q.12h. Swine: 22–38.5 mg/kg PO q.12h.
Injection	Vetisulid		Calves: 33–49.5 mg/kg IV q.12h.
Sulfadimethoxine			
Bolus or oral solution	Albon	Pfizer Animal Health	Cattle: 55 mg/kg PO initially, then 27.5 mg/kg PO q.24h.
Sustained release bolus	Albon SR		Cattle: 137.5 mg/kg PO q.96h.‡
Injection	Albon Injection		Cattle: 55 mg/kg PO initially, then 27.5 mg/kg IV q.24h.
Tilmicosin injection	Micotil 300	Elanco Animal Health, Indianapolis, Ind.	Beef cattle: 10 mg/kg SC q.3d.‡ Swine: contraindicated
Tylosin injection	Tylan 200	Elanco Animal Health	Beef cattle and nonlactating dairy cattle: 17.6 mg/kg IM q.24h. Swine: 8.8 mg/kg IM q.24h.

*Doses for feed additives often vary with the intended use and are not covered here. See manufacturer's recommendations.
†Many dosages exceed manufacturer's recommendations and prolonged withdrawal times may be necessary.
‡Label directions restrict the number of doses that may be administered. Repeated doses may produce prolonged withdrawal times.

is a prodrug that is converted to ampicillin by esterases. It is used as an intramammary infusion.

Extended-Spectrum Penicillins

The extended-spectrum penicillins are very effective against a variety of gram-negative pathogens, including *Pseudomonas* spp. Carbenicillin, the first extended-spectrum penicillin to be introduced, has been replaced by the more efficacious agents ticarcillin and piperacillin. Each can be given by IV or IM injection three to four times per day. Their cost is usually prohibitive in the treatment of most food animals, but they may be considered in individual valuable animals.

Cephalosporins

First-Generation Cephalosporins

The cephalosporins are divided into first, second, and third generations based on their spectrum. Like the narrow-spectrum penicillins the first-generation cephalosporins are effective against many gram-positive bacteria. Unlike the case of penicillin G, most staphylococci are sensitive to these drugs and a moderate number of gram-negative bacteria are susceptible. Indeed, one of the few intramammary infusions with a reasonable gram-negative spectrum is cephapirin (the only first-generation cephalosporin approved in food animals). Though active against many obligate anaerobes, enough resistance to the cephalosporins is encountered to make other agents preferred when anaerobic organisms are suspected, particularly *Bacteroides* infections. Cephalexin or cefadroxil could be given orally to swine or preruminant calves but this is only occasionally done in clinical practice. If the individual cephalosporin is not tested, then in vitro susceptibility to cephalothin can be extrapolated to these drugs. Cefazolin, the most commonly used injectable first-generation cephalosporin, has found some use in food animal medicine. In most diseases, however, cefazolin would be deemed inferior to the approved drug, ceftiofur. By comparison, cefazolin has an inferior gram-negative spectrum and a shorter elimination half-life, requiring much more frequent dosing than ceftiofur.

Second-Generation Cephalosporins

Second-generation cephalosporins have an enhanced gram-negative spectrum compared to first-generation drugs. Notable injectable second-generation cephalosporins are cefoxitin and cefotetan, which, unlike most cephalosporins, have an excellent obligate anaerobic spectrum. This subclass of antibiotics is, however, seldom used in food animal medicine.

Third-Generation Cephalosporins

The third-generation cephalosporins have a greatly extended gram-negative spectrum although they are not always effective against *Pseudomonas*. Most cephalosporins cross barriers rather poorly. Because of low protein binding (only free drugs cross membranes) and the high sensitivity of many organisms, the injectable third-generation cephalosporins such as cefotaxime have found a preferred use in treating bacterial meningitis in humans and small animals. Their frequent dosing interval and more particularly their cost often prohibit use in most food animals.

Ceftiofur is often classified as a third-generation cephalosporin based on its chemical structure, although some argue that it does not fit the categorization well due to pharmacokinetic and spectrum differences. At present, it is the only approved parenteral cephalosporin in veterinary medicine. It has excellent activity against most gram-negative bacteria, nonenterococcal streptococci, and *Fusobacterium*. The drug may also be effective against some staphylococci. The enterococci and *Pseudomonas* are usually resistant. Resistance is not uncommon in clostridia and *Bacteroides* spp.[29] Unlike cefotaxime, ceftiofur and its active metabolite, desfuroylceftiofur, are highly protein bound. The disadvantage of this binding is that less free drug is available to diffuse across membranes and hence ceftiofur does not cross the blood-brain barrier in the healthy animal. The advantage, however, is that the binding acts to extend the elimination half-life of the drug allowing for less frequent dosing (e.g., once daily). This binding may also produce higher free and total drug concentrations at infection sites where there are increased protein concentrations (e.g., exudates).[30] Ceftiofur is unique among antimicrobials in that it has no milk or slaughter withdrawal requirements. By virtue of its high probability of bacterial sensitivity, ceftiofur is a valuable antibiotic in many diseases and fills a unique niche due to its lack of slaughter withdrawal requirements in allowing treatment of food animals while still maintaining slaughter salvage as an option. The lack of withdrawal requirements is not to imply that if an animal is slaughtered within a few hours of receiving a dose of ceftiofur, that no drug is present. Rather, it has been shown that any residues present have minimal public health significance. It is prudent, however, to point out that antimicrobial inhibition screening tests on urine or kidney tissue may show some residue if taken within a few hours of dosing. Likewise, while ceftiofur treatment of lactating dairy cattle at label doses does not usually trigger the standard *Bacillus stearothermophilus* disk assay, the Lactek cef or Lactek B-L (Idetek, San Bruno, Calif.) milk antibiotic screening tests, the drug may occasionally be detected at the first postdosing milking by more sensitive immunoassays such as the Charm Test II (Charm Sciences, Malden, Mass.) which detect inactive ceftiofur metabolites at extremely low concentrations.[31] This is of particular importance in mass treatment of a dairy herd.

Tetracyclines

The tetracycline antibiotics have one of the broadest antimicrobial spectra. They are effective against mycoplasmas (as an alternative to macrolides or lincosamides), spirochetes, and rickettsiae for which they remain the drug of choice. Regarding conventional bacterial infections, it is important to contrast the difference in the terms "broad spectrum" and "susceptibility pattern." It is true that a variety of gram-positive, gram-negative, and anaerobic bacteria can be susceptible to the tetracyclines. It is more important to realize that a high degree of resistance to these drugs exists. While the tetracyclines are used extensively for mild to moderate infections, they should be selected with caution as an empirical first choice in most serious bacterial infections. Most *Pasteurella* spp., staphylococci, and obligate anaerobes (except *Fusobacterium*) have too high an incidence of resistance for the drug to be a good first choice. Streptococci and *Haemophilus* organisms tend to have a moderate degree of resistance, allowing for some tetracycline use, although other antibiotics are usually preferred. Thus, without an in vitro susceptibility test, only rickettsial, mycoplasmal, leptospiral, and perhaps *Moraxella bovis* infections can be treated with a high degree of confidence in their responsiveness to a tetracycline.

The tetracycline family includes tetracycline hydrochloride, chlortetracycline, oxytetracycline, and for small animals, doxycycline and minocycline. Though some staphylococci have been reported to be more susceptible to minocycline, generally cross-resistance among the tetracyclines is complete and hence susceptibility profiles can be extrapolated between drugs. Chlortetracycline is too irritating to be given by injection and is used primarily as a feed additive for growth promotion or disease prevention. Likewise, tetracycline hydrochloride is used as a feed additive, although it has been given IV in an extra-label manner.

By far, the predominant tetracycline used in food animal medicine for disease treatment is oxytetracycline. It is approved in three concentrations for injection at 50, 100, or 200 mg/mL. The first two products contain propylene glycol as the vehicle, while the last contains polyvinylpyrrolidone (PVP). The three products may be given IV or IM (significant tissue necrosis may occur when given IM), and some of the 200 mg/mL products are approved for SC use. The 200 mg/mL products, sometimes known as "long-acting oxytetracycline," have a repository effect where a single IM injection at 20 mg/kg produces concentrations effective against sensitive pathogens (e.g., anaplasmosis) for 3 days. This prolonged action does not occur if the product is given IV or if administered at the conventional IM dose of 6 to 11 mg/kg. The muscle soreness associated with repeated IM injections, as well as injection site trim loss at slaughter, make IV injection for some clinicians a desirable route of administration. Rapid IV administration can, however, result in acute collapse of the animal due to chelation of blood calcium which causes arrhythmias, or vehicle-associated release of histamine leading to peripheral vasodilation and hypotension. Slow administration or dilution of the drug into sterile water or saline usually avoids this adverse reaction. Though death can occur from collapse, most animals usually recover spontaneously. Mild hemolysis and hemoglobinuria are sometimes seen with IV administration, most likely due to the vehicle tonicity. As tetracyclines chelate to divalent and trivalent ions (i.e., calcium, magnesium, aluminum) they should not be administered orally with dairy products, antacids, nor be diluted in IV solutions containing these ions. Tetracycline, chlortetracycline, and oxytetracycline are moderately lipid-soluble and can achieve therapeutic concentrations across many cell membranes, particularly if inflammation is present. The human tetracyclines minocycline and doxycline, which are much more lipid soluble than the older agents, are not used in food animal medicine at present.

The tetracyclines are not normally considered nephrotoxic, although they tend to promote catabolism and hence increase the nitrogen load to the kidneys. Some conditions, however, are synergistically nephrotoxic with tetracyclines. Methoxyflurane anesthesia in humans receiving tetracycline therapy has been associated with nephrotoxicity. More important, endotoxemia with high-dose oxytetracycline therapy (e.g., 20 mg/kg b.i.d.) has been reported to cause severe kidney injury experimentally and in clinical cases of *Pasteurella* pneumonia and coliform mastitis.[32] If tetracycline therapy is to be used in such patients it is prudent to use label doses and maintain good hydration, if not fluid diuresis. Use of outdated tetracycline products may result in a Fanconi-like syndrome with associated severe tubular damage. Idiosyncratic tetracycline hepatotoxicity associated with pregnancy has been reported in humans and the bitch, though it has not been recognized in large animals.

Sulfonamides

Prontosil, a prodrug that is metabolized to sulfanilamide, ushered in the age of modern antimicrobial therapy when patented in 1932.[33] Because sulfonamides are totally synthetic in origin rather than from a microorganism, they are technically antimicrobials rather than antibiotics. Sulfonamides, sometimes referred to as "sulfa drugs," are often stated to have a broad spectrum. This is true in the sense that they can be effective in a variety of gram-positive and gram-negative infections, but

resistance is extremely common. Though *Fusobacterium* spp. infections can be treated with sulfonamide therapy, most other obligate anaerobes are quite resistant. Because of the high incidence of resistance by most bacteria, sulfonamides are usually a poor choice for treating most serious bacterial infections unless a culture and sensitivity test has indicated in vitro susceptibility. Even then, therapeutic failure can occur, particularly in diseases associated with large amounts of purulent debris which tends to inactivate the sulfonamide (see earlier comments under Selection Criteria: Local Activity). Barring sensitivity tests that report otherwise, cross-resistance between sulfonamides should be assumed. The oral sulfonamides are effective against coccidia and this represents a common use in many species, as does growth promotion and the prevention of susceptible infections.

All sulfas work by competing with PABA for dihydropteroate synthase in bacteria that cannot use preformed folic acid.[34] Most sulfonamides are extensively protein bound and hence often have long elimination half-lives. Because of this, priming doses are typically employed to achieve rapid steady-state therapeutic concentrations. This protein binding, along with other physiochemical characteristics, tends to restrict most sulfonamides to the extracellular fluid space and therefore these drugs are not considered good choices to cross most membranes or enter phagocytes (see note on sulfadiazine under Potentiated Sulfonamides).

Older sulfonamides have been associated with crystalluria as their major toxicity. Though still a consideration, most sulfa drugs in common use in the United States are less prone to this problem provided adequate hydration is maintained. Urinary acidification will increase the precipitation of sulfonamides and is best avoided when using this class of antimicrobials. Although hypersensitivity reactions to any drug can occur, this side effect seems to have a higher incidence for the sulfonamides. It is thought that sulfonamides can act as a hapten to sensitize the immune system against certain body tissues. Though not reported in large animals, sulfonamide-associated keratoconjunctivitis sicca and polyarthropathies have been reported in the dog. Sulfonamides must be given IV or orally as they are too irritating to be given IM or SC. Because they have been linked experimentally to thyroid hyperplasia, and in the case of high-dose sulfamethazine to thyroid neoplasia, extra-label use of sulfonamides is prohibited by the FDA in lactating dairy cattle as a precaution to minimize sulfonamide residues in the milk supply.[35]

Potentiated Sulfonamides

If a sulfonamide, which works by competing with PABA, is combined with a dihydrofolic acid (DHFA) reductase inhibitor such as trimethoprim or ormetoprim, a synergistic blockade of the folic acid pathway occurs. This results in a greatly enhanced spectrum of activity for this combination known as a potentiated sulfonamide. Many gram-positive and gram-negative organisms resistant to sulfonamides are susceptible to potentiated sulfonamides. Most obligate anaerobes also are susceptible in vitro although their efficacy in vivo is sometimes questioned, perhaps because of local environmental factors inactivating the sulfonamide portion of the combination. Coccidiosis is also treatable in monogastric animals using this drug combination. Potentiated sulfonamides are considered by many to be the drug of choice in the treatment of nocardiosis, although the need for adequate drainage, high doses, and long duration of therapy make the treatment difficult at best. (Note that no adequate treatment has yet been found for nocardial mastitis.)

Trimethoprim is a relatively lipid-soluble antibiotic that crosses most membranes well. Though most sulfonamides cross membranes poorly, sulfadiazine (the sulfonamide usually com bined with trimethoprim) is less protein bound than other sulfa drugs and can cross some barriers, including the blood-brain barrier to some degree. Though sulfadiazine and trimethoprim used singly are bacteriostatic, the combination is bactericidal. Potentiated sulfonamides are presently available only in oral form in the United States where their use in food animals is extra-label. In Canada they are approved for food animals in oral and injectable forms.[36] Though well absorbed orally in monogastric animals, including swine, trimethoprim does not reach measurable plasma concentrations in ruminants because of rapid metabolism or ruminal degradation. Without the synergy between the two drugs, the remaining sulfadiazine concentration is too small to be therapeutic. As such, oral use in cattle is restricted to preruminant calves.

Potentiated sulfonamides pose almost no risk of crystalluria because the dose of the sulfonamide is reduced due to its synergistic action with trimethoprim or ormetoprim. Though trimethoprim and ormetoprim have a very high selectivity for bacterial DHFA reductase, the mammalian enzyme can be affected. As such, bone marrow suppression can be seen in patients receiving the drugs at high or prolonged dosages. Frequent complete blood counts to check for anemia, leukopenia, and thrombocytopenia are prudent if prolonged use is undertaken. Should bone marrow suppression occur, folinic (preferably) or folic acid can be given to antagonize this toxicity. Toxicities seen in small animals include diarrhea due to floral disruption, hypersensitivities, keratoconjunctivitis sicca, polyarthropathies, and hypothyroidism.

Macrolides

The three macrolide antibiotics approved for veterinary use in the United States are erythromycin, tylosin, and tilmicosin. They can be quite effective against many gram-positive cocci and are considered by many to be the drugs of choice against mycoplasmal infections. They generally have little activity against most gram-negative pathogens, although *Pasteurella*, *Haemophilus*, and *Campylobacter* may be sensitive. Tylosin and erythromycin have been reported to be effective against some spirochetes, including *Treponema hyodysenteriae* and *Leptospira* spp., respectively.[36, 37] In leptospirosis the carrier state may not be cleared and other agents are preferred. Though some obligate anaerobic activity exists, resistance is quite common and these drugs should not be relied upon for most obligate anaerobic infections.[38] Bacterial cross-resistance to the macrolides is common.

As a result of ion trapping, high concentrations of macrolides accumulate in many tissues and substances, including milk, the prostate, lung, and phagocytes. These drugs do not cross the blood-brain barrier, even with inflammation. The macrolides are removed primarily by hepatic processes, although therapeutic concentrations are achieved in the urine. Though not commonly used for urinary tract infections, urine alkalization tends to promote their antimicrobial potency.

Erythromycin use in food animals is restricted to an IM formulation. While used for a variety of infections, including gram-positive mastitis (severe cases when a systemic antimicrobial may be required), the tissue irritation associated with this product can be severe. This side effect has greatly limited the use of injectable erythromycin.

Tylosin has found great utility in the swine industry, orally or by IM injection, particularly for mycoplasmal pneumonia. The premix is approved for low-level use in beef cattle to reduce the incidence of hepatic abscesses. The injectable product is also approved for IM administration in beef cattle, though injection site irritation limits its use.

Tilmicosin has greater activity against *Pasteurella* spp. than do the other macrolides, with susceptibility for bovine isolates tested at 90% and 78% for *P. haemolytica* and *P. multocida*, respectively. It is also active against *Haemophilus* spp. Tilmicosin is available as a repository formulation for SC use in beef cattle where one injection provides 3 days of therapeutic lung concentrations against *P. haemolytica*. Some local tissue reaction may occur at the injection site but this is manageable. Because milk residues have been detected 1 month or more post injection, the drug should not be used in dairy cattle.[39] IM administration is ill-advised as it results in significant tissue irritation. Intravenous administration of tilmicosin is contraindicated and IV use is not without risk for the other macrolides. Tilmicosin is uniquely cardiotoxic and should not be given to goats or horses. Though too toxic for injection in swine it has been approved as a feed additive for treating porcine respiratory disease due to *Actinobacillus pleuropneumoniae* and *P. multocida*.

Florfenicol

Florfenicol is related to the well-known antibiotic, chloramphenicol, and has many of the same properties. It lacks however, the *p*-nitro structure of chloramphenicol, thought responsible for the development of aplastic anemia in humans, and hence does not pose the public health hazard associated with chloramphenicol. A dose-dependent reversible bone marrow suppression can be seen with high dose or prolonged use, but is unlikely to be encountered in most dosage regimens employed in food animals.

Though only approved in cattle for the treatment of bovine respiratory disease due to *P. haemolytica*, *P. multocida*, or *Haemophilus somnus*, it has in vitro activity and is likely to be effective against most gram-positive and gram-negative bacteria. Some organisms resistant to chloramphenicol are sensitive to florfenicol, although *Pseudomonas* and *Serratia* are usually resistant. Though the activity of the drug against obligate anaerobes is not addressed in the literature, it is likely to be quite effective.[40]

Though perhaps slightly less lipid soluble than chloramphenicol, florfenicol crosses membranes easily and will penetrate well into all tissues, including reasonable penetration into the CNS where concentrations are 25% to 50% of plasma concentrations. Approximately 70% of the drug is excreted unchanged by the kidney, with hepatic metabolism playing a smaller role in elimination than with chloramphenicol.[41] Whether florfenicol acts as a P450 enzyme inhibitor, as does chloramphenicol, is unknown. Residue depletion studies in lactating dairy cattle and veal calves have not been done and therefore the label warns against the use of florfenicol in these animals. Possible diarrhea, inappetence, and decreased water consumption are listed as transient signs following dosing.

Florfenicol is approved in Mexico for oral use in swine to treat and control respiratory disease due to *A. pleuropneumoniae* and *P. multocida*. Whether florfenicol can be given orally to ruminants is unknown, but as chloramphenicol is destroyed when given by this route it is probable that florfenicol would likewise be destroyed. The injectable product for IM administration in the neck of beef cattle uses organic vehicles, including *N*-methyl-2-pyrrolidone, to provide a repository effect. Though some tissue irritation can occur, this formulation allows for a dosing interval of 48 hours. The drug can be given IV, but no repository effect occurs if administered by this route.

Fluoroquinolones

At this writing there are no United States–approved fluoroquinolones for cattle or pigs. Furthermore, whether fluoroquinolones should be approved for use in food animals has been a matter of considerable controversy. They are considered such valuable antibiotics in human medicine that many public health officials have expressed concern that their use in food animals would rapidly increase the incidence of bacterial resistance among human pathogens. A key issue in this argument is whether bacterial resistance is spread vertically (mutation of an organism and its subsequent replication) or horizontally (R factor plasmid transmission). Because of the ability of horizontal transmission to disseminate drug resistance across bacterial genera, this method clearly has a much larger impact on bacterial populations. Most studies to date have indicated that spread of resistance to the fluoroquinolones is a vertical process. If so, these drugs may well be released for use in cattle and swine, although restrictions on their extra-label use are anticipated. Regardless, the veterinarian should be acquainted with this important class of antibiotics and the following information is offered.

The fluoroquinolone antibiotics have a number of desirable characteristics. Though obligate anaerobic bacteria are uniformly resistant and streptococcal organisms have a high incidence of resistance, the majority of gram-negative pathogens are quite sensitive to the drug. In humans and small animals the fluoroquinolone antibiotics have allowed for treatment of serious gram-negative infections that previously would have required aminoglycoside therapy. Most *Staphylococcus* spp., mycoplasmas, and some rickettsial organisms are sensitive to fluoroquinolones.

Enrofloxacin is perhaps the fluoroquinolone best known to veterinarians in the United States because of its extensive use in small animal medicine. It is approved in Europe for dogs, cats, swine, and cattle. This bactericidal drug is highly lipid soluble and crosses all membranes easily. In most species enrofloxacin is partially biotransformed to ciprofloxacin, an active metabolite. Elimination is primarily renal. The drug is well absorbed following IM or SC administration.[42] Enrofloxacin is well absorbed orally in most species and is one of the few antibiotics absorbed orally in ruminants (although bioavailability is reduced compared to that in monogastric animals). Whether this is true of other fluoroquinolones remains to be determined. The primary toxicity reported has been arthropathy from cartilaginous injury in young, rapidly growing animals, although this does not seem to be a major concern in calves.[43]

Aminoglycosides

The aminoglycoside antibiotics approved in the United States for parenteral or intrauterine use in nonfood animals include kanamycin, gentamicin, and amikacin. Gentamicin is approved orally and for injection (one dose) in pigs up to 3 days of age, and orally in weanling pigs for 3 consecutive days. Apramycin is approved for oral use in pigs as a water and feed additive. Apramycin is actually an aminocyclitol rather than an aminoglycoside; however, it shares many of the residue and toxicity concerns associated with the aminoglycoside family.

Minimal absorption occurs following oral administration (< 10%). Parenteral administration is required to treat nonenteral infections, an extra-label use in food animals. Once in the central circulation the aminoglycosides are restricted primarily to the extracellular fluid space. Elimination is by renal mechanisms. These drugs bind avidly to the renal proximal tubules and in addition to causing nephrotoxicity are associated with prolonged slaughter withdrawals (after parenteral administration of gentamicin, an 18-month slaughter withdrawal is commonly recommended in cattle). The aminoglycosides can also be ototoxic and can rarely cause a neuromuscular blockade resulting in respiratory arrest, particularly if given rapidly IV.

Because of residue concerns, two veterinary associations have

recommended that parenteral aminoglycosides not be used in food animals. In the rare instance of a valuable individual animal with an infection resistant to other antimicrobials, these drugs could be employed, as they are not technically banned by the FDA. This would, however, require strict adherence to prolonged withdrawal recommendations for the animal according to AMDUCA requirements. Properties of the aminoglycosides can generally be extrapolated across most species and the reader is referred to other texts should such therapy be anticipated.[44, 45]

Spectinomycin

Spectinomycin is an aminocyclitol antibiotic, as are the aminoglycosides. Though spectinomycin is similar in many respects to the aminoglycosides, it lacks the toxicity and long residues associated with aminoglycoside use. Though the drug may have some activity against gram-positive organisms, its primary spectrum and use are against gram-negative bacteria. Spectinomycin has some activity against mycoplasmal organisms and is used in the poultry industry for this purpose. *Pseudomonas* and obligate anaerobic organisms are generally resistant.[46]

Spectinomycin is approved for use in the pig and in poultry for treatment of certain enteric infections, including colibacillosis. It is, however, poorly absorbed orally and parenteral injection is required to treat nonenteral infections. Spectinomycin crosses membranes poorly and is largely restricted to the extracellular fluid space. Elimination is almost entirely renal. Unlike the aminoglycosides, there is no nephrotoxicity or ototoxicity noted with its use. The water-soluble oral product has historically been used for injection in an extra-label manner to treat bovine pasteurellosis and other gram-negative organisms. An injectable product for use in cattle is currently undergoing regulatory review in the United States.

Lincomycin

Lincomycin was the forerunner of clindamycin, the preferred lincosamide (lincosaminide) in human and small animal medicine. Though clindamycin has the more proven anaerobic activity and is more bioavailable orally, lincomycin remains a useful drug in food animal medicine. A related drug, prilimycin, is available as a bovine intramammary infusion for use in clinical mastitis caused by susceptible bacteria.

Lincomycin is a narrow-spectrum antibiotic with excellent activity against a variety of gram-positive bacteria and serpulinal organisms such as *T. hyodysenteriae* and *Serpulina pilisicoli*. It has, however, no gram-negative activity. The activity of lincomycin against obligate anaerobic bacteria remains somewhat speculative, as it is largely untested. Sensitivity testing of obligate anaerobic bacteria was not well refined when lincomycin was released and by the time the technique was perfected most in vitro sensitivity tests used clindamycin as the prototype lincosamide. It is believed that, by allowing for differences in potency and pharmacokinetics, the activity of lincomycin parallels that of clindamycin and therefore the drug should have excellent activity against most obligate anaerobes. It is also effective against mycoplasmal organisms. Lincomycin is effective against swine dysentery caused by *T. hyodysenteriae* and has been reported to have some activity against *Leptospira pomona*. Cross-resistance has been reported with the macrolide antibiotics.

Lincomycin is moderately lipid-soluble, but ion trapping allows this weak base to concentrate in many tissues, including respiratory, prostate, bone, and joint tissues. Very high concentrations are achieved in milk. It is, however, not a preferred drug for most CNS infections. Elimination is renal and hepatic.

Lincomycin is available in oral and injectable forms for use in the pig and the dog. Because of its anaerobic spectrum even small doses of lincomycin administered orally to cattle have resulted in severe diarrhea and side effects. This finding has been misconstrued to imply that parenteral use is also contraindicated. In actuality, although diarrhea can occur following parenteral use, this is rare and the drug is surprisingly well tolerated when given IM to cattle. The drug causes minimal tissue irritation at the injection site.

Tiamulin

Tiamulin is a diterpene bacteriostatic antibiotic that inhibits protein synthesis at the 50s ribosomal subunit. Its spectrum of activity is primarily gram-positive, but it is also active against mycoplasmal organisms and some spirochetes. While a few *Haemophilus* spp. and some *E. coli* and *Klebsiella* strains may be sensitive, the activity of the drug is quite poor against most gram-negative organisms. It is approved in the United States as a water and feed additive for use in pigs weighing less than 250 lbs (114 kg) for the treatment of swine dysentery associated with *T. hyodysenteriae* and swine pneumonia due to *A. pleuropneumoniae*. Tiamulin is well absorbed following oral administration to pigs and has relatively few side effects. The drug is extensively metabolized and is a P450 enzyme inhibitor. Accordingly, it has been reported to decrease the metabolism of certain drugs, including ionophores whose coadministration may lead to toxicity.

Carbadox

Carbadox is a unique antimicrobial effective against a variety of organisms, although it is more active against gram-negative bacteria. It is approved in swine as a feed additive for the control of swine dysentery associated with *T. hyodysenteriae* and the control of enteric salmonellosis. It is also used for improved weight gain and feed efficiency. Carbadox should not be fed to pigs weighing more than 75 lbs (34 kg).

Rifampin

Rifampin is best known as an antimycobacterial drug but also has excellent activity against a variety of gram-positive bacteria. Gram-negative bacteria are usually resistant. Because of its high lipid solubility it has a reputation for use in *Staphylococcus* and *Rhodococcus* infections involving severe abscessation or for use across tissue barriers. More specifically, it has been used in humans for *Staphylococcus aureus* osteomyelitis or endocarditis. Because resistance develops quickly if used as a single agent, rifampin must be combined with another antimicrobial to which the bacteria are sensitive. The drug is well absorbed orally in monogastric animals and is about 40% absorbed in sheep. Rifampin penetrates nearly all tissues, including the CNS, and undergoes extensive metabolism. A dose of 20 mg/kg PO (orally) every 24 hours has been suggested for sheep and cattle with Johne's disease, although it appears to be palliative rather than curative. Since hepatic microsomal enzyme induction occurs with continued use, the dose may need to be increased.[47] Though results have been conflicting, high-dose long-term use of rifampin in one strain of mice resulted in an increased incidence of hepatomas. Because of this suspected tumorgenicity, use of rifampin in food animals may best be restricted to the rare valuable animal that can be excluded from human food production.

Bacitracin

Bacitracin is a narrow-spectrum antibiotic effective against most gram-positive bacteria and some spirochetes. It is used in many topical preparations and orally, where it is poorly absorbed. It is approved in the United States as a water or feed additive to control swine dysentery and to reduce liver abscesses in feedlot cattle. It is also approved for administration to pregnant sows for control of clostridial enteritis caused by *Clostridium perfringens* in suckling piglets.

Virginiamycin

Virginiamycin is a mixture of two antibacterial components with synergistic bactericidal activity toward gram-positive pathogens. It is used orally to control swine dysentery, treat necrotic enteritis due to susceptible *C. perfringens* in poultry, and to reduce the incidence of liver abscesses in feedlot cattle. The drug is used in the swine, poultry, and feedlot industries to improve weight gain or feed efficiency.[48]

Novobiocin

Novobiocin can have some activity against a few gram-negative organisms but is used mostly for its gram-positive spectrum, particularly against staphylococci. Its main use in food animals is in synergistic combination with penicillin G as an intramammary infusion for staphylococcal mastitis.

Polymyxin B

Polymyxin B acts as a detergent to destroy the cytoplasmic membrane of bacteria. It has excellent activity against gram-negative pathogens, including *Pseudomonas*, but no activity against gram-positive bacteria. The ability of polymyxin B to bind endotoxin has sparked a great deal of interest in its use in treating severe endotoxemia. Unfortunately, parenteral administration often results in nephrotoxicity or neurotoxicity, which limits its use primarily to topical products. Relative to a proposed benefit against endotoxemia, the drug has been used as an extra-label intramammary infusion in coliform mastitis. In one experimental study the benefits, however, were not dramatic.[49] It is approved for use in a combination intramammary product in Canada.

REFERENCES

1. Hirsh DC, Ruehl WR: A rational approach to the selection of an antimicrobial agent. J Am Vet Med Assoc 185:1058–1061, 1984.
2. Owens WE, Ray CH, Watts JL, et al: Comparison of success of antibiotic therapy during lactation and results of antimicrobial susceptibility tests for bovine mastitis. J Dairy Sci 80:313–317, 1997.
3. Cox HU, Luther G, Newman S, et al: Comparison of antibiograms determined by disk diffusion and microdilution methods for selected gram-negative bacilli. Am J Vet Res 42:546–551, 1981.
4. Hirsh DC, Indiveri M, Jang SS, et al: Changes in prevalence and susceptibility of obligate anaerobes in clinical veterinary medicine. J Am Vet Med Assoc 186:1086–1088, 1985.
5. Watts JL, Yancey RJ, Salmon SA, et al: A 4-year survey of antimicrobial susceptibility trends for isolates from cattle with bovine respiratory disease in North America. J Clin Microbiol 32:725–731, 1994.
6. Burrows GE: Systemic antibacterial drug selection and dosage. Bovine Pract 15:103–110, 1980.
7. LeFevre PG: Principles of permeation and distribution. *In* Knoefel

PK (ed): Absorption, Distribution, Transformation, and Excretion of Drugs. Springfield, Ill, Thomas, 1972, pp 5–38.

8. Prescott JF, Baggot JD: Antimicrobial susceptibility testing and antimicrobial drug dosage. J Am Vet Med Assoc 187:363–368, 1985.

9. Rebhun WC, deLahunta A: Diagnosis and treatment of bovine listeriosis. J Am Vet Med Assoc 180:395–398, 1982.

10. Houang ET, Hince C, Howard AJ: The effect of composition of culture media on MIC values of antibiotics. In Russel AD, Quernel LB (eds): Antibiotics: Assessment of Antimicrobial Activity and Resistance. New York, Academic Press, 1983, pp 31–48.

11. Burrows GE: Gentamicin. J Am Vet Med Assoc 175:301–302, 1979.

12. Benitz AM: Future development in the aminoglycoside group of antimicrobial drugs. J Am Vet Med Assoc 185:1118–1123, 1984.

13. Applegate J: Clinical pharmacology of sulfonamides. Mod Vet Pract, August 1983, pp 667–669.

14. The International Antimicrobial Therapy Cooperative Group of the European Organization for Research and Treatment of Cancer: Efficacy and toxicity of single daily doses of amikacin and ceftriaxone versus multiple daily doses of amikacin and ceftazidime for infection in patients with cancer and granulocytopenia. Ann Intern Med 119:584–593, 1993.

15. Forrest A, Nix DE, Ballow CE, et al: Pharmacodynamics of intravenous ciprofloxacin in seriously ill patients. Antimicrob Agents Chemother 37:1073–1081, 1993.

16. Cohen SN: Combinations of antibiotics—An introductory review. In Klastersky JK, Jawetz E (eds): Clinical Use of Combinations of Antibiotics. New York, Wiley, 1975, pp 1–10.

17. Lepper MH, Dowling HF: Treatment of pneumococcic meningitis with penicillin compared with penicillin plus aureomycin. Arch Intern Med 88:489–494, 1951.

18. Mathies AW, Leedom JM, Ivler D, et al: Antibiotic antagonism in bacterial meningitis. Antimicrob Agents Chemother 7:218–224, 1967.

19. Nicoletti P, Milward FW, Hoffman E, et al: Efficacy of long-acting oxytetracycline alone or combined with streptomycin in the treatment of bovine brucellosis. J Am Vet Med Assoc 187:493–495, 1985.

20. Eckhoff GA: Mechanisms of adverse drug reactions and interaction in veterinary medicine. J Am Vet Med Assoc 176:1131–1133, 1980.

21. Wenzel RP: Preoperative antibiotic prophylaxis. N Engl J Med 326:337–339, 1992.

22. Code of Federal Regulations Title 21, Part 530, Animal Medicinal Drug Use Clarification Act of 1994: Federal Register; 61(217):57731–57746, 1996.

23. Mercer HD, Teske RH, Long PE, et al: Drug residues in food animals—II; plasma and tissue kinetics of oxytetracycline in young cross-bred swine. J Vet Pharmacol Ther 1:119–128, 1978.

24. Threlfall EJ, et al: Epidemic in cattle of Salmonella typhimurium DT104 with chromosomally integrated multiple drug resistance. Vet Rec 134:577, 1994.

25. Endtz HP, et al: Fluoroquinolone resistance in Campylobacter spp isolated from human stools and poultry products. Lancet 335:787, 1990.

26. Smith HW: Antibiotic-resistant Escherichia coli in marketpigs in 1956–1979: The emergence of organisms with plasmid-borne trimethoprim resistance. J Hyg 84:467–477, 1980.

27. Clarke CR, Burrow GE, Ames TR: Therapy of bovine bacterial pneumonia. The Vet Clin North Am Food Anim Pract 7:669–694, 1991.

28. Lopez A, Kadis S, Shotts E: Enterotoxin production and resistance to antimicrobial agents in porcine and bovine Escherichia coli strains. Am J Vet Res 42:1286–1288, 1982.

29. Samitz EM, Jange SS, Hirsh DC: In vitro susceptibilities of selected obligate anaerobic bacteria obtained from bovine and equine sources to ceftiofur. J Vet Diagn Invest 8:123–124, 1996.

30. Clarke CR, Brown SA, Streeter RN, et al: Penetration of parenterally administered ceftiofur into sterile vs Pasteurella haemolytica–infected tissue chambers in cattle. J Vet Pharmacol Ther 19:376–381, 1996.

31. Kausche FM, Robb EJ, Alaniz G, et al: Safety of dairy milk from cattle treated with ceftiofur sodium (Naxcel/Excenel sterile powder) administered intramuscularly at 1.0 mg ceftiofur/kg body weight. J Vet Pharmacol Therap 20(suppl 1):294, 1997.

32. Lairmore MD, Alexander AF, Powers BE, et al: Oxytetracycline-associated nephrotoxicosis in feedlot calves. J Am Vet Med Assoc 185:793–795, 1984.

33. Weinstein L: Antimicrobial agents: sulfonamides and trimethoprim-sulfamethoxazole. In Goodman LS, Gilman A (eds): The Pharmacological Basis of Therapeutics. New York, Macmillan, 1975, pp 1113–1129.

34. Smith JT: Bacterial resistance to antifolate chemotherapeutic agents mediated by plasmids. Br Med Bull 40:42–46, 1984.

35. Littlefield NA, Gaylor DW, Blackwell BN, et al: Chronic toxicity/carcinogenicity studies of sulfamethazine in B6C3F1 mice. Food Chem Toxicol 27:455–463, 1989.

36. US Pharmacopeia Drug Information. Vol 1: Drug Information for the Health Care Professional. September Update. Rockville, Md, US Pharmacopeia Convention, 1997.

37. Prescott JF: Leptospirosis. In Howard JL (ed): Current Veterinary Therapy 3: Food Animal Practice. Philadelphia, WB Saunders, 1993, pp 541–546.

38. Dow SW, Jones RL: Anaerobic infections—part II: Diagnosis and treatment. Compend Contin Educ Pract Vet 9:827–840, 1987.

39. Helton-Groce SL, Thomson TD, Readnour RS: A study of tilmicosin residues in milk following subcutaneous administration to lactating dairy cows. Can Vet J 34:619–621, 1993.

40. Varma KJ: Personal communication. July 31, 1997.

41. Nuflor Technical Monograph. Kenilworth, NJ, Schering-Plough, 1996, p 16.

42. Kaartinen L, Salonen M, Alli L, et al: Pharmacokinetics of enrofloxacin after single intravenous, intramuscular, and subcutaneous injections in lactating cows. J Vet Pharmacol Ther 18:357–362, 1995.

43. Copeland D: Personal communication. July 1997.

44. Freeman CD, Nicolau DP, Belliveau PP, et al: Once-daily dosing of aminoglycosides: Review and recommendations for clinical practice. J Antimicrob Chemother 39:679–686, 1997.

45. Anaizi A: Once-daily dosing of aminoglycosides: A consensus document (revised April 25, 1977). Available at: http://www.cpb.vokhc.edu/pkin/consensus/ODACD.html#top.

46. Cuerpo L, Livingstone RC: Spectinomycin. Residues of some veterinary drugs in animals and foods. Monographs prepared by the forty-second meeting of the joint FAO/WHO expert committee on food additives. FAO Food Nutr Pap 41:1–86, 1994.

47. St-Jean G, Jernigan A: Treatment of Mycobacterium paratuberculosis infection in ruminants. Vet Clin North Am Food Anim Pract 7:793–804, 1991.

48. Rogers JA, Branine ME, Miller CR, et al: Effects of dietary virginiamycin on performance and liver abscess incidence in feedlot cattle. J Anim Sci 73:9–20, 1995.

49. Ziv G, Schultz WD: Influence of intramammary infusion of polymyxin B on the clinicopathologic course of endotoxin-induced mastitis. J Am Vet Med Assoc 44:1466–1480, 1983.

50. Rasmussen F: Mammary excretion of sulfonamides. Acta Pharmacol Toxicol 15:139–148, 1958.

51. Stowe CM, Sisodia CS: The pharmacologic properties of sulfadimethoxine in dairy cattle. Am J Vet Res 24:525–535, 1963.

52. Ziv G, Shani J, Sulman FG: Pharmacokinetic evaluation of penicillin and cephalosporin derivatives in serum and milk of lactating cows and ewes. Am J Vet Res 34:1561–1565, 1973.

53. Ziv G, Sulman FG: Distribution of aminoglycoside antibiotics in blood and milk. Res Vet Sci 17:68–74, 1974.

54. Ziv G, Sulman FG: Serum and milk concentrations of spectinomycin and tylosin in cows and ewes. Am J Vet Res 34:329–333, 1973.

55. Sisodia CS, Stowe CM: The mechanism of drug secretion into bovine milk. Ann N Y Acad Sci 111:650–661, 1964.

56. Ziv G, Sulman FG: Penetration of lincomycin and clindamycin into milk in ewes. Br Vet J 129:83–90, 1973.

57. Rasmussen F: Renal and mammary excretion of trimethoprim in goats. Vet Rec 87:14–18, 1970.

58. Rasmussen F: Mammary excretion of benzyl penicillin, erythromycin, and penethamate hydriodide. Acta Pharmacol Toxicol 16:194–200, 1959.

59. Jacoby GA, Archer GL: New mechanism of bacterial resistance to antimicrobial agents. N Engl J Med 324:601–612, 1991.

60. Neu HC: Overview of mechanism of bacterial resistance. Diagn Microbiol Infect Dis 12(suppl 4):109S–116S, 1989.

61. Denver LA, Dermody TS: Mechanisms of bacterial resistance to antibiotics. Arch Intern Med 151:886–895, 1991.

62. Lynch MJ, Drusano GL, Mobley HLT: Emergence of resistance to imipenem in Pseudomonas aeruginosa. Antimicrob Agents Chemother 31:1892–1896, 1987.

■ Anthelmintic Therapy

Robert M. Corwin, D.V.M., Ph.D.

Anthelmintic drugs are designed for the effective removal of helminth parasites. These helminths include nematodes, cestodes, and trematodes. The effectiveness or efficacy of an anthelmintic drug is a measure of the percent reduction of helminth parasites in the host animal following drug delivery. Usually there is one parasite species targeted, namely, the target species, for example, *Ostertagia ostertagi* of cattle. To be considered truly efficacious, 90% or more of that worm burden must be removed. Often the target parasite species is one of a complex and is deemed most important from a clinical, subclinical (economic), or pathophysiologic appraisal. *Ostertagia*, the cattle abomasal worm, is part of the parasitic gastroenteric complex (PGE) of cattle, and is considered the most important worm parasite of cattle on a worldwide basis. Thus it serves as the target species for testing the efficacy of the newer generations of anthelmintic drugs.

Efficacy is determined by controlled-critical studies in which experimentally or naturally infected cattle are necropsied at a specific time after drug treatment, and the *O. ostertagi* parasites remaining in the abomasa of treated vs. nontreated animals are then compared. Quantitative fecal examination to determine number of eggs per gram (epg) prior to and following treatment is not a measure of efficacy. This observation is less reliable because of variability in egg production per parasite species during the different parasitic phases in the host and with changes in host physiologic conditions.

A spectrum of activity also must be established both in terms of number of parasite species affected, the degree of removal of each, and the stages eliminated, for example, larval (usually fourth stage, L4) vs. adult (A). For the cattle PGE, there are a number of trichostrongylid species which include *Haemonchus*, *Ostertagia*, *Trichostrongylus*, *Cooperia*, and *Nematodirus*, also the lungworm *Dictyocaulus*, the strongylid *Oesophagostomum*, perhaps the whipworm *Trichuris*, and the tapeworm *Moniezia*. In the past 30 years, drugs developed and marketed have shown exceptional activity against many if not all these worm species, especially against their adult stages. Some also have larvicidal activity which is especially important for *Ostertagia ostertagi* infections in which the inhibited fourth stage larva (iL4) and the emergent fifth stage (L5) or immature stage can be devastating in a sequela of pathophysiologic changes. Thus, anthelmintic drugs with a broad spectrum of activity, including larvicidal, are desirable, have been developed, and are marketed. Note that there is not the desirability to have 100% removal, as there is the need for the presence of a small number of parasites to stimulate the immune system of the host animal for better control of reinfection.

Safety, as determined by the therapeutic index, is of paramount importance. This is monitored by changes in feed consumption; loss of weight or depressed weight gain and scouring; aberrant nervous behavior; chronic debilitation; reproductive abnormalities such as fetal anomalies, abortion, and stillbirths; and acute to chronic death. If there has been evidence of teratogenicity, mutagenicity, and so on, then avoidance of a certain period during gestation is stated. The newer generation of anthelmintic drugs is quite safe as indicated by a factor of a dose greater than 3 to greater than 100 times the recommended dose. Any potential toxic problems at dose levels higher than recommended and for administration during times of stress, especially during breeding and pregnancy or physical debilitation or for a given breed such as *Bos indicus*, must be listed. Tissue residue as a food safety factor consists of retention of the drug and its metabolites in meat, milk, and excreta. And withdrawal times are given for each of these more recently

approved drugs, whereas this might not be stated for older compounds.

The response of individuals and herds or flocks to administration of an anthelmintic drug should be monitored by overall appearance and conditioning, presence or absence of adverse reactions, and by fecal egg count reduction (FECR) in a 3- to 5-week period following treatment. Variability in response might be due to (1) stage of parasite development at the time of treatment; (2) climatic conditions or seasonality; (3) drug metabolism and kinetics; (4) physical and immunologic condition; (5) nutritional status; (6) genetics of the host and of the parasite; and (7) parasite resistance to drugs.

1. Newer drugs are more likely to have larvicidal as well as adulticidal effects, including activity against inhibited or dormant and migrating larvae. Post-treatment examination of fecal samples is necessary to determine this effect. Be aware that under natural field conditions reinfection does occur, but also consider prepatent periods of 2 to 4 weeks dependent upon parasite species and dormancy of larvae, namely, *Ostertagia ostertagi* of 14 to 18 weeks.

2. Seasonality varies per geographic region, by husbandry, and with climatic conditions each year. Precipitation, temperature, forage and soil type, conventional vs. intensive rotational grazing, and stocking rate per given season are major influences in maintenance of pasture contamination and possible infection rate. Strategic deworming programs for livestock have been recommended based on target parasite species, climatic conditions, and herd management. For beef cow and calf production, cows should be dewormed following the calving season, that is, just prior to turnout onto summer pasture; spring calves by midsummer; and all stock at weaning in late fall. For a fall calving operation, cows should be dewormed prior to overwintering and all stock in the spring prior to summer pasturing. Yearling spring calves and fall calves, grazed as stockers, should be dewormed in the late spring, and if on intensively grazed summer pasture, again in the summer. All backgrounded stock brought into a feedlot should be dewormed (including a flukicide) upon arrival. These programs should greatly reduce *Ostertagia* populations, including inhibited larvae.

For sheep and goats, deworming is necessary at or prior to breeding and at lambing or kidding or just prior to summer turnout. All sheep in the flock or goats in the herd need to be dewormed at 3- to 4-week intervals when forage is lush, the temperature warm, and precipitation adequate for forage growth. *Haemonchus contortus* is the target species.

Swine likewise should be dewormed at or just prior to farrowing, at weaning, and at breeding. Target parasites include *Ascaris suum*, *Trichuris suis*, and *Oesophagostomum* spp.

3. The pharmacokinetics of a given drug varies according to host species, breed, and individual. However, most of the modern generation of anthelmintics are quite effective on one administration.

4. Certainly the best-conditioned animal should respond positively to a well-designed drug and well-conceived program. If the animal metabolizes poorly or is immunodeficient, poor response will be observed regardless of these efforts. Observe others in the herd to appreciate the overall effect. Those animals with nutritional deficiencies due to metabolic abnormalities or inexperience with a given ration will not respond to the best of drugs.

5. Selective breeding of cattle, sheep, and goats has been and is underway to establish breeds and lineage within a breed for response to parasite infection. There also appear to be phenotypic expressions of host resistance or susceptibility of individuals. Differences have been demonstrated in genetic response of drug metabolism, for example, some breeds are more susceptible to organophosphates or to higher-than-recommended dose levels of a given drug.

6. Strains of parasites respond differently to their environment, outside and within the host, and to given drug classes. Physical factors such as ensheathment of the parasite, response to sudden environmental changes, for example, cold stress, escaping immune response, and ability to metabolically avoid otherwise effective drugs, are described for given species and strains.

7. Resistance of parasites to anthelmintic drugs has been documented and is being monitored in countries such as Australia and New Zealand where stock are dewormed more intensively. This phenomenon has also been observed in the United States since the late 1980s. *H. contortus* of sheep and goats is involved most frequently but *Ostertagia* of cattle and *Oesophagostomum* of swine are also capable of resistance development. When egg counts are made from fecal samples of treated animals, those with resistant parasite species will show a lessened response or increasing number of eggs over time in spite of continued drug use. To avoid development of drug resistance in a parasite population, classes of compounds should be alternated each year and their activity monitored. Do not alternate within a given class such as with albendazole and fenbendazole in the benzimidazole group.

A number of factors confuse the issue of anthelmintic resistance, namely, poor or inadequate administration, poor scheduling, and use of a drug not targeted for a given species of parasite. Another consideration is identification of the species involved, for example, there are a number of trichostrongylid species with eggs of similar morphometrics. With the exception of *Nematodirus* spp., eggs and larvae need to be cultured to the infective L3 stage for specific identification. *Cooperia* spp. are more numerous in population size, seemingly more drug-tolerant, and therefore epg alone does not substantiate resistance. The following description of anthelmintic drugs is presented alphabetically by class of compounds: avermectins, benzimidazoles, imidazothiazoles, organophosphates, tetrahydropyrimidines, and miscellaneous. A chemical description, mode and spectrum of activity, dose level and mode of administration, possible adverse effects, therapeutic index, and approved host use are included. Compounds not readily available or no longer marketed are listed at the end.

AVERMECTINS

The avermectins are derived from fermentation products of the soil microorganism *Streptomyces avermitilis* and as such are antibiotics. Their antimicrobial activity is insignificant but some possess anthelmintic and ectoparasiticide properties. Those avermectins approved for use in the United States include ivermectin and doramectin.

The mode of action of avermectins does not involve a single mechanism. Rather, it is presumed that the entire class of compounds acts by modulating chloride channels and increasing their permeability to chloride ions. The influx of chloride ions inhibits electrical activity of the nerve cells and paralyzes the parasite. The initial mechanism of action was believed to be release of γ-aminobutyric acid (GABA), an inhibitory neurotransmitter which causes paralysis and slow death of target parasitic nematodes and certain arthropods.

Avermectins are not effective against tapeworms, flukes, and protozoans, such as coccidia, because they do not possess GABA. In the mammalian host, GABA is present only in the central nervous system and would be unaffected by ivermectin in the normal healthy animal because of the blood-brain barrier. *Ivermectin* (Ivomec) was the first avermectin approved and marketed as an anthelmintic for livestock, including cattle, sheep, and swine. It is available in several formulations: a solution for subcutaneous injection in cattle and hogs, a solution as a topical pour-on for cattle, a solution as a drench for sheep, and as a semisolid in a bolus for sustained release for cattle.

Ivermectin was first approved and marketed as a 1% solution for subcutaneous injection in cattle only. The recommended dose level for cattle is 200 μcg/kg and this is effective for the treatment and control of *Haemonchus placei*, *Ostertagia ostertagi* (adults [A], L4, and iL4), *Ostertagia lyrata*, *Trichostrongylus axei*, *Trichostrongylus colubriformis*, *Cooperia oncophora*, *Cooperia punctata*, *Cooperia pectinata*, *Oesophagostomum radiatum*, *Nematodirus helvetianus* (A only), *Nematodirus spathiger* (A only), the lungworm *Dictyocaulus viviparus* (A and L), and ectoparasites such as the cattle grubs *Hypoderma bovis* and *Hypoderma lineatum*, the sucking lice *Linognathus vituli* and *Haematopinus eurysternus*, and the scabies mites *Psoroptes ovis* and *Sarcoptes scabiei* var. *bovis*. The injectable formulation is not to be administered by intramuscular or intravenous injection. Doses greater than 10 mL should be divided between two injection sites in the neck region. Each milliliter of ivermectin per 110 lb or 50 kg body weight will provide the recommended dose of 200 μg/kg. Observation should be made of treated cattle for injection site reactions such as swelling and discomfort, which may progress to clostridial infection. As with any grubicide, proper timing of treatment by geographic region is necessary to avoid bloat, paralysis, and possible death due to disintegration of grubs in esophageal and spinal cord sites.

In safety studies, toxic signs appeared only with doses exceeding 30 times the recommended dose. The recommended dose does not affect breeding performance of bulls or cows. Cattle must not be treated within 35 days of slaughter. Because a withdrawal time has not been established for milk, ivermectin should not be used in dairy cows of breeding age.

Ivermectin (Ivomec Pour-On), a pour-on for cattle only, is a topically applied, systemically active parasiticide, consisting of a 0.5% solution of ivermectin and is applied at a rate of 0.5 mg/kg of body weight. It is formulated for external application only. Each milliliter of Ivomec Pour-On contains 5 mg of ivermectin, sufficient to treat 22-lb body weight. It should be applied along the topline in a narrow strip from withers to tailhead.

Ivomec Pour-On is approved for the removal of *Ostertagia ostertagi* (including L4), *Haemonchus placei*, *Trichostrongylus axei*, *Trichostrongylus colubriformis*, *Cooperia* spp., *Strongyloides papillosus*, *Oesophagostomum radiatum*, *Trichuris* spp., *D. viviparus*, *Hypoderma bovis*, *Hypoderma lineatum*, *S. scabei* var. *bovis*, *L. vituli*, *Haematopinus eurysternus*, *Damalinia bovis*, *Solenopotes capillatus*, and the horn fly *Haematobia irritans* (up to 28 days). Cattle must not be treated within 48 days of slaughter for human consumption. Ivomec Pour-On should not be used in dairy cows of breeding age as a withdrawal time in milk has not been established.

Ivermectin was approved in late 1996 as Ivomec Sustained Release (SR) Bolus. This bolus contains 1.72 g of ivermectin and is packaged as 12 boluses per carton. The Ivomec SR Bolus for cattle is a unique design consisting of an external semipermeable membrane allowing rumen fluid to reach the osmotic driver which in turn expands against a barrier that separates ivermectin from the driver and with expansion causes the release of ivermectin through a port screen. The ivermectin semisolid formulation contains 1.72 g of ivermectin. A density element provides sufficient weight to ensure that the bolus stays in the reticulorumen and is not regurgitated or passed through the gastrointestinal tract. Only a balling gun of specific dimensions will successfully deliver the bolus. Ivermectin is continuously released for a period of 135 days. The spectrum of activity is similar to that of other ivermectin formulations.

One Ivomec SR Bolus is given to cattle weighing at least 275 lb (125 kg) and not more than 660 lb (300 kg) on the day of administration. Calves must be ruminating and greater than 12 weeks of age. Administration to calves weighing less than 275 lb may result in esophageal injuries, including obstruction or perforation with associated complications, including fatalities. The Ivomec SR Bolus was specifically designed for use in cattle and is not intended for use in other species. It is not to be administered within 180 days of slaughter and is not to be given to dairy cows of breeding age. Ivermectin is also approved for use as a fixed combination product with clorsulon (a flukicide cited below). This product was initially labeled as Ivomec F but recently was relabeled as Ivomec Plus. It is available in three ready-to-use packages; a 50-mL pack with sufficient solution to treat 10 head of 550 lb (205 kg) cattle, a 200-mL bottle with sufficient solution to treat 40 head of 550 lb (205 kg) cattle, and a 500-mL bottle with sufficient solution to treat 100 head of 550 lb (205 kg) cattle. This is an injectable parasiticide for the treatment and control of external and internal parasites of cattle, including the adult liver fluke. It is to be given only by subcutaneous injection at a dose of 1 mL/110 lb (50 kg) body weight. This volume will deliver 10 mg ivermectin and 100 mg clorsulon.

Ivermectin has no measurable effect against flukes but relies upon the activity of clorsulon to kill adult *Fasciola hepatica*. Activity is the same as for single-entity ivermectin formulations against all nematode and arthropod parasites listed above.

In 1990, ivermectin (Ivomec Sheep Drench) as a 0.08% solution with 3% benzyl alcohol was approved and marketed for sheep only. It is available in 4.8-L containers, ready to use as a free-flowing solution with any standard drenching equipment. Administration is 0.2 mg/kg orally or 3 mL/26 lb; this appears to be much more than the cattle dose, but note the percent solution of each preparation. In sheep, ivermectin is effective against the adult and L4 stages of gastrointestinal worms *Haemonchus contortus*, *Ostertagia circumcincta*, *Trichostrongylus axei*, *Trichostrongylus colubriformis*, *Cooperia curticei*, *Nematodirus spathiger*, *Nematodirus battus*, *Oesophagostomum columbianum*, the lungworm *Dictyocaulus filaria*, adults only of *Haemonchus placei*, *Cooperia oncophora*, *Strongyloides papillosus*, *Oesophagostomum viviparus*, *Trichuris ovis*, and *Chabertia ovina*, and all larval stages of the nasal bot *Oestrus ovis*. Do not administer within 11 days of slaughter. As with dairy cows, do not administer to milking ewes. Other animal species should not be given Ivomec Sheep Drench.

Ivermectin (Ivomec Swine Injectable) is available for swine in two formulations, a 0.27% solution for grower-feeder pigs at 1 mL/20 lb body weight and a 1% solution for adult pigs at 1 mL/75 lb body weight, both given by subcutaneous injection in the neck region. This delivers 300 μg/kg body weight and is effective in the removal of *Ascaris suum* (A, L4), *Oesophagostomum* spp. (A, L4), *Metastrongylus* spp. (A), *Hyostrongylus rubidus* (A, L4), *Strongyloides ransomi* (A), *Haematopinus suis*, and *Sarcoptes scabiei* var. *suis*. Withdrawal is 18 days prior to slaughter.

Warning: Do not give ivermectin to other animal species not approved as cited above. Fatalities have occurred with livestock formulations given to dogs.

Precaution: Do not expose containers of ivermectin to ultraviolet light as this breaks down the drug; heat and freezing do not affect the product.

Environmental impact: Ivermectin binds to the soil and is inactivated over time. However, free invermectin may affect fish and waterborne organisms adversely so that contamination of lakes, streams, and ponds by runoff from feedlots, and so on, must be avoided. Dispose of used containers in an approved landfill or by incineration.

Doramectin was approved in mid-1996 and became the second avermectin available for cattle. It has the same broad-spectrum activity as ivermectin. Doramectin, the active ingredient in Dectomax, induces a rapid, nonspastic paralysis in nematodes and parasitic arthropods (cf. mechanism of action above for avermectins).

Doramectin 1% injectable solution has an oil-based carrier of sesame oil and ethyl oleate and is packaged in an amber-colored glass vial contained inside a polycarbonate shield. Glass is nonporous to oil-based formulations and the amber color prevents ultraviolet light from degrading the product. The recyclable polycarbonate shield holds the bottle during use and has a predrilled hole for easy hanging during administration with automatic multiple dose equipment.

Dectomax injectable solution is a ready-to-use colorless to pale yellow, sterile solution containing 1% w/v doramectin. It is formulated to deliver the recommended dosage when given by subcutaneous or intramuscular (this IM route differs from ivermectin) injection at the rate of 1 mL/110 lb of body weight and is well tolerated at both injection sites. It is formulated to deliver the recommended dose level of 200 μcg/kg body weight by either the subcutaneous or IM routes.

The spectrum of parasitic activity includes adults and L4 of the gastrointestinal roundworms, including *Ostertagia ostertagi* (including iL4) for up to 21 days, *Ostertagia lyrata*, *Haemonchus placei*, *Trichostrongylus axei*, *Trichostrongylus colubriformis*, *Trichostrongylus longispicularis* (A only), *Cooperia oncophora*, *Cooperia pectinata* (A only), *Cooperia punctata*, *Bunostomum phlebotomum* (A only), *Syrongyloides papillosus* (A only), *Oesophagostomum radiatum*, and *Trichuris* spp. (A only), as well as the lungworm *Dictyocaulus viviparus*, the eyeworm *Thelazia* spp. (A only), the grubs *Hypoderma bovis* and *Hypoderma lineatum*, sucking lice *Haematopinus eurysternus*, *Linognathus vituli*, and *Solenopotes capillatus*, and mange mites *Psoroptes bovis* and *Sarcoptes scabiei*. For grubs, appropriate timing is important. For most effective results, cattle should be treated as soon as possible after the end of the heel fly season.

A single administration of doramectin at 10 or 25 times its label dose is well tolerated by cattle with no adverse effects with respect to clinical condition or weight gain. Further, no pathologically significant changes occurred in any of the hematology and clinical chemistry valves. Occasional postdose salivation was observed in some of the test animals given multiple doses at 10 to 25 times label dose levels. Metabolism data suggest that the liver is the most likely target tissue for doramectin in cattle. Dectomax administered at three times the recommended dose caused no adverse reproductive effects and can be safely administered to breeding cows and bulls. It is not to be used in dairy cows over 20 months of age. A withdrawal period has not been established for this product in preruminating calves. Do not use in calves to be processed for veal. Cattle must not be slaughtered for human consumption within 35 days of treatment.

Doramectin is a high-molecular-weight, nonvolatile drug and therefore will not pass into the atmosphere during manufacture or use. Doramectin is excreted into the environment in low concentrations by cattle treated for internal and external parasitic infections. Doramectin binds strongly to soil and manure particles and is naturally degraded by soil microorganisms. Doramectin has extremely low aqueous solubility and this, coupled with its preferential binding to soil and manure, ensures that only extremely low concentrations will be found in surface waters. Furthermore, these concentrations tend to rapidly decline because doramectin, like other compounds from the avermectin class, is degraded by sunlight. As the Dectomax label indicates, free doramectin may adversely affect fish and certain waterborne organisms on which they feed. Therefore, exercise care when disposing of Dectomax containers.

BENZIMIDAZOLES

There are three benzimidazole carbamate anthelmintic drugs now approved and marketed for livestock. Thiabendazole was the progenitor of this group with later analogues collectively called substituted benzimidazole carbamates. Thiabendazole is no longer marketed in the United States. The substituted benzimidazoles are albendazole, fenbendazole, and oxfendazole. Benzimidazoles are poorly soluble and therefore are usually given by mouth. They are especially effective in ruminants because of slow transit time through the rumen. Benzimidazoles bind to tubulin molecules and disrupt cell division. They also inhibit fumarate reductase blocking mitochondrial function in the parasite, which depletes glycogen reserves and causes parasite death. Each may have specific but different activities as well.

Albendazole (Valbazen) is the most recently approved of this group for cattle only in the United States, where it is not approved for use in sheep, goats, or swine. It differs from the other benzimidazoles in being effective in killing adult liver flukes, *Fasciola hepatica*, at 8 weeks post infection, as well as for all parasitic stages of *Ostertagia ostertagi* (including iL4), and adult and L4 stages of *Haemonchus contortus* and *Haemonchus placei*, *Trichostrongylus axei*, *Nematodirus spathiger*, and *Nematodirus helvetianus*, *Cooperia punctata* and *Cooperia oncophora*, *Bunostomum phlebotomum* (A), *Trichostrongylus colubriformis* (A), *Oesophagostomum radiatum* (A), *Dictyocaulus viviparus* (A, L4), and *Moniezia* spp. (scolices and segments). Albendazole is administered as an 11.36% suspension in an oral drench at 10 mg/kg or 4.54 mg/lb. It has no overt toxic effects at 4.5 times the highest recommended therapeutic dose level and it is tolerated at 7.5 times the recommended therapeutic dose. At 2.5 times the highest recommended therapeutic dose, it had no significant effect on pregnancy, incidence of stillborn calves, or condition of calves at birth. However, since an adequate margin of safety for administration during breeding or early gestation has not been established, albendazole should not be administered during the first 45 days of pregnancy.

Fenbendazole (Panacur, Safe-Guard) was approved for use in cattle in the United States in 1983. The dosage approved was 5.0 mg/kg which is effective in the removal of adult *Haemonchus contortus*, *Ostertagia ostertagi*, *Trichostrongylus axei*, *Trichostrongylus colubriformis*, *Bunostomum phlebotomum*, *Nematodirus helvetianus*, *Cooperia* spp. *Oesophagostomum radiatum*, and the lungworm *Dictyocaulus viviparus*. Subsequent approvals provide label indication for removal of immature stages of most gastrointestinal nematodes at 5 mg/kg and removal of inhibited L4 of *Ostertagi* and the tapeworm *Monezia* spp. at 10 mg/kg. Fenbendazole is available as a 10% suspension and in a multidose 10% paste cartridge. Withdrawal is 8 days prior to slaughter. Feed grade formulations of fenbendazole are also available. The Safe-Guard/En-Pro-Al Blocks provides fenbendazole in a dose of 5 mg/kg over a 3-day consumption period. Cattle must not be slaughtered within 11 days following the last treatment. A 20% type A fenbendazole premix is also available to be mixed in the complete feed for a 1-day treatment providing 5 mg/kg. The premix can also be used to manufacture medicated crumbles, pellets, and cubes. A fenbendazole free-choice mineral mix is also available. The total dose of 5 mg/kg should be consumed over a 3- to 6-day period. Cattle must not be slaughtered within 13 days following the last treatment. In 1996, approval was given for use of fenbendazole formulations (Panacur, Safe-Guard) in dairy cattle of breeding age. There is no milk withdrawal period and no milk discard. All nine nematode parasites in lactating dairy cattle are effectively removed.

For swine, fenbendazole was introduced in the United States in 1984. At a total dose of 9 mg/kg over a 3- to 12-consecutive-day period, it is effective in removal of the large roundworm *Ascaris suum* (A and L in the liver, lung, and intestine), the nodular worms *Oesophagostomum dentatum* and *Oesophagostomum quadrispinulatum*, the small stomach worm *Hyostrongylus rubidus*, the whipworm *Trichuris suis* (A and L in the intestinal mucosa), the kidney worm *Stephanurus dentatus* (A and L), and the lung-

worm *Metastrongylus apri* and *Metastrongylus pudendotectus*. Fenbendazole is available as an 8% premix. There is no slaughter withdrawal time in pigs when used as labeled.

Fenbendazole has a broad margin of safety: 100 times the recommended dose for cattle is not toxic. It can be used safely in all breeding animals and concurrently with vaccines, growth implants, and organophosphate treatments in cattle and with feed additive antibiotics in swine without adverse effects.

Oxfendazole suspension (Synanthic) is administered at 2.5 mg/kg body weight either by oral dose or by intraruminal injection. It is approved for use in beef and nonlactating dairy cattle. It is effective against *Haemonchus* spp., *Ostertagia ostertagi*, *Cooperia* spp., *Oesophagostomum radiatum*, *Bunostomum phlebotomum*, *Dictyocaulus viviparus*, and the tapeworm *Moniezia benedini*. The withdrawal period is 7 days before slaughter.

Clorsulon (Curatrem) is a flukicidal drug commercially available for control of *Fasciola hepatica* in cattle. It is a 4-amino-6-trichloroethenyl-1,3-benzenedisulfonamide which inhibits glycolytic pathways of flukes. It has greater than 99% efficacy against adult *F. hepatica* and 94% against stages over 8 weeks of age in the bile ducts. It is administered as an oral drench (1-qt container) at 7 mg/kg body weight with an 8-day withdrawal period and can be used in conjunction with other anthelmintics. Commercial recommendations are that in the northern United States, cattle should be treated in the fall following freezing and again in late winter or early spring, and in the southern United States in late fall and in late spring to reduce adult *F. hepatica* populations and consequently egg production and pasture contamination.

IMIDAZOTHIAZOLES

Levamisole (Tramisol, Levasole) is the *l*-isomer of *dl*-tetramisole and was approved for use in cattle, sheep, and swine in the United States in the late 1960s and early 1970s. It is available as a phosphate salt for subcutaneous injection in cattle, as a hydrochloride salt in an oral gel for cattle, as oral boluses for cattle and sheep, as a soluble powder for drenching cattle and sheep, as a pour-on for cattle, and for drinking water for pigs.

In cattle, levamisole is indicated for the removal of the gastrointestinal nematodes *Haemonchus*, *Ostertagia*, *Trichostrongylus*, *Cooperia*, *Nematodirus*, *Bunostomum*, and *Oesophagostomum*, and the lungworm *Dictyocaulus viviparus*. At 8 mg/kg, it is highly effective against adult forms of these parasites and less so against immature stages. The withdrawal period is 2 days for oral administration, 7 days for injection, and 9 days for the pour-on. It is not to be used in dairy cows of breeding age.

The approved dose for sheep formulations is 8 mg/kg for removal of *Haemonchus*, *Ostertagia*, *Trichostrongylus*, *Nematodirus*, *Bunostomum*, *Oesophagostomum*, and *Chabertia*, and *D. viviparus*. Withdrawal of treatment for sheep is 3 days.

For swine, levamisole is recommended at 8 mg/kg for removal of *Ascaris suum*, *Oesophagostomum*, *Strongyloides*, *Stephanurus*, and *Metastrongylus*. A withdrawal time of 3 days must be observed. Levamisole has a narrow margin of safety with slight muzzle foaming occurring in cattle given two times the subcutaneous injection dose recommended, with occasional swelling at the site of injection. Usually reactions disappear in a short time. It is not contraindicated in pregnant animals.

ORGANOPHOSPHATES

Dichlorvos (Atgard) is formulated in a polyvinyl chloride resin that adds stability to and delays release of the drug, thus reducing its toxicity and enhancing overall delivery to the gastrointestinal tract. It is approved for use in swine only of the food-producing group. Formulations include Atgard as resin pellets in a litter pack to be added to the ration at the time of use and Atgard C and XLP-30 for bulk feeds. Dichlorvos is indicated for the removal of adult and immature *Ascaris suum, Oesophagostomum* spp. *Trichuris suis,* and *Ascarops strongylina.* Dichlorvos added to the feed and administered shortly after mixing is approximately 17 mg/kg as a single treatment and may be repeated in 4 to 5 weeks. Atgard C given for a single treatment is 479 g/ton feed or 348 g/ton for 2 consecutive days. For pregnant sows, XLP-30 is fed at 334 to 500 g/ton for the last 30 days of gestation, providing 1 g/head/day.

Dichlorvos is generally safe in swine, although softening of stools may occur occasionally and at a dose too high organophosphate toxicosis may be seen. This drug should not be used with other cholinesterase inhibitors. When mixed with complete feeds, feeds must not be pelleted and must remain dry. There are no withholding requirements for slaughter of treated pigs.

PIPERAZINE

Generic piperazine salts have been available since the 1930s. Salts include adipate, citrate, hydrochloride, phosphate, sulfate, and tartrate. The efficacy of these is similar. Piperazine is available in powder for drinking water and as a premix for feed. It is primarily a swine anthelmintic with moderate efficacy in removal of *Ascaris suum* and *Oesophagostomum* at a single dose of 110 mg/kg. Herd treatment is accomplished with 0.2% to 0.4% piperazine in feed or 0.1% to 0.2% in water. All medicated feed or water should be consumed in 8 to 12 hours; therefore fasting or withholding water overnight may be useful prior to treatment. Retreatment is recommended after 2 months. Drug withdrawal times have not been established for swine. It has a wide margin of safety and can be used during pregnancy.

TETRAHYDROPYRIMIDINES

In the United States, *morantel* tartrate (Rumatel) is commercially available for beef cattle as an oral bolus or as a medicated premix. The premix is added to complete feeds to provide 0.968 mg/100 kg of morantel tartrate. This anthelmintic is safe and effective for lactating cows with zero milk withholding, young calves, and replacement heifers. At 9.68 mg/kg (4.4 mg/lb), mature *Haemonchus, Ostertagia, Trichostrongylus, Cooperia, Nematodirus,* and *Oesophagostomum radiatum* are removed. Do not use with severely debilitated cattle. Do not mix in feeds containing bentonite. Withdrawal prior to slaughter following treatment is 14 days.

Pyrantel tartrate (Banminth) is approved for use as a swine premix. It is recommended for addition to the ration at 800 mg/T (22 mg/kg) for a single treatment in removal of *Ascaris suum* and *Oesophagostomum* spp. or at 96 g/T (2.6 mg/kg) for a 3-day treatment for removal and prevention of *A. suum* and prevention of *Oesophagostomum* spp. Pyrantel is also supplied as a fixed combination product with carbadox for swine weighing up to 34 kg. With pyrantel only, withdrawal prior to slaughter is 24 hours, and with carbadox, 10 weeks.

Pyrantel does have some cholinergic activity, but there is no evidence against its use with other cholinergic drugs. It is safe to use during the growth phase and pregnancy.

MISCELLANEOUS

Anthelmintics once used often but now infrequently or not at all include thiabendazole, organosphosphates such as coumaphos and haloxon, and phenothiazine and hygromycin. For information about these, refer to *Current Veterinary Therapy: Food Animal Practice*, volume 2 or 3.

■ External Parasiticides
Robert G. Arther, Ph.D.
James A. Shmidl, D.V.M., M.S.

External parasiticides are compounds used for the control of arthropod pests of livestock including diptera (flies, mosquitoes), lice, mites, and ticks. They are more commonly referred to as animal insecticides. Generally, external parasiticide products for livestock are regulated by the Environmental Protection Agency (EPA). Some of these products also have activity against internal as well as external parasites (e.g., avermectins). They are considered drugs and are therefore regulated by the Food and Drug Administration (FDA).

External parasiticides may be required to treat animals with severe infestations that result in clinical disease or to prevent the spread of vector-borne diseases within a herd. However, more insidious production losses frequently occur from lower pest infestation levels that exceed an economic threshold without obvious clinical signs.

The use of external parasiticides should be combined into a program along with biologic, physical, and cultural control methods (i.e., integrated pest management) to reduce the dependence on pesticides alone and to manage the development of insecticide resistance. A well-designed program to control external parasite pests will improve herd health, increase meat and milk production, improve profitability for the producer, and prevent the public health or public nuisance problems frequently associated with some of these pests.

BOTANICAL AND CHLORINATED HYDROCARBON COMPOUNDS

The first products used for control of external parasites of food-producing animals were botanically derived extracts, including rotenone, nicotine, and natural pyrethrins. These compounds had limited application and usefulness for insect control. The first highly effective compounds for insect control were the chlorinated hydrocarbons, including DDT, lindane, methoxychlor, and toxaphene. DDT received widespread use in the 1940s and 1950s with dramatic success. The use of DDT coincided with the beginning of the modern era of agriculture which achieved a tremendous increase in agricultural productivity. DDT was also used during this time with great success against mosquitoes for malaria control, human body lice that carry typhus, and fleas that transmit plague.

The chlorinated hydrocarbon insecticides, although highly effective, had serious ecologic and toxicologic shortcomings. They were chemically stable and slow to degrade in the environment. In addition, insecticide residues accumulated in the body fat of exposed animals. A phenomenon known as "biologic magnification" was observed with DDT and other related compounds in which residues in the lowest organisms in the food chain were passed on to the next higher organism in the food chain when they were consumed. For instance, an aquatic insect with DDT residue was eaten by a fish, which in turn was consumed by a larger fish, which was eaten by a bird. Each succeeding organism in the food chain accumulated a greater DDT residue than the organism it consumed. In some cases this accumulation process created toxic manifestations at the top of the food chain. The accumulation of DDT in tissues was detrimental to various species of wildlife and was particularly disastrous for certain raptors such as eagles and hawks, causing population reduction as a result of decreased eggshell thickness. DDT was banned in the United States in 1973, and the other chlorinated hydrocarbons have been withdrawn from the market since that time.

ORGANOPHOSPHATE COMPOUNDS

Introduction of organophosphate compounds subsequent to the chlorinated hydrocarbons provided the agriculturist and the veterinarian with effective alternatives for pest control on plants and animals. The neurotoxic action of these compounds is through inactivation of acetylcholinesterase in the synaptic nerve cleft. Organophosphate compounds are systemic in action, that is, they are translocated in the body of the plant or animal. Dermal application of a systemic organophosphate compound may also control parasites in remote anatomic locations such as migrating stages of *Hypoderma* larvae (cattle grubs).

Organophosphate toxicity in mammals produces clinical signs which may include diarrhea, salivation, dyspnea, vomiting, miosis, frequent urination, and bradycardia. The most important indicator of exposure to organophosphate compounds in animals or humans is through measurement of acetylcholinesterase depression in plasma or red blood cells. Atropine is the most effective antidote to organophosphate intoxication. An elevated atropine dose is required for bovines, and product labels should be consulted for dosage directions. The compound pralidoxime (2-PAM) may also be used in combination to reactivate acetylcholinesterase.

Application of organophosphates to cattle infested with grubs in the later phase of their migration occasionally induces an adverse host-parasite reaction due to toxins released from dead larvae in the esophagus or spinal region. This reaction may be manifested by bloat, salivation, ataxia, and posterior paralysis. While this host-parasite reaction may resemble symptoms of organophosphate toxicity, atropine is contraindicated. Epinephrine and anti-inflammatory steroids may be used to reduce the severity of these reactions.

Organophosphate compounds are rather unstable after application and do not accumulate in the environment. They are rapidly metabolized and eliminated in the body. The re-registration process by EPA has effectively eliminated many products because of environmental issues or economic considerations.

PYRETHRINS AND PYRETHROIDS

Pyrethrins consist of a mixture of several closely related insecticidal substances recovered from flowers belonging to the genus *Chrysanthemum* (sometimes referred to as "natural pi"). Pyrethrins quickly paralyze and kill insects by disrupting sodium and potassium ion transport in nerve membranes. Their insecticidal activity is greatly enhanced with the synergist piperonyl butoxide and commonly these compounds are formulated in combination. Pyrethrins have little residual activity because the compounds are rapidly degraded in the presence of sunlight, oxygen, and moisture.

Pyrethroids are synthetic products similar to pyrethrins which have greater insecticidal activity, are chemically more stable, and have greater residual activity. The synthetic pyrethroids have favorable mammalian toxicology profiles although they are all very toxic to fish. Fenvalerate and permethrin are both synthetic pyrethroids which became available in the 1970s and have been used extensively for external parasite control on livestock in various formulations including ear tags, pour-ons, and sprays. Permethrin has also demonstrated repellent activity. Newer pyrethroid insecticides, including cyfluthrin, lambdacyhalothrin,

and zetacypermethrin, have greater potency and photostability than their older counterparts.

Pyrethroids occasionally induce a skin sensation transient following application known as "paresthesia," characterized by numbness, prickling, and tingling. Livestock may display head tossing, tail twitching, restlessness, and irritability. Dairy cattle appear to be more prone to this reaction than beef breeds. These symptoms generally subside within 48 hours of treatment without intervention. Although this reaction can occur with any pyrethroid, it is observed more frequently with the newer pyrethroids.

ENDECTOCIDES

Endectocides are potent and persistent therapeutic agents with systemic activity against nematode as well as arthropod pests of livestock. Avermectins, a group of macrocyclic lactone compounds produced by fermentation of the soil-dwelling actinomycete *Streptomyces avermitilis*, are the most important endectocides in use today for livestock. Ivermectin, a semisynthetic derivative of avermectin B_1, and doramectin, a derivative of avermectin A_1, are approved for livestock in the United States and other avermectin derivatives are currently under development. The avermectins act on the arthropod nervous system to stimulate release of the neurotransmitter γ-aminobutyric acid (GABA) from nerve endings and enhancement of the binding of GABA to its receptor. This action increases the flow of chloride ions into the nerve cell with hyperpolarization and elimination of signal transmission.

While avermectin compounds are used principally for therapeutic and prophylactic treatment of gastrointestinal nematodes, their activity against external parasites is also important and some of the formulations have significant roles for use in the management of insecticide resistance.

AMITRAZ

Amitraz is a formamidine compound that kills lice, ticks, and mange mites on livestock by inhibition of monoamine oxidase. Amitraz has been used successfully in parts of the world for control of organophosphate or pyrethroid-resistant ticks. Amitraz has little or no activity against flies and is toxic to horses.

INSECT DEVELOPMENT INHIBITORS

The insect development inhibitors consist of several different chemical compounds that interfere with the development of insect eggs, larvae, or pupae. Methoprene is a juvenile growth hormone analogue that interferes with development of insect larvae. Diflubenzuron is a chitin synthesis inhibitor which interferes with the formation or deposition of chitin within developing eggs or larvae. Tetrachlorvinphos, an organophosphate, prevents the development of fly larvae. Insect growth regulants are available in various formulations (feed additive, combined with mineral supplements, or by bolus) for continual use during the fly season. The active ingredients are eliminated in the manure to control the development of immature stages of fecal breeding flies. These products have no effect on adult flies.

TREATMENT METHOD OPTIONS

Active ingredients have been formulated into a number of products for application by a variety of treatment methods. A product and method of application must be selected that will control the parasite without causing undue stress to the host animals. Pour-on products are formulated to be poured along the top of the back of the animal. They are easy to use and have become a popular method for treating cattle for grubs (*Hypoderma* spp.) Some of these products are also approved for the control of lice on cattle and swine. The avermectins are also available as pour-on formulations.

Solutions for dip vat use and whole-body spray (applied with a high-pressure sprayer) have similar uses, advantages, and disadvantages. These treatment methods are effectively used for ticks, flies, grubs, lice, and mange control. The dip vat is an effective application method and is used in cattle feedlot operations and tick control programs. Whole-body sprays, although still used, are not as popular as they were earlier. The main disadvantage of both treatment methods is their use during severe cold weather.

The back rubber is one of the oldest "self-treatment" methods used for applying parasiticides to cattle or swine. There are several types on the market. This application method has several advantages, one of which is ease of application, because infested animals tend to seek out and use a back rubber. The disadvantage of the back rubber is that it must be serviced regularly so that proper dispensing of the parasiticide is ensured.

Dust bags have generally the same advantages as the back rubber but are usually more effective because they require less servicing and dispense the parasiticide more consistently when used by cattle. Dust bags are especially effective for horn fly and lice control. They may be hung where cattle are forced to dust themselves, as in gateways to pastures, or they may be located where cattle congregate and use them at will.

The introduction of injectable and pour-on avermectin formulations has provided alternatives to older, conventional methods. Market figures show wide acceptance because of their spectrum of activity and convenience.

In determining what product or treatment method to use, several considerations need to be made. It is obvious that the treatment of choice should be effective in the control of the parasite, cause no untoward stress in the host, and be easy to apply and economical.

Tables 1 through 6 list common products used for external parasite control on cattle, sheep, goats, and swine. The products are listed by trade name and the common (generic) name of the active ingredient. These tables are not intended to be an all-inclusive listing of products for the noted indications but are only representative. Be sure to study product labels before use. Labels are frequently revised for necessary changes to use instructions, restrictions, product claims, and meat or milk withdrawal times.

INSECTICIDAL EAR TAGS AND HORN FLY CONTROL

Horn flies (*Haematobia irritans*) are the most economically important ectoparasite of range cattle in North America. Insecticidal ear tags containing the synthetic compounds permethrin and fenvalerate were first introduced to the market for horn fly control in the early 1980s. Initially these tags were highly effective and resulted in dramatic reduction of horn flies. The tags were convenient and provided a long duration of efficacy. This favorable situation only lasted for a few years, however, when pyrethroid resistance began to develop and these tags first started to fail against horn flies in areas of the southeastern United States. Pyrethroid resistance has now been documented throughout most of the United States and the use of pyrethroid ear tags has been implicated in the development of resistance. The use of DDT in the 1940s and 1950s for fly control is believed to have predisposed horn fly populations to pyrethroid

resistance development since both compounds have similar mechanisms of activity. Ear tags containing organophosphate insecticides have been introduced to help manage pyrethroid-resistant horn flies. While cross-resistance occurs within the pyrethroid family of insecticides, cross-resistance with organophosphate insecticides has not been indicated.

Pyrethroid tags may be used to control pyrethroid-susceptible horn flies, face flies, and lice. The newer pyrethroid ear tags will control horn flies with low to moderate levels of pyrethroid resistance, but use of pyrethroid tags alone in these situations will intensify the resistance level and eventually these tags will also begin to fail.

The following recommendations have been formulated by veterinary entomologists for the management of pyrethroid-resistant horn flies.

1. Rotate the use of pyrethroid and organophosphate ear tags.
2. If pyrethroid resistance is confirmed, do not treat with any pyrethroid formulation at any concentration or with any formulation.
3. Do not treat cattle in the spring before fly numbers exceed an excessive threshold level (generally accepted as 200 flies per animal).
4. Treat with insect development inhibitors (bolus or feed additives).
5. The greatest economic damage from horn flies is from decreased weight gains of young animals. Therefore, separate mature cows from growing calves with lactating cows and only treat animals in the growth mode.
6. Use supplemental treatment with sprays, dusts, pour-ons, or back rubbers (using organophosphate insecticides) at periodic intervals when fly numbers are excessive.
7. Use a late-season control method with alternative chemistry to reduce the over-winter fly stages (diapause).
8. Remove ear tags in the fall or when they fail.

INTEGRATED PEST MANAGEMENT

Integrated pest management (IPM) is the selection, integration, and implementation of various biologic, physical, and chemical methods to control pests and maintain infestations below an economic threshold. IPM frequently involves the use of two or more different pest management procedures concurrently to attack different stages of a pest life cycle.

IPM has been successfully developed for agronomic and horticultural crops and to some extent in the poultry industry. More recently these concepts have been adapted for livestock since many of the principles are the same. Some examples of methods that can be used in addition to direct animal treatments as an integrated approach to control of many livestock pests include culling "chronic or carrier" lice-infested cattle from the herd, drainage of wet areas in stockyards to reduce breeding areas of diptera, and disposal of manure, spilled feed, and decaying hay where stable flies breed. Manure management practices can be implemented to increase the populations of natural predators that attack egg, larval, or pupal stages of fecal breeding flies. Some of these predators are also commercially available to augment existing populations (e.g., beneficial parasitic wasps such as *Muscidifurax* and *Spalangia* spp.). Veterinarians can apply the concepts of IPM as a proactive approach to maintain pest levels below an economic threshold rather than rely solely upon drugs or insecticides to treat animals after clinically significant pest problems emerge.

A successful IPM program provides benefits that include improved feed efficacy and milk production, decreases the reliance upon insecticides alone, manages pesticide resistance problems, and reduces the social and public health nuisance concerns that are frequently caused by livestock pests.

Text continued on page 48

Table 1
INSECTICIDE SPRAYS AND DUSTS FOR EXTERNAL PARASITE CONTROL ON CATTLE

Trade Name	Active Ingredient	Company	Pests	Application	Withdrawal Period Before Slaughter (Days)	Comments
Co-Ral 1% Dust	1% coumaphos	Several different suppliers	Horn flies, lice; aids in reducing face flies	Dust bag or shaker can	0	Apply no more than 2 oz per animal; repeat as necessary but not more than once every 14 days
Co-Ral Emulsifiable Livestock Insecticide	11.6% coumaphos	Bayer Corp., Shawnee Mission, KS 66201	Grubs, horn flies, face flies, lice, ticks	Spray or back rubber	0	Restricted-use pesticide; for retail sale and use by certified applicators
Co-Ral Flowable Insecticide	42% coumaphos	Bayer Corp., Shawnee Mission, KS 66201	Scabies, horn flies, lice, ticks, screwworms	Spray or dip	0	A & PHIS (USDA)-approved pesticide for federal eradication programs
Co-Ral Livestock Insecticide Spray	5.8% coumaphos	Bayer Corp., Shawnee Mission, KS 66201	Horn flies, face flies, lice, ticks	Spray or back rubber	0	Use lower dilution rate for lactating dairy cattle
Co-Ral Wettable Powder	25% coumaphos	Bayer Corp., Shawnee Mission, KS 66201	Horn flies, lice, ticks, grubs, screwworms, mites	Spray or dip	0	Treat lactating dairy cattle only at lower dilution
Drycide	0.25% permethrin	Hess and Clark, Inc., Ashland, OH 44805	Horn flies, lice	Shaker can	0	
Del-Phos	11.6% phosmet	Schering-Plough Animal Health, Kenilworth, NJ 07033	Lice, ticks, horn flies, sarcoptic mange mites	Spray or back rubber	3	Do not treat lactating dairy animals within 28 days of freshening
Prolate	11.6% phosmet	Sandoz, Des Plaines, IL 60018	Horn flies, lice, mange, ticks	Spray or back rubber	1	
Rabon 3% dust	3% tetrachlorvinphos	Boehringer-Ingelheim, St. Joseph, MO 60060	Horn flies, lice; aids in reduction of face flies	Dust bag	0	For beef and dairy cattle
Rabon Wettable Powder	50% tetrachlorvinphos	Boehringer-Ingelheim, St. Joseph, MO 60060	Horn flies, lice, ticks	Spray	0	For beef cattle
Ravap E.C.	23% tetrachlorvinphos + 5.3% dichlorvos	Boehringer-Ingelheim, St. Joseph, MO 60060	Horn flies, lice, ticks; aids in control of face flies	Spray or back rubber	0	For beef and lactating dairy cattle
Taktic E.C.	12.5% amitraz	Hoechst-Roussel Agri-Vet Co., Somerville, NJ 08876	Ticks, scab and mange mites, lice	Spray	0	For beef and lactating dairy cattle
Vapona Feedlot—4 lb Concentrate	41.4% dichlorvos	Durvet, Inc., Blue Springs, MO 64014	Horn flies, stable flies, face flies, mosquitoes	Spray	1	For beef and dairy cattle; do not treat Brahman or Brahman cross cattle

A & PHIS (USDA), Animal and Plant Health Inspection Service (U.S. Department of Agriculture).

Table 2
INSECTICIDE POUR-ON FORMULATIONS FOR EXTERNAL PARASITE CONTROL ON CATTLE

Trade Name	Active Ingredient	Company	Pests	Application	Withdrawal Period Before Slaughter (Days)	Comments
PYRETHROID PRODUCTS						
Atroban Delice Pour-on Insecticide	1% permethrin	Schering-Plough Animal Health, Kenilworth, NJ 07033	Horn flies, face flies, lice	Pour-on	0	Approved for lactating dairy cattle
Boss Pour-on Insecticide	5% permethrin	Schering-Plough Animal Health, Kenilworth, NJ 07033	Lice, horn flies, face flies; aids in control of horse flies, stable flies, mosquitoes, black flies, ticks	Pour-on	0	Approved for lactating dairy cattle
Brute Pour-on for Cattle	10% permethrin	Y-Tex Corp., Cody, WY 82414	Pyrethroid-susceptible horn flies, lice; aids in control of face flies, stable flies, horse flies, deer flies, house flies, mosquitoes	Low-volume pour-on	0	Approved for lactating dairy cattle
Cylence Insecticide	1% cyfluthrin	Bayer Corp., Shawnee Mission, KS 66201	Horn flies, face flies, biting lice, sucking lice	Low-volume pour-on	0	Approved for lactating dairy cattle
Durasect long-acting Livestock Pour-on	1% permethrin	Pfizer Animal Health, Exton, PA 19341	Horn flies, face flies, lice; aids in control of stable flies and horse flies	Pour-on	0	Approved for lactating dairy cattle
Ectrin Insecticide	10% fenvalerate	Boehringer-Ingelheim, St. Joseph, MO 64506	Horn flies, lice, ticks, face flies, stable flies	Pour-on or spray	1	May also be applied as a dilute spray
Expar pour-on insecticide	1% permethrin	Schering-Plough Animal Health, Kenilworth, NJ 07033	Lice, horn flies, face flies; aids in control of horse flies, stable flies, mosquitoes, black flies, ticks	Pour-on	0	Approved for lactating dairy cattle
Permectrin CD Pour-on	10% permethrin	Boehringer-Ingelheim, St. Joseph, MO 64506	Lice, horn flies; aids in control of face flies, horse flies, stable flies, deer flies, house flies, black flies, mosquitoes	Pour-on	0	Approved for lactating dairy cattle
Saber Pour-on Insecticide	1% lambdacyhalothrin	Schering-Plough Animal Health, Kenilworth, NJ 07033	Horn flies, lice	Low-volume pour-on	0	Do not apply to lactating or dry dairy cows; not recommended for veal calves; do not apply to the face of beef cattle or calves
Synergized Delice Pour-on Insecticide	1% permethrin + 1% piperonyl butoxide	Schering-Plough Animal Health, Kenilworth, NJ 07033	Lice, horn flies, face flies; aids in control of horse flies, stable flies, mosquitoes, black flies, ticks	Pour-on	0	Approved for lactating dairy cattle
ORGANOPHOSPHATE PRODUCTS						
Lysoff pour-on	7.6% fenthion	Bayer Corp., Shawnee Mission, KS 66201	Lice, horn flies	Pour-on	21 (single treatment)	Dilute with water before use; do not use in female cattle of breeding age
Spotton Cattle Insecticide	20% fenthion	Bayer Corp., Shawnee Mission, KS 66201	Cattle grubs; aids in control of lice	Low-volume pour-on	45	Do not treat dairy cattle of breeding age
Tiguvon Cattle Insecticide Pour-on	3% fenthion	Bayer Corp., Shawnee Mission, KS 66201	Cattle grubs, biting and sucking lice	Pour-on	35 (single treatment)	Do not treat lactating dairy cattle
Warbex famphur Pour-on for Cattle	13.2% famphur	Schering-Plough Animal Health, Kenilworth, NJ 07033	Cattle grubs; reduces lice infestations	Pour-on	35	Do not treat lactating dairy cattle or within 21 days of freshening; do not treat Brahman bulls

41

Table 3
INSECTICIDE EAR TAGS FOR EXTERNAL PARASITE CONTROL ON CATTLE

Trade Name	Active Ingredient	Company	Pests	Application	Withdrawal Period Before Slaughter (Days)	Comments*
PYRETHROID PRODUCTS						
Atroban Extra Insecticide Ear Tags	10% permethrin + 13% piperonyl butoxide	Schering-Plough Animal Health, Kenilworth, NJ 07033	Horn flies, face flies, Gulf Coast ticks, spinose ear ticks; aids in control of lice, stable flies, house flies	2 tags/animal	0	Approved for beef and lactating dairy cattle
Cutter Gold	10% cyfluthrin	Bayer Corp., Shawnee Mission, KS 66201	Horn flies, Gulf Coast ticks, spinose ear ticks; aids in control of face flies	2 tags/animal	0	Approved for beef and lactating dairy cattle
Ectrin Insecticide	8% fenvalerate	Boehringer-Ingelheim, St. Joseph, MO 64506	Horn flies, face flies, Gulf Coast ticks, spinose ear ticks; aid in control of lice, stable flies, house flies	2 tags/animal	0	Approved for beef and lactating dairy cattle
Excalibur Ear Tags	10% lambdacyhalothrin + 13% piperonyl butoxide	Schering-Plough Animal Health, Kenilworth, NJ 07033	Horn flies, face flies	2 tags/animal	0	Not for use on lactating dairy cattle
Expar Extra Insecticide Ear Tags	10% permethrin + 13% piperonyl butoxide	Schering-Plough Animal Health, Kenilworth, NJ 07033	Horn flies, face flies, Gulf Coast ticks, spinose ear ticks; aid in control of lice, stable flies, house flies	2 tags/animal	0	Approved for lactating dairy cattle
Gard Star Plus Insecticide Ear Tag	10% permethrin	Y-Tex Corp., Cody, WY 82414	Horn flies, face flies, Gulf Coast Ticks, spinose ear ticks; aid in control of lice, stable flies, house flies	2 tags/animal	0	Approved for lactating dairy cattle
Python Insecticide Ear Tags	10% zeta cypermethrin + 20% piperonyl butoxide	Y-Tex Corp., Cody, WY 82414	Horn flies, face flies, lice, Gulf Coast ticks, spinose ear ticks; aids in control of house flies, stable flies, black flies, small horse flies	1 tag/calf; 2 tags/ mature animal	0	Approved for beef and lactating dairy cattle
Saber Extra Ear Tags	10% lambdacyhalothrin + 13% piperonyl butoxide	Schering-Plough Animal Health, Kenilworth, NJ 07033	Horn flies, face flies	2 tags/animal	0	Not for use on lactating dairy cattle
ZetaGard Insecticide Ear Tag	10% zetacypermethrin + 20% piperonyl butoxide	Y-Tex Corp., Cody, WY 82414	Horn flies, face flies, lice, Gulf Coast ticks, spinose ear ticks, aids in control of house flies, stable flies, black flies, small horse flies	1 tag/calf; 2 tags/ mature animal	0	Approved for beef and lactating dairy cattle

Table continued on following page

ORGANOPHOSPHATE PRODUCTS

Product	Active Ingredient	Manufacturer	Pests Controlled	Tags		Remarks
Bova Gard Insecticide Ear Tag	21.4% diazinon	Y-Tex Corp., Cody, WY 82414	Horn flies (including pyrethroid-resistant populations), Gulf Coast ticks, spinose ear ticks; aids in control of face flies, lice, stable flies, house flies	2 tags/animal	0	Not for use on lactating dairy cattle
Commando Insecticide Ear Tag	36% ethion	Boehringer-Ingelheim, St. Joseph, MO 64065	Horn flies (including pyrethroid-resistant populations), Gulf Coast ticks, spinose ear ticks; aids in control of face flies, lice, stable flies, house flies	2 tags/animal	0	Approved for use on beef and lactating dairy cattle
Cutter Blue Insecticide Ear Tag	20% fenthion + 15% piperonyl butoxide	Bayer Corp., Shawnee Mission, KS 66201	Horn flies (including pyrethroid-resistant populations); aids in control of face flies	2 tags/animal	0	Approved for beef and lactating dairy cattle
Cutter One Insecticide Ear Tag	40% diazinon	Bayer Corp., Shawnee Mission, KS 66201	Horn flies (including pyrethroid-resistant populations), Gulf Coast ticks, spinose ear ticks; aids in control of face flies, lice, stable flies, house flies	1 or 2 tags/animal	0	Not for use on lactating dairy cattle
Diaphos Rx Insecticide Ear Tag	30% diazinon + 10% chlorpyrifos	Y-Tex Corp., Cody, WY 82414	Horn flies (including pyrethroid-resistant populations), Gulf Coast ticks, spinose ear ticks; aids in control of face flies, lice, stable flies, house flies	1 or 2 tags/animal	0	Not for use on lactating dairy cattle
Dominator Insecticide Ear Tag	20% pirimiphos-methyl	Schering-Plough Animal Health, Kenilworth, NJ 07033	Horn flies (including pyrethroid-resistant horn flies); aids in control of face flies	2 tags/animal	0	Not for use on lactating dairy cattle

Table 3
INSECTICIDE EAR TAGS FOR EXTERNAL PARASITE CONTROL ON CATTLE *Continued*

Trade Name	Active Ingredient	Company	Pests	Application	Withdrawal Period Before Slaughter (Days)	Comments*
ORGANOPHOSPHATE PRODUCTS						
Patriot Insecticide Cattle Ear Tags	40% diazinon	Boehringer-Ingelheim, St. Joseph, MO 64065	Horn flies (including pyrethroid-resistant populations), Gulf Coast ticks, spinose ear ticks; aids in control of face flies, lice, stable flies, house flies	1 or 2 tags/animal	0	Not for use on lactating dairy cattle
Rotator Insecticide Ear Tags	20% pirimiphos-methyl	Schering-Plough Animal Health, Kenilworth, NJ 07033	Horn flies (including pyrethroid-resistant horn flies); aids in control of face flies	2 tags/animal	0	Not for use on lactating dairy cattle
Terminator Insecticide Ear Tag	20% diazinon	Boehringer-Ingelheim, St. Joseph, MO 64506	Horn flies (including pyrethroid-resistant horn flies); aids in control of face flies	2 tags/animal	0	Not for use on lactating dairy cattle
Warrior Insecticide Cattle Ear Tag	30% diazinon + 10% chlorpyrifos	Y-Tex Corp., Cody WY 82414	Horn flies (including pyrethroid-resistant populations), Gulf Coast ticks, spinose ear ticks; aids in control of face flies, lice, stable flies, house flies	1 or 2 tags/animal	0	Not for use on lactating dairy cattle
PRODUCTS CONTAINING PYRETHROIDS PLUS ORGANOPHOSPHATES						
Double Barrel Insecticide Ear Tags	6.8% lambdacyhalothrin + 14% pirimiphos-methyl	Schering-Plough Animal Health, Kenilworth, NJ 07033	Horn flies, face flies	2 tags/animal	0	Not for use on lactating dairy cattle
Max-Con Insecticide Ear Tags	7% cypermethrin + 5% chlorpyrifos + 3.5% piperonyl butoxide	Y-Tex Corp., Cody, WY 82414	Horn flies, face flies	2 tags/animal	0	Not for use on lactating dairy cattle

*All insecticide ear tags must be removed before slaughter.

Table 4
ENDECTOCIDES AND INSECT DEVELOPMENT INHIBITORS FOR EXTERNAL PARASITE CONTROL ON CATTLE

Trade Name	Active Ingredient	Company	Pests	Application	Withdrawal Period Before Slaughter (Days)	Comments
Dectomax	1% doramectin	Pfizer Animal Health, Exton, PA 19341	Sucking lice, mange mites (*Psoroptes bovis, Sarcoptes scabiei*), cattle grubs	Injectable	35	Not for use in female dairy cattle 20 months of age or older; also controls internal parasites
Eprinex	0.5 eprinomectin	MSD AGVET, Rahway, NJ 07065	Sucking lice, biting lice, mange mites (*C. bovis, S. scabiei*), cattle grubs, horse flies	Pour-on	0	For beef and dairy cattle; 0 milk discard and 0 tissue withdrawal
Ivomec 1% Injection for Cattle	1% ivermectin	MSD AGVET, Rahway, NJ 07065	Sucking lice, mange mites (*P. bovis, S. scabiei*), cattle grubs	Injectable	35	Do not use in female dairy cattle of breeding age; also controls internal parasites
Ivomec Pour-on for Cattle	0.5% ivermectin	MSD AGVET, Rahway, NJ 07065	Sucking lice, biting lice, *S. scabiei*, cattle grubs, horn flies	Pour-on	48	Do not use in female dairy cattle of breeding age; also controls internal parasites
Ivomec SR Bolus	1.72 g of ivermectin	MSD AGVET, Rahway, NJ 07065	Mange mites, sucking lice, cattle grubs, ticks	Sustained-release bolus	180 (after treatment)	Do not use in female dairy cattle of breeding age; also controls internal parasites
Moorman's IGR Cattle Concentrate	0.40% methoprene	Moorman Manufacturing Co., Quincy, IL 62305	Horn flies	Feed premix	0	For control of fly larvae in manure
Rabon Oral Larvicide	7.76% tetrachlorvinphos	Boehringer-Ingelheim, St. Joseph, MO 60060	Horn flies, face flies, house flies, stable flies	Feed premix	0	For control of fly larvae in manure; may be used for beef and lactating dairy cattle
Vigilante Insecticide	9.7% diflubenzuron	Hoechst-Roussel Agri-Vet Co., Somerville, NJ 08876	Horn flies, face flies; aids in control of house flies, stable flies	Bolus	0	For beef and dairy cattle

Table 5
SOME COMMON PRODUCTS USED FOR EXTERNAL PARASITE CONTROL ON SHEEP AND GOATS

Trade Name	Active Ingredient	Company	Pests	Application	Withdrawal Period Before Slaughter (days)	Comments
Atroban 42.5% EC	42.5% permethrin	Schering-Plough Animal Health, Kenilworth, NJ 07033	Horn flies, face flies, house flies, scabies, mites, ticks, lice	Spray	0	No label directions for goats
Atroban Delice Pour-on Insecticide	1% permethrin	Schering-Plough Animal Health, Kenilworth, NJ 07033	Keds, lice	Pour-on	0	No label directions for goats
Atroban 11% EC Insecticide	11% permethrin	Schering-Plough Animal Health, Kenilworth, NJ 07033	Horn flies, face flies, house flies, mange mites, ticks, lice, sheep keds	Spray	0	May be used for lactating dairy goats
Co-Ral 25% Wettable Powder	25% coumaphos	Bayer Corp., Shawnee Mission, KS 66201	Horn flies, lice, ticks, screwworms, fleeceworms, keds, scabies (*Psoroptes bovis*); sheep only	Spray or dip	3	Do not treat lactating dairy goats
Dryzon WP	50% diazinon	Y-Tex Corp., Cody, WY 82414	Keds, lice	Spray	14	No label directions for goats
Ectrin Insecticide	10% fenvalerate	Boehringer-Ingleheim, St. Joseph, MO 64906	Lice, keds	Spray or pour-on	2	Repeat at 30-day intervals for sheep and nonlactating goats
Expar Pour-on Insecticide	1% permethrin	Schering-Plough Animal Health, Kenilworth, NJ 07033	Keds, lice	Pour-on	0	No label claims for goats
Ivomec Sheep Drench	0.08% ivermectin	MSD AGVET, Rahway, NJ 07065	Nasal bots	Drench	11	No label directions for goats; also controls internal parasites
Permectrin II	10% permethrin	Boehringer-Ingelheim, St. Joseph, MO 64506	Flies, lice, ticks	Spray	0	No label directions for goats

Table 6
SOME COMMON PRODUCTS USED FOR EXTERNAL PARASITE CONTROL ON SWINE

Trade Name	Active Ingredient	Company	Pests	Application	Withdrawal Period Before Slaughter (days)	Comments
Atroban 11% or 42.5% EC Insecticide	11% or 42.5% permethrin	Schering-Plough Animal Health, Kenilworth, NJ 07033	Lice, mange mites	Spray	5	
Co-Ral Dust	1% coumaphos	Bayer Corp., Shawnee Mission, KS 66201	Lice	Dust	0	Bedding may be treated
Co-Ral Emulsifiable Livestock Insecticide	11.6% coumaphos	Bayer Corp., Shawnee Mission, KS 66201	Lice	Spray	0	
Co-Ral Livestock Insecticide Spray	5.8% coumaphos	Bayer Corp., Shawnee Mission, KS 66201	Lice	Spray	0	Repeat as necessary
Co-Ral Wettable Powder	25% coumaphos	Bayer Corp., Shawnee Mission, KS 66201	Lice, flies, ticks, screwworms	Spray	0	
Decto MAX	1% doramectin	Pfizer Animal Health, Exton, PA 19341	Lice, mange mites	Injectable	24	
Del-Phos Emulsifiable Liquid	11.6% phosmet	Schering-Plough Animal Health, Kenilworth, NJ 07033	Lice, mange mites	Spray	1	
Drycide	0.25% permethrin	Hess and Clark, Inc., Ashland, OH 44805	Lice	Shaker can	5	
Ectrin Insecticide	10% fenvalerate	Boehringer-Ingelheim, St. Joseph, MO 60060	Lice, mange mites	Spray	1	Repeat in 14 days if necessary
Ivomec 1% Injection for Swine	0.27% or 1.0% ivermectin	MSD AGVET, Rahway, NJ 07065	Lice, mange mites	Injectable	18	Also controls internal parasites
Ivomec Premix for Swine	6 g ivermectin/kg	MSD AGVET, Rahway, NJ 07065	Lice, mange mites	Medicated feed	5	7-day treatment duration; also controls internal parasites
Permectrin II	10% permethrin	Boehringer-Ingelheim, St. Joseph, MO 60060	Lice, mange mites	Spray or dip	5	
Prolate	11.6% phosmet	Sandoz, Des Plaines, IL 60018	Lice, mange mites	Spray	1	
Rabon 3% dust	3% tetrachlorvinphos	Boehringer-Ingelheim, St. Joseph, MO 60060	Lice	Dust	0	
Rabon Oral Larvicide	7.76% tetrachlorvinphos	Boehringer-Ingelheim: St. Joseph, MO 60060	House flies, stable flies	Feed premix	0	For control of fly larvae in manure
Taktic E.C.	12.5% amitraz	Hoechst-Roussel Agri-Vet Co., Somerville, NJ 08876	Lice, mange mites	Spray or dip	3	Do not treat more than 4 times/year

RESPONSIBLE USE OF INSECTICIDES

Modern chemistry has provided veterinarians with highly effective external parasiticides and it is important that these products be used according to label recommendations. These products have been reviewed and approved by regulatory authorities ensuring the products are effective as labeled, safe to the host species, and will not result in an unacceptable milk or meat residue. Every product should be used solely for the animal species for which it is labeled and only the prescribed label dose should be applied for that specific parasitic infestation. Adherence to all label recommendations is the professional responsibility of every veterinarian who uses or recommends the use of any animal medication.

■ Practical Immunology

Darrell Farmer, D.V.M.

The livestock industry has an interesting and colorful history. Westward expansion in the United States was brought about by rugged men and women with vision and the courage and innovative spirit to bring their dreams to reality.

Rangelands in the West were ideal for livestock production, but it soon became apparent that the market for their product was in the eastern population centers. Military contracts were also an important source of income, but they were to the north. Trail drives to strategic points on the railroads farther to the north were initiated and the rest is history. This bit of history is illustrative of an industry that is continually evolving. The way we feed, breed, and market cattle has changed tremendously over the last 125 years.

In the late 1940s and 1950s, American consumers developed a taste for grain-fed beef and farmer-feeders in the Corn Belt were leaders in the livestock feeding industry. I grew up in Kansas in a farm-feeder environment where livestock purchases were made as far away as Texas and New Mexico to obtain cattle that would perform well in the feedlot.

In the 1960s, large commercial feedlots were developed in western Kansas, eastern Colorado, and the Texas panhandle in a triangular area from Amarillo to Lubbock and westward to Clovis, New Mexico. This was an ideal location, with good weather and abundant supplies of grain.

The feedyard influence encouraged procuring cattle from every imaginable environment. The drastic changes in environment and management that occurred as cattle moved from the producer to the feedlot soon made it obvious that traditional management methods were no longer adequate and changes were needed.

Intensive management practice in the feedlot industry produces a great deal of stress which affects the health of the animal in many ways. Stress weakens the animal's natural body defenses, allowing various disease processes to develop. High-density populations also make it possible for communicable diseases to spread rapidly.

In the 30 years from the 1960s to the 1990s, the industry has invested countless hours and millions of dollars in research attempting to solve the problems encountered with cattle in the feedlot.

The virus respiratory diseases—infectious bovine rhinotracheitis, bovine virus diarrhea, parainfluenza type 3, bovine respiratory syncytial virus, and the bacterial organism *Haemophilus somnus*—were unknown before the 1950s. Extensive research and better diagnostic procedures have made it possible to identify the causative organisms and produce vaccines against them. The role of *Pasteurella haemolytica* and *Pasteurella multocida* in the respiratory disease complex has been investigated extensively

and with much progress. Further investigation is needed to clarify the many questions remaining.

Bovine respiratory disease is one of the most serious problems found in feedlot cattle. Intensive research has increased our knowledge of the immune system and pharmaceutical companies have invested large sums of money to provide better animal health products for the livestock industry to use in combating this problem.

We must prepare the animal for the stress encountered in the feedlot by beginning at the producer level to stimulate the immune system at a time when stress is minimal and the animal is able to produce a maximal response to immunizing agents utilized in a good animal health program.

Initial efforts to solve health problems in the livestock feeding industry were centered primarily on the feedlot itself. Promiscuous use of various drugs, often without professional supervision, produced erratic results and ultimately led to complaints about the quality and safety of the products.

Beef industry leaders became concerned with the continued decline in per capita consumption of beef and began developing strategies to improve quality and regain market share. The National Beef Quality Audit in 1991 was a result of that concern. The results labeled cattle as too fat, too big, and too inconsistent.

The Beef Quality Audit also caused the livestock industry to honestly and fairly investigate retailer concerns about blemishes caused by injection of various health products. Concerns by consumers about quality, safety, and consistency were also addressed. The conclusion reached as a result of the extensive efforts of those working to solve the bovine respiratory disease problem in the livestock feeding industry can be summed up in one phrase: prevention at the producer level.

Past experience with attempts to prevent disease in the feedlot have led us to realize that to be effective, we must perform the procedure at the producer level where stress is minimal and there is ample time for development of a good immune response by the immune system of the animal.

The pork and poultry industries are major competitors of the beef industry for the consumer dollar and they have been very successful. Serious consideration of these three industries causes us to realize that genetics, nutrition, and animal health are major areas of management common and paramount in importance to all. While each industry has its unique aspects and special management concerns, all are intensive management operations and therefore conducive to stress.

Concentration of the genetic pool, standardized preventive health procedures, and strict biosecurity by the pork and poultry industries have enhanced production and minimized health problems by the use of vertical integration.

The formation of the Beef Improvement Federation in 1986 and the development of expected progeny difference (EPD) has helped producers improve the performance of cattle available to feeders. To underscore the effectiveness of their efforts, the beef industry produced approximately the same tonnage of beef in 1996 with an inventory of 103 million cattle as it did in 1975 with 132 million cattle. Weaning and yearling weights increased by 20% over the same period, and feedyard performance has improved to the point where 5×5 cattle (five lb of gain coupled with feed conversions of 5 lb) are realistic goals for producers.

The primary focus of the beef industry to this point has been PRODUCTION. The Beef Quality Audit in 1991 demonstrated the need to be concerned about PRODUCT.

Extensive research and effort by the animal health product industry has provided many quality products for the prevention and treatment of disease. There is the promise of products in the future that are less invasive (more animal-friendly) with even greater effectiveness. Current products and those of the future are highly sophisticated. Each has unique properties requiring special consideration to produce maximum effect. The professional expertise of the veterinarian is a must for the producer in planning an animal health program now and in the future.

The Beef Quality Assurance Task Force is a direct result of the Beef Quality Audit of 1991. One of its prime objectives is to educate producers about the seriousness of the correct use of animal health products and ways to be a part in helping the industry as a whole produce a product that meets the needs and expectations of the consumer.

The diverse nature of livestock producer units presents a special challenge. It is possible that larger units may be able to vertically integrate as the poultry and pork industries have done. Smaller operations will modify in a way that is financially feasible.

Vaccines requiring individual application and booster immunizations within 3 weeks are a problem for large ranching operations in the western states simply because gathering cattle for repeat injections (booster shots) is logistically impossible. Improved vaccines which stimulate the immune system aggressively enable vaccines given at branding time in the spring to produce an anamnestic response when vaccines are given at weaning time in the fall.

Formulation, packaging, and delivery systems designed for less stress on the animal and environmental safety are major research and development goals for animal health companies today. Delivery systems for vaccines will evolve toward mass administration through feed or water. Vaccines will become even more effective, longer-lasting, and less reactive with each other, allowing less frequent administration of vaccine combinations.

In summary, the concept of risk management has become very important to the producer and will involve closer cooperation between producer and veterinarian as they work to prevent disease and improve production efficiency while protecting the quality of the beef product.

Neonatal Disease and Disease Management

Consulting Editor
Elaine Hunt, D.V.M., Diplomate, A.C.V.I.M.

■ Neonatal Immunology

Victor S. Cortese, D.V.M., Diplomate, A.B.V.P.

The field of neonatal immunology is going through a revolution both in human and veterinary medicine. New and advanced methods for accessing immune status and function are being widely used to reevaluate some of the old beliefs about the young animal's immune system. While still in its infancy, these new studies are shedding light on a mysterious and critical time in the immunologically frail newborn.

DEVELOPMENT OF THE PRENATAL IMMUNE SYSTEM

The immune system of all species of mammals begins development fairly early in gestation. As the fetus grows the immune system goes through many changes as cells appear and become specialized. In general, the shorter the gestation period, the less developed the immune system is at birth.[1] However, the fetus does acquire immunocompetence while in utero and is able to produce an immune response to many diseases (Table 1). The

best example is the ability of the bovine fetus to mount an antibody response to bovine virus diarrhea virus. For these types of diseases, precolostral titers from the neonate can be used for diagnostic determination of fetal exposures. The primordial thymus can be seen in both fetal lambs and calves between days 27 and 30 as an epithelial chord.[2, 3] As a percentage of body weight, the thymus reaches its maximum size near midgestation, then rapidly decreases after birth. Actual regression of the thymus begins around puberty and the extent and speed with which it regresses will vary by husbandry practices and genetics.

The cells that initially infiltrate the thymus are of unknown origin, but thymic development and differentiation of thymocytes into specific CD cell lines occur during gestation. Some of this development and differentiation can occur in secondary lymphoid organs as well. B cells, by contrast, develop and differentiate in the fetal bone marrow. There is a steady increase in peripheral lymphocytes throughout gestation. The majority of these circulating fetal lymphocytes are T cells. At the same time that lymphocytes are developing in the fetus, development and expansion of other white blood cell populations is occurring.

THE NEONATAL IMMUNE SYSTEM

The immune system is fully developed, albeit immature, in the neonate. Susceptibility of the newborn to microbes is not due to any inherent inability to mount an immune response but to the fact that its immune system is unprimed.[4] Although there are higher numbers of phagocytic cells in the neonate, the function of these cells is decreased (these deficiencies are found, in calves, up to 4 months of age).[5] Complement attains 12% to 60% of adult levels at birth. Complement will not reach adult levels in calves until they are 6 months of age. There is a slow maturation of the immune system in mammals. As an animal approaches sexual maturity and begins to cycle, the immune system also matures. In cattle, most immune system maturity is seen by 5 to 6 months of age. For example, T cells (CD4+, CD8+, and T cell antigen receptor 2) do not reach peak levels until the animal is 8 months of age.[6] This does not mean a young calf cannot respond to antigens, but the response will be weaker, slower, and easier to overcome. For all practical purposes, this immaturity leads to moderation of disease rather than prevents infection. Since in our food-producing mammals (cattle, pigs, sheep) the placenta is of the epitheliochorial type, there is no transplacental transfer of antibodies or white blood cells. Therefore an important component of the newborn food animal's defense mechanism is colostrum.

COLOSTRUM

Colostrum is the most important example of passive immunity. Defined as the "first" secretions from the mammary gland

Table 1	
SEQUENTIAL DEVELOPMENT OF THE IMMUNE SYSTEM IN THE BOVINE FETUS	
Gestation (Days)	**First Appearance of Immune-Related Events**
42–60	Lymphocytes of thymus, spleen, and peripheral lymph nodes
78	Lymphocyte reaction to phytohemagglutinin
90	Complement
100	Lymphocytes of mesenteric lymph nodes
120	Antibody to parainfluenza 3 virus
130	IgM in blood and blood neutrophils
141	Antibody to parvovirus and *Anaplasma marginale*
145	IgG in blood and interferon in reaction to bovine virus diarrhea
162	Antibody to *Leptospira saxkoebing*
165–170	Antibody to infectious bovine rhinotracheitis virus
175	Lymphocytes of the gastrointestinal tract
190	Antibody to bovine virus diarrhea
243	Antibody to *Chlamydia*
Birth	Antibody to *Brucella abortus*
Birth	Cell-mediated response to *Mycobacterium bovis*, tetanus toxoid, and *Brucella abortus*

From Halliwell REW, Gorman NT: Veterinary Clinical Immunology. Philadelphia, WB Saunders, 1989, p 194.

present after giving birth, colostrum has many known and unknown properties and components. Constituents of colostrum include concentrated levels of antibodies, many functional immune cells (B cells, CD cells, macrophages, and neutrophils),[7] immune system substances such as interferon,[8] and many nutrients in concentrated forms.[9] The primary colostral antibody in most domestic species is IgG except in ruminants in which the primary antibody of colostrum is IgG1 (Table 2). The function of the various cells found in colostrum is still undergoing much research. The cells are known to enhance defense mechanisms in the newborn animal in the following ways: transfer of cell-mediated immunity, enhanced passive transfer of immunoglobins, local bactericidal and phagocytic activity in the digestive tract, and increased lymphocyte activity. Research in swine has shown higher absorption of these white blood cells when the sow is the true dam as compared to grafted piglets. Similar studies have not been done in ruminants. These cells are destroyed by freezing.

COLOSTRUM ABSORPTION

When food-producing mammals are born, the cells that line the digestive tract allow absorption of colostral proteins via pinocytosis. As soon as the digestive tract is stimulated by ingestion of food, the cells begin to change into cells that no longer permit absorption. By 6 hours after birth only approximately 50% of the absorptive capacity remains; by 8 hours, 33%; and by 24 hours, no absorption is available.[10] Colostrum transfer is a function of quality and quantity of the colostrum as well as the timing of colostral administration. In the Holstein breed, the first feeding should be a minimum of 3 qt (2.8 L) of colostrum. Also, colostrum high in red blood cells will make any scours caused by gram-negative bacteria worse. Colostral supplements are available, as well as products for oral or systemic administration that contain specific antibodies. Although feelings about their efficacy are mixed in colostrum-deprived animals they may have a significant value in decreasing mortality and morbidity.

MATERNAL ANTIBODY INTERFERENCE

One of the accepted beliefs is the ability of maternal antibody to block immune responses from vaccination. This has been based on vaccination followed by a titer evaluation in the vaccinees. It is clear from many studies that animals vaccinated in the presence of high levels of maternal antibody to the antigen, may not display increased antibody levels. However, recent studies have shown both the formation of B cell memory responses[11-13] as well as cell-mediated immune responses in the face of maternal antibody[14] when attenuated vaccines were used. Similar responses have been reported in laboratory animals.[15-17] It is clear from these studies that maternal antibody interference of vaccines is not as absolute as once thought and the immune status of the animal, the specific antigen, and the presentation of the antigen should be considered in designing vaccination programs when maternal antibody may be present.

IMPACT OF STRESS

Stress affects the neonate's immune system as it does older animals. There are several factors that affect the immune system that are unique to the neonatal animal. The birthing process has a dramatic impact on the newborn's immune system because of corticosteroid release. Furthermore, the newborn has an increased number of suppressor T cells. These factors, plus others, dramatically decrease systemic immune responses in the first week of life. Systemic vaccinations during this time may have other undesired effects[8] and should not be done. Other stresses should be avoided in the young calf to maintain immune system integrity in the immunologically frail newborn. Procedures such as castration, dehorning, weaning, and movement need to be considered as stresses and all have the potential to decrease immune system function temporarily.

VACCINATION

As discussed above, the vaccination of the young calf is being reassessed. Many types of vaccines are routinely used in veal, dairy beef, and dairy replacement heifers, as well as branding and turnout vaccines in beef calves. The effectiveness of the programs is an interaction of several factors, including the preparations (e.g., IBRV, infectious bovine rhinotracheitis virus vs. *Pasteuralla hemolytica*); the use of modified live or inactivated vaccines;), the age of the calf for some antigens; the presence of maternal antibody; other stress factors present at the time of vaccination; and timing of disease agent exposure. Vaccines utilizing the mucosal immune system have been tested and licensed for use in the young calf, including the newborn. These vaccines include modified live, intranasal infectious bovine rhinotracheitis–parainfluence virus 3 (IBR-PI-3) vaccines and modified live, oral rotavirus-coronavirus vaccine. Exact timing of early vaccination will vary somewhat by antigen and presentation. In human immunology, times in which antigen exposure may cause a predominance of IgE have been shown. Similar immune responses have not been shown in food animals. However, our research has shown that initial systemic vaccination for the three primary viral diseases (bovine viral diarrhea virus, IBRV, PI-3) has little impact when administered during the 3- to 5-week age window in dairy calves. This corresponds to the time frame in which maternal T cells are disappearing from the calf. However, if the calf is vaccinated before then, vaccination seems to work well (i.e., a 1- to 5-weeks-of-age vaccination program).[19] In general, vaccination in the young calf should precede anticipated or historical times of disease by at least 10 days, allowing the immune system to respond before exposure. If a booster dose is required, it should be administered at least 10 days before the anticipated problem. Vaccination against diseases which have a primary cell-mediated protective mechanism may be more likely to stimulate protection in the face of maternal antibody than those in which humoral immunity is the primary protective mechanism. Although in its infancy, the use of vaccination programs in young and neonatal food animals is gaining popularity and more research is needed to further define protection and timing.

Table 2
MAJOR ANTIBODY CLASSES AND CONCENTRATION OF COLOSTRUM AND MILK (mg/100 mL)

	Sheep IgA	Swine IgA	Cow IgA
Colostrum	100–700	950–1000	100–700
Milk	5–12	300–700	10–50
	IgG	**IgG**	**IgG**
Colostrum	4000–6000	3000–7000	3400–8000
Milk	69–100	100–300	50–750

SUMMARY

The neonatal immune system is a complex and interrelated system containing components from both the dam and the newborn. Although the system is capable of responding and conferring varying degrees of protection, it is the combination of passive and active immunity that provides protection, often in the form of reduced disease severity, to the neonate.

REFERENCES

1. Halliwell REW, Gorman NT: Veterinary Clinical Immunology, Philadelphia, WB Saunders, 1989, pp 193–205.
2. Jordan HK: Development of sheep thymus in relation to in utero thymectomy experiments. Eur J Immunol 6:693, 1976.
3. Anderson EI: Pharngeal derivatives in the calf. Anat Rec 24:25, 1922.
4. Tizard I: Immunity in the fetus and newborn. *In* Veterinary Immunology: An Introduction, ed 4. Philadelphia, WB Saunders, 1992, pp 248–260.
5. Hawser MA, Knob MD, Wroth JA: Variation of neutrophil function with age in calves. Am J Vet Res 47:152, 1986.
6. Hein WR: Ontogeny of T cells. *In* Goddeeris BML, Morrison WI (eds): Cell Mediated Immunity in Ruminants, Boca Raton, Fla, CRC Press, 1994, pp 19–36.
7. Riedel-Caspari G, Schmidt F-W: The influence of colostral leukocytes on the immune system of the neonatal calf. [I. Effects on lymphocyte responses (pp. 102–107). II. Effects on passive and active immunization (pp 190–194). III. Effects on phagocytosis (pp. 330–334). IV. Effects on bactericidity, complement, and interferon; synopsis (pp. 395–398).] Dtsch Tierarztliche Wochenschr 98:102–398, 1991.
8. Jacobsen KL, Arbtan KD: Interferon activity in bovine colostrum and milk. *In* Proceedings, 17th World Buiatrics, and 25th American Association of Bovine Practitioners Congress, vol 3, 1992, pp 1–2.
9. Schnorr KL, Pearson LD: Intestinal absorption of maternal leukocytes by newborn lambs. J Reprod Immunol 6:329–337, 1984.
10. Rischen CG: Passive immunity in the newborn calf. Iowa State Vet 2:60–65, 1981.
11. Parker WL, Galyean ML, Winder JA, et al: Effects of vaccination at branding on serum antibody titers to viral agents of bovine respiratory disease (BRD) in newly weaned New Mexico calves. *In* Proceedings, Western Section, American Society of Animal Science, 1993, p 44.
12. Kimman TG, Westenbrink F, Straver PJ: Priming for local and systematic antibody memory responses to bovine respiratory syncytial virus: Effect of amount of virus, viral replication, route of administration and maternal antibodies. Vet Immunol Immunopathol 22:145–160, 1989.
13. Pitcher PM: Influence of passively transferred maternal antibody on response of pigs to pseudorabies vaccines. *In* Proceedings of the American Association of Swine Practitioners, 1996.
14. Ellis JA, Hassard LE, Cortese VS, et al: Effects of perinatal vaccination on humoral and cellular immune responses in cows and young calves. J Am Vet Med Assoc 208:393–399, 1996.
15. Ridge JP, Fuchs EJ, Matzinger P: Neonatal tolerance revisited: Turning on newborn T cells with dendritic cells. Science 271:1723–1726, 1996.
16. Sarzotti M, Robbins DS, Hoffman FM: Induction of protective CTL responses in newborn mice by a murine retrovirus. Science 271:1726–1728, 1996.
17. Forsthuber T, Hualin, CY, Lewhmann V: Induction of T_H1 and T_H2 immunity in neonatal mice. Science 271:1728–1730, 1996.
18. Bryan LA: Fatal, generalized bovine herpesvirus type-1 infection associated with a modified-live infectious bovine rhinotracheitis/parainfluenza-3 vaccine administered to neonatal calves. Can Vet J 35:223–228, 1994.
19. Cortese VS, McGuirk S, Shields D, et al: Responses to viral vaccines in young dairy calves (unpublished manuscript).

▪ Colostrum and Passive Immunity

Allen J. Roussel, Jr., D.V.M., M.S., Diplomate, A.C.V.I.M.
Phillip R. Woods, D.V.M., Ph.D., M.R.C.V.S., Diplomate, A.C.V.I.M.

The immediate postparturient period is a challenging time in the life of a calf, lamb, kid, or pig. Survival requires immediate adaptation to a new, often harsh, environment. The newborn ruminant and pig are remarkably prepared anatomically and physiologically, but they are devoid of specific immunity. Failure of successful transfer of immunity from the dam to the neonate can significantly reduce the probability of survival and later productivity and economic value. The ability to manage the food animal neonate during this critical period is of paramount importance.

NEONATAL IMMUNITY

Specific protective immunity of the neonate is achieved primarily by passive immunity in the form of colostrum and leukocytes ingested shortly after birth. Food animal species do not have the luxury of passive immunity derived in utero because of syndesmochorial-epitheliochorial placentation, which does not permit the transplacental transfer of antibody.

The neonatal calf possesses a rather mature and functional immune system. In fact, the developing fetus is able to respond immunologically to a variety of infectious challenges such as parainfluenza 3 (PI-3) virus, infectious bovine rhinotracheitis (IBR) virus, and bovine virus diarrhea (BVD) virus. Although there is a capacity to respond immunologically to pathogens, the neonate is sometimes incapable of mounting a response quickly enough to protect itself against the massive infectious challenge it faces soon after birth. This is primarily due to a combination of hypogammaglobulinemia and immunologic naivete. The correlation between high rates of neonatal mortality and lack of passive immunity emphasizes the importance of colostrum administration in reducing neonatal losses.

CONTENTS OF COLOSTRUM

Colostrum has both nutritional and disease-preventing functions. Bovine colostrum has 20% to 25% total solids, being relatively rich (compared with milk) in immunoglobulins, casein, fats, and vitamins.

Colostral immunoglobulin (Ig) provides specific immunity against infection, IgG being the predominant antibody class in all farm animal species. IgA and IgM are present in colostrum in smaller but significant amounts. In pigs, as lactation progresses, IgA becomes the major antibody class in mammary secretions. Lactoperoxidase, lactoferrin, and lysozyme activity provide nonspecific protection against infection. Colostral immunoglobulins are protected from enzymatic digestion by the presence of a trypsin inhibitor.

In addition to the humoral and biochemical components, the cellular component of colostrum is a significant contributing part of the overall transferred immunity of the calf. Calves which receive colostral cells are better able to respond to immunologic challenge during the neonatal period than those that do not. The cellular component of colostrum is composed mostly of lymphocytes and monocytes, with a few neutrophils.

ALTERNATIVE TO FRESH COLOSTRUM

Stored frozen colostrum is problably the best substitute for fresh colostrum provided that it was of good quality when it was frozen. Colostrum may be frozen and thawed with little loss of Ig if it is not subjected to excess heat. Of course, the cellular components are lost in the process. A variety of colostrum substitutes are available. Many of the commercial products are named to suggest that their content is similar to that of colostrum. Unfortunately, the names may sound the same, but the products are quite different. Most do not have the protective qualities of fresh colostrum in establishing adequate passive immunity, particularly in regard to Ig content. Some products, particularly the spray-dried products, provide significant Ig and appear to provide protection from disease. These products are indicated when fresh colostrum is unavailable. Veterinarians should read the label carefully to determine the source and quantity of Ig contained in a "dose" of the product. It must contain about 50 g of IgG per liter to be comparable to colostrum.

FORMATION OF COLOSTRUM

Colostrum is primarily a product of the mammary gland. The elevated protein concentrations found in colostrum, compared with milk, are in part accounted for by elevated levels of Ig. In farm animals, colostral IgG is produced systemically and is selectively transferred by a receptor-mediated process into the mammary gland; as IgG accumulates in the mammary gland to 5 to 50 times the concentration in plasma, systemic concentrations of IgG can fall by 50%. IgA and IgM in colostrum appear to be produced both systemically and locally. The cellular components of colostral immunity are derived systemically (intramuscular vaccination of the dam results in the appearance of sensitized lymphocytes in colostrum) and from the secretory immune system of the mammary gland. A variety of factors are associated with the quality and quantity of colostrum produced, including the following:

1. *Breed and volume.* Dairy cows produce more colostrum than do beef cows, but the concentration of Ig in dairy colostrum is much lower. Therefore, much more dairy colostrum than beef colostrum is needed to confer adequate passive transfer. Volume and the resultant dilution are responsible for most, but not all, of the variation among breeds. Considerable variations in colostral IgG have been noted among breeds of sheep, and among rams within a breed.

2. *Parity.* It has been suggested that first-calf heifers produce less colostrum and of poorer quality than that of cows. However the results of several studies are contradictory. Cows and sows in their third or later lactation produce higher concentrations of Ig and more lacteal IgA, respectively.

3. *Nutrition.* An energy-deficient diet reduces the quantity of colostrum produced. In sheep and cattle, underfeeding during the third trimester of pregnancy results in a significantly reduced colostral yield after parturition. This is due to reduced prenatal accumulation of colostrum and a reduced rate of mammary gland secretion.

4. *Loss of colostrum.* Leakage of colostrum and preparturient milking reduce the total amount of colostrum available. Epidemiologic studies have shown leakage to be the major cause of low colostral Ig levels. Ig concentrations between the first two milkings after calving can drop by at least 50%. It is important to realize, however, that the Ig content of colostrum decreases rapidly post partum *even if the cow is not milked or nursed.*

5. *Vaccination status of dam.* High titers of specific Ig in the dam's colostrum are associated with a lower prevalence of neonatal disease and reduced shedding of infectious agents by the neonate, compared with nonvaccinated cohorts. Vaccination of sows against *Haemophilus sommus* 5 weeks and 2 weeks prior to farrowing results in a significantly reduced incidence of associated disease in their offspring. Vaccination of pregnant cows with bovine rotavirus or enterotoxigenic *Escherichia coli* vaccine confers protective immunity in their offspring to infection by those agents.

ABSORPTION OF COLOSTRUM BY THE NEONATE

Colostrum ingested by the food animal neonate is nonselectively absorbed from the gastrointestinal lumen by pinocytosis. The absorptive mechanism appears to be saturable because large quantities of colostrum are absorbed less efficiently than are smaller quantities. After about 24 hours of age, the ability to absorb colostral Ig is dramatically reduced to the point at which further administration of colostrum does not enhance serum Ig concentrations further. However, colostrum administered after Ig absorption has stopped has significant effects in neutralizing enteric pathogens.

Cellular immunity associated with lymphocytes and monocytes in colostrum appears to be functional in the neonate. Lymphocytes migrate across the neonatal gastrointestinal wall and are functional for a time.

Many factors affect the eventual passive immune status of the neonate. Environment and behavior of both dam and neonate play significant roles in the quality and total amount of colostrum absorbed. Factors affecting absorption include the following:

1. Some corticosteroids used to induce parturition are reported to reduce absorption of colostral Ig in the neonate.

2. Temperature stress reduces colostrum absorption by the neonate.

3. Calves that are delivered by assisted or induced parturition or by cesaren section or that are dysmature or premature have a slower and less efficient uptake of colostrum and subsequently lower IgG concentration.

4. Mothering and cow-calf bonding affect uptake of colostrum. Calves taken from their dam at birth absorb less colostral IgG compared with calves left with their dams for the first 24 hours, despite ingesting the same amounts of colostrum. Piglets weaned at 24 hours of age have reduced immunity compared with piglets weaned at 6 weeks of age.

5. Calves born in a stall may orient toward a dark corner instead of the udder, whereas at pasture the neonate has no such confusing and time-wasting options.

6. Poor udder and teat conformation (e.g., poorly developed teats on first-calf heifers and pendulous udders on old cows) may result in the neonate's inability to find the teat.

7. Calves born of dams fed protein-deficient diets tend to have low IgG concentrations, presumably due to low vigor which delays and may reduce suckling.

8. Calves that suckle absorb more IgG than do calves that nurse a bottle, which absorb more than calves that are force-fed by esophageal feeder. However, the difference is small and can easily be overcome by increasing the volume fed.

9. In more general terms, the later the neonate starts to suckle, the less chance it has to achieve its theoretically maximum absorption of colostrum.

FAILURE OF PASSIVE TRANSFER

Failure of passive transfer (FPT) is the absence of adequate concentrations of plasma IgG with the potential consequence of a diseased neonate. When management is good, not all or even most neonates with FPT will succumb to disease, but within a herd, a neonate with FPT is at significantly greater risk of death than its herdmates with adequate passive transfer. In a large study of dairy calves, it is has been shown that the risk of death is almost fivefold greater in calves with complete FPT. But when the death rate in calves with optimal passive transfer is 5%, over 75% of those with FPT survive Septicemia and diarrhea are the most common diseases to which susceptible neonates succumb, but the risk of morbidity and mortality continues in later life, at least in cattle.

Although critical to optimal growth, productivity, and economic return of a livestock-rearing operation, passive transfer and the consequences of FPT have perhaps been given too much importance in some situations. Reliance on the single value of neonatal serum Ig concentrations as an indicator of neonatal well-being or the cause of poor health and productivity is inappropriate because (1) protection against infectious agents is conferred by specific antibody titers, not total Ig concentrations, and (2) other factors, such as management and infectious challenge, contribute to the risk of disease. The protective effect of a particular Ig concentration in the neonate is modified by environment; elevated levels of ammonia in a piggery cause an increased prevalence of *Bordetella bronchiseptica* rhinitis in piglets. Some well-controlled studies have failed to show any significant association between passive transfer and neonatal health. It has been shown that nonspecific serum factors such as complement may be of much greater significance in the neonatal pig.

ASSESSMENT OF PASSIVE IMMUNITY

Adequacy of colostral transfer is most specifically assessed by measurement of serum Ig concentrations in the neonate. This value appears to correlate well with survival. Although the concentration value considered "adequate" varies among authorities, a serum IgG concentration of 1000 mg/dL is currently the standard for calves and our definition of FPT in calves is a serum IgG concentration less than 1000 mg/dL. Also, the results and recommendations in this discussion are based on samples obtained between 24 and 48 hours of age. Passively acquired Ig falls and active immunity begins to increase after birth, so samples collected after 48 hours do not necessarily reflect passive transfer status.

The single radial immunodiffusion test (SRID) is a simple, specific quantitative test, but the cost and the delay of 24 to 48 hours in obtaining a result limits its value as a field test on which to base immediate management decisions. This is the test against which most others are compared in recent studies, making it the "gold standard."

Refractometry is a simple, nonspecific test that measures total plasma or serum protein. The test assumes that the presuckle neonate has a relative hypoproteinemia that is corrected by adequate intake of colostrum. Either serum or plasma may be used, and studies using each have been published. The values obtained are roughly 0.5 g/dL greater when plasma is used because of the fibrinogen. In this discussion, all values are for *serum* protein. Total serum protein measured by refractometry shows a good correlation with quantitative Ig assays in normal calves and sick calves. In a large study of dairy calves, a value of 5.2 g/dL was the best single cutoff point, classifying over 80% of calves correctly. However, more useful information can be obtained by using a dual cutoff point. In a typical population of dairy calves where one third of the calves have FPT (Ig <1000 mg/dL), approximately 90% of calves with a serum protein of less than 5.0 g/dL have FPT, and 95% of calves with serum protein greater than 5.5 g/dL have adequate passive transfer.

The zinc sulfate precipitation test is a quantitative assay, but

is time-consuming and requires sophisticated instrumentation. It is possible to get a rough estimate of Ig concentrations by visual inspection of degree of turbidity. However, comparison of visual inspection results with SRID does not show a worthwhile correlation, and visual inspection of zinc sulfate turbidity alone cannot be relied on.

The sodium sulfite precipitation test is a simple, semiquantitative test that requires a minimal amount of equipment. The traditional system calling for three concentrations of sodium sulfite solution (14%, 16%, and 18%) appears to be unnecessary. Tyler and colleagues[1] described a test whereby 0.1 mL of serum is added to 1.9 mL of an 18% sodium sulfite solution and incubated at room temperature for 15 minutes. A positive test for FPT is defined as lack of turbidity sufficient to prevent the operator from reading newsprint through the tube. Using this method, 77% of calves with a positive test will have FPT, while 91% of those with a negative test will not.

The whole-blood glutaraldehyde coagulation test is available commercially in the United States. It offers the convenience of using whole blood instead of serum or plasma. There are dramatically conflicting reports in the literature of its effectiveness.

Serum γ-glutamyltransferase (GGT) activity is increased in neonatal calves following colostral absorption because of the high concentration of the enzyme in colostrum and the efficient absorption in the neonate prior to "gut closure." Although there is a correlation between serum IgG and serum GGT, evaluation of GGT seems to offer no advantage over simpler, less expensive tests for FPT.

COLOSTRUM MANAGEMENT

Evaluation of colostrum before it is administered to the neonate may be of value. There is a good correlation between colostral Ig concentration and neonatal serum Ig concentration. Refractometry has been reported as a simple and reliable method of estimating the quantity of Ig in colostral whey. In dairy calves it has been shown that reduced fecal shedding of rotavirus and *Cryptosporidium* is associated with more than 9 g/dL total protein of ingested colostrum.

The colostrometer has been shown to be of value in estimating the quantity of Ig in colostrum. There is a positive correlation between colostral specific gravity and colostral Ig concentration. A specific gravity of more than 1.050 implies a colostral Ig concentration of 50 g/L. Ideally, colostrum with an Ig concentration of 50 g/L should be used for administration to the newborn neonate. Colostrum with a specific gravity below 1.050 should not be used as the first-feeding colostrum, and is best saved and used in later feedings after gastrointestinal absorption of colostral Ig has stopped. Unfortunately, about 75% of poor colostrum will still be classified as adequate using this test. There is also a negative correlation between colostral Ig and the weight of the first milk. If possible, if the weight of the first milking is greater than 20 lb, it should not be used. In high-producing herds, it may be necessary to increase the cutoff to a higher weight in order to have adequate colostrum, but the principle still holds that the higher the volume, the poorer the colostrum. Pooling of colostrum is not recommended because large volumes of poor colostrum from one cow can dilute good colostrum from several cows, amplifying the effect of the poor colostrum over several calves. Also, diseases such as bovine leukosis, paratuberculosis, and caprine arthritis-encephalitis can be spread by infected colostrum. As a rule of thumb, 1 gal (3.8 L) of Holstein colostrum should be administered to calves by esophageal feeder as soon as possible after birth. As little as 1 L of beef cow colostrum may be adequate for a beef calf.

Although quantification of Ig concentrations appears to be

useful in managing herd health, it must be recognized that this is not an infallible tool. It is becoming more apparent that a sick neonate metabolizes Ig faster and thus requires higher concentrations of antibody for protection. It is also recognized that Ig with appropriate activity against relevant pathogens is required for protective immunity.

From a practical point of view, the astute veterinarian or owner will be able to make some basic estimates of the probability that adequate transfer of colostral immunity will occur. A checklist based on the following questions can be developed to evaluate the risk of FPT: Does the dam have a history of poor nursing ability? Is the conformation of the teats and udder adequate? What is the physical nature of the first postpartum mammary fluids? Did the dam have any significant leakage of colostrum prior to parturition? Is the neonate premature or dysmature, and did the dam have any illness during the last trimester of pregnancy?

CORRECTION OF FAILURE OF PASSIVE TRANSFER

Several strategies can be employed to correct FPT. The initial decision to be made is whether the neonate still has the capacity to absorb ingested colostrum. If the neonate is a potential FPT candidate and is less than 12 hours old, it is probably of value to administer an adequate amount of good-quality colostrum orally, preferably by a bottle and nipple: for example, a Holstein calf requires 3 to 5 L of first colostrum. Further colostrum feeds should be administered so that the neonate receives approximately 10% to 15% of its body weight in colostrum by 24 hours of age. Similarly, lambs should be bottle-fed to attain approximately 10% to 15% of body weight in colostrum at 24 hours of age.

Once the gastrointestinal tract no longer has the ability to absorb colostrum, the only way to achieve protective levels of passive systemic immunity is a plasma or serum transfusion. Ideally, cells should be separated, but when necessary, whole-blood transfusions can be used. Consideration must be given to the increased risk of disease transmission (e.g., leukosis, anaplasmosis) when using whole blood for transfusion. Plasma or serum at 40 mL/kg should be administered slowly, intravenously or intraperitoneally. Ideally, the plasma or serum should be from the dam or animals in the same herd, ensuring that the plasma has immunoreactivity to local environmental pathogens. This system is equally effective in calves, lambs, and kids. There is little information on its use in piglets. Commercially prepared bovine plasma is available, although the cost is prohibitive for many cattle. It is very important to be aware of the total amount of Ig a product contains. There are products available that when administered as directed provide woefully inadequate amounts of Ig.

MANAGEMENT TO OPTIMIZE PROTECTIVE IMMUNITY

Good maternal nutrition is important for allowing optimal intrauterine growth and adequate maternal immunity. A dairy cow body score condition of 3.0 or a beef cow body condition score of 5.5 in the last 2 months of pregnancy is recommended.

The dam should be kept in her normal environment during the last trimester to minimize stress and allow development of good environmental immunity. Vaccination of the dam at 7 and 9 months of gestation will produce a colostrum rich in vaccinal IgG. Vaccines used depend on the diseases affecting neonates in the locality. Cows may be vaccinated or receive boosters with

vaccines against IBR, BVD, bovine respiratory syncytial virus, PI-3, *Leptospira pomona*, *E. coli* pili, clostridia, rotavirus, and coronavirus. Care should be taken not to use abortigenic forms of the vaccine during gestation.

Cows need a dry period of 5 to 8 weeks before parturition in which to produce and accumulate adequate amounts of colostrum. It is best not to use milk from cows prior to parturition, since the titer of colostral IgG can fall dramatically as it is removed from the udder, presumably reflecting changing hormonal influences on the udder in the periparturient period.

Beef cows should calve in a dry, protected environment with good footing so that the calf is able to stand and nurse as soon as possible after birth. Dairy calves should be force-fed a gallon of good colostrum as soon as possible via esophageal feeder.

REFERENCE

1. Tyler JW, Hancock DD, Parish SM, et al: Evaluation of three assays for failure of passive transfer in calves. J Vet Intern Med 10:304–307, 1996.

■ Diarrheal Diseases of Neonatal Calves

Elaine Hunt, D.V.M., Diplomate, A.C.V.I.M.

Yearly calf mortality is thought to cause a net loss of up to $120 million to the American agricultural economy. Although failure of passive transfer of antibody is a major primary and secondary factor in these losses, diarrheal disease is still the primary cause of death in the neonatal bovine. The third edition of this book contains an extensive description of the most common etiologic agents of neonatal calf diarrhea, including diagnostic techniques, pathophysiology, and necropsy findings. The reader is encouraged to consult that edition (pp. 103–109). Common factors of therapy and prophylaxis are discussed herein as well as new and specific information concerning individual pathogens.

FACTORS PREDISPOSING TO ENTERIC DISEASE

The immunoincompetent calf requires massive quantities (150 to 300 g) of oral immunoglobulins to protect against enteric disease. Rapid depletion of local (enteric) colostral immunoglobulin results in onset of susceptibility to enteric pathogens; calves deprived of adequate colostrum can be expected to become susceptible even more rapidly. Early ingestion of colostrum is paramount; *calves fed within 1 hour of birth experienced significantly less diarrhea than those whose colostrum feedings were delayed.* This may be because specific IgG$_1$ antibody ingested on the first day of life persists for at least 5 days within the gut, apparently protected from the normal proteolytic activity of the intestine. This same antibody does not persist in the bowel lumen when calves are not fed colostrum until day 2. Absorbed antibody also is released slowly from the systemic circulation into the bowel, providing low-level immunity against enteric pathogens.

Overwhelming pathogen exposure will also predispose the calf to enteric disease. The significance of the sick calf as a "multiplier" of disease should not be overlooked—one calf with diarrhea is capable of contaminating its environment, locally depositing 10^{10} organisms per milliliter of liquid stool. Calving schedules often coincide with the onset of inclement weather and since many Canadian and U.S. cattle are also housed during this period we find large numbers of susceptible neonates confined with populations of older calves that are actively excreting pathogens. Smaller calves may find themselves competing for feed, warmth, dry bedding, and draft-free space. All these stress factors can be expected to contribute to the increased incidence of infectious enteritis, particularly during the winter months.

CONTROL OF PATHOGEN EXPOSURE

Good management practices should be implemented to avoid exposure to large numbers of enteric pathogens. The calving area must be as clean as possible; calving on open pasture is generally superior to calving in a stall. If a calving stall is necessary and the farmer is unlikely to clean it following each occupation, use inorganic bedding materials (e.g., clean sand), which are less likely to foster pathogen survival. Cleanliness of, and accessibility to, each dam's udder is imperative.

Adopt strategies to house or pasture the newborn in areas not previously contaminated by calves 2 to 21 days of age. For dairy calves, this translates to hutch rearing, except in the coldest months of the year. Use hutches constructed of inorganic materials and clean these religiously between calves; turn them upside down to allow sunlight to destroy pathogens. Hutches should be spaced well apart and moved frequently. For stationary hutches, maintain ground surface with rock and sand to facilitate drainage and drying of pathogen-rich excretions. If bedding is used inside the hutch, continually add new (dry) bedding to form a thick pad of water-permeable bedding. When the calf leaves the hutch, remove this pad with a front-end loader and allow the underlying ground prolonged exposure to sunlight.

If calves must be housed indoors, prevent nose-to-nose contact. House calves with suspected poor IgG status well away from other calves as these can serve as "pathogen multipliers." When calves first arrive in barns with concrete flooring, avoid cleaning with high-pressure hoses, as this serves to produce aerosol pathogens resulting in more widespread infections. All calves must have a dry, draft-free surface to lie on; disease risk is inversely porportional to liquid content of bedding.

If practical for beef herds, try to avoid small calving pens or pastures. Every effort should be made to reduce the calving interval to a compact period. Contact with older calves or ground contaminated by older calves results in high mortality rates at the end of prolonged calving seasons, so try to separate postparturient cows (and their calves) from those still gestating. Encourage farmers to breed to calve during warm dry months.

GENERAL THERAPEUTIC PRINCIPLES

The most important therapy for a calf with acute, severe diarrheal infection is properly maintained hydration and electrolyte and acid-base status. Depending on the severity of dehydration, intravenous, oral, or subcutaneous fluids can be administered. Calves in hypovolemic shock will benefit from immediate administration of 1 L of intravenous hypertonic saline (7% to 9%); this therapy should be followed by slow infusion of an alkalizing polyionic electrolyte solution and oral electrolytes.

Calves should be maintained on electrolyte feedings as much as possible, but new information suggests that *milk should not be removed from the diet during diarrheal episodes and we should be providing a greater total volume of fluid to the calf than we have in the past!* Calves kept off feed or fed primarily electrolyte solutions (even the high-energy solutions) emaciate rapidly. Calves

with coronavirus, *Cryptosporidium parvum*, or salmonellosis must receive milk during the protracted disease process; otherwise sick calves will starve to death before cessation of diarrhea. Work at Saskatoon and Wisconsin indicates that calves lose less weight, experience less hypoinsulinemia, have greater mucosal regeneration with less villus atrophy, sustain body muscle mass better, and maintain functional levels of gut digestive enzymes when allowed to drink milk during enteric infections. Calves normally receiving 8 pt of milk per day should continue to be fed milk at this rate and should also be supplemented with *2 to 10 pt of oral electrolytes per day* as well. Such calves may be expected to gain weight rather than lose it during the diarrheal phase. Since less than 1% of the body weight of the calf is fat, it is important to provide adequate caloric intake during the diarrheal phase.

Small (1 to 2 pt), frequent milk feedings may be particularly important in dual infections because enzyme activity increases in unaffected portions of the bowel as a compensatory mechanism to enhance the digestive process; therefore it is important to have a small quantity of nutrient available to these functional areas as frequently as possible.

For years we have also been concerned about the effect of alkalizing oral electrolyte solutions on abomasal rennin clot formation; for this reason, electrolyte solutions containing bicarbonate should not be mixed directly with whole milk. It is safer to use electrolyte solutions containing metabolizable base precursors (e.g., lactate or acetate), as these are unlikely to interfere with rennin clot formation. Work at Wisconsin suggests that rennin clot formation proceeds very rapidly (within about 10 minutes of arrival of milk in the abomasum) and that whole milk should be fed first and that bicarbonate-rich electrolyte solutions can be offered safely in 30 to 60 minutes. Calves fed milk replacers do not form a rennin clot owing to the large quantity of whey and other processed proteins in the product. Recommendations in this case are to wait 10 to 30 minutes after a milk replacer meal before following it with bicarbonate-rich electrolytes.

The *theory of strong ion difference* now suggests that (in acidosis) administration of sodium bicarbonate is less important than is total volume replacement with a solution containing sodium ion in excess of chloride ion. This theory holds that the benefit derived from sodium bicarbonate solution was primarily due to the presence of sodium rather than the alkalinization provided by bicarbonate ion. The advantage of strong ion solutions is that they may be mixed directly with whole milk without concern over interfering with rennin clot formation.

Electrolyte solutions also may contain probiotics (selected lactobacillus and *Streptococcus fecalis* cultures) to help establish a more normal competitive gut microflora. These are unlikely to be harmful. Oral solutions also may contain soluble fibers like pectin, gum arabic, guar gum, xanthum, agar carrageenan, citrus or apple pulp, alginate, or psyllium. These substances add fiber to the diet, and should increase the time necessary for foodstuffs to traverse through the bowel (theoretically increasing the opportunity for fluid resorption). Some such European products claim to bind cryptosporidial oocysts within the gel matrix created within the bowel, thus decreasing autoinfection. Although the character of the stool may improve with the use of these products, at present it is unknown if this is actually beneficial to the calf. Some early products were so successful that calves actually developed functional obstructions that were very deleterious.

In the future electrolyte solutions may be formulated to include constituents to enhance mucosal healing. Glutamine is presently being evaluated in Great Britain, Canada, and the United States; glutamine appears to play an important role in maintenance of a healthy and functional gut mucosa.

So-called coating agents are probably not detrimental to the calf with enteric disease. Doses as low as 20 mL orally every 6 hours have been reported to make the calves appear more comfortable during the course of disease.

Nonsteroidal anti-inflammatory agents (NSAIDs) have been used routinely by many practitioners for calves with enteric disease. There are arguments for and against the use of these agents. Calves treated with NSAIDs may feel better and begin eating, but NSAIDs have a serious potential for causing nephrotoxicity in dehydrated calves and are potentially ulcerogenic. For this reason, use of these agents is generally discouraged unless calves are endotoxic; NSAIDs are beneficial in these instances.

Use of antimicrobial agents is not warranted in calves with any of these diarrheal disorders (except enterotoxemia): the viral agents and crytosporidia are resistant to antibiotics; salmonella infections may be made more severe with antimicrobial therapy, and K99+ binding sites are lost by the time the calf reaches 72 hours of age so antibiotic therapy is unwarranted in enterotoxigenic coliform infections. Antibiotics should be relied upon only when there is evidence of, or potential for, systemic complications (bacteremia, navel infections, or infectious arthritis).

ROTAVIRUS DIARRHEA

Ubiquitous throughout neonatal bovine populations, rotavirus infection is characterized by diarrhea which may be voluminous, a rich yellow color, and pudding-like at onset, later becoming more watery. Calves may be affected as young as 12 hours of age but are more commonly 3 to 21 days old, although susceptibility is likely maintained until the virus is encountered. Systemic viremia does not occur, so calves appear bright until onset of weight loss; dehydration and acidosis develop. Different serotypes of rotavirus exist and may explain vaccine failure and variation in virulence. Serotypic similarity exists between human and bovine rotaviruses and a distinct *potential for zoonotic infection* does exist.

DIAGNOSIS

The new rapid enzyme immunoassay (ImmunoCard Rotavirus, Meridian Diagnostics, Inc., Cincinnati) costs about $8 a test, but appears to be the best option for the practitioner or regional laboratory wishing to offer this service. Also, the latex agglutination test (MERITEC Rotavirus, Meridian Diagnostics) lends itself well to rapid diagnosis and can be used by the practitioner. Electron microscopy is still offered by many diagnostic laboratories; immunofluorescent tests of tissues or feces are somewhat less sensitive.

Prophylaxis

The original vaccine developed to stimulate lactogenic immunity was criticized heavily; the killed vaccine (for rotavirus, coronavirus, and K99+ coliforms) presently available has not yet been evaluated rigorously by independent researchers in this country (it is worth noting that European reports have been more positive regarding vaccine success in the face of rotavirus infection). Using a different adjuvant, the vaccine now available is reported to result in a four-fold increase in antibody titers above those achieved by the previous vaccine.

Strict guidelines must be adhered to to avoid vaccine failure. The dam must receive a two-shot series the first time the vaccine is used; all animals must receive boosters within 40 days of calving. If the vaccination-to-calving interval exceeds 40 days, revaccination is necessary. Failure to provide rapid and adequate

access to colostrum will obviate any benefit derived from vaccination of the dam as transplacental transfer of antibody does not occur. Cross-species immunity has been reported when lambs were fed colostrum from vaccinated cows. Efforts by the English to produce a more efficacious vaccine have shown promising results. Extralabel use of the vaccine for the adult bovine is described in some veal houses, although ability of the calf to respond with any effective antibody is unlikely to occur until the calf is older (by which time it has already encountered the infection).

A modified live combination vaccine for the newborn is also available. Vaccine failures can be expected because the attenuated virus is neutralized by ingested colostrum. Because oral administration should occur at least 1 hour before colostrum ingestion, this product is prone to failure except in the hands of the most meticulous producer. Double-blind trials have not substantiated the usefulness of the product, possibly because colostral antibody neutralization frequently occurs.

Two products have been used to provide specific enteric antibody for the calf: one derived from bovine colostrum should now include rotavirus antibody (First Defense, ImmuCell, Portland, Maine) and one from hyperimmunized chicken egg yolk (Pro-body Gel, Jorgenson Laboratories, Inc., Loveland, Colo.). The latter is relatively inexpensive (35 to 50 cents per dose), but has only been marketed as a food additive in the United States. Studies by the Japanese show that a similar yolk-derived product has been very effective in providing prolonged protection against rotavirus challenge.

ENTEROTOXIGENIC *ESCHERICHIA COLI*

Enterotoxigenic *E. coli* (ETEC) is caused by encapsulated *E. coli*, a hardy organism that can persist for months in a dirty environment. About 90% of bovine ETEC is caused by strains that are positive for the K99+ pilus adherence antigen; strains carrying the F41 and FY adhesins are also capable of causing ETEC but are not as widespread. Differing serotypes are responsible for neonatal septicemia and mastitis. The original source of the infection may be the environment or the dam; the infected calf then contaminates the environment by producing up to 10^{13} infectious bacteria per 12-hour period.

Clinical Signs

Variable degrees of diarrhea and dehydration are manifest but the onset of "pineapple juice" diarrhea may be so acute and severe that dehydration and terminal collapse occurs in 7 to 12 hours. Calves are generally hypothermic and rarely over 5 days of age as K99+ binding sites are lost rapidly after birth.

Diagnosis

Gross and histologic examination of gut tissue collected immediately after death will demonstrate little other than a gas- and fluid-distended bowel with intact mucosa. The practitioner may culture the proximal duodenum in a calf dead less than 1 hour; the presence of large numbers of hemolytic coliforms is suggestive of this cause, but identification of specific serotypes is necessary to confirm ETEC. To demonstrate the presence of K99+ coliforms, a quick latex agglutination kit is available to test fresh feces from calves less than 5 days of age that have not received an oral K99+ antibody preparation (K-99 PILITEST VMRD, Inc., Pullman, Wash.).

Specific Therapy

A newly developed product (Immunoboost K, Vetrepharm Research, London, Ontario) has been reported to be helpful in ETEC. Calves that received this product intravenously had significantly lower mortality rates vs. those in controls. The product (which should soon be available in Canada) contains mycobacteria cell wall components and may have a protective nonspecific immunostimulation effect. Should this product prove to be efficacious, it may also be useful in other diseases of the neonatal bovine. It does not result in future false-positive reactions to other diagnostic tests for pathogenic mycobacteria.

Prophylaxis

A successful coliform vaccine has been developed that results in significantly elevated titers of K99 + -specific antibody in the pregnant dam. Yearly boosters are necessary within 40 days of calving; early and adequate colostrum ingestion is imperative. Oral administration of specific (K99 +) antibody is more expensive, equally effective, and must also be administered soon after birth. Very effective specific antibody preparations are available that are derived from colostral whey, hens' eggs, and horse sera, and are supplied in capsules, tubes, as a paste, in colostral supplements, and in small quantities of milk replacers. Proper hygienic precautions are still necessary; control or delay onset of concurrent viral infections if these are a contributing factor.

CORONAVIRUS INFECTION

Coronavirus causes a severe and long-lasting disease with high morbidity and moderate mortality in neonatal calves, even in the face of routine supportive therapy. Coronavirus infection is said to be less widespread than rotavirus infection.

Clinical Signs

Calves are commonly affected between 5 and 21 days of age. Severe depression is noted; diarrhea and dehydration progress through a course of 4 to 5 days, by which time the calf is often moribund. Dysentery is not a feature of this infection, but mild respiratory disease can occur when aerosol virus is inhaled and precedes the onset of enteric disease.

Diagnosis

Although fecal enzyme-linked immunosorbent assay (ELISA) kits exist in Europe and have been evaluated in Canada and the United States, kits are presently unavailable in the United States despite a growing need for them. Presently, diagnosis is achieved through electron microscopy of feces or immunofluorescent examination of chilled (not frozen) intestinal tissues (particularly the spiral colon). Blunted villi may also be detected on histopathologic examination or with the use of a dissection scope on ultrafresh tissues.

Prophylaxis

The combination coronavirus-rotavirus-ETEC vaccine was discussed in the preceding sections. This vaccine must be administered to the pregnant cow within 40 days of calving and the calf must receive colostrum! The vaccine may have some benefit, or at least delay onset of disease until the calf becomes a few days older and is more capable of dealing with enteric disease. Even if specific antibody is provided by colostrum, the half-life is about 72 hours in the gut. An oral specific antibody preparation is available, but the half-life of the antibody administered can be expected to be similarly short. The oral vaccine (modified live virus) is also available, but must be given prior to intake of colostral antibody. At least one product is available that provides specific local antibody derived from hyperimmunized bovine colostrum (ImmuCell).

A synergistic effect between coronavirus and prepatent coccidia infection has been demonstrated and may explain the duration and severity of disease previously attributed to coronavirus alone. If this is truly an important factor in the pathogenesis of coronavirus, perhaps specific anticoccidial therapy may become a significant factor in controlling morbidity and mortality previously associated with coronavirus infection.

CRYPTOSPORIDIOSIS

The significance of *C. parvum* as an enteric and important zoonotic agent is now well documented, particularly by the 400,000 people who developed this disease when oocysts contaminated the Milwaukee water supply. Infections can readily spread from calves to humans. Prevalence rates in 1- to 3-week-old calves on infected farms are often greater than 50% and more than 90% of farms are thought to harbor this coccidian. Persistent and fatal diarrheal infections can occur in humans and calves.

Clinical Signs

Clinical signs are often nonspecific and vary from anorexia and mild diarrhea to protracted, watery, nonresponsive diarrhea and debilitation; since this protozoan is refractory to conventional antimicrobial agents, therapy has no beneficial effect. Feces may contain blood on occasion, as well as bile, mucus, and undigested milk. Dehydration is not necessarily noted, but weight loss and emaciation are always a problem. Duration of diarrhea is 6 to 10 days; maximum oocyst detection occurs at 12 days of age.

Diagnosis

Day 12 of life is the optimal sampling time as a large percentage of naturally infected calves will be shedding oocysts on this day. Fecal diagnosis can be achieved through fecal floatation (do not use sugar solutions for floatation); slides are stained with Giemsa or acid-fast stains. Two excellent, rapid diagnostic techniques are available but require use of an epifluorescent microscope: direct rectal swab evaluation using auramine-O stain and fecal direct immunofluorescent assay (MERIFLUOR, Meridian Diagnostics).

Diagnosis in the dead calf is not enhanced by gross necropsy alone because gut lesions are relatively nonspecific: moderate enteritis with adherent mucofibrinous exudate is present in the lower small intestinal mucosa, sometimes involving the cecal and colonic mucosa. Microscopic examination of ileal mucosal scrapings or fixed tissue sections is a useful means of identifying infection in the recently dead calf. Multiple pathogen infections are common and contribute to the severity of the *C. parvum* infection; always check for other enteric pathogens.

Therapy and Prevention

Specific therapeutic and preventive measures against cryptosporidiosis are limited. Uptake of vitamin A is decreased in *C.*

parvum infection resulting in lowered liver levels of vitamin A during the infection, so supplementation may be advisable. An avian egg yolk–derived product with specific antibody against *C. parvum* has been described in Japan. Antimicrobial agents exist for humans but are prohibitively expensive (paromomycin and azithromycin).

The efficacy of available coccidiostats should be viewed with skepticism. Lasalocid did help prevent infection when it was administered at a dosage capable of causing mortality in 50% of calves treated. Five to ten times the label dose of decoquinate begun soon after birth was of some benefit, but administration at this level is impractical. Halofuginone lactate has received a great deal of praise in Europe as an effective control mechanism for cryptosporidial infection, but is not yet available in the United States.

Contaminated articles that cannot be effectively sterilized (nipples, bottles, halters, etc.) can be frozen overnight in a standard freezer to destroy oocysts. Oocysts are resistant to conventional disinfectants (including phenols, chloroform, perchloethylene, perchloracetic acid), even remaining viable after 30-minute acid immersion.

Prophylaxis

Hyperimmune bovine colostrum will suppress parasite development. For this reason, vaccine development is ongoing and will likely result in passive antibody protection in bovine colostrum as well as egg yolk.

Strict cleanliness is helpful in minimizing the severity of infection, but prior environmental contamination is difficult to overcome. Raising calves in hutches has been shown to diminish the severity of cryptosporidial infection.

Zoonotic Potential

Any human exposed to neonatal calves (unless previously infected) should be considered at risk of developing cryptosporidial infection. Physicians need to be apprised that opiate therapy is probably contraindicated in humans owing to the immediate infectivity of oocysts and the potential for superinfections when gut motility is disrupted.

CLOSTRIDIUM PERFRINGES TYPE C ENTEROTOXEMIA

Several manifestations of *Clostridium perfringens* infection are referred to as enterotoxemia. This is an acute or peracute non-contagious disease that often affects the healthiest, fastest-growing calves, yet is easily and inexpensively avoided.

Clinical Signs

Type C enterotoxemia results in development of an acute fatal hemorrhagic enteritis in calves less than 2 weeks of age. Frequently, those affected are offspring of cows producing large quantities of milk. Death may occur so rapidly that signs of abdominal pain or depression are never witnessed. If survival is prolonged, neurologic signs may prevail. Salivation and moderate increase in body temperature may occur, but hypothermia can be expected as signs of terminal endotoxemia develop.

Diagnosis

The diagnosis is generally made on the basis of necropsy. Necropsy may demonstrate extensive hemorrhage in the small intestine and mesenteric lymph nodes; jejunum and ileum can be expected to give evidence of extensive hemorrhage. Petechiae may be noted in abdominal organs, and edema and neuronal degeneration may occur in the brain. Mouse toxin inoculation is necessary to verify the presence of clostridial toxin.

Therapy

Because of the poor prognosis, therapy should be undertaken only in the most valuable animals and it must be vigorous. Hyperimmune serum, extralabel dosages of intravenous and intramuscular penicillin, massive fluid therapy, and NSAIDs for endotoxic shock may be successful if administered early and aggressively.

Prophylaxis

Prevention of deaths in newborn can be relatively certain through vaccination of the dam twice, followed by yearly boosters. Colostrum ingestion is a must. Passive immunity will last for about 3 weeks. Calves should then be vaccinated with toxoid (twice) to prevent type D enterotoxemia, which can be expected once the calf begins consuming large quantities of grain or milk. Colostrum-deprived calves can be treated with the endoserum, but this product is expensive and needs to be discarded after opening the bottle because bacterial contamination and proliferation is possible under the best of conditions.

SALMONELLOSIS

Salmonellosis is an enteric disease of cattle that is capable of high morbidity and mortality rates in neonates and adults alike and is a significant cause of economic loss in the food animal industry. The effects of salmonellosis are particularly severe in the neonate. The disease may cause signs of pneumonia, peracute septicemia, acute or chronic enteritis, meningitis, or infectious osteomyelitis or arthritis.

Clinical Signs

Salmonella typhimurium generally affects calves over 10 days of age. Sale barn calves are at great risk of developing this disease. The diarrhea is intractable, may result in metabolic acidosis and dehydration, and is characterized by a "septic tank odor" and by dysentery with chunks and flakes of fibrin or full fibrin casts present in the stool. Some calves may develop only enteric disease while others show multiple organ involvement. Survivors are often chronic carriers and suffer ill-thrift. *Salmonella dublin* may not result in diarrhea, but the calf may be depressed, show signs of ill-thrift, septicemia, meningitis, polyarthritis, osteomyelitis, fatal peracute pneumonia, or vasculitis-thrombosis and gangrene of the skin.

Diagnosis

The diagnosis is achieved in the living animal by submitting at least six 1-g fecal samples for enrichment culture (selenite tetrathionate broth) over a 2- or 3-day period; if a group of calves is affected, culture six different animals. Rectal biopsy cultures are usually not attempted in the neonate. Serum ELISA titers can be performed for a fee at the University of California, Davis, to identify *S. dublin* carriers. Results are subject to interpretation, but may also be useful for identifying carriers of other *Salmonella* spp.

Leukocyte anomalies occur in enteric and septicemic salmonellosis. Marked leukopenia and neutropenia can be expected. Neutrophil cytology may also be affected; toxic granulation may be abundant. The presence of fecal leukocytes on fibrin tags in the stool is supportive of *Salmonella* infection. Calves surviving several days consuming low sodium fluids (whole milk, water) can be expected to develop hyponatremia and are often hypoalbuminemic.

Necropsy specimens submitted for culture should include gut, gallbladder, and mesenteric lymph nodes for enrichment culture. A pseudodiptheritic membrane may be noted in the distal small bowel and large colon.

Prevention

Dairies with flush systems seem to struggle particularly with this infection. Surface water may have to be fenced off and pastures rested after flooding. Wild rodents and avian species may be associated with introduction of disease. Calf facilities should be disinfected between groups of calves whenever possible. Other risk factors include overcrowding, common calving areas, contaminated feed or water, septic tank overflow, and improperly handled farm waste.

Subunit vaccines have been used in very young calves to help protect against future endotoxin challenge in salmonellosis and pasteurellosis. Vaccination with J-5 vaccine at 2 to 3 days of age and 2 weeks later resulted in decreased risk of death in reasonably well-managed calves, but in an increased risk of death in poorly managed calves. Success of bacterins has been reported but needs further study. Measurerable antibody was detected in calves 1 to 3 weeks of age vaccinated with an experimental *S. dublin* mutant strain (modified live) vaccine.

BIBLIOGRAPHY

General References

Bolton JR, Pass DA: The alimentary tract. *In* Robinson WF, Huxtable CRR (eds): Clinicopathologic Principles for Veterinary Medicine. New York, Cambridge University Press, 1988, pp 163–193.
Curtis CR, Erb HN, White ME: Descriptive epidemiology of calfhood morbidity and mortality in New York Holstein herds. Prevent Vet Med 5:293–307, 1988.
Howard, JL (ed): Current Veterinary Therapy 2: Food Animal Practice. Philadelphia, WB Saunders, 1986.
Roussell AJ (ed): The Veterinary Clinics of North America: Food Animal Practice, Philadelphia, WB Saunders, 1990.
Semrad SD, Dubielzig R: Effect of phenylbutazone and repeated endotoxin administration on hemostasis in neonatal calves. Am J Vet Res 54:1339–1346, 1993.

Rotavirus Infection

Acres SD, Radostits OM: The efficacy of a modified live reo-like virus vaccine and an *E. coli* bacteria for prevention of acute undifferentiated neonatal diarrhea of beef calves. Can Vet J 17:197–212, 1976.
Archaumbault D, Morin G, Elazhary Y, et al: Immune response of pregnant heifers and cows to bovine rotavirus inoculation and passive protection to rotavirus infection in newborn calves fed colostral antibodies or colostral lymphocytes. Am J Vet Res 49:1084–1091, 1988.
Besser TE, Gay CC, McGuire TC, et al: Passive immunity to bovine rotavirus infection associated with transfer of serum antibody into the intestinal lumen. J Virol 62:2238–2242, 1988.
Burki F, Mostl K, Spiegl E, et al: Reduction of rotavirus-, coronavirus- and *E. coli*–associated calf-diarrheas in a large-size dairy herd by means of dam vaccination with a triple-vaccine. J Vet Med Br 33:241–252, 1986.

Castrucci G, Ferrari M, Frigeri F, et al: Experimental infection and cross protection tests in calves with cytopathic strains of bovine rotavirus. Comp Immunol Microbiol Infect Dis 6:321–332, 1983.
Castrucci G, Frigeri F, Ferrari M, et al: Neonatal calf diarrhea induced by rotavirus. Comp Immunol Microbiol Infect Dis 11:71–84, 1988.
DeLeeuw PW, Ellens DJ, Talmon FP, et al: Rotavirus infections in calves: Efficacy of oral vaccination in endemically infected herds. Res Vet Sci 29:142–147, 1980.
Ellis GR, Daniels E: Comparison of direct electron microscopy and enzyme immunoassay for the detection of rotavirus in calves, lambs, piglets and foals. Aust Vet J 65:133–135, 1988.
Grotelueschen DM, Duhamel GE, Lu W, et al: Possible vaccination failure in beef cow herds caused by infection with rotavirus distinct from the vaccine virus: Clinical observations. *In* Proceedings at the American Association of Bovine Practitioners, vol 1, 1992, pp 190–196.
Hall GA, Bridger JC, Parsons KR, et al: Variation in rotavirus virulence: A comparison of pathogenesis in calves between two rotaviruses of different virulence. Vet Pathol 30:223–233, 1993.
Haralambiev H, Georgiev G, Mitov B, et al: Application of an attenuated vaccine, RoCo-81, against viral enteritis of calves. Acta Vet Hung 35:469–473, 1987.
Heath SE, Naylor JM, Guedo BL, et al: The effects of feeding milk to diarrheic calves supplemented with oral electrolytes. Can J Vet Res 53:477–485, 1989.
Hussein HA, Parwani AV, Rosen BI, et al: Detection of rotavirus serotypes G1, G2, G3, and G11 in feces of diarrheic calves by using polymerase chain reaction–derived cDNA probes. J Clin Microbiol 31:2491–2496, 1993.
Ikemori Y, Kuroki M, Peralta RC, et al: Protection of neonatal calves against fatal enteric colibacillosis by administration of egg yolk powder from hens immunized with K99-piliated enterotoxigenic *Escherichia coli*. Am J Vet Res 53:2005–2008, 1992.
Killen JR, Hugill MC, Jones HL: Treatment of scour in lambs (letter). Vet Rec 122:494, 1988.
Kuroki M, Ohta M, Ikemori Y, et al: Passive protection against bovine rotavirus in calves by specific immunoglobulins from chicken egg yolk. Arch Virol 138:143–148, 1994.
Lee J, Babiuk LA, Harland R, et al: Immunological rersponse to recombinant VP8* subunit protein of bovine rotavirus in pregnant cattle. J Gen Virol. 76:2477–2483, 1995.
Mebus CA, Newman LE: Scanning electron, light and immunofluorescent microscopy of intestine of gnotobiotic calf infected with reoviruslike agent. Am J Vet Res 38:553–558, 1977.
Reynolds DJ, Morgan JH, Chanter N, et al: Microbiology of calf diarrhea in southern Britain. Vet Rec 119:34–39, 1986.
Runnels PL, Moon HW, Matthews PJ, et al: Effects of microbial and host variables on the interaction of rotavirus and *Escherichia coli* infections in gnotobiotic calves. Am J Vet Res 47:1542–1550, 1986.
Saif LJ, Smith KL, Landmeier BJ, et al: Immune response of pregnant cows to bovine rotavirus immunization. Am J Vet Res 45:49–58, 1984.
Schroeder BA, Sproule R, Saywell D: Prevalence of rotavirus in dairy calves as diagnosed by ELISA. Surveillance 12:2–3, 1985.
Snodgrass DR: Evaluation of a combined rotavirus and enterotoxigenic *Escherichia coli* vaccine in cattle. Vet Res 119:39–42, 1986.
Snodgrass DR, Terzolo HR, Sherwood D, et al: Aetiology of diarrhoea in young calves. Vet Rec 119:31–34, 1986.
Stiglmair-herb MT, Pospischil A, Hess RG, et al: Enzyme histochemistry of the small intestinal mucosa in experimental infections of calves with rotavirus and enterotoxigenic *Escherichia coli*. Vet Pathol 23:125–131, 1986.
Thurber ET, Bass EP, Beckenhauer WH: Field trial evaluation of a reo-coronavirus calf diarrhea vaccine. Can J Comp Med 41:131–136, 1977.
Twiehaus MJ, Mebus CA: Licensing and use of the calf scour vaccine. Proc Annu Meet US Anim Health Assoc 77:55–58, 1974.
Waltner-Toews DV: Dairy calf management, morbidity, mortality and calf-related drug use in Ontario Holstein herds. Dissertation Abstract Interna B 46:2589, 1986.
Waltner-Toews D, Martin SW, Meek AH, et al: A field trial to evaluate the efficacy of a combined rotavirus-coronavirus/*Escherichia coli* vaccine on dairy farms in southwestern Ontario. Can J Comp Med 49:1–9, 1985.

Enterotoxigenic *Escherichia coli*

Contrepois MG, Girardeau JP: Additive protective effects of colostral antipili antibodies in calves experimentally infected with enterotoxigenic *Escherichia coli*. Infect Immun 50:947–949, 1985.

Okerman L: Enteric infections caused by non-enterotoxigenic *Escherichia coli* in animals: Occurrence and pathogenicity mechanisms. A review. Vet Microbiol 14:33–46, 1987.

Rogan D, Behan W, Elrafih M, et al: Immunotherapy of calves infected with enterotoxigenic *Escherichia coli* (ETEC) by mycobacteria cell wall (MCW) immunostimulant/Immunoboost K. Presented at 77th Conference of Research Workers in Animal Disease, Chicago, 1996.

Williams Smith H, Huggins MB, Shaw KM: The control of experimental *Escherichia coli* diarrhoea in calves by means of bacteriophages. J Gen Microbiol 133:1111–1126, 1987.

Williams Smith H, Huggins MB, Shaw KM: Factors influencing the survival and multiplication of bacteriophages in calves and in their environment. J Gen Microbiol 133:1127–1135, 1987.

Coronavirus Infection

Clark MA: Bovine coronavirus. Br Vet J 149:51–70, 1993.

Heckert RA, Saif LJ, Hoblet KH, et al: A longitudinal study of bovine coronavirus enteric and respiratory infections in dairy calves in two herds in Ohio. Vet Microbiol 22:187–201, 1990.

Hoblet KH, Shulaw WP, Saif LJ, et al: Concurrent experimentally induced infection with *Eimeria bovis* and coronavirus in unweaned dairy calves. Am J Vet Res 53:1400–1408, 1992.

Rodak L, Babiuk LA, Acres SD: Detection by radioimmunoassay and enzyme-linked immunosorbent assay of coronavirus antibodies in bovine serum and lacteal secretions. J Clin Microbiol 16:34–40, 1982.

Wieda J, Bengelsdorff HJ, Bernhardt D, et al: Antibody levels in milk of vaccinated and unvaccinated cows against organisms of neonatal diarrhoea. J Vet Med Br 34:495–503, 1987.

Cryptosporidium parvum

Anderson BC: Cryptosporidiosis in Calves: epidemiologic questions, diagnosis and management. *In* Proceedings of the 14th Convention of the American Association of Bovine Practitioners, Nashville, 1982, pp 92–94.

Anderson BC: Moist heat inactivation of *Cryptosporidium* sp. Am J Public Health 75:1433–1434, 1985.

Campbell I, Tzipori S, Hutchinson G, et al: Effect of disinfectants on *Cryptosporidium* oocysts. Vet Rec 111:414–415, 1983.

Garber LP, Salman MD, Hurd HS, et al: Potential risk factors for *Cryptosporidium* infection in dairy calves. J Am Vet Med Assoc 205:86–91, 1994.

Gobel E: Diagnose und Therapie der akuten Cryptosporidiose beim Kalb. [Diagnosis and treatment of acute cryptosporidiosis in the calf.] Tierarztliche Umschau 42:863–869, 1987.

Lazo A, Barriga OO, Redman DR, et al: Identification by transfer blot of antigens reactive in the enzyme-linked immunosorbent assay (ELISA) in rabbits immunized and a calf infected with *Cryptosporidium* sp. Vet Parasitol 21:151–163, 1986.

Moon HW, Woode GN, Ahrens FA: Attempted chemoprophylaxis of cryptosporidiosis in calves. Vet Rec 110:181–182, 1982.

Ongerth JE, Stibbs HH: Prevalence of *Cryptosporidium* infection in dairy calves in western Washington. Am J Vet Res 50:1069–1070, 1989.

Quigley JD III, Martin KR, Bemis DA, et al: Effects of housing and colostrum feeding on the prevalence of selected infectious organisms in feces of Jersey calves. J Dairy Sci 77:3124–3131, 1994.

Redman DR, Fox JE: The effect of varying levels of DECCOX on experimental *Cryptosporidium* infections in Holstein bull calves. *In* Proceedings of the 26th Annual Meeting of the American Association of Bovine Practitioners, Albuquerque, 1993, pp 157–166.

Robert B, Ginter A, Antoine H, et al: Diagnosis of bovine cryptosporidiosis by an enzyme-linked immunosorbent assay. Vet Parasitol 37:9–19, 1990.

Sobich M, Tacal J, Wilcke BW, et al: Investigation of cryptosporidial infection in calves in San Bernardino County, California. J Am Vet Med Assoc 191:816–818, 1987.

Tilley M, Fayer R, Guidry A, et al: *Cryptosporidium parvum* (Apicomplexa: Cryptosporidiidae) oocyst and sporozoite antigens recognized by bovine colostral antibodies. Infect Immun 58:2966–2971, 1990.

Tzipori S, Campbell R, Angus KW: The therapeutic effect of 16 antimicrobial agents on *Cryptosporidium* infection in mice. Aust J Exp Biol Med Sci 60:187–190, 1982.

Tzipori S, Smith M, Halpin C, et al: Experimental cryptosporidiosis in calves: Clinical manifestations and pathological findings. Vet Rec 112:116–120, 1983.

Clostridium perfringens Type C Enterotoxemia

Fleming S: Enterotoxemia in neonatal calves. Vet Clin North Am Food Anim Pract 1:509–514, 1985.

Salmonellosis

Butler DG: Bovine salmonellosis. Bovine Proc 18:14–19, 1986.

Clarke RC, Gyles CL: Galactose epimeraseless mutants of *Salmonella typhimurium* as live vaccines for calves. Can J Vet Res 50:165–173, 1986.

Daigneault J, Thurmond M, Anderson M, et al: Effect of vaccination with the R mutant *Escherichia coli* (J5) antigen on morbidity and mortality of dairy calves. Am J Vet Res 52:1492–1496, 1991.

Roden LD, Smith BP, Spier SJ, et al: Effect of calf age and *Salmonella* bacterin type on ability to produce immunoglobulins directed against *Salmonella* whole cells or lipopolysaccharide. Am J Vet Res 53:1895–1899, 1992.

Scott P: Management of a salmonellosis outbreak in a cattle herd. In Practice 16:17–20, 1994.

Smith BP, Oliver DG, Singh P, et al: Detection of *Salmonella dublin* mammary gland infection in carrier cows, using an enzyme-linked immunosorbent assay for antibody in milk or serum. Am J Vet Res 50:1352–1360, 1989.

Wray C: Bovine salmonellosis: An update. Irish Vet J 46:137–140, 1993.

▪ Omphalitis and Its Sequelae in Ruminants

Thomas R. Kasari, D.V.M., M.V.Sc., Diplomate, A.C.V.I.M.
Allen J. Roussel, Jr., D.V.M., M.S., Diplomate, A.C.V.I.M.

The umbilical cord (umbilicus) of bovine, ovine, and caprine fetuses in utero consists of an outer amniotic membrane surrounding (1) two veins that fuse intra-abdominally to a single vein that returns blood from the placenta to the liver of the fetus, (2) two arteries that communicate with internal iliac arteries and carry blood from the fetus to the placenta, and (3) the urachus, a tubular structure connecting the urinary bladder with the allantoic cavity. Normally, at parturition, as the fetus is expelled from the pelvic canal of the dam, the umbilicus is torn a few inches from the body wall. In response to this tearing action, umbilical arteries usually constrict and retract into the abdomen to the level of the bladder, with only remnants of amniotic membrane left surrounding the externally exposed umbilical veins and urachus. The umbilical veins and urachus gradually close, and the remnants of amniotic membrane dry up and fall from the neonate within 1 week after birth.

Localized inflammation or infection of the contents of the umbilical cord external to the body wall is referred to as *omphalitis* (navel ill). *Omphalophlebitis*, *omphaloarteritis*, and *urachitis* are terms used to further describe the extension of inflammation or infection from the external umbilicus to the intra-abdominal segments of the umbilical vein, umbilical arteries, and urachus, respectively. More than one of these structures may be infected in the same animal.

Delineation of the extent of inflammation or infection to the external or intra-abdominal segments of the umbilicus is dependent on thorough palpation and other aids such as ultrasonography. Presenting clinical signs vary depending on the location of infection within umbilical structures. Furthermore, resolution of an umbilical mass via either surgery or medical treatment and overall prognosis are predicated on whether external or intra-abdominal involvement of these structures is present.

OCCURRENCE

Although surveys on the incidence of omphalitis in domestic ruminants are lacking, it is perceived by veterinarians to be a commonly encountered problem. Most health problems and deaths in calves, lambs, and kids from birth to 1 to 2 days of age are the result of dystocia, starvation, exposure, or predation. Pathologic and microbiologic conditions causing death are relatively minor in importance during this time. Postnatal infections become more important near the end of the first week of life when either diarrhea and pneumonia or omphalitis and septicemia occur.

Whereas most cases of navel ill in lambs and kids will be presented for examination by 3 months of age, enlargement of the umbilicus and clinical signs referable to navel ill in calves can be seen as early as 2 to 5 days after birth. However, if the umbilicus appears relatively normal and intra-abdominal segments of the umbilicus are involved, cases may be up to 3 months of age or older before presentation.

ETIOLOGY AND PATHOGENESIS

Infection of the umbilicus is presumed to occur soon after birth, often as a consequence of poor hygiene, hypogammaglobulinemia, and neonatal weakness. The lumina of umbilical veins, arteries, and urachus do not close immediately after birth, leaving a portal of entry for pathogenic bacteria. Provided the infection remains restricted to the external umbilicus, either localized cellulitis or an abscess with a thick fibrous capsule forms. The urachus is overwhelmingly the most frequently involved intra-abdominal umbilical remnant, followed by umbilical vein and, rarely, umbilical arteries.

Urachal involvement may remain localized to the urachal stalk, or infection may migrate retrograde to the bladder mucosa. Cystitis, as evidenced by signs of pollakiuria, stranguria, and dysuria in animals of any age, particularly those without any enlargement of the umbilicus, can be the first indication that a urachal stalk abnormality exists. The changes in frequency and nature of urination are thought to be the result of mechanical interference with normal filling and emptying of the bladder. The urachus anchors the apex of the bladder to the ventral abdomen which, in effect, stretches the bladder longitudinally and reduces the functional volume. The reduced holding capacity of the bladder allows smaller volumes of urine to stretch the detrusor muscles and stimulates frequent voiding of small amounts of urine. If a patent urachus accompanies umbilical swelling, the end of the umbilicus may remain moist, persistent dribbling of urine from this structure may occur, or fluid may dribble from the umbilicus concomitant with the act of urination.

Extensive omphalophlebitis often results in abscessation of the liver. Omphaloarteritis may promote the development of septicemia if bacteria gain entrance to arterial circulation through the umbilical arteries. However, the oropharyngeal mucosa appears to be the most important route of invasion of pathogens responsible for septicemia. The gastrointestinal and respiratory tracts can also be portals of entry for septicemic bacterial organisms.

The most important predisposing factor in the development of septicemia is failure of passive transfer (FPT). The quantity of immunoglobulin needed for protection of a calf depends on the number and virulence of the organisms to which the calf is exposed. Factors which predispose calves to FPT include (1) being born to primiparous dams; (2) being unable to rise soon after parturition (weakness at birth due to in utero infections or nutritional deficiencies, or extreme environmental conditions); (3) musculoskeletal or neurologic abnormalities; (4) dystocia; and (5) leaking of colostrum or poor udder or teat conformation. Bacteria isolated from umbilical masses and deeper structures are generally confined to those genera that have the capability to grow under anaerobic conditions. *Actinomyces pyogenes* (formerly *Corynebacterium pyogenes*) is probably the most frequently isolated pathogen. This bacterial organism has a propensity for abscess formation with a thick fibrous capsule. *A. pyogenes* may also be isolated as part of a mixed infection with coliforms, particularly *Escherichia coli*, or *Staphylococcus* spp., *Proteus* spp., *Streptococcus* spp., and *Enterococcus*. Less frequently reported bacterial isolates include *Salmonella dublin* and *Mycoplasma alkalescens*.

Although many of these same bacteria can be responsible for septicemia, *A. pyogenes* and *E. coli* account for approximately 80% of isolates from the blood and tissues of septicemic calves. Similar to umbilical masses, gram-positive and gram-negative bacterial organisms can (and often do) combine to cause toxemia and subsequent signs of septicemia in affected calves.

CLINICAL SIGNS

Ruminant neonates with omphalitis can show signs of disease as early as 2 to 5 days after birth. The umbilicus is enlarged, warmer than surrounding skin, and painful when palpated. The mass can be firm with pitting edema, if cellulitis is present, whereas fluctuance may exist if an abscess has developed. There should not be any intra-abdominal cylindrical structures coursing anteriorly or posteriorly from the body wall directly above the umbilicus. The umbilical stump may be dry, moist, or, less frequently, draining purulent debris. Tachycardia and tachypnea may be present owing to pain. Variable degrees of depression usually exist, resulting in a loss of appetite. Fever may be evident.

Calves appear to be more sensitive than lambs and kids to the effects of infection within the umbilical vessels and urachus. Calves with omphalophlebitis usually present at 1 to 3 months of age, most often for unthriftiness. The umbilicus may not be noticeably enlarged. The key diagnostic feature of this form of navel ill is that deep abdominal palpation detects a cylindrical structure 3 to 5 cm in diameter coursing from the umbilicus in the direction of the anterior abdomen. The animal may need to be restrained in lateral or dorsal recumbency to facilitate thorough abdominal palpation. Palpation usually elicits a painful reaction from the animal. Inappetence and a low-grade fever usually accompany omphalophlebitis along with variable degrees of depression. Dehydration and tachycardia may exist as a consequence of low-grade toxemia.

Omphaloarteritis will present a clinical picture very similar to that of omphalophlebitis, with the exception that abdominal palpation reveals a space-occupying mass above the umbilicus that courses in a dorsocaudal direction.

If urachitis is present, abdominal palpation will reveal findings identical with those of animals with omphaloarteritis. However, clinical signs of pollakiuria, dysuria, and stranguria, as well as changes in urine parameters consistent with cystitis (if a communicating urachal abscess is present), frequently accompany the palpatory findings. Unlike other umbilical remnant diseases that occur characteristically during the suckling period, urachal abnormalities can escape detection in cattle until after they are weaned or are yearlings. A urachal stalk abnormality that mechanically impedes urination normally has no untoward effects on body condition, appetite, and demeanor.

Various reported sequelae to omphalitis, omphalophlebitis, omphaloarteritis, and urachitis include septicemia as well as diffuse gangrene of the limbs, peritonitis, intestinal strangulation, and hepatic abscessation. Regarding septicemia, early clinical signs are weakness or lethargy. However, these signs may go unnoticed or be ignored. Rectal temperature, pulse, and respiratory rates are variable. Other signs reflect the body systems in which the bacteria localize. The central nervous system and ophthalmologic system appear to be most often affected. Signs referable to central nervous system disease (meningitis, encephalitis) may range from mild to profound depression, seizures, nystagmus, strabismus, opisthotonos, head tilt, and circling. Perhaps one of the most reliable indicators of sepsis in the calf is anterior uveitis, manifested by hypopyon, hyphema, aqueous flare, and synechia. The calf may even be blind. In some cases, petechial or ecchymotic hemorrhages, indicative of vasculitis and disseminated intravascular coagulation, are present. These are very serious negative prognostic indicators. Acute bovine virus diarrhea (BVD) infection with type II BVD virus (mostly) can also result in thrombocytopenia and hemorrhage from body orifices. Consequently, BVD should be considered also as a differential diagnosis when the latter striking clinical findings are observed. Diarrhea is seen occasionally but is not a consistent clinical finding in septicemic calves. Although not always clinically apparent, pneumonia is often found on postmortem examination. Lameness or joint effusion, or both, may result from septic arthritis and osteomyelitis, laminitis, or discospondylitis.

CLINICOPATHOLOGIC ABNORMALITIES

Clinicopathologic abnormalities that are specific or pathognomonic for navel ill do not exist. Neutrophilic leukocytosis with or without immature bands and hyperfibrinogenemia may be found and reflect the infectious nature of this disease. Mild anemia may coexist. If septicemia is present and the causative bacterial organism is gram-negative, particularly *E. coli*, disseminated intravascular coagulation may develop (thrombocytopenia, hypofibrinogenemia, prolonged prothrombin and partial thromboplastin times, and increased fibrin degradation products).

Many calves, lambs, and kids will also exhibit hypoproteinemia. Rather than low albumin concentrations, this is usually a reflection of immunoglobulin concentrations that do not sufficiently raise protein levels in the blood of these calves as a result of failure of passive gastrointestinal absorption of maternal immunoglobulins. Hypogammaglobulinemia is also a necessary prerequisite to development of septicemia.

Those animals with cystitis will show hematuria, pyuria, proteinuria, and bacteriuria. Serum concentrations of aspartate transaminase, alkaline phosphatase, and γ-glutamyltransferase may be elevated in instances when extensive liver abscessation is present as a sequela to omphalophlebitis.

DIAGNOSIS

Diagnosis of omphalitis, omphalophlebitis, omphaloarteritis, and urachitis is dependent on thorough abdominal palpation. The umbilical vein and arteries and the urachus are not palpable intra-abdominally in the normal animal. Consequently, palpable intra-abdominal structures emanating from the umbilicus should be viewed as abnormalities. A diagnosis of omphalitis or other umbilical remnant disease is warranted provided appropriate signalment and characteristic presenting signs accompany the palpatory findings.

The primary differential diagnosis to consider when an umbilical mass is observed in an umbilical hernia is complicated by other pathologic processes, including omphalitis. An uncomplicated umbilical hernia will be reducible, that is, the contents of the mass can be manipulated back into the abdomen through

the abdominal wall defect, whereas omphalitis will not respond in a similar manner. In the case of an umbilical hernia involving any or all of the remnants of the umbilical cord, manipulation of the contents allows partial reduction of the mass adjacent to the body wall through a distinct and uniformly smooth hernial ring except for the firm nonreducible portion of the mass associated with the umbilicus. Skin overlying the nonreducible portion is firmly attached to the mass. Depending on the direction in which the ventral component of the mass courses intra-abdominally, omphalophlebitis, omphaloarteritis, or urachitis should be considered.

Diagnosis of an umbilical abscess can be made by aspiration of purulent material from the mass with a large-bore needle. Ultrasonography should be considered if confusion exists over the composition of an umbilical mass or if the significance of an intra-abdominal structure originating from the umbilicus is unclear. A 7.5-MHz transducer is preferred for this procedure because of its improved resolution. Positive contrast cystography or intravenous contrast urography provides meaningful information if a urachal stalk abnormality is suspected. Normally, the urinary bladder is well within the pelvis; however, with urachal involvement, the bladder shows filling well outside of the pelvis and in a cranioventral direction. In older animals that are amenable to rectal palpation, immobility of the bladder may be detected with digital manipulation. If the umbilicus has a fistulous opening, radiopaque contrast material can be injected retrograde in an attempt to outline the affected structures.

The diagnosis of accompanying septicemia is usually based on clinical signs, and is strengthened if failure of passive transfer of maternal immunoglobulin is present. Definitive diagnosis is based on isolation of bacteria from the blood via blood culture.

Assessment of colostral immunoglobulin transfer will help substantiate the diagnosis as well as contribute to prognosis, to some degree. There is no "magic number" that guarantees that a particular calf has adequate immunoglobulin concentrations. Passive transfer is often classified as complete failure, partial failure, or adequate. One of the simplest and most accurate ways to assess survivability of calves is to measure total *serum* protein by refractometry. Although the value will be different for different farms and ranches, in general, less than 5.0 g/L indicates FPT and a greater probability of morbidity and mortality, and greater than 5.5 g/L indicates good transfer and a lesser probability of morbidity and mortality. The morbidity and mortality rate in calves with protein concentrations between 5.0 and 5.5 g/L depends greatly on management factors, environment, and pathogen exposure. Single radial immunodiffusion, zinc sulfate turbidity, sodium sulfite precipitation, glutaraldehyde coagulation, serum γ-glutamyltransferase concentration, latex agglutination, and protein electrophoresis are other techniques which can be used to assess adequacy of passive transfer in blood.

TREATMENT

Antimicrobial therapy can be quite beneficial in those cases in which cellulitis is present in the external umbilicus. However, antimicrobial therapy is imperative if septicemia is suspected. Examples of suitable antimicrobial drugs for *E. coli* and *A. pyogenes*, the two most common bacterial isolates for omphalitis and septicemia, are listed in Table 1.

When abscessation of the umbilicus has occurred, surgical drainage should be initiated. A stab incision is made in the most ventral aspect of the abscess; the cavity is drained and lavaged with a 7% iodine solution. Several days of this treatment may be necessary to achieve satisfactory resolution of the abscess. For cases that show signs of systemic toxemia associated with umbilical abscessation, antimicrobial therapy in addition to surgical drainage is recommended.

Table 1
ANTIMICROBIAL AGENTS WITH ACTIVITY AGAINST
Escherichia coli AND *Actinomyces pyogenes*

Drug	Route	Dosage
E. coli		
Ampicillin trihydrate	IM, SC	22 mg/kg b.i.d.
Amoxicillin trihydrate	IM	5.0 mg/kg b.i.d.
Ceftiofur	IM	2.2 mg/kg b.i.d.
Florfenicol	IM	20 mg/kg q.48h.
A. pyogenes		
Penicillin G		
Sodium salt	IV	50,000 IU/kg q.i.d.
Potassium salt	IV	50,000 IU/kg q.i.d.
Procaine	IM, SC	20,000 IU/kg s.i.d.
Erythromycin	IM	44 mg/kg s.i.d.
Ampicillin trihydrate	IM, SC	22 mg/kg b.i.d.
Amoxicillin trihydrate	IM	5.0 mg/kg b.i.d.
Ceftiofur	IM	2.2 mg/kg b.i.d.
Florfenicol	IM	20 mg/kg q.48h.

IM, intramuscular; IV, intravenous; SC, subcutaneous.

Infected intra-abdominal segments of the umbilicus are best managed by surgical correction. Urachal infections extending to the bladder require excision of the apex of the bladder and ligation of the umbilical arteries along with any external umbilical structures. Infection of the umbilical vein can be localized anywhere along its length or become diffuse and involve the liver with sequelae of abscessation. Localized omphalophlebitis that does not involve the liver can be managed by ligation and removal of the affected umbilical vein. Liver abscessation is best handled by marsupialization of the infected umbilical vein. This procedure entails securing the wall of the abscessed umbilical vein to the ventral body wall in the right paramedian area approximately 5 cm caudal to the xiphoid. Contents of the abscess are allowed to drain externally from the now patent umbilical vein stalk. The tract should be flushed daily with a 10% povidone-iodine solution until drainage ceases. When the umbilical arteries are involved, the treatment of choice is ligation and resection of the involved arteries along with any external umbilical tissue.

When an accompanying septicemia is suspected, early aggressive treatment with a broad-spectrum antimicrobial agent (see Table 1) is often the key to the successful outcome of a septicemic calf. When previous clinical experience or blood culture and sensitivity patterns suggest these drugs are not effective, the veterinarian may consider the use of aminoglycosides and potentiated sulfonamides. However, assumption of responsibility for extralabel drug usage and tissue residues must be considered. Combination therapy (e.g., penicillins or cephalosporins and aminoglycoside; potentiated sulfonamides and penicillin) will extend the effective spectrum of activity and may be synergistic in killing the microorganisms.

Antimicrobial therapy should be continued for approximately 10 to 14 days to minimize sequelae from possible sequestered bacteria in joints, meninges, and other organs. If clinical signs of septic arthritis or meningitis are detected, the duration of therapy should be extended for an additional time. Lavage of affected joints is an extremely beneficial (almost essential) part of therapy for septic arthritis. Endotoxemia caused by *E. coli* and other gram-negative organisms may contribute to the disease process. The use of nonsteroidal anti-inflammatory drugs such as flunixin meglumine or ketoprofen may mitigate the effects of endotoxin and provide analgesia if joints are involved. Although corticosteroids are also antiendotoxic, their immunosuppressive effects are probably undesirable. If steroids are chosen, only a

single dose should be given to the calf. Fluid therapy may be necessary to correct and maintain the hydration status of septicemic calves as well as correct acid-base and electrolyte abnormalities. Glucose supplementation may be indicated, as hypoglycemia can accompany gram-negative sepsis or may occur due to prolonged anorexia. Because septicemic calves typically are not acidotic, solutions with minimal alkalinization potential should be used.

Calves with septicemia should benefit from the administration of whole blood or plasma. However, the difficulty of administration, lack of availability, and high cost of these products often prohibit their use in the field. In addition, this exogenous source of immunoglobulin (and other components in blood) appears to be more effective when given prophylactically to a hypogammaglobulinemic calf than as a treatment to a sick septicemic calf. The administration of up to 50 mL/kg plasma (2 L to a large calf) is usually insufficient to adequately increase the concentration of immunoglobulin. If the calf is less than 24 hours old, administering colostrum (or commercially available dried colostrum products) may be of some benefit. Ancillary nursing care should include heat lamps when necessary, adequate nutrition, oxygen supplementation when necessary, clean dry stalls or bedding areas, and physiotherapy as necessary to prevent tendon contracture and pressure sores. If the calf develops complications associated with septicemia (e.g., septic arthritis, osteomyelitis) specific treatment for these conditions will need to be initiated.

PREVENTION

Infection of the umbilicus is presumed to occur soon after birth owing to the interaction of poor hygiene, neonatal weakness, and hypogammaglobulinemia. Consequently, improving hygiene in the maternity area, providing prompt attention and intervention to females experiencing dystocia, and ensuring adequate early ingestion of colostrum will decrease the potential for umbilical infection and septicemia. Although dipping the umbilical cord in tincture of iodine at birth is a time-honored procedure, there is no good supportive information that this antiseptic is effective in prevention of subsequent bacterial infection of the umbilicus.

BIBLIOGRAPHY

Kasari TR: Weakness in the newborn calf. Vet Clin North Am Food Anim Pract 10:167–180, 1994.
Trent AM, Smith DF: Surgical management of umbilical masses with associated umbilical cord remnant infections in calves. J Am Vet Med Assoc 185:1531–1534, 1984.

■ Solving Neonatal Pig Problems

Guy-Pierre Martineau, D.V.M.
Jean-Pierre Vaillancourt, D.V.M., M.Sc., Ph.D.

Many infectious and noninfectious diseases, as well as poor performances observed during the neonatal period, result from circumstances that were allowed to develop over a long period of time.[1] Such situations can rarely be solved overnight. It is important for the practitioner to make the grower understand this, because a good practitioner-grower partnership is needed to rectify neonatal problems. The following discussion offers a 'game plan' for practitioners as they tackle such problems.

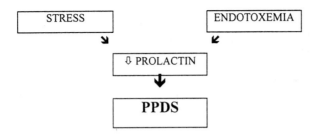

Figure 1
Schematic pathway leading to the postpartum dysgalactia syndrome (PPDS).

POSTPARTUM DYSGALACTIA SYNDROME

Clinical Importance

Postpartum dysgalactia syndrome (PPDS) is one of the main causes of endemic neonatal problems.[2] Clinically, one mainly observes an increase in the incidence of diarrhea or crushing (laid-on), and a reduction in piglets' growth. This syndrome is difficult to characterize because of its many different clinical manifestations.

Causes

Multiple causes exist (see Evolution and Risk Factors), many of them interactive. This complicates the diagnosis process and the development of effective control strategies. PPDS is often considered one manifestation of the MMA (mastitis-metritis-agalactia) syndrome. In fact, it is the other way around, the MMA syndrome being only a particular form of PPDS. The MMA syndrome is today probably its least frequent, but most severe form.

Bacterial endotoxins are an important component of the PPDS. They can easily be absorbed and reach the blood circulation (endotoxemia). Endotoxin-producing bacteria can be part of the sow's normal flora. In this case, the increase in endotoxin production comes from an excess multiplication of these bacteria (Fig. 1). Therefore, it is essential to identify the origin of this bacterial overgrowth. There are three major sites of bacterial multiplication: the urogenital tract, the mammary glands, and the digestive tract (Fig. 2). Hence, to be successful, the therapeutic and prophylactic approaches must target the affected site(s).

Pathophysiology

The secretion and excretion of colostrum is controlled by a complex hormonal mechanism. The essential point to remember is that stress-related hormones and endotoxins inhibit the liberation of prolactin, the main hormone triggering lactation.

Evolution and Risk Factors

A risk factor is an event or characteristic of the animals or their environment that has a significant impact on these animals' health. Some risk factors are well known (parity of the sow, piglet's weight at birth, etc.). To identify a risk factor, the practitioner must be in a position to compare the prevalence of this factor in affected herds or sows or litters and healthy ones. One such factor is colostrum intake by piglets. Colostrum is as much a source of energy as it is a source of immunoglobulins.[3] Any restriction in colostrum consumption, even for a limited period of time, will have pathologic (diarrhea) as well as production (reduced neonatal growth) consequences.

Significant risk factors are those associated with stress in sows and those responsible for bacterial growth and the production of endotoxins. These risk factors are numerous and are associated with specific clinical or pathologic entities (cystitis, metritis, vaginitis, constipation, and mastitis). In particular, water consumption by gilts and sows throughout gestation and lactation should not be overlooked, although in recent years much emphasis has been put on this issue to the detriment of other risk factors.[4]

Associated Clinical Signs

The clinical expression of PPDS may vary greatly from herd to herd. Clinical signs are rarely all present at the same time. Their sequence of appearance also varies depending on the herd. The main observations are:

- In sows: the fat sow syndrome (FSS), long farrowings, puerperal fever, anorexia; in particular, overweight sows exposed to high ambient temperatures are at higher risk of developing PPDS.
- In piglets: increase in the number of stillborn and low-viability piglets, neonatal diarrhea, higher incidence of laid-on piglets (crushing), and low growth rate, which is always present.
- The producer: too many manual interventions during farrowing, the systematic administration of many drugs to sows (antibiotics, oxytocin, prostaglandins) and to piglets (mainly antibiotics).

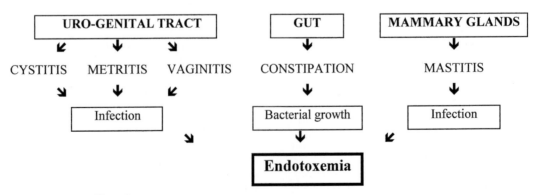

Figure 2
Schematic representation of the different pathways likely to produce endotoxemia.

General Approach

To be successful, an intervention must address all significant risk factors. Indeed, correcting a single factor is often not sufficient to bring long-lasting results.

Diagnosis

The PPDS is rarely at the top of most practitioners' differential diagnosis because it is more common to limit the diagnosis at the sow (cystitis, metritis, vaginitis, constipation, or mastitis) or piglet (neonatal diarrhea) level. It is also tempting to approach each problem separately (neonatal diarrhea, long farrowing, vulvar discharge, etc.). However, these are rarely individual problems. They are indeed linked to each other, and should be tackled as such.

Treatment

Therapeutic or prophylactic interventions limited to a single application (or a short series) are generally efficient only on a short-term basis. However, in the long run, they quickly incite producers to become dependent on the following interventions:

- Antibiotics for postpartum "fever" (often only a marginal hyperthermia), for mastitis, for vaginal infections, for uterine infections, or for neonatal diarrhea
- Oxytocin or prostaglandins for problems related to long farrowings or postpartum vaginal infections or uterine infections
- Systematic manual interventions during farrowing (systematic use of a thermometer for each sow after farrowing, uterine examinations, uterine washings, etc.)

NEONATAL PIGLET CRUSHING (LAID-ON)

Clinical Importance

Crushing represents, with low viability, one of the main causes of preweaning mortality. Indeed, 20% to 40% of all preweaning deaths occur by crushing. The incidence is highest during the first 48 to 72 hours of life. This is often a very frustrating problem for producers. In fact, crushed piglets are often healthy piglets (nearly two thirds of crushed piglets would have been viable).

Causes

There are three different kinds of crushing: (1) posterior crushing occurs when the sow sits (this type of crushing is normally minimized with modern farrowing crates); (2) anterior crushing occurs when the sow passes from a dog-sitting position to a laid-down position; piglets are then crushed by the thorax of the sow (this type of crushing is especially associated with lactation problems, piglets seeking, in vain, to suckle); finally, (3) lateral crushing occurs when the sow rotates, especially in farrowing pens (piglets, mainly during the first 24 hours of life, like to stay close to a natural source of heat, the mammary glands).[5]

Causes of crushing can be classified according to the origin of the problem (the sow, the piglet, or the environment) (Table 1). This classification does not exclude interactions. For example, overweight sows on a slippery floor will have a tendency to

| **Table 1** | | |
| **MAIN RISK FACTORS ASSOCIATED WITH A HIGH CRUSHING RATE** | | |
Origin of the Problem	**Main Risk Factors**	**Specific Characteristics**
Piglets	Weakness, competition	Weight, birth order, splayleg, splay-weak, congenital tremors, teat order
Sows	Locomotion, farrowing process, lactation, parity	Primary (leg weakness syndrome) and secondary (fat sow syndrome, slippery floor) locomotion problems, duration of farrowing, postpartum dysgalactia syndrome, old sows
Environment	Ambient temperature: impact on the sow, impact on the piglets; general comfort, farrowing crate	High temperature, low temperature, air drafts (slatted floor), stressful conditions (noise, sow manipulations, etc.); many characteristics with a weak cause-effect relationship

From Martineau G-P: Approche générale d'un problème de mort-nés. *In* Martineau G-P (ed): Maladies d'élevage des porcs. Paris, France Agricole, 1997, pp 286–289.

remain in a dog-sitting position, which can lead to anterior crushing. Weak piglets are also more at risk of being crushed during long farrowings, or when sows are affected with PPDS.

It is worth mentioning that in the not too distant past, much emphasis was put on crate design in an attempt to solve crushing problems (crate width, inferior bars, etc.). The importance of crate characteristics is now being questioned.

Diagnostic Steps*

1. *Quantification of the problem at the herd level.* In general, the higher the crushing rate and the higher the proportion of litters involved, the easier it is to identify risk factors. This, however, does not mean that the problem can easily be solved!

2. *Description of the evolution of the problem* to determine whether it is chronic or acute. This is an important, albeit often neglected step. When acute, one must focus on recent changes in the herd that may have triggered the problem. When chronic, factors that may have initiated the problem may no longer be present when it becomes clinically apparent (Fig. 3). Emphasis is put on factors that perpetuate the problem.

3. *Identification of sows* associated with the majority of crushings. Normally, the data analysis should start with an assessment of the parity distribution of crushings. Crushings are generally highest in sows of higher parities. Therefore, it is important to look at the demography of the herd. It is not unusual to observe that fewer than 20% of the sows are responsible for at least 80% of all crushings (20:80 rule).

4. *Determination of the age distribution of crushed piglets.* A low incidence of crushing may be considered "normal" during the first day of life (≤2.5%). However, any crushing occurring after the second day should not be considered acceptable. When this

*Adapted from Martineau.[6]

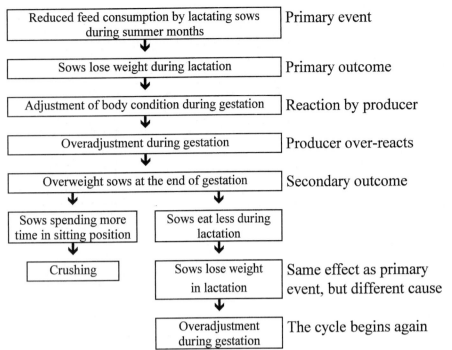

Reduced feed consumption by lactating sows during summer months	Primary event
↓	
Sows lose weight during lactation	Primary outcome
↓	
Adjustment of body condition during gestation	Reaction by producer
↓	
Overadjustment during gestation	Producer over-reacts
↓	
Overweight sows at the end of gestation	Secondary outcome

Sows spending more time in sitting position → Crushing

Sows eat less during lactation ↓ Sows lose weight in lactation — Same effect as primary event, but different cause ↓ Overadjustment during gestation — The cycle begins again

Figure 3

Example of a cascade of events leading to a recurring crushing problem.

happens, it is recommended to evaluate milk consumption by the crushed piglets to determine whether starvation is a significant component of the problem. When milk consumption is adequate, piglets are in good body condition. When starvation is a problem, piglets are weak, and their crushing is simply the final stage of a starve-out problem.

5. *Description and assessment of the environment* in the farrowing facilities in terms of comfort (microenvironment of the sows) *and the maternal quality of the sows.* It is often useful to compare the body condition of the sows at farrowing and at weaning when FSS is suspected.

6. *Categorization of the type of crushing:* posterior vs. anterior vs. lateral types. The producer should be required to note this information on the sow card when removing crushed piglets.

7. *Identification of risk factors* that would explain a higher incidence for one or two of the three types of crushing. For example, crushing and weakness of piglets at birth may have a common cause. Producers categorize correctly crushing as a cause of death in the first week post partum. However, if a high incidence is reported after 1 week of age, these cases may well be misreported.[7]

NEONATAL DIARRHEA

Most cases of neonatal diarrhea have a primary or secondary infectious origin. Diarrhea results from an imbalance between the piglet's immunity (the immune protection conferred by maternal antibodies via colostrum) and the infection pressure (the combined effect of the number of microbes in contact with individuals [viruses, bacteria, protozoa, etc.] and their virulence) (Fig. 4).

Low colostrum intake is a common risk factor (see Postpartum Dysgalactia Syndrome) associated or not with a high infection pressure. However, when confronted with neonatal diarrhea, it is often tempting to put the blame on the poor immunologic quality of the colostrum. Such colostrum is mainly produced by para I primiparous sows. It is not a frequent occurrence in older sows.

The clinicoepidemiologic description of neonatal diarrhea usually provides the information needed to determine its origin. This is why it is important to take the time to describe the problem. It is our opinion that in at least 80% of cases, it is possible to identify risk factors associated with inadequate colostrum intake or high infection pressure. Unfortunately, the descriptive component of a neonatal diarrhea investigation is probably the most neglected step in the diagnostic process, which diminishes the likelihood of implementing an effective long-term control program. Too often, it is assumed that the clinical portrait is the same for various causes, and that only the laboratory is in a position to come up with a valid diagnosis.

The clinicoepidemiologic description consists of obtaining accurate answers to the following questions: WHICH PIGS have WHAT, WHERE, WHEN, SINCE WHEN, HOW, and HOW MUCH?

WHICH piglets are affected? It is easier and, especially, more expeditious to assume that all piglets within a litter have diarrhea once diarrheal feces have been noticed on the floor or when piglets are soiled with diarrheal feces. How many piglets are really affected within a litter? And how many litters are really affected? These are key questions. If all piglets in a litter are affected, that may indicate that the causative agent is new in the herd or that sows are not immunized or that piglets did not have access to colostrum for a sufficient period of time. Piglets would then be affected from birth and not at 2 to 3 days of age. The characterization of the proportion of affected piglets and the age at the onset of diarrhea go a long way toward an assessment of the problem.

How to interpret the fact that only a few piglets in a litter are affected? This is, indeed, the most frequent case scenario. Is it because they have not suckled enough colostrum? Or that they suckled colostrum only a long time after the first-born piglets? Or that sick piglets are very small? Or that these piglets do not have access to a warm environment?

WHICH sows have affected litters? It is not unusual to be told that there is no parity effect or that the problem is limited to para I sows. Colostrum of low immunologic quality should result in neonatal diarrhea within 24 to 36 hours post partum

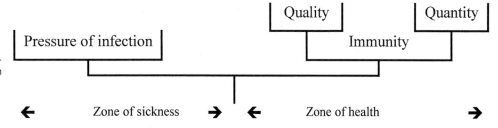

Figure 4
Schematic representation of the equilibrium between colostral protection (immunity) and infection pressure.

and not at 48 to 72 hours. Even in the case of primiparous sows, one should not conclude too quickly that these sows are not transmitting sufficient protection to their offspring.

WHAT type of diarrhea? The color and texture of piglet diarrhea, when associated with other clinical events, can provide valuable information on the specific agents involved in the problem (e.g., *Clostridium perfringens* type C or *Isospora suis*). Other characteristics may also be informative. For example, alkaline feces are indicative of hypersecretion (e.g., colibacillosis), whereas acidic feces are associated with malabsorption (e.g., transmissible gastroenteritis or less severe diarrhea associated with rotavirus).

WHERE does diarrhea occur in the farrowing section? Does diarrhea occur in all crates or is it more often seen in some of them, that is, close to openings, or in areas where the ventilation seems deficient? It is particularly important to pay attention to the location in relation to heat sources, air inlets, and the air distribution pattern. Air drafts are always very detrimental to piglets.

WHEN did diarrhea appear? Knowing when the first cases occurred may provide a helpful hint about likely risk factors. Many producers have noticed diarrhea appearing within the first 24 hours of life that then disappeared without any treatment. This diarrhea is probably a colibacillosis associated with a delay in colostrum intake. It is exceptional to observe viral diarrhea before 24 hours of age. Diarrhea due to the PPDS occurs mainly at 2 to 3 days.

SINCE WHEN does the problem exist? Is the problem new in the herd? Some diarrhea is seasonal, and can be quite predictable year after year. For example, clinical signs associated with intestinal coccidiosis (*I. suis*) are more severe during the warmer months of the year.

HOW did the problem evolve? It is essential to know the evolution of the disease. In particular, one must closely monitor any intervention. For example, antibiotics would be ineffective against viral diseases and coccidiosis.

HOW MANY litters are affected? Two attitudes are common among producers: In herds with endemic neonatal diarrhea, many producers will trivialize the problem as long as there is no or little mortality, even if growth is below the target value. In other herds, diarrhea may be an infrequent occurrence, but its presence is enough to push the producer to take extreme measures that often lead to catastrophic results. In both cases, it is important to determine with precision the number of affected litters, and because of the perceptions associated with the attitudes described above, practitioners should not rely exclusively on producers to obtain this information. Once obtained, it should be looked at with consideration of all clinical findings.

STILLBIRTHS

Clinical Importance

Stillbirths usually represent 5% to 10% of total born piglets.[8] This range is often considered an acceptable target. However, for the same percentage of stillbirths, notable differences may exist in the type of stillborn and the factors associated with their occurrence. The diagnostic approach needed to solve a stillborn problem is often underestimated. A meticulous assessment of the clinical picture is an essential step that may often, on its own, contribute to the identification of the main causes of risk factors.

Classification

Stillborn piglets fit in one of three categories:

Class I: Death occurred shortly before farrowing (antepartum stillborns).
Class II: Death occurred during parturition (intrapartum stillborns). The majority of stillborns fall in this category.
Class III: Death occurred just after farrowing; therefore, these may not be considered "true" stillborns; however, they are so weak at birth that they are not viable under the best of conditions and cannot survive past the first hour of life.

Pathophysiology

Whatever the category, stillborns should be completely developed at birth. Their lungs are collapsed in class I and II stillborns. At least a fragment of lung floats in class III stillborns, indicating that they breathed before death.

Microorganisms are commonly isolated from antepartum stillborns (class I). These microorganisms are often opportunistic agents such as *Streptococcus* spp., *Staphylococcus* spp., *Escherichia coli*, etc. They take advantage of the accidental contamination of the uterus following the premature opening of the cervix prior to parturition. Another possibility is bacterial contamination of the amniotic fluid causing an increase in the antepartum stillborn rate. In contrast, most intrapartum stillborns are sterile. Figures 5 and 6 highlight the main risk factors associated with an increase in the number of stillborns per litter.

Diagnostic Steps

1. *Identification of the stillborn category* (class I, II, or III). The hoof of class I piglets often appears immature. Class II piglets are usually covered with meconium because of hypoxia during parturition. The respiratory tract may also contain meconium. As mentioned above, the lungs of class III piglets float (when a fragment of the lung is placed in water) in contrast to the lungs of class I and II piglets.

2. *Quantification of the problem at the herd level* and characterization of its evolution over time (i.e., an acute increase, several fluctuations over time, or steady high rate). When an acute increase is observed, the focus of the investigation must be on any recent changes that may have occurred in the herd.

3. *Identification of other diseases* that may have occurred prior

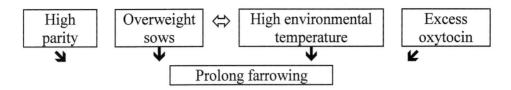

Figure 5
Main risk factors associated with intrapartum deaths due to a prolongation of farrowing.

to, or that may be concurrent with, the stillborn problem (neonatal mortality in liveborn piglets, reproduction problems, localized or systemic diseases).

4. *Identification of the sows from which the majority of stillborns have been recorded.* This starts with an assessment of the parity distribution. For example, stillbirths are generally more prevalent in older sows (higher heterogeneity of the litter, increase in the length of farrowing). Therefore, it is important to consider the demography of the herd. It is also necessary to verify if the increase in the number of stillborns is connected with an increase in some sows only (it is not rare to identify sows that will repeatedly produce numerous stillborns; these sows should be culled).

5. *Identification of risk factors* that would explain the preponderance of one or two of the three classes of stillborns. Because of the importance of intrapartum stillborns, the investigation is often focused on prolong farrowings.

6. *Laboratory investigation of piglets* typical of the observed problem. At least two piglets must be submitted for each problem.

NEONATAL ARTHRITIS AND POLYARTHRITIS

Clinical Importance

Arthritis and polyarthritis are frequent causes of lameness in nursing piglets. Although these diseases rarely reach epidemic proportions, they may have a major impact on production performances and, consequently, on production costs. Contrary to popular belief, such problems are even encountered in herds with high health status.

Cause

Several bacteria can be isolated from lesions (e.g., *Streptococcus suis*, *Streptococcus equisimilis*, other *Staphylococcus* spp., *E. coli*). These are opportunistic pathogens, always present in all breeding herds.

Pathophysiology

Most cases of polyarthritis follow a bacteremia or sometimes a septicemia. It is important to identify the reasons or factors that allowed these bacteria to overcome the defense mechanisms of one or two piglets (rarely more) within affected litters. Although relatively rare, some cases evolve from skin lesions (in splayleg piglets, for example, or after skin necrosis of the knees). A particular form, mainly observed in well-managed herds with high health status, is associated with the premature administration of iron (before 2 days of age) and in too large quantity ($\geq$ 200 mg), particularly in small piglets.[9] Indeed, an excess of iron leads to the saturation of iron-binding proteins, transferrins, providing free iron for bacterial growth.

Clinical Signs

Although early signs are not evident, lameness is the first clinical observation. Even when some articulations appear visually affected, pain is not always apparent in nursing piglets. However, after a few days, emaciation becomes obvious. Polyarthritic piglets are more sensitive to other infections (mainly digestive) because of reduced milk intake. These piglets are also more likely to be crushed by the sow.

Evolution and Risk Factors

The balance that allows piglets to be healthy is complex and delicate. Risk factors associated with polyarthritis are numerous, and so are its clinical expressions (severity of lameness, number of affected piglets, etc.). In most cases of polyarthritis, one joint is more affected than the others.

The fact that this disease occurs in well-managed herds benefiting from a high health status goes against the concept of high infection pressure. However, in this case, the early administration of a large quantity of iron largely contributes to the problem.

The total quantity of colostrum intake is another common risk factor (see Postpartum Dysgalactia Syndrome). One should also consider the underconsumption of colostrum by only a few piglets for a given litter (small or weak piglets, piglets born in

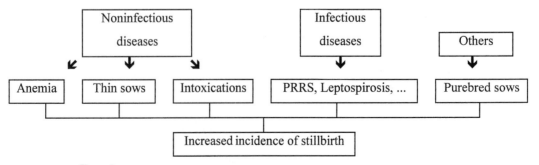

Figure 6
Risk factors associated with intrapartum deaths independent of the duration of farrowing.

the last third of the farrowing period). The quality of the colostrum may sometimes be an issue since, in healthy breeding herds, sows are not submitted to an important infection pressure (mainly para 1 sows).

Herd management is also an important factor. Given identical infection pressure and immunity, any management procedures creating portals of entry for bacteria may result in a higher incidence of polyarthritis. Note that any wounds can easily be infected: umbilical wounds, castration wounds, caudotomy incisions, gum lesions (caused by clipping of the teeth), various cutaneous traumas (tattoos, for example), including fights, are all potential portals of entry for numerous opportunistic agents.

General Approach

The first step is to describe the problem and not to merely observe the presence of arthritis (or polyarthritis). It is an essential step toward the identification of related risk factors. It is very uncommon that only one factor is responsible for such a disease. Small, usually isolated, epidemics are often seen in nursing piglets raised under excellent management and environmental conditions. This is, indeed, a source of great frustration for pig producers. The systemic treatment of all piglets with antibiotics a few days prior to the expected onset of the disease may provide short-term relief in these operations. Vaccines are ordinarily of poor value.

Diagnosis

The clinical diagnosis is generally easy. The pathologic diagnosis is not cause-specific. However, it provides an assessment of the magnitude of the problem and of the prognosis. Several joints may appear normal although they may already be the site of an infection. The etiologic diagnosis is needed to determine the appropriate antibiotic therapy and to ascertain the epidemiology of the disease. The most important diagnosis remains the clinicoepidemiological diagnosis: WHICH PIGLETS (small vs. normal weight; fostered vs. resident piglets; piglets from primiparous or multiparous sows) have WHAT (arthritis, polyarthritis, with or without large tumefactions), WHERE (in pens or crates, in some crates only), WHEN (age at onset), SINCE WHEN (acute or chronic problem), HOW (evolution of the problem, evolution after treatment), and HOW MANY (how many piglets in a litter, how many litters affected). This description is the first and the most important step in the identification of risk factors.

Note that congenital hyperostosis is an uncommon congenital abnormality that can mimic polyarthritis.

Treatment

Curative treatment is sometimes disappointing because it is necessary to treat early and to repeat injections for several days. The early identification of affected piglets is not always easy. Long-acting antibiotics may be useful.

REFERENCES

1. Vaillancourt J-P, Tubbs RC: Preweaning mortality. *In* Tubbs R, Leman A (eds): Vet Clin North Am Food Anim Pract 8:685–706, 1992.
2. Klopfenstein C, Farmer C, Martineau G-P: Diseases of the mammary glands and lactation problems. *In* Straw B, D'Allaire S, Mengeling W, et al. (eds): Diseases of Swine, eds. Ames, Iowa State University Press (in press).
3. Martineau G-P, Vaillancourt J-P, Broes A: Principal neonatal diseases. *In* Varley MA (ed): The Neonatal Pig: Development and Survival, Wallingford, UK, CAB International, 1995, pp 239–268.
4. Klopfenstein C, Bigras-Poulin M, Martineau G-P: La truie potomane, une réalité physiologique. Journees Rech Porc France 28:331–338, 1996.
5. Fraser D, Phillips PA, Thompson BK, et al: Behavioural aspects of piglets survival and growth. *In* Varley MA (ed): The Neonatal Pig: Development and Survival. Wallingford, UK, CAB International, 1995, pp 287–312.
6. Martineau G-P: Approche générale d'un problème de mort-nés. *In* Martineau G-P (ed): Maladies d'élevage des porcs. Paris, France Agricole, 1997, pp 286–289.
7. Vaillancourt J-P, Stein TE, Marsh WE, et al: Validation of producer-recorded causes of preweaning mortality in swine. Prev Vet Med 10:119–130, 1990.
8. Martineau G-P: Approche générale d'un problème d'écrasemenet de porcelets. *In* Martineau G-P (ed): Maladies d'élevage des porcs. Paris, France Agricole, 1997, pp 290–293.
9. Holmgren N: Polyarthritis in piglets caused by iron dextran. *In* Proceedings of the International Pig Veterinary Society. Bologna, Italy, 1996, p 306.

Herd Health Management

Consulting Editor
Terry J. Engelken, D.V.M., M.S.

■ Ovine Production Medicine

Marie S. Bulgin, D.V.M., M.B.A.

The goal of production medicine is to optimize the profitability of a livestock enterprise. This is accomplished by measuring critical production parameters and identifying areas in which improvements can be made. By combining all facets of veterinary medicine with some concepts of animal science and business principles, production medicine attempts to maximize profits within the constraints of the particular management system. In most instances, this is the maximization of pounds of lamb sold per production unit (ewe) at least cost.

Sheep producers make up a very diverse group. Many of these producers call veterinarians in only the direst of emergencies, whereas others expect the same medical treatment for their sheep as for their pets. However, the production medicine–oriented veterinarian, knowledgeable about sheep production and management, is usually able to offer some level of production medicine to meet most clients' goals. Maximizing pounds of lamb sold per ewe while minimizing cost, the goal of production medicine, should also be the goal of most clients.

MARKETING PRODUCTION MEDICINE

Marketing is the process of making skills and services known so that they are understood and desired by potential clients. This involves establishing a relationship of trust with a client, usually by the practice of traditional veterinary medicine. The producer must feel that your primary interest is to help him and that your knowledge is broad enough to qualify you to advise on animal breeding, management, nutrition, marketing, environmental impact, and record-keeping. This involves knowledge and awareness of the markets, new products, governmental regulations, and technologies affecting the industry. Taking the time to talk to your clients and to know their problems, as well as discussing markets and the sheep business, sets the stage for client's willingness to accept and pay for suggestions and recommendations affecting their whole enterprise.

A factor that often keeps veterinarians from the practice of production medicine is their own perception of the low value that producers place on the services rendered and the difficulty in quantifying their worth. To rectify this problem, work out on paper the saving or increase in profit to a client who becomes involved in your recommended production medicine program. This can help sell the program to the producer and, more important, it will give you, the practitioner, a clear sense of the program's practicality and real worth.

When setting fees, know that a certain percentage of time will be spent doing things that are difficult to bill. Charging by

the procedure has been effective in a traditional veterinary practice in which short tasks are being carried out but it doesn't fit well for production medicine. However, clients are accustomed to paying by the hour for other professionals, such as attorneys, accountants, and service providers. Billing for time spent in consultation as well as for definite tasks enables one to take the time to "talk" to the producer and allows compensation when working away from the farm (e.g., solving nutritional problems or reviewing records). Some veterinarians use different rates for different types of work. Define the services that will be provided on a scheduled basis for a set fee; extra services, such as necropsies or laboratory tests, can be billed as additional charges as they occur. A written contract will make clear exactly what is being provided and what payment is expected. A 1-year contract works well when certain goals of herd performance have been identified, and the function of the veterinarian is to help reach these goals. At the end of the year, herd performance gains are reviewed, and the contract is renewed, modified, or forgotten.

GOALS

The ewe has the most untapped potential of any of the food animals. Not only can she commonly produce more than one lamb per gestation, but she has the potential of having two gestations and of producing three-plus lambs per year, wool, and (new to the U.S. farm scene) milk. Furthermore, sheep are more efficient converters of agricultural waste and poor-quality forage than are cattle.

Table 1 suggests some minimal goals as a guide. Five parameters to consider when trying to increase lambs marketed per production unit are conception rate, embryonic and fetal losses, lamb losses, pounds of lamb/ewe sold, and number of gestations per year. To document the area in which change could improve production, a record-keeping system must be in place to monitor those areas.

To effect a change, special attention must be paid to all management periods: prebreeding and breeding, pregnancy, lambing, and lactation in the areas of disease control, nutrition, and genetics (choice of replacement breeding animals). Lambing more than once a year does not fit well into most management situations, but it can be very profitable when it does.

PREBREEDING AND BREEDING MANAGEMENT

Ideally, 90% of the lambing should be completed within 45 days. The most desirable (or profitable) time to have lambs born must be selected. Winter lambing makes use of idle time for

---

Table 1
PRODUCTION PARAMETERS*

Culling

Ewe culling due to problems other than age	<2%–3%
Ram culling due to breeding soundness	<5%–7%

Conception Rate (During September Through December, Northern Latitudes)

Number of mature ewes bred in 45 days	>90%
Number of mature ewes bred in 60 days	>95%
Ewes not lambing	<5%

Fetal Losses

Abortion rate	<1%
Stillbirth	<2%

Lamb Losses

Neonatal lamb losses	<12%†
Total lamb losses	<15%†

Weight Gains, 0–60 Days

Single lambs	>0.5 lb/Day
Twin lambs (added together)	>0.8 lb/Day

*Number of lambs per ewe is dependent on breed, season bred, and nutrition. However, 150% (at least) should be a goal.
†Percent of the total lambs.

---

crop farmers, allows selling of lambs during the traditional period of peak lamb prices (May and June) and before hot summer weather. However, the period of peak lamb prices for the late spring has recently appeared to be shorter in duration and more moderate in its peak. Spring lambing, on the other hand, allows for maximum use of grass and pasture and requires less labor and less elaborate lambing facilities. Ewes and rams tend to be more fertile later in the fall; thus, lambing percentages tend to be higher and lamb losses from inclement weather less likely. The decision regarding when to lamb should be based on breed of sheep, feed costs, lamb prices, weather, labor availability, markets, convenience, and lambing facilities.

An appointment should be set up for the client 180 days prior to the first day chosen for lambing (Table 2). This farm visit should encompass a casual look at the ewes and breeding soundness examinations for the rams. The ewes should be checked for individual ear-tag identification, as no efficient production program can be instituted without keeping individual records. The veterinarian may need to assist the client in performing condition scoring for both the ewe and the ram flock. Unless the ewes have been recently sheared, condition scoring (CS) must be done by actual hands-on palpation of ribs, vertebral processes, and tuber ischia. The animals are rated 1 to 5 according to the following criteria:

1. Extremely thin, emaciated.
2. Thin, but not emaciated. Tuber ischia are prominent; vertebral processes and ribs are easily felt.
3. Tuber ischia, vertebral processes, and last three ribs can be felt but are not prominent. Not fat, not thin.
4. Last three ribs can be felt with some difficulty. Tuber ischia and vertebral processes difficult to feel. The dorsum or back of the sheep is flat.
5. No bones can be palpated. There is an obvious trough down the middle of the back. The brisket is filled with fat and does not hang loose. Obese.

Ovulation rate appears to respond to short-term increased energy intake within a specific intermediate range of body condition (i.e., CS 2 to 3.5). Above and below this range, no additional positive or negative effect is seen.[1] For optimum ovulation and conception, the CS of ewes should be 2.5 approaching 3 (i.e., in a gaining mode during breeding time). Therefore, when breeding begins, the CS of the ewes should be

approximately 2.5, and they must be fed appropriately in the interim. When the rams are turned in, the ewes should be fed for a weight gain of 10 to 15 lb in 2 to 3 weeks' time. This procedure is called *flushing*.

It is not uncommon to find ewes to be too fat (CS 5), in which case they need to lose weight before breeding. Implantation failures and early embryonic deaths are reported to be more common in obese ewes early in pregnancy, but even more difficult to handle are related prolapses later in pregnancy and dystocias. Furthermore, depending on the feed source, having and keeping ewes in this condition may be an unnecessary expense.

The selenium status of the flock could be determined at this time. Previous history of white muscle disease or known selenium status of the area may indicate that selenium supplementation is needed. Otherwise, three to five ewes should be bled into heparin- or EDTA-containing tubes for either glutathione levels or selenium analysis. If blood selenium levels are less than 0.1 ppm or glutathione levels are less than 2.0 mmol/L, supplementation with 90 ppm of selenium in loose salt will give positive results in weight gain, fetal and newborn health, and general flock health. Many so-called selenium salts are not supplemented with the maximum selenium concentration by law (90 ppm). The veterinarian should make it a point to check

---

Table 2
VACCINATION AND WORMING SCHEDULE

30 Days Before Breeding
1. Condition score and separate culls
2. Vaccinate ewes and ewe lambs for *Campylobacter* spp. and *Chlamydia* abortion
3. Deworm, pour-on if necessary
4. Breeding soundness examinations on rams
5. Adjust nutrition
6. Ear tag

21 Days Before Breeding
1. Turn in vasectomized rams

Breeding Time
1. Remove vasectomized rams
2. Turn in breeding rams

30 Days Prior to Lambing
1. Crutch or shear ewe
2. Vaccinate for enterotoxemia C and D
3. Vaccinate for *Escherichia coli*, tetanus, *Clostridium septicum* if desired
4. Adjust nutrition
5. Deworm
6. Start coccidiostats in salt
7. Treat individuals for nasal discharge

Birth
1. Iodine navels
2. Check udders and milk of dam
3. Isolate dam and lamb(s)
4. Make sure lamb nurses
5. Record birth statistics
6. Weigh lamb (optional)

First Week of Life
1. Dock and castrate
2. Ear tag

3–4 Weeks of Life
1. Vaccinate for enterotoxemia C and D
2. Supply coccidiostat in feed or salt for lambs
3. Selenium supplementation if necessary—salt or injections

6–8 Weeks
1. Vaccinate for enterotoxemia C and D
2. Weigh lambs if possible

Weaning
1. Choose replacement ewe lambs
2. Vaccinate replacement ewe lambs with abortion vaccine

mineral concentrations in trace mineral salt mixes, with special attention to copper concentrations as well. Sheep require less copper than most other animals and usually get more than enough in their diets. Never recommend trace mineral formulations with copper concentrations greater than 30 ppm for sheep.

This is the time to cull all ewes that are not fully productive. The owner should examine teeth and udders of all ewes and remove those ewes that are found to have problems. In farm flocks, front teeth, or even their lack, do not usually indicate problems, but hard masses that can be palpated on the mandibles through the skin indicate tooth abscesses and osteomyelitis. Unexplained weight loss and chronic health problems such as foot rot, ovine progressive pneumonia, or caseous lymphadenitis should be recognized and taken care of or the ewes should be culled. The cause of excessive culling (2% to 3% over the number culled for age) should be identified and steps taken to rectify the problem in the upcoming year. Ewes that are kept and replacement ewe lambs should be vaccinated, dewormed, and treated for lice and keds if necessary (see Table 2).

Breeding soundness examination (BSE) often reveals 5% to 10% of young "normal rams" to be infertile or sterile due to factors other than infection. Some of these are probably genetic. Without a BSE, this infertility goes undetected in multi-sire operations. One good ram can cover for several less-than-adequate rams. A fertile ram with good libido can service at least 100 ewes in 45 days under natural breeding systems. However, keeping unnecessary ram power, or rams that are not doing an optimal job, is expensive. Kimberling has estimated an annual maintenance cost of $175 and $225, excluding purchase price, for $200 and $300 rams, respectively.[2] In single-sire flocks, the importance of identifying an infertile ram before breeding season is obvious.

The BSE should begin with a good general physical examination. Rams should have a CS of 3 to 3.5. Feet should be trimmed if needed, and teeth, eyes, and prepuce should be checked. Ulceration of the prepuce (pizzle rot) should be treated at this time, and the scrotal contents should be palpated and measured. Any rams with hernias, epididymitis, or extremely soft or atrophied testicles should be culled. Although rams with abnormally small (Table 3) but normal-feeling testicles are generally fertile, productivity is limited. Daughters of early-maturing ram lambs with large scrotal circumference (>30 cm) at 9 months of age are more early-maturing and productive than daughters of later-maturing rams with small testicle size (<28 cm). If epididymitis is discovered in any ram, all rams passing the semen examination should be bled for the *Brucella ovis* serum enzyme-linked immunosorbent assay (ELISA). Rams with epididymitis and rams testing positive on the ELISA must be culled. For more detailed control methods for epididymitis and/or *B. ovis* see Bulgin[3] and Kimberling and co-workers.[4]

A vasectomized or epididymectomized ram introduced into the flock 2 to 3 weeks before the start of breeding season will stimulate the onset of estrus and advance the breeding season by a couple of weeks. A silent heat generally occurs within 6 days of the introduction of the ram, and a peak number of ewes will simultaneously come into estrus some 18 to 20 days later.

Rams with epididymitis should not be chosen for vasectomies or epididymectomies. The causative agents of epididymitis reside in the bulbourethral and secondary sex glands as well as the epididymis, and they can be transmitted to the ewes via servicing.

MANAGEMENT OF THE PREGNANT EWE

The most common causes of fetal wastage are infectious agents. *B. ovis* transmitted by rams, and bluetongue transmitted by the *Culicoides* gnat (common in some areas of the United States during breeding and early gestational periods) can cause early abortion and implantation failures. *Campylobacter* spp., usually associated with late abortions, also cause early abortions and weak lambs. Toxoplasmosis and *Chlamydia* spp. cause late abortions, stillbirth, and weak lambs. Border disease virus causes weak lambs, hairy lambs, and lambs that appear premature. A history of abortions, stillbirths, mummified fetuses, and/or nonpregnant ewes usually indicates an infectious disease in the flock. However, diagnosis after the fact is difficult, and proceeding with a good disease control program is the best way to attack the problem.

Use of *B. ovis* ELISA-negative rams for breeding and vaccinating ewes against *Campylobacter* spp. controls losses from those two organisms. Vaccine against bluetongue serotype 10 is commercially available*; however, it gives no protection against other serotypes. Vaccines against other serotypes of bluetongue are also available in some states, but as of this writing they cannot be taken across state lines. Use of insect repellent sprays, fly tags, and elimination of muddy areas in which the vector (*Culicoides*) breeds seems to help. The use of cattle vaccines against border disease (bovine viral diarrhea) has not been shown to be effective.

Eliminating intact, female barn cats can reduce the threat of toxoplasmosis and feeding of tetracycline, 200 mg/head/day, for 30 days before lambing will control *Chlamydia* problems in most cases.

Pregnancy testing of ewes with real-time ultrasound 45 to 60 days after the breeding season is now an accurate, practical, and economic practice. It can be utilized to discover whether "dud" stud rams or early embryonic death is a problem in a flock. More than 3% to 4% open ewes would indicate a problem.

---

*Colorado Serum Co, 4950 York St, Denver, CO 80216.

Table 3
BREEDING SOUNDNESS CRITERIA FOR RAMS

	Score*								
	8	7	6	5	4	3	2	1	0
Scrotal circumference (cm)†									
<12 mo	>32		30		29		28		<25
12–18 mo	>36		34		32		31		<30
>18 mo	>39		37		35		33		<32
Spermatozoa motility (% normal)	—		—	>80	>60	>50	>30	>20	>20
Morphology (% normal)	>90	>80	>70	>60	>50	>40	>30		>20

*Excellent, >16; satisfactory, 8–16; unsatisfactory, <8, or >5 WBCs per high-power field, or epididymitis in one or both testicles.
†Scrotal circumference normally decreases by 1 to 2 cm during anestrous periods.

Possible causes to rule out would include ram fertility, nutrition, or disease.

Used routinely, ultrasound examination would allow culling of noneconomical production units in the flock. The average cost of feeding and maintaining a farm flock ewe is $65 to $85 per year. Kimberling and associates calculated that the cost of keeping a nonproducing ewe vs. a producing ewe is $80 over the cost of feeding her.[4] Ewes carrying twins and triplets may also be identified, if desired, for special care or feeding. In very productive flocks, ultrasound might allow a producer to sell off ewes having only single fetuses. Under farm flock conditions, when the cost of maintaining a ewe is between $65 and $85, it requires 1.3 to 1.6 lambs marketed per ewe to pay for the ewe's maintenance. Thus, pregnancy testing can help ensure that the lamb crop is adequate to pay the bills. Kott and Padula give details involving instruments and techniques.[6]

PRELAMBING MANAGEMENT

Twenty to 30 days before the beginning of lambing season, three very important activities should be scheduled: shearing or crutching, veterinary care (vaccination, worming, and control of *Coccidia* and *Pasteurella* spp.), and nutritional adjustment (see Table 2). This is an excellent time to schedule a second examination of the ewe flock and to look over the lambing facilities, particularly if the owner is a novice.

Shearing or Crutching

Winter shearing is practiced by a few producers with great success; however, shelter will need to be available in case of unexpected inclement weather immediately after shearing. Crutching, or the removal of wool from around the vulva and udder, is an important disease management practice for the control of both *Escherichia coli* scours and *Coccidia* spp. infections in the lambs. Furthermore, it allows the producer to observe both the swelling of the vulva and enlargement of the udder, which are signs that lambing will occur within 1 to 3 weeks. The ewes can then be separated from the others for increased feeding and attention.

Veterinary Activities

Some form of coccidial control should be instituted at this time. Coccidiostats such as lasalocid* or decoquinate* can be mixed into salt (2 lb of 15% lasalocid premix per 50 lb of salt or 2 lb of 6% decoquinate premix per 50 lb of salt) and offered on a free-choice basis to the ewes until lambing. Coccidial numbers shed by the ewes into the environment are vastly decreased, thus reducing the dose to the newborn lamb.

Vaccination of the ewe flock at this time ensures having maximum levels of specific antibodies in the colostrum. Protection of the young lambs against *Clostridium perfringens* is imperative in any flock, whereas other diseases such as *E. coli* scours and tetanus can be of importance in individual flocks with previous histories of those diseases.

If white muscle disease has been diagnosed in the flock or in the area, or the area in which the feed was grown, supplementation with selenium in the salt at this time is advisable. It will not interfere with the use of decoquinate or lasalocid. The injectable selenium products are labeled against use in late pregnancy in the ewe.

The heavy nasal discharge seen in ewes during this time of the year may be caused by *Oestrus ovis*, the nasal bot fly larva. Such discharge is generally laden with *Pasteurella* spp. and is a source of early *Pasteurella* infection of neonatal lambs, which is transmitted as the dam licks them off. Individual treatment of these ewes with ivermectin† and long-acting oxytetracycline† usually alleviates the problem.

Nutritional Adjustment

In the third trimester of pregnancy, the time of 75% of fetal growth, the ewes may require dietary adjustment. The veterinarian can be of great help in planning and balancing diets. The utilization of least-cost nutritional computer programs makes this job exceptionally easy, but it can also be done using the tables found in *Nutrient Requirements of Sheep*.[7] The previous flock production history usually dictates current flock nutrition management unless multiparous ewes have been identified with real-time sonography. If so, the flock can be separated according to fetal numbers and fed exactly what they need for the number of fetuses. Proper nutrition at this time is necessary for vigorous lambs and optimal lactation at parturition.

LAMBING MANAGEMENT

Lambing management is well covered in Gates' book *A Practical Guide to Sheep Disease Management*,[8] which should be recommended reading for the producer. A barn sheet for recordkeeping is a must. Lambs need to be identified, weighed (optional), and recorded. Birth weights are called for in most computer programs designed to evaluate ewe productivity. Neonatal lamb deaths should not exceed 10% to 12%, but many management and disease problems quickly cause neonatal losses to soar.

Because on-farm necropsy of aborted fetuses is seldom helpful, producers can mail aborted fetuses directly to the diagnostic laboratory for culture. Some laboratories accept frozen fetuses for culture, whereas others prefer them fresh. Know if the laboratory is capable of diagnosing *Chlamydia;* then let the producer know how to store, package, and mail fetuses and placentas to the laboratory that your research indicates will do the best job. Be sure that the producer knows that the placenta is by far the most useful specimen for diagnosis.

Abortion control is dependent on vaccination for *Campylobacter* and the use of tetracycline in feed or water prior to lambing to control *Chlamydia*. Chlamydial vaccines are not particularly reliable. Thus, if a flock has a history of *Chlamydia* abortion, tetracycline should be administered in feed or water at the rate of 250 mg/head/day 3 to 4 weeks prior to the onset of lambing. It should be continued for at least 60 days.

Because aborting ewes continue to excrete the infectious agent for several weeks, they should be immediately separated from the pregnant ewes. The area contaminated by the fetus and fluids should be disinfected and the fetus and placenta removed and destroyed. Disinfecting can be done by burning a bale of straw at the site, throwing lime on the spot, or pouring household bleach liberally over the area.

The newborn lamb is not able to maintain its body temperature in the face of extreme environmental temperatures for the first 36 hours of life. More than a half hour of exposure to cold or wet weather rapidly leads to hypothermia, hypoglycemia, weakness, and death. Lambs with temperatures below 100°F should be tubed with colostrum and warmed. The use of a hair dryer is probably the best method for warming hypothermic lambs. Warm water baths are effective, but the warmed wet lamb tends to cool off again while drying, and the identifying

---

*Cleared for use in sheep in the United States.

†Not cleared for use in sheep in the United States.

odor of the lamb is washed off. Many ewes then reject the lamb on its return. Giving 20 mL of 5% dextrose solution subcutaneously helps supply needed energy while the lamb is warming. Two to 4 oz of thawed or fresh cow, goat, or ewe colostrum definitely increases survival of lambs inadequately supplied by their mothers. Udders of the periparturient ewe should always be checked and stripped, verifying that a full-appearing udder is not actually "hard bag," the mastitic form of ovine progressive pneumonia (OPP). Ewes with abnormal milk should be milked out and treated immediately with an intra-mammary dry cow mastitis product or a long-acting oxytetracy-cline injection. This procedure should be repeated at least twice a day until signs abate. *Staphylococcus aureus* is one of the most common agents causing subclinical infection and is also commonly implicated in gangrenous mastitis. *Streptococcus agalactiae*, *S. uberis*, *E. coli*, *Pasteurella multocida*, and *P. haemolytica* are also found in subclinical, acute, and generalized mastitis. The advent of sheep dairying in this country has revealed that subclinical mastitis in the sheep is common. The California mastitis test (CMT) is a simple procedure to check for subclinical mastitis in any flock. The test needs to be conducted at least 5 days after lambing, as colostrum will give a positive reaction on the CMT. Weaning management so far has been the only practical control method for ovine mastitis (see discussion of weaning).

Although starvation is the primary cause of neonatal lamb death on most farms, its cause must be identified. Exposure, trauma (being laid upon or mashed by an unfriendly ewe), and in utero disease all render weak lambs unable to get up to suck.

Diarrhea, which occurs during the first 3 days after birth, is generally caused by enterotoxic *E. coli*. *Clostridium perfringens* type C, *E. coli*, and *Pasteurella* septicemia can also cause death this early, but are less common. *E. coli* diarrhea and *Pasteurella* septicemia and pneumonia are generally spread by the ewes.

Diagnoses of most neonatal lamb problems can be made on gross necropsy and the producer should be encouraged to either bring dead lambs to you or to save them and have them necropsied on a biweekly visit to the farm. Dead lambs younger than 60 days of age cool rapidly. If they are kept cool and away from predators, they will remain in good necropsy condition for several days. Older sheep with functional rumens, particularly those with heavy fleeces, deteriorate rapidly. Six to 8 hours is usually the maximal allowable time between death and necropsy.

In the case of *E. coli* scours or very early pneumonia, antibiotics can be used prophylactically. One dose of an antibiotic, such as trimethoprim-sulfamethoxazole* or spectinomycin,* given orally within the first 12 hours after birth is extremely effective.

Docking and castration should be done early; 2 or 3 days of age is probably best, particularly when elastrators are used. Elastrators are very popular with producers due to ease, reduction of secondary infections and weight loss, lack of bloodshed, and elimination of any possibility of herniation and of fly strike in warmer weather. Tetanus, which has been associated with their use, can easily be prevented by the use of tetanus toxoid in the ewes prior to parturition. However, colostral antibodies last only for 4 weeks or so; thus elastrators should not be used after this time unless tetanus antitoxin is given prior to the procedure. See Table 2 for vaccination schedules. If dams were not vaccinated for clostridial infections before lambing, lambs should be vaccinated earlier, at 1 or 2 weeks of age.

Lambs should be weighed sometime before weaning to evaluate both the milking ability of the ewe and the growth potential of the lambs. Average daily gain is a simple parameter to measure ewe productivity for culling purposes and for choosing replacement breeding stock. It can also indicate the presence of a flock problem. Single lambs should gain at least 0.5 lb/day, and twin lambs together should average at least 0.8 lb/day. Fast-growing, early-maturing "mutton" breeds should do much

better. If a large number of lambs are gaining less than 0.5 lb/day, energy and protein nutrition, mineral supplementation, and/or disease may all be implicated.

Maximizing Pounds of Lambs for Sale

In many farm flock situations, marketing lambs as early as possible has been economically advantageous. Generally, the earlier in the year the lambs go to market, the higher the price. Additionally, the producer has more free time and lambs have less time for problems to develop. In this case, concentrate feeding should be started at about 3 weeks of age, when lambs begin to nibble at solid feed. Subclinical coccidial infections, probably present in all lambs, interfere with optimal weight gains and should be controlled in any lamb feeding situation. Lasalocid† may have a further advantage over other coccidiostats because of improving feed efficiency. Sulfa drugs, the most effective agents for treatment and the most expensive, should be reserved for treatment of clinical cases.

Weaning

Weaning of lambs may be early (at 3 to 4 weeks of age, when ewes are to go in the milking string or to be bred back for twice-a-year lambing); late (at 6 to 9 months, in range or pasture management systems); or at 60 to 90 days (for early marketing). Lambs weaned at 6 to 9 months usually go straight to market weighing 110 to 120 lb, depending on breed and feed. Lambs weaned at 60 days or 60 lb can be grown out and fattened on pasture, on concentrates in the feedlot, or on such things as turnips, onions, ensilage, and on aftermath of grass seed, alfalfa, sugar beets, and/or other crops.

Management of ewes at this time to reduce milk production will help a great deal in the prevention of mastitis. This is especially important when weaning lambs at 3 to 4 weeks, as ewes should be at the peak of their milk production. Two days before weaning, remove feed from ewes. A creep should be available for lambs. The day of weaning, water should be taken away from the ewes as well. It is best to leave the lambs in the area with which they are familiar and to remove the ewes. Water can be supplied to the ewe the day after the lambs are taken away, then 1 to 2 lb of straw or very poor-quality hay made available to the ewes on day 4 and for the rest of the week. At the end of the week, the ewes' udders should be examined by palpation for evidence of heat, hardness, or pain. If any of these are present, the ewe should be treated immediately for mastitis. Lopsided udders are usually evidence of subclinical mastitis in the smaller half of the udder. These should be cultured and treated with either dry cow intramammary infusion or an intramuscular injection of a long-acting antibiotic. In fact, all dairy ewes should be so treated.

On a high-concentrate diet, 60- to 90-day-old coccidia-free healthy mutton-type lambs are able to approach or surpass gains of 1 lb/day, particularly when started at 3 weeks of age. Gains of creep-fed lambs will slump, however, if placed on high-roughage feeds after weaning, due to the immaturity of the rumen at this age. Internal parasites, specifically helminths, can reduce gains or even cause clinical problems if lambs are placed on pasture or have been pastured before weaning with their dams.

Management of early weaned lambs is a little trickier, as they cannot utilize roughage well at 3 to 4 weeks of age, and a highly digestible protein substitute for the dam's milk must be fed if the lambs are going to do well. Soybean meal is very palatable to lambs and is probably the protein supplement of choice. Milk pellets are excellent but expensive; however, they may be cost-effective in small amounts. Because the immature rumen cannot

---

*Not cleared for use in sheep in the United States.

handle fiber well, rolled corn is usually used because of palatability and digestibility.

Most diseases of the feedlot lamb are diet- and management-related. Urolithiasis, for example, is related to the calcium-phosphorus ratio in the diet, which should optimally be 2 to 3:1 for prevention. In high-concentrate diets, it will be necessary to add calcium, usually in the form of limestone. Ammonium salts for acidifying urine may also be added in the form of ammonium chloride or ammonium sulfate as 1% of the diet. Sodium chloride may be added as 1% to 2% of the diet as well, to increase water intake and decrease crystal formation in the bladder. Availability of water is of utmost importance, particularly when salt is added to the feed.

Polioencephalomalacia may be caused by a thiamine deficiency exacerbated by the high demand for thiamine in the metabolism of carbohydrates, low amounts of thiamine in mixed feeds, and/or presence of thiaminase-producing bacteria in the rumen. Addition of thiamine in the total diet at a concentration of 0.05 lb of thiamine per ton will usually eliminate cases of polioencephalomalacia. However, high levels of sulfates in feed or water have also been shown to cause a non–thiamine-responsive polioencephalomalacia in lambs and steers.

Rectal prolapse is most often seen in females late in the feeding period. Coughing exacerbated by upper respiratory disease or dusty conditions and straining caused by enteritis (coccidia, *Salmonella* spp., acidosis) are also associated with prolapse. Prevention is difficult and is usually directed at the control of coughing or enteric problems. Leaving tails shorter than 2 to 3 inches when docking has long been associated with rectal prolapse; nevertheless, short docks are still favored for show animals.

Pneumonia is most often caused by *Pasteurella haemolytica* and is very similar to the shipping fever complex seen in cattle in that stress, viruses, and *Mycoplasma* spp. are considered to be initiators. It is commonly seen at commercial feedlots in young lambs recently weaned and transported. Sheep tend to carry the organisms in the nose and/or tonsils. Stress appears to reduce the animal's normal defense mechanisms, allowing these opportunistic organisms access to the lung. Antibiotics in the feed or water are helpful if the organism is susceptible. However, lambs in new surroundings sometimes will not eat or drink for the first few days. Availability of running water and familiar feeds or any innovative enticements to eat or drink will reduce stress and disease. *Pasteurella* spp. are well known for becoming resistant to antibiotics, so necropsies and cultures are warranted when treatments do not work. Vaccination of lambs with live virus cattle products against infectious bovine rhinotracheitis (IBR), parainfluenza virus type 3 (PI₃), and bovine respiratory syncytial virus (BRSV) has, when given before shipping, conferred some protection against disease. In a controlled study, 35% of nonvaccinated lambs suffered from pneumonia during their stay in the feedlot, vs. 18% of the vaccinated lambs.[9]

Enterotoxemia is prevented by vaccination against *C. perfringens* types C and D. However, sporadic sudden deaths have been seen in vaccinated lambs on high-concentrate diets. Many producers have attributed these to failure of enterotoxemia vaccine. However, they can also be due to acidosis or grain overload. Diagnosis is relatively simple in the dead lambs by checking rumen pH using pH paper. Normally, rumen pH in lambs on high-concentrate diets is found to be around 6.5, whereas rumen pH in those dead of acidosis will be around 4.5 to 5.5. Although acidosis may be due to sudden changes in feed, it often occurs unrelated to any identifiable form of management change or error. Addition to the diet of more roughage, lasalocid, or buffers (e.g., sodium bicarbonate and calcium carbonate) can often reduce these losses.

Problems of Dry Ewes

Normally, dry ewes are problem-free and require little effort in management, other than the attention given to ensuring they reach the CS needed for later breeding. This is a good time, however, to tackle and eliminate foot rot if it is endemic in the flock. The *Sheep Production Handbook*[10] outlines the steps required for control of foot rot.

If ewes are grazing green pastures, internal parasites can be a problem. Periodic fecal checks for ova are a service that the production-oriented veterinarian can provide. Keeping track of parasite load is the only way to fashion a strategic worming program. Managed intensive grazing alone does not eliminate the need to deworm.

Unexplained weight loss during the dry period may also be due to endemic disease in the flock such as ovine progressive pneumonia (OPP), caseous lymphadenitis, Johne's disease, or scrapie. Osteomyelitis of the mandible or maxilla may also be responsible for weight loss and can result from grass awn–contaminated pasture or hay. Awns invade the intradental spaces between gum and teeth, initiating infection and even loss of teeth. Affected ewes are unable to ruminate effectively.

Some diseases of dry ewes are much more acute. Blue-green algae, copper and nitrate toxicosis, fluke infestation leading to Black's disease, and bluetongue can all occur in late summer. In these diseases, weight loss is generally not a sign.

Producers should be encouraged to have necropsies done on any dead animals. Certainly they should be performed if more than 3% of the flock is affected. If affected animals do not die, then several animals should be sacrificed and a diagnosis arrived at.

Diagnosis of OPP or caseous lymphadenitis should lead to implementing some means of control. Blood testing for OPP is available, and culling of affected ewes (if not many are affected) is relatively simple. However, separation of animals with positive and negative findings, taking lambs from mothers before sucking, and testing twice a year may be in order for producers to rid the disease from a flock that is heavily infected.[11]

Because the blood test for caseous lymphadenitis (*Corynebacterium pseudotuberculosis*) is not routinely available at most laboratories, and the specificity of the test still leaves a little to be desired, control is still elusive. At this time, vaccination* is probably the control method of choice.

OTHER CONSIDERATIONS IN PRODUCTION MEDICINE
Records

Production medicine requires good dependable records to identify the areas of management that require change for optimization of production. In smaller flocks, hand-kept records are adequate. However, owners of large flocks with more than 100 ewes may want to go to a computerized system. Some producers have their own program or are subscribing to computerized records. Several breed associations are encouraging members to subscribe. Computerized records should keep track of the pounds of lamb and wool each ewe in the flock has produced, compare the production of young ewes with that of older ewes, record health problems or other variables determined by the producer or the veterinarian to be important, and compare performance of lambs from various sires. It should also compute the average daily gain of lambs adjusted for sex and type of birth (e.g., single, twin). Productivity of the ewes and rams should be ranked to allow the culling of the poorer producers and their offspring and to choose offspring of the higher producers for replacements. Most extension agents have information about computerized production programs for sheep.

Replacement Ewe Lambs

Ewe replacements, preferably those from outstanding production ewes, need to be identified at weaning or soon after and

---

*Not cleared for use in sheep in the United States.

separated from the feeder lambs. Although high-concentrate diets with adequate protein contribute to fast growth rates, it is not beneficial to fatten replacement ewe lambs. Not only will losses from rectal prolapses be more likely, but as the udder fills with fat, milk-producing tissue is crowded out, and milk production of the ewe lamb is reduced.

Ewe lambs, however, should be supplemented enough to guarantee a size adequate for breeding in the late fall (two-thirds of their mature body weight). Ewe lambs that breed and conceive as ewe lambs have been found to be more productive throughout their entire lifetime, even when not counting the progeny from the first pregnancy. Ewe lambs selected on the basis of the dams' production should be the best ewes in the flock, and their offspring from production-selected sires should prove to be the future best lambs in the flock. Thus, breeding ewe lambs speeds up the genetic improvement of the flock.

Ewe lambs usually do not breed until they reach 60% to 70% of their mature body size. They require additional nutritional supplementation during breeding, pregnancy, and the year after they lamb if they are to breed back and reach their potential mature size. The duration of estrus is shorter for ewe lambs than the older females and rams tend to show a preference for the more mature females. Ewe lambs in heat tend to make little or no attempt to approach the ram, but will accept service. Thus, ewe lambs need to be kept apart from the ewes for both breeding and feeding.

LAMBING MORE THAN ONCE A YEAR

For flocks that are *not* composed of Dorsets, Polypays, Finnsheep, Merinos, Rambouillets, or other breeds with a long breeding season, lambing in the fall becomes a matter of artificially inducing estrus. In general, this is not practical. However, there are special cases in which producers enlist the aid of the veterinarians to fool nature. Intravaginal pessaries (sponges) or controlled internal drug-release (CIDR) dispensers utilizing a synthetic progesterone are available and are used extensively outside the United States. Producers from the United States often obtain them. They are extremely useful for inducing early mating of 9- to 11-month-old female lambs after reaching an adequate body weight, increasing the number of lambings a year by mating ewes in the spring to facilitate the practice of artificial insemination (AI) or synchronizing lambing.[12]

The synthetic progesterone has some adverse effects on the survival of spermatozoa in the female genital tract, which makes it necessary to mate animals during the second half of heat (36 to 48 hours after initiation). Sponges are placed in the vagina for 10 to 12 days (a longer time reduces fertility). This treatment does not work well on lactating ewes, as only 15% to 20% will become pregnant.

Subcutaneous implants have also been used. Norgestomet (Searle) is used outside the United States, but Syncro-Mate B* (Ceva), which is available in the United States for synchronizing estrous cycles in cows, has been used with moderately good results.[13] The 6-mg Syncro-Mate B implant must be cut in half for use in sheep and implanted over the cartilage of the ear, from which it can easily be removed. The injectable norgestomet-estradiol valerate that is included in the packaging is not required. Removal of the implant at the end of 10 to 12 days results in an onset of estrus in 24 hours. Cattle show a decrease in fertility if bred on the first heat, but breeding on the second heat results in an increased pregnancy rate. It may be similar in ewes. The conception rate with implants appears to be reduced 10% compared with that of sponges, but the prolificacy is about the same in adult ewes. Unfortunately, the implants are not as

effective in lambs unless pregnant mare serum gonadotrophin (PMSG) injections are given when implants are removed.

The prostaglandin products (dinoprost tromethamine,* cloprostenol sodium*) used for synchronizing heat cycles of cattle have been used for synchronizing estrus in the cycling ewe. They will not initiate estrus during anestrus. As in the cow, for best results, two injections are required 11 days apart. Breeding on the first heat (which occurs 12 to 48 hours later) often causes a decrease in lambing percentage. For optimum lamb numbers, it may be better to breed the ewes on the second heat, 17 to 18 days after the second injection. The dose is usually a third to a quarter of that used in cows.

Light is the primary environmental factor controlling the natural onset of estrus. Cycling for most breeds usually begins 8 to 10 weeks after the longest day of the year, and this can be very variable depending on the breed. Polypays, Finnsheep, Dorsets, Merinos, and Rambouillets are U.S. breeds having the longest breeding season, and individuals of those breeds may show a great deal of flexibility for breeding during the anestrus period. However, fertility generally is greatest during the middle of the breeding season for all sheep, both rams and ewes.

Artificial alteration of illumination can alter the breeding season. Estrus is triggered by decreasing light exposure to 10 hours. To utilize light for initiating estrus, fluorescent lights are recommended (1 ft of bulb per 10 ft² of floor space). The ewes are exposed to 18 to 20 hours of light for 60 days, after which the light is reduced to 10 to 12 hours; estrus should then occur within several days. The rams require the treatment as well. Fifty percent to 60% of the ewes should conceive. Outdoor exposure using mercury vapor lamps has also been reported to work.

The STAR sheep accelerated management system was developed at Cornell University for taking advantage of the sheep's potential for two gestations a year without using hormones.[15] It requires the use of a breed with a long breeding season (in their program they utilize Dorset and Finnsheep breeds). By exposing the dry flock to a ram or rams known to breed "out-of-season," for five equally spaced 30-day periods, five back-to-back lambing-lactation cycles are produced annually. The shortest interval between lambing for each ewe is 7.2 months, with a second chance at 9.6 months and a third at a 12-month interval. In addition to increasing ewe productivity and improving feed utilization, the STAR system can maximize use of lambing and feeder lamb facilities, reduce risk, even out cash flow and labor requirements, and, most important, allow a year-round supply of young, efficiently grown lambs. Veterinarians and producers interested in this system should contact the Animal Science Department at Cornell University (Ithaca, NY).

SCRAPIE CERTIFICATION PROGRAM

Scrapie, a recognized sheep disease for more than 250 years, became a public health concern recently owing to its assumed relationship to bovine spongiform encephalopathy (BSE). Present in the United States since 1947, scrapie has been diagnosed in some 850 flocks as of 1996. Although it is a disease primarily reported in Suffolk sheep, it has been reported in Cheviots, Corriedales, Dorsets, Hampshires, Finnsheep, Merinos, Shropshires, Montadales, Southdowns, Rambouillets, and a Cotswold.[15]

The agent is thought to be a protein, called a *prion*, believed to be spread at lambing through the birthing fluids. The disease takes at least 2 to 4 years to manifest; the most well-known sign is itching. However, signs may vary widely among individuals. The most consistent signs are progressive weight loss, hind end weakness, recumbency, and inevitable death in 2 to 5 months. No live animal test for the disease has yet been developed.

*Not cleared for use in sheep in the United States.

Confirmation requires histopathologic examination of brain tissue or, more recently, a test for the specific protein in the brain.

Due to lack of a live animal test, scrapie eradication has been difficult to address. However, in 1993 the Scrapie Voluntary Certification Program was initiated and is administered by the United States Department of Agriculture (USDA). This program is based on good records, diagnosis of all adult deaths, and closing the flock to all but other certified sheep. After a 5-year "observation" period, and annual checks by a federal veterinarian, the flock progresses through several levels of certification. A scrapie-free certification is given if no evidence of scrapie-induced disease is found. The flock remains certified scrapie-free unless scrapie is identified as originating from the flock or it leaves the program.

Veterinarians need to become familiar with the signs of scrapie and cultivate a high degree of suspicion when faced with the diagnosis of a CNS, wool loss, or locomotor problem of slow onset, long duration, and inevitable death in adult sheep older than 2 years. If in doubt, contact your Federal Veterinary Services Office.

In the meantime, a movement by packing houses is in progress to require signed statements from lamb sellers that guarantees that the lambs originated from a scrapie-free flock.[15] Sheep breeders who plan to stay in business should probably give some thought to or be encouraged to join the Voluntary Scrapie Program. Drawbacks are the need to procure rams from certified flocks and record-keeping. However, the records needed are less extensive than are required for good flock management.

Recent research has suggested that genetics play a part in whether a sheep will become clinically infected, how quickly signs of scrapie will appear, and how long the animal will take to die. Two sites on the chromosomes of Suffolk sheep appear to affect the susceptibility of the breed to scrapie.[16] These are referred to as codon 171 and codon 136. At site 171, one of three genes can be present: Q, R, or H. The scrapie-infected sheep in the United States have been found to be QQ. The R gene apparently confers immunity to clinical scrapie; thus, it is presently believed that QR, RR, and RH animals are resistant. In a sampling of 500 Suffolk sheep, 54% were QQ and 43% carried the R gene. Only 4% were RR.

Gene A or V is found at codon 136. Gene V is associated with a high susceptibility to strain A of the scrapie agent. Information from other countries suggests that gene V will override the resistance conferred by R to this particular scrapie strain. Not many U.S. Suffolks have the V gene, nor has strain A of scrapie been found yet in the United States. All the scrapie-affected sheep in the United States that have been tested so far have been AA QQ. Many Suffolk breeders are testing their breeding animals and selecting for those with the R gene. Testing requires only a tube of EDTA blood and costs approximately $35.* Unfortunately, the research has not been done on other sheep breeds in the United States.

REFERENCES

1. Gunn RG: The influence of nutrition on the reproductive performance of ewes. *In* Haresign W (ed): Sheep Production. Kent, England, Butterworth, 1983, pp 103–104.
2. Kimberling CV: The cost associated with maintaining a *Brucella ovis* (ram epididymitis) infected ram flock. *In* Proceedings of the Western Regional Coordinating Committee 46 meeting (Ram Epididymitis and Footrot). Reno, Nev, 1987, pp 14–18.
3. Bulgin MS: Epididymitis in rams. Vet Clin North Am Food Anim Pract 6:683–690, 1990.
4. Kimberling CV, Schweitzer D, Butler J, et al: A new way to eradicate ram epididymitis. Vet Med 82:424, 1987.
5. Kimberling CV: Just one more chance: Does it make cents? *In* Proceedings of the American Association of Small Ruminant Practitioners and Western Regional Coordinating Committee 46 meeting. Corvallis, Ore, 1990, p 87.
6. Kott RW, Padula RF: Pregnancy diagnosis and fetal number determination in sheep. *In* Proceedings of the American Association of Small Ruminant Practitioners and Western Regional Coordinating Committee 46 meeting, Boise, 1989, pp 29–37.
7. Subcommittee on Sheep Nutrition, Committee on Animal Nutrition, Agriculture National Research Council: Nutrient Requirements of Sheep, ed 6. Washington, DC, National Academy Press, 1985.
8. Gates N: A Practical Guide to Sheep Disease Management. Moscow, Idaho, News-Review Publishing Co, 1985, pp 9–22.
9. Hansen DE, McCoy RD, Armstrong DA: Six vaccination trials in feedlot lambs for the control of lamb respiratory disease complex. Agri-Pract 9:19, 1995.
10. SID, Sheep Production Handbook. Sheep Industry Development Program, Dept I, 200 Clayton St, Denver, CO 80206.
11. Bulgin MS: Ovine progressive pneumonia, caprine arthritis-encephalitis, and related lentiviral disease of sheep and goats. Vet Clin North Am Food Anim Pract 6:691–704, 1990.
12. Wheaton JE, Calson KM, Windels HF, et al: Use of controlled internal drug release (CIDR) dispensers for controlled breeding of sheep. *In* Proceedings of the Out of Season Breeding Symposium. Ames, Iowa, 1992.
13. Youngs CR: Utilization of norgestomet (Syncro-Mate-B) implants for out of season breeding of sheep. *In* Proceedings of the Out of Season Breeding Symposium. Ames, Iowa, 1992.
14. Magee B: STAR accelerated lambing system. *In* Proceedings of the American Association of Small Ruminant Practice and Western Regional Coordinating Committee 46 meeting, Corvallis, Ore, 1990, p 47.
15. Wilson SI: Scrapie Update. Livestock Conservation Institute, Bowling Green, Ky, 1996.
16. O'Rourke KI, Melco RP, Mickelson JR: Allelic frequencies of an ovine scrapie susceptibility gene. Anim Biotechnol 2:155, 1996.

■ Production Medicine and Health Problems in Goats

Bruce M. Olcott, D.V.M., M.S., M.B.A.

The 1990s have been a tumultuous decade for the North American goat industry. The reason for the tumult was the arrival of the South African Boer goat. The result of this new entry was the beginning of the incorporation of the meat goat industry into mainstream agriculture. This change in the industry provides great opportunities and challenges for us veterinarians.

Goat production can be divided into the following sectors: dairy, meat, fiber, and pet, with weed control an important sideline of most goat production systems. Goats have tremendous potential to produce meat, milk, and fiber; however, the industry is plagued by health issues that limit production efficiency. There is great potential for improvement of disease control through cost-effective herd health programs.

CAPRINE HERD HEALTH PROGRAMS

Herd health programs have to be tailor-made to fit individual herds and will depend on the herd size, the purpose of having the herd, and the production goals of the owner. For the most part goats are managed in small groups of 5 to 50 animals. Purebred sales, showing, Four-H projects, and production of milk and meat for home use are the major reasons for keeping these small herds. Small herds tend to have high nonproductive-productive ratios. Large commercial herds may have more than

---

*Genecheck, 400 E Horsetooth Rd, Fort Collins, CO 80521, or University of Minnesota, Dr. James Mickleson, Rm 295, AS/Veterinary Medicine Bldg, 1988 Fitch Ave, St. Paul, MN 55101.

1000 head of goats. In general these herds are better managed than the small herds. However, when problems occur they occur on a larger scale. Cost-effective preventive programs are critical to large-scale goat raising.

Management practices contribute significantly to disease problems. Goat husbandry is very labor-intensive, and many herds are maintained by people who earn their living away from the farm. Disease problems can often be eliminated by correct management, with emphasis on proper sanitation, nutrition, and animal husbandry.

1. Kids and Weanlings
   a. Dry off kids immediately after birth and provide a warm, dry, clean environment. Kids are very susceptible to hypothermia. Kids may be removed from their dams at this time if they are to be bottle-reared.
   b. Dip or spray the kid's navel and soles of the feet with tincture of iodine immediately following birth.
   c. Clean the dam's teats and strip milk from each teat.
   d. Feed 2 oz of colostrum within 30 to 60 minutes of birth (by stomach tube if necessary) and provide colostrum for the next 3 to 4 days or for as many feedings as available.
   e. Examine kids for congenital defects.
   f. Disbud kids as soon as buttons can be detected, usually from 3 days to 2 weeks of age. Castrate male kids at the same time.
   g. If coccidiosis is a problem in the herd, treat with a coccidiostat beginning the second week of life.
   h. If nutritional muscular dystrophy is a problem, inject kids with vitamin E and selenium at 1 to 2 weeks of age and repeat in 4 weeks.
   i. At 1 month of age, vaccinate with *Clostridium perfringens* Types C & D Toxoid and with *Clostridium tetani* Toxoid. Repeat this in 2 to 4 weeks. Other optional vaccines may be started at this time.
   j. Begin nematode parasite control programs at 1 month of age. Monitor parasite egg counts and deworm as necessary.
   k. Separate doe kids from intact buck kids before 3 to 4 months of age.
2. Does
   a. Check does for mastitis at freshening, at dryoff, and any time you are suspicious they may have mastitis. Use a strip cup and California Mastitis Test (CMT) paddle. Infuse glands of dairy goats with dry cow antibiotic products at the time of dryoff.
   b. Feet should be checked monthly and trimmed as needed. Routinely trim feet 1 month before the breeding season begins and 1 month prior to kidding.
   c. Vaccinate 1 month prior to the start of breeding for chlamydiosis, leptospirosis, and vibriosis if these diseases are important in your area or herd.
   d. Perform pregnancy tests on all does by ultrasound at 45 to 60 days postbreeding.
   e. Monitor fecal egg counts and deworm does as necessary. Routinely deworm at dryoff and again 1 month prior to kidding.
   f. Administer a booster dose of multivalent *Clostridium* vaccine including *Clostridium perfringens* Types C & D Toxoid and *Clostridium tetani* Toxoid 30 days before kidding.
   g. In deficient areas administer vitamin E and selenium to does 45 days and 15 days prior to kidding.
   h. Restrict calcium intake during the dry period and be sure does are not overconditioned upon entering the dry period.
   i. Provide plenty of exercise for periparturient does.
   j. Provide a clean, dry, draft-free area for the maternity pens or a well-drained pasture with shelter.

   k. Score body condition of does at midgestation, parturition, weaning, and prebreeding.
3. Bucks
   a. Administer vaccines to the bucks at the same time does receive them.
   b. Monitor fecal egg counts and deworm as needed. Routinely deworm the buck 1 month prior to the breeding season.
   c. Check feet monthly and trim as needed. Routinely trim feet 1 month prior to the breeding season and 1 month prior to the kidding season.
   d. Score body condition of bucks 1 month prior to the breeding season.
   e. Maintain high ratios of dietary calcium to phosphorus (2.0–2.5:1.0) and high levels of salt (up to 4%) in the diet of bucks. Make sure that drinking water is fresh and readily available.

This is a basic outline for herd health programs in the goat herd. Different production types (dairy, meat, fiber) require different programs. Individual herd needs will dictate modifications of this program.

VACCINATION PROTOCOL FOR GOATS

1. Enterotoxemia
   a. *Initially.* Vaccinate all adults and all kids over 1 month of age with *Clostridium perfringens* Types C & D Toxoid. Give a second dose of vaccine 2 to 4 weeks later.
   b. *Annually.* Give a booster dose to all adults once a year 2 to 4 weeks prior to the start of the kidding season.
   c. *Kids from immunized dams.* Vaccinate at 3 to 4 weeks of age with booster doses at 6 to 8 weeks and again at 6 months.
   d. *Kids from nonimmunized dams.* Vaccinate at 1 week of age, with a booster dose 3 to 4 weeks later, a second booster dose 3 to 4 weeks later, and a final booster dose at 6 months.
   e. *Antitoxin* is available for passive transference or treatment.
2. Tetanus
   a. *Initially.* Vaccinate all adults and kids over 1 month of age with *Clostridium tetani* Toxoid. Give a second dose of vaccine 2 to 4 weeks later.
   b. *Annually.* Give booster doses to all adults once a year 2 to 4 weeks prior to the kidding season.
   c. *Kids from immunized dams.* Vaccinate at 3 to 4 weeks of age and then give a booster dose at 6 to 8 weeks of age.
   d. *Kids from nonimmunized dams.* Vaccinate at 1 week of age with a booster dose in 3 to 4 weeks, a second booster dose in 3 to 4 weeks, and a final booster dose at 6 months of age.
   e. *Antitoxin* is available and should be used on nonimmunized goats prior to surgeries of any type (e.g., castration, dehorning, tagging) to provide temporary prophylaxis. Anaphylaxis is reported following the use of antitoxin.
3. Blackleg, Malignant Edema, Big Head, and Black Disease
   a. *Initially.* Vaccinate all adult animals in the herd and give booster doses 4 weeks later.
   b. *Annually.* Give booster doses to all adult animals 1 month prior to the kidding season.
   c. *Yearlings.* Give initial vaccine series to yearlings 60 days and 30 days prior to kidding. These are very unusual diseases of goats and prevention is probably not economically justifiable. Multivalent clostridial vaccines, including blackleg, malignant edema, overeating, and tetanus, are available and can be given to adult stock. Only overeating

and tetanus vaccines are given to kids to minimize the amount of injection site reactions.

4. Chlamydiosis
   a. *Initially.* Vaccinate all yearlings and adults 60 days and 30 days prior to the breeding season.
   b. *Annually.* Vaccinate all adults 2 to 4 weeks prior to the start of the breeding season.
   c. *Doelings.* Vaccinate 4 to 6 weeks prior to the start of the breeding season and again 2 to 4 weeks later.
   d. *Chlamydia* is a major cause of reproductive wastage in goats.

5. Vibriosis
   a. *Initially.* Vaccinate all yearlings and adults 60 days and 30 days prior to the breeding season.
   b. *Annually.* Vaccinate all adults 2 to 4 weeks prior to the start of the breeding season.
   c. *Doelings.* Vaccinate 4 to 6 weeks prior to the start of the breeding season and again 2 to 4 weeks later.
   d. *Vibrio* is not a major cause of reproductive wastage in goats.

6. Leptospirosis
   a. *Initially.* Vaccinate all yearlings and adults 60 days and 30 days prior to the breeding season.
   b. *Annually.* Vaccinate all adults 2 to 4 weeks prior to the start of the breeding season.
   c. *Doelings.* Vaccinate 4 to 6 weeks prior to the start of the breeding season and again 2 to 4 weeks later.
   d. Leptospirosis is not a major cause of reproductive wastage in goats.

7. Contagious Ecthyma
   a. *Initially.* Administer one dose of vaccine to all animals in the herd.
   b. *Annually.* Give booster doses to does and bucks 1 month prior to expected kidding.
   c. *Kids.* Vaccinate 2 to 4 weeks prior to weaning.
   d. *Yearlings.* Vaccinate 1 month prior to entry into the adult herd.
   e. Sore mouth vaccine is a virulent live virus vaccine. It is capable of surviving in the environment for years. Sore mouth vaccination is only recommended in herds which are already infected with the virus. Once the premises have been contaminated with vaccine virus or virus from a natural infection, vaccinations will be mandatory for subsequent generations. Immunity from the vaccine or disease will persist for 1 to 5 years. An alternative minimal vaccination program would consist of initial vaccination of the entire herd followed by annual vaccination of kids and new acquisitions.

A list of biologicals available for use on goats is presented in Table 1.

PARASITE CONTROL PROGRAMS

Of all the disease problems of goats parasitism is the most limiting factor for production. The greatest parasite problems are encountered with *Haemonchus contortus*. *H. contortus* has the ability to reproduce quickly, is a voracious bloodsucker, and has developed resistance to all of the currently marketed anthelmin-

Table 1
BIOLOGICAL AGENTS AVAILABLE FOR GOATS

Disease	Product Name	Manufacturer
Enterotoxemia	Ultrabac CD	Pfizer Animal Health
	Clostridium perfringens Types C & D Toxoid	Colorado Serum
	Fortress CD	Pfizer
Enterotoxemia and tetanus	*Clostridium perfringens* Types C & D–Tetanus Toxoid	Colorado Serum
	Bar-Vac CD/T	Anchor
	Fermicon CD/T	Bio-Ceutic
	Vision CD·T with Spur	Bayer
Enterotoxemia, malignant edema, blackleg, and tetanus	Covexin-8 Vaccine	Coopers
Tetanus toxoid	Tetanus Toxoid	Fort Dodge
	Tetanus Toxoid	Franklin
	Tetanus Toxoid	Colorado Serum
Tetanus antitoxin	Tetanus Antitoxin	Colorado Serum
	Tetanus Antitoxin	Fort Dodge
	Tetanus Antitoxin	Professional Biological
	Tetanus Antitoxin	Rhone Merieux
Overeating disease antitoxin	C & D Antitoxin	Anchor
	C-D Antitoxin	Bio-Ceutic
	Clostridium perfringens Types C & D Antitoxin	Colorado Serum
Contagious ecthyma	Contagious Ecthyma Vaccine	Texas Agricultural Experiment Station, Sonora, Tex.
	Ovine Ecthyma Vaccine	Colorado Serum
Campylobacter, Chlamydia	*Campylobacter fetus* Bacterin (ovine)/*Chlamydia psittaci* Bacterin	Colorado Serum
	Enzabort (EAE-Vibrio)	Colorado Serum
	Campylobacter fetus Bacterin	Colorado Serum
	Chlamydia psittaci Bacterin	Colorado Serum
	Escherichia coli Bacterin	Vineland
Foot rot	Footvax Vaccine	Coopers
	Volar	Bayer
Caseous lymphadenitis	Case-Bac	Colorado Serum
	Caseous D-T (overeating, tetanus, and caseous lymphadenitis)	Colorado Serum

tics. Control of parasitism in goats requires multifactorial programs of which treatment is only one component.[1] When anthelmintics are used make sure that appropriate withdrawals are used. A list of available anthelmintics with withdrawals is presented in Table 2.

PRODUCTION MANAGEMENT

The first component of a caprine production medicine program is the establishment of a record system.

Records

Animal records may be very simple in the case of the meat goat producer. These records may consist of only an adult head count and annual numbers of kids weaned. This allows the calculation of the net weaned kid crop (kids weaned/total number of does exposed to the buck/year). This provides an important indicator of profitability for the farm.

Records can be kept by hand on individual cards, on a home computer, or on a remote computer, as is done with Dairy Herd Improvement Association records. The need for extensive records increases with the intensity of production expected from the animals.

Identification

Individual animal identification is imperative if individual animal records are to be kept. This is usually in the form of a plastic ear-tag. Goats love to feed around briars, vines, and fences, all of which are excellent at tearing out plastic tags. A second identification will permit the animal to be identified should the tag be lost. Secondary identification can be done by tattoo on the ear or tail, a metal tag in the ear, a second plastic tag in the opposite ear, or freeze branding. In areas where goats are communally grazed, ear-notch systems are often used to identify the herd of origin of an individual goat.

Goals

Ultimately, productivity is determined by the goals of the owner. For goats kept primarily as pets, high levels of productiv-ity may be counterproductive to the owner's perceived life-style. For those who truly plan to generate income in the goat industry, the establishment of competitive goals of productivity is imperative. Practical goals for goat production are presented in Table 3.

Reproduction

Of all the individual production yardsticks used to evaluate the economic success of a goat operation, the most significant one is the level of reproductive efficiency. Goats have the ability to kid more than once per year and to produce multiple births. This ability is rarely exploited. It must be realized that in very harsh environments multiple kiddings and multiple births may not be desirable.

Doe

The doe is a seasonally polyestrous animal. The degree of this trait varies by breed and distance from the equator. Control of the estrous cycle in cycling can be obtained with the use of prostaglandin $F_{2\alpha}$ (Lutalyse Sterile Solution, Pharmacia & Upjohn) 5 to 10 mg or cloprostenol sodium (Estrumate, Bayer) 125 μg. Prostaglandin injection will result in estrus in 36 to 72 hours in cycling does. Injection with prostaglandin twice 11 days apart will result in estrus synchronization of randomly cycling does.

Does which are in seasonal anestrus can be brought into estrus by the use of progestagen implants. Implants are removed at 11 days and a luteolytic dose of prostaglandin is given at the same time. The only progestagen implant source in the United States is estradiol valerate–norgestomet (Syncro-Mate-B, Rhone Merieux). The recommended dose is one-half an implant placed subcutaneously in the ear or tail. Progestagen intravaginal sponges and controlled internal drug release formulations (CIDRs) are available in other countries.

Pregnant mare's serum gonadotropin (PMSG) is a critical hormone in programs designed to synchronize estrus in cycling does or to induce estrus in anestrus does. PMSG is not commercially available in the United States. P.G. 600 (Intervet) has been used successfully as a substitute for pure PMSG and is available in the United States. One program which has been successfully used in synchronizing estrus in transitional dairy goats is the following:[2]

Table 2				
ANTHELMINTIC PRODUCTS AND DOSAGES FOR GOATS				
Family	**Product**	**Dose**	**$/cwt**	**Slaughter Withdrawal**
Benzimadazoles	Thiabendazole (TBZ)	44 mg/kg	0.24	30 days*
	Fenbendazole (Safe-Guard)	5.0 mg/kg	0.25	6 days*
	Oxfendazole (Synanthic)	5.0 mg/kg	0.27	6 days†
	Albendazole (Valbazen)	7.5 mg/kg	0.30	27 days†
Avermectins	Ivermectin (Ivomec Sheep Drench)	0.2 mg/kg	0.55	56 days†
	Doramectin (Dectomax)	0.2 mg/kg	0.55	56 days†
	Eprinex (Eprinomectin)	0.1 mL/kg	0.60	0 days†
	Ivermectin (Ivomec Plus)	0.2 mg/kg	0.55	56 days†
Imidazothiazole	Levamisole (Levasole)	8.0 mg/kg	0.28	10 days†
	Morantel tartrate (Rumatel)	10 mg/kg	0.27	30 days*‡
Tetrahydropyrimines	Pyrantel pamoate (Strongid T)	25 mg/kg	1.00	30 days†

*Approved for use in goats with goat withdrawal time.
†Food Animal Residue Avoidance Databank (FARAD) recommendation (1996).
‡Available as a medicated mineral or feed only.
cwt, hundredweight.

Table 3
GOALS FOR GOAT PRODUCTION

Index	Goal	Definition
Cycling	>70%	Percentage of does found in estrus during the first 21 days of the breeding season
Mating	>95%	Percentage of does that are bred during the breeding season
Pregnancy	>95%	Percentage of does that become pregnant after 2–3 successive estrous cycles
Abortion	<5%	Percentage of does with visible abortions
Kidding	>90%	Percentage of mature does that kid following the breeding season
Reproductive proportion	1.5–2.0	Average number of kids born (alive and dead) per exposed doe per breeding season
Kid crop per doe per year	0.9–1.5	Number of kiddings/year divided by the number of does exposed to bucks
Stillbirth	<2%	Number of kids born dead or dead at <24 hr divided by the total number of kids born
Preweaning mortality	<10%	Number of kids alive at 24 hr of age and dead prior to weaning
Net weaned kid crop	1.25–1.5	Number of kids weaned/year divided by the number of does exposed to bucks/yr
Kid weight weaned per doe per year	35–65 lb	Kid weight weaned per exposed doe
Mohair per head per year	4–8 lb	Mohair removed per head/yr (highly variable)
Milk per doe per year	1000–5500 lb	Milk per doe/yr (highly variable)
Net income per doe per year	$0–$500	Dollars of income generated per doe/yr (highly variable)

1. Implant Syncro-Mate-B one-half implant in the tail for 9 to 13 days.

2. Inject P.G. 600 3.5 mL subcutaneously at 36 hours prior to implant withdrawal.

3. Inject Estrumate 125 μg intramuscularly at the time of implant removal.

Buck

It should be remembered that the buck is affected by photoperiod, may not be in rut, and may have poor-quality semen during the nonbreeding season. The buck can be stimulated by estrual or estrinized does. It may be necessary to administer gonadorelin (gonadotropin-releasing hormone; Cystorellin, Rhone Merieux) three times daily for 3 to 7 days to stimulate testosterone production and libido in the buck.[3]

Replacement Doelings

Replacement doelings are expected to kid as yearlings (12 months of age). This will require special nutrition or will result in the breeding of an undersized female who will never reach her optimal mature weight. In herds which kid only once a year, failure to breed the doeling at 7 months of age means that she will not be bred until 19 months of age and will kid as a 2-year-old.

Breeding Season

The breeding season varies depending on the distance from the equator. Goats in the southern United States may breed all year long. Goats in the northern United States may be in a seasonal anestrus from May until September.

OPTIMAL PRODUCTIVITY

In harsh environments (western United States open range) it is probably appropriate to breed only once a year and to kid during the peak forage season (spring). It may be unwise to select heavily for multiple births in this environment. In areas with more temperate weather, better pastures, and more inten-sive management, goats need to be managed for greater levels of productivity. Multiple breeding systems, as are used in sheep production (Cornell, Star), allow for multiple mating and kidding of does during the year. Under conditions of intensive management the production of twins more than once per year is highly desirable.

NUTRITION

In general, intensive feeding of goats is a little researched area. Nutritional supplementation of grazing goats is complicated by the fact that they do not go into a pasture and graze the predominant plant (grass). Instead they nibble on a shrub here and a vine there. They are very selective even to the extent of eating only newly sprouted leaves and plants. This makes it difficult to adequately predict the nutrient intake of goats on pasture. Body condition scoring (BCS) of goats is done using a 5-point system. Scores are assigned based on the presence or absence of lumbar musculature and sternal fat.[4]

INFECTIOUS DISEASE CONTROL AND PREVENTION

In most caprine operations disease appears to be the limiting factor to production. This is very different from the production limitations facing other animal industries. The majority of diseases affecting productivity are infectious or parasitic. Control and prevention of these diseases must be addressed by the herd health program. Contagious diseases of particular concern to the goat owner are listed in Table 4.

BIOSECURITY

The heart of a herd health program to prevent infectious diseases begins with the farm biosecurity program. It is much more cost-efficient to prevent the access of key diseases into the herd than it is to eliminate them later. The components of an effective biosecurity program include the following:

1. Prepurchase examination and testing
2. On-farm quarantine
   a. Incubation period

Table 4
CRITICAL CONTAGIOUS DISEASES OF GOATS

Caprine arthritis encephalitis (CAE)
  Prevent entry: Serotest all new purchases.
  Control: Isolate seropositive does and raise offspring on pasteurized milk.
  Goal: Eradication.
Caseous lymphadenitis
  Prevent entry: Examination of all new purchases for presence of abscesses. A serologic test is available but lacks sensitivity and specificity.
  Control: Cull affected animals or quarantine.
  Goal: Eradication.
Foot rot
  Prevent entry: Examine and treat feet of all new entries.
  Control: Trim feet, foot-bathe in 10% $ZnSO_4$, and treat with parenteral antibacterials.
  Goal: Eradication.
Johne's disease
  Prevent entry: Serologic testing of all new entries.
  Control: Serotest and cull all seropositive animals. Eliminate fecal oral transmission.
  Goal: Eradication.
Contagious ecthyma
  Prevent entry: Examine and quarantine all new entries.
  Control: Vaccinate.
  Goal: Prevention of clinical signs.
Pinkeye
  Prevent entry: Quarantine and examine the eyes and conjunctiva of all new entries.
  Control: Parenteral antibacterials.
  Goal: Prevent clinical signs.
Chlamydial abortions
  Prevent entry: Prevent entry of carrier animals during critical times (pregnancy).
  Control: Tetracyclines can be used to clear the carrier state and to halt abortion epizootics. A vaccine is available to confer longer-term resistance.
  Goal: Prevention of abortion.
Contagious mastitis
  Prevent entry: CMT and milk culture on all entering lactating does. Treat all entering dry does.
  Control: (1) Milk only clean and dry teats. (2) Use properly functioning machines. (3) Post milking dip all teats in an effective disinfectant. (4) Treat all teats of all does at dryoff. (5) Treat all new infections quickly with effective antibiotics and cull chronic cases.
  Goal: Minimize the number of new infections.
Parasitic disease
  Multiple drug–resistant *Haemonchus contortus*
    Prevent entry: Quarantine and deworm all new entries with several unrelated anthelmintics. Release from quarantine only with a negative fecal egg count.
    Control: Minimize the number of dewormings per year. Rotate drugs on an annual basis. Perform egg count reduction assays at every deworming.
    Goal: Minimize drug resistance.

  b. Retest period
  c. Pathogen elimination period
  d. Immunization period
3. Herd immunization

The appropriate sequence would be to buy a goat only from a herd with a known history of being free from important contagious diseases. Test the goat prior to purchase by physical examination and laboratory work. Transport the goat to the farm, but put it into a quarantine facility away from the herd to see if the goat is incubating any contagious disease. The goat should be quarantined for a minimum of 30 days. Retest the goat by physical examination and laboratory evaluation for the continued absence of contagious diseases. Treat the goat prophylactically with antibacterials and anthelmintics for the possibility of subclinical carrier states. Immunize the incoming goat for diseases which are present in the nucleus herd. Keep high levels of immunity in the nucleus herd in case there is a breakdown in the biosecurity system.

REFERENCES

1. Craig TM: Control of gastrointestinal nematodes of sheep and goats in North America. *In* Proceedings of Symposium on the Health and Disease of Small Ruminants, Kansas City, 1996, p 132.
2. Rowe JD, East NE: Comparison of gonadotropin for estrus synchronization in does. Theriogenology 45:1569, 1996.
3. Hill J: Goat reproductive management. *In* Proceedings of Symposium on the Health and Disease of Small Ruminants, 1996, p 114.
4. Smith MC, Sherman DM: Goat Medicine. Philadelphia, Lea & Febiger, 1994, pp 545–546.

BIBLIOGRAPHY

Baxendell SA: The Diagnosis of the Diseases of Goats. Sydney, Australia, Post-Graduate Foundation in Veterinary Science, University of Sydney, 1988.
Boden E: Sheep and Goat Practice. London, Bailliere Tindall, 1991.
Ensminger ME, Parker RO: Sheep and Goat Science. Danville, Ill Interstate Printers and Publishers, 1986.
Goat Advisory Practice. Refresher Course for Veterinarians. Proceedings 135. Sydney, Australia, Post-Graduate Committee in Veterinary Science, University of Sydney, June 1990.
Goat Health and Production. Refresher Course for Veterinarians. Proceedings 134. Sydney, Australia, University of Sydney, June 1990.
Nutrient Requirements of Goats: Angora, Dairy and Meat Goats in Temperate and Tropical Countries. Washington, DC, National Academy Press, 1981.
Smith MC: Advances in sheep and goat medicine. Vet Clin North Am Food Anim Pract 3:563–806, 1990.
Smith MC, Sherman DM: Goat Medicine. Philadelphia, Lea & Febiger, 1994.

■ Dairy Heifer Development and Monitoring

Thomas L. Bailey, D.V.M., M.S., A.C.T.
Julia M. Murphy, D.V.M.

Raising dairy replacement heifers is costly. In fact, if the dairy is divided into enterprises, replacement rearing is the second largest cost, after the cost of feed for lactating cows. The percentage will vary from farm to farm, but approximately 9% to 20% of the expenses incurred will involve rearing and developing replacement heifers. Before these heifers can return a profit to the farm, they will subtract dollars from cash flow. Therefore, heifers should represent a sound investment, as the impact on future herd profitability is great. Goals can be set and heifers monitored to develop a heifer that will calve at 24 months of age and weigh 613 kg (~1350 lb). These heifers should weigh approximately 556 kg (~1225 lb) postcalving, with a wither height of ~138 cm (54 in.) and a body condition score of between 3.25 and 3.5 (Fig. 1). Rearing goals should also include (1) having 80% to 85% of the heifers born reaching the lactating herd and (2) having heifers that will produce ~90 kg (~200 lb) more milk than last year's heifers. These goals are not only attainable but also cut expenses and increase profits for the dairy.

A successful replacement rearing program is not accidental. It must be a conscious effort with a priority placed on heifer rearing. Several factors can dramatically reduce replacement-rearing cost and increase potential profits for the producer: (1) adequate quality and quantity of colostrum; (2) proper nutrition, which feeds strategically for the growth and developmental periods of the heifer; (3) the use of genetically superior sires in an artificial insemination program; (4) monitoring weight, height, body condition score, and age at first calving; and (5) reducing heifer inventory numbers.

The cost of raising a heifer from birth to 24 months is between $1080 and $1300. Therefore, a heifer may be well into the second lactation before she starts to return on the investment made during rearing. Reducing the number of days to first calving and thereby reducing both feed costs in the nonproductive period and the total number of replacement heifers needed can decrease the total expenses and keep herd numbers at a desirable level. Figures have also shown that using top sires with high predicted transmitting ability (PTA) for breeding heifers can increase the potential milk yields and subsequently the potential income of the dairy. With heifers being the genetically superior animals on the farm, and since one third or more of the annual calf crop is coming from first-calf heifers, it is imperative that we encourage the use of superior genetics for future generations offered through the use of artificial insemination.

THE NEWBORN

Getting calves started correctly is the first step toward raising healthy replacements. Colostral management, good nutrition, and keeping young calves clean, dry, and comfortable are the keys to healthy replacements. Colostrum quality and quantity is the first step to a healthy calf. Colostrum can be easily collected, evaluated for immunoglobulin status using a colostrometer,* refrigerated for 4 to 5 days, placed in a −20°C freezer, or soured. Keeping track of colostrum quality with a colostrometer ensures that adequate levels of immunoglobulins (250 mg/dL) are present. However, colostrum should be at room temperature for an accurate reading on the colostrometer. Colostrum from older cows should be utilized and fed to calves born from first-calf heifers. This may be necessary, as first-calf heifers have not been exposed to numerous environmental pathogens and may not have the immunoglobulin level of older vaccinated cows. Thaw colostrum in warm water, as extremely high water bath temperatures can denature the protein content of immunoglobulins. Colostrum may be frozen for 6 to 12 months and should be properly labeled with the contributing dam's identification number, the date collected, and the immunoglobulin status of the colostrum. Colostrum should be hand-fed to ensure adequate intake of 8% to 10% of the calf's body weight in the first 12 hours of life: 2 L in the first 2 hours postbirth and an additional 2 L 6 to 8 hours later. An additional 4 L should be divided into two feedings to bring the total intake of high-quality colostrum to 8 L within the first 24 hours of age. Research has shown that if calves are left to nurse on their own, 25% to 40% of calves do not receive adequate intake of colostrum with protective immunoglobulin levels against primary digestive and respiratory pathogens.

Another valuable tool for assessing the colostrum management by farm personnel is to monitor immunoglobulin status with the routine use of either the refractometer† for total serum protein, the sodium sulfite precipitation test, the zinc sulfate turbidity test, or radial immunodiffusion test. Refractometer readings are made using serum from a calf between 2 and 10 days of age for accurate assessment of immunoglobulins. Serum protein readings should be above 5.5 g/dL and preferably 6 g/

---

*Colostrometer, Nasco, PO Box 901, Fort Atkinson, WI 53538.
†Reichert-Jung Model Refractometer, available from Fisher Scientific, 145 Delta Dr, Pittsburgh, PA 15238.

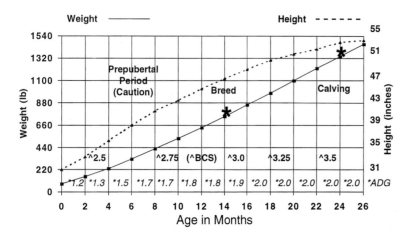

Figure 1

Heifer chart demonstrating optimal weight, height, average daily gain (ADG) and body condition score (BCS) by months of age. ADG stratified by months of age. BCS stratified by growth periods. (Charts may be obtained from the authors at the Virginia-Maryland Regional College of Veterinary Medicine.)

dL. If levels fall below 5.5 g/dL, calves are questionable for adequate protection. With levels below 5 g/dL, failure of passive transfer has occurred, and the calf is therefore susceptible to pathogens leading to calf diarrhea, joint-ill, and respiratory diseases. When levels of protective immunoglobulins fall below 5.5 g/dL, an evaluation of calf management should be performed with all associated farm personnel. Several other factors, primarily extremes in temperature and dystocia, can adversely affect immunoglobulin absorption and uptake.

Calves should have their navel dipped in an iodine solution. This practice should be repeated every 12 hours for three treatments, or until the navel cord appears dry. Navel dipping, however, aids only in decreasing the incidence of umbilical infections. A clean, dry, comfortable environment plays a much greater role in calf health. The primary objective of the calving and neonatal environment should be aimed at reducing the number of pathogens the calf is exposed to. If calf death is followed by a postmortem examination and joint-ill is found, virtually all cases can be traced back to inadequate colostrum and unsanitary calf-rearing facilities.

CALF NUTRITION

Calves should be maintained on whole milk or a quality milk replacer until calves are eating adequate amounts of grain to sustain rapid growth and rumen development. Whole milk, in general, can be found in one of three forms on the average dairy farm: extra colostrum or transition milk, nonsaleable milk (e.g., mastitic or antibiotic-tainted), and saleable milk. Of these, extra colostrum or transition milk is preferred because of its superior nutritional value, and because it cannot be sold. This milk can be preserved via fermentation or freezing.

Mastitic milk is an area of controversy in relation to safety and the "seeding" of mastitis-causing organisms, especially relative to *Staphylococcus aureus*. Mastitic milk should only be fed if it has the appearance of normal milk. Milk containing visual signs of purulent material, clots, or blood should not be fed to calves. As antibiotic-containing milk has been associated with slower growth and higher rejection rates, it is the least preferred form of supplementation, including milk replacer.

Milk replacers should be of the highest quality to mimic whole milk as closely as possible. To maintain growth levels, replacers should be 20% protein, a minimum of 15% fat (dependent on environmental temperatures), and less than 0.25% crude fiber. Producers may want to increase the fat level to 20% to 24% in cold climates for adequate energy intake. Periods of heat stress may be another time to increase the energy of the milk replacer. Calves will decrease intake during times of extreme heat, and feeding higher levels of fat will make a more energy-dense ration. The higher the crude fiber levels, the higher the plant origin in the milk replacer. Calves less than 1 month of age are incapable of digesting a higher amount of crude fiber and can have digestive upsets leading to diarrhea and dehydration.

Important information regarding a milk replacer's quality can be found by examining the feed tag. Protein, fat, and fiber levels, as well as the sources of protein and energy, should be scrutinized. Protein sources such as dried skim milk or whey products are preferred, whereas most vegetable sources such as soy flour and fish byproducts are considered inferior. Carbohydrate content should consist almost exclusively of lactose while either animal or vegetable fat can be used. Many milk replacers are medicated with antibiotics, but this often proves to be of little benefit. Other characteristics, such as the ease with which the powder mixes with water, are also important to evaluate. Calves should initially be fed 8% to 10% of their body weight divided into two feedings per day. As the calf grows the same

absolute volume of milk replacer should be maintained to encourage calf starter consumption and with clean, fresh water available at all times. Fresh water ad libitum encourages more grain intake leading to an earlier weaning. In several surveys of dairies, heifer age at freshening is often extended by 1 or 2 months because nutritional programs for nursing calves are below optimum.

Weaning should be dependent on the individual calf's eating habits and not a preset weaning age. Generally calves should be eating approximately 2.0% to 2.5% of their body weight in grain at the time of weaning. Hay and grain are both important in the development of rumen volatile fatty acids (VFAs). However, concentrate has been shown to play a more critical role in the formation of rumen papillae. Diets high in energy value result in the formation of greater concentrations of butyric and proprionic acids. These VFAs have a considerably greater effect than acetate on the formation of rumen papillae by stimulating blood flow to the rumen's mucosal layer, resulting in increased metabolic activity. As a calf's rumen size increases exponentially (eight times its birth size) by the eighth week of life, optimal levels of calf starter to be introduced during this time should reach approximately 3 lb per calf per day prior to weaning. If hay is fed to nursing calves it should be of the highest quality found on the farm for rumen development. Without a doubt, good-quality hay is effective in stimulating rumen growth and may aid in papillae development necessary for nutrient absorption. However, relative to dry matter intake being the limiting factor, grain is the more energy-dense ration, producing more butyric and proprionic acid for rumen growth and development.

If a Holstein heifer weighs 37 kg (80 lb) at birth and our goal is a 613-kg (1350-lb) heifer 24 months later at calving, she must gain an average of 0.75 to 0.79 kg (1.8 lb) per day. Groups of 10 to 12 heifers would be partitioned according to age and body weight to combat their competitive nature for feed. Formulation of heifer rations should be based on nutritional analysis of feed components. This is the single most important factor to guarantee heifers are fed for optimal weight gain as well as skeletal development. One recommendation for calves up to weaning is to feed an 18% crude protein ration, 75% total digestible nutrients (TDN), and 10% fiber. Rations after weaning can be about 16% crude protein and 5% crude fiber. Up to 5 months of age, calves should receive a third of their dry matter intake from forage and two thirds from grain. From 6 to 10 months, 75% of the dry matter can come from forage, since the rumen should be fully functional. Average daily grains should be monitored to not exceed those presented along the bottom of the chart in Figure 1 for their respective months of age.

Bunk management is essential to adequate growth and development. Bunk space is allocated according to the weight and size of the pen of heifers. Each calf requires 15 to 18 in. of linear bunk space up to approximately 410 kg (~900 lb). At approximately 454 kg (~1000 lb), bunk space should be increased to 2 linear ft of bunk space. Bunk space requirements are also dependent on the number of feedings per day, with once-a-day feeding requiring more linear feet of bunk space.

HEALTH

Both parasite control and the feeding of growth promotants improve feed efficiency and enhance growth. Regular deworming and treatment programs for internal and external parasites are essential to improve heifer performance. Coccidia control measures should be started in baby calves at 5 to 10 days of age and continue until 30 days prior to calving. Ionophores are effective as an aid in reducing coccidiosis and improving feed efficiency. Supplementation costs pennies per heifer per day, which is more than offset by decreasing the amount of grain

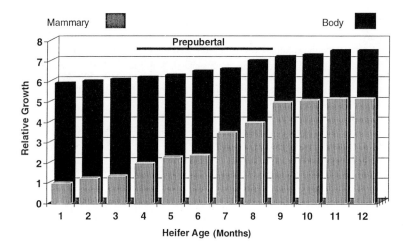

Figure 2

Relative growth rate of the mammary gland during the prepubertal period relative to body growth. (From Sinha YN, et al: Mammary development and pituitary prolactin level of heifers from birth through puberty and during the estrous cycle. J Dairy Sci 52:507–512, 1969.)

required per kilogram of gain or supporting adequate growth with lower-quality forage for older heifers. These products should be managed properly. However, the use of ionophores in confinement-reared heifers or those fed excessive rations may lead to overconditioning. This is especially important during the time calves are 3 to 9 months old, or the prepubertal phase of rapid mammary gland development (Fig. 2).

Cryptosporidiosis is perhaps one of the larger problems we face in nursing replacements today. It has been diagnosed on essentially every dairy farm in the United States. In our experience it strikes calves at approximately 8 days of age, causing a profuse diarrhea with subsequent dehydration. Morbidity is high, but mortality is low with the proper administration of fluids and supportive therapy. Therapy and vaccinations are now being tested to eliminate this problem, but at this time these products have not been adequately tested to advocate their use.

Vaccination programs in the heifer herd are tailored to protect against the specific diseases on individual farms. Most vaccinations are initiated at 4 to 5 months of age, when maternal protection gained from colostrum has subsided. These vaccinations are then repeated at 6 months of age to ensure peak immunity. Vaccinations should be repeated 45 days prior to breeding or at approximately 12 to 13 months of age. Many of the diseases that cause early embryonic death or infertility can be prevented through proper vaccination procedures. Injections are then repeated at 18 months of age and 45 to 60 days prior to calving for sufficient levels of immunoglobulins in the colostrum.

For an excellent schedule and review of the more common vaccinations administered to dairy replacement heifers, see "Dairy Replacement Rearing Programs" by M. L. Van Der Leek, G. A. Donovan, and R. K. Braun, in Howard's *Current Veterinary Therapy 3: Food Animal Practice*, 1993.

HEIFER PUBERTY

Heifers can become overconditioned. There is a critical period when overfeeding can have a detrimental effect on udder development. This begins at about 3 months of age and ends at puberty or approximately 9 months of age. This is referred to as the allometric period. During this period, udder development is 3.5 times that of other body systems' growth (see Fig. 2). Studies indicate that when overconditioning during this period occurs, mammary secretory or milk-producing tissue in the udder is greatly reduced. Temporary periods of rapid gain after puberty are acceptable and may allow compensatory adjustments for weight gain to reach 24-month targets.

The age heifers reach puberty is dependent on the plane of nutrition, and puberty may be delayed or accelerated. The time when heifers reach puberty can be long when heifers are fed low-energy diets which yield low average daily gains. When the age to puberty is longer, it is highly likely that the growth of mammary gland is also delayed compared to that of heifers that reach an earlier puberty. We should expect heifers to reach puberty at 40% to 50% of mature body weight, begin breeding by 14 to 15 months of age (Table 1) at about 50% to 60% of mature body size, and become pregnant and calve at 24 months. Heifers should start lactation with a postcalving weight of 556 kg (~1225 lb); therefore, they will need to add 23 kg (~50 lb) of body weight per month from birth to first calving or an average daily gain of 1.8 lb/day. Average daily gains of 1.3 lb/day are too low because they add only 18 kg (~40 lb) per month, resulting in a postcalving weight of 431 kg (~950 lb) (Fig. 3).

MONITORING AND GRAPHING HEIFER GROWTH

Charting heifer growth for body weight, skeletal development, and body condition scoring can evaluate performance and spot trends or problems in heifer management. These charts show stages of growth and development in partitioned groups and determine either decreased skeletal development, overconditioning, or underconditioning. All are good indicators of improper feeding or poor overall heifer management. The heifers depicted in Figure 4 show periods of poor development. Heifers

Table 1
RECOMMENDED BREEDING WEIGHT AND AGE

Breed	Weight [kg (lb)]	Age (mo)
Holstein	350–363 (785)	14–15
Brown Swiss	350–363 (785)	14–15
Milking Shorthorn	320–365 (750)	14–15
Guernsey	275–320 (685)	14–15
Aryshire	275–320 (685)	14–15
Jersey	250–295 (575)	13–14

From Van Der Leek ML, Donovan GA, Braun RK: Dairy replacement rearing programs. *In* Howard JL (ed): Current Veterinary Therapy 3: Food Animal Practice. Philadelphia, WB Saunders, 1993, p 152.

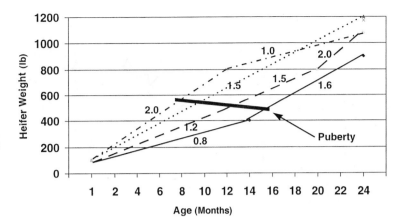

Figure 3

Age at puberty relative to varying average daily gains during growth periods of heifer development. (From Reid JT, et al: Effect of plane of nutrition during early life on growth, reproduction, production, health and longevity of Holstein cows: I. Birth to fifth calving. Cornell University Agricultural Experiment Station Bulletin No. 987, 1964.)

are failing to reach projected targets during the postneonatal and early prepubertal period. They are also falling below targets after breeding.

Below-adequate height is generally an indication of low protein in the diet. This generally occurs in heifers older than 7 months during the summer when grass pasture is of lower quality. Overconditioning heifers may indicate excessive corn silage diets or feeding high-energy rations, such as feeding refusal from the lactating cow ration. Body condition should be monitored to ensure adequate skeletal development (height) and body tissue mass. Heifers should be charted at least five times before they reach 2 years of age. This can be done at times of deworming, vaccinations, breeding, or pregnancy checks, so it is not an additional chore.

The period from pregnancy check to calving appears to be the time heifers are most neglected. Once breeding occurs and heifers are examined pregnant, they are often ignored until calving. Heifers should be monitored during this time for adequate weight and development at calving. In our experience, heifers typically fall below our target goals for average daily gain during the period of time between breeding and calving. Charting growth and height can ensure heifers are on target for our goals at breeding and calving (Table 2).

Heifers should be first weighed or girth-taped* and a height stick† used at 2½ to 3 months. This could coincide with the time calves are removed from the hutches and delegated to smaller partitioned groups. Frequently a 1-month delay in time to calving occurs during this first 3-month development period

and is reflective of poor nutritional and young stock management. The second measurement should be done as the calves are vaccinated for calfhood diseases and brucellosis at about 5 to 6 months of age. Measure again at 9 to 12 months of age to evaluate the critical period up to puberty, when calf development is so important for udder growth. A prebreeding graph will determine if development is on target for breeding at 352 kg (~775 lb) to 363 kg (~800 lb) with a height of 122 cm (~48 in.) or greater. A fifth measurement at 18 to 22 months is taken to ensure that heifer growth is adequate to meet our goals at calving. Heifer performance is often suboptimal at this time, but can be clearly demonstrated to producers with a simple chart of weights and heights in relation to optimal growth (see Fig. 4).

Body condition scoring is also a useful tool for determining how heifers are developing. Heifers should not be allowed to exceed a body condition score of 2.5 to 2.75 during the period of 3 months to puberty, as a higher score may lead to fat deposition in the mammary gland. After puberty and up to the time of prebreeding, a condition score of 2.75 to 3.0 is desirable for optimal fertility. At calving a body condition score of 3.25 to 3.5 is acceptable because overconditioning can lead to fat deposits in the pelvic canal and potential problems with dystocia.

ARTIFICIAL INSEMINATION IN HEIFERS

Research has consistently demonstrated that a good artificial insemination (AI) program will produce an annual genetic gain of at least 91 kg (~200 lb) of milk per heifer. Conception rates

---

*Weigh tape, Nasco, PO Box 901, Fort Atkinson, WI 53538.
†Height stick, Nasco, PO Box 901, Fort Atkinson, WI 53538.

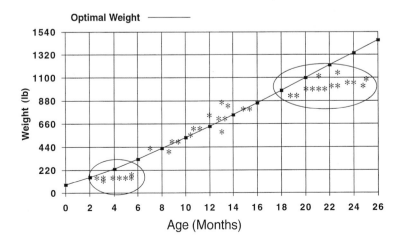

Figure 4

Replacement heifers *(asterisks)* plotted on the basis of weight in relation to months of age.

Table 2
MONITORING THE GROWTH RATE OF LARGE-BREED HEIFERS

Management Activity	Age (mo)	Weight [kg (lb)]	Height [cm (in.)]
Move to group pens	2	70 (154)	85 (34)
Brucella vaccination	6	170 (375)	100 (39)
Regrouping	10	255 (560)	125 (50)
Prebreeding	14	363 (800)	122 (48)
Precalving	24	613 (1350)	138 (54)

From Van Der Leek ML, Donovan GA, Braun RK: Dairy replacement rearing programs. *In* Howard JL (ed): Current Veterinary Therapy 3: Food Animal Practice. Philadelphia, WB Saunders, 1993, p 150.

decline with advancing age of the cow, but the biggest drop is from replacement heifers to first-lactation cows. Heifers have a 60% to 70% pregnancy rate across almost all herd management levels, while first-lactation-and-greater cows will have pregnancy rates of 40% to 50%. Another reason for breeding heifers to superior sires is that first-lactation heifers represent the highest number of calvings per lactation group on most farms. First-lactation heifers have 31.9% of the calves born, while second-lactation heifers have 25.1%, and third-lactation cows produce 18.6% of the calf crop. The remaining 24.4% is divided among the fourth-, fifth-, and sixth-or-greater lactation cows. Therefore, breeding to natural or inferior genetic sires puts approximately 32% of the herd's genetic potential at risk.

One major argument against the use of AI on many dairies is a question of calving ease. The most recent sire summary of Holstein sires demonstrates that of the top 100 Holstein sires, 38% are calving-ease sires. Sires with scores below the average of 9% difficult births are considered to be calving-ease sires. Calving-ease bulls may not always be the answer, as heifer development may be inadequate for calving.

Studies have also been conducted to determine the differential cost between maintaining a natural-service sire vs. an AI program. Although producers incur the added cost of semen, handling facilities, and labor for heat detection, researchers have indicated that AI provides cost savings. However, improved genetic progress remains the best reason to use AI. Mating to genetically superior sires generates three to four times the genetic progress compared with natural-service sires. A recent review of the U.S. Department of Agriculture (USDA) sire summary shows that active AI Holstein bulls' average PTA for milk, fat, and protein is greater than $180. This monetary figure indicates that when these bulls are utilized in an AI program, the progeny should produce $180 more milk per lactation than when bulls with $0 PTAs are used. The same summary indicated that natural-service sires are less than $0 to $10 PTAs. This would mean that if 25 heifers were mated to the active $180 PTA Holstein sires and 25 were mated to natural-service sires, the AI-produced offspring would potentially produce $4500 more from milk sales. Very few dairies have access to natural-service sires that can compare with the genetic progress available through AI. To provide adequate genetics for future generations in the herd it is generally recommended that service sires be above the upper 80th percentile (Table 3).

MASTITIS IN FIRST-CALF HEIFERS

Mastitis is the single most costly disease in the dairy industry and heifers are not immune. More emphasis is now placed on the heifer-rearing portion of the dairy enterprise to control replacement mastitis and high somatic cell counts when heifers enter the lactating herd. Heifers have generally been regarded as an uninfected population with regard to mastitis. Until recently heifers have been neglected and our aim has been in the direction of mature lactating cows for the control and prevention of mastitis-causing organisms. However, research conducted at the Mississippi State University College of Veterinary Medicine and Hill's Research Farm in Louisiana demonstrates the majority of first-lactation heifers on farms are infected prior to calving.

Control programs for heifers, as for mature cows, are designed to reduce the number of mastitis-causing organisms at the teat end, which replicate and gain entry to the gland tissue. These would include individual hutches for nursing calves to prevent suckling and the subsequent migration of organisms into the gland. This is especially important if mastitic milk is being fed to nursing calves. Some research has shown a consistently higher incidence of *S. aureus* mastitis in calves fed mastitic milk, even though these animals are segregated. The *S. aureus* organisms may be harbored in the tonsils and carried to the udder by a hematogenous route. Sanitation in the hutches and the environment where calves are later placed in small groups is of utmost importance. If hutches, lots, or pastures are filthy, damp, or muddy, the teat end is constantly exposed to a barrage of mastitis-causing organisms. Hutches should be well-bedded, clean, dry, and comfortable. Lots and pastures should be managed to prevent muddy areas in which heifers would be walking or lying down.

Fly control is another area of major concern. Flies can carry a number of mastitis-causing organisms on their feet and legs. Biting flies traumatize the teat ends, allowing pathogens to colonize and later enter the teat end. Therefore, during the fly season, effective procedures for control and prevention are very important. If sprays are used, emphasis should be placed on the mammary gland. Orally administered larvicides are also very effective in reducing the fly population. The area of the udder, and especially the teat end, should be routinely examined for

Table 3
TARGETS FOR A DAIRY REPLACEMENT REARING PROGRAM

Parameter	Target		
ME 305-day improvement	>100 kg (~200 lb)		
PTA of sire	Upper 80th percentile		
Calving-ease index of sire	<9%		
Body condition at calving	3.5 ± 0.25 (3.25–3.75)		
Calves dead in <24 hr (born dead or alive)	<8%		
Incidence of dystocia	<20%		
Incidence of mastitis at calving	<7%		
Incidence of blind quarters	<0.5%		
First-service conception rate	>65%		
Heat detection rate	>80%		
Culling for reproduction	<5%		
Culling for disease/poor growth	<2%		
Calves with enlarged umbilical stumps	<8%		
	0–60 days	**2–6 mo**	**6–24 mo**
Mortality	<5%	<2%	<1%
Diarrhea	<20%	<5%	<1%
Pneumonia	<5%	<5%	<2%
Pinkeye	<1%	<5%	<5%

ME, mature equivalent; PTA, predicted transmitting ability.
From Van Der Leek ML, Donovan GA, Braun RK. Dairy replacement rearing programs. *In* Howard JL (ed): Current Veterinary Therapy 3: Food Animal Practice. Philadelphia, WB Saunders, 1993, p 152.

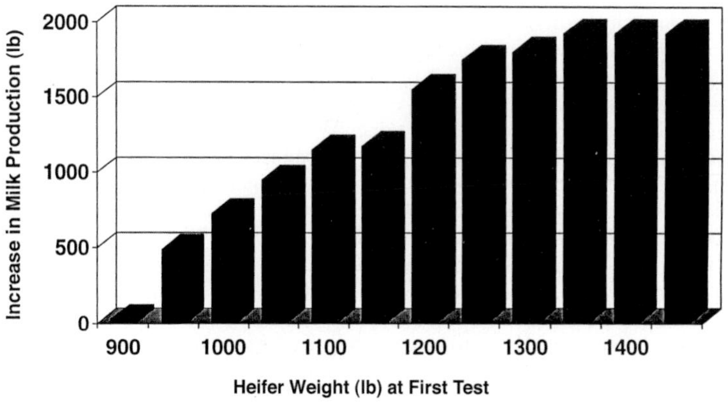

Figure 5

Increase in milk production relative to the increase in heifer weight at the first test day postpartum. (From Keown JF, et al: Freshen heifers at 1200 pounds. Dairy Herd Management, August 1986, p 18.)

fly-induced trauma and for cuts and lacerations that may lure flies to the teat ends. Flies can potentially transport mastitis from the lactating or dry cows to pregnant heifers. Therefore, heifers should be isolated from this source of potential infection before calving.

The use of teat infusion products into the mammary gland prior to first parturition may hold a promising future for prevention and control of heifer mastitis. Heifers utilized for research purposes have been infused at 60 days prior to calving with a dry cow infusion product. This appears to be efficacious in preventing or reducing the number of infected quarters. Extreme precautionary measures must be practiced to ensure strict sanitary procedures are used when infusing heifers, as mastitis-causing organisms can be introduced during this procedure. To date, there are no approved mastitis infusion products for precalving heifers. This would be categorized as extralabel drug use and can only be practiced under the direct supervision of a licensed veterinarian. Injectable products (extralabel use) are also being tested for the treatment and prevention of heifer mastitis, thus alleviating the problem of infusion. Vitamin E and selenium supplementation in heifers has also been shown to be effective in reducing the incidence of mastitis in conjunction with other preventive programs on the farm.

MILK PRODUCTION IN HEIFERS

Studies on the effect of weight and age at first calving on subsequent milk yields have demonstrated that weight at calving and not age played a more significant role in milk production and reproduction. Groups of heifers gaining 1.1 kg (~2.4 lb) per day after puberty and freshening at 19.7 months of age were compared with heifers calving at 26.9 months of age. First-lactation milk yields were significantly lower in the younger group, but there were no significant differences in the second lactation. A greater cumulative milk yield based on day of age was experienced at 36 months of age because the younger group was already into their second lactation. This would also significantly reduce the number of nonproductive months for replacement heifers. While calving at 19 months of age is not suggested, these studies illustrate how increased weight gain and earlier breeding can affect lifetime production and decrease the nonproductive months prior to calving.

Weight at calving has the most significant influence on increasing the first-lactation milk yield (Fig. 5). The only other time weight is more important is when the cow is sold as a cull cow. Keown and colleagues' studies presented data showing an increase in total first-lactation milk yields in heifers weighing 568 kg (~1250 lb) after calving as compared to lighter weight, 522-kg (~1150 lb) heifers. The heavier heifers produced 239 kg (~527 lb) more milk than the lighter heifers, whereas heifers

weighing 590 kg (~1300 lb) produced only 18.6 kg (~41 lb) more milk than the 568-kg heifers. The goal of 568 kg could be easily accomplished at a daily gain of 0.8 kg (~1.75 lb) per day during development. However, an additional gain of 22.7 kg (~50 lb) of body weight for 18.6 kg of milk may not be economically justifiable in the 590-kg heifers.

Heifers can calve at 24 months of age and have high milk production. Holstein herds in Wisconsin producing in excess of 10,000 kg (~22,000 lb) raise heifers that weigh 363 kg (~800 lb) at 13 months for breeding, calving at an average of 24 months, weighing 613 kg (~1350 lb). Furthermore, large heifers, weighing 568 kg after calving, are closer to their genetically determined mature size and need to grow less during their first lactation. This may help alleviate the syndrome known as "sophomore slump" or milk production depression after the second calving.

DECREASING HEIFER INVENTORY NUMBERS

Calving heifers at an older age has many disadvantages other than increasing their nonproductive life and delaying potential milk income. When heifers calve at ages greater than 24 to 25 months, larger heifer inventory must be maintained. Increasing the age at calving also increases the generation interval because of the delay in bringing genetically superior replacements into the herd. If the annual replacement rate is 33%, 33 heifers are needed per 100 cows per year. Assuming a 15% attrition for death loss, infertility, and selection within the heifer pool, approximately 38 heifers at 2 years of age will be needed. For every 1-month increase in the age at calving, an additional 4.2% increase in total heifer inventory numbers is needed to maintain adequate culling rates in the lactation herd. This figure takes into account the inventory of heifers from birth through calving. Therefore, if a herd is calving 28-month-old heifers at an average culling rate of 33%, we now need 89 heifers per 100 cows on the farm rather than 76 heifers. This equates to an increase of 16.8% in the total number of heifers consuming feed and needing management on a yearly basis.

HEIFERS IN THE LACTATING HERD

Heifers should be considered for replacements in the herd if milk production of the dam is above the herd average. Projected mature equivalent (ME) for heifers should be within 182 kg (~400 lb) to 227 kg (~500 lb) of that for second- and later-lactation cows. Despite this fact, data from the Raleigh Dairy Records Processing Center indicate that in 1996 the average heifer ME milk is within 454 kg (~1000 lb) of second- and later-lactation cows. If heifers were given the same opportunity to be fed equally, the same level of genetics applied to heifers as to mature cows, and culling pressure the same for heifers and later lactations, then we would expect the projected ME 305-day milk production to be the same. While heifers should be genetically superior, the same culling procedures have not been applied as in later-lactation cows. Since culling increases production faster than genetics, second- and later-lactation cows' projected ME for milk production should be within 227 kg (~500 lb) of that of heifers. The disadvantage of using ME as a measure of genetic progress is the 2- to 3-year lag period between conception and projected production records of progeny. Even though ME is not a true measure of genetics, it does measure genetic potential if all the other variables between parties are equal.

Another measure of potential genetic gain in the herd is the 305-day ME of this year's first-lactation heifers over that of the previous year. An average of greater than 91 kg (~200 lb) over that of last year's heifers is reasonable (see Table 3). Heifer peak milk should also be evaluated as to the genetic level of management. The goal for peak milk of first-lactation heifers would be expected to be 75% of the third-lactation-and-greater cows and 80% of peak milk production for second-lactation cows. Surveys of inadequately developed heifers on several farms have peak milk for heifers at 28 kg (~62 lb) to 29.5 kg (~65 lb), when second-and-greater-lactation cows are reaching 41 kg (~90 lb) to 45.5 kg (~100 lb). To meet targets, these heifers should have an additional 4.5 kg of peak milk. These farms had heifer inventories in the lactating herd of 35% to 47%. This type of production level was a direct result of inferior heifer development and a lack of heifer monitoring, resulting in decreased milk production. For every additional pound of peak milk, an increase in the total lactation of 91 kg (~200 lb) of milk can be expected. If these heifers were reaching this additional 4.5 kg (~10 lb) of peak, the potential exists for 909 kg (~2000 lb) of total lactation milk yield.

ECONOMICS OF DELAYED PARTURITION

The delay in first parturition of heifers can be costly. Projections range from a loss of $1 to $3 for every day in excess of 24 months of age parturition is delayed. If a herd is calving 50 heifers with an average calving age of 27 months, the potential loss in income is approximately $7500 per year. Returns from the transition period down to 24 months could also represent generated income. If, for example, the age at first calving is reduced from 27 down to 24 months, the dairy could expect 3 months' worth of additional heifers for potential sale. Of the 50 heifers previously needed, we can now reduce this number to 44 heifers needed to maintain our culling rate and additional heifers for selection. If they are sold at $1250 per heifer, the income would be $7500. It should be noted this is a one-time transition return and would not be expected in subsequent years if the calving age remained at 24 months. Dairymen should not anticipate reducing the age to calving in several months, as experience indicates this will probably take at least 18 to 24 months to decrease age at calving to our goal of 24 months.

In a microcomputer simulation model to evaluate management strategies for raising dairy replacements, Bethard demonstrated the effects of heat detection efficiency in replacements. This model looked at three heat detection rates (40%, 50%, 60%) at each of three conception rates (40%, 60%, 80%). Across all conception rates, improving heat detection efficiency from 40% to 50% reduced the total rearing costs by $39.72. The reduction was $16.22 when moving from a 50% to a 60% heat detection efficiency. This demonstrates that heat detection efficiency is proportionately more costly at lower heat detection rates, emphasizing the costs of poor heat detection. The sum of the two figures ($55.94) represents the decrease in rearing costs when improving heat detection from 40% to 60%. Across all heat detection and conception rates evaluated, total rearing costs for each heifer entering the milking herd decreased $2.80 for each percent increase in heat detection efficiency. Economics of heat detection aids that improve heat detection efficiency could be evaluated using this figure.

MARKETING HEIFER REPLACEMENT PROGRAMS

Marketing is informing clients and potential clients of your skills and services. Although this usually comes by way of the traditional practice of veterinary medicine (i.e., vaccination programs, dehorning, disease outbreaks, checking heifers for pregnancy, etc.), these procedures can be used to promote a production medicine program with an emphasis on heifer management. Disease outbreaks can often lead to monitoring of colostral absorption in neonates, and while vaccinating heifers an additional minute per heifer is all that is needed to tape or weigh and check height and body condition score on a random selection of heifers. With the aid of a growth chart and plotting points of heifer data, a diagrammatic picture can be presented to the producer in an appropriate manner. The phrase "a picture is worth a thousand words" and "a graph is worth $1000" is valuable if these heifer data are available in a fashion that is easily understood by the producer.

Improvement in the heifer program may be slow. In working with heifers, we inform producers that diligent work and a priority placed on heifer rearing will demonstrate their value in approximately 2 years. This takes into consideration that often the problem is in the early neonatal or early growth period. This means starting with the new group of neonates and developing them through to 24 months of age. It is important for consultants to prioritize problems on an economic basis and to consider the short- and long-term effects of any recommended changes on the total economic outlook of the dairy.

BIBLIOGRAPHY

Bailey TL: Economic considerations of dairy heifers. *In* Proceedings of the Society for Theriogenology. San Antonio, Aug 14–15, 1992, pp 56–59.

Bethard G: A microcomputer simulation to evaluate management strategies for rearing dairy replacements. PhD dissertation, Virginia Polytechnic Institute and State University, Blacksburg, Dairy Science Department, May 1997.

Braun RK, et al: Body condition scoring dairy cows as a herd management too. Compend Contin Educ Pract Vet 9:F192–F200, 1987.

Day JD: Optimizing heifer growth rates in high producing dairy herds. Compendium Continuing Educ Pract Vet 13:693–700, 1991.

Donovan GA, et al: Evaluation of dairy heifer replacement-rearing programs. Compend Contin Educ Pract Vet 9:F133–F138, 1987.

Fetrow J: Dairy production medicine software. University of Minnesota, St Paul.

Fetrow J, et al: Dairy herd health monitoring. Part II. A computer spreadsheet for dairy herd monitoring. Compend Contin Educ Pract Vet 10:75–80, 1988.

Fiez E: Sizing up heifer age. Dairy. January, 1989, pp. 6–8.

Fisher LJ, Hall JW, Jones SE: Weight and age at calving and weight change related to first lactation milk yield. J Dairy Sci 66:2167–2172, 1983.

Gardner CE, Johnson AP: Nontraditional opportunities for dairy practitioners. *In* Dairy Practice Management. Vet Clin North Am Food Anim Pract 5:575–581, 1989.

Gardner RW, et al: Accelerated growth and early breeding of Holstein heifers. J Dairy Sci 60:1941–1948, 1977.

Head HH. Heifer performance standards: Rearing systems, growth rates and lactation. *In* Van Horn H, Wilcox C (eds): Large Dairy Herd Management. Champaign, Ill, Management Dairy Science Association, American Dairy Science Association, 1992, pp 422–433.

Heinrichs AJ. Opportunities in replacement heifer growth. Dairy session III. *In* Proceedings of the American Association of Bovine Practitioners, 1991, pp 73–75.

Heinrichs AJ, et al: Standards of weight and height for Holstein heifers. J Dairy Sci 70:653–660, 1987.

Hoard's Dairyman: Raising Dairy Heifers. A Supplement. Nutrition Is the Key to Breeding Age Size. Fort Atkinson, Wisc, W. D. Hoard and Sons, 1990.

Hoffman PC, et al: Growth rate of Holstein replacement heifers in selected Wisconsin herds. *In* University of Wisconsin College of Agriculture and Life Sciences Research Report R3551, 1992.

James RE, et al: Heifer feeding and management systems. *In* Van Horn H, Wilcox C (eds): Large Dairy Herd Management. Champaign, Ill, Management Dairy Science Association, American Dairy Science Association, 1992, pp 411–421.

Keown JF, et al: Freshen heifers at 1200 lbs. Dairy Herd Management, August 1986, p 18.

Kirking GA, et al: AI: Easy and profitable. Dairy Herd Workshop, May 1991, pp 34–36.

LeBlanc MM: Management of calf herd programs. Vet Clin North Am 3:435–445, 1981.

Nickerson SC: Mastitis control in replacement heifers. Dairy session III. *In* Proceedings of the American Association of Bovine Practitioners, 1991, pp 76–78.

Reid JT, et al: Effect of plane of nutrition during early life on growth, reproduction, production, health and longevity of Holstein cows. 1. Birth to fifth calving. Cornell University Agricultural Experiment Station Bull. No. 987, 1964.

Serjsen K, et al: Influence of nutrition on mammary development in pre- and postpubertal heifers. J Dairy Sci 65:793–800, 1982.

Sinha YN, et al: Mammary development and pituitary prolactin level of heifers from birth through puberty and during the estrous cycle. J Dairy Sci 52:507–512, 1969.

Stobo IJF, et al: Rumen development in the calf, the effects of diets containing different proportions of concentrates to hay on rumen development. Br J Nutr 20:171–188, 1966.

Van Der Leek ML, et al: Dairy replacement rearing programs. *In* Howard JL (ed): Current Veterinary Therapy 3: Food Animal Practice. Philadelphia, WB Saunders, 1993, pp 147–153.

■ Dairy Production Medicine

Bruce L. Clark, D.V.M., Diplomate, A.C.T.

Dairy production medicine can be viewed as an evolving discipline within veterinary medicine.[1] This discipline is based on techniques and technologies developed over many decades and continues to adapt current technologies to provide a service that is primarily concerned with the production of milk by the most efficient means possible.

The historical development of individual animal medicine was based on a thorough understanding of physiology, pathophysiology, disease diagnostics, and therapeutics. As the concept of herd health became popular, the use of disease control programs utilizing developments in vaccines and anthelmintics expanded the role of the veterinarian on farms. Research and development in the management of mastitis and reproductive performance were also included in the herd health concept. As these programs became commonplace, the idea of risk management and disease prevention were an integral part of the management programs of more progressive dairy producers.

In the 1970s and 1980s, computer technology made great strides. The cost of maintaining records on computers was within the grasp of most producers. Advisors to such operations promoted these activities so that monitoring of performance and health could be accomplished more accurately. This provided a mechanism for evaluating the results of the management strategies developed for each operation. Rates of disease could be monitored with much less effort and disease control strategies adjusted as necessary. Individual and group production performance could be monitored and illustrated graphically so that critical evaluations could be conducted. From this activity, a list of strengths and weaknesses could be identified and programs targeted to address the areas that were likely to result in the highest return. Today, many producers develop teams of consultants to identify opportunities and to advise them on management strategies that may create greater efficiency. As illustrated in Table 1, production medicine veterinarians are essential members of such teams.

SKILLS AND ABILITIES

It is very difficult to compile a complete list of the skills and abilities required to be considered a dairy production medicine veterinarian. As the involvement of the veterinarian expands in an individual operation, new situations constantly develop that require specialized knowledge and abilities. An example of such a situation is the investigation of potential stray voltage and its possible impact on udder health and production performance on a particular farm. Therefore, a discussion of general areas is the only practical alternative.

Knowledge of dairy production systems is essential to the practice of dairy production medicine. The operation of a modern dairy farm is complex and involves many components, such as housing, crop management, and genetics. An understanding of the day-to-day management activities of a dairy farm is critical to the production veterinarian's ability to communicate effectively with management.

A strong background in individual animal medicine is also essential to the production veterinarian. Interaction of the animal, environment, and agents is a basic concept taught to veterinary students. The ability to evaluate individual animals and to diagnose individual animal diseases and an understanding of the complex nature of disease are critical in the development of prevention and control programs.

Principles of epidemiology are essential. An understanding of rates, disease risk factors, disease outbreak investigations, and levels of intervention is a central theme of many production medicine activities. Establishing rates of particular conditions is essential to an understanding of the current and historical situation on a dairy farm. An investigation of known risk factors for those conditions can be undertaken so that an effective control program can be implemented. The investigation process is based on a scientific process of disease investigation techniques[2] that have been developed. These techniques establish a procedural approach encompassing steps to be followed during the investigation. This stepwise approach may prevent the veterinarian from overlooking important areas.

Table 1
POTENTIAL MEMBERS OF MANAGEMENT TEAM*

◆ Veterinarian
◆ Nutritionist
◆ Forage specialist
◆ Milking equipment dealer
◆ Dairy records specialist
◆ Banker/accountant

*This list may be modified as needed.

Table 2
SKILLS IMPORTANT TO DAIRY PRODUCTION VETERINARIANS

Animal production systems
Epidemiology
Nutrition and feeding systems
Microcomputer record systems
Housing and cow comfort
Milk quality assurance
Individual animal medicine
Theriogenology
Biotechnology (bovine somatotropin, etc.)
Production economics
Residue avoidance
Presentation skills

Once the conditions that are limiting efficiency have been identified and investigated, an intervention strategy must be developed. Three levels of intervention are suggested. The first level of intervention addresses clinical disease and strategies for the treatment of sick animals. This level is related to individual animal medicine and the significant production losses that occur in affected animals. The second level of intervention addresses subclinical disease (e.g., subclinical mastitis). Methods for monitoring and controlling subclinical diseases are developed. Again, production losses occur, and effective strategies to minimize these losses can result in significant increases in efficiency. The third level of intervention addresses management of risk for disease. Vaccination and parasite control programs are examples of this level of intervention, but other strategies are necessary for such diseases as mastitis and noninfectious causes of abortion. This level of intervention is related to prevention of disease and prevention of production losses. Effective production medicine services should promote the development and implementation of all three levels of intervention.

Table 2 lists these and other skills necessary for the dairy production medicine veterinarian. A comprehensive review of all of these areas is beyond the scope of this article.

COMPONENTS OF A DAIRY PRODUCTION MEDICINE SERVICE

The components of a dairy production medicine service will vary from practitioner to practitioner. Table 3 is a suggested list of areas associated with most dairy production medicine services.

RECORD SYSTEMS

Effective record systems are an essential component of a production medicine service. Many different record systems are

---

Table 3
COMPONENTS OF A DAIRY PRODUCTION MEDICINE SERVICE

◆ Record systems
◆ Nutrition and feeding systems
◆ Cow comfort
◆ Udder health and milk quality
◆ Reproductive management
◆ Replacement rearing
◆ Disease control programs
◆ Economic analysis

---

available. The availability of support, ease of use, cost, and recommendations by other dairymen and consultants often determine which system is used on a particular farm. The basic types of systems currently used are manual record systems, dairy herd improvement (DHI) testing programs, and computerized on-farm systems. Individual computer programs are also available to access the various computerized record systems and create a standardized report format.

The ability to manipulate the data recorded in a computerized record system to develop information about a particular farm is important. This is obviously based on the individual practitioner's skill with a computer. The basic output of most record systems should provide management and analytical reports. Examples of management reports are heat expectancy lists and individual milk production reports for grouping and other purposes. Analytical reports provide information on herd trends and current performance. Examples of analytical reports are production reports stratified by lactation number and stage of lactation. The ability to convert data to graphs is also important so that a visual image of the data can be presented to the producer. An example of a set of reports for a specific farm is presented in Table 4.

NUTRITION AND FEEDING SYSTEMS

Many regional differences exist in types of feed ingredients and feeding systems utilized on dairy farms. The dairy production veterinarian must be familiar with these differences. Although a comprehensive discussion of dairy nutrition is beyond the scope of this article, a short discussion of the types of ingredients and types of feeding systems utilized on dairy farms will provide a basis for further study. Continuing education programs offered by the American Association of Bovine Practitioners and others provide excellent basic and applied information for evaluating and balancing dairy rations. The National Research Council publication[3] on dairy cattle requirements is an indispensable resource for the practicing production veterinarian.

Forages are the basis of any dairy ration. High-quality forage must be either grown on the farm or purchased from a reliable source. Forages can be in the form of hay, haylage, silage, and grazing. The physical form of the stored forages is as important as the nutrient content. A high-quality stored forage such as corn silage must have sufficient length to maintain rumen health if it is to be utilized in rations properly. Insufficient length of cut is often a consequence of efforts to create the best environment for fermentation and to maximize storage capacity within the silo. These types of problems often result in milk fat depressions and a higher than normal rate of foot and leg problems due to subclinical rumen acidosis. Forages also vary significantly

---

Table 4
EXAMPLE OF A SET OF MONTHLY ANALYTICAL REPORTS

Herd summary (rolling herd averages and current test day summary data)
Persistency stratified by lactation and days in milk
Yearly reproductive summary statistics
Rolling herd milk production graph (24-mo averages)
Average somatic cell score graph (24-mo averages)
Production averages stratified by lactation and days in milk
Udder health (LSCC) stratified by lactation and days in milk
Days to first breeding analysis stratified by days to first breeding
150-Day corrected milk production graph (24-mo averages)
Projected calving interval graph (24-mo averages)

in their nutrient and moisture content. Ration formulation using published averages of forage nutrient composition is unreliable and inefficient.

The concentrate portion of a dairy ration is composed of grains, minerals, vitamins, and specialized feed ingredients, and often includes by-products of grain-processing industries. The grains provide sources of energy and protein. Macrominerals and microminerals are usually provided in a pre-mix formulation that also includes the vitamin components of the ration. Specialized feed ingredients, such as rumen-protected fats, are often included for energy supplementation in rations for high-producing cattle. The byproduct feeds, such as cottonseed and distillers' grains, are often a good source of energy and protein at a cost that is beneficial to the dairy producer. Some byproducts can also function as a forage extender for farms with limited forage resources. Many production veterinarians work closely with professional nutritionists when working with specific producers. Other production veterinarians provide a complete nutrition-balancing program. Computer programs, such as the Spartan Dairy Ration Evaluation program available from Michigan State University, are an inexpensive tool for developing and evaluating rations for dairy farms.

Although it is important for the production medicine veterinarian to be familiar with ration balancing, it is also important to understand how the feed is prepared and delivered to the cows. There are many different types of feeding systems. Total mixed rations have become very popular since the late 1980s. Computer feeders are also utilized on many farms so that grain feeding can be adjusted to an individual cow's needs. The mixing and delivery of feed should be monitored frequently by management and by the production veterinarian to ensure that the cows are getting and eating the ration as developed. The evaluation should determine the feeding frequency as well as the physical form of the ration. The rumen health and potential risk of nutritionally related diseases can only be assessed with a complete understanding of the ration, ration ingredients, and feed delivery system.

COW COMFORT

A major limitation of production efficiency on many dairy farms is related to cow comfort. Cows are housed in many different types of systems within the United States. Many southern herds are housed primarily on pasture. Free stall and loose housing are also widely used, especially in the larger commercial dairy operations. Stanchion barn housing is common in northern areas of the United States. Each system has its advantages and disadvantages. Pastured cattle tend to have fewer foot and leg problems than cattle maintained primarily in total confinement facilities with concrete alleys. However, the ability to deliver feed to cattle in groups may be easier in total confinement operations. Other considerations are also important.

Environmental heat stress is a critical limitation to milk production in many areas of the United States. Facilities that provide adequate ventilation and cooling of cows during periods of heat stress are vital considerations when designing facilities. Strategies to control heat stress, such as cooling fans and sprinklers, are best implemented in total confinement facilities. Specific design recommendations for free stalls, fans, and sprinklers for dairy facilities are available from most state extension services. Due to the differences in humidity in the southern states vs. western states, different design considerations are important.

Bedding is another important consideration related to cow comfort. The bedding selected should provide a high degree of comfort without compromising health or milk quality. Sand is a common form of bedding utilized in free stalls. When properly maintained, it will provide good comfort and will not support high bacterial populations. However, sand has the potential for creating problems with current waste management systems, such as manure separators and lagoons. Dried manure and other organic bedding, such as wood shavings and sawdust, also provide a high degree of comfort but have the potential for supporting high populations of bacteria in humid regions of the country, resulting in udder health problems.

To maintain the most efficient production possible, feed intake of a properly balanced ration should be maximized. Cow comfort is a critical component of achieving maximum dry matter intake.

UDDER HEALTH AND MILK QUALITY

Udder health and milk quality constitute a major component of dairy production medicine. The regulatory requirements are developed by each state using the pasteurized milk ordinance as a guideline. These regulations establish the minimum standards for somatic cell count concentration and bacteria counts of milk. It is important to understand that these standards are the *minimum* standards for milk quality. The progressive dairyman should exceed these standards. The minimum standards in most states are a somatic cell count of 750,000 per milliliter or less and a bacteria count of 100,000 or less.

The National Mastitis Council is an excellent reference for current information related to understanding and maintaining acceptable udder health. Their membership has developed recommendations for controlling mastitis through proper milking techniques and proper milking machine function. Progress in mastitis research that is important in development and maintenance of udder health is reported during their annual meetings. The dairy production medicine veterinarian should participate and utilize this valuable resource.

The basic principles of disease control must be applied to controlling mastitis on dairy farms. An effective method of controlling mastitis is to control the number of new infections that occur and to decrease the duration of existing infections. New infections can be defined in many ways. A common method is to utilize monthly DHI somatic cell count data. The linear score discriminator for infected cows may differ, but a linear score value of 5 will be used for this description. (Some dairy practitioners, however, may prefer a linear score of 4.) At least 2 months' data are necessary to classify cows. A new infection will have a current test day linear score of 5.0 or above and a previous test day linear score of less than 5.0. A chronically infected cow will have a current test day linear score of 5.0 or above as well as a previous test day linear score of 5.0 or above. Rates of new and chronic infections of 6% or less can be achieved on most dairy farms. If rates are higher than desired, individual milk cultures of newly and chronically infected cows can be performed to establish the pathogens responsible for the infections. The resulting culture data can be utilized in developing a control program. Continuous monitoring of the DHI somatic cell count data should indicate the effectiveness of the control program.

Development of an effective mastitis control program should be based on the pathogens isolated from infected cows. Each individual pathogen has characteristics that must be considered when developing control strategies. For example, *Streptococcus agalactiae* is a contagious pathogen of the udder that is commonly spread from cow to cow during milking. It responds well to antibiotic therapy during lactation. A control program that addresses this particular pathogen must include strategies for preventing new infections as well as decreasing the duration of existing infections. Therefore, a thorough review of milking machine function and milking procedures would address prevention of new infections. Existing infections must be identified for antibiotic therapy so that the duration of infections can be decreased. Additional strategies, such as segregation of infected cows, may also be recommended based on practitioner experience and specific farm situations. Regardless, the basic concept of identifying and controlling new and chronic infections should be applied, and the results of the program should be monitored.

Periodic culture of bulk tank milk is also a useful technique for monitoring udder health. Bulk tank culture results quantify pathogen populations per milliliter of milk. This information should be considered in conjunction with individual cow culture results. The appearance of a particular pathogen within bulk tank milk at significant numbers should be reflected in the culture results of individual cows. If there is a discrepancy, a review of the investigation would be indicated. Although bulk tank cultures provide valuable information about the pathogens existing on a particular farm, multiple bulk tank cultures are probably more indicative of the true dynamics of mastitis on the farm. Some pathogens, such as *Staphylococcus aureus*, are intermittently shed from cows. A single bulk tank culture may not accurately reflect the significance of a specific pathogen.

Residue avoidance must be considered when developing mastitis control programs. Therapeutic strategies must include both the types of antibiotics and other drugs used on a particular farm and specific strategies to prevent drug residues in milk and meat. Proper identification of cows receiving treatment and adequate withholding times must be specified for each drug. Bulk tank milk testing kits for most approved antibiotics are available for on-farm use so that residues are more likely to be detected before milk is shipped from the farm. These test kits are also utilized on individual cows, although their accuracy when used in this manner may be questionable.

REPRODUCTIVE MANAGEMENT

Many production medicine programs begin with a reproductive management program. These programs consist of regularly scheduled visits to a dairy farm to perform examinations for pregnancy, proper postpartum involution, and evaluation of cows that fail to exhibit estrus. A reliable record system is utilized to establish a list of cows to be examined during each visit. The cows are then examined and results recorded. The results of each trip are reviewed with the farm manager to determine the efficiency of the reproductive management program. A vital component of any reproductive management program is accurate recording of reproductive events. Every calving, estrus, and breeding event must be recorded. The results of each reproductive examination must also be reported, especially pregnancies and pathologic findings such as cystic ovaries or pyometra. Accurate records are essential for proper evaluation of specific reproductive parameters. Reporting of reproductive data is often overlooked by a busy dairyman and must be encouraged by the dairy production veterinarian.

Many parameters have been developed for evaluating reproductive efficiency.[4] The most commonly utilized parameters are listed in Table 5. The voluntary waiting period is the stage of lactation during which cows become eligible for breeding. Common voluntary waiting periods range from 45 to 60 days. The interval selected is important to the dairy production veterinarian when evaluating other parameters. The goal for days to first service on a dairy farm is the voluntary waiting period plus half an estrous cycle, or about 12 days. This is due to the fact that as cows become eligible for breeding, estrus should occur within 21 days. If a group of cows are evaluated, the average interval to breeding should be in the middle of this interval, or about 11 or 12 days.

Days open is the average of the current days in milk for nonpregnant cows that have not been bred plus the days in milk at last breeding for cows that are pregnant or have a current breeding. Another way of thinking about days open is to artificially assume that all cows beyond the voluntary waiting period are pregnant. The days open for pregnant cows is the days in milk at their last breeding. The days open for cows that have been bred but not confirmed pregnant is the last breeding. The days open for cows that have not been bred is their current days in milk. The average of these values for each cow would be the herd's average days open. If you add the gestation length for cattle to the average days open, you get the best possible estimate of the average calving interval of the herd. This value should be less than or equal to the herd's calving interval goal. A reasonable goal for calving intervals is from 12 months to 13.5 months, depending on the production level of the herd. Higher-producing herds may have more difficulty achieving the "ideal" calving interval of 12 to 12.5 months. Lower-producing herds should be achieving a calving interval closer to this "ideal" calving interval. Services per pregnancy are the number of services, or breedings, required to establish a pregnancy. This value should be below 2.0.

Reproductive inefficiency in dairy herds is most commonly associated with failure to observe estrus. Procedures for observation of estrus should be established and monitored by the dairy production medicine veterinarian. Twice-daily observation for 1 hour of cows for estrus should be established in herds utilizing artificial insemination. These observations should occur during times when the cows are not being moved for specific purposes, such as milking. All personnel on the farm should be aware of the signs of estrus and should report cows in estrus to the appropriate person. The use of estrus detection aids, such as prostaglandins and heat mount detectors, are valuable adjuncts to regular heat detection but should not become the primary mechanism for determining when to breed cows.

Improper breeding technique and semen handling are also common reasons for poor reproductive efficiency. A thorough review of breeding technique should be conducted as part of an evaluation of poor reproductive efficiency. Procedures for evaluation of frozen semen are available from the Society for Theriogenology if semen viability is suspect.[5]

Through attention to detail and evaluation of reproductive records, most reproductive inefficiency problems can be resolved. Published rates of reproductive diseases can be compared to rates on a particular farm to determine whether specific intervention strategies are appropriate.

REPLACEMENT REARING

Replacement rearing is an often neglected area of dairy production management. The future success of a dairy operation is dependent on developing a quality replacement for the cows in the herd. The primary goal of replacement rearing is to maintain optimal weight gain and height from birth to first calving. It is also important to minimize morbidity and mortality. The development of the replacement heifer is commonly divided into

---

Table 5
COMMON REPRODUCTIVE PARAMETERS

- ◆ Average projected calving interval
- ◆ Average days to first service
- ◆ Services per conception
- ◆ Average days open

the phases listed in Table 6. Each phase has specific management requirements.

The interval from birth to weaning typically requires the most time per animal. The primary objective of this interval is to provide adequate colostral transfer of immunity, minimize stress, and provide for adequate development of the rumen. The majority of the problems that occur in replacements typically occur during this phase of development. The primary deficiency that occurs during this phase is inadequate colostral management. Each calf should receive 1 gallon of good colostrum as soon as possible after birth. The critical period is within 24 hours after birth. The only method that ensures that adequate colostrum has been obtained by the calf is hand-feeding of colostrum to each calf. The calf should then receive 1 gallon of milk or quality milk replacer until weaned. Starting at age 3 days, each calf should be offered a quality calf starter. It will typically take approximately 2 weeks for the calves to begin significant intake of this starter. Once the calves are eating an adequate amount of the calf starter, they can be weaned. In Holstein calves, 2 lb of calf starter intake is a reasonable guideline for weaning readiness. Housing during this phase should minimize stress. This will best be accomplished by providing housing that is clean and dry and does not allow direct contact with other calves.

The next phase of heifer development is from weaning to puberty. A ration developed for these calves should provide for a daily weight gain of about 1.8 to 2.0 lb/day. The rumen should be developed adequately at the beginning of this phase so that a good-quality forage can be utilized as a portion of the ration. In calves up to 6 months old, however, wet silage should be avoided. Initial vaccinations are given during this interval to protect the calf from diseases such as brucellosis. Specific guidelines for this and other phases of replacement rearing are covered in another section of this book.

The production veterinarian should implement a monitoring program that will provide a means of determining whether growth and development goals are being achieved. This should include actual weights if possible, but tape weights can be utilized if necessary. The height of the replacements should also be determined. These data should be compared to established standards for growth and development.

DISEASE CONTROL PROGRAMS

Disease control will continue to be the main responsibility of the veterinarian working with animal agriculture production units. The knowledge required to develop and implement effective disease control programs is the basis of a veterinarian's education. The ability to integrate this knowledge with the production efficiency demands of a modern dairy operation are a distinguishing attribute of a production medicine service. Vaccination and parasite control programs must be developed that address both existing and high-risk diseases unique to each dairy operation. Overutilization of financial resources to protect against diseases that have a very low risk of occurrence is inefficient. Failure to utilize health products that have a strong potential for enhancing health and productivity is also inefficient and potentially devastating. The dairy production veterinarian must develop disease control programs for all animals on a particular production unit. Many products cannot be used in lactating cattle, and the veterinarian must not only be aware of these limitations but must be capable of explaining the reasons for these restrictions whenever possible. Common infectious diseases, such as leptospirosis and bovine viral diarrhea, are usually included in most vaccination programs. Other procedures, such as routine deworming of lactating dairy cattle, may only be appropriate in selected herds. The production medicine veteri-

| Table 6 |
| **REPLACEMENT REARING PHASES** |
| ◆ Birth to weaning |
| ◆ Weaning to puberty |
| ◆ Puberty to breeding |
| ◆ Breeding management |
| ◆ Pregnant heifer management |

narian must make these judgments based on knowledge of the disease, diagnostic test results, and the risk factors for the existence of that disease in each herd.

ECONOMIC ANALYSIS

Many practicing dairy production medicine veterinarians have developed a cost of production analysis service. This activity is highly specialized and requires continuing education courses, such as are offered by the American Association of Bovine Practitioners. The objective of determining a farm's cost of production is to determine the areas that may require excessive economic resources. One of the difficulties associated with this process is the availability of cost-of-production guidelines or benchmarks. Regional differences as well as the variation in size of operations may make some published guidelines difficult to utilize.

SUMMARY

Dairy production medicine has gained recognition as a production-oriented service offered by veterinarians. It is a highly specialized area within veterinary medicine that requires skills and abilities specific to the dairy industry. The veterinarian often begins a production medicine service with a reproductive management program or a nutritional consulting service. These activities often lead to identification of other potential areas that need attention, such as udder health management, disease management, or production records monitoring. The development of a comprehensive production medicine program will develop as the veterinarian becomes more knowledgeable of a particular dairy. The training necessary to develop and implement services associated with production medicine have traditionally been acquired through independent study and continuing education programs offered by various organizations. Recently, veterinary colleges have begun to develop the specialized programs of study for veterinary students interested in production medicine.

REFERENCES

1. Radostits OM, Leslie KE, Fetrow J: Herd Health: Food Animal Production Medicine, ed 2. Philadelphia, WB Saunders, 1994.
2. Hancock DD, Wikse SE: Investigation planning and data gathering. Vet Clin North Am Food Anim Pract 4:1, 1988.
3. National Research Council: Nutrient Requirements of Dairy Cattle, 6th ed. Washington, National Academy Press, 1988.
4. Fetrow J, McClary D, Harman R, et al: Calculating selected reproductive indices: Recommendations of the American Association of Bovine Practitioners. J Dairy Sci 73:78, 1990.
5. Barth AD: Evaluation of frozen bovine semen by the veterinary practitioner. In Theriogenology Handbook. Hastings, Neb, Society for Theriogenology, B-9, 1993.

■ Breeding Season Evaluation of Beef Herds

Vincent Traffas, D.V.M.
Terry J. Engelken, D.V.M., M.S.

Reproductive efficiency is the single most important economic trait in a beef herd.[1] A review of the standardized performance analysis (SPA) data suggests that reproductive efficiency can be broken down into two separate functions: (1) the percent of females exposed that actually wean a live calf and (2) the calving distribution resulting from a breeding season of variable length. Reproductive efficiency is contingent on sire fertility, a sound overall herd health program, optimum nutrition, genetic makeup, ranch environment, and owner management. Because it is the interaction of all of these components that controls the potential for profitability, each of these must be considered individually to successfully evaluate the breeding season.

Many extensive and in-depth literature sources are available to the reader that address infectious causes of infertility in the beef cow.[2] Well-planned, cost-effective preventive health programs should be in place prior to the beginning of breeding season. Biosecurity is of equal importance in preventing venereal disease transmission. Reviews dealing with breeding soundness evaluations and the overall health management of beef bulls have been published.[3, 4] When reproductive failure occurs, these areas should always be investigated. However, it is not within the scope of this article to review these areas in detail. This treatise seeks to examine noninfectious causes of infertility that fall into the realm of management, environment, and/or genetics, which is a risk-factor approach to the multifactorial production disease of infertility. This approach centers around the very traditional role of the veterinarian in establishing pregnancy status after the breeding season is over.

As can be seen in Table 1, heritability estimates for general reproductive performance traits are low.[5] Therefore, management has a greater impact on fertility in beef cows than does heredity. Management risk factors involved in fertility or pregnancy status should be evaluated at the end of the breeding season. These risk factors include breed, age, weight, frame score, and body condition score (BCS) of the dam[6] and the sustained fertility of the sire or sire groups. These factors are key determinants in the causal pathway of fertility and are subject to owner manipulation. Reproductive performance can be used as a barometer to evaluate how well cow type fits the natural forage base of the ranch and the particular management style of the owner.

The basic steps in any disease investigation also apply to

Table 1
HERITABILITY ESTIMATES FOR BEEF CATTLE

Female reproduction	10%–20%
Mothering ability	20%–25%
Weaning weight	20%–25%
Feed conversion	30%–35%
Postweaning gain	35%–40%
Carcass quality grade	40%–50%
Carcass cutability	40%–50%
Yearling weight	60%–70%
Mature weight	60%–80%
Skeletal size	60%–80%

From Bolze RP: Beef cow genetics that will be profitable in the future. Cow-Calf Conference VI: Focus on Basics of Good Management. Manhattan, Kansas, Kansas State University, 1996, pp 3–21.

Table 2
INFORMATION CATEGORIES USED TO EVALUATE REPRODUCTIVE EFFICIENCY OF THE BEEF HERD

Breeding herd inventory
Sires utilized
Sire-to-female ratios
Pregnancy test results
Bull turnout dates
Length of the breeding season
Anticipated calving dates
Projected calving distribution
Herd averages
Range of herd variation
Variables affecting pregnancy status of individual dams
    Age
    Breed
    Weight
    Body condition score
    Frame score
    Bull performance

---

production diseases. This would include the collection of pertinent data as well as the compilation, analysis, and expert interpretation of these data. Finally, recommendations to correct inherent problems are discussed with the producer and a means of subsequent evaluation is put in place.

DATA COLLECTION

To successfully evaluate the reproductive performance and efficiency of a beef herd, information is needed that will define the herd as a single entity, which is then broken down into its component parts. The information gleaned should also clearly project or anticipate when events will occur in the ensuing calving season. Table 2 lists the information categories that are necessary to permit this kind of evaluation. The production data collected from the herd are based on the information needed to clearly define each of these components. The ultimate goal of any cow/calf operation should be profit. Anything that affects profitability should be monitored.

Pregnancy evaluation should be done as soon after the breeding season as is practical and possible. This enables a more accurate dating of the pregnancy and allows the practitioner to pick up clues as to why certain animals did not conceive. Load cells placed beneath the chute to weigh cows and a quick and simple way to measure hip height enable the practitioner to collect additional relevant data. Several different load cell manufacturers offer quality products to choose from. The reader is referred to any available beef industry trade journal in which listings for companies are found. Generally, electronic load cells are preferred because of their speed and reliability.

Several instruments specifically designed to measure hip height are available commercially. However, they tend to be cumbersome and greatly reduce the speed of the operator. This breaks one of the cardinal rules of data collection. The measuring device must be fast and accurate or it will be abandoned. A center rod can be mounted or fastened to the top of most chutes. A tape measure is fastened to the overhead rod so that it slides back and forth. This in turn allows the tape to be moved quickly to the point over the back of the animal so the measurement may be read. This distance, subtracted from the distance from the rod to the floor of the chute, is the animal's true hip height. This method is fast and efficient and can be adopted with minimal expense.

Owner _____ Date _____

Fall Worksheet—Pregnancy Checking

INVENTORY

Current

Females

  Adult cows _____

  2nd calf heifers _____

  Rep. heifers _____

Sires

  AI sires _____

  Nat serv _____

Calves

  Steers _____

  Heifers _____

Total acres allotted for summer grazing

Stocking rate

Length of grazing season Turnout _____ Removal date _____ Total days _____

Comments—Disease incidence and other problems _____

Alterations

Culling information (No. & causes)

_____

_____

_____

_____

_____

Death losses (No. & causes)

_____

_____

_____

REPRODUCTIVE INFORMATION

Natural service

  Start of breeding season _____

  Date bulls removed _____

Artificial insemination

  Synchronization programs _____

Total AI Cows _____

    Heifers _____

    2nd calf _____

First aid date _____ Last AI date _____

Cleanup bulls turned in _____

Date cleanup bulls removed _____

Figure 1

Inventory and reproductive information survey form. AI, artificial insemination.

It should be noted that the natural reaction of a cow with her head caught is to pull back. If in doing so she squats in the chute, an error is caused in the height measurement. Taking into consideration that one frame score is equivalent to 2 in., this error can be substantial. Hydraulic chutes are better at holding the cow and thereby enhance the accuracy of frame score measurement. However, one of the authors (V.T.) has found that the annual measurement of cows in the same herd has acceptable accuracy after several years, provided that the largest frame score is always recorded. When this kind of information is gathered initially, it is much easier to take accurate frame scores of replacement heifers that hold true after yearly measurement.

Many means are available to record data in the field, ranging from a laptop computer to a tablet of paper. The use of pre-printed forms enhances the speed and accuracy of data collec-

tion. These forms can be made up in tablets by most local print shops. It should be noted that unless data collection is fast and simple, it is likely that it will not be done or that its accuracy will be compromised.

Figure 1 details the inventory and reproductive information form. It is arranged in a survey format to collect information regarding actual cattle inventory and pertinent facts about the breeding season. If performance record-keeping is part of the veterinarian's services, the information is even more critical. Unidentified changes in inventory always add to the confusion between producer and veterinarian, and this is the easiest way to keep track of events occurring during the breeding season. This also provides the opportunity to examine problem areas that might not have been identified without collecting this information.

Data capture at the time of pregnancy examination is critical

PREGNANCY CHECK WORKSHEET

Owner _____   Date _____

Cow ID	Breed	Age	Wght	Frame	BCS	Status	Comments

Figure 2
Data sheet used at the time of herd pregnancy examination.

Breeding Season Evaluation

Owner   Joe Rancher
Date   09/23/96

Breeding Information
Inventory and Male-to-Female Ratios

No. of females checked   234
No. of adult females   167
No. of 2nd-calf heifers   32
No. of 1st-calf heifers   35

	No.	**Sires/Female**
No. of sires utilized	7	1 per 33
No. of sires for adult females	6	1 per 28
No. of sires for 2nd-calf heifers		Run with cows
No. of sires for 1st-calf heifers	1	1 per 35

AI Utilized
    Adults   No
    2nd-calf heifers   No
    1st-calf heifers   No

Pregnancy Testing Results

Bull turnout date for cows and 2nd calvers   05/18/96
Bull turnout date for 1st calvers   05/01/96
Length of breeding season for adults   60
Length of breeding season for 1st calvers   45

	No.	% Pregnant	No. Open	% Open
Overall	234	97	6	3
Adults	167	99	2	1
2nd Calvers	32	97	1	3
1st Calvers	35	91	3	9

No. of abortions   0
No. of diagnosed pregnancies but no calf   ?

1st Anticipated calving date for adults   02/25/97
1st Anticipated calving date for heifers   02/08/97

Figure 3
Breeding inventory and pregnancy examination report.

Table 3
PROJECTED CALVING DISTRIBUTION AND HERD STATISTICS REPORT

	Staging (Best Estimate of % Calving per Breeding Season Cycle)			
Heat cycle	1st	2nd	3rd	Late
Overall	61	25	12	2
Adults	57	27	14	2
1st-Calf heifers	91	9	0	0

	Population Statistics Performance Variables			
Averages	*Age, yr*	*Weight, lb*	*Frame Score*	*BCS*
Overall	4.50	1081	4.7	5.2
Adults		1183	5.0	5.0
2nd-Calf heifers		981	5.0	5.0
1st-Calf heifers		1052	5.0	6.0
Largest cow weight	1610 lb			
Smallest cow weight	754 lb			
Standard deviation	168			
Largest frame score	8.5			
Smallest frame score	2.0			
Standard deviation	1.1			

in evaluating the success of the breeding season (Fig. 2). The cow's identification number, breed or phenotype, age, weight, hip height, BCS, and pregnancy status are recorded. Bull assignment, pasture location, and additional comments are quickly recorded. The pregnancy status can be recorded by noting during which cycle of the breeding season the cow was bred. This facilitates the projection of the calving distribution for the following calving season, making compilation of data much easier. Additional comments to be recorded include information about soundness defects, udder abnormalities, or any other health problems in the recent history. It is also important to note any ovarian or uterine reproductive pathology found during the pregnancy examinations.

DATA ANALYSIS

Once data are collected they must be analyzed and summarized. There are many ways to accomplish this, but the use of computer spreadsheets greatly facilitates the task. The information is entered in database format, and if the spreadsheet is created correctly, the information in Figure 3 and Tables 3 through 8 can be easily generated and printed out. Information generated in any of these tables can be presented in a tabular or graphic format, depending on the preferences of the producer and veterinarian. At first glance, much of this information may not seem relevant to simple pregnancy checking of cows. Although a breeding season evaluation should determine pregnancy status first and foremost, a complete evaluation must take into account the costs involved in getting cows pregnant and the end point of the pregnancy: the sale of edible protein. Cost centers should be targeted, and the time schedule of herd events should be clearly defined.

At the time of pregnancy evaluation, inventories of breeding females and the bull battery can be evaluated (Fig. 3). Information concerning bull-to-cow ratios, bull turn-in dates, and breeding season length enables the practitioner to better understand pregnancy results. These factors can have a great impact on percent of cows pregnant and the calving distribution. Expenses associated with bull ownership can be quite high ($20 to $40 per exposed female) and are affected by purchase price, useful lifespan, and number of females covered.[7] If possible, bull

performance by pasture should also be evaluated. Pregnancy status should be defined for the whole herd as well as for each female group, and the results should be clearly illustrated. This enables producers to understand herd performance and the recommendations put forth by the practitioner.

Figure 3 demonstrates the degree of excellence that can be achieved when the cow type matches the environmental resources and the management style on the ranch. This producer consistently maintains one of the highest yearly pregnancy rates in the practice of one of the authors (V.T.) while maintaining one of the lowest feed costs per cow per year. Pounds of weaned calf per acre of grass utilized are above average. One remaining place for improvement in this herd is the bull-to-female ratios. Increasing the number of cows covered by each bull may lower breeding costs even further.

Table 3 illustrates the expected calving distribution for the herd and compares reproductive performance between the mature cows and first-calf heifers. This represents a very useful evaluation tool, because management and disease processes can dramatically affect calving distribution.[8] This in turn directly affects herd output, as older calves tend to be heavier at weaning.[9] This particular set of cows performed adequately, as evidenced by the number of females bred in the first 21-day period (first heat cycle). Additional information given in Table 4 allows comparisons of weight, frame score, and BCS among the different female groups. Examination of the range and standard deviation of particular traits allows the practitioner to evaluate female uniformity. Analysis of this type of data may show the producer a potential problem area and gives valuable insight to explain poor reproductive performance.

The reproductive performance exhibited in Table 3 is fairly typical for many cow/calf operations. The breeding season for the mature herd lasts 90 days and there is tremendous variation in cow weight and frame score. This rancher has done an excellent job of maintaining cow condition. The average cow weight and frame score is very acceptable, but the diversity and ranges show that this is not a uniform herd. This herd represents the end result of several years of this kind of monitoring and reporting. The rancher sold a major portion of his herd and was in the process of rebuilding with replacement heifers. These heifers were bred in a 45-day season with excellent results.

Table 4
PREGNANCY EVALUATION AS PER BREED OF COW

Breed	No. of Cows	Average Age, yr	Average Weight, lb	Average BCS	Average Frame Score	% Pregnant	% Open
Angus	69	4	1078	5.4	4.1	93	7
Angus x Hereford	29	5	1079	5.4	3.7	97	3
Charolais x British	12	6	1291	5.6	5.6	92	8
Simmental x British	8	10	1233	5.0	5.4	88	12
Saler x British	21	6	1150	5.2	4.9	100	0
Charolais	33	6	1303	5.4	5.5	85	15

Table 5
PREGNANCY EVALUATION AS PER WEIGHT OF COW

Weight, lb	No. of Cows	Average BCS	Average Frame Score	% Pregnant	% Open
<1000	23	5.2	3.3	87	13
1000–1099	55	5.3	4.1	96	4
1100–1199	57	5.5	4.5	95	5
1200–1299	27	5.4	5.1	93	7
1300–1400	23	5.3	5.8	87	13
>1400	13	5.5	5.7	92	8

Table 6
PREGNANCY EVALUATION AS PER AGE OF COW

Cow Age, yr	No. of Cows	Average Weight, lb	Average BCS	Average Frame Score	% Pregnant	% Open
2 (Heifers)	18	976	5.5	5.6	89	11
3	18	1115	4.9	5.4	72	28
4	11	1215	4.9	5.3	100	0
5	14	1285	5.4	5.0	100	0
6	9	1308	5.4	5.0	89	11
7	9	1332	5.2	5.4	100	0
8	8	1374	5.3	5.1	88	12
9	7	1314	5.2	5.1	100	0
10	1	1300	5.5	5.5	100	0
11	3	1183	5.3	4.7	100	0
≥12	3	1271	5.2	3.3	100	0

Table 7
PREGNANCY EVALUATION AS PER FRAME SCORE OF COW

Cow Frame Score	No. of Cows	Average Weight, lb	Average BCS	% Pregnant	% Open
<4	9	1189	5.4	100	0
4–4.9	22	1158	5.3	91	9
5.0–5.9	45	1215	5.2	98	2
6.0–6.9	23	1239	5.1	83	17
≥7.0	4	1204	5.1	50	50

Table 8
SUMMARY REPORT FOR INDIVIDUAL SIRE PERFORMANCE

Bull ID No.	No. Exposed	Average Female Age, yr	Average Female BCS	Average Female Frame Score	% Pregnant	% Open
AN74	1	9.0	5.0	4.5	0	100
LE92	126	8.4	5.3	3.8	92	8
MS92	43	4.0	5.2	4.2	88	12
PA92	18	6.9	5.3	3.7	100	0
RA92	49	3.1	5.2	4.2	94	6
RR92	134	7.6	5.2	3.9	93	7
UK92	13	5.3	5.3	3.6	92	8
WA92	58	6.8	5.1	4.0	98	2
OH92	39	3.0	5.4	3.9	97	3

Female breed and weight are related to age, frame score, BCS, and pregnancy rate as part of this analysis (Tables 4 and 5). This enables the practitioner to profile the cow type that matches the rancher's management and environment. As expected, there is a general trend for decreased reproductive performance when cows are larger-framed, heavier, and/or of a breed recognized for high milk production. The BCS across breed and weight is within acceptable limits, and the temptation exists to discount the impact of BCS on reproductive performance in this example. However, these data were collected at pregnancy examination, following a limited breeding season that may have occurred several months earlier. Even if larger cows enter the breeding season in thin condition, they may gain enough weight through the summer grazing period to obtain moderate condition by the time of pregnancy examination. Unfortunately, many of these cows may be open or late bred, and the producer is faced with increased costs associated with postcalving supplemental feed. When evaluating information concerning breed and frame score, it is also necessary to closely monitor precalving and prebreeding BCS to view the whole reproductive picture.

The association of dam age with pregnancy status is shown in Table 6. This analysis is used to illustrate performance differences between replacement heifers, cows nursing their first calf, and mature females. With a herd average-mature-cow weight of just above 1300 lb, the heifers are well on their way to reaching 85% of this value by the time they calve. The pregnancy rate, frame score, and BCS of this group are a reflection of proper development. The 3-year-old cows nursing their first calf show evidence of inadequate development or nutritional stress. With an average BCS of 4.9 and a 72% conception rate, management changes need to be made. These females are approximately 100 lb under target weights. The performance of the 6- and 8-year-old cows may be a reflection of their relatively small number. However, a breed effect should also be examined.

The evaluation of frame score (Table 7) illustrates a common phenomenon. The larger the cow size, the more difficult it is to maintain body condition and, consequently, the higher the open rate. This becomes more evident the sooner the cows are examined for pregnancy after breeding. When nutritional management fails to meet the requirements for maintenance and lactation, reproductive efficiency is compromised. This documentation also gives the practitioner an excellent opportunity to point out the critical relationship between the timing of breeding and calving with the growth curve of the predominant forage on the ranch. These events should be sequenced to allow the producer to take advantage of the surplus energy from forage and protein at a time when cow requirements for these

are high. This tends to optimize reproductive performance and minimize supplemental feed costs.

Pregnancy status should be evaluated for sire effects (Table 8). Female characteristics that may affect reproductive performance are also listed for each pasture. The number of females in each pasture is listed, and bull-to-female ratios of 1:40 are standard in this operation. Pregnancy rates were very good for this particular bull battery. This section may not reveal pertinent information provided that bulls passed a breeding soundness evaluation prior to turnout. However, in the event of poor pregnancy rates in certain female groups or pasture locations, the possibilities of bull injury must be evaluated. The offending sires can be identified and examined for evidence of physical abnormalities. If none are found, then mating behavior should be observed, or the bull-to-female ratio may need to be decreased.

RECOMMENDATIONS AND REPORTING

The examples illustrated in Figure 3 and Tables 3 through 8 were taken from herd reports in the practice of one of the authors (V.T.), and they are used to clarify this style of client communication. Although these examples are not all taken from the same herd, they do provide some insight as to how the variables listed in Table 2 have an impact on herd reproductive performance and how these factors can be communicated to the producer. This standard analysis is accompanied by written documentation of any suggestions or recommendations made to the producer. Each year's performance is compared to those of previous years to document the impact of the veterinarians' recommendations and management changes made by the producer. A track record is established that allows monitoring to take place. Goal-setting, based on economically achievable standards, automatically falls into place for all of these parameters. Not only have we measured what we have done, but we now can compare ourselves to the nation's cowherd.

Poor reproductive efficiency can be associated with a disease process, improper management, and/or a prolonged breeding season.[8, 10, 11] In these herds, any evaluation should target factors that affect pregnancy rate in the first 21-day period. Ideally, 65% to 70% of the females should conceive in the first 21-day breeding period. Seventy percent of the remaining females should become pregnant in the second breeding period. In a limited breeding season of 60 days, a producer should anticipate that a minimum of 4% to 6% of the exposed females will fail to become pregnant. This can be achieved in well-managed herds with lower feed expense compared to those in herds with less stringent demands and longer breeding seasons.

The number of females cycling at the beginning of the breeding season has the greatest impact on early conception rates. In those instances in which females are not conceiving early, herd profiling (see Tables 3 through 8) should offer some insight as to the reasons why. Utilizing a projected calving distribution and comparing the number of females found pregnant with the actual calving percentage should aid the practitioner in determining the timing of reproductive losses. This in turn gives focus to possible causes. Specific recommendations concerning vaccination protocols, heifer development, bull management, timing of the breeding season, and supplemental feeding and grazing needs can then be communicated to the producer.

As the environment becomes more harsh, cow size (weight and frame score) must be moderated if the cow is to breed efficiently. This is not to say that one breed is innately more fertile than another. If all classes of cattle are fed to meet their requirements (maintenance, lactation, reproduction), differences in productivity will be hidden. In most instances, once a female calves, cows are fed and grouped together. In the practice area of one of the authors (V.T.), an F1 English-bred female with a mature body weight of 1100 to 1150 lb will possess the most desirable reproductive efficiency. The natural forage base present will best support this type of cow in the beef herd. The "ideal" cow will vary from region to region across the United States and this type of analysis will identify her and document her performance to the producer.

The breeding season evaluation of the cow herd has another benefit as well. Once the ideal cow type is identified, her characteristics can then be reproduced in the replacement heifer program. Heifers are fed to reach a target of 65% of expected mature weight by first breeding. It is necessary to know the mature body weight of the cows producing these heifers to plan the feeding phase of the developmental program. Weights can be monitored and rations adjusted to maintain needed growth rates that will ensure heifers reach puberty prior to the beginning of the breeding season.

It has been suggested that an acceptable pregnancy rate for replacement heifers in a 45-day breeding season is 80% to 85%. Approximately 30% more than the anticipated number of replacements are needed to support this level of reproduction and culling. Because culling and replacement rates in beef herds constitute major expenses, heifers must be selected and developed to fit the ranch environment if the herd is to become more efficient. If these heifers are well developed and managed intensively through calving, their attrition rate can be less than 10% following their second breeding season. This represents a potential cost-savings for the operation.

Mismatches between the cow and the environment negatively affect calf performance as well. Cows calving in poor body condition exhibit prolonged postpartum intervals, have higher levels of dystocia, and produce less milk. Calves are born later in the calving season and are weaned at an earlier age and lighter weight. The producer will often extend subsequent breeding seasons in an effort to maintain pregnancy rates. This provides a calf crop that is extremely variable in both size and weight. This decreases the total value of the calves. Postweaning nutritional management of the cow and replacement heifer development are now much more complicated. With retained ownership through the feedyard, the effects of a prolonged calving season are also clearly evident. Days on feed and calf age greatly affect cattle grade and yield. Calves born over a 90-day calving season can offer a real challenge to feedyard management.

Nutritional management of a cow herd requires cost-effective supplemental rations that complement the forage base of the ranch. Inventories detailing the quantity and quality of a producer's feedstuffs, whether stored or grazed, are required. Because cows are typically managed in groups, variations in average cow weight, body condition, milk production, and pregnancy status are important considerations when making feeding recommendations. As the variability in the herd increases, efficiency decreases. For example, if all cows are fed together to meet the nutritional needs of heavier cows, the producer ends up overconditioning smaller cows and wasting feed dollars. Once these complicating factors of the nutritional program are realized and cost projections are made, feeding strategies can be developed.

There are usually both short- and long-term objectives associated with the feeding program. Following periods of severe grazing stress or nutritional mismanagement, a typical short-term objective is to recondition the breeding females so that they calve in moderate body condition. This situation is exacerbated if the cows are of an extreme frame score or milk-producing ability. This environmental mismatch is usually not detected until the time of pregnancy examination. Cows should be segregated and fed on the basis of BCS and required average daily gain (ADG). As a general rule, feed resources are better matched with animal needs if the herd is split into three groups. Replacement heifers should be developed separately. Young cows nursing their first calf can be grouped with the oldest cows. The mature cows, which make up the main body of the herd, represent the third group. Nutritional needs are then evaluated separately for each group.

A change in the timing of the breeding season and manipulation of cow type are two long-term objectives that can have a great impact on nutritional management. A delay in the onset of breeding to encourage late-spring calving is a viable alternative in situations in which annual supplemental feeding costs are deemed excessive. This recommendation can also be used to shorten a prolonged breeding season. The delay in bull turnout should be based on either the established median pregnancy or median calving date of the herd.[10–12] The objective is to give the forage on the ranch a chance to "catch up" with the nutritional requirements of the postcalving female. This will decrease the reliance on supplemental feed and should decrease input costs. Simply listing the dates that the breeding season began and the expected start of calving affords an opportunity to discuss the merits of matching forage growth with peak cow requirements.

Changing the genetic base of the cow herd to better match the ranch environment and managerial skill of the producer is a long-term proposition. It is not uncommon to find cow/calf operations that have moved toward larger females with higher levels of milk production in an effort to maximize weaning weight output. Weaning weights have typically increased, but pregnancy rates, especially in young cows, may eventually decrease in a linear fashion. As reproductive efficiency continues to fall, the practitioner is often called in to diagnose a reproductive pathogen and provide a quick fix for the problem.

Producers and practitioners must weigh this extra weaning weight against the added expense needed to feed this type of cow so that she will reproduce. This relationship will have a tremendous impact on replacement heifer development and culling rates. Pounds of calf weaned per exposed female must be monitored as a means of evaluating this balance. By tracking the measure over time, the practitioner can give the client valuable input concerning cow size and level of milk production that can be managed on the ranch.

SUMMARY

The determination of pregnancy via rectal palpation is more of an art than a science. In a limited breeding season, the need for accuracy in this art begins to decrease. It may be enough to know that the animal is pregnant. Veterinarians are not always needed for this task, as evidenced by the many "cowboy colleges" that demonstrate this art to any ranch hand who is willing to pay the tuition. Despite this, many veterinarians continue to cling to the performance of this service and try to protect it as part of their exclusive domain. Attempts to justify the expense of a breeding season evaluation to producers have centered around the economic justification of culling open cows to avoid feeding them through the winter. Opportunity costs are assigned to supplemental feed, and the expense-per-cow is calculated. It is then determined how many open cows need to be identified, so that savings in feed costs offset the cost of pregnancy evaluation.

The time-honored adage "you get what you pay for" still holds true. A percentage of producers pay more than they should to get what they have and then are uncertain about what they have purchased. Clear documentation of herd findings serves to clear up this uncertainty. The astute producer who realizes the economic importance of both the breeding season and the innate fertility of the herd has actively sought out this type of analysis and is willing to pay for it. The economic justification, in addition to feed savings associated with culling open cows, for a breeding season evaluation resides in the fact that the information generated is useful in decision-making.

If veterinarians provide this type of analysis, we elevate the art to a science. This science then elevates the practitioner into every consultative aspect of the modern cow herd. In addition to the traditional role of establishing preventive programs, genetic selection, nutrition and range management, replacement heifer development, cull cow management, sire fertility, and economic justification are areas in which the veterinarian should have input. For this role expansion to occur, a breeding season evaluation must emphasize why cows are open, and not simply how many are pregnant.

REFERENCES

1. Cunningham B: Evaluation of breeding herd. *In* Bailey C (ed): Guidelines for Uniform Beef Improvement Programs, ed 7. Colby, Kansas, Beef Improvement Federation, 1996, pp 5–11.
2. Barr BC, Anderson ML: Infectious diseases causing bovine abortion and fetal loss. Vet Clin North Am Food Anim Pract 9:343–368, 1993.
3. Chenoweth PJ, Spitzer JC, Hopkins FM: A New Bull Breeding Soundness Evaluation Form. Proceedings of the annual meeting of the Society for Theriogenology, 1992, pp 63–70.
4. Spire MF: Health management of beef bulls. Vet Med 90:777–788, 1995.
5. Bolze RP: Beef cow genetics that will be profitable in the future. Cow-Calf Conference VI: Focus on Basics of Good Management. Kansas State University, Manhattan, Kansas, 1996, pp 3–21.
6. Rice LE: The effects of nutrition on reproductive performance of beef cattle. Vet Clin North Am Food Anim Pract 7:1–26, 1991.
7. Kasari TR, Wikse SE, Jones R: Use of yearling bulls in beef cattle operations: I. Economic analysis and fertility assessment. Compend Contin Educ Practicing Vet 18:1244–1253, 1996.
8. Spire MF: Breeding season evaluation of beef herds. *In* Howard JL (ed): Current Veterinary Therapy 2: Food Animal Practice, ed 2. Philadelphia, WB Saunders, 1986, pp 808–811.
9. Engelken TJ, Lehman FD, Little RD, et al: Helping beef producers improve cow culling practices. Vet Med 88:1102–1107, 1993.
10. Engelken TJ, Spire MF: Management of large-producer cow/calf herds. *In* Howard JL (ed): Current Veterinary Therapy 3: Food Animal Practice, ed 3. Philadelphia, WB Saunders, 1993, pp 124–130.
11. Engelken TJ: Reproductive health programs for beef herds: Analysis of records for assessment of reproductive performance. *In* Youngquist RS (ed): Current Therapy in Large Animal Theriogenology. Philadelphia, WB Saunders, 1997, pp 451–456.
12. Mossman DH: Analysis of calving. *In* Proceedings of the J.D.

Stewart Memorial Refresher Course on Beef Cattle Production. University of Sydney, Australia, 1984, vol 68, p 201.

▪ Backgrounding and Stocker Calf Management

Robert A. Smith, D.V.M., M.S., Diplomate, A.B.V.P.
Donald R. Gill, M.S., Ph.D.

Backgrounding describes a management system by which cattle, generally recently weaned calves, are assembled from many sources and are kept for a period of time before they are placed in a feedlot. Knowledge of their history is often sparse to nonexistent. Stocker calves of similar ages are assembled and placed on forage, generally grass or small-grain pastures. When they are grown to a suitable size they are sold or shipped to a feedlot. Heifers intended for future breeding can also be handled in stocker operations.

Health management of calves in backgrounding or stocker programs can be among the greatest challenges facing the food animal practitioner. Calves in these programs have often been extremely stressed under the current management and marketing systems. Most are recently weaned, moved through auction markets in which they are exposed to many pathogens for the first time, commingled, and then transported long distances. At the backgrounding or stocker operation, the calves must establish a new social order, adapt to different feedstuffs, and frequently must acclimate to new weather conditions. The result is that the calves suffer from fatigue, dehydration, hunger, and psychological stress, which makes them quite susceptible to bovine respiratory disease and other stress-related diseases. Many calves have been given antibiotics before arrival. Morbidity in newly received calves is frequently 40% to 50%, and mortality is often 5% or more.

INSPECTION OF CATTLE

Shipment of calves should be scheduled so that they will arrive during daylight hours. This allows better inspection and evaluation of the calves as they are unloaded. Calves should be evaluated for sickness, lameness, injury, and quality. Arrival weights should be compared with purchase weights so that shrinkage can be calculated. If any calves are unacceptable, the seller or orderbuyer should be contacted immediately so that a solution to the problem can be negotiated. Delaying notification of the seller of problems noted at arrival is usually unrewarding.

PROCESSING

Proper handling and management of cattle during processing is essential to minimize stress, to reduce the risk of injury, and to detect sickness as soon as possible. The veterinarian plays a vital role in the success of this phase of the receiving program by providing detailed instructions to employees of the backgrounding yard or stocker operation on proper techniques to be used in processing calves, on the procedures to be performed, and on sanitation and the proper use and handling of vaccines and other drugs. The consulting veterinarian should provide a written processing protocol to both managers and their employees.

Processing should not be delayed for more than 24 to 36 hours after arrival. Longer delays result in higher rates of morbidity and do not take full advantage of the protection offered by vaccines or preventive medications. Each day that processing is delayed results in a 1% increase in morbidity. In many veterinary practices, facilities are available to process cattle before they are delivered to local backgrounding or stocker operations. This reduces the labor and facility requirements of the producer. The processing program will be influenced by the age of the calves, their origin and background, the weather, and facilities and personnel.

In general, cattle can be classified into one of three risk categories: (1) high-risk exposed; (2) high-risk not exposed; and (3) low risk.[1] The most common type of calves received into stocker operations are high-risk exposed. These calves are usually from small farms, have passed through one or more auctions, and are excessively commingled. It is not uncommon to take up to a week to assemble a load of calves for delivery. Many of these calves are sick on arrival, and the peak morbidity can occur during the first week after arrival. Vaccination programs do very little to reduce the initial wave of illness due to respiratory disease, because the onset of disease occurs before the immune system can respond to vaccines. Mortality can be very high in this class of stocker calves.

High-risk nonexposed calves are those purchased direct from the ranch or single-source calves purchased at auctions in truckload lots. The onset of illness usually occurs 2 weeks or more following arrival. Because morbidity is delayed, vaccination programs are more effective in preventing disease. It is important to understand that these calves are indeed high-risk; therefore, revaccination programs are important to maximize immunity prior to respiratory breaks.

Low-risk calves are those that have been vaccinated, weaned, and turned out for some period of time before shipment. These calves may originate from a ranch or may have been in a backgrounding yard prior to arrival. When properly managed and conditioned prior to arrival, calves in this category experience low morbidity and mortality rates.

Processing procedures to be considered for high-risk exposed calves are as follows:

1. Identify calves with tag or brand
2. Vaccinate with viral antigens for infectious bovine rhinotracheitis (IBR), bovine virus diarrhea (BVD), parainfluenza-3 (PI₃), and bovine respiratory syncytial virus (BRSV); modified live virus (MLV) vaccines are preferred
3. Vaccinate with clostridial bacterin/toxoid as needed
4. Vaccinate against leptospirosis as needed
5. Institute internal and external parasite control, based on origin of calves, season of year, and any available laboratory information
6. Implant with growth-promoting hormones
7. Perform castration or banding of bull calves. If banding is done, immunization against tetanus is highly recommended
8. Tip horns
9. Revaccinate with viral respiratory vaccines 7 to 10 days following processing when using MLV vaccines, or at 14 days following processing if killed virus vaccines are used

In addition to this standard processing, metaphylactic treatment, or mass medication, of high-risk exposed calves may be indicated.[2] As a rule of thumb, metaphylaxis should be considered when the projected morbidity or pull rate for respiratory disease is 25% or greater. The estimation of the morbidity rate is based on the history of calves previously received from a given source and the appearance of the calves at arrival and just prior to processing. Options for medicating the calves include injection, water medication, and FDA-approved feed additives.

Metaphylactic treatment with injectable antimicrobials is often the best choice when receiving high-risk exposed calves. Two options are available: (1) treat all calves at processing or (2) take the rectal temperature and selectively treat those with a temperature over 104.0°F and those showing clinical signs of respiratory disease, regardless of rectal temperature. Selective metaphylaxis is most successful when sufficient, highly skilled labor is available. Research has shown that metaphylactic treatment of calves reduces morbidity, mortality, and treatment costs, and markedly improves performance.

The rectal temperature of calves just unloaded from trucks is not a reliable indicator of illness. The rectal temperature is most useful if calves are rested overnight, with water and hay made available, and they are worked early in the morning, quietly and in groups small enough to complete processing within 1 hour of leaving the pen.

Calves not treated with metaphylactic antimicrobials at processing may benefit from later treatment if there is a 10% or greater pull rate on two consecutive days or if feed intake markedly decreases.

Processing procedures to be considered for high-risk nonexposed calves are as follows:

1. Identify calves with tag or brand
2. Vaccinate with viral antigens IBR, BVD, PI₃, and BRSV; MLV vaccines are preferred
3. Vaccinate with clostridial bacterin/toxoid as needed
4. Vaccinate against leptospirosis as necessary
5. Institute internal and external parasite control, based on origin of calves, season of year, and any available laboratory information
6. Implant with growth-promoting hormones
7. Perform castration or banding of bull calves. If banding is done, immunization against tetanus is highly recommended
8. Tip horns
9. Revaccinate with viral respiratory vaccines 10 to 14 days following processing

As mentioned previously, calves in this risk group usually do not become ill with respiratory disease until 14 days or more following arrival. Revaccinating at 10 to 14 days following arrival provides booster immunizations on a timely basis and allows for maximum priming of the immune system before booster vaccinations are administered. Vaccines are more effective in preventing respiratory disease in this risk group than in high-risk exposed calves.

Pasteurella haemolytica is the primary bacterial agent that causes pneumonia in stocker calves. It may be beneficial to administer a newer-generation *P. haemolytica* bacterin/toxoid to calves in this risk group. Research has shown that the use of a *P. haemolytica* bacterin/toxoid may reduce mortality due to pneumonia. Because of their cost, products with a single injection label are preferred.

Haemophilus somnus bacterins have been commonly used in receiving programs for stocker calves. Few data are available to support their effectiveness, and many of these products contain high levels of endotoxins, which may cause serious setbacks in calves receiving them.

Taking the rectal temperature of fresh high-risk nonexposed calves at processing is usually not worthwhile. Likewise, metaphylactic treatment with injectable antimicrobials at processing is usually not cost-effective because the onset of illness due to respiratory disease occurs so much later in the receiving period. If some calves have begun to show illness by the time they are scheduled for revaccination, it may be helpful to take the rectal temperature when the calves are revaccinated and to treat those with a rectal temperature greater than 104.0°F. This procedure should reduce the number of calves becoming sick with respiratory disease once they are turned out onto pasture.

Processing procedures for low-risk calves are as follows:

1. Identify with a tag or a brand
2. Vaccinate with IBR, BVD, PI₃, and BRSV booster; MLV vaccines are preferred

3. Vaccinate with clostridial bacterin/toxoid and leptospirosis bacterin only if vaccinations have not been given on the ranch or in the backgrounding yard

4. Institute internal and external parasite control based on previous treatment history

5. Implant with growth-promoting hormones; avoid reimplantation within 60 days of any previous implantation

6. Tip horns

7. Castrate or band any calves remaining as bulls

The pregnancy rate of stocker heifers is usually less than that of feeder heifers, primarily because stocker heifers are younger. The pregnancy rate in stocker heifers can be significant. Those large enough can be palpated and abortion can be effected with an approved luteolytic agent. Abortion can be accomplished in smaller heifers of unknown background by injecting each heifer in the group. Injection with prostaglandins without palpation can be highly effective because stocker heifers are usually in an early stage of pregnancy owing to their age. Prostaglandins should not be administered to high-risk heifers for at least 21 days following arrival, as the stress of abortion and the prostaglandins have been shown to increase the mortality rate from respiratory disease.

NUTRITION

No standard nutritional programs exist for receiving cattle into backgrounding or stocker operations because of the wide diversity of programs for which the cattle are used. In some cases diets must be composed of the feeds native to the area in which the cattle will be grazed or fed. In most areas of the United States "native grass hay" is a major component of receiving diets. It is important to know the nutrient composition of these hays, as they vary greatly in different parts of the country. The protein content should always be known. Cattle being received for placement on feed are handled differently than those received for grazing programs. While diets vary, the nutritional requirements for a given weight and class of cattle do not and are dependent on the gain potential of the diet.

In 1996 the National Research Council (NRC) added a chapter to *Nutrient Requirements of Beef Cattle*,[3] on the implications of stress. The biggest problem with newly received or sick cattle is that stress and disease may reduce feed intake. Reductions of 50% have been reported with respiratory disease and fever. After the onset of bovine respiratory disease it sometimes takes 10 to 14 days for intake to return to normal. It is suspected that energy deficiency in cattle may depress the immune system. However, the feeding of high-energy (high-starch) diets has been shown to increase the incidence of respiratory disease. Most commercial receiving diets are composed largely of roughage products and are relatively low in energy. It is possible to formulate diets that are low in starch and higher in energy, and these diets often result in lower cost gains during an extended receiving period.

Protein requirements are likely not different for stressed or sick cattle than for normal cattle. The problem in most stressed or sick cattle is reduced protein intake due to low feed intake. When the diet is made up of low-protein roughage products, lack of protein leads to decreased microbial activity in the rumen, which in turn reduces turnover rate, which slows feed intake. It is possible in normal animals to achieve as much as a 25% to 30% increase in intake of lower-protein grass hays by supplementation with small amounts of protein, such as soybean or cottonseed meal. It appears that the rumen organisms are responding to amino acids from these proteins, because the same effect is not observed with nonprotein nitrogen supplementation. Protein supplementation of newly arrived cattle can be manipulated to solve many of the nutritional deficiencies seen in stressed or sick cattle. Thousands of cattle have been received on a diet consisting of free-choice native prairie grass hay plus 2 lb/day of a 38% to 42% protein supplement. Usually the major ingredient in the supplement is soybean meal, but cottonseed meal, sunflower meal, peanut meal, and canola meals have also been used at various locations. The key is to develop a palatable high-protein supplement.

Forming the supplement into small pellets (³⁄₁₆ to ¼ in.) increases both intake and constancy of intake in calves. Even the most stressed cattle, when received, are easily able to consume 2 lb of the supplement daily from the day of arrival. The logic of this approach is that a high-protein supplement contains an abundance of the nutrients that will aid the rumen bacteria in accelerating the digestion, and thus the intake, of the grass hay. Because the protein concentrates are relatively high in protein, potassium, phosphorus, and the trace minerals, they provide a high percentage of these nutrients in the diet even when intake of the hay is low. The supplement is easily fortified to provide about 30,000 IU of vitamin A and 400 IU of vitamin E per day. Bovatec,* Deccox,† or Rumensin‡ should be added for the prevention of coccidiosis.

In most cases, cattle received for grazing programs are received on diets of low-protein grass hays or pastures. However, if a high-protein hay, such as alfalfa hay, is used, a palatable low-protein supplement can be formulated. In either case it is desirable to feed a small amount of palatable supplement containing additives and vitamins, because offering feed is an easy way to help detect sick animals.

Table 1 shows an example of a high-protein supplement fed at a rate of 2 lb/day to cattle being fed 6%- to 7%-protein prairie hay. The complete chemical composition of the diet (hay plus supplement) was calculated, and three of the trace minerals (zinc, selenium, and copper) were to be added to achieve the NRC recommended levels. The example supplement contains monensin at a level of 100 mg/lb.

It is easy to accelerate gains of newly received cattle in the later parts of the receiving period with higher-concentrate diets. Studies have consistently shown that when gains are increased from about 1 lb/day to more than 2 lb/day, about 60% of the increased gain may be lost during the normal grazing period. Rate of gain in receiving programs for cattle in the feedlot or going to the feedlot can be higher without consequence unless ownership changes. Many cattlemen make the mistake of thinking cattle can be "cheapened back" while they are in a receiving lot. A backgrounding lot is a very labor-intensive operation compared to a commercial feedlot. The extra labor required during the receiving period (especially during high morbidity) is costly. The nonfeed costs in a backgrounding lot can easily be twice those of a commercial feedlot.

TREATING SICK CALVES

About 88% of sickness and death loss in stocker calves is due to "shipping fever" or bovine respiratory disease (BRD). In most stocker operations, the incidence of BRD is significant despite aggressive preventive medicine programs. Stocker calves usually have a more favorable case-fatality rate, or pull-to-dead ratio, than feeder cattle.

The single most important factor that has an impact on treatment response is early pulling and treatment of sick calves. Typical clinical signs of BRD are depression, off feed, and "laying around." Most calves will cough softly when disturbed.

---

*Hoffmann-La Roche, Inc., Paramus, NJ 07652.
†Rhone-Poulenc Animal Nutrition, Atlanta, GA 30350.
‡Elanco Animal Health, Indianapolis, IN 46285.

Table 1
COMPOSITION OF FEED SUPPLEMENTS

Feed Name	Percent
Soymeal 44	73.042
Cottonseed meal	25.001
Salt	1.500
Rumensin 80*	0.127
Vitamin A–30,000	0.110
Vitamin E–50%	0.088
Selenium 600	0.110
Zinc sulfate	0.018
Copper sulfate	0.005

Nutrient	As Fed Composition
Nem, Mcal/cwt	74.71
Neg, Mcal/cwt	50.16
TDN, %	72.78
Fat, %	1.28
Crude fiber, %	7.81
Crude protein, %	42.16
Potassium, %	2.06
Calcium, %	0.14
Phosphorus, %	0.80
Magnesium, %	0.37
Sulfur, %	0.39
Cobalt, ppm	0.25
Copper, ppm	27.9
Iron, ppm	185.4
Manganese, ppm	34.2
Selenium, ppm	0.89
Zinc, ppm	121.2

*Bovatec or Deccox can be substituted for Rumensin.
Nem, net energy for maintenance; Neg, net energy for gain; Mcal/cwt, megacalories per hundredweight; TDN, total digestible nutrients.

About 10% will have an increased respiratory rate. Depression is the most significant and consistent clinical sign, characterized by lowered head and ears, lying down, inattentiveness to pencheckers, self-isolation, and moving more slowly than normal calves.

Moving sick calves to a hospital area with a chute is preferable to roping the calves. Roping calves places undue stress on sick calves. Once calves are in the chute, the rectal temperature should be taken and recorded and a tag with a unique number should be placed in the calf's ear. Most calves suffering from BRD will have a rectal temperature greater than 104°F.

The selection of antibiotics to treat BRD should be based on clinical response (treatment records) of treated animals, culture and antibiotic sensitivity testing, necropsy findings, and results of clinical treatment trials published in the literature.[4] Samples for culture and antibiotic sensitivity testing should only come from untreated calves showing clinical signs of BRD. In the end, clinical response rates with a particular antibiotic are the most important determinants of a drug's effectiveness. This makes periodic careful reviews and analysis of treatment records very important.

Calves with BRD should be treated so that therapeutic tissue levels of antibiotics are maintained for a minimum of 3 days. Research has shown that about 25% of calves require 5 days' treatment for successful recovery. If the calf's condition worsens during treatment, the course of therapy should be changed. As long as the calf continues to improve, the same course of therapy should be continued until the calf is recovered (generally 3 to 5 days).

Realistic goals for the treatment program should be established. Time of year, cattle source, and type and level of management influence target goals. In general, response rates to the first course of therapy should be 80% or greater. Case-fatality rates should be 5% or less.

Calves that are pulled too late, are sick on arrival, or are suffering concurrent disease (e.g., viral diseases, coccidiosis, or salmonellosis) respond poorly to treatment. A review of the history of the calves, necropsy examination, and diagnostic laboratory assistance help to explain treatment failures.

Ancillary therapy for BRD is commonly used. There is, however, little evidence to support the use of vitamins, antihistamines, or antipyretics.[4] They add to the cost of treatment, increase the risk of injection site blemishes, and contribute to discomfort due to injection site pain. Of more value than adjunct therapy is the purchase of fresh calves, good penchecking, an aggressive and well-planned antibiotic program, good nutritional management, and proper hospital management.

Proper hospital management is an essential component of a successful treatment program. Unsanitary pen conditions, overcrowding, and improper feeding all contribute to increased relapse rates. Hospital pens should be well drained and a minimum of 150 ft² of space should be allocated to each calf. Pens should be bedded during periods of inclement weather. Sick cattle from a single origin should be returned to their home pen after treatment or should have a sick pen of their own.

Sick calves do not eat normal amounts of feed, and it is easy to offer too much feed, so that leftover feed becomes stale. Leftover feed should be removed daily. Waterers should be cleaned on a daily basis.

TURNING CALVES OUT

Calves need to be kept in receiving pens until they stop walking the fence and the period of peak morbidity has passed. It is desirable to move calves to small traps as soon as practical. Grass traps reduce crowding, reduce the spread of viruses and bacteria, and provide a more comfortable environment.

The decision to turn calves out requires careful management consideration. The goal is to turn them out as quickly as possible, but they must remain accessible for prompt treatment if they become ill. As a rule, plan to closely observe yearlings for at least 2 weeks and high-risk calves for at least 28 days.

QUALITY CONTROL

The stocker calf is part of the food chain. It is imperative that stocker operators have a beef quality assurance program in place to avoid injection site blemishes in the valuable cuts of meat, especially those from the "top butt" and rounds. Research has shown that scar tissue caused by intramuscular injections given to calves as young as 50 days persists until slaughter. Feedlots, packers, and consumers are demanding that the highest-quality product be offered, and stocker operators must meet that expectation. To satisfy this demand, injectable products labeled for subcutaneous use should be used whenever possible. If an injectable product must be given by the intramuscular route, it should be administered into the muscles of the neck.

Chemical or antibiotic residues must also be considered. Calves treated with animal health products in accordance with label directions must not be marketed until the FDA-approved withdrawal time has expired. When products are used in an extra-label manner, the withdrawal period recommended by the Food Animal Residue Avoidance Databank (FARAD) should be observed. All prescription products and products used in an extra-label manner should be used only when a valid veterinarian-client-patient relationship exists and a written prescription or drug order has been issued.

Complete records are necessary in any stocker operation, not only for legal reasons but also as a useful source of management information. It is important to maintain processing records, including processing maps and individual treatment records. Calves treated for disease conditions should be identified individually.

An ongoing employee training program is an essential part of a quality control program. Training programs are available through the extension service, veterinary clinics, and nutritional consulting services. Employees should be trained in beef quality assurance programs, sick cattle detection, treatment programs, disease processes, record-keeping, and use of animal health products. Informed employees are better and more effective employees.

CONCLUSION

Consultation with backgrounders and stocker operators is still in its infancy; however, opportunities for increasing productivity and profits abound. Data regarding economic benefits of veterinary consultation input are lacking and are sorely needed. Producers are inundated with information, but the information received is often biased or is not based on good factual research.

Management of the feeding program and management of the health program is probably more important to success than the selection of products used. A well-planned, scientifically based health and nutrition program executed by well-trained, motivated people offers the best pathway to success. Do not be afraid to change, but base any changes on an analysis of records and scientifically documented information.

REFERENCES

1. Deyhle CE Jr: Processing, handling, penriding, pulling sick cattle and sampling procedures. *In* Abin RC, Thompson GB (eds): Cattle Feeding: A Guide to Management, ed 2. Amarillo, Trafton Printing, 1996, pp 182–189.
2. Smith RA: Metaphylactic treatment of bovine respiratory disease: When is it appropriate? *In* Advances in Therapeutics: Problems and Perspectives. Proceedings of the Elanco Satellite Seminar held at the 19th World Buiatrics Congress, Edinburgh, 1996, pp 43–54.
3. National Research Council: Nutrient Requirements of Beef Cattle, rev ed 7. Washington, DC, National Academy Press, 1996.
4. Smith RA: Therapeutic management of the bovine respiratory disease complex. *In* Bovine Respiratory Disease: Sourcebook for the Veterinary Professional. Trenton, NJ, Veterinary Learning Systems, 1996, pp 49–56.

■ Development of Replacement Heifers

Lawrence E. Rice, D.V.M., M.S.

HEIFERS' INFLUENCE ON THE HERD

Economics dictate that replacement heifers first calve at 2 years of age. They have 1.2 more pregnancies and wean 0.9 more calves in a lifetime than those that first calve at 3 years of age.[1] Nevertheless, some low-input–low-outcome operations may calve heifers at 3 years of age. Also, some operations that have spring and fall calving may calve heifers first at 30 months of age. Marginal analysis is an economic comparison of alternatives and the variables that have an impact on the alternatives.

Using marginal analysis, one study showed that many variables, such as feed and grazing costs, labor, pregnancy rates, dystocia rates, weaning weights, and calf prices, alter the advantage of calving at 24 months rather than at 30 or 36 months.[2] This analysis emphasized the importance of managing costs, accurately estimating reproductive rates, and hitting reproductive goals for a heifer development program to be successful.

The success of managing heifers through the second calving will determine the success of the adult cow herd. To emphasize this concept, let us examine a hypothetical herd drawn from observation of many herds. The example herd has 100 cows that calve during a period of approximately 4 months. The owner adds 10 replacement heifers that calve relatively early during the calving season. The owner also retains selected dry cows (cows that failed to wean a calf during the current calving season) to maintain enough pregnant cows. With the exception of the dry cows, which are fat, the cows are in moderate to thin body condition at calving in the late winter and spring. Nutrition improves following calving, especially as new pasture improves, and cows gain weight during the breeding season. Approximately 100 cows and 15 to 20 replacement heifers are bred to maintain 100 pregnant females for the next calving season. Pregnant replacements are pastured and fed with the adults. The calving pattern has been similar for many years (Table 1).

The long calving season in this herd can be traced to the management of heifers, cow body condition, and leaving the bulls with the herd until weaning. Note that 7 (70%) of the heifers calved in the first 42 days of the calving season but only 41 (46%) of the cows calved during the same period. If the time of replacement heifer calving represents the future calving patterns, 70% of the cows in this herd should also calve in the first 42 days. However, first-calf heifers require approximately 20 days more postpartum rest to manifest cycling rates and conception rates comparable to those of cows. In this case, the second calving actually sets future calving patterns.

This chapter describes procedures for 3-year control of replacement heifers and also reviews the onset of puberty in beef heifers and the onset of postpartum estrus in beef cows. These events are greatly influenced by genetics and the environment. Selection and management are key factors in achieving economic control of reproduction in a beef herd. A good understanding of reproductive physiology and endocrinology is necessary for veterinarians to advise producers about selection for and management of reproductive efficiency.

ONSET OF PUBERTY

First, what are the endocrine events associated with the onset of puberty? Apparently the prepubertal hypothalamus and anterior pituitary are extremely sensitive to the negative feedback of gonadal steroids. Minute steroid levels prevent the release of gonadotropins that are necessary for the onset of estrual activity. During prepubertal development in heifers, estrogen becomes less effective in inhibiting luteinizing hormone (LH) secretion, finally becoming more effective in causing LH secretion through positive feedback as puberty approaches. A theory gaining credibility is that hypothalamic and pituitary activity are controlled by a pulse generator in the central nervous system.[3] The activity of the pulse generator can be modified by a large variety of internal and external stimuli, such as genetics, gonadal hormone levels, photoperiod, pheromones, and nutritional status. The negative feedback mechanism of the gonadal steroid is probably mediated through the pulse generator. Puberty would be reached following changes in the pulse generator, which would increase the frequency and amplitude of episodic gonadotropin-releasing hormone (GnRH) and gonadotropin release, resulting in estrus and ovulation.

Table 1
CALVING PATTERN IN 90 ADULT COWS AND 10 HEIFERS

Calving Group* (Day of Calving Season)	1 (21)	2 (42)	3 (63)	4 (84)	5 (105)	6 (126)	Total
First-calf heifers, No. of calves	3	4	1	1	1	—	10
Adult cow, No. of calves	14	27	27	13	6	3	90
Total	17	31	28	14	7	3	100

*Each calving group represents consecutive 21-day periods.
Adapted from Rice LE: Nutrition and the development of replacement heifers. Vet Clin North Am Food Anim Pract 7:27–41, 1991.

Bovine ovaries are responsive at an early age (3 months) to gonadotropins, so exogenous follicle-stimulating hormone (FSH) and GnRH will stimulate ovulation, but cyclic function cannot be maintained. Studies have shown that up to 20% of heifers may have an anovulatory estrus (nonpubertal estrus).[3] Apparently follicular development and estrogen secretion cause behavioral estrus, but there is a failure of ovulation. Puberty is only one step in sexual maturation, as it has also been reported that fertility at pubertal estrus is lower than at the third estrus following puberty.

As in the anestrous ewe, the prepubertal heifer requires a priming level of progesterone to act synergistically with estrogens for estrus and ovulation to occur. One study showed progesterone levels to be very low in prepubertal heifers, but two distinct prepubertal elevations and declines were observed followed by LH peaks after the progesterone level returned to baseline. Pubertal estrus and ovulation soon followed.

Methods for induction of estrus in prepubertal heifers have been reported with varied success. The most reliable is the use of progesterone priming for 9 days with a progestogen implant, such as norgestomet (Syncro-Mate-B).[3] The hypothesis is that exogenous hormone induction works only when heifers are in a physiologic state that allows the hypothalamus to respond to progesterone priming. Young or lightweight heifers fail to respond, and there are reports of an increase in prepubertal estrus. I think that these methods will not advance the onset of puberty more than one cycle (20 days). Simply put, if pubertal estrus and ovulation are not imminent, hormonal stimulation will not significantly advance the onset of cyclic activity.

Photoperiod and the presence of a male markedly influence the onset of puberty in seasonal breeders. Although domestic cattle are not seasonal breeders, these factors have some effect on the onset of puberty in heifers. Fall-born heifers or heifers exposed to 18 hours of light have been reported to reach puberty approximately 30 days earlier than spring-born heifers or heifers exposed to natural light.[3] Reproductive performance in zebu cattle (*Bos indicus*) is more influenced by seasonality than in European breeds (*B. taurus*). Zebu cattle have a lower preovulatory LH surge in winter than in spring or summer, and first service conception rates are dramatically reduced in the winter. Anestrus and prepubertal estrus have been reported to be higher in winter than in summer among young zebu females.

Results of bull exposure for prepubertal heifers are varied, sometimes enhancing the onset of puberty and sometimes having no effect. The positive results have occurred when heifers gaining in excess of 1.5 lb/day were exposed to intact sterile bulls ("gomer bulls") for 60 to 90 days prior to the breeding season.[3] The message is clear. Inherent fertility and feeding to achieve target weights before the breeding season are really responsible for the success of such minor enhancements as bull exposure or induction of puberty.

POSTPARTUM REPRODUCTIVE PHYSIOLOGY

Probably the most important endocrine event associated with the onset of estrus in the postpartum cow is the establishment of episodic pulsatile LH secretion. As a cow approaches the first postpartum estrus, frequency and amplitude of the LH release increase just as in the prepubertal heifer, which is followed by waves of follicular development and atresia. The pulsatile LH release is reestablished by the 10th to 15th day after calving in nonsuckled healthy cows. Suckled cows, however, have a much later and highly variable onset of episodic LH release patterns. Some suckled cows return to estrus by 30 days postpartum, but others may not cycle until the calf is weaned.[4] Part of the variability can be explained by the postpartum interval, but major factors are nutritional status and body condition. Energy restriction during late gestation results in thin body condition at calving and extends the postpartum anestrous interval. Cows that are in good body condition (body condition score [BCS] ≥5) at calving and that maintain condition after calving overcome the suckling inhibition earlier in the postpartum period.

Research indicates that endogenous opioid peptides may be responsible for the anestrus observed in suckling beef cows.[5] Opioids such as β-endorphin and methionine-enkephalin decrease LH levels in humans and laboratory animals. In cows, the proposed action is that suckling apparently increases the opioid levels, which in turn inhibits GnRH release. Early weaning or 48-hour calf removal theoretically reduces opioid levels, and cows that are physiologically responsive resume cycling.

Calf removal is a management tool sometimes used to increase cycling at the beginning of the breeding season, but results are inconsistent. Thin cows (BCS <5) respond poorly. It may be that the energy-suckling interaction is influenced by both endogenous opioids and energy-dependent growth factors (e.g., insulin-like growth factor). Evidence suggests that the "quality" of a maturing follicle and its oocyte may be influenced by the microenvironment (e.g., nutrition, disease) to which it was exposed as a primordial follicle in the previous weeks or months.[6] It is theorized that the microenvironment influences growth factors that are responsible for the progression of primordial follicles to gonadotropin-responsive antral follicles. It is apparent that health and nutritional status in the prepartum period greatly influence the quality of follicular and oocyte development months prior to the eventual maturation of the oocytes.

Recent research conclusively shows the futility of trying to shorten the postpartum interval in young, thin cows by improving the BCS after calving (Table 2).[7] Cows with a BCS of 5 or greater are all cycling by 80 to 90 days postpartum. Cows that are in poor condition (BCS ≤4) at calving do not cycle until 110 to 140 days postpartum, even if they are fed high-energy supplements to improve BCS by two points. Cows that calve in good body condition cannot be permitted to lose weight between calving and breeding. Cows that lose weight during the breeding season have lower conception rates than those that gain or maintain weight. Understanding the physiologic limitations of the first-calf heifer's returning to estrus after calving is of utmost importance in managing replacements.

SELECTION

The onset of puberty is a highly (40% to 50%) heritable trait that is altered by the environment. Evidence suggests that early puberty can be selected through proper sire selection. Bulls with large testicles at 15 months of age reach puberty earlier than those with small testicles, and their half-sib heifers also reach puberty earlier. The heritability of bull scrotal size is very high (67%). The correlation coefficient between bull scrotal size and age of heifer at puberty is −0.71, which means that as bull scrotal size increases, the age of the heifer at puberty is reduced.[8] Selection pressure can also be put on the heifers by breeding them for only 30 to 45 days, identifying the pregnant heifers through early pregnancy diagnosis, and sending the open ones to the feedlot. Heifers that reach puberty and breed early are more likely to have a shorter postpartum interval as cows.

Other genetic traits may influence the onset of puberty. Breeds historically selected for milk production reach puberty earlier than breeds of similar size that are not selected for milk.[1] In general, crossbred heifers reach puberty at younger ages and heavier weights than straightbred heifers. Crossbred heifers also tend to have higher first-service conception rates and increased calf crop.

A procedure suggested to select for early puberty is yearling reproductive tract scoring (RTS) by rectal palpation. Colorado State University developed a five-point scoring system to aid in selecting pubertal yearling heifers for breeding that ranges from 1 (uterine horn diameter <20 mm with no palpable follicles) to 5 (uterine horn diameter >30 mm with a corpus luteum on an ovary). In one study, heifers with a yearling RTS of 3 or greater conceived sooner in the breeding season and had higher pregnancy rates than those with an RTS of 1 or 2.[8] Another study had similar results, except only heifers with an RTS of 1 had lower conception and pregnancy rates.[9] In both cases, heifers with an RTS of 1 or 2 represented a very small portion of the herds (<10%) and were below target weights. I believe that if the objective of early puberty is to have a favorable impact on herd fertility, proper bull selection, culling on the basis of not meeting target weights, and early pregnancy diagnosis following a 30- to 45-day early breeding season is just as objective and is more practical and cost-effective.

Pelvic area has been the maternal trait most frequently associated with dystocia in first-calf heifers.[10] However, studies show that calf birth weight accounts for more than twice as much of the variability in dystocia rate as does dam pelvic area. Several statistical and epidemiologic analyses have been performed to predict dystocia or calving ease from prebreeding or precalving values such as dam pelvic area and estimated calf birth weights. The scientific data raise questions concerning the accuracy and cost-effectiveness of using dam pelvic area as a culling tool to prevent dystocia.

Some producers who have used pelvic area measurements in heifer selection regularly claim that the prevalence of dystocia decreased for the first few years after implementing the practice. When the practice of measuring pelvic area is undertaken, other management factors (e.g., nutrition, sire selection, short calving season) are often included, which may be equally responsible for decreasing dystocias. A 1993 Nebraska survey showed that veterinarians thought culling heifers with small pelvic areas reduced calving problems for their clients.[11] There was doubt as to the singular importance of doing pelvic area measurements as opposed to the more total herd management approach undertaken in the replacement program.

In the last 25 to 30 years, genetic selection has produced larger cattle with larger pelvic areas, heavier birth weights, and, sometimes, an increase in dystocia rates. Selecting for the largest pelvic area alone will also result in increased frame scores and birth weights. At this writing, a shift has occurred toward favoring more moderate-sized cows as a result of the relative inefficiency of large cattle in less-than-favorable environments. Integrated resource management–standardized performance analysis (IRM-SPA) shows that the herds with the heaviest weaning weights are not the most profitable. Within a breed or line, the largest-frame score cattle also tend to reach puberty later, and first-service conception rates may be lower in adequately developed very large frame score heifers.[1] One advocate of selection for desirable pelvic area recommends culling both the bottom and top 10% pelvic area sizes, thereby eliminating extremes.[11]

The veterinarian needs to consult with each producer concerning the cost-effectiveness of RTS and pelvic measurements. Type of producer, type of cattle, producer goals, and many other factors will influence these decisions. A large commercial producer who has ample numbers of heifers might minimize costs of heifer development with good forage and pasture management, meeting target weights, and breeding for 30 days with calving ease bulls. The most cost-effective culling procedure would be based on early pregnancy diagnosis. Producers who cannot attain that level of management might benefit from using RTS and pelvic area measurements to cull late-maturing and/or high-dystocia-risk replacements.

Table 2
PREDICTED NUMBER OF DAYS FROM CALVING TO FIRST HEAT AS AFFECTED BY BCS AT CALVING AND BCS CHANGE AFTER CALVING IN FIRST-CALF BEEF COWS

| | BCS Change After Calving to Day 90 | | | | | | |
BCS at Calving	−1	−0.5	0	0.5	1	1.5	2
3	189	173	160	150	143	139	139
4	161	145	131	121	115	111	111
5	133	116	103	93	86	83	82
5.5	118	102	89	79	72	69	66

BCS, body condition score (1 = emaciated; 9 = obese).
Adapted from Lalman DL: Influence of early lactation energy balance on postpartum interval, milk production and metabolic hormone concentration in thin primiparous beef heifers, doctoral dissertation, University of Missouri, Columbia, 1996.

NUTRITION

The most easily controlled (and most costly) factor in heifer management is nutrition. Heifers should be fed to reach a weight that will ensure puberty at 13 to 15 months of age. Low average daily gain (ADG) from weaning to breeding has been reported to delay the onset of puberty. One study showed heifers with ADGs of 0.6 lb, 1.0 lb, and 1.5 lb had cycling rates of 7%, 31%, and 83%, respectively, at the beginning of the breeding season. Pregnancy rates during the first 40 days of breeding were 40%, 83%, and 80%, respectively. Depending on weaning weights, days from weaning to breeding, and target weight at breeding, an ADG from 1.25 to 1.50 lb should meet the growth requirements for most yearling replacement heifers.[12]

High-quality forages such as small-grain pastures, legume-grass mixture pastures, Sudan grass–sorghum hybrid pastures, and other improved pastures will meet the protein and energy requirements of heifers from weaning through breeding. The availability of these forages is limited to geographic areas and seasons that favor their production at a reasonable cost. In some areas in which wheat pastures are utilized for heifer development, the heifers are removed from the very nutritious pastures 4 to 8 weeks before breeding. This may result in sufficient weight loss (depending on the next feeding regimen) to seriously reduce conception rates or even to stop cycling. A study that evaluated the effect of weight loss in cycling yearling heifers showed those that lost more than 0.5 lb/day for 2 months tended to stop cycling, whereas heifers that lost less than 0.5 lb/day tended to continue cycling.[13] Heifers that became anestrous did not resume cyclicity until 4.5 weeks after feeding of a high-concentrate ration, with a weight gain of 2.4 lb/day. Such losses must be avoided.

Supplementation with available hay or silage or provision of a complete mixed ration is often necessary. In all circumstances, target weights must be determined, average daily gain calculated, rations balanced, and weight gains monitored. Apparently it is not necessary that ADGs be uniform, and catch-up gains are satisfactory. One study showed that heifers on pasture and protein supplement with less-than-desirable ADGs in late fall and early winter can be fed high-energy rations in late winter and early spring to achieve compensatory gains and reach target weights by breeding season.[14] The cycling rates for the spring high-energy group were in excess of 70% at the beginning of breeding compared with less than 10% for the control pasture heifers.

Feed additives and growth stimulants influence growth rate and the onset of puberty.[12] Replacement heifers fed an approved ionophore from weaning through breeding had higher ADGs and reached puberty at an earlier age in several studies. However, no difference was noted in first-service conception rates or pregnancy rates. Some reports indicated that in addition to improved ADGs, ionophores enhanced pituitary response to GnRH and ovarian response to gonadotropins. The mechanism is unknown, but the data clearly indicate that the inclusion of an ionophore in replacement heifer rations enhances the onset of puberty.

Growth-stimulating implants improved growth rates in replacement heifers. Whereas all implants improved growth rates and increased pelvic areas at 1 year of age, there was no increased pelvic area or decreased dystocia at calving. However, aberrant cycling rates and reduced pregnancy rates were often associated with the use of growth implants at ages over 4 months. Apparently one-time implantation in 2-month-old nursing heifer calves does not harm reproduction, but implantation before 45 days of age and reimplantation at weaning must be avoided.

CONTROLLED 3-YEAR HEIFER PROGRAM

A controlled 3-year heifer program should be used to set the calving pattern for the cow herd.[12] Control the first two calvings, and management of the cow herd is much easier thereafter. What is the controlled 3-year heifer program? (1) Breed 13- to 15-month-old virgin heifers for 42 days; 85% of the heifers should be cycling and bred during the first 21 days and 95% should be cycling by the end of 42 days. Eighty-five percent of the heifers bred are likely to become pregnant. (2) Two-year-old heifers nursing their first calves should be cycling at a rate of 85% to 95% during the first 42 days of the regular breeding season, and 85% or more should be pregnant at the end of 63 days' breeding. Even if the producer elects to calve at 30 or 36 months of age, these reproductive rate goals should be set.

To accomplish these breeding goals, three growth requirements must be achieved during the following specific times:

1. First year (from birth to breeding): Heifers should obtain 65% of their mature weight to ensure 90% cycling at 13 to 15 months of age.

2. Second year (from first breeding to first calving): Pregnant replacement heifers that have been properly managed should have a BCS of 6 and achieve about 85% of their adult body weight at calving. Heifers that are poorly fed during the last trimester will not conceive early the next breeding season and often will have increased dystocia rates due to small pelvic areas and weakened conditions. Excessively fattened heifers may have increased dystocia rates due to internal pelvic fat but will not have heavier birth-weight calves than will properly managed heifers. Producers relate protein to increased dystocia, but data would indicate excess protein has no effect on dystocia.[10] Oklahoma studies showed no difference in dystocia rates or birth weights between heifers on wheat pasture, drylot grain ration, or native winter pasture with protein supplementation. The wheat pasture heifers and drylot heifers calved at BCS 6.0 to 6.8, and the winter pasture heifers calved at BCS 5.0 to 5.7. A study in Kansas showed similar results using different levels of alfalfa feeding to provide 150%, 100%, or 75% of the daily protein requirement. The only difference was that the lowest protein intake resulted in longer postpartum anestrus. Finally, protein malnutrition can be a cause of weak calf syndrome.

3. Third year (from second breeding to second calving): Heifers should reach 95% of their mature weight at 3 years of age. During all these years, replacements must be maintained as a separate herd.

The following steps are required to establish a 3-year controlled heifer program:

1. Select approximately 1.3 times as many heifers as will actually be needed for replacements. These heifers should be selected on the basis that they will be between 13 and 15 months of age at the beginning of the heifer breeding season. Zebu breeds may require 3 to 6 months longer to reach puberty.

2. Weigh heifers at weaning, and if wide ranges occur between the smaller and the larger heifers, they should be divided into two feeding groups to reach their desired weight by breeding time. Calculate the necessary ADG to reach the desired breeding weight and feed to achieve that gain. The addition of approved levels of an ionophore to the ration will improve ADG and enhance the onset of puberty. User-friendly computer programs are available that greatly simplify ration balancing.*

---

*NRC Nutrient Requirements of Beef Cattle. National Academy Press, 2101 Constitution Ave NW, Lockbox 285, Washington, DC 20055 ($34.95). Grower program for stockers and yearlings and Balancer program for prepartum and postpartum heifers and cows. Cooperative Extension Service, Department of Animal Science, Kansas State University, Manhattan, KS 66506 ($50.00 each).

3. Weigh a random sample of the heifers every 30 days to check growth rates. Yearling weight is critical because high-energy rations between then and breeding can be used to achieve compensatory gains in below-target-weight heifers.

4. It may be necessary to cull approximately 10% of heifers at 1 year of age as being undesirable for replacement breeding. Twelve to 14 months of age is a good time for RTS or taking pelvic measurements, if these are part of the program. This also is the proper time for booster immunizations, such as for infectious bovine rhinotracheitis (IBR) and bovine viral diarrhea (BVD) and, when recommended, vibriosis and leptospirosis immunizations.

5. The breeding season should not exceed 40 to 45 days. Depending on management practices, some operations may start breeding heifers 21 days before breeding the cows, but others may breed heifers with the cows. Well-grown replacement heifers are ideal candidates for estrus synchronization, which facilitates a short breeding season. Preferably, breeding should be by artificial insemination, using semen from a progeny-tested bull proved to be an "easy-calving" bull. The use of such a bull, by artificial insemination or natural service, will reduce the dystocia rate.

6. The heifers may be tested for pregnancy as early as 35 days following the end of the breeding season. Once the pregnant replacement heifers have been selected, their growth rate should be maintained at BCS 6 and they should reach 85% of mature cow size at calving. Adverse conditions such as drought, storms, or parasitic infestation cause heifers to be thin and weak at calving. A good manager develops "what if" plans for such situations to avoid wasting 2 years of work, as happened in the example herd as described in Table 1.

7. Heifers with a BCS of less than 5 to 6 at calving that do not maintain weight after calving have prolonged postpartum intervals to first estrus. Although all efforts should be made to prevent such an occurrence, it does happen, and remedial procedures can be taken. Early weaning of calves (8 weeks of age) can markedly improve reproductive performance of thin (BCS <5) first-calf beef heifers. In an Oklahoma study of a 90-day breeding season, heifers nursing calves had a 58% pregnancy rate as compared with 97% in heifers that had calves weaned early.[12] The calves were weaned on a high-energy/high-protein starter ration without encountering sickness, and they weighed the same at weaning age as the nursing calves. Economic analysis indicated early weaning would be the most cost-effective way to salvage a reproductive program that would be set back by an unfavorable environment.

SUMMARY

After having been on a controlled heifer replacement program and short breeding season for 3 to 5 years, the entire herd will develop a short calving season, resulting in more weaned calf weight per cow exposed to breeding. The key ingredients are selection and nutrition management. Proper sire selection and female culling create reproductive traits that remain in the herd throughout generations. The best management cannot create performance beyond the genetic potential, and aids such as ionophores and bull exposure cannot replace good nutritional management.

Obviously, the benefits continue through subsequent calvings, emphasizing the importance of managing the replacement heifers for 3 years, through their second breeding and calving.

REFERENCES

1. Spire MJ: Managing replacement heifers from weaning to breeding. Vet Med 92:182–191, 1997.

2. Lehman FD, Engelken TJ, Little RD, et al: A logical method for comparing beef heifer development strategies. Vet Med 88:1094–1101, 1993.

3. Kinder JE, Robertson MS, Wolfe MW, et al: Management factors affecting puberty in the heifer. *In* Fields MJ, Sand RS (eds): Factors Affecting Calf Crop. Boca Raton, Fla, CRC Press, 1994, pp 69–89.

4. Rice LE: The effect of nutrition on reproductive performance of beef cattle. Vet Clin North Am Food Anim Pract 7:1–26, 1991.

5. Short RE, Staigmiller RB, Bellows RA, et al: Effect of suckling on postpartum reproduction. *In* Fields MJ, Sand RS (eds): Factors Affecting Calf Crop. Boca Raton, Fla, CRC Press, 1994, pp 179–187.

6. Stevenson JS: Update of reproductive endocrine function in the bovine female. Proceedings of the Annual Meeting of the Society of Theriogenology. Kansas City, 1994, pp 38–49.

7. Lalman DH: Influence of early energy balance on postpartum interval, milk production and metabolic hormone concentration in thin primiparous beef heifers, doctoral dissertation. University of Missouri, Columbia, 1996.

8. Brinks JS: Genetic influences on reproductive performance of 2-year-old beef heifers. *In* Fields MJ, Sand RS (eds): Factors Affecting Calf Crop. Boca Raton, Fla, CRC Press, 1994, pp 45–54.

9. Patterson DJ, Bullock KD: Using prebreeding weight, reproductive tract score and pelvic area to evaluate prebreeding development of replacement beef heifers. Proceedings of the Beef Improvement Federation. Sheridan, Wyo, 1995, pp 174–177.

10. Rice LE: Dystocia-related risk factors. Vet Clin North Am Food Anim Pract 10:53–68, 1994.

11. Deutscher GH: Beef heifer development: Selection, pelvic measurements and dystocia. Proceedings of the Annual Meeting of the Society for Theriogenology. Kansas City, 1994, pp 68–75.

12. Rice LE: Nutrition and the development of replacement heifers. Vet Clin North Am Food Anim Pract 7:27–41, 1991.

13. Vizarra JA, Wettemann RP: Relationship between body weight changes in postpubeal heifers and cessation of luteal activity, Animal Science Research Report P-933. Oklahoma State University, Stillwater, Okla, 1993, pp 351–353.

14. Marston TT, Lusby KS, Wettemann RP: Effects of Different Supplements and Limited Drylot Feeding on Replacement Heifer Development, Animal Science Research Report P-933. Oklahoma State University, Stillwater, Okla, 1993, pp 100–106.

■ Standardized Performance Analysis

Edward D. Hamilton, D.V.M., M.Agr.

This chapter does not cover the history of integrated resource management (IRM) or standardized performance analysis (SPA). The reader may refer to Hamilton for a better understanding of the development of the IRM concept and SPA. The reader may use information in the following pages as a reference for both production (SPA-P) and financial (SPA-F) measurements encountered in SPA. Definitions, calculations, and interpretation are included. Implementation issues and key records are discussed.

TIME LINE

A key to an accurate SPA-P analysis is good cattle inventory records. Reconciled inventory numbers can be very challenging. The best way to ensure accurate production information is to use a time line (Fig. 1). Production information spans at least 2 years, and sometimes 3. A time line reduces the confusion caused by the production overlap. The time line depicted in Figure 1 provides the appropriate adjustments to the exposed female breeding number. The calf crop weaned for the SPA report is determined by the weaning that occurs during the fiscal year of the analysis.

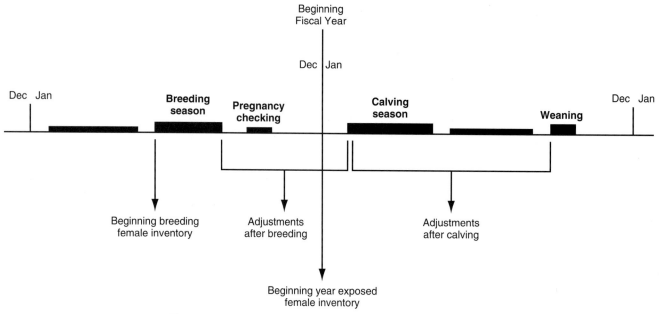

Figure 1
Standardized performance analysis (SPA) time line for spring-calving herds.

RECORDS REQUIRED

Two major problems are usually encountered by the person making a first attempt to complete an SPA. The first is frustration at a lack of records or at the format of the records, and the second is lack of a basic understanding of financial statements. If these problems are overcome, the decision-making process is enhanced.

A first attempt at completing an SPA should focus on the process involved and not on the accuracy of the numbers. If records do not exist or if the format is incorrect, adjustments can be made to complete the process. For example, cow inventory numbers are important in the analysis, but adjustments may be required to reconcile cattle numbers. A time line is very helpful in tracking inventory numbers. Calves weaned during the fiscal year make up the group of interest for the analysis. The breeding inventory number is the number of cows bred during the prior breeding season. Inventory measurements can be primary or secondary. The following primary inventory numbers correspond to the SPA-EZ (an easier, shorter version of a complete SPA) form depicted in Figure 2.

1. Number of Females Exposed. This is the number of females in the breeding herd. Some adjustments must be made. Do not include females exposed but not intended to be calved. Females transferred out of the breeding herd during breeding should not be included. Females transferred into the breeding herd during breeding should be included.

2. Number of Pregnant Females or Pairs Transferred Out of Herd. You should only include known pregnant females or females that have calved and have been removed as a pair (with live calf) before weaning.

3. Number of Females (Pregnant or Pairs) Transferred into the Herd After Breeding. You should only include known pregnant females or females that have a live calf at side at the time of purchase/transfer.

4. Adjusted Exposed Female Inventory. This is an inventory of exposed females that results from the beginning inventory plus all adjustments. This is the divisor for weaning percentage and other reproduction and production measurements.

5. Number of Calves Weaned. This is a head count of all calves actually weaned during the weaning period. Do not include nursing calves removed before weaning as a cow-calf pair. Purchased grafted calves require some adjustments. The number of purchased grafted calves weaned should not be included in the reproductive measurements (calving percentage, weaning percentage). However, purchased grafted calves that are weaned are included in the revenue and pounds weaned sections. If purchased grafted calves are a part of this analysis, you will need to adjust item 5 before calculating the weaning percentage in item 9. Item 5 may be entered based on sex of calves or as the total of all calves.

6. Total Pounds Weaned. Enter the total pounds weaned by calf sex or all calves. Include the weight of the purchased grafted calves. Do not include the weight of calves removed as pairs (not weaned). The weight should be determined at the time of weaning. These values may be determined by multiplying item 7 by item 5.

7. Average Weaning Weight. Enter the average weaning weight per calf by sex of calf or all calves. These values may be determined by dividing item 6 by item 5. If the weight for purchased grafted calves is included in item 6, then the herd count of calves weaned (item 5) must be adjusted to include purchased grafted calves.

8. Average Price per Pound of Calves. This value should be determined from the net weaned calf revenue divided by the total pounds weaned (item 6). The net weaned calf revenue should include the net value of all weaned calves sold, a non-cash value for all retained calves at weaning, and a base value for all replacement calves weaned.

9. Percent Weaned Calves. (Item 5 divided by item 4) times 100 equals weaning percent. Do not include purchased grafted calves in item 5.

10. Total Dollar Value of All Calves Weaned. Item 8 times item 6. The value of purchased grafted calves weaned and the value at weaning of all retained calves should be included. This is the net value of the weaned calf crop.

11. Pounds Weaned per Exposed Female. Item 6 divided by item 4. This measurement includes the actual weaning weight of all weaned calves (include purchased grafted calves) in item 6. Item 4 is the adjusted exposed female count.

12. Total Acres. This is the total adjusted acres for grazing and raised feed land used by the cow-calf enterprise. This includes both owned and leased acres for grazing and raised feed land. The acres are adjusted for use by other enterprises. For example if a stocker enterprise utilizes some of the same acres used by the cow-calf enterprise, then the acres shared by the two enterprises must be proportioned to each of the enterprises.

13. Total Breeding Females. This is the size of the cow herd. This determined by the head count of all *exposed* females, both mature cows and replacement heifers, still in the herd on the first day of the fiscal year. This represents the number of exposed females on the beginning balance sheet.

If records are incomplete, one should use the best number available. That might be the number of calves weaned or the number of females checked for pregnancy. Adjustments can be made in both directions along a time line to estimate the additional inventory numbers required. Initially, it is more important to become familiar with the analysis process than to be concerned with totally accurate numbers. Completing the process

enables one to develop questions, which in turn determine the information that will be relevant to a particular operation over time. Attention can then be directed toward acquiring and maintaining these records more accurately.

SPA-P GUIDELINES

SPA examines the cow-calf enterprise as a system rather than a series of individual animals. SPA looks at not only the production variables (SPA-P), but also the financial statements (SPA-F), and the environment in which production occurs. In other words, the veterinarian is collecting and analyzing a more complete history of the production unit. The more historical information the veterinarian has, the more complete his or her understanding, and the more valuable the recommendations.

It must be understood that a SPA report is historical and summary information. It should be the foundation or baseline from which to evaluate future performance. The SPA report indicates problem areas, but it does not provide specific answers. If a problem area is identified by a SPA report, a more detailed evaluation should be completed to develop an understanding of

Name:	Location of ranch (state)		
Address:	Location in state (circle one)		
Address:	North West	North Central	North East
Fiscal yr. Herd ID:	South West	South Central	South East
Phone number:	Bull turn out date: / /		
Days in breeding season:	Beginning calving season: / /		
Preg check date: / /	Weaning date: / /		

<u>Cows</u>

1. Exposed females (number of females in breeding herd exposed)   _____

2. Pairs or pregnant females sold/transferred out of herd before weaning   _____

3. Pairs or pregnant females purchased/transferred into herd before weaning   _____

4. Adjusted exposed female inventory (line 1 minus line 2 plus line 3)   _____

<u>Calves</u>

	Steers/Bulls	Heifers	All Calves
5. Total head of calves weaned	_____ hd	_____ hd	_____ hd
6. Total pounds of calves weaned or (line 7 times 5)	_____ lb	_____ lb	_____ lb
7. Average weight of calves weaned or (line 6 divided by line 5)	_____ hd	_____ hd	_____ hd
8. Average price per pound (value) of calves	$/lb _____	$/lb _____	$/lb _____

<u>Total</u>

9. Percent weaned calves [(line 5 divided by line 4) times 100]   _____ %

10. Total dollar value of all calves weaned (line 8 times line 6) $ _____

11. Pounds weaned per exposed female (line 6 divided by line 4)   _____ lb/hd

12. Total acres (grazing plus hay plus aftermath)   _____

13. Total breeding females (number of exposed females [mature plus replacement] on premises at beginning of fiscal year)   _____ hd

Figure 2
SPA-EZ production inventory and calculations.

Table 1
SELECTED ANIMAL PRODUCTION PARAMETERS UTILIZED IN THE SPA-P ANALYSIS

Pregnancy % = [(No. of females exposed diagnosed as pregnant/No. of females exposed) × 100]

Pregnancy loss % = [(No. of females diagnosed as pregnant that failed to calve/No. of females diagnosed as pregnant) × 100]

Pregnancy loss % = (Pregnancy % − calving %)

Calving % = [(No. of calves born/No. of females exposed) × 100]

Calf death loss based on exposed females = [(No. of calves that died/No. of exposed females) × 100]

Calf death loss based on calves born = [(No. of calves that died/No. of calves born) × 100]

Calf crop or weaning % = [(No. of calves weaned/No. of females exposed) × 100]

Female replacement rate = [(Raised replacement heifers exposed for 1st calf + purchased replacement heifers and breeding cows exposed)/No. of females exposed] × 100

Calving distribution = [(Cumulative no. of calves born by 21, 42, and 63 days and those after 63 days of the calving season/total No. of calves born) × 100]

Actual weaning weight for steer/bull calves = (Total weight of weaned steer and bull calves/total No. of weaned steer and bull calves)

Heifer calf weaning weight = (Total weight heifer calves weaned/total No. of heifer calves weaned)

Average weaning weight = (Total weight of weaned calves/total No. of calves weaned)

Pounds weaned per exposed female = (Total pounds of calf weaned/total No. of females exposed)

---

the problem and make recommendations for improvement. The following paragraphs outline the SPA-P guidelines. The guidelines are listed in Tables 1 and 2, and the computation equations are provided.

Pregnancy Percentage

Pregnancy percentage is a good indicator of breeding performance in the herd. If the measure computed is lower than the average of similar operations, it may indicate that the nutritional program is inadequate, that bull power or fertility is inadequate, that disease causing early embryonic death is present, or that a mismatch has occurred between herd genetics and the environment (e.g., feed resources and management style). The meaning of this percentage is greatly enhanced if it is kept by female age group, because rebreeding is often only a problem within certain age groups (e.g., females exposed for a second calf).

Table 2
FORAGE AND LAND PRODUCTION PARAMETERS UTILIZED FOR SPA-P

Grazing and raised feed acres per exposed female = (Grazing acres + raised feed acres/total No. of exposed females)

Grazing acres per exposed female = (Grazing acres/total No. of exposed females)

Raised feed acres per exposed female = (Raised feed acres/total No. of exposed females)

Crop aftermath acres per exposed female = (Crop aftermath acres/total No. of exposed females)

Raised/purchased feed fed per breeding cow = (Total pounds of raised and/or purchased feed fed/No. of breeding females)

This value will only be available to production systems that routinely diagnose pregnancy through rectal palpation procedures. However, for small herds, good heat checking can determine which animals are not pregnant without rectal palpation, and this percentage can be calculated.

Pregnancy Loss Percentage

Pregnancy loss percentage is a good indicator of reproductive performance. If the measure is higher than the average for similar operations, it may indicate late-pregnancy reproductive disease problems that cause abortions. This measure may signal a potential problem before it becomes serious. Feedstuff quality groups may possess nutritional inadequacies, or there may be a management problem with the females. Rectal palpation requirements are the same as for the pregnancy percentage values. Accuracy is reduced if only a portion of the total herd is tested for pregnancy. The exposed females not tested may have a higher or lower pregnancy rate.

Calving Percentage

Calving percentage is a good indicator of breeding performance and gestation management in the herd. If the measure is lower than the average for similar operations, it may indicate that the nutritional or grazing program is inadequate, that bull power or fertility is inadequate, that disease causing embryonic death is present, or that a mismatch between herd genetics and the environment exists. This value does not indicate in what manner the calf crop is born. The calving distribution will illustrate how calves are grouped by birthdate.

Calf Death Loss

Calf death loss can be very useful in evaluating the herd health program, calving environment, nutritional program, and genetic selection program. A more accurate analysis of calf death loss would include age of calf at death, age of dam, and cause of death. Abortions before calving should be included in the pregnancy loss percentage. Purchased grafted calves should not be included in the calf death loss based on calves born measurement.

The type of operation, extensive or intensive, should be considered when a comparison is made using this measure of performance. The age makeup of the cow herd could influence calf death loss and must be considered when comparisons are made between herds. Calf death loss at birth vs. death loss during the suckling period is not distinguished here. Calf death loss records should include those calves lost at birth and any that die up to weaning.

Calf Crop or Weaning Percentage

Calf crop or *weaning percentage* measures the reproductive rate of the herd. As reproductive rate has been shown to be a major factor in profitability, it is probably the most important single measure of production performance. Because reproduction is largely a function of nutrition, it is an excellent indicator of the adequacy of the nutritional program. Additionally, it is an excellent indicator of how well the cows are matched to the resources. The adequacy of the herd health program used and any disease problems can be evaluated, in part, by this measure.

This measure does not, however, account for excessive use of feed and nonfeed inputs. Calf crop percent may not correlate highly to economic performance in cases in which cull marketing decisions are made prior to times of high-input costs when the measure is compared to that in herds in which this practice is not followed.

Female Replacement Rate Percentage

Female replacement rate percentage is a good indicator of herd replacement rate and cow longevity. If this percentage is higher than the average of similar operations it may indicate that the herd has reproductive problems or that it is in an expansion phase. Generally, a high percentage will mean higher herd costs and lower productivity per cow because a larger portion of the herd consists of first- and second-calf females. Also, if this percentage is high, it may mean that the current genetic type does not match the resources, thus causing higher-than-normal culling rates and heifer retention. A low percentage may indicate that the herd is in a liquidation phase.

Market fluctuation, more than production, may cause this percentage to vary. Farmers or ranchers with herds in either an expansion or liquidation phase will find this percentage hard to compare and less valuable.

Calving Distribution

Calving distribution is another measure of reproductive performance. Calf weaning weight and uniformity of the calf crop is greatly affected by calf age. This measure is very useful in evaluating the adequacy of nutrition during crucial reproductive periods, bull power, herd health, and heifer development programs. It is most useful if calculated by age of females, because the distribution for certain groups, particularly second-calf heifers, is often much lower than for mature cows. Additionally, separate calculations by age of females may be necessary for meaningful comparisons when yearling heifers are bred prior to the cow herd.

Calving distribution, however, cannot be used in extensive grazing environments in which accurate counts of the number of calves born may be difficult to obtain. A controlled breeding season is very important in analyzing production data. A year-round breeding season and calving season is very difficult to evaluate. The goal should be to have the calving distribution skewed to the beginning of the calving season.

Actual Weaning Weights

Actual weaning weights may be difficult to interpret, but they must be assessed to measure productivity and performance. The best use of this measure of performance is to establish gross revenue for the operation and to evaluate the effect of changes in the breeding program or management. Also, because the environment and feed supply greatly affect weaning weights in any year, long-term trends are more useful than yearly changes. Because producers calve and wean calves at different times and ages, actual weaning weights are not standardized to age. However, including average age weaned in the data serves as a guide in interpreting weaning weights for comparative purposes.

Because of differences in pasture production and management, it can be difficult to compare weaning weights between operations. This is especially a problem when comparing fall vs. spring calving herds in which calf weaning age may differ by 3 months. In situations in which two calving seasons are used, it is best to do a separate analysis for each season.

Weaning weights are greatly affected by annual environmental conditions. For example, high and low levels of moisture or extremes in temperature, which are beyond the manager's control, can influence weaning weights more than all controlled management factors. Thus, producers should avoid placing too much emphasis on the weights for any single year and should concentrate on long-term trends. Users of this measure must remember that higher weaning weights normally mean higher gross revenue but not necessarily increased profit. Increased profit is also dependent on calf crop and production costs.

Pounds Weaned per Exposed Female

Pounds weaned per exposed female combines into one figure the herd reproduction rate, calf death loss, and genetics for growth and maternal traits. From a herd production standpoint, this is probably the best measure of performance. This measure is a tool to assist producers in managing the tradeoffs between growth rate and reproductive rate. In other words, concentrating on improving the number of pounds weaned per cow exposed should be more profitable than emphasizing either calf crop or weaning weight separately.

Because this measure is a combination of the measures used to analyze reproduction and production, it has some of the limitations of each these measures. Age at weaning and distribution of calving can influence this value a great deal, making it more valuable as a measure for an individual operation than for comparison between farms or ranches. The number of females exposed must be adjusted for the same factors that were used in the calf crop percent calculations. Purchased grafted calves should be included in this measurement. Do not include calves sold while still nursing their dams or pairs transferred out.

Grazing, Raised Feed, and Crop Aftermath Acres per Exposed Female

Grazing, raised feed, and crop aftermath acres per exposed female (see Table 2) is a measure of the primary input in the cow-calf enterprise: forage and land. These measures also provide a description of the production system that the producer can monitor. Differences in acres of the grazing and feed sources are most valuable for the same operation over time. Farms or ranches in the same area can be a useful comparative analysis. However, these values have limited use in comparing different regions for land with different production capacity. Acres of land do not reflect forage production quality or differences in production.

Adjusting for the time that land is used for grazing or growing another crop requires judgment. Land having more than one use, such as corn grain production and stalk grazing, should be adjusted to the time actually used for grazing. Consistency between years is important. Adjustments in grazing time must be made when supplemental feeding and grazing are simultaneous, based on the portion of cow requirements being met by grazing. As a primary input, management of forages has an important impact on production costs.

Raised/Purchased Feed Fed per Breeding Cow

Raised/purchased feed fed per breeding cow is an excellent indicator of efficient resource use and cost control (see Table 2). Because harvested and purchased feed represent a major expense in most operations, this measure, when compared with that of other operations within a region, can indicate either a strength or weakness in herd nutritional management.

This measure would include feed fed to replacement heifers and bulls that support the cow-calf enterprise. Higher-than-average feed needed per breeding female could indicate over-feeding, below-normal pasture production or use, above-normal feed wastage, below-normal use of aftermath grazing, below-average feed quality, or above-average female replacement rates.

Herds with larger grazing resources will have smaller harvested/purchased feed use. Use caution when comparing this measure between herds. This measure is useful when kept over a period of time for an individual operation, so progress can be measured. The type of feed can vary greatly in energy and protein density from ranch to ranch or year to year, making comparison less accurate. This measure is difficult to measure in herds in either an expansion or a liquidation phase.[1]

SPA-F GUIDELINES

Balance sheets contain a list of all assets and liabilities assigned to an enterprise. Balance sheets are dated for a specific point in time: the first and last day of the fiscal year (Fig. 3). If the use of the asset is shared by another enterprise, then its value must be prorated between the enterprises based on use. Assets are categorized as either current or noncurrent (Table 3). The value of the asset should be its book value (original cost less accumulated depreciation) or base value (accumulated cost). Balance sheets determine the value of assets on both a cost basis and a fair-market-value basis.

The most difficult balance sheet input consists of inventory values. These include feed and cattle inventories. Inventories include stored feed and livestock numbers. Inventories should be valued at market value and cost. The value of the current and noncurrent liabilities can be obtained from the loan payment schedules. The following discussion refers to the second page of the SPA-EZ form given in Figure 3.

14. Feed Inventory. Feed inventory should include all feed in inventory (raised and purchased) on hand at the date of the balance sheet. The raised feed should be valued at its accumulated cost basis. If its cost value is not available, use its fair market value. If the types and quantity of feed are available, show the detail. The pounds of roughage should be calculated on an air-dried basis.

15. Prepaid Expenses. These are expense items that have been paid for but not received and not used by the enterprise.

Assets	Beginning of the Year			End of the Year		
Current assets Feed inventory	Pounds	Total Value		Pounds	Total Value	
Roughage	_____	_____		_____	_____	
Grain/concentrate	_____	_____		_____	_____	
Protein supplement	_____	_____		_____	_____	
Salt/minerals	_____	_____		_____	_____	
14. Total feed inventory		_____			_____	
15. Prepaid expenses		_____			_____	
16. Cash (checking, savings, etc.)		_____			_____	
17. Misc.		_____			_____	
18. Total Current Assets		_____			_____	
Non-current assets						
19. Machinery and equipment		_____			_____	
20. Real estate, buildings, and improvements		_____			_____	
Breeding Cattle	Head	Base Value	Total	Head	Base Value	Total
21. Replacement heifers (1-yr-olds)	_____	_____	_____	_____	_____	_____
22. Bred heifer (2-yr-olds)	_____	_____	_____	_____	_____	_____
23. Mature cows	_____	_____	_____	_____	_____	_____
24. Bulls	_____	_____	_____	_____	_____	_____
25. Other non-current assets (horses, etc.)			_____			_____
26. Total non-current assets			_____			_____
27. Total assets			_____			_____
			(line 27a)			*(line 27b)*
Liabilities						
28. Current liabilities (accounts/notes payable, accrued interest, accrued taxes, etc.)			_____			_____
29. Non-current liabilities (machinery, real estate, livestock, etc.)			_____			_____
30. Total liabilities			_____			_____

Figure 3
SPA-EZ cost-basis balance sheet.

Table 3
FINANCIAL TERMS AND RATIOS UTILIZED BY SPA-F

Current assets and liabilities = Assets realized in cash, sold, or
   consumed + liabilities discharged + obligations due on demand
   within 1 yr from balance sheet date
Cost value of purchased breeding livestock = Cost of the animal −
   accumulated depreciation
Net farm income = Return to farmer for unpaid labor, management,
   and owner equity
Current ratio = Total current farm assets/total current farm liabilities
Working capital = Total current farm assets − total current farm
   liabilities
Debt/asset ratio = Total farm liabilities/total farm assets
Equity/asset ratio = Total farm equity/total farm assets
Rate of return on farm assets = (net farm income from operations +
   farm interest expense − owner withdrawals for unpaid labor and
   management)/average total farm assets

They will be listed as a current asset. An example would be feed that was paid for before the end of the year but not in the beginning year feed inventory.

16. Cash (Checking, Savings, etc.). This is the checking account balance on the date of the balance sheet as well as any savings accounts assigned to the enterprise.

17. Miscellaneous. All current assets not listed above should be entered here. Only list the value assigned to the cow-calf enterprise.

18. Total Current Assets. This is the total of the current assets listed above.

19. Machinery and Equipment. Enter the book value of all equipment and machinery used in the enterprise. If the equipment is used by more than one enterprise, proportion the value across the enterprises involved.

20. Real Estate, Buildings, and Improvements. Enter the cost basis for the real estate and the book value for the improvements and buildings. Proportion the value to the amount utilized by the enterprise. For example, if the grazing acres are used by both a cow-calf enterprise and a stocker enterprise at the proportions of 70% and 30% respectively, then the cost value of the grazing acres should be a 70/30 proportion also.

The breeding cattle inventory (see Fig. 3) includes all females and males in the herd on the date of the balance sheet. If possible, break this down by age of animal. For example, a replacement heifer would have a different value than a mature cow. Purchased animals should be valued at their book value (original cost less accumulated depreciation), and raised animals should be valued at a base value. The base value for raised animals should approximate the accumulated cost to get the animals to that point. The base value should not change from year to year after it has been established. For example, if it has been established that for a given herd replacement heifers should be valued at $450 each, bred heifers valued at $550, and mature cows valued at $650, then these same values should be used each year and not changed over time or with changing market conditions.

21. Replacement Heifers (1 Year Olds). Enter the head count and the base value of the raised replacement heifers for the date of the balance sheet. The total value should include the total value (using base value concept) of the raised replacement heifers plus the book value of the purchased replacement heifers.

22. Bred Heifers (2 Year Olds). Enter the head count and the base value of the raised bred heifers for the date of the balance sheet. The total value should include the total value (using base value concept) of the raised bred heifers plus the book value of the purchased bred heifers.

23. Mature Cows. Enter the head count and the base value of the raised mature cows for the date of the balance sheet. The total value should include the total value (using base value concept) of the raised mature cows plus the book value of the purchased mature cows.

24. Bulls. Enter the head count and the base value of the raised bulls for the date of the balance sheet. The total value should include the total value (using base value concept) of the raised bulls plus the book value of the purchased bulls.

25. Other Noncurrent Assets (Horses, etc.). Enter the book value of all other noncurrent assets not listed above.

26. Total Noncurrent Assets. This is the total value of all noncurrent assets.

27. Total Assets. This is the total value of all assets assigned to the cow-calf enterprise.

Liabilities are the debts incurred by the enterprise. Proportion the debts according to the proportion used by the cow-calf enterprise. The debts are categorized into current and noncurrent liabilities (see Fig. 3).

28. Current Liabilities. Enter the total of all accounts due, notes payable, accrued interest, accrued taxes, and current part of noncurrent debt.

29. Noncurrent Liabilities. Enter the total noncurrent debt. This would include the noncurrent part of debt on, for example, equipment, real estate, livestock, and machinery that is utilized by the cow-calf enterprise.

30. Total Liabilities. This is the sum of current and noncurrent liabilities.

Deferred taxes and opportunity cost are not included in the SPA-EZ analysis. This analysis is a pre-tax financial analysis. The complete SPA analysis is needed to address these and other more detailed issues.

Income statements contain a list of revenues and expenses (Fig. 4). These are then adjusted for accrual changes to place in the correct time period. The income statement accounts for both cash and noncash items. The primary revenue items are the value of the weaned calves, gain or loss on culled animals, and increases in value of raised replacement animals. Expenses should be only those incurred by the cow-calf enterprise. The best starting place is with the financial instruments that everyone must keep, the Internal Revenue Service (IRS) tax schedules. Schedules F and the depreciation schedule are used. Adjustments must be made to these instruments to make them useful in managerial decision-making.

31. Weaned Calves. The value of the weaned calf crop is given in item 10. This should be net amount less the cost of selling. Remember to include base value of replacement animals, non-cash value of retained animals, and value of purchased grafted calves. Values are determined at weaning.

32. Gain/Loss on Culls. The gain/loss on culls must be determined from the value shown on the beginning balance sheet for that animal. The gain/loss is the net market value received less the value used on the beginning balance sheet (base value and/or book value). Enter the head count culled by category, the total market value received, and the total base value. Animals on the beginning balance sheet that die during the fiscal year will be shown as a loss in this section. The amount of the loss will be the value of that animal on the beginning balance sheet.

33. Change in Base Value. Enter the head count from the ending balance sheet that changed categories (animals that were on the beginning balance sheet and ending balance sheet). Enter the base value used on the beginning balance sheet and the ending balance sheet. Subtract the total for ending base value from the total for beginning base value. The change in base value is the difference between the established base values. For example, if replacement heifers, bred heifers, and mature cows

Revenue

31. Weaned calves (see production calculations line 10) $ _____

32. Gain/loss on culls

	Head	Total Market Value	Total Base Value	Total Difference
Mature cows	_____ hd	$ _____	$ _____	$ _____
Heifers	_____ hd	$ _____	$ _____	$ _____
Bulls	_____ hd	$ _____	$ _____	$ _____
				$ _____ Total

(line 32)

33. Change in base value*

	Head	Total Beginning Base	Total Ending Base	
	_____ hd	$ _____	$ _____	
	_____ hd	$ _____	$ _____	
Total change in base value		_____ Total	_____ Total	Total $ _____ Difference

(line 33)

34. Other non-calf revenue $ _____

35. Total revenue $ _____

   *See balance sheet lines 22 & 23 for base values.

Expenses (Cash and non-cash)

Purchased feed, supplement, and mineral $ _____

Lease/rental $ _____

Labor, management, family living (paid and unpaid) $ _____

Veterinarian/medicine $ _____

Interest $ _____

Other (fuel, supplies, taxes, insurance, repairs, etc.) $ _____

Depreciation $ _____

Change in inventories/accounts $ _____

36. Total expenses $ _____

(line 36)

37. Annual cow cost (line 36 divided by line 13) $ _____

38. Non-calf revenue adjusted expenses (line 36 minus lines 32, 33, & 34) $ _____

39. Calf breakeven (line 38 divided by line 6) $ _____ per lb

40. Net income per cow ([line 35 minus line 36] divided by line 13) $ _____ $/hd

41. Total net income (line 35 minus line 36) $ _____

42. Year average asset value ([line 27a plus 27b] divided by 2) $ _____

43. ROA ([line 35 minus line 36 plus interest] divided by line 42) times 100 $ _____ %

Figure 4

SPA-EZ financial information and calculations for completion of the income statement.

are valued at $450, $550, and $650, respectively, the change in base value is $100 for each category. If a replacement heifer is on the beginning balance sheet at $450, this heifer would be on the ending balance sheet as a bred heifer at $550. Thus, there is a $100 increase in base value that is recognized as non-cash revenue on the income statement. The calculation requires multiplying the head count on the ending balance sheet that moved to the next age category (from beginning balance sheet) times the change in base value (i.e., $100). Total change in base value of each category is summed in item 33.

34. Other Non-calf Revenues. Sum all miscellaneous revenues that are allocated to the cow-calf enterprise. Accrual adjust-

ments to revenue are included in this item. For example the beginning accounts receivable is subtracted from the ending accounts receivable, and the difference is included in item 34.

35. Total Revenue. This is the sum of revenues (items 31 through 34) with accrual adjustments.

Proportion expenses to different enterprises if multiple enterprises exist. For example, only charge the cow-calf enterprise for the purchased feed that was used by that enterprise. Do not charge for purchased feed that was used by the backgrounding enterprise. Categorize expenses if possible (see Fig. 4). Include in the *labor, management, family living* category an expense for the labor that family members contributed to the cow-calf enterprise. The value should approximate the amount that would have been paid to a non-family member to perform the same job. The depreciation expense includes all depreciation (e.g., equipment, machinery, livestock) allocated to the enterprise based on its utilization by the enterprise (check balance sheet allocations). The original cost, the depreciation method used, and its salvage value must be known to calculate depreciation of an asset. Depreciation is a method of allocating use over time.

Changes in inventories/accounts are accrual adjustments that are very important to the analysis. The changes are calculated from the beginning and ending balance sheet differences for each category. For example, if the beginning balance sheet value for feed inventory is $50,000 and the ending balance sheet value for feed inventory is $30,000, then there is a decrease in feed inventory of $20,000 (change in inventory). This decrease (negative change) in inventory would be added to the income statement as a positive number to show an increase in expenses. This logic should be followed for asset accounts such as inventories, accounts receivable, and notes receivable. A decrease in a liability account, such as accounts payable, notes due, interest due, or taxes due, would require a negative expense (decrease in expenses) on the income statement.

Net farm income is calculated on a pre-tax basis and matches revenues with expenses incurred to create those revenues. It provides for a close approximation of matching revenues with the expenses incurred to create those revenues. If the income statement is prepared using cash-basis accounting, then both beginning and ending accrual adjusted balance sheets are needed to make the necessary adjustments for changes in inventories, accounts receivable, accounts payable, prepaid expenses, and accrued expenses.

Tax-based depreciation methods are likely to be utilized by many preparers of financial statements. The form of business organization can cause problems for interpretation of this amount. A corporation will include operator labor payments as a labor cost in its tax-based records unless adjustments are made. Interfarm comparability must be made with caution whenever different forms of business organization are represented.

36. Total Expenses. This is the sum of all expenses with accrual adjustments.

37. Annual Cow Cost. Item 36 divided by item 13.

38. Non-calf Revenue Adjusted Expenses. Item 36 minus items (32 plus 33 plus 34).

39. Calf Break-Even. Item 38 divided by item 6.

40. Net Income per Cow. (Item 35 minus item 36) divided by item 13.

41. Total Net Income. Item 35 minus item 36.

42. Year Average Asset Value. (Item 27a plus 27b) divided by 2.

43. Return on Assets (ROA) %. [(Item 35 minus item 36 plus interest) divided by item 42] times 100.

SUMMARY

The SPA methodology integrates production values with the associated financial and economic cost and returns. This allows for the analysis of the whole enterprise system. The production measures that are required for integration with financial measures are beginning fiscal year breeding inventory, total pounds of weaned calves produced, and total number of acres allocated to the cow/calf inventory.

The beginning fiscal year breeding female inventory value is the divisor for the financial and economic measure to give the per head measurements. The total pounds weaned is the divisor for the financial and economic per-hundredweight measures.

The total acres allocated measure is the divisor for the financial and economic per-acre measurements. These units of production measurements are essential for integration of production and financial information.

BIBLIOGRAPHY

Hamilton ED: Standardized performance analysis. Vet Clin North Am Food Anim Pract 11:199–213, 1995.

McGrann JM: Integrated Resource Management (IRM) Standardized Performance Analysis (SPA) Handbook. College Station, Texas, Texas Agricultural Extension Service, Texas A&M University, 1994.

Recommendations of the Farm Financial Standards Council: Financial Guidelines for Agricultural Producers (rev ed). Farm Financial Standards Council, 1995.

■ The Bovine Practitioner's Role in Beef Quality Assurance

Donald E. Hansen, D.V.M., M.P.V.M.

BACKGROUND HISTORY

In the mid-1980s, beef consumption by Americans decreased substantially in some areas and plateaued in others. By the late 1980s, beef consumers became more health conscious and expressed concern about the relationship between red meat diets and diseases of overconsumption. There were additional public misgivings about potential drug and chemical residue contamination of beef products as well as a perception that using antibiotics in food animals might be responsible for increased antibiotic resistance to pathogens associated with foodborne illness in humans. These public apprehensions and perceptions about the safety of beef products sparked industry leaders to investigate ways to address public regard for beef product quality.[1]

During this same period, industrial business enterprises, particularly automobile manufacturers, were experiencing stagnation and/or downward trends in annual sales. Their marketing experts determined that unit price was only part of the reason for the trend. The other reason was consumer belief that foreign cars were better constructed. The quality of U.S. cars had slipped, and consumers were unhappy about it. To reverse the trend, U.S. manufacturers began developing and implementing quality assurance and total quality management concepts into their management schemes. The success of these programs hinged on establishment of a team approach wherein responsibility for the quality of the final product was shared by all who had a part in constructing the automobile.[2]

By 1990, all cattle industry leaders recognized the importance of developing and implementing quality assurance standards for meat and milk products that would not only enhance product quality but also augment their images. They concluded that the best approach included veterinarian, producer, and feeder and packer participation for complete success.[3] However, the means used to gain participation differed between the dairy and beef groups.

The beef industry, under the combined leadership of the National Cattlemen's Beef Association (NCBA), the American Veterinary Medical Association (AVMA), and the American Association of Bovine Practitioners (AABP), followed the automobile industry's concept of bottom-up team building and developed ways to induce producer-driven quality assurance programs for beef production systems and encouraged their spread throughout the country.[3] By 1994, virtually all states had some form of beef quality assurance program in operation. Currently, beef quality assurance programs aim at a spectrum of quality aspects of the finished carcass, including drug and chemical residue avoidance, reduction of injection-site damage in back and rump muscles, reduction of tissue damage from bruises, and reduction of excessive fat trim.[4] A number of quality deficits in mature cows and bulls, such as advanced lameness, inadequate muscling in cows, heavy live-weights in bulls, and low dressing percentages, are also included.[5]

By comparison, the dairy industry, after a 1-year voluntary trial, embraced top-down regulatory methods to assure quality in the milk supply by expanding the regulations of the Pasteurized Milk Order (PMO). The PMO ultimately governs on-the-farm aspects of producing grade-A milk by regulating standards for all shipment of milk. The PMO was changed in 1992 to control and restrict antibiotic storage, labeling, and use in U.S. dairies, and it required preprocess testing of bulk milk for antibiotics.[6] The dairy industry also developed a voluntary, producer-veterinarian–driven program aimed at drug residue avoidance in dairy-beef animals, which has been widely distributed since 1991.

The newest efforts toward overall quality and wholesomeness of meat products have been directed at reducing the number and prevalence of zoonotic pathogens on finished carcasses. These efforts have been sparked by recent outbreaks of food-borne illness involving specific human pathogens found in hamburger and other meat products. At present, reduction and control steps are being regulated by federal law at slaughter facilities throughout the country. In the near future, the beef industry will be called on to initiate efforts directed at reducing and/or controlling specific pathogens in animals at production facilities, such as feedlot, backgrounding, and cow/calf operations. Current methods for pathogen reduction at beef production centers are not well developed or are theoretical. As research continues, practical prevention and/or reduction methods may be developed that can be applied at various production levels in the beef industry.

This article addresses current quality assurance issues, including drug and chemical residues, injection-site and bruising blemishes, slaughter of non-ambulatory animals, lameness and other physical defects in animals, and carcass traits and quality assurance for marketing mature animals.

WHAT IS THE BOVINE PRACTITIONER'S ROLE IN QUALITY ASSURANCE EFFORTS?

First, a practitioner must be convinced of the legitimacy of industry and public concerns for strengthening and sustaining quality in beef products. In a survey conducted among consumers in July 1996, 83% of those surveyed believed that food safety was a very important issue. In fact, food safety concerns were ranked nearly equal with the importance of crime prevention, safe drinking water, and health and nutrition issues. Further, 81% of respondents said they believed most or all of the information they got from the media regarding food safety issues. And 67% believed that rules governing food safety were not tough enough. Issues of greatest concern to respondents were bacteria in food (85%), food handling and preparation (82% each), pesticide residue (78%), drug residue (75%), and hormones in food (67%).[7]

The red meat industry is trying to remain sensitive to consumer demands for its product. The competition raised by poultry and swine products for market shares of meat sales is stronger than ever before. If the market share of red meat is to remain competitive, the industry must establish and maintain high quality standards for its product. Decreased public confidence in red meat products causes reduced consumption, the cost of which trickles back along the production chain until it

comes to rest at the producer's gate. For example, in 1996, overall beef consumption dropped immediately following an announcement by a very popular television talk show host that she would no longer eat hamburger. Her statement was prompted by the revelation that some U.S. cattle rations included animal protein. Nevertheless, beef consumption remained down for the remainder of the year, resulting in a 2% ($700 million) loss in sales for 1996. On the production side, live-cattle prices remained low for a prolonged period. In another instance, cattle futures prices plummeted immediately following a news release that falsely stated that two people in the Midwest had died from "mad cow disease" (bovine spongiform encephalopathy).

In the big picture, veterinarians and their cattle clients have a vested interest in the continued viability and strength of consumer demand for meat products. Ultimately, they share the responsibility of ensuring to the public that high standards of wholesomeness and quality are being met. No matter what segment of the cattle industry is represented by the veterinarian's client (cow/calf, backgrounder, or feeder operation), all veterinarians must realize they are producing or handling an animal destined for human consumption. A healthy old cow is certain to become food as soon as she is placed on the to-be-sold list. A bull travels the same road as soon as he fails to meet the breeding demands of the operation.

Bovine practitioners are encouraged to join or lead the efforts to magnify the quality of food produced by their clients. Practitioners may lay the groundwork for this endeavor by consistently reminding clients of quality assurance issues and by educating clients about industry quality concerns and encouraging them to participate in the effort to amplify the goodness of the animals they sell.

Drug and Chemical Residue Avoidance

Violative residue avoidance is the main focus in quality assurance programs for all food animal species. For most fed cattle sent to slaughter, contamination from drug or chemical residues may be a moot issue, as the annual incidence of violative residues in that group remains at or near zero.[8] However, the incidence of violative residues in young slaughtered calves and slaughtered cows continues to be problematic for the industry.[8] Scientific evidence of actual human illness resulting from drug residues in meat is scant, and some existing reports may be equivocal. However, the public and physician perceptions of personal harm from residues in meat and milk continue.[7] Although federal agencies, the NCBA, and veterinary associations continually strive to reassure consumers about the security of meat products, concerned activists persistently assert to the government and the public that illegal, cavalier, and/or uncontrolled drug and/or chemical use is pervasive in some sectors of the cattle industry. According to Food and Drug Administration (FDA) reports, in 1991, 8% of violative drug residues in marketed cows resulted from treatment advised by a veterinarian, whereas 63% of violative residue followed owner treatment. By comparison, in 1995, only 2% of violative drug residues in marketed cows resulted from treatment advised by a veterinarian, whereas 43% resulted from an owner's failure to read and/or follow label directions for proper use of drugs or to observe approved withdrawal times. This provides clear evidence that close work between veterinarians and their cattle-producing clients could lower the incidence of violative residues and thus help assure dependability of safety of beef.

Veterinarians have the opportunity to be proactive on the residue-avoidance issue by always communicating clear and complete drug-use instructions that include appropriate identification of treated animals and observation of established withdrawal times. Bovine practitioners must continue to strive to be in the forefront of the residue-avoidance effort both as individuals and as members of a profession. The "us-against-them" attitude (veterinarians and clients against regulatory agencies responsible for wholesomeness of food products) is disappearing. In its place is an attitude of acceptance of everyone's responsibility in ensuring consistent quality of the product through the production chain. Many veterinarians and producers are reassessing drug uses and choices for food animal patients in efforts to ensure that they comply with current state and federal regulations, including accurate animal identification and record-keeping.

Of course, the first step in avoiding drug residue contamination of meat commodities is to prevent occurrence of diseases that require use of drugs considered to be harmful to the consumer. Disease prevention and the bovine practitioner's role in providing advice about it are vital parts of all quality assurance programs. However, when prevention fails and disease occurs, or when drugs and chemicals are used in disease prevention, the following guidelines are recommended for veterinarians and their clients to minimize the risk of violative drug residue in an animal at slaughter.

1. Follow label directions for dosage and administration.
2. Use discretion when choosing to prescribe products in an extra-label manner.
3. Use appropriately extended withdrawal time for extra-label drug use.
4. Identify and/or separate all treated animals.
5. Keep records of animal identification, product name, treatment dosage, and dates used.

For a more complete discussion of this topic, readers are encouraged to read *Prevention and Management of Drug and Chemical Residues in Meat and Milk* by H. Dwight Mercer in the last edition of this book (p. 39). For questions about use, efficacy, and/or withdrawal times for specific products, readers are encouraged to contact personnel at a Food Animal Residue Avoidance Databank (FARAD) office for assistance.

INJECTION-SITE TISSUE DAMAGE

Research has shown that when certain products are injected into or near muscle tissue they produce damage at the site and in surrounding tissue. They may cause abscessation in the short

term, and most cause a meat toughening scar in the long term. Tissue damage from highly irritating products is grossly evident at processing months after administration and is cut out of the carcass when it is discovered. Common injectable products known to cause detectable muscle lesions at 180 days or more postinjection include certain clostridial bacterins, oil-based virus vaccines and bacterins, macrolide antibiotics, long-lasting oxytetracycline, and injectable vitamin and mineral products.[9] In one study, even 10 mL of sterile saline caused measurable muscle damage, which was detectable after 180 days[9] (Fig. 1). Increased toughness extends up to 3 in. beyond the outer margins of the infused material. In a 1997 NCBA audit of more than 10,000 top sirloins sampled from processors throughout the country, injection-site blemishes were detected in 7.5% of the carcasses and required an average of 6 oz to be trimmed out around the blemish. This represents a decrease from 22% and a 12.9-oz trim-out found in the 1991 audit. However, when the 1997 data are extrapolated to include the total pounds of top sirloin butts retailed in the United States, the loss from injection-site blemishes is more than 1.2 million lb of wasted meat with a retail value of more than $3 million. See Figure 2 for injection-site blemish summary history.

Practitioners should be aware of potential adverse reactions from administration of intramuscular products.[11] Cervical intramuscular vaccination caused granulomatous inflammation that resulted in spinal cord compression and paralysis in a group of 3- to 5-month-old dairy heifers. Seven of 50 heifers (14%) in this group developed a progressive neurologic deficit. Three affected heifers were evaluated clinically, but results were nondiagnostic. Symptomatic therapy did not slow progressive worsening of the clinical picture. Five heifers (10%) died or were euthanized after becoming tetraplegic, and three of these underwent necropsy. Gross and histopathologic changes were similar in all three cases.

Epaxial muscle on the right side of the neck between C4 and C6 was pale, firm, and friable with extension of the soft tissue reaction through intervertebral foramina at either C4–5 or C5–6. Grossly visible compression of the spinal cord by the resultant granuloma was evident in one calf at necropsy.

Histopathologic examination in all cases showed focal, segmentally severe, wallerian degeneration of spinal cord segments immediately beneath the epidural granulomas. Affected muscle was neurotic and was expanded by numerous granulomas surrounding variable-sized optically clear spaces. One granuloma contained a hair shaft.

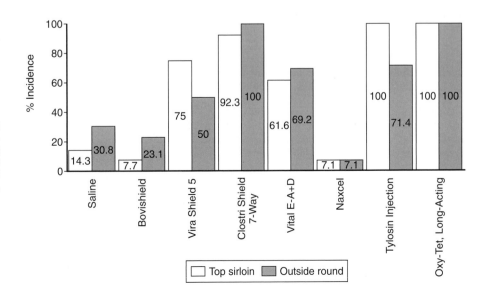

Figure 1

Incidence of injection-site lesions at 180 days post-treatment associated with intramuscularly injected products into calves at weaning time. (Data from George MH, Ames RA, Glock RG, et al: Report to the National Cattlemen's Beef Association, Englewood, Colo, 1997.)

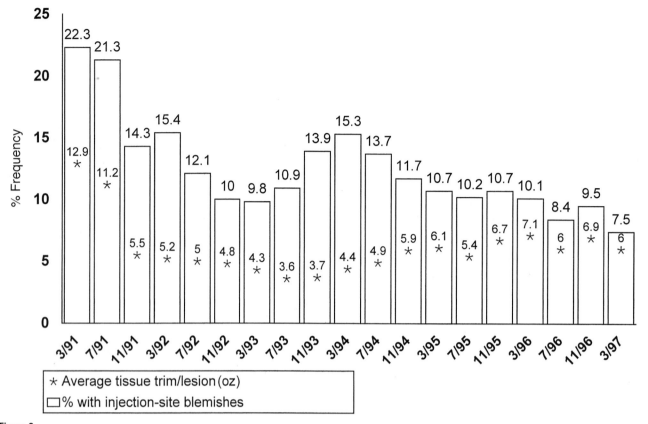

Figure 2
Injection-site audit summary of results from 1991 to 1997. Bars represent percent of sampled top sirloins with detectable injection-site lesions and the average tissue trim/lesion in ounces (*). (Data provided courtesy of the National Cattlemen's Beef Association, Englewood, Colo, 1997.)

Aerobic and anaerobic cultures of affected muscle were negative. Stains for fungi, microbacteria, and bacteria were negative. The combination of the histologic appearance, localization of the gross lesions, the presence of the hair shaft deep within the epaxial muscle, and negative culture and stain results led to the conclusion that these granulomas were the result of an injection-site (foreign body) reaction.

Questioning of the owner revealed that all 50 heifers in this group had been vaccinated in the cervical musculature 15 days prior to the onset of clinical signs. Each calf received three different oil-adjuvant bacterins for a total of 9 mL of vaccinal product. This case illustrates the risk of losing individual animals if a large volume of an irritating solution is administered close to the cervical spine.

With their unique understanding of the mechanics of abscess and scar formation, veterinarians are in a good position to affirm the reported damage and to support recommendations for use of injectable materials that eliminate tissue damage in expensive cuts of meat as well as to help avoid adverse reactions from improper injection technique or from overloading a site with product. In addition, practitioners could encourage reduction in the overall use of intramuscular routes in favor of effective subcutaneous routes for delivery of injectable inventories. The following are some basic methods recommended by beef quality assurance programs to address this problem:

1. Administer injectable products by the subcutaneous route whenever the product label and/or good medicine practices allow.

2. Use sharp, sanitary needles, between 16 and 18 gauge and 1.0 to 1.5 in. long, for all intramuscular injections.

3. For adult animals, inject no more than 10 mL of product per site and separate injection sites by at least 4 in. For calves and lightweight cattle, reduce the volume of product per site and maintain separation of sites.

4. When injecting product by the intramuscular route, place injection into muscles in front of the shoulder region.

5. Change needles often (i.e., every 10 to 15 animals) or whenever the syringe needs to be refilled.

6. Avoid giving injections when animals are wet and/or when injection sites are covered with dirt, mud, manure, or other potentially contaminating material.

DAMAGE FROM BRUISING

Quality assurance audits have addressed this issue, and reports by industry list tissue damage from bruises as a quality concern in feeder cattle and in non-fed cattle as well.[4, 5] Depending on the severity of the original injury, damaged muscle may be unhealed at time of slaughter, resulting in a significant lesion that requires cut-out and removal of 3 to 4 lb of damaged tissue per site.[5] A 1995 audit revealed that 52% and 25% of mature cows and bulls, respectively, presented for slaughter with major bruises, 54% and 19.5% of cows and bulls, respectively, had medium bruises, and 31% and 7.4% of cows and bulls, respectively, had minor bruises. The combined loss from bruised tissue cut-out was approximately $61 million in retail sales for 27 million lb of meat product (Fig. 3). In addition to the obvious quality issue involved with bruised tissue, a concern about animal well-being may exist as well. Rough handling of cattle, particularly during procedures requiring the use of a squeeze chute and head catch, is likely to escalate the incidence of severe bruising of the shoulder muscles. Leading the way in the effort to reduce the incidence of carcass bruises, an increasing number of feedlot employees are being persuaded by both managers and veterinarians to place emphasis on maintaining a quality carcass in place of trying to establish processing speed records.[12] Reduction of injection-site lesions, bruised carcasses, and drug residues is part of the quality assurance program.

Recommendations for reduction of bruised carcass damage include the following:

1. Using good management practices when moving cattle into and/or through restricted passageways.

2. Controlling animal movement into and through squeeze chutes in a manner that minimizes body collisions with head catch gates and/or tail gates.

3. Removing or covering sharp objects and edges in alleyways, chutes, gate openings, and other areas used for cattle passage.

4. Removing or tipping horns on cattle to minimize bruising from purposeful or accidental butting.

5. Encouraging safe transportation methods that minimize rough handling.

NON-AMBULATORY ANIMALS PRESENTED FOR SLAUGHTER

The quality issues involved in presenting non-ambulatory animals (occurs primarily in marketed adult cattle) for slaughter involve actual animal product quality and potential animal well-being concerns as well. In addition, non-ambulatory animals present a picture to the viewing public that affects their perception of meat quality in general. In view of the meat industry's effort to enhance actual product quality and public perception, continuing to send non-ambulatory animals through public slaughter channels should be discouraged. For animals that are non-ambulatory before shipment, the veterinarian's examination may determine whether the animal is suitable for wholesome slaughter. For animals that may be suitable, private slaughter or discreet arrangements for commercial slaughter may be made.

What about animals that become non-ambulatory while in transit to a slaughter facility? The practitioner can be proactive about this issue by discussing factors that cause animals to become non-ambulatory in transit. In some cases the situation can be avoided altogether. Sometimes the producer or client may be unaware of factors that lead to this predicament, but with good advice he or she can make more informed decisions.

Veterinarians can counsel clients to market animals before they become so emaciated or lame that they are at high risk of being injured, knocked down, and/or developing transport tetany while in transit. (See discussions on lameness and quality assurance.) Separating aggressive animals (e.g., bulls) from one another or excessively large animals from smaller ones while in transit may also reduce the risk. Discussion of other contributing factors, such as proper loading and careful driving, should not be overlooked in discussions with clients. In cases of doubt, an appropriate examination of animals by a veterinarian before shipment may detect those at high risk of becoming "downer cows" during subsequent transportation. Following detection of high-risk animals, the veterinarian may apprise the client of other options.

LAMENESS AND OTHER PHYSICAL DEFECTS

About 9% of all adult beef cattle are presented at slaughter with ocular neoplasia (extreme to severe), actinomycosis (lumpy jaw), or a disabling lameness (Table 1). These quality defects resulted in an estimated $5 million loss from carcass and partial tissue removals at slaughter in 1996. As described for non-ambulatory animals, cattle with advanced diseases as mentioned here present an image at auction markets and slaughter plants that affects the viewer's perception of quality wholesome meat. Much of this loss and negative public impact is avoidable.

Disease prevention programs that are designed for the individual client should consider sire and dam combinations that meet the producer/client production goals and reduce the risk of ocular neoplasia for the herd (by selective breeding for pigmented periocular skin). Follow-up disease monitoring and treatment protocols may be designed to detect neoplasia at earlier stages at which effective therapy might extend the pro-

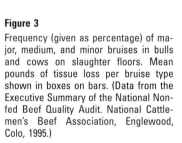

Figure 3

Frequency (given as percentage) of major, medium, and minor bruises in bulls and cows on slaughter floors. Mean pounds of tissue loss per bruise type shown in boxes on bars. (Data from the Executive Summary of the National Non-fed Beef Quality Audit. National Cattlemen's Beef Association, Englewood, Colo, 1995.)

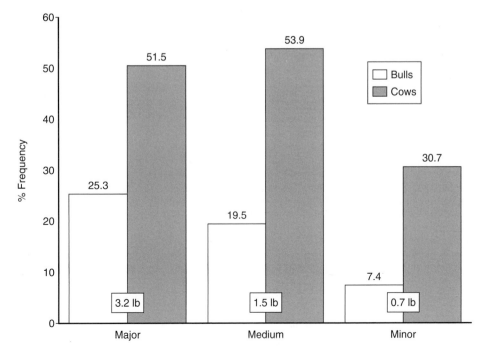

Table 1
FREQUENCY OF DEFECTS FOUND IN BEEF CATTLE AT SLAUGHTER PLANTS

Defect	Frequency
Muscling score too low (scores of 1 or 2)	81.9%
Fat color too yellow	48.5%
Fatness score too high (scores of 4–9)	34.6%
Horns	24.2%
Disabled cattle	4.3%
Bovine ocular neoplasia	3.6%
Lumpy jaw	1.9%

Data from the Executive Summary of the National Non-fed Beef Quality Audit. National Cattlemen's Beef Association, Englewood, Colo, 1994.

ductive life of the affected animal or allow earlier marketing of animals with minimal ocular lesions.

Although prevention of actinomycosal infections may not be very effective, a well-designed disease monitoring program might detect lesions at an earlier stage, during which drug therapy is more efficacious. Also, early disease detection may allow marketing of the affected animal before chronic infection causes excessive weight loss and/or before the lesion becomes very invasive.

Quality deficiencies from severe lameness should be considered at two levels: (1) lameness due to noninvasive, noninfectious injury and (2) lameness related to infection. Sometimes noninvasive, noninfectious injuries, such as joint dislocation and tendon or muscle rupture, may be treated conservatively until the severity of swelling and lameness subsides. If the animal has had access to an adequate ration, weight loss can be minimized as well. With the effects of its injury thereby reduced, the animal is a better market prospect in terms of quality and profit. When medically and economically feasible, these cases should receive appropriate therapy and nutrition before being marketed.

In situations in which therapy is not possible or is economically infeasible, the practitioner should determine, for the client, whether the animal's injury would alter its acceptability as wholesome food for human consumption. If in the practitioner's assessment the animal is acceptable for human consumption, it should be slaughtered immediately to minimize suffering and further deterioration of quality. Again, keeping public perception in mind, custom or on-the-farm slaughter might be the best decision. If the animal is deemed unfit for consumption, it should be humanely and immediately euthanized.

Animals with lameness from an infectious process, such as foot or joint abscesses, should not be sent to slaughter with the hope of being found acceptable for human consumption. From a quality assurance and animal welfare point of view, the animal should be either treated medically to remove the infectious agent or euthanized humanely.

All of the issues raised by this topic require and encourage the participation of a competent and confident bovine practitioner. These scenarios demand crucial decisions that need to be made in a timely manner and/or planned for in advance. The bovine practitioner is the vital key in the cattle producer's overall quality assurance program.

QUALITY ASSURANCE FOR ANIMALS MARKETED WHEN THEY ARE FULLY MATURE

Meat products from slaughtered mature cows and bulls represent approximately 20% of total U.S. beef production.[13] Con-

trary to the popular belief that nearly all non-fed cattle are converted to ground beef, packers save and sell 89% of the rounds and 40% of the top sirloin butts from non-fed cattle. In addition, revenues from sales of cows and mature bulls account for as much as 30% of a producer's annual income.[5] Choosing which animals to be marketed is done on the basis of the individual animal's production capacity and/or utility in relation to overall producer goals and expected economic return for keeping or selling the animal. Given the importance to beef markets and individual producers, decisions on marketing cows and mature bulls can have an impact on both. This section will discuss carcass quality defects commonly found in cows and mature bulls at slaughter that can be affected by management decisions made before marketing.

Two extremes in carcass defects account for the greatest revenue losses and are the most frequently found in the mature non-fed cattle presented at slaughter: being too thin or too fat. Inadequate muscling or low muscling scores were found in 67% of cows and 15% of bulls at slaughter. Excess external fat or too-high carcass weights were detected in 62% of bulls and 28% of cows at slaughter. These combined defects accounted for 52% of the more than $448 million in revenue lost to the beef industry from noncorrected quality defects in non-fed cattle.[5] Table 1 gives summary statistics on extreme trait carcasses surveyed at slaughter.

To address this area of quality assurance, veterinarians are encouraged to discuss various marketing strategies with their clients. Prices for slaughter cows and bulls are traditionally lowest in October to December and highest in February to April. For thin, inadequately muscled cows, the marketing plan could include options to feed thin cows to improve their carcass traits before selling. Short-term feeding plans range from 30 to 100 days. For cows whose thinness is detected in the fall, one option is to feed a ration developed for maximum gain for 30 days, to market animals in better condition and at higher weight. Another option is to feed thin animals inexpensively for minimum gain through the winter months and then to place them on a maximum-gain ration and market them during the early spring when prices increase. Of course, the economic returns from feeding cows depend on feed costs and price at selling, so the producer who chooses to raise value in the animals through holding and feeding incurs some amount of increased risk.

For cattle of excessive carcass size and/or weight (e.g., mature bulls), the marketing strategy should be to sell sooner. The same is true for cattle with excessive external fat, such as the open cow that has lost her calf or missed being sold the previous year. In many areas, producers are paid less money for these animals than they receive for better-conditioned cattle. Depending on the price deduction incurred for these cattle, one option could be to hold fat cattle over on inexpensive feed until they have attained a more balanced condition.

Overall strategies and recommendations for marketing non-fed cattle include the following:

1. Prevent residues and injection-site lesions by ensuring responsible administration and withdrawal of all animal health products.

2. Effect meat product quality monitoring and managing of non-fed cattle by marketing them before they become too fat, too lean, too light, too heavy, too thinly muscled, or emaciated.

3. Reduce bruises by dehorning; by correcting deficiencies in facilities, transportation, and equipment; and improving handling.

4. Minimize condemnations by monitoring herd health and marketing non-fed cattle with physical disorders in a timely manner.

5. Decrease hide damage through strategic parasite control methods and use of new methods for owner identification of

non-fed cattle; use brand sites that minimize hide damage and discourage the use of multiple brands on one animal.

6. Enhance beef wholesomeness by encouraging practices that reduce bacterial contamination of carcasses.

7. Encourage on-farm euthanasia of disabled cattle and of those with advanced bovine ocular neoplasia.

Bovine practitioners are encouraged to join and/or direct efforts to enhance the quality of their clients' food products. Veterinarians may show the way in this endeavor by consistently reminding clients to observe drug and chemical withdrawal times, directing and/or encouraging discretionary use of drugs, advocating the use of sanitary injection techniques, and emphasizing recommended injection sites and dosage loads per site. Practitioners may also guide or take part in educating clients about the other industry quality concerns mentioned here and may encourage clients to participate in the effort to reduce the prevalence of quality defects in the animals they sell.

REFERENCES

1. National Cattleman's Association: Task Force Report, Beef Safety Assurance. National Cattleman's Association, Englewood, Colo, 1987.
2. Deming WE: Out of the Crisis. Cambridge, Mass, MIT Press, 1986.
3. Wilkes W: Quality Comes to America. Address to the Annual National Cattleman's Convention, 1991.
4. Dexter DR, Cowman JB, Morgan RP, et al: Incidence of injection-site blemishes in beef top-sirloin butt. J Anim Sci 72:824, 1994.
5. Grant E: The National Non-fed Beef Quality Audit. Englewood, Colo, Beef Promotion and Research Board, 1994.
6. Hentschl A, Green V, Hoffsis G, et al: Milk and Dairy Beef Residue Prevention Protocol. Stratford, Iowa, Agri-Education, 1991, pp 1–38.
7. Bodensteiner C: Fourth Annual Food Safety Survey, conducted by CMF&Z Public Relations, an affiliate of Young & Rubicam. July 1996.
8. Paige JC: Analysis of tissue residues. FDA Vet 11:9–12, 1996.
9. George MH, Ames RA, Glock RG, et al: Incidence, Severity, Amount of Tissue Affected and Effect on Histology, Chemistry and Tenderness of Injection-Site Lesions in Beef Cuts from Calves Administered a Control or One of Seven Compounds. In Report to the National Cattleman's Beef Association, Englewood, Colo, 1997.
10. George MH, Heinrich PE, Dexter DR, et al: Injection-site lesions in carcasses produced by cattle receiving injections at branding time. J Anim Sci 73:3510, 1995.
11. Paralysis after vaccination. DVM News, South Dakota State University Extension Service, Vol. 10, No. 4, July/Aug 1996.
12. Huston PL: Quality Assurance and Residue Avoidance in Midwest Feedlots. Proceedings of the 23rd Annual Convention of the American Association of Bovine Practitioners, Indianapolis, 1990.
13. Lambert C: Industry Facts: Beef Economics. In Beef Promotion and Research Board, Cattle and Beef Handbook. Englewood, Colo, 1996.

■ Management Programs for Developing Beef Bulls

Glenn H. Coulter, Ph.D., P.Ag.*
John P. Kastelic, D.V.M., Ph.D.*

Unlike the dairy breeder or feedlot operator, the beef breeder derives his or her entire income from calves born into the herd, making fertility unquestionably the most important trait to be considered in a breeding program. Economically, reproductive merit is five times more important to the cow-calf producer

*For the Department of Agriculture and Agri-Food, Government of Canada. © Minister of Publick Works and Government Services, Canada, 1998.

Table 1
GENETIC CORRELATIONS BETWEEN TESTICULAR MEASUREMENTS OF SIRE AND REPRODUCTIVE TRAITS IN FEMALE PROGENY

Female Traits	No. (%) of Favorable Correlations	Average Coefficient
Age at first breeding	24 (100)	− .77
Age at first calving	22 (92)	− .66
Pregnancy rate	22 (92)	.66

Adapted from Toelle VD, Robison OW: Estimates of genetic correlations between testicular measurements and female reproductive traits in cattle. J Anim Sci 60:89, 1985.

than growth performance and 10 times more important than product quality (e.g., carcass quality),[46] at least until value-based marketing becomes a reality. These figures refer to the relative importance of these traits for the beef herd in total. When discussing the bull component alone, an additional aspect must be incorporated into the model, that of the male-to-female ratio at breeding. Whether considering the 1:10,000+ ratio of the artificial insemination sire or the 1:25 to 1:40 ratio of the herd bull used for natural service, fertility is much more important in the bull than in any individual female. This is adequate justification for placing much greater emphasis on the fertility of our beef bulls.

Little to no selection pressure has been placed on the fertility of the world's beef bull population. Multiple-sire breeding, used routinely by commercial breeders, has made it difficult to identify subfertile sires. Estimates of the proportion of unselected beef bulls in North America that are deficient reproductively range from 20% to 40%. Many more are barely adequate. Some breeders in North America have become preoccupied with growth rates and frame scores when selecting bulls to the extent that the single most economically important trait, bull fertility, has been overshadowed and often forgotten. When selecting beef bulls, fertility must be given first priority.

GENETIC ASPECTS

Generally, the heritability of reproductive traits in cattle is considered to be low. However, this refers to measures of reproductive performance such as conception or calving rate. In fact, the heritability of reproductive traits known to influence fertility in the bull is relatively high. This is particularly true for anatomic traits such as the degree to which the sheath of a bull is attached to the abdomen, or the presence of a scrotal frenulum that tends to hold the posterior side of the scrotum high (almost horizontal in severe cases). The heritability of testicular size is moderate to high, with most estimates at approximately .5. Large variation in testicular size of bulls of the same age within a breed, coupled with the high heritability of the trait, provides considerable opportunity for improving the testicular size of bulls within a herd, or breed, through selection.

The greatest long-term benefits of using bulls with above-average testicular size may come from positive carryover effects to their female progeny. High negative genetic correlations ($r = −.71$ and $−1.07$, respectively) are found between testicular size in bulls and age at puberty in half-sib heifers or daughters.[7, 27] This implies that the use of a sire with above-average testicular size for his age and breed will result in female progeny that reach puberty at a younger age, cycle more regularly, and consequently have greater lifetime productivity. Results from a North Carolina study[45] (Table 1) not only confirm the findings of the two previous studies but indicate a high positive genetic correlation between bull testicular size and pregnancy rate of female progeny ($r = .66$). A 1-cm increase in a sire's scrotal circumference (SC) measurement is reported[43] to result in a $-.796$ day change in age at puberty, and a $-.826$ day change in age of first calving of female offspring. A phenotypic correlation coefficient of $r = .98$ has been reported between eight breed means for SC measurements of bulls and age at puberty of heifers.[31] These relationships suggest that SC measurements and puberty are essentially the same trait. Since puberty in females is favorably associated with subsequent reproduction,[47] selection for larger SC measurements should improve the reproductive potential of the cow herd.

Testicular consistency, as measured by the tonometer, is known to be associated with seminal quality and has a moderate heritability of about .34.[22] Some sperm abnormalities (e.g., knobbed acrosome defect[25] and the Dag defect[29]) have been reported to be inherited as recessive traits. Others are speculated to be the result of genetic deficiencies, but specific modes of inheritance have not as yet been identified.[3] Heritability estimates of seminal quality traits, such as progressive sperm motility and the proportion of spermatozoa with primary and secondary abnormalities in young beef bulls, have generally been inconsistent and low to moderate in size (range, $-.05$ to .44). Estimates of primary sperm abnormalities were most consistent, ranging from .30 to .44.[1, 26, 44] Heritability estimates of behavioral traits such as serving capacity or libido are generally higher at about .5 to .6.

Heritability estimates of growth performance traits such as rate of gain, weight per day of age, and the efficiency of feed conversion are moderate at about .4. Anatomic traits such as feet and leg conformation, which are extremely important to the longevity of the beef bull, are very high and easily influenced through selection. Similarly, carcass traits such as dressing percentage, rib eye area, and marbling are generally considered to be moderate to high.

Genetically, the best bulls in a herd from a reproductive, growth, and quality aspect should be the top yearlings. Maximal genetic progress can be made by use of these young beef bulls in a breeding program. Unfortunately, the difficulty comes as a result of these yearlings' not having any progeny or extensive records of performance. This necessitates a strong evaluation and selection program for young beef bulls. In contrast, the use of more mature beef bulls may be more predictable, but, less genetic progress will likely be made for all traits.

BULL MANAGEMENT

Beef bulls, used predominantly for natural service throughout the world, are exposed to a greater range of environmental and management factors than are dairy bulls. Most environmental or management practices that diminish the inherent quality of a bull's semen are mediated through either temperature-sensitive or hormonal mechanisms. Little is known about the basic mechanisms involved in the interaction between supporting Sertoli cells and dividing and differentiating germ cells. More is known about the effects of the environment and management practices on seminal quality in beef bulls. A general premise that applies is that the degree of injury to the testes is proportional to the severity and duration of the environmental or management-mediated insult. Exposure of the testes or epididymides to a minor but prolonged insult can often have a detrimental effect on seminal quality. Such an insult may not be easily identified.

Nutrition

Nutrition of the beef bull is one factor that may have prolonged effects. Diets adequate in protein, vitamins, minerals, and energy appear to hasten the onset of puberty in beef bulls. However, the feeding of high energy diets to postpubertal beef bulls is of no benefit to reproductive capacity, including seminal quality, and may result in substantial harm to reproductive potential. Feeding a medium level of dietary energy (limit-fed alfalfa-straw cubes, in a 70:30 ratio) to Hereford and Angus bulls from weaning (6 to 7 months of age) to 12 months of age[12] resulted in 52% greater total epididymal sperm reserves than for bulls fed a high energy diet (60% barley, 10% oats, 10% beet pulp, and 20% alfalfa-straw cubes). Similarly, Hereford and Angus bulls fed a medium energy diet from weaning to 15 months of age[13] had a 12% greater daily sperm production per gram of testicular parenchyma than bulls fed a high energy diet. Bulls in the medium energy diet groups, at 15 months of age, had 76% greater caput-corpus epididymal sperm reserves for Herefords in year 1, and 89% greater caput-corpus epididymal sperm reserves for both breeds in year 2, and 52% greater cauda epididymal sperm reserves than high energy diet bulls. Seminal quality was not assessed in this experiment.

Experiments were also conducted on Hereford and Angus bulls fed medium or high energy diets from weaning through 24 months of age.[18] In the first year, Hereford bulls fed the medium energy diet had 300% greater total epididymal sperm reserves than bulls fed the high energy diet. Angus bulls did not differ. In the second year, Hereford and Angus bulls fed the medium energy diet had 55% and 16% greater total epididymal sperm reserves than comparable groups of bulls fed the high energy diet. Seminal quality of bulls fed the high energy diet was inferior to that of bulls fed the medium energy diet, particularly with respect to progressive sperm motility and the incidence of spermatozoa in which a crater defect of the head was present.

In a study conducted in Kansas,[40] three different levels of dietary energy were fed to Hereford and Simmental bulls for a 200-day period followed by 10 days' adjustment to a roughage diet, 38 days on pasture, and then reproductive capacity was assessed. No effect of dietary energy was observed on seminal characteristics or serving capacity of either breed. However, it should be noted that although there was no significant effect of level of dietary energy, the proportion of progressively motile spermatozoa (29.2%), the incidence of morphologically abnormal spermatozoa (54.4%), and aged acrosomes (36.3%) in the Herefords suggest that all Hereford bulls may have been affected detrimentally by the diets fed. The mean backfat thickness for the three Hereford dietary groups (nine bulls each) were 6.1, 7.2, and 10.4 mm. The mean backfat thickness for Hereford and Angus yearling bulls of similar age fed medium and high energy diets in the Lethbridge Research Centre (Lethbridge, Alberta) study were 0.5 (n = 61) and 7.1 mm (n = 42), respectively (no breed differences were observed). Although seminal quality was not assessed in the Lethbridge study, clearly the medium energy diet fed was substantially lower in dietary energy than the lowest energy level fed in the Kansas study. This may account for the apparently conflicting results.

In a 3-year field study[19] of multiple-sire breeding under range conditions, 277 crossbred beef bulls were examined prior to the breeding season and the effects of physical soundness, testicular development, seminal quality, and both sexual and social behavior on fertility were determined. A regression model was developed that accounted for 29% of the total variance in fertility. One of the five traits making a contribution to the model was backfat thickness. The mean backfat thicknesses for 1-, 2-, and 3-year-old bulls were 1.6 (n = 116), 1.5 (n = 126), and 1.9 mm (n = 35), respectively (range, 0 to 7 mm). Even with these relatively low levels of backfat thickness, a negative relationship was observed between backfat thickness and beef bull fertility under multiple-sire, range-breeding conditions. As backfat increased, fertility declined. Most evidence indicates that feeding high energy diets to young beef bulls reduces sperm production, seminal quality, and ultimately bull fertility.

The exact mechanism by which the feeding of high energy diets affects seminal production and quality is not known. However, circumstantial evidence indicates the probable involvement of impaired thermoregulation, and possibly a stress-induced hormonal imbalance. It appears that the decreased fertility is due to the deposition of fat both within the scrotal tissue overlying the testes and epididymides, and fat deposited in the neck of the scrotum over the pampiniform plexus. Research by one of us (G.H.C., unpublished data) suggests that although the feeding of high vs. medium levels of dietary energy to young beef bulls has no effect on the amount of lipid present within testicular parenchyma, bulls fed the high energy diet had 34% more total scrotal lipid than bulls fed the medium energy diet (13.7 vs. 10.2 mg lipid per gram scrotal tissue). The correlation coefficient between total scrotal lipid and epididymal sperm reserves was −.26. The corresponding coefficient between backfat thickness and epididymal sperm reserves was −.38. As highly insulative lipid is deposited within the scrotal tissue, it may reduce the radiation of heat from the scrotal surface, thereby increasing testicular temperature. This may reduce sperm production and in some cases seminal quality. One study[14] indicates that yearling beef bulls fed high vs. moderate energy diets have a lower scrotal surface temperature gradient (3.4°C vs. 3.9°C) as measured by infrared thermography.

Deposition of lipid or fat in the neck of the scrotum immediately over the pampiniform plexus may have an even greater detrimental effect on normal scrotal-testicular thermoregulation. The pampiniform plexus is generally associated with testicular thermoregulation as a countercurrent heat exchange mechanism. However, in the normal bull it also facilitates the radiation of considerable heat energy from the surface of the neck of the scrotum. Deposition of fat within the neck of the scrotum, which is very common in beef bulls fed high energy diets, may dramatically impede if not virtually eliminate this component of the thermoregulatory mechanism.

An additional mechanism that may impair testicular function in bulls fed high energy diets is stress. Perhaps in obese bulls the stress from extra body weight and its effects on feet and legs may increase corticoid production that may suppress the production or release of gonadotropin-releasing hormone (GnRH). A lack of GnRH would prevent the release of luteinizing hormone (LH) which is essential to testosterone production from the Leydig cells. Very preliminary data comparing LH and testosterone levels in fat vs. thin bulls suggests that a hormonal mechanism may play a role in reduced fertility (G.H.C., unpublished data). Other stresses, such as the trucking of bulls over long distances, or the foreign environment of the show circuit, may also have a similar influence on the bull's endocrine system, thereby resulting in reduced seminal quality.

Other Environmental Factors

Other environmental factors that can have a detrimental effect on testicular function and seminal quality include scrotal frostbite, scrotal sunburn, severe attack of the scrotum by biting arthropods, severe dermatitis, and numerous diseases or infections that result in increased core body temperature. These conditions all result in increased scrotal-testicular temperature that cannot be compensated for through normal physiologic, thermoregulatory mechanisms. Some of these factors can be prevented or at least mitigated by proper management practices.

Infections in the bull, particularly those that are prolonged and that raise core body temperature, can have a detrimental effect on fertility. One common infection of beef bulls that has a two-pronged, negative effect on fertility is foot rot. Not only

does the bull have considerable physical difficulty in breeding estrous females but the elevated body temperature associated with the infection tends to result in reduced seminal quality and impaired fertility. If treated immediately, impaired seminal quality is generally short-lived, lasting only 1 to 2 weeks. Other conditions within the scrotum such as testicular tumor, abscesses, orchitis, and varicocele will have a more dramatic, prolonged effect on testicular temperature, as well as a more severe detrimental effect on seminal quality. These conditions may result in irreversible damage to the testicles and permanently impair seminal quality. If recovery occurs, it will likely be over months or possibly even years. Some cattlemen believe that antibiotics can have a detrimental effect on seminal quality. However, to our knowledge, there are no antibiotics currently licensed for use in cattle in North America that have such an effect.

BULL SELECTION FOR REPRODUCTION

From a reproductive perspective, limited selection can be made in weaned bull calves over and above the selection of the calf's parents. One trait that some selection pressure can be applied to in these calves is testicular size. It has been suggested[48] that beef bulls entering a 140-day growth performance test that have an SC measurement of less than 18 cm will have a high risk of ending the test with an SC measurement of 30 cm or less as yearlings. To have nearly 100% probability of ending a 140-day growth performance test with an SC measurement of 30 cm, it has been reported[39] that Angus, Simmental, and Zebu-derived bulls need an SC measurement of 23 cm at the beginning of a growth performance test, while continental breeds (other than Simmental) and polled Hereford bulls need an SC measurement of 26 cm. In our opinion, the reproductive capacity of beef bulls can only be assessed adequately following puberty, no sooner than 1 year, and preferably at 14 to 16 months of age.

BREEDING SOUNDNESS EVALUATION

Four aspects of a beef bull must be evaluated to determine its reproductive potential. These are (1) testicular and scrotal development; (2) ability to physically breed females; (3) seminal quality; and (4) bull reproductive behavior. All are of equal importance and all must be adequate before normal fertility can be expected. To conduct an effective breeding soundness evaluation it is essential to have good cattle working facilities that include a head gate and squeeze chute in an area approaching room temperature. An alternative is to transport beef bulls for evaluation to a veterinary clinic.

Testicular and Scrotal Development

The first activity that must be carried out in conducting an evaluation of testicular and scrotal development is a thorough palpation of scrotal contents to ensure that they are normal. First, one must make sure that the testes are not in any way adhered to the scrotum. The testes must be free and able to move unimpaired within the scrotum to facilitate thermoregulation. This can be checked by palpating the testes upward within the scrotum toward the abdominal wall. Adhesions between the testes and scrotum may result from physical injury, or moderate to severe scrotal frostbite. Testes should be uniform in size.

Any significant asymmetry in testicular size is an indication of potential problems.

Testes should be uniform in consistency, both between the testes, and from the dorsal to the ventral pole of each testis. Testicular consistency should be firm, but not hard. The normal testis is a resilient organ, which, when compressed and released, will spring back to its original form. Testes should be neither mushy, nor feel as if they are soft on the surface and have a hard core. Both hard and soft spots on a testis should be noted. Soft testicular consistency is indicative of testicular degeneration and is often related to reduced sperm production, poor seminal quality, and subfertility or sterility.[42] Testicular consistency as measured by a tonometer[23] has been demonstrated to be correlated with the proportion of normal spermatozoa (r = .61 to .74), motility of spermatozoa after ampule freezing (r = .64 to .95), and fertility (60- to 90-day nonreturn to estrus; r = .67) in Holstein bulls of different ages.[24] Similar relationships would be expected in beef bulls.

Orientation of the testes within the scrotum may also be important, although there are limited data to establish whether aberrant orientations cause fertility problems, or are merely a blemish. Two such abnormal orientations are one testicle being held higher than the other, and the rotation of one or both testes to different degrees around their long axes. If one testis is held slightly higher than the other, few problems would be expected. However, if one testis is held quite high, this testis may not be able to move adequately within the scrotum to permit normal thermoregulation. Rotation of one or both testes around their long axes is reasonably common. The normal orientation is for the body (corpus) and the tail (cauda) of the epididymis of each testis to be adjacent to each other in the middle of the scrotum. One or both testes may rotate up to 180 degrees or more. The significance of this rotation is not clear. The concern is that a severe rotation could cause a torsion of the vascular cone that may influence normal blood flow to the testes, thereby impairing thermoregulation. Because of the lack of data as to how these conditions affect fertility, a clear recommendation cannot be made. At the least, the condition should be considered an undesirable blemish.

In addition to the testes, the epididymides of both testes should be palpated to ensure that they are normal. The head (caput) of the epididymis varies as to its prominence as it covers the dorsal pole of the testis. Any asymmetry, or lumps, within the caput epididymides should be noted. The body (corpus) of each epididymis should be palpated to ensure that it is present and that no obvious abnormalities are present. This can be accomplished by palpating each testis to the top of the scrotum while palpating the corpus on the contralateral testis. The cauda epididymis is the site of most epididymal problems. Normal cauda epididymides vary considerably as to the tightness of their attachment to the testes. In some cases they will seem almost detached from the testes, while in others they will be so tightly attached that considerable care must be taken to be sure that they are actually present. The cauda epididymis should be firm in consistency, but not hard. A hard, or hard and enlarged cauda, is indicative of epididymitis. In some cases, one cauda will feel normal, while the other is very small, flaccid, tightly attached, and difficult to palpate. This may be the result of a segmental aplasia of the epididymis that usually occurs in the corpus. This condition prohibits any spermatozoa produced within that testis to reach the exterior, making the bull functionally a one-testicle bull. Obviously, such an individual should be culled. The condition is generally unilateral and can occur on either side. It has been our experience that the testis with the affected epididymis will eventually degenerate, becoming very soft and flaccid. Infrared thermography can be used effectively to assist in the diagnosis of this condition.

Testicular size or the amount of sperm-producing tissue is estimated through the use of the SC measurement. The SC measurement can be used to predict accurately the amount of potential sperm-producing tissue within the testes. Regression and correlation coefficients calculated between SC measurements and paired testes weight range from r = .91 through r = .98 for young beef bulls.[16, 36, 41] Therefore, the larger the SC measurement, the greater the potential sperm production.

The technique recommended for taking SC measurements is that of the Society for Theriogenology.[2] A consistent SC measurement technique is essential if comparisons are to be made among bulls for selection purposes or if minimum standards are applied as an eligibility criterion for bull growth performance test stations or shows. The testes are palpated firmly into the lower part of the scrotum so that they are side by side and scrotal wrinkles that might inflate the measurement are eliminated. Second, the thumb and fingers of one hand are placed on the sides of the scrotum cradling the testes rather than grasping either the front and back or neck of the scrotum. The latter two techniques of stabilizing the testes and scrotum introduce error. Third, the looped scrotal tape is slipped up over the testes-scrotum and contracted around the largest circumference. Moderate tension is placed on a sliding tape with the thumb until moderate resistance is provided by the testes-scrotum. Little compression of the testes-scrotum will occur in bulls with normal testes, while in bulls having a thick, fat scrotum or soft testes, compression may be substantial. Finally, the circumference is read. Once a reading is taken, the procedure is repeated to confirm the result.

The largest source of variation among operators taking SC measurements is the amount of tension placed on the conventional SC measuring tape prior to taking a reading. "Moderate tension" is interpreted differently by different operators. A new SC measuring tape (Coulter Scrotal Tape) is now available that minimizes this source of error. It has a spring that places exactly the same amount of tension on the measurement tape every time an SC measurement is taken, regardless of the operator.

The tape is applied in a similar fashion to conventional SC measuring tapes. The major difference is that while the testes-scrotum is being steadied by the operator's other hand, the button is released, and the tape is allowed to be pulled slowly and gently toward the posterior of the scrotum by the constant tension spring. When the tape comes to rest, the reading is taken. Caution must be exercised not to snap the tape, which will introduce error into the measurement and may cause discomfort to the bull. The tape is again fixed with the button and slid off the bottom of the scrotum. The measurement should then be repeated to ensure consistency.

A consistent SC measurement technique is essential if comparisons are to be made among bulls for selection purposes, or if minimum standards are applied as an eligibility criterion for bull growth performance test stations or shows.

Effects of Age on Scrotal Circumference

Bull age is the factor that has the greatest effect on testicular development in young bulls from 6 through 36 months of age. Young bulls (6 through 16 months of age) exhibit very rapid testicular growth and there is a tremendous range in testes size in bulls of the same age within a breed.[20] Paired testes weight in bulls of the same age may vary by as much as 550 g. This amount of testicular tissue represents a potential sperm production of over 8 billion spermatozoa per day. This pattern of testicular development is similar for all breeds.

Age Adjustment of Scrotal Circumference

Age adjustment factors for SC measurements in yearling beef bulls have been derived from 3409 measurements of SC taken

Table 2
AGE OF DAM ADJUSTMENT FACTORS FOR YEARLING BEEF BULLS (*BOS TAURUS*)

Age of Dam (yr)	Adjustment Factor (cm)
≥5	+0.0
4	+0.4
3	+0.8
2	+1.3

Adapted from Lunstra DD, Gregory KE, Cundiff LV: Heritability estimates and adjustment factors for effect of bull age and age of dam on yearling testicular size in breeds of bulls. Theriogenology 30:127, 1988.

on Aberdeen Angus, Blond D'Aquitaine, Charolais, Hereford (horned and polled), Limousin, Maine Anjou, Shorthorn, and Simmental bulls upon completion of their 140-day growth performance tests in western Canada (G.H.C., unpublished data). The SC-age relationship was examined as a linear function and the resulting adjustment coefficient was 0.028 cm/day of age. Large variation in testicular size of bulls of the same age within a breed, coupled with the high heritability of the trait, provides considerable opportunity to improve the testicular size of bulls within a herd or breed through selection.

SC measurements have been adjusted both on an age and body weight basis. SC measurement is a more accurate predictor for establishing when a bull reaches puberty than either age or body weight regardless of breed or breed cross.[34] Therefore, SC measurement in yearling beef bulls is essentially a measure of age at puberty. If the primary reason for adjusting SC measurements is to increase the accuracy of selection for age at puberty in bulls and the correlated response in age at puberty in heifers, then adjustment for age, not weight, would seem appropriate. Furthermore, body weight is not purely an environmental effect as it is influenced by genetics.[6] Published age adjustment factors for SC measurements taken upon completion of growth performance tests as yearlings range from .024 to .026 cm/day for Hereford bulls,[6, 30] .028 to .032 cm/day for nine (G.H.C., unpublished data) and twelve[35] Bos taurus breeds, and .041 cm/day for Brangus bulls.[30] Hereford bulls fed high energy diets during growth performance testing require a higher adjustment factor of .032 cm/day.[6] All adjustment factors are in relatively close agreement.

Age of Dam Adjustment of Scrotal Circumference

Several reports[6, 30, 35] have recommended age of dam adjustment factors for SC measurements of yearling beef bulls. Although some differences occur among the studies as to the magnitude of the adjustment factor for a particular age of dam,

there is general agreement that the SC measurement of bulls from 2-year-old dams requires the greatest upward adjustment, followed by bulls from 3- and 4-year-old dams. Adjustment factors from one study based on 12 breeds[35] are shown in Table 2. These age-of-dam effects may be the result of differences in calf body weight. Age-of-dam adjustment should be added to the SC measurement only after the SC measurement has been adjusted to 365 days of age.

Recommended Minimum Scrotal Circumference

Recommended minimum SC measurements[21] by age are outlined in Table 3. These minimums fall within the guidelines of the Society for Theriogenology. Cattlemen selecting herd sires should seriously consider selecting bulls having SC measurements substantially greater than the minimums listed. The objective should be to select superior bulls, not those barely adequate. Bulls having an SC measurement less than these minimums may on occasion produce an acceptable semen sample. However, such bulls have limited sperm-producing capacity and would be expected to be of unsatisfactory fertility under moderate to heavy breeding pressure.

Breed Effects on Scrotal Circumference

Bull breed also influences testicular development.[21] Table 4 shows the effect of breed on SC for yearling bulls measured on completion of a 140-day, growth performance test and for 2-year-old bulls presented for sale at spring show-sales.[21] SC increases from 2 to 3 cm between 1 and 2 years of age for most breeds. The difference in SC between yearlings of the extreme breeds (Simmental and Limousin) is 5.7 cm. This represents about 194 g of testicular tissue or the potential to produce an additional 2.9 billion spermatozoa per day. This example illustrates the effect breed can have on testicular size and consequently sperm production.

Effects of Growth Rate on Scrotal Circumference

Genetic correlations between SC measurements and growth traits in young bulls are favorable. Correlations between SC measurements and birth weights are negative to low[6, 30, 44] ($r = -.04$ to .18), indicating that bulls with larger SC measurements can be selected without substantially increasing birth weights and subsequent calving difficulty. Both weaning weights ($r = .00$ to .86) and yearling weights ($r = .10$ to .68) have low to high correlations with SC measurements.[6, 28, 30, 37, 44] Yearling height was also positively correlated ($r = .36$ to .40) with SC

Table 3
MINIMUM SCROTAL CIRCUMFERENCE (CM)

Age (mo)	Simmental, Gelbvieh	Angus, Charolais, Maine Anjou	Hereford, Shorthorn	Limousin, Blond D'Aquitaine, Salers
12–14	33	32	31	30
15–20	35	34	33	32
21–30	36	35	34	33
>30	37	36	35	34

Adapted from Coulter GH, Mapletoft RJ, Kozub GC, et al: Scrotal circumference of two-year-old bulls of several beef breeds. Theriogenology 27:485, 1987.

Table 4

EFFECT OF BREED ON SCROTAL CIRCUMFERENCE (CM) OF BEEF BULLS: COMPARISON OF 1- VS. 2-YEAR-OLDS

Breed	1-Year-Olds		2-Year-Olds	
	No. of Bulls	Scrotal Circumference ± SE	No. of Bulls	Scrotal Circumference ± SE
Simmental	401	36.0 ± 0.2	543	38.7 ± 0.1
Aberdeen Angus	260	33.9 ± 0.1	630	37.2 ± 0.1
Maine Anjou	311	33.7 ± 0.2	—	—
Charolais	607	33.1 ± 0.1	506	36.3 ± 0.1
Hereford (horned)	614	32.9 ± 0.1	3769	36.1 ± 0.0
Shorthorn	147	32.5 ± 0.2	233	34.9 ± 0.1
Hereford (polled)	332	32.3 ± 0.2	2174	35.6 ± 0.1
Blond D'Aquitaine	115	30.7 ± 0.5	—	—
Salers	255	30.4 ± 0.2	—	—
Limousin	276	30.3 ± 0.3	80	32.1 ± 0.3

Adapted from Coulter GH, Mapletoft RJ, Kozub GL, et al: Scrotal circumference of two-year-old bulls of several beef breeds. Theriogenology 27:485, 1987.

measurements.[6, 30] However, a moderate negative correlation has been noted between maternal weaning weight and direct yearling height[17] ($r = .-34$), suggesting that selection of bulls superior in height may diminish the maternal ability of their daughters. Positive genetic correlations between direct effects for weaning weight and maternal effects for SC measurements and maternal effects for weaning weight and direct effects for SC measurements (.21 and .20) suggest that selecting bulls with larger SCs will not decrease, but may enhance, the maternal value of a bull.[30] It appears that selecting bulls with larger SC measurements will not decrease, and may enhance, growth performance.

The relationship between body growth rate during 140-day growth performance tests and testicular development at 1 year of age was examined in 1770 bulls of six breeds.[17] SC appeared to be moderately correlated with body weight in young beef bulls even when age was held constant. Growth rate, as measured by average daily gain (over the 140-day test), or weight per day of age (WPDA), was not positively correlated with SC. Results emphasize the need for independent evaluation of reproductive potential and growth potential in young beef bulls. Emphasis on one trait will not ensure a positive response in the other.

Experiments conducted at North Carolina State University[45] suggest that testicular size is controlled by different physiologic systems at about 6 months of age (weaning) and as yearlings. At weaning, testicular size is a reflection of general body size or weight. Between weaning and 1 year of age, the testes come under the influence of gonadotropic hormones. By 1 year of age, differences in testicular size are believed to depend more on the prevailing hormonal system than on differences in body weight. Therefore, the selection of the heaviest calves at weaning may not provide adequate testicular size by breeding age.

Effects of Scrotal Circumference on Seminal Quality

The probability of a beef bull having satisfactory seminal quality increases dramatically as SC measurements increase until an SC measurement of about 38 cm is attained.[8] For example, of the 155 bulls having an SC measurement of 32 cm, only 23% were considered to be satisfactory in that size group (Fig. 1). In contrast, 88% of the 136 bulls with an SC measurement of 38 cm were classified as satisfactory. Seminal quality improved little above 38 cm of SC.

Potential Effects of Conformation on Scrotal Circumference

Another aspect of beef bull selection worth consideration is the selection of bulls having a very "extreme" conformation. In our opinion, the reproductive capacity of these bulls should be given particular attention. This type of bull, on average, tends to reach sexual maturity slower than a bull with more conventional conformation. Recent research results suggest that the female progeny of these bulls will likely have a similar tendency. If breeders select an "extreme" or "steerlike" conformation, they should be particularly careful not to inadvertently select a "steerlike" hormonal system.

Relationship Between Scrotal Circumference and Bull Fertility

Results from a field trial indicate that as SC measurements increased in young beef bulls used for multiple-sire, natural

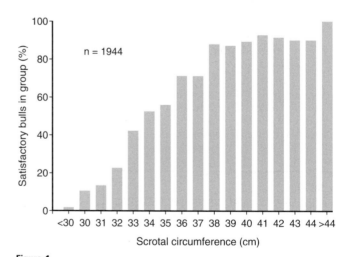

Figure 1

Proportion of bulls having satisfactory seminal quality in each scrotal circumference size group. (Adapted from Cates WF: Observations on scrotal circumference and its relationship to classification of bulls. In Proceedings of the Annual Meeting of the Society of Theriogenology, Cheyenne, Wyo, 1995, p 9.)

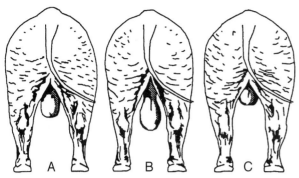

Figure 2

Three scrotal shapes commonly seen in beef bulls are the straight-sided scrotum *(A)*, the normal scrotum *(B)*, and the wedge-shaped scrotum *(C)*. Scrotal shapes *A* and *C* are the least desirable. (Adapted from Cates WF: Observations on scrotal circumference and its relationship to classification of bulls. *In* Proceedings of the Annual meeting of the Society of Theriogenology, Cheyenne, Wyo, 1995, p 9.)

service under range conditions, fertility also increased.[19] SC made a highly significant, positive contribution to the predictive model. It should be emphasized that, in this field trial bull age and SC measurements were confounded. In general, as bull age increased, so did SC. The precise effects of these two traits on bull fertility cannot be separated. A note of caution should be expressed here. Although expected bull fertility increases with testicular size as measured by SC, the effect of selection of bulls with extreme SC on their fertility and that of their progeny is unknown. For example, little benefit may be realized in the selection of 2-year-old bulls with an SC measurement greater than 40 or 42 cm. This suggested upper limit to SC measurement may vary with breed.

Scrotal Shape

Scrotal shape also has an influence on testicular development and function.[8] There are three basic scrotal shapes in beef bulls. These are (1) the "normal" or "bottle-shaped" scrotum, (2) the "straight-sided" scrotum, and (3) the "wedge-shaped" scrotum. Bulls having a normal scrotum with a distinct neck (Fig. 2, bull B) generally have the best testicular development. Testes are located in the scrotum as spermatogenesis only occurs within a narrow temperature range several degrees cooler than core body temperature. The testes move closer to, or away from, the body wall to compensate for environmental temperature. The normal scrotal configuration permits adequate temperature compensation. Often the testes of bulls with straight-sided scrota (see Fig. 2, bull A) are only moderate in size. The straight-sided neck of the scrotum is generally the result of fat deposits which may impair proper thermoregulation. As bulls mature and lose condition, they will often develop a more normal scrotum. Wedge-shaped scrota (see Fig. 2, bull C) are pointed toward the bottom and tend to hold the testes close to the body wall. Bulls with this scrotal configuration have undersized testes that seldom produce seminal of adequate quality. Bulls with wedge-shaped scrota should be avoided.

Ability to Physically Breed Females

There are numerous anatomic deficiencies and defects that can prevent or impair a bull from effectively breeding females. Good feet and legs are essential if a bull is to travel over extensive, rough terrain. Eyesight must be good to assist in the

identification of estrous females. To discuss all potential anatomic abnormalities and breeding problems is not possible here. Instead, the dramatic effect one such defect can have on herd fertility will be illustrated. The defect is the spiral deviation of the penis. This defect has received almost no consideration in the evaluation of reproductive potential of North American beef bulls. Australian researchers[5] indicate that bulls in 60% of herds examined were affected and that 1% of horned bulls and 16% of polled bulls had the defect. There is no reason to believe the prevalence of the spiral penile deviation would be any less in North America. Spiral penile deviations are most often found in bulls 3 to 6 years of age. The detrimental effect of this defect on fertility is shown by the mating trial summarized in Table 5. The spiral penile deviation cannot be diagnosed at the time of electroejaculation. In fact, electroejaculation can induce a similar penile configuration that may not occur at all during natural service. Cattlemen must watch the breeding activity of their bulls to ensure the absence of this defect.

Seminal Quality

Semen-testing of young beef bulls (11 to 13 months of age) should be exercised with caution. Seminal quality in young bulls has been demonstrated to improve, often dramatically, for up to 16 weeks following puberty.[33] Puberty will occur at different ages and body weights depending on the breed, management, and genotype of the individual bull. Puberty is often defined as the first time a bull produces an ejaculate with at least 50×10^6 spermatozoa per milliliter with at least 10% progressively motile spermatozoa. An SC measurement of 26.1 cm at puberty is relatively constant among breeds differing widely in age and weight at puberty.[34] Cattlemen should be advised to semen-test their young bulls at 14 to 16 months of age to avoid the potential early culling of a bull that may have adequate seminal quality 2 months later.

Two often overlooked aspects of semen evaluation of beef bulls that must be given attention by the veterinarian are (1) the quality, adjustment, and cleanliness of microscopes used for the evaluation, and (2) maintaining the appropriate temperature for all surfaces that semen comes in contact with while conducting an evaluation. Microscopes used for seminal evaluation must be of adequate quality, have sufficient power (oil immersion objective for morphologic examination), and maintained in an appropriate manner to ensure an accurate evaluation. Similarly, sufficient care should be taken to prevent the temperature-shocking of the seminal sample, particularly in cool to cold climates. When the weather is cool, it is critical to use a water jacket containing warm water that surrounds the collection vessel. Transfer pipettes, slides, and the microscope stage should be warm enough to prevent the effects of cold shock on sperm

Table 5
SPIRAL PENILE DEVIATION IN AUSTRALIAN BEEF BULLS: MATING TRIALS

Bull No.	Mounts Affected (%)	Females Exposed	Pregnancy (%)
1	100	26	3
2	100	60	3
3	80	30	33
4	50	54	43
5	0 (normal)	58	87

Adapted from Blockey MA de B, Taylor EG: Observation on spiral deviation of the penis in beef bulls. Aust Vet J 61:141, 1984.

motility. Under cold conditions, serious consideration must be given to moving bulls to the practitioner's facilities.

Prior to electroejaculation, fecal material should be removed from the rectum. This provides an opportunity to conduct a rectal examination of the bull's internal organs. A common problem in young beef bulls that can be diagnosed at this time is seminal vesiculitis. Vesiculitis results in the seminal vesicles becoming enlarged, sometimes two to three times their normal size, and quite turgid to the touch. In severe cases, palpation of the infected seminal vesicles may be quite painful to the bull. Some controversy exists as to whether treatment is effective or whether the condition will correct itself in time. Generally, bulls with severe seminal vesiculitis cannot be recommended for use. Seminal vesiculitis can also be detected by the presence of white blood cells in the ejaculate.

The two most important factors to be examined in the semen are the proportion of motile spermatozoa and their morphology. In the field trial referred to earlier,[19] bull fertility decreased significantly as the number of spermatozoa with primary defects increased. In this trial, neither the number of secondary defects nor the proportion of normal acrosomes contributed significantly to the variance in bull fertility. A third factor, the concentration of spermatozoa in an ejaculate is difficult to assess when the seminal sample is collected by electroejaculation.

Protrusion of the penis during electroejaculation also provides an opportunity to check the bull for conditions such as a retained frenulum, penile warts, and hair rings. Retention of the penile frenulum is usually an indication of immaturity in a bull. The separation of the penis from the prepuce is a normal process that occurs with age. In some cases separation is incomplete. Many practitioners simply cut the frenulum, but this practice should be reconsidered as it may result in the inadvertent selection of slower-maturing bulls.

Penile warts are more common and seem to have a greater prevalence when young beef bulls are maintained together in a group. If the warts are narrow-based, they can usually be simply cut off. Care must be taken, however, because considerable hemorrhaging may occur. Bulls having untreated penile warts should not be used for natural service as this will usually result in a painful experience for the bull which may reduce or stop sexual activity.

Penile hair rings are another problem often seen in group-housed bulls. It has been suggested that hair rings result from bulls riding each other. Attention to the presence of a hair ring is important as the ring may constrict the penis and in severe cases has been known to amputate the end of the penis. Usually the hair ring can be simply slid off the penis.

Positive results from a seminal evaluation, even in yearling bulls, indicate a moderate to high probability of acceptable fertility, while negative results are not conclusive, particularly if the bulls involved are young or sexually rested. Subsequent evaluations of bulls with poor seminal quality should be carried out at 3- to 4-week intervals. If the results do not improve, the breeder can be fairly sure that the bull is infertile and should be culled. Seminal evaluations need to be conducted as close to the breeding season as possible. However, the breeder must allow enough time to retest bulls if necessary. All bulls should be tested before every breeding season, as injuries, frostbite, or other problems may have reduced the bull's seminal quality since the previous evaluation.

Bull Reproductive Behavior

In our opinion, this aspect of bull evaluation is in its infancy, but at least one comprehensive review is available.[9] The use of restrained heifers or cows that may or may not be in estrus raises ethical and animal welfare issues that need to be discussed

Table 6
RELATIONSHIP BETWEEN A BULL'S SERVING CAPACITY AND HERD FERTILITY*

Serving Capacity	First Estrus Conception Rate (%)	Pregnancy Rate (%)
0–2	4–40	4–67
3–5	55–68	89–93
6–11	62–78	90–100

*Twenty-three bulls were exposed to 35 to 40 heifers for 10 weeks.
Adapted from Blockey MA de B: Serving capacity and social dominance of bulls in relation to fertility. In Proceedings of the First World Congress on Applied Animal Ethology, Madrid, 1978, p 523.

with the client. To date, much of the research on sexual behavior of beef bulls used for natural service has been conducted in Australia. Early research indicated value in measuring behavioral traits in beef bulls[4] (Table 6). This study examined the relationship between the number of services in a 40-minute yard test and field fertility. Although there was no substantial difference in fertility between bull groups of high and medium serving capacity, there was a significant reduction in fertility in the low serving capacity group.

A more recent study by scientists at Clay Center, Nebraska,[32] tested libido and fertility in eight Hereford bulls at 16 and 40 months of age. At each age, bulls were libido-tested six times during a 21-day period by exposure to restrained, ovariectomized, estrus-induced females (30 minutes per test). As yearlings, four bulls exhibited high libido and four bulls exhibited low libido. Each bull was fertility-tested by exposure to 50 cycling females for 21 days. The results are summarized in Table 7. Not only did the high libido bulls have more services than the low libido bulls, but the pregnancy rate was also superior. This was true both in the yearling bulls and after the same bulls matured, although the differences were more pronounced in the young bulls. The higher fertility rate of the mature bulls compared to the same bulls as yearlings should also be noted.

Both studies described here showed improved fertility of medium to high libido or serving capacity bulls compared to those with low libido or serving capacity. Both of these studies used single-sire matings to determine fertility. Results from the Lethbridge field trial[19] that examined behavioral factors that might be important to bull fertility for multiple-sire breeding under range conditions indicated that two traits contributed significantly to the variance in bull fertility. As the total number of mounts counted in two 20-minute exposures to cull females on different days increased in excess of that required to service the

Table 7
CHANGES IN LIBIDO-FERTILITY RELATIONSHIPS

Bull Age (mo)	No. Services/Libido Test		Pregnancy Rate (%)	
	High Libido	Low Libido	High Libido	Low Libido
Yearling (16)	3.9	0.3	58	15
Mature (40)	3.5	1.6	74	58

Within traits $P < 0.5$ in mature bulls; $P < .01$ in yearlings.
Adapted from Lunstra DD: Changes in libido-fertility relationships as beef bulls mature. J Anim Sci 59 (suppl 1):351, 1984.

test females, bull fertility decreased. Mounting behavior in the testing situation not associated with the servicing of females may be indicative of a lack of experience, physical inability to breed (possible feet and leg or spinal problems), or other deficiencies which are later reflected in reduced fertility. In contrast to mounting behavior, increased numbers of services was indicative of higher fertility, but only to a degree, at which point fertility then began to decline. Both a low number of services and a very high number of services were associated with poor fertility. Low numbers, or no services, during testing is likely predictive of low breeding activity under field conditions. Very high serving activity may have resulted in sperm reserve depletion through the servicing of some females many times, reducing the probability of conception for others. Bulls servicing females an intermediate number of times during the prebreeding season test had the best fertility in the field. Other sexual behavior traits measured, as well as social dominance order, did not make a significant contribution to the variance in bull fertility in this trial.

Research results from both Australia and Lethbridge indicate that the mixing of bulls of different ages (e.g., yearlings with 2-year-olds or 3-year-olds) may reduce the number of progeny from the younger bulls and may reduce overall herd fertility. Body weight and age are two factors that have a substantial influence on social dominance order. More information is needed to sort out the importance of, and relationships among, behavioral traits.

The single most important aspect of reproductive behavior of beef bulls that must be impressed upon the cattleman is that they must carefully monitor the breeding activity of their bulls. The fact that a bull is mounting estrous females does not necessarily mean that they are being bred. Cattlemen must recognize the differences between mounting, copulation, and ejaculation. Many do not know the difference, nor do they pay adequate attention. Only careful observation will allow defects such as spiral penile deviations to be detected. Use of a comprehensive evaluation and selection program for reproductive potential in young beef bulls, coupled with optimal management, will increase the probability that highly fertile sires will be available for natural service in a beef breeding program.

NEW EVALUATION TECHNOLOGIES

Infrared Thermography

Infrared thermography (IRT) is a relatively new, noninvasive, radiologic technique that provides a pictorial image of a viewed object's infrared emissions. To obtain a pictorial image (thermogram), a scanner converts electromagnetic energy (heat) radiated from an object into electronic video signals. These signals are amplified and displayed as a gray-level image on a screen. Abnormalities are recognized by analysis of the thermograms and identification of areas of increased or decreased object surface temperature from the norm. The presence of pathologic abnormalities may be associated with thermal abnormalities of either increased or decreased skin temperature, providing the basis for diagnosis.

Maintenance of a specific temperature range within the testes of the bull is essential for normal sperm production. Adverse effects of elevated testicular temperature on sperm production, seminal quality, and subsequent male fertility are well documented. For this reason, the ability to monitor scrotal-testicular temperature would be expected to contribute to our understanding of, and ability to evaluate, scrotal-testicular function. Purohit and co-workers[38] conducted a study establishing the normal thermographic pattern of the bull scrotum and its contents, and compared some clinical conditions for diagnostic differentiation of scrotal and testicular diseases. In the normal thermogram of a bull, a temperature gradient of 4 to 6°C occurs from the base to the apex of the scrotum with a constant, symmetrical thermal pattern. In pathologic conditions, lack of symmetry has been observed in cases of unilateral lesions.

Inflammation of one testis increased ipsilateral scrotal infrared emission temperature by 2.5 to 3.0°C above the contralateral side. If both testes had inflammation and hyperemia, then an overall increase in scrotal temperature of at least 3°C was shown, along with a 2 to 3°C reduction in temperature gradient. Further, it has been reported[10] that sperm defects increased and progressive sperm motility decreased in the bull as the scrotal surface temperature gradient decreased.

Ultrasonography

Ultrasonography, using a real-time linear ultrasound scanning method, can be used to visualize the composition and orientation of organs within the scrotum of the bull. Results of experiments conducted at Lethbridge[11] indicate that the use of ultrasonography as a diagnostic tool in the beef bull has no discernible effects on either sperm production or seminal quality. This technology has been used to demonstrate some types of testicular pathologic conditions in situ. Ultrasonography has detected mineralized inclusions within the testicular parenchyma that displace normal sperm production and impede sperm transport (G.H.C., unpublished data). Further, ultrasonography permits the observation and measurement of blood vessel diameter in the neck of the scrotum. Enlarged vessels may alter blood flow that will disturb sensitive testicular thermoregulation mechanisms, similar to varicocele in the human.

SUMMARY

Proper development of the young beef bull is critical to the profitability of the cow-calf enterprise. Management and selection of bulls to optimize their reproductive potential is essential to maximize productivity. Generally, little selection pressure has been placed on reproductive traits of our beef bull population. Although the heritability of herd fertility is usually considered to be low, traits associated with reproductive capacity in the beef bull generally have a moderate to high heritability. Bulls exposed to suboptimal environmental conditions and management practices are likely to not achieve their inherent reproductive potential. The extent of the reduction in reproductive potential is usually directly proportional to the severity and duration of the environmental insult.

The four aspects of a beef bull that must be evaluated to determine reproductive potential are (1) testicular and scrotal development; (2) ability to physically breed females; (3) seminal quality; and (4) bull reproductive behavior. All are of equal importance and all must be adequate before normal fertility can be expected. New techniques that show promise in assisting in the evaluation of reproductive capacity are infrared thermography and ultrasonography of the scrotum and its contents. Strive for fertility first.

REFERENCES

1. Abadia D, Brinks JS, Carroll EJ: Genetics of seminal traits in young beef bulls. Proc West Sect Am Soc Anim Sci 27:30, 1976.
2. Ball L, Ott RS, Mortimer RG, et al: Manual for breeding soundness examination of bulls. J Soc Theriogenol 12:1–65, 1983.
3. Barth AO, Oko RJ: Abnormal Morphology of Bovine Spermatozoa. Ames, Iowa State University Press, 1989.

4. Blockey MA de B: Serving capacity and social dominance of bulls in relation to fertility. *In* Proceedings of the First World Congress on Applied Animal Ethology, Madrid, 1978, p 523.

5. Blockey MA de B, Taylor EG: Observation on spiral deviation of the penis in beef bulls. Aust Vet J 61:141, 1984.

6. Bourdon RM, Brinks JS: Scrotal circumference in yearling Hereford bulls: Adjustment factors, heritabilities and genetic, environmental and phenotypic relationships with growth traits. J Anim Sci 62:958, 1985.

7. Brinks JS, McInerney MJ, Chenoweth PJ: Relationship of age at puberty in heifers to reproductive traits in young bulls. Proc West Sect Am Soc Anim Sci 29:28, 1978.

8. Cates WF: Observations on scrotal circumference and its relationship to classification of bulls. *In* Proceedings of the Annual Meeting of the Society of Theriogenology, Cheyenne, Wyo, 1975, p 9.

9. Chenoweth PJ: Libido testing. *In* Morrow DA (ed): Current Therapy in Theriogenology 2, Philadelphia, WB Saunders, 1986, pp 136–142.

10. Coulter GH: Thermography of bull testes. *In* Proceedings of the 12th Technical Conference on Artificial Insemination and Reproduction, National Association of Animal Breeders, Milwaukee, 1988, p 58.

11. Coulter GH, Bailey DRC: Effects of ultrasonography on the bovine testis and semen quality. Theriogenology 30:743, 1988.

12. Coulter GH, Bailey DRC: Epididymal sperm reserves in 12-month-old Angus and Hereford bulls: Effects of bull strain plus dietary energy. Anim Reprod Sci 16:169, 1988.

13. Coulter GH, Carruthers TD, Amann RP, et al: Testicular development, daily sperm production and epididymal sperm reserves in 15-month-old Angus and Hereford bulls: Effects of bull strain plus dietary energy. J Anim Sci 64:254, 1987.

14. Coulter GH, Cook RB, Kastelic JP: Effects of dietary energy on scrotal surface temperature, seminal quality, and sperm production in young beef bulls. J Anim Sci 75:1048, 1997.

15. Coulter GH, Foote RH: Bovine testicular measurements as indicators of reproductive performance and their relationship to productive traits in cattle: A review. Theriogenology 11:297, 1979.

16. Coulter GH, Keller DG: Scrotal circumference of young beef bulls: Relationship to paired-testes weight, effect of breed, and predictability. Can J Anim Sci 62:133, 1982.

17. Coulter GH, Kozub GC: Relationship between testicular size and body growth rate in yearling beef bulls. *In* Proceedings of the American and Canadian Societies for Animal Science, 1982, p 345.

18. Coulter GH, Kozub GC: Testicular development, epididymal sperm reserves and seminal quality in two-year-old Hereford and Angus bulls: Effects of two levels of dietary energy. J Anim Sci 59:432, 1984.

19. Coulter GH, Kozub GC: Efficacy of methods used to test fertility of beef bulls used for multiple-sire breeding under range conditions. J Anim Sci 67:1757, 1989.

20. Coulter GH, Larson LL, Foote RH: Effect of age on testicular growth and consistency of Holstein and Angus bulls. J Anim Sci 41:1383, 1975.

21. Coulter GH, Mapletoft RJ, Kozub GC, et al: Scrotal circumference of two-year-old bulls of several beef breeds. Theriogenology 27:485, 1987.

22. Coulter GH, Rounsaville TR, and Foote RH: Heritability of testicular size and consistency in Holstein bulls. J Anim Sci 43:9, 1976.

23. Hahn J, Foote RH, Cranch ET: Tonometer for measuring testicular consistency of bulls to predict semen quality. J Anim Sci 29:483, 1969.

24. Hahn J, Foote RH, Seidel GE Jr: Quality and freezability of semen from growing and aged dairy bulls. J Dairy Sci 52:1843, 1969.

25. Hancock JL: The spermatozoa of sterile bulls. J Exp Biol 30:50, 1953.

26. Hughes ST: Breeding soundness traits in beef bulls, Ph.D. dissertation, Colorado State University, Fort Collins, 1987.

27. King RG, Kress DD, Anderson DC, et al: Genetic parameters in Herefords for puberty in heifers and scrotal circumference in bulls. Proc West Sect Am Soc Anim Sci 34:11, 1983.

28. Knights SA, Baker RL, Gianola D, et al: Estimates of heritabilities and of genetic and phenotypic correlations among growth and reproductive traits in yearling Angus bulls. J Anim Sci 58:887, 1984.

29. Koefoed-Johnsen HH, Anderson JB, Andersen E, et al: The Dag defect of the tail of the bull sperm. Studies on the inheritance and pathogenesis. Theriogenology 14:471, 1980.

30. Kriese LA, Bertrand JK, and Benyshek LL: Age adjustment factors, heritabilities and genetic correlations for scrotal circumference and related growth traits in Hereford and Brangus bulls. J Anim Sci 69:478, 1991.

31. Lunstra DD: Testicular development and onset of puberty in beef bulls. *In* Beef Research Program Progress Report No. 1, US Meat Animal Research Center ARM-NC-21, 1982, p 26.

32. Lunstra DD: Changes in libido-fertility relationships as beef bulls mature. J Anim Sci 59(suppl 1):351, 1984.

33. Lunstra DD, Echternkamp SE: Puberty in beef bulls: Acrosome morphology and semen quality in bulls of different breeds. J Anim Sci 55:638, 1982.

34. Lunstra DD, Ford JJ, Echternkamp SE: Puberty in beef bulls: Hormone concentrations, growth, testicular development, sperm production and sexual aggressiveness in bulls of different breeds. J Anim Sci 46:1054, 1978.

35. Lunstra DD, Gregory KE, Cundiff LV: Heritability estimates and adjustment factors for the effect of bull age and age of dam on yearling testicular size in breeds of bulls. Theriogenology 30:127, 1988.

36. Madrid N, Ott RS, Rao Veeramachaneni DN, et al: Scrotal circumference, seminal characteristics, and testicular lesions of yearling Angus bulls. Am J Vet Res 49:579, 1988.

37. Neely JD, Johnson BH, Dillard EU, et al: Genetic parameters for testes size and sperm number in Hereford bulls. J Anim Sci 55:1033, 1982.

38. Purohit RC, Hudson RS, Riddell MG, et al: Thermography of the bovine scrotum. Am J Vet Res 46:2388, 1985.

39. Pratt SL, Spitzer JC, Webster HW, et al: Comparison of methods for predicting yearling scrotal circumference and correlations of scrotal circumference to growth traits in beef bulls. J Anim Sci 69:2711, 1991.

40. Pruitt RJ, Corah LR: Effect of energy intake after weaning on the sexual development of beef bulls: 1. Semen characteristics and serving capacity. J Anim Sci 61:1186, 1985.

41. Rao Veeramachaneni DN, Heath EH, Ott RS, et al: Changes in basal lamina of seminiferous tubules associated with deranged spermatogenesis in the bull. Am J Vet Res 48:243, 1987.

42. Roberts SJ: Veterinary Obstetrics and Animal Diseases Theriogenology. 3rd ed. Ithaca, NY, Author, 1986, pp 752–893.

43. Smith BA, Brinks JS, Richardson GV: Relationships of sire scrotal circumference to offspring reproduction and growth. J Anim Sci 67:2881, 1989.

44. Smith BA, Brinks JS, Richardson GV: Estimation of genetic parameters among breeding soundness examination components and growth traits in yearling bulls. J Anim Sci 67:2892, 1989.

45. Toelle VD, Robison OW: Estimates of genetic correlations between testicular measurements and female reproductive traits in cattle. J Anim Sci 60:89, 1985.

46. Trenkle A, Willham RL: Beef production efficiency. Science 198:1009, 1977.

47. Werre JF, Brinks JS: Relationship of age at puberty with growth and subsequent productivity in beef heifers. Proc West Sec Am Soc Anim Sci 37:300, 1986.

48. Wittier WD, Bowen MJ, Eller AL: Relationship between starting and ending scrotal circumference for bulls in 140-day test-of-gain programs. *In* Proceedings of the 23rd Annual Convention of the American Association of Bovine Practitioners, Indianapolis, 1991, p 151.

■ Feedlot Production Medicine Programs

Karen C. Rogers, D.V.M., M.S.
Bruce W. Hoffman, D.V.M.
Delbert G. Miles, D.V.M., M.S.

Production medicine demands a margin of separation between disease challenge and resistance, regardless of the facet of the industry. Resistance levels exceeding disease challenge precludes disease (Fig. 1). However, when resistance levels are

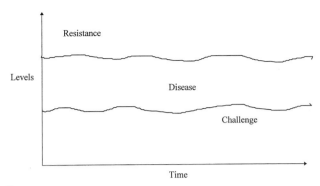

Figure 1

A healthy animal. (Adapted from Richey EJ: Marketing Healthy Calves That Remain Healthy. Gainesville, University of Florida, Florida Cooperative Extension Service, 1992, circular 1037.)

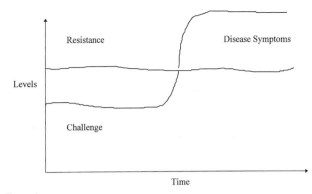

Figure 3

An increase in disease challenge causing symptoms of disease. (Adapted from Richey EJ: Marketing Healthy Calves That Remain Healthy. Gainesville, University of Florida, Florida Cooperative Extension Service, 1992, circular 1037.)

lowered or disease challenge is raised or both, the two intersect, and a disease state (and often a loss of production) results (Figs. 2 and 3). One of the goals of the industry is to raise resistance through preventive management (e.g., enhancing maternal antibodies, colostrum, and immunization) (Fig. 4). Management tools to reduce disease challenge include the judicious use of medications, parasite control, sanitation and hygiene, and removal of diseased and carrier animals from the herd. A proactive or preventive approach, rather than a reactive one, aids in increasing resistance levels, reducing challenge, and increasing monetary returns.

In an industry whose profit margins are often low, the challenge has become one of maximizing production while keeping production costs as low as possible. This is especially true as it relates to respiratory disease. Bovine respiratory disease (BRD) remains the most costly infectious disease facing stocker and feedyard operations. A survey of 59 feedyards representing 38.6 million cattle between January 1990 and May 1993 acknowledged BRD to account for 44.1% of all dead cattle. Digestive diseases (bloat, acidosis, and coccidiosis) represented 25.9%, and other diseases (skeletal, urogenital, CNS, and unknown) represented 28.6%. BRD costs the industry as much as $1 billion per year and kills more feedlot cattle than other diseases. Production losses are realized through poor performance, labor costs, and medicine costs, not just death losses.

Major advances have been made in respiratory vaccines, pharmaceuticals, and management systems; however, reluctance to adopt newer technology and advances prevents the industry as

a whole from moving forward. It is therefore prudent that management practices be implemented and honed to reduce production losses.

Preconditioning programs have gained increased acceptance and are growing in popularity as alliances are being formed. Feedlot operators have come to realize that much of their grief can be prevented or reduced through precision management prior to arrival of cattle at the stocker operation or feedlot. Preconditioning programs may specify certain vaccination programs, weaning, castration, dehorning, or a certain degree of feed bunk adaption. All of these are done to reduce the level of stress when an animal reaches the lot. It is no secret to the feedlot manager that differences exist in cattle sources. Well-managed herds may decrease morbidity and/or mortality, whereas poorly managed, low-input operations or poor genetics may have a disastrous effect. The feedlot operator realizes this, and this may in turn be reflected in the purchase price.

Intense management also strives to maximize performance through reduced illness. The most obvious economic losses resulting from BRD are death loss and medicine cost. In the summary reports of the Texas A&M Ranch to Rail Program, medical costs for sick calves ranged from $20.76 to $37.90/head. Calves sold for salvage are also a significant loss; the cost of these may range from $240.00 to $307.00/head. The hidden costs are reduced performance. The difference in average daily gain (ADG) among calves that remain healthy vs. those that become ill can be substantial. In a 28-day receiving period, a difference of 0.5 lb/day in ADG has been reported. This differ-

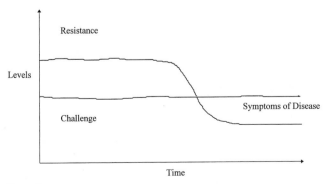

Figure 2

A decline in animal resistance causing symptoms of disease. (Adapted from Richey EJ: Marketing Healthy Calves That Remain Healthy. Gainesville, University of Florida, Florida Cooperative Extension Service, 1992, circular 1037.)

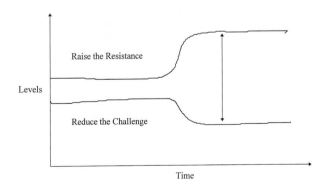

Figure 4

Decreasing opportunity of disease through increased resistance and decreased disease challenge. (Adapted from Richey EJ: Marketing Healthy Calves That Remain Healthy. Gainesville, University of Florida, Florida Cooperative Extension Service, 1992, circular 1037.)

ence tends to decrease over the course of the feeding period, but the difference persists between treated and untreated cattle. Thus, if performance is to be maximized, maintenance of health must be a top priority.

ARRIVAL PROGRAM

The arrival program may vary on the basis of the origin and background of the cattle received as well as on weather conditions at the feedyard, transportation shrink, sex of the cattle, and design of facilities. Regardless of the source, calves should be observed immediately off-truck for injuries and health status. Cattle that are unacceptable should be rejected and the seller contacted. Truckers should assume the responsibility for cattle that are trampled or badly injured during transit.

Shrinkage is the weight lost between purchase and delivery of the cattle. Generally, shrinkages of 2% to 6% can be attributed to loss of ingesta (extracellular fluid) in the form of feces and urine. Greater than 7% shrinkage represents intracellular loss of fluid from the animal's muscles, organs, and tissues. Small shrinkage is rapidly replaced by regaining fill; however, large shrinkage takes considerably more time to replace and is often associated with higher morbidity and possible mortality. These calves often require more intensive management. Unweaned fleshy calves and calves off of lush pasture tend to suffer the worse shrinkage.

After the load has been accepted, calves should be placed in receiving pens with free access to good-quality long-stem hay and fresh water. The importance of fresh water cannot be emphasized enough; cattle that don't drink don't eat, and become ill.

Bawling calves, whether from a country source or salebarn, normally have not been exposed to waterers. Thus, it is important to entice the calves to drink by strategic placement of the waterers in the pen or allowing them to overflow to provide the sight, sound and smell of running water. Hydrants or hoses can also be placed on the waterer such that a mist is sprayed into the air, allowing it to be seen. Lowering bunk cables for the calves may prevent escapes, because they will do a great deal of walking and bawling until they rest. It is often advisable that in extreme weather or in wet conditions calves in poor flesh be bedded in an area of the pen with wood chips to prevent hypothermia and to alleviate some of the stress.

Mill feed may be placed on top of the hay. The hay should help entice the cattle to the bunk and fill the cattle up. Typical starter rations should contain approximately 40% to 60% grain.

Backgrounded cattle are not quite as restless as bawling calves, and some have experienced drinking out of waterers. These cattle do not pose as much of a problem, but free access to fresh hay and water should be provided.

Yearlings may provide a little more of a challenge because many may be bunk broke or are already very aggressive eaters. These cattle need to be filled up on hay so that they do not consume ration too readily and become acidotic.

Generally cattle are allowed to rest overnight in the receiving pens prior to processing. Optimally they should be processed within 24 to 36 hours after arrival. This allows them time to replenish transit losses and reduce fatigue. Cattle can also be observed to go from a random pacing of the fenceline to a resting state. Once they become methodical about seeking out feed and water, they are ready to be processed.

Delays exceeding 36 hours after arrival jeopardize animal health. For each day that processing is delayed, a 1% increase in morbidity can be seen. This delay also compromises the ability of the animal to respond to vaccinations and medications because it allows the disease process to progress.

The receiving facilities should not add to the stress of the animal. Tubs and chutes should be free of sharp objects and allow for good footing. Pen size is not critical, but 60 to 120 ft²/head is usually sufficient. Because the new arrivals are probably not aggressive yet, 12 in. of bunk space per head is normally adequate.

PROCESSING

Knowing the origin and history of the calves is desirable in formulating a processing program. This is often not possible, however, because salebarn calves can have a variety of origins, and prior treatment and/or vaccination history status may vary.

Regardless of source and history, proper handling and management is an essential component to the success of the calves as stress and injuries create added cost. Key components necessary for successful immunization are an immunocompetent animal and effective vaccine. Vaccine failures may arise from inattention to detail. Various products and combinations are available for vaccination against the major respiratory viral (infectious bovine rhinotracheitis [IBR], bovine viral diarrhea [BVD], bovine respiratory syncytial virus [BRSV], parainfluenza-3 [PI₃]) and bacterial agents (*Pasteurella* spp.). The particular agents used may depend on incidence and geographic location. Other procedures performed during processing may include treating for internal and external parasites, giving clostridial vaccines, horn tipping, banding bulls, implanting with growth-promoting hormones, and checking for pregnancy. It is imperative that any cattle demonstrating lameness, sickness, or other injury be investigated further and possibly be sorted off prior to processing. Cattle that are injured or extremely lame may be salvaged for slaughter or treated without having to experience long withdrawal times from products used in processing.

Processing crews, whether in house or custom, can enhance or adversely affect the success of an animal health program. Proper handling of vaccines is critical. For maximum effectiveness, no more vaccine should be reconstituted than can be used within 1 hour. Transfer needles should be used to make the process easier and more sanitary. Extremes in temperature should be avoided, especially when using modified live viral (MLV) vaccines, which are heat and light labile. A portable cooler with ice packs aids in keeping the reconstituted vaccine viable on warm days. Equally important is keeping the mixture from freezing such that quantity and suspension continue to be delivered adequately. Brand and serial numbers used should be recorded on processing records in case a problem arises in the future. The animal should be adequately restrained to prevent processor and animal injury. Intramuscular and subcutaneous injections are best given in the triangular musculature of the neck. This avoids carcass blemishes and tenderness problems in the more expensive cuts of meat. Research has shown that products administered at weaning and branding persist throughout the feeding period and can be found at slaughter 300 days later. Needles for subcutaneous injection should be 16- or 18-gauge and should be ½ to ¾ in. long. Intramuscular injections require a 16- to 18-gauge 1- to 1½-in. needle, depending on the size of the animal. Sanitation is also extremely important because burred and dirty needles can introduce bacteria, which could negate product viability and/or create abscesses. Needles should be changed between every 15 to 20 head, or sooner if they become dirty or bent. The use of disinfectants to clean needles needs to be avoided with MLV vaccines as this can deactivate the vaccine. Injecting through manure or wet hides may increase the risk of infection at the site. Only clean, unused needles should be used to refill syringes.

DIAGNOSES AND THERAPEUTICS

Pen riders, or pen checkers, play an integral part of any animal health program. They must demonstrate dexterity in horsemanship, have a sincere interest in the well-being of the cattle, and have an innate sense of cattle handling. Cowboys can be trained to ride pens and spot compromised cattle, but the best pen riders demonstrate dedication and an inherent ability to do what is in the best interest of the cattle.

Training sessions with the pen riders on basic lung pathology and pathogenesis of interstitial and bronchopneumonia are valuable. Additionally, they should be trained in spotting other common feedlot diseases. Videos on animal handling and pen-riding basics also serve as a good refresher course for the veterans and a starting point for the rookies. Cattle should be evaluated for disease daily and twice daily in newly received calves or problem pens. These two groups should be given priority and ridden first or in the early morning, especially on hot days. Because the pen riders are exposed daily to inclement conditions, it is in the best interest of the feedyard to keep the crew motivated. Untimely or missed pulls are costly, as response to therapy and performance are ultimately jeopardized.

Cattle psychology and animal handling need to be given special consideration when facilities are designed or remodeled. Motivation and crew compliance are enhanced by good facilities and ease of working conditions. Facilities should augment the flow of cattle by providing good lighting such that shadows are minimized, noise is reduced, and adequate footing is established to prevent slippage, toe abscesses, and other injuries. Safety for both crew and cattle should be foremost. The use of circular crowding areas and working chutes takes advantage of the cattle's tendency to circle toward the outside of a curved passage. This encourages cattle to move in a more continuous flow toward the squeeze chute. Enclosed sides that keep humans and objects from view also enhance this design. Hospital chutes should ideally allow both calves and yearlings to be treated by having an adjustable-width bottom. Proper restraining capability, which allows accessibility of the head and neck for treatment, is also an important consideration.

As many treatment regimens are probably in existence as are feedyards. Some are based on historical preference and perceived success, whereas others are random and constantly changing. It is the authors' opinion that the better programs are those in which decisions are based on sound scientific data and well-conducted clinical trials. Regardless of approach, consistency should be maintained to evaluate efficacy. It is also difficult to assess a treatment regimen in which compounding of drugs and the use of more than one antimicrobial at a time occurs.

Once cattle are taken to the hospital, the temperature should be taken regardless of disease condition, with the exception of cattle in severe distress. Underlying conditions such as respiratory disease can be revealed in cattle pulled for other causes, especially bullers. The decision of whether to administer treatment to cattle is generally based on appearance and rectal temperature of 104°F or greater. Response to therapy is highly correlated with the timeliness of pulls. Cattle that are missed in the pens for a few days generally carry lower temperatures, and recovery is delayed or poor. Choice of therapy may be immaterial if lung pathology has progressed to a state in which drug penetration into consolidated tissue is reduced or inhibited. Drug rotational systems are beneficial because drug penetration and spectrum of activity varies with the stage of respiratory disease.

Nutritional status of incoming calves affects the immune system, which may drastically effect response to therapy. Trace minerals, such as copper, zinc, and selenium, and vitamin E play an integral role in disease resistance of the animal. When these levels are low or unavailable owing to factors such as high sulfate levels in the water, morbidity and/or mortality may be much higher than expected.

The following diseases represent those most commonly encountered in the feedlot.

Respiratory (Pneumonia) – "Shipping fever" is the most common disease of feedlot cattle and is characterized by signs such as depression and/or oculonasal discharge, gauntness, and possibly dyspnea.

Respiratory (Chronic) – Cattle demonstrate more advanced signs of pneumonia (i.e., severe dyspnea, rough hair coat, gauntness, and weakness).

Atypical Interstitial Pneumonia – This condition has a sudden onset, and the response to therapy is poor. Open-mouth breathing with an increased abdominal effort on expiration is often noted. The condition may actually be a digestive disorder. Recent evidence suggests a possible relationship of pneumotoxins produced from ruminal gases (hydrogen sulfide and/or ammonia).

Honker Syndrome – This condition is generally seen in heavy cattle during the last two-thirds of the feeding period; it is characterized by marked tracheal hemorrhage and edema resulting in loud expiratory and guttural sounds. Increased incidence is seen in hot weather and dusty conditions.

Diphtheria – Most commonly seen in calves and characterized by strenuous noisy breathing. *Fusobacterium necrophorum* is most commonly implicated as the cause of necrosis of laryngeal cartilage.

Acidosis – Highly acidic condition in the rumen and bloodstream with rumen pH ranging from high 4s to less than 6, but varies considerably with the severity. It is caused by rapid consumption or overconsumption of readily fermentable feed, resulting in excessive lactic acid production. Typical signs are staggering, slight bloating, "bubbly" feces, and sunken eyes.

Bloat – Characterized by excessive accumulation of gas in the rumen and reticulum produced by mircroflora. Two forms are gas bloat and frothy bloat, with the latter being the most common in feedlot cattle owing to concentrated slime, which is a product of a high-concentrate diet.

Coccidiosis – Characterized by bright red bloody scours and spread by ingestion of feces. Increased incidence in areas of contaminated bedding.

Foot Rot (Infectious Pododermatitis) – Characterized by swelling in the interdigital spaces. Increased incidence in muddy conditions. Response to therapy good if caught early in disease process.

HOSPITAL MANAGEMENT

Considerable ground in animal health can be gained or lost in the feedyard's hospital. It takes a dedicated and highly motivated individual to maximize treatment response. A well-designed and effective treatment program can fail miserably in the hands of the wrong individuals. Although this is one of the most critical areas in the feedyard, facilities are often less than optimal and space severely limited so that health is compromised. This is especially true during times of heavy pulls, as occurs during the fall run of calves. Ideal facilities generally have three to four hospital pens through which the animals can be rotated on a daily basis. Cripple pens and convalescent pens are also desirable in providing a less competitive environment when cattle need more time for recovery before returning to the home pen. Pen densities should not become so tight that bunk space is less than

12 in./head. The tub, snake, and chute should be free of jagged metal so that injuries are not incurred in coming through the hospital system. Adequate footing should be provided to prevent slippage. Belting or tire tread may be placed in the snake or in front of the chute to help alleviate some of these problems. Caution should be taken not to sort go-homes in areas containing smooth-surfaced concrete, if possible. Excessive pivoting and spinning in these animals potentiates toe abscesses. A surface of manure or an adequate layer of sand will help decrease their occurrence.

Hospital chutes equipped with scales allow for more accurate delivery of therapeutic drugs, potentially increasing efficacy of the product or reducing drug cost. Running water, preferably with hot water availability, is also valuable for maintaining a clean working environment and performing minor surgeries. Generally, the more desirable the working facilities, the better the care delivered to the animals. Educating the animal health crews can be achieved through regular training sessions and demonstrations by the consulting veterinarian. It is essential to the success of the program that therapeutics be handled properly and administered by their intended route, volume, and frequency. Necropsies are especially desirable to determine cause of death, which may be different than the antemortem diagnosis.

Proper identification and accurate records of individuals coming through the hospital is critical to guarantee quality assurance. The veterinarian providing health recommendations and services must remain acutely aware of the need to constantly caution against the slaughter of animals with potential drug residues.

Proper injection technique, site, needle size, and aseptic practices also helps reduce carcass blemishes and tenderness problems. Recent work conducted by Colorado State University researchers have determined the effect that different biologic and antimicrobial agents have on muscle tenderness. Even sterile saline injected intramuscularly decreased muscle tenderness 3 in. away from the injection site.

"Realizers" can represent a significant percentage of the feedyard population and consist of cattle with ailments such as chronic pneumonias, downers, cripples, and "poor doers." They are frustrating, costly, and pose a definite management problem. Not only do realizers occupy valuable pen space in the hospital while awaiting withdrawal, but also they are inefficient in utilization of ration. Daily maintenance requirements are often barely met, leaving little energy for gain. If available, one of the best management decisions is to place selected individuals on a paddock of grass and let nature take its course. Cattle often find a new will to live, and performance may exceed gains achieved under feedlot hospital conditions.

Hospital bunk management requires special attention as head count can vary greatly throughout the day, and a constant supply of fresh feed and water is imperative. Hay should also be available at all times to help entice the cattle to the bunk. Because compromised cattle are normally poor eaters, it is essential the ration be energy and nutrient dense. Rations consisting of an intermediate energy level are utilized. Acidosis is generally not a problem with new cattle, as the hay helps buffer the rumen.

RECORD-KEEPING

Record-keeping systems do not need to be complex; rather, they need to be current and accurate. The basic information that should be recorded when an animal comes through the hospital is the lot number, hospital identification number, date of treatment, diagnosis, drug administered, and volume of drug. Temperature and weight are desirable for future reference. The size of the feedyard normally dictates the type of system that is utilized. Cards are normally used in smaller operations, whereas laptop computers that can be carried to each hospital catch are utilized in larger ones. Regardless of system used, animals need to be positively identified and records accurately maintained so that cattle are not realized or sent prematurely to slaughter before completing drug withdrawal. Different computer programs are available through some of the larger pharmaceutical distributors and are valuable for tabulating data quickly.

Records that are beneficial to maintain on the computer are the success/failure, morbidity/mortality and drug withdrawal records. The success/failure record readily assesses treatment response for different diagnoses and therapies. The morbidity/mortality reports can signify where problems lie, such as problem pens of cattle, pen riding or hospital deficiencies, or treatment compliance failures. In essence, it summarizes the number of animals being treated for various reasons, identifies stage of feeding period, days to retreatment, treatment regimen, and treatment response. It is also beneficial to be able to call up data for certain lots of cattle that are going to be shipped and check withdrawal times prior to shipment.

NECROPSY

The practice of performing necropsy of animals should not be limited to recovering losses solely for insurance purposes (e.g., storms, electrocution/lightning) but should be utilized as a vital tool in fine-tuning a feedlot program. It is essential that all fatalities undergo necropsy to determine the type and extent of lesions and probable cause of death. Ideally, the animal should be observed in the pen and/or hospital prior to moving so that clues to cause of death may be obtained. This information can be extremely important prior to implementation of feed or therapeutic changes and to preempt incorrect decisions. Valuable information can be gleaned by taking samples for histopathologic analysis, culture and sensitivity, or virologic or toxicologic analysis when the circumstances warrant closer scrutiny.

Routine necropsies also offer the advantage of being an instructional tool for feedlot personnel. Necropsies provide the veterinarian a great opportunity to discuss disease processes and treatment failures and to end disputes between different crews (e.g., digestive vs. respiratory loss). Training crews to perform necropsy and diagnose certain conditions allows adequate records to be maintained. Technique is not as important as being able to spot normal from abnormal findings. However, this is only accomplished if a thorough examination is performed. Pulling two ribs back and looking into the chest cavity ("peek-a-boo" necropsy) can be deceiving and should be avoided. Training the crews to separate the dead animals into three groups (respiratory, digestive, and other) allows the consulting veterinarian to readily assess problems occurring at the feedyard. Crews, with practice, should be able to differentiate between types of pneumonia (i.e., bacterial/viral [bronchopneumonia] vs. allergic pneumonia [interstitial]) and to have a relatively good idea of chronicity (acute vs. chronic pneumonia).

NUTRITIONAL CONSIDERATIONS

The type of nutritional program and diet fed during the first 2 to 4 weeks after arrival at a feedyard can significantly affect morbidity, mortality, performance, and cost of gain. Intake patterns can vary considerably, and it may take 10 days for preshipment levels to be achieved and up to 3 weeks for normal consumption to occur. One cannot expect to maximize performance without compromising animal health. Optimal animal health is achieved by high-roughage starting diets; however, decreased rates of gain are to be expected. The negative effects of feeding high-concentrate diets can be partially overcome by feeding hay with the concentrate for 3 to 7 days after arrival. Silage in starter rations has also been associated with higher morbidity, and its use should be avoided.

Table 1
PERFORMANCE AND HEALTH DURING 28-DAY RECEIVING STUDY

Diet Supplement	Ad Lib Hay 1.5 lb, 40% CP	Ad Lib Hay 2 lb, 40% CP	Ad Lib Hay 4 lb, 20% CP	Limit Hay and Low Starch
Feed, lb/day	13.2†	13.7†	16.0*	12.4‡
Hay, lb/day	11.7*	11.7*	12.0*	1.3†
Supplement, lb/day	1.5§	2.0‡	4.0†	11.1*
Gain, lb/day	.77†	.81†	1.05†	1.85*
Feed/gain	27.3	29.6	27.4	7.3
Gain/feed (×100)	5.7†	5.7†	6.5†	14.9*
Morbidity, %	32.7	30.4	12.9	21.6

CP, crude protein.
*,†,‡,§Means with different superscripts differ ($P < .05$).
From Gill DR, Van Koevering M, Owens F: High Concentrate–Low Starch Starting Diets. Stillwater, Okla, Oklahoma State University, Animal Science Research Report, 1994.

Restrictive intake programs in calves during the first 3 weeks after arrival in which intake is limited to 1.7% to 2% of body weight are showing promise in decreasing morbidity. For the program to be successful, adequate bunk space must be maintained, because the calves remain extremely aggressive at the bunk. Restrictive programs offer the advantage of spotting compromised cattle more easily, as the healthy cattle charge the bunk during feeding while the ill cattle stand in the rear of the pen.

Work by Gill and co-workers (Table 1) compared the effects of feeding a diet high in roughage with a diet high in concentrate but low in starch (distiller's grain). The high-concentrate low-starch diet resulted in higher gains without incurring higher morbidity and mortality. Starch is thought to be responsible for the acidification of rumen fluid and rapid volatile fatty acid (VFA) production. Some researchers believe that dietary upsets can result in higher cortisol levels and subsequent immunosuppression, resulting in higher morbidity.

The importance of trace minerals in rations cannot be overemphasized. Table 2 presents the typical mineral requirements for feedlot cattle. Numerous variables effect the requirements of minerals for feedlot cattle (i.e., age, production level, weather, and ration ingredients). Newly received cattle, especially calves, do not consume much feed, so rations need to be nutrient dense. Overt clinical signs of a deficiency are not generally exhibited; however, deficiencies can be realized through inadequate response to vaccines and drug therapy. Supplementation may take several days to a few weeks for deficiencies to be corrected once intake is adequate. Trace minerals in rations must therefore be formulated according to actual consumption rather than theoretical intake.

The most common mineral deficiencies in cattle diets are zinc and copper. Diets may need to be adjusted for cattle according to area of origin, as other minerals consumed may interfere with bioavailability. Documentation of deficiencies can be easily obtained at necropsy by the collection of liver samples. Mineral interactions must also be taken into consideration and accounted for (e.g., high sulfate levels in water may tie up copper).

CONCLUSION

Prevention of disease through management practices in the feedlot increases survivability and performance and maximizes monetary returns. Enhancing the immune system by minimizing stress; providing proper vaccinations, therapeutics, and dietary supplementation; and using proper animal husbandry practices all aid in increasing an animal's ability to cope with disease and increase disease resistance.

BIBLIOGRAPHY

George MH, Ames RA, Glock RG, et al: Incidence, severity, amount of tissue affected and effect on histology, chemistry and tenderness of injection-site lesions in beef cuts from calves administered a control compound or one of seven chemical compounds. Proc Meet Acad Vet Consult 24:82–115, 1996.

Gould D: Hydrogen Sulfide and Its Relationship to Polioencephalomalacia (PEM) and AIP Syndrome. Proc Meet Acad Vet Consult 24:1–14, 1996.

Grandin T: Handling and processing of feedlot cattle. *In* Albin RC, Thompson GB (eds): Cattle Feeding: A Guide to Management. Amarillo, Trafton Printing, 1990, pp 51–61.

Smith RA, Gill DR: Unpublished data, Oklahoma State University, 1989.

Texas A&M ranch to rail summary report. College Station, Texas, Texas A & M University, 1992–1993.

Texas A&M ranch to rail north/south summary report. College Station, Texas, Texas A & M University, 1993–1994.

Texas A&M ranch to rail north/south summary report. College Station, Texas, Texas A & M University, 1994–1995.

Vogel GJ, Parrott C: Mortality survey in feedyards: The incidence of death from digestive, respiratory and other causes in feedyards on the Great Plains. Compend Contin Educ Practicing Vet 16:227–234, 1994.

Table 2
MINERAL REQUIREMENTS FOR FEEDLOT CATTLE

Mineral	Finishing Cattle	Stressed Cattle
Calcium, %	0.5–0.8	0.6–0.8
Phosphorus, %	0.3–0.4	0.4–0.5
Potassium, %	0.6–0.8	1.2–1.4*
Magnesium, %	0.2–0.3	0.3–0.4*
Sodium Chloride, %	0.1–0.5	0.2–0.5
Sulfur, %	0.05–0.15	0.08–0.15
Copper, ppm	6–10	10–15
Iron, ppm	50–100	100–200
Manganese, ppm	20–50	30–50
Zinc, ppm	50–75	75–100
Cobalt, ppm	0.1–0.15	0.15–0.20*
Selenium, ppm	0.1–0.2	0.20–0.30*
Iodine, ppm	0.2–1.0	0.2–1.0

*Values determined by research.
From Hutcheson DP: Minerals for feedlot cattle. Agri-Pract, 8:3–6, 1987.)

Dietary Management

Consulting Editor
Dee Griffin, D.V.M., M.S.

■ Growth-Promoting Implants and Feed Additives in Beef Cattle Production

Robert T. Brandt, Jr., Ph.D., M.S.

The use of growth stimulants and feed additives to promote rate and efficiency of growth was discussed in the third edition of this book. It is the purpose of this revision to briefly update products currently available for use, describe their modes of action, and offer suggestions for their use in field applications. The reader is referred to the manufacturers of individual products, feed companies, or animal health product suppliers for more detailed information on product applications, forms of administration, dosage, and warnings.

Efficacy and Safety

Products used to enhance animal production and health generally fall into one of two categories from a regulatory standpoint. Compounds that are "generally recognized as safe" (GRAS) are naturally occurring substances (e.g., buffers, some fermentation and plant extracts, yeasts) and are not regulated by the Food and Drug Administration (FDA) unless therapeutic claims have been made for their use. The FDA has recently ruled that *competitive exclusion products*, or products that contain beneficial microbes or agents that inhabit the gastrointestinal tract preferentially to pathogens, are subject to regulation and INAD (investigational new animal drug) approval. Compounds that do not fall into the GRAS category are regulated by the FDA and have undergone extensive research to prove their effectiveness and safety when used at approved levels, and they do not result in residues that pose any potential human health hazard. Thus, when used properly, products available for food animal production are effective and safe. Problems arise when products are administered improperly or not used at approved levels or when withdrawal times are not observed. Thus, it is the responsibility of every professional involved in the livestock production industry to make knowledgeable, prudent recommendations to producers with respect to animal health and growth-promotion products. Recent changes have been made in administration sites, withdrawal periods, or new uses for some products, which are addressed in this chapter.

Anabolic Growth Promotants

An anabolic compound, by definition, is one whose use results in constructive metabolism (i.e., lean tissue growth). It is important to remember that protein accretion (muscle growth) is an extremely dynamic process and is in a constant state of flux. Two metabolic processes occur continuously and simultaneously, namely, protein anabolism and protein catabolism. Thus, net protein growth per unit of time is the difference between the amount of protein formed and that broken down. It follows that net protein growth rate can be increased by processes or compounds that increase protein anabolism or decrease protein catabolism. Anabolic compounds apparently affect both anabolic and catabolic rates. Although not fully elucidated, it appears that the net effect of estrogenic compounds is an increase in protein synthetic rate, whereas the net effect of androgens is a reduction in protein turnover (catabolism).

Mode of Action

Estrogenic Compounds

Estrogens are phenolic steroids synthesized primarily by the ovary but also by the testes and the adrenal cortex. The primary role of estrogen is in female reproductive function and development of secondary sex characteristics, but research has shown that estrogens and compounds with estrogenic activity improve growth rate and feed efficiency when administered to beef cattle. The precise mode of action of estrogens and compounds exhibiting estrogen-like activity is unclear. The primary mechanism classically thought to be responsible for growth promotion from estrogens in ruminants was by an effect on the anterior pituitary. It has been shown that growing-finishing cattle treated with estrogen or estrogen-like compounds exhibit heavier pituitary weights, greater cell size and number of acidophiles (which produce and secrete growth hormone [GH]), and higher blood plasma concentrations of GH when compared to nontreated control animals. GH (as well as insulin) increases nitrogen retention and muscle growth rate, apparently by increasing amino acid uptake and/or protein synthesis by muscle cells. More recently, however, Hancock and Preston[6] and Wagner and associates[13] demonstrated that estradiol (E_2) and GH were additive in anabolic response. Further, estrogen receptors have been identified on skeletal muscle, and E_2 may influence hepatic GH receptors to increase binding of GH. Therefore, it appears that the anabolic response to E_2 may consist of some combination of direct stimulation of E_2 receptors and indirect effects of increased GH production, increased hepatic binding of GH, and production of somatomedins (e.g., insulin-like growth factor II), and/or other mechanisms. Zeranol (Ralgro), originally isolated from mold growth, is not an estrogen, but it exhibits some estrogenic properties when administered to animals. As with estrogens, zeranol increases pituitary weight and plasma GH concentration.

Androgens

Trenbolone acetate (TBA) is a synthetic androgen used in commercial implants, and it possesses approximately eight to ten times the anabolic activity of testosterone. Similar to estrogens, the definitive mode of action has not been elucidated, and it may occur through both direct and indirect mechanisms. Administration of TBA results in a reduction of both protein synthesis and degradation, with a greater reduction in degradation, resulting in increased net protein accretion. Muscle cells contain androgen receptors, which may be directly stimulated by circulating androgens. Androgens may also affect animal growth indirectly as a result of effects on other hormonal systems. Androgens have been shown to displace corticosteroids from their receptors and to downregulate corticosteroid receptors. This may be beneficial to protein accretion, because corticosteroids are catabolic. Androgens have also been reported to reduce plasma thyroxine levels, which would theoretically reduce maintenance energy expenditures by the animal and improve efficiency.

Available Anabolic Products

Since 1991, eight new implants have been introduced for use in the United States, bringing the total number of implants currently on the U.S. market to 18 (Table 1). Six of the 18 implants are generic estrogenic products, and it is anticipated that more generic products will be available in the near future. Implants dramatically improve rate and efficiency of growth and reduce the cost of beef production, but they may have some undesirable effects on carcass quality (reduced marbling), and animal behavior (increased secondary sex characteristics). Therefore, generic entries into the marketplace should be accompanied by sufficient research not only to document equivalency to the pioneer product, but also to characterize the magnitude of undesirable side effects.

Implants listed in Table 1 contain estradiol (or estradiol benzoate), trenbolone acetate, zeranol, or a combination of estradiol and trenbolone acetate. It is important to recognize that there is a wide variance in implant form (active agent), dose, and approved use. For calculation of equivalent estrogenic dosage between implants, estradiol benzoate contains approximately 72% estradiol by weight. Therefore, an implant with 10 mg of estradiol benzoate contains approximately 7.2 mg of estradiol. Further, research has shown that zeranol contains approximately 33% of the estrogenic activity (milligram per milligram) of estradiol.

The effective payout time for maximal growth promotion for the implants listed in Table 1 is approximately 70 to 100 days, with the exception of Compudose, whose life is 150 to 170 days. All implants listed in Table 1 have a 0-day withdrawal.

Proper Implant Location and Technique

All implants currently available should be administered subcutaneously in the middle third of the back of the ear. It was previously recommended that Ralgro be implanted close to the base of the ear. It is critical that implants be administered in the proper location (middle of the ear) to achieve maximum response, minimize the development of secondary sex characteristics and related problems (e.g., udder development, raised tailheads, riding activity, vaginal prolapse), and eliminate the potential for residues in meat removed from the head and neck regions of the carcass.

Proper implantation technique requires skill, patience, and common sense. Implants listed in Table 1 made by different

Table 1
ACTIVE INGREDIENTS AND APPROVED USES FOR CURRENTLY AVAILABLE ANABOLIC IMPLANTS

Trade Name	Active Ingredient(s)	Sex*	Growth Phase†
Synovex-C	10 mg of estradiol benzoate 100 mg of progesterone	S,H	S
CALF-oid	10 mg of estradiol benzoate 100 mg of progesterone	S,H	S
Component-C	10 mg of estradiol benzoate 100 mg of progesterone	S,H	S
Ralgro	36 mg of zeranol	S,H	S,G,F
Compudose	24 mg of 17β-estradiol	S,H‡	S,G,F
Synovex-S	20 mg of estradiol benzoate 200 mg of progesterone	S	G,H§
Implus-S	20 mg of estradiol benzoate 200 mg of progesterone	S	G,F§
Component-S	20 mg of estradiol benzoate 200 mg of progesterone	S	G,F§
Synovex-H	20 mg of estradiol benzoate 200 mg of testosterone propionate	H	G,F§
Implus-H	20 mg of estradiol benzoate 200 mg of testosterone propionate	H	G,F§
Component-H	20 mg of estradiol benzoate 200 mg of testosterone propionate	H	G,F§
Ralgro Magnum	72 mg of zeranol	S	F¶
Finaplix-S	140 mg of trenbolone acetate	S	F¶
Finaplix-H	200 mg of trenbolone acetate	H	F¶
Revalor-G	40 mg of trenbolone acetate 8 mg of estradiol benzoate	S,H	P
Revalor-S	120 mg of trenbolone acetate 24 mg of estradiol	S	F¶
Revalor-H	140 mg of trenbolone acetate 14 mg of estradiol	H	F¶
Synovex Plus	200 mg of trenbolone acetate 28 mg of estradiol benzoate	S	F¶

*S, steer; H, heifer.
†S, suckling; G, growing; F, finishing; P, pasture.
‡Heifer approval is for growing-finishing feedlot heifers only.
§For use in animals weighing 400 lbs or more.
¶For use in feedlot animals.

companies have an applicator (implant gun) or applicators unique to the particular line of products. Thus, familiarity with the applicator is needed. For most applicators, the needle should be inserted to the hub into the middle third of the ear between the skin and cartilage and between major veins. The needle should then be withdrawn approximately 1 cm to create a cavity in which to deposit the implant. The implant should be deposited carefully, taking care not to crush the implant pellets. The needle is then withdrawn and the wound gently pinched shut to prevent excessive bleeding and the loss of a portion of the pellets that make up the implant. The needle of the applicator should be wiped clean with an antiseptic solution between animals to minimize the risk of infection and walling off of the implant. It cannot be overemphasized that proper technique and sanitation, not the speed with which animals are processed, are critical to realizing the profit potential afforded by implants. Net returns from implants range from $10 to $20 per head in suckling and growing situations and up to $50 or more per head in the feedlot. Improperly placed, walled-off, or missing implants result in the loss of this profit in addition to the cost of the implant.

Performance Responses to Implants

It is important to understand that the magnitude of improvement in rate and efficiency of gain is dictated by protein and energy adequacy of the diet. This point is illustrated in a summary of stocker grazing studies to evaluate Compudose efficacy in Table 2.

Therefore, up to a point, implant response increases with increased plane of nutrition. Animals at a maintenance level of intake (zero gain) will not respond to estrogenic implants with faster growth rates; in fact, they will likely lose weight. It is recommended that implantation be deferred to a later growth phase in animals on very limited planes of nutrition (e.g., some wintering programs) that result in less than 0.25 lb of daily gain.

Suckling Calves

Implants cleared for use in suckling calves are Ralgro, Synovex-C, CALF-oid, Component-C, and Compudose (steers only). The bulk of available information indicates that implants can increase weaning weights by an average of 10 to 20 lb, despite a large degree of variation between reports. It is likely that much of the variation in implant response between studies is the result of differing pasture conditions (forage quality and availability), and milking ability of the dams used. A growing body of evidence[1] also suggests that response to calfhood implants is linked to age and/or weight of the calf. For greatest growth response, implants should not be administered at birth but should be given at 2 to 4 months of age (e.g., at branding).

Considerable debate exists concerning the merit and risk of using implants in heifer calves that may be used as replacements in the breeding herd. Kansas (Simms[10]) and Missouri (Morrow and associates[9]) data clearly indicate that inserting implants in heifers at birth, but *not* at 2 to 5 months of age, dramatically reduces fertility in yearlings. Cycling occurred in heifers that were given implants at birth, but they did not conceive. Implantation *once* during the suckling phase at age 2 to 5 months has generally had little or no effect on fertility. Although some studies (Simms[10]) have demonstrated increased pelvic size at weaning for implanted heifers, little or no difference is noted in pelvic size at first calving between implanted and nonimplanted heifers. Therefore, a single calfhood implant at 2 to 5 months of age, although perhaps not counterproductive to fertility, may have little if any benefit for heifer reproductive performance. Compudose is not approved for use in suckling heifers and should be avoided altogether for replacement females.

Growing Cattle

Stocker cattle grown on high-roughage diets in drylot or grazed on pastures generally display increased weight gain in response to implants. Responses to estrogenic implants have been well documented through the years. Revalor-G is a new, low-dose implant for use in pasture cattle. Comparative re-

Table 2
IMPLANT RESPONSE IN GRAZING TRIALS AS AFFECTED BY AVERAGE DAILY GAIN (ADG) OF CONTROL CATTLE

No. of Trials	Control ADG	ADG in Cattle With Implants	Improvement Over Control, %
9	1.16	1.26	8.6
5	1.22	1.39	13.9
10	1.33	1.54	15.8
5	1.45	1.72	18.6

Adapted from Compudose Technical Manual. Indianapolis, Elanco Products, 1982.

Table 3
THREE-TRIAL POOLED SUMMARY OF THE EFFECTS OF SYNOVEX-S, RALGRO, OR REVALOR-G ON AVERAGE DAILY GAIN (LB/DAY) OF STOCKER STEERS

Treatment	Location* Virginia	Oklahoma	Kansas	Mean	% Increase†	Range‡
Control	1.16¶	1.44‖	1.69‖	1.43‖	—	—
Synovex-S	1.22¶	1.65§,¶	1.87§	1.58¶	10.5	5.2–15.2
Ralgro	1.36§	1.57¶	1.95§	1.63§,¶	14.0	7.0–17.2
Revalor-G	1.37§	1.71§	1.90§	1.66§	16.1	12.4–18.8

*Total number of steers (and primary grass type) were 300 (orchard grass), 304 (Bermuda grass), and 480 (tallgrass prairie) for Virginia, Oklahoma, and Kansas, respectively. Trials averaged 94 days in length.
†Percentage increase in daily gain vs. control.
‡Range in percentage increase vs. control.
§,¶,‖Means in a column with different superscripts differ (P < .05).
From Revalor-G Technical Bulletin No. 5, Hoechst Roussel Vet, Somerville, NJ.

sponses of grazing steers implanted with Revalor-G to the conventional stocker implants of Ralgro or Synovex are shown in a three-trial pooled summary in Table 3. All implants promoted significant increases in average daily gain compared to nonimplanted animals. Revalor-G promoted gain to a greater extent (P<.05) than Synovex-S, with Ralgro being intermediate and not different from either Synovex-S or Revalor-G. The range in response across different sites compared to that in nonimplanted animals was more narrow for Revalor-G than for Ralgro or Synovex. More information of this type is needed, because consistency of implant response across a variety of cattle types and grazing situations (forage quality and availability) is one important determinant of implant recommendations.

Carryover Effects From Previous Implants Into the Feedlot

It is important to be able to predict how previously implanted cattle will perform when placed in the feedlot and given another implant. Several studies have shown that the added weight gain achieved from implanting stocker cattle on grass will be maintained through the finishing period. Table 4 shows results from a 2-year trial that was conducted to evaluate the effects of pasture implanting on feedlot and combined pasture-feedlot performance and production economics. Results show that administering a pasture implant resulted in increased grazing gain and beef-per-acre, which was more pronounced for intensively grazed steers compared to those allowed season-long grazing. Increased gains on pasture carried over through the finishing phase (steers fed to a constant back-fat thickness). Implanting pasture cattle tended to reduce feed efficiency in the feedlot, where all cattle were reimplanted. Fankhauser and co-workers[4] also reported that implants inserted during the grazing phase reduced feed efficiency during the feedlot phase, although a report by Kuhl and others[7] showed no effect of implantation during grazing on feed efficiency in a subsequent finishing period. Even with slightly lower feedlot feed efficiency, production economics (see Table 4) suggest that implantation during the grazing phase increases net returns in a retained ownership, grazing-finishing system.

Finishing Cattle

Finishing cattle respond dramatically to implants, regardless of whether they have received an implant in previous growth

Table 4

EFFECT OF GRAZING SYSTEM AND PASTURE IMPLANT ON GRAZING AND FINISHING PERFORMANCE OF STOCKER STEERS (2-YEAR SUMMARY)

Item	Intensive-Stocked*		Season-Long*	
	Control	Implant†	Control	Implant†
Pasture phase				
On weight, lb	612	612	612	612
Off weight, lb‡	725	749	818	827
Gain, lb‡,§	113	137	204	216
ADG, lb¶	1.59	1.93	1.41	1.49
Beef/acre, lb¶	56	68	51	54
Feedlot phase				
Final weight, lb‡,**	1158	1179	1238	1257
ADG, lb‡	3.78	3.77	3.32	3.39
DMI, lb/day‡,§	21.9	22.6	20.9	21.9
Feed/gain‡	5.78	6.03	6.33	6.51
Carcass traits				
Hot weight, lb‡,**	735	748	786	798
Dressing, %‡	62.4	62.0	63.4	64.1
Back fat, in.	.42	.40	.41	.43
% choice	66	54	58	55
Returns††				
$ per head	14.68	21.04	4.06	5.95
$ per 100 acres	734.00	1052.00	101.50	148.75

*Intensive-stocked steers grazed 71 days (2 acres/head); season-long grazed 145 days (4 acres/head).
†Implanted with Synovex-S; season-long steers reimplanted after 70 days on pasture.
‡Grazing system effect ($P < .05$).
§Pasture implant effect ($P < .05$).
¶Grazing system times pasture implant interaction ($P < .05$).
**Pasture implant effect ($P < .10$).
††Stockers, $74/cwt; finished steers, $64.50; receiving cost, $40/head; interest, 9%; pasture cost, $13/acre plus $11.50 (intensive stocked) or $23.00 (season-long) for minerals, labor, etc.; feed, $130/ton; pasture implants; $1/dose.

phases. In a summary of 37 research trials in which a multitude of different implant products and strategies were used, Duckett and colleagues[3] reported that compared to nonimplanted cattle, feedlot cattle given implants had increases in daily gain, feed efficiency, and hot carcass weight of an average of 18%, 8%, and 5%, respectively. Quality grade or percent choice was reduced by an average of 6%. Several factors need to be considered in establishing feedlot implant programs to meet the performance and carcass merit goals of the producer. These include the target market for finished cattle (live selling vs. grade and yield, formula, or grid selling), and sex, age, and breed type of the animals to be fed.

The target market for finished cattle will be the primary determinant of how aggressive (number and dose of implants administered over the feeding period) the implant program should be. An example of feedlot implant programs based on marketing goals is presented in Table 5. A trade-off is generally made between performance enhancement and quality grade. It should be remembered that the more aggressive an implant program, the greater the gain and feed efficiency, but the trend for reduced quality grade will be magnified.

Sex of the animal will also play a large role in the selection of a feedlot implant program. Performance responses to implants in heifers are about 65% of those observed in steers. More important, sex of the animal will dictate which products are appropriate to use. Table 1 shows that a variety of estrogenic implants are available in heifer and steer formulations. Steer and heifer formulations for implants with trenbolone acetate (Finaplix), or trenbolone acetate and estradiol (Revalor) are available. Synovex Plus and Ralgro Magnum are currently ap-

proved for use in feedlot steers only. Programs for heifers can be planned from Table 5 by substituting appropriate zeranol and E_2 products from Table 1, or appropriate E_2 plus trenbolone acetate products (Revalor-H or Finaplix-H). Maximum response to Finaplix-H in heifers is observed when melengestrol acetate (MGA) is fed.

Age and weight of the animal (calf vs. yearling), and days on feed are also important considerations in the selection of a feedlot implant program. Typically in animals placed on feed as calves, the response to two implants of E_2 plus trenbolone acetate is not significantly greater than use of one E_2 plus trenbolone acetate as the terminal implant, with E_2 or zeranol as the initial implant. This is not the case with short yearlings, in which maximum gain and feed efficiency can be obtained by using E_2 plus trenbolone acetate twice, at 70- to 90-day intervals. It is reiterated, however, that more aggressive implant programs result in greater reductions in quality grade (marbling). It is also important to remember that reimplanting at narrow intervals (<50 days) can result in a higher expression of secondary sex characteristics, as well as reduction of carcass quality grade.

Secondary Sexual and Carcass Effects of Implants

Bullers

The incidence of riding behavior (bullers) can be increased by the use of implants in cattle. It is important to recognize,

Table 5

IMPLANT PROGRAMS FOR FEEDLOT CATTLE

Aggressive Implant Program

Superior performance in terms of average daily gain (ADG) and feed efficiency (F/G) is the main goal, and high-quality grade is not a priority in *yearling cattle**:

Initial implant	60–80 days	Reimplant	60–80 days	Slaughter
∧		∧		∧
E_2 + TBA		E_2 + TBA		

Intermediate Implant Programs

Improved performance in terms of ADG and F/G and possible slight depression of quality grade is acceptable:

Initial implant	>60 days	Reimplant	70–120 days	Slaughter
∧		∧		∧
Zeranol† or E_2		E_2 + TBA		

Conservative Implant Programs

A modest improvement in ADG and F/G is the goal but high-quality grade is required:

Option 1

Initial implant	No reimplant 100–130+ days			Slaughter
∧				∧
E_2 + TBA				

Option 2

Initial implant	>60 days	Reimplant	100–130+ days	Slaughter
∧		∧		∧
Zeranol† or E_2		E_2 + TBA		

*The use of two E_2 + TBA has been shown to be more effective in yearling cattle than in calves.
†Research indicates a positive correlation with the use of zeranol in the initial 60–75 days of the feeding period with 1) reduced incidence of bullers and 2) final USDA Quality Grade, when Revalor-S is the terminal implant.
E_2, estradiol; TBA, trenbolone acetate.
Adapted from Revalor-S Technical Bulletin No. 12, Hoechst Roussel Vet, Somerville, NJ.

however, that seldom are implants the primary factor involved, and management strategies need to be developed on a case-by-case basis to minimize the incidence. The primary cause of bulling behavior is the establishment of a social hierarchy within the pen, particularly if cattle are put together and/or are brought in from pasture to confinement. Poor implantation technique that results in a large number of crushed, walled-off, or missing implants will result in animals within the pen having different blood levels of hormones, which may exacerbate the problem. Other contributing factors to high buller rates include the following: phytoestrogens of greater than 40 to 50 ppm in feed sources (e.g., some legumes); fungal estrogens in some moldy feedstuffs; hot, dry, and windy conditions (which may allow increased amounts of pheromones from urine and feces to circulate in the air); reimplantation done too soon (<50 days) after a previous estradiol implant; and inadequate water trough or feedbunk space. Sick, injured, or weak animals appear to be the first to be ridden. Masculine behavior from improperly castrated bulls or high levels of trenbolone acetate, which has three to five times the androgenic activity of testosterone, may also be causative factors.

Vaginal Prolapses

The incidence of vaginal prolapses is sometimes increased in female cattle given estradiol implants. As with bullers, there may be contributing factors (e.g., reimplanting too soon following a previous implant, consumption of phytoestrogens or fungal estrogens). It has been speculated, but not proved, that trenbolone acetate–containing implants may reduce the incidence of prolapses in heifers, presumably through anti-estrogenic effects on the reproductive tract.

Dark-Cutting Carcasses

The industry-wide occurrence of dark-cutting beef carcasses is approximately 0.8% to 5%, depending on the survey. Although the biochemistry, physiology, and histology of dark-cutting beef carcasses have been well-documented, the cause remains elusive. Pre-slaughter stressors (commingling, too large a load size, rough handling or loading, rapid climatic changes, long waits behind the packing plant) have been associated with depletion of muscle glycogen, increased postmortem muscle ultimate pH, increased water-binding capacity by muscle fibers, and dark-cutting beef. Historically, peak incidence of dark-cutting carcasses occurs in March through April and again in August through September, coinciding with periods of wider fluctuation in daytime-nighttime temperatures. Extensive reviews on dark-cutting beef (Morgan,[8] Smith and colleagues,[11] and Tatum[12]) indicate that implants are not a primary causative agent. However, when other significant stressors are present, implants may interact to increase the incidence. It appears that pre-slaughter handling and management practices to minimize stress are the best approaches to reducing the problem of dark-cutting carcasses.

Advanced Carcass Maturity

Beginning Jan 31, 1997, changes were made to the U.S. Department of Agriculture (USDA) grading system so that B-maturity beef carcasses (approximate chronological age, 30 to 42 months) with only small or slight degrees of marbling were discounted from the choice and select grades into the standard grade. The economic impact, although quite large on an individual-animal basis (≥$20/cwt of carcass), was expected to be rela-

tively small (1.5% to 2%) on the total fed cattle slaughter mix, with heiferettes and aged cattle (e.g., of Mexican origin) being most greatly affected. Among other factors, concern over the effect of implants on skeletal maturity came to the fore. A review of 74 trials[8] indicated that feedlot implants increased skeletal maturity an average of approximately 15% within a maturity grade. For example, if nonimplanted animals have a maturity score of A[40], then implanted animals would be expected to have a maturity score of about A[55]. The increase, although modest, is associated more with estrogenic implants. Use of implants with trenbolone acetate does not further increase maturity. The practical implication is that implants given to animals on the A-B maturity score border may result in a slightly higher incidence of standard-grade carcasses at slaughter. However, unless a very high percentage of a given pen is affected, a slight increase in standard carcasses will not offset the economic advantages in gain, feed efficiency, and carcass weight obtained from using implants. Although a number of factors may affect the more rapid onset of maturity (e.g., chronic administration of estradiol throughout the animal's life, excessive mineral supplementation) there is at this time a paucity of information on management strategies to circumvent it.

Feed Additives

Feed additives are essential to livestock production to enhance animal health and well-being, accelerate growth, and reduce the cost of production. Each additive offers specific benefits. Feed additives used for enhanced production can be generally divided into six categories: (1) growth-promoting ionophore and non-ionophore antibiotics, (2) antibiotics for liver abscess control, (3) coccidiostats, (4) estrus suppressants, (5) buffers, and (6) others. The reader is referred to the *Feed Additive Compendium*,[5] which provides annually updated information on feed additives and their approved uses.

Growth-Promoting Ionophore and Non-ionophore Antibiotics

Ionophores

Ionophores are carboxylic polyether antibiotics that depress or inhibit the growth of specific ruminal microorganisms. The precise mode of action of ionophores on altering ruminal microflora is unknown, although it is probably related to their facilitation of passage of numerous monovalent and divalent actions through hydrophobic lipid membranes. However, the net results of ionophore additions to ruminant diets are well known. These include the following:

1. Improvements in ruminal and whole-animal energetic efficiency, which is accomplished mainly by an alteration in ratio of ruminal volatile fatty acids (VFAs), resulting in a greater production of propionate, the only glucogenic VFA from rumen fermentation. Methane production is lowered, resulting in increased fermentation efficiency. Research also shows that ionophores may reduce the maintenance energy requirement of cattle.

2. Enhancement of animal health. Ionophores are coccidiostatic, but they may also aid in the reduction of bloat (by reducing methanogenesis) and acidosis (by modulating feed intake). Reduction in the incidence and severity of coccidiosis and digestive disorders results in improved animal performance.

3. Reduction in ruminal protein degradation. This protein-sparing effect is most important from a practical standpoint for growing cattle fed a low-quality, high-roughage diet that is

marginally deficient in protein. Because of reduced ruminal proteolysis, ionophores may also aid in reducing the incidence of tryptophan-induced pulmonary emphysema ("fog fever") by reducing the ruminal conversion of tryptophan to the toxic 3-methyl-indole.

4. Increased lipid content of ruminal microorganisms. It is unknown whether this is the result of microbial lipid synthesis acting as a hydrogen sink or the result of ionophores selecting for bacterial populations that synthesize a greater amount of lipid. However, increased de novo lipid synthesis may increase weight gain (grazing cattle) and feed efficiency (feedlot cattle) in animals that are fed ionophores.

The three ionophores cleared for use in ruminant animal production are laidlomycin propionate (Cattlyst), lasalocid sodium (Bovatec), and monensin sodium (Rumensin). The following text outlines FDA-approved use levels, indications for use, and approved combinations with other feed additives.

Laidlomycin: Finishing Cattle

Label. Feed continuously at a rate of 5 g/ton (30 to 75 mg/head/day) for improved feed efficiency and increased rate of weight gain, or at 5 to 10 g/ton (30 to 150 mg/head/day) for improved feed efficiency only.

Lasalocid: Finishing Cattle

Label. For improved feed efficiency, 10 to 30 g/ton in complete feed. Feed continuously to provide not less than 100 nor more than 360 mg/head daily. For improved rate of gain and feed efficiency, use 25 to 30 g/ton of complete feed (250 to 360 mg/head daily).

Combinations Allowed. (1) Lasalocid (25 to 30 g/ton) plus oxytetracycline (7.5 g/ton, to provide 75 mg/head of oxytetracycline daily). For improved feed efficiency and increased rate of weight gain and reduction of the incidence and severity of liver abscesses. (2) Lasalocid (25 to 30 g/ton) plus melengestrol acetate (MGA; 0.25 to 0.50 mg/head daily) fed continuously for increased weight gain, improved feed efficiency, and suppression of estrus in beef heifers fed in confinement for slaughter.

Lasalocid: Growing Cattle

Label. Feed continuously at a rate of not less than 60 mg nor more than 200 mg daily for increased weight gain of pasture cattle (stockers, feeders, slaughter cattle, beef and dairy replacement heifers).

Lasalocid: Coccidiosis

Label: Cattle. Feed continuously at a rate of 1 mg per 2.2 lb of body weight, up to a maximum of 360 mg/head daily (800 lb of body weight) for the control of coccidiosis caused by *Eimeria bovis* and *E. zuernii*. Feed only to cattle weighing up to 800 lb.

Label: Sheep. Feed continuously to provide not less than 15 mg nor more than 70 mg/head daily (20 to 30 g/ton) for the prevention of coccidiosis caused by *E. ovina*, *E. crandallis*, *E. ovinoidalis*, *E. parva*, and *E. intricata* in sheep maintained in confinement.

Monensin: Finishing Cattle

Label. For improved feed efficiency, 5 to 30 g/ton in complete feed. Feed continuously to provide not less than 50 nor more than 360 mg/head daily.

Combinations allowed. (1) Monensin (5 to 30 g/ton) plus tylosin (Tylan) (8 to 10 g/ton) for improved feed efficiency and the reduction of incidence of liver abscesses. (2) Monensin (5 to

30 g/ton) plus MGA (0.25 to 0.40 mg/head daily) for increased rate of weight gain, improved feed efficiency, and suppression of estrus in heifers fed for slaughter.

Monensin: Growing Cattle

Label. For increased rate of weight gain in stocker cattle and dairy and beef replacement heifers weighing more than 400 lb on pasture. Feed continuously at a rate of 40 to 200 mg/head daily in not less than 1 lb of feed. After the fifth day, 400 mg can be offered every other day in not less than 2 lb of feed.

Monensin: Cows

Label. Feed 50 to 200 mg/head daily in a minimum of 1 lb of feed for improved feed efficiency. Feed can be restricted to 95% of normal requirements when 50 mg of monensin is fed, and to 90% at 200 mg. Clearance is for mature, reproducing beef cows in drylot or on pasture.

Non-ionophore Antibiotics

Two new non-ionophore antibiotics have received recent approval for use in beef cattle to enhance rate and/or efficiency of gain. Bambermycins (Gainpro) is a high-molecular-weight (1582 g/mol) antibiotic that is not absorbed by the gastrointestinal tract. It is a fermentation product of a variety of *Streptomyces* spp. Research results indicate that bambermycins increases ruminal volatile fatty acid production, reduces methane production, and may enhance nutrient absorption in the lower gut. Another interesting aspect of bambermycins, according to published reports, is that it may reduce populations of *Escherichia coli* and *Salmonella* bacteria in the lower gut.

Virginiamycin (V-Max) is a peptolide antibiotic of high molecular weight, which is apparently not absorbed by the gastrointestinal tract. Similar to ionophores, V-Max increases the molar proportion of propionate in the rumen. Additionally, research indicates that V-Max reduces ruminal lactic acid production and may enhance nutrient uptake by the gut. V-Max also reduces the incidence of liver abscesses in feedlot cattle.

Bambermycins: Pasture and Stocker Cattle

Label. Feed continuously at a rate of 4 to 20 g/ton (10 to 20 mg/head/day) for increased rate of weight gain.

Bambermycins: Finishing Cattle

Label. Feed at a rate of 1 to 4 g/ton (10 to 20 mg/head/day) for increased rate of weight gain and improved feed efficiency.

Virginiamycin: Finishing Cattle

Label. Feed continuously to cattle fed in confinement for slaughter at a rate of 11 to 16 g/ton (70 to 240 mg/head/day) for improved feed efficiency, 13.5 g/ton (85 to 240 mg/head/day) for reduction of the incidence of liver abscesses, or 16 to 22.5 g/ton (100 to 340 mg/head/day) for increased rate of weight gain.

Field Comparisons of New Products to Existing Products

Use of feed additives that have been cleared by the FDA for some time were discussed in the third edition of this book. This section makes some comparisons between new products and established products with which the industry has had considerable experience.

Table 6
SEVEN-TRIAL COMPARISON OF GAINPRO, BOVATEC, OR RUMENSIN ON GRAZING PERFORMANCE OF STOCKER CATTLE*

Location	Investigator	Pasture Type	Length, Days	No. of Animals	Average Daily Gain, lb/Day			
					Control	*Gainpro*	*Bovatec*	*Rumensin*
Illinois	Faulkner	Fescue	112	128	1.87‡	2.07†	1.86‡	1.82‡
Kansas	Vanzant	Native pasture	112	80	1.75§	2.09†,‡	1.89‡,§	2.12†
Missouri	Lalman	Fescue	118	77	2.11	2.15	2.10	2.32
Nebraska	Rush	Wheatgrass	113	96	1.35‡	1.65†	1.59†	1.53†
Oklahoma	McCollum	Bermuda	112	80	1.61†	1.62†	1.67†	1.39‡
Texas	Rouquette	Ryegrass	112	72	2.38	2.42	2.35	2.48
Virginia	Wray	Orchardgrass	113	267	1.12§	1.38†,‡	1.23‡,§	1.46†,‡
Summary				800	1.74§	1.91†	1.81†,§	1.87†,‡
Extra gain vs. control, lb/day					—	.17	.07	.13

*All cattle fed 2 lb of supplement daily. Feed additive levels (mg/head/day) were Gainpro (20), Bovatec (200), and Rumensin (150).
†,‡,§Means in a row with different superscripts differ (P < .05).
From Gainpro Technical Bulletin No. 14, Hoechst Roussel Vet, Somerville, NJ.

Bambermycins (Gainpro) was recently approved for use in pasture and stocker cattle as well as in feedlot cattle. A pooled summary of seven studies of pasture cattle is presented in Table 6. All animals in this study received 2 lb of supplement per head daily, containing either no feed additive, 20 mg/head of Gainpro, 200 mg of lasalocid (Bovatec), or 150 mg of monensin (Rumensin). Overall, Gainpro resulted in a significant (P<.05) improvement in rate of gain when compared to results with no medication or to lasalocid. In addition, the consistency of response appeared to be greater for Gainpro.

Virginiamycin (V-Max) is a new antibiotic for use in finishing cattle. As previously discussed, V-Max has approved claims for improved rate and efficiency of gain and for the reduction of the incidence of liver abscesses. Table 7 presents a 12-trial summary that compares V-Max (17.5 g/ton, dry matter [DM] basis) to Rumensin plus Tylan (28 and 10 g/ton, respectively, DM basis), or to nonmedicated controls fed conventional finishing rations. Both products were very effective in improving feed efficiency when compared to that of control animals, but the data favor V-Max over Rumensin plus Tylan in some eco-

nomically important performance and carcass variables. Cattle fed V-Max had higher rates of gain and tended to have better feed efficiency than those fed Rumensin plus Tylan. Improved rates of gain for the cattle given V-Max resulted in heavier carcass weights and a trend toward increased dressing percentage when compared to weights in cattle given Rumensin plus Tylan. Both Rumensin plus Tylan and V-Max reduced the incidence of liver abscesses; however, Rumensin plus Tylan was more effective. The incidence of total and A+ (severe) liver abscesses in this summary was high. Feeding and feedbunk management practices should be taken into account when deciding which feed additives to use for optimal performance.

Laidlomycin propionate (Cattlyst) is a new ionophore that has been approved for improved weight gain and feed efficiency in finishing cattle. It is similar in structure and ruminal effects to the other approved ionophores, monensin and lasalocid. Table 8 shows results of a six-trial summary comparing performance and carcass traits of finishing cattle fed no ionophore, Cattlyst (11.1 g/ton, DM basis), or Rumensin (33.3 g/ton, DM basis).

Feeding Cattlyst resulted in significant improvements in rate

Table 7
TWELVE-TRIAL COMPARISON OF VIRGINIAMYCIN (V-MAX) TO MONENSIN (RUMENSIN)/TYLOSIN (TYLAN) IN FINISHING RATIONS

Item	Treatment*			Contrast†		
	Control	*RT*	*VMax*	*RT-C*	*VMax-C*	*RT-VMax*
Performance						
ADG, lb	3.70	3.76	3.86	.1224	.0002	.0057
DMI, lb/day	21.68	21.13	21.45	.0029	.1599	.0513
Feed/gain	5.91	5.65	5.59	.0001	.0001	.1895
Carcass traits						
Hot wt, lb	776	782	789	.0732	.0011	.0061
Dressing %	61.68	61.73	61.88	.6554	.0912	.1807
KPH fat, %	2.13	2.12	2.13	.65	.95	.68
Back fat, in.	.46	.47	.49	.39	.0011	.0061
Ribeye area, in.²	13.10	13.12	13.22	.88	.1894	.2204
Yield grade	2.74	2.77	2.83	.40	.0187	.0884
Marbling score	430	435	438	.1308	.0228	.38
Liver abscesses,						
Total, %	33.4	13.6	26.7	NA	NA	NA
A and A−, %	20.7	10.8	17.5			
A+, %	13.7	2.8	9.2			

DMI, dry matter intake; KPH, kidney, pelvic, and heart fat.
*Rumensin/Tylan (RT) and V-Max (VMax) were fed at 28/10 and 17.5 g/ton of dry matter, respectively.
†Contrasts of Rumensin/Tylan vs. control (RT-C), V-Max vs. control (VMax-C), and Rumensin/Tylan vs. V-Max (RT-VMax), respectively.
Data from Dr. A. C. Brake, personal communication, 1997.

Table 8

SIX-TRIAL SUMMARY OF PERFORMANCE AND CARCASS TRAITS OF FINISHING STEERS AND HEIFERS FED LAIDLOMYCIN (CATTLYST) OR MONENSIN (RUMENSIN)

Item	Treatment*		
	Control	Cattlyst	Rumensin
Performance			
Daily gain, lb	3.50‡	3.66§	3.43‡
DM intake, lb/day	21.04‡	20.91‡	20.04§
Feed/gain	6.04‡	5.75¶	5.87§
Carcass traits			
Hot weight, lb	736‡	746§	729‡
Dressing, %	63.2	63.2	63.2
Ribeye area, in.²	12.90	12.85	12.70
Back fat, in.	.54‡,§	.55‡	.52§
KPH fat, %	2.31	2.32	2.32
Yield grade	2.99	3.07	2.97
Quality grade†	4.05	4.07	4.03

*Cattlyst and Rumensin fed at 11.1 and 33.3 g/ton of dry matter (DM), respectively.
†Quality grade: 3, select; 4, low choice; 5, average choice.
‡,§,¶Means in a row with different superscripts differ ($P < .05$).
Adapted from Cattlyst Technical Manual, 1994. Syntex Agribusiness.

of gain and feed efficiency compared to those of either control cattle or those fed Rumensin. These data also show that cattle fed Cattlyst had feed intakes similar to those of control cattle, whereas feed intakes of cattle fed Rumensin were significantly depressed. The reader is cautioned that the level of Rumensin used in these studies, although within the range approved for use by FDA, is higher than that typically fed by the commercial feedlot industry. This may have some impact on interpretation of the data in Table 8.

Antibiotics for Liver Abscess Control

Liver abscesses can occur in finishing cattle as a result of receiving high-grain diets. Low ruminal pH can result in sloughing of ruminal papillae and abrasions to ruminal epithelial tissue. Ruminal bacteria can then gain entry into the portal blood system and are transported to the liver. The most common bacterial species isolated from liver abscesses have been *Fusobacterium necrophorum* and *Actinomyces pyogenes*. If they are severe enough, abscesses can reduce performance (Table 9) and increase carcass trim (e.g., if open abscesses are found or if the liver becomes adherent to the diaphragm).

Table 9

EFFECT OF LIVER ABSCESS SEVERITY ON FINISHING CATTLE PERFORMANCE

Item	Liver Score*			
	0	A−	A	A+
No. of cattle	362	50	35	60
Daily gain, lb	2.63	2.73	2.59	2.32
Daily feed, lb DM	18.55	18.60	18.22	17.88
Feed/gain	6.94	6.71	6.94	7.63

*0, no abscesses; A−, one or two small abscesses or abscess scars; A, 2 to 4 well-organized abscesses, generally <1 in. in diameter; A+, 1 or more large, active abscesses and inflammation of liver tissue.
From Brink D, Lowry S: How should efficiency of feed utilization be evaluated? Nebraska Beef Cattle Report. Lincoln, University of Nebraska, 1985, pp 19–20.

Severe abscesses may reduce gain and increase feed requirements by 10%. These data, in agreement with those of other studies, indicate that a moderate degree of abscessation (scores of A−, A) does not negatively influence feedlot performance. Antibiotics have been shown to improve rate and efficiency of gain in feedlot cattle. This is probably primarily accomplished through a reduction in the incidence of severe liver abscesses, but beneficial alterations in gut microflora may also be involved.

Tylosin

Label. Feed continuously at a rate of 8 to 10 g/ton (60 to 90 mg/head/day) for the reduction of liver abscesses caused by *F. necrophorum* and *A. pyogenes*. Also cleared to be fed in combination with MGA, or monensin plus MGA. Animals must not receive more than 90 mg/head/day of tylosin when fed in these combinations.

Oxytetracycline

Label. Feed continuously at a rate of 75 mg/head/day to reduce the incidence and severity of liver abscesses. Cleared to be fed in conjunction with lasalocid.

Virginiamycin

Label. Feed continuously at a rate of 13.5 to 16 g/ton (85 to 240 mg/head/day) for the reduction of the incidence of liver abscesses.

Coccidiostats

Coccidiostats are primarily used in receiving rations to aid in the prevention or treatment of coccidiosis. Survey data indicate that approximately 75% of all cattle in the United States harbor pathogenic coccidia. Clinical outbreaks can be caused by environmental and management stressors such as weather changes, auction barn commingling, trucking, processing, and ration changes. Readily detectable clinical signs of coccidiosis include diarrhea, hemorrhaging, and dehydration. Subclinical cases may also cause performance losses as a result of damage to intestinal lining, which can decrease nutrient absorption.

Prevention. Amprolium, marketed under several trade names, is approved for use in beef and dairy calves at 227 mg/100 lb of body weight for a 21-day period to aid coccidiosis prevention. Use of amprolium requires a 24-hour withdrawal before slaughter of any animals. Decoquinate (Deccox, Rhone-Poulenc) is approved for use at 22.7 mg/100 lb of body weight. Deccox should be fed for 28 day in a preventive program. As previously discussed, the ionophores lasalocid (1 mg/kg of body weight) and monensin (10 to 30 g/ton) are approved for the prevention and control of coccidia caused by *E. bovis* and *E. zuernii*.

Treatment. Amprolium is approved for treatment of coccidiosis at 454 mg/100 lb daily, with a treatment period of 5 days.

Estrus Suppressants

The only estrus suppressant currently available commercially is melengestrol acetate (MGA), which is a progestational steroid similar in structure and function to progesterone. Unlike progesterone, MGA is orally active in suppressing estrus and promoting growth. There is no evidence that progestins directly stimulate growth. Rather, it is thought that the stimulatory response is a function of an elevated baseline level of estrogen production in the animal resulting from the maintenance of mature follicles on the ovaries. Long-acting implants containing progestins are in various stages of development. The main advantage of such an implant over orally administered drug is that implants would allow males and females to be fed together in backgrounding and growing-finishing situations.

Feedlot Heifers. Suppression of estrus in feedlot heifers is desirable to prevent losses from injury resulting from riding behavior, and because riding and chasing increases energy requirements and may reduce performance. Generally, feeding MGA increases rate and efficiency of gain by 3% to 7%. The response is additive to that from ionophores, and MGA is cleared to be fed at a level of 0.25 to 0.40 mg/head daily in combination with monensin, or at a level of 0.25 to 0.50 mg/head daily in combination with lasalocid.

Estrus Synchronization. Synchronization of estrus in beef heifers can shorten the breeding season and allow concentration of labor during breeding and calving in addition to increasing the practicality of artificial insemination. Kansas State University studies (L.L. Corah, personal communication, 1995) showed that feeding MGA at 0.5 mg/head daily for 14 days, followed by injection of prostaglandin F_2 17 days later, resulted in 908/1451 heifers (62.6%) responding to synchronization. Response rates ranged from 33% to 95% at 11 locations. Locations with low response rates were also those with a high number of prepubertal heifers.

Buffers

Buffers resist change in ruminal pH and theoretically should be beneficial in maintaining health and high levels of performance in ruminants fed finishing diets. Feed additives that have been used as buffers include sodium bicarbonate, sodium sesquicarbonate, limestone, sodium bentonite, and magnesium oxide. Response in animal performance to buffers, however, has been extremely variable. This is in contrast to dairy cattle, in which buffers have proven extremely useful in maintaining animal health and high levels of milk production. The routine use of buffers in beef cattle diets does not appear to be cost-effective.

Other Feed Additives

Other feed additives are available that claim to enhance performance of ruminant animals. Most are composed of naturally occurring GRAS compounds that are not FDA-regulated unless therapeutic label claims are made.

Sarsaponin

Marketed as Sevarin, sarsaponin is an extract of the yucca plant. The active ingredients and mode of action have not been identified. Because it is not regulated, it can be included in any feeding program. The manufacturer recommends a rate of 0.5 g/head daily to be fed in conjunction with monensin or lasalocid. Controlled research studies have shown no consistent performance benefit from sarsaponin-ionophore combinations.

Yeasts

Several products are commercially available that contain yeasts and/or fermentation extract. Studies have shown that these products sometimes increase fiber digestion. Large improvements in cow milk production have also been reported when these products are used. Performance responses in growing animals have generally been variable and small, although yeasts may be beneficial in very high-roughage diets. It is doubt-ful whether these products would be beneficial for animals fed high-grain diets, as few or no fungi normally exist in the rumen under these conditions.

Probiotics

Probiotic is a term used for products containing "beneficial" microorganisms. A number of products are available for oral administration (pastes and gels), intraruminal injection, or as feed-additive preparations. Most contain either *Lactobacillus* spp. (primarily *L. acidophilus*) or *Streptococcus faecium*. In addition, many contain vitamins, trace minerals, and various "growth factors."

The conceptual basis for use of probiotics stems from the fact that beneficial strains of bacteria naturally inhabit the gastrointestinal tract of mammals, and are believed to play an important role in regulating the growth of *E. coli* and other pathogens along the digestive tract. Further, it has been observed that restriction of feed and water to laboratory animals resulted in reductions in lactobacilli and yeast, with a concomitant increase in coliform bacteria and *Salmonella*. Thus, there has been great interest in the therapeutic value of lactobacilli and *S. faecium* for stressed animals.

Studies with poultry, swine, and preruminant calves have shown significant declines in fecal excretion of coliform bacteria and corresponding improvements in health and performance with lactobacillus supplementation. However, a review of the available literature shows generally no response in functioning ruminants. In the few studies that have shown a response, it is difficult or impossible to ascertain whether the response was the result of the probiotic or the nutritional supplement (vitamins and/or trace minerals) included in the particular preparation.

Lack of response in ruminants may be the result of (1) lack of sufficient viable microbial counts in the preparation, (2) low ruminal survivability, or (3) host species specificity for colonization (e.g., it has been observed that only lactobacilli indigenous to rats will attach to rat gastrointestinal epithelium). Until research is conducted to demonstrate site and mode of action of the various probiotic preparations, no firm basis exists on which to recommend their routine use.

REFERENCES

1. Brandt RT Jr: Factors affecting release rates and blood levels of hormones from steroidal implants. Proceedings of the Oklahoma State University Implant Symposium, Tulsa, 1997. Stillwater, Okla, Oklahoma Agricultural Experiment Station, Publication P-957, pp 34–39.
2. Brink D, Lowry S: How should efficiency of feed utilization be evaluated? Nebraska Beef Cattle Report. Lincoln, University of Nebraska, 1985, pp 19–20.
3. Duckett SK, Wagner DG, Owens FN, et al: Effects of estrogenic and androgenic implants on performance, carcass traits, and meat tenderness in feedlot steers: A review. Professional Animal Scientist 12:205–214, 1996.
4. Fankhauser TR, Kuhl GL, Drouillard JS, et al: Influence of implanting grazing steers with Ralgro or Synovex-S followed by Synovex Plus or a Ralgro/Synovex Plus reimplant program in the feedlot on pasture/finishing performance and carcass merit, Report of Progress No. 783. Cattlemen's Day, Kansas State University, Manhattan, Kansas, 1997, pp 38–42.
5. Feed Additive Compendium. Minnetonka, Minn, Miller Publishing Co, 1997.
6. Hancock DL, Preston RL: Interaction between 17-β estradiol (E2) and recombinant bovine somatotropin (bST) in the anabolic response of feedlot steers. J Anim Sci 67(suppl 1):215, 1997.
7. Kuhl GL, Milton CT, Stokka GL, Brandt RT Jr: Comparative performance of grazing steers implanted with Revalor-G, Ralgro, or Synovex-S, and subsequent finishing performance and carcass merit. J Anim Sci 75(suppl 1):233, 1997.

8. Morgan JB: Implant program effects on USDA beef carcass quality grade traits and meat tenderness. Proceedings of the Oklahoma State University Implant Symposium, Tulsa, 1997. Stillwater, Okla, Oklahoma Agricultural Experiment Station, Publication P-957, pp 147–154.

9. Morrow R, Brooks A, Fairbrother T, et al: Effects of implanting with Ralgro on growth and reproductive performance of beef heifers, Animal Science Report No. 103. Missouri Agricultural Experiment Station, University of Missouri, Columbia, 1983, p 52.

10. Simms DD: Ralgro implants in suckling calves and growing cattle. Proceedings of the Management for Growth Conference, Orlando, Fla, 1985, p 177.

11. Smith GC, Tatum JD, Morgan JB: Dark cutting beef: Physiology, biochemistry, and occurrence. Monograph prepared by the Meat Science Program, Department of Animal Sciences, Colorado State University, Fort Collins, 1993.

12. Tatum JD: The effects of anabolic implants on beef quality traits. Meat Focus Int 2:71–74, 1993.

13. Wagner JF, Cain T, Anderson DB, et al: Effect of growth hormone (GH) and estradiol (E$_2$B) alone and in combination on beef steer growth performance, carcass and plasma constituents. J Anim Sci 66(suppl 1):283, 1988.

■ Ration Management in Feedlot Cattle

Robbi H. Pritchard, Ph.D.

The first and most critical aspect of ration management is getting cattle started on feed properly. When starting cattle there are three basic classes of cattle that must be addressed. There are bawling calves that know nothing about feedbunks and milled feed and are extremely disoriented by their relocation into the feedyard. There are cattle that know how and are ready to eat milled feed. Most (but not all) yearlings fit into this category. Calves weaned and retained at the ranch or in a backgrounding yard may also fit into this group. The third group is cattle that do not feel well enough to eat. They may or may not be bunk-broke, which exacerbates the problems of ration management. Each of these classes of cattle requires different diets and management to optimize performance. These issues are discussed before concerns with keeping cattle on feed are reviewed.

STARTING CATTLE

Bawling Calves

It is important for the cattle feeder to realize that bawling calves and cattle removed from extensive range production systems do not recognize feedbunks or milled feed. They make no association between these sights and food. The first step is to cultivate that association, which is the root purpose of providing long grass on feedlot arrival. Obviously, if recognizable food is provided at a location other than the feedbunk its role in starting cattle becomes compromised.

There is little nutritive value in the long prairie hay used to entice eating. It is realistic to assume that dry matter intake (DMI) by naive calves will be 0.75% of body weight (BW). This is 4 lb of dry matter (DM) for a 550-lb calf. This same 550-lb calf requires 8.8 lb of prairie hay to maintain body weight. Protein will also be inadequate. Clearly then, the primary role of long grass hay is to entice cattle to the feedbunk and to eat. A secondary role is to provide support for the mechanical components of ruminant digestive physiology, that is, to stimulate mastication, salivation, and rumination. Once that is accomplished, a more nutritionally dense diet is required. This is

readily accomplished by delivering milled feed on top of the long hay. It is recommended that the long hay enticement be continued until most of the calves have learned to use the feedbunk (3 to 5 days).

A good benchmark for starting 550-lb calves is that they will be consuming 9 lb of DM on the seventh day after arrival and that this will climb to 14 lb DMI on the 14th day. In order to achieve positive energy and nitrogen balances necessary to support the immune system and minimal growth on day 7, this diet must contain 54 Mcal net energy for gain (NE$_G$)/cwt. This translates into a 60:40 concentrate-roughage diet. When the DMI of this diet reaches 14 lb (on day 14), the average daily gain (ADG) on that day will be 2.73 lb. The DMI should be that high to help replenish the body reserves and weight lost between weaning and the seventh day in the feedlot when we finally reached a maintenance level of DMI.

The energy density of the diet and the DMI must be in proper proportion during this period. If the DMI is lower than the target level, energy and nutrient density should be increased.[3] If the DMI is greater than these benchmarks, energy density should be reduced. Too much fermentable carbohydrate intake at this point will lead to digestive disorders that precipitate other health problems.[4]

Yearlings

Typical yearlings know how to eat and aggressively seek feed once they are rested from their trip to the feedlot. Feeding roughage to these animals is necessary to take the edge off their appetite, since aggressive intake of grain would lead to obvious digestive disorders. Most people are familiar with adapting this class of cattle to high grain diets by gradually reducing dietary roughage over 25 to 30 days. Four or five different diets are used in this adaptation process. Cattle are managed to allow ad libitum consumption and we are using roughage to control grain intake. In large commercial cattle feeding, roughage handling is expensive and presents logistic challenges. Another disadvantage is that this system causes the rumen microflora to go through multiple adaptations over a prolonged period of time. Ruminal inefficiencies occur because of this, and digestive disorders are not eliminated.

By using scales to accurately quantify feed deliveries, using multiple feedings each day, and including ionophores, we can accelerate the step-up to high grain diets. Ration step-up can be completed in 7 to 14 days in some commercial feedlots. Peak DMI is achieved only after cattle are adapted to the final diet.

Stressed Cattle

These cattle have high nutrient demands but limited motivation to eat. Diets need to be palatable and relatively dense in nutrients. Bunk space is critical since the more lethargic cattle lack the motivation or strength to compete for feed. Providing 16-in. bunk space and feeding at least three times each day will keep feed fresh and available for all of the cattle. It is important to be aware of processing schedules and feed grade medications and their proper use when feeding these cattle. As cattle in this pen respond to therapy, their appetites will increase. It is critical that management avoid allowing these cattle to overconsume feed.

KEEPING CATTLE ON FEED

In a normal pattern, DMI climbs during the initial 25 to 40 days on feed and then reaches a plateau. Once this plateau is achieved, the DMI increases only slightly with additional time on feed and increasing BW. The DMI level at the plateau is apparently a reflection of the initial BW.[5] As a result, a 1000-lb calf-fed steer (initial BW, 600 lb) may have a DMI plateau of 19 lb, while a 1000-lb long yearling (initial BW, 800 lb) may have a DMI plateau at 23 lb. The key to good ration management is to sustain this plateau and avoid cyclic DMI patterns.

Cyclic DMI patterns cause poor gain efficiency[1] and are presumed to contribute to metabolic disorders. There are economic incentives to maximize DMI, which prompt the cattle feeder to continually try to increase feed deliveries. Changing weather conditions will intermittently involve increased appetites among steers. This combination of events causes cattle to be offered and to consume increasing amounts of feed. Eventually, physiologic tolerances are exceeded and feed consumption drops to levels below the plateau. Cattle may never learn to avoid this phenomenon. If they do, we see a new, lower plateau established. This condition is commonly referred to as "stall-out" or "burned" cattle.

Avoiding cyclic feed deliveries requires making feed calls and deliveries based on a historical base of daily feed records. Some yards will use running averages of the previous 7-day and 3-day feed deliveries. Other yards will look at the previous 4- to 7-day daily deliveries. In either situation, a feed delivery change of greater than 10% is a sign of problems. Both systems temper their feed delivery based on the quantity and condition of carryover feed in the bunk, the behavior demonstrated by the cattle, and prevailing environmental conditions.

For these systems to work, feed deliveries must be accurate. That involves more than just pounds delivered. Feed batches must be accurately proportioned and properly mixed and delivered. When high-moisture feeds are used or commodity piles are exposed to the elements, it is necessary to frequently monitor the DM content. Under these conditions monthly feed moisture determinations will not be adequate for maintaining formulation integrity. It is necessary for feed schedules to remain firm. Variations of feeding time by more than 15 minutes will affect intake patterns. Feeding cattle later in the day is not harmful[2] so long as the schedule is consistent.

The fermentability of the diet dictates how stringent the feed management program must be. Dietary roughage concentrations of greater than 25% create a cushion allowing considerable flexibility in management. This is especially true when feeding whole shelled corn or dry rolled corn. Adding corn gluten feed to the diet also reduces cattle sensitivity to feeding management. High-moisture corn is very rapidly fermented. Cattle become very sensitive to feeding management on these diets. This contributes in part to the lower DMI that occurs when wet corn is substituted for dry corn. Wet corn, rolled barley, and steam-flaked corn are comparable in this respect. Wheat is the most sensitive grain to feed.

CONCLUSION

Tradeoffs in ration management are unavoidable. Most steps taken to improve growth efficiency increase cattle sensitivity to feeding management. Variation in feeding schedules, quantities of feed delivered, and actual formulation delivered are the principle concerns in assessing the level of the feeding management. An effective program will match the diet formulation with the type of cattle and level of management available.

REFERENCES

1. Bierman SJ, Pritchard RH: Effect of feed delivery management on yearling steer performance. Presented to Midwestern Section of the American Society of Animal Science, 1977, p 92.
2. Knutsen JS, Vetos JJ, Pritchard RH: Effect of morning, evening or twice daily feeding on yearling steer performance. SD Agri Exp Station Beef Rep Cattle 14:45, 1994.
3. Lofgreen GP, Stinocher LH, Kiesling HE: Effects of dietary energy, free choice alfalfa hay and mass medication on calves subjected to marketing and shipping stress. J Anim Sci 50:590, 1980.
4. Pritchard RH, Mendez JK: Effects of preconditioning on pre- and post-shipment performance of feeder calves. J Anim Sci 68:28–34, 1990.
5. Thornton JH, Owens FN, Gill DR: Feed intake by feedlot beef steers: Influence of initial weight and time on feed. Oklahoma Agricultural Experiment Station miscellaneous publication. MP 117:320, 1985.

■ Protein Supplementation in Beef Cattle Diets

Todd Milton, Ph.D.

ANIMAL REQUIREMENTS AND PREDICTION MODELS

Until recently, the protein requirements of beef cattle have been expressed on a crude protein (CP) basis.[41] The publication *Nitrogen Usage in Ruminants*[42] proposed a rationale for expressing protein requirements on a metabolizable protein (MP) basis. Recently, the publication *Nutrient Requirements for Beef Cattle*[43] was revised to predict animal requirements on the basis of MP. Metabolizable protein is defined as the true protein absorbed from the small intestine, which is derived from microbial crude protein (MCP) synthesis and dietary undegraded intake protein (UIP).

Metabolizable protein systems have two basic advantages over traditional CP systems. First, a CP system assumes that all protein sources are degraded equally in the rumen and that all CP is converted to MP with similar efficiency across diet types. Second, there is a greater amount of information concerning UIP and MCP synthesis with the MP system. This allows more accurate and useful information for evaluating diets with respect to satisfying the requirements of both the ruminal microorganisms and the host animal protein requirements. Summation of the degradable intake protein (DIP) and the UIP of feedstuffs will give the CP concentration of any diet. A representation of an MP system is provided in Figure 1. Obviously, the success of an MP system is highly dependent on accurate prediction of MCP synthesis and UIP of a given dietary situation.

Microbial Crude Protein Synthesis

Microbial crude protein production is an important source of MP in all beef cattle diets. Studies conducted in Arizona[68]

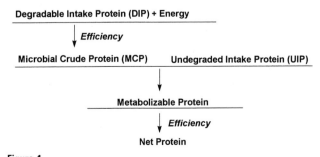

Figure 1

A metabolizable protein system.

demonstrated that at least 50% of the MP supply is derived from MCP in steers fed high-grain diets. In other diets, such as low-quality forages, MCP supplies essentially all the MP to the host animal. Therefore, the efficiency with which MCP is synthesized in the rumen is important to an MP system. The direct correlation between ruminal available energy and microbial protein synthesis has been well established and reviewed.[10, 70] Researchers in Iowa suggested that MCP synthesis was related to dietary concentration of total digestible nutrients (TDN) (0.13 × TDN)[8]; however, estimating MCP production from TDN and utilizing a standard value for bacterial efficiency can lead to an overestimation of bacterial protein production. In general, ruminal microbes derive energy from carbohydrates such as starch, cellulose, and hemicellulose. Feed ingredients such as fat supplies no energy, and protein supplies little energy to ruminal bacteria, but these ingredients are included in dietary TDN values. Additionally, fermented feeds like corn silage supply less energy to ruminal microorganisms because a portion of the carbohydrate has been fermented to organic acids. An approach to differentiate between energy available for the host animal (e.g., net energy for maintenance and gain) and energy available to ruminal microbes remains elusive, however. Estimates of ruminal carbohydrate digestion may improve the estimate of MCP synthesis from diets.

The value 13% of TDN represents a good estimate of MCP production for mixed diets typically containing greater than 50% and less than 70% of TDN. Efficiency of MCP synthesis with diets outside of this range are lower than 13% of dietary TDN, but for different reasons. Increasing the dietary TDN concentration above 70% is generally associated with high-grain diets, which reduce ruminal pH. Low ruminal pH reduces bacterial efficiency,[42, 60] resulting in a lower supply of MCP than predicted using the value of 13% suggested previously.[8] Experiments from Nebraska suggest that for a finishing diet containing 10% roughage, the efficiency for dietary TDN to be converted to MCP is 8% rather than 13%.[64] These reductions in bacterial efficiency also would reduce the DIP requirement of this high-grain diet, because DIP requirements are considered equal to MCP production.

Similar to high-grain diets, low levels of dietary TDN with lower-quality forages have resulted in lower microbial efficiencies.[19, 30] Slow rates of passage of digested material are often associated with intake of low-quality forages. Greater amounts of digestible energy are utilized for microbial maintenance, and cell lysis is increased in the ruminal environment.[60] Thus, efficiency of MCP synthesis is lower than 13% of TDN. In experiments conducted with growing steers fed low-quality forages, microbial efficiency averaged approximately 7.8% of the total-tract digestible organic matter.[19] Work conducted in Nebraska has demonstrated that the DIP requirement for gestating cows grazing winter range is 4% of the dietary organic matter.[22] This value translates into a microbial efficiency of 7.1% of the total digestible organic matter. The value obtained for cows grazing low-quality forage is similar to the values obtained from growing steers individually fed low-quality forages. Other estimates suggest that microbial efficiency ranges from 5% to 11% for beef cattle fed low-quality forages.

These differences in microbial efficiency associated with diet type, more specifically dietary TDN concentration, firmly suggest that a static efficiency value for MCP synthesis is inadequate for predicting MCP production for all segments of beef production. Workers at Cornell have proposed a model that simulates ruminal fermentation.[60] This model utilizes digestion rates for carbohydrate and protein degradation to predict microbial protein synthesis. In this approach, factors such as ruminal pH, rate of passage of digested material, and nitrogen recycling are also incorporated to predict MCP synthesis and DIP requirement. This approach corrects the limitations of using TDN and a constant bacterial efficiency in predicting MCP synthesis and subsequent MP supply. However, knowledge of digestion rates for various feedstuffs and methods to accurately define these digestion rates remain limited. The consequences of using an inaccurate value for microbial efficiency are overestimation of the MCP supply and DIP requirement and underestimation of the UIP requirement and MP supply.

Metabolizable Protein Requirements

Maintenance. Previous protein systems have included a factorial approach for predicting protein requirements.[41] Metabolic fecal, urinary, and scurf nitrogen losses were considered in the protein (nitrogen) requirement for maintenance. Distinguishing between fecal nitrogen losses associated with MCP originating from hindgut fermentation and those representing true metabolic fecal loss is problematic. Hindgut fermentation removes urea nitrogen from the blood, and this nitrogen is incorporated into MCP and excreted in the feces. Therefore, urea that would have been excreted as endogenous nitrogen in the urine is excreted in the feces. Consequently, diet digestibility influences the MP requirement. The net effect of this approach is an overestimation of the MP requirement, particularly when cattle are consuming low-quality forages because of the large amount of hindgut fermentation that is typically associated with these diets.

Nitrogen balance data suggest that the maintenance requirement for protein is 3.8 g of MP/kg of metabolic body weight (BW$^{0.75}$).[73] This estimate, derived from nitrogen balance, would include fecal, urinary, and scurf losses. Animal growth experiments have also demonstrated 3.8 g of MP/kg of BW$^{0.75}$ to be required for maintenance.[80] Calculation of the MP required for maintenance using metabolic body weight eliminates the effect of diet type and digestibility on metabolic fecal nitrogen, and subsequently the overestimation MP required for maintenance. The subcommittee on beef cattle nutrition has chosen to incorporate this change in the seventh, revised edition of *Nutrient Requirements of Beef Cattle*.[43]

Requirements for Production. The MP requirement for weight gain is based on net protein (NP) required for a given level of gain. The efficiency of MP in conversion to NP is an important component of the MP system (see Fig. 1). The National Research Council (NRC)[42] assumes that MP is converted to NP with an efficiency of 50%. Data from recent experiments suggest that the efficiency with which MP is converted to NP decreases as body weight increases.[1, 80] These data predict that 78% of MP will be converted to NP for a 50 kg steer, whereas in a 500 kg steer, an efficiency of approximately 25% would be achieved.[1] The net effect is that using these data,[1] MP requirements were doubled for the 500 kg steer, compared with the prediction using the NRC data.[42] The equation produced from these recent experiments was developed using steers weighing 300 kg or less[1, 80]; nevertheless, NRC[43] used these data to include the following equation in their latest revision:

$$\text{\% efficiency of MP to NP} = 83.4 - (0.114 \times EQEBW)$$

where *EQEBW* represents kilograms of equivalent shrunk body weight. This equation is used for animals weighing 300 kg or less; 49% of MP is considered to be converted to NP for steers weighing more than 300 kg. This value is the product of two different efficiencies. First, metabolism of protein absorbed from the small intestine is less than 100% efficient unless the MP contains an ideal mix of amino acids. It is unlikely that any diet or supplemental UIP source fed to beef cattle provides a mixture of ideal amino acids. The biologic value of the MP supplied constitutes the second component of the efficiency of MP to

NP. Undegradable intake protein sources vary in their amino acid composition and digestibility and, thus, their biologic value. Microbial crude protein has a relatively high biologic value and has a constant amino acid composition across diet types.

Metabolizable protein requirements for daily gain are based on the requirement of NP as previously discussed. The NP protein requirement for gain is based on the amount of protein deposited in the empty body (carcass) of beef animals. Protein deposition is the multiple of the rate of gain and the chemical composition of the gain. Composition of tissue gain in the carcass depends on the physiologic maturity and rate of live weight gain. It is generally well accepted within the scientific and industry communities that net energy intake above the maintenance needs of the animal (NE_g) is deposited as either protein or fat. Thus, having the ability to predict composition of gain is important in calculating the NP and subsequent MP needs of cattle. Composition of gain at a given empty body weight varies with frame size, mature size, sex, and, to some extent, breed. Previously, cattle frame score was used to predict protein requirements for these differences.[41] Models developed more recently have used a scaling approach to adjust for differences in weight at similar body composition.[43] The approach implemented in the *Nutrient Requirements of Beef Cattle*[43] uses standard reference weights for different final body compositions based on the percentage of body fat and average marbling score. In this publication, carcasses with *trace*, *slight*, and *small* amounts of marbling are considered to be 25.2%, 26.8%, and 27.8% fat, respectively, and standard reference weights of 435, 462, and 478 kg, respectively. Using these standard reference weights, the equivalent shrunk body weight can be determined for calculation of NP protein requirements. For example, a steer is predicted to achieve grade *choice* at 550 kg (final shrunk weight) and initially weighs 300 kg. Using the equations described, this steer would have an initial equivalent shrunk body weight of 261 kg [(478/550) × 300]. Assuming this steer consumes 2.25% of its body weight of a high-grain diet containing 66 Mcal/kg of NE_g, then 4.9 Mcal of energy are available for gain [(300 kg × 0.0225)/0.66]. The predicted weight gain for this steer would be 1.34 kg/day ($13.91 × 4.9^{0.9116} × 255^{-0.6837}$).[43] The NP calculated for the initial equivalent shrunk body weight of the steer is 160 g/day [NP = 268 − (29.4 × [4.9/1.34])], where NP = 268 − (29.4 × [retained energy/weight gain]).[43] The NP requirement (160 g/day) is now divided by the efficiency of conversion of MP to NP for this equivalent body weight, which is 54% (determined from the preceding equation). This value of MP required for gain [286 g/day; (160/0.54)] is added to the MP required for maintenance (274 g/day). Thus, the total daily intake of MP required for this steer weighing 300 kg is approximately 560 g/day. By using equivalent shrunk body weight and standard reference weight, the need for MP is adjusted for differences in frame, sex, and mature weights for the current weight of the animal. With this approach adopted by the *Nutrient Requirements of Beef Cattle*,[43] the requirement for MP for any given body size can quickly and easily be determined.

PROTEIN SUPPLEMENTATION STRATEGIES IN BEEF CATTLE DIETS

Once animal requirements have been established for a given level of production, it is important to have useful information on protein sources that are available for incorporation into diets. With the exception of vitamins, minerals, and some other unique ingredients, all feedstuffs contain some level of protein. The most common method of measuring the protein in feedstuffs is to determine the nitrogen concentration and multiply this by 6.25 to arrive at crude protein (CP). With the use of more sophisticated protein models, the value of knowing the

CP concentration has decreased. With MP models, knowledge of the amount of protein degraded in the rumen and that escaping ruminal degradation is much more useful information. Using the principals of an MP system, the remaining discussion concentrates on the usefulness of common protein supplements in beef cattle diets.

Nonprotein Nitrogen in Finishing Diets

Feedlot Performance and Dietary Urea Concentration. Because of its low cost and ease of incorporation into finishing diets, urea is the predominant source of non-protein nitrogen utilized in finishing diets. Feed grade urea typically contains 45% nitrogen (dry matter [DM] basis), and therefore dietary protein concentrations can be increased with minimal displacement of grain in finishing diets. Urea can satisfy the ruminal DIP requirement as ammonia and subsequently provide MP as MCP.

Numerous experiments have evaluated the use of urea in high-grain diets; however, most have compared urea to natural, degradable protein sources, making interpretation of the optimal concentration in finishing diets difficult to determine. Early reviews suggested that urea can be effectively utilized if it is not more than one third of the total supplemental protein or 1% of dietary DM.[55, 69] These estimates have little empirical data to support them, and finishing diets utilized today are considerably different than those used to derive these estimates of maximal urea supplementation. In addition, these estimates give little consideration to the amount of urea required to satisfy the nitrogen (DIP) requirement associated with ruminal fermentation.

Researchers at Iowa State[8] provided a model to predict the optimal dietary urea concentration based on dietary TDN and DIP content. The term *urea fermentation potential* (UFP) was used to describe this model and was calculated as:

$$UFP = (0.1044 × TDN − RDEGP)/2.8$$

where *RDEGP* is the amount of ruminal degradable protein of the basal diet before urea supplementation, and TDN is expressed as a percentage. Other experiments have utilized a regression approach based on ruminal ammonia and dietary TDN concentrations to predict the usefulness of NPN in various diets.[56] However, both the UFP system[8] and the relationships established by regression[56] have little empirical data for their support.

Improvements in average daily gain (ADG) or gain efficiency (average daily gain/feed intake, or G/F) were not evident when dietary urea was increased above 0.7% of the dietary DM in steers fed a medium-energy growing-finishing diet.[74] Performance was maximized with a dietary urea concentration below that predicted by the UFP system (1.0% DM basis).[8] Likewise, no improvements in steer performance were noted when urea was used to increase the dietary CP concentration above 11% in finishing diets based on dry-rolled corn.[6] Recent experiments conducted in Iowa observed no improvement in ADG or G/F when the dietary urea concentration was increased from 1.04% to 1.97% of the dietary DM for steers fed diets based on dry-rolled corn; concentrations of urea below 1.04% were not included in this study.[78] Results from experiments designed to evaluate increasing dietary concentrations of urea indicated that the dietary urea concentration required for maximal feedlot performance was near 0.9% of the dietary DM in dry-rolled corn–based finishing diets.[37, 64] In those experiments, the UFP system predicted that the dietary urea concentration required to obtain maximal performance was greater than 1.5% of the dietary DM. Clearly, the UFP system overestimated the optimal dietary urea content in these studies. This overprediction of optimal urea level probably is related to the oversimplification of the relationships among dietary TDN concentration, MCP synthesis, and microbial efficiency, as discussed previously. In addition, the UFP system does not account for recycling of nitrogen into the ruminal ammonia pool. With steers fed low-protein diets, approximately 40% of microbial nitrogen was derived from nitrogen that had been recycled back to the rumen.[7]

Using the model provided by NRC,[43] Milton and coworkers[37] determined that the MP requirement of steers in their experiment was met by the diet containing no supplemental urea (control diet). This was a result of the high ruminal escape of corn proteins (65%) in that diet.[42] Although the predicted MP requirement was satisfied by the control diet, both ADG and G/F were enhanced by the addition of 0.9% urea to the diet, suggesting that the DIP requirement must be satisfied even though MP requirements were satisfied or in excess. In their experiment, the DIP requirement was near 6.7% of the dietary DM (1.07% nitrogen [N]). This requirement for DIP was near that determined in experiments conducted in Nebraska (6.8%).[64] Studies in which steam-flaked corn and steam-flaked barley are fed have also evaluated the usefulness of urea in finishing diets.[84] Assuming that steam-flaked corn contains 65% and barley contains 40% ruminal escape protein, the DIP requirements were near 7.0% and 6.0% percent of the dietary DM, respectively, for these diets. The model developed by NRC[43] predicts similar dietary urea concentrations to satisfy the DIP requirements for the diets fed in these experiments.

Microbial Protein Synthesis and Ruminal Fermentation. In typical feedlot diets, much of the MP supply (usually greater than 50%) is derived from MCP exiting the rumen.[43, 68, 80] Therefore, identifying the appropriate dietary urea concentration to maximize MCP synthesis is necessary. In addition, ruminal microorganisms require nitrogen in the form of ammonia or amino acids and peptides, or both, for optimal fermentation of energy-yielding substrates.[60] Flows of MCP to the small intestine were maximized when the dietary urea concentration reached approximately 1.1% of the dietary DM, but increases in ruminal ammonia concentrations were evident only when urea exceeded this level in low and medium energy density diets.[25, 67] Increasing the dietary urea concentration above that which provided maximal MCP production would result in reduced ruminal nitrogen efficiency and, subsequently, wastage of nitrogen and increased cost with no benefit to the host animal.[56, 62]

In contrast, increases in MCP synthesis have not been evident with urea supplementation of high-grain diets based on dry-rolled corn[37] or steam-flaked corn.[84] In finishing steers fed steam-flaked barley–based diets, 0.4% dietary urea produced a significant increase in the MCP flow to the small intestine.[84] This improvement only resulted in a 6 g/day increase in MCP flow, however, compared with the basal diet, which contained no supplemental nitrogen. In the companion feedlot experiments accompanying these metabolism studies, performance was maximized by the addition of 0.8% urea (DM basis) to the diet.[37, 84] The experiments reviewed suggest that improvements in performance associated with urea supplementation of high-grain diets are not fully explained by increased MCP production and MP supply. Lack of increased MCP synthesis with urea supplementation of high-grain diets may be related to nitrogen recycling when cattle are fed highly fermentable diets.[27] Additionally, a deficiency of amino acids or peptides, or both, available to the rumen microorganisms may limit microbial growth because of the high ruminal escape protein fractions associated with most feed grains[58]; this hypothesis will be discussed later. More importantly, the usefulness of urea in high-grain finishing diets is most likely associated with increased energy availability to the animal by increasing ruminal digestion of starch and organic matter and not increased MCP flow to the small intestine.

Nutritional dogma from several years in the past considers the usefulness of urea in finishing diets to be that urea-nitrogen is incorporated into MCP and subsequently meets the host animals protein needs. In experiments conducted at Roulette Institute of Research, urea enhanced ruminal fermentation of organic matter in lambs fed diets based on rolled-barley.[36, 46, 47] In experiments conducted using duodenally fistulated steers, dietary urea supplementation up to 1.0% increased ruminal and total tract digestion of organic matter and starch.[37, 84] Microbial protein production was not increased by urea supplementation in these studies.[37, 84]

Ruminal metabolism experiments provide additional support to the argument that urea enhances energy utilization in high-grain diets. In steers fed dry-rolled corn–based diets, total volatile fatty acid concentrations increased as the dietary urea level increased from 0 to 1.5% of the dietary dry matter.[37] Additionally, molar proportions of acetate and predicted methane production were 9% and 17% lower, respectively, for steers fed diets supplemented with 1.2% urea compared to those supplemented with 0.8% or 1.6% urea.[84] The concentration of ruminal ammonia necessary for maximal MCP synthesis has been estimated to be 1.6 mmol/L. However, increasing the ruminal ammonia concentration above 1.6 mmol/L numerically enhanced total VFA production.[67] These responses in ruminal digestion of starch and in animal performance challenge the theory that ruminal ammonia concentrations above those required for maximal MCP synthesis are of little benefit in high-grain diets.

Urea can be used effectively to meet the ruminal DIP requirement of cattle fed high-grain diets. However, MCP synthesis is probably not increased when urea-nitrogen is the sole source of supplemental protein in high-grain finishing diets. Increases in cattle performance with urea supplementation most likely are responses to enhanced ruminal fermentation (increased energy utilization) and not increased MP supply. The optimal concentration of urea for diets based on dry-rolled or steam-flaked corn is near 1.0% of the dietary dry matter. Grain sources such as barley, wheat, and high-moisture corn may reduce the amount of urea needed to meet the DIP requirement. The protein fraction of these grain sources has a higher ruminal degradability, thus reducing the need for supplemental DIP.

Natural Protein Supplementation of Finishing Cattle

Natural protein supplements contain both ruminally degradable and escape protein fractions. Like urea supplementation, the ruminally degradable fraction can supply ammonia to the microbial population. Unlike urea, the ruminal degradable protein fraction of natural proteins also can supply a source of amino acids, peptides, and other nutrients ("growth factors") to the microbial population. The ruminal degradability of these natural protein sources varies based on natural characteristics of the protein and processing conditions, such as heat. Natural protein sources are generally classified as high or low ruminal escape protein sources. Protein sources arising from oil seed production, like soybean meal and cottonseed meal, are extensively degraded in the rumen, whereas those arising from corn milling industries that are dried by heat (e.g., corn gluten meal) and animal byproducts that are heated during processing (e.g., blood meal, meat and bone meal, and fish meal) are typically classified as high ruminal escape proteins.

Degradable True Protein Supplementation

Feedlot Performance. Supplementation of high-grain diets with degradable true protein sources has been shown to increase the rate or efficiency, or both, of gain relative to supplementation with only urea (Table 1). The summary given in Table 1 does not include a complete listing of experiments evaluating the effects of urea or degradable true protein on feedlot performance, but includes those studies that evaluated urea or degradable true protein at equal dietary protein concentrations. Most of the experiments listed in Table 1 involved diets based on dry-rolled corn, which constituted 80% or more of the dietary DM, and diets were fed for an average of 96 days across all experiments.

Averaged across experiments, daily gains increased 7.6%, daily dry matter intake increased 2.73%, and gain efficiency was enhanced 4.0% for cattle fed diets supplemented with degradable true protein (soybean meal) relative to those fed urea-supplemented diets at equal dietary protein concentrations. Advantages for soybean meal supplementation in daily gain ranged from −8.9% to +20.5% and in conversion efficiency from −10.0% to +16.6% for diets containing less than 15% dietary CP. More consistent was the increase in dry matter intake when diets were supplemented with soybean meal as compared with urea.

In studies that provided interim data (divided into the first and second half of the feeding period), supplementing high-grain diets with soybean meal significantly[38, 53, 74] or numerically[6, 35] improved both ADG and G/F during the initial phase of the feeding period relative to urea supplementation. Further, rate and efficiency was enhanced by soybean meal supplementation during the final phase of the feeding period.[35, 38]

Because of the high cost of degradable true protein sources relative to that of urea, other experiments have directed efforts toward supplementing high-grain diets with a combination of urea and degradable protein. In experiments conducted in Iowa, dietary CP concentrations were increased from 11.5% (1.04% urea) to 14.0% by replacing urea and dry-rolled corn with soybean meal at 5.6% or 10% (DM basis).[78] Daily gains of steers fed soybean meal at 5.6% or 10% of the dietary DM (both diets, 14% CP) were 5.6% and 8.5% higher, respectively, than those of steers fed no soybean meal. Gain efficiency increased 6.4% with the addition of 5.6% soybean meal relative to the diet containing 1.04% urea, but no further advantage was noted for increasing soybean meal supplementation to 10% of dietary DM. Feeding higher levels of soybean meal may have reduced the energy density of the diet. Steers fed steam-flaked corn–based diets containing 13% CP and supplemented by a combination of urea and soybean meal gained faster and were more efficient than those supplemented with urea or soybean meal alone; the mix of supplemental nitrogen that provided optimal performance was 33% soybean meal and 67% urea (N basis).[20] Other experiments conducted in South Dakota reported that responses to supplementing finishing diets based on dry-rolled corn with a 50:50 blend (N basis) of urea and soybean meal were intermediate compared with response to diets supplemented with urea or soybean meal alone.[53]

Carcass characteristics, other than carcass weight, are rarely changed to any great extent when the diets of finishing cattle are supplemented with urea, soybean meal, or a combination of the two. Consistently, carcass weights were increased, in response to more rapid gains, when the diets of finishing cattle were supplemented with soybean meal or a combination of urea and soybean meal, compared with supplementation with urea alone. This confirms that the increases in ADG attributed to degradable protein supplementation are not associated with digestive tract fill, but rather with increases in tissue gain.

The reviewed performance experiments substantiate the response to degradable true protein sources in high-grain finishing diets. It can be concluded that feedlot performance can be enhanced by supplementation with soybean meal alone or a combination of urea and soybean meal compared with supple-

Table 1
EFFECT OF UREA OR DEGRADABLE, TRUE PROTEIN SUPPLEMENTATION ON DAILY GAINS AND CONVERSION EFFICIENCY OF CATTLE CONSUMING HIGH-GRAIN FINISHING DIETS

| Reference | Dietary CP, % | Feedlot Performance | | | | Degradable, True Protein, % Different From Urea | | |
| | | Urea | | True Protein | | | | |
		ADG	G/F	ADG	G/F	ADG	DMI	G/F
6	11.0	1.45	.20	1.32	.18	− 8.9	+ 2.7	− 10.0
	13.0	1.43	.20	1.48	.20	+ 3.5	+ 2.7	0
	15.0	1.23	.20	1.40	.21	+ 13.8	+ 6.4	+ 5.0
	17.0	1.29	.19	1.58	.22	+ 22.5	+ 4.4	+ 15.8
63	10.7	1.36	.108	1.64	.126	+ 20.5	+ 3.2	+ 16.6
82	11.0	1.00	.106	1.10	.103	+ 10.0	+ .9	− 2.8
51	10.5	1.51	.128	1.61	.134	+ 6.6	+ 2.2	+ 4.6
35	—	1.49	.154	1.56	.162	+ 4.7	− 1.4	+ 5.2
74	10.8	1.29	.135	1.47	.145	+ 13.9	+ 6.3	+ 7.4
66								
Calves (207 DOF)	12.5	1.39	.161	1.36	.150	− 2.2	+ 3.0	− 7.3
Yearlings (164 DOF)	12.5	1.42	.144	1.54	.151	+ 8.5	+ 3.0	+ 4.8
52	11.3	1.93	.187	2.05	.197	+ 6.2	+ .3	+ 5.3
53	12.0	1.90	.188	1.99	.193	+ 4.7	+ 2.1	+ 2.7
	13.0	1.92	.193	2.02	.198	+ 5.2	+ 2.1	+ 2.6
84	11.5	1.39	.188	1.41	.190	+ 1.4	+ .7	+ 1.1
38	11.5	1.25	.128	1.36	.139	+ 1.1	+ 0.5	+ 8.6
	13.5	1.24	.133	1.46	.145	+ 17.4	+ 6.7	+ 9.0
Average response to degradable, true protein						+ 7.6	+ 2.7	+ 4.0

ADG, average daily gain in kg/day; G/F, gain/feed; DMI, dry matter intake; DOF, days on feed; CP, crude protein.

mentation with urea only. The most economical approach often is a combination of urea and a degradable protein source.

Degradable True Protein

Nitrogen Flow to the Small Intestine and Nutrient Digestion. Research has demonstrated that certain ruminal microbes may prefer amino acids or peptides to ammonia as a nitrogen source, particularly those microbes involved in the fermentation of nonstructural carbohydrates.[58] Because typical feed grains (corn and grain sorghum) contain proteins that are largely resistant to ruminal degradation, supplying degradable true proteins to high-grain diets may benefit both MCP production and the fermentation of starch and organic matter.

In general, flows of non-ammonia nitrogen to the small intestine are increased with the provision of degradable true proteins in high-grain diets. Typically, flows of MCP account for approximately 40% to 50% of this increase in non-ammonia nitrogen flow. Steers consuming dry-rolled corn–based diets supplemented with soybean meal had 14% greater flows of MCP compared with those consuming diets supplemented with urea only.[15] In addition, MCP synthesis was stimulated when cottonseed meal or dehydrated alfalfa meal was added to dry-rolled corn diets containing urea.[85] These responses would suggest that microbial protein synthesis can be enhanced by providing protein sources susceptible to ruminal degradation in high-grain diets and that this response is not limited to soybean meal only.

Evidence supports the conclusion that peptides and amino acids rather than "unidentified growth factors" are largely responsible for increases in MCP synthesis. In vitro[31, 32, 33, 58] and continuous culture experiments[2, 18] have demonstrated enhanced microbial growth with the addition of amino acids and peptides to mixed rumen bacteria cultures with ammonia as the sole nitrogen source. Further, microbial growth was higher with the addition of 10 mg/L of peptides than the corresponding amount of free amino acids.[2] When adequate carbohydrates are available for production of ATP, as with cattle fed high-grain diets, a larger portion of amino acids transported into the cell can be directly incorporated in MCP.[59] Further, when amino acids are incorporated into MCP, it is necessary that all amino acids be available for protein synthesis to occur.[2] There is still debate as to whether starch-fermenting bacteria prefer amino acids or peptides as their nitrogen source.

From the previous discussion, it is apparent that supplementation of high-grain diets with degradable protein increases both MCP and feed protein flows to the small intestine in feedlot cattle relative to urea supplementation only. Metabolizable protein models[8, 43] typically predict that the MP requirement is met or often exceeded with typical dry matter intakes of cattle consuming high-grain diets. Assuming that these predictions are correct, increases in MP supply associated with degradable protein supplementation may not explain increased feedlot performance, particularly those improvements that take place during the latter phase of the finishing period, when predicted MP requirements are considerably less than predicted MP intakes. It has been suggested that degradable protein (amino acids and peptides) is necessary for optimal fermentation of high-starch diets.[77] Total-tract starch digestibility in cattle was increased by the addition of degradable true protein to a high-grain diet.[61, 79] The addition of 10% (DM basis) cottonseed meal to diets based on dry-rolled or steam-flaked corn already containing 0.8% urea reduced fecal starch concentrations by 35% in finishing heifers.[3] A typical explanation for the improvement in total tract starch digestion is a reduction in total starch intake. Assuming that dry matter intake was similar across grain sources for urea- or cottonseed meal–supplemented diets, it seems unlikely that a 10% replacement of the grain source with cottonseed meal

would translate into a 35% reduction in fecal starch concentrations. Furthermore, heifer diets supplemented with additional cottonseed meal were 6.5% more efficient than those supplemented with only urea. These data provide additional support to the hypothesis that degradable true protein is required for optimal utilization of high-starch diets.

The digestive site responsible for these improvements in starch digestion could not be determined from the previous experiments. Including fish meal in diets based on dry-rolled corn already containing urea to supply 0%, 25%, 50%, or 75% of the supplemental protein increased ruminal digestion of starch 19% and total tract starch digestion 6.2% with the first increment of fish meal.[72] These data suggest that peptides or amino acids liberated from the degradable fraction of fish meal enhanced ruminal fermentation of starch.

Ruminal Escape Protein Supplementation on Feedlot Performance

Supplementation of high-grain diets with degradable true protein enhances daily dry matter intake, daily gain, and gain efficiency of feedlot cattle (see Table 1). Because these protein sources contain both degradable and escape protein fractions, it becomes difficult to determine whether performance responses are associated with increased MP supply (both MCP production and feed protein escape) or whether degradable protein sources enhance fermentation and subsequent energy supply to the host animal. In addition, improvements in genetics, nutritional management, growth stimulants, and feed additives have increased daily gain of cattle in the feedlot during the past several years. Based on the hypothesis that cattle requirements for protein have increased, many researchers have evaluated higher MP supplies in finishing diets.

Several protein sources are reported to have a high degree of ruminal escape protein, including blood meal (82%), corn gluten meal (86%), fish meal (68%), feather meal (69%), meat and bone meal (70%), brewer's dried grains (61%), and distiller's grains (68%). Protein sources such as these, when used on combination with urea to supply ruminal ammonia, offer a means of increasing the MP supply to cattle. Studies conducted using ruminal escape protein sources in combination with urea have demonstrated their usefulness in increasing the nonbacterial protein flowing into the small intestine relative to diets supplemented with degradable protein.[9, 75] Protein supplementation programs using ruminal escape protein and urea can be provided to ruminants at a cost lower than that of diets containing degradable protein.[28] This economic difference is a result of most ruminal escape protein sources containing a much greater protein concentration than typical degradable protein sources (e.g., blood meal, 90% CP, versus soybean meal, 54% CP).

Performance responses of cattle consuming high-grain diets supplemented with ruminal escape protein sources are summarized in Table 2. Comparisons between rumen degradable and escape protein sources are summarized also.

Supplementation of high-grain diets with a combination of blood, meat and bone, and feather meals significantly increased the rate and efficiency of gain in one experiment.[86] However, the lightweight steers (198 kg initial body weight) were fed experimental diets for only 84 days. In all other experiments, cattle fed diets supplemented with ruminal escape protein provided little if any improvement in feedlot performance relative to those fed diets supplemented with urea alone. Predominantly, studies feeding low protein diets based on corn cobs have demonstrated a beneficial response to ruminal escape protein relative to urea or degradable true protein supplementation in growing steers.[16, 17, 71] Because supplementing high-grain diets with rumi-

Table 2
EFFECT OF RUMINAL ESCAPE PROTEIN ON FEEDLOT PERFORMANCE IN CATTLE FED HIGH-GRAIN DIETS

Reference	Supplemental Protein	ADG, kg/Day	SEM	Gain/Feed or Feed/ Gain	SEM
65	Urea only	1.54	.03	.170	.003
	Urea + BM:FTM	1.58		.176	
66	Urea only	1.42	.05	.144	.006
	SBM only	1.53		.151	
	Urea + BM	1.49		.151	
	Urea + FTM	1.50		.153	
86	Urea only	1.34	.09	5.10	.25
(1993), light-weight calves (84 DOF)	Urea + BM, MBM, and FTH	1.52		4.99	
52	Urea only	1.89	.04	5.20	.09
	Urea + SBM	1.93		5.13	
	Urea + BM:CGM	1.89		4.98	
76	Urea only	2.01	.12	5.14	.12
	Urea + BM:CGM	2.02		5.06	
	Urea + SBM	2.17		4.90	
53	Urea only	1.92	—	.193	—
	Urea + BM:FTH	1.93		.193	
	SBM only	2.02		.198	
39	Urea only	1.69	.05	.146	.003
	Urea + BM:CGM	1.68		.151	
	Urea + SBM	1.76		.156	
	SBM only	1.72		.158	
	SBM + BM:CGM	1.68		.152	
	SBM + SBM	1.72		.160	

SBM, soybean meal; BM, blood meal; MBM, meat and bone meal; FTH, feather meal; CGM, corn gluten meal; ADG, average daily gain; SEM, standard error of the mean; DOF, days on feed.

nal escape proteins rarely results in a performance advantage above urea supplementation alone, it can be concluded that the combination of MCP production and ruminal escape of grain proteins is adequate to satisfy the MP requirements of finishing cattle.

Some experiments (summarized in Table 2) also demonstrated that supplementing high-grain diets with a combination of urea and soybean meal or soybean meal alone enhanced both ADG and G/F relative to both the combination of urea plus ruminal escape proteins and urea only supplementation.[39, 53, 76] These responses provide further evidence that a source of degradable true protein is required to optimize fermentation (energy utilization) of high-grain diets.

Basal Diet and Supplemental Nitrogen Interactions

Dietary Roughage Source. Roughage sources vary in their dietary nitrogen concentration and ruminal degradability and, therefore, may alter the response to supplemental nitrogen in high-grain diets. Assuming a steer consumes 10 kg of feed daily that contains 10% of either alfalfa or prairie hay, the hay intake would be 1 kg/day. If alfalfa hay contained 2.9% nitrogen that was 72% rumen-degradable, then the roughage source would provide 21 g of nitrogen to the microbial population. If prairie hay contained 0.8% nitrogen that was 50% rumen-degradable, then the roughage source would provide only 4 g of nitrogen to the microbial population. It seems reasonable to consider that the dietary roughage source has the potential to alter the dietary level of non-protein nitrogen needed to satisfy DIP requirements. Additionally, the degradable nitrogen fraction of

roughage sources like alfalfa hay can also supply peptides and amino acids to ruminal bacteria.

Dietary Grain Source. The dietary grain sources provided approximately 65% to 75% of the dietary protein in finishing diets.[28] Grain proteins differ in their physical structure (e.g., corn versus wheat) and can be altered by processing conditions that utilize heat (e.g., steam flaking); therefore, the ruminal escape of protein differs among grain sources. Without consideration of heat processing, grain sources commonly utilized in finishing diets can be ranked by the proportion of ruminal escape protein as: grain sorghum > corn >> high-moisture corn > barley ≥ wheat. Studies directly comparing the interaction between grain source or processing method and supplemental protein strategy are limited. Responses to degradable protein (soybean or cottonseed meals) supplementation were of greater magnitude in steers fed high-moisture corn than in those fed steam-flaked or whole shelled corn diets.[34] When steers were fed high-moisture corn, ruminal escape protein supplementation tended to increase gain efficiency (10.4% improvement), whereas gain efficiency for steers fed dry-rolled corn was the same between protein sources.[65] In addition, increased rate and efficiency of gain in steers fed barley-based finishing diets were observed when diets were supplemented with a combination of animal byproduct proteins.[44] Experiments to examine the interactions between basal diet ingredients and supplemental protein sources are needed to further optimize supplementation programs for finishing cattle.

SUPPLEMENTATION OF LOW-QUALITY FORAGE DIETS

In many phases of beef production, low-quality forage is the predominant energy source available to grazing beef animals. In particular, the beef cow is required to utilize low-quality forage for 3 to 6 months of each year, depending on location. These forages are high in cell wall content and deficient in protein. In general, protein concentrations are typically below 7% of the dietary dry matter in these low-quality forages.[12] Forages containing greater than 7% to 9% (DM basis) protein usually supply enough protein to meet the requirements of the mature cows grazing them. However, for growing beef animals, such as steers or first-calf heifers, the protein concentration of these forages may not meet requirements. The discussion of this section is limited to low-quality forages.

Energy supplementation of beef cows consuming low-quality forage has been ineffective in improving the energy status of the animal.[34] This information provides additional support that protein is the first limiting nutrient in beef cattle consuming low-quality forages. Protein supplementation appears to both satisfy the MP need and increase the energy status of the animal. This increase in energy status is accomplished by two mechanisms. First, increased forage intake and digestion are common when supplemental protein is fed with low-quality diets, compared with nonsupplemented control diets. The second possible mechanism is enhanced utilization of metabolizable energy. Providing supplemental protein to beef cattle consuming low-quality forage has proven the be an economical approach to improve forage utilization and, subsequently, animal performance.

Degradable intake protein is the protein fraction generally viewed as the first limiting nutrient in low-quality forage diets. Once the DIP requirement is satisfied, synthesis of MCP can meet the MP needs of mature cows. Validation that the DIP fraction of protein that is first limiting is provided by researchers in Kansas.[24] Pregnant cows were offered supplements containing high, moderate, or low levels of UIP, while DIP concentration was constant across the three diets. Providing additional protein in the form of UIP did not increase calf birth weight or decrease the cow weight loss over the supplementation period. For growing beef animals, additional MP in the form of UIP may have to be supplied to support weight gain. In general, performance expectations are low if low-quality forages is the primary feedstuff in the diets of growing beef animals or first-calf heifers. In these situations, both energy and protein are supplemented to satisfy animal requirements to achieve higher levels of performance.

Supplementation of the diets of beef cattle under range conditions can be costly. Since DIP is in most cases the first limiting nutrient, the level and source of DIP needed to meet DIP requirement is economically important. Experiments have demonstrated that forage intake and digestion are maximized when DIP intake reaches approximately 4 g/kg of metabolic body weight.[29] By expressing this value as a percentage of the digestible forage intake, the DIP requirement can now be estimated as a percentage of the total digestible organic matter in the diet. In the previous experiment, the percentage of digestible organic matter intake was measured to be 36%.[29] Therefore, the DIP requirement would be approximately 11% of the total digestible intake [(4/36) × 100 = 11%]. This value agrees closely with that calculated from a large database using forages less than 7% CP.[12] This relationship suggests that the DIP requirement needed in the supplement changes as forage intake, digestibility, and DIP concentration of the forage change. If a forage contains 60% digestible organic matter, then the supplement would need to contain approximately 5.9% DIP on a dry matter basis. Conversely, if a forage contains 40% digestible organic matter, then the supplement would need to contain 3.9% DIP on a dry matter basis. These estimates are calculated in the following manner: 60 × 0.11 × 0.90 = 5.9, where 60 = organic matter digestibility of the forage, 0.11 = DIP requirement expressed as a percentage of the digestible organic matter, and 0.90 assumes the forage contains 90% organic matter (10% ash). By using these equations, the amount of a given protein supplement required to meet the animal's need can be calculated. For example, cows consume about 1.8% of their body weight in low-quality forage when digestibilities are between 50% and 60%. Therefore, a cow weighing 1100 pounds will consume approximately 20 pounds of dry forage. If the digestibility of the forage is 50%, then the digestible dry matter intake is 10 pounds daily. Based on the previous method of determining the DIP requirement, this cow would need approximately 1.1 pounds of DIP to maximize utilization of this forage (10 × 0.11). If the protein supplement being used was soybean meal, which contains 54% protein on a dry matter basis, and 80% of the protein is in the form of DIP, then this cow would require 2.6 pounds of soybean meal (DM basis) daily to meet the DIP requirement. This amount is calculated as 1.1/0.54 = 2.04; 2.04/0.80, where 1.1 is the pounds of DIP required, 0.54 is the percentage of protein in soybean meal, and 0.80 is the proportion of soybean meal that is degraded in the rumen. This method of determining the supplement amount to meet the DIP requirement for beef cattle consuming low-quality forage is valid for any protein supplement in which the total protein concentration and the proportion of that protein concentration degraded in the rumen are known.

Use of Nonprotein Nitrogen in Low-Quality Forage Diets

Similar to the scenario with growing and finishing diets, economics are responsible for the use of nonprotein nitrogen (NPN) as a source of DIP in supplements for beef cattle consuming low-quality forages. All sources of DIP are degraded largely to ammonia in the rumen before incorporation into MCP. Thus, it seems logical to consider that NPN can be an effective DIP source in low-quality forage diets as well.

Urea and biuret are two common sources of NPN used in supplementation strategies for beef cattle consuming low-quality forages. Similar in nitrogen concentration, the rate of hydrolysis of biuret to ammonia in the rumen is slower than that of urea. Both urea and biuret contain about five to seven times the concentration of nitrogen than commonly used degradable protein sources of plant origin (e.g., soybean meal). However, in addition to supplying DIP, plant protein sources also supply energy, vitamins, and minerals. Because neither urea or biuret contain these other nutrients, they need to be considered in the evaluation of supplements containing NPN sources.[49] Of great importance is the sulfur concentration of the supplement when NPN sources are utilized. Sulfur is necessary for synthesis of microbial protein, specifically for the synthesis of the amino acids methionine and cystine. Data from Australia[23] suggest that the dietary nitrogen-to-sulfur ratio needs to be 10:1 to avoid limitations in MCP synthesis. As in high-grain diets, NPN supplementation will be of little benefit unless the ammonia is converted into MCP.[56]

Because NPN-based supplements influence the energy status of the animal, their effect on forage intake and digestion becomes important. As observed with supplements containing degradable true protein, supplements containing NPN also stimulate intake and digestibility of low-quality forages. Forage intake increased 34% compared with animals receiving no supplemental DIP when urea was used as the supplemental DIP source.[40] Additionally, experiments comparing NPN supplementation with nonsupplemented control diets suggest that forage digestibility increased an average of 15% (range, 4.5–55%).[29] Likewise, MCP synthesis and efficiency of MCP synthesis (grams of microbial nitrogen per kilogram of fermented organic matter) is also increased with NPN supplementation, as compared with nonsupplemented control diets.[29] This increase in digestion and subsequent increase in forage intake would enhance the energy status of beef cattle consuming low-quality forages. The increase in MCP supply, from the increased fermentation of forage, will now satisfy the animal's requirement for MP.

The previous discussion demonstrates the usefulness of NPN in terms of digestion and MCP synthesis. From these metabolism experiments, it is apparent that NPN may be fed as the only DIP source or at least supply a portion of the DIP in the supplement. However, the performance of beef cattle grazing low-quality forage provides more meaningful data to production situations. In general, supplements containing only NPN will decrease body weight losses compared with no supplemental protein. Most experiments have evaluated replacement of plant protein sources with NPN. In these trials, the performance of beef cows whose diets are supplemented with NPN typically lags behind that of cows whose diets are supplemented with only degradable true protein sources when supplements are formulated to contain similar levels of CP.[50, 57] These differences in performance typically include increased body weight and body condition losses with NPN compared with all natural protein supplementation. Data concerning pregnancy rate are limited. Pregnancy rate of mature cows and first-calf heifers were shown to be reduced by approximately 10 percentage units when NPN replaced protein sources of plant origin in the supplements[14]; however, this decline was not statistically significant. Other experiments recently conducted in Kansas report no negative impact on pregnancy rate when urea supplied up to 40% of the DIP in supplements.[29] Although some differences exist in cow weight loss, calf daily gains and weaning weights are not different between cows whose diets are supplemented with NPN and those whose diets are supplemented with natural protein. An optimum ratio of NPN and true protein most likely exists for supplementation programs of cattle consuming low-quality forage. That ratio remains elusive based on performance data with mature cows.

In agreement with studies conducted with mature cows, weight gains of growing cattle are generally greater with true protein sources than NPN when they consume low-quality forage.[11, 45, 54] Some fraction of all true protein sources escapes ruminal degradation, however. Thus, the MP supply may be enhanced by an increase in both MCP synthesis and greater amount of UIP when supplements contain true protein rather than NPN. This increase in UIP supply explains a portion of the improved performance of growing cattle. Mature cows have a low MP requirement because little net tissue gain is deposited as protein. Conversely, a large amount of tissue gain is in the form of protein in growing cattle that consume low-quality forage.

Nonprotein Nitrogen Toxicity and Acceptability

Large amounts of NPN can be toxic when ingested during a short period of time.[21] Experiments conducted in Kansas demonstrated that cattle dosed with 0.5 g of urea/kg of body weight showed signs of urea toxicity.[4] The symptoms of urea toxicity include restlessness, dullness, muscle tremors, frequent urination, rapid respiration, tetany, and eventually death if untreated. A common treatment is to drench the animal with acetic acid. Addition of acid to the rumen contents supplies hydrogen ions, which bind free ammonia. Ammonia readily diffuses across the ruminal wall, but when sufficient hydrogen ions are present for NH_4, the absorption of ammonia across the ruminal wall greatly decreases. Thus, free ammonia (NH_3) is the toxic form of urea in cases of overconsumption. The incidence of urea toxicity is therefore closely related to the amount of carbohydrate available for ruminal fermentation. Cattle consuming high-grain diets most likely will never experience urea toxicity under normal feeding conditions. Additionally, with cattle consuming low-quality forage, grain, grain byproducts, and molasses are often carriers of the urea and other supplemental nutrients. These carriers contain carbohydrate that is rapidly fermented in the rumen, and thus aids in the prevention of urea toxicity. Other compounds like phosphoric acid added to liquid supplements not only prevent overconsumption but aid in slowing the absorption of free ammonia across the ruminal wall. Problems with urea toxicity are generally not a concern with normal supplementation strategies for cattle consuming low-quality forage.

An item of concern is the acceptability of NPN-based supplements in grazing cattle. Because supplements are fed at low level, NPN concentrations can become relatively high (10% to 20% of supplement DM). Regardless of how well NPN satisfies the DIP requirement, if animals refuse to consume appropriate amounts of supplement, the inclusion of NPN has little value. Palatability experiments have demonstrated a decline in supplement intake with increased urea concentration.[48] Some researchers have suggested that because of the low acceptability of urea, the upper limits of inclusion are approximately 30% to 40% of the supplemental protein.[13] However, improvements in supplement technology, such as pressed blocks and liquids, may eliminate the concerns with acceptability of high NPN range supplements.

Frequency of Supplementation

Delivering supplements to beef cattle in range situations is an expensive process with respect to time, labor, and equipment. In many cases, several miles are traveled daily to deliver supplements. If the frequency of supplementation could be reduced without negative impacts on animal performance, reduced labor and equipment cost may enhance profitability. Experiments conducted in Kansas have evaluated supplementing cows daily or three times weekly.[5] Supplements contained 20% protein and consisted of 74% grain, 23% soybean meal, and 3% molasses (DM basis). Cows fed supplements three times weekly lost more weight by calving time than those supplemented daily, but this total difference in weight loss was only 24 pounds and was not a large difference from a biologic standpoint, which was reinforced by the lack of change in body condition score during the supplementation period. The ability of ruminants to conserve nitrogen via nitrogen recycling back to the rumen allows for these types of supplementation strategies. More recent experiments evaluated supplementation frequency when urea constituted 30% of the total protein concentration of the supplements.[81] Intake of low-quality forage was unaffected by supplementing daily or on alternate days (every two days). Total-tract organic matter and neutral detergent fiber digestions were reduced when supplements were fed on alternate days compared with supplementing on a daily schedule. This reduction in forage digestibility appeared to be greater with supplements containing urea than with supplements containing only true protein. These data suggest that when high levels of NPN are included in a supplementation program, daily intake might support greater performance than less frequent supplementation. High NPN supplements could be provided daily in a milled or pelleted form or by a continuous access system like liquid supplements. Although digestion was reduced by less frequent supplementation of the supplements containing urea, data evaluating supplementation frequency on animal performance using high NPN supplements are limited.

REFERENCES

1. Ainslie SJ, Fox DG, Perry TC, et al: Predicting amino acid adequacy of diet fed to Holstein steers. J Anim Sci 71:1312, 1993.
2. Argyle JL, Baldwin RL: Effects of amino acids and peptides on rumen microbial growth yields. J Dairy Sci 72:2017, 1989.
3. Barajas R, Zinn RA: Interaction protein supplementation and corn processing method on growth performance and fecal starch in feedlot heifers [abstract]. J Anim Sci 74(suppl 1):291, 1996.
4. Bartley EE, Davidovich AD, Barr GW, et al: Ammonia toxicity in cattle: I. Rumen and blood changes associated with toxicity and treatment methods. J Anim Sci 43:835, 1976.
5. Beaty JL, Cochran RC, Lintzenich BA, et al: Effect of frequency of supplementation and protein concentration in supplements on performance and digestion characteristics of beef cattle consuming low-quality forages. J Anim Sci 72:2475, 1994.
6. Braman WL, Hatfield EE, Owens FN, et al: Protein concentration and sources for finishing ruminants fed high-concentrate diets. J Anim Sci 36:782, 1973.
7. Bunting LD, Boling JA, MacKown CT: Effect of dietary protein level on nitrogen metabolism in the growing bovine: I. Nitrogen recycling and intestinal protein supply in calves. J Anim Sci 67:810, 1989.
8. Burroughs WA, Trenkle A, Vetter RL: A system of protein evaluation for cattle and sheep involving metabolizable protein (amino acids) and urea fermentation potential of feedstuffs. Vet Med Small Anim Clin 69:713, 1974.
9. Cecava MJ, Merchen NR, Berger LL, et al: Intestinal supply of amino acids in sheep fed alkaline hydrogen peroxide-treated wheat straw-based diets supplemented with soybean meal or combinations of corn gluten meal and blood meal. J Anim Sci 68:467, 1990.
10. Clark JH, Klusmeyer TH, Cameron MR: Symposium: Nitrogen metabolism and amino acid nutrition in dairy cattle; microbial protein synthesis and flows on nitrogen fractions to the duodenum of dairy cows. J Dairy Sci 75:2304, 1992.
11. Clanton DC: Non-protein nitrogen in range supplements. J Anim Sci 47:765, 1978.

12. Cochran RC: Developing optimal supplementation programs for range livestock. In: 50 Years of Range Research. Kansas Range Field Day, 1995, p 58.

13. Fonnesbesck PV, Kearl LC, Harris LE: Feed grade biuret as a protein replacement for ruminants: A review. J Anim Sci 40:1150, 1975.

14. Forero O, Owens FN, Lusby KS: Evaluation of slow-release urea for sinter supplementation of lactating range cows. J Anim Sci 50:532, 1980.

15. Garrett JE, Goodrich RD, Meiske JC, et al: Influence of supplemental nitrogen source on digestion of nitrogen, dry matter and organic matter and on in vivo rate of ruminal starch digestion. J Anim Sci 64:1801, 1987.

16. Goedeken FK, Klopfenstein TJ, Stock RA, et al: Hydrolyzed feather meal as a protein source for growing calves. J Anim Sci 68:2945, 1990.

17. Goedeken FK, Klopfenstein TJ, Stock RA, et al: Protein value of feather meal for ruminants as affected by blood additions. J Anim Sci 68:2936, 1990.

18. Griswold KE, Hoover WH, Miller TK, et al: Effect of form of nitrogen on growth of ruminal microbes in continuous culture. J Anim Sci 74:483, 1996.

19. Hannah SM, Cochran RC, Vanzant ES, et al: Influence of protein supplementation on site and extent of digestion, forage intake, and nutrient flow characteristics in steers consuming dormant bluesteam-range forage. J Anim Sci 69:2624, 1991.

20. Healy BJ, Brandt RT Jr, Eck TP: Combinations of nonprotein nitrogen and natural protein affect performance of finishing steers fed flaked corn diets. KS Agri Exp Sta Rep Prog 727:34, 1995.

21. Helmer LG, Bartley EE: Progress in the utilization on urea a protein replacer for ruminants: A review. J Dairy Sci 54:25, 1971.

22. Hollingsworth-Jenkins KJ, Klopfenstein TJ, Adams DC, et al: Ruminally degradable protein requirement of gestating beef cows grazing winter sandhills range. J Anim Sci 74:1343, 1996.

23. Hume ID, Bird PR: Synthesis of microbial protein in the rumen: IV. The influence of the level and form of dietary sulfur. Aust J Agri Res 21:315, 1970.

24. Jones TJ, Cochran RC, Olson KC, et al: Influence of post-ruminal protein supply on gain and forage intake of beef cows consuming dormant, tallgrass-prairie forage. J Anim Sci 72(Suppl 1):353, 1994.

25. Kang-Meznarich JH, Broderick GA: Effects of incremental urea supplementation on ruminal ammonia concentration and bacterial protein formation. J Anim Sci 51:422, 1981.

26. Kellaway RC, Leibholz J: Effects on nitrogen supplements on intake and utilization of low-quality forages. World Anim Rev 48:33, 1983.

27. Kennedy PM, Milligan LP: The degradation and utilization of endogenous urea in the gastrointestinal tract of ruminants: A review. Can J Anim Sci 60:205, 1980.

28. Klopfenstein TJ, Stock RA, Britton RA: Relevance of bypass protein to cattle feeding. Prof Anim Scientist 1:27, 1985.

29. Koster HH: An evaluation of different levels of degradable intake protein and nonprotein nitrogen in intake, digestion, and performance by beef cattle fed low-quality forage. Ph.D. Dissertation, Kansas State University, 1995.

30. Krysl LJ, Branine ME, Cheema AU, et al: Influence of soybean meal and sorghum grain supplementation on intake, digest kinetics, ruminal fermentation, site and extent of digestion, and microbial protein synthesis in beef steers grazing blue gramma rangeland. J Anim Sci 67:3040, 1989.

31. Maeng WJ, Baldwin RL: Factors influencing rumen microbial growth rates and yields: Effect of amino acid additions to a purified diet with nitrogen from urea. J Dairy Sci 59:648, 1976.

32. Maeng WJ, Baldwin RL: Factors influencing rumen microbial growth rates and yields: Effects of urea and amino acids over time. J Dairy Sci 59:643, 1976.

33. Maeng WJ, Van Nevel CJ, Baldwin RL, et al: Rumen microbial growth rates and yields: effect of amino acids and protein. J Dairy Sci 59:68, 1976.

34. Martin SK, Hibberd CA: Intake and digestibility of low-quality native grass hay be beef cows supplemented with graded levels of soybean hulls. J Anim Sci 68:4319, 1990.

35. Martin JJ, Owens FN, Gill DR, et al: Protein sources for steers fed steam flaked, high-moisture, or whole shelled corn grain. Oklahoma Agric Res Rep MP-107:114, 1980.

36. Mehrez AZ, Ørskov ER: Protein degradation and optimum urea concentration in cereal-based diets for sheep. Br J Nutr 40:337, 1978.

37. Milton CT, Brandt RT Jr, Titgemeyer EC: Urea in dry-rolled corn diets: Finishing steer performance, nutrient digestion, and microbial protein production. J Anim Sci 75:1415–1424, 1997.

38. Milton CT, Brandt RT Jr, Titgemeyer EC: Effect of dietary nitrogen source and concentration in high-grain diets on finishing steer performance and nutrient digestion. J Anim Sci 75:1415–1424, 1997.

39. Milton CT, Brandt RT Jr, Titgemeyer EC: Effect of degradable and escape protein and roughage type for finishing yearling steers. J Anim Sci 75, 1997 (submitted).

40. Minson DJ: Forage in Ruminant Nutrition. San Diego, Academic Press, 1990.

41. National Research Council: Nutrient Requirements of Beef Cattle, ed 6. Washington, DC, National Academy Press, 1984.

42. National Research Council: Ruminant Nitrogen Usage. Washington, DC, National Academy Press, 1985.

43. National Research Council: Nutrient Requirements of Beef Cattle, ed 7. Washington, DC, National Academy Press, 1996.

44. Nelson ML, Martin EL: Escape protein supplementation of steers consuming barley finishing diets [abstract]. J Anim Sci 74(Suppl 1):278, 1996.

45. Nelson AB, Waller GR: Urea in winter supplements for range beef cattle [abstract]. J Anim Sci 21:387, 1962.

46. Ørskov ER, Fraser C, McDonald I: Digestion of concentrates: 2. The effects of urea or fish-meal supplementation of barley diets on the apparent digestion of protein, fat, starch, and ash in the rumen, small intestine and the large intestine, and the calculation of volatile fatty acid production. Br J Nutr 25:243, 1971.

47. Ørskov ER, Fraser C, McDonald I, et al: Digestion of concentrates in sheep: 5. The effect of adding fish meal and urea together to cereal diets on protein digestion and utilization by young sheep. Br J Nutr 31:89, 1974.

48. Owens FN, Lusby KS, Mizwicki, et al: Slow ammonia release from urea: Rumen and metabolism studies. J Anim Sci 50:527, 1980.

49. Owens FN, Zinn R: Protein metabolism of ruminants. In Church DC (ed): The Ruminant Animal: Digestive Physiology and Nutrition. Prospect Heights, IL, Waveland Press, 1993, p 227.

50. Pate FM, Sanson DW, Machen RV: Value of molasses mixture containing natural protein as a supplement to brood cows offered low-quality forages. J Anim Sci 68:618, 1989.

51. Pendlum LC, Boling JA, Bradley NW: Plasma and ruminal constituents and performance of steers fed different nitrogen sources and levels of sulfur. J Anim Sci 43:1307, 1976.

52. Pritchard RH: Effect of supplement crude protein source and dietary crude protein levels on feedlot performance of yearling steers. South Dakota Beef Rep. 94-3:6, 1994.

53. Pritchard RH: Evaluation of crude protein sources and levels for high growth potential yearling steers fed high energy diets. South Dakota Beef Rep. 95-9:30, 1995.

54. Raleigh RJ, Wallace DJ: Effect of urea at different nitrogen levels on digestibility and on performance of growing steers fed low quality flood meadow roughage. J Anim Sci 22:330, 1963.

55. Reid JT: Urea as a protein replacement for ruminants: A review. J Anim Sci 12:955, 1953.

56. Roffler RE, Satter LD: Relationship between ruminal ammonia and nonprotein nitrogen utilization in ruminants: I. Development of a model for predicting nonprotein nitrogen utilization by cattle. J Dairy Sci 58:1880, 1975.

57. Rush IG, Johnson RR, Totusek R: Evaluation of beef cattle range supplements containing urea and biuret. J Anim Sci 42:1297, 1976.

58. Russell JB, Sniffen CJ, Van Soest PJ: Effect of carbohydrate limitation on degradation and utilization of casein by mixed rumen bacteria. J Dairy Sci 66:763, 1983.

59. Russell JB, Onodera R, Hino T: Ruminal protein fermentation: New perspectives on previous contradictions. In Tsuda T, Sasaki Y, Kawashima R (eds): Physiological Aspects of Digestion and Metabolism in Ruminants: Proceedings of the Seventh International Symposium on Ruminant Physiology. San Diego, Academic Press, 1991, p. 681.

60. Russell JB, O'Connor JD, Fox DG, et al: A net carbohydrate and protein system for evaluation of cattle diets: I. Ruminal fermentation. J Anim Sci 70:3551, 1992.

61. Rust SR, Owens FN, Gill DR, et al: Corn moisture, protein concentration, and Rumensin and digestion by feedlot steers. Oklahoma Agric Exp Sta MP-104:55, 1979.

62. Satter LD, Slyter LL: Effect of ammonia concentration on rumen microbial protein production in vitro. Br J Nutr 32:199, 1974.

63. Schmidt SP, Jorgensen NA, Benevenga NJ, et al: Comparison of soybean meal, formaldehyde treated soybean meal, urea and starea for steers. J Anim Sci 37:1233, 1973.

64. Shain DH, Stock RA, Klopfenstein TJ, et al: Level of degradable nitrogen in finishing diets. Nebraska Beef Cattle Rep MP 61-A:35, 1994.

65. Sindt MH, Stock RA, Klopfenstein TJ, et al: Effect of protein source and grain type on finishing calf performance and ruminal metabolism. J Anim Sci 71:1047, 1993.

66. Sindt MH, Stock RA, Klopfenstein TJ, et al: Protein sources for finishing cattle as affected by management system. J Anim Sci 71:740, 1993.

67. Slyter LL, Satter LD, Dinius DA: Effect of ruminal ammonia concentration on nitrogen utilization by steers. J Anim Sci 48:906, 1979.

68. Spicer LA, Theurer CB, Sowe J, et al: Ruminal and post-ruminal utilization of nitrogen and starch from sorghum grain-, corn-, and barley-based diets by beef steers. J Anim Sci 62:521, 1986.

69. Stangel HJ: Urea and Non-protein Nitrogen in Ruminant Nutrition. New York, Allied Chemical Corp, 1963.

70. Stern MD, Hoover WH: Methods for determining and factors affecting rumen microbial protein synthesis: A review. J Anim Sci 49:1590, 1979.

71. Stock RA, Merchen NR, Klopfenstein TJ, et al: Feeding value of slowly degraded proteins. J Anim Sci 53:1109, 1981.

72. Streeter MN, Mathis MJ: Effect of supplemental fish meal protein on site and extent of digestion in beef steers. J Anim Sci 73:1196, 1995.

73. Susmel P, Spanghero M, Stefano B, et al: Digestibility and allantoin excretion in cows fed diets differing in nitrogen content. Livest Prod Sci 36:213, 1993.

74. Thomas EE, Mason CR, Schmidt SP: Relation of feedlot performance and certain physiological responses to the metabolizable protein and urea content of cattle diets. J Anim Sci 58:1285, 1984.

75. Titgemeyer EC, Merchen NR, Berger LL: Evaluation of soybean meal, corn gluten meal, blood meal and fish meal as sources of nitrogen and amino acids disappearing from the small intestine of steers. J Anim Sci 67:262, 1989.

76. Trenkle A: Comparison of protein supplements for yearling steers implanted with estradiol and trenbolone acetate. Iowa State Beef Rep AS-625:33, 1994.

77. Trenkle A: Effects of controlling feed intake on feeding alfalfa or soybean meal protein on performance of steers implanted with estradiol and trenbolone acetate. Iowa State Beef Rep AS-630:92, 1995.

78. Trenkle A: Response of finishing steers implanted with estradiol and trenbolone acetate to varying concentrations of dietary urea and soybean meal. Iowa State Beef Rep AS-630:85, 1995.

79. Veira DM, Macleod GK, Burton JH, et al: Nutrition of the weaned Holstein calf. II. Effect of dietary protein level on nitrogen balance, digestibility, and feed intake. J Anim Sci 50:945, 1980.

80. Wilkerson VA, Klopfenstein TJ, Britton RA, et al: Metabolizable protein and amino acid requirements of growing beef cattle. J Anim Sci 71:2777, 1993.

81. Woods BC, Cochran RC, Mathis CP, et al: The effects of supplementation frequency and amount of urea in dry supplements on intake and digestibility of low-quality tallgrass-prairie forage by beef steers. Kansas Agri Exp Sta Rep Prog 783, 1997.

82. Young AW, Boling JA, Bradley NW: Performance and plasma amino acids of steers fed soybean meal, urea, or no supplemental nitrogen in finishing rations. J Anim Sci 36:803, 1973.

83. Zinn RA: Characteristics of ruminal and total tract digestion of canola meal and soybean meal in a high-energy diet for feedlot cattle. J Anim Sci 71:796, 1993.

84. Zinn RA: Protein level, source, and non-protein nitrogen for feedlot cattle. In Proceedings of the Plains Nutrition Council Symposium, Amarillo, Texas, 1995, p 16.

85. Zinn RA, Owens FN: Site of protein digestion in steers: Predictability. J Anim Sci 56:707, 1983.

86. Zinn RA, Owens FN: Ruminal escape protein for lightweight feedlot calves. J Anim Sci 71:1677, 1993.

▪ Nutritional Management of Livestock Grazing Range and Pasture Lands

M. M. Kothmann, M.S., Ph.D.
R. T. Hinnant, M.S.

Animal nutrition is based on empirical estimates of the nutrient requirements of animals and the nutritive value of feeds. The nutritive value of feeds consumed in mixed diets is considered to be additive and independent of the kind of animal consuming them; however, these assumptions and the empirical estimates derived from pen-fed animals are frequently inappropriate for nutritional management of grazing animals. Grazing animals are not fed a ration; they select a diet from the forage available. It is difficult to determine the nutritive value of grazed diets because animals select varying combinations of plant species and plant parts which differ in nutritive value. Supplements, which usually represent only a small fraction of the total diet, may affect both intake and digestibility of the grazed forage; thus, their effects are not additive. Supplements should be formulated to alleviate specific nutrient deficiencies and complement intake and utilization of grazed forage. Expensive processed or harvested feeds should only be provided as substitutes for the less expensive grazed forage if the quality or quantity of forage is too low to support a supplemental feeding strategy. Many nutritional problems of grazing animals result from ineffective management practices that limit the quantity or quality of forage and that provide inappropriate supplemental feeding strategies.

Grazing management can enhance or reduce the quality of the diet. Grazing plans should be developed to make efficient use of the forage produced. Grazing management must consider factors such as stocking rates, season of grazing, grazing methods, plant species available, and kinds and classes of animals best suited to the forage resource. Grazing management should consider long-term maintenance or improvement of perennial forage stands, as well as nutrition of the animal. The Grazing Manager (TGM)[3] is an effective software tool to assist grazing managers with organizing resources, developing grazing plans, and monitoring grazing.

This discussion examines animal, vegetation, environmental, and management factors that affect the nutritional status of grazing animals. Topics include (1) resource characteristics, (2) forage growth, (3) diet selection, (4) intake regulation, (5) grazing management, (6) forage quantity and quality, (7) supplemental feeding strategies, and (8) water requirements.

FORAGE RESOURCES

The same principles apply to nutrition of livestock grazing on both range and pasture lands, but management practices may differ. Pasture consists of monocultures or simple mixtures of plant species selected for local adaptation, quality, and yield. Cultural practices used to maintain the productivity of pasture lands include selecting plant materials, establishing new stands, fertilization, weed control, harvesting and storing excess production, and grazing management.

Rangelands consist of complex mixtures of naturally occurring plant species, including grasses, forbs, and shrubs. The manager's ability to apply intensive cultural practices to vegetation management is generally limited by inherently low productivity of the sites. The forage resource is managed with limited inputs to assure sustained yield. It is difficult to use expensive cultural inputs to re-establish rangeland vegetation that has been depleted through improper management. Grazing management is the primary tool used to alter competitive relationships and manipulate vegetation on rangelands. Brush management is the primary cultural practice applied to rangelands and this may be in the form of prescribed burning.

FORAGE GROWTH

Forage grows in response to environmental and management inputs. Forage quality is strongly influenced by maturity. Forages that depend primarily on the C_3 metabolic pathway are classified as cool-season and those that utilize the C_4 pathway are classified as warm-season. Cool-season species have greater frost tolerance and lower optimal temperatures for growth than warm-season species. Cool-season species are in the reproductive growth phase during spring when warm-season species are initiating rapid vegetative growth. Cool-season plants do not grow well at temperatures above 30°C. Warm-season forages require higher temperatures than cool-season species.

Warm-season forages—for example, Bermuda grass (perennial) or sorghum (annual)—begin production early in the summer and continue to grow until either the temperature becomes too low or moisture becomes limiting. Cool-season forages initiate growth during late summer or early fall and may provide some grazing prior to and during winter if there is adequate moisture. Their growth rate typically slows during the coldest period of the winter and then increases rapidly as temperatures rise and light intensity and duration increase in spring. The plants become reproductive during spring. Growth rate declines as the temperature increases during late spring. In warmer climates, cool-season forages may be dormant during the summer. Perennial and annual cool-season forages follow the same general growth pattern except annuals die during the reproductive phase and regenerate from seeds in the fall. Perennial cool-season forages maintain live vegetative shoots or buds during the summer dormant period if they can access soil moisture. Cool-season perennials exposed to high temperatures and light intensities die if soil moisture is depleted.

Pastures

Forages produced on tame pastures usually require additional inputs of nutrients. High levels of inputs produce high-quality forage which needs to be used efficiently. Forages may be grazed and surplus forage harvested and stored as silage. Tame pasture forages are almost always grazed seasonally during the primary vegetative growth period. If forages are allowed to mature prior to grazing or harvest, their nutritive value declines greatly. Thus, intensively managed pastures receiving costly inputs must be utilized intensively to recover the nutrients while the forage is near peak quality.

Rangelands

The species which grow on rangelands are determined by natural selection as influenced by the soils, climate, and availability of propagules. Past use and management affect the composition and production, but current environmental conditions play a major role. The manager needs to be able to identify the kinds of plants that are present and to understand their responses to environmental conditions and management interventions. Large year-to-year variation in environmental conditions on many rangelands make planning difficult.

Many rangelands support a mixture of both warm- and cool-season forages. Warm-season grasses, produced in the summer, can be deferred for grazing through dormant periods. Forages produced in the fall can be stockpiled for winter grazing, but spring growth of cool-season forages cannot be saved as standing hay for summer grazing. The warm-season component begins growth during the period when the cool-season component is fully reproductive. Diverse rangeland vegetation can provide a stable grazing resource throughout the year. Periods of maximal growth rate will provide maximum nutrient availability. Animal production cycles should be planned and managed to match the maximum nutrient demand with the periods of maximum production.

DIET SELECTION

It is well documented that livestock graze selectively on range and pasture lands. Both animal and forage attributes affect diet selection. Animal attributes include species, class of animal, productive function, prior conditioning, and experience. Forage factors affecting diet selection include chemical composition (both positive and negative attributes) and physical characteristics such as texture, pubescence, or the presence of spines. Preference is a relative value referring to the choices animals make among feeds. Palatability relates to acceptability of the feed and is measured by intake. Preference and palatability are closely related and are frequently used interchangeably in the literature. Absolute values for preference and palatability cannot be assigned to feeds. Relative rankings of preference may be useful, but care must be exercised in making comparisons between different cases. Certain expressions of forage preference are similar for all kinds of livestock. Animals prefer leaf over stem and live over dead forage. Dietary preferences reflect selection of diets having nutritive value higher than the average of the forage available. Heavy grazing pressures will force increased utilization of lower-quality forage, reducing the nutrient intake of the animal.

The effects of chemical composition of the forage on diet selection are not simply expressed since many chemicals interact with the animal's senses during the grazing process. Plant components such as crude protein (CP), phosphorus, carotene, and moisture content and digestibility of forage have been positively associated with preference. Lignin, cellulose, cutin, silica, cell walls, alkaloids, and various terpenes and essential oils have been negatively associated with preference. Simple classifications of plant palatability based on limited chemical characteristics such as CP, crude fiber, or digestibility are inadequate when applied to diverse kinds of forages and animals.

Broad generalizations can be made about dietary preferences of cattle, sheep, and goats for forage classes on rangelands; however, these are subject to considerable variation in specific cases. Forage classes are generally selected in proportion to their ability to provide green foliage, with grasses utilized most heavily by cattle, forbs by sheep, and browse by goats. Seasonal shifts in dietary preferences are common to all range livestock. These shifts reflect the changing phenology, composition, and growth rates of forage species.

Secondary plant compounds that cause toxic effects reduce preference. If toxic effects are acute and rapid, poisoning can occur before the animal learns to avoid the plant. Offspring develop conditioned preferences and learn feeding patterns from their mothers. This is an advantage for locally adapted animals. When livestock are moved to new environments and introduced to new forages, especially on rangelands, they require a period of adaptation and learning. Under severe conditions where there are numerous toxic species, animals newly introduced to the environment may not survive, although indigenous animals thrive there.

The average forage quality on many ranges is not adequate

to support livestock production and only by allowing the animals to graze selectively can livestock production be sustained economically. On pastures where the average forage quality is adequate, selective grazing can "stratify" the forage by removing green leaves first, leaving stems and dead leaves, which are not of adequate quality to support desired levels of livestock production. To avoid this problem on tame pastures, forage can be utilized at an immature stage or can be strip-grazed, forcing utilization of all the forage during 1 or 2 days. This maintains the average nutrient intake at an acceptable level and prevents several days of luxury consumption followed by several days of deficient intake which may occur with longer grazing periods in rotation grazing. If the average forage quality will not support the desired level of animal production, reducing the level of use will provide a higher-quality diet.

INTAKE REGULATION

Selective grazing is advantageous to the animal but causes a variety of problems for grazing management. On rangelands, the major problems caused by selective grazing are related to species and area selectivity. Most rangelands support diverse floras with species varying in palatability. Also, topography may be steep and rough with large paddocks encompassing a variety of soil types. Distance from water to forage may be in excess of 2 miles. All of these factors accentuate selective grazing. Grazing management on rangelands is primarily directed toward alleviating the problems caused by selective grazing. Adjustments of stocking rates and season of grazing and development of specialized grazing methods are commonly used to alleviate problems of *species-selective* grazing. Development of additional water and fencing and strategic location of mineral supplements and feed grounds are primary methods directed to reduce problems of *area-selective* grazing.

Animal Units

Pastures and rangelands are grazed by different kinds and classes of animals, each requiring different amounts of forage. The "animal-unit" (AU) is a concept designed to provide a standard expression of the forage demand by different kinds of grazing animals, since adding numbers of sheep and steers and cows does not provide a useful figure. An *animal-unit* has been defined as a constant forage demand rate. The value suggested for the constant varies with 8 or 12 kg/day being most common. The "animal-unit-equivalent" (AUE) for any animal may be calculated by dividing that animal's forage demand (in kilograms) by the selected demand rate constant. The number of animals multiplied by this AUE will give the number of AUs.

To calculate stocking rates, the time factor must be incorporated by multiplying the number of AUs by the number of days they grazed on an area giving animal-unit-days (AUDs). The total number of AUDs grazed on an area during a year is the stocking rate. AUDs may be converted to animal-unit-months (AUMs) or animal-unit-years (AUYs) by dividing by 30.5 or 365, respectively.

The AU and AUE should not be confused with substitution ratios or competition indices used for different kinds of animals on ranges. Different kinds of animals have different dietary preferences and grazing behavior. For example, goats and deer will utilize more browse and steeper, rougher topography than cattle. However, cattle will utilize relatively level grasslands more efficiently than goats or deer. Thus, the suitability of rangelands for different animal species varies with vegetation, topography, and other factors. The purpose of the AU is simply to express the total forage demand in common units. The suit-

ability of any given range for different kinds of animals must be determined and substitution ratios worked out independently of the AUE.

GRAZING MANAGEMENT

Grazing management should always be one of the first nutritional considerations of the livestock manager. Primary considerations are to select the proper season for grazing; the proper stocking rate; a suitable kind, class, and breed of animal; and the most appropriate grazing method.

Season for Grazing

There are two important principles which should be considered when making decisions regarding season for grazing. First, animal production is greatest when forage is grazed soon after it is produced and before it has matured. Second, to obtain range improvement through plant succession, the desirable forage species must be allowed to reproduce. Thus, when range improvement is an important goal, there will need to be some reduction in animal production to achieve the improvement. It is obvious that, on tame pastures and rangelands in good condition where range improvement is not an objective, the grazing plan can be designed to maximize economic returns from animal production. Tame pastures should be fully utilized during the growing season. There is no logical reason to defer use of most tame pastures during the growing season and utilize them during the dormant season. These expensive forages should be grazed to harvest the maximum amount of nutrients for high levels of animal production.

Rangelands generally provide the flexibility in forage systems where they are combined with tame pastures. This means that the tame pastures are grazed when they provide the most nutrients and the rangelands are used to fill the gaps. This not only utilizes the most expensive forage most efficiently, it also can promote range improvement by providing growing season deferment for rangelands. However, it is important that the amounts of production from range and tame pasture be properly balanced to prevent overutilization of the range. In mixed systems, excessive amounts of tame pastures can result in greater numbers of animals than the rangeland can support for the remainder of the year.

Range sites may differ significantly in their suitability for grazing during different seasons. Cool-season herbaceous forage and evergreen browse will generally provide better grazing during fall, winter, and early spring, whereas warm-season forages are best suited to use during late spring, summer, or fall. Large pastures with a mix of sites allow animals to rotate their grazing seasonally. Smaller pastures, which contain less variation in vegetation, may require the use of seasonal adjustments in grazing to match the seasonality of the forage.

Stocking Rates

As stocking rate increases, gains per animal decrease, but gains per acre increase (Fig. 1). This relationship is only linear to the point where forage availability begins to limit intake. Further increases in stocking rate beyond that point will reduce both gains per animal and gains per acre. This general relationship applies to all grazing lands, although the rate of decline in animal production per head varies among forage types and stands. The optimal stocking rate will lie in the range between the rate producing maximum gain per head and the rate producing maximum gain per acre. Within this broad range of stocking

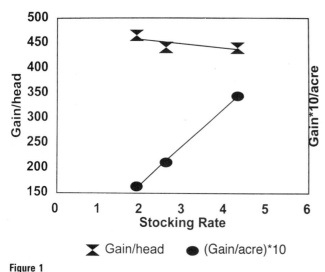

Figure 1

Relationship between stocking rate and calf production per head and (production/acre) *10. Stocking rate is expressed on a normalized scale of 0 to 6 with 6 representing the stocking rate that would produce complete use of all grazable forage. Markers represent means for light (2), moderate (3), and heavy (4.5) stocking rates over a period of 8 years. (Data from Kothmann MM, Mathis GW, Marion PT, et al: Livestock Production and Economic Returns from Grazing Treatments on the Texas Experimental Ranch. College Station, Tex, Texas Agricultural Experimental Station, B-1100, 1970.)

rates, the optimum will shift with changing economic conditions. When costs associated with an individual animal (variable costs) are high relative to fixed costs, the stocking rate should be adjusted to improve gain per animal. This is the general situation on rangelands, if land values are excluded from fixed costs. Stocking rates should be shifted to increase gain per acre when fixed costs are high relative to variable costs. This situation may be more common on tame pasture with high levels of inputs than on rangelands.

Site potential (e.g., land use capability class) generally differs between tame pastures and rangelands. Intensive cultural practices are applied to maintain the productivity of tame pastures where the land is capable of sustaining intensive agriculture. Because of low site potential, many rangelands are not capable of sustaining intensive agriculture. Heavy stocking rates designed to maximize animal production per unit of land cause deterioration of both vegetation and soil conditions on rangelands.

Our field experience indicates that on perennial rangelands, approximately one fourth of the total usable forage produced can be consumed by grazing animals under proper stocking. If estimates of annual forage production are available, a moderate stocking rate for perennial rangelands can be set by allowing four times as much forage per animal as its predicted forage demand. Allowing two times the predicted demand will result in heavy stocking. Significantly higher levels of stocking are possible on annual ranges and tame pastures than on perennial rangelands.

The best procedure for arriving at the correct stocking rate is experience combined with records of animal production and vegetation trends. A computer decision aid, The Grain Manager (TGM),[3] provides a method for monitoring grazing and the balance of forage production and demand. This decision aid simplifies this most important and difficult task of matching animal demand to fluctuations in forage production.

TGM is designed to be used and calibrated by ranchers. There are only six parameters in the model and values for these are determined by the on-site user. At the beginning of the year, the manager enters a grazing plan and evaluates the projected forage balance for the coming year. During the year, forage and animal conditions are monitored and entered into TGM. Monitoring data are used to update the plan and to improve the accuracy of the initial estimates for the model parameters. Information can be obtained and the program may be purchased by contacting M.M. Kothmann, Dept. of Rangeland Ecology & Management, Texas A&M University, College Station, TX 77843–2126; telephone: (409) 845–5575; fax: 409–845–6430; e-mail: m-kothmann@tamu.edu.

Rotational Grazing Methods

Selective grazing results in the most desirable forage components and the most accessible areas of the range receiving the most frequent and intensive grazing. This may result in reduced vigor and productivity of these components, and invasion of undesirable species. Thus, the effect of continuous stocking, especially at heavy stocking rates, is a decline in productivity of the resource. Grazing methods have been designed to offset the effects of selective grazing and to enhance range improvement by promoting secondary plant succession.

The components of a grazing method are the number of pastures and herds of livestock and the length of grazing and rest periods for each pasture. Livestock are restricted to a portion of the land to allow the vegetation on the remaining land in the system to grow for a period of time without grazing. Livestock are rotated among pastures to provide scheduled periods of grazing and rest for each pasture.

Grazing method design requires an understanding of three basic concepts of grazing management. (1) *Stocking rate (SR)* is cumulative forage demand per unit area of land. It is determined by the number of animals, forage demand rate per animal, time of grazing, and total land area. (2) *Stocking density (SD)* is determined by the number of pastures per herd and the SR. (3) *Cumulative grazing pressure (CGP)* is the ratio of cumulative forage demand to cumulative forage supply. It is determined by the length of the grazing periods and the SR and SD.

Both SD and CGP can be changed in a rotational grazing method without changing SR, but changes in SR will always affect SD and CGP. Increasing SD results in more uniform spatial distribution of grazing but will not affect selection for species or plant parts. Concentrating animals on smaller portions of the land; that is, more pastures and fewer herds, may accentuate species-selective grazing by increasing the ratio of forage demand rate to forage growth rate. Increasing CGP reduces diet quality; thus, reducing the length of grazing periods should improve animal performance if animal handling stress is not greatly increased by more frequent handling. Long ungrazed periods which allow significant amounts of forage to mature between grazing periods will reduce animal production. However, long ungrazed periods are required to allow desirable species to reproduce and promote range improvement. With all of these factors to consider, the design of a successful rotational grazing method which meets both plant and animal requirements is not a simple exercise.

Animal production from rotational methods seldom exceeds levels obtained from continuous stocking at the same SR. The primary reasons for using rotational stocking methods are to facilitate livestock management and achieve vegetation management objectives. Unless significant benefits can be anticipated in one or both of these areas, use of rotational stocking methods may not be justified.

FORAGE QUALITY AND AVAILABILITY

The quality of a forage is judged by its nutritive value, which is the ability of the feed to support animal production functions. The nutritive value of forage depends upon its nutrient content, the amount the animal will consume (intake), and the balance of nutrients relative to the animal's requirement. Crude protein and organic matter digestibility are the primary forage analyses used to assess quality; however, these analytic procedures do not provide highly accurate predictions of nutritive value of forages since they do not consider intake. Empirically based equations for prediction of animal performance work well within a forage species and location, but generally cannot be extended to other kinds of animals, kinds of forages, or locations. Variation in nutritive value exists among forage classes, within a forage class, between individual plants within a species, between leaf and stem fractions within a plant, and between live and dead fractions. The influences of forage classes, maturity, availability, and environment on forage quality will be discussed.

Nutrient Content

The nutritional components of forage have been empirically grouped into cell contents and cell walls. Cell contents contain most of the protein, digestible minerals, and soluble carbohydrates. The nutrients in the cell contents are readily accessible to the microbes in the rumen and are digestible by the animal. Cell walls provide only energy in the form of volatile fatty acids obtained from microbial digestion of cellulose and hemicellulose. Digestion is slower and more variable than for cell contents. The digestibility of cell walls depends on the availability of ammonia and an acceptable level of pH for rumen microbes, which produce cellulase.

Forage Classes

Forages are classified in many different ways. All have some nutritional significance, but none have general nutritional significance. Classifications include herbaceous (grasses and forbs) and woody (browse), cool-season and warm-season, perennial and annual, toxic and nontoxic, antiherbivory or palatable. Grasses include annual and perennial members of the family Poaceae. Forbs are herbaceous annual and perennial dicots and monocots other than grasses. Browse consists of perennial woody shrubs and vines utilized as forage by grazing animals. Characteristic differences exist among classes and within classes.

Warm-season perennial grasses have the lowest CP, the highest proportion of cell walls, and the lowest average digestibility. Legumes have the highest CP and digestibility, with cool-season annual and perennial grasses being intermediate. Total dry matter production and forage quality follow inverse trends. Cost per pound of forage produced tends to vary directly with forage quality.

The nutritive value of forages varies seasonally. Warm-season grasses generally cannot provide adequate digestible energy to meet the requirements of high-producing animals, such as lactating dairy cows or young growing animals, whereas a high-quality legume pasture may. Thus, it is usually preferable to graze animals with lower requirements—for example, mature beef cows, on warm-season perennial grasses and to utilize higher-quality legume and cool-season annual grass pastures for animals having high requirements—for example, growing stock or high-producing lactating cows.

Mixtures of forage classes can be an asset. Monocultures may be high-producing pastures, but their growth is usually seasonal; thus, when growth stops, stock must either be moved to pastures with different seasonality or fed stored feeds. Pastures that contain a mixture of forage classes are more likely to provide some high-quality forage year-round, reducing the need for supplementation. For example, desert ranges in the intermountain region of the western United States support primarily grass-shrub communities with few forbs. They are grazed primarily by dry ewes and cows during the winter when forage quality is relatively low and animal requirements are low. Animal diets contain a mix of grasses and browse. Diets consisting of all browse would be deficient in energy, but would contain adequate levels of CP, phosphorus, and carotene to meet the maintenance requirements of dry cows and ewes. Diets composed of all grasses would contain adequate energy but would be deficient in CP, phosphorus, and carotene. Where animals could select from both grasses and browse, the need for supplements is reduced.

Legumes are the only forbs that have received significant attention as forage species for seeded pastures. Evaluation of the nutrient content of some common weed species, for example, redroot pigweed (*Amaranthus retroflexus*), common lamb's quarters (*Chenopodium album*), and common ragweed (*Ambrosia artemisiifolia*), revealed that their nutrient composition and digestibility were equivalent to that of high-quality alfalfa (*Medicago sativa*). Thus, some of the common weed species found in stands of perennial forages growing in fertile soils do not decrease the nutritive value of hay or pasture if utilized prior to maturation. However, generalizations are not possible when comparing forage quality of "weed" and crop species. Some weed species contain high levels of secondary compounds that significantly reduce their nutritive value. Comparisons must be based on specific examples where species and environmental conditions are described.

Maturity

As plants mature, forage quality declines. Several factors contribute to this decline. Initial growth of forage consists primarily of green leaves with high proportions of cell contents and highly digestible cell walls. As plants mature, the proportion of cell contents decreases and the cell walls become more lignified and less digestible. Growth and senescence occur simultaneously in plants. During the growing season, new leaves are produced and older leaves die and accumulate as standing dead forage. As the plants mature, they become reproductive and stem growth increases. Thus, during the early part of the growing season, pastures have a higher proportion of green leaves, and as the stand matures, the proportions of stem and dead leaf increase and their nutritive value declines.

Warm-season perennial grasses, for example, love grasses, Bermuda grass and Bahia grass, are highly digestible at initiation of growth in the spring, but forage quality declines rapidly from spring to summer as plant maturity increases. However, the rate of decline varies among species and varieties. Varieties selected for improved forage quality, such as Coastal Bermuda grass, maintain higher digestibility, but also reach a low point in midsummer when soil and air temperatures are high. High temperatures increase maintenance respiration of the plant which reduces cell contents and promotes growth of cell walls. The decline in forage quality also may result from lower growth rates of leaves and accumulation of stem and dead forage. As the growth rate slows, the average age of live-leaf standing crop increases. Late summer rains during most years, combined with reduced temperatures, produce fall growth, which increases forage quality. Fall forage growth frequently is lower in digestible energy than spring growth, probably as a result of lower light intensities and shorter day length. Fall growth may have greater proportions of stem and reproductive parts in the standing crop.

Grazing alters the quality of forage standing crop by changing the relative proportions and average age of plant parts in the standing crop. It may also alter plant growth rates, either increasing or decreasing production depending on the intensity, frequency, and time of grazing and the environmental conditions. Consumption of live forage by grazing reduces the amount that senesces, resulting in less dead standing crop. It also retards phenologic development of plants, promoting vegetative growth over reproductive growth. Apical meristems may be removed, promoting growth of secondary tillers and increasing the leaf-stem ratio of the standing crop.

Availability

Average daily gain of grazing animals is related to both quality and quantity of forage. These relationships were examined for six warm-season perennial grasses (Fig. 2). When dry matter digestibility (DMD) of forage was greater than 60%, gains of yearling heifers were not affected until forage availability fell below 500 kg/ha. As average digestibility of the forage declined, the relation between gains and availability changed. There was an asymptotic relationship between animal gain and mean pasture availability for all qualities of forage. A 4 to 6 in. mean height of green leaves was required for cattle to obtain maximum intake. Even small increases in green forage, when availability was below 500 kg/ha, resulted in significant increases in gain per animal. Critical heights and standing crops differ among kinds of animals. The critical heights and weights for forage vary for species having different growth forms and stands of different densities, but the management implications are similar.

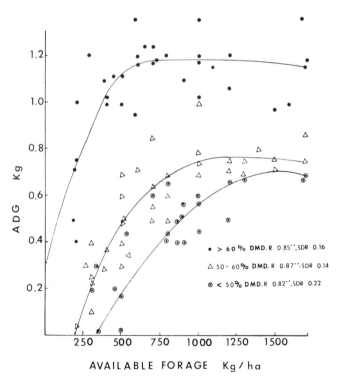

Figure 2

Polynomial regressions, $Y = a + bX + cX^2 + dX^3$, between animal performance (Y) and available forage (X) on warm-season grasses for three ranges of dry matter digestibility (DMD) (SDR = standard deviation from regression). (From Duble RL, Lancaster JA, Holt EC: Agron J 63:795, 1971.)

Variation in forage quality is often confounded with amount of standing crop. Quality of standing crop is relatively homogeneous during early growth when forage is primarily young live leaf and digestibility is high. As forage matures, standing crop usually increases, but average digestibility of standing crop declines and variability increases. Since animals select the highest-quality forage first, the obvious conclusion is that stands of uniformly high-quality forage can be grazed more closely with less effect on animal performance than more mature stands that contain greater proportions of dead leaves and stems. The relative amounts of each forage quality component in the stand affects the relationship between animal performance and standing crop. Where the quality of forage in the standing crop varies significantly and forage growth rates are low, animal performance will be much more sensitive to grazing intensity.

Environment

Many environmental factors may affect forage quality, but only temperature, light intensity, moisture, fertility, senescence, and leaching will be considered here.

In temperate regions, the effects of temperature, light intensity, and moisture give rise to predictable seasonal changes in forage growth and quality of standing crop. High light intensities combined with cool temperatures and adequate water and nutrients increase water-soluble carbohydrate content, whereas high temperatures and drought will lower CP and soluble carbohydrates and increase cell walls. In temperate regions spring grass has high CP and low fiber content; summer grass has low CP and high fiber content; autumn grass has high CP and average fiber content. Low light intensities and reduced water availability and high soil nitrate can result in accumulation of NO_3 in plants, which can result in poisoning of animals. In tropical regions forage quality is affected primarily by variations of moisture, stage of maturity, species, and fertility.

Optimal levels of temperature and light intensity vary between temperate cool-season and tropical warm-season grasses. Cool-season grasses and forbs (including legumes) are cold-hardy and optimal temperatures for growth are below 25°C. Warm-season plants grow only during the frost-free periods and optimal temperatures are above 25°C.

Seasonal changes in light and heat produce the seasonal growth patterns for cool- and warm-season species. Low light intensities and temperatures restrict plant growth during the winter. During spring, light intensity and temperature both increase, improving conditions for plant growth. During summer, temperature may be above the optimum for plant growth, and water is frequently limiting. During fall, light intensity and temperature both decrease. Limited water availability may restrict plant growth during any season.

Increasing soil fertility primarily increases growth rate and dry matter production, although some changes in chemical composition of forage have been reported. Changes in chemical composition can also result from differences in the relative proportion of plant parts (e.g., leaf, stem, and inflorescence) and in stage of maturity. High levels of soil nitrogen increase the leaf-stem ratio and retard plant maturity. CP content increased, but digestibility of kleingrass (*Panicum coloratum*) and Bermuda grasses did not change in response to nitrogen fertilization (Table 1). These data were based on forage harvested at the same stage of maturity. Fertilization generally improves animal production by increasing forage growth rates (i.e., reducing average leaf age), increasing forage density and standing crop, and increasing the leaf-stem ratio.

Leaching is an important factor that reduces the nutritive value of mature forages. Young, actively growing plant tissue is relatively immune to loss of mineral nutrients and carbohydrates

Table 1

EFFECT OF NITROGEN FERTILIZATION ON CRUDE PROTEIN (CP) CONTENT AND ITS LACK OF EFFECT ON DRY MATTER DIGESTIBILITY (DMD)

Texas*						Homer, Louisiana†			Oklahoma‡		
Kleingrass			Coastal Bermuda			Coastal Bermuda			Coastal Bermuda		
N (lb/acre)	CP (%)	DMD (%)	N (lb/acre)	CP (%)	DMD (%)	N (lb/acre)	CP (%)	DMD (%)	N (lb/acre)	CP (%)	DMD (%)
25	5.9	56.1	25	6.7	53.8	0	10.4	51.4	0	11.5	64.9
100	6.6	57.1	100	7.6	54.8	600	15.8	53.1	400	18.4	66.0
200	9.8	55.8	200	10.6	53.4	1200	16.9	52.1	1400	18.9	65.0
300	10.8	57.4	300	10.8	55.1	—	—	—	—	—	—

*One application 6 weeks prior to cutting. Data from Buentello JL, Ellis WC: *In* Proceedings of the 24th Annual Texas Nutrition Conference, 1969.
†Six applications 4 weeks prior to cutting. Data from Rainwater WA, Ellis WC, Oliver WM: Abstract. J Anim Sci 38:214, 1974.
‡Four applications. In vitro data from Webster JE, Hogan JW, Elder WE: Agron J 57:323, 1965.
From Ellis WC, Lippke H: Texas Agricultural Experiment Station Research Monograph RM-6C, 1976.

by leaching, whereas tissues approaching senescence and fully mature tissues are very susceptible to leaching. Potassium, calcium, magnesium, and manganese are the inorganic nutrients leached from live plants in largest quantities. Minerals most resistant to leaching are iron, zinc, phosphorus, and chloride. Of the major organic constituents, carbohydrates are most likely to be leached from live plant material. Quantitative losses of proteins, amino acids, and organic acids from live plant material are slight.

Another major loss of nutrients from foliage as plants mature occurs through translocation. The major elements, nitrogen, potassium, and phosphorus, and nonstructural carbohydrates are readily mobilized and translocated from senescing plant tissues. In addition to the effects of translocation and leaching which reduce levels of nutrients in cell contents, the digestibility of cell walls also declines with advancing maturity. Thus nutrient levels are always low in dead tissue. In humid regions, it generally is not feasible to use standing dead forage because its nutritive value is too low. In arid regions where leaching is minimal, standing dead forage may be used if the nutrients lost during senescence are supplemented. In dry climates, warm-season forage which is killed by frost while it is still in an immature vegetative state during the fall can provide a good-quality standing hay during winter.

EVALUATING FORAGE QUALITY

Nutritional evaluation of forages should consider energy, protein, and minerals. Both the levels and balance of nutrients need to be considered. Levels of protein and energy in range forages have a moderately high positive association. The gross energy content of forages expressed on an organic matter (OM) basis varies little across forage species or with plant maturity. However, the digestibility and metabolizability of gross energy to support animal production varies greatly among plant species and maturities.

Crude fiber, lignin, cellulose, CP, cell contents (acid detergent fiber), and cell walls (neutral detergent fiber) are chemically determined components which have been used to fit regression equations to predict forage quality, forage intake, and animal performance. Best results are obtained when these regression equations are used only within the plant species and locations from which data were obtained. Lack of fit increases greatly when the equations are extended from warm- to cool-season grasses, from grasses to forbs and browse, or when they are used at different locations or for a different kind of animal.

In vitro techniques provide a more direct estimate of the digestible energy content of a forage than use of regression equations. However, considerable variation may occur between different "batches" or analyses with in vitro techniques. Therefore, it is advisable to include a standard forage of known digestibility with each batch to correct for this variation. To convert digestible organic matter (DOM) to digestible energy (DE), Jeffery[2] developed the equation $DE = -0.218 + 4.92\ OMD$ ($r = .939$), where OMD is the coefficient of digestion for OM and DE is in units of kilocalories per gram. This equation can also be used to convert total digestible nutrients (TDN) to DE.

Most commercial laboratories utilize near-infrared reflectance (NIR) to provide nutritional analyses. This procedure involves the use of regression equations to relate the composition of samples analyzed by wet chemistry procedures to the reflectance spectrum of the feed. This technique provides a rapid procedure to evaluate samples, but caution must be exercised that the calibration set is appropriate for the samples being analyzed. Most calibration sets are based on harvested forages and single feeds. Analysis of range diets consisting of mixtures of grasses, forbs, and shrubs with NIR may result in significant errors if not properly calibrated.

Protein may be evaluated as total CP, digestible protein (DP), degraded intake protein (DIP), or undegraded intake of protein (UIP). DIP and UIP refer to the fractions of dietary CP that are degraded and undegraded, respectively, in the rumen. The relation between the percentage of CP in the diet and digestible CP in the diet was determined to be linear (Fig. 3). The estimated true digestibility of dietary CP was 94% and metabolic fecal nitrogen was 3.26 g/100 g of dry matter (DM) consumed. The relationship between CP in the diet (x) and its digestion coefficient (y) was determined to fit the general form $y = a + bx^{-1}$. Fitting 361 observations from South Africa by the least squares technique produced a realistic equation (Fig. 4).

These data indicate that using DP adds little information to using CP as a measure of the protein content of the diet of grazing animals. Although the true digestibility of CP in the diet does not vary greatly, the fraction that is soluble and degraded to NH_3 in the rumen varies widely among feeds. Little research work has been reported on DIP and UIP values for range forages. The following section was prepared by Kent Mills of Ezell-Key Grain Co., Inc., Sales and Nutrition, P.O. Box 1062, Snyder, TX 79550. He has been evaluating the use of analytically measured DIP and UIP for formulating supplemental feeding programs for range livestock in western Texas over the past 5 years. His program includes chemical analyses of hand-plucked

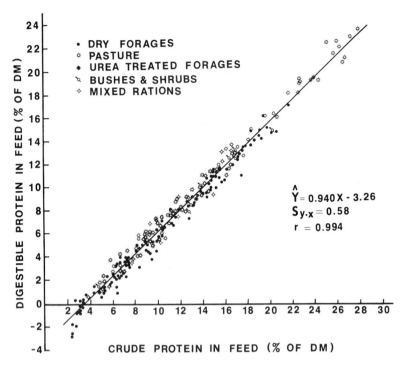

Figure 3

Relationship between the crude protein and apparently digestible crude protein concentration of feeds. (From van Niekerk DGH, Smith DWWQ, Oosthuysen D: Proc S Afr Soc Anim Prod 6:108, 1967.)

simulated diet samples for levels of DIP and UIP in addition to other analyses. He uses these values in a nutritional model he adapted for use with beef cows, sheep, and goats in the western Texas region.

Degradable Protein in Western Texas Native Forages*

DIP and UIP values for native forages are still in the development stage. The Northeast Dairy Herd Improvement Association (DHIA) Forage Analysis Laboratory in Ithaca, New York, has been analyzing for degradable protein since March 1993 using a *Streptococcus griseus* method developed by Cornell University. Using DIP data from this method has allowed development of more accurate and economical feeding programs for livestock in western Texas.

Degradable protein, being that protein faction that is available to the microorganisms in the rumen, affects forage intake. The size and activity of microbial populations in the rumen are dependent on the amounts of nitrogen and energy that are available to them. Optimizing the NH_3-to-energy balance in the rumen enhances microbial activity. More microbial activity increases fiber digestion and forage intake.

Other than during periods of lush growth, DIP values in simulated diets from western Texas rangelands have been in the range of 45% to 50% for cattle, 40% to 50% for sheep, and 30% to 40% for goats (Table 2, Fig. 5). Degradable protein levels in immature rapidly growing forages may reach as high as 70%. However, as the plants mature, the DIP level declines. Higher temperatures may contribute to the decreasing degradability of the proteins since roasting (heating to a temperature of at least 130°F) will decrease the degradability of the protein in soybeans. However, whether heat is an influence in declining DIP levels of forages has not been pursued or proved. Secondary compounds, especially in browse plants, may play a significant role in binding proteins so they are not available in the rumen.

This may explain why goat diets are much lower in degradable protein than cattle and sheep diets.

Whether a low DIP level results in a ruminal NH_3 deficiency depends on, among other things, the total level of protein in the forages. Rumen microorganisms need roughly 13% of the animal's DOM intake as DIP. Therefore, the amount of DIP required for a particular animal depends on both the energy-to-protein balance of the forage and the amount of forage that is consumed. A cow in late gestation that is eating 22 lb/day of forage organic matter with 59% TDN would need 7.67% of the total diet to be DIP to meet her ruminal requirements. However, recycled nitrogen may contribute as much as 30% to 50% of the total protein intake available to the rumen microorganisms, which lessens the dietary DIP requirement. As a rule of thumb, if the total protein in the forage is less than 7%, degradable protein is less than 50% of the total protein, or forage intake is restricted by availability, cattle performance can be enhanced by the addition of a supplement high in degradable protein.

Sheep and goats have higher total protein requirements per pound of intake than cattle. Also, the browse and forbs preferred by sheep and goats are lower in DIP than the grasses preferred by cattle. Thus, sheep and goats generally have a greater need for degradable protein supplementation than cattle. Goats, with DIP levels from 30% to 45% of the total protein intake, may have DIP deficiencies that restrict intake at total protein levels below 9%. Sheep performance can be improved with DIP supplementation at total protein levels below 8.5%. However, these recommendations must be modified by the type of diet that the sheep and goats are eating. Since sheep and goats can be more flexible than cattle in the plants they consume, there is more variation in the DIP values of their diets. If they are eating more grasses and less forbs and browse, the degradable protein values will be higher, more like those of cattle diets. In these cases, ruminal protein deficiencies will not occur at the same levels of crude protein mentioned above.

Supplementing to correct degradable protein deficiencies requires that supplements be evaluated based on their DIP levels as well as their CP. Where there is sufficient energy intake from the forage for rumen microorganism synthesis, urea or

---

*This section prepared by Kent Mills, B.S.

associated equivalent protein products are economical supplements to provide ruminally available nitrogen. The energy intake is critical, and if not available from the forage, supplemental energy must be fed. Of the "natural" proteins, soybean meal is highest in degradable protein, with values of 65% to 80% based on the National Research Council's (NRC) *Nutrient Requirements of Beef Cattle.*[5] Cottonseed meal, more readily available in Texas, has a degradable protein level of 57%. Grains will vary in the degradability of their protein based on the type of processing they have received. Grinding and flaking enhance the rumen passage rate, and as the rate of passage increases, DIP decreases.

Determining DIP requirements and supplementing to correct deficiencies in ruminal protein is still experimental. However, as more work is done, the confidence level in the values received from the laboratory analyses increases. Also, the performance of the livestock supplemented based on these levels indicates that the values received are reliable. Working with DIP values has helped to identify reasons for variable performances of livestock grazing under apparently similar forage conditions. The main effort of ruminant nutrition for livestock on native pastures should be to meet the nitrogen needs of rumen microorganisms to maximize intake and microbial fermentation of forages. Understanding and using DIP values is a critical first step.

NUTRIENT INTAKE FROM GRAZED FORAGE

Nutrient intake is a function of the amount of feed an animal consumes and the content and availability of the nutrients in

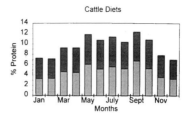

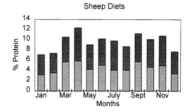

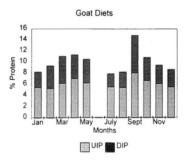

Figure 5

Average monthly crude protein content of hand-plucked forage samples simulating diets of cattle, sheep, and goats from rangelands in western Texas. Total protein is partitioned into degradable intake protein (DIP) and undegradable intake protein (UIP). (Data from Kent Mills, Ezell-Key Grain Co., Inc., Sales and Nutrition, P.O. Box 1062, Snyder, TX 79550.)

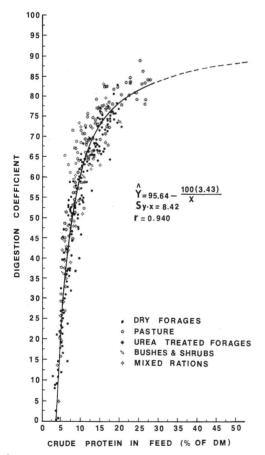

Figure 4

Relationship between the crude protein concentration of feeds and its apparent digestibility. (From van Niekerk DGH, Smith DWWQ, Oosthuysen D: Proc S Afr Soc Anim Prod 6:108, 1967.)

the feed. The amount of forage a grazing animal will consume is a function of the availability and quality of the forage, the kind of grazing management applied, and the kind, class, and physiologic status of the animal. We have already considered some of the factors affecting nutrient content of forages and the process of diet selection by the animal. Understanding the relationships among plant and animal components in range and pasture systems is vital to providing proper nutrition for grazing animals.

Intake of forage varies with species, maturity, and plant part. Digestibility is a useful indicator of intake and nutritive value within a forage class, but is not valid when comparing grasses with legumes or leaves with stems. Voluntary intake of sheep was 13.7% higher for legumes averaging 53.2% OMD than for grasses averaging 63.0% OMD. Voluntary intake was 28% greater for legumes having the same percent OMD as grasses. The legume diet had a shorter retention time (17%) and a higher amount of OM (14%) in the rumen than the grass diet of equal or greater digestibility. There was a close relation ($r = .96$) between daily intake of digestible OM and retention time in the rumen. Whereas it is commonly assumed that digestibility, rate of passage, and rumen volume control intake, these data indicate that intake control is centered elsewhere and digesta load and rate of passage are functions of intake.

Animals have been shown to regulate consumption of certain minerals and energy relative to their requirements. The level of metabolically available protein is critical to determining the energy demand of an animal. Animals generally select diets to maximize protein and energy intake and to maintain a balance

Table 2
MONTHLY ANALYSES OF FORAGE SAMPLES HAND-PLUCKED TO SIMULATE DIETS OF CATTLE, SHEEP, AND GOATS GRAZING ON RANGELANDS IN WESTERN TEXAS DURING THE PERIOD 1993–1996*

Month	Sample No.	Protein (%)	Degradable CP (% of CP)	NEm (Mcal/lb)	NEg (Mcal/lb)	Ca (%)	P (%)	K (%)	Mg (%)	S (%)	Cu (ppm)	Zn (ppm)	Mn (ppm)	DM (%)
					Cattle Data (3/93–2/97)									
Jan	74	7.21	46.49	0.470	0.214	0.616	0.081	0.466	0.100	0.123	11.5	31.3	83.0	88.32
Feb	46	7.06	48.04	0.471	0.215	0.596	0.073	0.401	0.091	0.113	11.3	32.8	74.6	90.32
March	29	9.21	50.82	0.505	0.251	0.618	0.109	0.738	0.114	0.143	10.5	31.8	69.3	79.00
April	12	9.21	48.92	0.519	0.268	0.585	0.115	0.716	0.098	0.134	9.5	28.3	59.3	79.21
May	5	11.78	51.72	0.540	0.292	0.568	0.162	1.314	0.122	0.158	13.6	30.6	59.0	66.00
June	6	10.70	48.97	0.548	0.298	0.533	0.142	1.282	0.130	0.140	9.7	28.2	63.7	82.75
July	17	11.34	49.67	0.548	0.298	0.576	0.154	1.378	0.144	0.223	8.0	24.2	59.7	68.96
Aug	44	10.34	50.98	0.545	0.298	0.585	0.129	1.330	0.143	0.154	14.2	29.5	62.0	72.72
Sept	14	12.31	54.91	0.520	0.269	0.578	0.165	1.574	0.146	0.184	13.4	36.0	64.1	66.63
Oct	54	10.80	49.74	0.527	0.278	0.724	0.132	1.266	0.146	0.163	11.9	30.9	65.4	67.86
Nov	50	7.80	46.46	0.496	0.243	0.717	0.090	0.810	0.134	0.129	13.3	32.4	75.7	80.74
Dec	57	6.97	47.63	0.488	0.233	0.621	0.083	0.534	0.106	0.111	11.4	31.4	67.3	87.44
Total	408													
					Sheep Data (3/93–2/97)									
Jan	18	7.05	44.56	0.467	0.212	0.683	0.077	0.392	0.077	0.109	10.7	32.2	90.7	87.06
Feb	11	7.35	47.99	0.482	0.227	0.637	0.071	0.364	0.071	0.102	11.0	34.5	76.0	88.21
March	8	10.50	53.84	0.514	0.264	0.608	0.120	0.800	0.088	0.155	7.5	30.1	66.0	72.68
April	4	12.33	47.80	0.568	0.320	0.783	0.125	1.175	0.123	0.165	9.0	34.3	56.8	65.28
May	1	9.00	46.70	0.590	0.350	1.110	0.120	1.270	0.140	0.160	11.0	26.0	58.0	89.70
June	3	10.17	50.13	0.513	0.263	0.723	0.117	1.033	0.130	0.157	10.3	31.0	62.7	66.87
July	4	9.78	41.55	0.563	0.313	0.750	0.120	1.120	0.143	0.133	14.8	38.8	68.0	87.05
Aug	5	8.66	47.36	0.520	0.266	0.542	0.106	0.842	0.100	0.116	14.6	39.8	72.2	89.36
Sept	4	11.23	51.05	0.523	0.273	0.635	0.130	1.058	0.115	0.148	10.5	38.0	61.3	68.20
Oct	12	10.07	46.63	0.516	0.262	1.000	0.110	1.010	0.143	0.148	15.3	40.7	80.8	68.33
Nov	11	10.77	46.16	0.517	0.263	0.933	0.118	0.961	0.138	0.163	10.8	32.5	91.9	67.73
Dec	17	7.68	44.27	0.511	0.260	0.787	0.087	0.517	0.101	0.106	11.3	31.2	84.2	81.38
Total	98													

Table 2
MONTHLY ANALYSES OF FORAGE SAMPLES HAND-PLUCKED TO SIMULATE DIETS OF CATTLE, SHEEP, AND GOATS GRAZING ON RANGELANDS IN WESTERN TEXAS DURING THE PERIOD 1993–1996* *Continued*

Month	Sample No.	Protein (%)	Degradable CP (% of CP)	NEm (Mcal/lb)	NEg (Mcal/lb)	Ca (%)	P (%)	K (%)	Mg (%)	S (%)	Cu (ppm)	Zn (ppm)	Mn (ppm)	DM (%)
						Goat Data (5/93–1/97)								
Jan	23	8.21	33.01	0.525	0.275	1.091	0.097	0.567	0.115	0.115	9.4	28.7	72.4	73.74
Feb	11	9.32	42.83	0.550	0.300	1.034	0.105	0.597	0.105	0.110	7.6	26.6	68.9	66.08
March	8	11.03	43.53	0.556	0.308	0.969	0.129	0.895	0.114	0.163	6.4	27.1	52.3	60.48
April	7	11.30	37.86	0.599	0.354	1.073	0.127	1.179	0.144	0.154	9.7	30.9	51.9	62.20
May	2	10.50	40.35	0.585	0.335	0.920	0.140	1.290	0.165	0.140	19.0	28.5	42.5	56.40
June	0	0.00	0.00	0.000	0.000	0.000	0.000	0.000	0.000	0.000	0.0	0.0	0.00	0.00
July	3	7.87	28.97	0.530	0.280	0.783	0.097	1.010	0.133	0.127	12.3	24.0	43.0	65.13
Aug	6	8.20	33.80	0.532	0.280	1.092	0.092	0.868	0.153	0.107	8.7	24.0	50.5	68.80
Sept	4	14.85	45.40	0.523	0.268	0.898	0.180	1.430	0.185	0.188	7.0	33.0	57.5	36.13
Oct	15	10.84	38.04	0.578	0.332	1.337	0.129	1.287	0.179	0.155	11.4	30.9	61.8	53.03
Nov	15	9.46	35.41	0.535	0.287	1.319	0.111	0.855	0.156	0.131	8.6	27.8	66.2	56.56
Dec	13	8.65	35.06	0.538	0.287	1.252	0.092	0.575	0.177	0.117	8.4	27.5	72.5	65.47
Total	107													

*CP, crude protein; DM, dry matter; NEm, net energy for maintenance; NEg, net energy for grain.

173

of these nutrients that matches their physiologic requirements. Secondary plant compounds (e.g., tannins) that increase metabolic losses of nitrogen reduce intake.

The level of metabolizable protein available determine the animal's energy demand, which then regulates intake. Legumes and leaves provide significantly higher levels of metabolizable protein than do grasses and stems, respectively; therefore, they support greater intakes. This metabolic hypothesis is proposed as an alternative to the hypothesis of physical control of intake.

GRAZING MANAGEMENT AND NUTRIENT INTAKE

Nutrient intake of grazing animals is influenced by the standing crop and growth rate of available forage relative to the forage demand rate. Total standing crop, measured at one point in time, is not an adequate indicator of forage availability over a period of days or weeks. Since animals graze selectively, standing crop should be evaluated by species or groups of similar species and separated by leaf and stem to identify the sources and extent of nutritional heterogeneity (Fig. 6). Growth rates of leaf and stem of the various species should also be estimated. Three general conditions exist for the relationship between forage growth rate (FGR) and forage demand rate (FDR): FGR > FDR, FGR = FDR, FGR < FDR

If FGR exceeds FDR, standing crop will increase and animals will graze selectively for green foliage. This produces optimal animal performance as long as the availability of the new growth is not hindered by an accumulation of mature or dead forage. Under this condition, nutrient intake will not be sensitive to the duration of grazing periods in rotational systems. However, selective grazing increases nutritional heterogeneity of the stand. If the grazing season on ranges is longer than the growing season, then periods when FGR is less than FDR will occur. This results in reduced forage quality with resultant change in nutrient intake of animals.

When FDR exceeds FGR, standing crop will decline. Selective removal of live leaves results in dead leaves and stems contributing a greater proportion of the standing crop, and sensitivity to grazing pressure increases. The impact on nutrient intake will depend on the nutritional heterogeneity of the standing crop and the kind, class, and physiologic status of the animal.

If nutritional heterogeneity is high, selective grazing will result in a progressive decline in nutrient intake, until low forage availability results in a sharp drop in intake. If the forage quality of the standing crop is uniform—for example, it contains a high proportion of green leaves—nutrient intake will be relatively constant until it is restricted by low availability, at which point it will decline sharply. This generally describes the pastures where the data for Figure 1 were collected.

Nutrient intake is sensitive to standing crop below some critical level. Above that level, there is no relationship between nutrient intake and standing crop. On tame pastures, grazing should be deferred until standing crop is above the critical level; then FDR should be set equal to FGR. When FGR is equal to FDR, standing crop should be stable. A continuous stocking strategy offers an efficient approach to maximizing nutrient intake from grassland pastures which produce primarily vegetative tillers. Pastures having species which produce primarily culmed tillers or legumes with elevated apical meristems may be utilized more effectively with rotational grazing methods. Grazing on tame pastures generally does not allow for accumulation of forage for use during periods when growth declines.

On most rangelands, the grazing season is significantly longer than the growing season and growth rates vary throughout the season. FGR may greatly exceed FDR for short periods. However, for much of the year FDR will exceed FGR on rangelands grazed yearlong. Seasonal use of rangelands (e.g., early intensive grazing) can significantly increase animal production per unit area. However, shortening the grazing season requires that alternative forage resources be provided to cover the period when the rangeland will not be grazed.

SUPPLEMENTAL FEEDING STRATEGIES

Livestock grazing on green, actively growing forage generally obtain adequate levels of most nutrients unless intake is limited by low availability. When animals are forced to utilize mature or dormant forage, nutrient deficiencies may be expected. Distinction should be made between nutritional problems resulting from limited forage supply and those related to concentrations of nutrients or toxins in the forage.

Supplemental feeding is the practice of providing limited

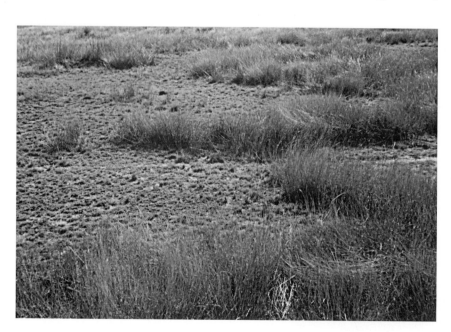

Figure 6
Selective grazing is a major problem in range utilization. Animals graze some plants too closely while leaving other plants undergrazed. This results in inefficient utilization of the forage and leads to deterioration of the range.

amounts of feed containing concentrated levels of specific deficient nutrients. Sometimes supplemental feeding is confused with emergency or maintenance feeding. Emergency feeding is practiced to meet the total requirement of animals on range or pasture when forage is temporarily unavailable for grazing, as when covered by snow. Maintenance feeding is required when pastures are overstocked and forage availability drops below levels which restrict intake, resulting in a DM deficiency. In emergency and maintenance feeding situations, the objective is generally to feed a balanced ration to carry animals through a stress period. This section examines the role of supplemental feeding of livestock on range or pasture. Maintenance feeding of animals on rangelands is not recommended because it results in environmental degradation and is seldom economical. Forage shortages should be addressed by reducing animal demand to match the supply, by increasing the forage supply, or by a combination of these measures.

Vitamins and Minerals

Significant body reserves of some nutrients, such as vitamin A and energy, may be accumulated by grazing animals. However, there are small body reserves of most minerals, protein, and water, and the animal's dietary requirements must be met on a regular basis. Supplementation of minerals and vitamins is not considered in detail in this chapter. Vitamin A is the only vitamin commonly deficient in diets of range livestock. Following periods of grazing green forage, body reserves may be adequate for 90 to 120 days. Synthetic vitamin A is added to most commercial range supplements and it may also be supplied by injection. Sodium and phosphorus are the minerals which are most widely deficient and provision should be made to supply them. Sodium should be provided throughout the year. Phosphorus should be provided whenever livestock are grazing mature or dormant vegetation. Phosphorus is required yearlong in many regions with phosphorus-deficient soils.

Green forage contains high levels of potassium. However, potassium may be deficient in diets of cattle grazing mature dormant forage. Potassium is highly mobile in plant tissue. It is removed during senescence and is readily leached from mature forage. Deficiency symptoms (reduced intake) may be observed within 2 weeks.

Protein and Energy

Protein- and energy-providing diets are both commonly deficient during certain periods of the year on rangelands. Whenever protein is deficient, animal production will be greatly reduced and digestion of the energy-providing components in the forage will be reduced. Growth will be reduced in stocker animals and reproduction and lactation will be reduced in breeding stock. However, if cows and ewes are provided protein and minerals with an adequate supply of forage, they can draw on body reserves of fat to meet a portion of the energy needs for lactation and reproduction. This strategy presumes that adequate fat stores are present.

The principle of utilizing periods of high-quality forage to store energy reserves for later periods of deficiency has great economic importance. If animals are stocked too heavily or otherwise managed during the growing season to prevent accumulation of energy reserves, costly supplemental feeds will be required to maintain body condition during the dormant season. Body condition of cows at calving can also be manipulated by adjusting the weaning date. Earlier weaning reduces nutrient demand and promotes storage of energy reserves. The livestock management calendar should be set to obtain an optimal match of the animal's nutrient requirements with the seasonal cycles of forage availability and quality.

Average daily gains of sheep and cattle decline as vegetation on spring and summer ranges matures; however, gains of lambs and calves decline much less than gains of ewes and cows. This is a common occurrence in the production of lambs and calves from rangelands and represents an important principle. It is not always possible to meet the total energy requirements of lactating cows or ewes from grazed forage, nor will the forage meet the nutrient requirements of young, growing animals. However, the cow or ewe meets the nutrient requirements of the young animal through conversion of forage and fat reserves to milk. When energy-providing intake of the cow or ewe is below its requirement, fat can be mobilized to support lactation if adequate protein is available. It is usually much more economical to store fat in the cow or ewe during periods when high-quality forage is available than it is to feed it as a supplement during periods of deficiency.

Not only is it expensive to supplement energy-providing diets, but intake and digestibility of forage are negatively affected by supplements containing large amounts of grain. Both intake and digestibility are enhanced by the addition of protein-rich supplements to roughage diets low in nitrogen. The greater the protein deficiency in the forage, the greater the increases in intake and digestibility of forage in response to protein supplements. The addition of supplements containing large amounts of starch depresses fiber digestion and forage intake.

Studies evaluating protein (cottonseed and soybean meals) vs. energy-providing (corn and barley) supplements for sheep on desert winter range in Utah showed that protein supplement increased daily intake of range forage, but grain supplements had no effect or tended to decrease daily intake of forage. The total quantity of digestible protein consumed daily in the supplement and the range forage was actually decreased by feeding corn or barley in some trials. High-protein supplements substantially increased the levels of metabolizable energy consumed by the sheep. Corn supplements slightly increased metabolizable energy in the daily ration, but barley actually reduced daily intake of energy because of reduced daily forage intake and depressed fiber digestibility. It was concluded that range livestock producers could benefit more from feeding a protein supplement such as cottonseed meal or soybean meal than from supplements such as corn and barley because protein supplements enhanced the value of range forage and produced better livestock responses.

Nonprotein nitrogen (NPN) may provide an economical substitute for part or all of the supplemental protein required by range livestock. Suggestions and guidelines for use of NPN supplements can be found in two publications: the NRC's *Urea and Other Nonprotein Nitrogen Compounds in Animal Nutrition*,[8] and *Non-Protein Nitrogen in the Nutrition of Ruminants*, published by the Feed and Agriculture Organization of the United Nations.[4]

WATER REQUIREMENTS

Water consumption by adult livestock of medium weight in a temperate climate may range from 7 to 17.5 gal/day for beef cattle and from 1 to 4 gal/day for sheep and goats.[6] As a general rule, cattle require 8 to 10 gal/day, sheep require 0.75 to 1.0 gal/day, and horses require 10 to 12 gal/day. However, these figures should be adjusted depending on ambient temperature. To account for the amount that will be lost by evaporation, cattle and horses should be allowed 12 to 15 gal/day and sheep 1.0 to 1.5 gal/day.

Sources of water include streams, springs, wells, and stock ponds (earthen tanks). The dependability of a water system should be judged during the dry season. The most common problems related to watering systems include poor distribution of watering places, not having enough water at each place, and poor water quality.

Reducing water intake reduces DM intake. The water-to-DM ratio in the rumen remains relatively constant when water intake is restricted. The animal adjusts to reduced water intake through a reduction in moisture excreted in urine and feces and by reducing DM intake. For this reason cattle should never go longer than 48 hours without water. Reduction of water consumption has also been reported to cause a reduction in CP digestibility.

All mineral elements essential as dietary nutrients are present to some extent in water and it is generally believed that elements in water solution are available to the animal as much as if they were consumed in dry feed or mineral blocks. Water may contribute part of the animal's requirement of S, I, Ca, Cu, Co, Fe, Mn, Zn, and Se,[7] but the amount contributed is subject to a great deal of variation depending on the kind and class of livestock, amount of water consumed, and the concentrations of these minerals in the water. In addition, the difference between the minimum requirement and the level at which toxic effects may occur is very small in some cases. For these reasons the NRC suggests that water not normally be relied upon as a source of essential minerals.[6] Of greater importance are the physical, chemical, and biologic properties of the water and their effects on water palatability and animal health.

There are a variety of substances that may be suspended or dissolved in livestock water that influence palatability or may be potentially harmful. These include inorganic elements and their salts, biologically produced toxins, parasitic or disease-carrying organisms, and manmade pollutants, particularly fertilizers and pesticides. Concentrations at which these substances render water undesirable are subject to many variables. Turbidity caused by suspended particles of clay and organic matter does not appear to be an important factor in itself with regard to palatability or animal health. Both short- and long-term effects and interactions with other substances must be considered.[7] Substances found in quantities not toxic to the consuming animal may accumulate within the animal to levels undesirable for those who consume livestock products. These factors make it difficult to determine safe levels for toxic substances.

Salinity problems are more universal in scope and are more likely to be encountered by the stockman. Total salt or mineral content (also expressed as total dissolved solids), while not indicating a single contaminating substance, is a common measurement that carries significance in determining livestock water quality. Highly mineralized water can cause physiologic disturbances (and even death) in animals. Even small salt concentrations can result in a decrease in palatability.

From time to time watering places may become infested by blooms of blue-green algae that produce toxins seriously affecting livestock. Toxicity of these blooms is extremely variable depending upon which species and strains of algae are present, types and numbers of associated bacteria, growing conditions, animal health, and amount of toxin consumed. Livestock poisonings have also been observed following rapid decomposition of algal blooms. This may be due in part to botulism poisoning resulting from anaerobic conditions accompanying decomposition. Algae can be controlled by use of 1 ppm of copper sulfate added to the water.

The purity of water consumed by livestock has far-reaching implications and there are many ways in which livestock water can become contaminated. Certain contaminants may affect livestock directly through losses by death, gains, or reproduction. They may also contaminate milk and meat to the point that human consumption is undesirable. It is necessary to understand the possible hazards to ensure an adequate supply of good-quality drinking water for livestock.

REFERENCES

1. Effects of Environment on Nutrient Requirements of Domestic Livestock. Washington, DC, National Academy of Sciences, 1981.
2. Jeffery H: Assessment of faecal nitrogen as an index for estimating digestibility and intake of food by sheep on *Pennisetum clandistinum* based pastures.
3. Kothmann MM, Hinnant RT: The Grazing Manager and Grazing Management Stock Adjustment Templates, rev II. College Station, Tex, Texas Agricultural Experimental Station Computer Software Documentation Series MP-1760, 1994.
4. Non-Protein Nitrogen in the Nutrition of Ruminants. Rome, Feed and Agricultural Organization of the United Nations, 1968.
5. Nutrient Requirements of Beef Cattle, ed 7. Subcommittee on Beef Cattle Nutrition, Committee on Animal Nutrition, Board on Agriculture, National Research Council, 1996.
6. Nutrients and Toxic Substances in Water for Livestock and Poultry. Washington, DC, National Academy of Sciences, 1974.
7. Proposed Criteria for Water Quality, vol I: Water for Livestock Enterprises. Washington, DC, US Environmental Protection Agency, 1973.
8. Urea and Other Nonprotein Nitrogen Compounds in Animal Nutrition. Washington, DC, National Academy of Sciences, 1976.

■ Mineral Supplementation of Beef Cattle: Rangeland and Feedlot

John C. Doyle, II, M.S., D.V.M., Ph.D.
Norbert K. Chirase, M.S., Ph.D.
J. E. Huston, Ph.D.

Beef cattle production relies primarily on forage (pastures and rangeland) for breeding and growth, which may be followed by grain feeding (feedlot). Market prices for beef (live and carcass specifications) and grain commodities determine the weight and age at which an animal is entered into a feedlot and an abattoir. The limitations imposed on livestock production are several, but foremost are the animal's genetic potential and nutrient supply. Recognition of limitations within any production system is required to maximize efficiency. One of the tenets of nutrition is that none of the nutrients acts in isolation, but that all nutrients interact within metabolic pathways to maintain homeostasis and promote productivity. Major and trace minerals are required in mammalian cells in numerous biochemical functions. An inadequate supply of any one can cause a malfunction of the system.

The diversity of environments in which cattle are grazed creates uncertainty in the prediction of mineral imbalances. Diets vary in amount and quality but satisfy most of the basic physiologic nutrient requirements of livestock. Deficiencies that commonly occur seldom produce simple, well-defined malfunctions. Marginal deficiencies or imbalances may totally escape notice as a management problem yet lead to subtle reductions in productivity that have a major negative impact on the economics of an enterprise.

Mineral deficiencies can be classified into the following categories:

Primary—The element is not present in adequate quantities, as observed through classic clinical signs (e.g., milk fever, grass tetany).

Secondary—The mineral is unavailable because of antagonistic interactions, resulting in toxicity of major or trace minerals and organic compounds that alter the biologic process (e.g., copper vs. molybdenum/sulfur, phytate vs. phosphorus).

Tertiary—The animal is in a negative balance because excretory losses arising from disease situations (e.g., parasitism, stress) exceed amounts ingested.[121]

Supplementation minimizes the disparity between pastures and animals' requirements. The nutrient demands of a cow/calf unit result from maintenance, pregnancy, lactation (colostrum and milk), and weight gain. Mineral supplementation should be considered essential, because inadequate consumption of various elements may limit the productivity of animals on pasture.

Feedlot production is dependent on grain as a primary energy and protein source for growth. Mineral deficiencies are not commonly observed under feedlot conditions; however, this does not preclude the possibility that supply of some minerals may be insufficient for varied phases of growth and breed. The animal's retained mineral nutrient tissue status (in muscle, liver, bone) on entry to the feedlot has a greater impact on initial health (immune status and structural integrity) than elements consumed during the first few days on the feedlot. A nutrient deficiency is difficult to overcome when animals initially fail to consume adequate quantities of feed. The best nutritional management practice for animals destined for feedlots is implemented during the growing phase.

The immunologic status and structural integrity of cattle arriving at the feedlot are influenced by various imposed stressors, including commingling, feed or water deprivation, weaning, exposure to infectious agents, weather changes, castration, dehorning, vaccination, dipping, and deworming. This predisposed or imposed physiologic stress can lead to nutritional deficiencies of both macrominerals and microminerals. Macromineral nutrition in feedlot cattle could be limited by depressed feed consumption as a result of stress. Seven trace minerals have been recognized as essential for the health and performance of feedlot cattle.[97, 125–127, 129] These minerals are cobalt, copper, iron, iodine, manganese, selenium, and zinc.

A single nutrient input becomes the metabolic output of a multitude of compounds that are utilized in subsequent inputs for various processes. The metabolic processes of lactation, maintenance, reproduction, growth, and immune function are given priority in terms of the energy component of the animal's diet. Efficiency of function, however, is predicated on the entirety of available nutrients. As knowledge of metabolic processes is advanced, introduction of nutritional inputs are best made in a sensible form.

AVAILABILITY OF NUTRIENTS FROM PASTURE PLANTS AND GRAINS

Ruminant nutrition includes two unique metabolic systems, the animal cellular physiology and the ruminal microbial population. Cellulose (structural carbohydrate) is the most abundant carbohydrate in the world, yet may be used only by microbes. Ruminant microbial fermentation includes the conversion of both structural and nonstructural (e.g., sugar, pectin, and starch) carbohydrates to volatile fatty acids (VFA) and synthesis of microbial protein. As ruminal fermentation is modified (e.g., forage vs. grain diet), the bioavailability of various elements is changed. This is because of the reduced digestibility of forages in grain diets. The principal function of the major minerals (calcium, sodium, chlorine, phosphorus, potassium, magnesium, and sulfur) in the ruminal microbial population is in the regulation of physicochemical properties, including osmotic pressure, buffering capacity, redox potential, and dilution rate. Microbial fermentation and animal tissue cellular function (i.e., glucose oxidation) utilize trace elements as catalysts in enzyme systems and as metalloenzymes. Natural protein sources (e.g., cottonseed meal, soybean meal) provide a high level of phosphorus and trace minerals that are partially soluble in the rumen, with a higher fraction available to the small intestines.

Pasture

Nutrients that animals derive from pasture plants and grains include energy (primarily from carbohydrates), proteins, various vitamins and vitamin precursors, and variable amounts of the different minerals. Grazing animals are in a dynamic nutrient flux. Nutritional requirements are in a constant state of change with the stage of production,[118] as are forage nutrients with the season.[71] Cows gain or lose tissue (fat and protein) depending on whether intake of nutrients exceeds or is exceeded by the requirements for on-going metabolic processes. Aligning the animal's major nutrient requirements with that of forage growth may provide adequate supplies of energy and protein, but some minerals are at minimal levels in the leaves of growing forages[93] and may not satisfy the animal's total requirements.

Nutrient deficiencies are observed when feedstuffs fail to provide adequate quantities of elements for animals. An audit of forage samples of 18 U.S. states showed that total forage mineral content (i.e., copper, manganese, zinc, cobalt, selenium, iron, and molybdenum) was theoretically insufficient to support optimal health and production.[33] A survey in Alberta, Canada, of plants located in dry-land saline sites observed zinc, copper, selenium, sodium, manganese, and potassium levels to be well below minimum requirements for beef cattle, whereas other elements (i.e., sulfur, magnesium, aluminum, iron, and molybdenum) exceeded maximum tolerable levels.[109]

The translocation of minerals from the soil, through the forage, and finally to the grazing animal does not necessarily proceed without interruption. Seasonal rainfall, climate, day length, and geologic pasture variations have major influences on the levels of plant minerals. Calcareous soils tend to prevent uptake of phosphorus and other individual or groups of minerals owing to high chelation properties.[21] Therefore, soil analysis may lead to erroneous conclusions regarding forage content. Different plant species growing on similar soil types and under similar environmental conditions exhibit differences in mineral content.[85] Hartmans[61] reported that copper levels within the soil and plants showed no correlation with copper status of the animal. The presence of minerals in plant matter does not ensure their availability to the consuming animal.

Mineral analysis of feedstuffs determines elemental concentration; however, bioavailability is more difficult to assess. Absorption of plant minerals will vary with the extent of ruminal fermentation of large molecular compounds followed by changes of pH throughout the digestive tract.[13] Utilization of minerals from the plant is dependent on their location within the plant cell, as follows:

1. Highly soluble and rapid release
2. Slow release as cell walls and protein components are degraded
3. No release

Copper is accumulated in the rapid-release fraction, as are calcium, magnesium, potassium, and phosphorus, whereas zinc is in the slow-release fraction. As the neutral detergent fraction (i.e., structural carbohydrates) of the diet increases, apparent absorption of manganese, zinc, iron, and copper decreases.[106, 157] This may be attributed to the high negative charge of fiber, which attracts cations. The rate of forage mineral release in the rumen is greater for potassium, magnesium, and sodium than for calcium and zinc. Phosphorus and copper availability vary depending on the forage species.[47, 137] Manganese and copper were found within the soluble plant fraction of alfalfa and Sudan hays and, along with zinc, became weakly bound to insoluble ruminal residue.[39] Minerals from high-quality forages (low structural carbohydrate fraction) tend to be released extensively for animal metabolism.

Absorption of a majority of minerals by the ruminant occurs at the upper region of the gastrointestinal tract (magnesium absorption occurs within the rumen). Thus, minerals are exposed to ruminal fermentation (microbial metabolism), acidic conditions of the abomasum, and followed by neutralization with entry into the small intestines. Trace elements that are cations may share similar absorptive pathways and are known to interact with each other. An excess of one trace mineral may saturate membrane-bound or intracellular carriers that two elements have in common and inhibit the absorption of the other element.[67]

Fermentation of organic matter in the rumen can either increase or decrease the biologic availability of minerals. Fiber sources are negatively charged and thus potentially antagonistic to cations. Binding agents such as phytate and oxalates may reduce the availability of some elements (i.e., phosphorus, calcium, zinc, and copper).[171] On hydrolysis of phytate (inositol hexaphosphoric acid) during ruminal fermentation, phosphorus is released for absorption.[106] The presence of copper, molybdenum, and sulfur in the rumen results in the formation of copper thiomolybdate, a nonabsorbable copper compound.[157] Thus, total trace minerals within plant material may not coincide quantitatively with those that are biologically available for the consumer (ruminal microbe or animal).

Feedlot

Grain variety, cultivar, processing method (e.g., steam flake vs. tempering or dry rolled), and ionophore dictate the availability of various nutrients for animal metabolism in feedlots. The mineral content of grains varies significantly and may have an impact on overall performance in feedlot situations. In feedlots in which grains are obtained from multiple sources throughout the year, the influence of a single grain cultivar nutrient source (i.e., superior or inferior nutrient content) is minimized. The roughage contribution of bioavailable minerals from high-grain diets is low because of depressed fiber digestibility.

Animal utilization of minerals from forage and grains is dependent on solubilization or release of the mineral element from the feedstuff and absorption of the released mineral.[51] The concentration of phosphorus in wheat, barley, and oat grains from soils low in available phosphorus are approximately 50% to 60% of those from fertile soils.[166] The phosphorus concentrations can be raised from 0.25% to 0.45% by superphosphate applications that subsequently increase the grain yields. Underwood[166] reported that wheat grain from zinc-deficient soils in Western Australia averaged only 16 ppm zinc, compared with 35 ppm from the same soil fertilized with zinc oxide. In wheat grain, mean selenium concentrations in the United States have been reported to be 0.80 and 0.05 ppm from soils high and low in selenium, respectively.[146] The mineral content of grains may depend on the soil in which they were grown as well as several other factors. The need to supplement feedlot diets with minerals is dependent on the requirements of the cattle fed as well as the source of dietary grain and protein meals.

FEED INTAKE, RATE OF PASSAGE, AND STRESS

Any nutrient deficiency influences overall animal performance; therefore, the complex neurohormonal regulation of dietary intake is critical. The animal's dietary intake and digestion are influenced by thermal, visceral, and osmo-, chemo-, and mechanico-receptors. Animals attempt to consume adequate

feedstuffs to meet or exceed energy requirements. An increased intake generally is accompanied by an increased rate of passage, with a decreased "digestion coefficient." Thus, intake determines the amount of nutrients consumed and influences nutrient digestibilities. The "absorption coefficient" of several elements is dependent on the animal's attempts to maintain homeostatic control through the demands of production. Diets possessing lower energy content (forage-based) are consumed at higher quantities with slower rates of passage than high-energy (grain-based) diets, which depress feed intake.

The "threshold of environmental stress" on animals can be measured through *temperature-humidity index* and *wind chill factor*.[59] These are indicators for extreme hot and cold weather conditions that impose physiologic stress on animals and may serve as an indicator for changes in dietary management.

Thermal stress has a pronounced effect on the animal's respiration rate, skin evaporation rate (sweating), body temperature, feed intake, and digestibility of various feedstuffs.[59, 96] One physiologic response to hyperthermia is sweating, which increases skin loss of sodium, potassium, magnesium, calcium, and chlorine.[79] An increased respiration rate (i.e., cooling—saliva loss with panting) may also modify mineral turnover. The heat-stressed animal fed a diet low in digestibility encounters a slower rate of passage and reduction in energy consumption.[29] A critical aspect of feeding animals in hot environments is to maintain the highest energy intake possible, which may require modifying the roughage source or level of concentration, or both, in the diet. Water availability (consumption) and air convection (position in pen) currents are used by animals in hot weather for cooling.

Exposure of ruminants to cold environments elicits a variety of physiologic responses that involve minerals. Exposure below the lower critical temperature results in an increased metabolic rate to compensate for heat loss and is accompanied by increased voluntary intake and increased rumen motility. Kennedy and coauthors[84] observed a consistent depression (10.2% vs. 4.4%) of apparent digestibility of calcium when animals were exposed to cold temperatures. Exposure to moderately cold temperatures failed to depress plasma magnesium concentrations in fed ewes but did act synergistically with starvation to induce hypomagnesemia.[164]

Many stresses, such as weaning, castration, deprivation of feed and water, transit, environment, and pathogenic disease, can alter the appetite of feedlot cattle. Hutcheson and Cole[76] reported that during the first week of arrival, healthy calves consumed 1.55% of their body weight in feed, whereas those that were diseased only consumed 0.90% of their body weight. Hence, an increased nutrient density is necessary to compensate for the decrease in feed intake and disease or stress. One of the basic principles of feedlot operation is "if one can keep a stressed animal eating (i.e., consuming adequate quantities of nutrients), one can save it." To compensate for the depressed feed intake during the initial phase of the finishing period, increasing the densities of nutrient (energy, protein, minerals, and vitamins) in the diet has been found to improve performance[76] and weight recovery rate.[26]

Feed and nutrient intake are the primary determinants of weight gain (muscle and fat deposits) and animal performance. Animals entering the feedlot are "shrunk" and stressed to varied degrees, which compromises health. An indicator of feed energy consumption for animals starting on feed can be calculated through a multiple of maintenance energy consumed (MMEC).

$$MMEC = \frac{\text{Feed intake (as fed [kg])} \times \%DM \times NE_m \text{ (Mcal/kg)}}{BW^{0.75} \times 0.077 \text{ (for } Bos\ taurus)}$$
$$\text{or } BW^{0.75} \times (0.077 \times 0.9) \text{ (for } Bos\ indicus)$$

where "as fed" is the weight of the feed including dry matter and moisture; DM equals dry matter (e.g., no moisture); and NEm is the net energy required for maintenance.

An MMEC value of 1.0 indicates that animals are maintaining entry weight, whereas greater values, of 1.7 to 2.1, infer gain and possible change from introduction diet to second dietary energy level. This method monitors energy intake against animals of varied weight classifications, body condition score, and days on feed. As animals increase total body fat content (>28%), energy and feed consumption becomes depressed.

REPRODUCTIVE PERFORMANCE: TRACE ELEMENTS

An important economic loss to a cow/calf operation is the non-pregnant cow; therefore, maintaining acceptable reproductive performance is essential. Early embryonic mortality loss (conception to day 40) in cattle has been estimated at 75% to 80%.[12] Research has identified several trace elements that affect reproductive efficiency during early embryonic development. Low copper and magnesium levels during the breeding season increased the number of services for conception and the rate of early embryonic mortality in lactating dairy cows.[80] Delayed and suppressed estrus has been associated with low copper and zinc intake.[65, 102] Elevated levels of manganese (53 ppm vs. National Research Council requirement of 40 ppm) significantly reduced days to conception (16 vs. 34 days) in first-calf heifers and cows.[38] Supplementation of copper, manganese, zinc, and cobalt influenced liver concentrations and increased numbers of animals exhibiting estrus by 45 days after calving and palpable ovarian structures.[163]

Body condition at calving to the end of the breeding season is clearly associated with return of estrus and conception,[45] but frequently unexplained departures from this generalized cause-and-effect relationship (well-conditioned animals that do not exhibit estrus nor breed) have been noted.[70] Mineral supplementation (phosphorus, copper, manganese, and zinc) on native pasture increased reproductive performance of lactating beef cattle possessing uniform body condition scores without altering serum or liver values.[40] The liver values of these beef cows were within physiologic norms, which may suggest an inadequate tissue response or lack of elemental mobilization to recipient reproductive tissues, or both. Uterine tissue regeneration is mandatory for reproductive response in the postpartum cow. The increase in physiologic response in reproduction to trace mineral supplementation may have been attributed to satisfying the immune system trace element requirements.

The ovum prior to implantation (day 14) is totally dependent on a dynamic oviduct and uterine environment for proper osmolality, nourishment, and antioxidant protection for blastomere division to progress.[141] One of the roles of trace minerals in reproductive performance may be at the endometrium level.[41] The differences of endometrial tissue element levels (elevated at day 1 and depressed at day 12) denote the dynamics of metabolism under hormonal influence. Similar observations have been identified with high levels of copper and zinc dismutase (antioxidant enzymes) in the uterus of pregnant animals.[78] Nutrient inputs fluctuate in copper, manganese, and zinc levels within the endometrium to a greater degree than observed with serum and liver levels. The multiple roles that copper, manganese, and zinc serve within the endometrium are presently unknown; however, their functions are both nutritional and protective (detoxification of uterine environment) for developing ovum.

WEIGHT GAIN: TRACE ELEMENTS

Animals that possess a genetic potential for rapid growth (large frame) have a higher nutrient requirement for production.

These animals generate greater quantities of beef on a per head basis, but many times the cow/calf operator has not realized true genetic potential because of nutritional limitations. Young growing animals generally encounter energy and protein deprivation under pasture conditions rather than a limitation of major or trace minerals. The weight gain observed with mineral supplementation may be a direct result of fulfillment of a physiologic deficiency, or it may result indirectly from the added minerals' stimulating an increase in forage consumption, which provides greater quantities of metabolizable energy and protein. Mineral supplementation (e.g., salt, phosphorus, calcium, and cobalt) is well recognized to stimulate feed intake for animals under grazing conditions. The use of selenium and cobalt rumen boluses has shown a response in certain geographic regions where these specific trace element deficiencies are encountered.[89, 132]

Pasture

A weight gain response was observed when a balanced mineral supplement was fed to young animals (150–200 kg) on pastures with marginal to deficient copper supplies.[72] Increased condition scores (6.0 vs. 4.5), weights (approximately 73 kg difference), and serum copper values were observed when supplemental copper was fed to lactating cows on marginally copper-deficient pastures.[39]

Feedlot

Different trace minerals (zinc, copper, manganese) and their sources (organic vs. inorganic) have been reported to influence feed intake and animal performance in feedlots.[11] Organic trace mineral supplementation on finishing diets was shown to influence feed intake, daily gain, and carcass quality (i.e., grades and marbling).[57] Hematocrit and plasma concentrations of zinc and copper were not altered with trace mineral supplementation.[44]

The use of anabolic agents (e.g., hormone growth promotants, steroid implants) has greatly influenced beef production in both pasture and feedlot situations. Anabolic agents are observed to enhance absorption and retention of nitrogen and minerals (i.e., calcium, phosphorus, magnesium, and zinc) from the diet.[55, 60, 69] Animals consume greater quantities of feed, grow faster (i.e., increase frame score), and deposit greater quantities of protein more efficiently.[49] The biologic attributes of anabolic agents may affect the levels of nutrients observed in feedlot waste.

IMMUNE FUNCTION: TRACE ELEMENTS

Nutritional deficiencies that depress structural and metabolic functions of the immune system create *immunocompetent defects*. The complexity of the immune system's *acquired response* is based on cellular and humoral function, whereas the *immediate response* function is phagocytic. The bone marrow is the production site of lymphocytes, which migrate to primary lymphoid organs that regulate and differentiate these cells. Cellular immunity is mediated through lymphocytes that mature within thymus, accumulate in lymph nodes (and other lymphoid tissues), and await a specific antigen to react as T-lymphocytes. Cell-mediated immunity is important in killing virus, bacteria, protozoan-infected cells, and tumor cells. Cytotoxic T-cells destroy target cells through binding and release of cytotoxic proteins (perforians), which disrupts membrane integrity, resulting in osmotic rupture. Another mechanism is through release of interferon-γ and lymphotoxins, which activate and stimulate macrophages to phagocytize organisms.

Humoral immunity lymphocytes are processed in intestinal lymphoid tissues and migrate to thymus independent areas to become B-lymphocytes. The B-lymphocytes produce antibodies, which are differentiated by immunoglobulin proteins (i.e., IgG, IgA, IgE, IgM, IgD). The antigen-induced production of antibodies involves a complex interaction of a number of cells.

The immune system's immediate response implements polymorphonuclear neutrophils (neutrophils and macrophages) that phagocytize pathogens via enzymatic degradation. Macrophages are also involved in processing antigens for T-cell function. Phagocytized pathogens are destroyed by lysosomes via free radicals (OH^-), superoxide radicals (O_2^-) and hydrogen peroxide (H_2O_2, potent oxidant) production. These potent oxidants are nonspecific and may destroy membranes of neutrophils and adjacent tissues (polyunsaturated phospholipids in biologic membranes) when adequate antioxidants are not present for protection. Hence, the role of antioxidant enzymes (i.e., zinc and/or copper superoxide dismutase [SOD]) is to protect tissues from oxidants.

A functional immune system requires nutrient inputs for cellular production and maintenance. Of primary importance are major tissues (e.g., bone, thymus, lymph nodes) that provide the physical sites and primary cellular tissues for immune function. The cellular tissue metabolic activity requires:

1. Energy for protein synthesis and cell replication.
2. Protein or amino acids for antibodies, complement, and cytokines.
3. Minerals: macrominerals (i.e., calcium and phosphorus) involved in membrane integrity and cellular function, trace minerals (i.e., zinc, copper, selenium) in antioxidant enzyme activity.
4. Vitamins A and D used in cellular differentiation, and vitamin E as an antioxidant to protect cellular membranes from polyunsaturated fatty acids.

Nutrient deficits can contribute to functional impairment, yielding a nonresponsive immune system.

Trace minerals have been shown to be involved in disease deficient processes.[53] Immune deficiencies evolve as either *immunocompetent defects* during primary tissue development (e.g., small thymus) or *immunosuppression*, a consequence of the metabolic effects of glucocorticoid and epinephrine release during periods of stress (e.g., transport, weather). Depression of the immune system is associated with nonresponsive medical therapy (i.e., vaccination, antibiotics, anthelmintics) of calves or older animals on pasture and in feedlots.

Chromium

Chromium has been reported to improve performance and immune status in stressed animals. Supplemental chromium fed to stressed calves in corn silage–based diets with soybean meal or urea-corn premix decreased serum cortisol and increased serum IgM and total immunoglobulins.[23] A study on transit-stressed calves evaluated the effects of chromium yeast on performance, morbidity, serum cortisol, and immunocompetence.[116] This study reported a 27% increase in average daily gain (ADG), decrease in morbidity, increase in primary antibody titers to human red blood cells (HRBC), decrease in serum cortisol, and an increase in IgG_1 concentrations at day 14. In these studies, supplemented chromium was 1 ppm (i.e., difficult to quantify). A subsequent study on efficacy of organic chromium supplementation on stressed calves with different protein sources observed no advantage in animal performance or morbidty.[99] Studies of calves fed diets supplemented with different sources of chromium (chromium chloride, chromium yeast, or chromium nicotinic acid) indicated that chromium nicotinic acid and chromium yeast affected immune response (intradermal injection of phytohemagglutinin [PHA]) and chromium nicotinic acid affected insulin-related functions.[83] Currently, more research is required

to determine whether the immunomodulatory properties of chromium sources are functionally related to its role with glucose tolerance factor (GTF).

Copper

Copper's various functions in the immune system include synthesis of copper and zinc superoxide dismutase (SOD-antioxidant enzyme), ceruloplasmin, lymphocyte replication, development of antibodies, neutrophil production, and phagocytic and killing ability. Deficiencies of copper have been associated with increased T-cell infections, inhibited T-cell mitogen response, decreased phagocytic activity, and pro-inflammatory effects.[94]

Pasture

Copper responsive therapy of calves exhibiting clinical signs of diarrhea (scouring) has been designated as "scouring disease" and "peat scours" in some regions of the world. This is associated with depletion of cytochrome oxidase and pathologic atrophy of the epithelium of small intestines.[48] Cytochrome oxidase functions in the terminal steps of oxidation metabolism, and copper-SOD acts within the defense mechanism against superoxide radicals.

Feedlot

Copper deficiency alters the acute-phase protein (ceruloplasmin) response to viral infections such as bovine herpes virus-1.[8] Injections of copper-glycinate in animals prior to transport (18 days) was reported to increase plasma copper levels as well as morbidity.[151] At the feedlot, these calves were challenged with an infectious bovine rhinotracheitis virus (IBRV), which lowered feed intake 30% and depressed body weight 6.9% when compared with steers not injected. This study indicated that parenteral copper was detrimental to the recovery rate of IBRV-stressed animals. Animals fed dietary copper source were observed to have lower weight gains 28 days after IBRV challenge ($P < .03$) when compared with steers fed either sulfur-molybdenum or copper-sulfur-molybdenum supplemented feedlot diets.[64]

Manganese

Manganese's role in immune function has not been well demonstrated in cattle. Supplementation of organic zinc and manganese prior to shipping to the feedlot is beneficial to the health of feedlot steers.[27] Steers fed zinc and manganese oxide before and after transit had the lowest recovery rate, whereas the zinc methionine and manganese methionine combinations provided best improvement in recovery. The zinc methionine and manganese oxide combination supplement was intermediate in alleviating feed intake depression, body weight loss, and rectal temperature elevation.[1] These results provided evidence that there existed synergism between an organic zinc and supplemental manganese in stressed calves.

Selenium

Selenium is recognized for its functional role in selenium-dependent glutathione peroxidase (antioxidant), reducing hydrogen peroxide and lipid hydrogen peroxides. Deficiency is associated with observed decreases in T-lymphocyte blastogenesis, neutrophil random migration, chemotaxis, phagocytosis, killing potential, and depressed antibody production of IgM and IgG.[90]

Pasture

Dietary restriction of cows prior to calving and during lactation affects the level of selenium in colostral antibodies and neonate tissues.[2] Other studies[16, 58] have reported a decrease in microbial activity of neutrophils isolated from selenium-deficient cattle.

Feedlot

Parenteral selenium alone or in combination with parenteral vitamin E increased serum selenium levels and improved immunocompetence (i.e., quadratic increase in IgG titers in response to *Pasteurella haemolytica* vaccination) in steers. However, animal performance and health were not affected.[43]

Zinc

Zinc deficiency is associated with atrophy of thymus. Zinc functions in immunity through protein synthesis, membrane stabilization (against endotoxins), superoxide dismutase (SOD; antioxidant enzyme), production maintenance of epithelial tissues, lymphocyte replication, and antibody production. Deficiencies impair cytotoxic T-cell activity, B-cell activity, natural killer cell activity, antibody-dependent and -independent antigens, delayed hypersensitivity, and corticoid production.

Pasture

Animals fed various sources of zinc (organic and inorganic) from birth to weaning have been observed to benefit in performance before and after stress, with subsequent feeding.[150]

Feedlot

Steers identified to be seronegative for IBRV and parainfluenza virus type 3 (PI$_3$) were fed organic or inorganic zinc sources to determine the influence on their immune response.[152] The greatest desirable IBRV antibody titers were reported in steers fed zinc methionine when compared with control steers, with zinc oxide–fed steers having intermediate titers. On day 14, 33% of control and 23% of zinc oxide–fed steers tested seronegative for IBRV, whereas only 10% of the zinc methionine–fed steers tested seronegative. Feeding organic zinc provided a more rapid titer response in steers with initial low titer values, but not in steers with initial titer values greater than 10. This suggests that bioavailability of organic zinc supplements may have an impact on the immune response during disease. A relationship between changes in rectal temperature and body weight (BW) due to IBRV infection in feedlot steers has been reported.[26, 27] The general pattern of daily BW changes indicated that dietary zinc methionine and manganese methionine combination tended to reduce BW loss in steers challenged with IBRV compared with steers fed a control diet or a zinc oxide and manganese oxide combination diet.

BREED INFLUENCES

Various breeds have been shown to exhibit differences in mineral requirements. The first established mineral requirements were constructed from controlled research studies from several breeds (primarily English) of cattle. Many crossbred and exotic breeds of cattle possess a greater genetic capacity for increased frame size. The 1996 Beef NRC tables report that animals of varied frame size possess different energy and protein requirements for gain. Several researchers have observed a greater copper requirement for Holstein calves and Simmental and Charolais cattle (i.e., large frame) than for medium-frame beef breeds such as Angus.[112, 172] Blood, liver, and bile samples were collected from nine breeds of cows fed different energy levels for 3 to 5 years and evaluated for copper and zinc concentrations. Both breed and feed intake affected liver zinc concentrations ($P < .05$). Limousin cows had the highest levels of liver

zinc, whereas Angus cows had the lowest. Liver zinc concentrations increased with increased daily feed intake. Liver copper concentrations were highest in Limousin, Simmental, and Charolais breeds at the lowest liver weights, whereas Hereford, Angus, and Red Poll breeds had the lowest liver copper levels at the lowest liver weights. However, copper concentrations generally decreased as liver weights increased.[91] Liver copper levels were similar across the range of liver weights for Gelbvieh, Pinzgauer, and Braunvieh cows.

MINERAL CONTENT OF WATER

The most important physiologic aspect of water as a nutrient is the quantity consumed. Depression of water consumption by contaminants (organic or inorganic compounds) is of more importance than an imposed mineral imbalance. Animals respond to heat stress with increased water consumption (i.e., 10% BW). Deprivation or reduced water intake depresses dry matter (DM) intake, resulting in lowered productivity. Cattle that are moved to different locations should be provided the best quality water for the most rapid rehydration on arrival.

Water treatment processes (i.e., filtration, ion exchange, or ozonization) can significantly improve water quality through removal of mineral contaminants (e.g., sulfur removal improves copper availability) or increased oxygen concentration or both. Improving water quality may improve consumption and livestock performance. Water quality is monitored through the concentrations of elemental compounds in solution. This concentration of dissolved elements is referred to as *total dissolved solids*. *Salinity* describes the total ionic concentration of salt (soluble sodium, calcium, magnesium, potassium salts) in water. The term *hardness* is related to the concentration of divalent cations (calcium and magnesium).

The elemental concentration of water may contribute to, but is generally inadequate to meet, the dietary requirements of ruminants. However, water may contain elements that exist at antagonistic or toxic levels. Water sources that provide high levels of sodium or calcium bicarbonate can increase the incidence of urinary urothiliasis (increase cations) in feedlot animals.[42] Antagonistic levels of sulfur and molybdenum in solution can interfere with copper metabolism. Substances and elements may vary in toxicity depending on the nature of the suspension (solid or solution) and the chemical forms in which they exist. *Total dissolved solid* content of water is a valuable tool in detecting elemental excesses that may impose depressed consumption or mineral imbalances.

Electrolyte and antibiotic therapy administered via water before and after transit stress to animals has been evaluated by many individuals with varying degrees of success. A common problem of implementing water as a carrier is associated with the failure of the animal to consume adequate volumes (i.e., limited by palatability) for rehydration followed by limited feed intake. This may be a result of inaccurate concentrations (i.e., dosage and/or evaporation rate) or the animals' not being accustomed to an elevated water mineral content. Supplementation of an ingredient via water source requires daily monitoring of volume consumed by the animals. Several minerals (i.e., copper and salt) are observed to be more toxic when presented in solution than in feed.[24, 124]

Supplementation of electrolytes may be successful under well-managed situations (i.e., monitoring concentrations and cleaning troughs). Beneficial effects of electrolyte therapy have been observed in feedlots and abattoirs. The physiologic shift caused by stress of electrolytes (i.e., decreased blood P$_{CO_2}$ and hydrogen ion and increased chloride) prior to slaughter influences meat quality (e.g., dark, firm, and dry meat). Improving electrolyte or glucose balance via water source for bulls 18 to 20 hours before slaughter coincided with improved meat quality traits and carcass yields.[144] A subsequent investigation of an electrolyte and glucose combination supplied via water source for bulls prior to slaughter (i.e., 0, 12, 24, or 36 hours) showed lower weight loss (1.5%) in the live animals and higher cold carcass weights (2.2 to 7.6 kg) for 12 to 36 hour groups, respectively.[145]

MINERAL IMBALANCES

Mineral deficiency signs can be perplexing because the observed conditions usually involve more than one mineral and can be combined with protein and energy malnutrition, parasitism, toxic plants, and infectious diseases. The animal's circulation attempts to maintain a consistent level of essential protein-mineral moieties (i.e., enzymes) to satisfy various tissues' metabolism. As physiologic function is altered, tissue demand is modified. Clinical signs often suggestive of gross mineral imbalances are observed as ill thrift in the presence of ample forage production. Mineral nutrition disorders range from acute deficiency or toxicity, characterized by well-marked clinical signs and pathologic changes, to mild and transient conditions difficult to diagnose (e.g., unthriftiness, unsatisfactory growth, low reproduction). Rarely does a gross mineral deficiency express itself, but when it does, it can be easily diagnosed and corrected. Thus, the most costly loss in production is the subclinical illness or disease that exists within a production unit.

DETECTION OF MINERAL IMBALANCES

The energy and protein requirements of animals should be satisfied for production prior to an evaluation of a mineral deficiency. A deficiency is best confirmed with response to specific supplementation of a bioavailable element. It is important to recognize limitations of clinical and pathologic data when attempting to "profile" animals.

The term *deficient* or *toxic area* (seen on geographic maps) is given to a region in which these entities are encountered more frequently. This does not imply that all plants or animals in the region have deficiencies or toxicities. The detection of mineral imbalances is derived from the combination of clinical, pathologic, and biochemical status of the animal and chemical analysis of the diet.

Tissue-mineral concentrations portray the contribution of the animal's total environment in meeting its requirements. Unfortunately, no mineral concentration of any one tissue will predict true animal status. As the animal's physiologic requirements are challenged, various tissue demands are modified. Animal-tissue concentrations are valuable indicators of mineral status but are greatly influenced by many factors. Whole blood, serum, and plasma are used widely in mineral research, yet only values that are significantly and consistently above or below "normal" range provide suggestive, but not conclusive, evidence of dietary excess or deficiency of a particular element. Precautions must be taken in interpreting blood mineral data collected under less than optimal conditions. Extraneous causes for elevated serum or plasma mineral values include collection contaminants (red silicone stoppers for blood collection tubes contribute zinc), stress, hemolysis, temperature, and serum separation time.[50] Stress and disease can dramatically alter blood concentrations, retention, and excretion of both major and trace minerals.[26, 27] Interpretation of blood mineral data from animals that have been stressed can be erroneous. It may appear that these animals have several mineral deficiencies, when they are physiologically responding to stress through modifying various moieties involved in im-

mune function to protect the body. Trace mineral deficiencies and excesses can depress immune function.[11]

Hair is a poor indicator of animal mineral status, since calcium, phosphorus, and copper levels in hair do not reflect dietary intake. On the other hand, zinc and selenium concentrations do exhibit some variation with the diet. Chronic consumption of heavy metals such as lead, arsenic, and cadmium has been reflected in hair assays. Enzyme assays for ceruloplasmin (copper) and glutathione peroxidase (selenium) are used regularly as a correlation of mineral status. Liver has been a traditional organ tissue collected for analysis of cobalt, copper, and zinc. Interpretation of elemental levels can be confounded by collection location, fat quantity, and tissue damage (parasitic migration and/or abscesses). Various breeds possess varied metabolic requirements, as observed when different breeds were grazed on the same pasture and liver copper and zinc concentrations were found to differ within breed.[91]

CATION/ANION DIFFERENCE

The animal's physiology attempts to maintain electrical neutrality of the body under fluctuating inputs of hydrogen ions and carbonate. Recognition and implementation of dietary cation/anion difference (DCAD) has been well demonstrated in dairy cattle through reduction of milk fever and ruminal stasis, improved postpartum uterine involution, ketosis, and total milk production. The complete formula of primary elements is expressed as milliequivalents:

$$mEq = [(\%Na + \%K + \%Ca + \%Mg) - (\%Cl + \%SO_4 + \%H_2PO_4 + \%HPO_4)]/100 \text{ g DM}.$$

The abbreviated equation or a common calculation is as follows:

$$DCAD \ mEq = [(\%Na/0.023) + (\%K/0.039)] - [(\%Cl/0.0355) + (\%S/0.016)].$$

The cation/anion difference has not been considered in beef production. However, implementing a *dietary electrolyte balance* (DEB) of 15 to 30 mEq/100 g of DM was shown to be beneficial to growing cattle on silage and feedlot concentrate diets.[138, 139] Calculation:

$$DEB \ mEq = (\%Na/0.023 + \%K/0.039 - \%Cl/0.035).$$

Feeding high cation diets (excessive bicarbonate supplementation through feed or water) can result in increased incidence of urinary urolithiasis in feedlot situations.[42]

Anionic compounds include ammonium sulfate, calcium sulfate, magnesium sulfate, ammonium chloride, calcium chloride, and magnesium chloride. A cation compound is sodium bicarbonate.

MAJOR ELEMENTS

Salt (Sodium and Chloride)

Sodium, chlorine, and potassium function to maintain osmotic pressure and regulate acid-base equilibrium for rumen microbes and animal cells. Both sodium (cation) and chlorine (anion) are involved with cellular function in basic metabolism, nutrient uptake, transmission of nerve impulse, and muscle contraction. Sodium is found in much lower quantities than chlorine in natural feedstuffs. The requirement of sodium is between 0.06% and 0.10% of the diet.[118] The chlorine requirement for beef cattle is presently unknown, yet its function is necessary for the formation of hydrochloric acid in gastric juices and activation of amylase.

Pasture

The highest physiologic requirement for salt is in lactating cows because of secretions in the milk. Sodium deficiencies are most likely to occur in animals that are growing, exposed to high environmental temperatures, and grazing pastures with high potassium content (rapidly growing forages). Beef cattle seek out salt; hence, it is an important component for many free-choice supplements. Along coastal regions or areas with high-sodium plant levels, salt-based supplements are not readily consumed, and an alternative intake enhancer may be required (e.g., protein meals, fat, dried yeast products, or molasses) to achieve adequate intake. Caution is recommended when using salt to restrict the intake of protein supplements. When forages are limited (drought conditions), energy-deficient animals can consume enough salt to be toxic (approximately 2.2 g/kg of body weight), especially when water is limited.[124] Salt is found to be toxic in water when at a concentration of greater than 1.25%.

Feedlot

The inclusion of salt in feedlot diets is traditionally held at approximately 0.20% to 0.25%. This increases water consumption (increased renal activity) and maintains feed intake during varied weather conditions. Minimizing salt excretion in manure is best achieved through recognizing the contribution from feed ingredients and water.

Potassium

Potassium functions primarily at the cellular level, maintaining osmotic pressure (major cation of intracellular fluid), acid-base equilibrium, water balance, muscle contractions, nerve impulse transmission, and some enzymatic reactions. In contrast to sodium, it is not stored in the body in appreciable amounts and must be supplied daily. Beef cattle requirements for potassium are between 0.6% and 0.7%.[118]

Pasture

Potassium supplementation has been shown to lessen gestating cow weight and body condition loss, increase calf weight gain, and improve reproductive performance.[158, 159, 169] The highest physiologic requirement of potassium is in the lactating cow for secretion in the milk. Forages are high in potassium (1% to 4%) during the growing season, but when dormant may contain inadequate levels (<0.5%) for grazing animals.[87] High potassium levels in plants (small grain pastures) can be antagonistic to magnesium absorption, predisposing to grass tetany.

Feedlot

Cattle subjected to the stresses of marketing and shipping encounter many metabolic changes. This weight loss or "shrink" is a result of body (i.e., tissue) and digestive tract water excretion. When excretion exceeds 8% of body weight, intracellular water losses and acute potassium deficiency could occur. Potassium supplemented at 1.3% in the receiving feedlot diet for the first 14 days lowered mortality rate and increased performance.[77] Potassium deficiencies are likely when high-producing animals (lactating dairy cows or feedlot animals) are fed high grain diets (grains contain less than 0.5% potassium).

Supplemental sources of available potassium include potassium chloride, potassium bicarbonate, potassium sulfate, and potassium carbonate.

Calcium and Phosphorus

Calcium and phosphorus constitute 70% of all mineral elements in the body and are vital to almost all tissues. Calcium functions in skeletal formation, blood clotting, cardiac rhythm, neuromuscular transmission, membrane permeability, and enzyme activation. The homeostatic concentration of calcium in the blood comes from bone. Phosphorus is a constituent of bone, red blood cells, muscle, and nerve tissue. It functions in buffering systems during the process of energy exchange. A severe limitation of phosphorus is reflected as a general impairment of health, yet does not directly relate to reproductive performance.[22]

Pasture

The 1996 Beef NRC separates calcium and phosphorus requirements for maintenance, growth, pregnancy, and lactation. In general, cattle requirements are 0.18% to 1.04% calcium and 0.18% to 0.70% phosphorus for growing heifers and steers, and 0.22% to 0.70% calcium and 0.17% to 0.37% for lactating heifers and cows. Either calcium or phosphorus, or both, can be deficient for the grazing cattle. Forages tend to have higher calcium and lower phosphorus content. Phosphorus deficiencies are the most widespread and of greatest economic importance of all mineral deficiencies for grazing cattle.[103, 167]

Energy, protein, and phosphorus levels tend to move in parallel in many pasture situations. The adequacy of these components within plants may or may not satisfy animal production requirements. When high animal production requirements (lactation, reproduction) are synchronized with plant growth (growing season = high energy and protein concentrations), phosphorus content can be near maximum for the soil or plant yet fail to meet the animal's requirements.[105]

Levels of calcium and phosphorus in free-choice mineral mixes that are commercially available are generally in a 1.5:1 to 1:1 ratio. A 2:1 ratio is considered adequate for the total diet, but the high calcium level that usually occurs in low-quality forages makes a low calcium:phosphorus ratio in the supplement preferred. The dietary calcium:phosphorus ratio can be as high as 7:1 as long as the animal consumes its minimal phosphorus requirement.[135] Some phosphorus sources are not palatable and, at high levels (e.g., 14%) within a supplement, may be economical but poorly consumed. In a free-choice supplement, the phosphorus concentration can be 6% to 8% when forages are 0.2% phosphorus or higher. When forages are below 0.2%, a mineral supplement containing 8% to 10% phosphorus would be more efficacious.[104] Higher concentrations of both calcium and phosphorus should be used when forage concentrations are low and when the animal's physiologic requirements are high (e.g., lactation).

Feedlot

Feedlot diets generally contain greater calcium levels than required (0.70% to 0.85%). The feed intake response to higher calcium levels may be attributed to buffering, DCAD, or ingredient interactions (e.g., wheat, fat).[15]

The biologic availabilities of calcium and phosphorus in mineral supplements vary with chemical source. Sources of calcium with high bioavailability include monocalcium phosphate and dicalcium phosphate. Calcium sources with intermediate bioavailability are calcium carbonate (e.g., from ground limestone, oyster shells), defluorinated rock phosphate, and dolomitic limestone. Phosphorus sources with high bioavailability are monocalcium phosphate, phosphoric acid, and sodium phosphate. Phosphorus in defluorinated rock phosphate and dicalcium phosphate is intermediate in bioavailability.

Magnesium

Magnesium is found in both the skeleton (60% to 70%) and soft tissues and functions in numerous enzyme systems. The most critical function under practical conditions is its involvement in neuromuscular activity. Low dietary intake results in grass tetany (hypomagnesemia).

Pasture

Hypomagnesemia usually occurs on immature pastures with high potassium content, and the incidence may be related to the requirements of different breeds.[56] The digestibility of magnesium was higher for Brangus, Brangus x Holstein, Angus, and Hereford x Holstein than for Hereford, Hereford x Jersey, Brangus x Hereford, Jersey, and Holstein cows. The magnesium requirement is 0.10% to 0.25%,[118] with potentially higher levels required for lactating cows. Older animals are more prone to grass tetany because of their inability to mobilize sufficient magnesium from the bone under higher metabolic requirements (lactation). Animals exposed to pastures where grass tetany may be a problem should be treated prophylactically (i.e., magnesium and/or inclusion of lasalocid in mineral supplement) during that time period.

Feedlot

Ionophore (e.g., monensin, lasalocid, laidlomycin and salinomycin) interactions are commonly identified with Mg[176] through increased fermentation or improved absorption.[77]

The bioavailabilities of magnesium are high for carbonates, hydroxide, oxides, and sulfates.[4, 37] High-magnesium supplements (8% to 14% magnesium with 100 to 200 g/day consumption) used to prevent hypomagnesemia are successful only if adequate intake is achieved. Toxicosis can occur with total diet supplementation of magnesium at levels greater than 2.4%.[133] Magnesium is an unpalatable mineral and requires formulation with ingredients (e.g., molasses, protein meals, grains) that induce intake. A complete mineral supplement should contain a minimal level of magnesium (>1%).

Sulfur

Sulfur is an essential component of amino acids (methionine and cysteine), vitamins (thiamine and biotin), hormones (somatostatin and oxytocin), and sulfate polysaccharides (chondroitin). It is involved in numerous metabolic functions including carbohydrate and fat metabolism, protein synthesis and metabolism, endocrine function, blood clotting, and acid-base balance of intracellular and extracellular fluids.

Pasture

Sulfur is not commonly given as a supplement under pasture conditions because of its elemental antagonistic properties. It has been observed to improve weight gains for young cattle grazing forage sorghum with elevated levels of prussic acid (cyanogenetic glucosides).[133] High sulfur contents in water have been shown to depress consumption as well as inhibit absorption and metabolism of copper by the formation of copper sulfide.[118]

Feedlot

Sulfur compounds are commonly used in the form of anionic salts to balance cation/anion difference for feedlot beef and dairy diets. Supplementation with sulfur was shown to be beneficial in feedlots when high levels of urea were used in the ration (nitrogen-to-sulfur optimum ratio 13.5:1 to 15:1).[13] High levels of ammonium sulfate supplementation in feedlots or pasture situations have been associated with polioencephalomalacia.[34, 42] The proper concentration of sulfur in the diet is between 0.08% and 0.15%. The maximum tolerable level is 0.4%.[118]

TRACE ELEMENTS

Chromium

Chromium functions as a component of the glucose tolerance factor (GTF), potentiating insulin.[80] Increased urinary losses of zinc and chromium have been reported with market transit stress, fasting, and IBRV infection.[123] Investigations have shown improved immune responses (vaccination, challenged and unchallenged with IBRV antigen) and additional growth rate (stressed and nonstressed) in cattle.[23, 82, 116, 117] Standardized investigations of chromium requirement have been inconclusive. Investigated levels of supplementary levels range from 0.2 to 1.0 mg/kg of DM, with a 70 day study at 4.0 mg/kg of DM showing no ill effects. Supplementation with organic compounds of chromium produced higher biologic response than with inorganic sources (chromium polynicotinate, chromium yeast, chromium chelate vs. chromium chloride).[83]

Cobalt

Cobalt is required for the synthesis of cobalamin (vitamin B_{12}), which is needed by both microorganisms and animal tissues. Vitamin B_{12} is involved in methyl malonyl-CoA isomerase, which is required for hepatic metabolism to glucose. Vitamin B_{12} is also required for the enzyme that catalyzes the recycling of methionine from homocysteine and normal liver folate (i.e., co-enzyme) metabolism. The majority of the cobalt is stored within the muscle (43%) and bone (14%), with small amounts distributed in organ tissues. These stores are not readily passed to the rumen for microbial synthesis of B_{12}. Of the ingested cobalt, only 3% is converted to B_{12} within the rumen.[149] Depletion of vitamin B_{12} results in a gradual loss of appetite, followed by anorexia, loss of muscular mass, anemia, and death.

Pasture

Cobalt deficiency occurs in many tropical and semitropical countries. A nervous disorder in cattle and sheep known as phalaris staggers occurs on pastures that contain a perennial grass *Phalaris tuberosa*. This grass contains compounds that affect cobalt requirement.[101] Clinical to subclinical signs of deficiencies are often difficult to distinguish from general malnutrition or starvation. A rapid and practical assessment of whether deficiency exists is through supplementation.

Feedlot

Basal feedlot diets consisting of 84% corn, sorghum, wheat, or barley were analyzed for cobalt and compared with the requirements of finishing cattle; the corn and sorghum diets indicated a shortage of 0.02 and 0.03 ppm, respectively.[129]

Generally, legumes are higher in cobalt than grasses. Oilseed meals are also good sources of cobalt, whereas cereal grains are poor sources. Cobalt is required in the diet at 0.10 ppm.[118] Supplemental sources for cobalt that are effective include carbonate, chloride, sulfate, and organic forms.

Copper-Molybdenum

Copper imbalances are almost as prevalent as phosphorus deficiencies as limiting factors for grazing livestock in many regions of the world.[100, 104, 171] This is a commonly observed problem in grazing areas with alluvial soils. Copper acts as a synergistic element for iron absorption and in hemoglobin formation. Ceruloplasmin is a copper protein that is synthesized in the liver and binds to transferrin (iron transport protein). The liver also metabolically controls non–direct reacting copper in plasma.[20] Achromotrichia, keratinization deficit, and nervous disorders also have been associated with copper imbalances. The reduction in lysyl oxidase (copper protein) activity reduces strength of cardiac and arterial tissues and can lead to aortic aneurysms with rupture. Other enzymes that contain or require copper are cytochrome oxidase, uricase, tyrosinase, glutathione oxidase, catalase, ascorbic acid oxidase, and oxaloacetate decarboxylase.

Pasture

Copper deficiencies have been categorized into four circumstances:

1. Elevated levels of molybdenum (>20 mg/kg).
2. Low copper and high levels of molybdenum (<2:1 ratio).
3. Low copper concentration (<5 mg/kg).
4. Normal copper and molybdenum concentrations with high intakes of soluble protein (i.e., ruminal production of copper sulfide which is unavailable).[171]

Liver copper values of pregnant cows decrease during the last 4 months of gestation due to elemental partitioning to the fetus,[39] and the liver copper content of the bovine neonate is greatly elevated over that of the dam.[66] Younger animals are observed to possess a greater affinity for copper absorption than older animals. Stressed or sick animals and animals receiving anabolic steroids usually have elevated serum copper and depressed zinc values.[57, 73] Copper deficiency has been associated with sudden death in cattle in Australia and Cuba.[168]

General recommendations for copper supplementation can not be made without reference to other elements that exist within the diet and to the breed of animal. Copper absorption is inhibited by numerous compounds, including phytates, lignin, calcium carbonate, iron, zinc, cadmium, sulfur, molybdenum, and silver. Elevated levels of molybdenum interfere with copper absorption through the formation of a copper-molybdenum (copper thiomolybdate) complex. The formation of copper sulfide reduces copper absorption. A copper-to-molybdenum ratio of 2:1 is needed, and lower ratios result in an imbalance.[114] When molybdenum forage levels are greater than 1 ppm, copper supplementation is probably needed. The recommended level of copper supplementation is 10 ppm when antagonistic elements are minimal.[118] Molybdenum is not required in supplements under most conditions.

Feedlot

An increase in plasma copper and its carrier ceruloplasmin have been reported to occur at the time of bacterial and viral diseases.[26] The role of copper in cattle disease is not well defined but does increase after viral infection.[27] Feedlots diets consisting of 84% corn, sorghum, barley, or wheat on a dry matter basis had a copper shortage of 7.50, 7.50, 6.65, and 2.40 ppm, respectively.[129] When 0.3% of each diet was supplemented with a trace mineral premix from 10 different sources, diets were still deficient in copper. Ironically, these diets provided more selenium and iron than required. Feedlot cattle that are stressed or diseased consume about 0.9% of body weight in dry matter, which may result in inadequate copper intake.

The suggested dietary concentration of copper is 10 to 15 ppm; however, when the low feed intake (1.55% of body weight in healthy cattle and 0.9% of body weight in morbid cattle) during the first 14 days after arrival at the feedlot is considered, the recommended concentration in receiving rations is best modified to 16 ppm.[76]

The use of injectable copper on grazing cattle (113 days)

showed no influence on weight gain. These animals were finished in a feedlot (207 days); treated animals' live-gain (27 kg/head) and carcass (13 kg/head) weights were reported to be depressed.[143] The chemical form of copper in the diet and associated dietary ingredients influence the availability of copper to animals.[40, 85, 86, 113, 119] When 1 kg of grain was used as a carrier for supplemental phosphorus, copper levels became elevated within the endometrium, suggesting an increase in the bioavailability of copper. Organic copper compounds tend to be more readily available than copper sulfate. Bioavailability of copper as an organic compound was greater than copper as a sulfate for calves fed high molybdenum diets.[86] Larger animals fed high molybdenum diets supplemented with (1) no copper, (2) copper sulfate, or (3) copper proteinate found no differences in liver copper reserves for supplemented groups; however, the copper proteinate group had a 16.8% higher weight gain.[174] Both copper sulfate and copper chloride are good inorganic sources. Copper sulfate is more toxic in solution than in dry diet form.[24]

Iodine

Iodine is required for the synthesis of active thyroid hormones (thyroxine and triiodothyronine) that regulate energy metabolism. Thyroxine functions as the transport form and as the feedback regulator of the thyroid gland. The dietary requirement of iodine is influenced by the efficiency of the thyroid gland and the extent of iodine recycling. Iodine deficiencies may go unobserved for prolonged periods before thyroid gland enlargement (goiter) occurs. Interrelationships that affect iodine metabolism include high arsenic, fluorine, or calcium; deficient or high cobalt; and low manganese.[167]

Goiter can result from animals feeding on certain Cruciferae plants (e.g., kale, rape, cabbage, soybeans, flaxseed, peas, peanuts, and turnips) containing goitrogenic substances as well as their feeding on low iodine diets. Thiocyanate type goitrogens can be overcome by additional iodine, whereas thiouracil types can only be partially suppressed by supplementation. Overall, goitrogens increase the iodine requirement. The recommended level of supplementation of iodine is 0.5 ppm. Supplementation for diets containing 25% goitrogenic feeds require doubling the level of iodine.[111] Sources of supplemental iodine that include calcium iodide, sodium iodide, and potassium iodide (stabilized) are highly available to the ruminant, but are unstable because of oxidation. More stable forms of iodine sources include potassium iodate (stable or nonstable) or pentacalcium orthoperiodate. Ethylenediamine dihydroiodide (EDDI) is an organic complex that is used in supplements to treat foot rot and lumpy jaw. Current U.S. Food and Drug Administration (FDA) regulations set the maximum limit of iodine supplementation at 10 mg/head/day.

Iron

Iron is an essential component of hemoglobin, myoglobin, cytochromes, and other enzyme systems. Iron deficiency in humans and livestock is manifested by anemia.

Pasture

Iron deficiencies in adult cattle are rare compared with those in young calves with higher requirements. Hematopoietic imbalances in cattle are more commonly due to copper imbalances or parasitism. A copper imbalance impairs iron absorption.

Feedlot

Low serum iron values have been documented in bacterial infections[3] and in viral infections of monogastrics.[115] Iron may play a role in rumen function of stressed or sick feedlot cattle due to some requirements of rumen microorganisms.[107] Owens[130] concluded that the requirements of iron in feedlot cattle are usually met from a typical feedlot ration and normal water consumption (3.9 lb of water per lb feed). Iron content of water is specific for each location and may vary with region.

The dietary requirement of iron for ruminants is not well established. Iron absorption is reduced by high dietary levels of phosphorus because of the formation of an insoluble ferric phosphate and phytate. Excess divalent cations (e.g., copper, manganese, zinc, lead, and cadmium) can interfere with iron absorption because of competition for absorption sites in the intestinal mucosa.[167] The suggested requirement is approximately 50 ppm.[118]

Generally, iron is found at high levels in most forages and as a contaminant of many phosphorous sources (1% to 2%). Thus, high levels of supplementation with high iron compounds is not required when contaminated phosphorus sources are incorporated into the supplement. The divalent form of iron (ferrous) is more soluble than the trivalent form (ferric) and is absorbed to a greater extent. Ferrous sulfate has a higher bioavailability than ferrous carbonate. Iron oxide is biologically inert, but adds red coloration to a mineral supplement.

Manganese

Manganese is essential for normal bone development, reproduction, and central nervous system function of the newborn. The functional enzymes that manganese catalyzes include hydrolases, kinases, decarboxylases, and transferases. The manganese body pool is small and 25% to 50% of the body pool is ingested daily.[88] Antagonistic agents to manganese absorption include high levels of calcium and phosphorus and alkaloids of *Lupinus* plants.[62, 68]

Pasture

The manganese requirement for reproduction and normal calf development is higher than for growth.[6, 38, 136]

Feedlot

Feedlot research observed steer calves during recovery from stress (28-day period), supplemented with inorganic or organic sources of zinc and manganese. Feed intake and average daily gains were greater for calves fed the organic zinc and manganese supplements. Eight days after a virus challenge, all animals were in negative energy balance. However, steers fed organic sources were 11 kg/head heavier than steers in the control (oxide) group. The conclusion was that zinc and manganese supplementation and their chemical form could affect the recovery rate from both transportation stress and virus infection.[49] Other feedlot research showed that higher levels of organic manganese (80 vs. 50 ppm) depressed average daily gain.[74, 92]

The minimum requirement for manganese, approximately 40 ppm, is dependent on physiologic function.[118] The forms of manganese in decreasing order of bioavailability are organic, sulfate, oxide, and carbonate.[14]

Selenium

Selenium is a constituent of glutathione peroxidase, which aids in protecting cellular and subcellular membranes from oxidative damage.[140] As an antioxidant, it destroys peroxides prior to cellular membrane attack and overlaps the functions of vitamin E. Glutathione peroxidase functions in growth, reproduction, and tissue integrity. Other biochemical roles of selenium include adequate immune response, selenoprotein of mitochondria for spermatozoa, RNA synthesis, and prostaglandin synthesis, and fatty acid metabolism. Selenium exerts a protective function in binding with heavy metals such as arsenic, cadmium, mercury, and silver.[101, 167] Antagonistic agents to selenium absorption are high sulfur diets (legumes) and the previously mentioned heavy metals. The requirement of selenium is dependent on the animal's previous status, vitamin E status, lipids (rancidity yields peroxides), and antagonistic and agonistic compounds.[5]

Pasture

The clinical syndrome of selenium deficiency is white muscle disease (WMD) in young animals. Maternal supplementation during gestation and lactation (colostrum) determines the status of the calf.[2] Selenium boluses have been observed to increase weight gain and feed efficiency for steers fed hay known to be deficient in selenium.[122]

Feedlot

Selenium derived from grain sources (0.5 ppm) favors absorption and retention four to five times that of the selenite form.[104]

The 1996 NRC[119] recommended level of selenium supplementation is 0.10 ppm. Sources of selenium supplementation are sodium selenate and sodium selenite. Organic sources (selenomethionine and yeast containing selenium) are twice as available.[131]

Zinc

Zinc functions as a constituent and catalyst in several hundred enzyme systems (e.g., carbonic anhydrase) and is involved in nucleic acid metabolism, protein synthesis, and carbohydrate metabolism. Maintaining plasma concentrations of vitamin A requires zinc for its mobilization from the liver.[148] Zinc is distributed throughout the body and found in high concentrations in the prostate, pituitary gland, choroid, and iris of the eye. The zinc requirement of an animal is dependent on the animal's physiologic function. The requirement for growth is considerably lower than that for testicular development and spermatogenesis.[165]

Zinc deficiency results in numerous maladies that usually involve a deficit in epithelial functions (i.e., mucosal epithelial lining, keratinization, and hair growth). Inadequate zinc intake has been identified with adverse reproductive process in females from estrus to parturition, abortion, fetal mummification, lower birth weight, and altered myometrial contractibility with prolonged labor.[95, 102] Animals are unable to mobilize zinc stores rapidly when the diet is deficient[89, 110]; therefore, continuous supplementation may be advised in situations of marginal dietary zinc. High levels of zinc supplementation protect against hepatic damage caused by fungal toxins of *Pithomyces chartarum*[168] and *Phomopsis leptostromiformis*.

Pasture

Studies were conducted in which calves and cows were fed supplemental zinc methionine prior to shipment during the cow/calf phase and offered the same levels in the feedlot receiving diet. The studies showed a substantial benefit in performance and health of the zinc methionine–fed calves when compared with a zinc oxide–treated group.[26, 75, 153]

Feedlot

Supplemental zinc methionine fed to feedlot cattle resulted in increased carcass quality grades and higher marbling scores.[57] The response observed was due to either zinc or methionine. Other researchers have found the zinc methionine compound to be of benefit.[98, 142, 154, 160] These favorable responses from the organic form of zinc may result from an increase in feed intake.

The suggested level of zinc supplementation is 30 ppm[118] Sources of zinc that are highly available include organic, sulfate, and oxide forms.[81]

MINERAL BIOAVAILABILITY

The definition of *relative mineral bioavailability* refers to the estimated proportion of an ingested source of a trace mineral that is utilized or retained by the animal.[46] Elemental compounds vary in relative bioavailability. Compounds that are rumen soluble are readily complexed to various forms that may be less available for absorption at the level of the small intestines. Microbial requirements of rumen soluble trace minerals is unknown for various diet types.

The action of ruminal microbes may interfere positively or negatively with the biologic availability of a mineral or mineral complex. Therefore, the exact form of a mineral or mineral complex arriving at the lower gastrointestinal tract or area of absorption depends on its resistance to ruminal microbial metabolism and its effect on the chemical form of the mineral or mineral complex. With advanced technology and refined analytical techniques, many such observations will aid in understanding the role of organic trace elements in animal physiology.

Generally, the ruminal solubility of a mineral or mineral complex partly determines the extent of its metabolism. Lower ruminal pH increases solubility, whereas higher ruminal pH decreases solubility and absorption.[170] Studies cited earlier in the text indicated differences in the biologic availability of inorganic metal vs. metal organic forms for chromium, copper, zinc, and manganese.

The bioavailability of an essential organic trace element is defined as the proportion that is absorbed, transported to site of action, and converted to the physiologic active form.[155] Various forms of metal organic compounds include metal proteinase, metal amino acid chelate, metal (specific amino acid) complex, metal amino acid complex, and metal polysaccharide complex.[10] The different forms of organic metal compounds vary in structural characteristics, binding properties, charge, and solubility. Several of these compounds possess ruminal bypass ability, and hence are readily available for absorption at the small intestines. Specific metal-containing organic compounds are unique in animal and tissue response and are absorbed and metabolized differently than inorganic sources. The benefits of feeding these compounds include the following:

1. Decreased interactions (antagonistic reactions) with other elements and compounds that may inhibit absorption.
2. Modified absorption and blood transport mechanism of elements to specific tissues.
3. Decreased adverse effects of inorganics when excessive to rumen microbes and animals.
4. Decreased oxidation of vitamins in premixes.

A standardized chemical assay method (i.e., electrochemical) to determine organic compound effectiveness under physiologic conditions is not recognized at this time.

FEEDLOT WASTE: AN ENVIRONMENTAL ISSUE

Nutrients that exceeded the animal's requirements are excreted, hence a financial and potential environmental cost to the feedlot. The major environmental issues of concern include need for nutrient balance in relation to the use of manure and waste water application to crop or forage plants, soil quality, and surface and ground water quality. Nutrient or salt excesses may enter soil, water, and air. The premise of minimizing potential feedlot waste contaminants (i.e., nitrogen, phosphorus, salt) may be through reduction of excesses in nutrients. A sustainable waste management program recognizes pre-existing soil quality and uptake of waste nutrients by plants.

Concepts for Reuse and Disposal Areas for Feedlots

1. You cannot manage what you do not measure. Estimates of amount and form of manure, liquid effluent, nutrients, and soluble salts are required for management.
2. Total mass on a dry matter basis is almost invariably a better basis for waste estimation than concentration because it ensures mass is reserved.
3. The allowable application rate of any element to land is the sum of its removal in the crop grown, plus its storage in soil sinks, plus allowable leakages (i.e., leaching to ground water, soil erosion) from the system. For nitrogen, volatilization of ammonia is a major pathway.
4. Waste reuse and disposal areas will always have a use-life expectancy if soil storage is a major sink for a nutrient (e.g., phosphorus).
5. The waste reuse scheme should have sufficient flexibility to adjust for errors in the predicted effluent production.[52]

Nutrients

The following nutrients are reviewed because of potential ecological impact:

Dietary protein obtained from grain, urea, and ammonium sulfate that exceeds the animal's dietary protein requirements results in excess excretion of nitrogen, increases the animal's metabolic and energy requirements, and is expensive. Nitrogen forms include total Kjeldahl-nitrogen, ammonia-nitrogen, nitrite-nitrogen, and nitrate-nitrogen. The animal's metabolic waste products (ammonia-NH_3), are converted by aerobic bacteria (oxidized) to nitrites (NO_2^-), followed by nitrates (NO_3^-). These compounds are water soluble and may leach into ground water sources. Fresh feces and manure stored in anaerobic environments contain low levels of nitrate. Nitrate consumption has greater toxicity (methemoglobinemia) to ruminants than monogastrics (except infants).

A majority of manure phosphorus is contributed through grain and protein meal, with minor levels contributed by phosphate sources incorporated in growing diets. Phosphorus exists in inorganic and organic forms, and is differentiated through analysis of total phosphorus and orthophosphate. Inorganic phosphorus is composed of insoluble compounds (aluminium, iron, and calcium compounds) and orthophosphate compounds ($H_2PO_4^-$, HPO_4^{2-}, PO_4^{3-}, used for crop application). Organic phosphorus is less available to plants because it is bound in organic matter (i.e., humus, plant residues, and manure). The decomposition of organic material by soil microbes provides an excess amount of phosphorus (above microbial requirement), which becomes available to the plant. In the diet, organic phosphorus (i.e., derived from grain—phytin, nucleic acids) is partially converted to inorganic phosphorus in the rumen and recirculated via blood and saliva. Phosphorus is excreted through feces in both organic and inorganic forms. The average total quantity of phosphorus in manure on a mass balance basis averages 1.6% of DM.[173] Australian literature reports that the ortho-phosphorus constitutes 2.6% to 27.8%,[147] whereas American literature cites 28% to 63%[9] of phosphorus in manure; hese differences may be attributed to analytic technique.

Salt added to diets at 0.20% to 0.25% of dry matter stimulates water consumption, which maintains renal activities. Plants uptake inorganic salt during growth; however, its presence does not ensure availability. The salt contribution of diet (NaCl and plant) and water (especially underground) can exceed animal requirements for sodium. Salinity (soluble sodium, magnesium, calcium, potassium salts) is monitored through electrical conductivity (EC − dS/m) with a conversion factor to dS/m × 640 = mg/L salt. Excess salinity (i.e., soluble salt) and sodicity (i.e., sodium) are potentially the most toxic nutrients of feedlot waste to animals and plants.

Management

Managing pen surface area is an important aspect of animal performance as well as environmental impact. The surface manure is best harvested frequently, leaving a "pad" for cattle to stand on and minimize infiltration and absorption by maximizing run-off. Odor is an annoyance factor to people and has health implications (i.e., ammonia to animals). Fermentation of undigested feedstuffs in manure results in odor. Odor is 50 times greater for wet than for dry feedlot.

Rain water run-off (first 1 cm absorbed) contains a high level of organic and inorganic compounds. The concentration of this material is 10 to 20 times as strong as domestic sewage, thus requiring capture. This solution is high in salinity and nitrate-nitrogen, which are derived from diet and water sources. A contribution to pen soil moisture is pen stocking density (varies with animal size and pen surface condition). Cattle excrete approximately 23 L of moisture per day, which is an equivalent of 46 cm/year of rainfall for a 18.6 m² area.[162]

MINERAL SUPPLEMENTS

The objectives of a mineral supplementation program must be established when choosing a mineral supplement. Factors for consideration include physiologic stage of animal production, current diet, and the mineral imbalances that potentially might occur. These variables will change throughout the year, and it may be of benefit to develop a synchronized supplementation program.

Free-choice feeding refers to providing for voluntary consumption of the supplement. The most critical aspect of a free-choice mineral supplement is that it will be consumed in adequate quantities to meet production demands yet is not wastefully consumed. The characteristics of a "good" free-choice mineral supplement[101] are as follows:

1. Final mixture containing a minimum of 6% to 8% total phosphorus. In areas where phosphorus in forages is consistently lower than 0.20%, mineral supplements in the 8% to 10% range are preferred.
2. Calcium-to-phosphorus ratio, not substantially over 2:1.
3. Provide a significant proportion (i.e., 50%) of trace mineral requirements of cobalt, copper, iodine, manganese, and zinc. In known trace mineral–deficient regions, 100% of specific trace mineral requirements should be supplied.
4. Composed of high-quality mineral salts that provide the best biologically available forms of each mineral element, and avoidance or minimal inclusions of mineral salts containing toxic elements (e.g., phosphates containing high fluorine concentrations).
5. Formulated to be sufficiently palatable to allow adequate consumption in relation to requirements.

6. Backed by a reputable manufacturer with quality control guarantees as to accuracy of mineral supplement label.
7. An acceptable particle size, which will allow adequate mixing without smaller size particles settling out.
8. Formulated for the area involved, the level of animal productivity, and the environment (temperature, humidity, etc.) in which it will be fed and as economical as possible in providing the mineral elements used.

MINERAL REQUIREMENTS AND NEED FOR SUPPLEMENTATION

Mineral ranges were presented in relation to DM intake (ppm = mg/kg) to fulfill animal requirements. These ranges were obtained from controlled research studies from several breeds (primarily English) of cattle. Many of the crossbred and exotic breeds of cattle possessing a greater genetic capacity for production will have increased absolute requirements of all nutrients and at times may require higher concentrations in the dry matter. Stage of production and environmental conditions also will influence the animal's basic requirements; thus, these ranges should be used only as basic guidelines.

The numerous variables encountered within the animal, diet, and environment suggest the advisability of supplying supplemental minerals to guarantee against imbalances. Requirements for major elements (calcium, phosphorus, magnesium) can be predicted for production requirements with some confidence even under pasture conditions and are justified economically. The need for trace minerals is more difficult to predict from forage and animal tissue data. The economics of supplementation often cannot be proven even under carefully controlled research conditions. However, there is credibility to the argument, "to be sure is worth the minor expense required." Supplementing all of the trace minerals at 30% to 100% (100% when known deficiency exists and greater with known antagonisms) of the animal's daily requirement is an economic insurance policy against potential imbalances. The potential for toxicity is relatively minor in supplementing all of the trace minerals, and the cost is not excessive in relation to the potential production enhancement.

Excess dietary concentrations of certain elements may result in antagonistic deficiencies and subclinical to clinical toxicities. *Mineral Tolerances of Domestic Animals*[121] is a guide for assessing elemental concentrations that can potentially create problems. Elements possessing the greatest potential for toxicity are selenium in cattle and copper in sheep. If the history of the circumstance does not suggest these elements to be in dangerously high concentrations, it is probably advisable to supplement all minerals in moderation.

MINERAL SUPPLEMENT TAG

Concentrations of minerals are expressed as percent or gram-per-kilogram basis for major elements; trace elements may or may not be listed. The mineral tag should provide the various compounds used in the formulation to allow estimates of bioavailability and presence of intake enhancers. The following units of measurement are for the following calculations:

ppm = mg/kg 1 kg = 1000 g % = 10,000 mg/kg 1 lb = 454 g
1000 mg = g 1 kg = 2.2 lb 1 ton (short) = 2000 lb 1 oz = 28 g
1 MT (metric tonne) = 1000 kg   1 MT = 2205 lb

Commercial mineral packages have various levels of elements, which should be evaluated for efficacy. An example of contents follows:

$$\frac{\text{Animal requirement (g/day)}}{\text{Elements contents (g/kg)}} = \frac{\text{(kg) Mineral consumption required to}}{\text{meet animal daily requirement}}$$

Elemental Zn content: 0.3% or 3 g/kg (to convert % to mg/kg multiply by 10,000, i.e., $0.3 \times 10,000$ mg/kg = 3000 mg/kg or 3 g/kg)

$$\text{Animal Zn requirement: 30 ppm (30 mg/kg}$$
$$\times \text{ 10 kg DM consumption}$$
$$= \text{300 mg or 0.3 g/day)}$$

$$\frac{0.3 \text{ g/day}}{3 \text{ g/kg}} = \frac{0.1 \text{ kg consumption of mineral is}}{\text{required to meet daily requirement}}$$

Generally, commercial mineral supplements are formulated for a consumption level of 3 to 4 oz (85 to 113 g) on a per-head per-day basis. The total dry matter intake for cattle is approximately 2% of the body weight (will vary with forage quality).

For simplicity, an average body weight of 500 kg (10 kg of dry matter intake) will be used in the following calculations:

$$\frac{[\% \text{ element in mineral mix}] \times [\text{daily intake of mineral mix (g)}]}{\text{total daily dry matter intake (g)}}$$

$$= \% \text{ element of the total diet from mineral mix}$$

Example:

Mn in mineral mix (%) = 0.20

Daily intake of mineral mix (g) = 85

Total daily dry matter intake (g) = 10,000

$$\frac{0.2 \times 85}{10,000} = 0.0017\% \text{ or 17 ppm}$$

This mineral mix would provide 42.5% (17 ppm/40 ppm $\times$ 100 = 42.5%) of the manganese requirement.

To calculate for the percentage of a mineral compound to provide the desired concentration of mineral element:

$$\frac{\% \text{ element desired in mixture} \times 100}{\% \text{ element in available compound}} = \frac{\% \text{ element containing}}{\text{compound required}}$$

Example:

% Mn required = 0.40

% Mn in Mn sulfate = 27.00

$$\frac{0.4 \times 100}{27.0} = 1.48\% \text{ Mn sulfate required}$$

MINERAL CONSUMPTION

The hypothesis that animals eat what they need or have nutritional wisdom is erroneous. This belief stemmed from cattle with depraved appetites that consumed bones and improved their health. Because bones are good sources of phosphorus, an assumption was made that animals have the ability to select minerals required for their diet. A symptom should not be confused with a diagnosis (rabid animals usually have depraved appetites). Unhealthy animals with depraved appetites will consume many things that are not part of their normal diet (i.e., rocks, noxious plants, or anything else they can find in the pasture). Animals that have been deprived of adequate phosphorus intake can exhibit an initial craving for a mineral supplement (extreme, phosphorus intake 120 g/head/day) for several weeks (low phosphorus absorption coefficient). These animals are generally observed to be in low body condition because of insufficient energy and protein intake.

When given a choice of calcium carbonate or calcium carbonate mixed equally with dicalcium phosphate, animals failed to consume adequate amounts of the phosphorus-containing supplement to prevent aphosphorosis.[133] Lactating dairy cows failed to consume adequate amounts of dicalcium phosphate (offered free-choice) to meet their calcium and phosphorus requirements.[34, 42] Cafeteria-style mineral supplements (individualized elements in different containers) was not an effective means of mineral supplementation.[108] It was concluded that it was nutritionally and economically advantageous to supplement a complete mineral mixture.

Animals will select a palatable diet with little nutritional value in preference to an unpalatable nutritious diet, even to the point of death.[23] Domesticated animals are more responsive to the sensory qualities of feed than the nutritive quality.[116] A major problem with free-choice supplements on rangeland is obtaining sufficient intake among individual animals within a herd. Thus, the goal is to maintain adequate intake of mineral supplements throughout the year to meet the animal's physiologic requirements.

Factors affecting free-choice mineral intake have been cited by several authors.[82, 83, 117] Soil fertility has been correlated with mineral consumption. Animals consume less minerals on highly fertile soils, whereas on native or poor-quality pastures cattle tend to consume more minerals. Supplemental feeding of protein-energy supplements tends to decrease mineral consumption. The elevated salt concentration of plants and water will depress mineral intake if salt is used to enhance acceptance of the supplement. The added physiologic stress of lactation and gestation will increase mineral intake.

An important aspect of any free-choice mineral supplement program is to monitor intake on a regular basis by the producer. If the minerals are not being consumed in adequate quantities, a palatability factor or appetite stimulator may be mixed into the supplement. Palatability of a mineral supplement is the key to any mineral program. Salt is a very economical and palatable mineral used in many commercial mineral supplements. Alternatives to salt include protein meals, dried molasses, flavoring, fat, and yeast products.

MINERAL FEEDERS

Covered mineral feeders should be used to protect the minerals from the environment (water, wind, and other contaminants). Minerals can deteriorate in nutritive quality and palatability through changes in pH or oxidation (rancid). The mineral feeder should be at an accessible height and location for animals of all ages. If the mineral supplement is highly palatable, its location can be altered within the pasture to distribute animal movement. The act of moving a mineral trough would encourage monitoring mineral consumption for a pasture.

The following items apply to mineral supplementation:

1. Complete mineral supplements are best fed alone; salt may detract from adequate consumption to satisfy requirements. The phosphorus concentration of a mineral supplement is dependent on the quality of forage in the pasture and type of animal production (growth vs. lactation). Early forage growth contains higher levels of phosphorus than forage in mature or dormant stages. Thus, lower levels of phosphorus can be used in early

stages of growth and higher levels for mature and dormant stages.

2. Best cost of mineral supplements (price of phosphorus) does not assure optimal intake of the mineral supplement.

3. Growing forages yield higher levels of soluble carbohydrates, protein, and phosphorus but do not necessarily satisfy all mineral requirements.

4. Animals consume about 10% less from a mineral block than from a loose or textured form.

MEDICATED MINERAL AND FEEDLOT SUPPLEMENTS

Medication can be delivered to animals through feedlot diets or mineral supplements. Therapeutic dosages can be achieved when the level of consumption of the diet or supplement is known. Several classes of feed additives (anthelmintics, antifrothing agents, antibiotics, coccidiostats, and ionophores) are FDA approved for use in diets and mineral supplements. Prior to medicating a group of animals, it is beneficial to consult a feed compendium for regulated use and contraindications. Medicated supplements should be mixed and used for their indication to ensure the highest quality of stability of all ingredients to avoid potential misuse.

Information required for using medicated supplements includes the range of animal weights, number of animals, average consumption of the supplement, and required dose and concentration. Usually, medicated supplements should be formulated for maximal animal weight within the herd to ensure a therapeutic dose for heavier animals.

Pasture Mineral Supplement

Examples of calculations for medication, at a constant mineral consumption, required for a herd using minimum, average, and maximal animal weights are as follows:

D = Medicated dosage per day (active ingredient), mg/kg of BW: 20 mg/kg of BW or 0.02 g/kg of BW
A = Medication activity in feed additive, g/kg: 150 g/kg
BW = Body weight average: 400 kg
C = Herd average consumption of supplement, g/day: 200 g/day
% = Percent of feed additive in supplement

Then,

$$\frac{[(D \times BW)/A]}{C \times 100} = \frac{[(0.02 \text{ g/kg BW} \times 400 \text{ kg})/150 \text{ g/kg}]}{200 \text{ g/day} \times 100}$$

$$\% = 0.0267$$

$$300 \text{ kg} = 0.020\% \text{ vs. } 500 \text{ kg} = 0.033\%$$

When the average animal weight is used for inclusion of a feed additive (0.0267%), the heavier animals with similar consumption (0.033%) require a higher therapeutic dose. Medicated feed additives are established on a minimal concentration level for biologic response, with a broad dose range for safety from toxicity. Many feed additives are unpalatable at high concentrations, depressing intake (e.g., 50 g); thus, associated ingredients to mask any off-taste or flavor should be selected. It is advantageous for these supplements to be highly palatable and low in medication concentrations. This lowers potential excessive medication as well as the cost of the supplement. A dose of 1 g/head/day can be administered with 2% (50 g intake), 1% (100 g intake), and a 0.5% concentration (200 g intake). The inclusion of a protein meal in the 0.5% supplement would add

nutritional quality to the supplement. High supplement intake can be achieved with protein meals, dried molasses, bonemeal, dried yeast cultures, fat, and flavorings. Animals prefer salt, but it should be limited because changes in forage quality and environment cause inconsistencies in salt consumption.

Feedlot Supplement

Nutrient and medication densities of a diet are expressed on a dry matter basis (DMB) vs. "as fed." Diets containing high levels of moisture tend to vary more than dry diets; hence, there is a greater risk of error.

Calculation for diets expressed as g/MT or mg/kg (1 g = 1000 mg) dry matter:

D = Medication dosage: 20 g/MT
F = Feed dry matter contents: 78%
A = Medication of active ingredient: 20 g/kg
E = Medication quantity required: 0.78 kg

Then:
D × F = C/A = E

− 20 g/MT × 0.78 = 15.6 g/MT

− 15.6 g/MT/ 20 g/kg = 0.78 kg/MT of medication

Medication is hand mixed in 10 to 20 kg of ground grain or protein meal, followed by inclusion to the grain layer in the mixer (to increase dispersion in the ration).

Classes of Feed Additives

Anthelmintics (e.g., fenbendazole and phenothiazine) and coccidiostats (e.g., amprolium and decoquinate) should be used strategically during the year for maximal efficacy. Parasite resistance is a problem with many anthelmintics; thus, caution is warranted with type and use of an anthelmintic. Ionophores (e.g., lasalocid and monensin) must be fed continuously to promote increased rate of gain. These compounds have nutrient-sparing effects but cannot overcome pastures that are limited in available nutrients (low digestible energy and protein). Young animals' live weight gain can be improved on pasture (nutrients are not limited for animal requirements) through ionophore supplementation. Lasalocid has been shown to alleviate malabsorption of calcium and magnesium in ruminants, thus decreasing the incidence of hypomagnesemia on small grain pastures.

Anti-frothing agents (e.g., poloxalene, turcapsol, and laureth-23-enproal bloat block) are used in the prevention of legume and wheat pasture bloat. The efficacy of these compounds is based on adequate and continuous intake, which is sometimes difficult to obtain on good-quality pastures. Liquid supplements may be more advantageous in achieving continuous intake when mineral supplements are not consumed with regularity.

Vitamins in Mineral Supplements

The inclusion of fat-soluble vitamins (A, D, and E) in mineral supplements can be advantageous when forages are in the dormant stage and vitamins A and E may be limiting nutrients. Vitamins are relatively non-toxic, even when consumed at high levels. Most vitamins are readily oxidized, especially in the presence of several of the trace element compounds within a mineral supplement. Stabilized and protective coated vitamins are less susceptible to the effects of time, heat, and moisture. However, it is important that mineral supplements that contain vitamins be as freshly mixed as possible and protected from the environment.

Acknowledgments

The assistance of Ms. Sue Engdahl and Ms. Suzanne Chaney in editing and manuscript completion is gratefully acknowledged.

REFERENCES

1. Abbas F: Canyon, West Texas A&M University, masters thesis, 1994.
2. Abdelrahman MM, Kincad RL: J Dairy Sci 78:625–630, 1995.
3. Adams EB, Mayet FG: SS Med J, 30:38, 1966.
4. Ammerman CB, Chicco CF, Loggins PE, et al: J Anim Sci 34:122, 1972.
5. Ammerman CB, Miller SM: J Dairy Sci 58:1561, 1975.
6. Anke M, Groppel B, Reissig W, et al: Arch Anim Nutr 23:197, 1973.
7. Arnold GW: Proc Aust Soc Anim Prod 5:258, 1964.
8. Arthington JD, Corah LR, Belcha F: J Anim Sci. 74:211, 1996.
9. ASAE Standard data: ASAE D384.1. St Joseph, Mich, American Society of Agricultural Engineers, 1994.
10. Association of American Feed Control Officials. No. 57, p 150, 1996.
11. Basalan M, Secrist DS, Hill WJ, et al: J Anim Sci 74(Suppl 1): 752, 1996.
12. Betteridge K, Miller RB: Proceedings 28th American Association of Bovine Practitioners Annual Conference, Buffalo, NY, 1985.
13. Bird PR: Aust J Agric Res 25:631, 1974.
14. Black J: Gainesville, University of Florida, doctoral dissertation, 1983.
15. Bock BJ, Harmon DL, Brandt RT, et al: J Anim Sci 69:2211, 1991.
16. Boyne R, Arthur JR: J Comp Path 89:151, 1979
17. Bray AC, Till AR: In McDonald IW, Warner ACI (eds): Digestion and Metabolism in the Ruminant. Henniker, NH, University of New England Press, pp 243–260, 1975.
18. Bremner I: Br J Nutr 24:769, 1970.
19. Briggs M: Advances in Steroid Chemistry, 1985, p 68.
20. Buckley WT: Can J Anim Sci 71:155, 1991.
21. Buckman HO, Brady NC: The Nature and Properties of Soils, ed 6. New York, MacMillan, 1962.
22. Call JW, Butcher JE, Shupe JL: Am J Vet Res 47:475, 1986.
23. Chang X, Mowat DN: J Anim Sci 70:559, 1992.
24. Chapman HL Jr, Nelson SL, Kidder RW, et al: J Anim Sci 21:960, 1962.
25. Chester-Jones H, Fontent JP, Veit HP: J Anim Sci 68:4400, 1990.
26. Chirase NK, Hutcheson DP, Thompson GB: J Anim Sci 69(10):4137, 1991.
27. Chirase NK, Hutcheson DP, Thompson GB, et al: J Anim Sci 72(1):212, 1994.
28. Chirase NK: College Station, Texas A&M University, PhD Dissertation, 1988.
29. Collier RJ, Beede DK: In McDowell LR (ed): Nutrition of Grazing Ruminants in Warm Climates. New York, Academic Press, pp 59–70, 1985.
30. Coppock CE, Everett RW, Merrill WG: J Dairy Sci 55:245, 1972.
31. Coppock CE, Everett RW, Belyea RL: J Dairy Sci 59:571, 1976.
32. Coppock CE: Proc Cornell Nutr Conf Feed Manuf, pp 29–35, 1970.
33. Corah LR, Dargatz D: Beef Cow/Calf Health and Productivity Audit. In Report by National Animal Health Monitoring Systems, March 1996.
34. Cummings BA, Caldwell DR, Gould DH, et al: Am J Vet Res 56:1384, 1995.
35. Cunha TJ, Shirley RL, Chapman HL Jr, et al: Fla Agr Exp Sta Bull 683, 1964.
36. Cunha TJ: Anim Nutr Health 35:11, 1980.
37. Davenport GM, Boling JA, Gay N: J Anim Sci 68:3765, 1990.
38. DiCostanzo A, Meiske JC, Plegge SD: Minnesota Beef Cow-Calf Report. Minn Agr Exp Ser AG-Bu-2310, pp 27–30, 1985.
39. Doyle JC: College Station, Texas A&M University, PhD dissertation, 1989.
40. Doyle JC, Huston JE, Spiller DW: J Anim Sci 66:579 (Abstract), 1988.
41. Doyle JC, Huston JE, Thompson PV: Theriogenology 34:21, 1990.
42. Doyle JC: Unpublished data, 1994.
43. Droke EA, Loerch SE: J Anim Sci 67:1350, 1989.
44. Dubeski PL, Owens FN, Gill DR: Okla Agric Exp Sta Misc Publ MP-129:93, 1990.
45. Dunn TG, Ingalls JE, Zimmerman DR, et al: J Animal Sci 29:719, 1969.
46. Ellis GL, McDowell LR, Conrad JH: In Proceedings of the 17th Annual Conference on Livestock and Poultry in Latin America. Gainesville, University of Florida, 1983, p 841.
47. Emanuele SM, Staples CR: J Animal Sci 68:2052, 1990.
48. Fell BF, Williams RB, Mills CF: Res Vet Sci 18:274, 1975.
49. Ferrao JL: Canyon, West Texas A&M University, MS Thesis, 1995.
50. Fick KR, McDowell LR, Miles PH, et al: Methods of Mineral Analysis for Plant and Animal Tissue, ed 2. Gainesville, University of Florida, 1979.
51. Field AC: Proc Nutr Soc 40:267, 1981.
52. Gardner TP, Watts R, Tucker, et al: In Designing Better Feedlots, Queensland Dept Primary Industries, 1994.
53. Good R, West A, Hernandez G: Fed Proc 39:3098, 1980.
54. Gordon JG, Tribe DE, Grahman TC: Br J Anim Behav 2:72, 1954.
55. Greene LW: Unpublished data, 1987.
56. Greene LW, Solis JC, Byers FM, et al: Tex Agr Exp Sta Tech Rept No. 86–1, 1986.
57. Greene LW, Lunt D, Byers FM, et al: J Anim Sci 66:1818, 1988.
58. Gyang EO, Stevens JB, Olson WG, et al: Am J Vet Res 45:175, 1984.
59. Hahn GL: Symposium on Intake by Feedlot Cattle, July 1995.
60. Hardt PF, Greene LW, Lunt DK: J Anim Sci 73:55, 1995.
61. Hartmans J: In Hoekstra WG (ed): Trace Element Metabolism in Animals. New York, University Park Press, 1974, p 261.
62. Hawkins GE, Wise GH, Matrone G, et al: J Dairy Sci 38:536, 1990.
63. Heitzman RJ: Mode of action of anabolic agents. In Forbes FJM, Lomax MA (eds): Hormones and Metabolism in Ruminants. London, Agricultural Research Council, 1981, p 129.
64. Herd LD, Greene LW, Herd DB, et al: J Anim Sci (Suppl 1):261, 1993.
65. Herd DB: In Proc Florida Ruminant Nutr Symp, 1994, p 76.
66. Hidiroglou M, Knipfel JE: Can J Anim Sci 69:141, 1981.
67. Hill CH, Matrone G: Fed Proc Fed Am Soc Exp Biol 29:1474, 1970.
68. Howes AD, Dyer IA, Haller WH: J Anim Sci 37:455–458, 1973.
69. Hufstedler GD, Greene LW: J Anim Sci 73:3785, 1995
70. Huston JE: Unpublished data, 1988.
71. Huston JE, Rector BS, Merrill LB, et al: Nutritional Value of Range Plants in the Edwards Plateau Region of Texas. Tex Agr Exp Sta Bull 1357, 1981.
72. Hutcheson D: Unpublished data, 1986.
73. Hutcheson D: Unpublished data, 1988.
74. Hutcheson D: Unpublished data, 1989.
75. Hutcheson DP, Chirase NK, Spears JW: J Anim Sci 69(Suppl 1):552, Abst No. 858, 1991.
76. Hutcheson DP, Cole NA: J Anim Sci 62:555, 1986.
77. Hutcheson DP, Cole NA, McLaren JB: J Anim Sci 58:700, 1984.
78. Imig-Fenton J, Gunther JD, Link JE, et al: J Anim Sci 74(Suppl 1):228, 1996.
79. Jenkinson DM, Mabon RM: Br Vet J 129:282, 1973.
80. Kappel LC, Ingraham HH, Morgan EB, et al: J Dairy Sci 70:167, 1987.
81. Kegley EB, Spears J: J Anim Sci 70(Suppl 1):302, 1992.
82. Kegley EB, Spears JW, Brown TT: J Anim Sci 74(Suppl 1):621, 1996.
83. Kegley EB, Spears JW: J Anim Sci 73:2721, 1995.
84. Kennedy PM, Christopherson RJ, Milligan LP: In Milligan LP, Grovum WL, Dobson A (eds): Control of Digestion and Metabolism in Ruminants. Englewood Cliffs, NJ, Prentice-Hall, 1985, p 285.
85. Kincaid RL, Cronrath JD: J Dairy Sci 66:821, 1983.

86. Kincaid RL, Blauwiekel RM, Cronrath JD: J Dairy Sci 69:160, 1986.

87. Lander RQ Jr: Unpublished data, 1990.

88. Lassiter JW, Miller WJ, Pate FM, et al: Proc Soc Exp Biol Med 139:345, 1972.

89. Lee LH, Marston HR: Aust J Agric Res 20:905–918, 1969.

90. Levander O, Mertz W: In Trace Elements in Human and Animal Nutrition, ed 5. New York, Academic Press, 1986.

91. Littledike ET, Wittum TE, Jenkins TJ: J Anim Sci (Suppl 1):262, 1993.

92. Lomax DA: Lubbock, Texas Tech, MS thesis, 1990.

93. Loneragon JF: In Nicholas DJ, Egan AR (eds): Trace Elements in Soil-Plants-Animal System. New York, Academic Press, p 109, 1975.

94. Lukasewycz OA, Prohaska JR: Copper and the immune system. In Bendich A, Chandra RK (eds): Micronutrients and Immune Functions. Ann NY Acad Sci 587:147, 1995.

95. Maas J: Vet Clin North Am Food Anim Pract 3:633, 1987.

96. Mader TL, Gaughan JB, Young BA: J Anim Sci 74(Suppl 1):604, 1996.

97. Maller O: In Kare MR, Maller O (eds): The Chemical Senses and Nutrition. Baltimore, Johns Hopkins Press, 1967.

98. Martin J, Strasia C, Gill D, et al: J Anim Sci 65(Suppl 1):500 (Abstract), 1987.

99. Mathison GW, Engstrom DF: Can J Anim Sci 75:549, 1995.

100. McCosker T, Winks L: Phosphorus Nutrition of Beef Cattle in Northern Australia. Queensland Department of Primary Industries, 1994.

101. McDowell LR: Cobalt, iodine, and selenium. In McDowell LR (ed): Nutrition of Grazing Ruminants in Warm Climates. Orlando, Academic Press, 1985.

102. McDowell LR: Minerals in Animal and Human Nutrition. San Diego, Academic Press, 1992, p 282.

103. McDowell LR: In Smith AJ (ed): Beef Cattle Production in Developing Countries. Edinburgh, University of Edinburgh Press, 1976, p 216.

104. McDowell LR, Conrad JH, Ellis GL, et al: Mineral for Grazing Ruminants in Tropical Regions, 1983, p 60.

105. McLean RW, Hendricksen RE, Coates DB, et al: Phosphorus and Beef Production in Northern Australia Tropical Grassland. Queensland, Australia, Dept of Primary Industries, 24:197, 1990.

106. McManus WR, Anthony RG, Gout LL, et al: Aust J Agric Res 30:635, 1979.

107. McNaught ML, Owen EC, Smith JB: Biochem J 46:36, 1950.

108. Mertz W: Biol Trace Elements Res 32:3, 1992.

109. Miller JJ, Read BJ, Wentz DJ, et al: Can J Anim Sci 76:385, 1996.

110. Miller WJ: J Dairy Sci 53:1323, 1970.

111. Miller WJ: In Dairy Cattle Feeding and Nutrition. New York, Academic Press, 1979, p 74.

112. Mills CF: Biochem J 63:187, 1976.

113. Mills CF: Soil Sci 85:100, 1958.

114. Miltimore JE, Mason JL: Can J Anim Sci 51:193, 1971.

115. Mirand EA, Grose Jr JT: Nature Land 200:92, 1963.

116. Moonsie-Shageer S, Mowat DN: J Anim Sci 71:232, 1993.

117. Mowat DN, Chang X, Yang WZ: Can J Anim Sci 73:49, 1993.

118. National Research Council: Nutrient Requirements of Beef Cattle, 7th ed. Washington, DC, National Academy Press, 1996.

119. Nockels CF, DeBonis J, Torrent J: J Anim Sci 71:2539, 1993.

120. Nockels C: Academy of Veterinary Consultants. Proceedings March 11, 1993.

121. NRC: Mineral Tolerance of Domestic Animals. Washington DC, National Academy Press, 1980.

122. Nunn CL, Turner HA, Drake DJ: J Anim Sci 74(Suppl 1):294, 1996.

123. Orr CL, Hutcheson DP, Grainger RB, et al: J Anim Sci 68:2893, 1990.

124. Osweiler GD, Carson TL, Buch WB, et al: Clinical and Diagnostic Veterinary Toxicology, ed 3. Dubuque, Kendall/Hunt, 1985, p 167.

125. Owens FN: Beef magazine 24:98, April 1988.

126. Owens FN: Beef magazine 24:29, March 1988.

127. Owens FN: Beef magazine 24:38, May 1988.

128. Owens FN: In Fall Cattle Festival, Guymon, OK, 1986, p 22.

129. Owens FN: Southwest Nutrition and Management Conference, Phoenix, Arizona. Feb 24–25, 1994, p 29.

130. Pamp DE, Goodrich RD, Mieske JC: J Anim Sci 45:1458, 1977.

131. Pehrson B, Knutson M, Gyllensward M: Swedish J Agric Res 19:53, 1989.

132. Phillips JM, Brown AH, Parham RW: Lenexa, KS, Veterinary Medicine Publishers, 1988, p 20.

133. Plasto AW: In Mineral and Vitamin Nutrition of Queensland Cattle (excluding phosphorus), Queensland Department of Primary Industries, 1984.

134. Reid RL, Franklin MC, Hallsworth EG: Aust Vet J 23:136, 1947.

135. Rickets RE, Campbell JR, Weinman DE, et al: J Dairy Sci 53:898, 1970.

136. Rojas MA, Dyer IA, Cassatt WA: J Anim Sci 24:664, 1965.

137. Rooke JA, Akinsoyinu AO, Armstrong DG: Grass Forage Sci 38:311, 1983.

138. Ross JG, Speats JW, Garlich JD: J Anim Sci 72:1842, 1994.

139. Ross JG, Speats JW, Garlich JD: J Anim Sci 72:1600, 1994.

140. Rotruck JT, Pope AL, Ganther HE, et al: Science 18:954, 1973.

141. Rowson LEA, Lawson RAS, Moor RM, et al: Reprod Fertil 28:427, 1972.

142. Rust S: J Anim Sci 61 (Suppl. 1):482 (Abstract), 1985.

143. Sankoh FA-R, RJ Boila: Can J Anim Sci 67:1033, 1987.

144. Schaefer AL, Jones SDM, Tong AKW, et al: Can J Anim Sci 70:107, 1990.

145. Schaefer AL, Jones SDM, Tong AKW, et al: Livest Prod Sci 30:333, 1992.

146. Scott ML, Thompson JN: Poultry Sci 50:1742, 1971.

147. Sinclair S: Relationship between ration/drinking water consumption versus manure characteristics—Feedlot Survey. October, 1996.

148. Smith CJ, McDaniel EG, Fan FF, et al: Science 18:954, 1973.

149. Smith RM, Marston HR: Br J Nutri 24:857, 1970.

150. Spears JW, Hutcheson DP, Chirase NK, et al: J Anim Sci 69(Suppl 1):858, 1991.

151. Spears JW, Hutcheson DP, Chirase NK, et al: J Anim Sci 69(Suppl 1):859, 1991.

152. Spears JW: Plains Nutrition Council, 1988.

153. Spears JW, Hutcheson DP, Chirase NK: J Anim Sci 69(Suppl 1):552 Abst No. 859, 1991.

154. Spears J, Samsell L: J Anim Sci 63(Suppl 1):402 (Abstract), 1986.

155. Spears JW, Kegley EB, Ward JD: Proc. 52nd Minnesota Nutrition Conf, 1992.

156. Spears JW: Plains Nutr Council Rep, 1988, p 1d.

157. Spears JW: In Proceedings of the Grazing Livestock Nutrition Conference. Steamboat Springs, Colorado, 1991, p 138.

158. Stanton TL, Schultz DN: Prof Anim Sci 9:159, 1993.

159. Stanton TL, Schultz DN: Prof Anim Sci 10:150, 1994.

160. Stobart R, Medeivors D, Riley M, et al: J Anim Sci 65(suppl 1):500, 1987.

161. Strasia CA, Owens FN: In Great Plains Beef Cattle Handbook, GPE-1303, 1988.

162. Sweeten J: Academy of Veterinary Consultants, March 1993.

163. Swenson CK, Paterson JA, Ansotegui RP: In 57th Minnesota Nutrition Conference & Protiva Technical Symposium, 1996.

164. Terashima Y, Tucker RE, Deetz LE, et al: J Nutr 112:1914, 1982.

165. Underwood EJ, Somers M: Aust J Agric Res 20:889, 1969.

166. Underwood EJ: In The Mineral Nutrition of Livestock, ed 2. Farnham Royal, England, Commonwealth Agricultural Bureaux, 1981.

167. Underwood EJ: The Mineral Nutrition of Livestock. London, Commonwealth Agricultural Bureaux, 1981.

168. Vilda F, Southerland TM: An examination of the copper status in 'Nuerte Subita' (sudden death) in Cuban cattle, 1970.

169. Waggoner JW Jr, Kaltenbach CC, Smith WW, et al: Proc West Sec Amer Soc Anim Sci 30:284, 1979.

170. Waldron-Edwards D: In Skorya S, Waldron-Edwards D (eds). Intestinal Absorption of Metal Ions, Trace Elements and Radionucleids. London, Pergamon Press, 1971, p 381.

171. Ward GM: J Anim Sci 46:1078, 1978.

172. Ward JD, Spears JW, Gengelbach JP: J Anima Sci 73:571, 1995.

173. Westerman PW, Safley LM, Barkes JC, et al: In Proc 5th Inter Symp on Livestock Wastes, ASAE 13.8, 1985, p 295.

174. Wittenberg KM, RJ Boila, MA Shariff: Can J Anim Sci 70:895, 1990.

175. Zinn RA, Shen Y, Adam CF, et al: J Anim Sci 74:1462, 1996.

▪ Dairy Cow Nutritional Guidelines

Bill Mahanna, M.S., Ph.D.

The objective of this section is to provide a quick checklist of nutritional "rules of thumb" for early-lactation and transition cows. This section is not intended to be a review of basic nutritional concepts or the requirements for all classes of dairy animals. That goal can be accomplished through coursework, reading the help menus of ration balancing software, or accessing any number of university or industry Web sites via Internet searches on key words such as "dairy nutrition." This section is intended, however, to provide general ration guidelines commonly used by feed manufacturers, consultants, and extension personnel across North America for a class of dairy animals that arguably are the primary determinants of herd profitability.

Anticipating nutritional problems will be increasingly important as producers set goals for ever higher production. Rules of thumb will certainly not replace the specific nutritional advice given by competent nutritional consultants, but they can serve as a yardstick to help track areas of potential concern. If dairy rations differ greatly from these guidelines, the areas of discrepancy may be a good place to begin more detailed diagnostic analysis.

DRY MATTER INTAKE

Dry matter intake (DMI) is a key factor in maintaining high production, body condition (conducive to reproductive goals), and general systemic and ruminal health. Many factors affect DMI, including ration ingredients and palatability (including commodity feeds), water intake and quality, feedstuff digestibility, energy density of ration, frequency of feeding, feed processing, level of production, cow comfort (ideally, more than 30% of cows in a given herd are ruminating at any one time, and half of those are lying down), cow genetics, rate of passage of digested material, and forage quality. Consistency of ration ingredients is also an important component to keeping cows on feed and maintaining a consistently balanced ration.

1. Cows should reach maximum daily DMIs no later than 10 weeks post partum. Intake regression equations are driven by body weight, number of days in milk, production level, and body weight change. Do not overestimate body weight.

2. At maximum intake periods, cows should be eating at least 4% of their body weight (BW) per day at peak intake. Example: 1350 lb cow × 4% = 54 lb DMI/day.

3. Cows milked three times a day will eat about 5% to 6% more dry matter per day, and cows milked four times a day will eat about 9% to 10% more dry matter, compared with cows milked two times each day. Cows receiving bovine somatotropin (BST) can be expected to have a DMI similar to that of nontreated cows producing the same amount of milk per day.

4. Use a 4.0% fat-to-3.3% protein-corrected milk (FPCM) equation to adjust production for different composition yield.

$$FPCM \text{ (lb)} = \text{(lb of milk} \times 0.337) + [\text{(lb of milk)} \times (0.116 \times \%fat)] + [\text{(lb of milk)} \times (0.06 \times \%protein)].$$

Example: 55 lb of milk, 3.8% fat, 3.1% protein.

$$FPCM = (55 \times 0.337) + [(55) \times (0.116 \times 3.8)] + [(55) \times (0.06 \times 3.1)] = 53 \text{ lb of milk.}$$

5. Under normal feeding, estimate DMI in pounds as:

$$DMI \text{ (lb)} = [A] \times [0.02 \text{ (lb of BW)}] + [0.3 \text{ (lb of FCM/day)}] + [B(\text{lb gain per day})],$$

where A (days in milk adjustment) =

$$1.0 - [0.2 ((80 - DIM)/80)], FCM \text{ (4\% fat corrected milk)} = \text{(lb of milk} \times 0.4) + \text{(lb of milk} \times \%fat)15,$$

and B (gain adjustment) =
1.0 if the cow is gaining weight and 0 if it is losing weight.

BW stands for body weight; DIM stands for days in milk. Example: DMI for a 1350 lb cow yielding 100 lb of 4% milk, 70 days in milk, and losing weight =

$$[1.0 - [0.2(80 - 70)80]] \times [0.02(1350)] + [0.3(100)] + [0] = 0.975 \times 27 + 30 + 0 = 56.3 \text{ lb of DMI/day.}$$

6. For every 2 lb of expected milk production, cows should eat at least 1 lb of dry matter. Eating less than this causes excessive body condition loss, and the cows are more prone to metabolic disorders.

7. Forage dry matter consumption should be near 2% of the cow's body weight to ensure proper rumen health.

8. If possible, provide a separate milking and feeding string for heifers. First-calf heifers will spend 10% to 15% more time eating when housed separately from older cows.

9. Consider offering sodium bicarbonate free-choice as an early warning of "off-feed" problems.

10. The best total ration dry matter is between 50% and 75%. Wetter or drier rations limit consumption. If silage is fed heavily, expect DMI to decline 0.02% of BW for every 1% increase in *total* ration moisture above 50%. This change is due to wetter feeds fermenting longer, which increases acid levels and protein degradation products. Example: For a 1350 lb cow, 60% moisture ration − 50% upper limit = 10 × (0.02% × 1350) = 2.7 lb less DMI per day, causing up to a 5 to 6 lb decrease in daily milk production.

11. If using a total mixed ration (TMR) mixer with weigh scales, check silage moistures on a routine weekly basis with a microwave and gram scale to ensure inclusion of the proper amount of silage dry matter. Provide a chart in the feed room listing how much silage to add depending on silage moisture levels. Silage moisture changes can alter the forage-to-grain ratio of the ration, causing off-feed and lowered milk butterfat content.

12. If intakes are below normal, begin by checking the nonfiber (nonstructural) carbohydrate and fiber lengths and levels in the ration. Also check water intake and whether the feed is moldy.

13. Expect cows to reduce dry matter consumption about 3.3% for every 2.2°F rise in temperature over 75°F. Cows begin to experience heat stress when the temperature exceeds 80°F, relative humidity exceeds 80%, or the two added together exceed 140.

14. Provide clean water within 50 feet of the feedbunk. Expect cows to drink about ½ gallon for each pound of milk. Periodically check waters for stray voltage. If water tests indicate high bacterial counts, consider water chlorination.

15. Consider the feedbunk and manger design. Cows spend more time eating, waste less feed, and produce more saliva to buffer the rumen when forced to eat in a grazing-like (head down) position.

16. Feed at least 60% of the ration at night during hot weather.

17. Silage pH (acidity) should be less than 4.2 for corn or cereal silages and less than 5.0 for legume silages. Silages with higher pH (less acid) are more prone to excessive spoilage and poor bunklife.

18. Feeds with mold counts in excess of 10,000 colony-forming units (CFU) per gram may cause digestive upsets. Counts are of limited value unless the individual molds are identified. Mold growth does not automatically indicate that mycotoxins are present. Test for mycotoxins if dangerous levels of mold populations have been identified in the feed.

19. Feed should be available to cows at least 20 hours per day. High-producing cows will eat up to 12 meals per day, each averaging 23 minutes. Cows usually eat after milking; therefore, fresh feed should be available in the feedbunk following milking to encourage maximum feed intake. Adapt your feeding to the eating behavior of your cows. Try to manage so it takes less than 3 hours per day to feed cows.

20. Provide each cow 2 to 2.5 ft of bunkspace. As little as 1.2 ft per cow is adequate in well-ventilated facilities where TMRs are fed twice daily. Sweep feedbunks or mangers clean daily, especially during hot weather.

21. Encourage eating by sweeping up feed, routinely getting cows up to eat, and providing periods of light during evening hours.

22. Income over feed costs is a more important profitability measure than simply monitoring feed costs per hundredweight of milk.

PEAK PRODUCTION AND FEEDING FOR COMPONENTS

Peak, or summit, milk production levels set the pace for the entire lactation schedule. High-string cows are under considerable stress from production demands and body condition losses. They are also the group of cows whose reproductive status exerts a tremendous influence over the profitability of the dairy herd. The performance of these cows in terms of production of milk and components (milk yield, protein, and fat content) can be diagnostic of the general nutritional status of the entire herd. Maintaining a production balance between pounds of milk and components is also an important economic consideration in many dairy markets.

1. Cows should peak in milk production 8 to 10 weeks after calving.

2. First-calf heifers should peak within 75% the production of older cows.

3. For each extra 1 lb of milk at peak production, the average cow will produce 200 to 225 lb more milk for the entire lactation period. This suggests the importance of getting and keeping cows on feed.

4. If a cow's milk production is not peaking as expected, check protein levels. If it is peaking well but not persistent, check energy levels.

5. After peak, the milk production of heifers will drop about 0.2% per day and that of older cows will drop about 0.3% per day (or 3% every 10 days). Cows with high genetic potential tend to peak higher, reach that peak later, and show more persistency.

6. Use the adjusted corrected milk (ACM) equation to account for differences in average days in milk (ADIM), fat content of milk, and current age of the herd when comparing month-to-month trends in production. ACM = (0.432 × lb of milk) + (16.25 × lb of fat) + [(0.0029 × lb of milk) × (ADIM−150)]. Example: 55 lb of milk, 3.4% fat, and 111

ADIM. ACM = (0.432 × 55) + [16.25 × (55 × 0.034)] + [(0.0029 × 55) × (111 − 150)] = 48 lb of milk.

7. Summit milk yield (average of highest two milk yields during first three production tests) should be within 5 lb of the average milk yield of all cows less than 100 days past calving. Greater differences indicate problems with maintaining early lactation production.

8. Milk protein: fat ratios should be near 0.90 for Brown Swiss and Milking Shorthorns, 0.85 to 0.88 for Holsteins and Ayrshires, and near 0.80 for Guernseys and Jerseys. Higher values could indicate fat intake problems. Lower values could mean protein intake problems from too much fat or too little total or undegraded protein in the ration.

9. When the ration is changed to improve components, fat content will change the most, followed at a much lesser extent by protein, and lactose will hardly vary.

10. To maximize protein content, rumen bacterial growth must provide adequate protein and amino acid production in the small intestine. Watch protein ration levels (degradable intake protein [DIP], soluble intake protein [SIP], and undegraded (bypass) intake protein [UIP]) and rumen fermentable carbohydrates (non-fiber carbohydrate [NFC]). This will also help reduce protein intake problems associated with a fat-supplemented diet.

11. To boost fat content, maximize forage intakes and the digestibility of forages by harvesting the forage at its proper level of maturity. The better the quality of the forage, the larger the portion of the ration it will be able to provide. Also watch levels of "effective fiber" so that rumination is maintained to buffer the rumen.

12. To improve fat intake, balance the types of carbohydrates and their degradation rates. For example: barley is more quickly fermented in the rumen than corn. Monitoring ration fiber levels and feed sequencing can help offset potential rumen acidosis problems associated with rapidly degraded grains or commodity feeds.

13. To maintain fat content through the heat of the summer, encourage forage intakes by keeping feed fresh in the feedbunk and feeding more during cooler evenings; consider feeding additives such as direct-fed microbials and yeast cultures, which can improve forage intake and digestibility. Buffers can also compensate for reduced buffering from lowered forage intake during hot weather.

TARGETING PROTEIN LEVELS

The word "protein" is translated from Latin as "first in importance." This derivation is most appropriate considering the cost of protein and the fact that in the case of body condition loss, relatively less protein than energy is provided for milk production demands.

1. Provide 18% to 19% crude protein in the total ration. Excess protein is costly, will not significantly increase protein content, and may reduce reproductive efficiency.

2. Provide 60% to 65% DIP in the entire ration.

3. Provide SIP levels to equal about half (30% to 32%) of the DIP levels. This ensures readily available nitrogen for rumen bacterial growth.

4. Provide UIP levels of 35% to 40% in the total ration. The upper range is suggested if supplemental fat is being fed. Fat is minimally metabolized in the rumen, thus reducing nutrients for microbial growth. To make up for a reduction in microbial protein flow to the intestines, higher levels of bypass protein are required.

5. Blood urea nitrogen (BUN) levels exceeding 25 mg/dL (or milk urea nitrogen [MUN] levels over 20 mg/dL) may

indicate improper ration formulation for degradable and undegradable protein. Breeding efficiency may also be affected.

6. In corn silage or corn-based rations, restrict the use of corn by-product feeds as a source of undegraded protein. Consider animal or marine sources, heat-treated soybean products, dried brewer's grain, or synthetic sources to provide potentially limiting amino acids such as lysine and methionine. Commercial "blends" of protein sources attempt to prevent amino acid deficiencies.

7. For cows yielding over 75 lb of 4% fat-corrected milk per day (79 lb, 3.7%) consider providing 1 lb of protein from an animal or marine source to lower the risk of amino acid and peptide deficiencies.

8. Silages with nitrate levels up to 4000 ppm nitrate (N) should be diluted with other feeds to achieve 1000 ppm or lower concentration in the total ration.

FIBER FOR RUMEN HEALTH

Fiber is a double-edged sword. Too little affects rumen health and component yields and makes for a more expensive ration. Too much can serve to limit total dry matter intakes and slow down the rate of passage so critical to cows in early lactation. The inability of current regression equations to accurately assess the energy availability in forages and provide adequate "effective fiber" only serves to complicate the problem, especially in light of new technologies such as kernel processing of corn silage.

1. Forage dry matter consumption should be near 2% of the cow's body weight. Example: 1350 lb cow × 2% = 27 lb dry matter from forages.

2. Provide at least 19% to 21% acid detergent fiber (ADF) in the total ration. Levels at 17% are adequate for high corn silage–based rations or herds receiving total mixed rations.

3. Provide at least 28% to 30% neutral detergent fiber (NDF) levels in the total ration.

4. Make sure that the ration provides a minimum of 21% NDF in the total ration dry matter supplied by forages. Boost this to 24% if corn silage makes up more than one fourth of total forage dry matter. Example: If forages in the ration average 44% NDF, then 21%/44% = 48% of the total ration dry matter should come from forages.

5. Forage NDF should be about 0.9% of body weight. Example: 1350 lb cow × 0.009 = 12.15 lb of ration NDF supplied by forages.

6. Make sure that 65% to 75% of the total ration NDF is supplied by forages.

7. The *maximum* pounds of total ration NDF should be about 1.25% of BW. Example: 1350 lb cow × 1.25% = 16.8 lb NDF. 16.8 lb/total DMI = upper % NDF in the ration. 16.8 lb NDF/54 lb typical DMI = 31% upper limit for %NDF in the total ration. Exceeding these NDF levels may result in lower dry matter consumption.

8. Provide at least 5 lb per day of fiber that is over 1½ inches long. Underfeeding of "effective" fiber can cause off-feed and fat content problems.

9. Rumen pH should be above 6.0. A lower pH could limit fiber digestion and protein synthesis, and the potential acidosis could cause reduced feed intake.

10. Fiber particles should be long enough to stimulate 15 minutes of cud chewing time per pound of ration dry matter. This will provide a cow eating 50 lb of dry matter with 35 to 40 gallons of saliva to buffer the rumen environment.

11. Silages (unprocessed) should be chopped at ⅜ to ½ in. theoretical length of cut (TLC) to ensure that 15% to 20% of the silage particles are over ½ in. long. Finer chopped silages do pack better in storage structures, but high silage–based rations need adequate particle length to stimulate rumen buffering from cud-chewing.

12. If feeding kernel-processed corn silage at levels of over 40% of the forage dry matter, consider lengthening the chop on corn silage (½ in. or more by manipulating the shear bar or actually removing knifes) and shortening the chop on legume and grass silages (≤½ in.). This allows for more of the effective fiber to come from corn silage while improving the fermentation potential of haycrop silages.

13. Sodium bicarbonate, or its buffer equivalent, should be added at 0.75% of the total ration dry matter, especially in high-corn silage or high-moisture corn-based rations. Example: 50 lb dry matter × 0.75% = 0.375 lb or 6 oz.

MEETING ENERGY NEEDS

Energy is referred to as the "nebulous nutrient," and providing enough energy to allow cows the opportunity to express genetic potentials can be a major feeding problem. Energy has traditionally been relatively cheap in North America and, as such, is often abused in the ration. The extremes of overfeeding (from excessive challenge feeding) in early lactation or underfeeding (to reduce the "grain bill") can severely limit production, reproduction, and herd health.

1. Energy density of the top cow ration should be up to 0.78 megacalories (Mcal) net energy of lactation (NE-L) per pound of dry matter in rations containing no added fat, up to 0.80 Mcal NE-L for rations with added fat, and up to 0.82 Mcal NE-L for rations adding ruminally inert (bypass) fat.

2. If lead feeding, cows should be eating 6 to 8 lb of grain at calving. Boost concentrate 1 to 2 lb/day, from 3 days after freshening until the desired grain feeding levels have been reached.

3. Do not feed more than 5 to 7 lb of grain at any single feeding. This reduces the changes in rumen pH, which helps prevent off-feed problems.

4. Grain intake should generally not exceed 60% of ration dry matter.

5. If too much corn passes undigested into the manure, check grain level, extent of processing, and harvest maturity (harvest corn silage at one-third to two-thirds milkline unless using a kernel processor or rolling). Also check levels of DIP and SIP protein (important to rumen bacteria) and amount of fiber intake over 1½ in. long (important for the rumen mat).

6. Provide non-fiber carbohydrate (NFC) levels of 35% to 42% in the total ration. NFC (by difference) = 100 − (% crude protein + %NDF + %fat + %ash). Providing excess sugars and easily fermented carbohydrates can result in acidosis and fat test depression problems.

7. Provide between 25% and 35% starch in the total ration.

8. Consider feeding supplemental fat to cows yielding over 75 lb of 4% fat-corrected milk per day (79 lb, 3.7%). As production rises, it becomes more difficult for cows physically to consume enough feed to meet energy requirements. Older cows will generally respond better than 2-year-olds. Fat levels in excess of 5% to 6% of the ration are not recommended during the first 5 weeks of lactation. Supplement the first ¼ lb in the transition ration, up to 1 lb at freshening, and, if needed, additional fat after 5 weeks past calving.

9. Limit total fat to no more than 7.5% of the ration dry matter. Example: 4 lb of total fat in the ration divided by a typical DMI of 55 lb/cow/day = 7.2% fat in the ration. Too much fat interferes with fiber digestion, reduces microbial protein flow to the lower tract, and can result in lowered milkfat content.

10. Provide the same amount of fat in the ration as pounds

of milkfat produced. Example: 100 lb of milk per day × 4% fat = 4 lb of milkfat and 4 lb of total fat in the ration.

11. Provide one third of fat in ration from normal ration feeds, from oilseeds or fats, and one third from rumen inert (bypass) fats. Example: If 4 lb of fat are to be provided in the ration, about 4 lb × 33% = 1.3 lb of fat should be from oilseeds such as whole cottonseed or soybeans. If soybeans are 20% fat, then 1.3 lb/20% = 6.5 lb of whole soybeans in the ration. Any additional fat should be provided by commercially available inert sources because they bypass the rumen and are digested in the small intestine.

12. Boost calcium to 1% and magnesium to 0.3% of ration dry matter when feeding supplemental fat. Fats bind with calcium, reducing calcium and magnesium availability.

WATCH BODY CONDITION

Monitoring body condition is something that is intuitive to good dairy producers and their consultants. It is the research community that has only recently begun to quantify the importance of maintaining and replacing body condition in terms of production and reproduction economics and the efficiency of nutrient metabolism.

1. Cows should freshen with a body condition score (BCS) of 3+ to 4− (1 to 5 scale: 1 = thin; 5 = fat). This should prevent metabolic problems during early lactation. Second lactation "burnout," or "sophomore slump," is often due to a lack of condition on high-producing, first-calf heifers.

2. Cows should not lose more than 1 BCS (1 to 5 system) (or >2 lb/day) during early lactation to reduce ketosis and breeding problems. One point of BCS is equivalent to about 125 lb of weight.

3. One pound of body weight loss provides enough energy for about 7 lb of milk but only enough protein for about 3 to 4 lb of milk.

4. It requires 2.3 Mcal NE-L (or 2.5 lb shelled corn dry matter) to replace 1 lb of body weight loss. Use the tail end of the lactation period to replace lost body condition. The cow is most efficient at replacing weight while still milking and is less prone to fatty liver problems that can occur when trying to condition a diverse group of dry cows.

5. If necessary, grain can be supplemented in the dry period to improve the body condition of individual cows that are dried off in an underconditioned state. In larger dairies, two dry lots may be justified to separate dry cows with different energy requirements.

MINERALS AND VITAMINS

Although required in relatively small amounts compared with energy or protein, minerals and vitamins are a necessary part of the ration, from the perspective of production, reproduction, and cost per pound of nutrient fed.

1. Provide at least 1800 IU of vitamin A per pound of ration dry matter daily. Example: 54 lb DMI × 1800 IU/lb = 97,200 IU/day.

2. Provide at least 450 IU of vitamin D per pound of ration dry matter daily. Example: 54 lb DMI × 450 IU/lb = 24,300 IU/day.

3. Provide at least 7 IU of vitamin E per pound of ration dry matter daily. Example: 54 lb DMI × 7 IU/lb = 378 IU/day. Many consultants supplement vitamin E at levels of 500 IU/day to fresh cows and 1000 IU/day to dry cows. Higher dry cow supplementation may help prevent some of the 20% of new mastitis infections that occur during the dry period. Vitamin E

and selenium are vital for proper functioning of the immune system.

4. Provide 0.3 ppm of selenium in the ration dry matter. Parts per million can be converted to percent by moving the decimal point four places to the left. Example: 54 lb DMI × 454,000 mg/lb × 0.00003% = 7.4 mg of selenium per day.

5. Watch elevated potassium levels of over 1.0% in the total ration of dry cows fed grass-based rations due to binding of magnesium (tetany) and calcium mobilization interference causing milk fever, retained placenta, and "downer cow" problems at calving.

6. Provide elevated levels of potassium (1.5%), sodium (0.5%), and magnesium (0.35%) in the milking ration dry matter during heat stress.

7. Provide a nitrogen-to-sulfur ratio of 11 to 13:1 in the total ration to meet rumen bacterial needs.

8. Force-feed 1 oz of trace-mineralized salt for maintenance and 1 oz of salt for every 30 lb of milk to meet chloride requirements.

9. For early-lactation cows, consider 25% of the mineral supplementation in the form of chelates, especially copper, cobalt, manganese, and zinc (i.e., zinc methionine).

10. For milk fever–prone herds, limit the calcium intake of dry cows to less than 80 to 100 g/day (0.5% to 0.7% of ration dry matter) and limit phosphorus intake to less than 45 g/day (0.3% to 0.35% of ration). Hold the calcium-to-phosphorus ratio to less than 2:1 without exceeding phosphorus limits.

11. For herds with milk fever problems in which it is unfeasible to avoid feeding high-calcium dry cow rations, adjust the dry cow cation-anion balance to provide a negative level of milliequivalents (sodium + potassium − chlorine) per 100 g of ration dry matter. Anionic salts such as ammonium chloride, ammonium sulfate, and magnesium sulfate can be supplemented to keep dry rations high in anions like chloride and sulfur. Milking rations should strive for a positive 25 to 45 mEq level.

TRANSITION RATIONS

The transition ration, typically defined as "2 weeks before freshening," is the one ration most nutritionists would like to control because it sets the stage for the entire lactation. The goal is to (1) allow time for rumen papillae to adapt and grow as exposed to increasing levels of fermentable carbohydrate, (2) minimize postpartum metabolic disorders, (3) minimize "normal" DMI depression that occurs around calving time, and (4) increase DMI as rapidly as possible following parturition.

1. Cows typically decline in DMI by upwards of 30% at 5 to 7 days before calving. Most cows rapidly increase DMI (3 to 6 lb/day) for the first 3 weeks after calving.

2. Feed stable forages and grains and perhaps consider binding agents if moldy feed has been a problem.

3. Keep cows on feed (upward of 31 lb of dry matter per cow per day).

4. Closely monitor feed bunks.

5. Do not feed the exact lactation TMR because of problems associated with positive cation-anion balances, high potassium, buffers, and protein fractions out of balance. However, it is advisable to adjust the cow's diet to the basic lactation ration ingredients such as protein, grain, and forage sources.

6. Increase energy (0.66 to 0.72 NE-L), protein (14.5% to 15.5% crude protein), and UIP (35% to 38%) in the transition ration to begin preparing for high DMI during the lactation phase.

TOTAL MIXED RATION CONSIDERATIONS

Although the concept of TMR-based rations is well accepted in the dairy industry, their implementation and management is still a common question for consulting nutritionists. It is also important to impress on producers that a TMR will only be as good as the quality of the individual feed components. Forage quality, feed bunklife, and actual TMR intakes are still critical success factors.

1. Base mixer capacity on 60% to 70% of the struck level capacity, with a minimum requirement of 2.5 ft³ per cow, assuming two feedings per day. Recommended mixing time is 3 to 6 minutes. Do not overmix, which results in loss of effective fiber. Locate magnets at mixer discharge areas. Accurate scales are a must, and silage moistures should be monitored weekly. Several manufacturers have mixers with knives that permit the use of unchopped, long-stemmed hay.

2. Using a single-group TMR system in herds producing more than 20,000 lb of milk may offer advantages in feeding simplicity, labor, cow movement, and production potential but will result in more costly use of specialty ingredients and has the potential to overcondition some cows.

3. Having two milking groups and a single dry group is workable for most herds. This arrangement can also be easily adapted to a tie-stall barn by the use of a mechanized feed cart.

4. There should be no more than a 15% change in nutrient density between TMR groups, to prevent digestive upsets. Early-lactation cows will rebound from off-feed problems and re-establish production much more quickly and easily than mid-to late-lactation cows.

5. Cows moved to a new TMR group in later lactation usually drop in milk production more than cows moved in early lactation. A workable system, proven overseas, challenges all cows for 45 days to establish milk potential. High potential cows are maintained in the high group and low cows are shifted to a lower TMR group.

6. The range of cows within a TMR group should not exceed 20 to 25 lb of 4% fat-corrected milk (22 to 27 lb, 3.7%).

7. Balance TMR groups for milk production 30% above the actual average of a one-group system, 20% for a two-group system and 10% for a three-group system. This will challenge fresh cows and allow for replacing lost body condition in late-lactation cows.

8. The use of electronic, computer grain feeders has advantages, especially for one- or two-group systems; however, cow requirements must be continually updated and feeders must be serviced and monitored routinely for accuracy.

9. When making TMR group changes, move as many cows at one time as possible, overfeed slightly on move day, and move at night when activity is lowest to reduce stress.

10. With more than one TMR grouping, do not move cows solely based on production but also take into account body condition score, age, and breeding status. High-producing cows and 2-year-olds may need more time in the high string to allow for growth and replenishing of lost body reserves.

11. If TMR rations are correctly balanced for fiber and energy, move fresh cows directly into the high group at freshening. A transition dry cow ration can assist in making this period of ration and environmental changes less stressful.

12. University research shows no benefit of feeding legume- and grass silage–based rations more than once a day if the feed remains fresh in the feedbunk and crowded feedbunks are not an issue. If corn silage constitutes over 30% of the forage, rations should be fed two times per day, especially during hot, humid weather. Use of a research-proven silage additive can improve bunklife and palatability. Pushing up the TMR ration to cows three to four times per day can also help encourage consumption.

13. Offer the TMR up to a 5% to 10% refusal. Less refusal is acceptable if eating behavior is normal and the refusal looks similar to the original TMR mix. Bunk sweepings should be analyzed and then reblended as a base mix for other milking groups or heifers. Watch mixing time when reblending, as over-mixing can reduce feed particle size.

14. Do not overpredict a group's DMI when starting to feed a TMR. This will cause lower than required nutrient density in the ration. Start balancing a TMR with intakes set lower than estimated and raise feeding levels to a point of refusal.

15. In TMR herds with poor housing or environment, increase the energy density of the ration (with better forages or fats, not more grain) to near 0.81 Mcal NE-L per pound of ration dry matter to adjust for lowered intakes (3.5% of body weight). Reduce NFC to 30% and NDF to 25% in the total ration.

MANURE AS A DIAGNOSTIC TOOL

Spend time with any respected nutritional consultant and two things will become immediately obvious. They spend considerable time just looking at cows eating, walking, drinking, and performing the necessary biologic functions. They also spend time walking behind and amongst cows analyzing manure. Although it is as much art as science, the following practical guidelines provide bountiful insight for those willing to "learn from the cow."

1. Fresh manure pH should be in the range of 6 to 6.8. A pH below 6.0 is indicative of excess starch escaping the rumen and being fermented in the small intestines.

2. Ideally, there should be "three rings in every plop."

3. Firm manure can be indicative of low salt, low water, high fiber, or low protein intake.

4. Loose manure with dark color can indicate high protein or low fiber intake.

5. Loose manure with lighter color is reflective of acidosis (generally with bubbles from fermenting starch and lowered pH).

6. If there is excess grain in the manure, check on acidosis, effective fiber or rumen mat problems, slug feeding, or whether DIP-to-NSC ratios are out of balance.

7. Fiber in manure is a sign of drastic effective fiber or rumen mat problems, or both.

BIBLIOGRAPHY

Allen MS, Knowlton KF: Non-structural carbohydrates important for ruminants. Feedstuffs, April 17:13, 1995.

Allen MS: Troubleshooting silage-based ration problems: Rumen fermentation of fiber and starch. *In* Proceedings of NRAES National Silage Production Conference. Syracuse, NY, 1993, p 186.

Allen MS, O'Neil KA, Dado RG, Kohn RA: Variation in fiber content and fiber digestibility of corn forages. Minn Forage Counc Update XVII(4), 1992.

Barmore JA: Guidelines help us tailor our rations. Hoards Dairyman, Sept 25, 1995.

Chase LE: Nonstructural carbohydrates in dairy rations. Agri-Pract 12(3):37, 1991.

Chase LE: Personal Communication via DAIRY-L. May 1995.

Chase LE: Feeding programs for dairy cattle fed silage based rations. *In* Proceedings of NRAES National Silage Production Conference. Syracuse, NY, 1993, p 157.

Chase LE, Howard T, Shaver RA: TMR's gain popularity in stall barns. Hoards Dairyman, Sept 10, 1990, p 728.

Dhiman TR, Satter LD: Particle size and corn moisture content of corn grain and their effects on dairy cow performance. U.S. Dairy Forage Research Center research summaries for 1994, p 93.

Erdman R: Silage fermentation characteristics affecting feed intake. *In* Proceedings of NRAES National Silage Production Conference, Syracuse, NY, 1993, p 210.

Harrison JH, Johnson L, Xu S: Managing corn silage for maximum nutritive value. Proceedings of the Pioneer Hi-Bred Pre-Conference Symposium of the Cornell Nutrition Conference, Rochester, NY, 1996, p 29.

Harrison JH, Fransen S: Silage management in North America. NFIA Field Guide for Hay and Silage Management in North America. NFIA, West Des Moines, 1991, pp 33–67.

Holland C, Kezar W: Pioneer Forage Manual—A Nutritional Guide. Pioneer Hi-Bred International, West Des Moines, 1990.

Holter JB: Personal communications via DAIRY-L, March 1995.

Hoover WH, Miller TK: Balancing dairy cattle rations for total carbohydrates. In Proceedings of the Pacific Northwest Animal Nutrition Conference, Vancouver, BC, 1990, p 173.

Huntington GB: Ruminant starch utilization progress has been extensive. Feedstuffs, June 16, 1994.

Hutjens MF: Nutrient balance revs up dairy cows. Successful Farming, Sept:36, 1987.

Hutjens MF: More grain in manure. Hoards Dairyman, Nov 25:873, 1989.

Hutjens M: Put your feeding program to the acid test. Hoards Dairyman, July, 1990.

Hutjens MF: Dry cow care can boost milk 1,000 to 2,000 pounds. Hoards Dairyman, Sept 25, 1991, p 702.

Hutjens MF: Strategies to tackle this winter's poor production. Hoards Dairyman, Feb 10:102, 1994.

Hutjens MF: Whole kernels pass. Hoards Dairyman, Jan 25:59, 1994.

Kautz WP: Personal communications, 1994–1995.

Linn J, Martin N: Review of the 1992 crop situation. In Proceedings from the Four-State Applied Nutrition Conference. LaCrosse, Wisc, 1993, p 45.

Mahanna WC: Silage fermentation and additive use in North America. In Proceedings of NRAES National Silage Production Conference. Syracuse, NY, 1993, p 85.

Mahanna WC: When the cows don't like your silage. Hoards Dairyman, Oct 10, 1991.

Mahanna WC: Hay Additive Review. In Proceedings of the Tenth Annual Alfalfa Conference. University of Kentucky, Cave City, Ky, Feb, 27, 1990.

Mahanna WC: 100 Feeding thumbrules revisited. Hoards Dairyman, Sept 25, 1995.

Mahanna WC: Proper management assures high-quality silage and grain. Feedstuffs, Jan 10:12 & Jan 17, 1994, p 17.

McCullough M: Feeding quality silage. Anim Nutr Health, Sept/Oct, 1984.

Muck RE, Bolsen KK: Silage preservation and silage additive products. In NFIA Field Guide for Hay and Silage Management in North America. West Des Moines, NFIA, 1991, p 105.

Muck RE: Factors influencing silage quality and their implication for management. J Dairy Sci 71:2992, 1988.

Nelson CE: Microbiological status as a critical quality control parameter of feeds and grains. In Proceedings of NFIA Feed Ingredient Institute. Rosemont, Ill, Proceedings of a NFIA meeting, 1991.

Nocek JE: Considerations in balancing carbohydrates in dairy cattle rations. In Proceedings from Four-State Applied Nutrition Conference. LaCrosse, Wisc, 1991, p 115.

Nutrient Requirements of Dairy Cattle, ed 6 (rev). Update 1989. National Academy Press, Washington, DC.

Perkins B: Personal communications, Sept 1995.

Pioneer Hi-Bred International: Corn Management/Diagnostic Guide. West Des Moines, Pioneer Hi-Bred International, Inc., 1987.

Pitt RE: Silage and Hay Preservation, NRAES publication No. 5. Ithaca, NY, Cornell University, 1990.

Rosenbrook R: Personal communications, 1994–1995.

Ruppel KA: Personal communications, Oct 1996.

Ruppel KA: Management of bunker silos: Opinions and reality. In Proceedings of NRAES National Silage Production Conference. Syracuse, NY, 1993, p 266.

Russell JB, O'Connor JD, Fox DG, et al: The rumen submodel of the Cornell net carbohydrate and protein system. In Proceedings of 1990 Cornell Nutrition Conference, p 34.

Sapienza DA: Personal communications, May 1995.

Sawyer T: Personal communications, 1993–1996.

Schwartau C: Personal communications via DAIRY-L, Dec 1995.

Seglar B, Mahanna B: Mold and mycotoxin update. Internal communications posted on Pioneer Web Site (www.pioneer.com), June 1996.

Shaver RD: Kernel milkline stage at harvest and hybrid quality effects on the nutritive value of corn silage for lactating dairy cows. In Proceedings from the Four-State Applied Nutrition Conference. LaCrosse, Wisc, 1993, p 56.

Shaver RD: Forage particle length in dairy rations. In Proceedings of NRAES Dairy Feeding Systems Symposium. Harrisburg, Penn, 1990, p 58.

Sniffen C, Allhouse B, Gulley C: Particle size of high moisture corn. Wm. H. Miner Agricultural Research Institute Farm Report, May 1, 1995.

Switzky D: A carbohydrate balancing act. Dairy, Nov 10, 1988, p 18.

VandeHaar M, Bucholtz H, Beverly R, et al: Spartan Dairy Ration Evaluator/Balancer Users Manual, CP-012, version 2.01. Lansing, Mich, Michigan State University, 1992.

Van Soest PJ, Allen MS: Limitations of prediction systems for digestibility and ration balancing. In Proceedings of NRAES National Silage Production Conference. Syracuse, NY, 1993, p 196.

Van Soest PJ: Environment and forage quality. In Proceedings of the Pioneer Hi-Bred Pre-conference Symposium of the Cornell Nutrition Conference. Rochester, NY, 1996, p 1.

Webb KE: The potential impact of proteolysis in high protein silages on peptide absorption. In Proceedings of 1992 California Animal Nutrition Conference Technical Symposium, 1992.

Whitlow LW: Mycotoxin contamination of silages: A potential cause of poor production and health in dairy herds. In Proceedings of NRAES National Silage Production Conference, Syracuse, NY, 1993, p 220.

■ Analyzing Milk Diets for Calves

John Maas, D.V.M., M.S., Diplomate, A.C.V.N. and A.C.V.I.M.

The assessment of calf diets is a common task for veterinarians involved in dairy consultation practice and is sometimes necessary for veterinarians in beef practice. Guidelines for the nutrient content of milk replacers commonly include the following recommendations:

Crude protein: 15%–20%
Crude fat (ether extract): 10%
Crude fiber: <0.5%
Ash: <10%

Several recommendations state that whole milk or liquid milk replacer should be fed at 10% of body weight per day, i.e., a 40-kg (88-lb) calf should receive 4 L (4.2 qt)/day. These guidelines may aid in comparing calf milk replacers; however, they may not be adequate for providing thorough medical or nutritional advice. A calf milk replacer should be formulated to meet all of the calf's nutrient requirements. It should be considered as a complete food, supplying energy, protein, essential fatty acids, minerals, and vitamins. The veterinarian's responsibilities for calf nutrition and health are best met by comparing the nutrient requirements of calves with the total feeding program, particularly the milk replacer or whole milk.

The newborn calf's gastrointestinal system is equipped to digest milk, and the ability of the calf to utilize other nutrient sources requires time to develop. As a practical matter, when evaluating calves up to 3 or 4 weeks of age, one need only account for nutrients derived from milk or milk replacer for meeting the calves' nutrient requirements.

MEETING ENERGY REQUIREMENTS

The most important nutrient requirement to account for is energy, and this, by convention, is based on the digestible energy (DE) system. Daily energy requirements for a neonatal calf are 45 to 55 kcal of DE per kilogram of body weight (BW) for maintenance. The maintenance requirement for energy depends on ambient temperature, with higher requirements for cold temperatures. The energy requirement for growth averages 300 kcal of DE per 100-g gain in BW. Expressions of DE requirements are listed (Table 1).

For example, a 50-kg calf gaining 0.75-kg (1.65 lb)/day would have an energy requirement of 5 Mcal of DE per day (2.75 Mcal of DE maintenance + 2.25 Mcal of DE per 0.75-kg gain = 5.0 Mcal of DE). This example uses fresh, whole milk with the following nutrient analysis: dry matter, 12%; DE, 5.73 Mcal/kg (dry matter basis [DMB]); crude protein, 25.8% DMB; calcium, 0.89% DMB; phosphorus, 0.72% DMB; and magnesium, 0.08% DMB. The calf in this example has the following energy requirements:

$$5.00 \text{ Mcal of DE} \div 5.73 \text{ Mcal/kg} = \\ 0.87 \text{ kg of whole milk (DMB)}$$

Because this milk is 12% DM:

$$0.87 \text{ kg of milk (DMB)} \div 0.12 = \\ 7.3 \text{ kg of whole milk}$$

$$7.3 \text{ kg of milk} \div 50 \text{ kg of BW} = 14.6\% \text{ BW}$$

This 50-kg (110-lb) calf would require 7.3 kg (16.1 lb, or just over 2 gal) of whole milk to gain 1.65 lb/day. This is well above the 10% of BW often recommended.

MEETING PROTEIN REQUIREMENTS

The protein requirements, as digestible protein (DP), for a calf are 0.5 g of digestible protein per kilogram of BW for maintenance and 22 g/100 g of BW gain for growth. The protein in whole milk is about 97% digestible, and the protein in an excellent quality milk replacer is about 94% digestible, whereas digestibility of protein in a poor-quality milk replacer may be as low as 60%. Using the calf in the above example, a 50-kg calf would require the following to gain 0.75 kg/day:

$$\text{Maintenance: } 0.5 \text{ g/kg} \times 50 \text{ kg} = 25 \text{ g}$$

$$\text{Gain: } \frac{22 \text{ g of digestible protein}}{100 \text{ g of BW gain}} \times 7.5 \ (0.75 \text{ kg}) = 165 \text{ g}$$

$$25 \text{ g of DP (maintenance)} + 165 \text{ g of DP (gain)} = \\ 190 \text{ g of digestible protein}$$

$$190 \div 0.97 = 196 \text{ g of protein from milk}$$

The 0.87 kg milk (DMB) was 25.8% protein; therefore:

$$0.87 \text{ kg} \times 0.258 = 224 \text{ g of protein}$$

This exceeds the protein requirement of 196 g of protein by 28 g.

COMPARING MILK AND MILK REPLACERS

Tables 2 and 3 list additional nutrient requirements for the young calf. The following several considerations should be mentioned separately:

1. Whole milk is a good source of the water-soluble B vitamins. These are added to the formulation of milk replacers.
2. Colostrum is very high in vitamins A and E, if these have been adequate in the diet of the cow.
3. Magnesium and iron levels in whole milk are often low.

Table 1
DAILY DIGESTIBLE ENERGY (DE) REQUIREMENTS FOR A NEONATAL CALF (50 kg)

Maintenance	45–55 kcal of DE/kg of BW	2.5–2.75 Mcal of DE
Gain	300 kcal of DE/100-g BW gain	
0.5-kg daily gain	1500 kcal of DE	1.5 Mcal of DE
1.0-kg daily gain	3000 kcal of DE	3.0 Mcal of DE

BW, body weight.

Table 2
NUTRIENT GUIDELINES FOR CALVES ON MILK REPLACER OR WHOLE MILK DIETS

Digestible energy	
Maintenance	45–55 kcal/kg of body weight (BW)
Gain	300 kcal/100 g of weight gain
Digestible protein	
Maintenance	0.5 g/kg of BW
Gain	22 g/100 g of weight gain
Fat (ether extract)	20% (10% NRC)
Crude fiber	No requirement*
Calcium	0.7% (3.2 g/0.45 kg)
Phosphorus	0.5% (2.3 g/0.45 kg)
Magnesium†	0.07%
Potassium	0.80%
Sodium	0.10%
Sodium chloride	0.25%
Sulfur	0.29% (in amino acids)
Iron†	100 ppm
Manganese	40 ppm
Zinc	40 ppm
Copper	10 ppm
Iodine	2.5 ppm
Selenium	0.1–0.2 ppm
Cobalt	0.10 ppm
Vitamin A	3800 IU/kg DMB (42 IU/kg of BW)
Vitamin D	600 IU/kg DMB (6.5 IU/kg of BW)
Vitamin E	15–60 IU/kg DMB

DMB, dry matter basis.
*Milk replacer should be less than 0.5% crude fiber.
†Whole milk often has <0.07% magnesium and milk replacers usually has ≥0.07% magnesium. Whole milk is quite low with respect to iron content, and iron is added to replacers.

Table 3
DAILY VITAMIN REQUIREMENTS FOR A 45-kg CALF

Thiamine (B$_1$)	2.9 mg
Riboflavin	2.0 mg
Niacin	12 mg
Pyridoxine (B$_2$)	3 mg
Pantothenic acid	8.8 mg
Biotin	0.9 mg
Choline	1.17 g
Folic acid	0.7 mg
Inositol	234 mg
Cyanocobalamin (B$_{12}$)	31 mg

These requirements are usually met as the calf begins to eat solid foods, such as hay and grain. Magnesium and iron are added to milk replacers.

4. The selenium (Se) status of the calf at birth will be normal if the cow has had adequate Se intake. Milk is often low with respect to selenium, and milk replacers contain added Se.

As an example for analyzing a milk diet, consider the following hypothetical commercial milk replacer label with this information:

Crude protein: Not <25%
Crude fat: Not <12%
Crude fiber: Not >0.3%
Ash: Not >8.5%
Moisture: Not >9% (Note: If ash or moisture are not listed, assume 9% for each.)

Label feeding instructions: Feed 2 measuring cups (0.45 kg; 1.0 lb)/day to each calf (diluted in 1 gal of clean, potable water).

DIGESTIBLE ENERGY REQUIREMENTS OF A 90-lb (40.8-kg) CALF

We will determine how the requirements of a 90-lb calf gaining 1.5 lb (0.68 kg)/day are met using this milk replacer. First, let us calculate the DE requirements of this calf.

Maintenance: 50 kcal/kg of BW	2041 kcal of DE
Growth: 1.5 lb (0.68 kg) 300 × 6.8 (300 kcal/100 g of gain)	2040 kcal of DE
Total daily energy requirements (DE)	4081 kcal of DE

Next, determine the energy content in 1 lb of the milk replacer. For ease of calculations, we will first determine the energy (total energy) in 100 g of replacer. Remember, that 1 g of protein or 1 g of carbohydrate has approximately 4 kcal, and 1 g of fat has 9 kcal of energy.

The total energy in 100 g of milk replacer is calculated as follows:

$$\text{Protein: } 22 \text{ g} \times 4 \text{ kcal/g} = 88 \text{ kcal/100 g}$$

$$\text{Fat: } 12 \text{ g} \times 9 \text{ kcal/g} = 108 \text{ kcal/100 g}$$

$$\text{Nitrogen-free extract (NFE)*: } 48.2 \text{ g} \times 4 \text{ kcal/g} = 192.8 \text{ kcal/100 g}$$

$$\text{Total (of three calculations above): } 388.8 \text{ kcal/100 g}$$
$$4.54 \times 388.8 \text{ kcal/100 g} = 1765 \text{ kcal/lb or}$$
$$1.765 \text{ Mcal/lb}$$

Assume the energy in this milk replacer is highly digestible (i.e., 90%); thus, the values in Table 4 are derived as follows:

---

*NFE is a measure of the crude carbohydrate content of a food and is obtained by subtracting the total of moisture, ash, fiber, fat, and protein from 100. In the case of milk or milk replacer, NFE would be the lactose content.

$$\text{NFE} = 100 - (\text{moisture} + \text{ash} + \text{fiber} + \text{fat} + \text{protein})$$

$$= 100 - (9 + 8.5 + .3 + 12 + 22)$$
$$= 100 - 51.8$$
$$= 48.2 \text{ g/100 g}$$

Table 4
MILK REPLACER ENERGY CONTENT

Amount of Replacer	Total Energy	Digestible Energy
0.45 kg (1 lb)	1.765 Mcal	1.59 Mcal
0.90 kg (2 lb)	3.53 Mcal	3.18 Mcal

$$1.765 \text{ Mcal (total energy)/lb} \times .90 =$$
$$1.59 \text{ Mcal of DE/lb (estimated)}$$

The maintenance requirement of this calf is 2.041 Mcal of DE, and 0.45 kg (1 lb) of this replacer does not meet maintenance requirements. Thus, the label instructions are not adequate for the nutrition and health of the calf in this example. Additionally, the requirement for maintenance and growth of the calf in this example is 4.081 Mcal of DE, and this is not met by feeding twice the label recommendations. To meet the DE requirements for maintenance plus 1.5 lb gain, the following calculation is needed:

$$4.081 \text{ Mcal of DE} \div 1.59 \text{ Mcal of DE/lb milk}$$
$$\text{replacer} = 2.46 \text{ lb}$$

Thus, almost 2.5 lb of milk replacer per day is needed for the calf in this example to gain 1.5 lb (0.68 kg)/day. This level of weight gain is common in beef calves and dairy calves fed an adequate diet. It is important to remember that common disease conditions in calves increase the nutrient requirements, and this must also be accounted for. The other nutrient requirements (e.g., protein, minerals) can be calculated in a similar manner. If the moisture and ash content are not on the label, the assumption that each is about 9% of the total should be fairly accurate. Also, complete nutrient information (e.g., energy, protein, fat, moisture, ash, vitamin A, zinc) can often be obtained from the manufacturer.

With these simple tools, a veterinarian can quickly and easily evaluate a feeding program for young calves being fed milk or milk replacer. It will become readily apparent that many recommendations and "rules of thumb" are not very accurate when examined closely.

BIBLIOGRAPHY

Agricultural Research Council Working Party: The Nutrient Requirements of Ruminant Livestock. Old Woking, Surrey, England, Commonwealth Agricultural Bureau, 1980.
Medino M, Johnson LW, Knight AP, et al: Evaluation of milk replacers for dairy calves. Compend Contin Educ Pract Vet 5:S148–S154, 1983.
National Research Council: Nutrient Requirements of Dairy Cattle. Washington DC, National Academy Press, 1988.
Roy JHB: The Calf: Management of Health, ed 5, vol 1. London, Butterworths, 1990.

■ Dietary Management in Pigs

Robert C. Thaler, M.S., Ph.D.

Because feed constitutes approximately 65% of the total cost of swine production, a great deal of attention must be paid to the nutritional program of a swine operation. The goal of a successful swine feeding program is to provide all of the essential nutrients (amino acids, fatty acids, vitamins, minerals, and water) in the required amounts necessary to maintain proper growth and reproduction as economically as possible. The factor that makes this challenging is the pig's ability to utilize a great many feedstuffs, ranging from corn and soybean meal to alfalfa and sweet potatoes. However, by combining the different ingredients in the proper ratios, the goal can be achieved.

Other factors can also influence the effectiveness of a swine feeding program. Some of them include life-cycle stage, nonnutritive feed additives, feed intake, and proper feed processing. Sound management practices in these areas, along with the required amounts of amino acids, fatty acids, vitamins, minerals, and water, will ensure a successful swine dietary management program.

ESSENTIAL NUTRIENTS FOR SWINE

Protein

Traditionally, protein "requirement" is the requirement most people are familiar with when working with swine rations. However, pigs do not have a protein requirement per se; they have a requirement for 10 essential amino acids and a source of nonspecific nitrogen. The 10 essential amino acids that must be present in the diet are lysine, tryptophan, threonine, methionine, isoleucine, phenylalanine, arginine, histidine, leucine, and valine. In swine diets utilizing natural feedstuffs, the amino acids of concern are lysine, tryptophan, and threonine. Nonspecific nitrogen is used in the synthesis of nonessential amino acids and is usually supplied by transamination of excess amino acids in the diet. As a rule of thumb, as long as the requirements for all essential amino acids are met, the requirement for nonspecific nitrogen will also be met.

It is also critical that the essential and nonessential amino acids be present in the diet in a specific ratio for optimum performance. If the ratio of the amino acids is grossly out of line, an imbalance or antagonism could occur. Symptoms of an imbalance or antagonism include a reduction in feed intake and a concomitant decrease in growth. However, minor discrepancies usually do not inhibit performance, so various other feedstuff combinations will work so long as the requirements for the essential amino acids are met.

Because an "ideal protein" with all amino acids present in the correct amounts does not exist, various feedstuffs are mixed together to provide the most economical combination to meet the requirement. Typically, when comparing natural feedstuffs, a corn-soybean meal blend provides an amino acid ratio closest to those of the ideal protein. In fact, corn-soybean meal diets can be formulated on a protein basis. However, when using other feedstuffs, diets should be formulated on a lysine basis, making sure tryptophan, threonine, and all the other essential amino acids are present in adequate amounts for optimum performance.

With the use of commercially available synthetic amino acids, certain feedstuff combinations can supply an amino acid balance closer to the ideal protein concept, diet cost can be lowered by decreasing the amount of protein supplement used, and nitrogen excretion can be reduced. It should be remembered, though, that the pig can utilize only the L-isomer of most amino acids. The exceptions are that DL-methionine can completely replace L-methionine, and dl-tryptophan can replace approximately 85% of the L-tryptophan in a diet. All other amino acids must be present in the L-isomer to be utilized by the pig. At today's prices, lysine is the only synthetic amino acid that is routinely price-competitive. However, in certain diets (e.g., starter pigs) threonine, methionine, and tryptophan have a place.

Because the form of commercially available synthetic lysine is L-lysine hydrochloride, it is only 78% L-lysine. For example, 3 lb of L-lysine HCl provides only 2.34 lb of actual lysine. In corn-soybean meal diets, a general "rule-of-thumb" is that synthetic lysine can decrease percentage protein of a diet by 2% (e.g., 16% down to 14%) without other amino acids becoming limiting. This can be accomplished by replacing 100 lb of 44% protein soybean meal with 3 lb of L-lysine HCl and 97 lb of corn. The decision to make the switch should be based strictly on the cost of 100 lb of soybean meal compared with that of 97 lb of corn and 3 lb of synthetic lysine. However, greater amounts of synthetic lysine can be used if the levels of the other nine essential amino acids are being balanced as well.

Perhaps because protein sources are some of the more expensive components in a swine diet, the most common nutrient deficiency is amino acid. Amino acid deficiencies result in increased feed wastage, reduced growth, general unthriftiness, and, in the case of lactating sows, impaired milk production. At the other extreme, excess amounts of protein cause no ill effects, except perhaps a mild case of diarrhea. However, large excesses of individual amino acids can result in an imbalance, antagonism, or toxic response.

Amino acid and protein requirements throughout the life-cycle of the pig are shown in Tables 1 and 2. These values come from the *South Dakota–Nebraska Swine Nutrition Guide*, and represent the consensus of nutritionists from South Dakota, Nebraska, and seven national feed companies, as well as selected veterinarians and producers. The guide is designed for the top 10% of swine producers, and recommended levels are designed for optimum performance based on available research.

Other factors can also influence the amino acid requirements of pigs. Amino acid requirement is dependent on the type of response criteria measured. It takes higher levels of amino acids to achieve maximum carcass leanness than it does to achieve maximum gains. Another factor is gender effect. Because gilts and boars eat less feed and are leaner, they need higher amino acid concentrations than barrows for lean tissue accretion. This difference has led to the development of split-sex feeding. In this situation, barrows and gilts are sorted into different pens (e.g., rooms, barns) and fed diets containing different protein levels to market weight. This avoids underfeeding the gilts and overfeeding the barrows, which will then result in feed savings and reduced nitrogen excretion. Also, from a management standpoint, it makes it easier to market barrows at a lighter weight, before more fat accretion, and to market gilts at a heavier weight, to take advantage of their leaner carcasses. For sake of ease in sorting hogs, most producers utilizing a split-sex feeding program sort by sex going into the nursery and feed the hogs a common diet until the animals reach 80 lb, at which point they are fed separate diets. Tables 1 and 3 outline an example of a split-sex feeding programs for grow-finish pigs.

Phase feeding is another method to better meet pigs' actual nutritional requirements. Instead of feeding one grower and one finisher diet, it is more sound nutritionally, economically, and environmentally to break those two categories into at least two different diets per period to decrease the amount of time the animal is overfed and underfed. Instead of making a 2% drop in protein from the grower to finisher stage, phase feeding allows for 1% decreases or less, depending on the producer's management abilities. Many producers feed at least ten different diets from weaning to market. Tables 1 and 3 offer examples of four phase-feeding programs for grow-finish pigs.

With the current emphasis on lean animals, a wide range of genetics in the industry is based on lean-growth potential. Because a high lean-gain animal accumulates more protein (muscle) in a shorter period than does an average pig, it is only logical that the lean, rapid-growing–genotype pig has a greater amino acid requirement than does the "average"-genotype pig. Based on that, amino acid requirements are reported in Table 3

Table 1
NUTRIENT RECOMMENDATIONS FOR GROWING SWINE (AS-FED BASIS)*

	Starter 1/ Transition Diet	Starter 2 Diet	Starter 3 Diet	Grower 1 Diet	Grower 2 Diet	Finisher 1 Diet	Finisher 2 Diet
Body weight, lb	8–13	13–25	25–45	45–80	80–130	130–190	190–250
Feed intake, lb/day	.55	1.20	2.0	3.3	4.6	5.8	6.9
Nutrients, % of diet							
Lysine, total	1.55	1.25	1.15	.95	.85	.75	.60
Lysine, digestible	1.32	1.05	.96	.77	.69	.60	.47
Tryptophan	.28	.23	.21	.18	.16	.15	.12
Threonine	.97	.78	.72	.62	.55	.51	.41
Methionine	.42	.34	.31	.26	.23	.20	.16
Methionine + cystine	.78	.63	.58	.52	.47	.45	.36
Calcium	.90	.80	.75	.70	.65	.60	.55
Phosphorus, total	.80	.70	.65	.60	.55	.50	.45
Phosphorus, available	.58	.48	.40	.34	.30	.25	.21
Additions							
Minerals							
Salt, %	0–.4	0–.4	.25–.4	.25–.4	.25–.4	.25–.4	.25–.4
Copper, ppm	6–15	6–15	5–15	4–15	4–15	3–15	3–15
Iodine, ppm	.15–.5	.15–.5	.15–.5	.15–.5	.15–.5	.15–.5	.15–.5
Iron, ppm	100–150	100–150	80–150	60–150	50–150	50–150	50–150
Manganese, ppm	4–30	4–30	3–30	3–30	2–30	2–30	2–30
Selenium, ppm	.3	.3	.3	.3	.3	.3	.3
Zinc, ppm	100–150	100–150	80–150	60–150	50–150	50–150	50–150
Vitamins							
Vitamin A, IU/lb	1000–4000	1000–4000	900–4000	700–4000	700–4000	700–4000	700–4000
Vitamin D_3, IU/lb	100–400	100–400	90–400	70–400	70–400	70–400	70–400
Vitamin E, IU/lb	7.5–30	7.5–30	5–30	5–20	5–20	5–20	5–20
Vitamin K, mg/lb	1–3	1–3	1–3	1–3	1–3	1–3	1–3
Riboflavin, mg/lb	2–10	2–10	2–10	2–10	2–10	2–10	2–10
Niacin, mg/lb	10–50	7–50	6–50	5–50	4–50	4–50	4–50
Pantothenic acid, mg/lb	6–25	5–25	4–25	4–25	4–25	4–25	4–25
Choline, mg/lb	0–100	0–100	0–100	0–100	0–100	0–100	0–100
Biotin, mg/lb	0	0	0	0	0	0	0
Vitamin B_{12}, mg/lb	.01–.02	.01–.02	.01–.02	.005–.02	.005–.02	.005–.02	.005–.02
Folic acid, mg/lb	0	0	0	0	0	0	0

*Ranges for vitamins and minerals represent the lowest and highest levels required to elicit a response. Values within the range will support normal performance.

for the three different genotypes: high lean-gain, average lean-gain, and low lean-gain animals. Low lean-gain animals are defined as those that exhibit less than 0.55 lb of lean gain per day from 45 to 250 lb; medium lean-gain animals, between 0.55 and 0.70 lb lean gain per day; and high lean-gain animals, greater than 0.70 lb of lean gain per day. Based on available research, there appears to be no difference in requirements for the other nutrients, so they should be fed at the levels recommended in Table 1.

The formula to calculate lean-gain values is as follows:

$$\text{Lean gain/day (lb)} = \frac{\text{final lb of lean} - \text{initial lb of lean}}{\text{days on test}}$$

$$\text{Final lb of lean} = (\text{fat-free lean index}/100) \times \text{hot carcass weight}$$

$$\text{Initial lean weight (lb)} = (0.42 \times \text{live weight [lb]}) - 3.65$$

For example, if a group of pigs with an average initial weight of 45 lb was tested for 100 days and had a fat-free lean index (FFLI) of 45% and a hot carcass weight of 180 lb, the lean-gain growth rate would be 0.66 lb of lean gain per day.

$$\frac{([45/100] \times 180) - ([0.42 \times 45] - 3.65)}{100 \text{ days}} =$$

$$\frac{81 \text{ lb lean} - 15.3 \text{ lb lean}}{100 \text{ days}} = 0.66 \text{ lb/day}$$

It is essential to calculate the actual lean-gain potential of an entire group of animals to ensure they are receiving the proper level of amino acids. Feeding higher levels of amino acids or protein will not increase lean gain of an animal unless it has the genetic potential to do it. Feeding high lean-gain levels of amino acids to average lean-gain animals will just result in higher feed costs, no differences in carcass merit, and more nitrogen and phosphorus in the manure.

To be competitive, swine producers need to incorporate split-sex feeding, phase feeding, and genotype-appropriate feeding into their feeding programs.

Minerals

Swine require minerals for skeletal structure and metabolic function. Minerals are classified according to relative need into two groups: macrominerals and microminerals. Macrominerals are required in relatively large amounts, whereas microminerals are required in very small quantities. Commonly, the minerals added to grain-soybean meal–based diets include calcium, phosphorus, sodium, chlorine, iron, zinc, iodine, selenium, copper, and manganese. Traditional feedstuffs usually supply adequate

Table 2
NUTRIENT RECOMMENDATIONS FOR ADULT BREEDING SWINE (AS-FED BASIS)*

	Developing Gilt Diet	Gestation Diet	Lactation Diet				Breeding Boar Diet
	(230 lb to flushing)		21-Day Litter Weight, lb				
			<120		>120		
Feed intake, lb/day	6.0	4.0	10.5	12.0	12.0	14.0	5.5
Nutrients, % of diet							
Lysine, total	.70	.55	.80	.75	.95	.90	.70
Lysine, digestible	.56	.43	.64	.60	.77	.73	.56
Tryptophan	.14	.11	.16	.15	.19	.18	.14
Threonine	.47	.37	.54	.51	.64	.61	.47
Methionine	.19	.15	.22	.20	.26	.24	.19
Methionine + cystine	.42	.33	.48	.45	.57	.54	.42
Calcium	.75	.90	.90	.90	.90	.90	.75
Phosphorus, total	.65	.80	.80	.80	.80	.80	.65
Phosphorus, available	.41	.55	.55	.55	.55	.55	.41
Additions							
Minerals							
Salt, %	.4–6	.4–.6	.4–.6	.4–.6	.4–.6	.4–.6	.4–.6
Copper, ppm	5–15	5–15	5–15	5–15	5–15	5–15	5–15
Iodine, ppm	.15–.5	.15–.5	.15–.5	.15–.5	.15–.5	.15–.5	.15–.5
Iron, ppm	80–150	80–150	80–150	80–150	80–150	80–150	80–150
Manganese, ppm	10–30	10–30	10–30	10–30	10–30	10–30	10–30
Selenium, ppm	.3	.3	.3	.3	.3	.3	.3
Zinc, ppm	80–150	80–150	80–150	80–150	80–150	80–150	80–150
Vitamins							
Vitamin A, IU/lb	2000–5000	2000–5000	2000–5000	2000–5000	2000–5000	2000–5000	2000–5000
Vitamin D_3, IU/lb	200–500	200–500	200–500	200–500	200–500	200–500	200–500
Vitamin E, IU/lb	10–30	10–30	10–30	10–30	10–30	10–30	10–30
Vitamin K, mg/lb	1–3	1–3	1–3	1–3	1–3	1–3	1–3
Ribovlavin, mg/lb	2–10	2–10	2–10	2–10	2–10	2–10	2–10
Niacin, mg/lb	5–50	5–50	5–50	5–50	5–50	5–50	5–50
Pantothenic acid, mg/lb	6–25	6–25	6–25	6–25	6–25	6–25	6–25
Choline, mg/lb	250–500	250–500	250–500	250–500	250–500	250–500	250–500
Biotin, mg/lb	0–.2	0–.2	0–.2	0–.2	0–.2	0–.2	0–.2
Vitamin B_{12}, mg/lb	.007–.02	.007–.02	.007–.02	.007–.02	.007–.02	.007–.02	.007–.02
Folic acid, mg/lb	.25–1.0	.25–1.0	.25–1.0	.25–1.0	.25–1.0	.25–1.0	0–1.0

*Ranges for vitamins and minerals represent the lowest and highest levels required to elicit a response. Values with the range will support normal performance.

amounts of three additional macrominerals: magnesium, potassium, and sulfur. Levels of specific microminerals are sometimes altered in swine feeds in different geographic locations to eliminate a potential imbalance or deficiency. Generally, excess levels of minerals are not recommended, as they can create an imbalance. Dietary mineral levels that support maximum rate of growth and feed efficiency or that are necessary for maintenance and reproduction are shown in Table 1.

Calcium and Phosphorus

Calcium and phosphorus play major roles in bone mineralization and in vital metabolic reactions. Common feedstuffs of plant origin usually contain limited quantities of calcium and little available phosphorus. For example, corn contains only 0.03% calcium and 0.28% phosphorus. Phosphorus from plants is typically bound in phytates, which limits phosphorus bioavailability to 15% to 30%. Dicalcium phosphate, limestone, and bone meal are common feedstuffs used in fortification of swine diets with calcium and/or phosphorus.

The pig's daily need for calcium and phosphorus is fairly well defined. However, excess calcium competes with phosphorus for absorption, creating a need for a balanced ratio of calcium to phosphorus. A calcium-to-phosphorus ratio of 1:1 to 1.5:1 is acceptable for swine in all stages of production. A calcium or phosphorus deficiency, or a deviation from the accepted ratio, results in poor growth, lameness, and bone demineralization. High-milk producing sows frequently exhibit posterior paralysis, or downer sow syndrome, as a result of extensive bone demineralization. Improper dietary levels of calcium, phosphorus, or vitamin D in either gestation or lactation rations is regularly the cause of an increased incidence of posterior paralysis, but frequently a high level of production and physical stress following weaning are equally important in causing the syndrome. Recently, nutritionists have been formulating diets on the basis of available phosphorus instead of total phosphorus. Approximately a third of the phosphorus in grains is in the phytate form and is unavailable to the animal. However, inorganic sources, such as dicalcium phosphate, are readily available. Therefore, when using nontraditional feedstuffs it is a good idea to base the balance on available phosphorus. An acceptable calcium-to-available phosphorus ratio is 2:1. Research has shown that phytases make more of the phytate phosphorus in grains available to the animal, which can reduce the amount of dicalcium phosphate needed in the diet. Currently, it is not economical to feed phytases from the point of view of simply factoring in the cost of dicalcium phosphate. However, because phosphorus levels in manure have the greatest impact on the amount of land needed to utilize the nutrients in manure,

Table 3
NUTRIENT RECOMMENDATIONS (%) OF AMINO ACIDS FOR HIGH, MEDIUM, AND LOW LEAN GAIN SWINE (AS-FED BASIS)

	Grower 1 Diet (45 to 80 lb)		Grower 2 Diet (80 to 130 lb)		Finisher 1 Diet (130 to 190 lb)		Finisher 2 Diet (190 to 250 lb)	
	Barrow	*Gilt*	*Barrow*	*Gilt*	*Barrow*	*Gilt*	*Barrow*	*Gilt*
Feed intake, lb/day	3.3	3.3	4.7	4.5	6.2	5.5	7.2	6.6
High-lean gain*								
Lysine, total	1.00	1.00	.88	.93	.73	.88	.60	.69
Lysine, digestible	.81	.81	.71	.75	.58	.71	.47	.54
Tryptophan	.19	.19	.17	.18	.15	.18	.12	.14
Threonine	.65	.65	.57	.60	.49	.59	.41	.46
Methionine	.27	.27	.24	.25	.20	.24	.16	.19
Methionine + cystine	.55	.55	.48	.51	.44	.53	.36	.41
Medium-lean gain†								
Lysine, total	.95	.95	.83	.87	.69	.83	.56	.64
Lysine, digestible	.77	.77	.67	.71	.55	.67	.44	.50
Tryptophan	.18	.18	.16	.17	.14	.17	.11	.13
Threonine	.61	.61	.54	.57	.47	.56	.38	.43
Methionine	.26	.26	.22	.24	.19	.22	.15	.17
Methionine + cystine	.52	.52	.46	.48	.41	.50	.34	.39
Low-lean gain‡								
Lysine, total	.90	.90	.79	.83	.66	.79	.51	.58
Lysine, digestible	.73	.73	.64	.68	.52	.64	.40	.45
Tryptophan	.17	.17	.15	.16	.13	.16	.10	.12
Threonine	.58	.58	.51	.54	.44	.53	.34	.39
Methionine	.24	.24	.21	.22	.18	.21	.14	.16
Methionine + cystine	.49	.49	.43	.46	.39	.47	.30	.35

*>.70 lb of fat-free lean gain/day from 45 to 250 lb.
†.55 to .70 lb of fat-free lean gain/day from 45 to 250 lb.
‡<.55 lb of fat-free lean gain/day from 45 to 250 lb.

changing political pressures and the ultimate effect on land use may soon make it advantageous to routinely add phytases.

Sodium and Chlorine

Sodium and chlorine are extracellular electrolytes involved in nerve function. Chlorine is also the anion in hydrochloric acid secreted by the stomach. Both minerals are supplied in swine diets as white salt, so the requirement is usually listed as the percentage of salt in the diet. Salt additions are recommended to be 0.25% for pigs in starter, grower, and finisher phases and 0.5% for gestating and lactating sows. Sodium and chlorine deficiency reduces appetite and growth rates in swine. Swine can tolerate up to 2.0% salt provided that they have free access to water. Salt toxicity can result if access to water is limited or if the water contains salt. Symptoms of salt toxicity are nervousness, weakness, staggering, epileptic seizures, and death.

Iron

Iron is required by the body as a component of hemoglobin, myoglobin, and many other metabolic enzymes. Lack of placental transfer of iron does not allow for accumulation of substantial iron stores in the liver of the newborn pig. Also, the iron content of sow milk as lactoferrin is low, which leaves the young suckling pig susceptible to iron-deficiency anemia. Supplemental dietary iron can be supplied through many sources and methods. Sources of dietary iron include ferrous sulfate, ferrous fumarate, ferric chloride, ferric ammonium citrate, and ferric citrate. Swabbing the udder of the dam, providing clean (pathogen-free) dirt in the crate, oral gavage, and supplementing the sow diet while providing the pig access to her fecal material are feasible methods of supplying dietary iron to the young pig.

The most common method of supplying iron is by injection of up to 200 mg of iron dextran, iron dextrin, or gleptoferron. The injection should be made in the neck muscle instead of the ham to prevent paralysis and the staining of a primal cut of pork. Excess iron should not be administered, as unbound serum iron promotes bacterial growth in the blood. Also, a route of excretion of iron is via sloughing of intestinal epithelium, which can also encourage bacterial growth in the gut. Dietary iron levels of 3000 ppm or more are toxic, whereas a single oral dose of 200 mg of ferric ammonium citrate, ferrous sulfate, or ferric oxide can be toxic in the newborn.

Zinc

Zinc is involved either as a component or as an activator of many enzymes and at least two hormones: insulin and estrogen. Swine diets containing grains and plant proteins are low in available zinc and so require supplementation for prevention of a zinc deficiency. The symptoms of a zinc deficiency include parakeratosis, impaired reproductive function, and depressed growth, including growth following correction of the deficiency. The requirement for zinc is elevated by plant phytates, calcium, copper, cadmium, and histidine. The recommended level of zinc for normal growth is 100 to 150 ppm. However, recent research indicates that high levels of zinc (2000 to 4000 ppm) act like an antibiotic in the starter phase. High zinc levels have little effect in any other growth phase, and its effect is not additive with high levels of copper sulfate.

Iodine

Iodine is required as a component of the thyroid hormones. Similar to other minerals, such as iron and selenium, the concentration of iodine in feedstuffs is dependent on geographic location. Low iodine concentrations exist in the soil of the Great Lakes and Northwest regions of the United States. Hypertrophy of the thyroid, commonly called *goiter*, results from low dietary iodine concentrations or from substances in the diet, called *goitrogens*, that lower the availability of iodine. Feedstuffs such as rapeseed, soybeans, and peanuts contain moderately high concentrations of goitrogens. Common sources of iodine are calcium iodate, potassium iodine, and iodized salt. Swine have a high tolerance to iodine, but toxicity can occur at 400 ppm.

Selenium

Selenium is required by swine as a component of the antioxidant enzyme glutathione peroxidase. Therefore, the function of selenium is interrelated with the presence of vitamin E, polyunsaturated fatty acids, and other antioxidants. A deficiency of either vitamin E or selenium in swine diets results in similar deficiency symptoms, including sudden death, liver necrosis, pale skeletal muscle, and a mottled, dystrophic myocardium, frequently with edema and fluid buildup in the pericardial sac. The U.S. Food and Drug Administration approved selenium additions of 0.3 ppm in 1982, but diagnosis of vitamin E–selenium deficiency syndrome has continued to rise (for further discussion, see section below on vitamin E). Regional differences in the selenium content of soils may contribute to incidence of selenium deficiency or to isolated cases of toxicity.

Copper

Copper is required as a component of many enzymes involved in collagen, elastin, and myelin synthesis and for hemoglobin formation. Dietary copper levels of 125 to 250 ppm stimulate growth in starter pigs despite a copper requirement of only 6 ppm. The mechanism of the response has yet to be determined but is probably due to an antibacterial action in the gut. The growth response occurs in addition to the growth-promoting effects of other antimicrobials. Copper toxicity can occur when dietary levels exceed 250 ppm. Signs of toxicity include reduced feed intake, anemia, jaundice, increased serum and liver copper concentrations, and death.

Manganese

Enzymes involved in mucopolysaccharide formation and energy metabolism contain manganese. Consequently, a manganese deficiency can result in varied symptoms, such as slow growth, lameness, impaired reproductive function in adult swine, and ataxia in newborns. A corn-soybean meal–based diet will usually meet the pig's requirement of 10 ppm, although supplementation is still quite common. Manganese toxicity occurs with dietary manganese levels of 1000 ppm.

Vitamins

Vitamins are defined as organic compounds other than carbohydrate, protein, or lipids required by organisms in small quantities for normal growth, maintenance, or reproduction. Vitamins are generally classified according to their solubilities, being either fat or water soluble. The fat-soluble vitamins required by swine are vitamins A, D, E, and K. The water-soluble vitamins are the B-complex vitamins and ascorbic acid (vitamin C). The B vitamins include biotin, choline, folic acid, niacin, pantothenic acid, vitamin B_6, vitamin B_{12}, riboflavin, and thiamine. Generally,

vitamins are required as coenzymes in metabolic reactions. Recent work demonstrates that the reproductive performance of the sow can be improved with additional B vitamins (folic acid, riboflavin, and biotin) and β-carotene injections during gestation by improving the nutrition of the fetus. Generally, swine diets are supplemented with vitamins A, D, E, and K, riboflavin, niacin, pantothenic acid, choline, and vitamin B_{12}. A grain-soybean meal–based diet is considered to contain adequate, available concentrations of the remaining vitamins.

Vitamin A

The functions of vitamin A remain unknown, but lesions in the case of a deficiency suggest that vitamin A plays many diverse roles in the pig. Vitamin A deficiency results in defects in bone growth, resulting in incoordination and paralysis, poor vision due to impaired rhodopsin formation in the eye, keratinization of epithelial tissue resulting in defects in its growth, and maintenance and reproductive failure.

Plants do not contain vitamin A but they do contain its precursor, β-carotene. β-Carotene is oxidized in the presence of heat, moisture, and storage, so vitamin A is supplied in swine diets by an esterified form of retinol (retinyl palmitate or retinyl acetate), for stability in these conditions. The pig readily stores vitamin A in the liver, so vitamin A status is best quantified through determinations of retinol in both plasma and liver tissue. Serum retinol concentrations of less than 10 μg/dL or liver retinol concentrations of 10 μg/g in tissue indicate a deficiency state. High levels of vitamin A supplementation can cause hypervitaminosis A and can impair vitamin E status in the pig.

β-Carotene may play a role in reproduction independent of its conversion to vitamin A. β-Carotene injections have been shown to improve embryonic survival, resulting in larger litter sizes in the gilt and sow.

Vitamin D

Vitamin D functions to maintain calcium and phosphorus homeostasis. Consequently, deficiency symptoms include rickets, bone deformities, lameness, and osteomalacia. Exposure of animal to ultraviolet (UV) radiation converts 7-dehydrocholesterol to cholecalciferol (vitamin D_3) in the skin. Ingestion of ergocalciferol (vitamin D_2), the form that occurs in plants, is another means of supplying vitamin D. Swine diets are supplemented with either vitamin D_2 or vitamin D_3 owing to the limited exposure of the animal to ultraviolet radiation in confinement. In addition to the deficiency symptoms, low serum calcium and high alkaline phosphatase concentrations can be used to support a diagnosis of vitamin D deficiency.

Vitamin D toxicity results from a high level of vitamin D supplementation (33,000 IU/kg of feed). Elevated serum calcium concentrations and calcification of soft tissue are signs of vitamin D toxicity.

Vitamin E

Vitamin E functions as an antioxidant in intracellular membranes to prevent damage that occurs when membrane lipids become peroxidized. Vitamin E supplementation of grain-soybean meal–based diets rarely improves pig performance, although an increased incidence of mulberry heart disease and hepatic necrosis might result from lack of supplementation, presumably from peroxidation of lipids in these tissues. The requirement of vitamin E is independent of selenium, but it is higher with elevation of the level of peroxide in vivo and oxidation in the diet, such as occurs with stress and with ingestion of high levels of polyunsaturated fats and low levels of selenium and other antioxidants.

Vitamin E can be supplemented through injection of D-α-tocopherol or D-α-tocopheryl acetate in an emulsifiable base or by dietary supplementation with an esterified form, D- or DL-α-tocopheryl acetate. Tissue or serum α-tocopherol concentrations are good indicators of vitamin E status. Serum α-tocopherol concentrations less than 0.40 μg/mL or liver concentrations less than 0.80 μg/g of wet tissue may be pathologic evidence of a vitamin E deficiency. Epidemiologic evidence is contradictory concerning the modern condition of mulberry heart disease. This condition may not be a result of vitamin E and/or selenium deficiency.

Vitamin K

Vitamin K is required for normal blood clotting, but the requirement of the pig can be supplied by the concentrations of vitamin K in common feedstuffs. Field cases of a hemorrhagic syndrome associated with the feeding of grains contaminated with mycotoxins have been shown to be responsive to vitamin K supplementation. Bacterial synthesis of vitamin K and subsequent absorption also lower the need for supplemental vitamin K. Menadione is the synthetic form of vitamin K used in supplementation of swine diets.

Biotin

Common feedstuffs contain enough biotin to meet the requirement of the growing pig, but the bioavailability is poor in small grains. General biotin dietary supplementation in diets of gestating sows improves reproductive performance, but no single reproductive parameter has responded consistently to supplementation.

Choline

The choline requirement of the growing pig is supplied in natural feedstuffs. Because choline supplementation in gestating sow diets has been shown to increase the number of pigs born alive, choline is generally added to gestational diets. Signs of choline deficiency in newborn pigs include incoordination, fat infiltration of the liver and kidney, depressed hematocrit, and diminished weight gains.

Niacin (Nicotinic Acid)

The low niacin availability in common feedstuffs and the importance of niacin as a component of the coenzymes nicotinamide adenine dinucleotide (NAD) and NAD phosphate (NADP) mean that diets fed to all classes of swine should be supplemented with niacin. Common deficiency signs include diarrhea, anorexia, dry skin, anemia, and inflammation of the cecum and colon. Excess tryptophan can be converted to niacin at the rate of 50 mg of excess tryptophan to 1 mg of niacin.

Pantothenic Acid

Pantothenic acid is one of the few B vitamins not contained in sufficient quantities in grain-soybean meal–based diets to meet the requirement of the growing pig. A deficiency of pantothenic acid results in an unusual characteristic gait called *goose-stepping*, bloody diarrhea, anorexia, poor growth, and reproductive failure. Pantothenic acid is generally supplemented as either D- or DL-calcium pantothenate. The L-form, which results from the synthesis of the synthetic form of pantothenic acid, is not utilized by the pig, so the racemic mixture (DL-) contains only 0.46 mg of active pantothenic acid per milligram.

Riboflavin

Signs of riboflavin deficiency include poor growth, anorexia, cataracts, light sensitivity, and eye-lens opacities. In addition, riboflavin-deficient sows may resorb fetuses, farrow preterm, or discontinue cycling. Consequently, riboflavin given as a supplement to all classes of swine.

Vitamin B₁₂

The vitamin B_{12} requirement of the growing pig is estimated to be only 19 μg/day. However, the rapid decline in growth and anorexia observed in the case of a deficiency makes vitamin B_{12} a very important part of a balanced swine diet. No clear evidence exists that microbial synthesis and subsequent absorption of vitamin B_{12} will meet the pig's requirement, so supplementation is essential.

Folacin (Folic Acid)

The pig's folacin requirement for growth and maintenance is met by folacin from the feedstuffs and from bacterial synthesis in the hindgut. However, recent research has shown that folic acid supplementation (1.5 g/ton of complete feed) of gestation and lactation diets increases the number of pigs born alive and pigs weaned.

Fatty Acids

Fatty acids are obtained from the hydrolysis of fats and oils and are essential for the production of several hormones. Because pigs cannot synthesize certain fatty acids, such as linoleic and arachidonic acid, they must be provided in the diet. However, because arachidonic acid can be derived in vivo from linoleic acid, only linoleic acid is an essential dietary constituent. The current recommended level of linoleic acid in all swine diets is 0.1%.

Water

Water is probably the most overlooked essential nutrient in swine production. Deprivation of water results in depressed performance and death more rapidly than does a deficiency of any other nutrient. Pigs need approximately 2 to 2.5 lb of water (¼ to ⅓ gallon) for every pound of feed consumed. Water requirements for the various sizes of pigs are given in Table 4. Also, if nipple waterers are being used, the water flow rate for pigs weighing less than 40 lb should be 0.25 gal/minute (1 to 1.5 cups/minute) and 0.5 gal/minute (2 to 3 cups/minute) for pigs weighing more than 40 lb.

Not only must water be provided in adequate amounts for optimum performance, it must also be clean, good-quality water. Table 5 lists the maximum amounts in which various compounds can be present in water without affecting performance. Although little research has shown that water temperature affects the

Table 4
WATER REQUIREMENTS FOR SWINE

Animal Type	Gal/Head/Day
Sow and litter	8
Nursery pig	1
Growing pig	3
Finishing	4
Gestating sow	6
Boar	8

performance of swine, the recommended water temperature is 50 to 55°F.

NONNUTRITIVE FEED ADDITIVES

Nonnutritive feed additives are compounds added to diets in an attempt to enhance gain, feed efficiency, and reproductive efficiency. Commonly used feed additives include antibiotics, probiotics, flavors, organic acids, anthelmintics, copper sulfate, and enzymes. Although some of these compounds do enhance pig performance, not all of them have shown a consistent, positive effect.

Antibiotics, chemotherapeutics, and antibacterials are well-known feed additives that improve performance. These compounds are thought to affect various metabolic processes, nutrient-sparing in the small intestine, and/or suppression of subclinical or nonspecific diseases. Subtherapeutic use of antibiotics began in approximately 1950, and today more than 75% of all hogs receive antibiotics in their feed sometime during their lives.

The reason for the high usage rate of antibiotics is their effectiveness. However, the magnitude of response observed is dependent on several factors. The younger the pig, the greater the growth response observed. Daily gain and feed efficiency of starter pigs are improved by 16% and 6.5%, respectively, whereas for grower-finisher pigs they are improved by only 3.6% and 2.4%, respectively. Also, level of production affects the response because the slowest-gaining pigs show the greatest response when an antibiotic is added to the diet. Environment and health status also affect the magnitude of the response. Pigs housed in a poor environment and/or exposed to a high disease load show the greatest improvement to dietary additions of subtherapeutic levels of antibiotics. Antibiotics not only enhance growth performance, they have also been shown to improve reproductive performance. Conception rate, number of pigs born alive, weaning weights, and survival were increased when antibiotics were added at breeding or during lactation. To be fully effective, antibiotics must be matched against the patho-

Table 5
MAXIMUM AMOUNTS OF IMPURITIES ACCEPTABLE IN WATER

Compound	Maximum Concentration (ppm)
Nitrates	300
Nitrites	100
Sulfates	350
Total dissolved solids	4290
Iron	No limit

gens present on the farm. Also, it is a good idea to review antibiotic usage annually to ensure that they are still effective and economical to add. For further information on feed additives, usage levels, and legal requirements, consult the *Feed Additive Compendium.*

Two newer benefits of antibiotics are currently being researched. Certain antibiotics have been shown to improve carcass merit by either increasing loin eye area or decreasing fat accretion. There is also an indication that some antibiotics may have nitrogen-sparing activities. However, more research needs to be conducted before production recommendations can be made.

High levels of copper sulfate and zinc improve growth performance owing to their antibacterial properties. When copper is added at 125 to 250 ppm or zinc at 2000 ppm in the starter diet (1 to 2 lb addition of copper sulfate), gain and feed efficiency are substantially improved. Much like the response to antibiotics, the response to copper sulfate and zinc is age dependent. Grower pigs exhibit a smaller response than starter pigs, and finishing pigs show little if any response. However, it should be noted that the effects of copper sulfate and zinc are not additive at high levels. One negative factor associated with copper sulfate additions is dirty pens, but that is because copper turns feces black, so pens only appear to be dirty.

Anthelmintics are commonly added to swine diets to combat internal parasites. To get maximum parasite control, the anthelmintic that is used must be matched against the spectrum of parasites present in the operation. Also, the parasite control plan must be followed religiously for continuous control.

The response to probiotics and organic acids has been quite variable. These compounds are mainly used in the starter phase, but the results have been inconsistent. These additives should be used if the response to them can be documented in each individual operation. If not, they are not economical to use.

Enzymes can be effective in increasing the availability of certain nutrients. Phytases make more of the phytate phosphorus available in grains and β-glucanases make more of the energy in barley available. The decision to use either of these enzymes should be dictated by economics. Although the use of phytases can reduce the amount of dicalcium phosphate needed in diets, it still is not of enough benefit to be feasible economically. However, as phosphorus content of manure continues to grow in importance in regard to land application and acreage needed, it is reasonable to assume that phytases will be more commonly used in swine diets in the not-too-distant future. The use of β-glucanases is dependent on the price of barley and corn, and they should be used when appropriate. Most other enzymes have little economic benefit in swine diets.

Flavors have been promoted as being beneficial in swine diets. However, research indicates that they have little, if any, positive effect on pig performance.

LIFE-CYCLE STAGES

Nutrient requirements for the entire life cycle of the pig are listed in Tables 1 and 2. The pig requires specific amounts of nutrients, not percentages of nutrients. The requirements are listed in percentages to assist in ration formulation. However, so long as the pig is consuming at least the expected feed intake given, its nutrient requirements will be met. If the pig is consuming less feed than expected, the diet will not provide adequate levels of the essential nutrients.

There are basically five stages in the life cycle of the pig: starter, grower, finisher, gestation, and lactation (boars are included in the gestational feeding program). Besides meeting the nutrient requirements of the animal, other factors must be taken into consideration to guarantee proper performance. These factors are discussed individually under the appropriate growth phase.

Starter Phase

Starter pig diets are the most expensive and complex diets used in a swine operation. The main problem in this phase is feed consumption. Anything that inhibits feed consumption will adversely affect the young pig. A poor nutritional program in this phase could result in depressed performance for an extended period. Therefore it is critical that the proper nutritional program be used.

With the increased popularity of segregated early weaning (SEW) programs, weaning pigs at 7 to 10 days of age, an increase in *postweaning lag* has been observed. This is not surprising when you compare the pig's diet before and after weaning. Before weaning, the pig receives its feed in 16 equally spaced, highly digestible meals in liquid form. The diet is composed solely of milk products and is 30% protein, 35% fat, and 25% lactose on a dry matter basis. After weaning, the pig receives a low-fat, low-lactose, high-carbohydrate diet composed of grain and soybean meal in dry form. It follows, then, that the young pig does not start eating immediately and that performance is reduced.

To alleviate postweaning lag, researchers at Kansas State University have developed a five-phase feeding program. It is designed to initially provide the weaned pig with nutrients from sources it currently utilizes, such as milk proteins and sugars, and then to gradually switch over to a grain-soybean meal–based diet. The five-phase starter program, which vis dependent on weaning age, is as follows:

Early Weaning (5 to 21 Days)

1. *SEW Diet:* A very nutrient-dense diet (fed to pigs from 5 to 11 lb). Typical ingredients include whey, lactose, plasma, blood meal, fish meal, hi-pro soybean meal, corn, soy oil, lysine, methionine, and an antibiotic. It should be given as 1/8- or 3/32-in. pellets.
2. *Transition Diet:* Slightly less nutrient-dense than the SEW diet (fed to pigs from 11 to 15 lb). This diet contains less whey, plasma, fish meal, soy oil, and methionine, more corn, hi-pro soybean meal, and blood meal, and no lactose.
3. *Phase 2:* 1.25% lysine, whey-corn-soybean meal diet (fed to pigs from 15 to 25 lb).
4. *Phase 3:* 1.10% lysine, grain-soybean meal diet (fed to pigs >25 lb).

Traditional Weaning (>21 Days)

1. *Phase 1:* Intermediate between the SEW and transition diets (fed to pigs <15 lb).
2. *Phase 2:* 1.25% lysine, whey-corn-soybean meal diet (fed to pigs from 15 to 25 lb).
3. *Phase 3:* 1.10% lysine, grain-soybean meal diet (fed to pigs >25 lb).

It is important that only high-quality ingredients be used, especially in the SEW, transition, and phase 1 diets. It does make the diet more expensive, but it represents less than 1% of the feed necessary to get a pig to market weight. Most producers do not have the time or number of pigs necessary to justify manufacturing the SEW, transition, or phase 1 diets on their farms. They need to purchase the pelleted feed that meets the pigs' requirements from a reputable feed company. Phase 2 and

3 diets can and should be manufactured on the farm. For a complete list of nutrient specifications for starter diets, check the *South Dakota/Nebraska* or *Kansas State Swine Nutrition Guides.*

Grower and Finisher Phase

As mentioned in the protein/amino acid section, producers need to utilize phase, genotype-appropriate, and split-sex feeding programs. Phase-feeding programs begin in the nursery, genotype-appropriate programs begin at 45 lb, and split-sex programs begin at 80 lb. The specifics of the programs are described in Tables 1 and 3.

Because pigs at these stages are adjusted to grain-soybean meal–based diets, little has to be done to alter the diets under normal conditions. However, in times of heat and cold stress, dietary manipulations may improve pig performance.

If temperatures remain above 85°F (29.4°C) during both day and night, the grower and finisher pig will be in a heat-stressed condition. One symptom of heat stress is a reduction in feed intake in an attempt to reduce the heat produced during digestion. Because feed intake is depressed, the pig does not receive enough total nutrients on a daily basis to support normal performance. To alleviate the situation, the nutrient density of the diet can be increased. That way, although the pig is consuming less feed, it is still meeting its nutrient requirements. The recommended dietary changes in a heat-stress situation are to increase lysine concentration 0.1% with synthetic lysine and to add 3% fat to the diet.

In a cold-stress situation, the pig has a higher energy requirement owing to the increased energy requirement for maintaining body heat. In general, the pig meets its increased energy requirements by consuming more feed. Although fat is 2.25 times as energy dense as carbohydrates, it should not be added to the diets of cold-stressed pigs because it gives off less heat during digestion, and the cold stress is made even worse. Fiber additions are more practical in cold stress because a great deal of heat is produced during its digestion. However, the increased heat increment is not enough to offset the energy dilution of the diet, so performance stays approximately the same. The decision to increase fiber additions in cold stress should be based on economics, and the fiber content should be reverted to its original volume when the pig is back in a thermal-neutral environment.

Because a pig consumes the most feed during the grower and finisher phases, feed efficiency becomes an economically important factor. Feed processing, as is discussed later, has a tremendous impact on feed efficiency. Fat additions can improve feed efficiency and dust control. Wet feeders also improve performance in the grower and finisher phases, again perhaps through a reduction of dust. However, the use of wet feeders can result in up to a 40% reduction of water in the pit, which can lead to manure removal problems. Wet or wet/dry feeders should not be used in the starter phase owing to the nutrient-diluting action of water.

Lysine level must be adequate in these phases or carcass merit will suffer. If the producer is selling hogs on a carcass-merit basis, a higher lysine level can be fed, as the bonus for the leaner carcass should more than offset the additional cost of increasing lysine level. However, if the producer is marketing on a live-weight basis, there is no economic benefit to feeding higher levels of lysine. Again, the animal must have the genetic potential for higher amino acid levels to be effective.

Females identified as replacement gilts need to be switched to the gestation diet at least by the time they reach 175 lb. Because the gestation diet is higher in minerals and vitamins than the finisher diet, mineral stores, mainly calcium and phosphorus, will increase for later lactations.

GESTATING FEMALES AND BOARS

Nutrient recommendations for sows are shown in Table 2. Feed intake is probably the most important factor for animals in this phase. There is a very strong inverse relationship between gestational and lactation feed intake. Sows eating too much feed in gestation consume less feed in lactation, resulting in lower milk yields, greater loss of body condition, and subsequent reproductive problems. Feed needs to be limited to ensure that the animals do not become obese. This could lead to boars with low libido, increased farrowing problems, more crushing of pigs after farrowing, and a delay in estrus after weaning. However, emaciated animals cannot perform to their full potential either. One recommendation is to feed boars and gestating sows 4 lb of feed/day of a grain-soybean meal mix. This is adequate in a thermal-neutral environment, but if the animals are cold stressed, energy intake needs to be increased. Also, prebreeding condition and genotype affect feed utilization by the sow. Therefore, the best recommendation is to feed sows and boars according to their body condition, with an average to moderate condition being most desirable.

Several methods are available to limit-feed animals. One common method is floor feeding. In floor feeding, the sows receive, on average, the appropriate amount of feed. However, if there are dominant sows or differences in size of animals within the pen, the dominant and larger sows will overeat, whereas the smaller, more docile gilts will get what little feed is left. This results in both overfed and underfed animals in the same pen. The best way to limit-feed is with individual feeding stalls. Feed offered can be controlled on an individual basis, and the producer also has the opportunity to observe each animal every day. This leads to better management. Other alternatives include allowing ad libitum consumption of a high-fiber, low-energy diet or allowing ad libitum consumption of a traditional diet 1 out of every 3 days. The last two methods work well in certain situations but are not recommended as a general rule. Currently, computerized feeding systems are being used in the field, with mixed results. However, as the technologies continue to improve, computerized feeding will become more accepted.

Flushing (increasing energy intake by at least 50% prior to breeding) has been used to increase ovulation rate and, consequently, number of pigs born alive in gilts. However, sows benefit little from flushing. Also, timing of flushing is critical. Increasing feed intake needs to begin 10 to 14 days prebreeding and must stop immediately after mating. If the high plane of nutrition continues after mating, there is an increase in embryonic mortality, and the advantage of flushing is lost. Therefore, flushing only really works in a hand-mating or artificial insemination situation in which the exact breeding date is known and the female is returned to limit-feed. Flushing is not effective in sows or in a pen mating program.

As was previously mentioned, sows that gain too much weight during gestation can have problems in returning to estrus after weaning. This is because the more a sow eats during gestation, the less she will eat during lactation. If the sow is consuming less feed in lactation, body tissue is being catabolized to meet the nutrient requirements for milk production, and she loses a tremendous amount of weight, mostly body fat. This weight loss results in a delay or inability to return to estrus. Therefore, it is essential that gestating animals not be overfed so that subsequent performance is not adversely affected. Gestating gilts and sows should gain 125 and 75 lb, respectively, as a rule of thumb.

LACTATION

The goal in lactation is to maximize feed consumption for milk production and subsequent rebreeding. The addition of high-fiber feedstuffs to prevent constipation decreases energy intake and is not recommended. If constipation is a problem, chemical laxatives, such as potassium chloride or magnesium sulfate, should be added to the diet.

Lactational requirements are dependent on feed intake and level of production (see Table 2). High-producing sows (>120 lb litters on day 21 of lactation) have a higher nutrient requirement than do "conventional" sows, and sows with a lower feed intake require greater percentages of nutrients to meet the nutritional requirements.

Fat additions to increase energy density of the lactation diet have produced mixed results. In herds with a large number of pigs of light birth weight or a preweaning mortality rate greater than 15%, fat additions are beneficial. In those instances, sows should consume a total of 3 lb of fat spread over a period of 7 days before farrowing, and then at least 7% fat should be added to the lactation diet. However, if high mortality and light-weight pigs are not a problem, fat additions to the lactation diet are not economical.

If feed consumption is reduced due to heat stress, drip coolers will increase feed intake. Also, some producers have found that wet feeders enhance feed intake during lactation.

FEED PROCESSING

Even if a diet is properly formulated and nutritionally sound in concept, it must be processed before it reaches the pig. During processing, acceptable diets can become unacceptable. Feed is ground to increase surface area for improved digestion and improved mixing characteristics. The smaller the particle, the better the digestibility and feed efficiency, and the lower the incidence of segregation. However, if feed is ground too fine, problems such as gastric ulcers, increased dustiness, increased grinding costs, and increased feeder management will occur. The standard particle size recommended for all diets is 700 to 800 μm. To obtain this particle size, grind corn through a 3/32-in. screen, and grind all other grains except wheat through an 1/8-in. screen. Wheat needs to be coarsely ground or rolled to avoid turning to paste in the pig's mouth.

Roller mills provide a better grind than do hammer mills. Particle size is more uniform, there is less fines, and less energy is required. The main problem with roller mills is that the rolls must be adjusted for each different grain used. Three key components of successfully grinding feed with a roller mill are (1) a differential drive, with one roll moving 50% to 75% faster than the other roll to produce a shearing action; (2) the correct number of corrugations per inch to slice the grain; and (3) a spiral of 1 to 2 in. per every 12 in. of roller.

Pelleting will improve feed efficiency and decrease dust levels. However, due to the cost of pelleting, it is not usually economical except for nutrient-dense diets or expensive specialty diets.

Portable, on-farm grinder-mixers are responsible for a large number of nutritional wrecks when not used properly. Proper weighing of the feedstuffs presents one problem. Without a scale, it is difficult to add the correct amount of grain or soybean meal. This is especially true when the test weights of the feedstuffs vary. By simply adding an extra 10 bushels of corn to a finishing diet, the protein content is reduced from 14.4% to 13.1%. Also, without a set of scales, the grinder can be overfilled, resulting in a reduction in mixing efficiency. Therefore, scales will greatly reduce the chances of improper mixing.

Probably the most common mistake in on-farm mixing is inadequate mixing time. It is essential that the mixer run at the proper revolutions per minute for at least 15 minutes *after the last* feed ingredient is added. If it is mixed for a shorter time or at a lower number of revolutions per minute, the feed will not be properly mixed and performance could suffer. With a horizontal mixer, the minimum mixing time is 3 to 5 minutes. Also, if the grinder is worn, mixing time needs to be increased. Other common problems include the addition of 5- or 10-lb "add-paks." The smallest addition to a portable mixer should be 40 lb. Amounts less than 2% of the total batch (40 lb/ton) get hung up in augers and do not get mixed properly. Therefore, anything that has an inclusion rate of less than 40 lb/ton needs to be premixed with soybean meal or ground corn.

Sequencing ingredients during mixing is also critical to ensure proper mixing of all ingredients, especially those at a lower level. First, add half of the grain or all the soybean meal. Next, add all of the smaller inclusion-level ingredients. Finally, add the remaining corn or soybean meal, and then mix for the appropriate amount of time.

BIBLIOGRAPHY

Feed Additive Compendium. Minnetonka, Minn, Miller Publishing Co, 1996.

Kansas State University Swine Nutrition Guide. Cooperative Extension Service, Manhattan, Kansas, 1996.

South Dakota–Nebraska Swine Nutrition Guide. Lincoln, Nebraska Cooperative Extension EC 95–273–C ESS38, 1995.

■ Dietary Management in Sheep

F. C. Hinds, M.S., Ph.D.

Although traditional management systems of sheep impose conditions requiring attention be given to dietary concerns, today's intensive systems of production impose much greater stress on the need to properly formulate and manage the diet of sheep. Under traditional systems of management and production, sheep were allowed to graze more or less freely and thus exercise their skill at selective grazing. Often, sheep have been found to consume diets much higher in nutritive value than the average quality of total forage available to them. This results from their ability to selectively consume the more nutritious parts of the available plants. This is not to imply that sheep have "nutritional wisdom"—the ability to properly balance their daily nutrient needs if provided an assortment of feeds. But the sheep's ability to be reasonably selective in choosing what to eat does aid the shepherd in meeting the sheep's needs.

As systems of management have reduced the opportunity for selective intake by sheep, the shepherd must use greater and greater control in dietary management. During the harvesting and processing of feedstuffs, particle size is reduced. Generally, the greater the reduction in particle size, the less selectivity the sheep are able to practice. This physical change in the feedstuff can influence several factors that are discussed later. Also, today's production systems generally emphasize maximum growth rate of market animals, and this introduces diets high in feedgrains and other sources of concentrated nutrients. Diets high in concentrates present a very real challenge to proper dietary management, and to management in general, because the slightest error in judgment or execution can cause the death of a high percentage of the animals receiving a high-concentrate diet. Thus, it can be seen that the degree and skill of dietary management necessary to successfully provide the nutrients for optimal productivity are dependent on the system of management used.

When considering diets for sheep, it is important to realize that physical form, as well as chemical composition and availability, is important. Also, it is important to recognize that the sheep is not a one-component nutritional system. Under most conditions, consumed feedstuff is first exposed to billions of anaerobic bacteria and millions of protozoa. These microorganisms also have nutrient requirements, and because they come in contact with the feedstuffs first, they metabolize and utilize the nutrients to meet their needs. If there is a nutrient deficiency for an individual microbial species, a group of species, or the entire microbial population, their performance (i.e., cellulose degradation) is greatly, or in some cases completely, impaired. Thus, although it may not be realized, the microbial population's nutrient needs must be considered first, and if the nutrient needs of the microorganisms are not met, it is unlikely that the needs of the animal will be met. Although this article does not address rumen microbiology and its interaction with the nutrition of the ruminant, it is important that the reader recognize the very complex symbiotic relationship that exists. The nonmetabolized nutrients from the feedstuff, the byproducts of the anaerobic fermentation, and the microbial tissue per se are the materials that leave the rumen and reach the small intestine and, thus, are the materials available for enzymatic digestion.

In the formulation of diets for sheep it must be recognized that under normal conditions the microbial populations in the reticulorumen are capable of synthesizing sufficient quantities of all of the water-soluble vitamins (B vitamins) in addition to vitamin K. Thus, dietary sources of these vitamins need not be supplied except in unusual situations. Vitamins of importance as dietary additions are vitamin A and vitamin E. Vitamin D is rarely needed if animals have access to solar radiation or feedstuffs that have been irradiated during curing (e.g., sun-cured hay).

The microorganisms in the reticulorumen also synthesize as part of their own tissue all of the essential amino acids. These amino acids are made available to the animal as the result of enzymatic digestion of the synthesized microbial tissue in the abomasum and small intestine. Unfortunately, the quantity of protein synthesized by the microorganisms may not be large enough to meet the needs of rapidly growing lambs or heavy-milking ewes during lactation. Thus diets for these two types of sheep will need to provide sufficient supplementary protein (not nonprotein nitrogen) to ensure that, in addition to the microbial requirements, the animal requirements are met. Because some sources of protein are more readily degraded in the rumen than others, it could be beneficial to use sources of protein that are not readily degraded. Protein sources are often classified as high bypass (not readily degraded in the rumen) or low bypass (readily degraded in the rumen). Examples of high bypass protein sources are corn gluten meal, dried brewer's grains, blood meal, and fish meal. Soybean meal and cottonseed meal are normally considered low bypass protein sources. Care must be taken not to provide too high a level of high bypass protein and thus not provide enough rumen degradable protein to meet microbial needs. Approximately 40% to 50% rumen-degradable protein should be sufficient to satisfy microbial needs.

Much of the energy made available to the animal is the result of the fermentation that occurs in the reticulorumen and is provided in the form of volatile fatty acids (largely acetic, propionic, and butyric acids) that are in large part absorbed from the four stomach compartments. Generally, 50% or more of the energy available to the animal from feedstuffs consumed is in the form of volatile fatty acids. Because acetic and butyric acids are ketogenic, and only propionic acid is glucogenic, animals with a high demand for glucose (late gestation and peak lactation) need special consideration in satisfying their demand for glucose.

With the foregoing as a general background, the following is a more specific discussion of the life-cycle dietary management of sheep.

DIETARY MANAGEMENT OF LAMBS

Nutrient Needs

The newborn arrives with very little nutrient reserve except for small amounts of fat (energy) and protein (energy and amino acids) and must be provided with a highly concentrated source of nutrients. Normal colostrum contains large quantities of vitamins A and E as well as fats and protein. Thus, colostrum is not only vital from an immunologic point of view, it also provides the newborn lamb with essential nutrients. The need for lambs to receive colostrum is so important that special attention should be paid to the newborn in litters of three or more lambs. Because the leading cause of death in newborn lambs is starvation and resulting dehydration and hypothermia, it is important to make certain that all lambs have ample opportunity to nurse, especially within the first few hours following birth.

Vitamin A deficiencies in neonatal lambs are rare, but apparent vitamin E deficiencies (stiff limb disease or white muscle disease) are not uncommon. Milk-fed lambs are generally more susceptible to vitamin E deficiencies than are older lambs that have been weaned to dry feed, because vitamin E functions in the body as an antioxidant and helps to prevent peroxide formation in tissues as a result of the oxidation of (unsaturated) fats. Lambs consuming milk from the ewe receive more than 50% of their dietary energy in the form of fat in milk. This is a very high level of fat, and thus there is a need for high levels of vitamin E to prevent peroxide formation in tissues. As the lamb's digestive tract matures as a result of eating dry feed, and its reticulorumen begins to function like that of a "mature ruminant," two things reduce the stress on dietary vitamin E. First, the dry feed consumed will contain far less fat (3% to 5%); second, the microorganisms in the reticulorumen attack dietary fat and saturate it, thus removing the double bonds in the unsaturated fat that tend to readily form peroxides in the animal's tissues. As lambs begin to eat dry feed and begin to gain maximally, it is not uncommon to find the lambs that gain best show vitamin E–deficiency symptoms, such as stiff limbs and even heart failure during exercise. This situation likely represents the case in which a rapidly growing lamb simply outgrows its dietary supply of vitamin E and succumbs to the deficiency. Slow-growing lambs show the symptoms less often.

Not all vitamin E deficiencies are straightforward. Selenium is an essential element required in the protein that transports vitamin E in blood. Thus, any time that selenium is deficient, the gross symptoms will include those of vitamin E deficiency. Selenium deficiencies are fairly common and occur in areas with highly leached soils. The occurrence in affected geographic areas is generally well known, and preventive programs have been developed. Borderline areas exist in which selenium levels of feedstuffs are almost deficient, and in these areas (e.g., the Great Lakes states) symptoms of deficiencies are less frequent than in heavily affected geographic areas and are localized to one or several production units. Generally, deficiencies are related to specific soil conditions that reduce accumulation of selenium in plants and/or to the use of low-quality feed ingredients, e.g., hay and grain damaged in storage or stored for several years. Also, as in the case of vitamin E, rapidly growing lambs are more likely to have a problem than slow-growing lambs.

Treatment is best handled for the milk-fed lamb as an intramuscular (IM) injectable containing both vitamin E and selenium. Repeated treatments may be necessary. Lambs on dry feed can be treated initially using injectable products containing both vitamin E and selenium, but they must also receive a diet containing added vitamin E and selenium to prevent further occurrence of the problem. Whether the problem is only vitamin E or selenium deficiency can best be determined by using two different therapies on several animals—one consisting of only vitamin E and the other of both vitamin E and selenium—and by differential response, the cause of the deficiency is apparent.

Another dietary problem that may become more common is an iron deficiency in lambs younger than 1 month. This will occur most exclusively in confinement and especially where strict sanitation is practiced. Newborn lambs, like newborn piglets, obtain their iron as *contaminant iron* on their mother's udder. Within the first 21 to 28 days life, fetal red blood cells are replaced by adult red blood cells, and unless sufficient iron is available for synthesis of the adult cells, anemia results. Once lambs begin to consume dry feed (creep feed or eating with the ewes), iron nutrition is no longer a problem, but milk is a very poor source of iron. Again, the most rapidly gaining lambs will experience deficiencies and show gross symptoms of pneumonia (thumps). Closer observation will reveal anemia (pale vascular beds around the eyes similar to those found in older sheep with nematode infections). Serologic evaluation reveals very low hematocrit and hemoglobin levels. Treatment is best handled using injectable iron dextran similar to that used for baby pigs. One injection at 1 or 2 days of age will prevent occurrence. If a deficiency is encountered in lambs 21 to 28 days old, it is essential that iron be provided immediately, and this should be from the injectable source previously mentioned. In addition, care must be taken to reduce stress, especially that associated with exercise, environment, and disease, which may increase the oxygen needs of the animal. Some lambs may recover spontaneously, but it is likely that performance will have been reduced.

Although not a common practice, it is not unusual to find lambs being weaned from their dams at 24 or so hours of age and reared artificially. This will likely become more common as reproductive rates in ewes continue to increase and more intensive management is used. Several nutrition considerations are very important. The milk replacer used should be designed for lambs because of the high levels and quality of fat and protein used in formulation. Using dairy calf replacers will not allow for maximum performance because of low levels and quality of fat and protein. The management of the feeding program requires that the lamb receive colostrum, and following weaning it must be trained to use a nipple and the milk-dispensing system of choice. Untrained lambs should not be mixed with older trained lambs during the training period. The milk replacer should be fed cold (refrigerated) to avoid overconsumption and to reduce the rate of spoilage. A small amount (1.0 mL per 4 L of milk replacer) of formaldehyde can be added to milk replacer to further réduce the rate of spoilage. Once lambs are readily consuming milk replacer, provide them with a highly palatable preweaning feed. The preweaning feed can be specially formulated to meet all of the young lamb's needs, and it should contain about 90% concentrate and at least 20% crude protein, all from intact protein. A baby pig preweaning feed can be used instead of a special diet. It is also advisable to place a flake of high-quality alfalfa hay in the pen, because some lambs prefer to pick at roughage. The goal is to start lambs eating dry feed as early in life as possible, and thus to hasten rumen development in preparation for weaning. Lambs are best abruptly weaned from milk replacer once they are eating dry feed (no earlier than 24 days and generally at 28 to 35 days of age). On weaning, the lambs may experience a setback or check in growth, but by market weight, no difference in overall performance will be evident. Once the lambs are weaned, they should be maintained on a high-concentrate (80% to 90%) diet high in crude protein (20% to 25%) until they weigh 18 to 23 kg, at which time the protein level can be reduced to 15% to 17%. From this point, they are handled as any other weaned lamb.

Caution should be used in meeting a lamb's nutrient needs if an appropriate milk replacer is not available. Augmentation of cow's milk with table sugar or ingredients other than glucose or lactose may cause severe digestive upsets. The newborn lamb is equipped with digestive enzymes capable of degrading products commonly found only in milk, and carbohydrates other than glucose and lactose are not digestible until at least 3 weeks after birth. At that time, the lamb's digestive tract experiences a major change to the production of "adult enzymes." After this time, many oligosaccharides can be degraded by the enzymes produced in the abomasum, pancreas, and small intestine. Sucrose (table sugar), although readily fermented in the reticulorumen, cannot be digested by even "adult" enzymes in the small intestine, and is only useful to a lamb with an active fermentation in its reticulorumen.

The stomach of the newborn lamb must undergo major changes before it is able to assume adult function. The largest of the four compartments at birth is the abomasum. The development of "normal" compartment volumes (relative and absolute) and metabolic maturity of the tissues, as well as musculature of the compartments, are dependent on the consumption of dry feed and the presence of active fermentation. Early in life, lambs learn to eat from their mothers, and although the amounts of food are relatively small, they may start to eat dry feed as early as several days of age. During normal grooming of the lamb by the ewe and the lamb's consuming feed previously mouthed by adult sheep, the young lamb's reticulorumen is inoculated with the necessary microorganisms to establish "normal" fermentation. Once the lamb starts consuming dry feed and receives its inoculum, its stomach starts undergoing a major change that culminates in the rumen becoming by far the largest compartment. From a nutritional point of view, the lamb that is raised with access to dry feed will be essentially nonruminant in its nutrient needs (i.e., intact protein, B vitamins, and relatively simple energy sources) from birth to 3 weeks of age. From 3 to 8 weeks of age the lamb is in transition between its previous nonruminant and future ruminant states, and it must still be considered to be a nonruminant. After 8 weeks of age, lambs that have had access to dry feed have a sufficiently well-developed reticulorumen and omasum to be considered functional ruminants.

More common is the practice of rearing lambs on their dams and weaning them early, at 42 to 90 days of age. Although some sheepmen may wean lambs as early as 28 days of age, the more common age is 50 to 70 days. Because the lambs will be weaned onto dry feed at an early age, it is essential that a creep diet be provided. This diet should be available to lambs within the first week to 10 days of life. Because lambs generally learn to eat with the ewes, the best physical form for the diet (e.g., whole, ground, pelleted) will depend on what the ewes receive. Most research on creep diet composition indicates that it should be high in available energy (concentrates) but that it need not be high in protein or other nutrients. Apparently these other nutrients are not as limiting as energy; however, once the lambs are weaned, the level of crude protein must be 16% to 17% for optimum performance. Nonprotein nitrogen (urea, ammonium salts, and other sources) should not be substituted for intact protein until the lambs are within 3 to 4 weeks of market weight and finish. If urea is used, it should not make up more than 1% of the diet or one third of the total dietary crude protein or more than half of the supplemental crude protein. Once early-weaned lambs have gained two thirds of the weight from weaning to market weight, the crude protein level can be reduced to 14% to 15% of the diet, and during the last 3 to 4 weeks of finishing, 12% to 13% crude protein is adequate.

The available energy level of diets for early-weaned lambs must be high to ensure optimum performance. Although all-concentrate diets can be fed, slightly greater gains will be obtained if 10% ground forage is included in the diet. As much as 25% ground forage can be included in diets without a marked reduction in gain; however, levels of forage greater than 25%

will reduce gains. Diets high in available energy are especially important for lambs close to market weight and finish. Early-weaned lambs should be vaccinated against enterotoxemia (type D), although with proper management, losses to this disease should be minimized. From both labor and nutritional points of view, self-feeding a complete diet should be recommended. Clean water must be available at all times, and environmental stresses should be minimized.

Mineral Needs

The mineral nutrition of early-weaned lambs must be carefully controlled. Urinary calculi in males may occur because of excesses of several mineral elements. Most common in lambs fed high-concentrate diets are phosphatic calculi. Generally, a calcium-to-phosphorus ratio of 2:1 or greater will prevent the occurrence of urinary calculi. If this does not prevent calculi, the addition of ammonium chloride as 0.5% of the diet will give good results. Ammonium sulfate has been used to replace ammonium chloride, but results generally favor use of the latter. If the foregoing efforts do not prevent calculi, chemical analysis of the calculi per se as well as the feed and water should provide valuable information as to the type of calculi causing the problem.

Selenium, as mentioned previously, must be provided in adequate amounts to ensure optimal availability and use of vitamin E. In areas known to be selenium-deficient, mineral mixtures containing selenium should be added to all diets. It is not recommended that individual producers prepare their own selenium supplements. Selenium is very toxic, and small mixing errors could cause high death losses.

Although high dietary copper levels may not always cause a toxicity in market lambs, the improper supplementation of copper may ultimately cause death losses if ewes or rams are retained and used as replacements. Sheep are especially efficient at retaining absorbed copper and storing large quantities in their liver. Once copper in liver reaches "critical" levels, the liver releases the copper and a hemolytic crisis occurs, resulting in hemolysis. Few sheep survive the hemolytic crisis. In most cases, copper toxicity occurs because of the overfeeding of copper. Most commonly, trace mineral salt mixtures are fed free choice, or the trace mineral mixtures (fed free choice or mixed in complete diets) that are used have been developed for swine or poultry diets and may contain four or more times as much copper as in mixtures developed for use in sheep diets. Copper levels of finished diets should not exceed 7 to 11 ppm.

In addition to overfeeding copper, too-low levels of molybdenum and sulfate ion can cause normal copper levels to elicit a toxicity. Molybdenum can be used at low levels to increase the mobilization of copper from the liver, thus serving a therapeutic function. It should be emphasized that although molybdenum increases the rate of copper mobilization from the liver, the rate of reduction is relatively slow; thus, if molybdenum is used once copper toxicity is a problem, it does not rapidly reduce liver levels, and losses subsequent to therapy are not uncommon. If a toxic response is encountered or suspected, it is important to minimize stress and exercise, because sheep not experiencing a hemolytic crisis are very likely have elevated liver copper levels, which could force a crisis or exacerbate an existing one.

DIETARY MANAGEMENT OF WEANED LAMBS

If early-weaned lambs are to be retained as replacements, it is essential that growth, and not fattening, be encouraged. Ewe lambs should be removed from the fattening pen prior to reaching market weight and finish and placed on a diet containing half good-quality forage and half concentrate. Crude protein levels should be 12% to 13% of the diet. Ewes gaining about 0.10 kg/day, if past puberty, will have the highest productivity. Both high and low levels of available energy prebreeding reduce reproductive performance.

Ram lambs kept as replacements can be fed diets containing 25% roughage and 75% concentrate until such time as their growth starts to slow down, at which time diets containing 50% to 60% roughage should be fed. Again, overfeeding and underfeeding both may influence a ram's reproductive performance. Dietary crude protein levels should be 14% to 15% until growth slows, at which time 12% to 13% should be adequate. Again, copper nutrition as well as the phosphorus-to-calcium ratio must be watched, or valuable animals may be lost.

Conventionally reared lambs produced in the farm flock states may or may not receive creep feed while on pasture with the ewes. If creep is provided, it should be high concentrate and reasonably high (15%) in crude protein. Often, lambs are weaned once pasture becomes limiting, when the ewes need to be prepared for rebreeding, or when the lambs are ready for market. If not sent to market, or if sold to a feeder, such lambs are termed *feeder lambs*. Dietary management for feeder lambs is, contrary to many people's beliefs, rather similar to that for early-weaned lambs of comparable size. Levels of dietary roughage and protein should be similar to those for early-weaned lambs of similar size. In cases in which lambs have not received creep feed or feed other than pasture prior to weaning, it is essential to gradually introduce prepared feed to the lambs. Often hay is first fed on the ground and then in bunks, and finally small amounts of grain are introduced.

Caution must be used in changing levels and types of feeds, especially when introducing animals to new feeds. Both the animal and its digestive tract must adjust to dietary changes. All animals must have ready access to feed if hand-feeding is practiced. If not, dominant animals may overconsume and may experience lactic acidosis. Also, changes in level of concentrate, if elevated too abruptly, can cause many lambs to experience lactic acidosis. Changes should be gradual, allowing 2 to 3 days at any new level of grain feeding before further changes are made. The amount of change should be on the order of 0.23 kg of grain per period of change. Large amounts may cause problems. Dietary management is the key to prevention of lactic acidosis. Most lambs will experience slight digestive upsets, often caused by lactic acidosis, that result in a small depression in appetite and mild diarrhea. Often lamb feeders prefer to feed higher levels of roughage to reduce problems of enterotoxemia and lactic acidosis. The higher the level of concentrate in the diet, the greater the importance of proper dietary management.

Patience is required while introducing range lambs to fences, prepared feed, and tank water. Although preconditioning of lambs going to feedlots would be very helpful, this is not widely practiced; thus, problems arising from insufficient water and feed intake may be common. If dietary changes are made too abruptly, the time required for readaptation of the lambs to the feed will be greatly extended, because not only is time lost during which the animal is "off-feed," but the lamb will start over in increasing and adjusting its intake.

The adaptation of the microorganisms to specific feedstuffs is much like the animal's adjustment. Too-rapid change causes rapid growth of specific types of microorganisms, creating conditions that are inhibiting to the growth of other organisms essential in maintaining normality within the reticulorumen. Usually 8 to 10 days are required for the microorganisms to completely adjust to a major change (introduction of grain) in feedstuff. As with the animal, a gradual change will assist the microbial population in adjustment without major problems.

DIETARY MANAGEMENT OF ADULT SHEEP

Adult sheep moving from one productive function to another require the same care and attention in dietary management as lambs. Prior to the breeding season the ewe has a fairly low energy and crude protein requirement. Care must be taken on many native forages not to allow ewes to become too fat. As explained in discussing ewe lamb replacements, ewes that are too fat or too thin will not reproduce optimally. Stocking rate and grazing time both can be modified to influence ewe condition. Thin ewes must be carefully evaluated to be certain their condition is related to plane of nutrition and not to parasite load. The influence of parasites cannot be eliminated with adequate nutrients; one cannot feed around parasites.

Breeding

As the breeding season approaches, some sort of flushing program is valuable. Two to 3 weeks prior to turning the rams with the ewes, the ewes should either receive 0.23 or 0.34 kg of grain per head per day or be placed on fresh highly nutritious pasture that has been saved for flushing. Recent research indicates a 30% crude protein (no nonprotein nitrogen) fed at .23 kg/head/day is superior to .23 kg of corn per head per day as a supplement for flushing. Specific types of pastures in specific areas are notorious for causing breeding problems. In Ohio it is not uncommon to find ladino clover, Dutch White clover, and birdsfoot trefoil reducing early season conception rates of ewes. Elsewhere, alfalfa, birdsfoot trefoil, ladino clover, and Dutch white clover, among other legumes, have been known to cause reduced reproductive performance, largely because of estrogenic materials associated with the plant. The practice of flushing causes an increase in number of eggs ovulated per ewe. As the breeding season progresses and natural levels of ovulation increase, the response to flushing decreases. Flushing is not as effective late in the breeding season as early. Flushing (improved plane of nutrition) should continue through the first heat cycle for maximum benefit. Ewes in fat condition do not respond to the same degree as do ewes in average to thin condition.

During the first two thirds of gestation, ewes need to be in average condition and need not gain weight unless they are thin. Their nutrient requirements are low (the same as those for dry ewes). However, during the last third of gestation the available energy in the diet needs to be increased to the equivalent of 0.23 to 0.45 kg of grain per head per day. This is because of the rapid growth of fetal tissues and the concomitant increased demand for energy, largely glucose. In addition to the demand of the fetal tissues, the volume occupied by the fetal tissues in the peritoneal cavity reduces the capacity of the stomach, which makes it impossible for the ewe to compensate for the increased nutrient demand by increasing feed intake if only roughage is fed. If the available energy level in the diet is not increased, ewes carrying two or more lambs may develop ketosis or pregnancy disease. Ketosis is more likely to occur in fat than in thin ewes. Therapy is discussed elsewhere, but needless to say, unless attended, the lambs, and often the ewe, die. Prevention through proper dietary management is by far the most effective treatment, as therapy is often not always successful.

At lambing, it is important not to overfeed ewes. For the first 5 to 7 days, do not increase grain over that fed during late gestation. After that period, ewes with single lambs should be grouped separately from ewes with twin lambs. Separation of ewe and lamb pairs from singles will permit more effective feeding of both types of ewes. Ewes with twins may produce as much as 40% more milk than ewes with singles, and thus need more dietary crude protein and available energy. Large, heavy-milking ewes with twins may need as much as 1.1 to 1.4 kg of grain per day in addition to all of the high-quality hay they can eat. Ewes with single lambs should be fed from 0.7 to 0.9 kg of grain per day.

If lambs are going to be weaned early, the ewes must be properly dried up to reduce the occurrence of mastitis. One week prior to weaning the lambs, all of the grain should be removed from the ewe's daily ration. One day prior to weaning, all feed and water should be removed, and a day after weaning, only water should be allowed. Three to 4 days following weaning, provide some low-quality roughage (not pasture) and gradually increase to normal feed. This should dry up ewes with little trouble from mastitis. One further caution: do not milk ewes once the lambs have been removed; this will only further complicate matters.

OTHER DIETARY CONCERNS

Not all concerns related to dietary management are associated with the chemical composition of feedstuffs. Physical form of the diet—long hay, chopped hay, ground hay, or pelleted hay, and similar descriptions for grains—has a major influence on animal performance and behavior. From the animal's point of view, two factors are important. First, lambs and older sheep self-fed or hand-fed ground diets or feedstuffs (e.g., hay) often cough as a result of the dustiness of the diet. Although coughing is not good for any type of sheep, it is often found to be a serious problem with lambs just prior to reaching market weight and condition. Coughing, and thus dustiness of the diet, is closely linked to rectal prolapse, especially in lambs confined to feedlots. Rapidly growing lambs consume large quantities of feed, and as they consume feed their respiratory system is often irritated by the dustiness of the feed, and they cough. These coughs are often violent and prolonged. This entire situation puts undue stress on the anal sphincter and often causes eversions of the rectum. Unless attended to immediately, rectal prolapses will cause a sharp drop in lamb performance. Although much of the stimulus for prolapse is dietary and possibly environmental, there is clear evidence that a tendency to suffer prolapse can be genetic. Thus, any offspring or relatives of a sheep with prolapse should be carefully considered as candidates for culling.

The second problem with the physical form of diets is small particle size. Sheep, during their evolution, have developed the process of regurgitation and rumination into a highly efficient and important process of reducing particle size of fibrous materials found in the reticulorumen. From 8 to 12 hours/day may be spent ruminating. When man, through chopping and grinding, reduces the particle size of feedstuffs to a very small size, sheep are unable to regurgitate, and therefore do not ruminate. Because large amounts of time are normally spent ruminating, a sheep that receives feeds of small particle size that preclude rumination has much idle time, during which vices develop, such as wool-picking, cribbing, and metal polishing. Wool-picking represents the most serious of the vices because it may seriously decrease the performance of several sheep within the group. This vice is thought to occur through inquisitiveness expressed as a picking at particles on fleeces of penmates. Eventually and accidentally, wool, as well as feed particles in the fleece, is plucked by the picking sheep. Picking is not an act of aggression nor is it considered to be associated with mineral, vitamin, or protein deficiencies or imbalances. It occurs in all ages and classes of sheep once dry feed is consumed. It is of greatest concern in adult ewes, especially during the winter, when a denuded sheep may not be able to survive the ensuing environmental stress. The proper treatment includes isolation of the picked sheep and an increase in both the fiber level and particle size of the diet to allow normal regurgitation and rumination.

Metabolic Diseases

Consulting Editor
Thomas H. Herdt, D.V.M., M.S., Diplomate, A.C.V.N. and A.C.V.I.M.

■ Milk Fever (Parturient Paresis) in Cows, Ewes, and Doe Goats*

Garrett R. Oetzel, D.V.M., M.S.
Jesse P. Goff, D.V.M., Ph.D.

Milk fever (parturient paresis, hypocalcemia, paresis puerperalis, parturient apoplexy) is a nonfebrile disease of adult dairy cows, beef cows, ewes, and doe goats, in which acute calcium deficiency causes progressive neuromuscular dysfunction with flaccid paralysis, circulatory collapse, and depression of consciousness. Hypocalcemia in sheep and goats causes varying combinations of tetany and/or flaccid paralysis.

OCCURRENCE

Milk fever is one of the most common metabolic diseases of dairy cattle. About 6% of U.S. dairy cattle are affected annually. Annual incidence rate of clinical milk fever within herds may vary from 2% to 60%.

Approximately 75% of all cases of milk fever in dairy cattle occur within 24 hours of calving. An additional 12% occur 24 to 48 hours after calving. Some cases (about 6%) occur at the time of delivery and cause dystocia because hypocalcemia inhibits uterine contractility. Cases of hypocalcemia that do not occur in association with calving are termed *nonparturient hypocalcemia* rather than milk fever.

Subclinical hypocalcemia (depressed blood calcium concentrations but without clinical signs) affects about 50% of all adult dairy cattle. Subclinical hypocalcemia may lead to decreased dry matter intake after calving, increased risk of secondary disease conditions, decreased milk production, and decreased fertility later in lactation (Fig. 1). Therefore, efforts to improve calcium metabolism in fresh cows may have payoffs even in herds without clinical milk fever problems.

Breed, age, and milk production level are important risk factors for milk fever in dairy cattle. Jerseys and Guernseys are the most susceptible to milk fever; Holsteins and Brown Swiss are moderately susceptible; and Ayrshires and Milking Shorthorns are the least susceptible.

The incidence of milk fever generally increases with parity and with higher levels of milk production, regardless of breed. First-lactation dairy cattle almost never develop milk fever.

Hypocalcemia is quite rare in beef cattle, probably due to their much lower milk production per unit of body weight compared to that in dairy cattle. Milk fever incidence is also lower in sheep than in dairy cattle; however, it is possible for outbreaks of milk fever in pregnant ewes to affect up to 30% of a flock. High-producing doe goats have a similar incidence of milk fever as do dairy cattle.

*All of the material in this article is in the public domain, with the exception of any borrowed figures and tables.

ETIOLOGY AND PATHOGENESIS

Milk fever is caused by hypocalcemia that occurs as an animal's complex mechanism for maintaining calcium homeostasis fails during a sudden and severe calcium outflow. Sudden calcium outflow occurs most commonly at the time of the initiation of lactation. The calcium demand associated with colostrum production in dairy cows and dairy goats exceeds the total prepartum calcium requirements, including those associated with mineralization of the fetal skeleton.

In beef cows, ewes, and doe goats not challenged for milk production, the colostral demand for calcium is generally less than calcium demanded by the fetal skeleton. Thus, these animals are at greatest risk for primary hypocalcemia in late gestation. Dry matter intake (and thus calcium intake) decreases as parturition approaches, which compounds the challenge to calcium homeostasis. These factors are multiplied for ewes or does carrying two or more fetuses.

An animal's ability to adapt to hypocalcemia is influenced by a number of factors. An important determinant of milk fever risk is the acid-base status of the animal at the time of parturition. Metabolic alkalosis appears to alter the physiologic activity of parathyroid hormone (PTH) so that bone resorption and production of 1,25-dihydroxycholecalciferol (1,25-[OH]$_2$D) are impaired, thus reducing the animal's ability to successfully adjust to increased calcium demands.

Magnesium status is another factor influencing an animal's

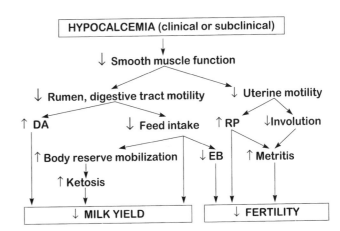

Figure 1
Early postpartum hypocalcemic cascade of events leading to decreased milk yield and fertility. DA, displaced abomasum; RP, retained placenta; EB, energy balance. (Adapted from Beede DK: Macromineral element nutrition for the transition cow: Practical implications and strategies. Proceedings of the Tri-State Dairy Nutrition Conference, Ohio State, Michigan State, and Purdue Cooperative Extension Services, Columbus, 1995, p 185.)

risk of hypocalcemia. Low blood magnesium levels can reduce PTH secretion from the parathyroid glands and can also alter the responsiveness of tissues to PTH. High dietary potassium reduces ruminal magnesium absorption. The effects of magnesium on calcium homeostasis are discussed further in this section under hypomagnesemic disorders. Excessive dietary phosphorus (>80 g/day) during late gestation is an additional risk factor for milk fever. When blood phosphorus concentration is in the range of 8 mg/dL, renal synthesis of 1,25-(OH)$_2$D is inhibited. Hypocalcemia may also be influenced by estrogen, which is a potent inhibitor of osteoclastic activity. Blood estrogen concentrations rise dramatically at the end of gestation and may blunt the effects of PTH on bone resorption.

CLINICAL PRESENTATION

The clinical effects of hypocalcemia in all species of livestock are broad, because calcium serves many critical physiologic functions. Calcium is required for release of the neurotransmitter acetylcholine, which mediates transmission of nerve impulses at the myoneural junction. Lack of acetylcholine release is the likely cause of flaccid paralysis in milk fever. In addition, hypocalcemia inhibits contractility of smooth and cardiac muscle, causing a variety of additional clinical signs in affected animals.

Some hypocalcemic animals show signs of hyperesthesia and tetany, especially during the early phase of hypocalcemia. This occurs because calcium affects membrane stability in peripheral nerves and muscle fibers. Hypocalcemia may initially speed impulse conduction or even allow spontaneous impulse production in peripheral nerves and muscle fibers. Animals initially affected with hyperesthesia and tetany often later lapse into flaccid paralysis as the hypocalcemia worsens and neuromuscular junctions become blocked. Tetany is generally more pronounced in sheep and goats affected with hypocalcemia than in cattle.

Whether tetany or flaccid paralysis is seen also depends on the relative activity of magnesium and calcium. Magnesium competitively inhibits calcium at the myoneural junction. High magnesium concentration at the junction prevents calcium from stimulating acetylcholine release and promotes flaccid paralysis. Low magnesium at the junction removes the calcium inhibition and promotes tetany, so long as the hypocalcemia is not severe.

Dairy Cattle

Clinical signs of milk fever in dairy cattle may be divided for convenience into three nondiscrete stages. Stage I milk fever is characterized by mild excitement and tetany without recumbency. Dairy cattle with stage I milk fever are typically excitable, nervous, hypersensitive, anorectic, and weak. They may shift their weight frequently and shuffle their hind feet. Physical examination during stage I milk fever often reveals tachycardia and slight hyperthermia due to increased muscular activity.

Stage II milk fever in dairy cattle is characterized by sternal recumbency due to flaccid paralysis. In contrast to the hypersensitivity and tetany of stage I, affected cows in stage II are depressed and paralyzed. The cow in stage II milk fever may also exhibit fine muscle tremors, particularly in the triceps muscles. Physical examination during stage II usually reveals rapid heart rate and decreased intensity of heart sounds due to reduced cardiac muscle contractility. Peripheral blood perfusion is poor, and the extremities of affected cows feel cold on palpation. Affected cows usually have lowered rectal temperature (35.6 to 37.8°C or 96 to 100°F), but the extent to which this occurs depends on ambient temperature. Impaired smooth muscle function due to hypocalcemia leads to clinical signs such as gastrointestinal atony, mild bloat, constipation, and loss of the

anal reflex. Pupils may be dilated and unresponsive to light owing to atony of the dilator pupillae muscle. Clinical signs of stage II generally last from 1 to 12 hours.

Dairy cows in stage III milk fever are laterally recumbent and progressively lose consciousness to the point of coma. They are often severely bloated at this stage as a result of lateral recumbency combined with profound gastrointestinal atony. Cardiac output becomes severely compromised, heart sounds may be nearly inaudible, and heart rate increases to 120 bpm or more. Cows in stage III milk fever do not survive for more than a few hours without treatment.

About 7% of all cases of milk fever in dairy cattle are nonparturient. In these cases, sudden calcium outflow associated with the onset of lactation is not the stimulus for hypocalcemia. Instead, any cause of severe stress or feed deprivation may be sufficient to cause a sudden shift in calcium balance and development of nonparturient hypocalcemia.

Beef Cattle

Milk fever in beef cattle is rare and is most likely to occur in late gestation under conditions of severe dietary mineral imbalances. If the mineral imbalances are chronic, then affected cows may present with clinical signs of osteoporosis rather than acute hypocalcemia with paresis. These problems are often corrected by simply increasing calcium and/or magnesium in the late-gestation diet. Occasional cases of nonparturient hypocalcemia may also occur in beef cattle.

Sheep

Milk fever in ewes is more likely to occur in late gestation rather than at the onset of lactation because ewes have a relatively larger fetoplacental unit (particularly ewes carrying multiple fetuses) and lower milk production than do dairy cattle. Hypocalcemia in ewes may reduce feed intake and lead to concurrent pregnancy toxemia. Milk fever in ewes is primarily characterized by flaccid paralysis; however, severe muscle tremors or tetany (similar to those due to hypomagnesemia) are frequently seen. Some affected ewes exhibit a stiff and uncoordinated gait before falling into rigid, sternal recumbency.

Goats

Milk fever may occur in doe goats either prepartum or postpartum because they have both the potential for high milk production and relatively large fetoplacental requirements associated with multiple births. The parturient form of milk fever predominates when goats are managed intensively for milk production. The prepartum form of milk fever predominates when goats are managed extensively and are not challenged for high milk production.

Clinical signs of milk fever in doe goats are similar to those in sheep and include both hyperesthesia with tetany and flaccid paralysis. Clinical signs in doe goats tend to be less severe than those observed in dairy cows. Goats may also be affected with nonparturient hypocalcemia.

CLINICAL PATHOLOGY

Milk fever is confirmed by low serum calcium concentrations. Clinical signs may begin as total blood calcium values fall below 7.5 mg/dL; however, more than half of all mature dairy cows will have total blood calcium concentrations below 7.5 mg/dL following calving without any evidence of clinical signs. Animals in stage I milk fever usually have mild hypocalcemia (5.5 to 7.5 mg/dL of calcium). Some animals are able to remain standing with total calcium concentrations as low as 5.0 mg/dL, although most become recumbent before this concentration is reached. Animals in stage II milk fever typically have total calcium concentrations of 3.5 to 6.5 mg/dL, and calcium levels may be as low as 1.0 mg/dL in animals with stage III milk fever.

Blood concentrations of phosphorus are typically below normal in milk fever, whereas magnesium concentrations are usually high. Phosphorus and magnesium abnormalities are further discussed elsewhere in this section.

Laboratory confirmation of the diagnosis of milk fever is often not necessary, as response to treatment is a useful and commonly used diagnostic method. Most cases of milk fever respond rapidly to a single parenteral treatment with calcium salts. It is good practice to collect a blood sample prior to initial treatment of cases of milk fever. If the animal does not respond to initial treatment, then an accurate diagnosis can be made from the pretreatment blood sample. Posttreatment samples are of very limited value in diagnosing milk fever because they are temporarily influenced by the calcium administered. It is important to rule out other possible causes of recumbency in parturient animals before initiating calcium treatment. The most important differential diagnoses are discussed in this section under the downer cow syndrome.

Milk fever must be diagnosed antemortem, because no gross lesions or histologic changes in affected animals are seen at necropsy. Urine obtained from the bladder will have very low calcium concentration, but this alone is not sufficient evidence to make a diagnosis. Postmortem blood samples cannot be used to assess calcium status.

TREATMENT

Milk fever should always be treated as promptly as possible, particularly if the animal is already recumbent. Stage I milk fever may be treated with either oral calcium supplements or intravenous calcium salts. Animals in stage II or III require immediate treatment with intravenous calcium salts. Animals affected with milk fever do not usually recover spontaneously, and 75% of all affected animals will eventually die if left untreated.

Standard intravenous treatment for cattle affected with milk fever is 500 mL of a calcium gluconate or borogluconate solution to provide 10.8 g of calcium. Intravenous calcium should always be administered slowly to prevent sudden cardiac arrest due to hypercalcemia. At least 12 minutes should be allowed for injection of intravenous calcium (8- to 12-g dose) into cattle. Adult sheep and doe goats affected with milk fever require only 50 to 100 mL of calcium solution intravenously.

The addition of phosphorus, magnesium, or potassium to milk fever treatment solutions may be beneficial. Therapeutic use of these electrolytes is discussed in other portions of this section.

In contrast, glucose added to treatment solutions may be detrimental because excretion of unneeded glucose in the urine causes increased excretion of much-needed phosphorus.

A precise calculation of the dose of calcium salts necessary to correct milk fever cannot be made because of the dynamic nature of calcium metabolism. The immediate total body calcium deficit in a dairy cow with milk fever is about 6 g, so a standard dose of 10.8 g of calcium should be adequate in many cases, although some large Holsteins may require more.

Approximately 60% of recumbent animals affected with uncomplicated milk fever will get up within 30 minutes after a single intravenous treatment with calcium salts. Another 15%

can be expected to rise within the next 2 hours. However, intravenous treatment only assists animals in getting through the temporary hypocalcemic crisis. Full restoration of normal calcium homeostasis usually requires 2 or 3 days.

Animals with unresponsive cases of milk fever should be reevaluated and re-treated at about 12-hour intervals until they recover, die, or are salvaged. About 10% of dairy cows with milk fever stay recumbent for over 24 hours but eventually recover. Management of nonresponsive milk fever cases is covered in this section under the downer cow syndrome.

Cases of stage I milk fever may be treated by administering calcium via a slowly absorbed route. For example, subcutaneously administered calcium is gradually absorbed over a period of several hours. Solutions containing glucose should never be given subcutaneously, because they often cause tissue destruction, abscess formation, and/or sloughing at the site of injection.

Calcium provided by oral dosing is also gradually absorbed. A variety of oral calcium salt preparations are now available. They typically contain between 25 and 100 g of calcium as either calcium chloride or calcium propionate. They work by rapidly raising calcium in the intestine to such a high concentration that a proportion is passively absorbed. For example, about 4 g of calcium will be absorbed and enter the bloodstream of a cow given an oral solution containing 50 g of calcium chloride. Calcium chloride also rapidly causes a compensated metabolic acidosis, which improves the animal's own calcium homeostatic mechanisms. However, high or repeated doses of calcium chloride can cause uncompensated metabolic acidosis, which is undesirable. Calcium chloride is irritating and may cause transient erosions in the mouth, esophagus, rumen, and abomasum of some cows. Calcium propionate is less irritating. Care must be taken during administration of any oral calcium supplement to avoid laceration of the pharyngeal region or aspiration of the solution. Typical doses of oral calcium supplements will increase blood calcium concentrations by 1 to 3 mg/dL within 30 minutes of administration. Blood calcium levels return to baseline values by 6 to 12 hours posttreatment.

About 25% to 40% of dairy cows with milk fever that respond favorably to initial intravenous calcium therapy will relapse into hypocalcemia within 12 to 48 hours. Animals with prepartum milk fever have an even greater relapse rate. Older cows are at greatest risk for a hypocalcemic relapse.

Incidence of hypocalcemic relapses in dairy cattle may be reduced to only 5% to 10% of the total cases by administration of an additional 500 mL of 23% calcium gluconate subcutaneously at the time of initial treatment with intravenous calcium. Calcium is apparently slowly released from the subcutaneous depot and sustains the treated animal through the surge of calcitonin release that follows intravenous calcium administration. Oral calcium supplements may also be used to prevent hypocalcemic relapses.

PREVENTION

Dietary Calcium Restriction

Calcium deficient diets (<15 g of calcium per day) fed for at least 10 days before calving will greatly reduce the risk of milk fever. However, such diets are difficult to formulate, and can therefore be impractical. See the third edition of this book for a more complete discussion of calcium-deficient prepartum diets for prevention of milk fever.

Acidification Through Diet

The effect of diet on acid-base balance is more important in controlling milk fever than is calcium intake. Diets fed prior to parturition that evoke an acidic response in the animal reduce milk fever risk, whereas diets that evoke an alkaline response increase it.

The potential of a diet to cause either alkalosis or acidosis can be estimated by calculating the dietary cation-anion difference (DCAD). Dietary electrolytes can be classified as either cations (positively charged) or anions (negatively charged). Inorganic ions that are highly dissociated in aqueous solutions influence acid-base status. Important dietary cations are sodium (Na), potassium (K), calcium (Ca), and magnesium (Mg); important dietary anions are chloride (Cl), sulfur (S), and phosphorus (P).

Several methods of calculating DCAD have been utilized, including the following equations:

$$\text{DCAD (mEq)} = (\text{Na} + \text{K} + .15\,\text{Ca} + .15\,\text{Mg}) - (\text{Cl} + .20\,\text{S} + .3\,\text{P}) \quad (1)$$

$$\text{DCAD (mEq)} = (\text{Na} + \text{K}) - (\text{Cl} + \text{S}) \quad (2)$$

$$\text{DCAD (mEq)} = (\text{Na} + \text{K}) - (\text{Cl}) \quad (3)$$

Note that the units are given in milliequivalents and the values are usually expressed on the basis of 100 g or 1 kg of dietary dry matter. The first equation takes into account new data on the bioavailability of all of the potential strong ions. Theoretically it should be the most accurate, but it is new and has not been widely applied. The second two equations are used more commonly. The equations used to calculate DCAD and the units used to express it vary among ration evaluation software programs.

Low-DCAD diets cause metabolic acidosis and reduce the risk of milk fever. A diet can have a low DCAD because it is low in cations, high in anions, or a combination of both. Typical diets fed to dry cows will have an DCAD (using equation 2 above) of about +50 to +250 mEq/kg of diet dry matter. In common feedstuffs, potassium is the most variable of the ions in the DCAD equation, and it is usually the most important determinant of DCAD in unsupplemented feed. A good first step in formulating a low-DCAD prepartum diet is to reduce dietary potassium to less than 1.5% of diet dry matter. However, removing potassium from a diet can be difficult, owing to its presence in forages, in which, depending on soil conditions, levels may be high.

Once the cation content of a prepartum diet has been reduced as much as possible by diet selection, anions can then be added to further reduce DCAD to the desired end point. Anion sources include anionic salts (any mineral salt high in chloride and sulfur relative to sodium and potassium) and mineral acids (hydrochloric or sulfuric acids). Optimal acidification generally occurs when anions are added to achieve a final DCAD (using equation 2 above) between −50 to −150 mEq/kg of dry matter.

Monitoring urinary pH after feeding supplemental anions may be a direct and useful approach to establishing the optimal dose of anions within a dairy herd. An advantage of this approach (over relying on calculated DCAD alone) is that it accounts for inaccuracies in mineral analyses and for unexpected changes in forage mineral content. Mean urinary pH can be evaluated by obtaining urine from a group of at least six animals near parturition. When acidification is optimal, mean urinary pH values will be between 5.5 and 6.5. Mean urinary pH values below 5.5 indicate overacidification and suggest that the DCAD could be increased. Conversely, urinary pH values greater than 6.5 reflect inadequate acidification and suggest that a lower DCAD is required for optimal milk fever prevention. Because variations in urinary pH related to time after feeding may be significant, most accurate results will be obtained by collecting urine samples at a standard time, preferably within a few hours of feeding.

Some uncertainty exists regarding the optimal dietary calcium concentration that should be used when low-DCAD diets are fed. Limited evidence suggests that low-DCAD diets work best in dairy rations that provide at least 120 g of daily calcium per cow per day.

Prophylactic Calcium Administration

Prophylactic treatment of cows with intravenous and/or subcutaneous calcium gluconate immediately after calving may reduce the risk of milk fever. Oral calcium supplements may also be used to prevent milk fever. Treatment with four doses of an oral calcium supplement (given prior to calving, at calving, 12 hours postcalving, and 24 hours postcalving) reduces the risk of clinical and subclinical milk fever in dairy cows by about half. This protocol works best when at least one dose of oral calcium can be administered prior to calving.

BIBLIOGRAPHY

Goff JP, Horst RL: Effects of the addition of potassium or sodium, but not calcium, to prepartum rations on milk fever in dairy cows. J Dairy Sci 80: 176–186, 1997.
Jardon PW: Using urine pH to monitor anionic salt programs. Compend Cont Educ Practicing Vet 17:860, 1995.
Oetzel GR: Use of anionic salts for prevention of milk fever in dairy cattle. Compend Cont Educ Practicing Vet 15:1138, 1993.
Oetzel GR: Effect of calcium chloride gel treatment in dairy cows on incidence of periparturient diseases. J Am Vet Med Assoc 209:958, 1996.

■ Phosphorus Deficiency*
Jesse P. Goff, D.V.M., Ph.D.

Phosphorus deficiency is fairly common in grazing ruminants, especially those fed on poor-quality pastures. With the exception of rickets and postparturient hemoglobinuria, the clinical problems associated with phosphorus deficiency are general and nonspecific. For a discussion of postparturient hemoglobinuria, an uncommon problem of sheep and cattle, see "Postparturient Hemoglobinuria" in the last edition of this book (p. 323).

OCCURRENCE

The most common of the phosphorus deficiency syndromes is unthriftiness and poor growth, with poor reproductive and lactation performance in females. In arid areas of the world, where soil fertility is low, infertility and poor growth resulting from inadequate phosphorus intake affects nearly all animals. In more temperate areas, phosphorus deficiency is observed in animals subsisting on overly mature forages or on crop residues, such as corn stalks. Sheep may be more resistant to phosphorus deficiency than are cattle.

ETIOLOGY AND PATHOGENESIS

Phosphorus is a component of phospholipids, phosphoproteins, nucleic acids, and energy-transferring molecules such as adenosine triphosphate (ATP). Phosphorus is an essential component of the acid-base buffer system. It is second only to calcium as the major component of bone mineral.

Plasma inorganic phosphorus concentration is normally be-

---

*All of the material in this article is in the public domain.

tween 4 and 8 mg/dL. Phosphorus exists in blood serum and other body fluids in organic and inorganic forms. Clinicopathologically, inorganic phosphorous, or phosphate, is usually all that is measured. In mature ruminant animals, the major phosphorus requirement is for salivary buffering, milk production, and fetal skeletal development. Salivary secretion is substantial. Much, but not all, of salivary phosphorus is reabsorbed.

Ruminants, unlike monogastrics, are able to use phytate phosphorus, a major source of phosphorus in plants. Plasma phosphorus concentrations are well correlated with dietary phosphorus absorption. Phosphorus absorbed in excess of needs is excreted in urine and saliva.

Rickets and Osteomalacia

Rickets is a disease of young, growing animals in which the cartilaginous matrix at the growth plate and the osteoid matrix formed during bone remodeling fail to mineralize. In adults (no active growth plates), the term *osteomalacia* is used to describe the failure of osteoid matrix to mineralize. Failure to supply phosphorus in the diet will result in low plasma phosphorus concentrations, which will not support bone mineralization.

Chronic Hypophosphatemia

Animals fed diets containing less phosphorus than necessary to meet physiologic needs suffer hypophosphatemia and all the physiologic consequences of impaired reproduction, failure to grow, inappetence, and unthriftiness. Milk production, but not phosphorus content, will decline.

Acute Hypophosphatemia

Beef cows fed a diet marginal in phosphorus will have chronic hypophosphatemia (plasma phosphorus, 2 to 3.5 mg/dL). In late gestation, plasma phosphorus can decline precipitously in these animals as the growth of the fetus accelerates and removes substantial amounts of phosphorus from the maternal circulation. Affected animals often become recumbent and are unable to rise, although they appear fairly alert and may eat feed placed in front of them. Cows carrying twins are most often affected. Plasma inorganic phosphorus concentration in these recumbent animals is often less than 1 mg/dL. The disease is usually complicated by concurrent hypocalcemia, hypomagnesemia, and, in some cases, hypoglycemia (see Pregnancy Toxemia later in this section).

At the onset of lactation, production of colostrum and milk draws large amounts of phosphorus out of extracellular phosphorus pools, depressing blood phosphorus concentrations. In addition, cows that develop milk fever have blood phosphorus concentrations that are even further depressed. Plasma inorganic phosphorus concentrations in cows with milk fever are often between 1 and 2 mg/dL. Plasma phosphorus concentrations usually increase rapidly following treatment of the hypocalcemic cow with intravenous calcium solutions. Restoring normocalcemia decreases parathyroid hormone secretion, which reduces urinary and salivary loss of phosphorus and stimulates resumption of gastrointestinal motility, which in turn allows absorption of dietary phosphorus and reabsorption of salivary phosphorus secretions. Protracted hypophosphatemia in some cows appears to be an important factor in some nonresponsive milk fever cases. Unlike typical cases of milk fever, plasma phosphorus levels in these cows remains low, despite successful treatment of the hypocalcemia. Why plasma phosphorus remains low is un-

clear. (For further discussion, see Downer Cow Syndrome later in this section.)

CLINICAL SIGNS

Moderate, chronic hypophosphatemia, with plasma phosphorus between 2 and 4 mg/dL, causes subtle decreases in animal performance. With more severe hypophosphatemia, performance of the animals becomes very poor, and feed intake is depressed. The reduction in feed intake is often accompanied by pica. Recumbency and paresis are associated with plasma phosphorus concentrations below 1 mg/dL.

Rickets and Osteomalacia

Young, growing animals with rickets exhibit joint pain and reluctance to move. Growth rate is greatly depressed. Affected animals have narrow chests, and the costochondral joints are enlarged and readily palpable. Adult animals with osteomalacia exhibit joint pain and lameness.

CLINICAL PATHOLOGY

Adult animals with plasma phosphorus concentration between 2 and 4 mg/dL are likely to perform poorly and, with time, develop osteomalacia. Plasma phosphorus concentration in young, growing animals should be between 5 and 8.5 mg/dL. Otherwise, growth impairment and rickets develop. Animals recumbent as a result of hypophosphatemia have plasma phosphorus concentrations below 1 mg/dL (often closer to 0.5 mg/dL). Hypocalcemia, hypomagnesemia, and hypoglycemia are often concurrently present in these animals.

Bones from animals with chronic phosphorus deficiency show a reduction in bone ash content. The ratio of calcium to phosphorus in the bone is not significantly altered.

Cows with postparturient hemoglobinuria exhibit true hemoglobin in the urine. The packed cell volume of blood will be reduced, and Heinz bodies will be readily observed in blood smears. Many of the animals also suffer from concurrent copper and/or selenium deficiency.

DIAGNOSIS

Clinical signs coupled with low plasma phosphorus concentration help in the diagnosis of phosphorus deficiency. Animals that have been exercised prior to blood collection may have falsely high plasma phosphorus concentrations. Also, if more than 12 hours have passed from sample collection until serum removal, the phosphorus concentration will be falsely elevated. Rickets is always accompanied by hypophosphatemia. Bones of rachitic animals tend to bend without breaking. Bone lesions are the only postmortem lesion that is pathognomonic of phosphorus deficiency. Vitamin D deficiency causes hypophosphatemia and hypocalcemia, even when dietary content of these minerals is normal. The presence of more than 10 ng of 25-hydroxyvitamin D per milliliter of plasma will rule out vitamin D deficiency. Hemoglobinuria in early-lactation cows is suggestive of phosphorus deficiency, but other nutritional and infectious causes of hemoglobinuria must be ruled out.

TREATMENT
Recumbent Cows

Beef cows in late gestation and dairy cows that remain recumbent following treatment for milk fever are often hypophosphatemic. Some of these "downer cows" will benefit from intravenous administration of phosphate to restore normal plasma phosphorus concentrations. Sodium monophosphate is a soluble form of phosphate that can be administered intravenously (30 g of sodium monophosphate in 300 mL of distilled water). Calcium salts cannot be included in these solutions, as insoluble calcium phosphate salts will form. Commercial preparations containing phosphorus often utilize more soluble hypophosphite salts, so that addition of calcium or magnesium to the solution will not cause a precipitate to form. Unfortunately, hypophosphite salts are not biologically functional, and the response to treatment is disappointing.

Intravenous sodium monophosphate treatment will maintain normal plasma phosphorus concentration for only a short time (6 to 10 hours). In most cases, these animals also require oral administration of sodium monophosphate (0.5 kg in warm water administered as a drench or via stomach tube). Bone meal or dicalcium phosphate may also be used (0.5 kg), but they are only poorly soluble and difficult to administer. A cocktail that includes calcium, magnesium, and an energy source, as well as phosphorus, can benefit the recumbent cow. A recipe we have used is 0.5 to 0.75 kg of calcium propionate, 0.35 kg of magnesium sulfate (Epsom salt), 0.75 kg of sodium monophosphate, and 0.5 L of propylene glycol dissolved in 6 L of warm water administered via stomach tube as a means of supplementation for recumbent cows. Calcium chloride (0.25 to 0.35 kg) can be substituted for calcium propionate.

Rickets and Osteomalacia

Animals with rickets and osteomalacia will, with time, recover once dietary phosphorus is supplied to the animal, providing the disease has not progressed to the point of irreparable joint damage.

PREVENTION

Phosphorus deficiency is a possibility whenever animals are on pasture that consists of less than 0.25% phosphorus. Heavily lactating dairy cows and ewes may develop phosphorus deficiency when pasture contains less than 0.35% phosphorus. Grains serve as good sources of phosphorus. In addition, mineral sources of phosphorus can be easily incorporated into the grain. Daily ingestion of 80 g of sodium monophosphate, 100 g of bone meal, or 100 g of dicalcium phosphate will prevent phosphorus deficiency in almost every case. Dicalcium phosphate is the most commonly used source of phosphate in the United States, and free choice supplementation of dicalcium phosphate can often prevent phosphorus deficiency in most of the herd if it is made readily accessible. Intake of dicalcium phosphate is often enhanced if mixed 1:1 with salt. Defluoridated phosphate, along with lesser amounts of ammonium polyphosphate and phosphoric acid, are also used in grain as phosphorus supplements.

Improving pasture phosphate is an option in some areas, and it often has the added benefit of improving forage yield. However, the price of phosphate fertilizer and the size of the area to be treated often renders this approach impractical in areas where phosphorus deficiency is endemic.

BIBLIOGRAPHY

Reinhardt TA, Horst RL, Goff JP: Calcium, phosphorus, and magnesium homeostasis in ruminants. Vet Clin North Am Food Anim Pract 4:331–350, 1988.

Underwood EJ: Calcium and phosphorus. In Underwood EJ (ed): The Mineral Nutrition of Livestock, 2nd ed. Slough, England, Commonwealth Agricultural Bureau, 1981, p 31.

■ Ruminant Hypomagnesemic Tetanies*

Jesse P. Goff, D.V.M., Ph.D.

Extracellular magnesium is vital to normal nerve conduction, muscle function, and bone mineral formation. Hypomagnesemia generally leads to hyperexcitability, tetany, convulsion, and, too often, death. Hypomagnesemia is often accompanied and complicated by hypocalcemia and hypophosphatemia.

OCCURRENCE

Hypomagnesemic tetany is most often associated with beef cows and ewes in early lactation that are grazing in spring or fall on lush pastures that are high in potassium and nitrogen and low in magnesium and sodium. This is the most common situation, and it is often referred to as grass tetany, spring tetany, grass staggers, or lactation tetany. Ewes suckling more than one lamb and higher-producing cows are at greatest risk. Magnesium cannot be mobilized from tissues to maintain plasma magnesium concentration, so it must be ingested continually. Conditions associated with hypomagnesemia as a result of feed restriction include transport (transport tetany) or sudden exposure to inclement weather. Hypomagnesemia can also develop in late gestation, often in association with and complicated by inadequate energy intake. This syndrome is sometimes referred to as *winter tetany* and is seen in animals subsisting on crop residues such as corn stalks or straw. Animals grazing wheat pasture (wheat pasture tetany) or other early-growth cereal forages can develop hypomagnesemia with concurrent severe hypocalcemia, resulting in a clinical picture that closely resembles milk fever. Hypomagnesemia can also occur in calves, especially if they are fed only milk or milk replacer beyond the first 2 months of age (milk tetany). Hypomagnesemic tetany can reach epidemic proportions on some farms, affecting nearly 20% of cows and ewes in early lactation on some pastures, although death losses of 2% to 3% are more commonly observed.

ETIOLOGY AND PATHOGENESIS

Bovine and ovine plasma magnesium concentrations are normally between 1.8 and 2.4 mg/dL, and 2.2 and 2.8 mg/dL, respectively. Blood and extracellular fluid magnesium is in equilibrium with and similar to magnesium concentration in cerebrospinal fluid (CSF), although changes in CSF magnesium concentration lag behind changes in plasma magnesium concentration, as the blood-brain barrier slows diffusion.

The tetany characteristic of hypomagnesemic disorders is the result of intracellular, cellular membrane, and extracellular metabolic effects of magnesium. Tetany is the result of the following factors:

1. Lower central and peripheral nervous membrane potential.
2. Excessive acetylcholine release at myoneural junctions.
3. Sustained myofibril contractions due to reduced intracellular adenosine triphosphatase (ATPase) activity.
4. Hypocalcemia due to hypomagnesemic influences on parathyroid function and vitamin D metabolism.

Despite the physiologic importance of magnesium, no hor-

---

*All of the material in this article is in the public domain.

monal mechanism is concerned principally and directly with magnesium homeostasis. Constant absorption of ingested magnesium is necessary to maintain normal plasma magnesium concentration. Dietary magnesium absorbed in excess of needs is excreted in the urine. The renal threshold for magnesium is 1.8 mg/dL in cows and 2.2 mg/dL in sheep. At plasma magnesium concentrations below these levels, little or no magnesium will be detected in urine. Maintenance of normal plasma magnesium concentration is nearly totally dependent on dietary magnesium absorption, which essentially occurs only in the rumen of ruminants.

Magnesium absorption from the rumen is dependent on the concentration of magnesium in solution in the rumen fluid and the integrity of the magnesium transport mechanism, which is a sodium-linked active transport process.

The soluble concentration of magnesium in rumen fluid is dependent on the following factors:

1. Dietary magnesium content.
2. Rumen pH, which affects magnesium solubility.
3. Presence of unesterified, long-chain fatty acids, which can form insoluble magnesium salts.
4. Presence of plant dicarboxylic acids, which form insoluble magnesium complexes. However, the role of these complexes in hypomagnesemic tetany is unclear.

Factors affecting magnesium transport across the rumen epithelium include the following:

1. Dietary sodium-to-potassium ratio. High dietary potassium can interfere with the sodium-linked transport of magnesium across the rumen wall.
2. Availability of lush, high-moisture pastures that increase the rate of passage of material from the rumen.
3. Dietary aluminum concentration, although this is controversial.
4. Dietary energy availability, especially in the form of nonstructural carbohydrates, which tend to increase magnesium availability.

CLINICAL SIGNS

Cattle

The clinical signs in affected cows depend on the severity of hypomagnesemia. The disease progresses more rapidly and tends to be more severe if it is accompanied by hypocalcemia, which is often the case. Both beef and dairy cows are usually affected 1 to 3 weeks into lactation, especially if they are on pasture. Moderate hypomagnesemia (between 1.1 and 1.8 mg/dL) is associated with reduced feed intake, nervousness, and reduced milk fat and total milk production. This can be a chronic problem in some dairy herds that often goes unnoticed. It can also predispose the animals to milk fever.

When plasma magnesium levels fall below 1.1 mg/dL, twitching is sometimes seen in the muscles of the face, shoulders, and flanks. Cows become restless and irritable and rumen motility is reduced. Affected animals may separate themselves from herdmates and take on a spastic, stiff-legged gait. Frequent urination and bellowing are common. Some animals become aggressive. The animals are particularly sensitive to sound. Blowing a car horn and forced movement of the cows often initiates the appearance of tetany in cows with more than moderate hypomagnesemia.

As hypomagnesemia progresses, tetanic spasms of the muscles become more common and eventually cause the cow to stagger and fall. Clonic convulsions quickly follow, with chomping of the jaws and frothy salivation. Affected cows usually lie with the head arched back and the legs paddling. The heart rate can approach 150 bpm and the heartbeat is often audible without a stethoscope. Respiratory rate approaches 60/min and the rectal temperature rises and can approach 40.5°C (105°F) as a result of the excessive muscular activity; the eyelids flutter and marked nystagmus is present. The animal may rise after several minutes, and the convulsive episodes may be repeated several times before it finally dies.

Hypomagnesemic tetany in calves is clinically similar to that in adult cows, and it is often accompanied by moderate hypocalcemia.

Ewes and Goats

Affected ewes are generally hypocalcemic as well as hypomagnesemic. They are usually in the second to fourth week of lactation and are often suckling more than one lamb. Affected ewes are generally depressed, stand with their heads down, and are reluctant to move. As hypomagnesemia and hypocalcemia progress, they suffer tetany and clonic convulsions, just as cattle do. The clinical signs in goats are similar to those observed in cattle.

CLINICAL PATHOLOGY

Plasma or serum magnesium concentrations below 1.8 mg/dL in cattle and below 2.2 mg/dL in sheep are considered to be low and indicative of inadequate magnesium absorption. Plasma magnesium concentrations below 1 mg/dL are indicative of a risk of development of tetany. Plasma calcium concentrations are often low as well, generally between 5 and 7.5 mg/dL. Cerebrospinal fluid magnesium concentrations less than 1 mg/dL are responsible for the clonic convulsions seen in animals with hypomagnesemic tetany. Blood samples obtained during or shortly after an episode of tetany may have near normal levels of magnesium as a result of muscle damage and leakage of magnesium from intracellular pools. The CSF magnesium concentration remains low during tetany and also can be a reliable indicator of magnesium status for up to 12 hours after death. Vitreous humor magnesium concentrations less than 1 mg/dL are also found in animals with tetany and can be a reliable indicator for 24 to 48 hours after death, provided that environmental temperatures have not exceeded 23°C. Aqueous humor has not proved reliable as a sample. Urine magnesium concentration is nearly undetectable in animals that are hypomagnesemic.

Animals in tetany, or that have just had a tetanic episode, often exhibit hyperkalemia (potassium, >7 mEq/L) and elevated serum aspartate aminotransferase (AST) and creatine phosphokinase (CPK) activity as a result of muscle cell damage and leakage.

DIAGNOSIS

A diagnosis is often made after one or two animals have already died of hypomagnesemic tetany. There are no pathognomonic necropsy lesions associated with hypomagnesemic tetany. A history of sudden death in early-lactation cows and ewes grazing on fast-growing cool-season grass or green cereal crop pasture is diagnostic in many cases. The CSF and urine magnesium concentrations may be of some aid postmortem. Blood analyses will confirm low plasma magnesium concentrations in herdmates.

Dairy herds grazing pasture and having suboptimal milk fat and total milk production may have mild hypomagnesemia. A response to supplementation is the most satisfactory confirmation of diagnosis. In growing calves, 43 calcium atoms are incorporated into bone for every magnesium atom (71 mg of calcium per 1 mg of magnesium). Bone formed during chronic magnesium deficiency will have a calcium-to-magnesium ratio of greater than 100.

TREATMENT

Animals exhibiting hypomagnesemic tetany need immediate treatment. Slowly injecting 500 mL (50 to 100 mL for ewes) of a solution of calcium borogluconate (8 to 10 g of calcium) and magnesium hypophosphite, magnesium borogluconate, magnesium chloride, or magnesium gluconate (1.5 to 4 g of magnesium) intravenously, is the safest and most effective general recommendation. Intravenous administration of solutions containing only magnesium increases the risk of respiratory failure as a result of medullary depression. The risk of cardiac failure during treatment is also reduced by addition of calcium to the intravenous solutions. In addition, most hypomagnesemic animals suffer from hypocalcemia, and solutions containing magnesium with no calcium will not effect a recovery. Treatment of these animals can be challenging, as insertion of the intravenous needle often initiates a tetanic episode. Some veterinarians use intramuscularly administered tranquilizers or sedatives, such as acepromazine, to reduce the risk of injury to the cow and to themselves from continuous clonic convulsions. Intravenous administration of tranquilizers has been associated with sudden hypotension and death. Response to therapy can be disappointing, and success is related to the interval between onset of tetany and treatment. To avoid initiation of tetany and convulsion, cows should not be stimulated to rise for at least 30 minutes after treatment. Cattle that will recover do so 1 hour after treatment, when CSF magnesium concentration returns to normal. Many of these cows suffer relapse and require further treatment within 12 hours.

The rate of relapse can be reduced with the following treatments:

1. Subcutaneous injection of 100 to 200 mL of a 20% to 50% magnesium sulfate solution. The stronger solutions are essentially fully saturated and hyperosmotic, and no more than 50 mL should be injected in any one site to avoid tissue damage.

2. Magnesium enemas, 60 g of magnesium chloride or 60 g of magnesium sulfate dissolved in 200 mL of water, administered into the descending colon. This treatment increases plasma magnesium concentration within 15 minutes. It can cause some mucosal sloughing, especially if more highly concentrated solutions are used.

3. Oral administration of magnesium salts can be given to provide longer maintenance of plasma magnesium concentration once the animal has regained good esophageal reflexes so that the risk of aspiration pneumonia is reduced. Drenching the cow with a slurry of 100 g of magnesium oxide in water has been reported to be effective. This provides 50 g of magnesium to the animal. Addition of 50 g of calcium carbonate, 100 g of dicalcium phosphate, and 50 g of sodium chloride may enhance the effectiveness of the slurry; especially if hypocalcemia and hypophosphatemia accompanied the hypomagnesemia. The addition of sodium may enhance ruminal magnesium absorption. Alternatively, 200 to 400 mL of a 50% magnesium sulfate solution can be administered by drench. Magnesium sulfate is more available for absorption than is magnesium oxide. Slurries can be difficult to administer. Gel formulations containing magnesium in comparable concentrations are also available commercially.

PREVENTION

If hypomagnesemic tetany has occurred in one cow or ewe in a herd or flock, steps should be taken immediately to increase magnesium intake to prevent further losses. Getting an additional 10 to 15 g of magnesium into each pregnant cow, 20 g of magnesium into each lactating beef cow, and 30 g of magnesium into each lactating dairy cow each day will usually prevent further cases of hypomagnesemic tetany. The problem with prevention is getting the extra magnesium into the animal.

Individual drenching of cows at risk is effective but highly laborious. Addition of magnesium salts to grain supplements is practical in some situations. Most magnesium salts are unpalatable, making free-choice consumption ineffective. However, magnesium is readily accepted in grain concentrates. Including 60 g of magnesium oxide in just 0.5 to 1 kg of grain is effective. However, the expense of the grain and the problems associated with feeding concentrates to pastured cattle often make this option difficult to implement. Feeding mature grass or legume hay to the cows or ewes can often improve magnesium intake by increasing total dry matter intake of cattle on pasture. Hay is usually higher in magnesium content than are rapidly growing immature grasses. Hay is also lower in potassium and, therefore, presents less inhibition of ruminal magnesium absorption. Adding magnesium oxide (60 g/cow, mixed with water and molasses) to the hay, at the time of baling or just before feeding, can increase the effectiveness of this option. Unfortunately, cows with access to lush pasture may not eat enough hay unless they are confined for that purpose each day. Dusting of pasture foliage with magnesium oxide is also an approach that has been used to increase magnesium intake. Feeding ionophores, in situations in which they are legal, can increase dietary magnesium availability.

Adding 5 to 10 kg per 2000 L or 10 to 20 lb per 500 gal of magnesium sulfate·7H$_2$O (Epsom salts) or magnesium chloride·6H$_2$O to drinking water can be an economical means of supplementing magnesium if cows have access to no other water supply. Molasses licks and mineral blocks containing magnesium oxide and salt can help supply magnesium to animals at pasture if made readily available and if the animals learn to use the licks prior to parturition. A problem with many of these methods is that some cows in the herd may not voluntarily consume enough of the magnesium supplement and, on some tetanogenic pastures, cows that do not receive supplementation are often found dead.

Intraruminal magnesium-releasing boluses and bullets, which remain in the reticulum and release low levels of magnesium (1 to 1.5 g) each day for periods of up to 90 days, have been developed. These devices do not supply enough magnesium to raise blood magnesium levels substantially, although they may prove successful in some situations despite the low level of supplementation achieved.

Agronomic practices to increase forage magnesium content and reduce hypomagnesemic tetany are in various stages of development and show good promise.

BIBLIOGRAPHY

Fontenot JP, Allen VG, Bunce GE, et al: Factors influencing magnesium absorption and metabolism in ruminants. J Anim Sci 67:3445–3455, 1989.

Littledike ET, Goff JP: Interactions of calcium, phosphorus, magnesium and vitamin D that influence their status in domestic meat animals. J Anim Sci 65:1727–1743, 1987.

Mayland HF: Grass tetany. In Church DC (ed): The Ruminant Animal: Digestive Physiology and Nutrition. Prospect Heights, Ill, Waveland Press, 1988.

■ Hypokalemia Syndrome in Dairy Cows

Raymond W. Sweeney, V.M.D.

Hypokalemia in dairy cattle usually develops secondary to inappetence or other conditions, such as altered renal function or diarrhea. In such cases the hypokalemia is mild and associated clinical signs are not recognized, and the hypokalemia resolves when the primary problem is corrected. However, a clinical syndrome consisting of severe hypokalemia with associated weakness has been recognized in dairy cattle. In some cases, repeated treatment with glucocorticoids for ketosis may have predisposed the affected cows to hypokalemia syndrome.

OCCURRENCE

Hypokalemia syndrome tends to occur sporadically in adult lactating dairy cattle, although multiple cases have been reported in some herds. In one report of 10 cases, all cows had delivered a calf less than 30 days prior to development of hypokalemia. Most cows had a history of treatment for another primary illness such as mastitis, metritis, left displacement of the abomasum, or diarrhea. In that report, all cows had been treated for ketosis with dextrose and isoflupredone acetate, but others have reported cases in which corticosteroids have not been administered.

ETIOLOGY AND PATHOGENESIS

Hypokalemia can result from either of two common mechanisms: an imbalance of external potassium regulation or an imbalance of internal or intracellular potassium homeostasis. External potassium regulation involves the balance of potassium absorption from the gastrointestinal tract with potassium excretion in urine, feces, sweat, and saliva. Most dairy cattle are adapted to high oral intake of potassium owing to the high potassium content of many forages. A sudden reduction in potassium ingestion as a result of reduced appetite, such as might occur with ketosis, mastitis, or displaced abomasum, may contribute significantly to hypokalemia, as the renal capacity to conserve potassium may lag behind the reduced intake. In addition, exogenously administered corticosteroids may have some mineralocorticoid activity, and as such may induce kaliuresis and hypokalemia as undesirable side effects. Dexamethasone has been shown to have little mineralocorticoid activity, whereas isoflupredone acetate has mineralocorticoid effects, at least in dogs and humans.

Low dietary potassium intake due to anorexia in combination with increased urinary losses of potassium associated with mineralocorticoid activity of corticosteroids used to treat ketosis are presumed to be the cause of the profound hypokalemia seen in dairy cows with this syndrome. However, other factors may also play a role in hypokalemia, especially in cows that have no history of corticosteroid administration. Alkalosis, as commonly occurs in bovine gastrointestinal disturbances, results in renal potassium wasting. Additionally, internal potassium homeostasis is altered, with cellular uptake of potassium in exchange for hydrogen ions resulting in hypokalemia. Internal potassium homeostasis may also be altered by common treatments for ketosis, such as administration of insulin and glucose. Cellular uptake of glucose, enhanced by insulin, is accompanied by intracellular movement of potassium, and these treatments may contribute to hypokalemia.

Potassium is the principal intracellular cation, and depletion results in altered muscle cell membrane excitability and flaccid paralysis. Additionally, histologic lesions of hypokalemic myopathy have been observed in cows with this syndrome.

CLINICAL SIGNS

The predominant clinical sign in cows with hypokalemia syndrome is profound muscle flaccidity with recumbency. The animal may be unable to support the weight of the head, with the neck curved to the side or the head resting against the flank. Cardiac arrhythmias, such as atrial fibrillation and ventricular tachycardia, are commonly detected. The chief diagnostic exclusions include other common causes for recumbency, as covered in Downer Cow Syndrome in the following article.

CLINICAL PATHOLOGY

Severe hypokalemia is confirmed by laboratory measurement of plasma potassium concentration, which in most cases is below 2.5 mEq/L. Hypophosphatemia is a common concurrent finding and may contribute to muscle weakness. Depending on the weight of the cow and the duration of recumbency, mild elevation of serum creatine phosphokinase (CPK) activity may be found. There are typically no gross lesions at necropsy other than those associated with the primary problem (e.g., hepatic lipidosis in cases of chronic ketosis). Histopathologic examination of muscle tissue may reveal evidence of hypokalemic myopathy.

TREATMENT

Intravenous treatment with isotonic fluids supplemented with potassium chloride is usually not effective in correcting the condition without additional oral potassium chloride (KCl) supplementation. Intravenous fluids containing high concentrations of sodium may actually exacerbate kaliuresis. Intravenous administration of 5% KCl solution is recommended on the isoflupredone acetate package insert as a remedy for hypokalemia associated with administration of that compound. In my experience, oral administration of 60 to 120 g of KCl salt (2 to 4 oz/vol), up to 4 times daily in gelatin capsules, or as an aqueous solution administered by intraruminal tube, is more effective at correcting the hypokalemia than is intravenous potassium treatment. Supportive care, such as correcting other medical conditions, and proper nursing care for recumbent cows to prevent additional muscle ischemia should be given.

PREVENTION

Recognition of the risk factors for hypokalemia should alert the clinician to the need for potassium supplementation. Cows that develop inappetence, especially those that receive multiple doses of corticosteroids (e.g., isoflupredone acetate), should be monitored carefully for signs of hypokalemia, and consideration should be given to supplementation with KCl before hypokalemia develops.

BIBLIOGRAPHY

Sielman ES, Sweeney RW, Whitlock RH, et al: Hypokalemia syndrome in dairy cows. J Am Vet Med Assoc 210:240–243, 1996.

■ Downer Cow Syndrome

Victor S. Cox, D.V.M., Ph.D.

"Downer cow" is a term applied to the syndrome of recumbency and inability to rise in cattle. The typical downer is in sternal recumbency and unable to rise for no physically apparent reason. The syndrome has a variety of causes. Downer cows are usually alert, but variable degrees of alertness and depression are commonly seen.

OCCURRENCE

Downers are more common in dairy, as opposed to beef breeds, and are most common in the peripartum period. The reported incidence varies widely depending on the defining criteria. The occurrence of downers in dairy herds in Minnesota was found to be 21.4 cases per 1000 cow-years. In this group of downers, 33% recovered, 23% were slaughtered, and 44% died or were euthanized. A New York State study found the incidence of postpartum downers to be 1.1% in dairy cattle.

ETIOLOGY AND PATHOGENESIS

The causes of downer cow syndrome are many but can be broadly classified as systemic vs. local, or anatomic. Differentiating these is important for clinical management.

Systemic Causes

Systemic factors involve both metabolic and infectious problems which cause paresis or paralysis. These include hypocalcemia, hypophosphatemia, and hypokalemia, as well as such problems as endotoxemia due to infectious causes, such as mastitis. These diseases are discussed elsewhere in this section.

Anatomic Causes

Anatomic causes of downer cows usually occur secondary to systemic causes, but not always. Compression injury of the hind limbs is the most common of the anatomic causes. The predilection for hind limb, as opposed to forelimb involvement appears to occur because the sternum and brisket bear the weight of the forward part of the body in a recumbent cow. In contrast, cattle in sternal recumbency normally position one hind limb under the body, subjecting it to the entire weight and pressure of the hindquarters.

In experiments, healthy, nonpregnant cows were held in sternal recumbency under halothane anesthesia. Periods of sternal recumbency as short as 6 hours produced downers in half of the animals. Postmortem observation revealed both ischemic and hemorrhagic lesions of large muscle groups.

Gross lesions of the sciatic nerve were found in the region where the nerve wraps around the caudal aspect of the hip joint. Further distally, the common peroneal branch of the sciatic nerve was often damaged lateral to the stifle joint.

Calving paralysis, or preferably "maternal obstetric paralysis," is a common neurogenic cause of downer syndrome, especially in primiparous cows. Calving paralysis occurs when the obturator nerve or L6 root of the sciatic nerve is compressed by a large calf passing through the birth canal. The L6 root is vulnerable to fetal-induced compression at the site where it passes tightly across a ridge on the ventral part of the sacral wing.

Forelimb paralysis is an occasional cause of downer syndrome. Forelimb neurologic problems occur after lateral recumbency. While forelimb paralysis cases are often referred to as radial paralysis, brachial plexus compression between the shoulder joint and the rib cage is more likely. The problem can be prevented by pulling the downside forelimb cranially so the shoulder joint is not against the rib cage.

Hip luxation is the most common skeletal lesion in downer cows, but fracture of the femoral head or neck is also found. A thorough physical examination with manual manipulation is usually necessary to confirm a diagnosis of hip dislocation.

Other anatomic causes of downer cow syndrome include vertebral fractures, spinal abscesses, and neoplasia, especially lymphosarcoma, involving the spinal cord. These cases are usually sporadic and not associated with parturition.

SIGNALMENT AND CLINICAL SIGNS

The alert downer cow maintains an appetite although at a reduced level. Manure passage is less frequent than normal, and the feces are often relatively dry. Vital signs are usually in the normal range, but an increased respiratory rate and panting are also common and may be related to pain and struggling to rise. Dark urine, which may even be brown due to myoglobin breakdown, seldom lasts more than 2 or 3 days.

Downer cows usually assume the normal bovine sternal recumbency position. With time, abnormal postures and malpositions may occur. Crawling movements and attempts to rise are most common during the first few days of recumbency. With time urine scalding and decubital sores develop in the absence of aggressive nursing care.

CLINICAL PATHOLOGY

Serum concentrations of minerals and electrolytes, especially calcium, phosphorus, potassium, and magnesium, are helpful in differentiating systemic metabolic causes of downer syndrome from primary or secondary anatomic causes. Primary abnormalities associated with these minerals are covered in other parts of this section. Complete blood counts are also useful in differentiating infectious and endotoxic causes from anatomic causes.

Prognosis is important in the management of downer cows. The extent of muscle damage can be evaluated by serum creatine phosphokinase (CPK) activity, as this enzyme is fairly specific to muscle tissue. Unfortunately, this interpretation does not work well in application because CPK activity in the blood is short-lived, and hence the CPK activity changes rapidly with time after the initial muscle insult.

When blood samples were taken from cows subjected to anesthetic-induced recumbency for 6 to 12 hours, there was no significant difference in CPK activity values during the first 24 hours post anesthesia when cows that recovered were compared with cows that became downers. However, there were differences in serum CPK dynamics whereby cows that recovered peaked at 24 hours, while CPK values in cows that became downers continued to rise until 48 hours after induction of recumbency. After this, CPK values fell rapidly in the downer group even though they remained recumbent.

Due to the short half-life in blood, CPK activity falls rather than accumulates in the face of ongoing muscle damage. Therefore, there is no "magic number" CPK value for prognosis. CPK activity could be useful if one has a good estimate of how long a cow has been down before the sample is taken and the CPK values are compared with published experimental data for a similar duration of recumbency.

DIAGNOSIS

Diagnosis is aimed at determining the cause of recumbency, keeping in mind that anatomic lesions frequently develop secondary to systemic lesions. A proper diagnosis is the best means of arriving at an accurate prognosis. A good history is an important starting place. Important questions are: Is the condition associated with calving? If so, was there dystocia? How old is the cow? Does she have a history of milk fever? Was she treated for hypocalcemia? How long has the cow been down? Where did it go down? If the animal has been moved, by what means was it moved? Does the cow make attempts to rise or move? Have these attempts changed with time? Have attempts been made to lift the cow? By what means and for how long? Does the cow have an appetite? If treated for hypocalcemia, did she display signs of response, such as passing manure after calcium administration? What kind of nursing care has been given?

When a cow is lying in sternal recumbency, physical diagnostic procedures are difficult to perform. Hip clamps are useful for lifting the cow for physical examination. Hip clamps should always be well padded and used sparingly. As soon as the cow is lifted the limbs should be evaluated. Can the forelimbs bear weight and is there any strength in the hind limbs? Cows that will not attempt to bear weight on the forelimbs are often, but not necessarily, down due to systemic causes. The hindquarters can be lowered gradually and the strength of the hind limbs evaluated.

When the cow is supported by hip clamps, the hind legs should be carefully evaluated for neurologic, muscular, and skeletal lesions. Knuckling over on the fetlock is indicative of peroneal nerve damage. The cow should be evaluated from behind for asymmetry which would indicate a hip abnormality or lumbosacral luxation. A manual examination per rectum is helpful in diagnosing pelvic fractures or hip luxation, which are often manifest by crepitus or asymmetry. While the cow is lifted it is a good time to examine the udder and reproductive tract, especially the udder. It is beneficial to milk the cows to lessen the risk of mastitis and reduce intramammary pressure.

TREATMENT

Farm personnel should be encouraged to consider the downer cow as an emergency case which requires immediate attention to prevent further complications. First, the cow should be moved off concrete onto a comfortable, clean, dry, nonslip surface. A manure pack should be avoided to prevent mastitis. Fresh straw is acceptable, but difficult to keep clean. Sand as bedding is most satisfactory. Having enough help available after calcium treatment is advisable to provide manual assistance when the cow attempts to stand. If the cow must be moved more than several meters, then a sled made from a material such as plywood should be used. It is important that ropes or cables used to pull the cow be applied to the sled and not directly to the cow.

Treatment will vary depending on the diagnosis. The reader is referred to other parts of this text for descriptions of treatment of systemic problems such as hypocalcemia, hypophosphatemia, and toxic mastitis. Regardless of specific treatment, good nursing care is critical. The prognostic outlook for a downer depends not only on the status of the cow but also on the commitment of her caretakers. If a downer is not lifted, frequent rolling from side to side is important to prevent tissue damage due to compression. A variety of lifting methods have been used with downers to lessen tissue compressive damage. Hip clamps are dangerous and should be used for diagnosis only. They are less dangerous when combined with a movable cart and chest sling which will support the foreparts of the body. Abdominal slings are less harmful than hip clamps, but they put pressure on the abdominal viscera which in turn are pushed against the diaphragm making inspiration difficult. A good sling, however, will distribute some of the body weight to the sternum, making abdominal pressure less of a problem.

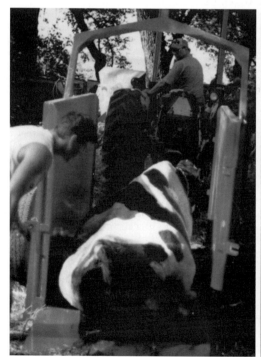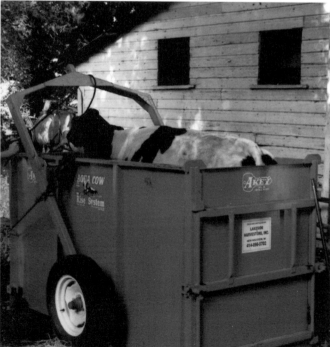

Figure 1
A downer cow being pulled into a flotation tank (left) and being floated (right).

The only method of lifting a downer without causing pressure damage is flotation. Commercially available flotation tanks have been enthusiastically received by dairy producers. Tanks are available with removable wheels, which allow easy transport. For loading into the flotation tank, the cow is manually positioned on a mat which is then pulled by a mechanical winch into the tank (Fig. 1, left). Once the cow is positioned in the tank, the ends are replaced and secured with turnbuckles. Leakage is prevented by wide rubber gaskets which seal the interface of side and end pieces (Fig. 1, right). Once sealed the tank is rapidly filled with warm water. About 700 gal are required to float a cow. The water can be heated by the sun in warm weather or a gas-fired boiler (optional with tank purchase) during cold weather. A 5-cm (2-in.)-diameter water supply is recommended to fill the flotation tank rapidly.

Flotation times should be at least 6 hours and times up to 24 hours have been useful. During the entire time of flotation it is important to maintain the water temperature at or near body temperature. After flotation, the water is drained, the tank ends removed, and the cow is encouraged to exit onto an adjacent nonslip surface.

There are two approaches to the management of downer cows. Either aggressive therapy, including lifting, preferably by flotation, or conservative therapy can be employed. Conservative therapy consists of providing good bedding such as sand or grass along with adequate nursing care such as rolling, but without lifting. In all cases, appropriate therapy for systemic disorders is required for recovery to occur.

If the client is unwilling to invest time and effort in proper management, euthanasia should be considered. A proper diagnosis is important so that time is not wasted on hopeless cases.

PREVENTION

The two most important factors in prevention of the downer condition are reduction of the risk of milk fever and provision of safe, nonslip calving areas. Prevention of milk fever is covered in another part of this section. As dry cows near the time of parturition it is best to move them into well-bedded calving stalls. Sand is an excellent and inexpensive bedding material for calving stalls. Close observation of cows will also aid in preventing downers. Prompt diagnosis and treatment of hypocalcemia, and skilled handling of dystocia will reduce the risk of downer cows.

BIBLIOGRAPHY

Correa MT, Erb HN, Scarlett JM: Risk factors for downer cow syndrome. J Dairy Sci 76:3460–3463, 1993.
Cox VS: Nonsystemic causes of the downer cow syndrome. Vet Clin North Am Food Anim Pract 4:413–433, 1988.
Smith BP, Angelos J, George LW, et al: Down Cows: Causes and Treatments. Proceedings of the American Association of Bovine Practitioners, 1997, pp 43–45.

■ Ketosis

Thomas H. Herdt, D.V.M., M.S., Diplomate, A.C.V.N. and A.C.V.I.M.
Brian J. Gerloff, D.V.M., Ph.D.

OCCURRENCE

Ketosis is generally a disease of dairy cows in the period from parturition to 6 weeks postpartum. Recent reports of lactational ketosis incidence range from approximately 5% to 16%. In some herds, ketosis can be a particular problem and can affect a large proportion of at-risk cows (i.e., those in early lactation). Ketosis is occasionally seen prepartum in dairy and beef cows, in which case the condition resembles pregnancy toxemia of ewes. Cows carrying twins and receiving low-energy diets are at increased risk of prepartum ketosis.

According to available reports, ketosis has a rather low heritability. The occurrence of ketosis in one lactation does not greatly increase the risk of development of the disease in a subsequent lactation. Age has little influence on ketosis risk, although in specific herds it may occur as a problem in one age group, but the age group affected is not consistent among herds. Dry cows and pregnant heifers that are overly fat are at increased risk of developing ketosis after calving.

Clinical ketosis is frequently associated with concurrent diseases, both infectious and metabolic. In many cases, ketosis may occur secondary to another disease. In other instances, ketosis may be the initial disease, or it may at least be a predisposing factor with respect to the occurrence of other diseases. This may be related, in part, to suppressed immune function associated with hyperketonemia, although other factors may also come into play.

Ketosis may be clinical or subclinical, and both forms are associated with reduced milk production and reduced reproductive efficiency. The economic impact of ketosis is derived from treatment costs, reduced milk production, a generalized increase in morbidity, and reduced fertility. The disease is seldom fatal, so death loss is not an important economic factor.

ETIOLOGY AND PATHOGENESIS

The initial event in the pathogenesis of all forms of ketosis is negative energy balance and the accompanying mobilization of non-esterified fatty acids (NEFAs) from adipose tissue. Negative energy balance is prevalent, perhaps universal, in dairy cows during the first 2 to 6 weeks of lactation, because feed intake does not keep pace with the rapid increase in energy demands for milk production. The occurrence of ketosis is determined by the metabolic fate of NEFAs. There is an indication that distinct metabolic types of ketosis might exist, dependent on hepatic patterns of NEFA metabolism.

Figure 1 illustrates two potential pathways of hepatic NEFA metabolism. With respect to metabolic disease development, ketogenesis and esterification are the most important pathways. NEFA entry into the ketogenic pathway predisposes to development of clinical ketosis, whereas entry into the esterification pathway favors fatty liver development. It is likely that glucose availability is an important factor in determining the relative activity of the two pathways of NEFA disposal. When glucose availability is very low, entry of NEFA into the ketogenic pathway is favored. With somewhat higher glucose availability, esterification and fat accumulation are favored. Thus, glucose availability, in addition to negative energy balance and NEFA mobilization, is an important factor in the pathogenesis of clinical ketosis.

Glucose supply is a constant metabolic challenge for ruminants, because fermentative digestion destroys most of the available carbohydrates in their diets. Early lactation is a particularly challenging period because of the high glucose requirement for milk production. Two factors determine glucose availability: (1) rate of gluconeogenesis and (2) availability of gluconeogenetic substrate. The metabolic type of ketosis that develops is probably dependent on which of these two factors is most adversely affected.

The first factor, rate of gluconeogenesis, may be impaired in those cases of ketosis that develop within the first week of

Blood NEFA

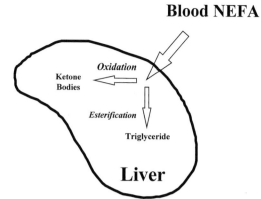

Figure 1

Metabolic pathways of nonesterified fatty acids (NEFAs) in the liver. After being absorbed by the liver, NEFAs can undergo esterification, resulting in triglyceride formation, or oxidation, resulting in ketone body formation. The consequence of high blood NEFA concentrations is determined by the relative activity of these two pathways: when ketogenesis predominates, ketosis is favored; when esterification predominates, fatty liver is favored. Glucose availability influences the activity of these pathways, with low glucose availability favoring oxidation.

lactation. Evidence suggests that hepatic fat accumulation prior to calving may interfere with gluconeogenesis. Thus, the progression of metabolic events in this type of ketosis is proposed to be (1) prepartum adipose lysis and NEFA mobilization, (2) NEFA esterification with fatty liver development, (3) reduced gluconeogenesis, (4) reduced glucose availability, (5) a shift in NEFA metabolism from esterification to ketogenesis, and (6) ketosis development. The term *periparturient ketosis* could describe this type of ketosis. Peripartum ketosis is reported to respond experimentally to glucagon administration, further suggesting that reduced gluconeogenesis plays a role in its pathophysiology.

Ketosis cases that develop later during lactation, near the time of peak milk production, may be of a different metabolic type. In this case it appears that availability of gluconeogenetic substrate is simply insufficient to meet the demands of milk production. This results in high NEFA concentrations, with a large portion of NEFA being directed into ketogenesis rather than esterification. *Peak-lactation ketosis* might be a suitable descriptive term for this condition. It is this manifestation of ketosis that fits the classical description of the disease in most older textbooks of veterinary medicine. This type of ketosis is reported to be nonresponsive to experimental glucagon therapy.

CLINICAL SIGNS AND SIGNALMENT

Cows that develop periparturient ketosis are frequently fat, whereas those that develop peak-lactation ketosis may be thin. The most common complaints at presentation include a sharp drop in milk production, a generally depressed attitude, and partial or complete anorexia. Slight dehydration may be evident, but vital signs are usually normal, and findings on physical examination are generally unremarkable.

Occasionally, marked central nervous system signs occur with ketosis. This has been referred to as *nervous ketosis*. The signs are quite variable and may include excitement and hyperesthesia, depraved chewing and licking (occasionally with self-mutilation), or abnormal gait (including hypermetria or ataxia).

CLINICAL PATHOLOGY

Clinical pathologic signs include hyperketonemia and ketonuria, hypoglycemia, and high blood concentrations of NEFA.

Values for these variables do not correspond closely with clinical signs, so exacting cut-off values are difficult to establish. Clinical cases are usually associated with plasma glucose concentrations less than 35 mg/dL and NEFA concentrations greater than 1000 μEq/L. Care must be taken in the interpretation of blood ketone body concentrations, as they may be expressed differently depending on the nature of the laboratory determination. Cases of clinical ketosis are usually associated with total ketone body (acetone, acetoacetate, and β-hydroxybutyrate) concentrations greater than 30 mg/dL. β-hydroxybutyrate concentrations alone are usually greater than 25 mg/dL. For quantitative determination of serum or plasma concentrations, β-hydroxybutyrate is preferable to acetoacetate or acetone because it is stable in the sample. It should be recognized, however, that commonly used semiquantitative methods (e.g., dipsticks) often measure only acetoacetate or acetoacetate plus acetone. The concentration of acetoacetate plus acetone usually constitutes only 10% to 20% of the β-hydroxybutyrate value, although this proportion increases in clinical ketosis. Urine ketone body concentrations are usually two to four times higher than blood concentrations, whereas milk ketone body concentrations are usually 40% to 50% of blood concentrations.

DIAGNOSIS

Diagnosis is usually based on clinical signs and the presence of detectable concentrations of ketone bodies in urine or milk. Field testing of urine and milk is done with semiquantitative methods based on visually discernible color changes. Dipsticks should be protected from moisture during storage to avoid false-negative results. The difference in ketone body concentrations between urine and milk make urine testing more sensitive but less specific than milk testing. Urine ketone body (acetoacetate) concentrations in peak-lactation ketosis are frequently very high (80 to 160 mg/dL) whereas those for periparturient ketosis will frequently be lower (20 to 40 mg/dL), as estimated by dipstick analysis.

Practical methods for diagnosis of subclinical ketosis have not been readily available in North America, although automated monitoring of milk acetone concentrations has been available in some Scandinavian countries. A recently developed dipstick method for estimation of β-hydroxybutyric acid in milk appears to be a practical means of monitoring for subclinical ketosis.* Milk concentrations of β-hydroxybutyric in excess of 1 to 2 mg/dL appear to be indicative of subclinical ketosis with associated risk of clinical ketosis, other diseases, reduced fertility, and impaired milk production.

TREATMENT

The prognosis and response to therapy are dependent on the type of ketosis. Peak lactation ketosis usually responds quickly to therapy, but relapses are common if the diet is not corrected. Periparturient ketosis responds less rapidly to treatment. Periparturient ketosis is closely associated with fatty liver, as discussed in "Fatty Liver in Dairy Cows" in this section.

Treatment is aimed at reducing ketogenesis and reestablishing glucose homeostasis. Bolus administration of 500 mL of 50% glucose or dextrose solution has been a standard treatment. Much of this dose is probably lost in the urine owing to the induction of serum glucose concentrations in excess of the renal glucose threshold. Nevertheless, the treatment is often effective. The high blood glucose concentrations associated with bolus intravenous (IV) infusion suppress both adipose NEFA release

---

*Ketolac BHB, Sanwa, Nagoya, Japan.

and hepatic ketogenesis, both favorable effects in ketosis therapy. The mechanisms of these effects are probably both insulin and non-insulin dependent. The major problem with bolus IV glucose therapy is that relapses are common. In situations in which it is practical, continuous IV infusion of glucose is beneficial. Fructose and sorbitol have been used as alternatives to glucose therapy. This sugar and sugar alcohol, respectively, are expected to supply glucose directly at the hepatic level. This is in contrast to the direct administration of glucose, in which the administered glucose would be available to all tissues.

Glucocorticoid therapy is also effective. Appropriate dosages of dexamethasone* and isoflupredone acetate† are 1.33 mg per 45 kg of body weight. Glucocorticoids do not appear to induce gluconeogenesis in ruminants, but rather they seem to affect glucose distribution and kinetics. This may be favorable in terms of ketosis therapy, because increased gluconeogenesis is usually associated with increased ketogenesis. Ketotic cows treated with glucocorticoids are less subject to relapses than are those treated with IV glucose therapy alone, although relapses can still occur. Due to the immunosuppressive nature of glucocorticoids, care should be observed in their administration to animals with infectious disease concurrent with ketosis.

Insulin, in conjunction with glucocorticoid therapy, may be more effective than glucocorticoids alone. Insulin is a powerful antiketogenic agent and also suppresses NEFA mobilization. It is important to provide a glucocorticoid or other agent, however, to counteract the hypoglycemic effects of insulin. A long-lasting form of insulin should be used. The usual dose is 200 to 300 IU per animal. Administration is repeated as necessary, usually at 24- to 48-hour intervals.

Several compounds, if administered orally, can serve as glucose precursors in ruminants. Of these, propylene glycol and salts of propionic acid have been most popular. Dosages of propylene glycol usually have been in the range of 250 to 400 g (approximately 8 to 14 oz), administered orally twice daily. Excessive dosage can result in incoordination and depression of consciousness.

PREVENTION

Prevention of peak lactation ketosis is directed toward maximizing energy intake and providing adequate glucose precursors. Feed intake is usually the most critical factor in determining energy balance of early-lactation dairy cows, so the first effort should be to maximize feed intake. This is achieved by making sure that feed is available nearly constantly, and that there is not excessive competition at the feed bunk. Rations should be well balanced for all nutrients, especially for carbohydrate components. Intake of insufficient amounts of starches and other nonstructural carbohydrates results in ration-energy densities that are too low to provide maximum energy intakes. In addition, nonstructural carbohydrates promote a relatively high proportion of propionate in the ruminal volatile fatty acids. Propionate is an important glucose precursor. However, excessive dietary nonstructural carbohydrates, relative to structural carbohydrates and effective fiber, can lead to rumen acidosis and reduced feed intake, thus reducing total energy intake. Thus, rations must be well formulated to provide maximum energy and sufficient effective fiber.

Forage quality for early lactation cows should be the best available. This promotes both energy intake and total feed intake. Fermentation characteristics of fermented forages can influence the incidence of ketosis. Hay crop forages ensiled at high moisture contents are prone to fermentation patterns that

produce butyric acid. In addition to being unpalatable to cows, much of the butyric acid is converted to β-hydroxybutyric acid as it is absorbed through the rumen wall. This enhances the total ketone body load on the animal and increases risk of ketosis.

The effect of dietary fat on the incidence of ketosis is unclear. Addition of fat to diets does increase their energy density. Dietary fat is absorbed in the form of chylomicrons and should not contribute substantially to blood NEFA concentrations. Fat, however, cannot contribute to glucose synthesis, so calories from fat do not directly improve glucose balance. There is speculation that provision of supplemental dietary fat may reduce the need for fatty acid synthesis in the mammary gland. This may indirectly improve glucose balance because glucose is an important energy source for fatty acid synthesis in the mammary gland.

The use of specific feed additives, such as niacin, propylene glycol, and ionophores, along with prevention of periparturient ketosis is discussed in "Fatty Liver in Dairy Cows" in this section.

BIBLIOGRAPHY

Foster LA: Clinical ketosis. Vet Clin North Am Food Anim Pract 4:253–267, 1988.
Herdt TH, Emery RS: Therapy of diseases of ruminant intermediary metabolism. Vet Clin North Am Food Anim Pract 8:91–106, 1992.
Holtenius P, Holtenius K: New aspects of ketone-bodies in energy-metabolism of dairy-cows: A review. J Vet Med 43(series A):579–587, 1996.
Schultz LH: Ketosis. *In* Larson BL, Smith VR (eds): Lactation: A Comprehensive Treatise, vol 2. New York, Academic Press, 1974.

■ Pregnancy Toxemia of Ewes

Joseph S. Rook, D.V.M.

Pregnancy toxemia is a metabolic disease that commonly affects ewes during late pregnancy. Terminology such as twin lamb disease, lambing sickness, lambing paralysis, or lambing ketosis is often used to describe the disease. Pregnancy toxemia is common in both range and farm flocks in the United States and can affect both overconditioned and thin ewes, usually pregnant with multiple fetuses. Ewes pregnant with a single fetus are occasionally involved. Clinical cases are typically limited to older ewes during their second or subsequent pregnancies. Pregnancy toxemia is seldom observed in bred replacement ewe lambs or in yearlings bred for their first pregnancy.

OCCURRENCE

Pregnancy toxemia in the ewe flock typically occurs during the last 2 to 4 weeks of gestation. Clinical cases usually follow a period of negative energy balance resulting in hypoglycemia, increased fat catabolism, ketonemia, and ketonuria in susceptible ewes. In commercial production systems a multitude of nutritional, metabolic, and management factors influence clinical expression of pregnancy toxemia. These include the following: (1) increased nutritional demands related to the developing fetal-placental unit; (2) reduced rumen capacity; (3) improper, declining, or interrupted feed supply; (4) management, environmental, transport, shearing, or predator stresses; (5) concurrent disease; and (6) individual ewe susceptibility. From a clinical standpoint, some authors divide the causes of pregnancy toxemia into four broad categories: (1) primary pregnancy toxemia, (2) fat-ewe pregnancy toxemia, (3) starvation pregnancy toxemia, and (4) secondary pregnancy toxemia. Primary pregnancy toxe-

---
*Azium, Schering Corporation, Union, NJ.
†Predef 2X, Pharmacia-Upjohn Company, Kalamazoo, Mich.

mia is common, resulting from a drop in the plane of nutrition during late pregnancy and/or management changes that create a brief period of fasting. Fat-ewe pregnancy toxemia results from an overconditioning of the ewe flock during early pregnancy, followed by a late gestational decline in nutrition. Starvation pregnancy toxemia involves excessively thin ewes whose condition usually results from mismanagement of feed resources or lack of availability of feed following periods of drought. Secondary pregnancy toxemia has a more sporadic occurrence and is the result of a primary concurrent disease in affected ewes.

Clinical cases of pregnancy toxemia occur sporadically, unpredictably, and at a low level in most flocks—independent of adequate management and feeding practices. Morbidity is usually quite low, involving less than 1% to 2% of the ewe flock, yet mortality rates often exceed 80% of affected animals. Furthermore, sporadic cases of pregnancy disease often involve animals with concurrent health problems (e.g., postshearing pneumonia, age-related poor dentition, lameness) initiating a cycle of partial or complete anorexia followed by fat catabolism and ketosis. Occasional cases of pregnancy toxemia, even in well-managed flocks, may also suggest that certain genetic lines or families may be predisposed to developing pregnancy toxemia. Therefore, offspring from affected ewes should not be retained for flock replacements.

Pregnancy toxemia can also occur as a flock problem and is usually characterized by the onset of numerous clinical cases during the last month of gestation. The majority of these cases occur during the last 2 to 3 weeks of gestation. When flock outbreaks occur morbidity is high, often involving 5% to 10% of the ewe flock. The mortality rate often exceeds 80% of untreated individuals and economic losses can be substantial. Flock problems usually result from improper feeding management decisions or sudden weather changes that generate nutritional, environmental, or psychological stresses that affect the pregnant ewe.

PATHOPHYSIOLOGY: DISRUPTION OF GLUCOSE HOMEOSTASIS

The pathophysiology of pregnancy toxemia is still not well understood. Research and clinical experience suggest that most clinical cases of pregnancy toxemia can be prevented by balancing the nutritional intake of the dam with the increased late gestational requirements of the fetal-placental unit. Late-gestation fetal growth and pregnancy requirements are substantial, about 1.5 times (ewe with a single lamb) to 2 times (ewe with twins) above maintenance requirements. Furthermore, 80% of fetal growth occurs during the last 6 weeks of gestation. During this time, the energy requirements of the fetal-placental unit are derived almost entirely from glucose and lactate, consuming nearly 30% to 40% of maternally produced glucose. Fetal energy (glucose) requirements increase at a time when rumen capacity is compromised by the developing fetus, placing additional stress on maternal glucose production. In addition, fetal uptake of glucose appears to be independent of blood glucose regulation in the dam. Thus, glucose requirements of the fetus are met at the expense of glucose homeostasis in the dam. Although it is often detrimental to the dam (and ultimately to the fetus), this prioritization of glucose supply is a safety mechanism that ensures short-term fetal viability, even in the presence of declining blood glucose concentrations in the dam. Failure of glucose homeostatic mechanisms in the ewe is thought to be the metabolic event that initiates pregnancy toxemia. However, this does not explain why some ewes develop low blood glucose levels (20 to 40 mg/dL) during late pregnancy but do not develop ketonemia, ketonuria, and clinical signs associated with pregnancy toxemia.

Although disruption in blood glucose homeostasis in susceptible animals appears to trigger symptoms associated with pregnancy toxemia, variability between individual animals in their susceptibility to pregnancy toxemia appears to result from individual differences in ability to maintain glucose homeostasis. Flock populations contain individuals that have varying susceptibility or resistance to pregnancy toxemia. Susceptible individuals exhibit impaired insulin function. Insulin-resistant animals may be unable to regulate glucose homeostasis during late pregnancy and may, therefore, be more susceptible to pregnancy toxemia than are animals with normal insulin sensitivity. It is theorized that constant fetal drain of glucose results in reduced insulin production, thus reducing the ability of pregnancy toxemia–susceptible animals to respond to fluctuations in blood glucose. Impaired intravenous (IV) glucose tolerance test results associated with pregnancy toxemia–susceptible individuals suggest that pregnancy toxemia may be very similar to insulin-dependent diabetes mellitus in humans. Genetic diversity in insulin resistance or sensitivity might explain the diversity of flock management conditions under which pregnancy toxemia occurs. It is not uncommon to observe long-established flocks with inadequate feeding practices that experience very few cases of pregnancy toxemia each spring. In these flocks, insulin-resistant individuals may have been naturally culled from the genetic pool.

CLINICAL SIGNS AND DIAGNOSIS

Pregnancy toxemia should be suspected whenever late-pregnant ewes exhibit neurologic signs of motor weakness and die within 3 to 10 days. Other disease considerations would include hypocalcemia, listeriosis, and meningeal worm infection. Clinical signs of pregnancy toxemia are characterized by anorexia, hypoglycemia, ketonemia, ketonuria, weakness, depression, incoordination, mental dullness, and impaired vision, followed by recumbency and death. Early clinical signs often go unnoticed, as affected ewes behave sluggishly and approach feeders with the remainder of the flock, yet fail to eat. As the disease progresses, affected ewes separate themselves from the flock; they appear blind and disoriented and often wander into objects or stand in the same area, failing to flee from approaching people or dogs. Affected ewes typically grind their teeth and appear constipated. In the later stages of the disease, weakness and mental dullness increase. Recumbency is common. Affected ewes will often stand when helped and will walk several steps before collapsing to a recumbent position. In the terminal phases of the disease, affected animals are unable to stand. Head pressing, muscle tremors, subtle convulsions, twitching of the lips, and star-gazing postures are often noted. Strong positive reactions on urine ketone body test strips and a ketone-body smell to the breath are also helpful diagnostic aids. Recumbency usually develops 3 to 4 days after observation of early clinical signs, followed by death in another 3 to 4 days.

Fetal death without parturition is a common complication in pregnancy toxemia. Recovery may result if the dead fetuses are expelled or if they are removed by cesarean section or corticosteroid-induced parturition.

TREATMENT

Prior to treatment of individual animals, practitioners should discuss treatment options, costs, and possible results with the producer. Many small flock owners fail to recognize the severity of the situation and, therefore, place unrealistic expectations on

Table 1
SUGGESTED BODY CONDITION SCORES (1 TO 5 SCALE) FOR THE EWE AT VARIOUS STAGES OF PRODUCTION*

Stage of Production	Suggested Body Condition Score
Maintenance	2
Breeding	2.5
Early gestation	2.5–3
Late gestation	3–3.5
Lambing	3.5
Weaning	2–2.5

*Note the increase in condition score as parturition approaches.

the veterinarian. Unless affected animals are valuable breeding stock, the potential economic value of the lambs, not the ewe, is of primary producer concern. Thus, most commercial producers will choose to medically support the ewe until parturition and recovery or death occurs. Prevention of pregnancy toxemia in the remainder of the flock is much more important and economically beneficial for the producer than is treatment of clinically ill animals.

Treatment should be aimed at correcting energy, electrolyte, and acid-base imbalances and dehydration and stimulating appetite. Treatment of recumbent ewes is difficult and frequently unrewarding. Multiple electrolyte, acid-base, and fluid imbalances are usually present. Animals of high value should receive IV replacement electrolytes, fluids, and glucose, based on serum chemistry profiles. An intensive treatment regimen calls for placement of an indwelling IV catheter for administration of fluids. Five to 7 g of glucose plus appropriate electrolytes should be administered intravenously every 3 to 4 hours. Additionally, 20 to 40 units of a repository insulin preparation should be administered intramuscularly at 48-hour intervals.

Traditional, less-intensive treatment of pregnancy toxemia includes oral drenching with 100 to 200 mL of propylene glycol solution or corn syrup 2 to 4 times daily. This is in addition to IV administration of 250 mL of 20% dextrose or 500 mL of 10% dextrose during the farm visit. B complex vitamins, with or without 50 to 125 mL of a 20% calcium borogluconate solution, are commonly administered subcutaneously or added to the IV fluid solutions. Recently developed oral calcium gel preparations may be safer than IV administration of calcium. Success of this treatment regimen depends on the severity of the condition at the time that treatment is initiated. If affected ewes are identified early in the course of the disease, repeated oral drenching with propylene glycol alone (or in combination with a commercial calf-scour oral rehydration solution) may be effective.

Treatment may also be aimed at removing the source of glucose drain on the dam. This usually involves removal of the lambs by cesarean section or by induction of parturition. In either case, treatment is usually directed at saving the life of the ewe at the expense of her lambs. Lambs that are born more than 7 days early seldom survive. Removal of the lambs should be reserved for the early stages of pregnancy toxemia, before the ewe's condition is irreversible and fetal death has occurred. A parenteral dose of 20 mg of dexamethasone sodium phosphate per ewe is commonly used to induce parturition. Lambing in healthy ewes usually occurs about 48 to 72 hours postinjection. Induction of parturition is quite variable and is often unreliable in advanced pregnancy toxemia.

PREVENTION

Flock problems with pregnancy toxemia can usually be prevented by designing a practical nutritional program tailored to the production requirements of the flock and the feeding system involved. However, feeding recommendations are only as effective as the producer's ability to comply with the recommendations. In most parts of this country sheep are forage-based animals, and as such they receive limited concentrate-type feeds. Concentrates, when fed at all, are generally limited to breeding, late gestation, and lactation (in winter-lambing systems) phases of production. Body condition scores (Table 1) should also be monitored to ensure (1) that ewes are not overconditioned during early gestation and (2) that the plane of nutrition rises during the second half of gestation. For specific recommendations see *Special Dietary Management in Lactation and Gestation* in the last edition of this book (p. 204).

BIBLIOGRAPHY

Bauman DE, Durrie WB: Partitioning of nutrients during pregnancy and lactation: A review of mechanisms involving homeostasis and homeorrhesis. J Dairy Sci 63:1514–1529, 1980.

Lynch GP, Jackson C: A method for assessing the nutritional status of gestating ewes. Can J Anim Sci 63:603–611, 1983.

Marteniuk JV: Pregnancy toxemia and ketosis of ewes and does. Vet Clin North Am Food Anim Pract 4:30, 1988.

Sigurdsson H: Susceptibility to pregnancy disease in ewes and its relation to gestational diabetes. Acta Vet Scand 29:407–414, 1988.

Wastney ME, Arcus AC, Bickerstaffe R, et al: Glucose tolerance in ewes and susceptibility to pregnancy toxemia. Aust J Biol Sci 35:381–392, 1982.

■ Fatty Liver in Dairy Cattle

Brian J. Gerloff, D.V.M., Ph.D.
Thomas H. Herdt, D.V.M., M.S., Diplomate, A.C.V.N. and A.C.V.I.M.

OCCURRENCE

Health problems in fat cows have been clinically associated with fatty infiltration of the liver and other organs. Clinical disease as well as subclinical effects of mild fatty liver have been described around the time of calving in all breeds of dairy cattle in all parts of the world. The clinical and subclinical problem usually occurs in obese dairy cattle within 1 to 2 weeks of calving. Clinical problems are usually apparent after calving, but they occasionally become evident prior to calving. The disease is unusual in primiparous cows, but it does occur. It is most common in mature, high-producing cattle. Mild cases of fatty liver are associated with reduced fertility and severe cases with increased culling, disease, and death.

ETIOLOGY AND PATHOGENESIS

The intrahepatic fat that accumulates in bovine fatty liver is primarily composed of triglyceride. Cattle do not synthesize fatty acid precursors of triglyceride in the liver; thus, fatty acids that accumulate as triglycerides in bovine fatty liver must be extrahepatic in origin. Fatty acids are stored as triglycerides in adipose tissue until mobilized. When they are mobilized in response to energy demand, adipose triglyceride is converted to non-esterified fatty acid (NEFA) and glycerol. The NEFAs are transported in the circulation bound to albumin. They can be extracted from the blood and used as an energy source by various tissues, including the mammary gland, liver, spleen, and muscle. However, the liver extracts a large portion of circulating NEFA because of its high blood flow and high NEFA extraction efficiency.

In the liver, these fatty acids can undergo partial or complete oxidation or reesterification to triglyceride, as discussed further in this section in "Ketosis." Esterified fatty acids remain in the liver as triglyceride until they can be oxidized or exported in lipoprotein particles. Secretion of triglyceride from the liver is a process requiring repackaging of the triglyceride in an envelope of cholesterol, phospholipid, and specific proteins.

Serum lipoprotein and cholesterol concentrations are low in cows with fatty liver, suggesting reduced hepatic lipoprotein output. However, it is clear that hepatic lipoprotein output is extremely low in all bovine liver, whether or not fatty liver is present. The metabolic machinery for hepatic lipoprotein synthesis and secretion appears to be rudimentary in the liver of adult cattle. Once fatty acids are taken up by the liver and reesterified to triglyceride, their removal is a very slow process. Thus, the major variable factor contributing to the accumulation of hepatic triglyceride in cows is an increase in circulating NEFA concentration, not a decline in lipoprotein output.

Fatty liver development can occur very rapidly. Within 48 hours, hepatic triglyceride levels can increase from less than 5% wet weight to more than 25%, under conditions of extreme adipose mobilization. Hepatic triglyceride accumulation usually begins prepartum and reaches maximum concentration in the immediate postpartum period. The lipid accumulation is triggered by the increasing serum NEFA concentrations observed at this time. The likely primary cause of increasing NEFA concentrations is declining dry matter intake (DMI). Serum NEFA concentrations are inversely related to DMI over the peripartum period. Declining DMI occurs in almost all cows as they approach parturition, but it is exacerbated in obese cows and also under conditions of environmental and nutritional stress. What triggers the decline in DMI is unknown. It may be related to endocrine changes that occur at parturition. Increasing estrogen concentrations just prior to calving, in particular, have been suspected as a possible cause, and the role of estrogen in the development of hepatic lipidosis has been investigated without yielding clear results. Reversing the prepartum decline in DMI by force-feeding has been shown to reduce the accumulation of hepatic triglycerides at day 1 postpartum. The hormonal milieu at parturition favors the allocation of body reserves away from adipose tissue (increasing growth hormone, decreasing insulin, increasing steroids), all fostering an increase in serum NEFA concentrations. The primary factor resulting in excessive NEFA concentrations, though, appears to be a profound decrease in DMI.

CLINICAL SIGNS

Clinical signs of fatty liver almost always include ketonuria, as might be expected given the close metabolic association between ketosis and fatty liver. Prepartum or postpartum cows affected by fatty liver frequently become extremely anorexic. In addition, they often develop other periparturient disease conditions that fail to respond to normal therapy. These conditions may include retained placenta, metritis, and mastitis. Fatty liver may also be associated with vague CNS signs, such as star-gazing. Without aggressive treatment, clinical fatty liver frequently progresses to weakness, recumbency, and death. Cows with severe fatty liver are at increased risk of culling and death. Affected animals are almost always initially obese (body condition score ≥4.0) at the outset of the dry period. However, weight loss leading to fatty liver is rapid, and at the time of clinical observation and treat-

ment, the cow's body condition may be normal or thin. As clinical fatty liver is frequently a herd-based problem, observation of obese dry cows and thin early-lactation cows is frequently a good clue that there may be some problems with fatty liver in the herd. In addition to severe clinical fatty liver, subclinical fatty liver in the first 3 to 5 weeks postpartum is a problem in many herds and is associated with economic losses, such as delayed postpartum return to estrus and reduced fertility.

Many herd operators can manage even obese cows through the peripartum period reasonably well, until an additional environmental stressor is added. For example, obese cows in a herd may calve and start their lactation in reasonably good health until the weather becomes hot and humid. The addition of heat stress may lead to severe clinical problems with fatty liver and increased rates of concurrent disease and death.

CLINICAL PATHOLOGY

Numerous experimental and clinical trials have demonstrated serum NEFA concentrations to be the blood parameter most reliably related to the development of fatty liver. Recent improvements in laboratory test kits have made determination of serum NEFA concentration a practical tool for diagnosis of excessive adipose mobilization, which is the underlying cause of fatty liver. In cows that develop fatty liver, serum NEFA concentrations are usually elevated several days prior to calving. Measuring serum NEFA concentrations in a group of cows from 1 week prepartum to 1 week postpartum can be a reliable indicator of excessive NEFA mobilization and can aid in making a presumptive herd diagnosis of fatty liver. Serum NEFA concentrations greater than 1000 μEq/L in lactating cows and greater than 325 to 400 μEq/L in prepartum cows should be considered abnormal.

Efforts to use serum concentrations of hepatic enzymes as a diagnostic aid for fatty liver have been mostly unrewarding. In advanced cases of fatty liver, the level of hepatic enzyme aspartate transaminase (AST) is usually elevated. Its correlation with hepatic triglyceride concentrations, however, is not consistent, and until severe hepatic cellular damage occurs in advanced cases of fatty liver, the relationship of liver triglyceride level with serum AST level is weak. Values above 100 units/L are consistent with the existence of fatty liver. Other hepatic enzyme and function tests have consistently shown correlation with the amount of liver triglyceride, but the correlations are small, and the predictive power of the serum or blood tests have been poor. Serum haptoglobin and sulfobromphthalein retention are indications of liver function that would fall into this category. Most of these tests of liver damage and/or function are consistently affected only in extremely advanced cases of fatty liver.

DIAGNOSIS

Clinical ketonuria within 1 week of calving accompanied by depression and/or other peripartum diseases with death loss should be considered presumptive evidence of fatty liver. For a definitive diagnosis, analysis of a liver biopsy for triglyceride or fat is the most reliable method with either an individual or a herd problem. Several quantitative methods of assessing hepatic fat content have been devised. They are compared in Table 1. A classification of severe fatty liver is necessary to substantiate a diagnosis of the clinical syndrome, as some degree of fatty liver is normal in all cows in early lactation. Moderate fatty liver associated with high production and subsequent poor reproduction may be of importance within a herd, but it should not be viewed as a significant clinical health problem.

Excessive fat mobilization and weight loss is necessary to

Table 1
CLASSIFICATION OF HEPATIC LIPIDOSIS

Severity	Histologic TG Content (% Volume)	Chemical TG Content (% Wet Weight)	Chemical TG Content (% Dry Weight)	Bouyancy in Solution of 1.055 Specific Gravity
Mild	0–20	<5.0	<15	Sinks
Moderate	20–40	5.1–10.0	15–30	Sinks
Severe	>40	>10.0	>30	Floats

TG, triglyceride.

produce the high serum NEFA concentrations and rapid hepatic triglyceride buildup associated with fatty liver. This usually involves obese cows. However, if weight loss has been rapid, a cow that is no longer obese may be clinically affected with fatty liver. Evidence of obese dry cows and thin early-lactation cows accompanied by high rates of early lactation metabolic disease, such as ketosis, retained placenta, and elevated cull rates, are strong indications of a herd fatty liver problem. Rate of weight loss is a more important component of the disease syndrome than is weight per se. Liver biopsies and/or postmortem findings should be utilized to verify a presumptive diagnosis.

TREATMENT

Traditional lipotropic agents, such as phospholipids and some amino acids, have not been demonstrated to be of great benefit in treatment of bovine fatty liver. These agents are intended to enhance lipoprotein production, but lipoprotein synthesis and secretion are inherently low in cows, and their rates probably cannot be substantially increased. Careful attention to protein and amino acid nutrition of cows with fatty liver is warranted, but it cannot be expected to have a large therapeutic effect.

Treatment attempts should be focused on reducing further NEFA mobilization and on providing a source of glucose and energy until liver function can improve. Daily administration of 500 mL of a 50% dextrose solution intravenously accompanied by 200 units of long-acting insulin, given once or twice 48 hours apart, can be a practical and effective treatment. In herds experiencing a clinical problem with fatty liver, it is important that this treatment be initiated early, before hepatic triglyceride accumulation becomes extreme and liver function is irreversibly compromised. Remember that hepatic triglyceride accumulation can occur very quickly. In herds with obese dry cows, urine should be monitored for ketone bodies beginning 1 week prior to calving. If ketonuria occurs, glucose therapy should be initiated. Glucose treatment may be required for 7 to 10 days. Our experience suggests that this aggressive treatment is frequently life-saving, although return to high performance does not often occur. Propylene glycol given orally as a glucose precursor is probably not as effective as parenteral glucose. Clinically, our impression is that parenteral administration of glucose is superior to oral administration of propylene glycol, possibly because propylene glycol metabolism depends on a healthy liver for its transformation to glucose. If propylene glycol administration at 10 to 12 oz/day is initiated early in the clinical course of triglyceride accumulation and ketonuria, it may be successful.

Force-feeding the anorexic, depressed cow with clinical fatty liver is an important and useful adjunct treatment. A slurry of a complete feed administered with a large-bore stomach tube has been a useful treatment in extreme cases. Some clinicians have suggested creating a rumen fistula to permit enteral feeding of

cows with fatty liver. All of these treatments are designed to provide energy and glucose to produce an endogenous or exogenous insulin surge and to reduce NEFA mobilization. We have been successful at saving many high-risk cows with these approaches, but many times the productive outcome has been disappointing. Prevention is a much better economic approach.

Systemic administration of glucagon appears to hold promise as a possible treatment, but at this point it is still experimental.

PREVENTION

Obesity in dry cows should be avoided. Most obese dry cows do not become obese during the dry period but rather during late lactation. This is particularly true for cows with extended lactation periods, such as those in whom establishment of pregnancy is delayed. In herds with breeding problems, particular attention needs to be paid to the body condition of late-lactation cows. Dry cows should be fed a diet to maintain weight, not lose weight. A weight-reduction program in late gestation can trigger excessive NEFA mobilization and fatty liver during the dry period.

Herd body condition scoring can be a useful tool to avoid problems with fatty liver. Dry cows and cows 3 to 4 weeks postpartum can be scored according to body condition. If the difference between condition scores of these two groups is 1.0 or greater, then excessive fat mobilization is occurring. Because NEFA mobilization and hepatic triglyceride accumulation is so closely tied to DMI, improving DMI the last 2 to 3 weeks before and the first 2 to 3 weeks after calving should be the top priority. This can best be accomplished by the formulation and delivery of a good "transition" ration to the cows. This ration should contain adequate digestible fiber, carbohydrate, and protein to allow rumen adaptation without inducing acidosis. Energy density should be intermediate between the dry cow diet and the peak lactation diet. (See the article "Special Dietary Management in Lactation and Gestation" [p. 204] in the last edition of this book for details.)

Recent Canadian research with the use of ionophores as an oral additive for the late gestation and early lactation cow has suggested some promise. In cattle with a body condition score (BCS) greater than 4.0, the addition of 6 mg of monensin to the diet beginning 3 weeks prepartum, either daily in the feed or as a slow-release bolus, resulted in decreased serum NEFA concentrations and a corresponding reduction in incidence of ketosis and improved milk production. The same benefit was not observed in thin cows. The use of ionophores is not approved for use in adult dairy cattle diets in the United States, and they cannot be used. However, they may hold some promise for future use.

Care to provide the peripartum cow with as stress-free an environment as possible is also important. Stress hormones significantly increase NEFA mobilization and have been suggested as a contributing cause in fatty liver. A quiet, clean place for calving is helpful. Providing comfortable, well-designed, well-ventilated stalls is particularly important. Attempts to improve the environment for the cow during the transition period should be very helpful in controlling fatty liver.

Niacin, or nicotinic acid, at pharmacologic doses reduces NEFA mobilization from adipose tissue. Six to 12 g/day, given orally, has been demonstrated to be of benefit in the treatment of experimental ketosis. Little or no research evidence confirms its use as a treatment or preventive agent for fatty liver, although its use is frequently advocated. Yeast products, or other probiotics, can be a useful additive in the transition diet to improve DMI and to help avoid excessive NEFA mobilization.

Fatty liver, both clinical and subclinical, is a disease of excessive NEFA mobilization from adipose tissue. Prevention and treatment efforts must focus on minimizing the adipose mobilization that normally occurs during the periparturient period. The objective is to prevent the downward spiral of declining DMI and increasing NEFA mobilization and hepatic triglyceride accumulation.

BIBLIOGRAPHY

Gerloff BJ, Herdt TH, Emery RS: Relationship of hepatic lipidosis to health and performance in dairy cattle. J Am Vet Med Assoc 8:845, 1986.

Grummer RR: Etiology of lipid-related metabolic disorders in periparturient dairy cows. J Dairy Sci 76:3882, 1993.

Physical and Chemical Diseases

Consulting Editor

Gary D. Osweiler, D.V.M., M.S., Ph.D., Diplomate, A.B.V.T.

■ Using Diagnostic Resources for Toxicology

**Gary D. Osweiler, D.V.M., M.S., Ph.D.,
Diplomate, A.B.V.T.**

The purpose of diagnostic toxicology is to provide consultation, suggestions, and interpretation regarding suspected toxicoses. When diagnostic assistance from a toxicologist is needed, a written or telephone history from the attending veterinarian is essential. A thorough pathologic examination may suggest other diagnoses or better focus on needed toxicologic tests. A complete history (including management and feed type) including symptoms and lesions, should be submitted with specimens for laboratory evaluation because there is no practical or cost-effective way to check for all possible poisons. In emergency situations, the laboratory should be alerted as early as possible.

SELECTING A LABORATORY

Generally, no single diagnostic or commercial laboratory can perform all possible analyses. If toxicologic needs are diverse and extensive, referring veterinarians should review the capabilities of several qualified laboratories from which they can request analyses as needed. Minimum expectations of a qualified laboratory should include the following:

1. A written schedule of fees and services.
2. Information about quality control programs and accreditation with recognized certifying agencies.
3. Information about the qualifications of the staff.
4. Use of modern analytical equipment.
   a. Major instrumentation should include ultraviolet and visible spectrophotometers, atomic absorption spectrophotometers, gas liquid chromatographs, high-performance liquid chromatographs, and fluorometers.
   b. Additional desirable capabilities are inductively coupled plasma element analysis, immunoassay, nuclear magnetic resonance imaging, and mass spectrometry.
5. Instructions in collection and preservation of samples and interpretation of the results in the context of the samples being analyzed and the source of the specimens.
6. Availability of a veterinary diagnostician for consultation and interpretation of results.
7. Documentation of normal or expected values for the tests performed.

SELECTING SPECIMENS FOR TOXICOLOGY AND CHEMICAL EVALUATION

Three main criteria are important in selecting the best specimens for diagnostic toxicology analyses. *Correct specimen selection* is essential to support the analyses requested, and may be affected by route of exposure, time since exposure, and dosage. A thorough history is needed to guide specimen selection and for developing a valid differential diagnostic list.

Analyses are directed toward exposure sites (skin and digestive tract), areas of metabolism and excretion (liver, kidney, urine), and accumulation in specific affected organs or storage sites (e.g., brain, fat, bone).

Specimens that should be submitted from a live animal include serum (clot removed; 5 mL), whole blood (in anticoagulant; 10 mL), urine (chilled; 50 mL), vomitus or feces (chilled or frozen; 200 g), and milk (if appropriate; 100 mL).

Specimens to be submitted from a dead animal include serum or whole blood (if available; 10 mL), urine (50 mL), liver (100 g fresh, thin slices fixed in formalin), kidney (100 g fresh, thin slices fixed in formalin); body fat (100 g), brain (divided by midsagittal section; submit one half frozen, one half fixed in formalin), rumen or stomach contents (200 g), ocular fluid (entire eyeball, or aspirate of aqueous or vitreous humor), bone (100 g).

Specimens should be free of chemical contamination and debris. Contamination of samples with hair, vomitus, dust, dirt, and so forth, may contaminate the sample and produce erroneous results. Frozen animal and tissue specimens for chemical analysis should be packaged to arrive at the laboratory while still frozen. Do not freeze whole blood samples, but keep them refrigerated. Serum, separated from the clot and not hemolyzed, may be frozen, especially for ammonia or hydrogen cyanide analysis. Package each specimen separately in clean glass or plastic containers that can be tightly sealed. Preservatives (e.g., formalin) should not be added unless there is a specific reason. If preservatives are added, include a sample of the preservative along with the specimen. Individually label each specimen (container) so it can be clearly identified. Samples for trace-level organic chemical analysis, such as pesticide residues or polychlorinated biphenyls (PCBs) should be put in glass containers, not plastic. Solid samples for this purpose may be wrapped in aluminum foil. On all toxicology cases involving a dead animal, submit both fresh and formalin-fixed tissues.

MAINTAINING PACKAGE INTEGRITY

For legal or insurance purposes, sealing of the package and transmittal procedures of the Federal Bureau of Investigation are recommended. Specimens are packed in a sealed box, and the history or other transmittal information should be in an envelope marked "invoice" which is then securely attached to the outside of the box. This entire package is covered with an outside wrapper and sealed with gummed paper or packing tape, then addressed to the laboratory, to the attention of a specific person if possible. Commercial carriers or hand delivery with a signature-acknowledged receipt at the laboratory may be useful for cases involving insurance or possible litigation.

FEEDS AND ENVIRONMENTAL SAMPLES

Sampling error or collection of a nonrepresentative sample is often a weak link in submitting feeds or forages for analysis. For grain and mixed feeds, multiple samples can be taken from a moving auger stream or by probe sampling of a bin. Mix samples thoroughly and retain a representative 2- to 4-kg sample for analysis. Holding back a duplicate sample until the original is received and processed by the laboratory provides additional security. Condensation and fungal growth during transport can be prevented by drying the sample to less than 14% moisture or by freezing. Cloth or paper bags promote less condensation and humidity than plastic bags.

Forage sample size should be at least 1 qt with all material cut to a length of 3 in. or less. Silage samples or green chop should be frozen to prevent mold growth or degenerative changes. For baled or loose hay, a Penn State forage sample or equivalent core sampling device should be used. Square bales should be sampled from the end of the bale the full length of the sampler tube, while round bales are sampled across the bale at the center.

Pasture and row crop samples should be selected from at least 8 to 10 locations in a W-shaped pattern within a field, with removal of forage from a 4-sq ft area at grazing height. Mix all collected forage and take a representative sample (2 to 4 kg) for analysis.

If bulk feed or forage is suspect, save enough for a potential test feeding in animals. Ten pounds or more may be required for a laboratory animal feeding trial, with several hundred pounds needed for feeding large animals. For a feeding trial or bioassay, contact the laboratory.

To collect water samples, let the hydrant or faucet run for a minute or more before collecting. Rinse the sample container with the water to be tested prior to collection. Containers should be sterile if microbiologic testing is requested. Water samples for organic chemical analyses should be in clean glass jars free of organic matter and with clean aluminum foil placed over the mouth of the jar before attaching the lid. Water samples should be refrigerated and shipped on ice as soon as possible.

INTERPRETATION OF RESULTS

Interpretation of significance of chemical data should be done carefully taking into consideration other evidence presented in the case. Positive chemical findings are not always evidence of intoxication nor are negative findings always indicative that toxicosis did not occur. For example, chlorinated hydrocarbon insecticides may accumulate to high levels in fatty tissues of animals without being associated with clinical signs. On the other hand, organophosphate insecticides and mycotoxins rapidly disappear from body tissues and their absence would not always rule out intoxication.

GUIDE FOR TOXICOLOGY SPECIMENS

Specimens required for diagnosis of common toxicants are listed in Table 1.

Table 1
GUIDE TO TOXICOLOGY SPECIMEN COLLECTION

Toxicants	Specimens
Alkaloids	Stomach contents, liver, urine
Ammonia	Whole blood, serum, rumen contents
4-Aminopyridine (avitrol)	Stomach contents, liver, bait
Anticoagulant rodenticides	Whole blood, liver, bait
Arsenic	Liver, kidney, urine
Brodifacoum	See Anticoagulant rodenticides
Calcium, phosphorus	Serum, feed
Carbon monoxide	Whole blood, fetal thoracic fluid
Carbamates	Whole blood, brain, rumen/stomach contents, feed
Cholecalciferol	Serum, kidney, bait
Chlorinated hydrocarbon insecticides	Brain, liver
Copper	Liver, kidney, serum, feed
Cyanide	Stomach/rumen contents, liver, whole blood, plant
Ethylene glycol	Serum, fixed kidney, stomach contents, bait
Fluoride	Urine, bone, feed
Gossypol	Feed, fixed heart
Herbicides	Stomach/rumen contents, liver, feed, water
Hormonally active compounds	Feed
Monensin, lasalocid	Feed, heart, skeletal muscle
Lead	Whole blood, liver, kidney
Magnesium	Serum, eyeball
Metaldehyde	Stomach contents, bait
Mycotoxins	Feed, urine (aflatoxin, ochratoxin)
Nitrate, nitrite	Eyeball, serum rumen contents, forage, water
Organophosphate insecticides	Whole blood, brain, rumen/stomach contents, feed
Oak	Fixed kidney, serum
Oxalates	Fixed kidney, forage
Petroleum, fuel products	Rumen/stomach contents, lung
Poisonous plants	Stomach/rumen contents, plant
Potassium	Serum
Salt, sodium	Brain (fixed, fresh), feed, eyeball
Selenium	Liver, serum, feed
Strychnine	Stomach contents, liver
Sulfonamides	Urine, kidney, feed
Urea	Rumen contents, serum, feed (freeze)
Vitamins A, E	Serum, liver
Yew	Rumen/stomach contents
Zinc	Serum,* liver

*Trace element tubes are recommended.

ANALYSIS FOR SPECIAL OR UNUSUAL TOXICANTS

The general specimen guidelines discussed above are usually suitable for detection of most toxicants; however, where special considerations for individual chemical analyses are required, users should establish a working knowledge of toxicants required for specific tests by the laboratories that they use routinely. If in doubt about sampling or analytical requests, contact the laboratory.

BIBLIOGRAPHY

Buck WB. Use of diagnostic laboratories. *In* Howard JL (ed): Current Veterinary Therapy: Food Animal Practice, ed 2. Philadelphia, WB Saunders, 1986, pp 335–341.

Osweiler GD. Toxicology. Philadelphia, Williams & Wilkins, 1996, pp 37–46.

Osweiler GD, Carson TL, Buck WB, et al. Clinical and Diagnostic Toxicology, ed 3. Dubuque, Iowa, Kendall Hunt, 1985, pp 52–66.

User's Manual. Ames, Veterinary Diagnostic Laboratory, Iowa State University, 1996.

Forensic and Legal Aspects of Food Animal Toxicoses

Farrel R. Robinson, D.V.M., Ph.D.

Veterinary practitioners are sometimes involved in legal disputes regarding their clients' cases, or as a witness or consultant in other legal proceedings.[1,2] The good part is that legal cases are often resolved before trial. The purpose of this discussion is to provide guidance to the practitioner in the preparation of cases for litigation, insight as to expectations of the legal setting, and tips on how the legal system works.

PRACTITIONER-CLIENT RELATIONSHIP

Practitioners may be asked by their clients to help resolve legal disputes. Owners often are quite certain that their evidence is adequate to collect damages when it is only the beginning of a long process of documentation and frustration. What appears to be a clear-cut solution may not be as simple as first thought; a clinical diagnosis or a laboratory report may not be enough evidence to support a case for litigation. It is in clients' best interests that the practitioner support their claims and the practitioner should be compensated for these professional services.

Practitioners need to keep factual detailed clinical records, accurate business records, and supporting documentation. A clinical problem must be documented by extensive laboratory work. Results of chemical analyses relating to a toxicologic problem are paramount. At a minimum, one must show that the chemical was *available to* the animal in question and that it was *present in* the animal in sufficient quantities to cause death. The opposing side will attempt to prove that the chemical was not toxic, or not toxic at the levels claimed, or that the animal died from some other cause.

It is important to record only factual information. One must avoid drawing conclusions based on speculation, and making disparaging comments. All records can be used as evidence and are legally available to both sides of a dispute. With telephone conversations, the date of the call, the name of the person(s) to whom you talked, and the general subjects discussed are sufficient.

WITNESS OF FACT OR AN EXPERT WITNESS

A practitioner usually serves as a witness of fact. Expert witnesses are expected to have a broad knowledge of a specific technical area, including the world literature, and be able to express an opinion based on this knowledge. A practitioner may serve as a consultant and assist in the preparation of a case for trial.

PRACTITIONER-ATTORNEY RELATIONSHIP

A veterinary practitioner must be candid with his client's attorney. The attorney should know all the facts and problems associated with each particular diagnosis prior to the trial. It is the veterinarian's responsibility to educate the attorney on the terminology, practices, client's management problems, and so forth. It is advisable not to offer information or answer the opposing attorney's questions unless the client's attorney is present.

ATTORNEY'S RESPONSIBILITIES

An attorney has a responsibility to put the best spin on the facts and does everything he can do, without breaking the law, to win the client's case. This means that the attorney will find errors in the interpretation of facts, logic, and testimony, and make the most of these errors. Attorneys can be very incisive and impolite to the opposing witnesses. The best witness is one who remains professional, reserved, and unaffected by the questioning attorney's demeanor. A witness should answer only the question asked and not offer any other information. Do not educate the opposing attorneys; that is the role of *their* witnesses and consultants.

THE DEPOSITION

A deposition is a recorded statement by a witness whereby the opposing attorney discovers what the witness knows and his or her professional opinions. An opposing attorney has the right to ask any relevant question and if the question is inappropriate, your attorney will object. After discussion of the objection, you may be directed to answer the question anyway. For the most part, a deposition is a boring, tedious proceeding.

A deposition begins with some routine questions about your qualifications, training, and so on, and proceeds to more substantive matters. The more incisive questions may be saved for the end of the deposition when your concentration wanes. Although a witness must answer all the questions, it is acceptable to say that you do not know the answer or do not remember the details. Attorneys like to test a witness's memory and memories are notoriously imperfect.

Do not invest an author with absolute authority. If you say that such and such author is *the* expert and that you agree with everything the author says, then the attorney will turn to a page in which the author contradicts your testimony. Attorneys like to confuse a given situation with alternatives to your diagnoses or opinions. Above all, do not offer more information than the question requires. Another potentially serious problem for the witness relates to compensation of clients for their losses. You should always avoid an answer which indicates prejudice or bias in favor of the client. You should explain that your testimony provides the facts of the case. The judge or jury decides if there is fault.

A potentially demoralizing question relates to payment for your services. An attorney may imply that your testimony is for sale and that you are being paid to testify for the client. Your answer should be straightforward, that is, that you are commonly compensated for your time and services and that you are an advocate of your evidence and opinions, rather than an advocate for the client. The client's advocate is the attorney. It is very important to avoid being paid on a contingency basis (which means that you get paid if your side wins); this is strictly forbidden since it implies bias and prejudice.

Depositions are more informal and relaxed than trials, but each recorded word in a deposition may be used in trial. It is during deposition that the opposing attorney recognizes your potential weaknesses, and will likely use that information at a trial.

THE TRIAL

After the deposition, you know the attorneys and the areas that they will cover in their questions and for which you should have studied. You must be sure of your facts and be prepared to present them in everyday English that the judge and jury can understand; avoid technical jargon and "weasel words." They will detract from your testimony. An attorney will prepare you for the trial; he or she will go over anticipated questions and make sure that you have a ready answer. You will not be told how to answer but you will be alerted to possible questions and pitfalls.

It is important to be professional, unharried, calm, and informative before judge and jury. You may need to educate the judge or jury on some technical points; this should be discussed with your attorney before you testify.

SUMMARY

The legal setting is much different from the professional veterinary atmosphere; it is a different ball game, so be prepared to follow your attorney's lead and do not be offended by some of the unwritten rules. For instance, it is common practice not to acknowledge members of the opposing side outside the courtroom. You ignore them; they ignore you. Remember that you are a witness and not the advocate; you are not to take sides or be an advocate of anything except your professional knowledge and opinions. The outcome of a trial should be of no interest to you since you are there only to present your testimony; it is up to the attorney to win or lose the case.

REFERENCES

1. Robinson FR: The bioscientist as an expert witness. Vet Hum Toxicol 37(suppl 1):1–36, 1995.
2. Rutherford L, Bone S: Osborn's Concise Law Dictionary, ed 8. London, Sweet & Maxwell, 1993.

■ Investigating Feed Problems

Thomas L. Carson, D.V.M., Ph.D.

The quality of the feed provided has a major impact on the health and performance of animals. In some cases feed-related problems may be included in a differential diagnosis or "rule-out" list when episodes of poor health and performance or even death occur. Careful evaluation of clinical evidence and animal specimens, finding the feed as the common denominator, and selection of representative feed samples and appropriate laboratory tests can help confirm the cause of the problem.

In addition, animal health problems associated with commercially prepared feeds or purchased feed ingredients may raise issues of liability and in some cases may lead to litigation for recovery of damages. Therefore, it is important to examine feed in a logical and scientific manner, being careful about labeling of samples, collecting feed tags, recording lot numbers, maintaining chain of custody, and using a reliable testing laboratory.

KINDS OF FEED PROBLEMS

Before looking at the evaluation of feed, it might be useful to briefly review some of the kinds of problems that have been associated with feed in the past. Some of the most basic feed problems leading to poor animal performance or health involve an imbalance or deficiency of nutrients, including protein, digestible energy, calcium, phosphorus, or microminerals. Errors in formulation or misinformation about nutrient requirements for specific animals are frequently responsible.

Contamination of feed with toxic compounds such as organophosphate insecticides, urea, ionophores, lead, selenium, copper, salt, or many other materials may have a disastrous outcome with a high death loss in exposed animals. These compounds contaminate feed through improper mixing of intended ingredients, malfunction of feed-formulating equipment, or accidental inclusion of toxic materials that may have been stored in the feed-mixing area that occurred as a contaminant of a feed ingredient.

Feed refusal or reduced consumption of feed by animals may be observed by producers. Deoxynivalenol (DON, vomitoxin) is recognized as causing this syndrome in swine, but frequently the cause of poor consumption or refusal may not be identified.

In addition, under specific growing or storage conditions, some fungal agents can produce mycotoxins, including aflatoxin, zearalenone, deoxynivalenol, fumonisin, ergot, and others. The clinical syndromes caused by these mycotoxins are characteristic for the species of animal involved. Many of these fungal toxins can be formed in the field prior to harvest with resulting contamination of feeds formulated with these grains. In addition, elevated moisture and temperature during storage can lead to saprophytic fungal growth in feed with resulting offensive odors, reduced palatability, and nutrient degradation.

Sometimes violative residues in meat, milk, or eggs have been traced back to contaminated feeds. Antibiotics, sulfonamides, or chlorinated hydrocarbon insecticides are included in the compounds producing these problems.

FEED HISTORY

When investigating possible problems associated with feed, several questions or kinds of information may be helpful. First, determine where the feed was formulated and by whom. The risks associated with a commercial feed mill are often different from an on-the-farm feed-mixing operation. The role of new employees, improperly functioning automated equipment, and the source of grain and other ingredients can affect the quality and safety of commercially manufactured feed. On the other hand, grinding, mixing, and formulating feed on the farm has its own unique risks. Feed ingredients and additives intended for one kind of livestock may be accidentally added to the feed for another species; records of feed formulations and mixing sequence may be unavailable or inadequate; the person doing the mixing may be inadequately trained or even a temporary worker; the source of grains is often a single source; and the risk of accidentally incorporating other chemicals used on the farm is always present.

An investigation of feed problems should also establish what feed was mixed just prior to the batch in question. Residual feed in a mixer can be a source of contamination to the following batch. Excess copper in sheep feeds and sulfonamides in swine feed are examples of batch-to-batch contamination from a feed mixer.

The time sequence between the mixing or delivery of new feed and the onset of animal health problems may be important circumstantial information. It is often enlightening to create a written time line to establish the chronology of the feed delivery or change and the clinical signs in the animals. Keep in mind that it may take a day or two for new feed in the top of a feeder to become available to animals. The investigation should determine what special constituents such as drugs, ionophores, mineral packs, distillers' byproducts, or other additives were incorporated into the feed and at what level. Finally, it should be established whether anything was unique or different about this particular batch of feed. Changes in personnel doing the mixing, location of the grinding or mixing, or the formula that was mixed can often be a clue to errors in formulation or accidental contamination.

SAMPLING

The care used in collecting the sample of feed for laboratory analysis has a direct effect on the accuracy of the analysis. The submitted sample must represent the average composition of the feed or grain sampled to make the analytic results valid. Identification and labeling of samples at the time of collection is also important. Mycotoxin analyses on whole grains represent special sampling considerations. Because mycotoxin concentrations are often high in a few individual kernels mixed throughout the grain, the odds of getting a representative sample are greatly increased when several subsamples are collected from multiple sites throughout the volume of grain. Recommended practice is to collect multiple small subsamples (use a grain probe in bins or feeders, or a container passed through a moving stream of grain or feed), mix these well, and then submit a composite of this pooled sample to the laboratory. The amount of feed submitted to the laboratory varies somewhat depending on the commodity being sampled. In general, a sample size of 2 lb of a ground, mixed feed is adequate for most analyses. When whole grains are being tested for mycotoxins, a sample size of 5 to 10 lb (~2.5 to 5.0 kg) may increase accuracy. Check with your analytic laboratory for their specific recommendations.

Dry feeds or grains can be shipped or stored for a short time in plastic bags or other closed containers. However, commodities that are not well dried should be shipped in cloth or paper containers to minimize condensation of moisture and secondary fungal growth. The integrity of high-moisture feeds would be maintained best by keeping the samples frozen during transit. Unfortunately, in some instances, the questionable feed has been consumed and no samples remain for testing. To guard against such predicaments, producers may want to consider retaining and freezing several pounds of each batch of feed for later analysis should the need arise.

LABORATORY EVALUATION

Examination of a feed sample by a laboratory can produce objective measurements that define the quality or defects of a feed, as well as how closely it matches the intended formulation. First, it is wise to physically examine the feed. A distinctive odor, an oily feeling, an abnormal color, or other characteristics should be noted. Problems of digestibility or gastric ulcers may sometimes be associated with the fineness of the grind (i.e., particle size) of the feed. A set of feed sieves (U.S. Standard or Tyler) can be used to measure the mean particle size as well as the distribution of particle size for a ground feed.

Analysis of a feed for some basic nutrients such as protein, digestible energy, salt, calcium, or other minerals will suggest how closely the feed matches the intended formulation or may show evidence of a misformulation. These analyses are relatively inexpensive and are readily available through commercial testing laboratories. In addition, quantitation of specific vitamins or drugs may be used as confirmation of an intended formula.

Specific chemical analysis of the feed for toxic contaminants like the organophosphate insecticides, ionophores, copper, selenium, and others should be based on the clinical signs and lesions observed in the affected animals. This analytic evidence is important for establishing a defect in the feed and supporting a diagnosis in the animals.

When mycotoxin contamination is suggested by the clinical syndrome associated with a feed, representative samples should be analyzed specifically for aflatoxin, zearalenone, fumonisin, or other specific mycotoxins in question. Because analytic methods for mycotoxins may vary among laboratories, it is helpful to be aware of the methods used when interpreting results. Some feed laboratories attempt to evaluate moldy feeds by determining a mold spore count. Results of these determinations are reported in colony-forming units (CFU) per gram of feed. In some instances, colonies are also identified by fungal genus. Although they may correlate with the sporulation (reproductive) stage of fungi, mold spore counts are not a good indicator of mold growth or toxin production, and should not be relied upon in place of actual mycotoxin analyses.

Another useful, but often underused tool for evaluating feeds is microscopy. A feed microscopist can identify individual feed ingredients, and may discover foreign materials, unknown components, or contaminants in a feed. A reasonably accurate estimate of the general formula of a feed can generally be determined by this method.

Some clinical situations may implicate the feed as a source of bacterial pathogens for the animals. In these cases feed can be subjected to bacterial culture methods for *Salmonella*, *Listeria*, or other organisms of interest.

Test-feeding a suspect ration to a small group of animals can on occasion serve as a bioassay or confirmation that the feed is the source of the problem. For example, the presence of a toxic amount of vomitoxin can be determined by experimental feeding of a few pigs and monitoring for reduced feed consumption or refusal.

SUMMARY

Evaluation of feed can be an important adjunct in the investigation of cases of poor animal health or death. However, to be of most value, results of feed examinations should supplement and correlate with the history, clinical signs, lesions, and laboratory evaluation of animal specimens. Selection of representative samples of feeds and appropriate laboratory testing can be valuable in these investigations.

■ Toxicologic and Quality Evaluation of Forages and Silages

William P. Kautz, D.V.M., Ph.D.

After dedicating considerable time and resources to plant, harvest, and store forages and high-moisture grains, the last thing a producer wants to see is moldy feed coming out of the storage structure. While the vast majority of molds are harmless, they still represent visible signs of spoilage and dry matter loss which can affect the energy, vitamin, and amino acid content of feeds. There is also the potential for reduced palatability and digestive upsets. Differences of opinion exist regarding the severity of problems caused by molds and mycotoxins in animal feeds. This is most likely due to the fact that the animal health and nutrition profession's knowledge of this area is still fairly limited.

Since the discovery of aflatoxin in 1961, over 300 different mycotoxins have been documented in the scientific literature. The levels of mycotoxins in livestock rations will increasingly be a concern as we continue to improve our ability to identify toxins and better understand their effects on production and reproduction. Environmental concerns are also surfacing which can lead to economic and legal implications centered around both livestock and human health.

OVERVIEW OF MOLD GROWTH

The conditions that generally favor mold growth include (1) moisture greater than 13%, (2) relative humidity in excess of 70%, (3) temperatures greater than 55°F, (4) readily available nutrients, (5) pH above 5, and (6) the presence of oxygen. Of these conditions, oxygen availability is the single most important factor that challenges silage management skills.

Other factors which contribute to mold growth in forages and grains include (1) early growing season stress, (2) late season harvest dates, (3) hot days coupled with cold nights, which causes heavy condensation, and (4) wet corn at harvest.

Moldy silages generally result from a series of bacterial and fungal interactions. Corn and cereal silages are generally more prone to mold growth than grass or legume crops. The spoilage process is usually initiated in corn by aerobic bacteria followed by an increase in yeast populations. Several species of yeast are able to metabolize lactic acid resulting in elevation of silage pH and a rise in temperature of the silage mass. These conditions, coupled with the presence of oxygen, produce conditions suitable for the growth of molds during the feedout phase. As a general rule, heavy loads of yeast do not cause reduced feed intakes, but the subsequent microflora growth from elevated pH can dramatically affect feed consumption.

Aerobic *Bacillus* species are significant in initiating spoilage because they are very resistant to low pH. These bacteria also produce spores which allows them to survive unfavorable environments. When conditions favor growth, *Bacillus* organisms become vegetative and multiply rapidly, producing enzymes that yield readily available nutrients that fuel the growth of other spoilage microflora.

Toxigenic and nontoxigenic molds compete in the environment for survival. Their energy for propagation is derived from protein, fat, and carbohydrates in feedstuffs. Dietary fat is affected more extensively than other nutrients. The likelihood of a toxigenic organism to produce toxins depends greatly on its ability to compete with nontoxigenic organisms also present in the silage mass.

MYCOTOXIN PRODUCTION

Most mycotoxins are produced when the organism is in the reproductive stage. The transformation from the vegetative stage of growth to the reproductive stage takes 10 to 14 days for most molds. The potential spoilage organisms are only exposed to oxygen for this long in very poorly managed storage structures. Thus, the majority of mold growth and especially mycotoxin production occurs in the field and only secondarily during storage and feedout. There have been reports of increases in toxin levels of stored feeds. This most likely occurs when the mold organism is introduced into the storage structure in the reproductive stage. Under these circumstances, toxin could be produced until the trapped oxygen introduced into the silo during filling is depleted. Environmental heating and cooling, especially in a damaged or poorly sealed storage structure, can allow continuous oxygen movement into the silage mass. This continual exposure to oxygen would also allow fungal organisms to go through the reproductive phase of growth with subsequent toxin production.

Several species of the *Fusarium*, *Penicillium*, and *Aspergillus* genera are the primary fungi with the potential to produce mycotoxins in corn. Other common genera such as *Mucor* and *Rhizopus* are common in corn but are not known to produce mycotoxins. *Diplodia maydis* is responsible for the common ear mold found in the eastern United States, but is not a known toxin producer. One of the most common producer concerns is that of smutted corn, caused by the organism *Ustilago maydis*. Research has shown no harmful effects on livestock consuming smutted corn. However, while many of the common molds do not produce known toxins, their presence may have a negative impact on palatability and nutrient availability and provide evidence that environmental conditions exist that could potentially support the growth of other unidentified toxin producers.

The primary mycotoxins produced by the *Fusarium* spp. include (1) deoxynivalenol (DON or vomitoxin), (2) zearalenone, (3) T-2, and (4) fumonisin. These molds grow well at 13% to 30% moisture over a wide range of temperatures. Of these toxins, DON and fumonisin are considered the least harmful to ruminants consuming silages that are infected. DON is commonly found in silages and high-moisture grains, while the others occur much less frequently. Fumonisin has been shown to be carcinogenic and has been linked to the death of horses consuming feed with as little as 5 to 10 ppm. Cattle tolerate from 50 to 100 ppm fumonisins with no demonstrated adverse effects.

Aspergillus spp. produce the aflatoxin compounds. These toxins are most commonly produced in hot, dry, and even drought conditions. Aflatoxin is a known carcinogen and as such interstate shipment of affected grain is controlled by Food and Drug Administration (FDA) regulations. Ruminants have the ability to degrade about 100 times more aflatoxin in the rumen than can be handled by monogastrics. However, transmission of aflatoxin to humans through milk consumption is a food safety issue.

DETECTION OF MYCOTOXINS

Requests for identification of molds and associated mycotoxins are on the rise for several reasons: (1) recent years of weather conducive to the growth of molds prior to harvest, (2) minimum or no-till soil practices that provide an environment that favors mold growth, (3) end-user demands for higher-quality forage, (4) availability and ease of use of on-farm rapid assay kits, and (5) increased production-related stress in animal production which makes animals more susceptible to the effects of low levels of mycotoxins.

Silages are considered to be heavily infested with molds when populations exceed 100,000 colony-forming units (CFU) per gram of fed material. Mold color is a poor indicator of mold identity, although the gray and black molds are considered less problematic than those that are white, pink, green, yellow, or blue. Mycotoxin concentrations are not well correlated with mold spore counts. Black-light screening tests do not effectively qualify or quantify specific mold populations and are a useful screening procedure only for aflatoxin. A general recommendation would be to submit a forage sample to a qualified laboratory for mold quantification and identification. Submit any forage sample that has large amounts of visible mold present and is suspected as a cause of a concurrent feed intake or health problem.

The physical presence of fungal growth may or may not indicate the presence of a mycotoxin. Likewise, a plant without visible fungal growth may be contaminated with mycotoxins. One of the challenges is the ability to culture the organisms in the laboratory. If samples are received with a heavy spore load, and the laboratory has the proper differential media to culture the spore, then identification and quantification are possible. However, if the mold did not sporulate and the vegetative mycelial fragments are injured by heat or drying, then culturing may be impossible. Toxin contamination in samples may be overlooked if laboratories subscribe to the protocol of requiring identification of toxin-producing colonies before they commit resources to quantify levels of potential toxins.

Producers can easily develop a mycotoxin detection program for screening grain. Reliable field ELISA (enzyme-linked immunosorbent assay) test kits for the detection of mycotoxins in grain are available at relatively low cost. At the current time, these tests should only be used as an initial screen for grain and should NOT be used on suspect forages. Low pH and other fermentation metabolites have been suspected as a cause of many false-positive results when these kits have been used on forages. In any event, any feed that is positive for mycotoxins with an ELISA test should be submitted to a competent laboratory for more extensive testing.

It is also important to remember that mycotoxin distribution in forages can be extremely uneven. It is critical to develop a sampling procedure which provides the best chance to determine the extent of the problem. A good rule of thumb is to sample several areas of the feed that do not appear visually to be affected, as well as sampling areas where there is visible mold present.

MANAGING MOLDS AND MYCOTOXINS

From a practical standpoint, producers should consider dilution of heavily contaminated feed with clean material. Silages with up to 100,000 CFU per gram of mold on an as-fed basis are generally considered safe for ruminants and can be fed undiluted. However, palatability may be a problem and dilution or slow adaptation to the feed may improve acceptance. If levels of contamination are between 1 and 5 million CFU/g, consider dilution of silage 1:1 with clean feed. Feed with counts in excess of 5 million CFU/g should be considered for discard or diluted by a factor of at least 1:2 with clean feed and fed to nonpregnant animals or other animals that are not under the stress of high production. If mycotoxin screens detect DON, zearalenone, or T-2 contamination, dilute the feed to a level of below 0.5 ppm. If diluting contaminated high-moisture grain with dry corn, screen the dry material to avoid the fines. In problem years, the fines can contain 5 to 10 times as much toxin as the rest of the material.

Various types of absorbents have been used successfully in recent years to "bind" mycotoxins found in forages. Traditional methods include the use of clays such as calcium or sodium bentonite at a level of 0.5% of the ration or 10 lb per ton. Other compounds that have been used are anticaking agents such as hydrated sodium calcium aluminosilicates at a level of 0.2 to 0.4 lb per cow per day. Inconsistencies exist in the ability of these compounds to bind specific mycotoxins. Research indicates that aluminosilicates bind aflatoxins, some zearalenone, but no DON. In spite of the research data, the use of these adsorbents has been generally successful in production units where mycotoxins have been detected at significant levels. Further research is needed to evaluate the mode of action of adsorbents in reducing the problems associated with moldy feeds.

Anhydrous ammonia at a level of 1.5% per ton of grain dry matter has been used by some producers to successfully detoxify corn grain infected with aflatoxin. This procedure has not been successful in detoxifying grain contaminated with *Fusarium* or *Penicillium* mycotoxins because differences in chemical structures prevent the ammonia-induced chemical reaction that neutralizes the toxin. The use of anhydrous ammonia has not been successful in detoxifying contaminated silages, nor is its use approved by the FDA for any feedstuff that will be shipped interstate.

PREVENTION OF MOLDS AND MYCOTOXINS IN FORAGES

As previously discussed, most experts agree that the majority of mycotoxins are produced in the field. Prevention, therefore, must be focused on seed selection, agronomic practices, and harvest management. In addition, cooperation from the weather is desirable. Prevention of additional mold growth in ensiled and baled forages must focus on careful management of harvest, storage, and feedout techniques.

Seed Selection

Growers should consult their seed supplier for disease resistance ratings in specific hybrids and varieties. Corn breeders and pathologists have been scoring inbreds and hybrids for mold resistance, but currently no hybrid can offer complete protection against mold growth. Therefore, growers should base hybrid and variety selection on the following criteria: (1) proper maturity for the average growing season, (2) a strong disease and stress tolerance package, (3) high ratings for resistance to lodging, (4) a moderate "staygreen" rating, and (5) high ratings for grain quality (kernel texture).

Agronomic Practices

No-till practices present a dilemma since they are environmentally desirable from a conservation standpoint. No-till fields may stimulate mold spore production and increase the inoculation risk. Growers may need to balance residue management with the potential for mold growth and potential mycotoxin production. In fields that are known to have produced contaminated forages it may be necessary to revert to conventional tillage for at least one growing season. Moldboard plowing or deep disking will facilitate the degradation of crop debris that serves as a growth medium for fungal organisms. The success of conventional tillage practices is dependent on the amount of time the crop residue is exposed to soil organisms. The amount of time needed is dependent upon soil temperature. Soils in northern climates should be fall-plowed, whereas in southern climates spring plowing may be adequate.

Fields in wet low-lying areas such as river bottoms are more prone to mold infestation and should be avoided. Judicious use of insecticides, when necessary, can prevent plant damage that would increase the chances for mold growth. Crop rotation has been suggested as a partial solution, but currently there is scientific debate about the efficacy of this practice. Rotation from corn to *Fusarium*-resistant crops is currently recommended, but current research may prove that this does not help.

Harvest Management

Growers should monitor maturity and moisture levels and harvest according to both crop and storage structure recommendations. *Fusarium* grows rapidly in feedstuffs testing 20% moisture, but is inhibited by moistures greater than 30%. High-moisture corn should be ensiled at greater than 25% moisture to assure the producer that oxygen will not penetrate the material and mold growth will be minimal. Corn harvested for dry bin storage should not exceed 12% moisture.

Storage and Feedout Management

Mold problems can be minimized in storage structures by adhering to some conventional recommendations designed primarily to minimize exposure of the material to oxygen. These include (1) harvesting at proper moisture, (2) chopping at the recommended theoretical length of cut, (3) filling the silo as rapidly as possible, (4) adequate distribution and compaction of the ensiled crop, (5) sealing bunkers with 4 to 6-mil plastic and covering with tires, and (6) use of a research-proven bacterial silage inoculant. Storage structures should be inspected annually for integrity. Doors and walls of tower structures should be kept in good repair to minimize the potential for oxygen penetration into the silage.

The storage of silage in plastic bags has become very popular. Bags present unique problems with regard to aerobic stability. Bags need to be filled uniformly to prevent large pockets of trapped air. Moisture levels are critical. If silage is put into bags too dry, the potential for oxygen penetration on feedout increases dramatically. Recommended moisture levels for silage stored in bags is 60% to 65%.

Slow or uneven feedout will create conditions favorable for growth of spoilage organisms. The utilization of storage structures should be based on the number of animals being fed. Producers should plan on removing at least 3 in. per day from tower structures and a minimum of 6 in. per day from bunkers to minimize problems associated with oxygen penetration into the silage mass. Bunker silos should be designed so that the producer can remove the proper amount of silage across the entire face on a daily basis. Special attention should be given to keeping the face of the silage clean and straight. Careful removal of feed from the bunker face will minimize air penetration into the silage mass. All loose feed dislodged from the face should be cleaned up and fed on a daily basis.

If feed does become moldy, the problems can be minimized by feeding forages and total mixed rations (TMRs) more often to minimize the exposure to oxygen. It is also important to clean augers, conveyors, mangers, and feedbunks more often when feeding moldy feed.

The use of propionic–acetic acid combinations on the face of bunker silos has been somewhat effective in holding additional mold growth in check. This may be beneficial in situations where the operator cannot get completely across the face of a silo in 1 day. This is a temporary fix and will not replace proper sizing and good face management. It should also be noted that many of the yeast organisms that initiate spoilage in corn silage are not affected by the acid products and heating may still occur on the silo face even after spraying with acid.

Several points should be considered when dealing with ensiled forages. Oxygen is the number-one enemy of quality silage! All available options to prevent oxygen penetration into the silage mass should be employed. Most molds common to silages do not produce mycotoxins but may affect palatability and energy content of the silage. Prevention is still the best option. The practice of good management techniques from seed selection all the way to feedout will minimize the chances for problems with spoiled feed.

BIBLIOGRAPHY

DiCostanzo A, Johnston LF, Murphy M: Effects of molds on nutrient content reviewed. Feedstuffs, Jan 16, 1995, pp. 17–20.
Kautz WP: Update on molds and mycotoxins. *In* Proceedings of Wisconsin Forage Council Annual Production and Use Symposium, Oshkosh, Wisc, Jan 23–24, 1996, pp 17–28.
Lindmeann MD, Blodgett DJ: Various clays provide alternative for dealing with aflatoxin. Feedstuffs, July 15, 1991, pp 15–16, 29.
May JJ: Respiratory problems associated with work in silos. *In* Proceedings of NRAES National Silage Production Conference, Syracuse, NY, Feb 23–28, 1993, pp 283–290.
Miller JD, Trenholm HL (eds): Mycotoxins in Grain-Compounds Other Than Aflatoxin. St Paul, Minn, Egan Press, 1995.
Nelson CE: Microbiological status as a critical quality control parameter of feeds and grains. *In* Proceedings of NFIA Feed Ingredients Institute, Rosemount, Ill, June 2–6, 1991.
Osweiler GD: Mycotoxin and livestock: What roles do fungal toxin play in illness and production losses? Vet Med 89–94, 1990.
Romer T: Resource Guide. Available from Romer Laboratories, Inc., 1301 Stylemaster Dr, Union, MO 63084.
Seglar WJ: Staff veterinarian, Pioneer Hi-Bred International, Inc. Personal communication, 1996.
Whitlow LH: Mycotoxin contamination of silages: A potential cause of poor production and health in dairy herds. *In* Proceedings of NRAES Nation Silage Production Conference, Syracuse, NY, Feb 23–28, 1993, pp 220–231.

■ Nonprotein Nitrogen–Induced Ammonia Toxicosis in Ruminants

John C. Haliburton, D.V.M., Ph.D., Diplomate, A.B.V.T.

Nitrogen is an essential dietary requirement for all ruminants. Dietary nitrogen can be provided in two basic forms: (1) natural plant protein, or (2) chemically synthesized nonprotein nitrogen (NPN). NPN may be simply defined as any source of nitrogen other than natural plant protein. The primary form of NPN used in ruminant nutrition is urea (see structural formula below), but other potential sources include various forms of ammonium salts and ammoniated feed products.

$$NH_2-\overset{\overset{\textstyle O}{\|}}{C}-NH_2$$

Rumen microbes degrade ingested plant proteins and ultimately reincorporate the nitrogen obtained from the plant protein into microbial protein. Rumen microbial metabolism of NPN liberates ammonia (NH_3) from the NPN source, combining the ammonia with carbohydrate-derived compounds to form amino acids which are incorporated into microbial proteins. Rumen microflora are very efficient in utilizing NPN for protein synthesis if they are preconditioned or adapted to receiving this form of nitrogen. However, when the amount of NPN consumed exceeds rumen microbial capacity to incorporate the released ammonia into protein, ammonia concentration in the rumen can reach toxic or lethal concentration.

MECHANISM OF ACTION

The toxicity of NPN compounds is due to the liberation and absorption of ammonia from the rumen producing a systemic hyperammonemia. Normal rumen pH generally ranges between 5.0 and 6.5, and in this pH range almost all of the ammonia produced in the rumen will be rapidly converted to the charged ammonium ion form (i.e., NH_4^+) with only a small fraction remaining in the uncharged NH_3 form. When ammonia is converted to an ammonium ion a hydrogen ion (H^+) is used in the reaction ($NH_3 + H^+ \rightarrow NH_4^+$). When hydrogen ions are incorporated into ammonia within the rumen, pH increases or becomes more basic. In rumen microbial degradation and metabolism of plant-derived proteins, hydrogen ions are also used in the production of ammonium ions; but the pH in the rumen remains unchanged because the slow rate of ammonia production allows the buffering system in the rumen to react to this change and maintain homeostatic pH conditions. In contrast, microbial metabolism of NPN compounds in the rumen involves a rapid rate of ammonia production, an equally rapid rate of conversion of ammonia to ammonium ion, and a concurrent rapid rate of hydrogen ion loss. With this rapid and extensive loss of hydrogen ions, the rumen buffering system is unable to maintain homeostatic pH conditions, resulting in an elevation of the rumen pH into the range of 8.0 to 9.0. When the pH reaches 8.5, the ammonium ion becomes unstable and reverts back to the uncharged ammonia molecule. Unlike the charged ammonium ion, which cannot leave the rumen, the uncharged ammonia molecule will be readily absorbed from the rumen into the blood. Blood ammonia is normally processed (i.e., detoxified) very efficiently by the liver, but in NPN-induced ammonia toxicosis the capacity of the liver to detoxify excessive ammonia absorbed from the rumen is exceeded and ammonia toxicosis ensues.

Urea is potentially the most toxic of all NPN compounds used in ruminant nutrition because the rumen contains the ureolytic enzyme urease. Urease produced by rumen microbes catalyzes or hastens the release of ammonia from urea. Therefore, urea is more toxic due to the enzyme-hastened release of ammonia within the rumen.

The potential toxicity of NPN compounds in ruminants is affected by feeding management. Animals preconditioned or adapted to dietary NPN sources are considerably more tolerant or resistant to NPN exposure. Preconditioning or adapting animals for the efficient and safe utilization of NPN requires an initial low level of exposure with a gradual and constant increase in exposure level over a period of 10 to 12 days. This permits rumen microflora to evolve and repopulate in type and density to species that are most efficient in processing NPN.

The toxic dose of urea in cattle not preconditioned or adapted to NPN intake is approximately 0.45 g/kg of body weight. In cattle adapted to NPN, the lethal dose of urea ranges from 1.0 to 1.5 g/kg of body weight.

CLINICAL SIGNS

In NPN-induced ammonia toxicosis, the onset of clinical signs may vary from one-half to 3 hours from the time of exposure. Early signs are changes in behavior such as restlessness, belligerence, and aggression. Muscle tremors, salivation, teeth grinding, bellowing, bloat, and convulsions are typical signs, and death often follows within 1 to 2 hours.

DIAGNOSIS

The knowledge that NPN was available to a group of acutely ill, dying, or dead cattle can be vital information in making a rapid and accurate presumptive diagnosis of NPN-induced ammonia toxicosis. This possibility should be determined when confronted with cattle showing the clinical signs described above. A quick but not always present indicator of NPN-induced ammonia toxicosis is the characteristic odor of ammonia emanating from the rumen of an affected or recently dead animal. Rumen fluid pH is a quick and easily obtained measurement in a clinically affected animal or one that died within the preceding 2 hours. The rumen pH will be 8.0 or higher in these animals. The rumen pH in animals dead for several hours following NPN-induced ammonia toxicosis may not be elevated since lactic acid production from rumen microbial carbohydrate metabolism continues after death and can cause rumen pH to

fall well below 8.0, especially in animals on a high-concentrate ration. Therefore, the diagnosis of NPN-induced ammonia toxicosis should not be ruled out on the basis of a low ruminal fluid pH.

Confirmation of NPN-induced ammonia toxicosis requires laboratory assistance. The preferred specimens for analysis may vary among laboratories, so the laboratory should be contacted prior to submitting specimens. Analysis of free ammonia concentration in whole blood, rumen, and vitreous fluids can be used for confirmation, but the diagnosis of NPN-induced ammonia toxicosis should not be based on rumen ammonia concentration alone. Although the rumen ammonia concentration in cases of NPN-induced ammonia toxicosis will usually be greater than 80 mg/dL, there are circumstances where this can occur and ammonia toxicosis has not. Cattle gazing winter wheat pasture will commonly have a rumen ammonia concentration in excess of 200 mg/dL and will not be affected by ammonia toxicosis. Elevated rumen ammonia concentration combined with an elevated blood or vitreous fluid ammonia concentration is the recommended criterion for confirmation of ammonia toxicosis. Analysis of the suspected NPN feed source should be done to confirm that the product is within the guaranteed label analysis.

Although NPN-induced ammonia toxicosis can be caused by an improperly formulated product, the problem is most often attributable to one of three management-related factors: (1) no preconditioning or adaptation to NPN sources, (2) inadequate mixing or improper dispensing of NPN products resulting in either a ration–NPN source separation or unrestricted consumption of NPN, and (3) errors in on-site NPN ration formulation resulting in excessive NPN exposure.

TREATMENT

There is no specific direct-acting antidote to ammonia toxicosis. The recommended protocol for treating NPN-induced ammonia toxicosis is to administer via ruminal infusion 2 to 6 L of 5% acetic acid (i.e., vinegar) to cattle or 0.5 to 1.0 L per animal in sheep and goats. This should be followed by a large volume of cold water. The rationale for this treatment is that the acetic acid lowers rumen pH, creating conditions favoring the conversion of free ammonia to the charged ammonium ion, thereby reducing any further absorption of ammonia. Cold water lowers the rumen temperature, which will slow the rate of ammonia release from urea.

PREVENTION

The most efficient service that veterinarians may offer the livestock producer in relation to NPN-induced ammonia toxicosis is their professional expertise on the proper, safe, and most efficient use of NPN sources in ruminant nutrition programs.

BIBLIOGRAPHY

Haliburton JC, Morgan SE: Non-protein nitrogen–induced ammonia toxicosis and ammoniated feed toxicity syndrome. Vet Clin North Am Food Anim Pract 5:237–250, 1989.
Urea and non-protein nitrogen. *In* Osweiler GD, Carson TL, Buck WB, et al (eds): Clinical and Diagnostic Veterinary Toxicology ed 3. Dubuque, Iowa, Kendall Hunt, 1985, pp 160–166.

■ Ionophore Toxicoses

Joe D. Roder, D.V.M., Ph.D., Diplomate, A.B.V.T.
C. Pat McCoy, D.V.M., M.S., Diplomate, A.B.V.T.

The carboxylic ionophores are open-chained oxygenated heterocyclic rings with a single terminal carboxyl group of moderate molecular weight (200 to 2000) that form lipid-soluble transport complexes with polar cations (K^+, Na^+, Ca^{2+}, and Mg^{2+}). The ionophores have a diverse antibacterial spectrum and are produced by saprophytic fungi, predominantly *Streptomyces* species.[1] The ionophores are anticoccidial and growth-promoting feed additives ubiquitous in animal production systems. The ionophores commonly used in the United States are lasalocid (Avatec, Bovatec, Hoffman-LaRoche, Nutley, N.J.), monensin (Coban 60, Rumensin 80, Elanco Animal Health, Indianapolis), narasin (Monteban, 45, Elanco), and salinomycin (Bio-Cox, Hoffman-LaRoche). Some other newly introduced ionophores include: laidlomycin propionate potassium (Cattlyst, Hoffman-LaRoche 50), for cattle, and semduramicin (Aviax, Pfizer Animal Health, Exton, Pa.) for broilers. In poultry, these compounds are used as coccidiostats. In cattle, ionophores improve feed efficiency, reduce the incidence of bloat and acidosis, prevent tryptophan-induced acute interstitial pneumonia, and are used for coccidial prophylaxis and treatment.[2]

Carboxylic ionophores mediate an electrically neutral exchange of cations for protons across cell membranes without using ion channels. This discharges electrochemical gradients across the intramitochondrial membrane, causing decreased adenosine triphosphate (ATP) production, increased ATP utilization (to maintain cation concentrations) with cell dysfunction and possibly cellular death.

TOXICOSIS

The ionophores currently approved for use are safe and efficacious at prescribed levels in intended species. Certain management situations increase the possibility of toxicoses due to overdose (mixing errors or premix consumption) or misuse in nontarget species (especially horses). Additionally, concurrent administration of other drugs (chloramphenicol, tiamulin, erythromycin, sulfonamides, and cardiac glycosides) can potentiate ionophore toxicosis.[2, 3] Ionophore toxicity differs by compound and the species affected. Monensin toxicosis is better described than toxicoses caused by other ionophores, probably because of the large market share, length of time on the market, and the sensitivity of the horse to this compound. Horses are more sensitive to ionophore toxicosis than other domestic species with LD_{50} (median lethal dose) values of 2.0 to 3.0 times, or 0.6 and 21.5 mg/kg, respectively, for monensin, salinomycin, and lasalocid. Broilers are generally the least sensitive species with acute oral LD_{50} values of 200, 44.3, and 71.5 mg/kg, respectively, for monensin, salinomycin, and lasalocid. Dietary monensin in excess of 150 g/ton of complete ration may cause moderate toxicosis in cattle.

DIAGNOSIS

Diagnosis of ionophore toxicosis is initially tentative without pathognomonic clinical signs and lesions. Any feed-related problem characterized by anorexia, ataxia, mortality, cardiomyopathy, myonecrosis, and congestive heart failure justifies a presumptive diagnosis of ionophore intoxication. Confirmation requires consideration of differential diagnoses and laboratory assays to determine the specific ionophore involved. Chemical analyses of feed (0.5 to 1.0 kg), liver, and gastrointestinal contents are most likely to detect the ionophore. The most common chemical analyses for ionophores use high-performance liquid chromatography (HPLC) and gas chromatography–mass spectrometry (GC-MS) with residue detection levels in the range of parts per billion. Some newer tests employ enzyme-linked immunosorbent or enzyme immunoassay techniques (ELISA or EIA) to detect ionophores in biologic samples.[4]

CLINICAL SIGNS

Anorexia is the most common clinical sign associated with consumption of toxic levels of an ionophore. In horses, other common clinical signs of toxicosis include sweating, restlessness, colic, weakness, cardiac irregularity, and dyspnea. In cattle, signs including anorexia, diarrhea, depression, ataxia, and prostration have been noted. In pigs, common clinical signs of intoxication include anorexia, ataxia, paraplegia, coma, and myoglobinuria. In poultry, clinical signs associated with toxicosis include leg weakness, posterior paresis, and incoordination.

Clinical Pathologic Changes

The clinical pathologic changes associated with ionophore intoxication indicate possible damage to muscle, kidney, and liver. Serum creatine phosphokinase (CPK) levels are commonly elevated in affected animals (especially myocardial isozymes). Pericardial fluid levels of lactate dehydrogenase (LDH) and CPK may be elevated in horses.[5] Kidney damage, especially of the proximal tubules, is expressed by increased serum urea nitrogen (SUN), acidic urine, and a markedly increased urinary phosphate clearance.[5] Serum Ca^{2+} and K^+ levels may decline to life-threatening levels in monensin-intoxicated ponies or horses.[2] Erythrocyte fragility is increased in affected horses with marked lysis at 0.5% salinity.[5]

PATHOLOGY

Cardiac and skeletal muscle are most often affected in ionophore toxicosis. In horses, the heart is predominantly affected, whereas in dogs and pigs skeletal muscle necrosis is noted primarily. In contrast, poultry, cattle, and rodents have equal distribution of cardiac and skeletal muscle lesions.[2] The gross lesions of ionophore-induced myonecrosis are pale, flabby myocardial tissue, dilated ventricles, yellow-white myocardial streaks, or hearts with petechiae and ecchymoses. Animals may die acutely with no gross pathologic changes.[2] Microscopically, ionophore-mediated necrosis is described as multifocal myocyte necrosis with variable inflammatory cell infiltrates and Purkinje system degeneration. Following ionophore-mediated damage to cardiomyocytes, injured tissue is replaced by fibrosis. The initial ultrastructural change is mitochondrial vacuolation caused by swelling and degeneration of the cristae. This is followed by extensive sarcoplasmic vacuolation, disrupted contractile proteins, pyknotic nuclei, and macrophage infiltration.

Recent reports suggest that in addition to myonecrosis some ionophores may cause a peripheral neuropathy in dogs[6] and broilers.[7] This syndrome is characterized by vacuolization and demyelination of the spinal cord and sciatic nerves with a concurrent reduction in nerve conduction velocity. These reports involved feeding lasalocid to a nontarget species (dog) and overfeeding broilers. This aspect of ionophore toxicosis warrants further research.

DIFFERENTIAL DIAGNOSIS

The differential diagnosis of ionophore toxicity should include other causes of myopathy. In cattle this should include vitamin E or selenium deficiency, gossypol, and some poisonous plants: coffee senna (*Cassia occidentalis*), coyotillo (*Karwinskia humboldtiana*), oleander (*Nerium oleander*), or white snakeroot (*Eupatorium rugosum*). In poultry the differential diagnosis includes nutritional myopathy, coffee senna, botulism, salt toxicosis, round heart disease, and viral arthritis. In horses, the differential diagnosis should include colic, blister beetle ingestion (cantharidin), white snakeroot, and azoturia.

TREATMENT AND PREVENTION

There are no specific antidotes to ionophore toxicosis, but removal of affected animals from medicated feed and administration of activated charcoal with a saline cathartic may reduce absorption and signs of intoxication. Symptomatic therapy, fluids, and electrolytes may be beneficial to the intoxicated animal. Potassium replacement may be necessary when serum levels fall below 2 mEq/L. Calcium channel antagonists are contraindicated as they cause increased mortality in monensin-intoxicated mice.[3] Horses surviving the initial episode of intoxication should be stall-rested for at least 6 weeks. These horses may never regain their previous level of athletic performance and may be prone to acute cardiac failure. Cattle recovered from acute ionophore toxicosis may also suffer unexpected acute cardiac failure, especially if exercised or stressed.

Producers should be reminded to control access to ionophore-supplemented rations by limiting feeding or thorough mixing to reduce the probability of adverse effects. Used properly, ionophores are safe and effective feed supplements.

REFERENCES

1. Pressman BC: Biological applications of ionophores. Annu Rev Biochem 45:501, 1976.
2. Novilla MN. The veterinary importance of the toxic syndrome induced by ionophores. Vet Hum Toxicol 34:66, 1992.
3. Mitema ES, Sangiah S, Martin T: Effects of some calcium modulators on monensin toxicity. Vet Hum Toxicol 30:409, 1988.
4. Mount ME, Cullor JS, Kass PH, et al: Monensin concentrations measured in feeder cattle using enzyme immunoassay. Vet Hum Toxicol 38:169, 1996.
5. Amend JF, Nicholson RL, King RS, et al: Equine monensin toxicosis: Useful ante-mortem and post-mortem clinicopathologic tests. Proc Am Assoc Equine Pract 31:361, 1985.
6. Safran N, Aizenberg I, Bark H: Paralytic syndrome attributed to lasalocid residues in a commercial ration fed to dogs. J Am Vet Med Assoc 202:1273, 1993.
7. Gregory DG, Vanhooser SL, Stair EL: Light and electron microscopic lesions in peripheral nerves of broiler chickens due to roxarsone and lasalocid toxicoses. Avian Dis 39:408, 1995.

■ Gossypol

Sandra E. Morgan, D.V.M., M.S.

Gossypol is the most prevalent toxic pigment found in cottonseed, which is widely used as a protein source for livestock. Gossypol is classified as a cardiotoxin and a sterility agent depending on the dose, duration of feeding, and age and type of animal consuming it. The most prevalent clinical signs are sudden death in apparently healthy animals or chronic poor-doers exhibiting dyspnea, anorexia, weight loss, occasionally hemoglobinuria, and death. For a more detailed description of clinical signs, necropsy lesions, histopathology, and historical background of this toxin, see Morgan.[1] Today, producers, veterinarians, and researchers are concentrating their efforts on finding the best utilization of an economical feed that is high in protein and fiber, without jeopardizing the health of those consuming it.

RESEARCH

The study of gossypol and its effects in cattle diets has been the topic of many discussions and research in recent years.[2–6] Varying age groups, beef vs. dairy, male vs. female, cottonseed meal vs. whole cottonseed, direct solvent vs. expander processing, free vs. total, are just some of the factors considered when gossypol is researched.[7] The complex nature of this molecule will continue to invite more research.

Four reproductively normal Brahman bulls averaging 20 months and 500 kg consuming 8.2 g of free gossypol per day in cottonseed meal for 11 weeks did not have clinical signs of gossypol toxicosis or decreased growth. They did have increased sperm midpiece abnormalities from week 3, less morphologically normal sperm from week 5, and lower sperm motility from week 9, with evidence of depressed sperm production by the end of the trial.[6]

Thirty-six sexually mature beef heifers were fed 0 to 20 g/day of dietary free gossypol for 2 months prior to breeding, and 18 mature beef cows were fed 10 g/day for 7 months. Both heifers and cows that received 10 g/day or more had increased erythrocyte fragility. However, although consumption of large quantities (10 g/day or more) of dietary free gossypol may result in certain clinically apparent signs of gossypol toxicosis, high levels of free gossypol consumption do not impair reproductive hormone secretion or fertility in bovine females, and levels of dietary free gossypol required to produce symptoms of gossypol toxicosis are well in excess of those typically fed to beef cattle via cottonseed or cottonseed byproducts.[7]

Whole cottonseed in sorghum silage–based diets for developing beef heifers was fed at two levels (0%, 7.5%, 15%, or 22.5% whole cottonseed with 1.04% free and 1.2% total gossypol, and 0%, 6%, 12%, 18%, or 24% whole cottonseed which contained 1.08% free and 1.15% total gossypol). Increasing cottonseed levels decreased the dry matter intake and average daily gain and affected rumen parameters in both studies, but the changes were minor at the lower levels.[8]

Plasma gossypol reflects the availability of gossypol in a ration. Dairy cows fed a total mixed ration with 15% good-quality, whole, linted cottonseed averaged 1.5 to 3.5 μg/mL plasma gossypol. Less than or equal to 5 μg/mL was considered the safe upper limit for plasma gossypol.[9]

For Holstein dairy calves 1 to 120 days of age, rations containing 200 ppm free gossypol in cottonseed meal were safe, 400 ppm was toxic, and 800 ppm resulted in death.[3]

PREVENTION

The best way to prevent toxicosis from occurring is to be knowledgeable about the toxin. Gossypol is in all cottonseed except the glandless variety that contains very low levels. If the feed is tested, it can be utilized most effectively; but this is time-consuming, expensive, and not always practical. If cottonseed is not tested it can be used in specific age groups at levels that have shown good results over the years, assuming average gossypol content from past experience. One study from 1977 to 1989 found gossypol in kernels with a mean of 0.89% (8900 ppm) and a range of 0.64% (6400 ppm) to 1.19% (11,900 ppm).[5]

The risk of feeding cottonseed can be reduced by alternating it with other protein sources so the cumulative effect will be interrupted, or whole cottonseed can be alternated with cottonseed meal (gossypol is more readily available in meal than the whole seed).[5]

TESTING

When testing the feed, whole cottonseed or cottonseed meal should be tested by itself, not mixed with other feeds. Proper sampling will help ensure a meaningful result. Twenty grab samples from a cottonseed pile at various locations and depths has been recommended.[5] These samples can be mixed in a trash can, then a 1-lb sample submitted to the laboratory. A laboratory should be used that is certified by the American Oil Chemists Society (AOCS) or the Association of Official Analytical Chemists (AOAC) for gossypol analysis. Gossypol testing laboratories report the results as free, bound, or total gossypol. Some researchers believe that since only the free form is toxic it is the only measurement that is needed. Others believe that the bound form can become unbound in the intestine so that total gossypol should be used. Most gossypol in the kernel is in the free form, so free and total gossypol should be similar. If only total gossypol analysis is requested, the cost of analysis is much less, but if cottonseed meal is used measurement of the free gossypol level may be warranted. Results are reported in parts per million which is milligrams of gossypol per kilogram of cottonseed. The interpretation of the results depends on (1) whether the gossypol level reported is from the kernel or whole seed, (2) whether the level reported is free or total gossypol, (3) whether the level is reported on an "as received" or a "dry matter" basis, and (4) whether the sample is a straight cottonseed product or a mixed feed. This level can be converted to milligrams of gossypol per kilogram body weight, or grams per head per day that an animal would consume if it ate a specified amount of a particular ration per day.[5]

Different methods of oil extraction used over the years have affected the amount of free gossypol in the cottonseed meal. The older screw-press method used heat, and more gossypol was in the bound or nontoxic form. The direct solvent method used in the past decade did not involve heat and more gossypol was left in the free or toxic form. Now, in most places, an expander process involves heat used before the solvent extraction, and free gossypol levels are less than they would be from direct solvent processing.

RECOMMENDATIONS

For Gossypol Levels That Are Unknown

With additional research, accurate margins of safety can be formulated for each age group and type of animal. At this time guidelines can only be based on historical usage, previous cases, and ongoing research. The following recommendations are for feeding cottonseed to beef cattle if it is not going to be tested.[2]

Beef Cows and Range Bulls

Based on studies of beef and dairy cows, feeding "normal" levels of cottonseed meal (2 lb per head per day of direct solvent extracted; 4 lb per head per day of expander processed; 4 lb per head per day of screw-press–processed meal; or 4 to 6 lb per head per day of whole cottonseed) should not pose any practical problems for fertility. These recommendations fall within typical levels fed in the industry.[2]

Young Bulls Being Grown or Developed for Breeding

Young developing bulls or show bulls are often kept on concentrate-based diets for many months where cumulative effects

of gossypol may build up. Whole cottonseed should be limited to 15% to 20% of the total diet for most cattle and to 10% or less for young developing bulls. Although little high free gossypol meal (0.3% or 3000 ppm) is now being produced, when used it should be limited to 5% of the total diet. Cottonseed meal from the old screw-press method and the more common expander process containing less than 0.1% or 1000 ppm can be used at levels up to 15% of the total diet. When using combinations of cotton products (hulls, meal, or whole seed), the combined concentration of gossypol will need to be considered. The total amount will depend on the proportion of each product used and its gossypol concentration.[2]

Embryo Transfer Programs

Again, to be cautious, producers with embryo transfer programs in which large sums of money are involved per animal may wish to use a conservative approach since other protein sources are available. The difference in protein costs would be minuscule in comparison with total expenses.[2]

Preruminant Calves

Preruminant calves (under 8 weeks of age to be safe), especially dairy calves, should not be fed gossypol-containing products until ongoing research establishes safe feeding levels.[2]

For Gossypol Levels That Are Known

Recommendations for feeding whole cottonseed (WCS) and cottonseed meal (CSM) that have been tested for gossypol were reported as the "Maximum Safe Level for Free Gossypol in the Total Diet for the following: cattle (preruminants)—100 ppm CSM and WCS, growing steers and heifers—200 ppm CSM, 900 ppm WCS; young developing bulls—150 ppm CSM, 600 ppm WCS; mature bulls (during breeding season, about 120 days)—200 ppm CSM, 900 ppm WCS; mature cows—600 ppm CSM; 1200 ppm WCS."[5]

More research is needed for lactating dairy cattle since they consistently eat high levels of concentrate and in general are more stressed, particularly in the summer.

DIAGNOSIS

Gossypol should not always be blamed for problems that occur when a ration contains cottonseed. Aflatoxins are commonly found in corn, cottonseed, and peanuts and can cause a variety of symptoms. Free fatty acids are a measure of rancidity in any oil seed. They can alter the rumen environment and bind calcium and magnesium. Toxic levels of monensin can cause cardiotoxic symptoms and lesions. Vitamin E and selenium affect the heart if concentrations are not in the normal range. Cardiotoxic plants should be ruled out. A diagnosis of gossypol toxicosis should be based on history, clinical signs, necropsy, and microscopic lesions, feed analysis, and ruling out of other cardiotoxins and sterility agents.

REFERENCES

1. Morgan SE: Gossypol toxicosis. *In* Howard JL (ed): Current Veterinary Therapy 3: Food Animal Practice. Philadelphia, WB Saunders, 1993, pp 331–332.
2. Lusby K, et al: "Recommendation statement" on feeding cottonseed

and cottonseed meal to beef cattle in Texas and Oklahoma. Cattle Research with Gossypol Containing Feeds. National Cottonseed Products Association, Memphis, Tenn, October 1991, pp 93–96.

3. Risco CA, Holmberg CA, Kutches A: Effect of graded concentrations of gossypol on calf performance: Toxicological and pathologic considerations. J Dairy Sci 75:2787–2798, 1992.

4. Randel RD, Chase CC, Wyse SJ: Effects of gossypol and cottonseed products on reproduction of mammals. J Anim Sci 70:1628–1638, 1992.

5. Rogers GM, Poore MH: Optimal feeding management of gossypol-containing diets for beef cattle. Vet Med October: 90(10):994–1005, 1995.

6. Chenoweth CA, Risco CA, Larsen RE, et al: Effects of dietary gossypol in cottonseed meal on aspects of semen quality and sperm production in young Brahman bulls. Bovine Pract, 29:51–52, 1995.

7. Gray ML, Williams GL: Effects of gossypol-containing diets on various hematologic, metabolic, endocrine and reproductive characteristics of beef females. Cattle Research with Gossypol Containing Feeds. National Cottonseed Products Association, Memphis, Tenn, October 1991, pp 63–78.

8. Poore MH: Whole cottonseed in sorghum silage-based diets for developing heifers. J Anim Sci 72:382, 1994.

9. Calhoun MC, Kuhlmann SW, Baldwin BC Jr.: Assessing the gossypol status of cattle fed cotton feed products. *In* Proceedings of the Pacific Northwest Animal Nutrition Conference, October 1995, pp 1–12.

■ Toxic Gases

Thomas L. Carson, D.V.M., Ph.D.

Several toxic gases present a potential risk to livestock. The most hazardous gases encountered in production animal medicine are hydrogen sulfide and ammonia from the decomposition of animal waste, carbon monoxide from inefficient combustion of carbon fuels, anhydrous ammonia from the escape of agricultural fertilizer, and nitrogen dioxide as a byproduct of ensiled forages.

The risk of potential animal loss or reduced performance from toxic gases is increased with the restricted atmosphere and artificial ventilation of confinement livestock facilities. Fortunately, even at the relatively low ventilation rates used during cold weather, concentrations of ammonia and hydrogen sulfide, the most dangerous gases from manure decomposition, usually remain below toxic levels. Under some circumstances, however, accidents, poor design, or faulty operation may result in insufficient ventilation and the concentration of poisonous gases in these structures.

The most important gases released by the decomposition of urine and feces either in anaerobic underfloor waste pits or in deep litter or manure packs are ammonia, carbon dioxide, methane, and hydrogen sulfide. In addition, organic acids, amines, amides, alcohols, carbonyls, skatoles, sulfides, and mercaptans, which account for the odors of manure decomposition, are also produced.

AMMONIA

Ammonia (NH_3) is the air pollutant most frequently found in high concentrations in animal facilities, especially where excrement decomposes on a solid floor. The characteristic pungent odor of ammonia can be detected by humans at approximately 10 ppm or even lower. NH_3 concentration in enclosed animal facilities generally remains below 30 ppm even with low ventilation rates, although under some circumstances levels of 50 ppm or higher may be achieved during long periods of normal facility operation.

Ammonia is highly soluble in water, and reacts with the moist mucous membranes of the eye and respiratory passages.

Excessive tearing, shallow breathing, and clear or purulent nasal discharge are common symptoms of aerial NH_3 exposure.

At concentrations less than 100 ppm, the primary impact of NH_3 is as a chronic stressor that can affect the course of infectious disease as well as directly influence the growth of healthy young animals. For example, in a series of experiments at the University of Illinois the rate of gain of young pigs was reduced by 12% during exposure to aerial NH_3 at 50 ppm and by 30% at 100 or 150 ppm. Aerial NH_3 at 50 or 75 ppm reduced the ability of young pigs to clear bacteria from their lungs. At 50 or 100 ppm aerial NH_3 exacerbated nasal turbinate lesions in young pigs infected with *Bordetella bronchiseptica*, but did not add to the infection-induced reduction in the pigs' growth rate. In another study, the reduced rates of gain of pigs exposed to 100 ppm aerial NH_3 (-32%) and that of ascarid infection (-28%) were additive when both stresses were present.

HYDROGEN SULFIDE

Hydrogen sulfide (H_2S) is a potentially lethal gas produced by anaerobic bacterial decomposition of protein and other sulfur-containing organic matter. This colorless gas with the distinctive odor of rotten eggs is heavier than air and may accumulate in manure pits, holding tanks, and other low areas in a facility. The sources of H_2S presenting the greatest hazard to livestock are liquid manure holding pits. Most of the continuously produced H_2S is retained within the liquid of the pit. However, when waste slurry is agitated to resuspend solids prior to being pumped out, H_2S is rapidly released. While the concentration of H_2S usually found in closed animal facilities (<10 ppm) is not harmful, the release of gas from manure slurry agitation may produce concentrations up to 1000 ppm or higher.

Humans can detect the typical odor of H_2S at very low concentrations (0.025 ppm) in air, providing a useful warning of its presence. However, at higher concentrations (150 to 250 ppm) H_2S presents a distinct hazard by paralyzing the olfactory response and neutralizing this warning signal.

H_2S is an irritant gas inducing local inflammation of the moist membranes of the eye and respiratory tract. The irritant action of H_2S is fairly uniform throughout the respiratory tract, although the deeper pulmonary structures suffer the greatest damage, often producing pulmonary edema.

At concentrations in air exceeding 500 ppm, H_2S must be considered a serious imminent threat to life, although spontaneous recovery is possible if fresh air is provided. A few deep breaths of over 1000 ppm H_2S can cause immediate collapse with respiratory paralysis. Unless artificial respiration is provided immediately, death results from asphyxia.

Management is key to preventing animal deaths from H_2S. When a manure is agitated, animals should be moved out of the building and maximum ventilation rates should be used. Immediate rescue of affected animals should not be attempted without a self-contained breathing apparatus or the rescuer may also be overcome by H_2S.

CARBON DIOXIDE

Carbon dioxide (CO_2) is an odorless gas present in the atmosphere at 300 ppm. It is given off by swine as an end product of energy metabolism and by improperly vented, though properly adjusted, fuel-burning heaters. It is also the gas evolved in the greatest quantity by decomposing manure. However, CO_2 concentration in closed animal facilities rarely approaches levels that endanger animals' health.

METHANE

Methane (CH_4), a product of microbial degradation of carbonaceous materials, is not a poisonous gas. It is biologically rather inert and produces effects on animals only by displacing oxygen in a given atmosphere, thereby producing asphyxiation. Under ordinary pressures a concentration of 87% to 90% CH_4 in a given atmosphere is required before irregularities of respiration and eventually respiratory arrest due to anoxia are produced. The danger inherent in CH_4 is its explosive hazard as concentrations of 5% to 15% by volume in air are reached.

CARBON MONOXIDE

Carbon monoxide (CO), a product of the inefficient combustion of carbonaceous fuel, is odorless and colorless and potentially lethal to all classes of livestock. The exhaust fumes of gasoline-burning internal combustion engines which can contain up to 9% CO may accumulate in garages, barns, and other closed structures to create toxic levels of CO. Poisoning also occurs when improperly adjusted and vented space heaters or furnaces are operated in tight, poorly ventilated buildings such as farrowing houses and other animal quarters.

Ambient background levels of CO are 0.02 ppm in fresh air, 13 ppm in city streets, and 40 ppm in areas with high vehicular traffic.

CO acts by competing with oxygen for binding sites on a variety of proteins, including hemoglobin, with which most of the compound is associated in the body. The affinity of hemoglobin for CO is some 250 times that for oxygen. When CO becomes bonded to the heme group, forming carboxyhemoglobin (COHb), the molecule's oxygen-carrying capacity is reduced with resulting tissue hypoxia. Acute CO poisoning occurs when COHb levels rise above 30% to 60% producing clinical signs of drowsiness, lethargy, incoordination, reduced mental and cardiac excitibility, dyspnea, coma, and death.

Moderate concentrations of CO (>250 ppm) in swine farrowing houses or lambing barns are capable of producing an increased number of stillborn fetuses. The clinical history generally associated with these stillbirths reveals (1) nonexistent ventilation, or inadequate ventilation due to blocked apertures of natural systems or reduction to minimal winter rates for mechanical systems, (2) use of unvented or improperly vented liquefied propane (LP) gas-burning space heaters, (3) a high percentage of near-term sows or ewes delivering dead fetuses within a few hours of being put in an artificially heated facility, (4) dams that appear clinically normal although the whole litter may be born dead, and (5) laboratory examinations for the detection of infectious causes of abortion that are negative.

Exposure to high levels of CO can be confirmed by actually measuring the CO level in the air or by measuring the percentage of COHb in the blood of the affected animal. In addition to these two valves, COHb concentration of greater than 2% in fetal thoracic fluid may be used as an aid in diagnosing CO-induced stillbirth in swine. Blood COHb levels may return to normal in as little as 2 hours once CO exposure has ceased and animals are breathing fresh air. Consequently, recovery time should be taken into account when interpreting COHb values.

ANHYDROUS AMMONIA

Anhydrous ammonia (gas-NH_3), used as an agricultural fertilizer nitrogen source, presents a unique risk of exposure to both animals and humans because of its use on farms and the fact that it is stored, transported, and applied under high pressure. Poisoning with gas-NH_3 is generally associated with gas release from broken hoses, failure of valves, and human error in operating the transport or application equipment. A large release of gas-NH_3 forms a white vapor cloud that may linger for several hours. In the atmosphere, gas-NH_3 rapidly combines with water forming caustic ammonium hydroxide. The moisture-rich membranes of the cornea, mouth, and respiratory tract are especially susceptible to damage from the resulting strong alkali burns. Acute death from laryngospasm and accumulation of fluid in the lungs can occur within a matter of minutes when the gas-NH_3 concentration is high. Animals surviving the initial exposure are frequently blinded from corneal damage and slough epithelium throughout the respiratory tract, and may not regain full productive status. Secondary bacterial invasion is a common outcome and generally affords a guarded prognosis.

NITROGEN DIOXIDE

Fermentation of ensiled corn and other forage containing elevated nitrate is the source of nitrogen dioxide (NO_2) presenting the greatest risk to livestock. NO_2 is a highly toxic gas with a bleachlike odor and a reddish-brown color. Most NO_2 forms during the first 2 weeks after harvested forage has been put in a silo, with the highest concentrations generally reached during the first 48 hours. Because NO_2 is heavier than air, it layers out on top of the silage within the silo and can gravitate down the access shute flowing into the silo room at the bottom of the shute and possibly the adjoining buildings, exposing animals in the feeding area.

NO_2 is a dangerous gas that can injure or kill livestock and humans. When NO_2 combines with water it forms highly corrosive nitric acid and can cause permanent damage to the lungs and respiratory tract because of the high moisture content of these tissues. Most humans can smell NO_2 at a concentration of 1 to 3 ppm, while membrane irritation is noted with 13 ppm. Mild to moderate irritation of the eyes and upper airways is experienced with from 50 to 150 ppm. The LD_{50} (median lethal dose) for NO_2 is 174 ppm for 1 hour. The health impact of NO_2 exposure is a function of both the concentration of the gas and the duration of the exposure. In general, short-term exposures to very high concentrations are much more toxic than exposure to lower levels for longer periods of time. Breathing moderate concentrations of NO_2 can cause coughing, choking, tightness in the chest, and nausea. Depending on the exposure, symptoms may subside in a few hours or persist for 1 to 2 weeks. In some cases a delayed phase of NO_2 poisoning characterized by pulmonary edema, tachycardia, fever, rales, and hypoxia is seen from 2 to 10 days after apparent recovery from the acute phase. Exposure to high concentrations can produce immediate death. Inhalation of sublethal doses may lead to chronic bronchitis or emphysema and in humans to the pulmonary condition known as silo filler's disease.

BIBLIOGRAPHY

Carson TL: Carbon monoxide–induced stillbirth. *In* Kirkbride CA (ed): Laboratory Diagnosis of Livestock Abortion, ed 3. Ames, Iowa State University Press, 1990, pp. 186–189.

Curtis SE: Environmental Management in Animal Agriculture. Ames, Iowa State University Press, 1983.

Dominick MA, Carson TL: Effects of carbon monoxide exposure on pregnant sows and their fetuses. Am J Vet Res 44:35–40, 1983.

Drummond JG, Curtis SE, Meyer RC, et al: Effects of atmospheric ammonia on young pigs experimentally infected with *Bordetella bronchiseptica*. Am J Vet Res 42:963–968, 1981.

Drummond JG, Curtis SE, Simon J: Effects of atmospheric ammonia on pulmonary bacterial clearance in the young pig. Am J Vet Res 39:211–212, 1978.

Drummond JG, Curtis SE, Simon J, et al: Effects of aerial ammonia on growth and health of young pigs. J Anim Sci 50:1085–1091, 1980.

Drummond JG, Curtis SE, Simon J, et al: Effects of atmospheric ammonia on young pigs experimentally infected with *Ascaris suum*. Am J Vet Res 42:969–974, 1981.

McMullen MJ, Hetrick TJ, Cannon LA: Ammonia, nitrogen, nitrous oxides, and related compounds. *In* Hadded LM, Winchester JF (eds): Clinical Management of Poisoning and Drug Overdose, ed 2. Philadelphia, WB Saunders, 1990, pp 1270–1280.

National Research Council Committee on Medical and Biologic Effects of Environmental Pollutants, Subcommittee on Ammonia: Ammonia. Baltimore, University Park Press, 1979.

National Research Council Committee on Medical and Biologic Effects of Environmental Pollutants, Subcommittee on Hydrogen Sulfide: Hydrogen Sulfide. Baltimore, University Park Press, 1979.

O'Donoghue JG: Hydrogen sulfide poisoning in swine. Can J Comp Med Vet Sci 25:217–219, 1961.

Osweiler GD, Carson TL, Buck WB, et al: Clinical and Diagnostic Veterinary Toxicology, ed 3. Dubuque, Iowa, Kendall Hunt, 1985.

■ Toxic Properties of Animal Wastes and Sewage Sludge Applied to Agricultural Lands

Robert H. Poppenga, D.V.M., Ph.D., Diplomate, A.B.V.T.
Daniel O'Brien, D.V.M.

Increasing generation of municipal sewage and animal wastes such as manure and poultry litter has created concern about appropriate and environmentally benign disposal methods. Disposal approaches to municipal sewage sludge have included ocean dumping, incineration, and land application.[1] Animal manure and poultry litter have been applied to land and incorporated into ruminant livestock feeds as sources of plant and animal nutrients, respectively. Because sewage and animal wastes can contain numerous organic, inorganic, and infectious contaminants, disposal of such materials generates interest because of possible adverse effects on human, animal, and environmental health. Veterinarians should be aware of the issues involved with sewage, manure, and poultry litter application to agricultural lands since it is likely that producers and their neighbors will raise questions concerning the safety of such practices. The following discussion focuses on potential risks to animal health and food safety from common contaminants found in sewage and animal wastes. Issues related to the presence of infectious agents in sewage and manure and the impact of land application of such materials on environmental quality are beyond the scope of this discussion.

MUNICIPAL SEWAGE

Municipal sewage is a mixture of liquids and solids derived from both domestic and industrial sources.[1] The presence of organic and inorganic pollutants in sewage varies considerably with location and time.[2] Initial treatment of sewage involves passage through screens which removes large debris. Wastewater is then directed to large holding tanks that allow heavier wastes to settle, creating sludge which is collected for further processing. Secondary sewage treatment involves the biodegradation of sewage by aerobic or anaerobic bacteria. A number of factors are important for proper microbial degradation of sewage, including the presence of appropriate amounts of nitrogen, phosphorus, and trace elements, and the right temperature and pH. Industrial sewage may be further treated by a variety of chemical and physical reactions for additional purification. Following treatment, sludge is dewatered by sedimentation, centrifugal separation, or filtration to reduce bulk prior to disposal. A variety of additives may be intentionally added during sewage processing.[1] Livestock manure is processed in several ways but, by and large, solids are separated from water; water is then available for recycling, and solids can be used as fertilizers or incorporated into ruminant feeds. Deep-stacked poultry litter, dried cage layer litter, and ensiled swine manure solids have been utilized in ruminant rations, as have municipal sewage products.[3] Poultry litter has higher concentrations of nutrients than manure from other livestock species and is also relatively dry and collectable. Thus, it has been widely used as a ruminant feed ingredient.

INDUSTRIAL CHEMICALS

Given the large increase in the use of synthetic chemicals by industry and in livestock feeds over the last several decades, it is not surprising that many of these substances can be found in sewage or animal wastes.[4] During sewage processing, contaminants may partition onto solids as a result of their hydrophobic and lipophilic nature. This adsorption can serve to concentrate contaminants in sludge. Although there are literally hundreds of possible contaminants in sludges or animal wastes, most studies have focused on possible health risks associated with several environmentally persistent organic compounds such as polychlorinated biphenyls, dioxin, and dioxin-like compounds and metals such as arsenic, cadmium, chromium, copper, lead, mercury, nickel, and zinc. Arsenic and copper are common poultry and swine feed additives while other metals originate primarily in municipal sewage from domestic and industrial sources. Concentrations of metals can reach relatively high levels. It is not uncommon for broiler litter to contain up to 300 ppm copper.[3]

HUMAN EXPOSURE TO TOXIC CONTAMINANTS

Of ultimate concern to veterinarians and producers is exposure of livestock to either potentially toxic concentrations of a contaminant or exposure of livestock to a nontoxic concentration that results in contamination of an animal product destined for human consumption. Given the diversity of contaminants in sewage and animal wastes and the large number of factors that may influence their persistence in the environment and, ultimately, their presence in animal food products, there is still much to be learned about the ultimate fate of many contaminants, particularly organic compounds. For example, poultry litter is removed from houses twice a year. It has been speculated that this allows time for microorganisms to degrade antibiotic residues in litter, although definitive studies are lacking.[3] Physical properties such as volatility and lipophilicity of contaminants, the source of sewage and its treatment method, surface or subsurface application methods, soil characteristics such as pH and organic content, crops grown on treated land, species of animal exposed to treated land or crops, and animal feeding and management factors can all influence the fate of contaminants.

FEEDING OF WASTE PRODUCTS

There have been numerous studies examining the potential effects of feeding sewage sludges, manure, and poultry litter directly to livestock.[5–10] Under the conditions of these studies there appears to be little adverse health effect on livestock from such practices. While modest increases in metal concentrations occur in some tissues, particularly liver and kidney, toxicoses are extremely unlikely when such products are fed as part of a nutritionally balanced ration. However, there is one case report of copper toxicosis in cattle fed chicken litter at 9 to 13.6 kg (dry matter) per cow.[11] Copper was detected in litter samples between 685 ppm and 920 ppm. Also, sheep have been intoxicated with copper from poultry litter.[12] There is at least some evidence that iron derived from sludges can result in iron toxicosis in livestock.[13] Perhaps of more concern is the accumulation of some metals, especially cadmium, in organs and muscle that exceed recommended human consumption levels.

The feeding of manure and poultry litter is regulated by individual states. Regulations generally follow guidelines established by the Association of Feed Control Officials which stipulate that manure be processed in such a way that no pathogenic organisms are present in the final product. In addition, for any material containing drug residues, at least a 15-day withdrawal period prior to slaughter or the use of milk and eggs for human consumption is recommended.[3]

WASTE-CONTAMINATED FORAGE

In addition to the direct feeding of sewage, manure, and poultry litter to livestock, studies examining the risk of feeding various forages grown on soil treated with such materials to livestock or allowing animals access to pastures where prior applications have occurred have been conducted.[14–18] Exposure to contaminants under such conditions is via incidental ingestion of soil, which can be substantial, or of plants that have taken up contaminants via their roots or via volatilization and absorption through foliage. As with the direct incorporation of sludge, manure, and litter into livestock rations, the risk to livestock is slight. The potential of contaminants in soil and crops to reach levels of concern in milk, meat, or other animal products intended for human consumption also appears to be slight, although environmentally persistent organics such as chlorobenzenes, chlorophenols, polychlorinated biphenyls and polychlorinated dibenzodioxins and dibenzofurans are of potential concern and warrant further study. Much more information is available concerning the tissue accumulation of metals. While some modest increase in metal concentrations have been noted, particularly for cadmium, the increases have occurred in organ tissues and not milk or meat. For example, goats fed corn silage grown on sludge-amended soil for 3 years had increased concentrations of cadmium in liver and kidney tissue but no increases in milk or meat.[19]

Because of concern about land application of contaminated sewage sludge, the Environmental Protection Agency (EPA) has promulgated regulations regarding sewage disposal and monitoring under the Clean Water Act. In addition, many states have their own regulations regarding the application of sludge to agricultural or reclaimed lands. Ceiling concentrations for several metals in sludge have been determined (Table 1). In addition, annual and cumulative pollutant loading rates have been established for most of the metals. The frequency of monitoring depends upon the amount of sewage applied to a given unit of land. Ultimately, sludge, manure, and poultry litters cannot be applied to land at rates that would exceed the amount of nitrogen needed by the type of vegetation grown on the land. Because of the lack of information regarding the fate of many organic chemicals, regulatory limits have not been established. If veterinarians or producers have questions about regulations in their own state, the environmental protection agency in that state should be contacted.

Table 1

CEILING LIMITS FOR METAL CONTAMINANTS IN SEWAGE AND ANNUAL AND CUMULATIVE LOADING RATES FOR LAND APPLICATION AS ESTABLISHED BY THE ENVIRONMENTAL PROTECTION AGENCY*

Metal	Ceiling Concentrations in Sewage Sludge (mg/kg Dry Weight)	Annual Pollutant Loading Rate (kg/ha/365-Day Period)	Cumulative Pollutant Loading Rate (kg/ha)
Arsenic	75	2.0	41
Cadmium	85	1.9	39
Copper	4300	75	1500
Lead	840	15	300
Mercury	57	0.85	17
Molybdenum	75		
Nickel	420	21	420
Selenium	100	5.0	100
Zinc	7500	140	2800

ha, hectare.

*Code of Federal Regulations, Part 503: Standards for the use and disposal of sewage sludge.

CONCLUSION

The present use of sewage, manure, and litter does not present a health risk for livestock. In addition, there would appear to be little risk to consumers of milk and meat. It will be important to continue to monitor land application of such materials for possible long-term environmental effects and to gather information concerning the ultimate fate of several persistent contaminants found in sludges and animal wastes.

REFERENCES

1. Kraut AG: Toxic hazards of sewers and wastewater facilities. *In* Sullivan JB, Kreiger GR (eds): Hazardous Materials Toxicology: Clinical Principles of Environmental Health. Baltimore, Williams & Wilkins, 1992, pp 600–603.
2. Mumma RO, Raupach DC, Waldman JP, et al: National survey of elements and other constituents in municipal sewage sludges. Arch Environ Contam Toxicol 13:75, 1984.
3. Council for Agricultural Science and Technology: Integrated Animal Waste Management, Task Force Report No. 128. Ames, Iowa, Council for Agricultural Science and Technology, 1996.
4. Duarte-Davidson R, Jones KC: Screening the environmental fate of organic contaminants in sewage sludge applied to agricultural soils: II. The potential for transfers to plants and grazing animals. Sci Total Environ 185:59, 1996.
5. Boyer KW, Jones JW, Linscott D, et al: Trace element levels in tissues from cattle fed a sewage-sludge amended diet. J Toxicol Environ Health 8:281, 1981.
6. Westing TW, Fontenot JP, McClure WH, et al: Characterization of mineral element profiles in animal waste and tissue from cattle fed animal waste. I. Heifers fed broiler litter. J Anim Sci 61:670, 1985.
7. Westing TW, Fontenot JP, Webb KE Jr: Characterization of mineral element profiles in animal waste and tissue from cattle fed animal waste. II. Steers fed cattle feedlot waste. J Anim Sci 61:682, 1985.
8. Sanson DW, Hallford DM, Smith GS: Effects of long-term consumption of sewage solids on blood, milk and tissue elemental composition of breeding ewes. J Anim Sci 59:416, 1984.
9. Sanson DW, Hallford DM, Smith GS: Effects of dietary sewage solids on feedlot performance, carcass characteristics, serum constituents and tissue elements of growing lambs. J Anim Sci 59:425, 1984.

10. Smith GS, Hallford DM, Watkins JB III: Toxicological effects of gamma-irradiated sewage solids fed as seven percent of diet to sheep for four years. J Anim Sci 61:931, 1985.

11. Banton MI, Nicholson SS, Jowett PLH, et al: Copper toxicosis in cattle fed chicken litter. J Am Vet Med Assoc 191:827, 1984.

12. Fontenot JP, Webb KE Jr, Buehler RJ, et al: Effects of feeding different levels of broiler litter to ewes for long periods of time on performance and health. Livestock Res Rep 1971–1972:145, 1972.

13. Decker AM: Heavy metals problem noted with sludge application to pasture. Food Chem News 12(11):20, 1978.

14. Fitzgerald PR, Peterson J, Lue-Hing C: Heavy metals in tissue of cattle exposed to sludge-treated pastures for eight years. Am J Vet Res 46:703, 1985.

15. Hogue DE, Parrish JJ, Foote RH, et al: Toxicologic studies with male sheep grazing on municipal sludge-amended soil. J Toxicol Environ Health 14:153, 1984.

16. Telford JN, Thonney ML, Hogue DE, et al: Toxicologic studies in growing sheep fed silage corn cultured on municipal sludge-amended acid subsoil. J Toxicol Environ Health 10:73, 1982.

17. Lisk DJ, Boyd RD, Telford JN, et al: Toxicologic studies with swine fed corn grown on municipal sewage sludge-amended soil. J Anim Sci 55:613, 1982.

18. Telford JN, Hogue DE, Stouffer JR, et al: Toxicologic studies with growing sheep fed grass-legume hay grown on municipal sludge-amended soil. Nutr Rep Int 29:1391, 1984.

19. Bray BJ, Dowdy RH, Goodrich RD, et al: Trace metal accumulation in tissues of goats fed silage produced on sewage sludge-amended soil. J Environ Qual 14:114, 1985.

■ Lead Poisoning

Stan W. Casteel, D.V.M., Ph.D., Diplomate, A.B.V.T.

The potential for lead poisoning remains an important concern. Centuries of mining and processing have resulted in the redistribution of lead in the environment, making it a ubiquitous multimedia contaminant. While concern over organic pollutants has declined somewhat in the 1990s, there is continuing interest in lead because it is neither degraded in the environment nor significantly metabolized. The ATSDR/EPA (Agency for Toxic Substances and Disease Registry/Environmental Protection Agency) Priority List for 1995 ranks lead at the top of the 20 most hazardous substances in the environment.[1]

SOURCES

The decline in use of leaded gasoline in the 1980s has largely removed used engine oil from consideration as a form of highly toxic lead; however, lead-acid batteries, leaded paint, and solder remain. Ashes from burned buildings painted with leaded paint are a less conspicuous, but hazardous, source of lead. Other less likely sources include lead objects such as spent lead shot and weights, lead-contaminated media associated with mining and affiliated industries, linoleum, grease, outdated lead arsenate pesticides, and various leaded materials found in refuse piles. Lead poisoning is an occasional complication of embedded bullets when contact occurs with certain body fluids capable of solubilizing lead. Lead projectiles invading joints and the pleural cavity are subject to solubilization by synovial fluid.[2]

ABSORPTION AND MECHANISM OF ACTION

Lead-containing material is commonly ingested, solubilized in the acidic environment of the stomach or abomasum, and absorbed similar to the way calcium is absorbed in the upper small intestine. The gastrointestinal absorption of multimedia sources of lead is influenced not only by physiologic factors within the digestive tract but also by chemical and physical variables such as chemical species, particle size, and matrix association. Finely divided, highly soluble forms of free lead are most readily absorbed from the gastrointestinal tract.

The basic mechanism of lead neurotoxicity appears to result from interference with some aspect of endogenous divalent cation, especially intracellular calcium, function.[3] Lead is also known to inhibit energy metabolism in brain capillaries of calves.[4] Results of this study also suggested a direct effect of lead on neuronal tissue.

Calcium is absorbed in the upper small intestine by a variety of energy-dependent and independent mechanisms. Active transport mechanisms for calcium in the gastrointestinal tract parallel increased calcium requirements for bone growth and maturation of other tissue. Calcium-binding proteins involved in these mechanisms have a similar, if not greater, affinity for lead.[5] This lead absorption mechanism is consistent with the greater absorption fraction of lead in immature animals. Estimates of the absorption fraction of soluble forms of lead in mature and immature animals are 8% to 10% in adults vs. 40% to 50% in juveniles.

CLINICAL SIGNS

Animal species differ in their sensitivity to lead, with cattle most commonly affected, partly due to their sheer numbers and to their propensity to lick, mouth, and ingest unusual materials. Mature cattle dosed with a mixture of lead sulfur and lead oxides at the rate of 2 mg/kg/day of lead in the diet for 28 days developed signs of plumbism.[6] At higher doses of lead, sudden death may occur in the absence of noticeable symptoms; however, signs of cerebrocortical dysfunction dominate the clinical picture of lead-poisoned cattle. Depression, cortical blindness, head bobbing, twitching of facial muscles and ears, rapid blinking, ataxia, circling, and head pressing are all symptomatic. Intermittent periods of extreme excitation and convulsions often end in death. Less sensational signs of gastrointestinal disturbance include anorexia, ptyalism, odontoprisis, rumen atony, and sometimes mild diarrhea.

Lead poisoning is rarely diagnosed in sheep and goats. The reasons for this are unclear, but probably reflect a limited population of small ruminants, reduced access to leaded materials, and a relative resistance to lead intoxication. Similarly, pigs are resistant to lead. Definitive reasons for their tolerance are unknown but may be related to a less permeable blood-brain barrier or cellular calcium homeostasis that is less sensitive to lead.

PATHOLOGY

Lead inclusion bodies are often found in proximal renal tubular epithelial cells and occasionally in hepatocytes. Calves dosed with 0.834 mg of lead per kilogram of body weight from lead acetate in a milk diet for 16 weeks did not show clinical signs of intoxication, but developed severe renal lesions.[7] Histologically, there were intranuclear inclusion bodies in proximal tubular cells, fibrosis, and periglomerular interstitial nephritis.

DIAGNOSIS

Diagnosis is based on signs of cerebrocortical dysfunction, anorexia, death in 24 to 96 hours, and chemical evidence of excessive exposure. In cattle, whole blood containing more than

0.35 ppm lead, or liver and kidney concentrations exceeding 10 ppm wet weight are diagnostic. Paradoxically, there is little accumulation of lead in the brain, suggesting either exquisite sensitivity of this organ or perhaps the involvement of cerebral ischemia in the development of the intoxication syndrome.

When essential, distinguishing sources of lead originating from different mining regions using stable lead isotope ratios is possible by matching the ratio (e.g., ^{207}Pb/^{206}Pb) found in tissues of poisoned livestock with that of suspect material.[8] Although this methodology has not been used in veterinary diagnostic medicine, the effectiveness of the technique has been demonstrated experimentally in pigs (author's unpublished data).

Like lead, causes of polioencephalomalacia (PEM), such as thiamine-responsive PEM and water deprivation, should be considered in the differential diagnosis of livestock showing cerebrocortical dysfunction. Toxicosis from ammoniated forage, and chlorinated hydrocarbon insecticides should be considered together with ketosis and hypomagnesemia when circumstances dictate.

TREATMENT

Calcium disodium ethylenediaminetetraacetic acid (EDTA) administered at 55 to 90 mg/kg body weight slowly intravenously (IV) or intramuscularly (IM) two times per day for 3 to 5 days, depending on the dose selected, is recommended for reducing the burden of lead in the toxic pool. Administration of EDTA in IV fluids is preferred to aid dehydrated animals and to facilitate excretion of the water-soluble chelate. At the same time, the IM administration of 2 mg/kg of thiamine HCl twice daily for up to 13 days is recommended to induce remission of nervous derangement more effectively than chelation.[6] Chelation therapy alone may increase the severity of clinical signs due to the redistribution of lead from bone and soft tissues (i.e., liver and kidney) to the central nervous system (CNS). Treatment should be followed by a 2- to 3-day rest period and reevaluation of the clinical condition. If improvement is insufficient, therapy can be repeated. Feeding of a zinc-containing mineral supplement to replenish chelation losses is a part of supportive care, especially when repeated therapy is required. When elevated blood lead concentrations persist, retention of leaded objects in the gastrointestinal tract or projectiles in synovial cavities should be considered for removal. Restricting further access to sources is essential. Reduction of bioavailable lead in contaminated soil may be accomplished with rock phosphate amendments.[9]

RESIDUES

A modicum of evidence addresses the issue of lead residues in edible tissues and milk. The absence of an accurate index of the body burden of lead and an incomplete understanding of lead toxicokinetics precludes establishment of slaughter withholding times for contaminated livestock. Cows dosed with lead for 28 days did not have significant lead residues remaining in skeletal muscle, liver, and kidney when slaughtered 68 to 110 days after exposure ceased.[6] Eight cows exposed, but not clinically intoxicated, to lead from lead-acid storage batteries for 2 days were monitored using blood and milk samples for 18 weeks.[10] Two weeks after exposure, the mean lead levels in milk and blood from six cows were 0.08 and 0.36 ppm, respectively. The half-life of blood lead was about 9 weeks. In eight acutely intoxicated cows that were emergently slaughtered, lead in skeletal muscle was 0.23 to 0.50 ppm wet weight. A significant portion of this lead can be attributed to blood perfusing the muscle.

REFERENCES

1. Agency for Toxic Substances and Disease Registry (ATSDR): Top 20 Hazardous Substances, ATSDR/EPA Priority List for 1995. Washington, DC, US Department of Health and Human Services, Public Health Service. Available at http://atsdr1.atsdr.cdc.gov:8080.
2. Meggs WJ, Gerr F, Aly MH, et al: The treatment of lead poisoning from gunshot wounds with succimer (DMSA). Clin Toxicol 32:377, 1994.
3. Chetty CS, Rajanna S, Hall E, et al: In vitro and in vivo effects of lead, methyl mercury and mercury on inositol 1,4,5-trisphosphate and 1,3,4,5-tetraisophosphate receptor bindings in rat brain. Toxicol Lett 87:11, 1996.
4. Ahrens FA: Effects of lead on glucose metabolism, ion flux, and collagen synthesis in cerebral capillaries of calves. Am J Vet Res 54:808, 1993.
5. Fullmer CS, Edelstein S, Wasserman RH: Lead-binding properties of intestinal calcium binding proteins. J Biol Chem 260:6816, 1985.
6. Coppock RW, Wagner WC, Reynolds JD, et al: Evaluation of edetate and thiamine for treatment of experimentally induced environmental lead poisoning in cattle. Am J Vet Res 52:1860, 1991.
7. Schraishuhn J, Kaufer-Weiss I, Weiss E: Light and electron microscopic studies of calf kidneys after exposure to subtoxic lead levels. Berl Munch Tierarztl Wochenschr 105:290, 1992.
8. Smith DR, Osterloh JD, Flegal AR: Use of endogenous, stable lead isotopes to determine release of lead from the skeleton. Environ Health Perspect 104:60, 1996.
9. Ma QY, Logan TJ, Traina SJ: Lead immobilization from aqueous solution and contaminated soils using phosphate rocks. Environ Sci Technol 29:1118, 1995.
10. Oskarsson A, Jorhem L, Sundberg J, et al: Lead poisoning in cattle—Transfer of lead in milk. Sci Total Environ 111:83, 1992.

■ Selenium Toxicosis

Merl F. Raisbeck, D.V.M., M.S., Ph.D., Diplomate, A.B.V.T.
Donal O'Toole, M.V.S., Ph.D., F.R.C.Path.
E. Lee Belden, Ph.D.

Selenium (Se) was first conclusively linked to naturally occurring disease during the 1920s by the Agricultural Experiment Stations of South Dakota and Wyoming. Despite six decades of research, many aspects of the natural history of selenium intoxication (selenosis) in livestock remain controversial. Classic descriptions, which are still frequently repeated in modern texts, attribute four discrete syndromes to selenium intoxication: (1) acute selenium poisoning, (2) experimental chronic selenosis, (3) alkali disease, and (4) blind staggers. It is likely that the neurologic condition described as "blind staggers" was, in fact, a potpourri of other maladies, especially sulfate-induced polioencephalomalacia, mistakenly attributed to Se.[1] The other three conditions most likely represent a continuum of the cytotoxic effects of Se in which target organs and thus clinical signs vary with dose and duration of exposure, species of animal, chemical form of Se, and so forth.

ACUTE SELENOSIS

Acute selenosis is usually the result of iatrogenic poisoning with nutritional supplements. Plants which accumulate sufficient Se to be acutely toxic are sufficiently unpalatable that animals will starve rather than eat them.[2] Acute selenosis may present as sudden death with few if any clinical signs. In most species clinical signs of acute Se intoxication involve the respiratory, cardiovascular, hematopoietic, and gastrointestinal systems.[3, 5–7] Affected animals exhibit lassitude, muscular weakness, ataxia, anorexia, and progressively worsening dyspnea beginning 1 to 24 hours after exposure. Abdominal pain is reflected in a stilted gait, tucked abdomen, or grinding teeth, or a combination of these. Heart rate and respiration are elevated, the pulse is weak, and animals are frequently cyanotic. Weakness progresses to prostration and coma and lethally poisoned animals usually die within 12 to 48 hours. Vomition is fairly common in swine and may occur in other species. Fever, polyuria, and hemolytic anemia have been reported, but are not always present. Diarrhea, if present, usually occurs in animals that survive the acute crisis.

Interestingly, many of the lesions of acute Se intoxication are similar to those of Se deficiency.[3, 4, 7] The most striking gross lesions are usually in the thorax. The heart may be pale or mottled and flaccid. Petechial to ecchymotic hemorrhages occur beneath the epicardium and endocardium and throughout the thoracic viscera. Marked hydrothorax, hydropericardium, and ascites are present and typically consist of a clear to yellow serofibrinous transudate. Lungs are wet, heavy, and often congested, with prominent septal edema and froth in airways. The gastrointestinal tract may be hyperemic, especially after oral exposure, and is usually edematous. Hepatic or renal damage, or both, are often present, but may not be grossly recognizable.

POLIOMYELOMALACIA

Flaccid paralysis or tetraplegia may occur after 5 to 30 days in swine.[8–10] Although there are widely scattered reports of neurologic lesions in other species, only swine consistently develop neurologic signs. The onset of signs may be sudden. Affected swine exhibit ascending paralysis or tetraplegia, but remain alert, have normal vision, and will eat if offered food. Very mildly affected animals may recover, but most do not. Clinical signs result from bilaterally symmetrical necrosis of the ventral gray horn of the cervical and lumbar spinal intumescences (poliomyelomalacia), combined in some pigs with lesions in specific brain stem nuclei. This lesion may be grossly visible in some cases, but is usually diagnosed histopathologically. Poliomyelomalacia usually occurs in the portion of a herd that survives an episode of acute intoxication and usually precedes or coincides with the occurrence of classic chronic selenosis or "alkali disease" in the same herd.

CHRONIC SELENOSIS

Alkali disease most frequently results from chronic (>30 days) exposure to seleniferous grains or forages. It may also be produced by inorganic Se salts (especially in swine) or by shorter exposures. The characteristic signs of alkali disease are bilaterally symmetrical alopecia and dystrophic hoof growth. Alopecia typically occurs on the nape of the neck and tail, but in severe cases may involve other parts of the body. The first signs of alkali disease in cattle, horses, and swine are lameness, erythema, and swelling of the coronary bands. These signs subside to be followed in a few days to 3 weeks by a circumferential crack parallel to and just distal to the coronet. Hoof separation and lameness progress apace until the damaged claw is displaced from underneath by new growth and sloughs. In some cases, the damaged claw is not shed but remains attached, resulting in an extended, upwardly curled toe. Affected animals become so lame they are unable to eat or drink and thus starve. Sheep are reportedly resistant to the epithelial effects of Se and experience only infertility when grazed on toxic pastures.[11] Although there are no definitive experimental comparisons, it is our opinion that species susceptibility to Se is, in descending order, swine, horses, cattle, sheep.

Se is immunotoxic in waterfowl and rodents.[12, 13] Recent experiments in our laboratory demonstrated that Se is also immunotoxic in ruminants, blocking primary antibody response to antigen administered while tissue concentrations were elevated.[14, 15] Immunotoxicity appears to require an Se dose just slightly less than that required for overt clinical toxicity. The practical significance of this observation remains to be determined under field conditions, but it suggests that animals chronically exposed to high dietary Se are at increased risk of infectious disease.

Several other syndromes, notably hepatopathy, anemia, infertility, teratogenesis, myocardial degeneration, and arthritis were attributed to chronic selenosis in the past.[11] The degree to which Se was directly responsible for these conditions and how much was secondary to starvation or recumbency is open to question and beyond the scope of this article. In our experience, these effects are rare in horses or cattle under field conditions. Nevertheless, veterinarians should be alert to the possibility that such effects may occur in herds with selenosis.

DIAGNOSIS

Diagnosis of Se intoxication rests on the traditional triad of clinical signs, biochemical and morphologic lesions, and chemical analysis. Tissue Se concentrations are less reliably predictive of damage than other toxicants. In general, inorganic Se is cleared more rapidly than Se from "natural" sources such as forages and grains. Natural Se (specifically selenomethionine) accumulates to greater concentrations in most tissues with chronic feeding, yet appears to be less available for either beneficial or toxic functions. Se may form biologically inert complexes with other elements in tissues which are diagnostically indistinguishable from biologically available forms.[16] Glutathione peroxidase activity, which normally increases with Se exposure, may briefly dip into the deficiency range in some horses and cattle near the onset of clinical signs.

Samples typically recommended for Se analysis include blood, liver, hoof, and hair. Each has advantages and disadvantages. Blood and hepatic Se are somewhat more ephemeral,[11] but elevated concentrations (greater than 1.0 ppm) usually persist past the onset of clinical signs in livestock.[17] Theoretically, Se deposited in hair or hoof is metabolically inert and thus is a more reliable long-term indicator of Se exposure than liver or blood.[11] Hair or hoof concentrations greater than 5.0 ppm suggest excessive Se exposure. Some caution is warranted, however, as hair and hoof Se content may be influenced by seasonal or nutritional influences on rate of growth, exogenous contamination, or anatomic location. It is not unusual to see a 10-fold or greater variation in Se concentration along a hair shaft or in different parts of a hoof (Fig. 1). Used judiciously, this variation in hair or wool Se can be helpful in approximating the temporal pattern of exposure as concentrations further from the follicle represent earlier exposures.

TREATMENT

There are no proven therapies for acute or subacute selenosis. Experimentally, antioxidants such as vitamin E lessen the cytotoxic effects of Se,[18] but this strategy has not been tested in food animals. Symptomatic and supportive therapy may be helpful in a few cases, but the prognosis for any animal showing signs of acute or subacute selenosis is poor. Uncomplicated alkali disease in horses has been successfully treated with palliative measures such as heart-bar shoes, therapeutic trimming, analgesics, nonsteroidal anti-inflammatory agents, and nursing care.[17] Clients should be emphatically warned that labor-intensive supportive

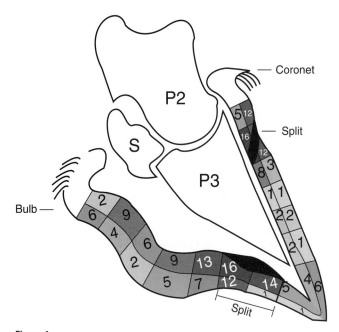

Figure 1

Selenium distribution in affected hoof. Schematic drawing of hoof of a horse 3 weeks after onset of lameness. Separation is denoted by *black* areas. Numerals denote selenium concentration in parts per million.

care will be required for several months and that animals will be very uncomfortable during most of this time.

Prevention consists of avoiding excess Se exposure. Total dietary concentrations as low as 5 ppm (dry matter) are potentially toxic. Se-containing mineral supplements should be avoided, if possible, in seleniferous areas. Flax-derived cyanogenic glycosides and organic arsenicals interfere with Se uptake experimentally, but have not been very successful under field conditions. Low dietary protein potentiates Se toxicity, but there is some question whether extremely high protein is protective. In situations where seleniferous vegetation is confined to "hot spots," these may be identified by chemical analysis and fenced out. Grazing may be timed to take advantage of seasonal variation in forage Se content. Published accounts from South Dakota indicate that highest concentrations occur in late spring or early summer[19] but this may not be true in all locations. There is anecdotal evidence of genetic adaptation by cattle to seleniferous ranges. Common sense thus dictates caution in introducing new bloodlines to affected herds. Selenosis is often exacerbated by other nutritional disorders (e.g., copper deficiency) endemic to arid grasslands. Before recommending management strategies to control selenosis, veterinarians should investigate the full spectrum of nutritional and toxic possibilities.

REFERENCES

1. O'Toole D, Raisbeck MF, Case J, et al: Selenium-induced "blind staggers" and related myths. A commentary on the extent of historical livestock losses attributed to selenosis on western US rangelands. Vet Pathol 33:104, 1996.
2. James LF, Panter KE: Selenium accumulators. *In* Howard JL (ed): Current Veterinary Therapy 3: Food Animal Practice, WB Saunders, Philadelphia, 1993, pp 366–366.
3. Blodget DJ, Beville RF: Acute selenium toxicosis in sheep. Vet Hum Toxicol 29:233, 1987.
4. Van Vleet JF, Meyer KB, Olander JH: Acute selenium toxicosis induced in baby pigs by parenteral administration of selenium–vitamin E preparations. J Am Vet Med Assoc 165:543, 1974.
5. Smyth JBA, Wang JH, Barlow RM, et al.: Experimental acute selenium intoxication in lambs. J Comp Pathol 102:197, 1990.
6. Ahmed KE, Adam SE, Idrill OF: Experimental selenium poisoning in nubian goats. Vet Hum Toxicol 32:249, 1990.
7. MacDonald DW, Christian RG, Strausz KI, et al.: Acute selenium toxicity in neonatal calves. Can Vet J 22:279, 1981.
8. Casteel SW, Osweiler GD, Cook WO: Selenium toxicosis in swine. J Am Vet Med Assoc 186:1084, 1985.
9. Wilson TM, Scholz RW, Drake TR: Selenium toxicity and porcine focal symmetrical poliomyelomalacia: Description of a field outbreak and experimental reproduction. Can J Comp Med 47:412, 1983.
10. Baker DC, James LF, Hartley WJ, et al.: Toxicosis in pigs fed selenium-accumulating *Astragalus* plant species or sodium selenate. Am J Vet Res 50:1396, 1989.
11. Olson OE: Selenium as a cause of livestock poisoning. *In* Keeler RF, Van Kampen KR, James LF (eds): Effects of Poisonous Plants on Livestock, New York, Academic Press, 1978, pp 121–133.
12. Fairbrother A, Fowles J: Subchronic effects of sodium selenite and selenomethionine on several functions in mallards. Arch Environ Contam Toxicol 19:836–844, 1990.
13. Koller LD, Exon JH, Talcott PA, et al.: Immune responses in rats supplemented with selenium. Clin Exp Immunol 63:570, 1986.
14. Schamber RA, Belden EL, Raisbeck MF: Selenium immunotoxicity. *In* Schuman G, Vance G (eds): Decades Later: A Time for Reassessment, Princeton, WV, American Society of Surface Mining and Reclamation, 1995, pp 384–393.
15. Raisbeck MF, O'Toole D, Schamber RA, et al.: Toxicologic effects of a high-selenium hay diet in captive adult and yearling pronghorn antelope (*Antilocapra americana*). J Wildlife Dis 32:9–16, 1996.
16. Goode AA, Wolterbeek HT: Have high selenium concentrations in wading birds their origin in mercury? Sci Total Environ 144:247, 1994.
17. Raisbeck MF, Dahl ER, Sanchez DA, et al.: Naturally occurring selenosis in Wyoming. J Vet Diagn Invest 5:84, 1993.
18. Csallany AS, Su L, Menken BZ: Effect of selenite, vitamin E and *N,N*'-diphenyl-*p*-phenylenediamine on liver organic solvent-soluble lipofuscin pigments in mice. J Nutr 114:1582–1587, 1984.
19. Olson OE, Jornlin DF, Moxon AL: The selenium content of vegetation and the mapping of seleniferous soils. J Am Soc Agron 34:607, 1942.

■ Aflatoxins*

Roger B. Harvey, D.V.M., M.S.

The aflatoxins (AF), a closely related group of polysubstituted bisfuranocoumarins, are secondary metabolites that may be produced by *Aspergillus* fungi on foods and feedstuffs during growth, harvest, storage, or transportation. They can cause death in humans and animals; however, the greatest economic impact comes from reduced productivity, suppressed immune function, teratogenic effects, and pathologic effects on organs and tissues. Consumption of AF-contaminated feeds has caused abortions in cows and death of calves that ingested AF-contaminated milk. Aflatoxins can induce hepatocarcinomas in laboratory animals and AF are suspected carcinogens for humans. All species of domestic animals are susceptible to the effects of AF, and the primary expressions of toxicity are hepatotoxicity and immunosuppression with secondary nephrotoxicity. Classic pathologic lesions from intoxicated animals consist of hepatocellular degeneration with bile duct hyperplasia.

There are four AF commonly identified in feed: AFB_1, AFG_1, AFB_2, and AFG_2, and this is also the generally accepted order of toxicity, with AFB_1 the most toxic. A toxic metabolite that is also carcinogenic, AFM_1 is secreted into the milk of lactating animals. With the exception of liver and kidney, residues of AF do not accumulate to any extent in edible tissues of domestic animals. The Food and Drug Administration (FDA) set the tolerance or action levels of AF in animal feeds and human foods at 20 ppb except milk, which is 0.5 ppb. While these are the legal limits for AF, exceptions have been made under published special FDA guidance levels when increased AF levels are allowed in animal feeds, depending on the species, age, and breeding status. Commodities most commonly associated with AF contamination in North America include corn, cottonseed, and peanuts. Increased incidences of AF contamination in feedstuffs are almost always associated with drought conditions during crop growth. There are species and age suseptibilities to the toxicity of AF with rainbow trout, ducklings, and turkey poults being the most sensitive. The order of sensitivity of domestic mammals from most to least sensitive are piglets; dogs, calves, foals, horses, and feeder pigs; finishing hogs and lambs; mature cattle; and mature sheep. Volumes have been written about AF since their discovery as the causative agent of turkey X disease in 1960, and excellent reviews on AF are included in Budine and Mertens, Coppock and Swanson, Council for Agricultural Science and Technology, Phillips et al., and Smith and Henderson.

If conditions are favorable for *Aspergillus* growth and subsequent AF production, it is reasonable to assume that conditions could be right for other mycotoxins to be produced and be present as co-contaminants of a feed. This does happen and researchers have investigated the interactive effects of dietary AF when combined with other mycotoxins. Generally speaking, when AF are fed with other mycotoxins the resultant toxicity is an additive response. Rarely is it a less-than-additive (antagonistic) response, but it is sometimes a greater-than-additive response. When 2.5 ppm AF was combined with 5 ppm diacetoxyscirpenol (DAS), or when 3.5 ppm AF and 4 ppm T-2 toxin were fed to broiler chicks, a synergism was noted for reduced body weight gain. The combined feeding of 2.5 ppm AF and 100 ppm fumonisin B_1 to growing barrows induced greater-than-additive responses for body weight, liver pathologic scores, serum biochemical alterations, and reduced immune function. Lambs fed 2.5 ppm AF and 5 ppm DAS had synergistic responses for reduced body weight, serum biochemical values, and hepatic lesions. When AF were combined with ochratoxin, T-2 toxin, deoxynivalenol, or DAS, the effects on growing swine were a primary expression of AF toxicity and the toxicity of the combination was not greater than would be predicted on the basis of each toxin's individual toxicity.

DIAGNOSIS

A diagnosis of acute aflatoxicosis would have to be based on clinical signs, the presence of AF in the feed or milk, and pathologic lesions. Although the same would be true of chronic aflatoxicosis, diagnosis is somewhat more difficult because the clinical picture is one of an unthrifty animal that could be reflective of a myriad of diseases. Immunosuppression, hepatic or renal dysfunction, clotting disorders, and possibly icterus are possible presentations with aflatoxicosis. Pigs are the most sensitive of the food-producing mammals. Taking a thorough clinical history may point to the possibility of a feed-related condition. Knowledge of the origin and history of grain or protein source is important because AF contamination is often associated with drought-stressed commodities. A thorough examination of feed storage facilities on the farm should also be included in the case workup and the presence of moldy feed, caked feed in bins or augers, or evidence of feed that has been exposed to moisture indicates the possibility of present or past fungal growth. On-farm mycotoxin analysis can be performed with enzyme-linked immunosorbent assay (ELISA)–based commercial test kits for AF. Both quantitative and qualitative kits are available, but the practitioner should recognize that they should only be used for the matrix intended (i.e., a single commodity) and not mixed feed. A composite sample of no less

than 5 kg should be collected (preferably with a probe) from various sites of the bulk feed container to be representative of the total lot. Whether tested on the farm or not, confirmation samples should be sent to an analytic laboratory. Testing with a black light or quantitating fungal spore counts in feed does not correlate well with mycotoxin content.

TREATMENT

There are no specific antidotes to or treatments for AF intoxication. Treatment is supportive and symptomatic. The practitioner should keep in mind that AF are hepatotoxins and treatments should be designed accordingly. The implicated feed should be removed and a mycotoxin-free ration that has been fortified with supplemental protein and limiting amino acids should be offered to animals. AF-contaminated milk from dairy cows should not be fed to nursing calves. Although animals many times will recover from aflatoxicosis once the feed is removed, they usually do not reach their full genetic potential.

PREVENTION

Grain and any other feedstuffs intended for animal feed should be tested for AF prior to ration formulation. This can be included as part of contract negotiations when purchasing bulk items. With the advent of test kits, such a stipulation should not add appreciably to the cost of feed. If feedstuffs are known to contain AF, several remedial treatments have been used to utilize the commodity for animals. Ammoniation of contaminated grain or cottonseed reduces AF content by approximately 90%. The only practical method employed in the United States is a low-temperature, low-pressure technique that uses anhydrous ammonia. There are human health risks and safety factors to consider with this process because of the danger of ammonia. Another successful remediation of AF has been the addition of adsorbent compounds such as hydrated sodium calcium aluminosilicate (HSCAS, NOVA SIL) or sodium bentonite to AF-contaminated feeds. Adsorbent compounds bind AF and prevent AF absorption in the gastrointestinal tract. The addition of 0.5% HSCAS has prevented toxicosis in swine, lambs, and poultry and reduced AFM_1 residues in milk of dairy cows and goats. Although these adsorbent compounds are not FDA-approved for this treatment, most enjoy a GRAS (generally *r*ecognized *a*s *s*afe) status and are routinely added to feeds as anticaking agents. An experimentally promising, but not yet available, technique for the destruction of AF involves the use of ozone to treat AF-contaminated commodities.

BIBLIOGRAPHY

Bodine AB, Mertens DR: Toxicology, metabolism, and physiological effects of aflatoxin in the bovine. *In* Diener UL, Asquith RL, Dickens JW (eds.): Aflatoxin and *Aspergillus flavus* in corn. Bull 279, Auburn, Alabama Agricultural Experiment Station, Auburn University, 1983, pp 46–50.

Coppock RW, Swanson SP: Aflatoxins. *In* Howard JL (ed): Current Veterinary Therapy: Food Animal Practice. Philadelphia, WB. Saunders, 1986, pp 363–367.

Council for Agricultural Science and Technology: Mycotoxins: Economic and Health Risks, Task Force Rep No. 116, Ames, Iowa, Council for Agricultural Science and Technology, 1989, pp 1–85.

Harvey RB, Edrington TS, Kubena LF, et al: Influence of aflatoxin and fumonisin B_1–containing culture material on growing barrows. Am J Vet Res 56:1668–1672, 1995.

Harvey RB, Edrington TS, Kubena LF, et al.: Effects of aflatoxin and diacetoxyscirpenol in ewe lambs. Bull Environ Contam Toxicol 54:325–330, 1995.

Huff WE, Harvey RB, Kubena LF, et al: Toxic synergism between aflatoxin and T-2 toxin in broiler chickens. Poult Sci 67:1418–1423, 1988.

Kubena LF, Harvey RB, Huff WE, et al: Efficacy of a hydrated sodium calcium aluminosilicate to reduce the toxicity of aflatoxin and diacetoxyscirpenol. Poult Sci 72:51–59, 1993.

Phillips TD, Sarr BA, Clement BA, et al: Prevention of aflatoxicosis in farm animals via selective chemisorption of aflatoxin. In Bray GA, Ryan DH (eds): Pennington Nutrition Series, Mycotoxins, Cancer, and Health, vol. 1. Baton Rouge, Louisiana State University Press, 1991, pp 223–238.

Smith JE, Henderson RS: Mycotoxins and Animal Foods, Boca Raton, Fla, CRC Press, 1991, pp 247–847.

■ Trichothecenes*

Roger B. Harvey, D.V.M., M.S.

The trichothecene mycotoxins are comprised of over 148 chemically related toxins that occur worldwide and may be produced by various species of fungi belonging to genera of *Trichoderma*, *Myrothecium*, *Cephalosporium*, *Verticimonosporium*, *Fusarium*, and *Stachybotrys*. By far, *Fusarium* is the most common producer of trichothecenes encountered in feedstuffs. The trichothecenes belong to a family of chemicals called "sesquiterpenoids" and can be divided into four groups, two known as "simple" trichothecenes and two known as "macrocyclic" trichothecenes. The simple trichothecenes are more prevalent in North America and the ones most commonly encountered with animal feed problems are T-2 toxin, diacetoxyscirpenol (DAS), deoxynivalenol (DON, vomitoxin), and nivalenol. The T-2 toxin occurs occasionally in the United States and Canada, but is better known for its association with "toxic alimentary aleukia" in humans of the Soviet Union in the 1940s caused by eating bread made from overwintered moldy grain. The T-2 toxin was reputedly used as a chemical warfare agent in Southeast Asia in the 1980s, and the macrocyclic mycotoxins have caused serious outbreaks of toxicoses in horses in Japan and eastern Europe. DON is a trichothecene frequently found in feedstuffs and is most commonly associated with chronic problems in livestock, primarily swine. Often zearalenone is a co-contaminant with DON. Both mycotoxins can be produced simultaneously by *Fusarium graminearum* in corn, wheat, or other cereal grains. DON at concentrations of 2 ppm or greater in the feed has been reported to cause reduced feed consumption and poor performance in swine. The susceptibility of swine to DON is highly variable, being dependent upon age, length of time exposed, and nutritional content of the ration. The T-2 toxin and DAS are caustic chemical compounds, and the signs associated with toxicosis, such as gastrointestinal irritation and cutaneous ulcerations, reflect this trait. Much has been written about trichothecene mycotoxins and excellent reviews for background information are contained in Beasley, Council for Agricultural Science and Technology, Prelusky et al., and Wannemacher et al.

Because multiple mycotoxins can coexist in grains and feedstuffs, researchers have questioned the interactive effects of mycotoxins in combination. Over 20 studies, conducted in my laboratory, indicated that trichothecenes act in an additive or less-than-additive manner when combined with other mycotoxins. Some notable exceptions were when 5 to 8 ppm of T-2 toxin and 5 to 15 ppm of DON were fed to broiler chicks or swine and toxic synergy was noted for decreased weight gain and increased pathologic lesions. When 100 ppm fumonisin B_1 and 4.5 ppm of DON were fed to growing swine, greater-than-additive effects were observed for reduced weight gain and relative liver weight.

---

*All of the material in this article is in the public domain.

DIAGNOSIS

Ideally, a diagnosis of trichothecene mycotoxicosis would come about because of presumptive clinical signs and lesions, and analyses of feed samples would show concentrations of mycotoxins at levels known to induce toxicosis. However, a diagnosis of trichothecene mycotoxicosis is difficult under the best of circumstances because of the vague clinical signs and nonpathognomonic lesions produced from either single or multiple mycotoxin exposure. Some of the animal disorders attributed to trichothecenes are reduced production and reproduction, emesis and diarrhea, immunosuppression, hematologic alterations, skin ulcerations, and bone marrow depression. Many of these effects have been observed during experimental feeding of trichothecene mycotoxins. Rarely do naturally contaminated feedstuffs have concentrations of mycotoxins sufficient to produce clear-cut signs or lesions described in laboratory studies. The practitioner should consider trichothecene mycotoxicosis in a differential diagnosis if decreased feed consumption or lack of gain, total feed refusal, sharply decreased milk production, or perioral cutaneous ulcerations are noted, particularly if conditions appear to be feed-related. Livestock instinctively will avoid most trichothecene-contaminated feed unless forced to consume it. Taking an accurate clinical history goes a long way toward diagnosis of any disease, and the origin of grain used in the ration can be very important. For example, knowledge of any adverse conditions conducive to fungal growth during growing, harvesting, or storage can be extremely important. Analysis of feed for mycotoxins has been simplified for the practitioner by the advent of field-expedient, user-friendly test kits employing enzyme-linked immunosorbent assay (ELISA) technology. Commercial qualitative and quantitative ELISA test kits are available for T-2 toxin and DON. The veterinarian should keep in mind that the kits are accurate only for the matrix intended, usually grain and not mixed feed. For more definitive results, a sample of feed, representative of that consumed at the time of or before the onset of signs, can be sent to a laboratory for mycotoxin analysis. Feed samples for laboratory analysis should be taken at random spots in the bin or container, preferably with a probe for a total of no less than 5 kg submitted. Fungal spore counts from feed do not correlate well with mycotoxin content; mycotoxins can be present with low spore counts or spore counts can be very high with undetectable mycotoxin concentrations. When interpreting results of trichothecene concentrations from laboratory analysis, the veterinarian should look carefully at DON content. Some mycotoxicologists view DON as a "marker" mycotoxin and its presence means that at one time, conditions were conducive for fungal growth, and it is possible that other undetected mycotoxins could be in the feed. Often, feeds with low concentrations of DON are associated with problems in herds or flocks that cannot be directly attributed to effects from DON.

TREATMENT

There are no specific treatments or antidotes for trichothecene intoxication. Treatment should be supportive and targeted at symptomatic signs. Animals should be removed from the causal diet and a mycotoxin-free feed substituted that is increased in protein or limiting amino acids. In cases of acute intoxication with extreme gastrointestinal irritation, activated charcoal may be indicated.

PREVENTION

Feedstuffs, particularly cereal grains, should be properly dried, stored, and handled to prevent mold growth, and generally speaking, overwintered or moldy grains should be avoided in ration formulation. With the advent of simple field test kits, it is suggested that routine mycotoxin testing be done on grains destined for animal feeds. If mycotoxins are detected, consultation with a toxicologist is recommended because mycotoxin-contaminated feed can sometimes be fed to less susceptible species with little or no effect. For example, DON-contaminated feed, while capable of inducing signs in growing swine, may not cause problems in beef cattle, sheep, or poultry. Moldy or mycotoxin-contaminated grains often have a nutritionally altered status and therefore may not be substituted into rations exactly as "normal" grain. Some supplemental ingredients may need to be added during formulation. To my knowledge, there are no chemical, biologic, or physical methods available to destroy trichothecene mycotoxins. Anecdotal information has it that sodium bentonite, hydrated sodium calcium aluminosilicate, or other adsorbent compounds added to DON-contaminated swine feeds reduce problems; however, I and others have exhaustively tested these compounds and find no efficacy for trichothecenes.

BIBLIOGRAPHY

Beasley VR: Trichothecenes. *In* Howard JL (ed): Current Veterinary Therapy 3: Food Animal Practice. Philadelphia, WB Saunders, 1993, pp 332–334.

Council for Agricultural Science and Technology: Mycotoxins: Economic and Health Risks, Task Force Rep No. 116, Ames, Iowa, Council for Agricultural Science and Technology, 1989, pp 1–85.

Friend DW, Thompson BK, Trenholm HL, et al: Toxicity of T-2 toxin and its interaction with deoxynivalenol when fed to young pigs. Can J Anim Sci 72:703–711, 1992.

Harvey RB, Edrington TS, Kubena LF, et al: Effects of dietary fumonsin B₁–containing culture material, deoxynivalenol-contaminated wheat, or their combination on growing barrows. Am J Vet Res 57:1790–1794, 1996.

Kubena LF, Huff WE, Harvey RB: Individual and combined toxicity of deoxynivalenol and T-2 toxin in broiler chicks. Poult Sci 68:622–628, 1989.

Prelusky DB, Rotter BA, Rotter RG: Toxicology of mycotoxins. *In* Miller JD, Trenholm HL (eds): Mycotoxins in Grain, Compounds Other Than Aflatoxin. St Paul, Eagan Press, 1994, pp 367–376.

Wannemacher RW Jr, Bunner DL, Neufeld HA: Toxicity of trichothecenes and other related mycotoxins in laboratory animals. *In* Smith JE, Henderson RS (eds): Mycotoxins and Animal Foods, Boca Raton, Fla, CRC Press, 1991, pp 499–552.

■ Zearalenone

Gary D. Osweiler, D.V.M., M.S., Ph.D.,
Diplomate, A.B.V.T.

SOURCES AND OCCURRENCE

Zearalenone is a mycotoxin produced on corn, wheat, barley, and milo by *Fusarium roseum (F. graminearum)*, the conidial stage of *Giberella zea*, as well as by some isolates of *Fusarium moniliforme*. Infected grain is commonly known by terms such as "pink ear rot" in corn, or "scabby" wheat or "tombstone wheat."[1] Zearalenone formation is favored by high-moisture conditions (grain with more than 20% moisture), and alternating high and low temperatures (45 to 70°F) typical of the North Central United States and Canada. Fungal infection and mycotoxin formation usually occur prior to harvest during maturation of the grain, and grains are often visibly affected with a pale, shriveled appearance, or a pink pigmentation. Zearalenone production is unlikely in stored grain unless storage moisture

exceeds 20%.[2] Concentrations in grain commonly range from 0.5 to 3.0 ppm.

MECHANISM OF ACTION

Zearalenone is a substituted resorcyclic acid lactone structurally similar to the anabolic agent zearalenol used to implant feedlot cattle.[3] It binds to cytosolic receptors for estradiol-17β forming a zearalenone-receptor complex which binds to nuclear estradiol sites on DNA. Zearalenone is weak estrogen with potency only one-fourth to one-half that of estradiol. It causes physical and behavioral changes typical of estrus, including uterine enlargement and edema with cellular proliferation and hypertrophy. Vaginal epithelial metaplasia changes cells from pseudostratified columnar to stratified squamous. Secretion and release of follicle-stimulating hormone (FSH) is inhibited, which interferes with preovulatory ovarian follicle maturation.

Zearalenone is absorbed from the gastrointestinal tract, metabolized to α- and β-zearalenol and excreted in bile, feces, and urine. Enterohepatic cycling prolongs retention of zearalenone after consumption stops, but detectable residues rarely persist more than a few days post exposure.[4]

CLINICAL EFFECTS

Effects of zearalenone are species-dependent, and reproductive toxicity varies widely among species. Approximate dietary concentrations causing clinical effects are as follows:

Prepubertal swine	**>1 ppm**
Sexually mature nongravid sows	**>3 ppm**
Pregnant sows (preimplantation)	**>30 ppm**
Immature boars	**>50 ppm**
Mature boars	**>200 ppm**
Virgin heifers	**>12 ppm**
Mature dairy cows	**>24 ppm**
Poultry	**>150 ppm**

In swine, the effects of zearalenone vary with when exposure occurs during the estrous cycle. Immature, prepubertal gilts experience signs commonly known as "vulvovaginitis" consisting of estrus with vulvar swelling, edema, and hyperemia; enlargement of mammary glands, tenesmus, and prolapse of the vagina or rectum, or both. Signs appear within 1 to 2 days after initial consumption of zearalenone and persist for 5 to 7 days post exposure. For mature sows, zearalenone early in the estrous cycle inhibits follicular development and induces signs of persistent estrous or nymphomania. Exposure during the middle of the estrous cycle in sows (days 11 to 14) causes persistence of functional progesterone-secreting corpora lutea leading to anestrus and pseudopregnancy. The estrous interval may range from 40 to 70 days from just a few days' exposure in the middle of the estrous cycle. Zearalenone given to pregnant sows 7 to 10 days post mating causes failure of implantation, and embryos do not survive beyond 21 days (i.e., early embryonic death).[1, 3] Limited amounts of zearalenone are secreted in the milk, but piglets farrowed to sows fed zearalenone may have signs of hyperestrogenism.[5]

Castrated male pigs develop enlargement of prepuce and nipples. Immature boars have reduced libido and retarded testicular development, whereas mature boars are not affected by zearalenone up to 200 ppm in the diet.[6]

Dairy heifers and mature cows may have infertility and reduced conception and vaginitis, and vaginal secretion may be increased. Mammary enlargement not related to lactation may occur in virgin heifers. Bovine infertility from zearalenone appears to be of very low clinical incidence and to not persist after exposure stops.[3]

DIAGNOSIS

Clinical signs of hyperestrogenism, nymphomania, or anestrus suggest zearalenone as a potential diagnosis. Functional corpora lutea in sows may be confirmed by analysis of plasma progesterone. Microscopic lesions of uterine and vaginal metaplasia and follicular atresia are characteristic lesions.

Detection of zearalenone residues in feces, body fluids, or tissues is generally not a reliable means of diagnosis. Instead, analysis of representative feed samples present at the time of initial exposure and clinical effects are the common means for confirmation of significant exposures. In some cases, for example, anestrus, effects may be apparent long after consumption of responsible feed has stopped, so retention and dating of samples from all diets fed is an essential management tool to confirm zearalenone toxicosis.

MANAGEMENT AND PREVENTION

If hyperestrogenism occurs, change the source of grain immediately, and acute signs should resolve within 1 to 2 weeks. Symptomatic or surgical treatment may be needed for vaginal or rectal prolapse and physical damage to external genitalia. Zearalenone-induced anestrus in sows responds to one 10-mg dose of prostaglandin $F_{2\alpha}$, or two 5-mg doses intramuscularly on successive days.

Alfalfa and alfalfa meal fed to swine at up to 25% of the diet may reduce absorption and increase fecal excretion of zearalenone, but this may be considered impractical.[1] Bentonite supplementation has been claimed to be useful, but available data are limited. Activated charcoal may bind zearalenone in the gastrointestinal tract and reduce enterohepatic cycling, but long-term feeding is not recommended.

Examine the diet for other sources of dietary estrogens (e.g., legumes) that could mimic some effects of zearalenone.

REFERENCES

1. Osweiler GD: Mycotoxins. *In* Leman AD, Straw BE, Mengeling WL, et al (eds): Diseases of Swine, ed 7. Ames, Iowa State University Press, 1992, pp 735–743.
2. Jimenez M, Manez M, Hernandez E: Influence of water activity and temperature on the production of zearalenone in corn by three *Fusarium* species. Int J Food Microbiol 29:417–421, 1996.
3. Diekman MA, Green ML: Mycotoxins and reproduction in domestic livestock. J Anim Sci 70:1615–1627, 1992.
4. Biehl ML, Prelusky DB, Koritz GD, et al: Biliary excretion and enterohepatic cycling of zearalenone in immature pigs. Toxicol Appl Pharmacol 121:152–159, 1993.
5. Vanyi A, Bata A, Glavits R, et al: Perinatal oestrogen syndrome in swine. Acta Vet Hung 42:433–446, 1994.
6. Ruhr LP: Zearalenone (F-2). *In* Howard JL (ed): Current Veterinary Therapy 2: Food Animal Practice. Philadelphia, WB Saunders, 1986, pp 380–381.

■ Fumonisins

Gary D. Osweiler, D.V.M., M.S., Ph.D., Diplomate, A.B.V.T.

SOURCES AND HISTORY OF OCCURRENCE

Fusarium moniliforme and *Fusarium proliferatum*[1, 2] fungi are ubiquitous in white and yellow corn worldwide, and have been identified as the source of the fumonisin mycotoxins, which cause equine leucoencephalomalacia (ELEM) and porcine pulmonary edema (PPE), respectively. Although many domestic animals are susceptible, natural outbreaks of clinical toxicosis from fumonisins have only been reported in swine and horses.[3–5] Drought stress followed by persistent rainfall or high humidity during maturity appears to produce fumonisins in damaged corn (Nelson PA: Personal communication, October 1989).

Fumonisins are water-soluble, heat-stable, alkaline-resistant aliphatic hydrocarbons with a terminal amine group and two tricarboxylic acid side chains. The number and position of hydroxyl groups on the aliphatic hydrocarbon determines the structure as FB1, FB2, or FB3.[6, 7] FB1 and FB2 are of approximately equal toxicity, but FB3 is much less toxic (Osweiler GD, et al: Unpublished data, 1993).

MECHANISM OF ACTION

Fumonisins inhibit the enzyme-mediated conversion of sphinganine to sphingosine which may interfere with cell cycle control function.[8, 9] The exact relationship of altered sphingolipid metabolism to swine and equine disease is currently under study.

Fumonisins are suspected human esophageal carcinogens in South Africa,[1, 6] and experimentally they act as tumor promoters leading to formation of precancerous liver nodules. In experimental swine, chronic fumonisin consumption results in esophageal hyperplasia and hepatic neoplasia.[10]

Acute porcine pulmonary edema appears associated with increases in pulmonary intravascular macrophages and increased pulmonary arterial pressure.[11, 12] These responses have been hypothesized to lead to pulmonary edema either by increased pulmonary hydrostatic pressure or by pulmonary capillary endothelial cell damage. Fumonisins are poorly absorbed orally and are excreted readily and rapidly in both bile and urine.[13]

TOXICITY AND CLINICAL SIGNS

For swine, cattle, and horses, there appears to be a variable latent period which is not proportionally shortened by increased dosage of fumonisins, and most species have some degree of hepatic damage.

Swine consuming more than approximately 120 ppm dietary fumonisins for 4 to 10 days develop acute PPE[14–17] with attack rates up to 50% and case fatality rates of 50% to 90%.[16] Survivors often develop subacute hepatic toxicosis in 7 to 10 days. More than 50 ppm causes mild liver lesions within 7 to 10 days, but concentrations of 25 ppm or less cause no apparent clinical effects. Mild microscopic hepatic lesions can be produced from diets as low as 23 ppm.[15] The serum sphingosine-sphinganine ration may be altered by feed concentrations as low as 5 ppm, although the clinical significance of this is not established.[15, 18] Signs include acute onset of dyspnea, cyanosis, weakness, and death. Once signs appear, death may occur in less than 4 hours.[14–18]

Dietary fumonisin concentrations of 75 to 120 ppm for 1 to

3 weeks cause icterus, reduced feed intake, weight loss, and occasionally diarrhea.[19] Clinical chemistry analyses reveal elevated serum concentrations of γ-glutamyltransferase (GGT), aspartate aminotransferase (AST), alkaline phosphatase (ALP), lactate dehydrogenase (LDH), cholesterol, and bilirubin.[14–19] Early increases in the serum enzymes and cholesterol are followed by sustained elevations of GGT and increasing concentrations of serum bilirubin consistent with development of clinical icterus. Transient reduction in lymphocyte blastogenesis and delayed titer response to pseudorabies vaccine have been observed.[19] Pregnant sows may abort from 1 to 4 days after the onset of acute signs,[16] probably as a sequela to fetal anoxia from severe pulmonary edema in the dam. Dietary fumonisin concentrations of 100 ppm FB1 in the last 30 days of gestation did not cause abortion, fetal abnormalities, or subsequent infertility in sows (author's unpublished data).

Cattle and *sheep* are mildly affected by dietary concentrations greater than 100 ppm, but fatalities do not occur.[20] Anorexia and mild reversible hepatic toxicosis occurs when the toxin is fed at greater than 200 ppm (Osweiler GD, Kehrli MA: Unpublished data, 1993). The toxins are rapidly excreted after intravenous or oral exposure.[21]

Horses are the most sensitive of the domestic animals, and dietary concentrations as low as 10 ppm for more than 30 days may cause fatal leukoencephalomalacia.[3, 5] Signs may develop acutely and proceed to death within 24 hours after many weeks of exposure with no evident clinical effects. Early *neurologic signs* of ELEM include intermittent anorexia and depression followed by incoordination, aimless walking, circling, repetitive motions, facial paralysis, dysphagia, blindness, and head pressing. Some animals may become belligerent and fractious.[3, 5, 22] Differential diagnoses include encephalomyelitis, rabies, lead poisoning, tansy ragwort (*Senecio* spp.) or yellow star thistle (*Centaurea solstitialis*). Death can occur suddenly, or clinical signs may persist from 1 day to a week. Hepatic damage and clinical icterus may precede the onset of ELEM and occasionally cause death before neurologic signs develop.

LESIONS

Lesions in swine are pulmonary edema and hydrothorax but no hemorrhage or cardiac necrosis. The thorax contains 200 to 350 mL of clear, cell-free, straw-colored transudate. Lungs are heavy and wet and do not collapse when the thorax is opened. Edema is mainly interstitial, and bronchioles, bronchi, and trachea are relatively clear. Microscopic lesions include acidophilic, fibrillar material in alveoli and interlobular lymphatics, hyalinized alveolar capillary thrombi, and increased numbers of pulmonary intravascular macrophages (PIMs) filled with osmiophilic material. Other acute PPE lesions are pancreatic necrosis and hepatosis characterized by disrupted hepatic architecture, increased mitotic figures in hepatocytes, and single-cell hepatic necrosis.[14–18]

DIAGNOSIS

Typical clinical signs and lesions, evidence of exposure to corn screenings, characteristic clinical chemistry changes, and elevated serum sphinganine-sphingosine ratios support a diagnosis of fumonisin toxicosis. The serum sphinganine-sphingosine ratio is a sensitive and unique indicator of fumonisin exposure, but analysis is currently not widely available. Many laboratories can detect and quantitate fumonisins in corn and feeds, but tissue analysis is not generally done.

TREATMENT AND MANAGEMENT OF FUMONISIN TOXICOSIS OR CONTAMINATION

There is no antidote to fumonisin toxicosis, and the very acute and massive damage of toxicosis in horses and swine make symptomatic and supportive therapy of little value. With delayed clinical signs, oral detoxification is usually not helpful. Liver damage may be reduced by appropriate supportive care. Analysis of corn or feeds for fumonisins will aid in identifying the source and estimating dietary risk. Contaminated corn should be cleaned and the good-quality grain reanalyzed to confirm decontamination.

REFERENCES

1. Scott PM: Fumonisins. Int J Food Microbiol 18:257–270, 1993.
2. Shephard GS, Thiel PG, Stockenstrom S, et al: Worldwide survey of fumonisin contamination of corn and corn-based products. J AOAC Int 79:671–687, 1996.
3. Ross PF, Rice LG, Osweiler GD, et al: A review and update of animal toxicoses associated with fumonisin-contaminated feeds and production of fumonisins by *Fusarium* isolates. Mycopathologia 117:109–114, 1992.
4. Ross PF, Rice LG, Plattner RD, et al: Concentrations of fumonisin B1 in feeds associated with animal health problems. Mycopathologia 114:129–135, 1991.
5. Wilson TM, Ross PF, Rice LG, et al: Fumonisin B1 levels associated with an epizootic of equine leukoencephalomalacia. J Vet Diagn Invest 2:213–216, 1990.
6. Bezuidenhoudt SC, Wentzel A, Gelderblom WCA: Structure elucidation of the fumonisins, mycotoxins from *Fusarium moniliforme*, J Chem Soc Chem Commun, 1988, pp 743–745.
7. Steyn PS: Mycotoxins, general view, chemistry and structure. Toxicol Lett 82–83:843–851, 1995.
8. Norred WP, Wang E, Yoo H, et al: In vitro toxicology of fumonisins and the mechanistic implications. Mycopathologia 117:73–78, 1992.
9. Ramasamy S, Wang E, Hennig B, et al: Fumonisin B1 alters sphingolipid metabolism and disrupts the barrier function of endothelial cells in culture. Toxicol Appl Pharmacol 133:343–348, 1995.
10. Casteel SW, Turk JR, Cowart RP, et al: Chronic toxicity of fumonisin in weanling pigs. J Vet Diagn Invest 5:413–417, 1993.
11. Haschek WM, Motelin G, Ness DK, et al: Characterization of fumonisin toxicity in orally and intravenously dosed swine. Mycopathologia 117:83–96, 1992.
12. Smith GW, Constable PD, Haschek M: Cardiovascular responses to short-term fumonisin exposure in swine. Fundam Appl Toxicol 33:140–148, 1996.
13. Prelusky DB, Trenholm HL, Savard ME: Pharmacokinetic fate of 14C-labelled fumonisin B1 in swine. Nat Toxins 2:73–80, 1994.
14. Colvin BM, Harrison LR: Fumonisin-induced pulmonary edema and hydrothorax in swine. Mycopathologia 117:79–82, 1992.
15. Motelin GK, Haschek WM, Ness DK, et al: Temporal and dose-response features in swine fed corn screenings contaminated with fumonisin mycotoxins. Mycopathologia 126:27–40, 1994.
16. Osweiler GD, Ross PF, Wilson TM, et al: Characterization of an epizootic of pulmonary edema in swine associated with fumonisin in corn screenings. J Vet Diagn Invest 4:53–59, 1992.
17. Colvin BM, Cooley AJ, Beaver RW: Fumonisin toxicosis in swine: Clinical and pathologic findings. J Vet Diagn Invest 5:232–241, 1993.
18. Riley RT, An NH, Showker JL, et al: Alteration of tissue and serum sphinganine to sphingosine ratio: An early biomarker of exposure to fumonisin-containing feeds in pigs. Toxicol Appl Pharmacol 118:105–112, 1993.
19. Osweiler GD, Schwartz KJ, Roth JR: Effect of fumonisin contaminated corn on growth and immune function in swine (abstract). Presented to Midwestern Section, American Society of Animal Science, Des Moines, Iowa, March 30, 1993.
20. Osweiler GD, Kehrli ME, Stabel JR, et al: Effects of fumonisin-contaminated corn screenings on growth and health of feeder calves J Anim Sci 71:459–466, 1993.

21. Prelusky DB, Savard ME, Trenholm HL: Pilot study on the plasma pharmacokinetics of fumonisin B1 in cows following a single dose by oral gavage or intravenous administration. Nat Toxins 3:389–394, 1996.
22. Step DL: Equine leukoencephalomalacia. Equine Pract 15:24–30, 1993.

■ Tremorgenic Mycotoxins

Francis D. Galey, D.V.M., Ph.D., Diplomate, A.B.V.T.

A variety of feedstuffs may contain mycotoxins that cause neurologic signs of ataxia and tremors as part of diseases often referred to as "staggers" syndromes. Staggers may be caused by a variety of pasture grasses and feedstuffs including perennial ryegrass (*Lolium perenne*) infested with *Neophytodium lolia*; Dallis grass (*Paspalum dilatatum*) infested with the ergot *Claviceps paspali*; Bermuda grass (*Cynodon dactylon*) for which the mold is unknown; *Phalaris* sp., which has tryptamine alkaloids and is not a mycotoxic disease; moldy walnuts (*Juglans* sp.) infested with a *Penicillium* sp.; and although not a forage, *Aspergillus* sp. in grain.[1, 3, 11–13] The toxins are alkaloidal, indole-based paxallines and include lolitrems (perennial ryegrass),[4] paspalitrems (Dallis grass), tryptamine alkaloids (*Phalaris*), penitrems (moldy walnuts), and aflatrems (*Aspergillus*).[1, 3, 6, 11–13] Although the mechanism of action of those toxins is not well understood, enhanced release of excitatory amino acid neurotransmitters has been implicated.[8]

The hazard associated with tremorgenic forages depends on the time of year, the climate, and species-specific grazing styles. The *Neophytodium lolia* of perennial ryegrass is found in highest amounts in the lower leaf sheaths of the plant. Thus it is most likely to cause staggers late in the season when the grass has been grazed low to the ground. Although all species are affected, sheep may be at greatest risk owing to their tendency to graze grass low to the ground.[3, 7, 10] In contrast, Dallis grass is hazardous when ergotized seed heads are grazed.[1] Thus, the portion of the season when animals, especially cattle, are exposed to the seeded portions of the grass is the time most likely to be associated with Dallis grass staggers. Penitrems are more of a hazard in the fall and winter when walnuts on the ground become moldy. Penitrem may also form on moldy dairy products such as cream cheese or yogurt. Thus, spoiled dairy products in feedstuffs may be a concern.

CLINICAL SIGNS

Although exposure may vary based on habits, once exposed to the staggers toxins, all species are sensitive. Perennial ryegrass and its seeds retain toxicity when dry.[4, 7] Signs of staggers appear within 7 days of initial grazing of staggers grasses and within hours of exposure.[3, 11] Initially, animals may appear to be normal when resting. A fine tremor may be noticed in the occasional animal. When stimulated, affected animals have a characteristic stiff, spastic gait, then spasms and tetanic seizures.[3, 10, 11] Ultimately, opisthotonos will appear, especially for the penitrems. Recovery from an episode may be rapid for perennial ryegrass, Dallis grass, and Bermuda grass staggers if animals are not stressed. The losses that do occur result from injuries, drowning, or becoming trapped during seizure episodes.[3] Epizootics tend to diminish by approximately 2 weeks after removal from the toxic forage. Perennial ryegrass endophyte may also produce ergovaline alkaloids similar to those produced by tall fescue (*Festuca*) infested with a related endophyte, *Neophytodium coenophialum*.[2] Some flocks of sheep along the northern coast of California have suffered apparent agalactia similar to fescue toxicosis in conjunction with staggers during the fall lambing period (personal observation).

DIAGNOSIS

Although lesions associated with staggers are usually minimal, degeneration of cerebellar Purkinje cells has been reported for longer-standing and severe cases of perennial ryegrass staggers.[9] Diagnosis of staggers syndromes requires ruling out other tremorgenic syndromes, identification of the grass or fungus, and when possible, identification of the toxin in the plant.[3] If forage toxins are not available for analysis, an extract of the forage can be bioassayed in laboratory animals.[3, 5]

TREATMENT AND PREVENTION

Treatment of staggers centers on prevention and largely involves grazing management and supportive care. In northern California, some producers have suggested feeding of additional magnesium to help control severity of clinical signs, but I am unaware of any published clinical trials in support of that suggestion. Despite the lack of specific treatment, animals with staggers need to be placed in a pasture where injury and drowning are unlikely. The most effective means of managing perennial ryegrass staggers is to provide alternative forage until new pasture growth is available. Mowing the seed heads will minimize effects of ergotized Dallis grass. Alternative forage also will aid treatment of Bermuda grass staggers. The environment should be cleaned up of moldy walnuts or spoiled dairy products to prevent penitrem A poisoning.

REFERENCES

1. Cole RJ, Dorner JW, Lansden JA, et al: *Paspalum* staggers: Isolation and identification of tremorgenic metabolites from sclerotia of *Claviceps paspali*. J Agric Food Chem 25:1997–2001, 1977.
2. Easton HS, Lane GA, Tapper BA: Ergovaline in endophyte-invested ryegrass pastures. N Z J Vet J 41:214, 1993.
3. Galey FD, Tracey ML, Craigmill AL, et al: Staggers induced by consumption of perennial ryegrass in cattle and sheep from Northern California. J Am Vet Med Assoc 199:466–470, 1991.
4. Gallagher RT, Cambpell AG, Hawkes AD, et al: Ryegrass staggers: The presence of lolitrem neurotoxins in perennial ryegrass seeds. N Z Vet J 30:183–184, 1982.
5. Gallagher RT, Hawkes AD: Estimation of neurotoxin levels in perennial ryegrass by mouse bioassay. N Z J Agric Res 28:427–438, 1985.
6. Gallagher RT, White EP, Mortimer PH: Ryegrass staggers: Isolation of potent neurotoxins lolitrem A and lolitrem B for staggers-producing pastures. N Z Vet J 29:189–190, 1981.
7. Hunt LD, Blythe L, Holtan DW: Ryegrass staggers in ponies fed processes ryegrass straw. J Am Vet Med Assoc 182:285–286, 1983.
8. Mantle PG: Amino acid neurotransmitter release from cerebro-cortical synaptosomes of sheep with severe ryegrass staggers in New Zealand. Res Vet Sci 34:373–385, 1983.
9. Munday BL, Mason RW: Lesions in ryegrass staggers in sheep. Aust Vet J 43:598–599, 1967.
10. Mortimer PH: Perennial ryegrass staggers in New Zealand. *In* Keeler RF, VanKampen KR, James LF, et al (eds): Effects of Poisonous Plants in Livestock. New York, Academic Press, 1978, pp 353–361.
11. Osweiler GD, Carson TL, Buck WB, et al: Clinical and Diagnostic Toxicology. Dubuque, Iowa, Kendall Hunt, 1985, pp 409–442.
12. Porter JK, Bacon CW, Robbins JD: Major alkaloids of a *Claviceps* isolated from toxic Bermuda grass. J Agric Food Chem 22:838–841, 1974.
13. Valdes JJ, Cameron JE, Cole RJ: Aflatrem: A tremorgenic mycotoxin with acute neurotoxic effects. Environ Health Perspect 62:459–631, 1985.

■ Ergotism

Thomas L. Carson, D.V.M., Ph.D.

Ergotism is an acute or chronic disease of livestock affecting primarily cattle and occasionally swine. The causative agents, *Claviceps* spp., are parasitic fungi that attack the developing ovary of various grasses, especially certain cereal grains. Rye is most commonly infected, but other cereal grains, including barley, triticale, wheat, and oats, are also infected. Ergot may be seen in common cool-season pasture grasses if they are overgrown and mature seed heads develop.

NATURAL OCCURRENCE

Infection and growth of the ergot fungus is promoted by warm, moist conditions and occurs through the open flowers of the grasses. Spores from fungal growth on the soil are spread by wind and serve as the primary infective source. The spores germinate and the fungus invades the embryo. Soon, a sticky spore-containing exudate known as "honeydew" exudes from the infected florets and is a source of infection to other grass flowers by insects that are attracted to the nectar-like secretion. As the seed head matures, the mass of fungal tissue enlarges to replace the embryo and form a sclerotium, a brownish-black elongated dry mass about three times the size of a normal seed kernel. The physical appearance of sclerotia is characteristic for each species of ergot. Many sclerotia fall to the ground before harvest and overwinter in the soil only to germinate as a source of spores in the spring. Sclerotia harvested with the grain are the common source of animal exposure.

The principal fungal species of veterinary importance are *Claviceps purpurea* and *Claviceps paspali*. Common cool-season grasses and small grains are invaded primarily by *C. purpurea*; Dallis grass (*Paspalum dilatatum*) is the usual host for *C. paspali*. *C. purpurea* is commonly associated with gangrenous ergotism and agalactia, whereas *C. paspali* causes a nervous syndrome known as paspalum staggers.

As ergot sclerotia are usually less dense than the grain they contaminate, a significant portion of ergot may be removed from cereal grains by cleaning with a gravity table. The screenings from such grain, heavily contaminated with sclerotia, become a hazard to livestock as they are mixed or milled into feeds. Once grinding or milling has occurred, ergot can be recognized only by microscopic examination or chemical analysis for ergot alkaloids. Ergotism is reported sporadically from many locations in North America. Morbidity within a herd is generally low, and unless exposure continues, recovery or salvage of affected animals is possible.

TOXICITY

The toxic effects of ergot are due to the ergot alkaloids in the sclerotia. The type and quantity of alkaloid vary with season, region, year, and type of grain. Generally, alkaloid content increases as grain reaches maturity. Ergot alkaloid concentrations are mainly from ergotamine and the ergotoxine group, and although quite variable, total ergot alkaloid concentration commonly ranges from 0.2% to 0.6% of sclerotia weight.

The dosage of ergot from feeds has traditionally been expressed as the percentage of ergot sclerotia by weight in a given grain. The toxicity of the ergot, however, may be subject to wide variability, depending on the amount of grain consumed by different animals, as well as the specific alkaloid content of ergot sclerotia. Approximately 0.5% of ergot in cattle rations is associated with reduced weight gain, poor feed consumption,

hyperthermia, agalactia, rough hair coat, and some nonspecific signs. Dietary contamination of ergot ranging between 0.3% and 1.0% for several weeks has been associated with gangrenous ergotism. Field case investigations and controlled studies support a recommendation that ergot levels should be kept below 0.1% in the grain portion of a ration to minimize risk to animals. U. S. Department of Agriculture tolerance for ergot sclerotia in grain is 0.3%.

PATHOGENESIS

Gangrenous ergotism is reportedly due to alkaloid-induced smooth muscle stimulation of arterioles. Natural ergot alkaloids produce α-adrenergic blockade and also antagonize 5-hydroxytryptamine. A rise in blood pressure results from peripheral vasoconstriction. Ergotamine is especially potent as a vasoconstrictor. Vasoconstriction results in congestion proximal to the lesion and ischemia distal to the arteriolar spasm. Endothelial swelling and degeneration develop in affected vascular beds. The combined effect of vasoconstriction and endothelial damage results in localized ischemia, vascular stasis, thrombosis, pain, lameness, and eventual necrosis or gangrene. Because venous and lymphatic drainage remain intact, the gangrene is "dry" in nature.

The hyperthermia syndrome produced in adult cattle is also likely the result of vasoconstriction which reduces blood flow to the skin and thus interferes with the animals' ability to dissipate body heat.

Agalactia from consumption of ergotized grain can occur in most classes of livestock. Swine appear to be highly susceptible. Ergot alkaloids decrease or prevent the prolactin surge that normally occurs in late gestation. Apparently they act at the hypophyseal level as a prolactin release inhibitor.

Nervous ergotism from *C. purpurea* is relatively rare. Intense vasoconstriction and cerebral ischemia are sometimes considered responsible for the neurologic signs seen in nervous ergotism occasionally associated with *C. purpurea*. Nervous ergotism in cattle consuming *C. paspali*–infected Dallis grass appears associated with a group of tremorgenic substances with neurotoxic properties expressed as paspalum staggers. One tremorgen has been identified chemically and named paspalinine. Paspalinine is similar to some of the tremorgens isolated from various species of *Penicillium* and *Aspergillus* (see Tremorgenic Mycotoxins).

CLINICAL SIGNS

Early typical signs of gangrenous ergotism in cattle are lameness or apparent pain or both. Hind limbs are often affected first. Swelling may occur just above the coronary band and extend upward past the fetlock. Affected cattle appear nervous and may walk with an ataxic or abnormal gait. Temperature, pulse, and respiration are sometimes increased, and milk production or body weight may drop drastically. Feed grains containing ergot alkaloids may be unpalatable and hence are eaten poorly or refused by animals. A toxic dose of ergot is difficult to establish owing to variability of alkaloid content. Any diet containing in excess of 0.25% ergot sclerotia should be considered suspect. On a body weight basis, 40 to 60 mg/kg of ergot alkaloid has been considered toxic. In sheep, there are reports of salivation, nausea, and diarrhea. Abortion is rarely reported as a consequence of ergot ingestion by ruminants. Field and experimental results are conflicting, but generally a strong case cannot be found for ergot-induced abortions.

A syndrome of hyperthermia and agalactia may be seen in dairy cattle consuming ergot-contaminated grain. Clinical signs in affected cattle include rapid and labored breathing, elevated rectal temperature (up to 107°F), open-mouth breathing with protruding tongue, excessive salivation, and reduced feed intake. Animals may appear to recover during the cooler nighttime hours, but then relapse during the heat of the day. In affected lactating cows, milk production drops by an average of 20% to as high as 50%. Serum prolactin levels are reduced. Recovered cows may have reduced fertility as indicated by an increase in days open and number of inseminations per conception.

In swine, feeding of ergot-containing grains often results in partial or complete feed refusal with decreased weight. Gangrene is infrequently reported, although I have seen several cases involving loss of margins of ears or tips of noses associated with ergot-containing grain and cold weather. A serious ergot-related problem in swine occurs in late gestation and early lactation. Gestation may be shortened by 3 to 5 days, and newborn piglets are smaller than normal, although abortion rarely occurs. When ergot is fed in the last 2 to 4 weeks of gestation, udder development does not occur, and lactation is inhibited or absent. The resulting agalactia can generally be differentiated from the MMA (metritis-mastitis-agalactia) complex by general good health of sows, lack of fever, and absence of congestive or inflammatory lesions of the udder. If affected sows are removed from the ergot-containing diet within a few days, many will lactate within 5 to 7 days. Usually this is not soon enough to prevent losses from starvation in piglets. The agalactia syndrome has been induced by diets containing from 0.1% to 1.0% ergot, but results vary greatly depending on alkaloid content.

The first signs of nervous ergotism are hyperexcitability and tremors that are intensified by excitement upon forced movement. At rest, the animals may stand with the rear legs extended and exhibit swaying motions. When made to run, they exhibit exaggerated flexure of the forelegs and incoordination that often becomes severe enough to cause the animals to fall. Once down, cattle usually lie for a short time, the severity of the signs decreases, and they regain their upright position and walk off slowly. In severely affected animals, extensor rigidity, opisthotonos, and clonic convulsions occur when they are down. When animals are left alone, the trembling and incoordination usually are minimal, and animals are able to move about slowly and graze.

CLINICAL PATHOLOGY AND LESIONS

There are no distinctive clinicopathologic lesions to confirm ergotism. Gross lesions of gangrenous ergotism may range from mild swelling, ischemia, and edema to severe ischemia, necrosis, and characteristic gangrene of the extremities that is sharply demarcated from unaffected tissue. The lesion is deep as well as superficial, and the entire appendage may slough. Microscopic lesions of necrosis, edema, endothelial damage, and thrombosis are seen.

There are no reports of clinicopathologic alterations in paspalum staggers. Apparently no characteristic gross or microscopic changes are associated with the disease.

DIAGNOSIS

The distinctive lesion of gangrenous ergotism should be differentiated from infectious pododermatitis (foot rot), fescue toxicosis, frostbite, trauma, and perhaps the vesicular diseases. Widespread hyperthermia, anorexia, and agalactia in dairy cows should be differentiated from fescue toxicosis and infectious disease. These syndromes should alert one to inspect the feed

and forage for the dark brownish-black ergot sclerotia. Samples of whole grain may be submitted to a seed laboratory where the ergot may be confirmed and quantitated. If grain has been milled, gross identification is nearly impossible. Representative feed samples should be submitted to a laboratory for microscopic or chemical analysis. Identification of ergot alkaloids or ricinoleic acid (in the absence of castor bean meal) is confirmatory of exposure to ergot. In swine, differentiation from mastitis or MMA syndrome is of most concern. Ergot-poisoned sows probably will respond poorly or not at all to parenteral oxytocin.

The diagnosis of nervous ergotism is based primarily on observing typical signs in cattle grazing pastures where mature sclerotia are present in the flowers of the grass. The problem usually occurs in late summer or early fall. Ryegrass staggers and Bermuda grass tremors have similar clinical manifestations. Differentiation rests primarily on the type of pasture to which the animals have access. *C. paspali* sclerotia on Dallis grass are rough-surfaced, nearly spherical, buff to brown, and 2 to 4 mm in diameter. The toxic fungal metabolites are found predominantly in the mature sclerotia.

TREATMENT AND PREVENTION

The only effective treatment for ergot poisoning is removal of the source. If agalactia is not advanced or if gangrene is not present, the prognosis is guarded to good.

Animals with gangrenous ergotism should be protected from cold, damp conditions, and if circumstances allow, hot packs should be applied to enhance circulation. Because little is known of the absorption and excretion of ergot alkaloids, specific therapy to enhance excretion cannot be recommended. A broad-spectrum antibiotic such as oxytetracycline hydrochloride (Liquamycin LA-200) at 6 to 11 mg/kg (3 to 5 mg/lb) or a long-acting penicillin combination such as benzathine penicillin G at 2000 units/lb (4400 units/kg) and procaine penicillin G at 2000 units/lb (4400 units/kg) should be used to control secondary infections.

Treatment of nervous ergotism consists in removing animals from affected pastures. Because death is generally accidental, care should be taken to avoid undue excitement in handling and moving cattle.

The time of greatest risk is in late summer or early fall when the pasture grasses have developed seed heads. Cattle may selectively graze grass heads containing sclerotia, thus obtaining a concentrated amount of toxic material. Control can be affected by grazing forage before it reaches the seed head stage or by clipping the heads as they form. Hay made from such pastures is potentially toxic, but sclerotia usually drop out as the hay is handled.

BIBLIOGRAPHY

Blood DC, Radostits OM, Henderson JA: Diseases Caused by Chemical Agents. Veterinary Medicine. London, Baillère Tindall, 1983, pp 1153–1156.

Burfening PJ: Ergotism. J Am Vet Med Assoc 163:1288, 1973.

Cole RJ, Dorner JW, Lansder JA, et al: Paspalum staggers: Isolation and identification of tremorgenic metabolites from sclerotia of *Claviceps paspali*. J Agric Food Chem 25:1197–1202, 1977.

Coppock RW, Mostrom MS, Simon J, et al: Cutaneous ergotism in a herd of dairy calves. J Am Vet Med Assoc 194:549–551, 1989.

Jang IH, Van der Tol I, Bryden WL, et al: Ergotism in dairy cattle: Effects of ingestion of ergots from *Claviceps purpurea*. Proc Nutr Soc Aust 12:169, 1987.

Jessup TM, Dent CHR, Kemp JB, et al: Bovine idiopathic hyperthermia. Aust Vet J 64:354, 1987.

Holliman A: Gangrenous ergotism in a suckler herd. Vet Rec 124:398–399, 1989.

Mantle PG: Ergotism in swine. *In* Wyllie TD, Morehouse LG (eds): Mycotoxic Fungi, Mycotoxins, Mycotoxicoses: An Encyclopedic Handbook. New York, Dekker, 1977, pp 145, 273.

Mantle PG, Mortimer PH, White EP: Mycotoxic tremorgens of *Claviceps paspali* and *Penicillium cyclopium:* A comparative study of effects on sheep and cattle in relation to natural staggers syndromes. Res Vet Set 24:49–56, 1977.

Osweiler GD, Carson TL, Buck WB, et al: Clinical and Diagnostic Veterinary Toxicology. Dubuque, Iowa, Kendall Hunt, 1985, pp 428–433.

Ross AD, Bryden WL, Bakau W, et al: Induction of heat stress in beef cattle by feeding the ergots of *Claviceps purpurea.* Aust Vet J 66:247–249, 1989.

Schneider DJ, Miles CO, Garthwaite I, et al: First report of field outbreaks of ergot-alkaloid toxicity in South Africa. Onderstepoort J Vet Res 63:97–108, 1996.

Young JC, Chen Z: Variability in the content and composition of alkaloid found in Canadian ergot: III. Triticale and barley. J Environ Sci Health B17:93–107, 1982.

■ Fescue Toxicosis

Larry A. Kerr, D.V.M., M.S.
William J. Kelch, D.V.M., Ph.D.

Tall fescue *(Festuca arundinacea)*, a major cool-season grass, is grown on approximately 35 million acres in the United States, primarily in the Southeast, and is used as forage for approximately 8.5 million cattle and 700,000 horses. Fescue is popular because it is adaptable to a wide range of soil and climatic conditions, is easily established, is persistent year after year, is tolerant of poor grazing management, and can be grazed throughout much of the winter. Nearly all the tall fescue in the Southeast is the Kentucky 31 variety.

Despite forage quality characteristics that compare favorably with other grasses, actual results for fescue have been disappointing because of the forage's toxic properties. These toxic properties, estimated to produce losses of $600 million per year, manifest themselves in cattle in three syndromes: (1) fescue foot, (2) poor performance (summer slump), and (3) fat necrosis. A single syndrome or combinations of all three may be observed in cattle ingesting toxic fescue over long periods of time. In mares, reproductive problems have included prolonged gestation, abortions, dystocia, thickened placentas, agalactia, large, weak foals, and high foal mortality.

In spite of extensive research, the toxic agent of fescue and the mechanism of action remain unknown. An association has been observed between fescue infested with an endophyte fungus, *Acremonium coenophialum*, and the toxic syndrome. Unlike most fungi, *A. coenophialum* grows inside the plant in the intercellular spaces and cannot be detected without special laboratory procedures. Some investigators speculate that this fungus may trigger the formation of various ergot, dizaphenanthrene, and pyrrolizidine alkaloids in the plant that adversely affect the ingesting animal's ability to form some essential hormones. Decreased circulating prolactin, progesterone, and melatonin, increased circulating estradiol-17β, and increased rectal temperatures have been demonstrated in animals ingesting endophyte-infested fescue grass and hay.

Prolactin is necessary for mammary gland differentiation leading to milk synthesis. It also influences body growth and reproductive functions. Ergot alkaloids, produced by *Claviceps* spp., are believed to stimulate dopamine receptors in the adenohypophysis and to antagonize serotonin receptors, decreasing prolactin concentrations by an unknown mechanism. Because the endophyte *A. coenophialum* is closely related to *Claviceps* spp. (family Clavicipitaceae), it may also produce toxic alkaloids. Ergot alkaloids such as ergovaline, ergonovine, and lysergic acid

amide could be responsible for all three syndromes of fescue toxicosis. Perloline, a dizaphenanthrene alkaloid, and ioline, a pyrrolizidine alkaloid, may also be involved.

CLINICAL SIGNS

Clinical signs of fescue toxicosis depend on which of the three syndromes is involved. Fescue foot usually occurs in late fall or winter, although it can occur any time. It is characterized by weight loss, lameness of the hind limbs, and gangrene of the feet, tail, and tips of the ears. Early signs include a tendency to shift weight from one rear foot to the other, a slight arching of the back, and soreness in the rear limbs. Often the left rear leg is the first affected. Knuckling of the pastern joint is sometimes observed early in the syndrome. As the condition progresses, reddening and swelling of the coronary band occurs, lameness worsens, and the animal becomes unthrifty and reluctant to move. In advanced cases, the swelling above the hoof becomes much more severe, and necrotic tissue is visible just below the swelling. Sloughing of the rear hooves often follows the appearance of this ischemic necrosis. In other cases, the tail switch or tips of ears may be lost. Emaciation is common in animals suffering moderate to severe signs because these animals are reluctant to move in search of feed.

Poor performance or summer slump appears to be the most common of the three syndromes and produces the most economic loss. Its occurrence usually corresponds to high environmental temperature and high humidity, though the condition may occur anytime animals are fed fungus-infested fescue grass or hay. This syndrome is characterized by reduced feed intake, decreased weight gain or an actual weight loss, decreased milk production, reproductive problems, failure to shed the rough winter hair coat, diarrhea, elevated body temperature, increased respiratory rate, photosensitization, and hypersalivation. Animals with summer slump spend less time grazing and more time in the shade or in farm ponds attempting to stay cool. Sheep are also affected by reproductive problems and a marked reduction in milk production. Conception rates in cattle and sheep may be significantly decreased when grazed on endophyte-infested fescue.

Fat necrosis or lipomatosis is the presence of necrotic fat in the abdominal or pelvic cavity. Necrotic fat is very hard, yellowish or chalky white, and often found in the mesentery surrounding the intestine in animals pastured on toxic fescue. This syndrome is probably much more common than presently recognized because few clinical signs are observed unless the fat masses exert physical pressure on a segment of intestine or gravid uterus. It has usually been associated with long-term ingestion of fungus-infested fescue that has been heavily fertilized with nitrogen or chicken litter. Digestive disturbances such as chronic bloating, decreased ruminations, reduced feed intake, weight loss, and scanty feces are often observed in affected animals. In severe cases, animals become emaciated and die, whereas others may become chronic poor doers. Large masses of necrotic fat may block the pelvic inlet and produce dystocia, making cesarean section necessary.

DIAGNOSIS

Diagnosis of fescue toxicosis depends on observing a clinical syndrome in affected animals similar to fescue foot, poor performance, or fat necrosis, and a history of having ingested fungus-infested fescue grass or hay for weeks or months. Serum prolactin concentrations may be helpful; a relationship apparently exists between serum prolactin and the appearance of signs of fescue toxicosis, particularly increased rectal temperatures.

Steers fed fungus-infested fescue hay have mean prolactin concentrations significantly lower than controls, and signs consistent with the poor performance syndrome.

Differential diagnoses of fescue foot include ergot and selenium toxicoses, foot rot, frostbite, and trauma. Differential diagnoses of the poor performance syndrome include molybdenum and chronic organophosphate toxicosis, internal parasites, and nutritional deficiencies. Differential diagnoses of fat necrosis include lymphoma, peritonitis, intussusception, and gastrointestinal blockage or torsion. Diagnosis of the last condition can sometimes be aided by the rectal palpation of large, hard masses in the abdominal or pelvic cavity and a history of having applied fertilizer or chicken litter to fungus-infested fescue grass. Except possibly for cases of fat necrosis, few or no gross or microscopic lesions are found at necropsy.

TREATMENT AND PREVENTION

Treatment of fescue toxicosis regardless of the syndrome involves removing animals from fungus-infested fescue grass or hay and placing them on a good alternative feed source. Those cattle with advanced fescue foot or with large masses of necrotic fat blocking the intestinal tract or uterus should be considered for slaughter. Many animals exhibiting poor performance signs will gradually return to normal when better forage is supplied.

Specific therapeutic alternatives are available and sometimes practical, particularly for valuable breeding horses and cattle. Dopamine antagonists such as domperidone and metoclopramide have been used to reduce reproductive problems, apparently by increasing prolactin levels depressed by the dopamine agonist activity of toxic fescue. Thiamine supplements have been shown to increase grazing time during hot weather for cattle grazing mixed toxic fescue and alfalfa pastures. The ammoniation of toxic fescue hay has, for unknown reasons, been shown to reduce its toxicity. Recent research suggests, though not yet conclusively, that ivermectin given at higher than anthelmintic doses may mitigate the effects of endophyte-infested fescue.

Fescue toxicosis can be prevented by grazing animals on alternative forages. However, because fescue is widespread in the Southeast, limiting consumption is usually not practical. If tall fescue is predominant, it should be tested for the presence and amount of endophyte fungus. Pasture may be lightly (less than 10%) or heavily (greater than 80%) infested. Because endophyte-infested fescue exhibits no external signs of the fungus, detection is dependent on either microscopic examination or serologic testing of plant tissue samples. The microscopic test involves staining thin slices of recently harvested seed or plant tissue and observing the fungus with the aid of a microscope. The serologic test uses an enzyme-linked immunosorbent assay based on an antibody reaction to the fungus in freshly harvested seed or fresh plant samples. Neither procedure distinguishes between live and dead fungus in seeds. Because the endophyte fungus is primarily seed-transmitted, a seed analysis before planting can help prevent spread of the toxic fescue. Although the fungus probably remains viable in stored seed for approximately a year, a greenhouse seeding and grow-out process is used to confirm by microscopic examination the viability of the fungus in seed and presence of infection in the seedling.

There are alternatives for managing toxic fescue pastures. One radical solution is to replace the fungus-infested fescue with fungus-free fescue, since individual cattle clearly perform better when grazing fungus-free fescue. However, infested fescue is hardier than fungus-free fescue and much more resistant to drought, overgrazing, disease, nematodes, and insects. In fact, overall carrying capacity (live weight per acre of pasture) of toxic fescue pastures may be superior to fungus-free pastures. Also, fungus-free pastures eventually become naturally reseeded by varieties that contain the toxic endophyte. Current research is aimed at fescue varieties which are infested at low levels, thereby being hardy, but with minimal untoward effects on grazing animals. In any case, pasture replacement, if contemplated, must be done realizing that many variables are at work: geography, climate, fescue variety, percent fescue infestation, feed supplementation practices and breed (Brahman cattle are more resistant to fescue toxicosis; some bloodlines of English and Continental breeds may also be resistant). The decision whether or not to replace pastures is very complicated; in most cases, it is probably not a good idea.

Other alternatives are available. Toxic fescue can be diluted, either in the pasture itself, by growing legumes such as clover with the fescue, or by providing supplemental hay or grain. While growing legumes with toxic fescue clearly mitigates the toxicosis, it is often difficult to maintain the legumes in the pasture since they are less hardy than the fescue. Toxic fescue grazing should, if possible, be minimized during the summer. The use of fungicides on fescue pastures and in animals grazing them has generally been unsuccessful.

BIBLIOGRAPHY

Cross DL, Redmond LM, Strickland JR: Equine fescue toxicosis: Signs and solutions. J Anim Sci 73:899–908, 1995.
Hemken RW, Bull LS, Boling JA, et al: Summer fescue toxicosis in lactating dairy cows and sheep fed experimental strains of ryegrass: Tall fescue hybrids. J Anim Sci 49:641–646, 1979.
Joost RE: *Acremonium* in fescue and ryegrass: Boon or bane? A review. J Anim Sci 73:881–888, 1995.
Kerr LA, McCoy CP, Boyle CR, et al: Effects of ammoniation of endophyte fungus-infested fescue hay on serum prolactin concentration and rectal temperature in beef cattle. Am J Vet Res 51:76–78, 1990.
Paterson J, Forcherio C, Larson B, et al: The effects of fescue toxicosis on beef cattle productivity. J Anim Sci 73:889–898, 1995.
Wallner BM, Booth NH, Robbins JD, et al: Effect of an endophytic fungus isolated from toxic pasture grass on serum prolactin concentrations in the lactating cow. Am J Vet Res 44:1317–1322, 1983.

■ Principal Toxic Plants of the Midwestern and Eastern States

Stan W. Casteel, D.V.M., Ph.D., Diplomate, A.B.V.T.

Chemical defenses orchestrated by plants serve an important role in their ability to limit intake by herbivores.[1] Intoxication of livestock by poisonous plants depends on the rate and quantity of ingestion. The amount of poisonous plant necessary to induce intoxication is usually expressed as a percentage of body weight of the animal. For example, a representative range of an acute toxic dose for livestock is typically 0.1% to 0.5% of body weight. This is equivalent to 1 to 5 lb of plant material for an animal weighing 1000 lb. Toxin concentration in a particular plant species varies with the stage of plant growth, and with environmental factors affecting growth such as rainfall, temperature, and soil type. Specific antidotes generally do not exist for plant toxins. Treatment is conditionally supportive, the primary goal in acute poisoning being to limit further absorption or enhance elimination of poisonous principles.

The palatability of poisonous plants compared to available suitable forage largely determines intake in many situations.[2] Other plant poisonings are often the result of poor pasture conditions and environmental changes such as freezing weather that influence palatability and toxicity of plants containing cyanogenic glycosides (see Table 10). Animals transported for long distances and denied feed and water during transit are particularly at risk when released into unfamiliar surroundings containing a heavy population of poisonous plants. Similar circumstances reduce the normal selective grazing habits of hungry livestock, leading to consumption of plants normally avoided. Contamination of harvested forage or grain also makes it difficult for livestock to avoid consumption of poisonous plants. Animals quartered in drylots or on barren ground in the winter are prone to ingestion of toxic shrubs or clippings when given the opportunity. Sudden death in livestock pastured adjacent to residential areas is cause for consideration of cardiotoxic ornamentals (see Table 2) such as oleander or yew.

Poisonous plants can be classified according to their predominant target organ. Clearly, some plant toxins affect more than one organ system while signs secondary to adverse effects on one organ system also may occur. For example, cardiotoxic plants often have an adverse effect on the gastrointestinal tract. Hepatotoxic plants typically induce gastrointestinal dysfunction such as diarrhea and central nervous system (CNS) derangement as a consequence of hepatic encephalopathy.

Adverse effects of plant toxins on blood or blood-forming organs (Table 1) usually can be detected by examination of a blood sample. Methemoglobinemia, induced by the rapid ingestion of a toxic quantity of a nitrate-accumulating plant, is indicated by the chocolate-brown color of a fresh blood sample. Definitive evidence of excessive exposure to nitrate is verified by chemical analysis of plasma or ocular fluid. The bone marrow–depressing effects of bracken fern are reflected by the pancytopenia identified during routine complete blood counts.

Intoxication by cardiotoxic plants (Table 2) includes signs of gastrointestinal upset in addition to signs of cardiovascular dysfunction. Weakness, trembling, dyspnea, collapse, and a variety of cardiac arrhythmias develop within hours of consumption and often terminate in death hours after onset. Livestock are commonly found dead prior to development of signs reflecting gastrointestinal disturbances such as colic and diarrhea. The

Table 2
PRINCIPAL PLANTS AFFECTING THE CARDIOVASCULAR SYSTEM

Plant Genus (Common Name)	Plant Recognition	Unique Effect(s)
Asclepias (milkweed)	Stems and leaves contain milky juice	Narrow-leaf species more neurotoxic, broad-leaf species more cardiotoxic; hazardous in harvested forage
Kalmia (laurel)	Evergreen shrub or small tree, leathery leaves	Weakness, colic, vomition, aspiration pneumonia common in survivors
Nerium (oleander)	Ornamental evergreen shrub	Diarrhea, cardiac arrhythmias, sudden death, myocardial necrosis, myocarditis, pulmonary edema
Persea (avocado)	Small tree	Guatemalan varieties especially toxic; acute onset of dyspnea, brisket edema, nonseptic mastitis
Rhododendron (azalea and rhododendron)	Deciduous or evergreen shrub	Weakness, recumbency, colic, vomition, aspiration pneumonia common in survivors
Taxus (yew)	Ornamental evergreen shrub	Sudden death, collapse, bradycardia, dyspnea, hypothermia
Veratrum (hellebore)	Coarse, erect, herbaceous	Bradycardia, hypotension, vomiting, diarrhea
Zigadenus (death camas)	Grasslike leaves, onion-like bulb	Weakness, hypotension, collapse, sheep may vomit, frothy oronasal discharge

Table 1
PRINCIPAL PLANTS AFFECTING THE BLOOD

Plant Genus (Common Name)	Plant Recognition	Unique Effects(s)
Allium (onions and garlic)	Strong-scented bulbous herb	Hemolytic effects in cattle with continuous ingestion for a week or more; icterus, hemoglobinuria, weakness, anemia
Pteridium (bracken fern)	Large fern	Onset of bone marrow depression in cattle 1–2 mo after consumption begins; fever, emaciation, leukopenia, thrombocytopenia, anemia, edema of larynx, dyspnea, anorexia, gastrointestinal and urinary bladder carcinomas, and hemangiomas
Sorghum (Johnson grass, Sudan hybrids)	Coarse grass family	Nitrate accumulation and cyanogenic glycoside production, especially in drought-stressed plants; blood bright red if cyanide and chocolate-brown if nitrate

stress of handling intoxicated livestock may increase the intensity of clinical signs or initiate collapse and death. When forced to move, cattle intoxicated by *Taxus* shrubs (Japanese yew, yew) may collapse to lateral recumbency as if shot by a gun. There are little or no data to support public health risk decisions related to residues of plant-derived cardioactive compounds. Consequently, disposal of contaminated carcasses or milk is recommended. Administration of activated charcoal in a palatable feed is an alternative to the stress-inducing method of intubation. Calcium-containing fluids are contraindicated for most cardiotoxic plant poisonings. Atropine is beneficial in cases of severe bradycardia.

Gastrointestinal upset is the most frequent consequence of poisonous plant ingestion (Table 3). Mucosal irritation usually leads to colic and diarrhea. Alternatively, some plants in this category inhibit protein synthesis (*Abrus, Ricinus, Robinia*) resulting in death of intestinal crypt cells and bloody diarrhea. Administration of fluids, gastrointestinal protectants, and laxatives is dictated by the particular clinical situation.

Photosensitized livestock (Tables 4 and 5) should be provided shade, broad-spectrum antibiotics to prevent secondary infections, and time for the integument to restore its protective barrier. Livestock with severe, chronic, progressive liver disease (see Table 5) have a poor prognosis.

Oak (acorn) poisoning is the most common cause of toxic nephropathy (Table 6) in cattle followed by pigweed in certain parts of the Midwest.[3] Clinical signs of oak poisoning in cattle reflect gastrointestinal and renal dysfunction, while pigweed

Table 3
PRINCIPAL PLANTS AFFECTING THE GASTROINTESTINAL TRACT

Plant Genus (Common Name)	Plant Recognition	Unique Effect(s)
Abrus (precatory bean)	Climbing vine mainly in Florida	Mastication of highly toxic seeds releases toxin causing severe gastroenteritis, bloody diarrhea
Aleurites (tung oil tree)	Small tree with milky sap and heart-shaped leaves	Ingestion of leaves or seeds induce bloody diarrhea, rumen atony, abomasitis 3–5 days following exposure
Euphorbia (spurges, poinsettia)	Woody plants or herbs with milky sap	Severe irritation of gastrointestinal tract including oral cavity; bloody diarrhea
Helenium (sneezeweeds)	Bitter-scented herb with filiform leaves	Gastroenteritis, bloating, vomiting in sheep, cattle, and goats; overgrazed pastures lead to consumption
Phytolacca (pokeweed)	Purple berries in grapelike cluster	Watery to bloody diarrhea, colic
Ricinus (castor bean)	Escaped ornamental	Toxic seed ingestion causes severe gastroenteritis within 12–48 hr
Robinia (black or yellow locust)	Leguminous tree to 75 ft	Bark, seeds, leaves toxic; diarrhea, cold extremities
Sesbania (coffee weed, bagpod)	Medium to large shrublike legume	Gastroenteritis 1–2 days after ingestion; hemolysis in some cases
Solanum (nightshade, bull nettle)	Annual and perennial herbs and shrubs; fruit is a berry	Intact glycoalkaloids induce irritation of the gastrointestinal tract; hydrolysis product (alkaloid nucleus) has a nervous system depressing effect

Table 4
PRINCIPAL PLANTS AFFECTING THE INTEGUMENT

Plant Genus (Common Name)	Plant Recognition	Unique Effect(s)
Fagopyrum (buckwheat)	Small grain crop mainly in northeastern United States	Photosensitization within 24 hr of ingestion, initial erythema, pruritus, photophobia, edema of ears, skin fissures, exudation of serum
Hypericum (St. Johnswort)	Erect perennial with yellow flowers; leaves appear perforated	Photosensitization within 24 hr of ingestion, initial erythema, pruritus, photophobia, edema of ears, skin fissures, exudation of serum

Table 5
PRINCIPAL PLANTS AFFECTING THE LIVER

Plant Genus (Common Name)	Plant Recognition	Unique Effect(s)
Crotalaria (rattlebox) Senecio (ragwort)	Pealike, yellow flower Yellow daisy-like flower	Both Crotalaria and Senecio induce delayed onset (2–8 mo) chronic progressive hepatopathy, subcutaneous edema, and occasional photosensitization
Eupatorium (white snakeroot)	Blooms in fall; small white flowers in cluster	1–2 wk duration of intermittent tremors, ataxia in cattle; photosensitization secondary to liver damage in goats
Lantana (lantana)	Escaped ornamental; showy flowers	Cholestatic liver disease and photosensitization in cattle
Microcystis (blue-green algae)	Blue-green algae on surface waters; cells the size of red blood cells	Intrahepatic hemorrhage, dissociation of hepatocytes; usually lethal within 24 hr; survivors may develop photosensitization
Cycas (false sago palm) and Zamia (coontie)	Tropical to subtropical, some ornamentals; coontie is native to Florida	Diarrhea, ascites, icterus, centrilobular necrosis
Xanthium (cocklebur)	Spiny capsule surrounds 2 seeds	Intoxication usually results from ingestion of 2-leafed stage of growth; cattle are blind, hypersensitive, and may convulse

Table 6
PRINCIPAL PLANTS AFFECTING THE KIDNEY

Plant Genus (Common Name)	Plant Recognition	Unique Effect(s)
Amaranthus (pigweed)	Flowers in dense spikes	Perirenal edema in swine and cattle from unidentified nephrotoxin; also accumulates nitrate and oxalates
Quercus (oak)	Hardwood trees	Consumption of buds or acorns for 1–3 wk induces rumen atony, constipation then bloody diarrhea, emaciation, renal failure, and typical perirenal edema
Rheum (rhubarb)	Considered a dangerous garden plant	Leaves contain toxic concentrations of soluble and insoluble oxalates; hemorrhagic gastroenteritis and oxalate nephrosis

Table 7
PRINCIPAL PLANTS AFFECTING THE MUSCULOSKELETAL SYSTEM

Plant Genus (Common Name)	Plant Recognition	Unique Effect(s)
Cassia (coffee senna, sicklepod)	Grooved stem; legume seed pod points upward or downward	Diarrhea, stiffness, ataxia, muscle fasciculations, recumbency; increased serum creatine phosphokinase and aspartate aminotransferase activities, myoglobinuria (coffee-colored urine)
Cestrum diurnum (day blooming jessamine)	Escaped ornamental in Florida	Vitamin D analogue responsible for soft tissue calcification; progressive weight loss, stiffness, hypercalcemia, calcification of tendons, ligaments, and major arteries

Table 8
PRINCIPAL PLANTS AFFECTING THE NERVOUS SYSTEM

Plant Genus (Common Name)	Plant Recognition	Unique Effect(s)
Aconitum (monkshood)	Hooded flower	Neuromuscular blocking action mostly responsible for weakness, bloating, collapse, sudden death
Aesculus (buckeye)	Small tree, fruit containing 1–3 large dark seeds with light scar	Emerging buds, leaves toxic in spring, seeds in fall; cattle show extreme incoordination, stiffness, falling to one side, and tetanic seizures; recovery likely with supportive care
Cicuta (water hemlock)	2–10 ft tall, stout hollow stem, horizontal plates in root	Root and new shoots most toxic and cause violent convulsions, running fits, then coma and death
Conium (poison hemlock)	3–6 ft tall, parsley-like leaves, purple-spotted stem	Nicotinic alkaloids stimulate, then depress; initial signs include hyperexcitability, tremors, ataxia, then depression, recumbency, respiratory paralysis
Delphinium (larkspur)	Backward spur on flower	Like monkshood, neuromuscular blocking action mostly responsible for weakness, bloating, collapse, sudden death
Gelsemium (yellow jessamine)	Climbing vine in woods and thickets of Southeast	Acute course of weakness, ataxia, convulsions, coma, and death within 48 hr

Table 9
PRINCIPAL PLANTS AFFECTING REPRODUCTION

Plant Genus (Common Name)	Plant Recognition	Unique Effect(s)
Astragalus and *Oxytropis* (locoweeds)	Erect or prostrate legumes, pealike flowers	Found only in the western portion of the Midwest and West, not in the East; decreased libido, abortion, stunted weak offspring, limb deformities
Conium (poison hemlock)	3–6 ft tall, parsley-like leaves, purple-spotted stem	Teratogenic in cattle, sheep, and goats; skeletal deformities, cleft palate when dams exposed early in gestation (e.g., day 50–75 in cattle)
Festuca (fescue) endophyte fungus–infected	Cool-season grass	Decreased fertility, dystocia, decreased milk production

Table 10
PRINCIPAL PLANTS AFFECTING RESPIRATION

Plant Genus (Common Name)	Plant Recognition	Unique Effect(s)
Sambucus (elderberry)	Bush up to 12 ft with red to purple berries	Cyanide released by rumen microbes blocks cellular respiration resulting in rapid onset of hyperpnea, dyspnea, weakness, muscle fasciculations, asphyxial convulsions, cherry-red blood
Perilla (perilla mint, purple mint)	Aromatic, square stem	Causes acute bovine pulmonary emphysema and edema, severe dyspnea
Prunus (chokecherry, cherry, plum)	Small-to-medium deciduous trees	Cyanide released by rumen microbes blocks cellular respiration resulting in rapid onset of hyperpnea, dyspnea, weakness, muscle fasciculations, asphyxial convulsions, cherry-red blood

poisoning is primarily renal. Pigweed is also a potential nitrate accumulator, but signs consistent with nitrate poisoning are readily apparent. Pigweed is usually a problem in drought situations while the incidence of oak poisoning from acorn ingestion seems to cycle every 3 to 4 years in conjunction with a heavy yield of acorns. When access to acorns cannot be controlled, cattle can be supplemented with rations containing 10% calcium hydroxide (hydrated lime) as a preventive. The addition of molasses may be required to enhance the intake of this somewhat unpalatable additive. Treatment of livestock poisoned by either oak or pigweed is seldom effective.

Grain sorghum contaminated with about 5% *Cassia* seeds by weight killed pigs and poisoned test chickens after 16 days of ingestion.[4] Like vitamin E–selenium deficiency, these plants induce a myodegenerative disorder in livestock. Treatment with vitamin E–selenium preparations is contraindicated in *Cassia* poisoning (Table 7).

Piperidine alkaloid–containing plants from *Conium* and *Nicotiana* genera are acutely neurotoxic (Table 8) to livestock and interfere with fetal development by suppression of fetal movement.[5] Cows exposed during gestation days 50 to 75 had calves with multiple congenital contractures (arthrogryposis and spinal curvature), a condition commonly referred to as crooked calf disease (Table 9). Periodic ultrasound during the gestational treatment period revealed severe inhibition of fetal movement suggesting that an adequate amount of fetal activity is necessary for normal development. Similarly, *Nicotiana glauca* (tree tobacco) may induce cleft palate and skeletal defects in cattle, sheep, and goats. In acute poisoning cases, sedatives are beneficial to hypersensitive or seizuring livestock.

Plants affecting both cellular and gross respiration (Table 10) can induce similar signs of oxygen deprivation. Plants containing cyanogenic glycosides prevent the utilization of oxygen by blocking electron transport, while *Perilla* mint poisoning hinders the exchange of gases across the respiratory membrane of the lungs. Livestock poisoned by cyanide-containing plants usually survive if still alive 2 hours after the onset of intoxication. Cattle poisoned by *Perilla* mint in contaminated hay or as dried plant material developed tachypnea or dyspnea with an expiratory grunt 12 to 72 hours after consumption commenced.[6] The duration of the intoxication may last for more than a week, but consumption of the seed stage of the plant may be lethal within 24 hours.

REFERENCES

1. Cheeke PR: A review of the functional and evolutionary roles of the liver in the detoxification of poisonous plants, with special reference to pyrrolizidine alkaloids. Vet Human Toxicol 36:240, 1994.
2. Ralphs MH, Pfister JA: Conditions of livestock poisoning and management strategies to reduce risks. *In* Colegate SM, Dorling PR (eds): Plant-Associated Toxins: Agricultural, Phytochemical and Ecological Aspects, Wallingford, UK, CAB International, 1994, pp 478–483.
3. Casteel SW, Johnson GC, Miller MA, et al: *Amaranthus retroflexus* (redroot pigweed) poisoning in cattle. J Am Vet Assoc 204:1068, 1994.
4. Flory W, Spainhour CB, Colvin B, et al: The toxicologic investigation of a feed grain contaminated with seeds of the plant species *Cassia.* J Vet Diagn Invest 4:65, 1992.
5. Panter KE, James LF, Gardner DR, et al: The effects of poisonous plants on embryonic and fetal development in livestock. *In* Colegate SM, Dorling PR (eds): Plant-Associated Toxins: Agricultural, Phytochemical and Ecological Aspects. Wallingford, UK, CAB International, 1994, pp 325–332.
6. Kerr LA, Johnson BJ, Burrows GE: Intoxication of cattle by *Perilla frutescens* (purple mint). Vet Human Toxicol 28:412, 1986.

■ Principal Toxic Plants of the Southwestern United States

Tam Garland, D.V.M., Ph.D.

It is a most daunting task to attempt to acquaint the reader with all of the toxic plants that occur on the ranges of the southwestern United States. Therefore, this discussion is confined to those plants that affect animal agriculture most frequently and most severely. Animal health, which is affected by toxic plants, has a direct economic impact on the producer with various forms of loss: decreased production of wool, fiber, and milk; reproductive problems; and animal deaths. The economy of the southwestern United States still relies heavily on animal agriculture and grazing of the rangelands by ruminants. It has been estimated that in some years loss due to animal deaths is as high as $100 million and probably averages $10 to $30 million per year in Texas alone.[1]

Plants that are toxic to livestock in Texas and adjacent states number over 130 species. There are plant species that do not occur in Texas but that may occur in New Mexico, Arizona, and southeastern California. There is some species overlap between areas in the Southwest, but to attempt to cover all of the toxic plants would be an impossibility. Consequently, an overview of the most important plants is presented here.

PLANTS AFFECTING THE RESPIRATORY SYSTEM

Perillia frutescens (Beefsteak Plant, *Perilla* Mint)

As a member of the mint family, *Perilla* mint has a characteristic square stem that aids in its identification. It is a plant that is native to Asia and found throughout much of the Southwest. It was originally imported into the United States as a garden plant and is now escaped and widespread. Its distribution includes northeastern Texas, southeastern Oklahoma, southwestern Arkansas, and northwestern Louisiana. The plant is generally green, but new growth and young plants may be more purple. Cattle and horses are most frequently affected, but sheep and goats may be affected also. Clinical signs are pulmonary emphysema and edema, and difficult breathing. Animals that succumb to this plant may have a mintlike odor in the gastrointestinal tract in addition to lesions of atypical interstitial pneumonia. Sheep may develop a straw-colored pleural fluid in the thorax with a typical minty odor.[2] Cattle do not develop this fluid in the thorax. However, all animals have gross and microscopic lesions. The plant is not generally grazed, unless by hungry animals or those unfamiliar with it. It causes problems both when grazed and when baled into hay. This plant contains the perilla ketones, egomaketone and isoegomaketone, which are substituted furans and the toxic agents of the plant. There is no good treatment for intoxication by *Perilla* mint.

Ipomoea batatas (Sweet Potato)

The sweet potato is capable of producing a 3-substituted furan that is toxic to both the lung and liver of several species of animals. Infection with the fungus *Fusarium solani* is regarded as one of the primary stressors that causes the plant to produce the 3-substituted furans as stress metabolites. Hence, it is commonly referred to as moldy sweet potato poisoning. Cattle are the animals most susceptible to this type of poisoning, although other animals are affected. Lesions are those of acute bovine pulmonary emphysema (ABPE). The sweet potato is a root and the ones that are not desirable for market are often fed to animals. It is when the root becomes infected with fungal pathogens that animals show signs of respiratory distress, often within 24 hours of consumption. Clinical signs in affected animals include anorexia, dyspnea, rapid breathing that becomes more labored, and death shortly thereafter. The lungs are heavy, wet, and emphysematous on postmortem examination. Microscopically, there is alveolar edema and trapped air.

Other stress metabolites that the sweet potato may produce may have an effect on the liver, producing hepatic cell necrosis. However, the liver lesions are generally not observed, since the bovine liver is more resistant to the longer-chain compounds.

Cynodon dactylon (Coastal Bermuda Grass)

Bermuda grass is a widely cultivated plant that is very adaptable where there is adequate moisture for its growth. This plant is native to Africa and has been introduced successfully in the warmer areas of the United States. The toxic agent of this plant is unknown, but its effects on cattle are well known. ABPE is acute and is seen when animals are allowed to graze lush pastures of Bermuda grass. ABPE does not seem to be associated with properly cured coastal Bermuda grass hay. Typically, the animals are not noticed to be in respiratory distress, unless there is forced exercise, such as moving the animals. Occasionally animals are suddenly found dead. Generally, there is pulmonary edema resulting in less elasticity of the lung. Inelasticity may cause right-sided heart failure from increased pressure of pumping blood into a less compliant lung. Treatment of pulmonary edema is difficult. Diuretics have been used in an attempt to decrease edema and ease cardiac function. Sedatives have been used in an effort to prevent cardiac oxygen deficiency. Animals that are not severely affected may recover if very slowly moved off the pastures. If animals can be slowly and carefully moved, low doses of atropine and antihistamines may be beneficial to the animals and may improve the likelihood of survival. If there is not a pasture that the animals can be put on, other than lush Bermuda grass, then the best recommendation is to put the animals onto an ionophore-containing feed such as monensin. It is important to recall that ruminants unaccustomed to ionophores may need to adjust slowly.

PLANTS AFFECTING THE LIVER

Lantana camara (Lantana, Large-Leaf Lantana)

This plant enjoys worldwide distribution, but in North America it is generally found in the southern region, from Florida to New Mexico and into Mexico. It is found as an ornamental or escaped ornamental and is cultivated as an outdoor annual, preferring sandy soils, waste areas, pastures, fields, and fencerows. If the plant is flowering it is easily recognized by two colors within the flower bloom. The flowers are small, tubular, and in tight flat-topped clusters. The center of the cluster is one color, such as yellow, and the outer edge of the cluster is a second color, such as red. The flowers range from yellow, pink, and orange, to bright red and include some hybrid colors of white and lavender or blue. The foliage and berries contain the toxic substance. The green berries have a higher concentration of toxin, lantadene A and B, which are polycyclic triterpenoids.

Poisonings occur most frequently among grazing animals, but all species, including humans, can be affected. In the bovine, as little as 1% of the animal's weight of plant material can result in toxicosis. A dose of 2% of body weight of plant material in sheep is lethal. Clinical signs appear approximately 1 day after consumption of a toxic dose. Acute signs include severe gastroenteritis with bloody or watery diarrhea, muscle weakness, rapid heartbeat, and dyspnea, conjunctivitis, reddening of the muzzle, and icterus. Death occurs within 3 to 4 days of consumption of a toxic amount.

More commonly the chronic form is observed. Clinical signs include photosensitization and jaundice due to hepatic dysfunction. Loss of appetite, dyspnea, conjunctivitis, and frequently severe constipation are evident. Death is usually from emaciation.

On postmortem examination there is evidence of gastroenteritis with some stasis. There are degenerative changes in a highly pigmented liver. Jaundice in a number of the tissues may be evident, particularly if photosensitization is present. The gallbladder may appear distended and paralytic.

Treatment may be unrewarding, especially in severe cases. However, supportive treatment is always indicated. Do not allow the animal any further access to the plant and move the animal out of the sun if there is photosensitization. Consider reinocu-

lating the rumen to help overcome the lack of gut motility. Perhaps the best treatment is prevention. Both herbicides and digging up the plant are very effective in eliminating it.

Senecio douglasi var. *longilobus* (Tansy Ragwort, Threadleaf Groundsel), *Senecio redillii* (Riddell's Groundsel, Wooly), and *Senecio glabellus* (Butterweed)

Senecio spp. in the Southwest all contain pyrrolizidine alkaloids and are usually range plants. Pyrrolizidine alkaloids are extremely hepatotoxic and affect primarily cattle and horses, while sheep and goats are slightly more resistant, requiring more plant material to become intoxicated. Hepatic insufficiency disease may occur as long as 6 months after removing animals from the infected pastures. Clinical signs that have developed in horses and cattle include cirrhosis,[3] jaundice, neurologic disturbances, continuous walking, head pressing, tenesmus, and frequent voiding of small amounts of bile-stained feces. In Texas, and some of the other southwestern areas, icterus and photosensitization are not clinical features. The disease is progressive. Postmortem examination reveals diffuse hepatic fibrosis, ascites with icterus, and in cattle distention of the gallbladder. Hepatic regeneration may be evident in some areas of the liver. There is no specific treatment and prevention is ultimately the best approach.

PLANTS THAT CAUSE PRIMARY PHOTOSENSITIZATION

Cooperia pedunculata (Rain Lily)

Cattle, sheep, goats, deer, and horses are affected by the small, native perennial forb, *Cooperia pedunculata*, belonging to the amaryllis family (Amaryllidaceae).[4] Rain lily arises from a large, usually black bulb. Its leaves are linear and a singular white to slightly flushed pink flower is produced. It grows well on native and improved pastures. In all animals that are affected, it produces a primary photosensitization, a condition that does not require liver damage. In horses, this is often referred to as "sand burn."

Light-skinned areas on various species, such as eyes, ears, nose, lips, udder, vulva, and lower legs, may become yellow to red early in the disease. Clinical signs may include kicking, scratching, switching the tail or shaking the head, rubbing against objects, licking and biting the affected parts, and tearing of the eyes. Other signs of primary photosensitization include erythema, pruritus, blister-like areas that peel and ooze, and corneal opacity. There may or may not be lameness, depending upon the pain around the coronary band of the hoof. These early signs may progress to swelling and pitting edema on the ears. Cracks may form in the skin with exudation of serum and edematous fluids. Scale formations and secondary infections can also occur. The swelling of the skin may subside in a few days leaving the skin in a necrotic state that very likely will slough. Animals may starve to death due to damage around the mouth and even reluctance to move to food or water.

Sensitivity and damage to udders of affected dams often result in calves or kids being unable to nurse. Although there have been no reports of adult cattle losses, large numbers of calves have died from rejection. Blindness in deer herds has resulted in a decrease in the deer population, another example of a negative economic impact in the area where this plant grows.

Photosensitization occurs from the ingestion of the dead or dry leaves of the plant. Livestock may consume the plant accidentally while grazing other available grasses or forbs. Deer may select rain lily as part of their diet during the fall and winter months, especially when there is limited forage available.

The best treatment is to eliminate direct exposure to sunlight. Placing sources of feed and water close to the animals may be necessary in severe conditions. If secondary infections become evident, then appropriate treatment will be necessary.

PLANTS THAT AFFECT THE NERVOUS SYSTEM

Eupatorium rugosum (White Snakeroot, Richweed, White Sanicle)

White snakeroot is an erect herbaceous perennial with stiff, generally branched stems. Most plants are 3 to 4 ft tall with opposite leaves, and 10 to 30 small, white, and composite flowers. It is easy to identify but is also easily confused with similar nontoxic *Eupatorium* spp.

This plant is distributed throughout the eastern United States and is prevalent in the eastern half of Texas. The plant's distribution stretches across Texas and produces most of its problems in the Edwards Plateau region of western Texas. The plant is also known to cause problems in the eastern United States. The plant prefers open-wooded areas and semishaded areas, but can become abundant following timber clearing.

The toxic principal is generally regarded as being trematol, an alcohol form, or tematone, the ketone form. The toxic substance remains in the dried plant after frost. It is a cumulative poison and repeated exposure to small amounts results in intoxication. The plant seems to remain succulent in dry weather and even after frost when it may be grazed more readily. Green plant material may be lethal to horses, cattle, and sheep with ingestion of 1% to 10% of the animal's body weight, either from ingestion at one time or in smaller successive doses. Goats, especially Angora goats, appear to be particularly sensitive, and the lethal dose may be less than that of other animals.

Since the toxins are secreted in the milk of animals consuming the plant, lactating animals are significantly protected while nursing animals are severely affected, as are nonlactating animals. This seems to be most noticeable in beef herds. During the period of western expansion of the United States this "milk sickness" was a problem for humans. It reportedly caused the death of Abraham Lincoln's mother. Pasteurization does not detoxify the milk, but dilution in modern dairies apparently provides some safety factor.

Clinical signs in horses may develop within 2 days to 3 weeks following ingestion of *E. rugosum*. Horses present signs consistent with congestive heart failure, including swelling of the ventral neck near the thoracic inlet. They also exhibit sweating, tremors, stumbling, hematuria, and severe depression.

In cattle the clinical signs include evidence of liver dysfunction, anorexia, weight loss, and photosensitization if they survive more than a few days. There may be some ataxia and tremors of the flank, neck, hind limbs, and face, which become more severe with exercise. The clinical signs may persist even after removing the animals from the plant. Similar clinical signs would be expected in goats. In Texas, Angora goats often present with severe liver dysfunction and photosensitization.

Treatment is supportive and nonspecific. It may be necessary to provide feed and water in extremely close proximity (under their noses) to affected animals. Remember to consider the need for vitamins, especially B vitamins. It may be necessary to tube-feed and to treat for ketosis. If possible, continue to milk the animals to enhance excretion of the toxic principle. In horses, symptomatic care may involve electrocardiographic monitoring.

Ease the stress on the animal by treating with fecal softeners and plenty of fluids.

Lesions are consistent with the clinical signs. In ruminants effects will probably include signs of photosensitization and lesions of hepatic lipidosis, congestion, and degenerative changes in the liver. In horses there will be myocardial degeneration, necrosis, and fibrosis. The pericardial sac is filled with straw-colored fluid. There is also likely to be some centrilobular degeneration with mild necrosis and fatty changes in the liver in horses.

Vicia villosa (Hairy Vetch), *Vicia sativa* (Common Vetch), *Vicia leavenworthii* (Leavenworth Vetch), *Vicia faba* (Faba Bean)

Vicia villosa is of primary importance and is an annual to biennial with stems spreading and villous and as long as a meter. The plant enjoys a wide distribution throughout the south central United States, South Africa, and the Mediterranean. It is prevalent in north central Texas and especially in Oklahoma. There are several species of vetch that have been associated with some toxicity, but the most consistent problem and well-documented cases involve *V. villosa*.

V. villosa affects cattle and horses primarily but may affect other ruminants. In cattle there are three syndromes. The first syndrome involves a nervous derangement with locomotor difficulty, convulsions, and death. The second syndrome is characterized by subcutaneous swellings of the head, neck, and body. There are herpetiform eruptions on the oral mucous membranes. The affected animals have a purulent nasal discharge, rales, cough, and congestion leading to cyanosis. These animals may develop alopecia and anorexia. Weakness and death follow 12 to 15 days of illness. The third syndrome is a dermatitis and is extremely important in the southwestern United States. The most notable clinical signs include dermatitis, conjunctivitis, anorexia, weight loss, increased temperature, and diarrhea that is often bloody. The dermatitis is associated with pruritus, a roughened hair coat, and thickened skin. Alopecia of the udder, tailhead, and neck appear first, and later the face, trunk, and limbs are involved. Frequently there are exudative crusts that may ooze a yellow fluid exudate and when the crusts are removed, the erythematous surface may erode and ulcerate. The dermal and gastrointestinal syndrome is recognized in horses.[5]

The syndrome occurs generally in the late spring when the plant is vigorously growing, and occasionally late in the season. The toxicosis may occur from consumption of vetch that is baled into hay. The onset of clinical signs is most often after 2 to 3 weeks of grazing, but occasionally may be as long as 6 weeks. From the first signs of illness until death can be as short as 3 days to as long as 5 weeks. Although the morbidity is commonly 6% to 8%, the mortality of those affected may be as high as 50%.

In addition to the histologic skin lesions, there may be macrophages, lymphocytes, and plasma cells, as well as giant cells and eosinophil infiltration in the heart, adrenal glands, kidney, thyroid, brain, and lungs. These organs may have gray or gray-yellow foci or streaks in them. The lymph nodes may be normal to markedly enlarged. There may be gray nodular formations in the cortex of the lymph nodes.

Perhaps the best treatment is prevention. Supportive therapy may be beneficial.

REFERENCES

1. Dollahite JQ: The need for training and research in toxicology. Southwest Vet 20:10–11, 1966.

2. Wilson BJ, Garst JE, Linnabary RD: Pulmonary toxicity of naturally occurring 3-substituted furans. *In* Keeler RF, Van Kampen KR, James LF (eds): Effects of Poisonous Plants on Livestock. New York, Academic Press, 1978, pp 311–323.
3. Cheeke P, Shull L: Alkaloids *In* Natural Toxicants in Feeds and Poisonous Plants. Westport, Conn, AVI Publishing, 1985.
4. Rowe LD, Norman JO, Corrier DE, et al: Photosensitization of cattle in southeast Texas: Identification of phototoxic activity associated with *Cooperia pedunculata*. Am J Vet Res 48:1658–1661, 1987.
5. Woods LW, Johnson B, Hietala SK: Systemic granulomatous disease in a horse grazing pasture containing vetch (*Vicia* sp.). J Vet Diagn Invest 4:356–360, 1992.

▪ Principal Poisonous Plants of the Western United States*

Lynn F. James, Ph.D.
Kip E. Panter, Ph.D.
Bryan L. Stegelmeier, A.V.M., Ph.D., Diplomate, A.C.V.P.
Dale R. Gardner, D.V.M., Ph.D.
James A. Pfister, M.S., Ph.D.

Approximately 835 million acres of rangeland are in the 48 contiguous states. Nearly 82% of these rangelands are located in 17 western states. Rangelands are of great economic importance to the livestock industry. They supply forage for millions of breeding cows, stocker cattle, and sheep yearlong; with proper management, this number could be increased. Poisonous plants are one of the serious impediments to the harvesting of forage on these ranges and pastures.

Poisoning of livestock by plants has been an important cause of economic loss to the livestock industry from the beginning of the grazing of livestock on western ranges. Losses are caused by death, chronic illness and debilitation, photosensitization, reproductive failure, abortions, and birth defects. Poisonous plants increase costs associated with management of rangelands and pastures. These costs include fencing, lowered forage production and utilization, altered grazing programs, nonuse of some infested range areas, and (in some cases) supplemental feeding programs and added medical expenses.

Losses of livestock due to poisoning by plants vary greatly from year to year and from region to region. Some poisonous plants grow only in localized and well-defined areas, whereas others seem to be ubiquitous. They all may be affected by environmental factors such as temperature and moisture, and as a result, may be more abundant and hazardous in one year than in another. Some plants are toxic only seasonally.

In considering poisonous plants or in attempting to diagnose or predict a poisonous plant problem, one should be familiar with the poisonous plants to be encountered and the conditions under which livestock may be poisoned by them. When conditions and circumstances become ideal for poisonous plant growth or for animals to overeat on these plants, the owners may suffer losses.

Management errors contribute to this problem. Management practices used by the range livestock industry in many cases are conducive to the poisoning of livestock by plants. For example, lupine is more toxic to cattle than to sheep on a weight basis; yet thousands of sheep, but few cattle, have died from eating this plant. Halogeton is equally poisonous to cattle and to sheep. Many sheep have died from halogeton poisoning, but relatively few cattle. The differences observed may be due to the way cattle and sheep are managed. Sheep are usually kept in large flocks and moved from place to place as deemed necessary by the sheepherder. Cattle, however, are left to move freely about

a range, limited only by fences and natural barriers. Sheep are normally given water and provided with new forage only when it is allowed by the herder, but cattle are usually free to search out water and forage as needed. Often sheep that are hungry may be driven through, bedded in, or unloaded from trucks into heavy stands of poisonous plants and thus exposed to plants that they would not normally graze.

Many poisonous plants are not palatable to livestock and are eaten only in stressful situations. Plants eaten under these conditions include death camas, copperweeds, milkweeds, and rubberweeds. Other plants such as lupine, halogeton, and greasewood are palatable and may form an important and beneficial part of a range animal's diet. We need to understand the conditions that cause a plant to change its role from a forage to a toxic plant. We need to recognize that plants with toxic properties do not always kill or otherwise harm animals when they are eaten. Death or serious damage occurs when excessive amounts of toxic plants are consumed in a short period of time.

Eliminating poisonous range plants where infestation is widespread is usually economically prohibitive and physically impossible. Furthermore, chemical or mechanical treatment may be undesirable because of the adverse effects on desirable plants; and often both methods are inadequate.

Medical treatment of livestock poisoned by plants is generally of little value because of the time interval between intoxication and treatment, and the number of animals involved may be large. Therefore, the most logical approach to prevention of livestock poisoning by plants is proper management—management should be concerned not only with the health of the livestock but also with pasture and range resources and environmental conditions. Resource people, such as veterinarians, county agents, and range managers, can render valuable assistance in the development of managerial procedures for the prevention of livestock poisoning by plants.

POISONOUS PLANTS

Lupine (*Lupinus* spp.)

Over 100 species and varieties of lupines grow in the United States and Canada. Most contain toxic quinolizidine or piperidine alkaloids and are poisonous to sheep and cattle grazing on mountain pastures. Large differences in alkaloid content and toxicity occur because of the species or variety, stage of growth, and location. Seed pods generally contain the highest level of alkaloids followed by young plants; the smallest amount of alkaloid in plants is found in the flower stage or after seed pod shatter. Lupine has been one of the most devastating of the range plants poisonous to sheep in the western United States. In recent years, poisoning has been less frequent owing to improved grazing practices, fewer sheep on mountain ranges, and a better understanding of the hazards of poisonous plants. The signs of poisoning in sheep include nervousness, depression, muscle fasciculation, ataxia, collapse, and eventually death from respiratory failure.

In the 1960s, lupine was shown to cause congenital skeletal birth defects in cattle and was referred to as "crooked calf disease." This continues to be a problem for cattle producers in the northwestern United States and western Canada. The quinolizidine alkaloid anagyrine was demonstrated to be the teratogenic alkaloid in the early studies; however, recent research has demonstrated that some of the piperidine alkaloids in lupine are potent teratogens. Piperidine alkaloids from *Lupinus formosus* induced skeletal birth defects and cleft palate in goats and cattle but the quinolizidine-containing *Lupinus caudatus* was only teratogenic in cattle. Sheep and goats are resistant to the quinolizidine alkaloids, whereas cattle are very susceptible. The skeletal defects are described as contracture-type defects involv-

*All of the material in this article is in the public domain.

ing the limbs, or arthrogryposis; spinal defects, including lordosis, kyphosis, and scoliosis; and rib cage depressions. Cleft palate and asymmetry of the head may also occur. The most susceptible period of gestation in cattle includes days 40 to 70; however, recent research has shown this period may extend to day 100 and the exposure period may be as short as 10 days. Cleft palate and moderate forelimb contractures occurred when pregnant cows were fed *L. formosus* and *Lupinus arbustus* from days 40 to 50 of gestation.

These birth defects may be prevented in cattle if grazing lupine-infested pastures is avoided during the seed pod stage and there is adequate quality feed available, thus not forcing the animals to consume less desirable lupines. Changing breeding seasons and avoiding lupine pastures during the 40th through about the 100th day of gestation will minimize lupine-induced birth defects.

Larkspur (*Delphinium* spp.)

Larkspur (*Delphinium* spp.) is one of the principal poisonous plants affecting cattle in the western range states. Larkspurs may be divided into three major groups: tall larkspur (2 m or 6 ft mature height), growing in moist, higher-elevation (>1800 m or 6000 ft) rangelands; low larkspurs (0.6 m or 2 ft), growing in foothill and mountain areas; and plains larkspur (1 m or 3 ft), growing primarily on the high plains of Wyoming and Colorado.

All species of larkspur are poisonous. Concentrations of the principal toxic alkaloids, methyllycaconitine, 14-deacetylnudicauline, and nudicauline, are generally highest in immature plants and decrease with maturity, except for seed pods. Cattle are generally poisoned when they ingest greater than 20 mg toxic alkaloids per kilogram of body weight. A typical 450-kg (1000-lb) cow would be poisoned on 1.1 kg (2.4 lb dry weight) of larkspur containing 8 mg toxic alkaloid per gram. Signs of poisoning appear within 2 to 7 hours, and include muscular tremors, staggering gait, periodic collapse, bloating, paralysis, and death. No diagnostic lesions are present. Treatment with physostigmine intravenously at 0.1 mg/kg body weight may be efficacious. Affected animals should not be stressed. Sheep and horses are much less susceptible to larkspur than are cattle.

Tall larkspur ranges may be grazed with low risk until larkspur elongates flowering stalks, because consumption is usually low or nil. Relative risk increases as consumption by cattle increases during flowering until larkspur pods begin to dry out. When pods begin to shatter in late summer or early fall, toxicity (hence risk) is usually low.

Cattle will graze low and plains larkspurs during any stage of growth but do so at some risk.

Other management options include herbicidal control, grazing sheep ahead of cattle to reduce larkspur density, using conditioned aversions to train cattle to avoid larkspur, and herding to keep cattle from dense patches.

Death Camas (*Zygadenus* spp.)

Death camas (*Zygadenus* spp.) is an herb with grasslike leaves and an underground bulb. The several species of death camas have various degrees of toxicity. Cattle, sheep, and horses are susceptible to death camas poisoning.

Death camas is one of the first plants to begin growth in the spring. Animals are usually poisoned at this time, when there is a shortage of good, desirable forage. Poisoning often occurs when a spring snow covers other forage and the death camas protrudes above the snow.

Signs of poisoning include increased respiration rates, exces-

sive salivation, apparent nausea, weakness and staggering, convulsions, coma, and death. No treatment is known for death camas poisoning. Severely poisoned animals usually die, whereas those less affected may recover. Animals poisoned on death camas should not be disturbed.

Prevention lies in preventing hungry animals from grazing areas infested with death camas in the early spring. As other forage becomes available, livestock are less likely to graze the death camas.

Hemlocks (*Cicuta* spp. and *Conium maculatum*)

Water hemlock (*Cicuta*) and poison hemlock (*Conium*) are common poisonous plants often confused with each other because of their similarities in name and appearance. Their toxins and modes of action are different.

There are four species of water hemlock recognized in North America and all are toxic. The toxin is a long-chain alcohol called cicutoxin. The clinical signs of poisoning include increased respiration, excessive salivation, nervousness, and tremors, with signs quickly progressing to severe intermittent grand mal seizures and eventually death. Severity of the clinical signs and time between ingestion and death depend on the amount of plant eaten. Tubers and roots or early-growth plant is most toxic, although recent field cases of poisoning implicated green seed as the cause of death in cattle. Early-growth plant and tubers are quite palatable in the early spring as growth often begins before other plants. Serum biochemical changes and gross and microscopic lesions are the result of the seizures and include elevated blood glucose, aspartate aminotransferase (AST), and lactate dehydrogenase (LDH) and lesions of skeletal and cardiac myodegeneration. Intravenous infusion of pentobarbital to control seizures will prevent death and the reported pathologic changes. Cattle, sheep, pigs, and humans have been poisoned with water hemlock.

There is only one species of poison hemlock in North America and poisoning has occurred in most livestock species and humans. Poisoning has also been reported in elk and wild geese grazing new-growth plants in the spring and in turkeys and chickens eating poison hemlock seed.

Conium maculatum toxins are simple piperidine alkaloids and include coniine and γ-coniceine as the predominant alkaloids. These alkaloids are also teratogens causing contracture-type skeletal defects and cleft palate in sheep, goats, cattle, and pigs similar to those described for lupine-induced crooked calf disease. Clinical signs of poisoning include nervousness, muscle fasciculations, ataxia, muscular weakness, collapse, and death. There are no pathologic lesions, but a "mousy" odor, similar to the smell of crushed plant or the pure alkaloids, is reported on the breath and in the urine of poisoned animals. Diagnosis of poisoning includes a history of ingestion, clinical signs, and chemical confirmation of coniine, γ-coniceine, or coniine-like compounds in the stomach contents, liver, or urine.

Poisoning from both plants may be prevented by controlling plant invasion with herbicides and avoidance of grazing in early spring before grasses begin to grow or in mid- to late summer when seed heads are green and more likely to be grazed. Conium frequently invades alfalfa fields and has caused poisoning in green chop, silage, and baled hay. The alkaloids are somewhat volatile, and drying and ensiling will reduce risk over time. Caution should be used when feeding contaminated hay or silage.

Halogeton (*Halogeton glomeratus*)

Halogeton (*Halogeton glomeratus*) is an annual plant that grows on the colder, arid, saline ranges of the West. The toxic principle is an oxalate that has been responsible for the death of many sheep and some cattle. This plant competes poorly with other vegetation, so ranges infested with halogeton should be expected to respond well to good range management practices. See the section on Oxalate Accumulators (this edition) for a more complete discussion.

Greasewood *(Sarcobatus vermiculatus)*

Greasewood *(Sarcobatus vermiculatus)* is an oxalate-producing shrub that grows in the colder, saline, arid, and semiarid regions of the western United States. It has been responsible for the deaths of numerous cattle and sheep.

Prevention of losses consists primarily of proper management. The plant sprouts from the crown and does not respond well to herbicides or burning.

Greasewood can form a useful part of the diet of sheep and cattle if it is properly managed.

Chokecherry *(Prunus virginiana)*

Chokecherry *(Prunus virginiana)* is a low-growing shrub or tree on the western ranges. It contains toxic amounts of hydrocyanic acid. When sheep or cattle graze considerable amounts of chokecherry, they may become poisoned.

Prevention of chokecherry poisoning in animals on western ranges involves proper management procedures. Ruminants can graze large amounts of chokecherry without harm. Poisoning occurs when they graze large amounts of plant rapidly. Therefore, hungry animals should not be allowed to graze chokecherry. Chokecherry is difficult to eliminate from the ranges.

Arrowgrass *(Triglochin spp.)*

Arrowgrass *(Triglochin spp.)* produces hydrocyanic acid under stressful conditions. Arrowgrass grows on wet, heavy, alkaline soil. Prevention involves keeping livestock from grazing this plant during drought or frost.

Selenium-Accumulating Plants

Several species of plants that grow on seleniferous soils accumulate selenium in such amounts that they become toxic to livestock grazing them. These plants are discussed under Selenium Toxicosis.

Ponderosa Pine *(Pinus ponderosa)*

Ponderosa pine *(Pinus ponderosa)*, when grazed by cows during the last trimester of gestation, can cause abortions. Ponderosa pine grows in all states west of the Great Plains, and in southwestern Canada and northern Mexico. The abortifacient toxin has been identified as isocupressic acid. This toxin is also found in *Pinus radiata* and Monterey cypress *(Cupressus macrocarpa)* grown in New Zealand, and lodgepole pine *(Pinus contorta)* in the United States; leaves or needles eaten from these trees may induce abortions in cattle.

Abortions can result when pregnant cows eat dry or green needles from standing trees, slash from cut trees, or needles from ground litter. Animals usually abort during the late fall, winter, and early spring. Factors apparently causing cattle to eat pine needles include sudden weather changes such as cold winds and snowstorms, hunger, changes in feed, and other stressful conditions. Cattle will eat ponderosa pine needles even when good forage is available.

There are generally few signs of impending abortions. A cow may show swelling of the external genital organs and filling of the udder if she grazes needles over a period of time before the abortion. Some animals may abort within 48 hours after they ingest pine needles, and other animals may abort as long as 2 weeks after they are removed from access to the needles. The abortion is characterized by weak parturition contractions, excessive uterine hemorrhage, and incomplete dilation of the cervix. The chances of calf survival increase when the abortion occurs near term.

Regardless of the stage of gestation, a persistent retained placenta is a constant finding after the abortion. Septic metritis often follows, body temperature increases, and, unless the animal is properly treated, generalized septicemia may follow. In acute cases, the cow appears to have toxemia and may die before or soon after she aborts. In such cases, there may be ecchymotic hemorrhages on the peritoneum, pleura, and viscera. There are no specific characteristic lesions in the aborted calves as a result of pine needle ingestion.

Although cattle may graze in areas with ponderosa pine during the critical stage of gestation and not eat the needles, there is always the risk that they may. Therefore, the best prevention currently involves keeping pregnant cows from grazing pine needles during the last trimester of gestation.

Broomsnakeweed *(Gutierrezia spp.)*

Broomsnakeweed *(Gutierrezia spp.)* is an herbaceous plant that branches close to the ground. The branches are topped by yellow composite flowers. The leaves are small, alternate, and filiform.

Signs of poisoning include anorexia, rough hair coat, listlessness, and loss of weight. The animal may develop diarrhea or may become constipated. There may be a vaginal discharge and also bloody urine.

Pregnant cows, principally in the last trimester of pregnancy, may develop signs of an impending parturition (e.g., swelling of the external genital organs and filling of the udder). Abortion will generally follow. Most cows have a retained placenta. The cow may die of a toxemia associated with the abortion. In excess of 60% of cows grazing broomsnakeweed may abort. The calves of those near term may survive but are small and weak and need extra care.

Cows grazing in excess of 20 lb of plant are at risk for an abortion. Cows grazing broomsnakeweed growing on sandy soils are more apt to abort than are cows grazing plants on limestone or hard soils. Cows are most apt to graze broomsnakeweed after a snowstorm or other adverse weather conditions and during times of forage shortages.

Sheep and goats also abort after grazing broomsnakeweed. Broomsnakeweed appears to be increasing in areas farther north.

Milkweeds *(Asclepias spp.)*

Milkweeds *(Asclepias spp.)* are perennial herbs that contain milky juice, stand erect, and have opposite or whorled leaf arrangements. The milkweeds are divided into two groups: the narrow-leaf milkweeds and the broadleaf milkweeds. Not all species of milkweeds are toxic. The principal poisonous species in the west are *A. labriformis, A. subverticillata, A. eriocarpa,* and *A. fascicularis. A. labriformis* is among the most toxic of range plants and contains cardiac glycosides (cardenolides) as its toxic principle. Milkweeds are unpalatable and usually eaten only by hungry animals. They may also be harvested with hay or green chop and thus cause poisoning as a contaminant.

The signs of poisoning include muscular incoordination, spasms, bloat, rapid weak pulse, respiratory difficulty, and death.

No treatment is known for animals poisoned on milkweed. Losses from milkweed can be reduced by maintaining ranges and pastures in good condition. Livestock that are hungry should not be allowed to graze in milkweed-infested areas. Milkweed should not be harvested with hay and other forages.

Horsebrush (*Tetradymia* spp.)

Horsebrush (*Tetradymia* spp.) is a shrub growing in the drier range areas of the West. These plants are principally a problem to sheep in the early spring.

Oak (*Quercus* spp.)

Oak (*Quercus* spp.) is poisonous primarily to cattle. Oaks of the West are low-growing shrubs or small trees. Oak grows in dense stands, and growth starts early in the spring. It is most toxic during the bud and early leaf stage. As the leaves mature, they decrease in toxicity. Large amounts of oak must be eaten for cattle to be poisoned. The toxins are tannins.

The signs of poisoning are rough hair coat, gaunt appearance, emaciation, edema, constipation or diarrhea, mucus or blood (or both) in the feces, dark-brown urine, and death.

Lesions include gastroenteritis and edema of the intestinal walls, subcutaneous edema, and ascites. The major lesion of oak poisoning is necrosis of the renal tubules.

Prevention consists of keeping cattle away from the oak brush during the period when oak is in the early bud stage, especially during times of feed shortage. This treatment may involve the development of a range or pasture free of oak brush.

Locoweed (*Astragalus* and *Oxytropis* spp.)

Locoweed intoxication or "locoism" results when animals continuously graze certain plants of the *Astragalus* or *Oxytropis* genera. Toxic North American species include *A. lentiginosus*, *A. mollissimus*, *A. earlei*, *A. wootoni*, *A. pubentissimus*, *O. sericea*, and *O. lambertii*. These locoweeds are legumes, pealike plants that grow early in the spring and late in the fall when other green feeds are not available. Locoweeds are generally eaten by livestock and wildlife in proportion to their availability and they remain toxic even when senescent or dried.

Clinical signs of locoweed poisoning become apparent when the animal has grazed the plant for several weeks. Signs of intoxication include depression, proprioceptive deficits, intention tremors, nervousness (especially when stressed), dull hair coat, emaciation, decreased libido, infertility, abortion, hydramnios, cardiovascular disease, and death. Though lacking gross lesions, intoxication results in characteristic histologic lesions of vacuolar degeneration of neurons and other parenchymatous cells. Most lesions develop within 4 or 5 days of poisoning and many resolve in 2 to 3 days. However, many neuronal lesions are permanent, and chronically poisoned animals often have behavioral and functional deficits. This makes the usefulness of many working animals questionable and possibly even dangerous. Additional work is needed to predict how poisoned animals will perform and to identify the pathogenesis of these permanent sequelae.

The diagnosis of locoweed poisoning is currently made by documenting exposure to the plant and identifying the characteristic clinical and pathologic changes of poisoning. Recently,

diagnostic tests using serum from living poisoned animals have been developed.

The locoweed toxin, swainsonine, is a potent inhibitor of lysosomal α-mannosidase and Golgi mannosidase II. This inhibition results in cellular vacuolation and abnormal glycoprotein metabolism similar to genetic mannosidosis of humans, Angus cattle, and cats, in which cellular α-mannosidase is defective. Swainsonine also alters glycoprotein production resulting in abnormal hormones, membrane receptors, and enzymes. As a result, locoweed poisoning has been associated with abnormal endocrine, reproductive, immune, and gastrointestinal function. All of these changes reduce animal efficiency, and production, and may make animals more susceptible to disease.

Swainsonine is rapidly absorbed from the gastrointestinal tract and is rapidly excreted in the urine, milk, and feces. The swainsonine clearance rate ($T_{1/2}$) from the serum of a chronically poisoned animal is about 20 hours while liver and kidney have a clearance $T_{1/2}$ of about 60 hours. This suggests that 5 days would be required to clear practically all the toxin from the animal and its tissues.

Timber Milk Vetch (*Astragalus miser*)

Timber milk vetch (*Astragalus miser*) and other *Astragalus* plants, such as *A. emoryanus*, *A. pterocarpus*, and *A. canadensis*, contain 3-nitro-1-propanol or 3-nitro-1-propionic acid as a toxic constituent.

Depending on the rate at which it is eaten by livestock, this group of plants may induce acute or chronic poisoning. Acute intoxication is characterized by nervousness, irregular gait, general body weakness, rapid weak pulse, coma, and death. Some animals may show indications of blindness. Lesions include lobular alveolar pulmonary emphysema, collapsed or constricted bronchioles, and interlobular edema. Some cases have widespread focal hemorrhage in the central nervous system.

Chronic intoxication is characterized by dullness, incoordination of the hind legs when walking, and goose-stepping. The animals may have cocked ankles and may fall when they run. There may be respiratory distress and posterior paralysis if the condition progresses to advanced stages. With proper care, poisoned animals may recover. However, animals poisoned by this plant usually die if they are not removed from access to the plant.

The postmortem lesions are not pathognomonic. The liver may be swollen, and the pericardial fluid may be increased; varying degrees of wallerian degeneration of the spinal cord and varying degrees of pulmonary emphysema are regularly observed.

Poisoning can best be prevented by not allowing animals to graze this plant over extended periods of time. Intoxication in areas where this plant is a problem seems to be more severe in periods of drought. Toxicity decreases as plants mature. Nursing cows are more often affected by this plant than are dry cows. Cows poisoned on this plant should be handled very carefully and should not be stressed.

Rayless Goldenrod (*Haplopappus heterophyllus*)

Rayless goldenrod (*Haplopappus heterophyllus*) is common in the dry rangelands of the Southwest. It is an erect, unbranched perennial shrub with yellow flowers that grows from 61 to 122 cm (2 to 4 ft) tall. The poisonous principle is thought to be tremetol, a higher alcohol. It is toxic to all classes of range livestock. If animals that are grazing this plant are not removed from it, they will die. The toxin is excreted in the milk, so the nursing offspring will be intoxicated before the dam.

The signs of poisoning are lassitude and depression, a humped-up posture, and stiff gait. The body may tremble, especially about the head and shoulders. Signs of poisoning may be accentuated by forced exercise. Postmortem findings are not characteristic. The liver may be pale, and the abomasum and intestines may be congested.

Eupatorium rugosum (white snakeroot) contains the same toxin as does rayless goldenrod. It has been shown that horses grazing white snakeroot may develop heart and skeletal muscle necrosis.

Prevention consists of eradication of the plants or not allowing livestock to graze them.

Sneezeweed *(Helenium hoopesii)*

Sneezeweed *(Helenium hoopesii)* grows on moist slopes and well-drained meadows at elevations from 1524 to 3048 m (5000 to 10,000 ft) throughout most of the 11 western states. Sneezeweed is an herbaceous perennial with yellow flowers, and it grows from 30 to 90 cm (1 to 3 ft) tall. It is primarily a problem in sheep. Sheep are poisoned after grazing the plant for about 10 days, most often in the late summer and early fall when better forage is gone or dried up.

Signs of poisoning are depression, stiffness, weakness, coughing, chronic vomiting (which leaves the area around the mouth stained green), and bloating. If the sheep are allowed to graze the plant until vomiting starts, they usually waste and die. Lambs poisoned by the plant are usually unthrifty and remain so.

The principal lesions of sneezeweed poisoning are gastroenteritis, edema of the stomach walls, excessive fluid in the pericardial cavity, and ascites.

Prevention consists of control of the plants or removing the sheep from sneezeweed-infested ranges at frequent intervals.

Rubberweed *(Hymenoxys richardsonii)*

Rubberweed or pingue *(Hymenoxys richardsonii)* is a perennial herb with yellow flowers that grows from 15 to 46 cm (6 to 18 in) tall. It grows principally on dry foothill areas from 1220 to 3048 m (4000 to 10,000 ft) of elevation. Rubberweed is principally a problem in range sheep. Heavy infestation of rubberweed indicates overgrazing. Signs of poisoning are salivation, anorexia, rumen stasis, apparent abdominal pain, uneasiness, weakness, and prostration. Lesions are associated with gastrointestinal irritation and hepatic degeneration.

Rubberweed is distasteful; therefore, sheep are poisoned primarily during trailing and during grazing of ranges heavily infested with the plant.

PREVENTION AND MANAGEMENT

Poisoning of livestock by plants that are part of their normal diet is uncommon. Livestock poisoning on the range usually becomes a problem because of a shortage of good forage or because of an increase in poisonous plants, which results when the more desirable plants have been completely grazed. In general, the prevention of loss from poisonous plants is often a problem of proper animal and range management. Many poisonous plants are distasteful to livestock but others may be palatable at different times of the year. Larkspurs, lupines, locoweeds, and others may be grazed extensively at certain times of the year. Some general rules for preventing livestock poisoning by plants are as follows:

1. Know the poisonous plants, especially those of local significance.
2. Know how poisonous plants affect livestock and the conditions under which they are toxic.
3. Avoid areas infested with poisonous plants during holding, trailing, or unloading of animals. If these situations cannot be avoided, special preventive procedures should be considered.
4. Avoid grazing hungry animals in areas infested with poisonous plants. Animals may become hungry by withholding feed or water and by overgrazing. Provide animals with water and adequate forage of good quality.
5. Provide adequate salt and mineral supplements.
6. Where possible, control or eradicate poisonous plants, especially from problem areas.
7. Develop and practice proper grazing procedures.
8. Keep the range in good condition. Avoid overgrazing.
9. Good management practices will prevent most cases of plant poisoning in livestock.
10. Know the conditions under which animals graze the poisonous plants you have to deal with and have a strategy to avoid the problem.

■ Oleander *(Nerium oleander)* Toxicosis

Francis D. Galey, D.V.M., Ph.D., Diplomate, A.B.V.T.

Oleander *(Nerium oleander)* is an ornamental, evergreen shrub native to the Mediterranean. The bush can grow to 20 ft tall and has leathery, lanceolate leaves that are long and narrow.[2, 4] The flowers are borne in terminal clusters of dark-red, pink, or white blossoms in the spring and early summer. The plant is commonly found in California and the southern portions of the United States.[4] Dried and fresh leaves of oleander are considered to be very poisonous to livestock because of cardiac glycoside toxins that can cause sudden death with gastroenteritis and heart failure. Other plants that contain similar cardiac toxins that are poisonous to livestock include *Rhododendron* spp. (also evergreen shrubs, e.g., azaleas), *Kalmia* spp. (laurels), *Pieris japonica* (Japanese pieris), *Digitalis* sp. (foxglove), and *Apocynum* (dogbane, less toxic). Related toxins include cardenolides (e.g., *Asclepias*, milkweeds), grayanotoxins, and bufadenolides.

All parts of the plant are toxic, including when dry as clippings. The dry clippings and dry leaves are a major cause of oleander poisoning in livestock.[2, 3] Although toxic when fresh, fresh plant is apparently not that palatable. Some of the other listed plants, such as the rhododendrons, may be grazed fresh or dry by livestock, causing toxicosis.

Oleander is extremely toxic. One leaf is potentially lethal to humans.[4] As little as 0.005% of their body weight in dried leaves may cause clinical toxicosis in cattle and horses,[4, 8] and 0.015% of body weight in sheep (two to three leaves).[4, 8] That dose is equivalent to about 10 to 30 g for cattle and 15 to 30 g for horses, or, in either case, a handful of leaves. Oleander toxin has been detected in milk from exposed cows. Therefore, milk and meat from animals exposed to oleander should not be consumed. The withdrawal time is not known for cattle, but at least 7 days should be allowed to pass before marketing milk or meat from those exposed animals.[9]

Oleander glycosides inhibit Na⁺,K⁺-ATPase which is essential to cardiac function, an effect that is similar to the digitalis glycosides.[2, 4] The onset of clinical oleander toxicosis is often delayed by several hours after ingestion. If a lethal dose is ingested, death usually occurs within 36 hours, although it may occur at any time between 45 minutes and 14 days[2, 5] (and personal observation).

The most common presentation of cardiac glycoside toxicosis is that the animals are found "suddenly" dead. If signs are observed, they are related to the gastrointestinal tract and heart. Ingestion of oleander plant material can cause mild abdominal pain, weakness, anorexia, rumen atony, and diarrhea.[2, 4, 5] Although bradycardia may be present initially, most commonly, the practitioner finds a weak, irregular, fast pulse with tachycardia, and a very wide variety of heart blocks and ventricular arrhythmias.[2, 4, 5, 8] Affected animals may also develop lethargy, uneasiness, mydriasis, tremors, increased urination, cyanotic mucous membranes, followed by excitement, intermittent convulsions, depression, dyspnea, and coma prior to death.

Postmortem findings included no lesions for some peracute cases. The most common lesions observed involve the heart.[3] Endocardial hemorrhage may be present, along with increased volumes of pericardial fluid and edema around cardiac vessels. Colon and cecal contents are often very watery. Lesions in the heart included subendocardial hemorrhages and multifocal myocardial edema, degeneration, and necrosis, especially in the subendocardium.[3]

Diagnosis of oleander toxicosis largely depends on identification of the plant, along with evidence of its consumption, and appropriate clinical signs and lesions. Identification of leaves in gastrointestinal contents can be aided by identification of characteristic venation pattern and stomata in leaves.[5] Ingesta, including rumen contents and cecal contents, can be tested in the laboratory for the presence of oleandrin to verify a diagnosis.[3]

Affected animals should be treated as for cardiac glycoside toxicosis. Exposed animals should be removed from the source. If very early, the gut should be evacuated using emesis or rumenotomy; otherwise, adsorption using cholestyramine resins[1] or activated charcoal is suggested.[6] Potassium therapy should be administered *only* if hyperkalemia (e.g., increased T wave elevations) is demonstrated to be absent.[1] As with other cardiac glycosides, calcium-containing solutions and quinidine should be avoided.

Atropine may be useful in treating bradyarrhythmias often observed in the first 24 hours.[1] Use atropine extremely carefully to avoid overatropinization with attendant gastrointestinal effects. Propranolol and lidocaine have been used to treat various tachyarrhythmias as they occur. Experimentally, the administration of anticardiac glycoside Fab antibodies has also been attempted in one case of oleander toxicosis in a human.[7]

Prevention is the most important aspect in oleander toxicosis. Trimmings from oleander bushes and hedges should always be promptly removed. Animals should be kept away from oleander bushes. Contamination of chaff or hay with oleander parts should be carefully avoided.

REFERENCES

1. Adams HR: Digitalis, other inotropic agents, and vasodilator drugs. *In* Booth NH, McDonald LE (eds): Veterinary Pharmacology and Therapeutics, ed 6. Ames, Iowa State University Press, 1988, pp 495–517.
2. Everist SL: Apocynaceae. *In* Poisonous Plants of Australia, ed 2. London, Angus & Robertson, 1981, pp 77–89.
3. Galey FD, Holstege DM, Plumlee KH, et al: Diagnosis of oleander poisoning in livestock. J Vet Diagn Invest 8:358–364, 1996.
4. Kingsbury JM: Poisonous Plants of the United States and Canada. Englewood Cliffs, NJ, Prentice-Hall, 1964, pp 264–267.
5. Mahin L, Marzou A, Huart A: A case report of *Nerium oleander* poisoning in cattle. Vet Hum Toxicol 26:303–304, 1984.
6. PoisIndex: Plants—Cardiac Glycosides. Denver, Micromedex, 1996.
7. Shumaik GM, Wu AW, Ping AC: Oleander poisoning: Treatment

with digoxin-specific Fab antibody fragments. Ann Emerg Med 17:732–735, 1988.
8. Szabuniewicz JD, McCrady JD, Camp BJ: Treatment of experimentally induced oleander poisoning. Arch Int Pharmacodyna Ther 189:12–21, 1971.
9. Galey FD, Holslege DM, Johnson BJ, et al: Toxicity and diagnosis of oleander (*Nerium oleander*) poisoning in livestock. *In* Gorland T, et al (eds): Proceedings of the Fifth International Symposium on poisonous plants, CAB International, Wallingford, UK (in press).

■ Hepatotoxic Plants

Stan W. Casteel, D.V.M., Ph.D., Diplomate, A.B.V.T.

The unique anatomic position and metabolic capacity of the liver make it particularly vulnerable to hepatotoxin exposure. Venous blood from the gastrointestinal tract flows through the liver before entering the systemic circulation. The portal blood supply from the gut makes up about 80% of the total liver blood flow, enhancing the concentration of ingested toxins in the hepatic blood. Besides this first-pass effect, the liver's prominent role in the biotransformation of xenobiotics increases its chances of injury from reactive metabolites.[1]

Signs of acute and chronic terminal liver disease are identical in cattle and usually remain subclinical until affected animals separate from the herd, become depressed, diarrheal, icteric, or photosensitized.[2] Signs of photosensitization are preceded by hepatobiliary dysfunction. Because of the liver's reserve and regenerative capacities, clinical evidence of disease may remain unapparent until 75% of the functional hepatic mass has been compromised.

PYRROLIZIDINE ALKALOID–CONTAINING PLANTS

Like most poisonous plants, hepatotoxic plants (Table 1) are more of a problem where suitable forage is limited, as in areas of the Southwest and West. Poisoning is also more likely when animals are transported and initially released or upon release from a drylot into infested areas. Plants containing pyrrolizidine alkaloids are responsible for a chronic progressive liver disease in livestock. From an economic standpoint, this is the most important class of hepatotoxic plants. *Senecio* spp. are a major problem in the Northwest and a lesser problem in the remaining West and Southwest. Species of *Cynoglossum* and *Amsinckia* are minor problems in the West, while *Crotalaria* is an occasional problem in the Midwest and Southeast. Goats and sheep are relatively resistant to *Senecio* spp. and can be used in the biologic control of the weed.[3] Consumption of from 0.5% to 5.0% of the body weight of cattle at a single feeding or divided over several days or weeks may induce chronic, progressive liver disease resulting in death months after exposure, with few clinical signs preceding terminal hepatic coma. More commonly, consumption occurs continuously or intermittently during the grazing season or from contaminated hay or silage.

Chronic disease is common following a characteristic delayed onset of from 2 to 8 months. Clinical disease or sudden death is consistently preceded by increased serum activities of glutamate dehydrogenase (GDH), serum alkaline phosphatase (SAP), and γ-glutamyltransferase (GGT).[3] Once the threshold for hepatic failure is exceeded, cattle are commonly found dead in the field; however, clinical signs of fulminant liver disease are sometimes seen and include depression, diarrhea, tenesmus, ascites, rectal prolapse, recumbency, coma, and death within 2 to 3 days of onset. Livers from affected cattle are typically firm, pale, and

Table 1
HEPATOTOXIC PLANTS OF THE UNITED STATES

Genus	Common Name(s)	Effect(s)
Pyrrolizidine al-kaloid plants		Chronic, progressive disease
Amsinckia	Fiddleneck	Delayed onset of 2–8 mo
Crotalaria	Rattlebox	Emaciation, photosensitization
Cynoglossum	Hound's tongue	Subcutaneous edema, diarrhea, tenesmus
Senecio	Ragwort	Terminal hepatic encephalopathy
Heliotropium	Heliotrope	Hypoproteinemia, hyperbilirubinemia
Echium	Pateron's curse	Increased activities of GDH, ALP, GGT
Symphytum	Comfrey	
Agave	Lecheguilla	Photosensitization, icterus, in sheep and goats
Eupatorium	White snakeroot	1–2 wk duration of tremors, ataxia in cattle; photosensitization in goats
Kochia	Summer cypress Mexican fireweed	Photosensitization in cattle
Lantana	Lantana	Bloody diarrhea and death, cholestasis, liver disease, photosensitization
Microcystis	Blue-green algae	Diarrhea, shock, dissociation of hepatocytes, intrahepatic hemorrhage
Nolina	Sacahuista	Photosensitization
Panicum	Kleingrass	Photosensitization and icterus, primarily in lambs and kids
Cycas	False sago palm, fern palm	Diarrhea, icterus, ascites
Zamia	Coontie	Centrilobular necrosis
Tetradymia	Horsebrush	Photosensitization in sheep
Tribulus	Puncture vine	Photosensitization in sheep
Xanthium	Cocklebur	Rapid onset of blindness, hypersensitivity, convulsions in cattle; swine are hypoglycemiac

GDH, glutamate dehydrogenase; ALP, alkaline phosphatase; GGT, γ-glutamyltransferase.

yellowish with petechial hemorrhages. Histologic changes include variable liver necrosis, biliary hyperplasia, megalocytosis, and fibroplasia. The prognosis for animals with advanced disease is poor. Low-protein, high-energy diets for moderately affected cattle are impractical and recovery is uncertain. The cinnabar moth has been a successful biologic control for *Senecio jacobaea* while herbicides, including clopyralid, chlorsulfuron, metsulfuron, 2,4-D, and picloram, provide excellent chemical control.[4]

OTHER HEPATOTOXIC PLANTS

Lecheguilla grows in arid regions of western Texas, southern New Mexico, and south into Mexico on dry hills, valleys, and along canyons. Sheep and goats are most frequently poisoned under normal range conditions, whereas cattle are occasionally poisoned under sparse range conditions. Sheep dosed with 0.23 to 0.46 kg of plant material daily for 9 to 12 days developed cholestatic liver disease resulting in icterus and hepatogenous photosensitization. Subacute to chronic lecheguilla intoxication diagnosed in a herd of Angora goats reflected clear evidence of

liver disease.[5] The diagnosis is based on evidence of lecheguilla consumption, clinical signs and lesions of hepatogenous photosensitization, icterus, and clinicopathologic evidence of cholestatic liver disease. Treatment is supportive. Preventing exposure to sunlight, administration of antibiotics, and provision of supplemental feed will aid recovery in animals not in an advanced stage of liver failure.

Lantana was introduced into the United States from its tropical habitat as an ornamental and now has escaped cultivation throughout many of the southern states and California. Lantana poisoning has been reported in cattle, sheep, goats, and buffalo.[6] Intoxication results from a single rapid ingestion of a large quantity of lantana. About 1% to 2% of body weight of the green plant is sufficient to induce intoxication in cattle and sheep. After reaching the liver, lantana toxins enter hepatocytes and are metabolized to more polar compounds, then are secreted into the bile. Bile canalicular membranes are subsequently damaged resulting in intrahepatic cholestasis and secondary photosensitization. Within 2 hours of ingestion of lantana foliage by livestock, anorexia and gut stasis occur followed by depression and photosensitization in the next 24 to 48 hours. Other signs of lantana poisoning include icterus, anorexia, dehydration, and sometimes bloody diarrhea in acutely poisoned cattle. Severe intoxication terminates in death in a few days. Diagnosis is based on evidence of lantana consumption, clinical signs and lesions of hepatogenous photosensitization, clinicopathologic alterations in liver function, icterus, dehydration, and constipation. Preventing continued absorption of the lantana toxins and general supportive measures are effective treatments. Doses of oral electrolytes and activated charcoal on the order of 2.0 to 2.5 kg for cattle and 0.5 kg for sheep have proved effective under experimental conditions. Treated animals usually show signs of recovery within 2 days. Alternatively, a rumenotomy may be performed to remove plant material. Repopulation with normal flora enhances recovery as rumen microbes are severely depleted in a static rumen. Treat photosensitized animals as mentioned above.

BLUE-GREEN ALGAE

Microcystis aeruginosa is a blue-green (BG) alga capable of producing potent hepatotoxins called microcystins. Ponds and lakes often become enriched with the nutrients necessary to allow the luxuriant growth of these microscopic plants. In late summer or early fall dry conditions often result in sufficient evaporation to concentrate the necessary nitrogen and phosphorus. Runoff from heavily fertilized fields or feedlots is the usual source. Most blooms are not hazardous to livestock,[7] but when intracellular microcystins reach sufficient concentrations and the downwind side of a body of water accumulates the bloom, the results can be disastrous. Lethal doses induce massive hepatic necrosis, intrahepatic hemorrhage, and hypovolemic shock. Liver weight as a portion of body weight may increase 60% or more.[8] Surviving animals may develop secondary photosensitization with markedly elevated serum GGT activity. Diagnosis is based on the occurrence of a visible blue or green scum on or just under the surface of the water, compatible gross and histologic changes, and microscopic identification of the cells in water samples.

FORAGE-INDUCED LIVER DISEASE OF CATTLE

Normally, excellent harvested forages such as alfalfa or red clover grass hay are sporadically associated with severe liver disease in cattle.[9] Conditions associated with the disease include feeding of legume (e.g., alfalfa or red clover) grass hay for 1 to 4 weeks, heavy rainfall during growth of the hay, and delayed harvesting (first cutting delayed 30 to 60 days). Symptoms include photosensitization, weight loss, elevated liver enzymes (especially GGT) in serum, icterus, and death, in some cases 2 to 8 weeks after withdrawal of the hay. Histologic examination of affected livers reveals mild to severe periportal fibrosis, mild biliary hyperplasia, and bile accumulation. The unknown toxin remains stable in hay for years.

REFERENCES

1. Moslen MT: Toxic responses of the liver. *In* Klaassen CD, Amdur MO, Doull J (eds): Cassarett and Doull's Toxicology: The Basic Science of Poisons, ed 5. New York, McGraw-Hill, 1996, pp 403–416.
2. Blythe LL, Craig AM: Clinical and preclinical diagnostic aids to hepatic plant toxicosis in horses, sheep and cattle. *In* Colegate SM, Dorling PR (eds): Plant-Associated Toxins: Agricultural, Phytochemical and Ecological Aspects, Wallingford, UK, CAB International, 1994, pp 313–318.
3. Craig AM, Pearson EG, Meyer C, et al: Serum liver enzyme and histopathologic changes in calves with chronic and chronic-delayed *Senecio jacobaea* toxicosis. Am J Vet Res 52:1969, 1991.
4. Whitson TD: Control of poisonous plants in the Western United States. *In* Colegate SM, Dorling PR (eds): Plant-Associated Toxins: Agricultural, Phytochemical and Ecological Aspects. Wallingford, UK, CAB International, 1994, pp 468–472.
5. Burrows GE, Stair EL: Apparent *Agave lecheguilla* intoxication in Angora goats. Vet Hum Toxicol 32:259, 1990.
6. Sharma OP, Makkar HPS, Dawra RK: A review of the noxious plant *Lantana camara*. Toxicon 26:975, 1988.
7. Beasley VR, Cook WO, Dahlem AM, et al: Algae intoxication in livestock and waterfowl. Vet Clin North Am Food Anim Pract 5:345, 1989.
8. Beasley VR, Dahlem AM, Cook WO, et al: Diagnostic and clinically important aspects of cyanobacterial (blue-green algae) toxicoses. J Vet Diagn Invest 1:359, 1989.
9. Casteel SW, Rottinghaus GE, Johnson GC, et al: Liver disease in cattle induced by consumption of moldy hay. Vet Hum Toxicol 37:248, 1995.

■ Nitrate Poisoning Associated With the Consumption of Forages or Hay

John C. Haliburton, D.V.M., Ph.D., Diplomate, A.B.V.T.

Nitrate poisoning associated with the consumption of forages or hay is a commonly encountered problem throughout North America. Although all species of domestic livestock are potentially susceptible to nitrate poisoning, cattle, sheep, and goats are unquestionably the animals most frequently affected. Although nitrate poisoning associated with the consumption of forages or hay occurs throughout North America, some regionally unique features of the syndrome include (1) differences in the types of native flora found and the cultivated forage crops produced and utilized within the region (i.e., relative risk of exposure to nitrate-accumulating plants), (2) variations in the type and nature of the livestock industry within the region (i.e., cow vs. sheep vs. goat production, meat or dairy production, range or stocker production), and (3) variations in climatic conditions during the growing, grazing, harvesting, and feeding periods in both forage and hay and animal production systems.

The sporadic accumulation of nitrate within the plant is explained by basic plant nitrate physiology. Nitrogen, in the form

of nitrate (NO_3), is absorbed from the soil through the root system, translocated within the plant, and converted through a series of chemical reactions to ammonia. Then the ammonia is incorporated into amino acids and the amino acids are converted into plant protein. The initial reduction of nitrate to nitrite ($NO_3 \rightarrow NO_2$) is a critical reaction that is completely dependent upon the nitrate reductase enzyme system (NRS). When the NRS activity is depressed, the rate of nitrate-to-nitrite conversion is decreased. The rate of NRS activity is affected by several factors. Genetic predisposition is a major factor reflected in the wide range of NRS activity among plant species. The NRS requires sunlight activation to reach its maximum rate of activity. Therefore, nitrate tends to accumulate in plants during the night and during prolonged periods of cloudy, overcast daytime conditions. Under low nutrient availability or extended periods of inadequate moisture (drought), the NRS activity of sorghum, Sudan, and sorghum-sudan hybrid grasses is considerably less than that of most other grasses. Under these conditions nitrate uptake from the soil continues, but the rate of nitrate-to-nitrite conversion is reduced, which leads to an accumulation of nitrate in the plant.

The highest nitrate concentrations are found in the stalk of the plant, with the lowest concentrations in the leaves. Nitrate concentration decreases significantly in the stalk from the ground to the top of the plant (Fig. 1).

There have been numerous publications identifying both native and cultivated plants that are known potential nitrate accumulators, and the reader is referred to the Bibliography for a listing of these plants. *Sorghum* spp., carelessweed, and lamb's quarter are commonly known as nitrate accumulators.

Ruminants are highly susceptible to nitrate compared with

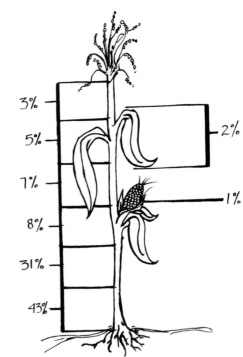

DISTRIBUTION OF NITRATE

3%
5%
7%
8%
31%
43%

2%
1%

PERCENT OF TOTAL NITRATE

Figure 1
Relative distribution of nitrate in a corn plant. Note that major portions of nitrate are in lower stems, with less in leaves and almost none in the seed.

monogastrics. When nitrate enters the rumen, it is rapidly converted to nitrite by the ruminal microflora; and then, through a series of reactions, nitrite is converted to ammonia and ultimately into protein by these organisms. When the amount of nitrate entering the rumen exceeds the microbial protein-assimilating capacity, poisoning may occur. The rumen microbes are capable of assimilating (i.e., detoxifying) an exceedingly high level of nitrate if they are acclimated by gradually increasing the nitrate exposure level.

Nitrate is converted to nitrite in the rumen and the nitrite is absorbed into the blood where it oxidizes the ferrous iron (Fe^{2+}) of hemoglobin to ferric iron (Fe^{3+}), thereby converting hemoglobin to methemoglobin. Methemoglobin is unable to transport oxygen. When 40% to 50% of the hemoglobin has been converted to methemoglobin, clinical signs develop, and when 80% to 90% has been converted to methemoglobin, death follows from anoxia. Antidotal therapy is directed toward converting the oxidized iron of methemoglobin back to the reduced iron of hemoglobin, thus restoring its oxygen-carrying capacity.

CLINICAL SIGNS

Owing to the rapidly lethal affects of nitrate, sudden death with no observed premonitory clinical signs is commonly associated with nitrate poisoning. When clinical signs are observed, they can occur within 30 minutes of feed consumption. Clinical signs characteristically begin with rapid breathing, restlessness, and apprehensive behavior. This may rapidly progress within minutes to dyspnea, weakness, ataxia, sternal recumbency, cyanosis, and terminal convulsions. Abortion due to fetal anoxia may follow in pregnant animals that have survived an acute episode of nitrate poisoning.

DIAGNOSIS

Although the clinical management histories may often allow a presumptive field diagnosis of nitrate poisoning, most cases require laboratory assistance in confirming the diagnosis and identifying the source of the nitrate. The preferred specimens for confirmational analysis may vary from laboratory to laboratory but will generally include one or more of the following: (1) an intact eye or the aspirated vitreous or aqueous fluid, (2) serum, (3) urine, and (4) samples of forage or hay.

TREATMENT

Because of the relatively short period of time between the onset of clinical signs and death, the veterinarian is seldom able to arrive on the scene in time to administer antidotal therapy. However, in those cases where therapy can be administered, a solution of 1% methylene blue in distilled water should be given intravenously at a dosage rate of 4 to 30 mg/kg body weight.

PREVENTION

The occurrence of nitrate poisoning associated with the consumption of forages or hay can be prevented by providing producers with the information and facts that will assist them in making sound feed utilization and animal management decisions. A typical nitrate poisoning scenario is the report of multiple acute deaths in stocker cattle soon after being given access to a large round bale of sorghum-Sudan hay during a bitter winter storm that has left a snow cover over any grazeable forages, thus causing the cattle to be without feed for 10 hours or more. Cattle under these conditions are highly susceptible to nitrate poisoning because they are (1) physiologically stressed by the inclement weather conditions (i.e., negative energy balance), (2) nutritionally stressed by the inability to graze due to the snow cover (i.e., hungry), and (3) unacclimated to high dietary nitrate intake. The most immediate concern is providing feed to the hungry and weather-stressed cattle. Feed-related management factors and factors that are generally not considered crop management factors are critical, yet subtle.

Forage/hay production–related factors involved in the prevention of nitrate poisoning must be addressed while the forage is still in the field approaching maturity. The producer should know that (1) plant nitrate concentration is in a continual state of change and can increase or decrease quickly as long as the plant is living and in a growing phase, and (2) forage should be sampled and the nitrate concentration determined immediately prior to the anticipated date of harvest. If preharvest analysis results indicate that the nitrate level is high, the producer may have the option of delaying the harvest and permitting the forage to continue to grow, thus allowing the nitrate level to potentially drop to a lower concentration. This is a viable option only if (1) the forage has not reached its maximum stage of maturity, and (2) favorable growing conditions exist. If the forage must be harvested, the producer may cut the hay at a greater height from the ground since the majority of the plant nitrate is in the lower stems (see Fig. 1). By increasing the height of the cut, more of the nitrate will be left in the field stubble, thereby reducing the nitrate concentration in the hay. Purchased forages or hay should be analyzed, preferably before the purchase but certainly before feeding. This will allow the maximum nitrate intake to be calculated and evaluated for the potential of causing nitrate poisoning. Under most circumstances, a level of 1.0% or less nitrate on a dry matter basis is within safe and acceptable limits for livestock consumption if animals are properly adapted to the forage. Under stress conditions, as described here, a maximum of 0.6% is recommended for dry, free-access hay.

As previously stated, feeding management decisions during the actual time of stress are equally as important as feed management. Hungry, stressed cattle will consume hay at a considerably faster rate than nonstressed cattle. Therefore, under stress conditions they should not be given free access to a potentially toxic nitrate-containing hay. Instead, a hay containing a low and safe level of nitrate should be provided to reduce appetite and produce a partial rumen fill. Hay containing a higher nitrate concentration can then be provided to complete the daily feed requirement with substantially less risk of nitrate poisoning. If hay containing a high nitrate concentration is fed daily in small but gradually increasing amounts, the animals can become acclimated to eating hay with a surprisingly high nitrate concentration without adverse affects. In addition to these strategies, a grain or some other high-energy carbohydrate supplement can be provided which will facilitate rumen microbial detoxification of nitrate and reduce the potential of nitrate poisoning.

A commercial product now available is a direct-fed or orally dosed rumen inoculum that contains propionibacteria. Propionibacteria are highly efficient at metabolizing nitrate, and once established in the rumen, they readily detoxify nitrate and reduce the potential of nitrate poisoning. This product, when used in conjunction with other preventive management strategies, may offer the producer, especially dairy operators, a greater latitude in their selection and utilization programs for forages and hay.

BIBLIOGRAPHY

Kingsbury JM: Poisonous Plants of the United States and Canada. Englewood Cliffs, NJ, Prentice-Hall, 1964, pp 42–43.

Osweiler GD, Carson TL, Buck WB, et al (eds): Clinical and Diagnostic Veterinary Toxicology, ed 3. Dubuque, Iowa, Kendall Hunt, 1985, pp 460–467.

■ Toxic Syndromes Associated With Sulfur

Merl F. Raisbeck, D.V.M., Ph.D., Diplomate, A.B.V.T.

Milton M. McAllister, D.V.M., Ph.D., Diplomate, A.C.V.P.

Daniel H. Gould, D.V.M., Ph.D., Diplomate, A.C.V.P.

Sulfur (S) is an essential element which exemplifies the dictum "Dose makes the poison." Essential for a variety of physiologic functions, it is extremely hazardous in excess. Common sources in animal production include sulfur-containing amino acids, notably cysteine and methionine, elemental sulfur ("flowers of sulfur"), or inorganic salts of sulfur oxides such as sodium sulfate (Na_2SO_4). Reduced forms of sulfur (sulfide, S^{-2}) are usually associated with insoluble pyritic ores in the environment and thus unavailable for ingestion. Hydrogen sulfide gas (H_2S), a highly toxic byproduct of septic systems and of oil and gas production, is an exception. Flowers of sulfur are still used as a folk remedy for parasites in many parts of North America. "Alkali" waters (heavily contaminated with sulfate salts) are a common problem in arid portions of the West and were documented to kill cattle as early as 1856.[1] Sulfate salts have been used to limit intake in self-feeding rations for cattle[2] and as urinary acidifiers. Pastured animals may be exposed to spills where elemental sulfur is used as a soil amendment. Many common feed ingredients such as sugar beet pulp and corn byproducts are rich in sulfur.

DIETARY SULFUR

Ingestion of elemental sulfur,[3] oxidized sulfur compounds,[4,5] or cruciferous crops such as turnips results in gastrointestinal H_2S production in ruminants and possibly in horses.[6] Depending upon the dose and other, as yet ill-defined dietary factors, sufficient H_2S may be produced to result in acute intoxication. There is disagreement as to whether gastrointestinal H_2S must first be eructated and then inhaled or whether sufficient H_2S is absorbed directly from the gastrointestinal tract to result in intoxication. Regardless of route, sufficient H_2S may be absorbed to cause peracute death. Animals which survive a few hours or days will exhibit some combination of incoordination, abdominal pain, blindness, cyanosis, and dyspnea. There may be convulsions before they become comatose and die.

If insufficient H_2S is produced to cause acute death, continued absorption may result in polioencephalomalacia (PEM) in ruminants.[2,4,5] Clinically, this condition is indistinguishable from cortical necrosis due to lead poisoning or thiamine deficiency. Sulfur-induced PEM may occur in animals which previously survived acute intoxication, or may occur in previously asymptomatic animals after 2 to 30 days on high sulfur diets.[2,3]

DIAGNOSIS

Sulfur intoxication is diagnosed on the basis of characteristic signs and lesions, a history of exposure to high dietary sulfur, normal blood thiamine, and elevated rumen sulfide concentrations. Animals which die peracutely may exhibit nothing on postmortem examination. Ruminants that die during the first 24 to 48 hours after exposure will exhibit pulmonary congestion and edema, inflammation of the upper gastrointestinal tract, ruminal hemorrhage, and the distinctive odor of H_2S in rumen contents. Since H_2S is volatile, the odor may not be apparent in samples that are not fresh. Samples for sulfide analysis may be preserved by adding 1 volume of 5% aqueous zinc acetate per volume of sample. The ruminal mucosa of animals receiving mineral supplements may be blackened as a result of metal sulfide deposits. Hepatic necrosis and hemorrhage have been reported. Later, gross lesions suggestive of PEM predominate. Cerebral swelling, if present, is indicated by flattened cortical gyri and by coning of the cerebellum as it is displaced into the foramen magnum. Laminar necrosis may be grossly evident in the cortical gray matter. These necrotic areas fluoresce under long-wave ultraviolet light. Conversely, damage may be insufficient to visualize grossly and will require histopathologic diagnosis.

Tissue sulfide analysis, while theoretically desirable, is not a reliable diagnostic tool at this time. Recently, the Drager method of atmospheric sulfide analysis has been adapted to monitor ruminal gas cap H_2S concentration.[7] Concentrations greater than 2000 ppm suggest a risk of PEM. While this method is potentially very useful, results should be interpreted with caution. At present the method is very new and suggested "diagnostic" concentrations may be revised as more experience is gained with the technique. Secondly, rumen H_2S production and loss is a dynamic process. Samples examined post mortem or after anorexia lowers dietary sulfur intake may not accurately reflect earlier peaks.

It is important that all dietary components (including water) be analyzed for sulfur and the cumulative contribution of each calculated. For example, a steer drinking 23 L of water containing 2500 ppm sulfate and eating 8 kg of hay containing 1000 ppm of sulfur ingests 27 g of sulfur (19 g from water and 8 g from hay) or about 0.34% total dietary sulfur. While it seems reasonable that various sulfur compounds contribute differently to overall gastrointestinal H_2S production, there is at present insufficient knowledge to utilize this information diagnostically. Thus, we recommend dietary analysis for total sulfur rather than specific forms such as sulfides, sulfates, etc. Total dietary sulfur greater than 0.4% is potentially hazardous to ruminants, but some individuals may tolerate more under certain circumstances.

PREVENTION

There are no practical therapies for respiratory H_2S intoxication beyond artificial ventilation, oxygen therapy, and supportive care. The first step in treating dietary sulfur intoxication is to identify and eliminate the sulfur source. In one report, survival of ewes poisoned by excess dietary sulfur was markedly improved by atropine therapy, although "no reasonable explanation" for this observation could be ascertained.[3] Sulfur-induced PEM is poorly responsive or nonresponsive to parenteral thiamine. Switching to an all-roughage diet improves survival if initiated before brain damage becomes too extensive. Oral iron administration was recommended, presumably to precipitate sulfide as insoluble iron sulfide,[8] but no evidence was provided as to the efficacy of such therapy.

Prevention of dietary sulfur intoxication consists primarily of avoiding excess dietary sulfur. If this is impossible, encouraging adaptation by gradually introducing new diets (including water) over 2 to 3 weeks seems to minimize losses. Supplemental dietary thiamine supplementation was not useful and actually increased the incidence of PEM associated with gypsum-based self-limiting rations (M.F. Raisbeck, unpublished observation). Low rumen pH increases sulfide production; thus animals on high-concentrate diets are more prone to intoxication than those on roughage diets. It was suggested that 50 ppm copper supplementation would tie up sulfide as metal sulfides in the gut and spare thiamine.[9] In our experience, precipitation strategies have not been very successful for either treatment or prevention.

REFERENCES

1. Burton RF: The city of the saints and across the Rocky Mountains to California. London, Longman, Green, Longman, & Roberts, 1861, pp 182–183.
2. Raisbeck MF: Is polioencephalomalacia associated with high sulfate diets? J Am Vet Med Assoc 180:1303, 1982.
3. Bulgin MS, Lincoln SD, Mather G: Elemental sulfur toxicosis in a flock of sheep. J Am Vet Med Assoc 208:1063, 1996.
4. Gould DH, McAllister MM, Savage JC, et al: High sulfide concentrations in rumen fluid associated with nutritionally induced polioencephalomalacia in calves. Am J Vet Res 52:1164, 1991.
5. McAllister MM, Gould DH, Hamar DW: Sulphide-induced polioencephalomalacia in lambs. Comp Pathol 106:267, 1992.
6. Corke MJ: An outbreak of sulphur poisoning in horses. Vet Rec 109:212, 1981.
7. Gould DH, Cummings BA, Hamar DW: In vivo indicators of pathologic ruminal sulfide production in steers with diet-induced polioencephalomalacia. J Vet Diagn Invest (in press).
8. Kandylis K: Toxicology of sulfur in ruminants. J Dairy Sci 67:2179, 1984.
9. Olkowski AA, Gooneratne SR, Rousseaux CG, et al: Role of thiamine status in sulphur induced polioencephalomalacia in sheep. Res Vet Sci 52:78, 1992

BIBLIOGRAPHY

Beke GJ, Hironaka R: Toxicity to beef cattle of sulfur in saline well water: A case study. Sci Total Environ 101:281, 1991.
Hamlen H, Clark E, Janzen E: Polioencephalomalacia in cattle consuming water with elevated sodium sulfate levels: A herd investigation. Can Vet J 34:153, 1993.

▪ Pyrrolizidine Alkaloid Toxicosis

Bryan L. Stegelmeier, D.V.M., Ph.D., Diplomate, A.C.V.P.

On a worldwide basis, the hepatotoxic plants containing pyrrolizidine alkaloids (PAs) are the most common poisonous plants and cause the greatest economic losses to the livestock industry. There are both native and introduced PA-containing plants in North America that have been reported to poison livestock and humans (Table 1). Many are invasive, noxious weeds that can infest open ranges and fields. Most are not palatable and livestock generally avoid eating them if there are other forages available. However, as these noxious weeds invade fields, they are often included in prepared feeds and grains which are then readily eaten by most animals. As a result, many poisonings occur as a result of contaminated feed. Human poisonings most often are a result of food contamination (often grain contamination) or when PA-containing plants are used for medicinal purposes.[1, 2]

Pyrrolizidine alkaloids are not directly toxic, but are metabolized into toxic pyrroles by the liver mono-oxygenase systems. These reactive pyrroles form adducts with numerous proteins and nucleic acids. PA bioactivation can be promoted or inhibited by treatments that alter hepatic microsomal activity (e.g., phenobarbital, chloramphenicol, SKF 525) depending on the alkaloid and the species. Less toxic metabolites are also formed in the liver as some of the PAs are oxidized to the N-oxide or hydrolysis of the ester side chain(s) (Fig. 1). Toxicity of the PA appears to be dependent on unsaturation within the necine base ring

and a branch, possibly with unsaturation in the ester side chain, as this promotes pyrrole formation. Alkaloids with a monocyclic diester side chain and sites of unsaturation are the most toxic.

Animal factors such as species, age, sex, and nutritional status also influence PA toxicity. Different animal species have vastly different susceptibilities to PA toxicity. Horses and cattle are very susceptible to PA intoxication and are the most commonly clinically poisoned animals. Sheep and goats are more resistant and they may safely graze PA plants in some situations. Species susceptibility has been speculated to be a result of differences in rumen PA metabolism, hepatic PA activation, or other factors influencing absorption and excretion. Age also plays a large role in determining response to PAs. Young animals are generally more susceptible to poisoning than aged adults. Neonatal and nursing animals have been reported to develop fatal hepatic disease while their lactating mothers were unaffected. Gender also plays a role as male rats are more susceptible to poisoning than females. This change has been directly linked to differences in hepatic PA metabolism. Many plant factors also contribute to toxicity. PA concentrations in plants vary with season, environment, plant phenotype, and site. As a rule, the plants are most toxic when beginning to flower; however, there are large variations in PA concentrations from year to year and from site to site. For example, the total alkaloid content in *Senecio riddellii* can vary from 0.2% to 18% of the plant dry weight. This makes it difficult to determine when a particular group of plants contains enough PA to be toxic. More work is needed to definitively determine the cause of these differences and to better detect or predict PA concentrations in plant populations. Cur-

Table 1
TOXIC PYRROLIZIDINE ALKALOID (PA)–CONTAINING PLANTS

Senecio spp. (family Compositae)	
S. jacobaea	Tansy ragwort
S. vulgaris	Common groundsel
S. riddellii	Riddell's groundsel
S. douglasii var. longilobus	Threadleaf or wooly groundsel
S. spartioides	Broom groundsel
S. integerrimus	Lamb's tongue groundsel
Other toxic *Senecio* spp.: S. pauperculus, S. confusus, S. plattensis, S. lobatus, S. ilicifolius, S. erraticus, S. burchellii, S. glabellus, S. cineraria, S. brasiliensis, S. alpinus, S. madagascariensis, S. lautus	
Crotalaria spp. (family Leguminosae)	
C. retusa	Crotalaria
C. spectabilis	Rattle pod, showy crotalaria
C. sagittalis	Arrow crotalaria, wild pea, rattlebox
(other toxic *Crotalaria* spp.: C. mucronata, C. incana, C. rotundifolia, C. burkeana, C. juncea, C. dura, C. equorum, C. globifera)	
Other PA-containing plants in the Boraginaceae family	
Cynoglossum officinale	Hound's tongue
Amsinckia intermedia	Tarweed, fireweed, fiddlenecks
Borago officinalis	Borage
Echium lycopsis (*E. plantagineum*)	Echium, Paterson's curse
Echium vulgare	Echium
Symphytum officinale	Comfrey
Heliotropium europaeum	Heliotrope

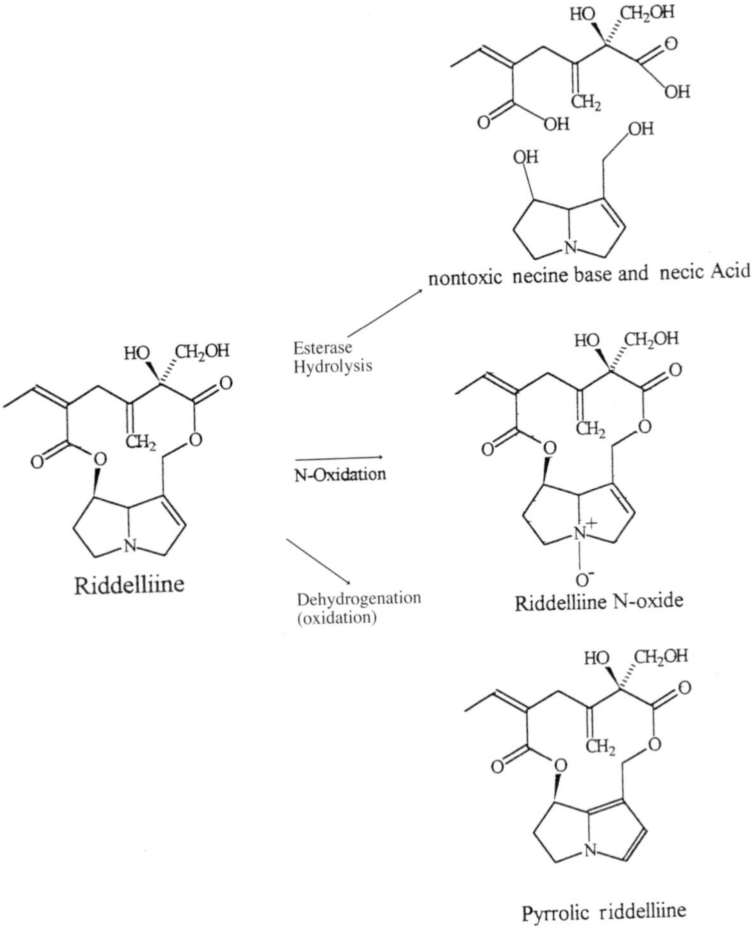

nontoxic necine base and necic Acid

Esterase
Hydrolysis

N-Oxidation

Dehydrogenation
(oxidation)

Riddelliine

Riddelliine N-oxide

Pyrrolic riddelliine

Figure 1
Structure and metabolism of pyrrolizidine alkaloids. Hydrolysis products and the N-oxides are generally considered nontoxic metabolites. The dehydrogenated pyrroles are toxic and quickly form adducts with proteins and nucleic acids.

rent recommendations are that one should recognize potentially toxic plants, know the susceptible species, and take necessary precautions to ensure that such animals are not exposed.[1]

As toxic pyrroles are principally generated in hepatocytes, most damage occurs in the liver. The clinical signs and progression of poisonings are dependent on dose. High doses result in extensive hepatocellular damage characterized by necrosis and hemorrhage. These animals show signs of acute liver failure such as anorexia, depression, icterus, visceral edema, and ascites. Many of these animals develop ulcerative gastrointestinal lesions, and rectal prolapse is common. Such cases are often diagnostic challenges as similar changes can be caused by a variety of other toxic, viral, and immunologic diseases. Fortunately, these cases have comparatively high concentrations of tissue-bound pyrroles that can be extracted and detected chemically. Lower PA doses result in less severe lesions that include focal hepatocyte necrosis (piecemeal necrosis), peribiliary fibrosis, and bile duct proliferation. With time, damaged hepatocytes develop into megalocytes. Animals poisoned at these levels often show no clinical signs and their serum biochemistries may be normal. The disease may progress resulting in cirrhosis and liver failure. These animals may present with clinical signs of photosensitivity, icterus, or increased susceptibility to other hepatic diseases such as lipidosis or ketosis. These animals generally have low levels of tissue-bound pyrroles making it difficult to confirm intoxication using chemical detection techniques. Some animals exposed to low PA levels may never develop liver disease. There is much evidence that low, chronic PA exposures have cumulative effects, but little is known of what dose or duration of exposure can be toxic, or if such subclinically intoxicated animals have impaired growth or productivity. More work is needed to better define these parameters, to identify markers

to predict how animals will progress after exposure, and to determine the fate and possible clearance of tissue-bound pyrroles in animals that recover. Although various treatments and diet supplements have been suggested, none have proved to be effective in livestock. Generally, poisoned animals that show clinical signs rarely recover. Subclinically poisoned animals are often hepatic cripples that are likely to perform poorly and be less efficient than normal animals.

As many signs of poisoning do not develop until months after exposure, it is often difficult to document exposure to PA-containing plants. Most diagnoses are made using histologic changes alone. As many of the histologic lesions of poisoning (liver necrosis, fibrosis, and biliary proliferation) are nonspecific and can be initiated by a variety of other toxic and infectious agents, PA intoxication may often be misdiagnosed. Chemical methods using spectrophotometry and gas chromatography and mass spectrometry can be used to detect tissue-bound pyrroles (PA metabolites).[3] These techniques are often inconclusive as they lack quantification and sensitivity. More sensitive diagnostic methods, including immunodiagnostics, are needed to definitively diagnose chronic, low-dose PA intoxication.

REFERENCES

1. Mattocks AR: Chemistry and Toxicology of Pyrrolizidine Alkaloids. Orlando, Fla, Academic Press, 1986.
2. Cheeke PR: Toxicity and metabolism of pyrrolizidine alkaloids. J Anim Sci 66:2343–2350, 1988.
3. Mattocks AR, Jukes R: Recovery of the pyrrolic nucleus of pyrrolizidine alkaloid metabolites from sulphur conjugates in tissues and body fluids. Chem Biol Interact 75:225–239, 1990.

Viral Diseases

Consulting Editor

James England, D.V.M., Ph.D.

■ Infectious Bovine Rhinotracheitis and Other Clinical Syndromes Caused by Bovine Herpesvirus Types 1 and 5

Fernando A. Osorio, M.V., Ph.D., M.S., Diplomate, A.C.V.M.

Bovine herpesvirus type 1 (BHV-1) was first recognized in the United States as an acute, febrile, highly contagious respiratory infection of cattle. This virus causes several different clinical syndromes, for example, rhinotracheitis and predisposition to bacterial bronchopneumonia, conjunctivitis, drop in milk production, abortion and lesions of the genital tract, and encephalitis. At least two different biotypes of BHV-1 are involved in the respiratory and eye form and in the genital form. The strains involved in most of the epizootic cases of encephalitis are considered to represent a type of bovine herpesvirus different from BHV-1.

ETIOLOGY

The upper respiratory tract form of BHV-1 infection is called infectious bovine rhinotracheitis (IBR) (also necrotic rhinitis or red nose). Because the virus also causes genital infections (infectious pustular vulvovaginitis [IPV] in the female and infectious pustular balanoposthitis in the male), BHV-1 has been also referred to as IBR-IPV. A third configuration of BHV-1 infection is the encephalitic form that typically affect younger calves. Virologic and antigenic studies indicate that an extensive degree of identity exists among the BHV-1 isolates recovered from these three distinct clinical forms. However, the use of restriction endonuclease analysis of the DNA genome (fingerprinting), shows that these isolates can be grouped in three different clusters. Thus three different BHV-1 biotypes were recognized: BHV-1.1 (the denomination for the IBR-related isolates), BHV-1.2 (for the IPV-related isolates), and BHV-1.3 (for the encephalitis isolates). Furthermore, more refined studies indicated that the polypeptide makeup and genetic sequence of the encephalitic isolates diverge significantly from those of the BHV-1.1 and BHV-1.2 isolates. Thus the encephalitic group of bovine herpesvirus isolates has been recently proposed as representative of bovine herpesvirus type 5 (BHV-5), a new type of bovine herpesvirus.

As is common to all herpesviruses, BHV-1 is sensitive to lipid solvents, heat, and acid, but persists for several days at 4°C and remains viable for years when it is frozen. The virus grows readily in different cell lines, while the only laboratory animal susceptible to BHV-1 or BHV-5 is the rabbit.

EPIZOOTIOLOGY

The differences in tropism observed between the BHV-1.1 and BHV-1.2 subtypes are probably determined by differences in cattle production systems and animal densities. In areas where there is a high concentration of cattle (i.e., a feedlot), the most important mode of transmission of BHV-1 is airborne and the most evident disease involves the respiratory tract. The respiratory infections are believed to be responsible for the spread of BHV-1 throughout all animals in a herd. In areas of lower cattle density, instead, venereal transmission becomes more evident, with concomitant genital disease but more restricted spread of the infection. While the respiratory forms of BHV-1 infections are common in North American feedlots, the genital forms of BHV-1 infection are frequent in European dairy and beef farms. The encephalitic forms caused by BHV-5 seem to be a consistent problem in certain areas of the world (e.g., Australia and South America), while very sporadic in others (North America and Europe). The increased incidence of encephalitic forms of BHV-5 infection in certain countries may respond to the absence in those countries of routine vaccination programs against BHV-1, which would otherwise mask the clinical expression of the infection by BHV-5. This cross-protection is due to the antigenic cross-reactivity between BHV-1 and BHV-5, which is fairly extensive.

The biology of infections caused by BHV-1 can be described as an interplay between acute forms of infection followed by establishment of latency in convalescent animals which then become carriers of the infection.[1] The acute phase of infection is characterized by evident clinical symptoms, abundant excretion of high titers of infectious virus, and frank spread of infection to naive animals. During that period extensive BHV-1 replication at the level of mucous membranes (the "portals of entry," i.e., the upper respiratory tract or genital mucosa) takes place. From there the BHV-1 can proceed, via peripheral nerve endings innervating the area, to those tissue sites where latency is established, mostly the neurons of the sensory ganglia, which are the trigeminal and sacral ganglia. The quiescent, latent BHV-1 may be reactivated in response to different stimuli (calving, stress, superinfections with other agents, treatments with dexamethasone and adrenocorticotropic hormone, etc.) and at different frequencies throughout the life of this carrier animal. The reactivated BHV-1 will travel back to the peripheral sites or portals of entry, where it can then be reexcreted and produce primary infection in susceptible contact animals. New outbreaks in feedlots and closed herds may result from excretion of virus from a latent carrier.

CLINICAL FORMS AND SIGNS

The infections caused by BHV-1 and related viruses are manifested in a variety of clinical presentations which can be grouped as (1) respiratory tract infections, (2) conjunctivitis, (3) genital tract infections and abortions, (4) central nervous system infections, and (5) fatal generalized disease of neonatal calves.[1]

Respiratory Tract Infections

This is the most common form of the disease in intensive production units and it was the first form of the disease to be recognized in the United States. The IBR may range from subclinical to very severe disease, with morbidity often approaching 100% and mortality as high as 10% in complicated cases. The respiratory illness has a sudden onset and the common initial symptoms include fever (40 to 41.5°C), salivation, rhinitis, conjunctivitis, loss of appetite, and dyspnea. The nasal mucosa is distinctly hyperemic, with abundant nasal discharge, initially serous and then mucopurulent. Lesions in the nasal path evolve from necrotic focal lesions to large, consolidated, frankly hemorrhagic areas that develop into diphtheric membranes. The breath of these animals is distinctly foul. In cases of advanced respiratory distress, the airways become blocked and the animals suffer respiratory distress with open-mouth breathing. If the case does not resolve promptly (5 to 10 days), the most common complication is secondary bacterial bronchopneumonia, with audible rales and coughing. The bacterial bronchopneumonia is generally the cause of death in these complicated cases.

Conjunctivitis

BHV-1-induced conjunctivitis may appear as a symptom associated with the respiratory form of the infection, but it can also be the principal or only symptom present. In those cases it is not uncommon that the infection is confused with pinkeye (infectious keratitis caused by *Moraxella bovis*). In addition, many times conjunctivitis is the main symptom that may precede, in 1 or 2 months, the abortion storms caused by BHV-1. Characteristics of BHV-1 conjunctivitis are the inflammation and edematous condition of the conjunctiva, which generally is bilateral. The discharge is initially clear but becomes mucopurulent upon bacterial involvement. Corneal opacities are not uncommon. These corneal opacities, in contrast with the lesions of pinkeye (which appear in the center of the cornea and spread centrifugally), are few and tend to originate in the corneoscleral line.

Genital Tract Infections and Abortions

The genital disease called coital exanthema has been known in Europe since the past century. The disease is most commonly associated with dairy cows and follows a typical venereal transmission. Two to three days after coitus, the animals may develop different degrees of fever, depression, anorexia, and frequent and painful micturition. In some cases the development of symptoms is not clearly associated with coitus. The vulva is distinctly edematous and hyperemic, with development of the typical herpetic pustules which coalesce into necrotic plaques and ulcers. The exudate, mucopurulent in character, is profuse. The condition resolves typically in 2 weeks, but other cases may become chronic. Similar mucosal lesions may develop on the mucosa of the penis and prepuce of bulls (infectious balanoposthitis).

These lesions are the source of infectious BHV-1 that contaminates the semen.

Under field conditions, abortions may occur in up to 25% of pregnant cows. While most cases of BHV-1 abortions involve expulsion of the fetus around the last third of gestation, the interval between infection and abortion can range from 7 days to several months, with expulsion of fetuses simultaneous with clinical signs of infection in the herd or as long as 100 days later. As is usually the case, the fetuses decompose easily and are not suitable for diagnostic work. When access to fresh fetal material is possible, intranuclear inclusion bodies are easily seen in tissues such as liver and adrenals. The stomach of aborted fetuses may present focal necrotic lesions.

Central Nervous System Infections

The existence of "variant strains of BHV-1" that for unknown reasons would invade the central nervous system of young animals was suspected by clinicians for a long time. The recently classified BHV-5 has been isolated from brains of fatal cases of nonpurulent meningoencephalitis in young calves of both dairy and beef cattle. The affected animals stay off feed and exhibit periods of excitement: incoordination, running, circling, and stumbling, followed by depression, recumbency, coma, and eventually death. It is important to note that, in addition to the frankly encephalitogenic BHV-5 isolates, some cases of encephalitis have been associated with infections with typical BHV-1. Latency of BHV-5 has also been demonstrated in animals that survived the acute phase of encephalitic forms of infection, as shown by experimental treatment with dexamethasone.

Generalized Disease in Neonatal Calves

This form is the consequence of BHV-1 infection in neonatal calves infected in utero during late gestation or shortly after birth. This severe, often fatal, form of infection is characterized by high temperature, anorexia, depression, and respiratory distress. Ocular discharge and diarrhea may be present. Necrotic ulcerative lesions may extend throughout the upper digestive tract. This generalized disease condition is simultaneous with or consecutive to abortion storms in the herd.

DIAGNOSIS

The clinical diagnosis of BHV-1 infection is based mainly on typical clinical signs and lesions in the upper respiratory tract and on the epizootiologic characteristics of the outbreak. Generally, IBR is suspected in cases of sudden outbreak of an upper respiratory infection and in cases of vaginitis and abortions. Characteristic gross lesions are the white plaques on the mucosal surface of the nasal cavity and vagina. At necropsy, inflammation of the trachea with a fibropurulent exudate loosely attached to the mucosal surface is characteristic of this disease.

A definitive diagnosis can only be obtained by laboratory procedures. BHV-1 is readily isolated in cell cultures from several infected tissues. Clinical specimens should be collected during the febrile, acute, phase of infection. The type of specimen to collect is determined by the form of disease. For ocular and respiratory forms of the disease, swabs containing ocular and nasal secretions are used. Vaginal and preputial swabs are the specimens of choice for diagnosing genital infections. Samples of several parts of brain (olfactory lobes, midbrain, cortex, etc.) are used to isolate BHV-5 from the encephalitic forms of BHV infection.

The rapid detection of BHV-1 has been traditionally approached by immunofluorescence. Tissue of aborted fetuses and neonatal calves that died from generalized infection, such as liver, spleen, kidney, lung, and adrenal glands, are the preferred sites. Histopathologic examination combined with immunohistochemistry (based on the use of BHV-1-specific monoclonal or polyclonal antibodies) has grown in popularity in recent years, due mostly to the powerful advantage of achieving a histopathologic diagnosis coupled with an etiologic confirmation. Histopathologic examination of the fetal liver often reveals intranuclear inclusion bodies in epithelial cells surrounding areas of necrosis.

The central nervous system infections caused by BHV-5 must be differentiated from lead poisoning and other infectious diseases such as listeriosis, pseudorabies, rabies, and *Haemophilus somnus* septicemia.

Traditionally, serum neutralization (SN) has been the most commonly used serologic assay to measure BHV-specific antibodies in serum. This procedure has the intrinsic requirement of testing paired serum samples. The first sample should be obtained during the acute stage of illness, and the second sample is taken 2 to 3 weeks later. An alternative to this requirement is the use of antibody capture enzyme-linked immunosorbent assays (ELISAs) for the detection of BHV-1-specific IgM, an indicator of acute infection by this virus. Because of the early appearance of the BHV-1 IgM after infection, which is simultaneous with the occurrence of acute clinical symptoms, this assay provides a way to accomplish serologic diagnosis of an acute BHV-1 infection using a single (acute) serum sample. Otherwise, serologic (SN or ELISA) titers on single serum specimens are of no diagnostic significance, except in those cases in which the complete absence of specific antibodies indicates that an (unvaccinated) animal is not a latent carrier of BHV-1. As is true for other herpesviruses, positive serologic status (in an animal that has not been exposed to vaccine) is a permanent indicator of latent infection. The recent advent of differential vaccines and diagnostic tests should now permit detection of latent carriers even in herds that have received BHV-1 vaccination.

While many BHV-1 ELISAs have been developed and applied on an experimental basis, no commercial or official kits of this test are available in the United States. However, a differential ELISA specific for BHV-1 glycoprotein E (gE) antibodies has been licensed in Europe, where steps for control and eradication of BVH-1 by application of differential BHV-1 vaccines are well advanced.[2]

The development of nucleic acid–based diagnostic tests for BHV-1 or -5, especially polymerase chain reaction (PCR) assays, has increased significantly the speed and sensitivity of BHV diagnosis. Particularly important has been the application of PCR to the detection of BHV-1 in semen, as well as the use of PCR to quantitate latent BHV-1, which now allows measurement of the effect of vaccination on the level of latency established by this virus.[3] The different subtypes, as well as single strains of BHV-1, can be identified by restriction endonuclease analysis of their DNA (fingerprinting).

TREATMENT

The infection of the upper respiratory tract by BHV-1 increases the colonization of the lower lung with bacterial pathogens, leading to the development of severe bronchopneumonia. The BHV-1 infection has a direct effect on the respiratory epithelium and, in addition, decreases alveolar macrophage function, which plays a central role in the establishment of effective lung defenses. While BHV-1 is the main triggering factor for these secondary bacterial complications, no specific anti-BHV-1 therapy has yet been described which could be of

use in clinical practice as a specific antiviral treatment for these infections. BHV-1 is perhaps the virus of cattle that has undergone the greatest number of experimental antiviral treatments. The list of drugs tested in the literature (with different levels of success) range from empirically identified phytotherapeutic agents to more complex clinical combinations of cytokines or immunomodulators. In spite of that, however, the most appropriate therapy against BHV-1 infection continues to be that which is directed to treat and control the secondary bacterial complications: early administration of antibiotics with supportive therapy. Management should be directed to minimize stress, isolate sick animals, and provide shelter, food, and water. The administration of corticosteroids is contraindicated in cases of bacterial bronchopneumonia, as these drugs will reactivate latent BHV-1 in cattle.

PREVENTION AND CONTROL

As is true for other herpesviruses that affect domestic livestock, such as pseudorabies virus vaccines have played a major role in the prevention and control of clinical BHV-1 disease. Management of clean herds without the use of vaccination requires extreme care in supervising the introduction of new animals into the herd and rigorous monitoring of the serologic status of the herd to prevent outbreaks. In addition, the establishment of latency contributes significantly to the difficulty of preventing the introduction of BHV-1 into clean herds. Biosafety is then a very important concept that applies both to the prevention of the introduction of BHV-1 into a herd or to the prevention of its dissemination, once the virus infection is established in the herd. In that respect, isolation of severely affected cattle tends to minimize contagion within the herd.

Several types of vaccines have been used worldwide since the characterization of BHV-1 as an etiologic agent.[2] In general, attenuated, modified live vaccines (MLVs) have been recognized to be superior to the inactivated, nonreplicating ones. These, called killed virus vaccines, are made with nonattenuated virus that is inactivated by chemical methods and combined with an adjuvant. The inactivated vaccines are not as immunogenic as, but are safer than, MLVs. Parenteral MLVs are not recommended for use in pregnant animals, while those MLVs licensed for intranasal delivery (i.e., temperature-sensitive mutants) are considered to be safe for use in pregnant animals. However, the parenteral vaccines have gained greater acceptance because they are easier to deliver than the intranasal types. Parenteral vaccines are commonly used in combination with other vaccines. Vaccination schedules vary according to the type of production and the practitioner's experience. In general, calves should be initially immunized with parenteral vaccines at 6 months of age, but they can be immunized as early as 2 to 4 weeks of age when using the intranasal vaccine. Boosters are generally recommended at 6 months and before breeding (heifers) or before entering the feedlot. A preconditioning program may typically require that feeder calves be vaccinated at weaning and at least 1 month before shipping. Annual vaccinations of adults are recommended because the time of protection conferred by the BHV-1 vaccines is accepted as being 1 year. Colostral-derived antibodies may last up to 5 months and they do interfere with vaccination.

In recent years, the need to harmonize the use of vaccination with the serologic diagnosis of BHV-1 infection has led to a renewed impetus for the development of "new-generation" BHV-1 vaccines.[2] Prior experience with pseudorabies virus vaccination programs has amply demonstrated the validity of the concept of differential vaccines, which are those vaccines that permit making a serologic distinction between vaccinated and naturally infected animals. There are currently licensed BHV-1 differential vaccines in Europe and the United States. These vaccines, of the MLV type for the most part (with one exception of gE-negative killed vaccine licensed in Europe), have been selected by classic methods or designed by genetic engineering.[2, 4] These vaccines carry a deletion in at least one gene that codes for the serologic marker antigen. BHV-1 vaccines with deletions of the gIII(IgC) or the gE glycoproteins have been licensed. In addition, a diagnostic companion test specific for gE antibodies has also been licensed in Europe (Idexx Co, Portland, Maine). Simultaneously with these releases, significant efforts are being made to develop new nonreplicating vaccines that are composed of a single immunogenic protein or "subunit," which is produced by different strategies of genetic engineering. The use of BHV-1 gIV(gD) and also gI(gB) glycoproteins as immunogenic subunits has been reported in the literature.[4] These subunit vaccines can be combined with differential diagnostic tests specific for glycoproteins other than the one used in the vaccine (i.e., with the gE ELISA). An apparent advantage of this type of differential vaccine is the higher safety of these products over that of the attenuated strains. One important aspect that remains to be solved for the market implementation of subunit vaccines is their cost-efficiency ratio, which seems to be significantly high. Such circumstances lead, in the case of pseudorabies, to abandoning the concept of subunit vaccines as a tool in the PRV eradication campaign, which is being accomplished based exclusively on the use of differential attenuated vaccines. An additional feature of the use of BHV-1 differential attenuated vaccine strains is that they can be used as vectors on which other viral antigens (such as bovine viral diarrhea virus or bovine respiratory syncytial virus glycoproteins) can be cloned, thus permitting simultaneous vaccinations against multiple antigens.

Although there are no reports of vaccines made exclusively with strains of BHV-5, it is fairly well accepted that, because of the extensive antigenic cross-reactivity between BHV-1 and BHV-5, the vaccines available for BHV-1 should be efficacious in protecting against BHV-5.

Currently, a number of countries, especially within the European Economic Community, are committed to eradication programs for BHV-1. Denmark and Switzerland have successfully eradicated BHV-1 without vaccination. It is anticipated that in countries with extensive cattle populations and with more complex cattle management practices, the eradication of BHV-1 will require the use of vaccines. The differential BHV-1 vaccines will then play an important role in these initial steps of the BHV-1 eradication campaigns.[2, 4]

PUBLIC HEALTH CONSIDERATIONS

None of the BHV-1 biotypes or BHV-5 are known to affect humans.

REFERENCES

1. Crandell RA: Selected animal herpesviruses: New concepts and technologies. *In* Cornelius CE, Simpson CF (eds): Advances in Veterinary Science and Comparative Medicine, vol 29. Orlando, Fla, Academic Press, 1985, pp 281–327.
2. van Oirschot JT, Kaashoek MJ, Rijsewijk FAM: Advances in the development and evaluation of bovine herpesvirus 1 vaccines. Vet Microbiol 53:43, 1996.
3. Galeota JA, Flores EF, Kit S, et al: A quantitative study of a deletion mutant bovine herpesvirus-1 differential vaccine in reducing the establishment of latency by wildtype virus. Vaccine 15:123, 1997.
4. Tikoo SK, Campos M, Babiuk LA: Bovine herpesvirus 1 (BHV-1): Biology, pathogenesis and control. *In* Maramorosch K, Murphy FA, Shatkin AJ (eds): Advances in Virus Research, vol 45. San Diego, Academic Press, 1995, pp 191–223.

■ Bovine Virus Diarrhea Virus and Mucosal Disease

Victor S. Cortese, D.V.M., Diplomate, A.B.V.P.

In the past several years bovine virus diarrhea virus (BVDV) infections have resurfaced as major problems for the cattle industry, particularly in North America. These problems include both high morbidity and mortality from acute BVDV infections,[1, 2] as well as the well-recognized syndromes associated with subclinical BVDV.[3] This has resulted in an increased awareness of acute BVDV infections and more diagnoses of BVDV in cattle with various clinical syndromes.[4, 5]

VIRUS CHARACTERISTICS

BVDV is a *Pestivirus* of the family Flaviviridae. It is a single, positive-stranded RNA virus and is highly mutable.[6] Currently there are two recognized biotypes of BVDV: cytopathic (CP) and noncytopathic (NCP). This is a laboratory differentiation based on the characteristics of the two types when grown in tissue culture. Replication of cytopathic strains results in death of target cells, whereas NCP strains reproduce without apparent damage to infected cells.[7] The majority of bovine virus diarrhea (BVD) field isolates are in fact NCP (approximately 95%). The NCP biotype is the natural state of the virus.[8] It is believed that all CP BVD strains arise from mutation of NCP strains. The NCP/CP designation does not relate to the virulence of the strain. Some of the virulent strains in vivo at this time are NCP in vitro. There are considerable antigenic variabilities of the surface proteins (gp53) of different BVDV isolates; therefore BVDV strains can also be classified phenotypically by the use of monoclonal antibody mapping procedures.[9, 10]

The type 1 vs. type 2 designation of BVDVs is based on genotypic differences in the 5′ untranslated region of the viral genome. It is now believed that the pestiviruses can be split into four distinct groups that share approximately 65% homology with each other. These include BVD type 1, true border disease in sheep, and hog cholera. The various *Pestivirus* groups can cause cross-infections and potential disease in any of the domestic and wild ruminants and swine.[11] These internal variations also contain surface variations that appear to be associated with each group. The type 1 vs. type 2 designation also does not correlate with virulence. There can be severe death loss with either division, depending on the strain.

DISEASE SYNDROMES

Subclinical Infections

The majority of BVDV infections are subclinical with little outright clinical disease apparent.[12] The severity of the infection is determined by the virulence of the strain and the susceptibility of the host. The infection may be completely inapparent as is often seen in adult cattle or may cause a severe disease bordering on the appearance of mucosal disease. The one constant that appears with these infections is immunosuppression. Again, the severity and duration of the immunosuppression appears to be tied to the strain infecting the animal. For example, neutrophil function is reduced for 3 weeks after the initial infection.[13] In most of these infections, if the animal is unexposed to other disease agents while undergoing immunosuppression, it will recover, but if there is another disease agent present, the mortality and morbidity rates can be greatly elevated.[14] Most endemic

BVD herds have the virus circulating subclinically, exhibiting only reproduction syndromes (see below).

Respiratory Tract Infections

The respiratory form of BVDV infection appears, clinically, much like infectious bovine rhinotracheitis. The trachea is the primary site of lesions and oral and tracheal ulcers may be seen. Reddening of the nares is often present. There can be a pneumonia in the anterior lung lobes but it is usually from secondary pathogens.

Digestive Tract Infections

Although severe diarrhea is usually associated with mucosal disease, many of the severe cases of acute disease involve the digestive tract. In our studies, diarrhea and nonresponsive fever (>104°F) are the most consistent signs with the particular type 2 challenge virus used. In both calves and cows the diarrhea may be bloody, and digestive tract ulcers, particularly of the Peyer's patches, are common.

Thrombocytopenic Syndrome

The newest syndrome to be described is the thrombocytopenic syndrome.[15] It has also been called the bleeder or hemorrhagic syndrome. In this syndrome the BVDV attaches to platelets and is found in the bone marrow. There is an accompanying decrease in destruction of thrombocytes. These animals may start with a mild diarrhea or anorexia with a slight fever. The first sign is often bleeding into the conjunctiva. If injected the calf will often bleed from the injection site for several hours or develop large hematomas. Hemorrhages are often found in or on the intestinal cavity or internal organs on postmortem examination. This is caused by several NCP type 2 strains and these animals are not persistently infected. Although originally thought to be primarily a disease of the Holstein calf, it has been seen in adult and beef cattle as well.

Reproductive Infections

The CP and NCP strains react most differently in the nonimmune pregnant cow. If a nonimmune cow is exposed to an NCP strain in the first trimester of gestation, early embryonic death, abortion, mummification, or persistently infected (PI) calves can result. If exposure occurs during the second trimester, birth defects, primarily involving nervous tissue, or occasionally persistent infection, is found. Infection during the last trimester usually has no effect on the fetus and the calf will be born with antibodies against BVD. Rarely, there is an overwhelming exposure which causes a late abortion (Fig. 1). PI cows can have all of the above fetal outcomes except that a PI cow cannot have an unaffected calf. Infections with CP strains cannot give rise to PI calves but can cause the other fetal problems.[16]

Persistent Infection

When BVD infection occurs before the immune system has fully developed, the calf learns to recognize that particular strain of BVDV as part of itself and never mounts an immune response against the strain of BVDV. They can mount immune responses to heterotypic BVDV antigen. PI calves can be born normal and constantly shed the virus or they can be born weak and die. These cattle are immunologically frail and have decreased immune function[17] and low survivorship. However, PI calves may appear normal and a low percentage can reach adulthood, breed, and have PI calves. They are also a constant source of viral shedding to the rest of the herd. The current persistent infection rate in the United States among cattle under 1 year of age is estimated at 1.5% to 2.0%.[18] In some herds, 10% to 50% of the calves may be carriers. Once an animal is PI, nothing can eliminate the virus or stop its shedding, although recent data have shown that virus shedding will vary by age, individual animal, and stress on the animal.[19]

Mucosal Disease

The exposure of a PI animal to a CP strain of BVDV can have three possible outcomes (Fig. 2). Mucosal disease is one of them. In order for mucosal disease to occur, a specific set of circumstances are required. First, the animal must be PI. Second, the animal must be exposed to another BVDV that is a CP strain. In mucosal disease, usually both strains can be isolated. Furthermore, new research indicates that this strain must be closely related to the NCP strain causing the persistent infection to consistently cause mucosal disease.[20, 21] More antigenically distinct CP BVDV strains can cause this fatal disease but not as consistently. This exposure may be from additions to the herd or from a PI animal spontaneously mutating to a CP strain. The result is explosive diarrhea and ulcers through the digestive

Figure 1

Outcome of BVDV persistently infected calves on exposure to a cytopathic BVDV strain.

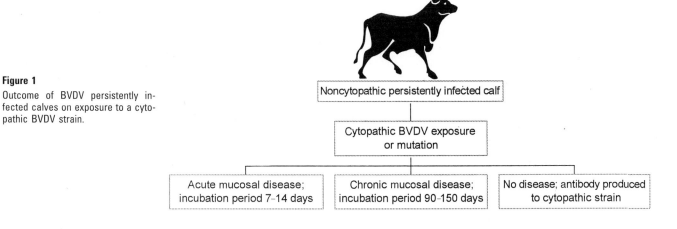

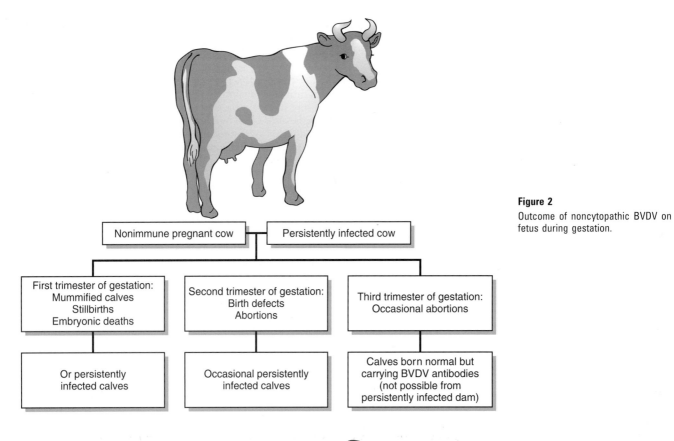

Figure 2
Outcome of noncytopathic BVDV on fetus during gestation.

tract. Mortality rates in cattle with mucosal disease are 95% to 100%.

Chronic Mucosal Disease

This form of BVD also requires persistent infection as a prerequisite. The animal again needs to be exposed to a CP strain. It appears that the strain is an intermediate in its antigenic relationship to the PI strain. A 3- to 5-month incubation period occurs that allows a recombination of the two strains and the chronic form to appear. The CP strain that is formed is antigenically different from the initial NCP or CP strain. These animals may begin with a lameness involving multiple feet or with a mild, nonresponsive diarrhea. The course of the disease is from 1 to 2 months and the mortality rate is very high with this complex also (>95%).

DIAGNOSIS

Diagnosis of BVD can be simple or difficult depending on the syndrome under investigation. Knowledge of the pathogenesis of the disease is important to determine the timing of sampling, the samples to be taken, and interpreting the results. Subclinical infections can be the hardest to diagnose and interpret. Furthermore, laboratory variation and strain variation to complicate the clinician's ability to correctly diagnose BVDV infections.[22] The diagnosis of subclinical BVD causing herd reproductive problems can be frustrating. The history will often give some clue. The most common history is that the herd has been experiencing a slow increase in reproductive problems manifested as early embryonic death with a few mummified calves or abortions. In some herds the first signs are a higher-than-expected number of weak and stunted calves or increased calf morbidity and mortality.

Virus Isolation

Virus isolation is still considered to be the diagnostic test of choice for many of the BVDV situations. It is the only way to adequately diagnose PI animals. In order to definitively diagnose a PI animal, the virus must be isolated twice from buffy coat or serum with a minimum of 4 weeks between the two samples. Serum or whole-blood samples from PI calves or calves undergoing mucosal disease and chronic BVD will usually yield positive viral isolation results, as will acutely infected animals if tested at the correct stage of the infection. Most acutely infected animals are virus isolation–positive for 3 to 10 days after exposure. Mononuclear cells from the buffy coat obtained from whole blood are the preferred sample. NCP strains are identified in cell culture by detecting viral antigen via immunofluorescence or immunoenzyme staining. Other samples that may be obtained for virus isolation include nasal swabs, semen, tissues (particularly lymphoid tissue), and smears from ulcerative areas.[23, 24]

If a large number of samples are to be tested, as for herd eradication programs or persistent infection screening, the microplate virus isolation technique may be used. The samples are incubated in microplate wells and viral antigen is detected using immunoperoxidase-labeled conjugate.[25] This method is usually quicker and less costly than traditional virus isolation techniques.

ANTIGEN DETECTION

Immunohistochemistry

Several immunohistochemical techniques are available for antigen detection from fresh or frozen tissue samples. The two most commonly employed methods of antigen detection are immunofluorescence and immunoperoxidase staining. There had been considerable debate on the accuracy of fluorescent antibody staining and it appears that immunoperoxidase staining, when available, is more accurate. This test also has the ability to be performed on fixed tissues.[26, 27] With either test the most important factor in diagnostic accuracy is the antibody(s) chosen for the detection of the antigen since BVDV antigen variability can affect the results if improper antibodies are chosen. Studies we have performed have shown most tissues have BVDV antigen following acute infection with BVDV when tested using immunoperoxidase staining techniques. New techniques, such as antibody capture enzyme-linked immunosorbent assays (ELISAs) and flow cytometry for detection of antigen, are generally used in research projects but may become commercially available.

Nucleic Acid Hybridization Probes

BVDV hybridization probes were initially used in research to prove the antigenic variability of BVDV isolates. Probes have been made from both the p80/125 protein region as well as the 5′ untranslated region (5′ UTR). Probes from the 5′ UTR have detected the widest range of BVDV isolates and have the highest level of detection. Detection of various BVDV strains ranges from 60% to 100%.[28] To date the use of hybridization probes is not common in diagnostic laboratories.

PCR Amplification

Polymerase chain reaction (PCR) amplification utilizes DNA oligonucleotides to bind to corresponding target sequences. These sequences must have a high degree of specificity for the infectious agent that is being detected. In PCR amplification, reverse transcription is followed by the PCR (RT-PCR). RT-PCR can detect from 100- to 1000-fold less virus than virus isolation.[29, 30] Furthermore, using PCR amplification, BVDV can be detected 12 to 14 days after infection. These two factors should make PCR detection at least as sensitive as virus isolation. PCR tests have been developed for detection of virus in serum, milk and both fixed and fresh tissues. This process of antigen detection will most likely become available at most diagnostic laboratories.

Serology

Serology can be difficult to interpret and often leads to overdiagnosis of BVDV problems in a herd. Virus neutralization (VN) is the most common serologic test performed for determination of BVDV antibody levels. No one standard reference strain is used by the various diagnostic laboratories so it is important to send paired samples to the same laboratory. This will also give different results on the same sample when sent to different laboratories. The antigenic variability of the infecting strains themselves leads to differences in serologic responses following infection. Often by the time a reproductive problem is diagnosed, the exposure has already occurred and no changes in titer are detected.

The antibody level of a single-sample titer can be useful for determining if further investigation is needed. This method is useful in unvaccinated herds, precolostral samples from calves, and samples from calves (before vaccination and after colostral antibodies have disappeared). The presence of BVDV VN antibody in these samples indicates exposure to the virus. It is difficult to interpret BVDV titers from single samples in vaccinated herds and usually the four- to eightfold increase in titer from paired samples is used to positively diagnose BVDV expo-

sures. Acute samples should be frozen and submitted at the same time as the convalescent sample to avoid differences in laboratory techniques. BVDV ELISA antibody testing has been done, but because extensive purification and preparation of the antigen is required, it has not gained widespread use.

PREVENTION AND CONTROL

In order to limit the risk of a BVDV infection occurring, a control program must contain two components. The first is to limit exposure of cattle to the BVDV. The second, and most controversial, involves implementation of a sound BVDV vaccination program.

Biosecurity

Many of the BVDV problems have arisen because of poor biosecurity on the farm. Most procedures that can be instituted are not unique to BVDV but should be considered for general disease control. Direct contact with infected animals is the most important method of transmission and BVDV is not transmitted by aerosol readily. Isolation of new arrivals or cattle returning from shows for 2 weeks will reduce the likelihood of an acutely infected animal shedding the virus. Limiting access to the facilities where animals are housed to employees will also help, although mechanical transmission is considered low in BVDV infections. Also, changing of needles between animals and maintaining fly control may also help in limiting transmission.

PI cattle constitute the hardest and often the most important control point in BVD biosecurity. It is believed that the most common source of BVDV spread is the PI animal and these cattle are often outwardly normal. Isolation of these animals for several weeks will not have any impact on virus shedding. To limit risk from PI animals, virus isolation can be performed on new additions to the herd, including breeding bulls. The animals should be kept in quarantine while awaiting the results of the test. If positive results are obtained, the animal can be culled or retested to confirm the PI diagnosis before culling.

Vaccination

Confusion exists regarding vaccination programs because of the increasing number of BVD problem herds being diagnosed and the myriad of BVDV vaccines available. Knowledge concerning the ability of different vaccines to protect against BVDV infection is increasing rapidly. Currently, all commercially available modified-live BVDV vaccines and most inactivated vaccines contain type 1 isolates. Recent studies have shown that VN antibodies stimulated by both inactivated and modified live BVDV vaccines can be neutralize a wide range of type 1 and type BVDV isolates.[31, 32] The duration of immunity afforded by the inactivated vaccines is dependent on the antigenic similarity between the vaccine strain and the wild-type virus to which the cow is exposed: The duration of cross-neutralizing ability to strains with only a few common proteins is less than 1 year.[33] ML vaccines stimulate neutralizing antibodies that cross-neutralize antigenically dissimilar strains for over 18 months following a single dose to mature animals[34] (author's unpublished data).

Clinical reports from Canada have shown the ability of both Modified live and inactivated vaccines to prevent acute disease. Studies are being performed to show the ability of the vaccines to protect against acute infection. Recent work has shown that a modified live BVDV vaccine can protect young calves against a virulent type 2 BVDV challenge.[35] Vaccination of calves with maternal antibodies is a source of debate. Studies have demonstrated the ability of modified live vaccines to stimulate immune responses when maternal BVDV-VN antibody levels were below 1:32.

There is nothing we can currently do to prevent mucosal disease or chronic BVD with vaccination or management except to minimize exposure, if possible.

Protection of the fetus is hard to obtain in vaccinated dams. It takes few viral particles to cross the placenta and cause fetal infection.[36] Several reproductive BVD studies have been performed. Most studies have used inactivated BVD vaccines and at least one study used a combination of an inactivated vaccine followed by a modified live BVDV vaccine. Birth of PI calves was the outcome assessed and the level of protection varied by study[37-39] (author's unpublished data).

There are advantages and disadvantages to both the inactivated and modified live vaccines. The advantages of inactivated vaccines include no possibility of reversion to virulence or genetic recombinations, contamination with adventitious agents, shedding of virus to contact animals, induction of immunosuppression, or mucosal disease. Disadvantages include greater cost, the requirement of two initial doses, longer time until peak immunity, shorter duration of immunity, and potential adverse reactions.

Advantages and disadvantages of modified live BVDV vaccines are opposite to those indicated for inactivated vaccines. One of the more common vaccination programs includes starting young stock with modified live vaccines and then switching to inactivated vaccines in adults.

When designing a vaccination program for BVDV several factors must be considered. The age of the animal, the syndrome to be protected against, the ability to work the animal, time until expected exposure, BVDV status of the herd, and management of the herd should all be factored in when designing the program.[40] Regardless of which vaccine is used, the label should be followed to obtain maximum benefit from the vaccine.

Herd BVDV Eradication

One option that is being exercised with increased frequency is herd BVDV eradication. In small herds, closed herds, or herds selling breeding stock, a program of virus isolation, culling, and annual vaccination is an attractive option for handling BVD problems. The entire herd can be tested or the young stock can be tested initially and then positive PI cattle followed up their family trees. In herd eradication programs it is important to continue testing for PI animals in newborn calves for 8 months after instituting the program to find PI calves that were in utero when the program was started. As cowside or in-clinic tests become available, this option may gain even more popularity.

SUMMARY

BVDV infection is being diagnosed with increasing frequency. The number of herds containing PI carriers may also be on the rise. A thorough understanding of this pathogen is required to diagnose and prevent disease syndromes in individuals and herds.

REFERENCES

1. Peracute bovine viral diarrhea reportedly spreading. J Am Vet Med Assoc 205:391–392, 1994.
2. Pollerin C, Vandershark J, Lecomte J, et al: Identification of a new group of bovine viral diarrhea virus strains associated with severe outbreaks and high mortalities. Virology 203:260–268, 1994.
3. Bolin SR: The current understanding about the pathogenesis and clinical forms of BVD. Vet Med October 1124–1132, 1990.
4. Brownlie J: The pathogenesis of bovine virus diarrhea virus infections. Rev Sci Tech Off Int Epizootiol 9:59, 1990.
5. Baker JC: Vet Clin North Am Food Anim Pract, 11:425–445, 1995.
6. Dubovi EJ: Molecular biology of bovine virus diarrhea virus. Rev Sci Tech Off Int Epizootiol 9:105–114, 1990.
7. Horzinek MC: Bovine virus diarrhea virus: An introduction. Rev Sci Tech Off Int Epizootiol 9:13–23, 1990.
8. Ernst PB, Baird JD, Butler DG: Bovine viral diarrhea: An update. Compendium Continuing Educ Pract Vet 5:S581–S589, 1983.
9. Corapi WV, Donis RO, Dubovi EJ: Characterization of a panel of monoclonal antibodies and their use in the study of the antigenic diversity of bovine viral diarrhea virus. Am J Vet Res, 51:1388–1394, 1990.
10. Bolin SR, Littledike ET, Ridpath JF: Serologic detection and practical consequences of antigenic diversity among bovine viral diarrhea viruses in a vaccinated herd. Am J Vet Res 52:1033–1037, 1991.
11. Loken T: Vet Clin North Am Food Anim Pract 11:579–596, 1995.
12. Duffel SF, Harness JW: Bovine virus diarrhea–mucosal disease infection in cattle. Vet Rec 117:240, 1985.
13. Roth JA, Kaeberle ML, Griffith RW: Effects of bovine viral diarrhea virus infection on bovine polymorphonuclear leukocyte function. Am J Vet Res 42:244, 1981.
14. Cravens RL, Ellsworth MA, Sorensen CD, et al: Efficacy of a temperature sensitive modified live bovine herpesvirus type 1 vaccine against abortion and stillbirth in pregnant heifers. J Am Vet Med Assoc 208:2031–2034, 1996.
15. Corapi W, et al: Thrombocytopenia and hemorrhages in veal calves infected with bovine viral diarrhea virus. J Am Vet Med Assoc 196:590–596, 1990.
16. Moennig V, Leiss B: Vet Clin North Am Food Anim Pract 11:477–489, 1995.
17. Brown GB, Bolin SR, Frank DE, et al: Defective function of leukocytes from cattle persistently infected with bovine viral diarrhea virus and the influence of recombinant cytokines. Am J Vet Res 52:381, 1991.
18. Houe H: Vet Clin North Am Food Anim Pract 11:521–548, 1995.
19. Brock K, Grooms DL: Impact of Bovine Viral Diarrhea Virus on Reproductive Performance. Presented at International Symposium on Bovine Viral Diarrhea Virus. A Fifty-Year Review. June 1996, Ithaca, NY.
20. Bolin SR: Vet Clin North Am Food Anim Pract 11:489–501, 1995.
21. Moennig V, Frey HR, Liebler E, et al: Reproduction of mucosal disease with cytopathogenic bovine viral diarrhea virus selected in vitro. Vet Rec 127:200–203, 1990.
22. Dubovi EJ: The diagnosis of bovine viral diarrhea infections: A laboratory view. Vet Med October 1133–1139, 1990.
23. Brock KV: Vet Clin North Am Food Anim Pract 11:549–563, 1995.
24. Evermann JF, Berry ES, Baszler TV, et al: Diagnostic approaches for the detection of bovine viral diarrhea (BVD) virus and related pestiviruses. J Vet Diagn Invest 5:265–269, 1993.
25. Afshar A, Dulac GC, Dubuc C, et al: Comparative evaluation of the fluorescent antibody test and microtiter immunoperoxidase assay for detection of bovine viral diarrhea virus from bull semen. Can J Vet Res, 55:91–93, 1991.
26. Ellis JA, West KH, Cortese VS, et al: Lesions and sites of viral replication following infection of young sero-negative calves with virulent bovine virus diarrhea virus type II. Vet Pathol (in press).
27. Haines DM, Clark EG, Dubovi EJ: Monoclonal antibody–based immunohistochemical detection of bovine viral diarrhea virus in formalin-fixed, parrafin-embedded tissues. Vet Pathol 29:27–32, 1992.
28. Brock K, Ridpath J, Deng R: Comparative hybridization and nucleotide sequence information form two noncytopathic isolates of bovine viral diarrhea virus. Vet Microbiol 36:69–82, 1993.
29. Lopez OJ, Osorio FA, Donis RO: Rapid detection of bovine viral diarrhea virus by polymerase chain reaction. J Clin Microbiol 29:578–582, 1991.
30. Hertig C, Pauli U, Zanoni R, et al: Detection of bovine viral diarrhea virus using the polymerase chain reaction. Vet Microbiol 26:65–76, 1991.
31. Bolin SR, Ridpath JF: Range of virus neutralizing activity and molecular specificity of antibodies induced in cattle by inactivated bovine viral diarrhea virus vaccine. Am J Vet Res 51:703, 1990.

32. Bolin SR, Ridpath JF: Specificity of neutralizing and precipitating antibodies induced in healthy calves by monovalent modified-live bovine viral diarrhea virus vaccine. Am J Vet Res 50:817–821, 1989.
33. Bolin SR, Littledike ET, Ridpath JF: Serologic detection and practical consequences of antigenic diversity among bovine viral diarrhea viruses in a vaccinated herd. Am J Vet Res 52:1033–1037, 1991.
34. Bolin SR: Vet Clin North Am Food Anim Pract 11:615–625, 1995.
35. Cortese VS, West K, Ellis JA: Clinical and immunological responses to type 2 BVDV challenge in vaccinated and unvaccinated calves. *In* Proceedings of the 19th World Buiatrics Congress, 1996, pp 610–614.
36. Ficken M, Jeevaraerathnam S, Wan Welch SK, et al: BVDV fetal infections with selected isolates. *In* Proceedings of the International Symposium on Bovine Viral Diarrhea Virus. A Fifty Year Review, June 1996, Ithaca, NY, pp 110–112.
37. Meyling A, Rensholt L, Dalsgaard K, et al: Experimental Exposure of Vaccinated and Non-Vaccinated Pregnant Cattle to Isolates of Bovine Viral Diarrhea Virus (BVDV). Slate Veterinary Institute for Virus Research 1985, pp 225–231.
38. Harkness JW, Roeder PL, Drew T, et al: The efficacy of an experimental inactivated BVD-MD vaccine. Agri Pest Infect Ruminants 233–250, 1985.
39. Kaeberle ML, Maxwell D, Johnson E: Efficacy of Inactivated Bovine Viral Diarrhea Virus Vaccines in a Cow Herd. Animal Science Leaflet R701. Ames, Iowa State University, 1990.
40. Schultz R: Certain factors to consider when designing a bovine vaccination program. *In* Proceedings of the 26th Annual Convention of the American Association of Bovine Practitioners 1994, pp 19–21.

■ Respiratory Disease of Cattle Associated With Coronavirus Infections

Johannes Storz, D.V.M., Ph.D., Diplomate, A.C.V.M.

The bovine respiratory disease complex remains an important cause of loss in the beef and dairy cattle industries. The multifactorial causes of this disease complex involve infections with viruses and bacteria as well as diverse stress factors. Viral infections with recognized etiologic roles are bovine herpesvirus type 1 (BHV-1), parainfluenza virus type 3 (PI-3), bovine respiratory syncytial virus (BRSV), and bovine viral diarrhea virus (BVDV). Modern vaccination programs with multiple, modified live virus vaccines and appropriate bacterial antigens have beneficial effects, but not all bovine respiratory disease problems have been controlled. Previous editions of this book highlighted concepts and pertinent information on the bovine respiratory disease complex. Recent investigations on currently prevailing viral respiratory tract infections of feedlot age cattle affected with respiratory distress yielded numerous unique coronavirus isolates as the most frequently detected viral agents.[1] The etiologic association of these respiratory bovine coronaviruses (RBCVs) with respiratory tract disease of cattle of different age groups is described below.

Enteropathogenic bovine coronaviruses (EBCVs) have been recognized as an important cause of diarrhea of neonatal calves to an age of up to 3 to 4 weeks.[2] This infection contributes to major losses resulting from diarrheal diseases among newborn calves. The virus replicates in the absorptive epithelial cells of the villi of the small intestine and in the superficial and crypt epithelial cells of the colon. Virus replication is cytocidal for infected cells and leads to loss of cellular functions prior to cell death, villus atrophy, dilated crypts, decreased numbers of goblet cells, and profuse watery diarrhea, often with fibrin casts.[3] The pathophysiologic changes associated with these lesions result in malabsorption, dehydration and acidosis, and electrolyte losses and imbalances, with ensuing death of severely affected calves.

Some of the EBCV-infected calves develop pneumoenteritis characterized by mild respiratory tract disease with nasal discharges, but these signs are overshadowed by the clinical picture of enteritis with diarrhea.

EBCVs were also found to be associated with cases of winter dysentery in adult cattle. Antigens to EBCV were demonstrated in intestinal lesions by immunohistochemical techniques. Virus isolation in HRT-18 cell cultures identified EBCV in diarrhea samples of adult cattle with this disease.[4] The lesions of the intestinal mucosa of these cattle are comparable to those seen in calves with EBCV-induced neonatal diarrhea. These cattle develop profuse watery diarrhea, become listless, lose weight, and have decreased milk production, which represents the major economic loss. The pathogenesis and control of neonatal diarrhea caused by EBCV in calves and descriptions of winter dysentery of adult cattle were presented in previous editions of this book.

EPIDEMIOLOGIC FEATURES OF RESPIRATORY BOVINE CORONAVIRUS INFECTIONS

A high rate of RBCV infections in nasal and tracheal specimens from cattle with signs of respiratory tract disease was detected.[1] These cattle were from ranches or had passed through sale yards and were shipped to feedlots or were involved in a livestock show. They came from Arizona, Arkansas, California, Kansas, Louisiana, Mississippi, Oklahoma, and Texas. Previously, coronavirus strains were isolated also from nasal samples of 4 of 16 calves with pneumoenteritis.[5] It was accepted that isolation of these coronaviruses was a difficult task with the types of cell cultures available in the past. Consequently, investigators attempted to detect coronavirus antigen by enzyme-linked immunosorbent assay (ELISA) or by immunofluorescent tests on samples of naturally infected calves or animals that had been inoculated oralpharyngeally with EBCV.[6, 7] Our investigations focused on isolation of the RBCV from such samples and included tests that also detected all other possible viruses known to be associated with respiratory tract infections of cattle to assess the currently prevailing viral infections. Surprisingly, 45 respiratory tract specimens collected from 136 cattle yielded RBCV. These viruses were only detected through the use of the G clone of human rectal tumor cells (HRT-18G).[1] Cell cultures permissive for the other bovine respiratory viruses yielded seven isolates of PI-3 and one strain each of BHV-1 and bovine adenovirus (BAV). A mixed infection involving RBCV and BHV-1 was observed in one case only. Coronaviruses were also isolated using this technique from tracheal washes as well as from lung tissues of young cattle with signs of a febrile pneumonia. Respiratory tract samples from 32 young cattle of a herd with protracted, chronic respiratory disease did not yield any virus isolates. A herd of 28 heifers and 31 bulls of the Charolais breed at the age of 6 to 8 months on winter pasture in Louisiana developed a rapidly spreading acute respiratory disease with nasal discharge and coughing, but they also had dark-brown watery diarrhea. They had been vaccinated at the time of weaning with a killed vaccine containing antigens to BHV-1, PI-3, BRSV, and BVDV, as well as five-way leptospiral, eight-way clostridial, and brucella bacterins. One of 15 nasal samples harbored BHV-1 and four had RBCV detected through virus isolation.

Seroepidemiologic investigations were reported on paired serum samples of three different cattle populations with respiratory problems involving a herd of 34 young cattle in Austria,[8] 196 cattle in Germany,[9] and 968 serum samples from cattle with respiratory disease in Ontario, Canada.[7] The Austrian herd shed coronaviruses in nasal secretions, and 18 of the 34 cattle seroconverted or had fourfold or higher increases in antibody titers, and two calves had rises in PI-3 antibodies. Serologic evidence of acute coronavirus infections was found in 16.8% of cattle with respiratory disease from 17 of 37 German herds with cattle older than 6 months.[9] The viral infectivity neutralization titers of the Canadian samples reached 1:4096 to 1:32,768 among cattle with pneumonia, which reflected seroconversion, or four-fold increases in titers of coronavirus antibodies in 17 groups.[7] Additionally, 26 groups with respiratory disease had antibody increases to coronavirus as well as other viral infections, 18 with BRSV, 8 with BVDV, 7 with PI-3, 6 with BHV-1, and 1 with BAV.[7] Investigations in England,[10] Ireland,[11] and India[12] furnished evidence of the association of coronaviruses with respiratory disease episodes of cattle.

CLINICAL SIGNS

The clinical signs of calves or young adult cattle from which RBCV strains were isolated, or in which coronaviral antigens were detected from respiratory tract samples, or where seroconversion and significant antibody rises were associated with respiratory disease episodes, can be differentiated into four clinical pictures: (1) Calves during the newborn phase up to about 4 weeks usually suffer from enteritis and diarrhea, but some develop signs of pneumoenteritis with shedding of virus in nasal secretions, which are serous to mucopurulent.[7, 12, 13] They cough and have higher respiratory rates, but the major clinical signs are determined by reactions to the gastroenteric infection. (2) A second condition can be differentiated in calves aged between 2 and 4 months. Increased seromucous discharges and coughing are observed, but the body temperatures vary within normal ranges; diarrhea and other adverse clinical signs are not observed. These calves usually have declining antibodies to EBCV.[8, 9] (3) Young cattle aged 5 to 13 months or older make up a third group with clinical signs of more severe respiratory disease.[1, 7-9] They have seromucous to mucopurulent nasal discharges with higher respiratory rates than normal and febrile pneumonia in the more severe cases. Diarrhea is usually not observed. The infection spreads rapidly through the herds, particularly among cattle stabled during the winter months or on winter pastures. This condition is called *Rindergrippe* or "cattle flu" in German-speaking countries, which describes the clinical picture quite accurately and implies a rapid spread and high mortality.[7, 9] The young cattle from which numerous RBCV strains were isolated after transport to feedlots had slight elevation of body temperatures to 41°C, with serous nasal discharges, increased respiration rates, and coughing.[1] (4) An epizootic of classical shipping fever in 105 cattle of a Texas feedlot is currently being investigated. These market-stressed cattle developed high fever, serous and mucopurulent nasal discharge, and other signs of respiratory distress 1 to 2 days after arrival in the feedlot. Seventy-two of the 105 cattle yielded RBCV strains by the G clone isolation method. Ten of these cattle died and all had RBCV infections. This virus infection was also detected in nasal swab samples collected from some of the cattle before vaccination and transport. Viruses with fusogenic properties and multiplying in bovine turbinate (BT) cell cultures were isolated from a few nasal samples of the 105 cattle. These viral isolates are being classified currently but do not have characteristics of BHV-1, BAV, or BVDV (Storz J, Purdy C, Loan R: Unpublished data, 1998).

PATHOLOGIC CHANGES IN RESPIRATORY TRACTS

Detailed pathologic and microbiologic investigations of 77 calves and young fattening cattle that died and were necropsied revealed 33 animals with lung lesions which consisted of suppurative or fibrinous bronchopneumonia in 14 cases, interstitial pneumonia in 8 cases, and interstitial and bronchopneumonia in 8 cases.[14] Bovine coronavirus antigen was detected as the only viral antigen in 37 animals. Eight of these cattle had diffusely consolidated lungs. These young cattle had died from naturally occurring infections and yielded only RBCV antigens in the mucous membrane samples. Diffuse consolidation was present throughout the lung lobes. The interalveolar septa were moderately to severely thickened and had infiltrations with mononuclear cells. Bronchioles and alveoles contained proteinaceous materials and harbored some desquamated epithelial cells. These changes were diffusely distributed throughout all lobes of the lungs.[14]

DIAGNOSIS

Clinical examination of calves and cattle with signs of respiratory disease does not give a clear indication of the actual infectious causes because of the similarity of clinical signs induced by different infections. Specific viral infections can only be identified through laboratory investigations. The most effective means for detecting and differentiating viral respiratory infections of cattle is a scheme devised in a recent investigation that included three specific cell culture types which are permissive for particular viruses, namely HRT-18G cells detecting RBCV and EBCV; Georgia bovine kidney (GBK) cells, highly permissive for BHV-1, PI-3, and cytopathic BVDV; and BT cells, which detect BRSV but also fastidious isolates of BAV and BVDV, while BHV-1 and PI-3 also multiply in these cells.[1] Bovine coronaviruses cannot be isolated from clinical specimens in GBK, BT, or several other types of cell cultures. The described diagnostic approach gives definitive answers about the prevailing acute viral respiratory infections of a specific clinical problem. This diagnostic scheme is more involved and specialized, but it has the power of revealing the frequency of currently prevailing bovine respiratory viral infections and furnishes viral isolates that can be further characterized. Additionally, RBCV or EBCV as well as other viral infections can be traced by sensitive capture ELISA or by detection of specific viral antigens through immunofluorescent testing of cells harvested with techniques of exfoliative cytology from nasal and other mucous membranes of cattle with respiratory tract disease.

Important information was generated by detailed serologic analysis through documentation of seroconversion or antibody titer increases associated with respiratory disease episodes. Significant increases in titers of viral neutralization antibodies as well as hemagglutination inhibition titers for RBCV were detected in herds where this infection prevailed.[7-9] Importantly, calves may have respiratory infections with RBCV and still have levels of corresponding antibodies. In attempts to clarify the role of RBCV infection in diverse respiratory disease cases, it is advisable to test fecal or diarrhea samples from affected cattle. This approach has not been followed sufficiently in past investigations of respiratory tract disease of calves. An excellent method of demonstrating EBCV infection of the intestinal tract is direct electron microscopic examination of diarrhea fluid or the use of immunoelectron microscopy. Antigen trap ELISAs, such as the Beldico Eli-vet bovine coronavirus antigen detection ELISA, are also useful.[7] Infections with EBCV also can be detected by immunofluorescence testing of frozen tissue sections from necropsy samples of affected cattle or isolation of EBCV in HRT-18G cells.

PROPERTIES OF THE RESPIRATORY BOVINE CORONAVIRUS

Bovine coronaviruses are enveloped viruses with a single-stranded, positive RNA genome of 31,000 bases coding for several nonstructural and five known structural proteins: the nucleopapsid (N) protein, the spike (S) glycoprotein, the membrane (M) glycoprotein, the small envelope (E) protein, and the hemagglutinin-esterase (HE) glycoprotein. Importantly, the S gene and the intergenic region between the S and E genes differ substantially between wild-type RBCV and EBCV strains. Some other characteristics that distinguish the RBCV from EBCV include the property that RBCV strains can be isolated and induce cell fusion in the first HRT-18G passage without the use of trypsin enhancement. Trypsin activation is essential to isolation of wild-type EBCV. In addition, the respiratory isolates have unusually high cell-fusing activities for HRT-18G cells, but other cultured cells are refractile. The RBCV isolates, unlike the EBCV strains and the modified strain used to vaccinate against enteric infections, have a restricted hemagglutination pattern. The newly isolated RBCV strains agglutinate only rodent but not chicken red blood cells which clearly distinguishes all of our RBCV isolates from the commercial vaccine strain of EBCV, which agglutinates both types of red blood cells.[1] These viruses multiply in polarized cells in culture and in epithelial cells of the nasal turbinates, trachea, and lungs.[15]

CONCLUDING PERSPECTIVES

The evidence of the etiologic association of RBCV with respiratory tract infections and diseases of calves as well as young adult cattle is strong. Highly sensitive viral isolation techniques of a recent investigation revealed that RBCVs were the most frequently occurring viral agents of the respiratory tract of cattle transported to feedlots and a livestock show involving cattle of eight states in the United States. Antigens of RBCV were demonstrated by fluorescent antibody tests in cells of nasal cavities, trachea, and lungs of calves and adult cattle with bronchopneumonia. Seroconversions and significant antibody rises were positively related to respiratory disease episodes of calves and young adult cattle in three major studies. Respiratory tract infections were induced in newborn calves and 6-month-old cattle following aerosol exposure to RBCV resulting in nasal shedding of virus and mild clinical signs. Viral isolation tests for RBCV and other known respiratory viruses of cattle detected 45 RBCV isolates as the most frequent viral respiratory infection followed by seven isolates of PI-3, two isolates of BHV-1, and one BAV strain. One case had RBCV and BHV-1. The infections of the test cattle were in early stages and not yet complicated by secondary bacterial infections.

Cattle developing respiratory clinical signs caused by RBCV infections are of weaning age and the age when they are transported in the United States to feeding establishments. Cattle arriving at feedlots after transport appear to be highly susceptible to RBCV infections. This observation has to be factored into programs of disease prevention. Current approaches to prevent EBCV infections leading to gastroenteritis in calves involve vaccinations of pregnant cows and passive colostral protection of newborn calves. The emergence of respiratory tract infections caused by RBCV at weaning and other production stages in the modern cattle industry may require strategically timed, active immunization with appropriate antigens to prevent this infection in stocker and feedlot cattle.

The successful and widely used vaccination with modified live viral vaccines against BHV-1, PI-3, BVDV, and BRSV infections probably creates immune pressures reducing the involvement of previously prevailing viral respiratory infections, which may explain the high rate of RBCV infections.

REFERENCES

1. Storz J, Stine L, Liem A, et al: Coronavirus isolation from nasal swab samples of cattle with signs of respiratory tract disease after shipping. J Am Vet Med Assoc 208:1452, 1996.
2. Mebus CA, Stair EL, Rhodes MB, et al: Neonatal calf diarrhea: Propagation, attenuation, and characteristics of a coronavirus-like agent. Am J Vet Res 34:145, 1973.
3. Doughri AM, Storz J: Light and ultrastructural pathologic changes in intestinal coronavirus infection of newborn calves. Zentralbl Vet Med 24:367, 1977.
4. Benfield DA, Saif LJ: Cell culture propagation of a coronavirus isolated from cows with winter dysentery. J Clin Microbiol 28:1454, 1990.
5. Jimenez C, Herbst W, Biermann U, et al: Isolierung von Coronaviren in der Zellkultur aus Nasentupferproben atemwegskranker Kälber in der Bundesrepublik Deutschland. J Vet Med B 36:635, 1989.
6. Heckert RAL, Sail J, Agnes AG: A longitudinal study of bovine coronavirus enteric and respiratory infections in dairy calves in two herds in Ohio. Vet Microbiol 22:187, 1991.
7. Carman PS, Hazlett MJ: Bovine coronavirus infection in Ontario. Can Vet J 33:812, 1992.
8. Mostl K, Burki F: Ursächliche Beteiligung boviner Coronaviren an respiratorischen Krankheitsausbrüchen bei Kälbern und pathogenetisch-immunologische Überlegungen hierzu. Dtsch Tierarztl Wochenschr 95:19, 1988.
9. Herbst VW, Klatt E, Schliesser T: Serologisch-diagnostische Untersuchungen zum Vorkommen von Coronavirusinfektionen bei Atemwegserkrankungen des Rindes. Berl Munch Tierarztl Wochenschr 102:129, 1989.
10. Thomas LH, Gourlay RN, Scott EJ, et al: A search for new microorganisms in calf pneumonia by the inoculation of gnotobiotic calves. Res Vet Sci 33:170, 1982.
11. McNulty MS, Brysson DG, Allan GM, et al: Coronavirus infection of the bovine respiratory tract. Vet Microbiol 9:425, 1984.
12. Rai RB, Singh NP: Isolation of coronavirus from neonatal calves with pneumoenteritis in India. Vet Rec 113:47, 1983.
13. Kapil S, Pomeroy KA, Goyal SM, et al: Experimental infection with a virulent pneumoenteric isolate of bovine coronavirus. J Vet Diagn Invest 3:88, 1991.
14. Appel G, Heckert HP, Hofman W: Über die Beteiligung von bovinem Coronavirus (BCV) am Rindergrippekomplex in Betrieben Schleswig-Holsteins. Tierarztl Umschau 47:296, 1992.
15. Lin XQ, O'Reilly KL, Storz J: Infection of polarized epithelial cells with enteric and respiratory tract bovine coronaviruses and release of virus progeny. Am J Vet Res 58:1120, 1997.

■ Bovine Respiratory Syncytial Virus

Herb Smith, D.V.M., Ph.D.
Neil Dyer, D.V.M., M.S., A.C.V.P.

Bovine respiratory syncytial virus (BRSV) was first recognized as causing or being associated with severe respiratory disease in cattle in 1970. There appear to be two closely related serotypes of the virus in cattle which are similar to a respiratory syncytial virus in sheep and may be identical to the serotype found in goats. The human respiratory syncytial virus has been recognized in infants and young children as the leading cause of life-threatening lower respiratory disease since the late 1950s.

During the 1970s, BRSV was isolated virtually worldwide and associated with bovine respiratory disease of varying severity in cattle of all ages and breeds. This prompted the development of various vaccines, both as a modified or inactivated virus and in combination with other agents of respiratory disease.[1]

The virus is a member of the family Paramyxoviridae and is classified with the pneumoviruses. It is a fragile, pleomorphic, easily inactivated virus that derives its name from the formation of characteristic masses of fused cells, or syncytia, in cell culture and in selected areas of affected lung. Much work has been done to develop an efficient enzyme-linked immunosorbent assay (ELISA) for BRSV, but efforts have met with variable success.

CLINICAL SIGNS AND LESIONS

The spectrum of clinical signs ranges from subclinical to life-threatening. The high incidence of antibody in cattle populations is indicative of widespread subclinical infection. Clinical signs include elevated temperature, hyperpnea, increased harshness in respiratory sounds, and spontaneous coughing that can vary from dry and nonproductive to moist. Coughing can often be easily induced. Nasal discharge in varying degrees is frequently present. Conjunctivitis may be seen, but is not a common feature. Most cases recover spontaneously, but severe cases may progress to death in spite of treatment.

Most efforts to infect calves experimentally have resulted in only mild or subclinical manifestations of disease, but some researchers have produced severe disease. It would appear there are differences in pathogenicity among virus isolates. In both naturally and experimentally infected calves, temperatures may reach 41 to 43°C (107 to 109°F), often without clinical signs of disease. Severe disease has been produced by concomitant infection with bacteria such as *Haemophilus somnus* or *Pasteurella* or another virus.[2] The virus is difficult to isolate because it is fragile, rapidly cleared, and often present in the posterodorsal portions of the lung rather than the anteroventral areas typically colonized in *Pasteurella*-type pneumonia.

The pathogenesis of BRSV-induced respiratory disease is unclear. A biphasic disease pattern is described. There is an initial, mild infection followed by a severe, often fatal episode characterized by emphysema. Immune-mediated factors are a likely explanation for some of these cases. The involvement of immunoglobulin E (IgE) in the interstitial pneumonia of feedlot cattle has been described. The association of BRSV with atypical interstitial pneumonia of feedlot cattle would support the hypothesis that immune mechanisms may be involved with severe disease. Recently, BRSV has been associated with bovine abortion.[3]

Postmortem examination of fatal BRSV pneumonia presents a variety of lesions, including consolidation of anteroventral lobes with varying degrees of emphysema and edema. Secondary bacterial infection is often evident, usually *Pasteurella hemolytica*–induced fibrinous pleuritis, but fatal pneumonia can be caused by a pure BRSV infection.

Microscopic features of respiratory tract lesions in fatal cases include necrotizing bronchiolitis, bronchiolitis obliterans, interstitial pneumonia, and edema with hyaline membrane formation. Syncytia with or without inclusions are frequently observed.

DIAGNOSIS

Serologic studies indicate that 40% to 50% of respiratory tract disease outbreaks in feeder calves involve BRSV. However, there are few salient features that would assist a clinician in making a presumptive diagnosis of BRSV-induced disease. Diagnosis is often made only by virus isolation, demonstration of a rise in antibody to the virus, or both. BRSV is difficult to isolate owing to its lability and because nasal swab samples are usually taken too late. Samples taken early in the clinical course, when temperatures are elevated, and before signs of severe respiratory disease appear, are most likely to be successful in yielding the virus. Many cell types support replication of BRSV.

Immunofluorescent techniques, both direct and indirect, and serum neutralization tests are used to detect antibody to BRSV. Recently a hemagglutination inhibition test has been described. By the time signs of severe respiratory disease are noted, the antibody levels may be quite elevated, causing inversion of the acute and convalescent serum titers. A number of animals in an outbreak should be sampled for meaningful serologic studies.

TREATMENT, PREVENTION, AND CONTROL

Conventional treatment with antibiotics and supportive therapy to combat secondary bacterial infections is usually successful. Where severe clinical manifestations exist (e.g., emphysema) and deaths occur within the infected herd, more vigorous therapy with antihistamines and corticosteroids, in addition to antibiotics and supportive therapy, may be necessary.

Conventional management practices, such as preconditioning to lessen stress coincident with weaning, are often helpful in disease prevention. Efficacy with vaccines has been observed, especially when vaccination is part of a total herd health program. Recent evidence of severe disease resulting from vaccine use concurrent with natural infection signals caution concerning indiscriminate use of biological agents.

REFERENCES

1. Ellis JA, Hassard LE, Cortese VS, et al: Effects of perinatal vaccination on humoral and cellular immune responses in cows and young calves. J Am Vet Med Assoc 208:393–399, 1996.
2. Potgieter LND, Helman RG, Greene W, et al: Experimental bovine respiratory tract disease with *Haemophilus somnus*. Vet Pathol 25:124–130, 1988.
3. Buote P, et al, quoted in Eugster AK: Bovine respiratory syncytial virus associated abortion in a dairy herd. Tex Vet, Feb 26–27, 1997.

■ Vesicular Stomatitis Virus in Swine and Cattle*

Beverly Schmitt, D.V.M., M.S.

Vesicular stomatitis (VS) is a sporadic disease of cattle, horses, swine, and wild ruminants in the United States. Clinical signs usually involve vesiculation of the mucosa of the gums, tongue, muzzle, and skin of the coronary band and interdigital areas. Economic losses from this disease result from decreased production in dairy cattle, restricted movement in livestock markets, and decreased trade due to trade barriers imposed by other countries.

VS is caused by vesicular stomatitis virus (VSV), a bullet-shaped virus that is a member of the family Rhabdoviridae, genus *Vesiculovirus*. Viruses of this family infect not only mammals and fish but also insects and plants. There are three serotypes of VSV: (1) New Jersey, (2) Indiana (subtypes Indiana-1, Indiana-2 [Cocal and Argentina strains], and Indiana-3 [Alagoas and Brazil strains]), and (3) Isfahan (subtypes Isfahan, Chandipura, and Piry). The New Jersey and Indiana-1 strains have been isolated from outbreaks of VS in the United States with the New Jersey strain identified as the causative agent in the outbreaks of 1982–1983 and 1995 and appearing with Indiana-1 in 1997. VSV is stable at a pH range of 4 to 10 and can survive in soil at 4 to 6°C for several weeks. VSV is an enveloped virus and can be inactivated by lipid solvents such as phenolics (Amphyl), quaternaries (Roccal-D), and halogens (chlorine).[1]

EPIZOOTIOLOGY

VSV causes disease in cattle and other ruminants, horses, swine, and humans. Experimental infections have been reported in other mammals such as opossum, rats, and laboratory animals (e.g., rabbits, mice, ferrets, hamsters). VS outbreaks in the United States have occurred sporadically throughout the last

---

*All of the material in this article is in the public domain.

two centuries. The interepizootic host has not been determined despite intensive research after each outbreak. The two serotypes most commonly seen in the United States, New Jersey and Indiana-1, are confined to the Western Hemisphere and annual epizootics that occur in Central America. Epizootics occur less frequently in temperate zones, and the disease usually disappears after the first frost. The transmission of VSV has not been completely elucidated, but insects are thought to play a major role. In the recent outbreak in 1995, clinical signs of VS were seen in horses in Arizona in May and New Mexico in June during the next 6 months the disease moved northward along river valleys into Colorado and Utah. This pattern of movement has been reported in previous outbreaks and appears to lend support to the theory of insect transmission of VSV. VSV has been isolated from black flies (Simulidae), phlebotomine sandflies, and *Culicoides*.[2, 3] Although replication of VSV has been demonstrated in Simulidae, it is believed that insects act primarily as mechanical vectors of VSV from animal to animal. Mechanical transmission has also been reported in dairy herds via milking machines and also among swine in close confinement, and it is believed that abrasions in the oral mucosa are important for contact transmission of VSV.

CLINICAL SIGNS

The incubation period for VS infection is short, ranging from 24 to 48 hours post infection with the development of fever and vesicle formation. Horses seemed to be the most susceptible species in the outbreak of 1995, developing vesicles or erosions on the lips, muzzle, and tongue and occasionally sloughing the dorsal epithelial surface of the tongue. Both cattle and horses may salivate excessively and refuse to eat. Oral lesions are also seen in cattle along with vesicles and erosions on the teats and interdigital areas. Clinical signs of VSV infection in swine may be inapparent or manifest with fever, salivation, and vesicles and erosions on the snout and tongue, coronary band, and interdigital spaces. Affected animals develop neutralizing antibodies that may persist for up to 8 to 10 years. However, reinfection can occur with a high titer of virus. There is no evidence of a carrier state of persistent infection with VSV in cattle, horses, or swine. Depending on the affected host species, the differential diagnosis must include foot-and-mouth disease (FMD), swine vesicular disease, vesicular exanthema, bovine viral diarrhea, rinderpest, malignant catarrhal fever, mycotic stomatitis, contagious ecthyma, photosensitization, trauma, and caustic agents.

DIAGNOSIS

Any vesicular disease of cattle or swine requires urgent attention because VS is indistinguishable from FMD. If horses and cattle on the same premises are affected with vesicular lesions, it is likely due to VSV; but combined infection with FMD could occur in cattle and should be ruled out. *State or federal veterinarians must be promptly notified of any suspected vesicular disease.* The collection of laboratory specimens is essential for differential diagnosis of vesicular disease. Specimens that should be collected from affected animals include epithelium of ruptured vesicles, vesicular fluid, and serum. Epithelium and vesicular fluid can be submitted on ice pack or in transport media such as buffered glycerol or TRIS-buffered tryptose broth. Laboratory tests include virus isolation, antigen capture enzyme-linked immunosorbent assay (ELISA), and competitive enzyme-linked immunosorbent assay (CELISA), serum neutralization, and complement fixation tests for antibody.

TREATMENT

Animals with lesions should be separated from unaffected animals and provided with separate waterers and feeders. New animals should be isolated from the herd until all clinical signs of VS have disappeared. Affected animals should be rested and provided with soft feed and water. Feed bunks should be cleared of rough feed and objects. Saliva-soaked feed and water sources should be destroyed or disinfected.[4] Cattle with lesions should have access to a high-energy feed source such as a molasses tank or soaked alfalfa pellets. Topical disinfectants and antibiotics may be used for skin and mouth lesions to prevent or treat secondary bacterial infections. Stabling of unaffected animals is recommended since it appears that pastured animals are more frequently affected by VS than animals in stables or barns.[5] In dairy herds, affected cattle should be milked last and the milking equipment disinfected. Disinfection of the bits of horse bridles should be encouraged.

PREVENTION AND CONTROL

Control measures for VS have traditionally included the quarantine of affected premises. Movement of cattle, swine, and horses from affected premises is prohibited until 30 days after the last clinical signs of the disease are evident, with the exception of animals going directly to slaughter. Movement of affected animals to livestock shows, fairs, and auction markets should be prevented to control the spread of the disease. During the 1995 outbreak, a 10-mile quarantine ring was put into effect around affected premises. In New Mexico, these rings were coalesced resulting in a quarantine of a large area in the central part of the state and with subsequent closure of auction markets in the area. In the 1997 VS outbreak these quarantines were limited to controlling movement from affected premises only. Insect control programs on affected and unaffected premises should be implemented in epizootic areas.

Vaccines for VSV have been available only during outbreaks and have been safety tested but not proved to be efficacious. A decrease in the severity of lesions due to VS was reported in vaccinated dairy herds during the outbreak of 1982. These vaccines have been used in affected states only.

PUBLIC HEALTH

VSV is infectious to humans and causes a flulike disease of 1 week's duration. Protective gloves should be worn when examining or handling an affected animal or specimens.

REFERENCES

1. Wright HS: Inactivation of vesicular stomatitis virus by disinfectants. Appl Environ Microbiol 19:96–99, 1970.
2. Francy DB: Entomological investigations of a 1982 vesicular stomatitis virus epizootic in Colorado, USA. *In* Proceedings of International Conference on Vesicular Stomatitis, Mexico City, 1984, Vol 1, pp 208–212.
3. Comer JA, Tesh RB, Govind BM, et al: Vesicular stomatitis virus, New Jersey serotype: Replication in and transmission by *Lutzomyia shannoi* (Diptera:Psychodidae). Am J Trop Med Hyg 42:483–490, 1990.
4. Thurmond MC: Vesicular stomatitis. *In* Third Annual Dairy Research Report, Department of Animal Science, University of California, Davis, 1984, pp 46–54.
5. Webb PA, Monath TP, Reif JS, et al: Epizootic vesicular stomatitis in Colorado, 1982: Epidemiologic studies along the northern Colorado front range. Am J Trop Med Hyg 36:183–188, 1987.

■ Bovine Leukemia Virus

Reginald Johnson, D.V.M., Ph.D., M.S.

The initial descriptions of leukosis in cattle appeared in the German medical literature in 1871. Reports of enzootic bovine leukosis (EBL) arising in virtually every eastern European country also appeared after World War II. European cattle that probably were infected with bovine leukemia virus (BLV) were imported from the shores of the Baltic sea to the United States at the end of the 19th century. Reports of EBL in the United States first appeared prior to World War II.

ETIOLOGY

Attempts to identify an infectious cause of bovine leukosis had failed for many years. A significant breakthrough came in 1969 when it was reported that the leukocytes of some cattle produced virus particles after being cultured for 2 to 3 days.[1] The particles were similar to particles from cells of other animal species with leukemia. The virus was isolated only in cows with adult lymphosarcoma, and from cows with persistent lymphocytosis, but not in cattle with the calf, thymic, and skin forms of leukosis. The virus was not isolated from cattle in EBL-negative herds. The transmissibility of the agent was confirmed after calves which were inoculated with cell cultures containing the virus became infected themselves and developed persistent lymphocytosis. Large-scale seroepidemiologic studies of the bovine population were conducted using serologic tests. The results of all of these early studies provided sufficient evidence to meet the virologic and seroepidemiologic criteria necessary for the establishment of a cause-and-effect relationship between BLV and EBL.

DESCRIPTIVE EPIDEMIOLOGY

A 1980 national study of BLV infection in Canada showed that 40% of its dairy herds and 11% of its beef herds were infected. The seroprevalence in dairy cattle was 18 times higher than it was in beef cattle (9.3% vs. 0.5%). BLV control programs have been established in member countries of the European Economic Community (EEC) since the 1980s. According to a 1987 report, the seroprevalence in the entire EEC cattle population rarely exceeds 0.5% to 1.5%. BLV infection has been reported by many other countries, but valid national estimates of seroprevalence are rare. In the United States, epidemiologic studies of BLV infection prior to 1996 had been restricted to a few states, small regions within those states, or single herds.[1] Seroprevalence varied among those herds from 0% to 95% of the cattle sampled.

An assessment of BLV prevalence in U.S. dairy operations was part of the National Animal Health Monitoring System's (NAHMS) Dairy '96 Study.[2] Between February and May of 1996, randomly selected dairy operations with at least 30 milk cows in 20 states representing 79% of the U.S. dairy cow population were contacted by federal or state animal health officials for voluntary participation in the study. Blood samples were collected from milk cows on 1006 operations and sent to the U.S. Department of Agriculture's (USDA's) National Veterinary Services Laboratories for BLV testing using the agar gel immunodiffusion (AGID) test.

Dairy '96 results showed that 89% of U.S. dairy operations had cattle that were seropositive for BLV. Herd prevalences in the West, Midwest, and Northeast were 87% to 89%, while the Southeast had a herd prevalence of 99%. Virtually all animals tested in some herds were seropositive. In the Southeast, the individual animal prevalence was higher than in other regions. Both herd and individual animal prevalence were slightly higher on operations with 200 or more cows than in smaller herds. In the Southeast, the within-herd prevalence was higher than in other regions, and it also was higher in herds with 200 or more cows. The within-herd seroprevalence was at least 25% in 75% of the positive herds.

CLINICAL SIGNS

The term *bovine leukemia virus* is somewhat misleading, since malignant lymphoma is the rule and frank leukemia the exception with BLV infection. The clinical signs associated with the deposition of solid tumors in cattle with EBL have been described previously (Table 1). Although the tumors originate from lymphoid tissue, they may be located in virtually every organ. The presence of a sign(s) is determined to a great extent by the location of the tumors. Enlargement of the external lymph nodes is common, but the internal nodes also may be enlarged in the absence of external involvement. The sublumbar and deep inguinal lymph nodes are common sites for tumors. The tumors very commonly invade the gastrointestinal tract, especially the abomasum, thus causing obstructions that lead to anorexia and weight loss. Tumors in the spinal cord result in neurologic disturbances. Clinical signs of myocardial failure are often associated with tumors in the myocardium. Exophthalmos results from tumors growing in the retrobulbar space.

Persistent lymphocytosis is an increase in the absolute lymphocyte count of at least 3 SD above the mean for a specific breed and age group of cattle from EBL-free herds. The lymphocytosis must persist for at least 3 consecutive months, and the cattle should have no detectable clinical manifestations of neoplastic lymphoproliferative lesions. *Persistent lymphocytosis* (PL) has been defined as a benign proliferation of B lymphocytes. The prevalence of PL in BLV-infected cattle was 33% according to one investigator.[2]

Table 1

PREVALENCE OF COMMON CLINICAL SIGNS OF ENZOOTIC BOVINE LEUKOSIS OBSERVED IN ONE GROUP OF HOSPITALIZED CATTLE AND ONE GROUP OF NONHOSPITALIZED CATTLE

Clinical Signs	Group 1* (%)	Group 2† (%)
Weight loss	Not known	80
Agalactia	Not known	77
Lymphadenopathy (enlargement)	58	58
Anorexia	62	52
Posterior paresis/ paralysis	16	41
Fever	Not known	23
Exophthalmos	9	20
Labored breathing	Not known	14
Gastrointestinal obstruction	19	9
Myocardial abnormality	64	7
Abnormal blood lymphocytes	63	Not known

*Data for group 1 collected from 298 hospitalized cattle.
†Data for group 2 collected from 1100 nonhospitalized (i.e., field) cattle.

MOLECULAR BIOLOGY

BLV and other retroviruses are called retroviruses because they all have a gene that codes for the enzyme reverse transcriptase.[3] This enzyme allows the viruses to convert their viral RNA into DNA and to integrate the viral DNA into the DNA of the target cells of their respective hosts, yielding a provirus. Similar to other retroviruses, the BLV provirus includes a long terminal repeat (LTR), *gag*, *pol*, and an *env* region. The *gag*, *pol*, and *env* regions contain the genetic information for the core proteins, the reverse transcriptase, and the envelope proteins, respectively. The major core proteins are p24, p15, p12, and p10. p24, the first recognized structural protein of BLV, has been purified, sequenced, and found to be distinct from the major core protein of most other retroviruses. The major glycoproteins of the envelope of BLV particles are gp51 and gp30. p24 and gp51 form the basis for the most commonly used, antibody-based diagnostic tests.

LABORATORY DIAGNOSIS

Historically, the diagnosis of BLV *infection* relied upon clinic pathologic study and serology for the detection of abnormal blood profiles and antibody response.[4] Cattle that developed *disease* and progressed to lymphosarcoma were diagnosed based on hematologic values or histopathologic findings. Owing to the uncertainties of foretelling which seropositive cattle will develop disease, the diagnosis of infection has become erroneously synonymous with the diagnosis of disease. It is important to use the most sensitive serologic assay when determining the infection status of cattle, since the results can be utilized to assist in epidemiologic studies and correlate seropositive status with disease conditions, establish control programs, and to screen cattle prior to sale or export.

The four most commonly used serologic assays for the bovine retroviruses are the agar gel immunodiffusion (AGID) assay; enzyme-linked immunosorbent assay (ELISA); Western blot (WB); and indirect fluorescent antibody (IFA), but not all are readily available commercially.[4] The AGID continues to be one of the most reliable indicators of BLV infection. This test correlates well with infection, and it has a high degree of specificity, due in part to the relative stability of the BLV genome. Although the AGID test is unable to detect low levels of BLV antibodies soon after infection, it has been shown to reliably detect antibodies within 2 to 4 weeks following experimental infection. In natural infection, where the dose of virus-infected cells may be low, it may take up to 12 weeks to detect antibodies.

While the AGID test will detect BLV-infected cattle, it cannot distinguish between passively acquired (colostral) antibodies and antibodies acquired through natural infection, and depending on the level of virus-infected lymphocytes, it may not detect infected cattle until several months after infection.[4] The AGID test is also less sensitive than several other serologic assays, such as the ELISA and radioimmunoassay (RIA), especially those that use monoclonal antibodies. The AGID test *does* have the advantages of being inexpensive and easy to perform, and it yields quick, clear, and easily interpreted results. These attributes outweigh some of the limitations of the test's sensitivity. Because of the diverse serologic assays available, a recommendation has been made to standardize BLV serologic assays using a known set of reference sera.

Although immunoassays have relied upon serum for the detection of antibodies, there would be advantages to testing other body secretions, such as milk and urine (e.g., ease of collection and a larger volume of substrate available for testing).[4] The disadvantages of assaying milk for BLV antibodies would be the large dilution factor, the interference by lactogenic proteins, and

the instability of antibodies in stored milk due to bacterial growth. Despite these problems, there are good reasons to utilize a milk-based antibody assay for BLV. For one thing, such a test would allow for cowside testing, which would be convenient and save time and money.

The application of flow cytometry and monoclonal antibodies directed to specific lymphocyte antigen markers appears to be a sensitive method of monitoring the abnormal proliferation of certain sets and subsets of B and T cells before the disease state occurs.[4] This early detection would allow valuable BLV-infected cattle to be used as embryo donors under strict management to prevent further transmission. These animals would be culled when clinical lymphosarcoma was predicted. This early detection would reduce the level of carcass condemnation, yet maximize the production of the animal in a herd. If early-detection tests become available, detection of later stages of BLV-induced lymphosarcoma would become somewhat academic. However, tests that identify later stages of BLV infection and disease by detecting tumor-specific antigens would still be useful in measuring an animal's response to antitumor therapy or to removal of a localized tumor.

CHEMOTHERAPEUTIC INTERVENTIONS

BLV infection is always persistent, and the tumors are eventually fatal. There are no published controlled *or* uncontrolled clinical trials in which currently available antiretroviral and antineoplastic drugs have been shown to be efficacious against BLV infection or tumors. New drugs are available to treat retrovirus infections in humans. Even if the drugs are shown to be efficacious against BLV, they probably never will be cost-effective for most animals in food animal practice, and only rarely cost-effective for the most valuable animals.

RISK FACTORS OF TRANSMISSION

Many potential modes of transmission of BLV have been investigated.[5, 6] The proportion of BLV infections attributable to specific routes of transmission in an individual herd varies substantially with management practices in the herd and the extent to which infection control measures are practiced. Hopkins and DiGiacomo's evaluation of risk factors for transmission is based on four aspects of bovine husbandry: (1) prenatal and periparturient period, (2) calfhood management, (3) breeding and reproductive management, and (4) conditions of housing and confinement.[6] A systematic evaluation of each of these aspects of a diary or beef operation will assist the veterinarian and producer in identifying modes of transmission and in tailoring an effective BLV control program.

Vertical transmission, either in utero or through colostrum and milk, accounts for a small proportion of infections. Iatrogenic horizontal transmission through procedures that augment the transfer of contaminated blood among cattle is a major route of transmission in many settings. This has been illustrated by high rates of BLV infection due to gouge dehorning with an unsanitized common instrument. The same may be true of invasive surgical procedures, vaccinations, injections, and rectal palpations. Contact transmission probably stems from a combination of natural sources of blood, exudates, and tissues that are present during parturition and which enter the susceptible host's body through mucosal surfaces or broken skin. Various aspects or periods of husbandry, the risk factors of concern during respective periods, and the qualitative and quantitative risks are presented in Table 2. *Quantitative* risk estimates are especially useful for measuring the strength of association between infec-

Table 2

QUALITATIVE AND QUANTITATIVE RISK OF TRANSMISSION OF BOVINE LEUKEMIA VIRUS (BLV) VIA 24 PRODUCTION PRACTICES RELATED TO SIX DIFFERENT ASPECTS OF HUSBANDRY

Aspect of Husbandry	Factor No.	Risk Factor	Odds Ratio/Relative Risk Qualitative	Quantitative (Point Estimate)
Prenatal period	1	Seropositive dam with persistent lymphocytosis	High	11.4 (1.7–75.1)
	2	Seropositive dam	Low	NA
	3	Semen	Low	NA
	4	Ova	Low	NA
Periparturient period	5	Colostrum	Low	NA
	6	Milk	Low	NA
Calfhood management	7	Gouge dehorner	High	NA
	8	Transfusion	High	NA
	9	Babesiosis vaccine contaminated with BLV	High	25 (17–36); 71 (51–100)
	10	IV injections: blood collection with common needle, syringe	High	NA
	11	IM, SQ, ID injections	Low	NA
	12	Castration	Low	NA
	13	Ear-tag	Low	NA
	14	Supernumerary teat removal	Low	NA
	15	Tattoo	Low	NA
	16	Saliva	Low	NA
Breeding and reproductive management	17	Rectal palpation with common sleeve	High	10 (1.7–62.4); 3 (1.1–6.8)
	18	Semen (artificial insemination)	Low	NA
	19	Semen (natural service)	Low	NA
	20	Ova and embryos (embryo transfer)	Low	NA
Housing and confinement	21	Close contact in high prevalence herds (i.e., >50%)	High	4.7 / 6.6 / 6.7
	22	Insects and arthropods	Low	NA
Miscellaneous	23	Open herd	High	NA
	24	Malignant lymphoma	High	46

NA, not available; IV, intravenous; IM, intramuscular; SQ, subcutaneous; ID, intradermal.

tion and exposure to a risk factor. Point estimates and the 95% confidence intervals for the point estimates of the *quantitative* risk are listed only if the authors provided the estimates, or if sufficient data were published to enable me to compute the estimates. Otherwise, only qualitative estimates are listed. A risk factor that has been qualitatively categorized as "low" is *not* intended to leave veterinarians with the perception that there is *no* or "zero" risk of transmission associated with that factor. An example of the correct interpretation of quantitative risk is as follows: A dairy cow that was vaccinated with a vaccine that was suspected to have been contaminated accidently with BLV was 25 times more likely to be seropositive than a cow that was not vaccinated with the vaccine, and one can be 95% confident that the point estimate for this odds ratio is between 17 and 36 (see Table 2, factor No. 9). Generally speaking, a point estimates that exceeds 4.0 indicates a strong association.

CONTROL, ERADICATION, PREVENTION

Results of the NAHMS's Dairy '96 study showed high prevalence and broad geographic distribution of BLV in U.S. dairy herds.[2] The high individual animal prevalence in seropositive herds indicates that culling alone will not be a cost-effective method for reducing BLV seroprevalence in those herds. Thus, control strategies in which culling and risk factor management are combined may be the only cost-effective methods for reducing the incidence of the infection in high-prevalence herds.[7] *Standards for Certification of Cattle Herds as Bovine Leukosis Virus*

Free was published by the Bovine Retrovirus Committee of the U.S. Animal Health Association. The state of New York is probably the only state that has allocated a significant number of resources to control BLV based on the current understanding of risk factors for transmission of BLV infection.

The New York State Department of Agriculture and Markets established a New York State Bovine Leukosis Virus Eradication and Certification Program (NYSBLVECP) in 1985.[8] The program was designed to assist producers in establishing a certified BLV-free herd. The list of management practices described below, a modification of the NYSBLVECP, is based on the premise that after an animal becomes infected with BLV, it will remain infected, and will *always* be a potential source of infection of other animals. Four of the practices are mandatory for all participants in the program. The nonmandatory practices should be selected on a farm-by-farm basis via consensus of the producer and veterinarian.

Mandatory and Nonmandatory Management Practices for Controlling BLV Infection in the Production Environment

Mandatory Practices

1. Sterile, disposable needles must be used on one animal only and then discarded in biohazard containers.
2. A different disposable obstetric sleeve must be used to

palpate each cow, or at least each cow that was seronegative on the last test.

3. Wash *first* and then disinfect any instruments that may be contaminated with blood. Many practitioners now avail themselves of at least two of the same instrument, soaking one set in a disinfectant while the other set is being used.

4. Use an electric dehorner rather than a gouge or a saw. Gouges and saws cause profuse hemorrhage and are difficult to sanitize.

Nonmandatory Practices

5. Develop a thorough insect vector control program.

6. Use artificial insemination.

7. Use a separate calving pen for each cow to reduce the exposure of susceptible animals to blood from infected cows.

8. Remove calves from their dams and raise them in hutches or a similar facility.

9. Calves from infected dams should not be permitted to contact other calves until their infectious status has been determined. A precolostral serum sample from highly valued offspring of infected dams should be tested. A positive test means that infection *already* has been acquired in utero.

10. If the prevalence of infection in the most recently tested 6- to 8-month-old calves is low (e.g., equal to in utero prevalence of 4% to 8%), colostrum probably is *not* a significant source of infection, and changes are *not* recommended.

11. If the prevalence of infection in the adult herd is low, feeding readily available colostrum from noninfected cows minimizes the risk of infection from colostrum. Thus, the calves can be tested much sooner than the usual 6 to 8 months of age, and their disposition can be determined at an early age, prior to large economic investments in them by the producer.

12. If the prevalence of infection in the adult herd is high (i.e., >60%), all calves should be fed frozen colostrum from infected cows. The purpose of freezing the colostrum is to reduce the infectivity of lymphocytes. The anti-BLV antibodies are intended to protect calves against postnatal infection.

13. Separate infected and uninfected animals to reduce close contact between them. Separation also facilitates processing of uninfected animals *before* infected animals. Herds may be tested for three reasons: (1) to distinguish infected animals from the population at risk of becoming infected during the initial phase of a control and eradication program, (2) to monitor progress toward the goal of eradication, and (3) to determine where there is horizontal transmission within the herd (e.g., bred heifers)[8] In the last case especially, additional management changes may be necessary to reduce the incidence of infection. The NYSBLVECP recommends a herd test semiannually. Assuming that an animal is not incubating BLV infection, the most that a producer can be assured of is that an animal was not infected on the date the sample was collected. Thus, a 6-month test interval (e.g., vs. 1 year.) favors rapid and accurate identification of newly infected animals followed by their separation from uninfected animals, and their removal from the herd if warranted.

ZOONOTIC IMPLICATIONS

Several epidemiologic studies have tried to show a relationship between human and animal leukemia or lymphoma.[9] In many of the studies the actual exposure to retroviruses is unknown. Based on the reported studies, retroviruses are not likely to be responsible for any significant occurrence of human disease, especially lymphoid malignancies. Although a definitive statement of no risk to human health is unwarranted, the evidence to date indicates that the risk to humans is low and perhaps nonexistent.

REFERENCES

1. Johnson R, Kaneene JB: Bovine leukemia virus: I. Descriptive epidemiology, clinical manifestations, and diagnostic tests. Compendium Continuing Educ Pract Vet 13:315, 1991.
2. USDA/APHIS/Veterinary Services: High Prevalence of BLV in U.S. Dairy Herds. Fort Collins, Colo, United States Department of Agriculture, 1997.
3. Johnson R, Kaneene JB: Bovine leukemia virus: III. Zoonotic potential, molecular epidemiology, and an animal model. Compendium Continuing Educ Pract Vet 13:1631, 1991.
4. Evermann JF, Jackson MK: Laboratory diagnostic tests for retroviral infections in dairy and beef cattle. Vet Clin North Am Food Anim Pract 13:87–106, 1997.
5. Johnson R, Kaneene JB: Bovine leukemia virus: II. Risk factors of transmission. Compendium Continuing Educ Pract Vet 13:681, 1991.
6. Hopkins SG, DiGiacomo RG: Natural transmission of bovine leukemia virus in dairy and beef cattle. Vet Clin North Am Food Anim Pract 13:107–128, 1997.
7. Johnson R, Kaneene JB: Bovine leukemia virus: IV. Economic impact and control measures. Compendium Continuing Educ Pract Vet 13:1727, 1991.
8. Brunner MA, Lein DH, Dubovi EJ: Experience with the New York State bovine leukosis virus eradication and certification program. Vet Clin North Am Food Anim Pract 13:143–150, 1997.
9. DiGiacomo RF, Hopkins SG: Food animal and poultry retroviruses and human health. Vet Clin North Am Food Anim Pract 13:177–190, 1997.

■ Bovine Spongiform Encephalopathy

Linda A. Detwiler, D.V.M.
Richard Rubenstein, Ph.D.

Bovine spongiform encephalopathy (BSE), widely known as "mad cow disease," is a chronic, degenerative disease affecting the central nervous system (CNS) of cattle. Worldwide, there have been more than 170,000 cases since the disease was first diagnosed in 1986 in Great Britain. BSE has had a substantial impact on the livestock industry in the United Kingdom. The disease has also been confirmed in native-born cattle in Belgium, France, Ireland, Luxembourg, the Netherlands, Northern Ireland, Portugal, and Switzerland. However, more than 95% of all BSE cases have occurred in Great Britain. BSE is not known to exist in the United States.

BSE belongs to the family of diseases known as the transmissible spongiform encephalopathies (TSEs). These diseases are caused by a transmissible agent that is yet to be fully characterized. They share the following common characteristics: (1) a prolonged incubation period of months or years; (2) a progressive debilitating neurologic illness that is always fatal; (3) when examined by electron microscopy, detergent-treated extracts of brain tissue from animals or humans affected by these diseases reveal the presence of scrapie-associated fibrils (SAFs); (4) pathologic changes are confined to the CNS and include vacuolation and astrocytosis, and (5) the transmissible agent elicits no detectable specific immune response in the host, which has inhibited the development of a live animal diagnostic test, and (6) is highly resistant to heat, ultraviolet light, ionizing radiation, and common disinfectants that normally inactivate viruses or bacteria. Specific types of TSEs include scrapie, which affects sheep and goats; transmissible mink encephalopathy; feline spongiform encephalopathy (FSE); chronic wasting disease of deer and elk; and kuru, Creutzfeldt-Jakob disease (CJD), Gerst-mann-Sträussler-Scheinker syndrome, and fatal familial insomnia, and new variant Creutzfeldt-Jakob disease (NVCJD), five diseases in humans.

ETIOLOGY

The clinical, pathologic, and molecular genetic features of BSE, as well as other transmissible spongiform encephalopathies, have led to speculation on the nature of the etiologic agent and the pathogenetic mechanisms of the disease. There are three main theories on the nature of the scrapie agent: (1) the *virus theory*, in which the virus would have to have unusual biochemical and biophysical characteristics that would help explain the remarkable physiochemical properties; (2) the *prion theory*, in which the agent is composed exclusively of the host-coded protein (PrP^c) that becomes partially protease-resistant (PrP^{BSE}), most likely through a post-transitional conformation change after infection. In this theory there are no non-host components of the agent; that is, a specific informational molecule (nucleic acid, e.g., RNA or DNA) is not present; and (3) the *virino theory*, which states that the agent consists of a host-derived protein coat, with PrP being one of the candidates for this protective protein, and a small noncoding regulatory nucleic acid.

All of the proposed theories have some degree of validity. Proponents of the virus and virino theories conclude that the existence of different scrapie strains unequivocally proves the existence of a nucleic acid component of the infectious agent which, as in conventional viruses, may undergo mutations responsible for phenotypic variations. The problem with these theories is that no agent-specific nucleic acid has been convincingly identified to copurify with infectivity.

It should be pointed out that the prion theory fails to explain (1) how the PrP of the infecting agents originally assumed the aberrant structure associated with infectivity, and (2) how the different structures originated as a function of the different strains. Although numerous scrapie strains can be differentiated in a single host (e.g., sheep), the PrP associated with these strains has not shown any biochemical and molecular differences. BSE seems to be caused by a single strain type. This BSE strain is different from historical or contemporary isolates from sheep or goats with natural scrapie, as determined by study of incubation periods and brain "lesion profiles" in mice.

Regardless whether the prion (PrP^{BSE}) is or is not the agent, the partially protease-resistant form is a marker of infection. There are currently a number of tests which may be used to detect the presence of the PrP^{BSE}.

EPIZOOTIOLOGY

There are different scientific hypotheses concerning the origins of BSE. The epidemiologic data suggest that BSE in Great Britain is an extended common-source epidemic involving feed containing TSE-contaminated meat and bone meal as a protein source. The causative agent is suspected to be from either scrapie-affected sheep or cattle with a previously unidentified TSE. Changes in rendering operations in the early 1980s—particularly the removal of a solvent-extraction process that included a steam-heat treatment—may have played a part in the appearance of the disease and the subsequent amplification of the agent in the food chain. In Great Britain the epidemic peaked in 1992–1993, with approximately 1000 cases being reported per week. In 1998 it remains on the decline with approximately 100 or fewer cases reported per week, indicating that control measures have been effective. Cases that have been detected in other countries appear to be a result of importations of live cattle or, more significantly, contaminated feed from Great Britain.

There is no evidence that BSE spreads horizontally, that is, by contact between unrelated adult cattle and from cattle to other species. New evidence suggests that maternal transmission may occur at an extremely low level. This study did not ascertain if this was the result of genetic factors or of true transmission. This level most likely would not perpetuate the epidemic under British farming conditions. Research continues in this area.

A TSE has been diagnosed in eight species of captive wild ruminants as well as exotic and domestic cats. There have been about 70 cases of FSE in Great Britain, one domestic cat in Norway, one in Northern Ireland, and one in Liechtenstein. The agent isolated from several of these cases is indistinguishable from BSE in cattle using strain typing in mice, suggesting that FSE is actually BSE in exotic and domestic cats. This also appears to be true for the other ruminants. Epidemiologic evidence suggests BSE-contaminated feed to be the primary source of infection in these species.

It has also been suggested that 25 cases (as of April 1998) of a variant form of CJD (NVCJD) in Great Britain and France may be linked to exposure to BSE before the introduction of a specified bovine offal (SBO) ban at slaughter in 1989. The SBO ban excluded from human consumption brain, spinal cord, and other tissues with potential BSE infectivity. NVCJD differs from the sporadic CJD in that the affected individuals are much younger, the clinical course of the disease is longer (13 months vs. 6 months), and, although brain pathology was recognizable as a spongiform encephalopathy, the lesion pattern was different, being composed of large aggregates of prion protein plaques. Research has found evidence to further support a causal association between NVCJD and BSE. Two significant studies published in the Oct 2, 1997 edition of *Nature* lead experts to conclude that BSE agent is highly likely to be the cause of NVCJD.

CLINICAL SIGNS

Cattle affected by BSE develop a progressive degeneration of the CNS. Affected animals may display changes in temperament, abnormalities of posture and movement, and changes in sensation. Specifically, the signs include apprehension, nervousness or aggression, incoordination, especially hind-limb ataxia, tremor and difficulty in rising, and hyperesthesia to sound and touch. In addition, many animals have decreased milk production and loss of body condition despite continued appetite. There is no treatment and affected cattle die.

The incubation period ranges from 2 to 8 years. Following the onset of clinical signs, the animal's condition gradually deteriorates until the animal becomes recumbent, dies, or is destroyed. This usually takes from 2 weeks to 6 months. Most cases in Great Britain have occurred in dairy cows (Friesians) between 3 and 6 years of age.

DIAGNOSIS

The diagnosis of BSE is based on the occurrence of clinical signs of the disease and currently must be confirmed by post-mortem laboratory testing. Histopathologic examination of brain tissue collected after the animal dies or is euthanized is the initial step in the diagnostic process. Bilaterally symmetrical vacuolar changes are usually seen in the gray matter neuropil of the brain stem giving the impression of a spongy brain. In addition, vacuolation or microcavitation of nerve cells is seen in the brain stem nuclei. Hypertrophy of astrocytes often accompanies the vacuolation. A diagnosis may also be made by the detection of SAFs using electron microscopy. Other supplemental tests are available to enhance the diagnostic capabilities for BSE. Research has shown that the partially protease-resistant form of the prion protein (PrP[BSE]) is found in the brain of BSE-infected cattle. There are two tests which may currently be used to detect the PrP[BSE]. These are immunohistochemistry and the Western blot technique. In the past, if the brain tissue was not harvested shortly after the animal's death, autolysis could make it very difficult to confirm a diagnosis. Both of these supplemental tests allow for the possibility of confirming a diagnosis of BSE even if the brain has been frozen or autolyzed.

The differential diagnosis for BSE includes rabies, listeriosis, nervous ketosis, milk fever, grass tetany, neoplasia, lead poisoning, and other toxicities or etiologic agents which affect the nervous system or musculoskeletal system of adult cattle.

TREATMENT, PREVENTION, AND CONTROL

There is no known treatment for BSE or any of the TSEs and there is no preventive vaccine. The introduction of BSE from foreign sources may be prevented by the implementation of import regulations prohibiting live ruminants and ruminant products (especially meat and bone meal and offal). Since the origin of BSE remains unknown, preventing a domestic epidemic of BSE would involve, at a minimum, the prohibition of feeing ruminant proteins to ruminants. The prevention program of any country should also include an active surveillance program for the early detection of BSE.

Agricultural officials in countries known to have BSE have taken a series of actions to control and hopefully eradicate BSE. These include making BSE a notifiable disease, prohibiting the inclusion of certain animal proteins in ruminant rations (the feed bans vary depending on the amount of BSE detected), and the depopulation of certain populations of cattle thought to be at higher risk as indicated by epidemiologic findings.

To minimize human exposure to the BSE agent, countries have established prohibitions on the inclusion of high-risk material in foods, pharmaceuticals, cosmetics, and so forth.

The US policy has been to be proactive and preventive. The US Department of Agriculture (USDA) has taken measures in surveillance, prevention, education, and response. Import restrictions have been in place since 1989 and active surveillance efforts began in 1990. BSE is a reportable disease. The USDA continually monitors and assesses all ongoing events and research findings regarding spongiform encephalopathies, as new information and knowledge may lead to revised conclusions and prevention measures. The Food and Drug Administration (FDA) has recently established regulations which prohibit the feeding of most mammalian proteins to ruminants.

BIBLIOGRAPHY

Bovine Spongiform Encepahlopathy in Great Britain: A Progress Report. London, UK Ministry of Agriculture, Foods and Fisheries, June 1997.
Bruce ME, Will RG, Ironside JW, et al: Transmissions to mice indicate that "new variant" CJD is caused by the BSE agent. Nature 389:498–501, 1997.
Collinge J, Sidle KCL, Meads J, et al: Molecular analysis of prion strain variation and the aetiology of "new variant" CJD. Nature 383:685–690, 1996.
Detwiler LA, Jenny AL, Rubenstein R, et al: Scrapie: A review. Sheep Goat Res J 12:111–131, 1997.
Hill AF, Desbruslais M, Joiner S, et al: The same prion strain causes vCJD and BSE. Nature 389:448–450, 1997.
Kimberlin RH: Bovine spongiform encephalopathy. Rev Sci Tech 11:347–390, 1992.
Wells GAH, Scott AC, Johnson CT, et al: A novel progressive spongiform encephalopathy in cattle. Vet Rec 121:419–420, 1987.
Wilesmith JW, Ryan JBM, Atkinson MJ: Bovine spongiform encephalopathy: Epidemiological studies on the origin. Vet Rec 128:199–203, 1991.
Wilesmith JW, Ryan JBM, Hueston WD, et al: Bovine spongiform encephalopathy: Epidemiological features 1985–1990. Vet Rec 130:90–94, 1992.
Will G, Ironside JW, Zeidler M, et al: A new variant of Creutzfeldt-Jakob disease in the UK. Lancet 347:921–925, 1996.

■ Caprine Arthritis-Encephalitis Virus

Donald P. Knowles, Jr., D.V.M., Ph.D.

The lentivirus caprine arthritis-encephalitis virus (CAEV)[1, 2] causes inflammation in synovial spaces, mammary gland, brain, and lung. Arthritis, the form seen most often clinically, is characterized by bilateral or unilateral swelling of carpal joints (Fig. 1). Mastitis is clinically recognized as diffuse swelling of the mammary gland with associated firmness. Encephalitis, which occurs most often in goats 1 to 5 months of age, presents as an ascending paralysis. An interstitial pneumonia, similar to that described for sheep infected with ovine progressive pneumonia virus (OPPV), has been found in goats infected with CAEV.

EPIZOOTIOLOGY

CAEV occurs worldwide, with the highest prevalence of infected goats occurring in industrialized countries. A 1981 serologic survey of 1160 goats from 24 states within the United States revealed that 81% of the goats tested were seropositive.[3] Other industrialized countries such as Canada, France, Norway, and Switzerland have CAEV prevalence levels of 65% or greater, and within individual infected herds, up to 100% of the goats may have CAEV antibody.[4] In contrast, Australia, New

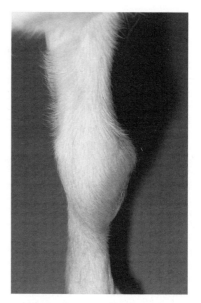

Figure 1

Carpus from a 5-year-old goat experimentally infected with CAEV as a kid. Notice marked periarticular swelling.

Zealand, and England have prevalence levels of 10% or less. Developing countries with no or low levels of CAEV-positive goats include Kenya, Mexico, Peru, Somalia, Sudan, South Africa, and Fiji.[4] Although serologic prevalence of OPPV or CAEV within a flock or herd can reach 90%, the majority of infected goats do not develop overt clinical disease. Clinical disease, as measured by swelling of the carpal joints, varies among herds and occurs in approximately 9% to 38% of seropositive animals. The incidence of clinical mastitis, encephalitis, and pneumonia caused by CAEV is not documented; however, the encephalitic form appears to be rare in the United States.

ETIOLOGY

CAEV is in the family Retroviridae and the genus *Lentivirus.* Other lentiviruses include equine infectious anemia virus, OPPV, feline immunodeficiency virus, bovine immunodeficiency virus, and the causative viruses of the acquired immunodeficiency syndromes of humans and nonhuman primates. Primary cultures of caprine synovial membrane, choroid plexus, and blood monocytes support CAEV replication.

TRANSMISSION

The major route of transmission for CAEV is via colostrum and milk from the doe to the newborn.[5] Contact transmission among adults, except during lactation, is not an efficient route of transmission. Intrauterine infection is rare, if it occurs at all, and transmission by aerosol has not been demonstrated. An understanding of the efficiency of transmission from the doe to the newborn is critical to the diagnosis of CAEV infection. Because anti-CAEV antibody cotransfers with virus during nursing, the finding of passively transferred anti-CAEV antibody in the neonate essentially indicates infection. Although in rare instances kids challenged with virus resist infection, from the standpoint of eradication programs, the presence of antiviral antibody in the milk or colostrum should be assumed to indicate that CAEV was also present and that transmission is likely to have occurred. No experimental evidence indicates that the presence of antiviral antibody in the milk impedes transmission.

PATHOGENESIS

Currently, of the multiorgan systems that CAEV affects, the pathogenesis of the arthritis is best understood. Carpal swelling can be detected as early as 6 months after experimental oral infection of newborn kids. In approximately 25% to 40% of experimentally infected kids, the course of the carpal swelling is progressive and characterized by recurrent episodes of active arthritis interspersed with periods of quiescence.[6] It appears that the goats, which eventually develop the most severe carpal arthritis, have recurrent episodes of periarticular swelling early in the disease course.

All evidence indicates that CAEV causes persistent infection in goats and that infection is for life. CAEV infects monocytes and macrophages in vitro and in vivo. Also CAEV replicates in cultures of microglial cells and synovial membrane cells. Both of these cells have characteristics of macrophages and have been shown to be targets of CAEV replication in vivo. Evaluation of synovial fluid from arthritic joints indicates that (1) there is a high concentration of immunoreactants, including cells and immunoglobulin, in the synovial fluid[7]; (2) a large amount of the synovial fluid antibody is specific for CAEV[7]; (3) virus can often be isolated from synovial fluid; (4) the isolation of virus from the synovial fluid correlates with the severity of arthritis as

measured by joint swelling; and (5) virus expressing antigenically variable neutralization-sensitive epitopes arises in joint fluid during chronic CAEV arthritis.[8] Additionally, goats challenged with CAEV during persistent CAEV infection or after vaccination with inactivated virus develop more severe arthritis than do uninfected or nonvaccinated goats.[9]

These observations support the hypothesis that CAEV arthritis is an immunopathologic process in which specific antibody and sensitized lymphocytes react with CAEV antigen in the synovial cavity. Furthermore, virus isolates expressing antigenically variable neutralization-sensitive epitopes and the immune response to these variants may contribute to periods of inflammation and progression of the arthritis.

CLINICAL SIGNS

Clinically, the arthritis caused by CAEV is characterized by bilateral or unilateral swelling of carpal joints (see Fig. 1). Clinical features of advanced disease are emaciation, rough and long hair coat, gait abnormalities, and carpal hygroma.[3]

The encephalitic form of CAEV infection is recognized most often in goats 1 to 5 months of age. Clinically, an ascending paralysis leads to recumbency. Even though recumbent, the goats are afebrile, alert, and maintain a good appetite. More severe signs include upward deviation of the head, twisting of the neck, and paddling movements of the feet. Regardless of the stage of progression, signs rarely if ever regress owing to the irreversible central nervous system damage.

The mastitis caused by CAEV presents as a diffuse swelling of the mammary gland with associated firmness. In some does, there is a marked acute swelling of the mammary gland that decreases with time; however, the mammary gland never completely returns to its original size or consistency. Experience with the experimentally infected herds indicates that the udder of nonpregnant does is susceptible to CAEV-induced mastitis. As is the case with arthritis caused by CAEV, there is wide variation in the eventual clinical severity of the mastitis.

An interstitial pneumonia, similar to that described for sheep infected with OPPV, is found in herds with a high prevalence of goats serologically positive for CAEV. Clinically, the pneumonia primarily affects adults, is insidious in onset, and progressive. The goats have histories of gradual weight loss and respiratory distress.

NECROPSY FINDINGS

Although the carpal joints are often the only joints with clinically apparent periarticular swelling, on histologic examination, the atlanto-occipital, fetlock (metacarpal) stifle joints, and atlantal and supraspinous bursae are also commonly affected. In joints with advanced disease, there is often discolored synovial fluid, marked thickening of the joint capsule, and periarticular mineralization. Articular cartilage usually remains intact. On histologic examination, the arthritis is characterized by a proliferative synovitis. There is synovial membrane hyperplasia, villous hypertrophy, and infiltration by lymphocytes, macrophages, and plasma cells (Fig. 2). In goats that develop severe disease, there is often fibroris, necrosis, and mineralization of synovial membranes and periarticular collagenous structures.[10]

In the encephalitic form of CAEV infection, gross lesions of the brain and spinal cord are sometimes visible as brown areas of softening; however, the lesions are often discernible only microscopically. On histologic examination, the inflammation involves primarily the white matter and meninges and is characterized by infiltrations of lymphocytes and demyelination.

The mastitis caused by CAEV is characterized histologically

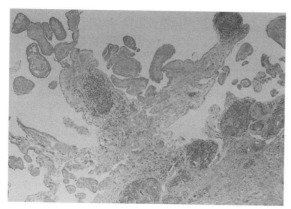

Figure 2

Radiocarpal synovium of CAEV-infected goat. Notice the synovial membrane hyperplasia, ischemic necrosis, and synovial and subsynovial cellular infiltrates (stain, hematoxylin-eosin).

by multifocal to diffuse periductal accumulations of lymphocytes, macrophages, and plasma cells.[11] In the more severe cases, affected parts of the mammary gland resemble lymphoid tissue.

Lungs affected by CAEV infection are swollen, firm on palpation, and have 1 to 2 mm gray foci on the cut surface. On histologic examination, the alveolar septa are irregularly thickened with lymphocytes and macrophages.[12] Lymphoid aggregates are present in some septa, usually adjacent to small vessels and bronchioles. Bronchial lymph nodes are often hyperplastic.

DIAGNOSIS

The most practical approach to confirming a diagnosis of CAEV infection is a combination of serology and clinical signs. Although a number of enzyme-linked immunosorbent assays (ELISAs) have been described for the detection of anti-CAEV antibody, the most widely used serologic test is the agar gel immunodiffusion (AGID) test. The sensitivity of the AGID test is dependent on the antigen used. When compared to the immunoprecipitation assay, the sensitivity of the AGID test for anti-CAEV antibody was 35% greater with CAEV antigen than with antigen from the related OPPV.[13] A question often raised concerning serologic detection of CAEV infections is whether antibody is an indication of persistent infection. Although instances have been reported in which goats were negative for anti-CAEV antibody and positive for viral nucleic acid, the majority of evidence indicates that once a goat is infected with CAEV, it is infected for life. The result of persistent infection is that a positive serologic test for CAEV indicates the goat is infected for life and is a continual potential source of virus transmission.

CONTROL AND PREVENTION

The important aspects of CAEV infection that must be considered in designing a prevention program are the following: (1) CAEV persists for life in the infected host; (2) a major route of transmission is to kids via colostrum and milk during nursing; (3) contact transmission among adults can occur; (4) there can be marked variability among individual goats in the time from infection to a positive serologic test. With consideration of these aspects of CAEV pathogenesis, a practical approach to preventing CAEV infection of newborn goats and reducing the prevalence of CAEV within a herd was devised.[5, 14] First, all kids must be immediately removed from the dam at birth, and there

should be no contact of the newborn kids with secretions of the dam. The kids should be isolated from infected goats and provided colostrum from known virus-free does. Colostrum from CAEV-positive does can be used if it is treated at 56°C for 1 hour. Further nutrition is goat milk from does free of virus, pasteurized cow milk, or pasteurized goat milk from infected does. Goats raised in this manner should be serologically tested for CAEV every 6 months, and those testing positive must be removed.

TREATMENT

With the current absence of a vaccine to prevent infection or a method to clear individual goats of CAEV, any treatment of clinical disease is only palliative. Management of caprine arthritis-encephalitis must be at the level of preventing transmission and reducing the prevalence of infected goats within a herd. Any attempt to reduce CAEV infection in a goat herd must take into account that a positive serologic result indicates a goat is infected for life and a potential, continual source for transmission of CAEV.

REFERENCES

1. Crawford TB, Adams DS, Cheevers WP, et al: Chronic arthritis in goats caused by a retrovirus. Science 207:997, 1980.
2. Cork LC, Hadlow WJ, Crawford TB, et al: Infectious leukoencephalomyelitis of young goats. J Infect Dis 129:134, 1974.
3. Crawford TB, Adams DS: Caprine arthritis–encephalitis: Clinical features and presence of antibody in selected goat populations. J Am Vet Med Assoc 178:713–719, 1981.
4. Adams DS, Oliver RE, Ameghino E, et al: Global survey of serological evidence of caprine arthritis-encephalitis virus infection. Vet Rec 115:493, 1984.
5. Adams DS, Klevjer-Anderson P, Carlson JL, et al: Transmission and control of caprine arthritis–encephalitis virus. Am J Vet Res 44:1670, 1983.
6. Cheevers WP, Knowles DP, McGuire TC, et al: Chronic disease in goats orally infected with two isolates of the caprine arthritis–encephalitis lentivirus. Lab Invest 58:510, 1988.
7. Johnson GC, Barbet AF, Klevjer-Anderson P, et al: Preferential immune response to virion surface glycoproteins by caprine arthritis–encephalitis virus–infected goats. Infect Immun 41:657, 1983.
8. McGuire TC, Norton LK, O'Rourke KI, et al: Antigenic variation of neutralization-sensitive epitopes of caprine arthritis–encephalitis lentivirus during persistent arthritis. J Virol 62:3488, 1988.
9. McGuire TC, Adams DS, Johnson GC, et al: Acute arthritis in caprine arthritis–encephalitis virus challenge exposure of vaccinated or persistently infected goats. Am J Vet Res 47:537, 1986.
10. Crawford TB, Adams DS, Sande RD, et al: The connective tissue component of the caprine arthritis–encephalitis syndrome. Am J Pathol 100:443, 1980.
11. Kennedy-Stoskopf S, Narayan O, Strandberg JD: The mammary gland as a target organ for infection with caprine arthritis encephalitis virus. J Comp Pathol 95:609, 1985.
12. Robinson WF, Ellis TM: The pathological features of an interstitial pneumonia of goats. J Comp Pathol 94:55, 1984.
13. Knowles DP, Evermann JF, Shropshire C, et al: Evaluation of agar gel immunodiffusion serology using caprine and ovine lentiviral antigens for detection of antibody to caprine arthritis–encephalitis virus. J Clin Microbiol 32:243, 1994.
14. Robinson WF, Ellis TM: Caprine arthritis–encephalitis virus infection: From recognition to eradication. Aust Vet J 63:237, 1986.

BIBLIOGRAPHY

Cheevers WP, McGuire TC: The lentiviruses: Maedi/visna, caprine arthritis–encephalitis, and equine infectious anemia. Adv Virus Res 34:189, 1988.

Clements JE, Zink MC: Molecular biology and pathogenesis of animal lentivirus infections. Clin Microbiol Rev, 9:100, 1996.

Knowles DP: Laboratory diagnostic tests for retrovirus infections of small ruminants. Vet Clin North Am Food Anim Pract 13:1–11, 1997.

McGuire TC, O'Rourke KI, Knowles DP, et al: Caprine arthritis–encephalitis lentivirus transmission and disease. Curr Top Microbiol Immunol 160:61, 1990.

Rowe JD, East NE: Risk factors for transmission and methods for control of caprine arthritis–encephalitis virus infection. The Vet Clin North Am Food Anim Pract 13:35–53, 1997.

■ Rabies in Food Animals

Deborah J. Briggs, Ph.D.

Rabies is a bullet-shaped RNA virus belonging to the family Rhabdoviridae, the same family to which vesicular stomatitis virus belongs. Rabies virus primarily attacks nervous tissue causing central nervous system (CNS) dysfunction which in turn leads to some type of abnormal behavior. There are two recognized clinical forms of the disease: paralytic or "dumb" rabies and furious rabies. Susceptibility to rabies infection is dependent upon the host, virus variant, dose of virus inoculum, and anatomic site of virus entry. Regarding large animals, cattle are considered to be highly susceptible; sheep, goats, and horses are moderately susceptible; and swine are the least susceptible to infection.[1] Cattle are at increased risk of exposure and infection to rabies because of their curious nature and the fact that they remain outdoors for most of their lives, thus increasing their opportunity to encounter a rabid animal. There are at least six rabies virus variants recognized in terrestrial mammals in the United States, which include the raccoon, North Central skunk, South Central skunk, gray fox, red fox, and Mexican dog/coyote virus variants.[2] All of these variants as well as numerous bat rabies variants can be transmitted to mammals.

EPIDEMIOLOGY

During a 5-year period (1991–1995), 778 cattle, 60 sheep and goats, and 7 swine were confirmed rabid in the United States.[2–6] The majority of cattle infected with rabies were located throughout the midwestern states of Iowa, Texas, Minnesota, North and South Dakota, or in the eastern state of New York. Skunk rabies is endemic throughout the Midwest where there is a high density of free-ranging cattle. In New York, rabies in cattle has risen significantly as the epidemic wave front of raccoon rabies continues to spread northward through the state. Cattle are naturally curious animals and most likely are exposed through a bite to their muzzle while investigating a rabid animal exhibiting unusual behavior.

More goats and sheep were confirmed rabid in Texas than in any other state. This is due to exposure from wildlife infected with rabies. The seven cases of swine rabies reported between 1991 and 1995 were all located in the eastern states where raccoon rabies is epidemic.

Rabies in food animals, as in other domestic animals, occurs as a result of "spillover" from the endemic rabies-infected species in a region.

PATHOGENESIS

Virus is introduced into a host through a break in the skin caused by a wound, bite, or (rarely) a scratch from a rabid animal. Virus can also enter the body through mucous membranes, and on *extremely* rare occasions, when there is a high concentration of virus in a confined area, through aerosol transmission. Virus multiplies at the site of the wound and enters the nervous system through exposed sensory and motor nerve endings. The virus travels centripetally along the peripheral nervous system to the CNS. When the virus reaches the brain, it multiplies rapidly and travels centrifugally to non-nervous tissues, including the salivary glands. Once it is present in the salivary gland, the virus is ready to be transmitted to the next host, generally through a bite wound inflicted to the skin.

The length of time that rabies virus remains infective in the environment is dependent upon several factors. Virus-infected saliva from a rabid animal is considered noninfectious once it is dried. In animals that have succumbed to rabies, virus inactivation occurs more rapidly at higher temperatures. In experimental studies conducted on brain tissue from dead animals, virus was inactivated after 1 day at 80°F and after 2 days at 52°F.[7] Otherwise the virus can be inactivated by ultraviolet (UV) light, heat, formalin, aqueous solutions of bleach, or most hospital disinfectants.[8]

CLINICAL DISEASE

The clinical manifestations of rabies are dependent upon the species infected, the virus variant, and the dose of inoculum. However, in almost every case, some type of behavioral change is noted in clinically ill animals and only on extremely rare occasions do animals survive infection. Three phases of disease are generally recognized in food animals: prodrome, excitation, and paralysis.[8]

Cattle

The rabies prodrome in cattle is similar to that described in other mammals. The initial signs include discomfort at the site of the infecting wound, separation from the herd, depression, and loss of appetite. In dairy cattle, a drop in milk production is frequently reported. Initial signs may go unnoticed and are of little diagnostic value unless there is evidence that exposure to a rabid animal occurred earlier. As the prodrome continues, pharyngeal paralysis and salivation may be misdiagnosed as "choke." Human exposure frequently occurs when the owner or veterinarian attempts to dislodge an apparent object from the animal's throat. As the disease progresses, rumination may cease, which in turn results in constipation, straining, and prolapse of the rectum. The three most commonly reported clinical signs of rabies in cattle are anorexia, cessation of rumination, and hypersalivation. Other classic signs of rabies in cattle include agitation, grating teeth, head pressing, depraved appetite, flaccid tail, and muscle twitching. Sexual excitement is not an uncommon event, especially among bulls, which may exhibit priapism. Paralysis of the throat muscles produces voice changes, resulting in a characteristic hoarse "bawl," which may or may not be followed by a "yawning" syndrome.

Although rabid cattle may charge inanimate objects or humans, they frequently do not exhibit furious rabies, but rather develop the paralytic form of the disease. Progressive paralysis usually begins in the hindquarters, causing incoordination and staggering. The affected animal may sit on its hindquarters, or fall and thrash about. Excessive salivation may or may not be accompanied by hydrophobia. Paralysis is followed shortly by coma and death. The duration of the disease from initial development of clinical signs to death is approximately 4 to 7 days. Survival for longer periods of time is unusual. The clinical signs described here are common in cattle infected with rabies and may occur singly or in combination. However, atypical rabies unaccompanied by any encephalitic signs has been reported in cattle.

Sheep and Goats

Rabies in sheep and goats is similar to rabies in cattle. Initially, animals exhibit depression, anorexia, agitation, excitation, muscle twitching, staring eyes, nystagmus, or hypersalivation. During the excitation phase, rams may demonstrate sexual stimulation. Rabid sheep and goats may charge and butt objects or humans, but generally do not try to bite. The disease progresses rapidly to the paralytic phase, resulting in incoordination, stumbling and falling, and paddling. The disease terminates in convulsions, coma, and death.

Swine

As mentioned previously, swine are rarely infected with rabies. This may be due to lack of exposure or to a lower degree of susceptibility. Swine have been reported to recover from the disease, producing neutralizing antibodies, with no history of vaccination. Clinical signs of rabies in swine include incoordination, fasciculation of neck muscles, trembling, anorexia, knuckling, hypersalivation, champing jaws, recumbency, coma, and death. During the excitation phase, swine may charge and attempt to bite and sows have been reported to kill their young. The duration of the clinical disease is between 2 and 6 days.

LABORATORY DIAGNOSIS

Historically, rabies was diagnosed by the presence of intracytoplasmic inclusions or Negri bodies in the brain of infected animals. In order to reduce the high number of false-negative results, it was necessary to allow the animal to progress through the clinical stages of the disease. Even so, Negri bodies were not present in 20% to 30% of the animals infected with rabies virus.[8] Currently, all rabies diagnostic laboratories in the United States confirm the presence of rabies virus using the fluorescent antibody technique (FAT). Many laboratories also test suspect tissue using the mouse inoculation test or in vitro virus isolation. FAT permits the diagnosis of rabies in animals early in the disease, thus reducing the potential for exposure from an animal exhibiting clinical rabies. In a diagnostic laboratory with appropriate quality controls, the FAT will confirm the presence of rabies antigen in nearly 100% of infected animals.

Animals suspected of having rabies should be humanely euthanized, avoiding damage to the head. The use of barbiturates and other injectable euthanasia solutions are acceptable and do not interfere with rabies diagnosis. Once the animal has been euthanized, proper handling of the tissue specimen is critical to an accurate diagnosis. Tissues should be refrigerated as soon as possible, should not be exposed to formalin, alcohol, or other preservatives, and should be hand-carried (in the case of human exposure) or shipped to the laboratory as quickly as possible. Decomposition of the specimen may make testing impossible. Although freezing does not interfere with rabies diagnosis, it may delay examination. Continued freezing and thawing of the specimen may inactivate the virus. After euthanasia, the head can be removed anterior to the first vertebra. If precautions are taken to avoid unnecessary exposure, the brain may be removed and sent to the laboratory in lieu of sending the entire head. The entire brain, or at least the cerebellum and brain stem, should be submitted to the diagnostic laboratory for testing. Once removed, the brain should be sealed in a crush-proof container and enclosed in at least two sealed plastic bags. The package should then be placed in a Styrofoam container with gel packs or ice packs. Wet ice should not be used because of the potential for leakage of infected fluid. The Styrofoam container should be sealed and placed in a cardboard box. Every rabies diagnostic laboratory requests specific information for surveillance and testing purposes. The minimal amount of data that should be sent with the specimen includes name and address of the submitting veterinarian or physician, species of animal, date and manner of death, vaccination status, location of incident, date and nature of human or domestic animal exposure, and names and addresses of contacts and owners. In the event that an animal is confirmed positive for rabies, local and state health officials should be notified immediately.

PREVENTION AND CONTROL

Rabies can be prevented in food animals either by eliminating exposure or by eliciting an immune response. Eliminating every potential for exposure to cattle and other food animals is unrealistic in areas endemic for rabies. On the other hand, vaccinating large herds may not be economically feasible. However, in areas where rabies is endemic and valuable livestock are at risk, or in cases where there is frequent interaction between livestock and humans, vaccination is a satisfactory solution to prevent the loss of a valuable animal. In the United States there are five rabies vaccines licensed by the U.S. Department of Agriculture (USDA) for use in cattle and six rabies vaccines licensed for use in sheep and horses.[9] There are no rabies vaccines licensed for use in goats or swine. The schedule for vaccinating cattle, sheep, and horses is identical. Animals should be vaccinated at 3 months of age and 1 year after primary vaccination, followed by yearly boosters. Vaccinating goats and swine off-label will in all likelihood produce an immune response. However, health officials may not recognize rabies vaccination in goats or swine as being legal or protective.

PUBLIC HEALTH CONSIDERATIONS

Cattle and other livestock are considered to be "dead-end hosts" as far as rabies infection is concerned. Vaccinated cattle, sheep, or horses that are exposed to a known rabid animal should be immediately revaccinated and observed for 45 days.[9] Unvaccinated livestock should be immediately slaughtered. Otherwise, the animal should be isolated and observed for 6 months. If the animal is slaughtered within 7 days of being exposed, the meat may be consumed provided that the area around the infecting wound is discarded. Federal meat inspectors will reject livestock for 8 months after the date of exposure. Tissues or milk from a rabid animal should not be consumed. However, eating cooked meat and drinking pasteurized milk from a rabid animal is not considered exposure. Since it is a rare event to have more than one animal in a herd succumb to rabies, it may not be necessary to quarantine the entire herd after exposure occurs. Public health officials should be consulted regarding the disposition of animals and humans exposed to rabies. All veterinarians and veterinary assistants should be vaccinated against rabies. For humans, the preexposure vaccine process consists of a series of three injections, given on days 0, 7, and 21 or 28.[10] Previously vaccinated humans at risk of exposure to rabies should have serologic testing performed every 2 years. Booster vaccinations should be given if antibody titers fall below 1:5 or in the event of an exposure. In the event of an exposure, public health officials should be notified.

REFERENCES

1. Beran GW: Rabies and infections by rabies-related viruses. *In* Beran GW, Steele JH: Handbook of Zoonoses, Section B: Viral, ed 2. Boca Raton, Fla, CRC Press, 1994, pp 307–357.

2. Krebs JW, Strine TW, Smith JS, et al: Rabies surveillance in the United States during 1995. J Am Vet Med Assoc 209:2031–2044, 1996.
3. Krebs JW, Holman RC, Hines U, et al: Rabies surveillance in the United States during 1991. J Am Vet Med Assoc 201:1836–1848, 1992.
4. Krebs JW, Strine TW, Childs JE: Rabies surveillance in the United States during 1992. J Am Vet Med Assoc 203:1718–1731, 1993.
5. Krebs JW, Strine TW, Smith JS, et al: Rabies surveillance in the United States during 1993. J Am Vet Med Assoc 205:1695–1709, 1994.
6. Krebs JW, Strine TW, Smith JS, et al: Rabies surveillance in the United States during 1994. J Am Vet Med Assoc 207:1562–1575, 1995.
7. Burkel MD, Andrews MF, Meslow EC: Rabies detection in road-killed skunks (*Mephitis mephitis*). J Wildl Dis 6:496–499, 1970.
8. Debbie JG, Trimarchi CV: Rabies. *In* Castro AE, Heuschele WP: Veterinary Diagnostic Virology: A Practitioners Guide. St Louis, Mosby–Year Book, 1992, pp 116–120.
9. Compendium of animal rabies control, 1997. J Am Vet Med Assoc 210:33–37, 1997.
10. Rabies prevention—United States, 1991. Recommendations of the Immunization Practices Advisory Committee (ACIP). MMWR 40 (RR-3):1–19, 1991.

■ Malignant Catarrhal Fever

Timothy B. Crawford, D.V.M., Ph.D.,
Donal O'Toole, M.V.B., Ph.D., F.R.C.Path.
Hong Li, D.V.M., Ph.D.

Malignant catarrhal fever (MCF) is a serious, globally distributed viral disease syndrome of certain susceptible ruminant species that has an intricate and as yet poorly understood epidemiology and pathogenesis. It is of greatest economic importance in domestic cattle breeds, but also can inflict serious losses in exotic and wild ruminants on game farms and in zoos. Certain other ruminant species are well adapted to the causative viruses, and serve as subclinical sources of transmission to susceptible species. The two most prominent reservoirs for MCF viruses are domestic sheep and wildebeest.

ETIOLOGY

There are at least two, and probably more, closely related viruses that are etiologically associated with MCF. They are classified in the subfamily Gammaherpesvirinae, the group that contains other important lymphotrophic herpesviruses such as Epstein-Barr virus of man and *Herpesvirus saimiri* of primates. Sheep and wildebeest (subfamily Alcelaphinae) provide the source of virus for most outbreaks of MCF in cattle. These sources represent the reservoir for the two major MCF viruses, which are closely related antigenically and genetically. However, their genomes can be readily distinguished by polymerase chain reaction (PCR) or restriction enzyme digestion, and the "lifestyles" of the two viruses within their respective reservoir hosts (sheep and wildebeest) appear to differ significantly from one another.[1, 2] Nevertheless the signs and lesions induced by these two strains of virus are indistinguishable.

The virus that is endemic in wildebeest can be isolated and propagated in vitro.[3] Considerably more is therefore known about this agent than about the one in sheep, which has never been successfully propagated. It was named acelaphine herpesvirus 1 (AHV-1) in reference to the wildebeests' subfamily. The agent that is endemic in sheep, though never isolated, has nevertheless been designated ovine herpesvirus 2 (OHV-2) on the basis of its antigenic and base sequence relatedness to AHV-1. It is referred to herein as the sheep-associated MCF virus (SA-

MCFV). The envelopes of these viruses are fragile, and thus close contact and cool, moist weather maximize the efficiency of transmission.

EPIZOOTIOLOGY

Most ruminant species are susceptible to infection with MCF virus.[4] The nature and impact of that infection, however, are variable, ranging from totally subclinical in well-adapted reservoir species, to rapidly lethal in species of high clinical susceptibility.

Reservoir Hosts

Almost all adult domestic sheep and wildebeest that are living under natural flock or herd conditions are infected.[3, 5] Though these two groups represent the source of most cases of MCF, other species are now known to harbor the virus, but the nature of the infection and the ability to transmit the virus are generally unclear. Exceptions include certain exotic species of sheep such as mouflons, and domestic goats, for which considerable evidence exists to implicate them in disease transmission. In the wildebeest, although transplacental infection occasionally occurs, AHV-1 usually passes from the dam to the newborn calf shortly after birth. Infection ensues, which results in active viral shedding to the environment in naso-ocular secretions, primarily during the first 3 months or so of life. Shedding ceases thereafter, presumably due to the emergence of an effective antiviral immune response. The calves are responsible for most cases of transmission to cattle.

The epizootiology of the sheep agent is somewhat controversial at present. Some reports suggest it is very similar to the wildebeest, in that infection occurs during the perinatal period.[6] Conversely, data from our laboratories indicate that the pattern varies somewhat from the wildebeest, in that most lambs appear not to be infected during the perinatal period, but several months later.[1] Recent data have shown that lambs weaned and removed from the flock at a sufficiently young age escape infection, and remain free of virus as long as they are not exposed to infected sheep.[2] Infection of lambs is predominantly horizontal, between flockmates. The site of viral shedding is apparently the nasopharynx, as it is in the wildebeest. More studies are needed in this area, to clarify the epidemiology of the infection in sheep.

Clinically Susceptible Hosts

These include many species belonging to the subfamilies Bovinae (cattle, buffalo, bison, gaur), Cervinae and Odocoilinae (deer, moose, elk, and reindeer, as well as duikers), and several other ruminant species. Only the basic outlines of the epizootiology of MCF are understood at present. Although the kinetics of some outbreaks can be explained, the frequent occurrence of puzzling epizootiologic patterns[7] is a humbling reminder of the meagerness of our current knowledge.

MCF is usually sporadic, with only one to a few cases occurring at a given time. Severe outbreaks with heavy losses are, however, not uncommon.[8–10] Whether transmitted from sheep or from wildebeest, the majority of, though not all, cases in cattle occur around the time of lambing or calving. The epizootiology of SA-MCF is as yet less well understood than that of wildebeest-associated MCF. Secretions from the neonatal wildebeest clearly are the predominant source of virus, but lambs have not yet been proved definitively to be the source of virus for most cases of SA-MCF. The ewes themselves or placental tissues are also potential viral sources. Clarification of this issue needs further study. Transmission is considered to be mostly due to direct contact with infected secretions or fluids, either by direct animal interaction or via fomites, including feeders, common water sources, birds, and caregivers.[3] Direct contact, however, is not absolutely necessary, as transmission sometimes occurs over short to moderate distances.[7, 8] Claims of aerosol transmission exist but are difficult to evaluate.

In addition to clustering during lambing season, significant numbers of cases of SA-MCF are also seen in late summer and fall, several months after the end of lambing season. Further, following removal of all sheep from the premises to quell outbreaks, cases may continue to occur for the next 3 or 4 months. Cases such as these apparently represent recrudescence of infections established earlier. Occasional transplacental transmission from cows to their fetuses has been reported with AHV-1.[3] The preponderance of the evidence suggests that clinically susceptible animals are dead-end hosts and do not transmit the virus horizontally to herdmates. What sometimes appear as epizootics of MCF probably represent multiple cases from common-source exposures.

Inapparent infections are not uncommon among clinically susceptible ruminants. Surveys[11] have shown that a minimum of 4% to 13% of cattle with no history of MCF-like disease are seropositive, as are similar percentages of whitetail and mule deer, elk, bison, and captive moose. These latent infections, under conditions not yet understood, sometimes reactivate, leading to acute disease. No figures are available on the probability of recrudescence or factors influencing its occurrence. In the absence of recrudescence, antibody can wane in these latently infected, clinically susceptible species until it can no longer be detected by current assays.[12]

PREVALENCE AND CASE FATALITY RATE

MCF is a significantly underreported disease. Probably 70% or more of bovine MCF cases are misdiagnosed, escape detection, or are simply not reported to laboratories. Recent detailed investigations in Switzerland revealed that only about 20% to 25% of cases of MCF are actually recognized (U. Müller-Doblies, personal communication, 1996). Lethal cases of MCF often are readily diagnosed clinically or by histopathology, but the subacute and chronic cases, which occur with some frequency,[12] often are never diagnosed, particularly if the animal recovers. Most descriptions of MCF include a very high case fatality rate.[13] Published estimates are based primarily on studies using parenterally inoculated AHV-1 virus,[3] and are probably too high for SA-MCF that is acquired by natural exposure. Improved diagnostic tools have recently enabled recognition of "atypical" cases that have historically gone undetected,[12] allowing a more realistic estimate of MCF lethality. A case fatality rate for SA-MCF of 50% to 70%, rather than the traditional 95% or greater is probably more accurate.

CLINICAL SIGNS

Clinical expression of MCF is quite variable, both as regards organ involvement and rapidity of progression. Classic descriptions of acute MCF divide the syndrome into "forms," for example, head and eye, alimentary, encephalitic, skin form, and so forth. These are arbitrary classifications, reflecting little of a fundamental nature. In significant outbreaks, several forms can often be seen on a single premise. Incubation periods are highly variable, ranging from 18 to over 100 days.[3, 14] Leukopenia may occur early in the disease but can be easily missed. MCF is basically lymphoproliferative, involving hyperplasia and perivas-

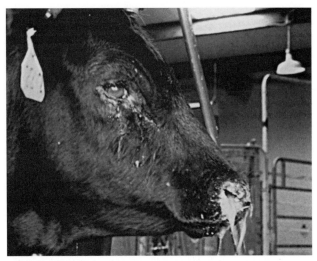

Figure 1
Heifer with acute MCF on third day of clinical signs. Animal has profuse nasal discharge and is blind from corneal edema.

cular accumulation of lymphocytes and other mononuclear cells, leading to inflammation and necrosis of serosal and mucosal surfaces and vessels, particularly medium-sized arteries (200 to 400 μm). The mechanism of lymphoproliferation and inflammation has not been worked out and has been the target of much conjecture. No viral antigen can be demonstrated in the lesions and no viral particles are evident ultrastructurally. Hypothesized mechanisms of damage include lymphoid dysregulation leading to proliferation of cytotoxic T cells and overproduction of tissue-damaging lymphokines, among others. Fundamental studies in this area are needed.

Fairly consistent signs of acute disease include prolonged high fever, salivation, lacrimation, photophobia, conjunctivitis, corneal edema, purulent nasal discharge, and generalized lymph node enlargement (Figs. 1 and 2). Corneal opacity, beginning as a fine line near the limbus and spreading centripetally, is almost pathognomonic if present.[3] Ocular involvement can progress to iridocyclitis, panophthalmitis, corneal ulceration, and staphyloma, particularly in cases that survive for longer periods[3, 12] (Fig. 3). Some animals, more commonly those with SA-MCF than wildebeest-associated MCF, exhibit extensive ali-

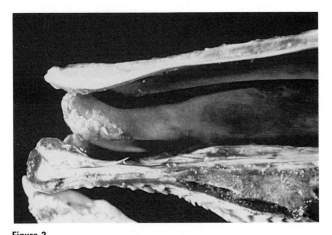

Figure 2
Sagittal section of the head of a heifer with acute MCF. The animal was exhibiting profuse nasal discharge. Note localized lesion on rostral aspect of turbinate.

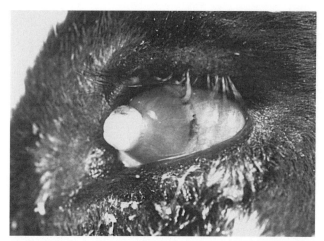

Figure 3
Prolapse of the iris in a heifer with MCF. This animal eventually recovered clinically.

mentary involvement, with oral, esophageal, and intestinal ulceration; diarrhea; and severe dehydration. Subclinical arthritis and synovitis are common, with lameness and cloudy or bloody synovial fluids being seen occasionally.[14] Skin involvement, consisting of hyperemia, or necrotic and hemorrhagic lesions of the muzzle, udder, legs, or between the digits, is commonly seen. Generalized vesicular ulcerative dermatitis occurs occasionally. Heavy encrustations of the muzzle may develop, which, if removed, leave a raw, bleeding surface. Also not uncommon is nervous system involvement, manifesting as tremors, ataxia, altered gait, circling, twitching of the ears, or aggressiveness.[3, 8] Some animals, particularly deer, die peracutely with few or no premonitory signs.

A significant proportion of cattle with SA-MCF will recover or survive for extended periods if provided with supportive therapy. Subacute or chronic debilitation may result, or the animals may recover with few residual effects.[9, 12] Animals with the chronic syndrome may develop a chronic obliterative arteriopathy,[15] with myointimal thickening in muscular arteries that may be apparent grossly (Fig. 4). They often will suffer permanent corneal scarring, leading to partial visual impairment or blindness due to destruction of corneal endothelium.[12] As with any herpesvirus, recovered animals remain infected indefinitely.

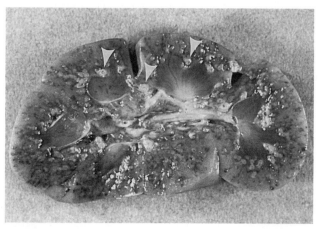

Figure 4
Kidney from a cow with chronic MCF. Note multiple petechial and ecchymotic hemorrhages *(dark spots)* and enlarged and thickened arteries, which are visible grossly *(arrowheads)*.

DIAGNOSIS

Typical acute cases of MCF can often be diagnosed clinically. A combination of high fever, salivation, profuse purulent nasal discharge, enlarged lymph nodes, and the characteristic bilateral corneal edema can be quite diagnostic. Often, however, the animals succumb before diagnostic signs develop, particularly in highly susceptible cervid species. On necropsy, one may observe swollen, hemorrhagic lymph nodes, tonsils, and Peyer's patches, erosions of the alimentary or nasal mucosa, or contrarily, few gross lesions may be found.[8] In these cases, histopathologic study often reveals the widespread lymphoproliferation and vasculitis, which may be highly indicative of MCF. Frequently, however, further criteria are needed to rule out bovine virus diarrhea (BVD) and mucosal disease, infectious bovine rhinotracheitis (IBR), or epizootic hemorrhagic disease (EHD) of deer. Morphologically, BVD in cattle, and EHD and bluetongue in deer can be particularly difficult to differentiate from MCF. The presence of florid necrotizing arteritis in medium-caliber vessels within multiple organs is, however, strongly suggestive of MCF.

Tests available for laboratory confirmation consist of serology, PCR, and viral isolation. Viral isolation is of little practical use in field diagnosis. Only the wildebeest strains can be cultivated in vitro; at present the sheep strains cannot. Moreover, isolation is too unreliable and takes too long to be of topical usefulness. However, efficient laboratory diagnostic tests are now available to detect the DNA of both AHV-1 and OHV-2 strains of MCF virus, and to measure anti-MCF antibody. Acute cases in susceptible species such as cattle are best confirmed by detecting viral DNA in the blood. All animals with acute MCF have high levels of viral DNA in circulating lymphocytes, which readily can be detected by PCR, using appropriate primers. The clinician should inform the laboratory as to which virus strain is suspected, sheep or wildebeest, so that the laboratory can use appropriate primers, many of which are strain-specific.[16] Submitting anticoagulated blood allows the laboratory to test both for DNA in the cells and for antibody in the plasma. At necropsy, the best tissue to submit for PCR is lymph node or spleen, although virtually any organ from acutely ill animals will yield positive results. PCR can also be conducted on DNA extracted from formalin-fixed, paraffin-embedded tissues, which is particularly useful for retrospective studies.[17]

Antibody testing in acutely ill animals can also be diagnostically useful. Serology is available at selected laboratories around the world. Polyclonal antibody assays such as immunofluorescence and conventional enzyme-linked immunosorbent assay (ELISA) are in use in some laboratories. They are useful, but suffer somewhat from a relative lack of specificity.[18] Highly specific assays based on monoclonal antibodies have recently become available,[5] representing a marked improvement in the reliability of MCF serology. One should bear in mind when interpreting serologic results that between 5% and 10% of normal cattle (and slightly lower percentages of deer, bison, and other susceptible species) are seropositive, and that about 25% of cattle with acute MCF die before producing detectable levels of antibody.[5] Thus the presence of antibody is proof of infection but not of etiology. One must also bear in mind that the significance of both serology and conventional PCR must be carefully interpreted in carrier species, in which a high proportion are naturally infected.

TREATMENT

As with most veterinary viral diseases, there is no specific treatment for MCF. General support with antibiotics, fluids, electrolytes, and topical treatment of corneal lesions may improve the recovery rate. In addition, a few reports exist of beneficial effects from the judicious use of corticosteroids.[15, 19] Corticosteroids will induce widespread necrosis in proliferating lymphoid populations in MCF. The benefits and cost-effectiveness of intensive treatment with corticosteroids, alkylating agents, antibiotics, or Vinca alkaloids have not been studied systematically owing to the difficulty and expense of reproducing the disease experimentally.

CONTROL

There is no vaccine for MCF; none of the published attempts to produce one have been successful.[3] Physical separation of carrier species (sheep, goats, wildebeest) from susceptible species is the only proven control measure available at present. The potential for recrudescence is always present in latently infected cattle or other susceptible species. Inclusion of a specific serologic examination for MCF antibody in a routine prepurchase examination to identify inapparently infected cattle, bison, or other susceptible species should be considered, to minimize the possibility of recrudescent cases. However, since there is little evidence that susceptible species shed infectious virus, even during active disease, the decision to remove all recovered or latently infected animals from the herd is difficult to justify.

REFERENCES

1. Li H, Shen DT, O'Toole D, et al: Investigation of sheep-associated malignant catarrhal fever virus infection in ruminants by PCR and competitive inhibition enzyme-linked immunosorbent assay. J Clin Microbiol 33:2048–2053, 1995.
2. Li H, Snowder G, O'Toole D, et al: Transmission of ovine herpesvirus 2 in lambs. J Clin Microbiol 36:223–226, 1998.
3. Plowright W: Malignant catarrhal fever virus. In Dinter Z, Morein B (eds): Virus Infections of Ruminants. New York, Elsevier, 1990, pp 123–150.
4. Heuschele WP: Malignant catarrhal fever: A review of a serious disease hazard for exotic and domestic ruminants. Zool Garten NF 58:123–133, 1988.
5. Li H, Shen DT, Knowles DP, et al: Competitive-inhibition enzyme-linked immunosorbent assay for antibody in sheep and other ruminants to a conserved epitope of malignant catarrhal fever virus. J Clin Microbiol 32:1674–1679, 1994.
6. Baxter SIF, Wiyono A, Pow I, et al: Identification of ovine herpesvirus-2 infection in sheep. Arch Virol 142:823–831, 1997.
7. Barnard BJ, Van de Pypekamp HE: Wildebeest-derived malignant catarrhal fever: Unusual epidemiology in South Africa. Onderstepoort J Vet Res 55:69–71, 1988.
8. Weaver LD: Malignant catarrhal fever in two California dairy herds. Bovine Pract 14:121–124, 1979.
9. Hamilton AF: Account of three outbreaks of malignant catarrhal fever in cattle in the Republic of Ireland. Vet Rec 127:231–232, 1990.
10. Collery P, Foley A: An outbreak of malignant catarrhal fever in the Republic of Ireland. Vet Rec 139:16–17, 1996.
11. Li H, Shen DT, Jessup DA, et al: Prevalence of antibody to malignant catarrhal fever virus in wild and domestic ruminants by competitive-inhibition ELISA. J Wildl Dis 32:437–443, 1996.
12. O'Toole D, Li H, Williams D, et al: Chronic and recovered cases of sheep-associated malignant catarrhal fever in cattle. Vet Rec 140:519–524, 1997.
13. Smith BP: Malignant catarrhal fever. In Smith BP (ed): Large Animal Internal Medicine (ed 2.) St Louis, Mosby–Year Book, 1996, pp 814–817.
14. Liggitt HD, DeMartini JC, McChesney AE, et al: Experimental transmission of malignant catarrhal fever in cattle: Gross and histopathological changes. Am J Vet Res 39:1249–1257, 1978.
15. O'Toole D, Li H, Roberts S, et al: Chronic generalized obliterative arteriopathy in cattle: A sequel to sheep-associated malignant catarrhal fever. J Vet Diagn Invest 7:108–121, 1995.
16. Baxter SIF, Pow I, Bridgen A, et al: PCR detection of the sheep-associated agent of malignant catarrhal fever. Arch Virol 132:145–159, 1993.
17. Crawford TB, Li H, Shen DT, et al: Diagnosis of sheep-associated malignant catarrhal fever by PCR on paraffin-embedded tissues. In Proceedings, 38th Annual Meeting of the American Association of Laboratory Diagnosticians, Reno, Nev, October 1995, p 52.
18. Heuschele WP, Seal BS: Malignant catarrhal fever. In Castro AE, Heuschele WP (eds): Veterinary Diagnostic Virology, St Louis, Mosby–Year Book, 1992, pp 108–112.
19. Milne EM, Reid HW: Recovery of a cow from malignant catarrhal fever. Vet Rec 126:640–641, 1990.

■ Foot-and-Mouth Disease*

Cecelia A. Whetstone, Ph.D.
Alfonso Torres, D.V.M., Ph.D., M.S.

Foot-and-mouth disease (FMD), a highly contagious, acute disease of domestic and wild cloven-hoofed animals, is characterized by fever, vesicular lesions, and subsequent erosions of the epithelium of the mouth, nares, feet, and teats. FMD is the number one foreign animal disease threat in the United States and is economically the most important virus disease of farm animals. Currently, FMD is not present in North and Central America or the Caribbean, but it is present in many South American countries, including Colombia, Peru, Venezuela, Bolivia, Ecuador, and northern Brazil. Argentina, the southern states of Brazil, and most of Paraguay are free of FMD, but vaccination is still heavily used as a control measure. Notably, Chile and Uruguay have been declared FMD-free countries. FMD has been eradicated from western Europe and several eastern European nations; however, it persists in Turkey, parts of Greece, and in several of the Balkan nations. Australia, New Zealand, South Korea, and Japan are free of FMD. All other countries in the world are considered infected. FMD continues to be the most significant disease affecting free trade in animals and animal products internationally.

ETIOLOGY

FMD is caused by an RNA virus, the sole member of the *Apthovirus* genus of the picornavirus family. There are seven distinct serotypes of FMD virus (FMDV), designated A, O, C, SAT-1, SAT-2, SAT-3, and Asia-1. In addition, there are more than 60 FMDV subtypes (A5, A24, O1, C3, etc.). Immunity is type- and even subtype-specific. Consequently, vaccination with some subtypes may not confer immunity against other subtypes from within the same serotype. Types A, O, and C virus occur in Europe, South America, Africa, and Asia, where Asia-1 also occurs. Types SAT 1 to 3 are generally limited to Africa. In recent years, O and A have been the predominant types associated with most reported outbreaks. FMDV may survive outside of the host for considerable periods of time in body fluids, animal products, and contaminated materials such as fodder and bedding, particularly in conditions of high relative humidity and low temperatures. The virus is destroyed by physical means such as high temperature, irradiation, or ultraviolet light and by chemicals such as formalin, sodium carbonate (4%), sodium hydroxide (1%), and citric acid (0.2%). A pH change below 6 or above 9 makes conditions for virus survival less favorable.

EPIZOOTIOLOGY

FMDV infects domesticated and wild cloven-hoofed animals, armadillos, rats, coypus, and elephants. Its greatest impact is on domestic cattle, swine, water buffalo, sheep, and goats. Horses

---

*All of the material in this article is in the public domain.

are not susceptible to FMDV infection, even experimentally. Except for a few rare laboratory infections, humans are not considered susceptible; thus FMD is not a public health concern. Dogs, cats, rabbits, mice, chinchillas, and guinea pigs are not susceptible to FMDV infection under natural conditions, but can be infected experimentally. South American camelids (llamas and alpacas) are susceptible under experimental inoculation but do not appear to be at high risk under natural field conditions. Mortality is low but morbidity is high; convalescence and virus shedding of affected animals may be protracted, and it is these features that make FMD important, particularly when the virus is introduced into a country that was previously free of the disease.

The primary route of infection is the respiratory tract by inhalation of infectious FMDV aerosols. Aerosols produced by infected animals contain large amounts of virus, and swine particularly shed the greatest amount of virus in respiratory aerosols. Large amounts of virus are excreted in the milk. FMDV is also transmitted by direct contact, by ingestion, by inoculation with contaminated vaccines, insemination with contaminated semen, and by contaminated fomites. FMDV does not survive in muscle tissue after postmortem glycolysis (due to pH below 5.9). This characteristic has permitted the international commerce of deboned and aged fresh or frozen beef from FMD-infected countries to FMD-free areas of the world. However, FMDV can survive a relatively long time in lymph nodes, bone marrow, and visceral organs where pH does not change much after death. Consequently, partially cooked or dry- or smoke-cured meat products are a high-risk commodity for the introduction of FMDV. After FMDV infection (even in the presence of vaccination) a large proportion of cattle and water buffalo can become carriers of the virus. Virus persists in and has been isolated from the pharyngeal region of carrier animals over 2 years after infection. Carrier animals, especially water buffalo, can be the source of FMD outbreaks. Clinical signs are well manifested in cattle and swine, but not in sheep and goats, in which lesions may be undetectable or nonexistent. Because of that, and because these small ruminants can become carriers, sheep and goats are considered to be silent amplifiers and potential carriers of the FMDV.

CLINICAL SIGNS AND LESIONS

In general, clinical signs of FMDV infection are most severe in cattle and swine, but outbreaks have been reported in swine while cattle in close contact did not develop clinical disease. Sheep and goats usually experience subclinical infections. Wild animals show a spectrum of responses from inapparent to severe disease or death.

Cattle

After a short postinfection incubation period of 2 to 4 days, there is fever, depression, loss of appetite, and marked drop in milk production. Infected cattle display a characteristic excess salivation and smacking of their lips, followed by the development of vesicles (blisters) on the lips, gums, tongue, nares, palate, teats, and even on the eyelids. Vesicles may also be found on the interdigital skin and coronary band of the feet, leading to severe and painful lameness (Figs. 1 and 2). When vesicles rupture, usually because of mechanical trauma, they leave eroded areas with serrated edges containing strands of vesicular epithelium. In most cases, vesicles in the tongue lift large segments of the tongue epithelium that slough, leaving large denuded areas. If vesicles develop in the more superficial layers of the stratified epithelium of the mouth, the outcome is not a

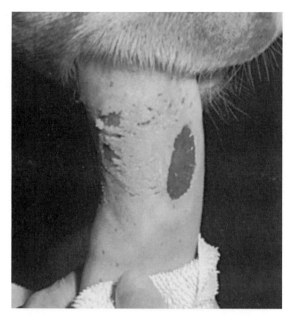

Figure 1
An eroded vesicular lesion and adjacent friable epithelium on a bovine tongue infected with foot-and-mouth disease virus.

vesicle but an erosive loss of the epithelium. It should be emphasized that the lesions of FMDV in cattle are identical to those observed in cases of vesicular stomatitis virus (VSV) infections, and cannot be differentiated by clinical observations. Lesions on the feet and within nasal cavities often become secondarily infected with bacteria, resulting in prolonged lameness and mucopurulent nasal discharge. Mortality is generally low in adults (1% to 5%) but quite high in young animals (20% to 50%), in which FMDV infection can produce a lethal necrotizing

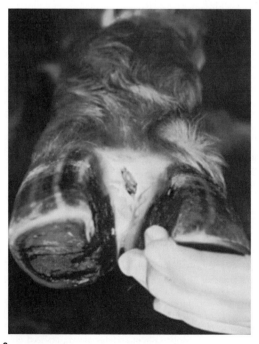

Figure 2
Ruptured vesicle on the foot of a cow caused by foot-and-mouth disease virus.

myocarditis. Although the virus does not cross the placenta, cattle may abort, presumably as a consequence of the fever. Morbidity in FMD outbreaks is extremely high and rapid, approaching 100% of susceptible animals. Affected animals become nonproductive or poorly productive for long periods. In endemic areas, where cattle may have partial immunity, the disease may be mild or subclinical.

Swine

In swine, lameness is often the first sign of infection. After a short 2- to 4-day incubation period, there is fever, depression, and loss of appetite. Foot lesions may become sufficiently painful to prevent the pig from standing. Vesiculation and separation of epithelium on the coronary band frequently lead to loss of the claw and prolonged lameness. Vesicles in the mouth are usually less prominent than in cattle, although large vesicles, which quickly rupture, often develop on the snout. Similar to cattle, mortality can be high in young animals owing to a necrotizing myocarditis. Lesions in swine caused by FMDV cannot be distinguished clinically from those caused by VSV.

DIAGNOSIS

Because FMD can spread very fast and has serious national and international trade implications, rapid diagnosis of FMDV infection, especially in countries that are free of the disease, is essential so that eradication can proceed as quickly as possible. Since other diseases, such as vesicular stomatitis, bovine papular stomatitis, bluetongue, infectious bovine rhinotracheitis, rinderpest, malignant catarrhal fever, and even chemical burns, can have similar clinical characteristics, all suspected cases of vesicular lesions need to be thoroughly investigated. When a vesicular disease is seen, it must be reported immediately to the appropriate government authority. Samples, usually including vesicular fluid, epithelial tissue from ruptured vesicles, blood in anticoagulant, serum, and, possibly, esophageal or pharyngeal fluids, are collected by government officials and submitted to the official vesicular disease laboratory for proper identification of the etiologic agent. Only laboratories with adequate biocontainment and trained staff are designated by individual countries, or groups of countries, to conduct diagnosis and research on FMD. Laboratory diagnosis is achieved by a variety of tests that include virus isolation and characterization, animal inoculation, and detection of serum antibodies, viral antigens, or viral nucleic acid.

PREVENTION AND CONTROL

Countries free of FMD have very active programs to prevent the introduction of FMDV into their territory, including active surveillance of borders adjacent to FMD-infected countries; border controls to interdict the entry of meat and meat products that could be contaminated with FMDV; and comprehensive animal importation protocols and quarantines. In these countries, FMD outbreaks are controlled by rapid slaughter of infected and exposed animals followed by destruction of infected carcasses (by burning or burying depending on the environmental circumstances). Countries with endemic FMD control the disease by vaccination campaigns using killed-virus vaccines containing the serotype and subtype virus(es) prevalent in the area. In endemic countries the introduction of a new FMDV serotype is controlled using the same procedures that countries free of FMD would use. Recent experiences in Uruguay and Argentina demonstrated that a control vaccination program that included greater than 90% of susceptible cattle every 6 months, or every year (depending upon the age of the animals and the number of vaccinations received), resulted in a drastic reduction in the number of outbreaks, and eventual eradication of FMD, even without routine vaccination of other susceptible species like sheep and swine.

■ Porcine Reproductive and Respiratory Syndrome

Kurt D. Rossow, D.V.M., Ph.D.
Christopher C.L. Chase, D.V.M., Ph.D.

Porcine reproductive and respiratory syndrome (PRRS) is a viral infection of swine characterized by abortion or premature farrowing in gilts or sows and pneumonia in neonatal, nursery, and grow-finish pigs.[10, 22, 53] First described in the United States in 1987 and in Europe in 1990, PRRS is now endemic in most swine-producing countries.[10, 22, 53] The causative agent, porcine reproductive and respiratory syndrome virus (PRRSV), is an RNA virus classified in the family Arteriviridae.[3, 38] The origin of PRRSV is unknown and swine are the only known mammalian host.

PRRSV infection occurs most commonly by exposure of mucosal surfaces to the virus but can also occur through bite wounds or multiple-use needles.[45] After infection, PRRSV replicates in macrophages, and pigs are viremic by 12 hours after infection.[44, 45] PRRSV replicates predominantly in pulmonary macrophages but also in macrophages of other tissues.[44, 45] The predilection of PRRSV for pulmonary macrophages results in interstitial pneumonia. PRRSV infection of macrophages in lymphoid tissue is important for virus persistence.[2] PRRSV transmission results from the emigration of infected macrophages or free circulating virus onto mucosal surfaces and contamination of body fluids.[45]

Persistent virus infection is defined by prolonged virus replication and does not imply immunologic tolerance. PRRSV can cause persistent infections in pigs exposed in utero or post farrowing.[1, 2, 59] Persistently PRRSV-infected pigs can remain viremic for up to 210 days, and in utero–exposed pigs can infect sentinel animals 120 days after farrowing. Persistent PRRSV infection may be lifelong for slaughter animals but lifelong persistence in breeding animals has not been demonstrated.

TRANSMISSION

Direct contact between infected and naive pigs is the main route of PRRSV transmission, and infection within a herd usually spreads slowly.[21] Aerosolization of PRRSV is commonly implicated as a route of transmission but has been difficult to demonstrate experimentally.[56] PRRSV has been isolated from or identified in serum (up to 210 days post infection [dpi]), semen (up to 92 dpi), saliva (up to 42 dpi), feces (up to 38 dpi), urine (up to 28 dpi), nasal swabs (up to 21 dpi), oropharyngeal swabs (up to 21 dpi), and oropharyngeal scrapings (up to 157 dpi).[2, 7, 43, 58, 59] All of these body fluids are potential sources of PRRSV for transmission.[45]

PRRSV vaccine and field strains can be shed in semen of intact and vasectomized boars.[7-9] The source of PRRSV in semen has not been identified but probably results from movement of PRRSV-infected monocytes or macrophages into semen. The fact that vasectomized and intact boars shed PRRSV indicates that virus shedding is not dependent on replication in reproductive tissue.[9] PRRSV can be identified in semen before seroconversion and after the cessation of viremia, indicating that virus isolation from serum and serologic testing are not adequate predictors of PRRSV status in the boar.[7]

The route of PRRSV infection of the fetus has not been identified. Infection of pregnant sows in their third trimester results in the reproductive syndrome of abortion or premature farrowing.[5, 30] Fetal PRRSV infection rarely occurs by intranasal infection of midgestation sows or by intravenous infection of first-trimester sows.[4, 30] However, fetuses in all stages of gestation can support replication of PRRSV when experimentally infected transplacentally.[4, 25] Postcoital intrauterine inoculation of PRRSV at or near the time of conception has little or no effect on reproductive performance, and 4– to 16–cell-stage pig embryos infected with PRRSV develop normally and do not support PRRSV replication.[26, 41] One report concluded that boar semen containing PRRSV has little or no effect on fertilization or conception but that transplacental infection occurs later, resulting in embryonic death prior to or at 20 days of gestation.[42]

PRRSV transmission via fomites under natural conditions has not been documented. PRRSV survived for 11 days in experimentally inoculated city water.[37] PRRSV can be isolated from muscle and although transmission is unlikely, it may be a reason for trade barriers.[29]

PRRSV infection has been limited to domestic swine with a single report of PRRSV infection and transmission in Muscovy ducks.[60]

CLINICAL SYNDROMES

The clinical presentation of PRRSV infection depends on the age of the pig infected and also on the pregnancy status and trimester of gestation of the infected sow or gilt. Coinfections with other viruses or bacteria may confuse or complicate the clinical presentation.

PRRSV transmission, infection, and induction of abortion within a herd of susceptible pregnant animals varies, resulting in a clinical presentation ranging from sporadic abortions to abortion storms.[1, 27] Fifteen percent of the breeding herd may escape initial infection with PRRSV, resulting in persistent populations of susceptible pigs.[15, 51] PRRSV-induced abortion may persist within a herd for periods ranging from 10 to 12 weeks up to 4 to 6 months.[1, 27] Reproductive failure resulting from third-trimester exposure of pregnant gilts or sows to PRRSV is characterized by late-term abortion or premature farrowing with stillborn fetuses, partially autolyzed fetuses, and mummified fetuses.[5, 27, 50] However, in one study experimental PRRSV infection of late-gestation sows resulted in delayed parturition.[32] Recent cases of PRRSV infection in PRRSV-vaccinated herds have been reported to induce abortion in all trimesters of pregnancy.[12] These observations conflict with prior experimental early and midgestation PRRSV infections.[4] Clinical signs in infected sows or gilts vary from none to inappetence, fever, lethargy, agalactia, red or blue discoloration of the ears and vulva, a postweaning delayed return to estrus, and less commonly, death.[20, 30, 49, 50]

Neonatal pigs infected with PRRSV in utero or at (or shortly after) birth develop a mild to marked increase in respiratory rate and distress, fever, inappetence, lethargy, and less commonly periocular edema, conjunctivitis, eyelid edema, blue discoloration of ears, cutaneous erythema, and central nervous system signs.[1, 10, 20, 27, 43, 45, 46] Clinical signs in PRRSV-infected neonatal pigs can vary markedly within and between litters. Mortality in neonatal pigs infected with PRRSV may approach 100%.

PRRSV infection in weaned pigs is characterized by fever, pneumonia, lethargy, failure to thrive, a marked increase in mortality from single to multiple concurrent bacterial infections, and a decreased rate of gain.[27, 43, 45] *Streptococcus suis*, *Haemophilus*

parasuis, *Pasteurella multocida*, *Bordetella bronchiseptica*, and *Salmonella cholerasuis* are common concurrent pathogens in PRRSV-infected lungs. PRRSV is a contributing agent to the porcine respiratory disease complex (PRDC) which also includes swine influenza virus and *Mycoplasma hyopneumoniae*. Subclinical PRRSV infections may occur in weaned pigs.

PRRSV infection in finishing pigs, boars, and unbred gilts or sows is frequently subclinical. If clinical signs of PRRSV infection occur, they usually include fever, lethargy, and inappetence.[18, 20, 36, 49] Some PRRSV-infected boars demonstrate a loss of libido, while most appear clinically unaffected.[16, 18, 39, 41, 48, 57] PRRSV seroconversion may be the only indication of infection in finishing pigs, boars, and unbred gilts or sows.[39, 41]

GROSS LESIONS

Gross lesions associated with PRRSV infection vary widely and may be dependent on the virus isolate, swine genetic differences, and stress factors (environment and endemic bacterial and viral flora).[19, 23, 45, 55] Lung lesions vary from none to diffuse tan consolidation and are commonly complicated by lesions resulting from concurrent bacterial infection.[10, 19, 20] Gross lung lesions from pigs with concurrent PRRSV and bacterial infection can be separate or intermixed. Multiple lymph nodes in a PRRSV-infected pig may be markedly enlarged.[45, 47] Infrequently there is subcutaneous edema, which is manifested most commonly as periocular edema and less frequently as dependent edema.[10, 43, 45] Fetuses from PRRSV abortions are late term and the body condition ranges from fresh to autolyzed.[5, 25] Umbilical cord hemorrhage has been reported to be a gross lesion of PRRSV infection.[24] However, umbilical cord hemorrhage is not specific for PRRSV infection because trauma at parturition can cause the same gross lesion.

DIAGNOSIS

A diagnosis of PRRSV infection is based on typical clinical signs, seroconversion, characteristic light microscopic lesions, and the demonstration of PRRSV by virus isolation, fluorescent antibody (FA) examination, immunohistochemistry, in situ hybridization, or polymerase chain reaction (PCR). The choice of specimens for diagnosing PRRSV infection is influenced by the clinical presentation. A serologic survey for anti-PRRSV antibodies is the most commonly used method to evaluate the PRRSV status of a herd. If the swine are not vaccinated with a PRRSV modified-live vaccine (MLV), the presence of anti-PRRSV antibodies indicates exposure, and subsequent tests should be directed at demonstrating characteristic lesions and identifying the virus with one of the aforementioned methods. If the swine herd is vaccinated with an MLV, serologic tests cannot differentiate between vaccine virus and field PRRSV isolates. In these cases, care must be taken to try to select pigs that have not been exposed to pigs vaccinated with an MLV, as vaccine virus can be transmitted to naive pigs, resulting in infection and seroconversion.[31] The most common serologic test used in the United States and Canada for the detection of anti-PRRSV antibodies is an enzyme-linked immunosorbent assay (ELISA) technique (HerdChek-PRRSV).[11] The ELISA technique will detect anti-PRRSV antibodies 9 to 13 days after infection and results are reported as a sample-to-positive (S/P) ratio.[11] S/P ratios greater than 0.39 indicate PRRSV exposure. S/P ratios from vaccinated or naturally infected animals can vary widely, and results should be interpreted as paired samples of the same individuals or comparison of samples from differently aged pigs. Other serologic techniques can be used to detect PRRSV seroconversion, but they are not widely used on a routine basis.[11] Thirty sera will provide a 95% degree of confidence for detecting a 10% PRRSV prevalence rate, while 10 sera will detect a PRRSV prevalence rate of 30% with the same degree of confidence.[11]

Most requests for PRRSV diagnosis are associated with clinical disease and therefore represent acute or subacute infections. Lung tissue should always be collected for the diagnosis of PRRSV infection because the virus can be recovered from lung or alveolar macrophages for up to 9 weeks post infection.[33, 45] The direct FA test, immunohistochemistry (detects virus antigen), or in situ hybridization (detects virus RNA) is used to demonstrate PRRSV in tissue sections.

Because young pigs infected with PRRSV have a prolonged viremia, frozen serum is an excellent sample for virus isolation. Tissues collected for virus isolation can include lung, lymphoid tissue, heart, and brain. Tissues collected for virus isolation must be kept refrigerated or frozen.

Modified-live PRRSV vaccine can be isolated from vaccinated pigs and the vaccine virus may also be shed.[6, 31, 34] Since PRRSV field isolates may coexist with PRRSV MLV in infected herds, sampling of nonvaccinees is important for identification of field strains. In addition, since PRRSV MLV grows as well or better in some cell culture systems, PRRSV isolates must be differentiated from vaccine virus. PRRSV restriction enzyme analysis can be used for differentiating PRRSV isolates.[35, 54] While PRRSV restriction enzyme analysis allows for a presumptive differentiation of vaccine virus from PRRSV field isolates, there will be isolates that are inconclusive by this test. Sequencing of PRRSV virus segments is another method of differentiating PRRSV vaccine from a field isolate, although sequencing is prohibitively expensive for routine cases.

Because of postmortem autolysis, PRRSV is infrequently isolated from fetuses.[52] Investigations of PRRSV-induced reproductive failure should include a serologic profile of affected gilts or sows and examination of serum and tissues from 3- to 5-day-old dyspneic pigs, in addition to fetuses. PCR testing of fetal tissue homogenates for PRRSV may prove to be more sensitive than virus isolation.

Both field and vaccine PRRSV are shed in boar semen.[6] Since PRRSV is shed intermittently in boar semen, two or three semen samples collected 1 week apart should be examined by the PCR technique.[5] Ten to 15 mL of boar semen or 50 mL of extended boar semen are required for PCR analysis. PRRS has been introduced into closed, PRRSV-naive swine herds with PRRSV-infected boar semen.

A diagnostic protocol for detecting persistently PRRSV-infected swine has not been formulated but will probably involve PCR testing of serum, buffy coats, or tonsil biopsies.[2]

The diagnosis of PRRSV infection is summed up in Table 1.

TREATMENT

There is no treatment for PRRSV infection. Nonsteroidal anti-inflammatory agents may lessen the severity of some clinical signs.

PREVENTION AND CONTROL

The most important part of a PRRSV control program is a laboratory-confirmed diagnosis of PRRSV infection with an appropriate corresponding clinical presentation. The diagnostic plan should try to determine when pigs are being exposed to PRRSV so intervention strategies can be designed to precede infection.

An important consideration in PRRSV control is the distinction between infection and disease. Vaccination will help decrease the clinical effects of PRRSV-induced disease but will not prevent infection. PRRSV MLV and field strains can coexist within a herd, and vaccination may not eliminate the PRRSV field strain from the herd.[46] Vaccination is not a substitute for biosecurity, and new PRRSV strains can be introduced into PRRSV-vaccinated herds.

If a swine herd is PRRSV-naive, then the goal of biosecurity is to prevent the introduction of PRRSV-seropositive animals or PRRSV-infected semen into a herd. PRRSV-seronegative animals from PRRSV-seropositive herds should still be considered as potential sources of PRRSV. Vaccinating naive herds with MLV is a decision based on the likelihood of PRRSV infection and what effect a positive PRRSV serostatus has on the producer's market (e.g., genetic stock vs. finishing operation).

Measures used to control PRRSV in infected herds include vaccination, all-in–all-out pig flow by building with disinfection, and 7 days downtime between groups, limiting cross-fostering to the first 24 hours post farrowing, and quarantine and acclima-

---

Table 1
DIAGNOSIS OF PORCINE REPRODUCTIVE AND RESPIRATORY SYNDROME VIRUS INFECTION

Pig Age	Clinical Signs	Diagnostic Specimens and Tests
Fetus/stillborn	Partially autolyzed or fresh fetus	Formalin-fixed (HI,IHC) and fresh (VI,PCR) lung, heart, liver, kidney, brain, spleen, and placenta; thoracic fluid (SE), stomach content; rule out other causes of abortion
Neonatal pig	Pneumonia, fever, inappetence, lethargy, high mortality	Serum (VI,PCR,SE); formalin-fixed and fresh lung (FA,VI,HI,IHC); fresh and formalin-fixed heart, brain, liver, lymph node (VI,HI,IHC); tissues to rule out other causes of illness/death
Nursery pig	Pneumonia with bacterial coinfections, fever, lethargy, increased mortality, inappetence, decreased weight gain	Same as neonatal pig
Grow-finish pig	Subclinical infection; clinical signs same as nursery pig	Same as neonatal pig
Sow	Subclinical infection, abortion, fever, inappetence, lethargy	Serum* (VI,PCR,SE), lung (FA,VI,HI,IHC), lymphoid tissue (VI,HI,IHC)
Boar	Subclinical infection, fever, ± changes in semen quality	Serum (VI,PCR,SE), semen (PCR), lung (VI,FA,HI,IHC), lymphoid tissue (VI,HI,IHC)

VI, virus isolation; SE, serology; HI, histopathology; PCR, polymerase chain reaction; IHC, immunohistochemistry; FA, fluorescent antibody test.
*Sows are viremic in the first few days of infection and are commonly not viremic at the time of abortion. Collect sow serum for virus isolation when sows are febrile and off feed.

tization of new stock prior to herd introduction.[13, 28] Vaccination protocols for the breeding herd generally recommend two pre-breeding vaccinations with PRRSV MLV and prebreeding booster doses in subsequent pregnancies. Another program recommends acclimating and vaccinating new arrivals, strict enforcement of quarantine and biosecurity measures, and no additional vaccinations in breeding or production pigs. Producers with poor quarantine and biosecurity measures will probably require more vaccination intervention to control losses from PRRSV infection. Vaccination of boars is an extralabel use and the vaccine virus may be shed in semen. Vaccinating gilts and sows in all parities with MLV in the face of an outbreak may lessen the clinical effects of natural infection, but MLV can also infect fetal pigs, resulting in stillborn and weak-born pigs.

The goal of PRRSV vaccination of neonatal, nursery, and grow-finish pigs is to establish immunity prior to natural infection. Vaccination protocols have been developed using intranasal (extralabel use) MLV at 2 to 5 days post farrowing, with intramuscular boosters at 14 to 21 days post weaning.[17] The efficacy of intranasal MLV has not been evaluated and the effects of colostral antibody on vaccination are unknown. Since pigs are commonly infected with PRRSV when commingled in a nursery, postweaning vaccination may not allow an adequate time period for the pig to develop vaccine-induced immunity. The effects of vaccination on persistently infected pigs have not been evaluated. The use of different modified live vaccines within a herd has not been evaluated, but exposure to different virus strains may better address the natural structural and genomic variation common to RNA virus populations.[14] PRRSV MLV may cause fever, inappetence, lethargy, and a slower rate of gain in nursery and grow-finish pigs. The benefits from PRRSV vaccination should be evaluated against the negative side effects.

Cyblue, a PRRSV-killed vaccine, is commercially available in Europe, but in one study vaccination had no influence on shedding of PRRSV in semen or the length of viremia.[36] Autogenous, killed PRRSV vaccines are used but have not been adequately evaluated for efficacy. Any vaccine that is not challenged will appear to work.

While all-in–all-out management and depopulation will not eliminate PRRSV infection, it does improve pig performance by reducing the exposure to bacteria that commonly complicate PRRSV infection.[13] All-in–all-out management will interrupt the continuous exposure of susceptible pigs to PRRSV. Vaccination of grow-finish pigs during an outbreak may lessen the clinical signs associated with infection by field virus.

Gilts and boars should be quarantined for 45 to 60 days prior to entry into the breeding herd. New pigs should be vaccinated in addition to acclimation with cull animals, because cohousing with cull animals will not guarantee PRRSV exposure. PRRSV titers in new pigs should be measured before quarantine and before introduction into the herd to evaluate vaccination and acclimatization procedures.

Control programs should be evaluated periodically to verify the effectiveness of the program and to monitor for changes in PRRSV circulation within the herd. PRRSV titers from groups of differently aged pigs should be monitored periodically for changes in comparison with previous groups. Because new gilts may not be exposed to the herd strain of PRRSV by farrowing, sera from nursery pigs of the new gilts may be a good sample for monitoring virus circulation.

REFERENCES

1. Albina E, Madec F, Cariolet R, et al: Immune response and persistence of the porcine reproductive and respiratory syndrome virus in infected pigs and farm units. Vet Rec 134:567, 1994.

2. Benfield DA, Christopher-Hennings J, Nelson EA, et al: Persistent fetal infection of porcine reproductive and respiratory syndrome (PRRS) virus. Proc Am Assoc Swine Pract 28:455, 1997.

3. Cavanaugh D: Nidovirales: A new order comprising coronaviridae and arteriviridae. Arch Virol 142:629, 1997.

4. Christianson WT, Choi CS, Collins JE, et al: Pathogenesis of porcine reproductive and respiratory syndrome virus infection in mid-gestation sows and fetuses. Can J Vet Res 57:262, 1993.

5. Christianson WT, Collins JE, Benfield DA, et al: Experimental reproduction of swine infertility and respiratory syndrome in pregnant sows. Am J Vet Res 53:485, 1992.

6. Christopher-Hennings J, Nelson EA, Benfield DA: Detecting PRRSV in boar semen. Swine Health Prod 4:37, 1996.

7. Christopher-Hennings J, Nelson EA, Hines RJ, et al: Persistence of porcine reproductive and respiratory syndrome virus in serum and semen of adult boars. J Vet Diagn Invest 7:456, 1995.

8. Christopher-Hennings J, Nelson EA, Nelson JK, et al: Detection of porcine reproductive and respiratory syndrome virus in boar semen by PCR. J Clin Microbiol 33:1730, 1995.

9. Christopher-Hennings J, Nelson E, Nelson J, et al: Identification of PRRSV in semen and tissue of vasectomized and non-vasectomized boars. Conf Res Workers Anim Dis 77:182, 1996.

10. Collins JE, Benfield DA, Christianson WT, et al: Isolation of swine infertility and respiratory syndrome virus in North America and experimental reproduction of the disease in gnotobiotic pigs. J Vet Diagn Invest 4:117–126, 1992.

11. Collins J, Dee S, Halbur P, et al: Laboratory diagnosis of porcine reproductive and respiratory syndrome (PRRS) virus infection. Swine Health Prod 4:33, 1996.

12. Collins J, Dee S, Halbur P, et al: Recent PRRS Outbreaks. Am Assoc Swine Pract Newslett, Jan 1997, p 1.

13. Dee SA, Joo HS, Polson DD, et al: Evaluation of the effects of nursery depopulation on the persistence of porcine reproductive and respiratory syndrome virus and the productivity of 34 farms. Vet Rec 140:247, 1997.

14. Duarte EA, Novella IS, Weaver SC, et al: RNA virus quasispecies: significance for viral disease and epidemiology. Infect Agents Dis 3:201, 1994.

15. Edwards S, Robertson I, Wilesmith J, et al: PRRS ("blue-eared pig disease") in Great Britain. Am Assoc Swine Pract Newslett 4:32, 1992.

16. Feitsma H, Grooten HJ, Schie FWV, et al: The effect of porcine epidemic abortion and respiratory syndrome (PEARS) on sperm production: Proc Int Congr Animal Reprod 12:1710, 1992.

17. Gillespie TG: Porcine reproductive and respiratory syndrome (PRRS) virus control by vaccination. Proc Allen D. Leman Swine Conf 22:163, 1995.

18. Gordon SC: Effects of blue-eared pig disease on a breeding and fattening unit. Vet Rec 130:513, 1992.

19. Halbur PG, Paul PS, Frey ML, et al: Comparison of the pathogenicity of two US porcine reproductive and respiratory syndrome virus isolates with that of the Lelystad virus. Vet Pathol 32:648, 1995.

20. Hopper SA, White MEC, Twiddy W: An outbreak of blue-eared pig disease (porcine reproductive and respiratory syndrome) in four pig herds in Great Britain. Vet Rec 131:140, 1992.

21. Houben S, Van Reeth K, Pensaert MB: Pattern of infection with the porcine reproductive and respiratory syndrome virus on swine farms in Belgium. J Vet Med B 42:209, 1995.

22. Keffaber KK: Reproductive failure of unknown etiology. Am Assoc Swine Pract Newslett 1:1–9, 1989.

23. Kristensen B: Possible influence of the parental MHC class I type on survival of offspring from sows with natural PRRS-virus infection. Int Symp PRRS 2:44, 1995.

24. Lager KM, Halbur PG: Gross and microscopic lesions in porcine fetuses infected with porcine reproductive and respiratory syndrome virus. J Vet Diagn Invest 8:275, 1996.

25. Lager KM, Mengeling WL: Pathogenesis of in utero infection in porcine fetuses with porcine reproductive and respiratory syndrome virus. Can J Vet Res 59:187, 1995.

26. Lager KM, Mengeling WL, Brockmeier SL: Effect of post-coital intrauterine inoculation of porcine reproductive and respiratory syndrome virus on conception in gilts. Vet Rec 138:227, 1996.

27. Loula T: Mystery pig disease. Agripractice 1223, 1991.

28. McCaw MB: McRebel PRRS: Management procedures for PRRS

control in large herd nurseries. Proc Allen D. Leman Swine Conf 22:161, 1995.

29. Magar R, Robinson Y, Dubuc C, et al: Evaluation of the persistence of porcine reproductive and respiratory syndrome virus in pig carcasses. Vet Rec 137:559, 1995.

30. Mengeling WL, Lager KM, Vorwald AC: Temporal characterization of transplacental infection of porcine fetuses with porcine reproductive and respiratory syndrome virus. Am J Vet Res 55:1391, 1994.

31. Mengeling WL, Lager KM, Vorwald AC: An overview on vaccination of porcine reproductive and respiratory syndrome. Proc Allen D Leman Swine Conf 23:139, 1996.

32. Mengeling WL, Vorwald AC, Lager KM, et al: Comparison among strains of porcine reproductive and respiratory syndrome virus for their ability to cause reproductive failure. Am J Vet Res 57:834, 1996.

33. Mengeling WL, Vorwald AC, Lager KM, et al: Diagnosis of porcine reproductive and respiratory syndrome using infected alveolar macrophages collected from live pigs. Vet Microbiol 49:105, 1996.

34. Molitor T, Shin J: Porcine reproductive and respiratory syndrome in boars: Porcine reproductive and respiratory syndrome in boars. Proc Allen D Leman Swine Conf 22:101, 1995.

35. Murtaugh MP, Elam MR, Kakach LT: Comparison of the structural protein coding sequence of the VR-2332 and Lelystad virus strains of the PRRS virus. Arch Virol 140:1451, 1995.

36. Nielsen TL, Nielsen J, Have P, et al: Examination of virus shedding in semen from vaccinated and from previously infected boars after experimental challenge with porcine reproductive and respiratory syndrome virus. Vet Microbiol 54:101, 1997.

37. Pirtle EC, Beran GW: Stability of porcine reproductive and respiratory syndrome virus in the presence of fomites commonly found on farms. J Am Vet Med Assoc 208:390–392, 1996.

38. Plagemann PGW: Lactate dehydrogenase-elevating virus and related viruses. In Fields BN, Knipe DM, Howley PM (eds): Fields Virology, ed 3. New York, Lippincott-Raven, 1996, pp 1105–1120.

39. Prieto C, Sanchez R, Martin-Rillo S, et al: Exposure of gilts in early gestation to porcine reproductive and respiratory syndrome virus: Vet Rec 138:536, 1996.

40. Prieto C, Suarez P, Bautista JM, et al: Semen changes in boars after experimental infection with porcine reproductive and respiratory syndrome (PRRS) virus. Theriogenology 45:383, 1996.

41. Prieto C, Suarez P, Martin-Rillo S, et al: Effect of porcine reproductive and respiratory syndrome virus (PRRSV) on development of porcine fertilized ova in vitro. Theriogenology 46:687, 1996.

42. Prieto C, Suarez P, Simarro I, et al: Insemination of susceptible and preimmunized gilts with boar semen containing porcine reproductive and respiratory syndrome virus. Theriogenology 47:647, 1997.

43. Rossow KD, Bautista EM, Goyal SM, et al: Experimental porcine reproductive and respiratory syndrome virus infection in one-, four-, and 10-week-old pigs. J Vet Diagn Invest 6:3, 1994.

44. Rossow KD, Benfield DA, Goyal SM, et al: Chronological immunohistochemical detection and localization of porcine reproductive and respiratory syndrome virus infection in gnotobiotic pigs. Vet Pathol 33:551, 1996.

45. Rossow KD, Collins JE, Goyal SM, et al: Pathogenesis of porcine reproductive and respiratory syndrome virus infection in gnotobiotic pigs. Vet Pathol 32:361, 1995.

46. Rossow KD, Collins JE, Shivers JL, et al: Porcine reproductive and respiratory syndrome virus infection characterized by marked neurovirulence. In Proceedings of North Central Conference on Veterinary Laboratory Diagnosticians, West Lafayette, Ind., June 10–11, 1997, p 3.

47. Rossow KD, Morrison RB, Goyal SM, et al: Lymph node lesions in neonatal pigs congenitally exposed to porcine reproductive and respiratory syndrome virus. J Vet Diagn Invest 6:368, 1994.

48. Swenson SL, Hill HT, Zimmerman JJ, et al: Excretion of porcine reproductive and respiratory syndrome virus in semen after experimentally induced infection in boars. J Am Vet Med Assoc 204:1943, 1994.

49. Swenson SL, Hill HT, Zimmerman JJ, et al: Artificial insemination of gilts with porcine reproductive and respiratory syndrome (PRRS) virus–contaminated semen. Am Assoc Swine Pract Newslett 2:19, 1994.

50. Terpstra C, Wensvoort G, Pol JMA: Experimental reproduction of porcine reproductive and respiratory syndrome (mystery swine disease) by infection with Lelystad virus: Koch's postulates fulfilled. Vet Q 13:131, 1991.

51. Terpstra C, Wensvoort G, van Leengoed LAMG: Persistence of Lelystad virus in herds affected by porcine epidemic abortion and respiratory syndrome. Proc Congr Int Pig Vet Soc 12:118, 1992.

52. Van Alstine WG, Kanitz CL, Stevenson GW: Time and temperature survivability of PRRS virus in serum and tissues. J Vet Diagn Invest 5:621, 1993.

53. Wensvoort G, Terpstra C, Pol JMA, et al: Mystery swine disease in the Netherlands: Isolation of Lelystad virus. Vet Q 3:121–130, 1991.

54. Wesley RD, Mengeling WL, Lager KM, et al: Differentiation of RespPRRS vaccine from field strains of porcine reproductive and respiratory syndrome virus by RT-PCR and enzyme restriction analysis. Annu Meet Am Assoc Vet Lab Diagn 39:54, 1996.

55. Wills RW, Fedorka-Cray PJ, Yoon KJ, et al: Synergism between porcine reproductive and respiratory syndrome virus (PRRSV) and *Salmonella cholerasuis*. Proc Am Assoc Swine Pract 28:459–462, 1997.

56. Wills RW, Zimmerman JJ, Swenson SL, et al: Transmission of porcine reproductive and respiratory syndrome virus: Contact versus airborne routes. In Proceedings of North Central Conference on Veterinary Laboratory Diagnosticians, Manhattan, Kans, June 14–15, 1994.

57. Yaeger MJ, Prieve T, Collins JE, et al: Evidence for the transmission of porcine reproductive and respiratory syndrome (PRRS) virus in boar semen. Swine Health Prod 1:7, 1993.

58. Yoon IJ, Joo HS, Christianson WT, et al: Persistent and contact infection in nursery pigs experimentally infected with porcine reproductive and respiratory syndrome (PRRS) virus. Swine Health Prod 4:5, 1993.

59. Zimmerman, Wills RW, Yoon KJ, et al: Persistent PRRS virus infection in experimentally infected swine. Conf Res Workers Anim Dis 75:243, 1994.

60. Zimmerman J, Yoon KJ, Wils R, et al: PRRS virus in avian species. Int Symp PRRS 2:29, 1995.

■ Porcine Parvovirus*

Prem S. Paul, B.V.Sc., Ph.D., Diplomate, A.C.V.M.
William L. Mengeling, D.V.M., M.S., Ph.D., Diplomate, A.C.V.M.

Porcine parvovirus (PPV) is ubiquitous in swine herds around the world. It is associated with reproductive failure characterized by embryonic death and resorption, fetal death and mummification, and a reduced number of liveborn pigs. Pregnant females have few if any clinical signs during acute infection, but PPV often crosses the so-called placental barrier to infect and affect part or all of the corresponding litter. Development and commercial availability of PPV vaccines have brought PPV-associated reproductive failure under control, as this disease is rarely observed in properly vaccinated herds. Because of the high financial risk from PPV-associated reproductive failure, vaccination of gilts and sows is generally considered to be highly cost-effective.

During the acute stage of infection, virus is transmitted via ingestion and inhalation of virus-laden secretions and excretions. PPV can remain infectious for months in a typical farm environment, and it is believed that this provides the primary reservoir for PPV between epizootics. PPV replicates in most mitotically active tissues, and a viremia is often detected 2 to 3 days after initial exposure.

The reproductive consequences of PPV infection depend on the stage of gestation at the time of exposure, and more specifically, the gestational age at which the conceptus is infected transplacentally. Infection of naive gilts and sows during about the first one third of gestation often results in embryonic death and resorption. If most or all of the litter is resorbed, pregnancy is terminated, and the affected female is likely to return to estrus. Infection about the second one third of gestation often results in fetal death and mummification (Fig. 1). Infection thereafter is usually without adverse effect. Although fetuses at about 70 days of gestational age and older are still susceptible to infection, they usually produce sufficient antibody to limit

*All of the material in this article is in the public domain.

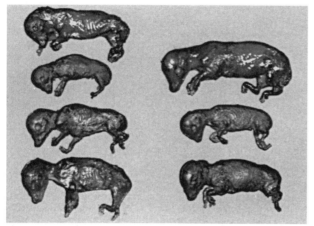

Figure 1
Mummified porcine parvovirus (PPV)-infected swine fetuses from a sow at 84 days of gestation. The sow was inoculated oronasally with virulent strain NADL-8 of PPV at 42 days of gestation. Note that all fetuses were dead and were positive for PPV antigen by immunofluorescence.

virus replication and virus-induced changes. As a result they are clinically normal at birth. When transplacental infection is early in gestation, and less than the entire litter is initially infected, virus can spread progressively in utero to some or all littermates. Therefore, members of such litters may present a spectrum of clinical consequences.

ETIOLOGY

PPV is a nonenveloped virus with a diameter of 20 nm. It agglutinates erythrocytes of a variety of species. However, guinea pig erythrocytes are most often used for tests based on hemagglutination (HA) and hemagglutination inhibition (HI). The genome of PPV is a single-stranded linear DNA with a size of 5 kb. The capsid of PPV is made up of three proteins: VP1 with a relative molecular mass (M_r) of 82.5 kDa, VP2 with an M_r of 65 kDa, and VP3 with an M_r of 62 kDa. VP2 is the major viral immunogen and is responsible for eliciting antibodies involved in HI and virus neutralization (VN).

PPV can be propagated in vitro in a variety of cell cultures of porcine origin. Although some established cell lines, for example, swine testicle cells, have been shown to support its replication, higher-infectivity titers are usually obtained in early-passage cell cultures, for example, secondary fetal porcine kidney cells. PPV replication depends on cellular DNA synthetic activity associated with mitosis. This requirement explains enhanced replication of PPV in mitotically active cell cultures in vitro and its predilection for embryonic and fetal tissues in vivo. PPV-induced cytopathologic changes in cell culture are characterized by cell rounding, pyknosis, and degeneration. Nascent viral antigens accumulate in the cell nucleus, where they can be detected by labeling procedures such as immunofluorescence microscopy. Comparison of viral isolates from different parts of the world by serologic tests such as HI, immunofluorescence, and VN have shown that PPV is antigenically conserved and that only a single serotype exists. Very minor differences in DNA fingerprints and pathogenicity have been observed between the prototype NADL-2 strain and two other laboratory-adapted PPV strains (Kresse and KBSH), while strain H-45, isolated from a diarrheal pig in Japan, appears to be distinct from the prototype PPV strain.

PPV is a very hardy virus and it is quite resistant to extremes of temperature and pH, to proteolytic enzymes, and to most of

the common disinfectants. It was found to be infectious after incubation for 4 hours at 56°C, and after more than 1 year at 37°C (when kept in otherwise sterile cell culture medium). However, PPV was inactivated at 80°C after 5 minutes. PPV was also inactivated at 37°C for 1.5 hours at pH 2, but it retained its infectivity after 9 hours at pH 3. Although PPV is resistant to most of the common disinfectants, it is easily inactivated by sodium hypochlorite.

CLINICAL SIGNS AND LESIONS

Acute infection of swine with PPV is usually subclinical or results in only a mild clinical response such as a low-grade fever and transient leukopenia. Maternal reproductive failure is usually not recognized until at least several weeks later, often not until the time of farrowing. The most common clinical features include an increased number of mummified fetuses with a corresponding reduction in the number of liveborn pigs. In addition, the interval of gestation may be prolonged for some affected females. Abortions are generally not observed with PPV infections.

A number of experiments have been performed to better define the pathogenesis of PPV-induced reproductive failure. Pregnant gilts are infected at selected times during gestation and tissues are collected at selected times thereafter. Under these conditions virus-infected and partially resorbed embryos have been observed. Affected fetuses typically go through a series of changes that begin with a hemorrhagic discoloration of tissues and an accumulation of serosanguineous fluids in the body cavities, and end with a marked dehydration (mummification) and a darkening of tissues that ranges from dark green to black. The latter stage is seen at the time of farrowing. Fetuses that are immunocompetent at the time of infection have tissue changes consistent with an immune response, such as endothelial hypertrophy and mononuclear cell infiltration. They may also have meningoencephalitis. Microscopic lesions in infected dams are mainly limited to mononuclear cell infiltration in the endometrium and lamina propria of the gravid uterus.

DIAGNOSIS

A herd history of a marked increase in the number of mummified fetuses is highly suggestive of PPV-induced reproductive failure. Such fetuses provide an ideal diagnostic sample because PPV antigen survives the mummification process and because viral antigen is typically present in high concentration throughout infected fetal tissues. Antigen is usually detected by immunofluorescence microscopy using cryostat-microtome sections of fetal lung (Fig. 2). The selection of lung is primarily based on its low background fluorescence and the ease with which it can be identified even in small mummified fetuses. The HA test (with the specificity of positive tests later confirmed by HI) may also be used to detect viral antigen in fetal lung and other tissues. Infectious PPV, like viral antigen, can survive the mummification process (although not as well as antigen). It may be isolated by inoculating tissue homogenates onto subconfluent (i.e., mitotically active) monolayers of primary or secondary cultures of porcine cells. Fetal kidney cells are most often used for this purpose. However, virus isolation is rarely attempted because it is more costly and time-consuming than detection of antigen. The presence of PPV in cell culture can be confirmed by demonstrating intranuclear immunofluorescence with PPV-specific antiserum, or by HI using specific antiserum and virus present in the culture medium. Nucleic acid probes, in situ hybridization, and the polymerase chain reaction method have also become available for the detection of PPV.

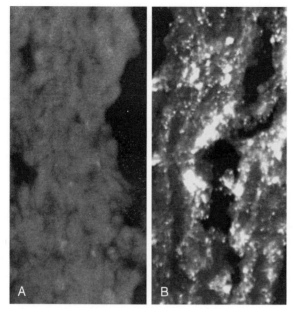

Figure 2
Lung section of an uninfected control (A) and mummified (B) pig infected with porcine parvovirus (PPV) and stained with fluorescein-labeled, anti-PPV immune serum. Note immunofluorescence in the infected but not in the uninfected lung.

Antibodies to PPV may be detected by tests such as HI, VN, or enzyme-linked immunosorbent assay. Because of the ease and reliability of HI, it is the serologic test of choice. The presence of antibodies is suggestive of passive or active immunity. Paired samples taken at 2-week intervals are ideally used to differentiate between passive and active immunity: passively acquired antibody titers decline, whereas active immunity titers either increase or remain the same. Unless antibody subclass can be determined, serology in adult animals is of limited use, as it indicates only that the animal has had a previous exposure to PPV. Treatment of serum with 2-mercaptoethanol (2-ME) in conjunction with the HI test can be used to differentiate recent from past infection, because IgM, the major antibody class present early after primary exposure, is sensitive to 2-ME while IgG is resistant to 2-ME treatment. Antibody to PPV in fetal serum or thoracic fluids is indicative of an in utero infection with PPV, because maternal antibodies do not cross the transplacental barrier in swine.

EPIZOOTIOLOGY

PPV is widespread in swine herds around the world. Almost 100% of adult swine over 1 year of age are seropositive for PPV in enzootically infected herds. Piglets are seronegative at birth unless infected in utero late in gestation. Piglets passively acquire antibodies through ingestion of antibody-enriched colostrum. Such antibodies generally persist from 3 to 6 months. The duration of passively acquired antibodies depends largely upon the initial titer. The duration of passive immunity and protection from PPV infection afforded by circulating antibodies suggests that gilts near breeding or early in gestation are at a high risk of PPV-induced reproductive failure.

PPV is very resistant to environmental conditions and is maintained for long periods in a contaminated environment. Virus infectivity may be a threat in a contaminated empty pen for at least 4 months. Virus-laden secretions and excretions are the main source of virus in the environment. Virus may also be transmitted via boar semen, embryos, and fomites.

TREATMENT

No treatment is available for PPV-associated reproductive failure.

PREVENTION AND CONTROL

Humoral immunity is the principal mechanism of immunity to PPV-associated reproductive failure. Circulating antibodies apparently neutralize PPV in blood and prevent transplacental infection. HI antibody titers of 1:80 or higher protect pigs from PPV infection, whereas lower titers do not. Natural infections with PPV result in high titers of circulating antibodies, and infected animals become immune to PPV infection. Although the duration of immunity is not known, it is believed to be lifelong.

Natural infection with PPV may be caused by feeding naive swine mummified fetuses that are suspected to contain infectious PPV, or by housing naive swine in a potentially PPV-contaminated environment. These practices neither ensure PPV exposure and immunity nor are they considered safe, that is, other pathogens may be transmitted by these same procedures. The most reliable method for inducing immunity and ensuring protection against PPV-induced reproductive failure is vaccination.

Inactivated and modified-live virus vaccines have been developed and shown to elicit anti-PPV antibodies and protect females against PPV-associated reproductive failure. Several chemicals, such as acetylethylenimine, binary ethylenimine, formaldehyde, and β-propiolactone, have been used as inactivants in the preparation of an inactivated vaccine. The most commonly used adjuvants are aluminum hydroxide or oil.

Commercial vaccines may include just PPV, or PPV in combination with other agents such as pseudorabies virus and *Leptospira* spp. Regular vaccination of gilts and sows before breeding is highly recommended. Because many gilts are exposed to PPV before they become sexually mature, the use of vaccine for these could be avoided by serologic testing. However, such testing is often more costly than vaccination. Interruption of vaccination may have devastating financial consequences resulting in mummy storms or large numbers of dams returning to estrus.

Passively acquired antibodies have been shown to persist for as long as 6 months. Because such antibodies can interfere with the development of active immunity, vaccination should be delayed until after their disappearance. This might be determined by serologic testing, but because testing is costly, the usual procedure is to wait as long as possible before vaccination, that is, 2 to 4 weeks before breeding if a single dose of vaccine is administered, or 6 to 8 weeks and 2 to 4 weeks before breeding if two doses of vaccine are administered. To ensure adequate protection during subsequent gestations, booster immunizations should be given prior to each breeding. Boars have been shown to shed PPV in semen during acute infection, and should therefore be immunized as well.

Based on the surveys of reproductive tracts and fetuses collected at abattoirs in 1977 and 1991, the current vaccination program appears to be effective in the control of PPV-associated reproductive failure. In the 1991 survey, 11 (11%) of the 101 litters with one or more dead fetuses and 100 (33%) of 302 dead fetuses tested positive for PPV. This was a major reduction from that observed in the 1977 survey, in which 46 (74%) of 62 litters with one or more dead fetuses and 392 (91%) of 432 dead fetuses tested positive for PPV.

PPV is difficult to eliminate from a swine herd because it is very resistant to the environment and most disinfectants. PPV-free pigs may be obtained from a herd that is enzootically infected with PPV, provided certain protocols are strictly followed. Cesarean-derived colostrum-deprived pigs may be obtained from multiparous sows with high serologic titers and raised in a clean PPV-free environment in a separate building. Alternatively, 2- to 3-week-old pigs with high passively acquired antibody titers obtained from multiparous sows can be raised in a clean PPV-free environment in a separate building. The buildings should be thoroughly washed, cleaned of all organic matter, and disinfected with chlorate-based disinfectants prior to moving the pigs into them. Access to these pigs and facilities should be restricted to personnel who work in the facility, with basic principles of security and disease control being followed. New stock must also be isolated prior to introduction into the herd.

BIBLIOGRAPHY

Mengeling WL: Porcine parvovirus. *In* Leman AD, Straw BE, Mengeling WL, et al (eds): Diseases of Swine, ed 7. 1992, pp 299–311.

Mengeling WL, Lager KM, Zimmerman JK, et al: A current assessment of the role of porcine parvovirus as a cause of fetal death. J Vet Diagn Invest 3:33–35, 1991.

Paul PS, Mengeling WL, Pirtle EC: Duration and biological half-life of passively acquired colostral antibodies to porcine parvovirus. Am J Vet Res 43:1376–1379, 1982.

Bacterial Diseases

Consulting Editors

M.M. Chengappa, D.V.M., Ph.D.
Derek Mosier, D.V.M., Ph.D.

■ *Haemophilus parasuis* Infection (Glasser's Disease)

Nonie L. Smart, D.V.M., Ph.D., M.Sc.

Haemophilus parasuis causes polyserositis and polyarthritis in susceptible pigs. This syndrome was first described in 1910, when K. Glasser described the sporadic occurrence of this disease in young, weaned conventionally raised pigs. More recently, outbreaks of Glasser's disease associated with high morbidity and high mortality have occurred in groups of specific pathogen-free (SPF) pigs of all ages. For this reason, Glasser's disease has taken on new importance in modern swine practice.

ETIOLOGIC AGENT

H. parasuis is a gram-negative coccobacillus which is a normal commensal organism of the upper respiratory tract of apparently healthy conventionally raised swine. There is some speculation that the presence of *H. parasuis* may predispose pigs to the development of enzootic pneumonia or atrophic rhinitis, but most culture-positive pigs have no apparent clinical signs of respiratory disease.

The fastidious nature of *H. parasuis* on culture often results in failure to isolate this organism from nasal swabs or at postmortem examination. To optimize the recovery of the organism from specimens, cultures should be incubated in an atmosphere containing 5% carbon dioxide, and on culture media containing V factor (NAD). Application of *Staphylococcus* sp. streak on a blood agar plate will usually provide sufficient NAD for growth. However, enrichment medium can also be used to encourage more vigorous growth of these bacteria. Since *H. parasuis* is easily overgrown by contaminants, the use of a selective agar containing antibiotics can increase the likelihood of recovery of the organism, especially from samples such as nasal swabs.[1]

There are few biochemical or phenotypic differences between isolates of *H. parasuis*, but many isolates can be differentiated on the basis of serologic[2] or DNA-based analysis.[1] There is a great deal of heterogeneity among strains, with at least 14 serovars described, although approximately 25% of isolates are not typable with this method. Several studies have shown that virulence differences do occur among *H. parasuis* strains. Some serotypes are more commonly associated with clinical disease,[2] whereas in experimental infections, other serotypes appear to be entirely nonpathogenic.[3, 4] However, the association between virulence and *H. parasuis* serotype is not fully understood.

PATHOGENESIS

In conventional pigs, Glasser's disease usually occurs sporadically in young weaned pigs. Affected animals may die, but more often they become unthrifty as the result of chronic sequelae. Because *H. parasuis* is widespread in conventional swine environments, young pigs are exposed to the organism at birth or shortly thereafter. Piglets are passively protected from Glasser's disease by maternal antibodies and develop active immunity at about 8 weeks of age. Piglets that receive inadequate or poor-quality colostrum or those that are stressed when maternal antibodies have decreased are at risk of developing Glasser's disease. In rare instances, large numbers of pigs may become affected with Glasser's disease. These outbreaks are usually traced to extreme environmental conditions, chilling, and mixing or transit, at or after weaning.

Glasser's disease in SPF pigs can have a quite different clinical picture. In situations in which SPF pigs have been exposed to conventional pigs (after sale of breeding stock or the mixing of fattening pigs), outbreaks of Glasser's disease with high morbidity and mortality have occurred in the SPF pigs, whereas the conventional pigs remained unaffected.[5] SPF pigs may not develop immunity to Glasser's disease because *H. parasuis* is often absent from the SPF environment. Thus, clinical disease in this group of pigs correlates with their first exposure to *H. parasuis* regardless of age. If *H. parasuis* is introduced into an SPF facility, a significant level of clinical disease is usually observed in baby pigs up to and including mature sows. In these instances, the outbreak will subside as animals that survive clinical and subclinical infection develop immunity to *H. parasuis*. In addition, there are some SPF herds which are infected with organisms identified as *H. parasuis*, but these strains do not appear to stimulate cross-protective antibodies against other field strains. For this reason, some culture-positive SPF pigs may still be susceptible to Glasser's disease when they are moved from SPF or minimal disease facilities.

CLINICAL SIGNS

Clinical signs usually begin 2 to 7 days after infection. For SPF pigs, this usually correlates with recent moving and mixing of these pigs with conventional pigs. The clinical course of Glasser's disease may range from peracute to chronic. In peracute cases, apparently healthy pigs may die within 12 to 24 hours. This syndrome is most common in SPF pigs. In less acute disease, inappetance, depression, pyrexia, coughing, dyspnea, and lameness involving one or more joints may occur. Joints may be hot and swollen and pigs may be reluctant to move. Incoordination, recumbency, and convulsions occur as the disease progresses and are usually followed soon by death. Recovered animals are often chronically lame or unthrifty.

NECROPSY

Lesions on postmortem examination vary depending on the clinical course of the infection and immune response of the pig.

When pigs die acutely, lesions may be negligible. When pigs have a longer disease course, fibrinous serositis and serous effusion may occur in the meninges, pleura, pericardium, peritoneum, and synovia. The extent of the lesions may range from mild to severe and they can occur singly or in combination. The latter necropsy picture is most common in conventional pigs, whereas SPF pigs are much more likely to die acutely with minimal postmortem lesions.

DIAGNOSIS

Diagnosis of Glasser's disease in SPF pigs is often based on a history of recent exposure of these pigs to conventional swine, the absence of postmortem findings, and (in some cases) isolation of *H. parasuis* from body fluids or tissues other than the respiratory tract. In conventional pigs, the postmortem findings are generally more characteristic of Glasser's disease. Gram-stained smears of fibrinous exudate may also be used to confirm the presence of gram-negative coccobacilli. Although serologic surveys are not used often, seroconversion of surviving SPF pigs could also be used to confirm exposure of pigs to *H. parasuis*.

Owing to its fastidious nature, *H. parasuis* may be difficult to isolate under standard laboratory conditions, even if fresh tissue specimens are cultured. Small, opaque, nonhemolytic colonies appear in 24 to 48 hours on blood or chocolate agar, and isolates which are enhanced by a *Staphylococcus aureus* feeder streak or NAD-impregnated disks can tentatively identify *H. parasuis* on the basis of the requirement for V factor. Since isolation of this bacterium is highly dependent on sample quality, as well as laboratory procedures, practitioners should recognize that a negative culture for *H. parasuis* does not necessarily rule out a diagnosis of Glasser's disease.

DIFFERENTIAL DIAGNOSIS

Conditions that mimic Glasser's disease include sudden death, septicemia, lameness, and diseases of neurologic dysfunction. Sudden death due to nutritional myopathy, gastric ulceration, salt toxicosis, and fibrinous pleuropneumonia can usually be differentiated at postmortem examination. Bacterial causes of septicemia such as beta-hemolytic streptococci, *Escherichia coli*, *Salmonella* spp., *Streptococcus suis*, or *Erysipelothrix rhusiopathiae* are usually recovered on routine culture. *Mycoplasma hyorhinis* causes a disease similar to Glasser's disease, but affected pigs are generally young, with lameness being the predominant clinical sign, and the overall mortality is low. Viral agents that cause nervous disease can usually be ruled out on the basis of clinical and histopathologic considerations.

TREATMENT

Antibiotic treatment of pigs affected with Glasser's disease is often unrewarding. Affected animals may not respond to therapy unless treatment occurs very early in the clinical course of disease, and survivors are often unthrifty. Parenteral use of antibiotics is more effective than oral administration, and antibiotics recommended for use include ampicillin, penicillin, tetracycline, and trimethoprim-sulfamethoxazole with penicillin. In outbreaks involving large numbers of SPF pigs, the impact of Glasser's disease within the herd may be reduced by vaccination of all susceptible animals, including pregnant sows and weaned pigs.

PREVENTION

In conventional pig facilities in which Glasser's disease is enzootic, attention should be given to management practices that will improve the quality of the environment for young pigs. These would include optimization of the transfer of immunity via colostrum. The effectiveness of vaccination under these circumstances has not been investigated.

SPF pigs of all ages should be immunized at least 3 weeks prior to anticipated exposure to conventional swine. All vaccinees should receive a booster dose 2 to 3 weeks after the initial inoculation. Either commercially available vaccines or a custom-prepared bacterin (containing *H. parasuis* strains known to be present at the destination) are usually quite effective in preventing Glasser's disease.[5, 6] Some strains elicit cross-protective antibodies, but this aspect of protection is not yet completely understood.[4] Pigs must be closely monitored upon arrival at new facilities, preferably isolated from the main herd, and integrated in a stepwise fashion. Prophylactic antibiotics in feed and water are often routinely used to introduce SPF pigs to conventional surroundings, but their effectiveness has not been proved. To prevent the entry of *H. parasuis* into an SPF facility, it is essential that these animals be maintained in strict isolation from conventional pigs.

REFERENCES

1. Smart NL, Miniats OP, MacInnes JI: Analysis of *Haemophilus parasuis* isolates from southern Ontario swine by restriction endonuclease fingerprinting. Can J Vet Res 53:319–324, 1988.
2. Rapp-Gabrielson VJ, Gabrielson DA: Prevalence of *Haemophilus parasuis* serovars among isolates from swine. Am J Vet Res 53:659–664, 1992.
3. Rapp-Gabrielson VJ, Gabrielson DA, Schamber GJ: The comparative virulence of *Haemophilus parasuis* serovars 1 to 7 in guinea pigs. Am J Vet Res 53:987–994, 1992.
4. Nielson R: Pathogenicity and immunity studies of *Haemophilus parasuis* serotypes. Acta Vet Scand 34:193–198, 1993.
5. Nielsen R, Danielson V: An outbreak of Glasser's disease. Studies on etiology, serology and effect of vaccination. Nord Vet Med 27:20–25, 1975.
6. Smart NL, Miniats OP: Preliminary assessment of a *Haemophilus parasuis* bacterin for use in specific pathogen free swine. Can J Vet Res 53:390–393, 1989.

■ Nonvenereal Campylobacteriosis

Roger Marshall, B.V.Sc., M.S., Ph.D.

The major problem associated with nonvenereal campylobacteriosis is diarrhea caused by *Campylobacter jejuni* and *C. coli* infection. The significance of *Campylobacter* as a cause of diarrhea has been debated over the years, and widespread distribution of these organisms among animals has made their etiologic role difficult to establish. The association of these bacteria with healthy animals does not mean that they do not contribute to disease, either on their own or in partnership with other microorganisms. The more recent definition of *C. cryophilia*, an aerotolerant *Campylobacter*, has made us realize that there may be more organisms in this genus with as-yet-undefined roles.

CATTLE

Etiology

C. jejuni and *C. coli* are associated with disease in cattle, but they have also been isolated from normal animals. Pure cultures of *C. jejuni* have been used to reproduce enteric disease in both milk-fed and ruminating calves as well as in adult cattle. Infection with *C. fetus* subsp. *fetus* can initiate clinical changes resembling those produced by *C. jejuni*. The distribution of these organisms is worldwide, but infection is uncommon when animals are kept at pasture or in feedlots. Clinical disease is still uncommon, but it is more likely when animals are housed and under a high standard of hygiene. This is presumably due to lower levels of acquired immunity as a result of a low level of challenge. The infection may occur in neonatal calves from the ingestion of milk that has become infected with feces containing *Campylobacter*, or as a result of *Campylobacter* mastitis. In older animals, ingestion of contaminated feed is a likely source.

Clinical Signs

Enteric disease due to *Campylobacter* spp. is generally regarded as mild and of minor clinical significance. Animals may be depressed and sometimes have an elevated temperature. The incubation period is 1 to 4 days, and the animals may remain affected for up to 16 days. Dark feces flecked with blood are also sometimes seen. In experimental infections, calves produced thick mucoid feces within 72 hours. In a number of clinical cases as well as in experimental studies, an associated mild pneumonia with coughing has been reported, and *C. jejuni* has been isolated from lung tissue. Clinical mastitis has been reported from which *C. jejuni* was isolated.

Diagnostic Features

Campylobacter may not be easily isolated from the feces owing to the intermittent nature of excretion and the efficiency of the isolation medium used. A rise in antibody titer against homologous organisms is consistently found in experimental infections, and it is assumed that this also occurs in natural infections. *C. jejuni* and *C. fetus* subsp. *fetus* are isolated from the mucosa of the ileum, cecum, colon (and sometimes gallbladder), jejunum, abomasum, and mesenteric lymph nodes of domestic animals. The ubiquitous nature of *C. jejuni* makes it difficult to determine the relevance of its isolation from the environment, from other animal sources, and even, on occasion, from pathologic samples. There is a great need for a technique to differentiate pathogenic from nonpathogenic strains. DNA studies have shown that there are a large number of genotypes within the species that can be differentiated by DNA fingerprinting and other genotyping methods. The degree to which these strains are species-specific in their ability to colonize, let alone produce disease, has not been defined.

Necropsy Findings

The ileum is the most frequently affected region of the intestine and it contains excess clear mucus and dark contents. The serosal surface of the ileum is pale, the walls are thickened and fleshy, and the mucosa is rough, granular, and slightly red. The jejunum may also be affected to a greater or lesser extent. The cecum and colon are usually grossly normal. Stunted villi, dilated crypts (often filled with inflammatory cells), dilated capillaries, and mononuclear cell infiltration in small intestinal mucosa present histologically, but these lesions are not specific to *Campylobacter* infection.

Treatment and Control

It is usually necessary to treat cases symptomatically; should antibiotics be deemed necessary, neomycin, erythromycin, or tetracyclines are usually effective. No control program is usually necessary, and diarrhea is mild and self-limiting. Prognosis is generally good. Clinical signs disappear in time, and the number of organisms that can be isolated from the feces gradually decreases. Control of this disease is based on preventing access of animals to infected animals and on reducing access to contaminated feed and environment.

Public Health Aspects

C. jejuni causes diarrhea in humans, and epidemiologic links have been made between bovine and human infection. Most of these infections have been due to consumption of unpasteurized milk and have resulted in large outbreaks. *C. fetus* subsp. *fetus* is also capable of producing an enteric syndrome in humans that is similar to that caused by *C. jejuni* but that is generally less severe. *Campylobacter*-like organisms can initiate lesions with features like those of *C. jejuni*. This organism may act in concert with other enteric disease agents and result in a disease that is more severe than either agent alone is capable of producing.

SHEEP
Etiology

Two species of *Campylobacter* have been isolated from the feces or intestinal tracts of sheep: *C. fetus* subsp. *fetus* and *C. jejuni*. *Campylobacter*-like organisms and *C. jejuni* are isolated from healthy grazing sheep and appear to be normal intestinal inhabitants. Distribution of the organisms is worldwide, but disease is uncommon. An animal infected with *C. fetus* subsp. *fetus* may suffer bacteremia. If the animal is pregnant, fetal septicemia with hepatitis, death, and abortion may follow. The consequences of *C. fetus* subsp. *fetus* infection are much less equivocal than are those that follow *C. jejuni* infection. There is little information on the degree of immunity that may develop as a result of natural infection with either species. The large number of serotypes may mean that the protective value afforded by any one serotype is specific and may provide little cross-protection for other serotypes. Little is known about the pathogenesis of *Campylobacter* enteritis in sheep; however, more is known about the abortion- and stillbirth-related aspects of the disease. *C. fetus* subsp. *fetus* is a well-recognized cause of abortion in ewes in late pregnancy. After ingestion of *Campylobacter* organisms, ewes may experience bacteremia for up to 1 to 2 weeks, during which time the placenta and the fetus become infected if the ewe is in late pregnancy.

Clinical Signs

In some field outbreaks of colitis and diarrhea, *Campylobacter*-like organisms have been isolated that may play a role, but this has yet to be substantiated. Blood-flecked feces, but not diarrhea, have been induced experimentally in ewes by giving *C. jejuni* orally. Abortion occurs in late pregnancy, and outbreaks are often cyclic in nature. This form of the disease often occurs during high-density grazing in winter. During an outbreak, aborted fetuses may be found, and affected ewes may have blood-stained perineal regions, with or without the presence of fetal membranes. Ewes rarely have systemic effects, but secondary metritis may develop and cause chronic ill health. *C. fetus* subsp. *fetus* may persist in uterine discharges for up to 6 weeks.

Transmission

During interepidemic times, the abortion-producing organisms are carried in the gallbladder and the intestines of sheep and are spread by fecal contamination of food and water. Carrion-eating birds, such as the North American magpie (*Pica pica*) and ravens (*Corvus corone corone*) in Britain, can spread the organism. Shepherds handling sheep at the time of an abortion outbreak may transfer the organism to healthy animals.

Diagnostic Features

Campylobacter spp. are found in the intestines, feces, and gallbladder. All clinical specimens should be kept at 4°C and cultured within 6 hours. In outbreaks of abortion, the etiologic agent must be distinguished from other possible causes, such as *Toxoplasma gondii*, *Chlamydia psittaci*, and *Listeria monocytogenes*. The number of ewes aborting and the necropsy appearance of the liver and cotyledons aid in diagnosis. *Campylobacter* can be readily demonstrated in a stained smear made directly from the fetal abomasal contents or from a cotyledon. The abortions usually affect only one or two ewes at the start of an outbreak, but this is followed by an abortion storm in which up to 20% of the flock can be affected. Even higher incidence rates occur if the flock has a large proportion of maiden ewes. The outbreak results in widespread contamination of pasture with the products of abortion, which leads to heavy contamination with *C. fetus* subsp. *fetus*. There is no venereal spread of the infection. Lambs are sometimes born alive, but they are weak and usually die within a few days. Affected ewes may produce insufficient milk to raise a lamb. A convalescent immunity may occur in ewes that will prevent subsequent infections for 2 to 3 years. Ewes that abort usually produce normal lambs in subsequent years. In a high proportion of aborted fetuses, pale areas of focal necrosis, up to 25 mm in size, often with reddened margins, appear in the liver. The cotyledons appear edematous, which is a general feature of abortion. The microscopic appearance of cotyledons is sufficiently characteristic that it should be submitted to the diagnostic laboratory to assist in the diagnosis.

In cases of enteritis, an increased fluidity of the colonic contents may be the only lesion. In severe cases, this may be accompanied by ascites, subcutaneous edema, and loss of adipose tissue. Histologically there is erosion of the cecal and colonic superficial epithelium and dilated glands containing necrotic debris. Some severe cases show deeper ulceration of the mucosa.

Treatment and Control

In abortion outbreaks, streptomycin (70 mg/kg of body weight) has been used as treatment. Elimination of the carrier state has been achieved by treatment with penicillin and streptomycin together or in conjunction with daily oral chlortetracycline. The success of such treatment is most effective when used early in an outbreak. The value of the sheep will determine if such expense is warranted. The enteric form of the disease is usually self-limiting and therefore requires no specific treatment or control program. A vaccine produced from a killed suspension of *C. fetus* subsp. *fetus* is available in some countries for control of abortion outbreaks, but to be effective it must be given before animals are infected. The success of the vaccine will depend on how well the field strains are represented in the vaccine and how early the vaccination program is started. If a diagnosis is made early enough, vaccination may be used to protect ewes that have not yet been exposed. Vaccination of a flock may have no effect if the outbreak has been in progress for 2 weeks or longer. Because of the sporadic nature of the disease, maintenance of the vaccination program beyond the year of the outbreak may not be justified. However, annual vaccination on a farm is recommended if abortions occur every year. As an alternative, only replacement ewes, especially young

ewes, can be vaccinated. The first dose is given before the rams are put out, and the second dose is given when the rams are withdrawn.

By the end of an outbreak, most ewes are likely to have been exposed to the organism and will have developed immunity. In these cases, vaccination is usually reserved for ewes that are newly added to the flock. Control of the disease is based on preventing access of sheep to the organism by reducing access to contaminated grass and other feeds. This may be achieved by reducing stocking density and, if possible, removing stock from contaminated pasture. Prompt recognition of the disease, isolation of aborting ewes, and prevention of mechanical spread on clothing and equipment is vital if an epidemic is to be avoided.

Public Health Aspects

The role of mutton as a source of *C. jejuni* infections in humans has not been seriously investigated, and so far no epidemiologic linkage has been established. Mouth-to-mouth resuscitation of weak lambs, however, can present a hazard and may be responsible for a condition known as *shepherd's scours*.

GOATS

Abortions due to *C. fetus* subsp. *fetus* or *C. jejuni* have been reported in goats.

PIGS

Etiology

The significance of *C. coli* and *C. jejuni* infections in pigs is unclear. These organisms are isolated worldwide, and young pigs become colonized by ingestion within the first few days of life, with the same strains colonizing either their dam or the pig that they are suckling. The discovery of *Serpulina (Treponema) hyodysenteriae* as the causal organism of swine dysentery relegated *C. coli* to the status of nonpathogen. However, large numbers of *C. coli* have been recovered from inflamed intestinal mucosa of young pigs without evidence of *Serpulina* spp. infection. Therefore, the possibility that *C. coli* can act alone or in concert with other potential pathogens to produce disease cannot be ruled out. Surveys have shown that 60% to 100% of postweaning pigs are infected with *C. coli*. Infected sows are the major source of infection for piglets.

C. jejuni is rarely isolated from pigs. Experimental oral inoculation of 7-day-old colostrum-deprived pigs, conventional suckling pigs, and conventional weaned pigs has been undertaken. Within 4 days of inoculation, both of the preweaned groups developed elevated temperatures and mucoid yellow diarrhea containing occasional flecks of blood; the mucosa was hyperemic, and the mesenteric lymph nodes were enlarged. No clinical signs were seen in the weaned animals.

Clinical Signs

Diarrhea supposedly resulting form *C. coli* infection is of varying severity but is usually mild. The significance of this infection is negligible or unclear.

Diagnostic Findings

Culturing the organism can be meaningless because its recovery is so common. A demonstrable serologic titer is likely to be more significant.

Infection causes mild to moderate inflammation of the small intestinal mucosa with possible enlargement of the draining lymph nodes. Nonspecific signs of enteric disease may occur, such as stunted villi, dilated crypts containing inflammatory cells, dilated capillaries, and mononuclear cell infiltration.

Treatment and Control

The diarrhea is usually self-limiting; therefore, control measures are usually not needed. Symptomatic treatment should be given; when necessary, neomycin, erythromycin, and tetracycline can be used. Prognosis is generally good, especially if fluid loss is controlled.

Public Health Aspects

Pork is considered a likely source of *C. coli* infection in humans. However, extensive biotyping, serotyping, or genotyping of pig isolates has not yet been undertaken to compare pig and human strains. At present, pork is generally considered to be a minor source of foodborne *Campylobacter* infections in humans.

BIBLIOGRAPHY

Bruere AN, West DM: The Sheep: Health, Disease and Production. Palmerston North, New Zealand, Foundation for Continuing Education of the NZVA, 1993.

Gumbrell RC, Saville DJ, Graham CF: Tactical control of ovine *Campylobacter* abortion outbreaks with a bacterin. NZ Vet J 44:61–63, 1996.

Jensen R, Swift BL: Diseases of Sheep, ed 2. Philadelphia, Lea & Febiger, 1982.

Nachamkin I, Blaser MJ, Tompkins LJ (eds): *Campylobacter jejuni*: Current Status and Future Trends. Washington DC, American Society for Microbiology, 1992.

Orr KE, Lightfoot NF, Sisson PR, et al: Direct milk excretion of *Campylobacter jejuni* in a dairy cow causing cases of human enteritis. Epidemiol Infect 115:15–24, 1995.

■ Bovine Venereal Campylobacteriosis

Richard L. Walker, D.V.M., Ph.D., Diplomate, A.C.V.M.

Bovine venereal campylobacteriosis remains an important cause of infertility, early embryonic death, and occasional midterm abortion in cattle. It is one of the most important venereally transmitted diseases of cattle and occurs in many countries worldwide. Economic losses incurred are the result of poor conception rates, increased culling due to infertility, shortened lactation periods, and increased management costs. Widespread use of artificial insemination, routine screening of bulls, and the addition of antibiotics to semen extenders have greatly aided in controlling the incidence of disease.

ETIOLOGY

Campylobacter fetus subsp. *venerealis*, the etiologic agent of bovine venereal campylobacteriosis, is a curved, motile, gram-negative rod that requires a microaerophilic environment for growth. There are two biotypes within this subspecies, biotype *venerealis* and biotype *intermedius*. These biotypes are differenti-

ated by detection of hydrogen sulfide production with lead acetate strips when organisms are grown in media containing cysteine. Biotype *intermedius* produces hydrogen sulfide, whereas biotype *venerealis* does not. Both biotypes cause disease; however, some evidence suggests that biotype *intermedius* is less pathogenic than biotype *venerealis*.

The other subspecies of *C. fetus*, *C. fetus* subsp. *fetus*, is a major cause of ovine abortions. It also causes sporadic abortions in cattle. Its main habitat is the intestinal tract of ruminants. Abortions are the result of bacteremia with localization in the gravid uterus. In some instances, the prepuce in bulls can become contaminated, and the organism can be transmitted through breeding. However, the importance of *C. fetus* subsp. *fetus* as a venereally transmitted agent is considered minimal. The isolation of *C. fetus* subsp. *fetus* does not have the herd implications or necessitate the intervention and treatment steps that are required with *C. fetus* subsp. *venerealis*. Other *Campylobacter* species and related organisms also cause occasional reproductive disease in cattle and must be differentiated from *C. fetus* subsp. *venerealis*. These include *C. jejuni*, *C. sputorum* subsp. *bubulus*, and *Arcobacter* spp.

OCCURRENCE

Bovine venereal campylobacteriosis exists in many countries around the world. The prevalence of disease is influenced by management and control practices. The true prevalence of disease is often unknown, either because of inadequate surveillance or because of the use of insensitive diagnostic techniques. Globally, biotype *venerealis* is widely distributed, whereas biotype *intermedius* is most common in the United States, South America, and parts of Australia. Some countries have specific requirements for testing for bovine venereal campylobacteriosis when animals or semen is imported.

Cattle are the primary host and main reservoir for *C. fetus* subsp. *venerealis*. Both dairy and beef cattle are affected. It is an obligate parasite of the bovine reproductive tract and does not survive for extended periods outside the host. Organisms can be recovered from the reproductive tract of both males and females. Colonization in bulls occurs on the penis and prepuce with the greatest concentration of organisms on the glans penis and fornix of the prepuce. Colonization in cows occurs in the anterior vagina, cervix, uterus, and oviducts. Cases of isolation from other species, including humans, have occasionally been reported.

PATHOGENESIS

Transmission is predominantly by the venereal route. Bulls serve as carriers and are the major means for transmitting the organism to cows. The transmission rate from an infected bull to uninfected cows is high, sometimes approaching 100%. Direct transmission between females is unlikely, as vulvar exposure alone does not result in disease. Infection, however, may be spread among cows through the use of poorly sanitized instruments utilized in reproductive procedures. Artificial insemination with contaminated semen is another means by which females can become infected. Infected bulls can infect other bulls through mounting when they are held in common areas. Also, spread from bull to bull can occur if semen collection equipment is not adequately cleaned between collections.

After exposure, colonization in cows occurs in the anterior vagina and cervix. Under the influence of progesterone, the infection spreads to the uterus and oviducts. The actual fertilization process and early embryo development are not directly affected by *C. fetus* subsp. *venerealis*. It is the inflammatory response in the uterus and oviducts that results in early embryonic death. The midterm abortions occasionally caused by *C. fetus* subsp. *fetus* are attributed, in part, to the reactions caused by heat-stable endotoxins.

Infected cows develop immunity and generally clear the organism over a period of 3 to 6 months from the time of infection. In the uterus, it is the production of IgG that leads to clearance through opsonization and phagocytosis. In the lower genital tract, IgA predominates and plays a role in immobilizing organisms and blocking adherence. Paradoxically, IgA production may block opsonization and promote persistent colonization of the lower genital tract. Some persistently infected cows harbor organisms for more than a year. Persistence in the cervicovaginal region in the presence of local immune response is, in part, due to antigenic changes in the organism that allow for avoidance of the host immune response. Specifically, antigenic variation in the S-layer, a regular array of high-molecular-mass surface proteins composing the outermost part of the cell envelope, results in expression of different immunodominant epitopes and persistence of the organism. Serum resistance and antiphagocytic properties of the S-layer have also been described and may be important in persistence.

The age of the bull influences susceptibility to, and persistence of, infection. Bulls younger than 3 years tend to be more resistant to infection and, if infected, can clear organisms within a few weeks. The increase in number and depth of crypts in the preputial epithelium of older bulls makes them more likely to become persistent carriers.

CLINICAL SIGNS

In females, the main clinical signs are related to infertility. The periods between estrus are frequently extended (27 to 53 days), and the number of repeat breedings increases. Typically, the average number of services per conception is extended to between 2.5 to 3.5. The herd profile soon after infection is one of low fertility. When the infection is newly introduced into a herd, as few as 20% of the cows become pregnant in some cases. Over time, the conception rate in the herd improves as infected animals clear the infection naturally. Eventually, the overall conception rate returns to normal; however, the succeeding calving period is extended. In chronically infected herds, reproductive problems are limited to newly introduced, previously unexposed animals. Infected cows show few signs of infection. It is uncommon to see any vaginal discharge, although a mucopurulent secretion is sometimes detected. Rectal palpation of the uterus does not reveal any abnormality. The infection in bulls is inapparent. Reproductive behavior is normal; however, bulls may appear thin and tired as a result of repeated breedings. Semen quality is unaffected.

Abortion resulting from *C. fetus* subsp. *venerealis* infection is uncommon. Fewer than 10% of the cows in an infected herd will abort a detectable fetus. Cows that abort are usually between the fourth and seventh month of gestation. Biotype *intermedius* appears to be associated with abortions more frequently than does biotype *venerealis*. If midterm abortions occur, there is usually a recent history of infertility in the herd.

PATHOLOGY

The pathology of bovine venereal campylobacteriosis is limited to the reproductive tract. In cows, a subacute, diffuse, mucopurulent endometritis with lymphocytic infiltration is common. Less commonly, salpingitis and cervicitis may be present. In bulls there are no gross or histologic changes associated with infection.

The aborted fetus may have fibrinous pleuritis, pericarditis, and peritonitis. Histologically, suppurative bronchopneumonia and interstitial hepatitis with neutrophilic infiltration are present. Autolytic changes may also be observed. The cotyledons of the placenta are pale and fluid-filled and have a yellow-brown discoloration. Necrosis of the chorionic epithelium, vasculitis with fibrinoid degeneration of vessel walls, and serofibrinous exudate with an infiltration of neutrophils and other inflammatory cells are observed. These lesions, however, are not pathognomonic for bovine venereal campylobacteriosis.

DIAGNOSIS

A clinical history of infertility or poor conception rate in a herd is the first suggestion that bovine venereal campylobacteriosis may be a problem. Other causes of infertility, including poor heat detection, problems with bull fertility, and bovine trichomoniasis, must also be considered. Bovine venereal campylobacteriosis should also be considered with the occurrence of second-trimester abortions. Confirmatory diagnosis must be made through laboratory evaluation. Laboratory diagnosis is performed by (1) isolation of the organism; (2) demonstration of positive-staining *Campylobacter*-like organisms in tissues of aborted fetuses, preputial scrapings, or vaginal washings using a direct fluorescent antibody test (DFAT); or (3) demonstration of *C. fetus* subsp. *venerealis* antibodies in vaginal mucus.

Isolation of *C. fetus* subsp. *venerealis* is difficult because of its fastidious nature; however, isolation provides a definitive diagnosis. Samples for isolation include semen, preputial secretions, vaginal mucus, tissues from aborted fetuses (e.g., abomasal fluid, liver), and fetal membranes. Cultures of preputial secretions are most rewarding when collected by scraping the mucosal surface with an insemination pipette, rather than by performing preputial washes, because the organisms tend to colonize deep in the preputial crypts. Culturing vaginal mucus is most useful diagnostically when samples are obtained early in the course of infection, before immunity develops. Collection should be performed around the time of estrus. The recovery rate from vaginal cultures drops substantially in chronically infected cows. From aborted fetuses, recovery is most easily made from abomasal fluid. Recovery attempts from fetal membranes can also be fruitful, but isolation is complicated by contaminating bacteria.

The handling of preputial scrapings or vaginal mucus samples requires special attention to optimize organism recovery. The transit time to the laboratory should be minimal. Ideally, samples should be received within 6 hours of collection to optimize recovery. Because this is often impractical, various transport enrichment media (TEM) have been described for transporting samples to the laboratory. Two commonly used media are Weybridge TEM and Australian TEM. Even under ideal conditions, recovery of *C. fetus* subsp. *venerealis* from preputial scrapings and vaginal washings is difficult. By sampling a number of animals in the herd, chances for recovering the organism are improved. Tissues from aborted fetuses should be shipped to the laboratory overnight and maintained at 4°C during shipment. Organisms are usually present in the abomasal fluid in such numbers that the recovery rate is high in cases of *C. fetus* subsp. *venerealis*–induced abortions.

Direct examination can be a useful adjunct to culture in the diagnosis of abortions caused by *C. fetus* subsp. *venerealis*. Organisms with *Campylobacter*-like morphologic characteristics and darting motility can be observed by direct examination of fetal abomasal contents using dark-field microscopy. Direct Gram's staining of abomasal contents for typical curved rods or S-shaped organisms is also helpful. *Campylobacter* species are more easily visualized by Gram's stain when counterstained with carbolfuchsin rather than the standard counterstain, safranin. Gram's stains and dark field examinations are generally not rewarding when performed on other types of samples.

Isolation of *C. fetus* subsp. *venerealis* requires plating on solid media. Filtering of samples and plating the filtrate on nonselective media is one method used for isolation. It has the advantage of using a noninhibitory medium, but it may actually decrease the number of organisms available for culture owing to the filtration process. Direct plating on selective media containing antibiotics is another commonly used method. A number of different antibiotics, including vancomycin, polymyxin B, and trimethoprim, are included in the media to suppress the growth of contaminating organisms. Amphotericin B can also be incorporated to control fungal contamination. Cultures for *C. fetus* subsp. *venerealis* are incubated in a reduced-oxygen environment, prepared either by purging anaerobe jars with a prepared gas mixture or by using commercially prepared gas-generating systems. An environment of 10% to 20% CO_2 and less than 5% O_2 is optimal.

Plates should be incubated at 37°C for at least 6 days before being discarded as negative. In most cases, colonies of *C. fetus* subsp. *venerealis* will be visible by 3 days. Colonies are round, raised, and 1 to 3 mm in diameter. Initially, they are clear, but they become opaque on further incubation. Conventional identification methods using specific phenotypic characteristics are most commonly employed for identification. Isolates of *C. fetus* subsp. *venerealis* are oxidase-positive, catalase-positive, and resistant to nalidixic acid (30-µg disks) but are sensitive to cephalothin (30-µg disks) and grow at 25 but not 42°C. Care must be taken to differentiate *C. fetus* subsp. *venerealis* from *C. fetus* subsp. *fetus*, which is phenotypically very similar and can also be recovered from aborted fetuses or from the prepuce of bulls as a result of fecal contamination. These two subspecies differ only in the ability of *C. fetus* subsp. *fetus* to grow in the presence of 1% glycine, whereas *C. fetus* subsp. *venerealis* does not. Cellular fatty acid profiles have also been used to differentiate the *C. fetus* subspecies, *venerealis* and *fetus*. Other methods, including protein profiling, nucleic acid probes, and polymerase chain reaction, are currently being investigated for diagnostic and identification purposes.

The DFAT can be used to examine vaginal mucus and preputial samples as well as tissues from the aborted fetus. The test is rapid and easy to perform and can differentiate *C. fetus* from other nonpathogenic *Campylobacter* species. It cannot, however, distinguish between the two subspecies of *C. fetus*. Because of the small number of organisms that may be present, repeat testing is recommended on negative vaginal mucus and preputial scrapings. Because there are sensitivity and specificity limitations, exclusive use of the DFAT should be accompanied by a strong clinical history supporting a positive diagnosis of bovine venereal campylobacteriosis.

Detection of specific antibodies is also used for diagnostic purposes. The vaginal mucus agglutination test is the most commonly used test. A vaginal mucus sample that causes complete agglutination at a dilution of 1:25 is considered sufficient to make a positive diagnosis. The test is most useful for evaluation on a herd basis. Because a substantial number of infected animals do not produce an adequate antibody response, the sensitivity of the test is too low for determination of an individual animal's infection status. Problems with specificity can occur as a result of contamination of samples with blood or as a result of unrelated inflammation. The response detected is also influenced by the stage of estrus during which the samples are obtained. An enzyme-linked immunosorbent assay (ELISA) for detection of IgA antibodies in vaginal mucus has also been described and appears to be very specific. Tests for the presence of antibodies in the serum are not used because of poor sensitivity and specificity.

TREATMENT AND CONTROL

If no treatment or control measures are employed, infection in a herd eventually becomes self-limiting. New entries into the herd, however, are susceptible to infection if natural breeding is continued.

Elimination of natural breeding and the use of artificial insemination is the best way to control bovine venereal campylobacteriosis. Because persistently infected cows are a source of infection for newly introduced bulls at subsequent breedings, artificial insemination should be continued for at least two breeding seasons after infection is detected. It is important that the semen used be adequately screened for *C. fetus* subsp. *venerealis* and that antibiotics be added to semen extenders to ensure that reintroduction of infection through contaminated semen does not occur.

Vaccination plays an integral part in many control programs for bovine venereal campylobacteriosis, especially when artificial insemination is not used. A number of *C. fetus* subsp. *venerealis* bacterins are commercially available. Some are combined with bacterins for *Haemophilus somnus* or *Leptospira* serovars. Initially, it is recommended that animals be vaccinated twice, 2 to 4 weeks apart, at least 30 days before breeding. Biannual vaccination is recommended following the initial vaccination series.

Vaccination of bulls plays a role both in the prevention of new infections and as a treatment for infected bulls. Elimination of the carrier state in bulls requires two vaccinations given 2 to 4 weeks apart. Higher than normal doses of vaccine may be required to eliminate the carrier state in bulls. Vaccination also plays a protective role when the bull serves only as a vehicle for mechanical transmission from an infected female to an uninfected female. The shorter the interval between when the bull is breeding an infected and an uninfected female, the less benefit vaccination has for prevention of mechanical transmission. The combination of culling infected bulls and vaccination of uninfected bulls accelerates control of disease in the herd. Vaccination of females results in a protection rate of up to 75%. Because of the potential for some cows to be persistent carriers, vaccination of cows is used in some programs as an additional control measure.

Treatment of infected animals with antibiotics may not be warranted if other control and treatment measures are employed. The lack of specifically approved antibiotics for treating bovine venereal campylobacteriosis requires the extra-label use of antibiotics if treatment is pursued. Uterine infusions with penicillin and streptomycin have been used to treat infected cows and may hasten recovery if treatment is performed early in the course of the infection. Antibiotic treatment of bulls has also been used with variable success. Topical treatment by deposition of antibiotic solution into the preputial cavity is the most efficient treatment. It requires closing the sheath opening after instilling the antibiotic solution and externally massaging the sheath for 5 minutes. The treatment is repeated two more times at 24-hour intervals. Treated bulls, however, remain susceptible to reinfection.

BIBLIOGRAPHY

Cipolla AL, Casaro AP, Terzolo HR, et al: Persistence of *Campylobacter fetus* subspecies *venerealis* in experimentally infected heifers. Vet Rec 134:628, 1994.

Clark BL: Review of bovine vibriosis. Aust Vet J 47:103–107, 1971.

Corbeil LB, Schurig GG, Duncan JR, et al: Immunoglobulin classes and biological functions of *Campylobacter (Vibrio) fetus* antibodies in serum and cervicovaginal mucus. Infect Immun 10:442–429, 1974.

Corbeil LB, Schurig GD, Bier PJ, et al: Bovine venereal vibriosis: Antigenic variation of the bacterium during infection. Infect Immun 11:240–244, 1975.

Hum S, Brunner J, McInnes A, et al: Evaluation of cultural methods and selective media for the isolation of *Campylobacter fetus* subsp *venerealis* from cattle. Aust Vet J 71:184–186, 1994.

Hum S, Quinn C, Kennedy D: Diagnosis of bovine venereal campylobacteriosis by ELISA. Aust Vet J 71:140–143, 1994.

▪ Proliferative Enteropathy of Pigs

Gordon H.K. Lawson, B.V.M.&S., B.Sc., Ph.D.
Steve McOrist, B.V.Sc., M.V.Sc., Ph.D.

The term *proliferative enteropathy*, or *proliferative ileitis*, is a pathologic description of a group of conditions with a common etiology and characteristic histologic changes of the intestine. The important microscopic features are the presence of proliferating immature enterocytes that contain *Lawsonia intracellularis* bacteria within the apical cytoplasm.

ETIOLOGY

In the past, much confusion surrounded the identity of the intracellular agent that is responsible for proliferative enteropathy, mainly because of the recovery of a variety of *Campylobacter* spp. from lesions and the morphologic similarity of these organisms to the intracellular bacteria. However, it has now been demonstrated that *L. intracellularis* is the intracellular organism that is the primary cause of proliferative change and typical disease, both in gnotobiotic pigs with commensal bacterial flora and in conventional animals.

The causal organism is an obligate intracellular bacterium that has only been grown in vitro in mammalian cell cultures, principally the rat enterocyte cell line IEC-18. Some genetic relation exists between these bacteria and *Desulfovibrio* spp.; however, this is of little veterinary significance, and the organism is distinct from all other intracellular bacterial species. *L. intracellularis* is a microaerophilic, curved, delicate, non–spore-producing gram-negative rod that retains carbolfuchsin when stained by the modified Ziehl-Neelsen method. All strains of the organism so far isolated have proved closely similar to the type species, and none shows any antigenic relationship with the numerous *Campylobacter* spp. that frequently contaminate the lesions of proliferative enteropathy.

PATHOLOGY

All cases of proliferative enteropathy demonstrate the same fundamental pathologic lesion of proliferating mucosa; however, a number of secondary changes may be superimposed on the underlying lesion that markedly alter both the clinical signs and the pathologic changes.

Affected intestinal crypt cells containing *L. intracellularis* continue to divide, which leads to a thickened mucosa made up of elongated, branched crypts. This histologic change can generally be appreciated grossly as a thickening of the mucous membrane. Lesions that consist of such a thickened proliferating mucosa without other significant intestinal change are described as *adenomatous* or *porcine intestinal adenomatosis*. The diseased mucosa may undergo further change, ranging from superficial destruction to deep coagulative necrosis; in the latter case, the affected mucosa is replaced by a yellow, cheesy exudate that retains the original form of the intestine. This pathologic presentation, when severe, is described as *necrotic enteritis*.

Animals that survive such necrotic change show a damaged, ulcerated mucosa with compensatory muscle hypertrophy, which

is visible as a thickened intestinal wall (*hosepipe gut*) and described as *regional ileitis*.

Some proliferative lesions culminate in acute blood leakage from the mucosal surface. These show the characteristic mucosal thickening together with a formed blood clot or free blood in the intestinal lumen, and are known as *proliferative hemorrhagic enteropathy*. The lesions of all of these conditions are most common in the lower ileum. Proliferative hemorrhagic enteropathy tends to be confined to the small intestine, whereas the other conditions may occur in the large bowel, with or without small intestinal involvement. The cause of these superimposed changes is not known, although immunocytologic differences and the occurrence of proliferative hemorrhagic enteropathy mainly in mature animals may suggest that this condition involves a more destructive immune response in the adult animal.

Necrotic enteritis may involve secondary infection of the primary proliferative enteropathy lesion.

OCCURRENCE

The disease occurs worldwide and has been present in pigs for many decades; however, it has only been since the commercial exploitation of high health production methods that the disease has made a dramatic and important impact on pig production. A high proportion of conventional herds (30% to 40%) have some clinical experience of the disease, and it is probable that infection is present, to some extent, in most herds of any size derived from unimproved stock.

Many minimal-disease or improved-health-status herds have suffered from the clinical effects of proliferative hemorrhagic enteropathy, which often has the characteristics of a highly contagious disease, with clinical signs in 12% to 50% of the adult herd and a mortality of approximately 50% in clinically affected animals. Although the hemorrhagic form of the disease may spread clinically from animal to animal, this condition can also affect single or small numbers of pigs, with nearby animals remaining unaffected. In certain countries, proliferative hemorrhagic enteropathy has been a continuing problem in boars and gilts involved in growth trials.

Most other manifestations of the disease are less dramatic than is the acute hemorrhagic form, and it is therefore less easy to evaluate their effect. Mortality in herds experiencing intestinal adenomatosis and/or necrotic enteritis may reach 1%, with some 0.89% to 2.5% of animals being detectably affected. Lesions can be present in animals presented for slaughter. The incidence of such lesions is generally low (0.7% to 1.63%), but occasionally a high proportion (40%) of pigs killed are affected.

CLINICAL SIGNS

Symptoms of proliferative hemorrhagic enteropathy are generally acute-onset intestinal blood loss with concomitant profound anemia in adult pigs. The hemorrhagic form of the disease mainly affects mature animals (older than 4.5 to 5 months), although on occasion all ages, including suckling pigs, may be involved. Unlike other forms of proliferative enteropathy, the clinical condition is not preceded by a period of wasting. Initial anemia is often sufficiently severe to cause sudden death without premonitory symptoms. Feces in affected animals contain blood, either altered or fresh, and may be diarrheic or formed but without free excess mucus. Vomiting may be present along with anorexia, but fever is not present other than as a slight or transient feature. Recovery takes place progressively over a period of about a week. Pregnant animals may abort, the majority within days of the onset of symptoms.

Adenomatosis or necrotic or regional ileitis can occur at any time in the fattening period and may appear as early as 6 weeks of age. The most prominent signs are those of loss of appetite and failure to gain weight. Affected animals become "hairy," have poor bodily condition, and show intermittent episodes of diarrhea. Such symptoms remain in evidence for up to 6 weeks, but most animals thereafter can regain appetite and subsequently make satisfactory progress to slaughter. Necrotic enteritis or regional ileitis is most commonly manifest as sudden death in previously unthrifty pigs; regional ileitis may terminate in intestinal rupture and peritonitis. Although adenomatosis may be apparent clinically, it may also be present as a subclinical entity, with depressed weight gain as the only manifestation.

DIAGNOSIS

Proliferative hemorrhagic enteropathy has to be differentiated from other enteric diseases demonstrating blood in the feces, notably swine dysentery, gastric ulcers, intestinal anthrax, warfarin toxicosis, salmonellosis, and certain mycotoxicoses. Only in gastric ulceration, warfarin poisoning, and mycotoxicosis is the anemia comparable in severity to that seen in proliferative hemorrhagic enteropathy.

Diagnosis of the wasting syndrome is more difficult, as a wide variety of specific and nonspecific conditions can cause failure to gain weight. The principal conditions that may cause confusion in diagnosis are spirochetal or other colitis, nutritional deficiencies (notably niacin or vitamin E deficiency in young piglets), other intestinal aberrations, and chronic respiratory disease.

Confirmation of diagnosis in the living animal can be achieved by demonstrating *L. intracellularis* in the feces by use of a PCR based on specific DNA primers derived from *L. intracellularis*. This test is sensitive and detects disease in animals with lesions but not low levels of infection. Other less sensitive tests are available that detect organisms in feces by an indirect fluorescent antibody technique using either specific monoclonal or polyclonal antibody as the primary reagent. Serum assays have been described, which use bacterial antigen extracted from the tissues of proliferative enteropathy cases, in either an ELISA or an immunofluorescence test. Both mainly detect short-lived IgM antibody, and positive results correlate well with the presence of lesions. Such tests are not available from all laboratories, but awareness of the condition and the availability of these procedures is rapidly becoming more widespread.

In the absence of such tests, confirmation depends on demonstration of typical lesions and the intracellular organism. A useful simple diagnostic aid is the staining of thin mucosal smears by the modified Ziehl-Neelsen technique. With care in preparation, these can clearly demonstrate the intracellular organism. Proliferative hemorrhagic enteropathy cases in animals found dead must be differentiated from the sporadic, frequent intestinal catastrophes described as *intestinal torsion* or *colonic bloat*. In the latter conditions the intestinal wall remains thin, the lumen is distended by gas, and the hemorrhagic contents are never clotted.

Although the presence of infection in a herd is often demonstrated by the presence of clinically affected animals, the infected status of herds free from clinical disease is more difficult to ascertain, and criteria for the identification of nonclinically infected herds have not been established.

TREATMENT

The recent identification of *L. intracellularis* as the etiologic agent of proliferative enteropathy has provided the means to evaluate the effectiveness of antibacterial agents in controlling the infection in both in vivo and in vitro studies.

Most current therapy is aimed solely at minimizing the clinical effects of the disease; controlled studies on the effects of therapy in the field are limited, and most clinical observations are confined to visual assessment of health and a cessation of mortality. In dealing with a disease syndrome expressed as a complex of pathologic lesions, some with superimposed secondary infection, it is often not clear whether the proliferative lesion or the secondary infection is being modified by treatment.

Our knowledge of the epidemiology of infection is poor. Clinical cases often occur after movement of animals; it may be uncertain whether this is clinical expression of a previously subclinical infection or whether infection has been acquired at the new location. The decision as to which is most likely is important in prescribing medication, even if it is sometimes impossible to assess accurately.

Treatment of acute hemorrhagic disease in breeding herds previously considered to be free of the disease requires a vigorous approach to therapy; treatment that is confined to clinically affected individuals or groups often does not prove satisfactory in controlling the infection. In these circumstances, whole-herd medication is often justified. Drugs often recommended for in-feed medication are tiamulin (150 ppm), chlortetracycline (400 ppm), or tylosin (100 ppm). It is likely that certain other macrolides are also active against *L. intracellularis* infections, but this awaits confirmation; in vitro sensitivity assays suggest that the aminoglycosides and aminocyclitols are likely to prove ineffective.

When acute disease occurs repeatedly in replacement breeding stock after incorporation into the main herd, the introduced animals should be "exposed" to infection for a period of up to 21 days. Animals are then treated with in-feed antibiotics, often chlortetracycline (100 ppm), sometimes in combination with other drugs (penicillin G [50 ppm], sulfamethazine [100 ppm]). Even with such a regimen, cases may be expected in treated animals following withdrawal of therapy; whether this is due to absence of exposure or recurrence of infection is not known. Pigs exposed to infection for longer than 21 days may develop symptoms before therapy can be initiated.

Growing or fattening pigs that are affected by the chronic disease (adenomatosis or necrotic enteritis) are often treated with high levels of in-feed antibiotics followed by continuous medication of the animals at risk at a lower or preventative rate with tiamulin (50 ppm), chlortetracycline (200 ppm), or tylosin (100 ppm). Such continuous medication of immature breeding stock may result in treated animals remaining susceptible to infection, with the very real danger of the reappearance of clinical disease on withdrawal of the drug.

A wide variety of other antibacterials have been used on farms in an effort to inhibit the disease, with effects being monitored by the presence of lesions at slaughter. Such reports have not been controlled, but they may be an indication of efficacy; halquinol and olaquindox, 60 to 120 ppm and 25 to 50 ppm, respectively, appeared useful, but both on occasion failed to control lesions for reasons that have not been investigated. This drug failure may indicate either that on-farm usage was not correctly carried out or that susceptibility of the intracellular organism may vary. Drug withdrawal periods before slaughter are of crucial importance, and withdrawal periods of more than 21 days may allow clinical cases to occur before slaughter. Not all drugs mentioned may be approved for use by national regulatory authorities.

CONTROL

Animals may be infected and asymptomatic. In experimental studies, the PCR test on feces has been shown to be sensitive and capable of detecting infection associated with proliferative enteropathy lesions. Knowledge of the epidemiology of infection and the suppressive effects of antimicrobials and growth promoters on fecal excretion is required before herds can be classified as noninfected on the basis of such tests. Cesarean-derived or similar herds that have never shown symptoms may be free from infection. Other animal species are affected by a similar disease caused by bacteria closely related to *L. intracellularis*, and hamsters and mice are susceptible to infectious material of swine origin. It is possible, therefore, that infection may be introduced into free herds by infected pigs, rodents, or other animals. Maintenance of a closed herd with elimination of rodents is, at the moment, the only advice that can be offered to exclude infection.

BIBLIOGRAPHY

Lomax LG, Glock RD, Hogan J: Porcine proliferative enteritis: Field studies. Vet Med 77:1777–1786, 1982.
McOrist S, Jasni S, Mackie RA, et al: Reproduction of porcine proliferative enteropathy with pure cultures of IS intracellularis. Infect Immun 61:4286–4292, 1993.
Rowland AC, Lawson GHK: Porcine proliferative enteropathies. *In* Leman AD, Straw BE, Mengeling WL (eds): Disease of Swine, ed 7. Ames, Iowa, Iowa State University Press, 1992.

■ *Escherichia coli* Infections in Farm Animals

John M. Fairbrother, B.V.Sc., Ph.D.

Escherichia coli is an important cause of disease worldwide and occurs in most mammalian species, including humans.

The most common clinical manifestations of *E. coli* infection are neonatal and postweaning diarrhea and edema disease in young pigs, neonatal diarrhea, dysentery, septicemia in young calves and lambs, and mastitis in adult cattle.

ETIOLOGY AND PATHOGENESIS

E. coli is a gram-negative, facultative anaerobic rod that is part of the normal intestinal flora and grows easily on most culture media. *E. coli* is classified into 150 to 200 serotypes or serogroups based on somatic (O), capsular (K), and flagellar (H) antigens. Only strains of a restricted number of serogroups are pathogenic and are classified into categories or pathotypes based on the production of virulence factors. The most important categories in farm animals are enterotoxigenic *E. coli* (ETEC); verotoxigenic *E. coli* (VTEC); attaching and effacing *E. coli* (AEEC); septicemic *E. coli* (SEPEC); and nonsepticemic extraintestinal *E. coli*. Strains causing hemorrhagic diarrhea in calves are both VTEC and AEEC. Enteroinvasive *E. coli* (EIEC) is rarely isolated from farm animals. Certain O serogroups are associated with specific disease manifestations in each animal species (Table 1).

Most *E. coli* organisms causing diarrhea in farm animals are ETEC. These strains produce fimbriae (pili), which mediate bacterial attachment to the small intestinal mucosa, and enterotoxins, which stimulate the secretion of water into the intestinal lumen and subsequently cause diarrhea. The most important fimbrial adhesins are F4 (K88), F5 (K99), F6 (987P), F41, F17, and F18 (F107).

Enterotoxins are classified as either STa, STb, or LT. The most important pathotypes, that is, combinations of fimbriae and enterotoxins, are listed in Table 1. F4-producing isolates

occasionally proliferate rapidly in the small intestine of young pigs and induce symptoms of shock and rapid death with the typical lesions of hemorrhagic gastroenteritis, congestion, and thrombi in the mucosa of the stomach and small intestine. These lesions probably result from rapid release of bacterial lipopolysaccharide from the intestine into the circulation.

AEEC attaches to and effaces the microvilli of small and large intestinal mucosa and has been associated with diarrhea in postweaning pigs and dysentery in young calves. Lesions range from mild and scattered through the large and small intestine to severe and involving mostly the cecum and colon. In pigs, lesions include light to moderate inflammation of the lamina propria, enterocyte desquamation and some mild ulceration, and light to moderate villous atrophy in the small intestine. In calves, lesions are often more severe and are most common in the colon. AEEC attaches intimately to the intestinal epithelial cell membrane by means of a bacterial outer membrane protein termed intimin or EPEC attaching and effacing (Eae) factor. In addition, calf isolates often produce verocytotoxin (VT) (or shiga-like toxin, SLT). These isolates tend to induce more extensive lesions of hemorrhagic colitis: edema, ulceration, and erosions in the large intestinal mucosa and consequently hemorrhage into the intestinal lumen. Edema disease in weaned piglets is caused by VTEC, mostly of serogroups O138, O139, and O141. These strains adhere to the small intestinal mucosa by means of the fimbrial adhesin F18 (F107), proliferate in the small intestine, and produce a variant of VT2, which enters the circulation and causes lesions associated with endothelial cell damage.

E. coli septicemia is most frequent in young animals with low maternal antibody levels and is caused by strains able to resist the bactericidal effects of serum complement and grow in body fluids with low available levels of iron. These strains usually possess the aerobactin iron acquisition system, belong to a restricted number of serogroups, and often produce the fimbrial adhesins F17, CS31A, or of the P, S, or AFA families. The role of these fimbriae in the pathogenesis of the disease is not yet well understood. Septicemic strains of *E. coli* often produce colicin V or cytotoxic necrotizing factor (CNF) 1 (pig) or 2 (calf). In contrast to enteric *E. coli* infections, *E. coli* mastitis is caused by a large variety of serotypes, similar to those present in the intestinal flora of adult cattle. A common characteristic of these strains is their ability to resist the bactericidal effects of serum complement. Following fecal contamination from the immediate environment of the cow, *E. coli* enters the teat and remains in the teat canal and lactiferous sinuses. The *E. coli* is either rapidly eliminated by infiltrating neutrophils with mild damage to the epithelial cells of the teat sinus or proliferates rapidly and causes more extensive epithelial damage in the secretory areas of the mammary gland, due to diffusion of endotoxin and possibly other cytotoxins. A wide variety of serotypes of *E. coli* may be involved in other extraintestinal infections such as wound or urinary tract infections.

CLINICAL SIGNS

The clinical signs of the disease depend on the virulence factors of the infecting *E. coli* and the age and immune status of the animals. ETEC causes severe watery diarrhea, followed by dehydration, metabolic acidosis, and death. In certain cases the infection may progress so rapidly that death occurs before the development of diarrhea. One or more animals in a group are affected. In calves, piglets, and lambs, neonatal ETEC diarrhea is mostly observed in the first few days after birth. In piglets, a less watery diarrhea is also observed in the first 1 to 2 weeks of age and postweaning, with low mortality and often decreased weight gain. Enteric colibacillosis complicated by shock occurs

Table 1
SEROGROUPS AND VIRULENCE FACTORS OF *Escherichia coli* CAUSING DISEASE IN FARM ANIMALS

	Disease	Serogroup	Virulence Factors
Pig	Neonatal diarrhea	O8, O45, O138, O141, O147, O149, O157	F4 (K88), F5 (K99), F6 (987P), F41, LT, STa, STb
		O8, O9, O20, O64, O101	F5 (K99), F41, STa
	Postweaning diarrhea	O8, O45, O138, O139, O141, O147, O149, O157	F4 (K88), F18 (F107), STa, LT, STb, VT, Eae
	Edema disease	O138, O139, O141	VT 2e (SLT IIv), F18 (F107)
Calf, lamb	Neonatal diarrhea	O8, O9, O20, O64, O101	F5 (K99), F41, F17, STa
	Septicemia	O8, O9, O15, O26, O35, O45, O78, O86, O101, O115, O117, O137	Aerobactin, Col V, CNF, P, CS31A, F17
	Hemorrhagic diarrhea	O5, O26, O103, O111, O118	VT1 (SLTI), VT2 (SLTII), Eae
Cow	Mastitis	Diverse	Endotoxin

in unweaned and recently weaned pigs and manifests as rapid death with some cutaneous cyanosis of the extremities, or less acutely with hyperthermia, diarrhea, and anorexia. In edema disease, recently weaned pigs die suddenly, sometimes with eyelid edema. In calves, hemorrhagic diarrhea due to VTEC is observed from 2 to 8 weeks of age. Symptoms may include dysentery, pyrexia, and depression and tend to be more chronic with less severe dehydration than observed in ETEC diarrhea. *E. coli* septicemia occurs in calves in the first few days of life and in lambs at 2 to 3 weeks of age. It is characterized by an acute generalized infection, sometimes with diarrhea, with signs of shock often followed by death. In some animals, the infection becomes localized causing polyarthritis and meningitis. *E. coli* mastitis affects lactating cattle and varies from very mild inflammation with some clotting of the milk and swelling of the gland to a very acute reaction with no early signs of inflammation in the gland, but a rapid buildup of *E. coli* and widespread damage to the udder, followed by signs of toxemia and possibly death. Chronic or recurrent mastitis may also occur.

DIAGNOSIS

In live animals, presumptive diagnosis of enteric *E. coli* infection is based on clinical history and signs, determination of fecal pH, and confirmation by culture of *E. coli* in the feces. Diagnosis is more definitive if the *E. coli* belongs to a pathogenic serogroup and is positive for the appropriate virulence factors by gene probe or polymerase chain reaction (PCR) or by various phenotypic assays such as agglutination, enzyme-linked immunosorbent assay (ELISA), or immunofluorescence for fimbrial antigens, and the infant mouse test, tissue culture assay, or pig gut loop test for the enterotoxins. Fecal material may also be tested directly for the presence of virulence factors.

On postmortem examination, diagnosis of enteric *E. coli* infection may be confirmed by demonstration of typical lesions and bacterial intestinal colonization on histopathology, immunoperoxidase, or immunofluorescence and by cultural identification of *E. coli* with the appropriate virulence factors or belonging to one of the pathogenic serogroups (see Table 1). Diagnosis of *E. coli* septicemia or extraintestinal infection can be confirmed by isolation in pure culture or in predominance in affected tissues of one of the pathogenic serogroups or *E. coli* possessing one or more of the appropriate virulence factors.

CONTROL OF *E. coli* DISEASE

Treatment

Treatment of *E. coli* disease is mostly aimed at removal of the pathogenic *E. coli* and should be rapidly instituted to be as

effective as possible. However, diagnosis of *E. coli* infection should be confirmed by culture and antibiotic sensitivity tests since antibiotic sensitivity varies greatly among *E. coli* isolates. A broad-spectrum antibiotic treatment could be used initially until the results of antibiotic sensitivity are known. Antimicrobial agents against which *E. coli* isolates have developed the least resistance are gentamicin, trimethoprim-sulfamethoxazole, cephalothin, amikacin and apramycin, ceftiofur, and enrofloxacin. However, isolates are becoming increasingly resistant to ampicillin, neomycin, kanamycin, spectinomycin, tetracycline, and sulfisoxazole. The route of administration depends on the type of infection and the choice of antibiotic. In *E. coli* diarrhea, oral administration is often more practical. If septicemia or a more generalized infection is present, parenteral administration is indicated. The main problem with the use of antibiotic therapy is the rapid development of antibiotic resistance by enteric bacteria and the depletion of the protective intestinal flora. Many *E. coli* isolates have multiple resistance to antibiotics. Alternative approaches to the treatment of *E. coli* diarrhea in calves include the use of antibiotics, such as tiamulin, to inhibit binding of ETEC to the intestinal epithelium. Also, glycoprotein glycans from the nonimmunoglobulin fraction of bovine plasma protects colostrum-deprived calves from ETEC challenge. In *E. coli* diarrhea, it is important to treat dehydration and acidosis. In mild cases, electrolyte replacement solutions should be given orally as soon as possible. In more severe cases, intravenous fluid therapy may be required. Drugs with antisecretory properties, such as chlorpromazine and berberine sulfate, may be useful for the treatment of diarrhea due to ETEC isolates. However, many of these drugs have undesirable side effects.

A potential treatment for gram-negative sepsis, such as *E. coli* septicemia, is the use of antiendotoxic drugs and antisera. Drugs that may help in treating symptoms of endotoxic shock include the cyclo-oxygenase inhibitor flunixin meglumine combined with dexamethasone and the lazarid drug tirilazad mesylate. The treatment of septic shock with antiserum against the endotoxin of the J-5 rough mutant strain of *E. coli* appears to delay the onset of clinical signs in experimentally produced *E. coli* septicemia but not to have an effect on the mortality rate in experimental or field conditions. In *E. coli* mastitis, intramammary antibiotic therapy may be administered, although in many cases the gland will be bacteriologically negative when clinical signs appear and hence therapy may be unnecessary. In cases of acute and peracute mastitis, supportive fluid and corticosteroid therapy may be beneficial to counteract the effects of dehydration and endotoxic shock.

Immunoprophylaxis

Early immunity to *E. coli* infection in young farm animals is provided by colostral antibodies. Failure to receive or absorb adequate colostral antibodies through the small intestinal wall within the first 24 hours after birth predisposes young animals to both enteric ETEC infection and to systemic *E. coli* infection. Immunoglobulin levels, particularly in calves, may be estimated by the zinc sulfate or sodium sulfite turbidity tests during the first 48 hours after birth. Immunodeficient animals can be treated with plasma from an adult animal originating from the same area and in contact with the same *E. coli* serogroups or with colostrum taken from an older cow in the herd and stored frozen until time of use. Oral administration of specific anti-F5 (K99) monoclonal antibodies or powdered egg yolk from hens immunized with F5 fimbriae to calves within the first 12 hours after birth appears to prevent intestinal colonization by F5-positive ETEC isolates.

Vaccination programs are helpful for the control of ETEC infections in young animals. Identification of virulence determinants important in the pathogenesis of ETEC diarrhea, particularly in neonates, has resulted in the production of more efficient vaccines. Vaccination of the dam prior to parturition is the most effective way of assuring the transfer of specific antibody in the colostrum for protection of neonatal animals. Bacterins containing strains representing the most important serogroups and producing the appropriate fimbrial antigens are commercially available for vaccination of farm animals. They are usually given parenterally 6 weeks and 2 weeks prior to parturition and have variable efficacy under field conditions. Recombinant DNA technology has enabled the production of large quantities of purified fimbrial antigens for use in parenteral vaccines for immunization of the dam. However, more widespread vaccination has led to a change in the bacterial population. For example, fewer F4-positive ETEC organisms are being isolated from neonatal piglets and F4-negative isolates from classic F4-positive serogroups are emerging. Recombinant DNA technology is being used to produce toxoid forms of the enterotoxins LT and STa. Conjugation of nonimmunogenic STa to carrier proteins has given protection under experimental conditions but has been less encouraging in the field. Addition of these components to fimbrial vaccines will provide protection against emerging ETEC with new fimbrial antigens in neonates and against ETEC commonly found in older pigs that lack known fimbrial antigens. Live autogenous oral vaccines, consisting of ETEC isolates from a particular herd, may be used. These are given to the dam 3 to 4 weeks before farrowing and offer good protection if the appropriate isolates are used. With the advent of recombinant technology, these vaccines will become less necessary. Oral or parenteral immunization of young piglets with live or killed ETEC vaccines may reduce the incidence of postweaning diarrhea and improve the growth rate of early weaned pigs. Parenteral vaccination of adult cows during the dry period with the J-5 rough mutant strain of *E. coli* appears to reduce the rate of clinical coliform mastitis in field trials. However, such vaccination does not appear to have any great effect on the severity of the clinical signs observed in experimentally induced disease.

Husbandry

A program for prevention of *E. coli* infection should be aimed at reduction of the numbers of pathogenic *E. coli* in the environment by good hygiene, maintenance of suitable environmental conditions, and provision of a high level of immunity. Because most pathogenic *E. coli* organisms in enteric infections belong to a limited number of serogroups, enteric *E. coli* infection could be eliminated from some herds.

Young farm animals should be maintained at an adequate temperature in an area free of draughts to reduce the effects of chilling on intestinal motility and resistance to enteric infection and septicemia. New animals should be quarantined to avoid

introduction of different pathotypes to which existing animals have very little immunity. Calving pens should be thoroughly decontaminated between batches of calves, to reduce the population of pathogenic *E. coli* in the immediate environment. It has been found that the longer calving houses are used, the greater the incidence of *E. coli* infection. Similarly, the design of farrowing crates is important to reduce contamination of young piglets. Use of the all-in, all-out system of farrowing with a period of rest and thorough disinfection between farrowings will reduce the incidence of enteric infection.

Careful attention to diet after weaning can reduce the incidence of postweaning diarrhea in pigs. A highly digestible, milk-based diet, fed in liquid form at regular intervals, reduces the incidence of postweaning diarrhea and results in improved growth rate.

The occurrence of *E. coli* mastitis is a direct reflection of poor hygienic conditions of winter housing. Thus, control measures should be aimed not only at regular teat-end decontamination, but at maintenance of clean bedding and disinfection of the immediate environment of the cow.

BIBLIOGRAPHY

Bertschinger HU, Fairbrother JM: *Escherichia coli* infections. *In* Straw B, Mengeling W, Taylor D, et al (eds): Diseases of Swine, ed 8. Ames, Iowa State University Press, 1998 (in press).

Butler DG, Clarke RC: Diarrhoea and dysentery in calves. *In* Gyles CL (ed): *Escherichia coli* in Domestic Animals and Humans, Wallingford, UK, CAB International, 1994, pp 91–116.

Gay CC, Besser TE: *Escherichia coli* septicemia in calves. *In* Gyles CL (ed): *Escherichia coli* in Domestic Animals and Humans, Wallingford, UK, CAB International, 1994, pp 75–90.

Hill AW: *Escherichia coli* mastitis. *In* Gyles CL (ed): *Escherichia coli* in Domestic Animals and Humans, Wallingford, UK, CAB International, 1994, pp 117–133.

Holland RE: Some infectious causes of diarrhea in young farm animals. Clin Microbiol Rev 3:345–375, 1990.

Wray C, Morris JA: Aspects of colibacillosis in farm animals. J Hyg Camb 95:577–593, 1985.

Zeman DH, Thomson JU, Francis DH: Diagnosis, treatment, and management of enteric colibacillosis. Vet Med 794–802, 1989.

■ *Actinomyces suis* Infection

Scott Dee, D.V.M., M.S., Ph.D., Diplomate, A.C.V.M.

In 1957, an anaerobic diphtheroid bacterium was isolated from cases of cystitis and pyelonephritis in swine herds in the United Kingdom and classified as *Corynebacterium suis*. It has since been reclassified into the genus *Eubacterium*, and more recently into the genus *Actinomyces*.

The prevalence of urinary tract infections induced by *A. suis* is worldwide, and it has increased as intensive management practices have changed the pigs' environment. It has been isolated from the pen floor of 10-week-old pigs and is a normal inhabitant of the preputial and vaginal tracts. Transmission to the sow was initially thought to occur during breeding; however, *A. suis* has been isolated from the vaginal tract of piglets immediately postparturition. The organism is piliated, which allows improved adhesion in the vagina, whereas the short, wide urethra of the sow may enhance accessibility to the urinary tract.

A. suis–induced cystitis and pyelonephritis is much more prominent in older sows (6+ parity) housed in gestation stalls owing to the higher incidence of fecal contamination of the perineal region, lack of exercise, reduced water availability, and infrequent urination. Urine stagnation leads to an elevation in urinary pH, enhancing the organism's growth. The organism produces urease, which splits urea, releasing ammonium ions that damage bladder epithelial cells and further elevates urinary pH. The elevated pH also initiates calculus formation. These changes predispose the kidney to pyelonephritis in a fashion similar to that of bovine *Corynebacterium* renal infection.

CLINICAL SIGNS

A. suis infection affects the kidneys, ureters, and bladder, producing acute or chronic renal failure. In the acute phase of infection, the animal is anorexic and unwilling to rise. Pus or blood may be present in the urine. Mortality can be high (up to 100%) if the infection is not treated immediately. If the animal survives the initial infection, it can suffer severe weight loss and manifest polyuria and polydipsia. Typically, the sow becomes a repeat breeder with subsequent poor reproductive performance secondary to loss of condition and is culled.

DIAGNOSIS

The presence of an acutely sick sow with hematuria should place *A. suis*–induced cystitis-pyelonephritis at the top of the differential list. Other causes of acute mortality in sows include mesenteric torsion, bacterial septicemia, endometritis, and coliform mastitis; however, hematuria is not commonly found with these conditions. Chronic weight loss secondary to renal disease can result from leptospirosis, *Stephanurus dentatus* infection, and a variety of toxicoses, such as from long-term gentamicin use or cadmium, citrinin, ochratoxin, or pigweed poisoning. Other potential causes of chronic weight loss, such as malnutrition, locomotor problems, parasitism, ulcers, pneumonia, or intestinal diseases (e.g., ileitis or dysentery) should also be considered. Finally, diseases such as African swine fever and hog cholera are capable of inducing glomerulonephritis and subsequent renal failure.

PATHOLOGY

Pathologic changes associated with *A. suis* infection are striking. Inflammatory reactions on the mucosal surface of the bladder may be hemorrhagic, purulent, or necrotic. The bladder wall is thickened, and deposits of granular material may be present in the lumen. The urine is usually red-brown and has a foul odor. The ureters may increase in size up to 1 to 1.5 cm in diameter. Unilateral or bilateral pyelonephritis may occur with the cortical, medullary, and pelvic regions distended with pus, blood, or foul-smelling urine.

MICROBIOLOGY

Isolation of *A. suis* to support the initial diagnosis is important. For enhancement of growth, anaerobiosis is required. If cultures are to be taken in the field, a small opening (1.25 cm in length) should be made in the bladder wall; the culture should be taken and placed immediately into anaerobic transport medium (Cary-Blair). To attempt the highest possible isolation rate, portable incubators, culture media, and anaerobic jars can be carried to the necropsy site. If tissues are to be taken to the laboratory, the neck of the bladder should be tied off with umbilical tape and one kidney should remain unopened.

The preferred medium is Columbia colistin-nalidixic acid (CNA) agar, which consists of Columbia agar with 5% sheep red blood cells as well as colistin sulfate (10 mg/L), nalidixic acid (15 mg/L), and metronidazole (50 mg/L). It is commer-cially available and minimizes gram-negative contaminants. The anaerobic environment is maintained with the use of gas-pack jars, and incubation should be carried out at 37°C for 5 to 7 days.

Morphologic features on blood agar are unique. Gray, pin-point, smooth-edged colonies, 1 mm in diameter, can be seen after 48 to 72 hours of incubation. Over the next 24 to 48 hours, the morphologic character changes to flat, dry, opaque colonies, 4 to 5 mm in diameter, with serrated edges. There is no hemolysis. Gram's staining reveals gram-positive rods with typical corynebacterial morphology. The organism is urease-positive and catalase-negative, and it ferments maltose, xylose, arabinose, and starch. Glucose and sucrose fermentation is variable. Gelatin hydrolysis, Voges-Proskauer, and methyl red tests are negative, as are nitrate reduction and esculin hydrolysis. Urinalysis indicates a severe bacteriuria ($\geq 10^5$/mL), proteinuria, hematuria, and pyuria. The pH can rise to 8 to 8.5, and the primary calculi produced are magnesium ammonium phosphate, calcium oxalate, apatite, calcium phosphate, and urate.

TREATMENT

If acute *A. suis* infection is recognized early, treatment can be successful. It is important to choose an antibiotic that is effective against the pathogen, nontoxic to the renal system, and active at an alkaline pH. Antibiotics known to be effective are ampicillin, penicillin, tetracycline, and the cephalosporins. Because of their safety, efficacy, and primary route of excretion being the urinary tract, the drugs of choice are ampicillin or penicillin. Although both are active at an alkaline pH, ampicillin has the greater spectrum of activity. A veterinarian-client-patient relationship is necessary for the use of this drug in swine in the United States. Acutely sick animals have been effectively treated with 11 mg/ kg of ampicillin, given twice daily, or penicillin, given as a daily intramuscular injection for 3 to 5 days. The withdrawal times are 21 days and 7 days, respectively. Other antibiotics, such as the tetracyclines, have been reported to be effective but are known to be nephrotoxic, and their activity is reduced at an alkaline pH. With the chronic form, the prognosis for full recovery is poor. Sows often become repeat breeders, and culling is the most cost-effective measure, rather than long-term therapy. If the affected females are of significant value, proper therapeutic measures should be taken and the sows rested for an entire estrous cycle.

Large-scale outbreaks of urinary tract disease are rare; however, water-soluble ampicillin is approved for use in swine, and water consumption is not usually a problem. The withdrawal time is 24 hours, and free-choice water should be available at all times. Feed-grade antibiotics are rarely cost-effective. Affected animals are anorexic, and the bioavailability of certain antibiotics, such as penicillin, is reduced owing to degradation in the gastrointestinal tract.

Infusion of boar preputial sheaths with penicillin or tetracy-cline has been reported as a means of controlling the problem. This practice may be helpful in reducing bacterial numbers short term, but long-term "flushing" programs have no value. With the high prevalence of *A. suis* on today's modern hog farm, it is better to control bacterial buildup and prevent the problem from occurring.

PREVENTION

Elimination of *A. suis* is not practical; therefore, the factors that increase the animal's susceptibility to the problem must be recognized. Proper hygiene in breeding and gestation is critical for control of all forms of urogenital disease. Manure should be removed regularly from behind the sow stalls, and gestation stalls should be washed and disinfected as groups are moved to farrowing. Breeding pens should be washed and disinfected on a daily basis. The phenols, formaldehyde-based or quaternary ammonium compounds, have been shown to be effective against *A. suis*, and the quaternary compounds are preferred because of the minimal skin irritation produced.

When utilizing hand mating, the producer should wear plastic gloves to reduce contamination. Fecal material on the vulva or prepuce should be wiped off with a paper towel before mating takes place. Walking behind sow stalls daily to look for discharges and to examine the level of fecal contamination and monitoring urine for pus or blood are good diagnostic tools for determining the level of urinary tract infection on the farm. The routine monitoring of urinary pH is also helpful in detecting acute infection.

Proper hygiene during farrowing is important as well. When assisting in farrowing, producers should wear plastic sleeves that are well lubricated and they should wash the sow's perineal region before entering the reproductive tract. Sows should be treated one time with benzathine penicillin (11 mg/kg) after such measures have been taken.

Proper design of gestation stalls is also important. The 2 m-long stall should include *at least* 1.0 m of slats under the sow. Gang slats of 10 cm in width with 2.54 cm gaps improve manure removal. New slat designs look promising, particularly those with slats that run perpendicular to the sow, with the gap space increasing in width toward the back of the stall. The solid portion of the floor should be gently sloped to allow for ease of water and urine runoff. The trough should be inlaid, *not raised*, to prevent excessive wetness in the stall after drinking.

Maximizing water consumption is necessary to induce frequent urination and flushing of the bladder. Fresh water should be made available at all times. Frequent watering and twice-a-day feedings will help the sows spend more time on their feet. Reducing feet and leg injuries will also help to promote frequent activity in the stall.

Nutritional modifications may also help water consumption, particularly by increasing salt content in the ration. Gestation diets should run 0.35% to 0.5% salt. Acidifying the urine through the addition of citric acid has been demonstrated to produce significant ($P<.0001$) reductions in urinary pH and urine bacterial concentration. In this report, citric acid was administered for 14 consecutive days postweaning at a level of 57 g per sow daily.

In conclusion, good management and proper building design for ensuring a high level of hygiene and a comfortable living environment still remain the best defense against *A. suis*–induced urinary tract disease in swine.

BIBLIOGRAPHY

Dee SA, Carlson AR, Corey MM: New observations on the epidemiology of *Eubacterium suis*. Compend Contin Educ 2:345–348, 1993.

Dee SA, Tracy JD, King V: Using citric acid to control urinary tract disease in swine. Vet Med 89:473–475, 1994.

Jones JET: *Eubacterium (Corynebacterium) suis*. In Leman AD, Straw BE, Mengeling WL, et al (eds): Diseases of Swine, ed 7. Iowa, Ames, Iowa State University Press, 1992, pp 643–645.

▪ Nocardioses

John A. Lynch, D.V.M., M.Sc., D.V.Sc.,
Diplomate, A.C.V.M.

DEFINITION

Nocardioses are noncontagious, pyogranulomatous infections caused by exogenous nocardioform bacteria. Numerous genera, species, and subtypes are now included in this group. *Nocardia asteroides* and *N. farcinica* are the most frequently reported veterinary isolates. Other species are being increasingly implicated as sporadic pathogens as identification techniques become refined. The pathogenic nocardioforms are globally distributed soil organisms. They have been found in higher prevalence in African and North American soil than in that of other continents that have been studied. Nocardioses are recognized worldwide and may occur as isolated cases or in epizootic proportions. Infection follows traumatic or iatrogenic implantation of foreign material, inhalation, or wound contamination. The form called *bovine farcy* is largely restricted to Africa, Asia, and the Middle East. Nocardial mastitis can cause economically significant losses in cattle and goat herds from repeated ineffective therapy, lost production, and lost genetic potential from culling. Human infection is not a zoonosis.

CLINICAL SIGNS

Typically, nocardiosis occurs as a localized infection; however, fever and other systemic signs may be present. The site of infection is dependent on the route of entry of the organisms. Response to antimicrobial drugs is consistently poor, despite in vitro tests, when disease is advanced.

Mycetoma (Including Bovine Farcy)

Mycetoma is characterized by tumefaction, draining sinuses, and granule formation as a result of traumatic inoculation of soil organisms, usually at a distal site in a lower limb. Bovine farcy is a specific, severe form involving subcutaneous lymphatic spread of *N. farcinica* to local lymph nodes, with or without concurrent infection with *Mycobacterium farcinogenes*.

Pneumonia

This rare form occurs in calves younger than 6 months or in goats. Inhalation is the presumed route of entry.

Abortion and Infertility

Nocardial abortion, which is also rare, has been described in cattle and swine. It can originate from contamination of the genital tract during obstetric manipulations. Fetal death follows from either placental necrosis or fetal septicemia. Uterine nocardiosis has been described as a cause of repeat breeding in cattle.

Mastitis

This is the most frequent clinical form of disease in food-producing animals, predominantly affecting mature cattle and goats. Major epizootic outbreaks occurred in France, Switzerland, and Canada in the late 1980s. *N. farcinica* was presumptively identified as the causative species in the Canadian epizootic outbreak. This ascending infection may occur as acute mastitis with fever and malaise, a chronic nonresponsive form, or a subclinical or preclinical infection. Heifers that have not received intramammary infusions are rarely affected.

Septicemia

Septicemic disease is infrequent, but it has been described and confirmed histologically. It usually follows prolonged localized disease. Sudden death after chronic nocardial mastitis is reported sporadically, but histologic confirmation of postulated nocardial septicemia is seldom documented.

CLINICAL PATHOLOGY AND NECROPSY LESIONS

In all forms of this disease, a chronic granulomatous tissue reaction with intermittent drainage through sinuses or natural orifices is typical. Mycetomas have a distal limb distribution, affecting skin and subcutaneous tissues. Bovine farcy is a nodular, suppurative dermatitis with granulomatous involvement of lymphatics and regional lymph nodes. In isolated or multiple nocardial mastitis, caseating granulomas with a lobular distribution may be present. These are often large and involve the dorsal portions of affected glands and supramammary lymph nodes. Only one gland is usually involved. Glandular secretions are initially watery with flakes, granules, or clumps. Thick, flocculent pus exudes in chronic cases. Leukopenia with a left shift may be present. Somatic cell counts for clinically infected quarters are generally 1 to 8×10^6 cells/mL, and California mastitis test scores are routinely $3+$. Branching, filamentous, modified acid-fast bacilli can be observed in secretions or tissues.

DIAGNOSIS

Specific diagnosis of nocardial mycetoma or farcy requires microscopic examination or laboratory culture for differentiation of the condition from eumycotic mycetoma, sporotrichosis, or bacterial cellulitis due to other agents. Index cases of nocardial mastitis in herds require similar laboratory assistance for etiologic differentiation from infection due to *Staphylococcus aureus*, *Actinomyces pyogenes*, atypical mycobacteria, or fungi. Because of sporadic shedding of the organism, subsequent cases may be more accurately diagnosed in herds on the basis of clinical findings, persistently high somatic cell counts, and abnormalities of the milk, unless serial cultures are performed. Accurate identification of the species and even the genus of the isolated nocardioform bacterium is difficult. Initial growth takes 48 to 72 hours, producing a small, chalky colony that develops a waxy, orange pigment and embeds in the agar. On microscopic examination, a mixture of gram-positive cocci, bacilli, and branching forms are present. *Nocardia* retain the modified acid-fast stain. In vitro susceptibility testing is of marginal value in directing therapy. It can be a useful adjunct in the identification of nocardioforms to the level of both genus (*Nocardia* is kanamycin resistant, rifampicin resistant, and sulfadimethoxine susceptible) and species (cefamandole, carbenicillin, and gentamicin susceptibility varies with the species). Demonstration of selected preformed enzymes, fatty acid profiles, and ribotyping are often required, in addition to conventional biochemical and cultural characteristics, to make species identification.

TREATMENT

Potentiated sulfonamides are most commonly recommended and they have proved effective in treating nocardial pneumonia. The prognosis for all nocardioses should be guarded to poor.

Treatment of nocardial mastitis rarely results in complete elimination of the organism, although temporary remissions in late lactation and intermittent negative cultures are common. Once the infection is confirmed, the animal should be shipped to slaughter at the earliest convenience. Most isolates are susceptible to tetracyclines, erythromycin, and potentiated sulfonamides, as well as some of the new cephalosporins, fluoroquino-

lones, and potentiated aminopenicillins. The use of these drugs by the recommended route and dosage may alleviate systemic or more severe local reactions sufficiently to maintain a cow until parturition. Repeated intermittent therapy, cessation of secretion with sclerosing agents (such as 500 mL of 2% formalin), or even mastectomy may be considered for exceptionally valuable cows. Whereas early diagnosis might allow a more satisfactory response to treatment, most cows appear to become infected during dry-treatment infusion, and clinical infection is not recognized until 1 to 2 months into lactation. Thus, the infection is generally in an advanced, chronic stage when initial therapy is instituted. Only rigorous attention to hygiene and relentless culling of all clinically affected or culture-positive animals appears to be effective in achieving long-term elimination of the problem from infected herds. At the time of diagnosis of the index case, producers should be advised of the frustrating nature of the disease, the insidious and persistent character of the infection in herds, and the potential for substantial economic loss if an aggressive control program is not strictly maintained.

PREVENTION

Considerations relative to prevention are largely restricted to nocardial mastitis. *Nocardia* is an environmental cause of mastitis, rather than a contagious cause. However, it is common to find multiple cases in herds. This may be a result of simultaneous or sequential exposure to the same contaminated source, rather than to true cow-to-cow transmission. Infected cows do provide a nidus of infection in herds. Contaminated multidose intramammary products or teat dips have been incriminated or suspected as sources. Isolation of the organism from such products retrospectively is difficult, owing to a variety of biologic factors, and incrimination of a specific product may require the application of carefully controlled epidemiologic studies. Blanket dry-cow therapy and the use of neomycin-based dry-cow infusions have been identified as significant risk factors in infected herds. Selective dry-cow therapy and the exclusive use of individually packaged, sterile, nonirritant intramammary infusions are advisable in known infected herds. Strict attention to aseptic infusion techniques must be reinforced. Teat dips containing dodecylbenzene sulfonic acid or nonylphenoxypolyethanol-iodine complex have greater in vitro efficacy against *Nocardia asteroides* than does chlorhexidine acetate, with or without emollient. The activity of disinfectants against nocardioforms is variable, but chlorine at 100 to 400 ppm for 5 to 60 minutes is reported bactericidal for mastitis isolates. Infected, suspected, or recently introduced cows should be milked last and isolated if possible.

This is an extremely disconcerting problem for producers because of the significant economic impact on individual affected herds, the lack of response to therapy, and the need to take control measures that contradict those advocated for control of contagious mastitis pathogens. An empathetic, patient, and informative approach is required to assist producers in the management of this disease.

BIBLIOGRAPHY

Laroque L, Malik SS, Landry DA, et al: In vitro germicidal activity of teat dips against *Nocardia asteroides* and other udder pathogens. J Dairy Science 75:1233–1240, 1992.

Manninen KI, Smith RA, Kim LO: Highly presumptive identification of bacterial isolates associated with the recent Canada-wide mastitis epizootic as *Nocardia farcinica*. Can J Microbiol 39:635–641, 1993.

Ollis GW, Schoonderwoerd M, Schipper C: An investigation of risk factors for nocardial mastitis in central Alberta dairy herds. Can Vet J 32:227–231, 1991.

■ Dermatophilosis

D.H. Lloyd, B.Vet.Med., Ph.D., F.R.C.V.S.,
Diplomate, E.C.V.D.

DEFINITION

Dermatophilosis is a seasonal proliferative and exudative skin disease, principally affecting mammals, that occurs throughout the world. The disease is also known as streptothricosis and, in sheep, as lumpy wool or mycotic dermatitis. The term *strawberry foot-rot* is used to describe an ovine syndrome involving the distal limbs in which concurrent infection with parapoxvirus (contagious ecthyma) occurs. Oral dermatophilosis has been described in cattle, buffaloes, cats, and humans. Subcutaneous lesions have been reported in cattle, lizards, and humans.

INCIDENCE

Subclinical infection is common in endemic areas, particularly in sheep. Clinical disease is usually associated with wet weather, and morbidity may be 100%. In African cattle, a higher incidence is seen in mature animals and males; however, in South America, infection is more prevalent in young animals. Considerable breed variation occurs in susceptibility. Zebu cattle are generally more resistant than *Bos taurus*, but West African N'dama and Muturu breeds are highly resistant. In sheep, the disease is more prevalent in fine-wooled breeds; lambs younger than 5 week old are particularly susceptible.

ETIOLOGY AND PATHOGENESIS

The causative organism, *Dermatophilus congolensis*, is an aerobic, gram-positive, filamentous bacterium normally found only in the epidermis. Its infective stage is a motile coccoid zoospore that is attracted toward breaks in the stratum corneum and germinates to form a mycelium that proliferates within the living epidermis. The mature mycelium becomes divided into packets of zoospores, which remain in the scabs formed by epidermal hyperkeratosis and can survive for long periods. On wetting, the zoospores are released and may initiate new infections. During dry weather, spontaneous recovery occurs in most animals, but the disease may persist in small chronic lesions, commonly on the ears. Scabs that remain attached to the coat may also act as reservoirs of infection. Transmission of the disease may be by contact or through the agency of ticks and flies, which may abrade the skin surface and inoculate the causative organism. Skin susceptibility is increased by trauma, heavy rainfall, exposure of unpigmented skin to sunlight, malnutrition, and concurrent disease. The immunosuppressive effects of infestation with the tick *Amblyomma variegatum* are associated with severe infections in cattle and goats.

Dermatophilus infection at sites other than the skin generally occurs in young or debilitated animals. In pigs, tonsillar infection with a *Dermatophilus*-like organism has been described, and isolation of *Dermatophilus* spp. from the skin of farmed saltwater crocodiles and of a new species, *D. chelonae*, from skin lesions of turtles has been reported.

IMPORTANCE

Hides and skins from diseased animals are unsuitable for use as leather; fleeces containing scabs are downgraded. The disease may cause decreased milk production and reduced fertility in dairy cattle. Performance of draft cattle may be greatly impaired. More severely affected animals suffer from cachexia and death. In Kenya and the Sudan, dermatophilosis of camels is a problem, particularly of calves, and appears to impair heat resistance.

CLINICAL SIGNS

The disease is first recognized when exudation and incipient scab formation mat the hairs, forming the characteristic "paintbrush" lesions. As the lesions develop, thick, dense scabs are formed, adjacent affected sites coalesce, and 50% or more of the body may be affected. Acute, generalized infection may occur in as little as 2 weeks, or the disease may extend progressively over periods of months or years. Mild infections may heal within 2 weeks in dry conditions and often pass unnoticed. Moist lesions in the fleeces of sheep are predisposed to fleece-rot and fly-strike.

The lesions can vary greatly in appearance and may occur on any part of the body. On haired skin, the scabs form flat plaques or horn-like projections; but on relatively hairless areas, such as the perineum, where wetting occurs, the scabs tend to be lost and the skin may become thickened, convoluted, and secondarily infected with other bacteria. In early lesions, hairs are found protruding from the scabs, but these disappear subsequently. The undersides of the scabs are typically concave and are covered with yellowish exudate when removed. The underlying skin has a red, coarsely granular, and often hemorrhagic appearance. On healing, the scabs separate from the skin but remain attached to the hairs.

Oral lesions in buffaloes and bulls appear as erosions or as raised granulomatous lesions affecting the palate, lips, and dorsal surface of the tongue. Subcutaneous and lymph node abscesses have been associated with *D. congolensis* infection in cattle, sheep, and a goat.

CLINICAL PATHOLOGY AND NECROPSY LESIONS

D. congolensis occurs as branching filaments composed of multiple rows of gram-positive cocci in stained smears obtained from freshly removed scabs; motile zoospores may be observed in emulsified preparations from such scabs. In chronic or secondarily infected lesions, the organism may not be readily found. In granulomatous oral, subcutaneous, and lymph node lesions, club-forming granulomas very similar to those in actinomycosis may occur.

Disease may be associated with a decrease in the serum albumin-to-globulin ratio; enlargement of lymph nodes and toxic changes in the liver and spleen may also be found. Concurrent disease, leading to other pathologic signs, may be present. Serum antibodies produced in response to infection are not protective, but serologic tests may be used to identify subclinical infection.

DIAGNOSIS

Diagnosis is based on the characteristic appearance of the skin lesions and demonstration of the causative organism in scabs or skin specimens. The seasonal nature of the disease and its association with humid conditions may assist in diagnosis. It should be differentiated from other skin conditions leading to scab formation on the skin. Bovine sarcoptic mange may produce a similar clinical condition, and fleece-rot may be confused with the disease, although the typical scabs of dermatophilosis are not present. Infections of the muzzle may be confused with contagious ecthyma and *peste des petits ruminants* in sheep and malignant catarrh or mucosal disease in cattle. Concurrent infection with these diseases may occur. Lesions at sites other than the skin usually occur in association with skin infection and in young or debilitated individuals.

TREATMENT

The objectives are to halt invasion and reinfection of the epidermis. In ruminants, invasion can be stopped by intramuscular injection of penicillin and streptomycin (or dihydrostreptomycin), either as a single dose (70,000 IU of penicillin and 70 mg of streptomycin per kilogram of body weight) or in five daily injections (5000 IU of penicillin and 5 mg of streptomycin per kilogram). Long-acting oxytetracycline (20 mg/kg) given as a single injection is also effective in most cases in cattle. Alternatively, 5-day treatment with tetracycline, chloramphenicol (which is unapproved for use in food animals in the United States), or spiramycin, at normal therapeutic levels, can be substituted. Successful treatment leads to separation of scabs from the skin surface; however, under wet conditions, reinfection may occur. Cases already advanced before treatment may fail to respond.

Topical therapy is less effective, but it may succeed in mild or early cases. Sprays containing 0.3% to 1% copper or zinc sulfate or cresols have been used. Sulfate dip (potash alum) may control the disease in sheep. In camels, topical use of 1% potassium-aluminum solution is reported to be effective.

Changes in management that will promote spontaneous recovery of ruminants include bringing animals into dry conditions and eliminating *A. variegatum* (see next section).

PREVENTION

The disease in sheep can be prevented by dusting the fleece with potash alum or aluminum sulfate during the wet periods of the year. These substances can also be used in the control of the disease as 1% solutions for dipping. The disease may be minimized by changes in management. Shearing should not be carried out during wet weather, and dipping or jetting should be avoided when fleeces are long. Cuts and abrasions after shearing may be disinfected by dipping in 0.5% zinc sulfate solution. Outbreaks in young lambs may be avoided by lambing during dry weather.

In cattle, control depends on the identification and elimination of predisposing factors such as ectoparasitic attack (ticks, flies, midges), abrasions due to thorny vegetation, concurrent disease, malnutrition, and other stress factors. When *A. variegatum* infestation occurs, it should be eliminated. In endemic areas, breeding for resistance and introduction of less susceptible breeds should be considered; DNA markers of resistance and susceptibility to dermatophilosis have been developed in Brahman zebu cattle in Martinique. Intradermal vaccination with live cultures of *Dermatophilus* reduces the incidence and severity of the disease, but effective preparations for field use are not yet available.

Eradication of the infection is generally impracticable owing to the widespread nature of the disease and the difficulty in identifying subclinical infections.

PUBLIC HEALTH SIGNIFICANCE

Dermatophilosis is a zoonotic disease, and care should be taken in handling infected animals.

BIBLIOGRAPHY

Ambrose NC: The pathogenesis of dermatophilosis. Trop Anim Health Prod 28:29S, 1996.
Hart CB, Tyszkiewicz K: Mycotic dermatitis in sheep: III. Chemotherapy with potassium aluminum sulfate. Vet Rec 82:272, 1968.
Ilemobade AA: Clinical experience in the use of chemotherapy for bovine dermatophilosis in Nigeria. Prev Vet Med 2:83, 1984.
Lloyd DH: Dermatophilosis: A review of the epidemiology, diagnosis and control. Proceedings of the CTA/CARDI Agricultural Seminar, Improving Health and Nutrition, Antigua, 1990. Trinidad, Caribbean Agricultural Research and Development Institute.

■ Systemic Mycoses

John F. Prescott, Vet.M.B., Ph.D.

The agents that cause systemic mycoses of food-producing mammals are part of the microbial flora of the external or internal environment. Those inhabiting the external environment, which constitute most of the organisms to be considered, are of low virulence. Animals are constantly exposed via the respiratory or intestinal route without adverse effects. Whether the agents assume a pathogenic role depends on developments that change the host-environment equilibrium, such as (1) a physiologic derangement in the animal (e.g., hormonal changes caused by advanced pregnancy or certain pituitary tumors or other immunosuppressive events); (2) an abnormal increase in the abundance of the fungi in the immediate environment (e.g., moldy feed and bedding or antibacterial therapy that removes competitive bacteria); and (3) the introduction of fungal cells by routes other than the respiratory or alimentary tract (e.g., mammary glands, wounds, or the uterus). The bulk of systemic mycoses are therefore sporadic, occurring most often in individual animals or in groups of animals subjected to comparable predisposition or exposure. Confirmation of these diseases involves pathologic, histopathologic, and cultural diagnosis. Special fungal stains include Wright's, Giemsa, silver, and periodic acid–Schiff (PAS) stains; in addition, yeasts—but not molds—stain with Gram's stain. Fungal hyphae and large yeasts may be readily seen on wet-mount examination.

Treatment is rarely attempted or successful in food animals, and antimycotic drugs have limited use. The proven means of dealing with systemic mycoses in food-producing mammals are largely confined to preventive measures instituted when the cause has been established by diagnostic tests.

ETIOLOGY

The most important mycotic syndromes recognized in food animals, primarily bovine abortion and mastitis, can be caused by a variety of fungal agents. With the exception of some of the *Candida* spp. (especially *C. albicans*) and, possibly, *Rhinosporidium seeberi*, all the fungi involved are free-living saprophytes of dead or decaying organic matter.

Aspergillus

Aspergillus spp. are common molds found in virtually every habitat. They grow as branching filaments (hyphae) with frequent subdivisions. They develop pigmented fruiting bodies at their free ends with chains of spores. The color and structure of the fruiting bodies are characteristic for each species. The most common species that affects animals is *A. fumigatus*. Septated hyphae can be demonstrated in unstained wet mounts, in

Giemsa- or Wright's-stained fixed smears, and in stained sections of pathologic material. Their presence in lesions justifies a provisional diagnosis of aspergillosis.

Zygomycetes or Phycomycetes

The Zygomycetes or Phycomycetes, also called mucoraceous fungi, are as abundant and cosmopolitan as *Aspergillus*. They differ in that there are few or no subdivisions in their usually broader hyphae, the only structures found in tissue. The fruiting bodies, which develop in culture, are spherical or oblong vesicles (sporangia). The shape of the sporangia, their support stalks (sporangiophores), and their relation to other hyphal features are important in determining genus and species. The genera important in animal diseases are *Mucor*, *Rhizopus*, *Absidia*, and *Mortierella*. A zygomycotic infection is suggested by the presence of broad, readily collapsing and twisting, nonseptate hyphae in smears or sections.

Histoplasma

Histoplasma capsulatum is a saprophytic fungus concentrated in the east central United States, but endemic foci are known in many parts of the world. *H. capsulatum* is dimorphic; fungi occur as molds in their saprophytic phase and as yeasts in their tissue phase. The yeasts can be demonstrated in Giemsa-, Wright's-, PAS-, or silver-stained smears or sections within phagocytic cells of infected hosts. At room temperature, these yeasts grow into the mold phase again, producing characteristic thick-walled spores. At 37°C they grow as yeasts. Demonstration of the two phases is required for definitive identification.

Coccidioides

Coccidioides immitis, the agent of coccidioidomycosis, is another dimorphic fungus confined to certain parts of the Western Hemisphere in which soil and climate favor its growth. All authentic instances of disease in all humans and animals are traceable to these areas. In the United States, they occur in parts of California, Arizona, New Mexico, and Texas. The saprophytic phase of *C. immitis* is mycelial, which is also the form in which the fungus grows on agar plates at either room temperature or 37°C. In the parasitic phase, after inhalation or, rarely, traumatic introduction, the arthrospore is transformed into a spherical structure (spherule, sporangium) in which nonbudding endospores develop. On liberation from the mature spherule, endospores may be disseminated to other tissues, in which another cycle of sporangium and endospore formation can be initiated. Culturing the sporangial phase on the usual media results in reversion to the filamentous mold form. The spherules can be demonstrated in wet mounts of bronchial washes or exudate and in stained sections of tissue.

Cryptococcus

Cryptococcus neoformans is encountered only in the yeast form. The organism lives in soil, its growth being enhanced by bird feces. On morphologic examination, *C. neoformans* is a spherical cell that reproduces by budding. The most striking feature is the presence of a mucoid capsule of varying thickness.

Candida

Candida spp., of which *C. albicans* is most prevalent in infections, is normally present on the mucous membranes, especially of the alimentary tract. Infections are most commonly endogenous. *Candida* spp. are basically yeasts that propagate by budding. The predominant cell shape is oval, and buds may be single or multiple. Under altered nutritional and atmospheric conditions, *Candida* spp. form mycelium by spore germination or pseudomycelium by cellular elongation and filament formation. This is also characteristic of *Candida* in its invasive phase, when it is actively growing in tissue rather than on mucus-containing membranes. *Candida* in its yeast, mycelial, and pseudomycelial forms is readily demonstrable in Gram's-stained smears of infected material.

Rhinosporidium seeberi

Most cases of infection are in tropical or subtropical climates. The pathogen has never been convincingly cultured on artificial media. In the parasitic state, it forms large vesicles, up to several hundred micrometers in diameter, in which endospores are generated. Their large size and anatomic predilection for the nasal mucosa differentiate them from the spherules (sporangia) of *Coccidioides immitis*. The natural reservoir of the agent is unknown.

Prototheca

Prototheca spp. are algae devoid of chlorophyll. They resemble yeasts superficially in that they are basically unicellular nucleated organisms enclosed by rigid cell walls. They undergo endosporulation, forming a sporangium from which, through internal cleavage, a new crop of organisms is produced and eventually liberated. Sporangia are readily demonstrated in unstained exudates and in culture suspensions as spherical to oval bodies, about 20 μm in diameter, containing a variable number of endospores. They stain with special fungal stains. They grow readily on common isolation media. Colonies resemble those of yeasts, being white to off-white and of creamy consistency. Microscopic examination demonstrates the characteristic pattern of spherical to oval cells at varying stages of endosporulation.

All of the agents mentioned are potentially pathogenic to humans under much the same conditions as for animals. The noncontagious nature of the diseases makes transmission from infected animals to humans a rather minor concern.

GENITAL INFECTIONS AND ABORTIONS

Incidence

The most prominent mycotic problem in food animals is abortion. Whereas fewer than 40% of all abortions in cattle can be associated with an infectious agent, fungal agents are blamed for about 2% to 30% of this total. The rate varies from year to year and from place to place. Fungal agents rank among the leading causes of bovine abortion, competing in the United States with viral abortion due to infectious bovine rhinotracheitis virus and in Europe with various bacteria, including *Brucella abortus* and *Leptospira* spp. Mycotic abortion in other food animal species is rare.

Etiology

A wide variety of fungal species have been implicated. *Aspergillus fumigatus* accounts for about two thirds or more of all mycotic abortions. It is followed in frequency by the zygomycotic fungi (*Mucor*, *Rhizopus*, *Mortierella*, and *Absidia*).

Epidemiology

The source of infection in most cases is external. Fungal spores are present in varying amounts in the feed and air, and the alimentary and respiratory tracts are portals of infection.

Genital infections may develop from commensal flora of the vagina or from contaminated semen. Breeding problems as a result of this type of infection involve yeasts more often than molds and are manifested in failures to conceive. Semen used for artificial insemination has repeatedly been shown to contain yeasts. In occasional instances, such contamination has been related to breeding problems, metritis, and even early abortion. Although various fungi of preputial origin have been demonstrated in semen, an important source of the fungi is semen extenders and other additives.

Mycotic abortions may occur at any time of gestation beginning in the third month, but they are most common in later pregnancy. The seasonal incidence shows a peak during winter. The circumstances responsible are (1) confinement in stables, with greater likelihood of prolonged respiratory exposure to suspended spores in high concentration; (2) the use of harvested feeds in which fungal growth has occurred, and, often, (3) the prevalence of animals in the advanced stages of pregnancy. Other predisposing factors may include steroid use, antibacterial drugs in the feed, and increased feeding of stored rather than fresh feeds. For example, in some studies, moisture and pH of hay and of silage have been related to mold infestation. High-moisture hay or moldy or rotten silage commonly contains common saprophytic fungi. In the outcome of exposure, quantitative aspects are of great importance, because abortions in cattle have frequently been related to the use of obviously moldy feed.

Pathogenesis

Most bovine mycotic abortions are the result of generalized infections via the respiratory and alimentary routes. Manifestations in these systems (e.g., granulomas in the lung and ulcers in the stomach) are usually subclinical but lead to bloodborne dissemination. Localization in the placenta results in placentitis, necrosis, and hemorrhage, with eventual separation of the chorion from the maternal placental tissue by an exudate in which fungal hyphae abound. Penetration of tissue and blood vessels is thought to be aided, at least in the case of certain fungi, by necrotizing enzymes. Attempts to account for the placental localization of fungi have revealed substances in tissue extracts of cattle that stimulate germination of fungal spores and growth of fungi. The chemical nature of such substances has not been adequately defined, nor is it necessarily the total explanation of the abortion process.

Clinical Signs and Pathology

Clinically, there are few features that differentiate mycotic abortions from other abortions at the same stage of pregnancy. In the majority of cases, no general illness is present in the aborting cow, although fatal, fulminating pneumonia after *Mortierella wolfii* infection has been reported in New Zealand, which was followed within 1 to 5 days by fulminating and ultimately fatal pneumonia in the majority of affected animals. Such systemic complications by *M. wolfii* abortions are not common elsewhere.

The aborted fetuses may be grossly normal. A variable percentage (2% to 25%) have ringworm-like skin lesions in which fungal elements can be demonstrated. They are concentrated in the head and neck region. Such lesions are observed with *Aspergillus*- and Zygomycete-induced abortions. Internal lesions of the fetus may include general lymphadenitis, dehydration, and emaciation. Mycotic colonization of lungs, liver, spleen, and brain may occur. Grossly recognizable mold colonies may be floating in the abomasal or amniotic fluid.

The most significant and the striking lesions of mycotic abortion are necrotizing hemorrhagic placentitis, manifested grossly by brownish discoloration and swollen necrotic placentomes with thickened edges distorting the structure into a cup-like shape. There is much adventitious placentation and thickening of intercotyledonary areas. The cotyledons adhere firmly to the maternal caruncles, so that retention of the placenta is very common. On microscopic examination, the basic lesion is one of vasculitis, with hyphal invasion of the vessel walls, especially when zygomycotic agents are involved. Thrombosis, hemorrhage, necrosis, and inflammation with neutrophilic components predominating follow. Microscopic fetal lesions include bronchopneumonia and, where skin lesions are present, necrotizing epidermitis.

Extragenital lesions in the cows consist of pyogranulomatous nodules in various internal organs, particularly lung and kidneys. In cases of fatal pneumonia described as an abortion sequela to *M. wolfii*, a fibrinohemorrhagic process is evident.

Diagnosis

The diagnosis of mycotic abortion rests on the demonstration of fungi in association with significant lesions. The mere demonstration or, even less conclusively, culture of fungi from specimens obtained after abortions or from genital tracts does not constitute adequate evidence of a causative role for the fungi. The ubiquity of fungi and the almost invariable contamination of placenta and fetus before examination render the presence of fungi in such material very likely. Fungi must be demonstrated as integral parts of the lesions before their etiologic significance can be fully established.

For pathologic examination, placental tissues, especially cotyledons, should be submitted. If the entire fetus cannot be promptly forwarded to a laboratory, skin lesions, lymph nodes, lung, and stomach—with its contents securely tied off—should be forwarded. Duplicate tissue samples can be placed into 10% formalin. The stomach contents may be preserved for microscopic examination by addition of 1 part formalin to 9 parts fluid. Fungi do not tolerate putrefactive tissue changes well, nor do they benefit from freezing.

Treatment and Control

To date, no specific control measures are available. A reasonable preventive step is the elimination of moldy feeds and, as far as possible, removal of animals from moldy environments. Most cows that survive an episode of fungal abortion return to breed normally without special treatment.

MYCOTIC MASTITIS

Incidence

The incidence of mycotic mastitis ranges from about 1% to 10% of total mastitis of infectious origin. These figures may have little relevance to individual herds, in which outbreaks, usually triggered by some management factor, may involve the majority of milking cows. A large variety of fungal agents have been implicated. The most frequent are the yeastlike fungi, particularly *Candida* spp. and *Cryptococcus* spp. Rare genera are *Hansenula*, *Pichia*, *Rhodotorula*, *Torulopsis*, *Trichosporon*, and *Saccharomyces*. Mold mastitis is rarely encountered, but *A. fumigatus* has been incriminated in a greater number of instances in recent years, particularly in Europe. *Pseudallescheria boydii* has been implicated on occasion, and there is growing awareness of the alga *Prototheca* (usually *P. zopfii*) as a cause of mastitis.

Epidemiology

Like all mastitis, mycotic mastitis is decisively influenced by management factors. Two aspects of dairy routine are particularly pertinent: (1) milking hygiene and (2) the use of antimicrobial drugs, especially by intramammary infusion. Inadequate milking hygiene may permit the passage of mastitis-producing agents from one mammary gland to another, converting a basically fortuitous, sporadic infection into a transmissible disease of potentially epidemic proportions. Mycotic mastitis as a herd problem is related to machine milking and other practices involving rapid successive contact of udders with persons or equipment capable of acting as vehicles of transmission. Heavy contamination of feedstuffs with molds or yeast may also lead to herd problems.

The use of antibacterial drugs can play a part in the production of mastitis in two possible ways. First, it can provide the mechanical means of introducing fungal spores into the gland, because these are abundant in the environment, including on the skin of the udder. Yeasts have also been found in freshly opened antibiotic preparations, which suggests contamination during manufacture. Second, some antimicrobials are suspected of stimulating fungal growth and depressing certain host-defense factors. For example, tetracycline has been described as having both of these effects with regard to *Candida albicans*. Circumstances surrounding mycotic mastitis outbreaks frequently include preceding or ongoing antibacterial intramammary therapy, but moldy or yeast-contaminated feed may also be implicated.

Clinical Signs, Pathogenesis, and Pathology

Fungal mastitis has no consistent peculiarities to distinguish it from bacterial mastitis. Reduced milk flow, swelling, and greater firmness of the affected gland are observed, along with varying abnormalities in the appearance of the milk and positive results of the California mastitis test. Fevers with "spiking" temperatures may occur, but they have not been correlated with demonstrable fungemia. The duration and course of the disease are highly variable, depending on the infecting agent and the size of the infecting dose. The most severe fungal mastitis is caused by *Cryptococcus neoformans*, which can extend over weeks and months, lead to complete suppression of milk flow, and leave glands with diminished or lost milk-secreting ability. By contrast, infection with other yeasts (*Candida* spp.) takes a more benign and, frequently, self-limiting course. Whenever herds undergoing outbreaks of fungal mastitis have been investigated, a large proportion of infected but clinically normal animals were identified, even when *Cryptococcus neoformans* was present. The pathologic changes evoked by yeasts are pyogranulomatous reactions. The acute phase is characterized by neutrophilic and eosinophilic exudates. Histiocytic infiltration and granuloma formation follow. In gross appearance, edema predominates early, with granulomatous foci and fibrotic changes occurring in advanced lesions.

In *A. fumigatus* mastitis, which is rare, a chronic progressive course is usually observed, with suppurative lesions predominating at necropsy. Protothecal mastitis, although ranging from acute to chronic to inapparent, also appears to follow a progressive, irreversible course eventuating in the destruction of the infected gland.

Diagnosis

In the absence of specific clinical criteria, the demonstration of the causative agent by direct microscopic findings and culture is a requirement for establishing a diagnosis of fungal mastitis. The manner of collection, promptness of handling, and method of processing determine results. The presence of fungi (e.g., *Candida* spp.) in the environment, on the skin, and even in the teat canal and sinus would render the isolation of small numbers of the organisms of doubtful significance. However, finding yeast cells in fresh milk by direct microscopic examinations of fixed stained smears indicates the presence of considerable numbers and points to infection. *Candida* cells are readily stained by Gram's stain and appear as predominantly purple, often budding, ovoids. Cryptococcal cells do not show any consistent staining patterns with Gram's stain and are apt to be overlooked.

Both *Candida* and *Cryptococcus* will grow on most common culture media, including blood and Sabouraud agar either at room temperature or at 37°C. Several days should be allowed for colonial growth to develop. The specific identification of the yeast is based on morphologic and physiologic tests. Several simple commercially available systems of yeast identification exist for clinically prominent species. Hyphal fragments can be demonstrated in centrifuged mammary secretions by wet mounts in 15% potassium hydroxide. *A. fumigatus* grows well on blood agar and most other common media and is identified on the basis of fruiting-structure morphology. Demonstration and culture of *Prototheca* spp. have been described earlier.

Treatment and Control

No established treatment presently exists for fungal mastitis, and many cases may resolve spontaneously in 2 to 4 weeks. In fact, no intramammary antimycotic drug has been approved to date for use in the United States. Recommendations followed in Europe include intramammary nystatin ointment, 3 g given on 3 successive days, or nystatin solution, 250,000 units in 2.5 mL given on at least 2 successive days but to no more than two quarters at one time, because of the toxic local and systemic effects that the aqueous solution may elicit. Clotrimazole is also suggested and may be preferable, and it can be used as ointment or as aqueous solution, 100 to 200 mg/quarter in 10 to 20 mL, given two to four times at 24-hour intervals. Another drug that has been suggested for treatment of *Candida* mastitis is intramammary natamycin given as 2.5% or 5% solution in 20 or 10 mL, respectively, on three successive days.

In vitro test results showed yeasts isolated from bovine mastitis to be most susceptible to clotrimazole. Results varied with regard to other antimycotics, including miconazole, nystatin, and flucytosine. One study rated ketoconazole next best to clotrimazole, and this and other imidazoles, such as enilconazole, may also be suitable for local treatment.

Treatment of *Prototheca* mastitis with most antibacterial antibiotics is ineffective. Strains are, however, sensitive to nystatin, with a proportion sensitive to polymyxin B, amphotericin B, and gentamicin. No accounts have been published on their use in treatment. Approaches to control have usually involved repeated cultural examination for identifying infected cows, which are then immediately culled. This approach is combined with environmental, especially water, hygiene.

No recommendations are available, based on adequate field or experimental studies, concerning the treatment of mastitis due to molds.

OTHER MYCOSES

Aspergillosis

Sporadic clinical aspergillosis in cattle, sheep, and swine as either isolated cases or limited outbreaks has been reported from all parts of the world. Primarily young animals or debilitated animals are involved. Either the respiratory or alimentary tract is affected and constitutes the likely portal of infection. General cases with lesions in kidney, liver, and lungs are also sometimes observed.

Massive exposure to moldy feed and bedding, rumen acidosis, and extended administration of antimicrobial drugs have been found to be associated with infection. Subclinical aspergillosis has been shown to be widespread in cattle, with both pulmonary and intestinal localizations reported. Several instances of fatal infections in newborn animals, especially lambs, point to the likelihood of prenatal exposure.

Acute cases exhibit hemorrhagic, necrotic lesions associated with vasculitis and thrombosis. More chronic cases are characterized by granuloma formation and fibrosis. Eosinophils may be prominent in association with the lesions and in the circulating blood. The agent occurs as septate filaments, 2 to 3 μm in diameter, fairly regular in outline, and generally branching at acute angles. In progressive pulmonary aspergillosis, cavitation may occur, with the fungus growing freely in the lumen of the cavities, producing cottony, aerial mycelia, complete with pigmented fruiting bodies. A frequent feature of chronic and subclinical aspergillosis is the presence of "asteroid" bodies, that is, hyphal nests surrounded by radiating acidophilic projections.

Zygomycoses

Systemic infection with Zygomycetes occurs primarily in cattle, but it also occurs in swine. Reports of infections in sheep are extremely rare. The genera involved are mainly *Mucor*, *Absidia*, and *Rhizopus*. Many cases are based on histopathologic findings only, so that no genus, let alone species, identification is possible. A noteworthy incidence of *Mortierella* infections has been reported, mainly from New Zealand.

The epidemiology of these infections, like that of aspergillosis, is related to acidosis, inappropriate diet, and concurrent infection due to other fungi, bacteria, or viruses. Unusually concentrated exposure to the agents is also thought to play a part. Gastrointestinal tract involvement predominates, especially in pigs. Several cases of neonatal encephalitis have been observed in cattle.

Reports of zygomycotic infections, especially in young animals, describe acute signs and lesions more often than is the case with aspergillosis. Gastrointestinal tract disturbances are frequently the first sign, including anorexia and mucosanguineous diarrhea. Ruminal atony, bloat, and colic have been observed in affected cattle. Other forms affect mainly the lymph nodes of the intestinal tract or thorax. The gross lesions in the gastrointestinal tract are ulcerations of the stomach and intestine. Any part of the stomach can be involved. In ruminants, the rumen and abomasum are the usual sites. Depending on the acuteness of the condition, hemorrhagic, necrotic, suppurative, or nodular granulomatous features will predominate, in that order. Vasculitis constitutes the basic lesion, affecting either arteries or veins;

it is initiated by hyphal invasion of the vessel wall. Thrombosis and vascular disintegration follow, causing hemorrhage, necrosis, and suppuration, all of which are grossly observable. In the form that produces lymphadenitis, the only lesions may be granulomas in the nodes, which range from a few millimeters in diameter to those that have replaced all recognizable lymph node tissue. The lymph node lesions resemble those of tuberculous change. Hyphae are apparent and are distinguishable from those of *Aspergillus* spp. by their larger size (up to 7 μm), their irregular outline, their relative lack of septa, and their greater tendency to branch to right angles.

In swine, gastric zygomycosis has been reported infrequently as a cause of mucosal or transmural hemorrhagic ulcers, sometimes in pigs as young as 1 week old. Predisposing factors may include liberal use of antibiotics in piglets or their dams. In older pigs, zygomycosis is sometimes associated with submandibular and mesenteric lymph node granulomas. No successful treatment has been established.

Candidiasis

Most *Candida* infections have been encountered in cattle and swine. The localization, other than in bovine mastitis, has been predominantly in the alimentary tract from the mouth to the intestine. Septicemic and pneumonic infections are seen rarely.

The source of the causative agents may be the mucous membranes of the animals themselves, which contain *C. albicans*, or the skin and external environment, which contain other *Candida* spp. The prolonged use of broad-spectrum antibacterial drugs is frequently a factor in initiating clinical candidiasis. The disruption of the normal microbial balance in the digestive tract produces the overgrowth by the yeasts. In some cases, massive prolonged exposure to contaminated feed has been implicated in the absence of, or in addition to, antibiotics predisposition.

The common clinical form of candidiasis is thrush and enteritis in calves and young pigs. Thrush is an ulcerative pseudomembranous inflammation of the mucous membranes of the mouth, esophagus, and stomach (rumen). The process in the intestine is similar, but it is not usually referred to as thrush. Clinical signs reflect the location of the process; inappetence, excessive salivation, and vomiting occur in oral and upper digestive tract infections. Intestinal infections are also characterized by diarrhea.

Lesions are those of ulcerative inflammation with varying amounts of overlying fibrinous exudate. As long as the process is relatively superficial, the yeast forms of *Candida* predominate. With invasion of deeper tissue, pseudomycelial and mycelial structures replace the yeasts.

Confirmation of candidiasis requires demonstration of *Candida* spp. in significant numbers in association with compatible lesions. The recovery of *Candida* from oral or rectal swabs and even from tracheobronchial washings does not establish the diagnosis. Overgrowth without significant pathogenic activity is a distinct possibility with these fungi. Finding a preponderance of filamentous forms is much more suggestive of a disease. Microbiologic observations must be evaluated in the light of pathologic and clinical evidence.

The agents of candidiasis are readily cultured on common media over a wide range of temperatures. A few reports of successful treatment of clinical candidiasis have been published, especially from the United States. Experience in Europe showed favorable results with oral nystatin and amphotericin B in isolated instances. Control measures should be directed at removing underlying causes.

Histoplasmosis and Coccidioidomycosis

Instances of clinical histoplasmosis in livestock are extremely rare. Existing reports concern cattle and pigs. Respiratory lesions were present in all 6 cases but 1, in which the lesions were in the liver. Among food-producing mammals, only cattle are infected with *C. immitis* to any significant extent. The infection is quite common in endemic areas but invariably subclinical and evident only at post-mortem examination, when thoracic lymphadenitis and small lung lesions may be noted. Coccidioidomycosis in sheep has been reported. The infection is of no economic importance in livestock.

Mycotic Nasal Infections

A variety of fungi have been implicated in nasal infections. Among food-producing animals, only cattle have been involved. The lesions are nasal granulomas and polyps, which lead to respiratory distress of varying severity. Best known among the polyp-forming infections is rhinosporidiosis, a disease mostly seen in tropical and subtropical climates but occasionally seen in the United States. Polyps, pedunculated or not, form in one nostril. They are soft and pink and bleed readily. The whitish specks they contain are the spherules (sporangia) previously mentioned. Treatment is through surgical excision. A report from Argentina refers to cures in nine cases after treatment with calcium, isoniazid, and 60% sodium iodide.

Bovine granulomas, with and without polyp formation, have been found to be associated with infections by pigmented saprophytic fungi (pheohyphomycosis). Some of these infections were accompanied by fairly widespread involvement of skin and lymph nodes. The agents included, among other black (dematiaceous) fungi, mainly *Drechslera rostrata* and *D. spicifera*. The lesions have been described as mycetomas, and allergy is assumed to be involved by many workers. No medical treatment is known.

Blue-Green Algae

Blue-green algal intoxication causing fatal hepatotoxicity has been described in cows drinking water contaminated with the algal bloom of *Microcystis* spp.

ANTIFUNGAL DRUGS

Medical treatment of deep mycosis in food animals is a virtually unexplored field, in part because antifungal drugs suitable for such treatment are relatively new and have not been adequately tested in food-producing mammals. It is to be expected that this situation will change and that drugs presently in use on humans and companion animals will be utilized on meat and dairy stock. A brief characterization of the types of drugs used on fungal infections is therefore appropriate. Present antifungal drugs fall into three chemical categories.

1. The polyenes are represented by nystatin (Mycostatin*) and amphotericin B (Fungizone*). They are characterized by limited solubility in water and poor absorbability from the gastrointestinal tract. They are also quite toxic. Nystatin is useful only for topical application or intestinal infection, mostly of yeasts. Amphotericin B, which is at present the mainstay of antifungal therapy in humans, is given by intravenous injection. Systemic amphotericin B has not been used in food animals. Natamycin is effective against a wide range of filamentous fungi

and yeasts. It is poorly absorbed and is therefore not useful in systemic infections, but it has been used effectively in the treatment of mycotic mastitis.

2. A more recently introduced antimycotic is flucytosine (Ancobon†), which is readily absorbed from the gastrointestinal tract and is generally well tolerated. Its usefulness so far has been confined largely to the treatment of infections due to yeast-like fungi, particularly candidiasis and cryptococcosis. A further limitation to the use of flucytosine is the existence of resistant strains of these yeasts in nature and the common emergence of resistance in the course of treatment. Susceptibility tests are advisable for establishing the appropriateness of this drug in each instance in which its use is considered.

3. The most recent additions to the antimycotic armamentarium are the various imidazole derivatives, for example, miconazole (Monistat‡), clotrimazole (Lotrimin§), fluconazole (Diflucan¶), and ketoconazole (Nizoral‡). Some of these drugs (e.g., miconazole) can be used both topically and systemically, whereas others are for topical use only (e.g., clotrimazole). The imidazole derivatives have a rather broad spectrum of activity and affect both yeasts and mycelial fungi. They are effective when administered orally. Resistance has not been a major problem so far. The drugs also inhibit dermatophytes. Their toxicity is much less than that of amphotericin B.

BIBLIOGRAPHY

Aalbaek B, Stenderup J, Jensen HE, et al: Mycotic and algal bovine mastitis in Denmark. APMIS 102:451, 1994.
Anderson KL, Walker RL: Sources of *Prototheca* spp. in a dairy herd environment. J Am Vet Med Assoc 193:553, 1988.
Elad D, Shpigel NY, Winkler M, et al: Feed contamination with *Candida krusei* as a probable source of mycotic mastitis in dairy cows. J Am Vet Med Assoc 207:620, 1995.
Johnson CT, Lupson GR, Lawrence KE: *Mortierella wolfii* abortion in British cows. Vet Rec 127:363, 1990.
Katamoto H, Shimada Y: Intra-arterial and intramammary injection of miconazole for bovine mastitis caused by *Aspergillus fumigatus*. Br Vet J 146:354, 1990.
Kirk JH, Bartlett PC: Bovine mycotic mastitis. Comp Contin Educ Pract Vet 8:F106, 1986.
Reed WM, Hanika C, Mehdi NAQ, et al: Gastrointestinal zygomycosis in suckling pigs. J Am Vet Med Assoc 191:549, 1987.

■ Swine Mycobacterial Disease

J. Glenn Songer, Ph.D.

ETIOLOGY

In the early 1900s, the etiologic agents of tuberculosis in swine were often *Mycobacterium bovis* or *M. tuberculosis*, perhaps reflecting the prevalence of these organisms in humans. The rise to prominence of *M. avium* began during the second quarter of the century and has gradually overtaken *M. bovis* and *M. tuberculosis* in importance as a cause of mycobacterial disease in swine. During the past 15 years, isolation from swine of mycobacteria other than *M. avium* has been uncommon. The human opportunist pathogens *M. kansasii*, *M. xenopi*, and *M. fortuitum* have been isolated, as has *M. chelonei*. The last is of potential significance to human health because the same organism has been isolated from prosthetic heart valves prepared from swine. *M. paratuberculosis*, the cause of Johne's disease, and *M. microti*, the vole bacillus, have also been isolated from pigs.

Pig-to-pig transmission may be a factor in the spread of tuberculosis, apparently because of shedding in feces of *M.*

avium from lesions in the intestinal wall. This means of spread is probably of relatively little significance because infection is not maintained in a herd after an external source is eliminated. Infection of the lungs, mammary glands, and uterus also occurs and may represent a means of dissemination. However, the major sources of infection are chickens or other birds and the feeding of improperly processed food waste.

Soil contaminated by chickens with tuberculosis may also be a reservoir of *M. avium*. In addition, the disease has been associated with wood shavings used for bedding. The incidence may be more than 50%, and serovars of *M. avium* recovered from swine can often be isolated from wood shavings as well. The organism survives for long periods in wood shavings (at least 4 years under natural conditions) and may multiply under appropriate conditions. Seasonal variation in moisture and temperature correlates with the incidence of tuberculosis in some herds.

SIGNIFICANCE

In contrast to the progressive disease caused by *M. tuberculosis* and *M. bovis*, *M. avium* rarely produces clinical signs in pigs. Some have suggested, with good reason, that the disease be called *swine mycobacteriosis* rather than tuberculosis. Estimates of the prevalence of swine tuberculosis have been based on the rate of detection of lesions at slaughter. On this basis, the prevalence is 0% to 5% in all hogs slaughtered under federal inspection and costs the pork industry an estimated $2 million annually. It is likely that false positives (caused by infection with organisms such as *Rhodococcus equi* and the occurrence of culture-negative, "healed" lesions) and false negatives (caused by the presence of *M. avium* in lymph nodes in the absence of lesions) influence these figures.

The possibility for transmission of *M. avium* infection from pigs to humans is the basis for current meat inspection regulations. In the past, swine tissues with gross lesions compatible with tuberculous were trimmed and discarded. However, a regulation adopted in 1972 in the United States calls for cooking (170°F, 30 minutes) of all carcasses that contain at least two isolated tuberculous lesions; these carcasses are designated "passed for cooking." The absence of cooking facilities in many processing plants requires that passed-for-cooking carcasses be condemned. There is no evidence to support a role for infected swine as a source of infection in humans (even those with acquired immunodeficiency syndrome).

PATHOGENESIS

Based on the high proportion of pigs with lesions developing in lymph nodes associated with the digestive tract, *M. avium* is probably most often acquired by the ingestion of contaminated feed. The organism apparently associates with epithelial cells of the digestive tract, occasionally multiplying there in an intracellular location and often being engulfed by macrophages in the subepithelial space. Lesions develop after transport to the regional lymph nodes (usually cervical or mesenteric). Susceptibility may be greatest during the neonatal period.

DIAGNOSIS

The typical absence of clinical signs of *M. avium* infection requires that the disease in swine be diagnosed by demonstration of compatible gross and microscopic lesions and by isolation and identification of *M. avium*. The tuberculin skin test may be a useful herd test, but its relative lack of sensitivity and specific-ity suggests that it should be used judiciously. No other diagnostic test is in common use.

Gross lesions of *M. avium* infection are typically nodular, white to yellow, and up to 10 mm in diameter. Diffuse fibrosis with proliferation of epithelioid and giant cells is a distinctive characteristic, and caseous exudate is usually seen. Calcification is common, but mainly in lesions that are no longer infected. Lesions are not usually pathognomonic for infection by a given *Mycobacterium* species, and bacteriologic culture is recommended.

THERAPY

No vaccine is available, and no antimicrobial agents have demonstrated efficacy in prophylaxis or therapy.

PREVENTION AND CONTROL

Direct and indirect contact between pigs and domestic or wild birds should be controlled. Housing of hogs in old poultry buildings should only follow thorough cleaning and disinfection with a phenol-based disinfectant or a 2% to 3% cresylic acid solution. Quaternary ammonium disinfectants are not effective. Equipment such as farrowing crates and feeders must also be disinfected. Decontamination of infected soil is not practical.

Many producers have experienced no significant problems while using wood shavings as bedding, but others have been forced out of business because of economic losses in slaughter hogs. Thus the use of wood shavings for bedding (especially in farrowing buildings) should be eliminated. If wood shavings are used, they should be kept dry during storage. Shavings from kiln-dried lumber may be less likely to contain *M. avium* than shavings from green lumber. Improperly processed food waste or other material that might contain pathogenic mycobacteria must not be fed to pigs. When possible, breeding stock should be purchased from tuberculosis-free herds.

If a source of infection can be found and eliminated, the producer's best alternative may be to wait out the approximate 6-month period until all exposed pigs have been slaughtered. Alternatively, infected herds may be depopulated, but the source of infection must be found and removed. If infected gilts are retained, lesions may regress before the pigs are eventually sent to slaughter.

BIBLIOGRAPHY

Gardner IA, Hird DW: Environmental source of mycobacteriosis in a California swine herd. Can J Vet Res 53:33–37, 1989.
Margolis MJ, Hutchinson LJ, Kephart KB, et al: Results of using histologic examination and acid-fast staining to confirm a diagnosis of swine mycobacteriosis made on the basis of gross examination. J Am Vet Med Assoc 204:1571–1572, 1994.

■ Bovine Tuberculosis
Janet B. Payeur, D.V.M., M.P.H., Ph.D.

Tuberculosis is a chronic infectious disease caused by certain pathogenic acid-fast organisms in the genus *Mycobacterium*. It is usually characterized by the chronic formation of nodular granulomas, known as *tubercles*. However, tuberculosis can sometimes assume an acute, rapidly progressive course.

ETIOLOGY

The etiologic agents of mammalian tuberculosis, classified as members of the *Mycobacterium tuberculosis* complex, are *M. tuberculosis, M. bovis, M. microti,* and *M. africanum.* The cause of bovine tuberculosis is *M. bovis,* otherwise known as the bovine tubercle bacillus. It has one of the broadest host ranges of all known pathogens. *M. bovis* has been isolated from domestic and feral cattle and swine, goats, sheep, horses, cats, dogs, fennec foxes, deer, bison, buffalo, badgers, possums, hares, ferrets, coyotes, antelopes, Arabian oryx, camels, llamas, alpacas, humans, and nonhuman primates.

EPIDEMIOLOGY

Tuberculosis caused by *M. bovis* is a zoonotic disease with a complex epidemiologic pattern that includes the transmission of infection within and between farm animal and wildlife populations. Bovine tuberculosis exists in all parts of the world. Zoonotic infection with *M. bovis* was a major cause of human tuberculosis before the introduction of programs for its control and elimination, which included milk pasteurization, tuberculin testing, and adequate meat inspection. In the United States in 1917, before the test and slaughter tuberculosis eradication program was initiated, the infection rate of bovine tuberculosis was approximately 5% in cattle.

During the 10-year period from Oct 1, 1987, to Sept 30, 1996, *M. bovis* represented 78% of the mycobacterial isolates from cattle specimens submitted to the National Veterinary Services Laboratories in Ames, Iowa, for tuberculosis examination. During the same period, *Mycobacterium avium* represented 95% of the mycobacteria isolated from swine. During the 6-year period from Oct 1, 1990, to Sept 30, 1996, *M. bovis* and *M. avium* represented 42% and 30% of the mycobacterial isolates from cervid specimens.

Although tuberculosis has been reduced to a low sporadic occurrence in U.S. cattle, 7 infected cattle and 4 infected cervid herds were reported during fiscal year 1996. From Jan 1, 1991, to Sept 30, 1996, there were 31 infected cervid herds and 31 infected cattle herds in the United States. The infection rate in 1996 was less than 0.001% in cattle and bison.

Hosts shed *M. bovis* in respiratory discharges, feces, milk, urine, semen, and genital discharges. When infection occurs by inhalation, a lesion is often found at the point of entry and in the draining lymph node, subsequently leading to localized lesions in the upper respiratory and pulmonary lymph nodes and in lung parenchyma. When ingestion is the route of entry, alimentary lesions are rare, but lesions may be present in the tonsils and pharyngeal, mesenteric, mediastinal, or bronchial lymph nodes. Additional lesions may then disseminate from the primary areas to other areas. In calves, the mode of infection may be by ingestion via milk. Lesions can occur in the intestinal wall, mesenteric lymph nodes, and liver and spleen and secondarily in the lungs. Occasionally, intrauterine infection has resulted from coital transfer.

PATHOGENESIS

Mycobacterial virulence factors seem to reside in the lipid components of the cell wall. Mycosides, phospholipids, and sulfolipids apparently protect tubercle bacilli against phagocytic killing. Glycolipids cause a granulomatous response and enhance the survival of phagocytosed mycobacteria. Wax D and various tuberculoproteins induce a delayed hypersensitivity reaction that can be detected by the tuberculin test. Infection is usually via the respiratory and intestinal tracts. In previously unexposed animals, local multiplication of the mycobacteria occurs, and resistance to phagocytic killing allows continued intracellular and extracellular replication. Infected host cells and mycobacteria can reach local lymph nodes and from there may pass to the thoracic duct with general dissemination.

After the first week, cell-mediated immune reactions modify the host response to enable activated macrophages to kill some mycobacteria. The aggregation of macrophages contributes to the formation of a tubercle, and a fibrous layer may encompass the lesion. Caseous necrosis occurs at the center of the lesion and may progress to calcification or liquefaction. Once cell-mediated immunity is established, lymphatic spread is retarded but occurs by contiguous extension or via the erosion of bronchi, blood vessels, or viscera. T-lymphocyte–mediated reactions cause tissue damage. Hematogenous dissemination may produce miliary tuberculosis in animals such as deer. This involves multifocal tubercle formation in an organ or on the serosal surface of a cavity.

DIAGNOSIS

Because of the chronic nature of the disease and the variable localization of the infection, which causes a multiplicity of signs, tuberculosis is difficult to diagnose clinically and is usually found only at necropsy. The etiologic agent must be isolated and identified to confirm a diagnosis of tuberculosis. Identification by culture requires specialized media incubated at 37°C aerobically for 4 to 8 weeks. The addition of 0.4% sodium pyruvate stimulates mycobacterial growth, whereas glycerol inhibits it and should not be included in the primary media. Mycobacteria are nonmotile, nonsporing, aerobic, and oxidative. Microscopically, *M. bovis* is an acid-fast rod 0.2 to 0.6 μm by 1 to 10 μm in size, sometimes with branching and cording.

Clinical Signs and Lesions

The signs of tuberculosis in animals usually vary with the distribution of tubercles in the body. Clinical evidence of disease may not become apparent in chronic cases until the terminal stages of disease. In cases with progressive pulmonary disease, the animals may show signs of dyspnea with an associated cough.

The alimentary form is unusual. There are few signs, but diarrhea may occasionally occur. Bloat can arise through enlargement of the mediastinal and bronchial lymph nodes.

Mammary involvement tends to be rare but may result in udder induration and supramammary lymph node enlargement. The udder form can be a serious hazard because it is a potential source of tuberculosis for humans and calves. The uterine form is uncommon; swelling of various lymph nodes can occasionally be seen, and abortion occurs infrequently.

A generalized form of tuberculosis can occur with signs following calving. There is a progressive loss of weight with a variable appetite. Rectal temperature may vary but is usually around 39.7°C (103.7°F). The animals are more docile than normal, but still bright and alert.

Immunodiagnosis

Cell-mediated hypersensitivity, acquired through infection, can be demonstrated systemically by fever, ophthalmically by conjunctivitis, or dermally by local swelling when tuberculin or its purified protein derivative (PPD) is given by the subcutaneous, conjunctival, or intradermal route, respectively. The official tuberculin tests (United States) for cattle, bison, and dairy goats are the caudal-fold test, the comparative cervical test, and the single cervical test.

1. Caudal-fold or single cervical test: In cattle and bison, an intradermal injection of 0.1 mL (5000 tuberculin units) of U.S. Department of Agriculture (USDA) PPD bovis is made in the caudal-fold region with observation and palpation at 72 ± 6 hours. A firm swelling indicates a positive reaction. In cervids, an intradermal injection of 0.1 mL of USDA PPD bovis is made in the midcervical region with observation and palpation at 72 ± 6 hours. A firm swelling indicates a positive reaction. In cattle known to have been exposed to *M. bovis*, a single cervical test of 0.1 mL (10,000 tuberculin units) of PPD bovine cervical tuberculin is injected in the neck region with observation, palpation, and postinjection measurements at 72 ± 6 hours.

2. Comparative cervical test: In cattle, bison, and cervids, an intradermal injection of 0.1 mL each of biologically balanced USDA PPD bovis (1 mg/mL protein) and USDA PPD avian (0.4 mg/mL protein) tuberculins is made at premeasured sites on the midcervical region with observation, palpation, and postinjection measurement at 72 ± 6 hours. The responses are recorded and plotted on the comparative cervical test scattergram, and classification is made according to the zone in which the animal's data are plotted on the scattergram. A positive test implies past or present infection and requires that the reacting animal be slaughtered and undergo necropsy. Lesions are often not found on necropsy.

Several in vitro laboratory tests developed in recent years are used in conjunction with tuberculin skin tests. These include the lymphocyte transformation test, serologic tests for circulating antibodies (such as an enzyme-linked immunosorbent assay), and interferon-γ assays using whole blood.

The blood tuberculosis test has been used in cervids as a clarifying test for suspects on the single cervical test and as an alternative to the comparative cervical test. It consists of a battery of tests using the lymphocyte transformation test, enzyme-linked immunosorbent assays using three antigens (PPD bovis, PPD avium, and the *M. bovis*–specific protein MPB70), and a test for serum haptoglobins, the presence of which indicates a systemic inflammatory process.

Pathologic Necropsy Findings

Tuberculosis is characterized by a tuberculous granuloma that has a yellowish color and is caseous, caseocalcareous, or calcified in consistency. Occasionally, the granuloma may be purulent. The caseous center is usually dry and firm and covered by a fibrous connective tissue capsule of varying thickness. In recent years, calcification has been seen less commonly. The lesions may be small enough to be missed by the unaided eye or so large as to involve the greater part of an organ. Bronchopneumonia may occur in instances of lung lesions, and there may be little evidence of fluid accumulation microscopically. Lesions may be situated in any of the lung lobes and cause productive pneumonia. In time, organisms are carried via the sputum and cause lesions in the bronchotracheal tree and regional lymph nodes.

When tubercle bacilli enter the body, they are usually immediately phagocytized by neutrophils. Subsequent destruction of the neutrophils by multiplying mycobacteria stimulates the accumulation of epithelioid cells that engulf the neutrophils and mycobacteria. The bacilli are not destroyed; they multiply within the epithelioid cells and apparently produce a toxic substance that destroys adjacent cells. This causes an area of caseous necrosis and the beginning of a tubercle. More epithelioid cells encircle the necrotic area, and in the center of the tubercle, the cellular nuclei disappear and structural detail is lost.

A number of epithelioid cells fuse to form multinucleated giant cells. These cells are often present in tuberculous lesions, but they are also present in granulomatous lesions of other chronic inflammatory diseases. Acid-fast bacilli may be demonstrated throughout a lesion within epithelioid cells and giant cells and in necrotic debris. Granulation tissue forms and is usually surrounded by a zone of lymphocytes and fibroblasts, frequently near a blood vessel.

TREATMENT AND CONTROL

Treatment of bovine tuberculosis in cattle and bison is usually not allowed in the United States and other countries because of the chronic nature of the disease, its potential zoonotic effects, and the cost of treatment. Isoniazid has been used prophylactically to control tuberculosis in zoos and animal parks with variable success. Disadvantages of using isoniazid include a poor success rate (up to 25% refractory cases), the threat of emergence of drug-resistant strains, secretion of isoniazid in the milk, and the danger of relapse when treatment with the drug is withdrawn. *M. bovis* is sensitive to isoniazid, streptomycin, para-aminosalicylic acid, rifampin, and thiacetazone. Control in Canada, the United States, Mexico, Australia, New Zealand, and many countries in Europe involves tuberculin testing and slaughter of reactors.

Decontamination of Infected Premises

M. bovis is killed by sunlight, but it is resistant to desiccation and can survive in a wide range of acidic and alkaline conditions. It may remain viable for long periods in soil that is moist and warm. In cattle feces, *M. bovis* can survive for as long as 8 weeks.

After depopulation of all animals on the premises, manure, litter, hay, straw, and other accumulated extraneous material should be removed from the environment and burned. The stables, building, and barnyard structures should be brushed, scraped, and washed down with a pressurized water spray. Within several days, a disinfectant should be applied under high pressure to saturate the same structures. The two preferred disinfectants are a cresylic compound and sodium orthophenylphenate. When depopulation is carried out because of tuberculosis, the premises are not repopulated for at least 30 days.

Eradication Programs

Rules governing the use of tuberculin tests in eradication programs vary from country to country. In the United States, only officially trained state, federal, or accredited veterinarians are allowed to administer the tuberculin skin test for cattle, bison, or cervids. The rules and regulations are published by the USDA as the Bovine Tuberculosis Eradication Uniform Methods and Rules (Feb 3, 1989) and the Tuberculosis Eradication in Cervidae Uniform Methods and Rules (May 15, 1994). Blood obtained from cervids for the blood tuberculosis test must be collected by state, federal, or accredited veterinarians and sent to an approved laboratory for testing.

PUBLIC HEALTH CONCERNS

Tuberculosis (*M. bovis*) in domestic and captive exotic animals provides a potential source of infection for humans. Veterinarians and animal technicians involved in necropsies of animals suspected of being tuberculous must be extremely careful to follow appropriate procedures. Carcasses should be incinerated immediately after aseptic removal of tissue for culture and histopathologic examination. The area where necropsies are performed should be decontaminated with a suitable disinfectant. All utensils and instruments should be autoclaved or treated with cresylic compounds, and adequate ventilation should be maintained.

In outbreaks in which *M. tuberculosis* or *M. bovis* has been confirmed, every effort should be made to protect caretakers from exposure to infected animals. Protective clothing and boots should be used in the contaminated area. Suitable safety masks and goggles should be worn for protection from aerosol transmission. Animal handlers known to be tuberculin negative should receive periodic tuberculin skin tests at 6-month intervals. Where there is evidence of direct exposure, the caretakers should receive tuberculin tests at 90-day intervals; chest radiography should be performed on individuals with positive reactions. The antituberculous drugs used for treating *M. tuberculosis* infection are also used for treating *M. bovis*.

Human infections with *M. bovis* have been mainly associated with outbreaks of tuberculosis in dairy cattle, but some have been related to contact with domestic animals or farm-reared captive wild animals. Tuberculous lesions caused by *M. bovis* have been observed in extrapulmonary tissue, which suggests that ingestion of unpasteurized milk or dairy products is the major source for humans. The absence of infected cattle and the pasteurization of milk have all but eliminated human infection with *M. bovis* in the United States.

TUBERCULOSIS IN WILDLIFE

Numerous wildlife species are capable of being infected by *M. bovis*, and the source is usually considered to be infected domestic livestock or humans. This organism may also cycle within wild populations over time and become endemic in certain wildlife species, whereas in other species, individual animals are incidentally infected. Bovine tuberculosis has an almost worldwide distribution. In free-living wildlife, it has been documented in the following areas: Africa—endemic in cape buffalo, lechwe, kudu, and warthogs and incidental in black rhinos, gray duikers, springboks, elephants, and giraffes; Europe—endemic in cervids and badgers; the Americas—endemic in wood bison in isolated populations and incidental in captive cervids, free-ranging white-tailed deer, and mule deer and coyotes; New Zealand—endemic in brush-tailed possums and incidental in mustelids and wild pigs; and Australia—endemic in feral water buffalo. In wildlife, transmission usually occurs either by inhalation of droplet nuclei or by ingestion of contaminated material. Both positive and negative results of tuberculin skin tests in wild species are very difficult to interpret.

BIBLIOGRAPHY

Biberstein EL: Mycobacterium species: The agents of animal tuberculosis. *In* Biberstein E, Zee YC (eds): Review of Veterinary Microbiology. Boston, Blackwell, 1990, pp 202–212.

Carter GR, Chengappa MM, Roberts AW, et al: Essentials of Veterinary Microbiology. Baltimore, Williams & Wilkins, 1995, pp 205–213.

Fraser CM, Bergeron JA, Mays A, et al (eds): Tuberculosis. *In* The Merck Veterinary Manual. Rahway, NJ, Merck, 1991, pp 367–371.

OIE Manual of Standards for Diagnostic Tests and Vaccines, ed 3. Paris, 1996, pp 267–275.

O'Reilly LM, Daborn CJ: The epidemiology of *Mycobacterium bovis* infections in animals and man: A review. Tubercle Lung Dis 76(suppl 1):1–46, 1995.

Payeur JB, Jarnagin JL, Marquardt JM, et al: Laboratory Methods in Veterinary Mycobacteriology. Ames, Iowa, USDA, 1993, pp 14–37, 49–115.

Quinn PJ, Carter ME, Markey BK, et al: Clinical Veterinary Microbiology. London, Wolfe, 1994, pp 156–169.

Thoen CO, Steele JH (eds): *Mycobacterium bovis* Infection in Animals and Humans. Ames, Iowa, Iowa State University Press, 1995, pp 145–157.

Thoen CO, Williams DE: Tuberculosis, tuberculoidoses, and other mycobacterial infections. *In* Beran GW, Steele JH (eds): Handbook of Zoonoses, ed 2. Boca Raton, Fla, CRC Press, 1994, pp 41–59.

USDA: Bovine Tuberculosis Eradication Uniform Methods and Rules, Effective February 3, 1989. Washington, DC, USDA, Animal and Plant and Health Inspection Service publication No. 91-45-001.

USDA: Tuberculosis Eradication in Cervidae Uniform Methods and Rules, Effective May 15, 1994. Washington, DC, USDA, Animal and Plant and Health Inspection Service publication No. 91-45-005.

■ Paratuberculosis (Johne's Disease)

Michael T. Collins, D.V.M., Ph.D.

GENERAL DESCRIPTION

Paratuberculosis, commonly known as Johne's disease, is a chronic wasting disease primarily affecting ruminants. The disease is caused by infection of the small intestine with *Mycobacterium paratuberculosis*. Officially the name is *M. avium* subsp. *paratuberculosis* because of its close genetic relationship with *M. avium* (the cause of avian tuberculosis); however, most authors continue to refer to it as *M. paratuberculosis*.[1] Unlike *M. avium*, *M. paratuberculosis* does not produce the siderophore (iron-binding molecule) mycobactin, grows much more slowly in vitro, and is an obligate parasite that replicates only inside macrophages of infected animals.

Paratuberculosis occurs in a wide range of domestic and wild ruminants. Among domesticated species, paratuberculosis is most common in dairy cattle, sheep, and goats. The disease occurs worldwide with the possible exceptions of Western Australia and Sweden. Paratuberculosis in farm-raised deer and elk may be an emerging disease problem. It has been reported in free-ranging wildlife and can become a significant problem in zoologic collections, particularly when diverse animal species are commingled. Paratuberculosis also occurs in camelids: camels, llamas, and alpacas. Sporadic infections in pigs, horses, wild rabbits, nonhuman primates, and humans have also been described.

For unknown reasons, young animals are more susceptible to infection with *M. paratuberculosis* than are adults. However, with high doses, even adult animals can become infected. Infection occurs following the ingestion of *M. paratuberculosis*–contaminated milk, water, or feed. In utero infection can occur, particularly during the latter stages of infection when the bacterium disseminates and infects multiple internal organs.[2] Offspring born to infected dams and suckled naturally until weaning have a high likelihood of becoming infected because *M. paratuberculosis* is excreted in milk by infected animals.[3, 4] For animal species typically managed by hand rearing of neonates, for example, dairy cattle, feeding of whole milk rather than artificial milk replacer is associated with rapid dissemination of the infection in a herd.

Following ingestion, *M. paratuberculosis* is taken up by macrophages in gut-associated lymphoid tissue, particularly Peyer's patches in the terminal ileum and occasionally the tonsils. There, intracellular multiplication of the bacterium induces a diffuse granulomatous tissue reaction. From the primary sites of infection, spread of *M. paratuberculosis* via the lymphatics to regional lymph nodes results in systemic infection. Infection dissemination probably occurs shortly before or at the time of onset of clinical signs because only a limited host tissue reaction occurs in tissues from which *M. paratuberculosis* can be isolated, such as the liver, spleen, and lung.

CLINICAL SIGNS

Cattle

Persistent diarrhea that is unresponsive to treatment, rapid weight loss in the presence of good appetite, and absence of fever are the signs that are typical of Johne's disease in cattle. Most often the disease occurs in 3- to 5-year-old cattle. However, as the infection spreads and affects a steadily increasing percentage of cattle in the herd each year, clinical signs in animals less than 3 years old can occur, presumably because the infection pressure (dose of bacteria that calves are exposed to) rises over time and higher doses cause more rapidly progressive infections.

Once the presence of paratuberculosis in a herd is confirmed, recognition of infected animals by clinical signs becomes easier, and more subtle signs of the disease, for example, rough, lackluster hair coat and depressed milk production, are noticed by herd owners. None of the clinical signs mentioned are unique to Johne's disease, however, and there is a risk of overdiagnosis if only clinical signs are relied on. The differential diagnosis should include chronic local peritonitis, liver abscessation, helminth parasitism, winter dysentery, pyelonephritis, and chronic salmonellosis.

Sheep, Goats, and Other Animals

Johne's disease in ruminants other than cattle is most often recognized as a chronic wasting disease that is only sometimes accompanied by diarrhea. For this reason and because the progressive weight loss is often undetected owing to the animal's hair coat, diagnosis of Johne's disease from clinical signs alone is difficult. Johne's disease should be included in the differential diagnosis for any ruminant or pseudoruminant (camelids) with poor body condition. Confirmation of the diagnosis can be made only by laboratory tests.

DIAGNOSIS

Cattle

A fast, accurate, inexpensive test to confirm a clinical diagnosis of Johne's disease in cattle is the absorbed enzyme-linked immunosorbent assay (ELISA). A positive test is invariably correct. However, approximately 15% of the cattle with clinical signs of Johne's disease may test negative for serum antibodies. The agar gel immunodiffusion test is less sensitive, and the complement fixation test is less specific. Acid-fast staining of fecal sample smears is another method for rapid confirmation of a clinical diagnosis. This technique requires some experience, however, and is less sensitive and specific than ELISA testing. A DNA probe for *M. paratuberculosis* is commercially available, but although faster and equally specific as fecal culture, it has lower sensitivity and higher cost.[5] Cattle with clinical Johne's disease have a grossly thickened ileum. Histopathologic examination with acid-fast staining of ileum and mesenteric lymph nodes is definitive for a diagnosis of Johne's disease.

Diagnosis of cattle in the preclinical stages of *M. paratuberculosis* infection is challenging because of the extended period of time when animals are infected but not shedding the bacterium in feces or producing serum antibodies. For this reason, in a paratuberculosis control program to select animals for culling, tests must be repeated every 6 to 12 months and only those animals repeatedly testing negative are likely to be free of the infection. Culture of fecal samples is the most widely used test, but it has the disadvantages of being expensive and requiring 16 weeks to perform. Testing for serum antibodies by absorbed ELISA is faster and less expensive, but it is somewhat less sensitive than fecal culture.[6, 7]

Detection of infected herds (herd-level diagnosis) rather than infected individual cattle is most important to control spread of the disease among herds. The absorbed ELISA has high herd-level sensitivity and is thus effective in discriminating between infected and noninfected herds. Owners of noninfected herds should keep the herd closed or, if necessary, only buy replacement cattle from ELISA-negative herds.

Sheep, Goats, and Other Animals

For clinical diagnosis confirmation or disease management at a herd level, ELISA, fecal culture, and acid-fast smears of fecal samples work as well in goats as they do in cattle. Unlike cattle, the ileum of infected goats is not usually as obviously thickened and gross pathology is limited to slight enlargement of mesenteric lymph nodes.

Agar gel immunodiffusion is the preferred serologic test in sheep. Culture of *M. paratuberculosis* from sheep is more difficult than from cattle because sheep strains of the organism are more fastidious. Similar to goats, ileal thickening is not common and gross pathology is generally limited to extreme cachexia. Histopathologic examination with acid-fast staining is the best method of diagnosis.[8]

For other animal species, serologic tests have yet to be developed and validated. Culture of fecal samples is the only antemortem diagnostic test available, and necropsy with histopathologic testing provides the most definitive diagnosis. In deer, *M. paratuberculosis* can cause caseous granulomatous lesions that are easily confused with tuberculosis.

TREATMENT

Long-term antimicrobial therapy with antituberculosis drugs results in improved body condition and somewhat prolonged life of infected animals. It does not cure the infection.

PREVENTION AND CONTROL

Prevention of infection is the most effective way to manage paratuberculosis. Because *M. partuberculosis* is an obligate pathogen, maintaining herds and flocks as closed populations and only introducing new genetic material by artificial insemination or embryo transfer will ensure that infection remains excluded. When the addition of new animals to a herd or flock is unavoidable, they should originate from a herd or flock that at least has tested negative (whole-herd test) in the previous 12 months and preferably from one that is certified to be free of paratuberculosis based on multiple animal herd tests. Many states in the United States as well as Australia have certification programs for cattle. Similar programs for other animal species are being developed.

Control of paratuberculosis in infected herds or flocks is by (1) identifying and culling the infected animals and (2) instituting husbandry measures that limit the opportunities for infection transmission. Both strategies must be used to achieve control in a reasonable period of time, e.g., 5 years. Vaccination of cattle herds has not proved effective in preventing infection, although it decreases the incidence of clinical disease.

Test-and-cull programs should use fecal culture together with serologic tests when possible. Use of both types of tests on the entire adult herd or flock increases the probability of detection of infected animals. To control the cost of testing, serologic examination and culture can be done on an alternating basis at intervals of 6 to 12 months. All test-positive animals should be culled. For faster elimination of the infection, the last offspring born to test-positive animals should also be culled.

Husbandry changes are primarily directed at limiting contact of neonates with potentially infected adult animals. Prompt removal of neonates from their dam, as well as hand rearing them with artificial milk replacers, is critical for control inasmuch as *M. paratuberculosis* is excreted in the milk of infected animals. Because there are no effective artificial colostrum replacements, colostrum for neonates should be obtained only from test-negative dams. Pasteurization of colostrum can reduce but not totally eliminate the chance that the colostrum contains viable *M. paratuberculosis*. Young animals, particularly those being raised as herd or flock replacements, should remain isolated from the adult herd as long as possible. The "window of susceptibility" is not well defined, but for cattle it is best to ensure that calves have no contact with the adult herd for at least 6 and preferably 12 months. This includes shared feed bunks, water troughs, and pastures. Manure runoff from areas where adult animals reside must also be kept away from young herd replacements.[9]

ZOONOTIC CONCERNS

Mycobacterium paratuberculosis has been isolated sporadically from individuals with Crohn's disease, a chronic, incurable, granulomatous, inflammatory bowel disease of unknown cause. Since the discovery in 1989 of a genetic element unique to *M. paratuberculosis* known as IS900, molecular methods to search for the organism in patients with Crohn's disease have been applied by several laboratories worldwide. Most such studies report that intestinal and lymph node tissue from such patients test positive for *M. paratuberculosis* significantly more often than does tissue from control individuals. This does not indicate a causal relationship between Crohn's disease and *M. paratuberculosis*. However, *M. paratuberculosis* is being actively investigated as the etiology or an important cofactor in the pathogenesis of Crohn's disease. If proven to have zoonotic potential, the way *M. paratuberculosis*–infected animals and herds or flocks are managed will probably be dramatically changed.[10-14]

REFERENCES

1. Thorel M-F, Krichevsky M, Levy-Frebault VV: Numerical taxonomy of mycobactin-dependent mycobacteria, emended description of *Mycobacterium avium*, and description of *Mycobacterium avium* subsp. *avium* subsp. nov., *Mycobacterium avium* subsp. *paratuberculosis* subsp. nov., and *Mycobacterium avium* subsp. *silvaticum* subsp. nov. Int J Syst Bacteriol 40:254–260, 1990.
2. Sweeney RW, Whitlock RH, Rosenberger AE: *Mycobacterium paratuberculosis* isolated from fetuses of infected cows not manifesting signs of the disease. Am J Vet Res 53:477–480, 1992.
3. Sweeney RW, Whitlock RH, Rosenberger AE: *Mycobacterium paratuberculosis* cultured from milk and supramammary lymph nodes of infected asymptomatic cows. J Clin Microbiol 30:166–171, 1992.
4. Streeter RN, Hoffsis GF, Bech-Nielsen S, et al: Isolation of *Mycobacterium paratuberculosis* from colostrum and milk of subclinically infected cows. Am J Vet Res 56:1322–1324, 1995.
5. Whipple DL, Kapke PA, Andersen PR: Comparison of a commercial DNA probe test and three cultivation procedures for detection of *Mycobacterium paratuberculosis* in bovine feces. J Vet Diagn Invest 4:23–27, 1994.
6. Collins MT: Diagnosis of paratuberculosis. Vet Clin North Am Food Anim Pract 12:357–371, 1996.
7. Sweeney RW, Whitlock RH, Buckley CL, et al: Evaluation of a commercial enzyme-linked immunosorbent assay for the diagnosis of paratuberculosis in dairy cattle. J Vet Diagn Invest 7:488–493, 1995.
8. Dubash K, Shulaw WP, Bech-Nielsen S, et al: Evaluation of an agar gel immunodiffusion test kit for detection of antibodies to *Mycobacterium paratuberculosis* in sheep. J Am Vet Med Assoc 208:401–403, 1996.
9. Collins MT: Clinical approach to control of bovine paratuberculosis. J Am Vet Med Assoc 204:208–210, 1994.
10. Grant IR, Ball HJ, Neill SD, et al: Inactivation of *Mycobacterium paratuberculosis* in cows' milk at pasteurization temperatures. Appl Environ Microbiol 62:631–636, 1996.
11. Thompson DE: The role of mycobacteria in Crohn's disease. J Med Microbiol 41:74–94, 1994.
12. Millar D, Ford J, Sanderson J, et al: IS900 PCR to detect *Mycobacterium paratuberculosis* in retail supplies of whole pasteurized cows' milk in England and Wales. Appl Environ Microbiol 62:3446–3452, 1996.
13. Mishna D, Katsel P, Brown ST, et al: On the etiology of Crohn disease. Proc Natl Acad Sci USA 93:9816–9820, 1996.
14. Chiodini RJ: Crohn's disease and the mycobacterioses: A review and comparison of two disease entities. Clin Microbiol Rev 2:90–117, 1989.

■ *Actinobacillus suis* Infection

Brad Fenwick, D.V.M., M.S., Ph.D., Diplomate, A.C.V.M.

Sporadic outbreaks of *Actinobacillus suis*–related disease in pre-weaning or early nursery pigs have been recognized for more than 20 years. Originally, *A. suis* was believed to be a commensal of the oropharynx of pigs and an environmental contaminant. It was considered an opportunistic pathogen of low virulence that was capable of causing clinical disease only in immunologically compromised pigs (including neonates), in those with contaminated wounds, and, occasionally, in those with mastitis. More recently, *A. suis* has emerged as a pathogen of growing and finishing pigs. Typically, disease outbreaks involve minimal-disease herds subject to one or more advanced production methods (i.e., all-in all-out, early weaning, multi-site). In some herds, *A. suis* is the dominant pathogen in grow-finish pigs and is responsible for a significant proportion of the disease-related reduction in herd profitability.

EPIDEMIOLOGY AND PATHOGENSIS

A high percentage of swine herds are infected with *A. suis*, yet clinical disease is relatively rare. The primary reservoir of *A. suis* within a herd is the sows. Under conventional production systems, which utilize continuous-flow production and wean pigs at ages ranging from 21 to 35 days, piglets become infected prior to weaning, but they rarely develop clinically evident disease because of the protection provided by colostral antibodies. In these herds, clinical disease is most likely to occur in piglets that did not receive adequate amounts of colostrum (preweaning disease) or are exposed after colostral protection has been lost (nursery disease).

The emergence of *A. suis* as a pathogen in older pigs is related to production systems designed to reduce or prevent transmission of pathogens from the sows to piglets. Prominent among these are all-in all-out stocking, early weaning (at less than 18 days), and multiple-site production. These systems produce a higher percentage of pigs that have not been exposed to *A. suis* and, thus, have no immunity. Subsequent exposure to *A. suis* at an older age may result in clinical disease.

A. suis colonizes the tonsils, where it localizes in the crypts and, less frequently, the parenchyma. Systemic invasion by *A. suis* is characterized by bacteremia with widespread vasculitis. Although the virulence factors of *A. suis* are not well characterized, it is generally assumed that *A. suis* has the normal complement of factors that allows colonization, avoids innate immune responses, damages host tissues, and induces an inflammatory response. The fact that bacteremia is a major component of the pathogenesis of *A. suis* suggests that it has mechanisms to avoid complement-mediated lysis and phagocytosis.

Like a number of related bacteria, *A. suis* produces at least one cytotoxin/hemolysin of the RTX type. As a group, the RTX toxins damage host cells by forming pores in their membranes. The toxin produced by *A. suis* is genetically, structurally, and immunologically similar to the toxins produced by *A. pleuropneumoniae*. The toxin-neutralizing antibody titer that follows recovery from an infection with *A. suis* may be responsible for the cross-protective immunity between *A. suis* and *A. pleuropneumoniae*.

CLINICAL SIGNS

The clinical signs related to *A. suis* infections vary widely. Sporadic cases of abortion, metritis, and mastitis have been reported. More commonly, clinical signs associated with *A. suis* are an outbreak of septicemia and deaths; clinical signs are not observed in many cases because the pigs are found dead. Disease in suckling or recently weaned pigs occurs most frequently in herds that are maintained by conventional production methods. Clinical disease occurs sporadically and involves one or more pigs in a litter. A number of litters may be involved over a period of several weeks.

Clinical disease in grow-finish pigs typically involves high–health status herds. Disease outbreaks are frequently related to the repopulation of existing facilities or reestablishment of a new herd using pigs from more than one source. In this situation, the most typical history is that one or more pigs are found dead. The other pigs in the pen are not clinically ill, and treatment may not be warranted, as the disease typically has a low clinical morbidity but high mortality rate. Nevertheless in some high–health status herds, *A. suis* is a significant cause of mortality in this phase of production.

In gilts, sows, and boars, clinical signs related to *A. suis* infection are more likely to be noticed, and pigs of this age are rarely found dead. Here again, clinical disease is much more frequent in high–health status herds, and it may follow the introduction of new breeding stock. As with grow-finish pigs, only a few pigs in any one group develop overt clinical disease.

In those cases in which clinical signs are recognized, they are not specific for *A. suis*. The clinical signs related to nonlethal infections are often overlooked because they are mild, transient, and nonspecific. These may include mild diarrhea, mild to moderate pneumonia, anorexia, and low-grade fever. An occasional abortion may occur. Clinical signs typically diminish in a few days without the need for treatment. In terminal cases, clinical signs are related to septicemia, vasculitis, and shock. Some cases may show severe respiratory distress, cyanosis, multifocal cutaneous petechial hemorrhages, neurologic signs, and vascular congestion of the ventral skin and ears. In adult pigs, it is not uncommon to see multifocal, sharply demarcated, raised, red skin lesions, which resemble those associated with erysipelas.

NECROPSY AND LABORATORY DIAGNOSIS

Given the variety of clinical signs associated with *A. suis* infections, it follows that the lesions are equally variable and nonspecific. The lesions induced by *A. suis* are generally related to acute septicemia, vasculitis, and shock. The pigs are in good condition and may have eaten within the past few hours. The most consistent lesion is multifocal necrohemorrhagic pneumonia, which is randomly distributed throughout the lung and lacks a recognizable airway orientation. It is not uncommon for the diaphragmatic lung lobes to be severely involved. Given the septicemic nature of *A. suis*, it is common to also have widespread petechial hemorrhages on serosal surfaces, serofibrinous pericarditis, pleuritis, peritonitis, and arthritis. Lymph nodes and the spleen may also be enlarged. In adult pigs, and less frequently in grow-finish pigs, cutaneous infarctions are common.

Given that *A. suis* can mimic the clinical signs and pathologic lesions induced by a number of other bacterial diseases, it is critical that efforts be made to confirm the diagnosis by isolating the microorganism. In young pigs, the differential diagnosis should include *Haemophilus parasuis*, *Streptococcus suis*, and *Salmonella*. In grow-finish pigs, *A. pleuropneumoniae* is the important differential diagnosis, because the clinical signs of acute death associated with severe focal pneumonia with pleuritis are hallmarks of both diseases. In older pigs, the focal dermal vascular thrombosis requires that erysipelas be considered.

A. suis can be readily isolated, often in pure culture, from characteristic lesions. In addition, because of the bacteremic nature of *A. suis* infections, the organism can be isolated from many tissues, including liver, spleen, skin, and blood. *A. suis* is a pleomorphic gram-negative bacterium that does not require X or V factor for growth on blood agar. On blood agar, the colonies are smooth and pale yellow to gray and are surrounded by a prominent zone of β-hemolysis. The biochemical characteristics of *A. suis* are variable and thus can be difficult to distinguish from *A. lignieresii* and *A. suis*–like and *Pasteurella*-like strains. It is generally more important to differentiate *A. suis* from biotype 2 strains of *A. pleuropneumoniae*, which do not require nicotinamide adenine dinucleotide, and thus do not form satellites around *Staphylococcus* sp. The most reliable method of making this distinction is by genetic analysis using DNA probes specific for *A. pleuropneumoniae*.

Different serotypes of *A. suis* are not recognized. Attempts to develop a serologic test to identify pigs that have been infected with *A. suis* have not been successful. In large part, this is related to cross-reactions with *A. pleuropneumoniae* and, possibly, other bacteria. Hemolysin neutralization assays for the type 1 hemolysin of *A. pleuropneumoniae* may be used to test pigs for previous *A. suis* infection if the herd is negative on enzyme-linked immunosorbent assay to the type 1 toxin–producing serotypes of *A. pleuropneumoniae* (serotypes 1, 5, 9, 10, and 11).

TREATMENT AND PREVENTION

For treatment to be successful, clinical disease must be recognized early and injectable antibiotics given without delay. In most cases, death occurs so rapidly that there is rarely an opportunity to use antibiotics. Many of the isolates are sensitive to a wide variety of antibiotics. Nevertheless, in some areas a substantial portion of the *A. suis* strains isolated from pigs with clinical disease are resistant to penicillin and tetracycline. The value of feed or water antibiotics as a means of preventing clinical outbreaks of *A. suis* in nursery or grow-finish pigs is uncertain. In herds in which *A. suis* causes only sporadic disease, the use of vaccines is not practical. In herds with repeated disease outbreaks, autogenous vaccine may be of value.

It is reasonable to assume that in *A. suis* infection, as in the case of many other infectious diseases, management practices and environmental conditions influence its transmission as well as the potential that it will cause clinical disease. Given that clinical disease occurs with the same or even greater frequency in high–health status herds (with excellent facilities) as it does in herds that are managed more conventionally, the role of environmental factors are of less concern. More likely, production systems that limit the transmission of diseases from sows to piglets and segregate subpopulations of pigs by age alter the immunologic status of the herd. For example, when administered incorrectly, early weaning systems produce a large number of disease-free pigs, but they also allow a few pigs to become infected. Under the correct conditions, the healthy carrier pig may subsequently transmit *A. suis* to the immunologically naive pigs in the herd, resulting in a clinical disease outbreak. Introduction of disease-free replacement gilts into endemically infected sow herds may result in clinical disease in the gilts. In the same fashion, introduction of healthy *A. suis* carrier pigs into an *A. suis*–free herd can result in disease outbreaks. Ultimately, successful prevention of *A. suis* depends on avoiding the mixing of pigs with different disease and immunologic status.

BIBLIOGRAPHY

Burrows LL, Lo RYC: Molecular characterization of an RTX determinant from *Actinobacillus suis*. Infect Immunol 60:2166–2173, 1992.

Kamp EM, Vermeulen TMM, Smits MA, et al: Production of Apx toxins by field strains of *Actinobacillus pleuropneumoniae* and *Actinobacillus suis*. Infect Immunol 62:4063–4065, 1994.

Mair NS, Randall CJ, Thomas GW, et al: *Actinobacillus suis* infection in pigs: A report of four outbreaks and two sporadic cases. Comp Pathol 84:113–119, 1974.

Miniats OP, Spinato MT, Sanford SE: *Actinobacillus suis* septicemia in mature swine: Two outbreaks resembling erysipelas. Can Vet J 30:943–947, 1989.

Odin M, Helie P: *Actinobacillus suis* in swine in southwestern Quebec. Can Vet J 34:634, 1993.

Sanford SE, Josephson GKA, Rehmtulla AJ, et al: *Actinobacillus suis* infection in pigs in southwestern Ontario. Can Vet J 31:443–447, 1990.

Sanford SE: *Actinobacillus suis* septicemia in piglets. Can Vet J 28:654, 1987.

Yaeger MJ: *Actinobacillus suis* septicemia: An emerging disease on high-health herds. Swine Health Prod 3:209–210, 1995.

Yaeger MJ: An outbreak of *Actinobacillus suis* septicemia in grow/finish pigs. J Vet Diagn Invest 8:381–383, 1996.

■ Actinobacillosis

Robert D. Walker, M.S., Ph.D.

OVERVIEW

Actinobacillosis, a disease of numerous animal species, including humans, is caused by bacteria belonging to the genus *Actinobacillus*. Bacteria belonging to this genus are fastidious, facultative, anaerobic, pleomorphic gram-negative rods. In addition, they are nonmotile and non–spore-forming. There are 12 species of bacteria belonging to *Actinobacillus*, seven of which have been associated with disease in animals. The pathogens are *A. capsulatus*, *A. equuli*, *A. lignieresii*, *A. pleuropneumoniae*, *A. seminis*, *A. suis*, and *A. ureae*. *A. actinomycetemcomitans*, which is most commonly associated with periodontal disease but may also cause epididymitis in rams, has been classified as *Haemophilus*

actinomycetemcomitans based on DNA-DNA hybridization studies. Because of the species-specificity and the nature of the infections caused by *A. pleuropneumoniae* and *A. suis*, these organisms are described in separate sections. Three new species have recently been identified: *A. minor*, *A. porcinus*, and *A. indolicus*. These organisms are part of the normal flora of the upper respiratory tract of pigs. Their role in disease has not yet been defined.

Bacteria belonging to the genus *Actinobacillus* may be part of the normal flora of the respiratory, alimentary, or genital tracts of numerous animal species throughout the world. When disease occurs it is usually sporadic and develops when an event occurs that adversely affects the animal's natural defenses, allowing the organism to grow in body sites other than on mucous membranes. This event may be as simple as a tooth abscess or a penetrating wound through the oral mucosa, for example, *A. lignieresii* causing "wooden tongue" or soft tissue infections in the jaw of cattle. Less frequently, disease may arise from exposure to an overwhelming number of organisms.

Actinobacillus lignieresii

A. lignieresii has a worldwide distribution and has been isolated from disease processes in cattle, pigs, chickens, horses, dogs, and humans. It is part of the normal flora of the alimentary canal of cattle and sheep.

The most frequent lesions are in cattle and consist of multiple, hard, granulomatous abscesses in soft tissues of the head and upper alimentary canal and associated lymph nodes. The frequent involvement of the tongue has led to the term "wooden tongue." Other tissues that may be infected by this organism include the pleura, lungs, liver, udder, lymph nodes, and subcutaneous tissues. Abscesses usually begin as firm nodules that eventually ulcerate and discharge a viscous, white to faintly green exudate. This exudate may contain small (less than 1 mm) grayish white granules. In sheep, lesions are present in the skin (especially around the head), lungs, testes, and mammary glands, but not the tongue. In pigs, an *A. lignieresii*–like organism may occasionally be isolated from abscesses in the udder.

A. lignieresii relies on a break in the integrity of the epithelial cell lining of the alimentary canal to cause disease. Such breaks can occur with the feeding of coarse feeds such as dry haylage. Once the bacterium has been allowed to penetrate into otherwise sterile tissues, local abscesses develop. From these abscesses the organism may, on rare occasions, spread to other body sites through the lymphatics (most common route), by hematogenous spread, by injection, or by aspiration into the lungs. Once in the lungs, *A. lignieresii* may cause multiple abscesses.

Diagnosis of actinobacillosis is usually made with the isolation of the etiologic agent from granulomatous lesions in conjunction with clinical signs and physical examination. Specimens for culture should be collected by aspiration from closed lesions, transferred to a sterile container, and transported to the laboratory on ice. Purulent material from the abscesses may contain small (less than 1 mm) grayish-white, sulfur-like granules. When the granules are digested in 10% sodium hydroxide, crushed and then Gram-stained, gram-negative rods and coccobacilli may be seen under microscopic examination under oil immersion.

Prevention of infections caused by this organism is restricted to attempts at minimizing injuries to the mucosa of the upper portion of the alimentary canal by avoidance of coarse feed that may cause injury. Treatment, when initiated early in the disease process, may prove to be successful if used aggressively. This should include surgical debridement, when possible, topical iodines or potassium iodine administered orally, or antibacterial agents, such as erythromycin, streptomycin, or tetracycline, to which the organism may be susceptible and which are approved for use in the affected animal species. Chronic infections generally do not respond well to therapy. The use of iodine products in animals that are destined for the human food chain is discouraged.

Actinobacillus equuli

A. equuli has been isolated from the intestinal tract as well as the mucous membranes of the upper respiratory tract and vagina of carrier animals. Specific virulence factors have not been identified. However, the capsular material may contribute to the organism's ability to evade phagocytosis and destruction by phagocytic cells and may also play an active role in tissue destruction. Disease usually occurs as a result of an immune dysfunction in the host. In pigs, *A. equuli* has been isolated from piglets with septic arthritis and older animals with endocarditis. This organism has also been isolated from the lungs of calves and rabbits with pneumonia, although this is not a very common occurrence.

Actinobacillus seminis

The taxonomic placement of *A. seminis* is unknown. Recent studies have shown that it is genetically unrelated to *Actinobacillus* or *Haemophilus*. It occurs primarily as a pathogen of sheep in which it has been associated with epididymitis and seminal vesiculitis in rams, mastitis in ewes, and purulent polyarthritis in lambs.

Other, less frequently encountered species of *Actinobacillus* include *A. capsulatus*, which has been isolated from synovial fluid in rabbits with septic arthritis, and *A. ureae* (formerly *Pasteurella ureae*), which has been associated with upper respiratory tract infections in humans and abortions in pigs caused by members of the genus *Actinobacillus*. Because the diseases described above rarely occur as outbreaks, prevention strategies, such as vaccination programs, have not been warranted.

Treatment of infectious disease processes caused by bacteria in this genus may differ depending on specific circumstances, that is, bacterial species, host species or body site peculiarities, but has traditionally included topical or systemic iodine. More recently, with increased concerns over food safety, the use of these products in dairy cows has been discouraged. In general, members of the genus *Actinobacillus* are susceptible to streptomycin, sulfonamides, ampicillin, and tetracyclines in vitro. However, consideration should always be made for the agent-drug environment in vitro vs. in vivo. In vivo, the antibacterial agent may not reach therapeutic concentrations at the site of infection either because of poor diffusibility or inactivation at the site of infection due to pH, purulent exudate, or other factors. If any of the above-listed antibacterial agents are to be used, they should be used in a manner that optimizes their pharmacodynamic potential, that is, maintaining concentrations of ampicillin above the minimum inhibitory concentration (MIC) of the pathogen for the majority of the dosing interval, or dosing streptomycin so as to produce high serum-MIC ratios after the abscess has been surgically debrided.

BIBLIOGRAPHY

Gyles CL, Thoen CO (eds): Pathogenesis of Bacterial Infections in Animals. Ames, Iowa State University Press, 1993, pp 126–128.
Lo RYC: Molecular characteristics of cytotoxins produced by *Haemophilus, Actinobacillus, Pasteurella*. Can J Vet Res 54:S33–S35, 1990.
Mandell GL, Bennett JE, Dolin R: Principles and Practice of Infectious Diseases, ed 4. New York, Churchill Livingstone, 1995, pp 2280–2288.
Müller K, Fussing V, Grimont AD, et al: *Actinobacillus minor* sp. nov., *Actinobacillus porcinus* sp. nov., and *Actinobacillus indolicus* sp. nov, three new V factor–dependent species from the respiratory tract of pigs. Int J Syst Bacteriol 46:951–956, 1996.
Mutters R, Pohl S, Mannheim W: Transfer of *Pasteurella urea* Jones 1962 to the genus *Actinobacillus* Brumpt 1910: *Actinobacillus urea* comb. nov. Int J Syst Bacteriol 36:343–344, 1986.
Potts TV, Zambon JJ, Genco RJ: Reassignment of *Actinobacillus actinomycetemcomitans* to the genus *Haemophilus* as *Haemophilus actinomycetemcomitans* comb. nov. Int J Syst Bacteriol 35:337–341, 1985.
Quinn PJ, Carter ME, Markey BK, Carter GR: Clinical Veterinary Microbiology. London, Wolfe, 1994, pp 144–151.
Walker RD: Actinobacillosis and actinomycosis. *In* Howard JL (ed): Current Veterinary Therapy 3: Food Animal Practice. Philadelphia, WB Saunders, 1993, pp 534–537.

■ Actinomycosis

Robert D. Walker, M.S., Ph.D.

OVERVIEW

Actinomycosis is a subacute or chronic disease caused by bacteria belonging to the genus *Actinomyces*. There are 11 species of bacteria belonging to *Actinomyces*, five of which have been associated with disease in animals: *A. bovis, A. hordeovulneris, A. israelii, A. pyogenes, A. suis,* and *A. viscosus*. Of these, only *A. bovis, A. pyogenes,* and *A. suis* are considered to be pathogens in food animals, although other species, on rare occasions, may be isolated from polymicrobial infectious processes. *Actinomyces pyogenes* has recently been renamed *Arcanobacterium pyogenes*. However, because everything else about this organism remains the same, it will still be covered in this section and referred to as *Actinomyces pyogenes*.

Actinomyces spp. are gram-positive, nonacid-fast pleomorphic rods that may appear as coccobacillary forms (primarily *A. pyogenes*), straight or slightly curved rods, or filaments that exhibit true branching. Most species grow best under anaerobic conditions at 35 to 37°C, with carbon dioxide being required for maximal growth. *A. pyogenes, A. naeslundii,* and *A. viscosus* are microaerophilic or facultative anaerobes.

Except for *A. suis*, the species of *Actinomyces* that have been associated with infectious disease in domestic animals are considered to be part of the normal flora, primarily of the nasopharynx and oral cavity, of the animal species in which they cause disease. *A. pyogenes* may also be found as normal flora on the skin and reproductive tracts of cattle. The habitat of *A. suis* is unknown, although it is suspected that trauma due to the action of the teeth of the suckling pigs is thought to provide both the inoculum and the tissue injury necessary for actinomycosis of the mammary gland of pigs.

Disease generally develops when the organisms gain access to sterile tissue beyond the confines of the mucous membranes on which it has colonized. In food animals, *A. bovis* and *A. pyogenes* account for most cases of actinomycosis, although *A. suis* may be a frequent isolate from chronic granulomatous and suppurative mastitis in sows. In cattle, the predominant lesion associated with actinomycosis involves bony tissues of the head, "lumpy jaw," which is generally associated with *A. bovis*, although *A. israelii* has also been isolated from some lesions. Actinomycosis is often part of a polymicrobial infection involving pyogenic aerobic and anaerobic bacteria.

Actinomyces spp. are not highly virulent pathogens. Rather they are endogenous oral commensals that produce chronic infections that spread contiguously in a slow and progressive manner along anatomic barriers once they are introduced into soft tissues as a result of traumatic or surgical injuries. These infections are characterized by suppurative granulomas, which in the case of *A. bovis* form external sinuses that discharge characteristic sulfur-like granules. A cytotoxin produced by *A. pyogenes* has been identified, but other virulence factors have not been described. However, it has been demonstrated that *A. viscosus* secretes a product that is chemotactic for neutrophils and stimulates host immune cells to release mediators of inflammation. Attempts to establish animal models of actinomycosis is enhanced by coinoculation with other organisms, most notably *Eubacterium corrodens*.

Because of the sporadic occurrence of actinomycosis and the habitat of the organisms associated with this disease, there is no specific prevention program that can be implemented. Successful treatment is dependent on the etiologic agent and the stage of the infection when treatment is initiated. In general, therapy is much more successful when initiated early in the disease process and involves surgical debridement and drainage.

Actinomyces bovis

Actinomycosis caused by *A. bovis*, or sometimes *A. israelii*, is a chronic, suppurative, granulomatous infection that is frequently referred to as "lumpy jaw." It is most frequently seen in cattle and is characterized by pyogenic lesions, with interconnecting sinus tracts containing granules (usually 1 to 3 mm in diameter) composed of microcolonies of the bacteria embedded in the tissue. Infections by this organism in other animals are rare but may include lumpy jaw in sheep and goats and fistulous withers and poll evil, associated with *Brucella abortus*, in horses. *A. bovis* is part of the normal flora of the oral cavity of the animal species in which it causes disease. Thus, most infections are endogenous in origin.

Infection caused by *A. bovis* occurs following an injury to the oral mucosa which allows the bacterium into deeper, sterile tissues. Once the organism has penetrated into these tissues, it spreads to contiguous areas along tissue planes, with resultant nodules and abscesses. Whereas the organism often infects bony tissues of the head (primarily mandible and maxilla), it may sometimes cause suppurative granulomatous disease in adjacent soft tissue. As the infectious process continues, it becomes a chronic progressive infection with hard, tumor-like masses. Nodules may coalesce, forming sinuses, many of which may open at the skin to discharge pus that contains sulfur-like granules. Depending on the severity of the infection, organisms may be ingested or aspirated with resultant visceral or pulmonary actinomycosis, respectively. Infection may also spread hematogenously resulting in abscesses at other body sites, including mammary tissue.

The pathogenesis of *A. bovis* infections has not been clearly elucidated. It is suspected that pathogenesis may be related to the inability of the host to remove organisms and the toxicity of their metabolic products once they have been introduced into deeper tissues, thus stimulating a granulomatous reaction. Many infections caused by *A. bovis* are polymicrobial and the other organisms present may also contribute to the pathogenesis of the disease process.

Diagnosis of lumpy jaw and related diseases may be made clinically in conjunction with a microscopic examination of the pus from the nodules or discharge from the draining tracts. Sulfur-like granules in the exudate may be examined by transferring them to a glass slide. The addition of 10% sodium hydroxide digests the purulent material around the granules, which may then be gently crushed under a coverslip. A Gram's stain of the crushed granule will reveal pleomorphic gram-positive club-shaped rods and filaments radiating from the center of the granule with examination under oil immersion. Confirmation may be made by isolation of *A. bovis* from granules or infected tissues by routine culture techniques.

Treatment of lumpy jaw and related diseases in other animal species is generally unsuccessful unless it is initiated early in the disease process and treated aggressively. For successful therapy, treatment should include surgical debridement and prolonged (weeks to months) antimicrobial chemotherapy. The drug of choice for the treatment of actinomycosis in food animals is penicillin, administered parenterally, although tetracyclines have also been used successfully. Because of the potential for mixed infections, some investigators believe that ampicillin or amoxicillin have an advantage over penicillin because of their broader spectrum. Sodium iodide solution administered intravenously or injected locally into the tumorous masses has also been used, and potassium iodide administered orally has been recommended. However, the use of these products in animals destined for the human food chain is discouraged.

Arcanobacterium (Actinomyces) pyogenes

A. pyogenes (formerly *Corynebacterium pyogenes*) is a commensal of cutaneous and mucosal surfaces of cattle and other animal species and has been associated with many pyogenic disease conditions in many animal species, including cattle, sheep, goats, and pigs. These include pneumonia and mastitis in cattle, peritonitis and pleuritis in pigs, and various forms of suppurative lesions in other animals, including sheep and horses. It has also been reported in rabbits. It is most commonly isolated from pyogenic infections in cattle, sheep, and pigs.

The mechanism by which *A. pyogenes* gains access to infected body sites has not yet been elucidated. *A. pyogenes* produces an exotoxin with cytolytic properties. However, it is unclear what role this toxin plays in abscess formation. It has been suggested that it may contribute to generalized symptoms associated with actinomycosis and contribute to *A. pyogenes*–induced abortions. More recently a hemolysin molecule has been demonstrated in a cell-free supernatant of *A. pyogenes*. Whether or not the hemolysin is a virulence factor or protective antigen of *A. pyogenes* remains to be studied. The results of another recent study suggest that macrophages may play a role in the dissemination of *A. pyogenes*. However, because of the slow growth rate of *A. pyogenes* and lack of potent virulence factors, there might also be a need for the presence of foreign material or a reduction in vascularization, as would occur following an injury or aspiration, for soft tissue infections to develop. On the other hand, flying insects have been identified as vectors for summer mastitis and pustular dermatitis in cattle. Under these circumstances, disease may be related to the introduction of high numbers of organisms.

Because *A. pyogenes* is frequently present in association with other bacteria, including anaerobes such as *Fusobacterium necrophorum* and *Porphyromonas (Bacteroides) asaccharolyticus*, bacterial cultures are usually necessary to confirm its presence in a disease process. The only sources from which *A. pyogenes* is usually recovered in pure culture are aborted ovine or bovine fetuses, septic arthritis, mastitis, and, occasionally, abscesses in cattle. Routine culture procedures are adequate for the recovery of *A. pyogenes*, provided the primary isolation medium is supplemented with a protein source such as serum or blood.

Penicillin is the drug of choice for infections caused by *A. pyogenes* in pure culture. For mixed infections in which the other organisms may not be susceptible to penicillin, ampicillin, amoxicillin, tetracycline, and potentiated sulfonamides have been used successfully. To ensure success, antimicrobial chemotherapy should be initiated early in the disease process and be accompanied by surgical excision and drainage whenever possible. As the disease process continues, the diffusion of any antimicrobial agent into the site of infection decreases, especially in the absence of surgical intervention. In infections with a copious amount of purulent exudate, sulfa drugs will be less effective than in treating infections with very little exudate.

Of the remaining species of *Actinomyces*, only *A. suis* has been isolated with some frequency from food-producing animals. This organism has been isolated from udders of swine with pyogranulomatous mastitis. *Actinomyces israelii* has, on rare occasions, been isolated from cattle and pigs with actinomycosis.

BIBLIOGRAPHY

Gyles CL, Thoen CO (eds): Pathogenesis of Bacterial Infections in Animals. Ames, Iowa, Iowa State University Press, 1993, pp 126–128.

Lo RYC: Molecular characteristics of cytotoxins produced by *Haemophilus, Actinobacillus, Pasteurella*. Can J Vet Res 54:S33–S35, 1990.

Mandell GL, Bennett JE, Dolin R: Principles and Practice of Infectious Diseases, ed 4. New York, Churchill Livingstone, 1995, pp 2280–2288.

Potts TV, Zambon JJ, Genco RJ: Reassignment of *Actinobacillus actinomycetemcomitans* to the genus *Haemophilus* as *Haemophilus actinomycetemcomitans* comb. nov. Int J Syst Bacteriol 35:337–341, 1985.

Quinn PJ, Carter ME, Markey BK, et al: Clinical Veterinary Microbiology. London, Wolfe, 1994, pp 144–151.

Ramos CP, Foster G, Collins ND: Phylogenetic analysis of the genus *Actinomyces* based on 165 RNA gene sequences: Description of *Arcanobacterium phocae* sp. Nov, *Arcanobacterium bernardiae* comb, Nov, and *Arcanobacterium pyogenes* comb. Nov. Int J Syst Bacteriol 47:46–53, 1997.

Walker RD: Actinobacillosis and actinomycosis. *In* Howard JL (ed): Current Veterinary Therapy 3: Food Animal Practice. Philadelphia, WB Saunders, 1993, pp 534–537.

■ *Corynebacterium* Species Infections

J. Glenn Songer, Ph.D.

THE *Corynebacterium renale* GROUP

The *Corynebacterium renale* group includes *C. renale, C. cystitidis,* and *C. pilosum,* organisms that cause cystitis and pyelonephritis in cattle and posthitis in sheep and goats. These organisms are piliated and nonmotile and can be distinguished biochemically. *C. renale* is Christie, Adkins, Munch-Peterson (CAMP)–positive because of the production of an extracellular protein called *renalin.*

Pyelonephritis

Pyelonephritis, caused by *C. renale* and its relatives, is a widespread but intermittent problem. Herd incidence greater than 5% is apparently uncommon, and a rate nearer 1% is typical. One quarter to one third of the cases may be fatal, and frequent relapses require additional treatment. Members of the *C. renale* group are normal residents of the reproductive tract of cattle, and thus transmission may be venereal. These organisms also survive well in soil, possibly facilitating indirect transmission.

Colonization of the genitourinary tract is pilus mediated, and animals are predisposed to infection by anatomic anomalies, physical damage, and obstruction of the urinary tract. Ascending infection ultimately results in cystitis and pyelonephritis. These organisms are rapidly urease positive in vitro, and the action of this enzyme in vivo leads to the production of ammonia, which causes mucosal inflammation. Cows with basic urine pH are at greater risk of the development of pyelonephritis, possibly related to pH-mediated suppression of antimicrobial defenses.

The clinical manifestation of acute pyelonephritis usually includes fever; anorexia; polyuria, hematuria, or pyuria; and abnormal posture, the hallmark of which is an arched back. If undiagnosed, infections can become chronic, with resultant weight loss, anorexia, and decreased milk production.

Rectal palpation (to detect left kidney infections) and vaginal examination (as a more sensitive measure of ureteral enlargement) can contribute to the diagnosis of pyelonephritis, and proteinuria and hematuria are useful diagnostic findings. Bacteria are sometimes isolated from urine, but *Escherichia coli* and other gram-negative bacteria are more likely to be found in chronic cases. Gross pathologic characteristics include multifocal kidney abscessation, dilated and thickened ureters containing purulent exudate, and cystitis.

Penicillin (at least 20,000 IU/kg) or trimethoprim-sulfamethoxazole (16 mg/kg) administered intramuscularly (IM) twice daily for at least 3 weeks is the recommended treatment. About 1 week after termination of antibiotic therapy, urine should be examined by bacteriologic culture to detect recurrent cases. In the absence of urogenital anomalies, the prognosis is good.

Posthitis

Posthitis (pizzle rot, sheath rot) is a preputial ulcerative dermatitis occurring primarily in entire and castrated sheep and goats. The etiologic agents are *C. pilosum* and *C. cystitidis,* which can normally inhabit the prepuce of these animals. Diets high in protein favor the production of alkaline urine (a significant risk factor for the development of posthitis) because of the excretion of urea in concentrations as high as 5%. Bacterial urease acts on the urea to produce ammonia, which may ulcerate the skin of the prepuce and predispose the animal to secondary bacterial infection. Wethers grazing rich pastures are clearly prone to the development of posthitis, as are breeding rams and bucks ingesting high-protein forage and ewes (in which the disease takes the form of ulcerative vulvovaginitis) exposed to diseased rams at breeding. Mild ulcers at the preputial orifice usually develop 1 to 2 weeks after a dietary change and, if unattended, may spread into the preputial mucosa with subsequent crusting, swelling, and pain. Painful urination may mimic urolithiasis. Pooled urine and purulent exudate inside the prepuce may lead to necrosis, the development of sinus tracts draining through the prepuce to the skin, and ultimately, chronic scarring of the preputial orifice. Sequelae include fly strike and, occasionally, obstructive uremia and death.

Diagnosis is based on the history, feeding practices, and examination of lesions. Posthitis should be included in the differential diagnosis along with urolithiasis, contagious ecthyma, and ulcerative dermatosis (lip and leg disease). The painful stance adopted by blocked males with urolithiasis is similar to that seen in animals with moderate posthitis, but in the former, other signs indicative of urethral blockage will be seen and ulcers will be absent. Lesions of contagious ecthyma typically involve the face and mouth; ulcerative dermatosis is venereally transmitted and usually manifested as an epidemic, with ulcers developing on the face, prepuce, penis, vulva, and feet. Flock morbidity with ulcerative dermatosis can be high and is not necessarily associated with high-protein feeding. The morbidity rate with posthitis is rarely more than 20%, and the disease is often sporadic; it is always associated with a history of high-protein feeding. *Campylobacter cystitidis* and *C. pilosum* may be cultured from preputial swabs of the early ulcers of posthitis.

Treatment begins with a reduction of total protein in the ration to 11% to 12%, typically by switching from legume hay to grassy or mixed hay. Mild lesions resolve spontaneously within a few weeks. In those requiring treatment, the wool should be clipped from the preputial opening and an antibacterial ointment or spray applied (5% copper sulfate solution flushed into the prepuce twice per week, penicillin-based ointments, 90% alcohol). Systemic penicillin (>20,000 mg/kg, IM, daily for 3 or more days) may be useful in animals that are severely affected.

If scarring and phimosis have occurred, a V-shaped section of the scarred portion of the prepuce should be surgically removed. Administration of a short-acting anesthetic such as xylazine (200 µg/kg IM for sheep, 10 µg/kg IM for goats) should be followed in 10 minutes by ketamine (5 mg/kg intravenously [IV]). No part of the penis should remain exposed, and the wound should be closed with a nonabsorbable suture.

Prevention and control require avoidance of long-term high-protein diets, and this may call for careful selection of pasture seedings. Legume and hay pastures are more appropriate for lactating ewes and does. The prepuce of wethers or individual rams and bucks with recurrent problems may be infused several times annually with an antiseptic solution, with the intent of reducing the number of resident coryneforms. It may also be good practice to clip the long wool or mohair from around the preputial opening.

Corynebacterium pseudotuberculosis

C. pseudotuberculosis (*C. ovis*) is a gram-positive diphtheroid that causes caseous lymphadenitis (CLA) in sheep and goats and ulcerative lymphangitis in cattle and horses. The latter condition is sporadic in nature, except in geographically limited areas, but CLA is an economically significant disease worldwide. All isolates of the organism produce a toxic phospholipase D that damages cell membranes, which is an obligate requirement for virulence. The ability of *C. pseudotuberculosis* to survive in phagocytes allows it to multiply in lymph nodes, with resultant chronic abscessation.

A prevalence of 30% to 50% in affected herds and flocks is not unusual, and the rate typically increases with advancing age. Lambs and kids are rarely affected beyond certain specific epidemiologic conditions (e.g., shearing and dipping of lambs with groups of infected ewes). Economic losses caused by CLA arise from deaths (often following development of the *thin ewe syndrome*), carcass condemnations at slaughter, decreased wool and milk production during at least the first year of disease, decreased value of hides, and decreased reproductive performance.

Typical clinical signs and bacteriologic culture of abscesses allow unequivocal establishment of a diagnosis. *Actinomyces pyogenes* and *Staphylococcus aureus* may be isolated with *C. pseudotuberculosis* or appear in pure culture from similar-appearing abscesses. The thin ewe syndrome, as well as its equivalent in goats, may result from infection by other conditions (e.g., internal parasitism, ovine progressive pneumonia, caprine arthritis-encephalitis, and paratuberculosis). The excellent sensitivity and specificity of an enzyme-linked immunosorbent assay may allow the assay to be used for management of the disease by allowing detection of animals with internal abscesses or inapparent disease and screening of new introductions.

Transmission occurs primarily through direct contact with contaminated shears, sheep dip, feeders, and feed. Recent findings suggest that congregation of sheep during shearing and dipping provides opportunities for aerosol transmission of *C. pseudotuberculosis* from lung abscesses to shearing wounds and abrasions. Organisms entering superficial tissues in this manner undergo phagocytosis and are transported to regional lymph nodes, where uncontrolled intracellular multiplication leads to abscess formation. Phospholipase D aids in the dissemination from primary to secondary sites, and anti-phospholipase D antibodies are protective. A role for phospholipase D in chronicity is probable but has not yet been demonstrated. Caseous lymphadenitis is characterized by chronic abscessation of peripheral lymph nodes. Abscesses are lamellar and filled with thick caseous exudate that may be slightly greenish. Extension to internal lymph nodes, particularly those associated with the lungs, occurs at a variable rate and may be involved in transmission.

Infected animals should be isolated and the abscesses lanced, with the contents collected to prevent environmental contamination. The abscess should be flushed with 2% iodine or 30% hydrogen peroxide, and if it is large, it may be packed with rolled gauze soaked in 2% iodine. A portion of gauze is removed daily to facilitate drainage and proper healing. If not packed, the abscess should be cleaned with chlorhexidine or iodine soap and then flushed with iodine or peroxide. Antibiotic therapy is not generally recommended because of poor penetration of antibiotics into the abscess. If needed for a specific clinical condition, penicillin is the antibiotic of choice.

The often difficult clinical diagnosis of CLA, as well as the poor prognosis for recovery, suggests the need for implementation of control measures. Regular disinfection of shearing blades in a cold sterilization solution is recommended. Fomites with the potential to cause wounds should be removed from the environment, and chronically infected animals should be culled. Two commercially available vaccines are Caseous DT (Colorado Serum Co, Denver) and Glanvac (CSL, Parkville, Victoria, Australia), both of which are sold as combination products with clostridial toxoids. Efficacy can be 70% to 90% with natural challenge. Vaccination will not often eliminate the disease from a herd, but it may decrease both the incidence and prevalence of the disease.

BIBLIOGRAPHY

McNamara PJ, Bradley GA, Songer JG: Targeted mutagenesis of the phospholipase D gene results in decreased virulence of *Corynebacterium pseudotuberculosis*. Mol Microbiol 12:921–930, 1994.

Sheldon IM: Suspected venereal spread of *Corynebacterium renale*. Vet Rec 137:100, 1995.

■ Leptospirosis*

Carole A. Bolin, D.V.M., Ph.D.
John F. Prescott, Vet.M.B., Ph.D.

Leptospirosis is an economically important zoonotic bacterial infection of livestock that causes abortions, stillbirths, and loss of milk production. Many aspects of leptospirosis in farm animals are poorly understood, in part because of difficulty in diagnosis, complexity of the host-leptospire relationship, and changing patterns of infection. Leptospirosis in livestock is largely a hidden disease that may cause considerable frustration in diagnosis and control. It should be considered a series of separate infections caused by individual serovars within a particular host, rather than a single disease with a common epidemiology, host response, and means of control.

ETIOLOGY

Leptospirosis is caused by infection with the spirochete *Leptospira*. The pathogenic leptospires were formerly classified as members of the species *Leptospira interrogans*; the genus has recently been reorganized and pathogenic leptospires are now identified in seven different species of *Leptospira*. Leptospiral serovars are recognized, and approximately 200 different serovars of *Leptospira* have been identified throughout the world.

---

*All of the material in this article is in the public domain.

Leptospires are slender spirochetes that do not stain with usual bacterial stains and are difficult to isolate in the laboratory. Serotyping to categorize isolates into serovars is increasingly being replaced by the simpler and more informative technique of genotyping.

In particular regions, different leptospiral serovars are prevalent and are associated with one or more maintenance hosts, which serve as reservoirs of infection (Table 1). Maintenance hosts are often wildlife species and sometimes domestic animals and livestock. The serovar behaves differently within its maintenance host species than it does in other incidental ("accidental") host species. A maintenance host relationship is characterized by the following: efficient transmission between animals, a relatively high incidence of infection, production of chronic rather than acute disease, and persistent infection in the kidney and sometimes in the genital tract. Diagnosis of maintenance host infections is often difficult because of a relatively low antibody response against the infecting serovar and the presence of few organisms in the tissues of infected animals. By contrast, an incidental host relationship is characterized by relatively low susceptibility to infection but high pathogenicity for the host, production of acute disease, sporadic transmission within the host species, and a short renal phase of infection. Diagnosis of incidental host infections is less problematic because of a marked antibody response to infection and the presence of large numbers of organisms in tissues of infected animals.

This distinction in behavior between animal species as either maintenance or incidental hosts is not absolute.

TRANSMISSION

Transmission among maintenance hosts often involves direct contact with infected urine, placental fluids, or milk. In addition, the infection can be transmitted venereally or transplacentally. Infection of incidental hosts is more commonly indirect, by contact with areas contaminated with urine of maintenance hosts. Environmental conditions are critical in determining the frequency of indirect transmission. Survival of leptospires is favored by moisture, moderately warm temperatures (optimal, around 28°C), and neutral or mildly stagnant water; survival is brief in dry soil or at temperatures lower than 10°C or higher than 34°C. Therefore, leptospirosis occurs most commonly in the spring, fall, and early winter in temperate climates and during the rainy season in the tropics.

PATHOGENESIS

Leptospires invade the body after penetrating exposed mucous membranes and water-softened skin. After a variable incubation period (4 to 20 days), leptospires circulate in the blood for up to 7 days. During this period, leptospires enter and replicate in many tissues including the liver, kidneys, lungs, genital tract, and central nervous system. Agglutinating antibodies can be detected in serum soon after the leptospiremia begins, and presence of antibodies coincides with clearance of the leptospires from the blood and most organs. Leptospires remain in the kidney and may be shed in the urine for a few weeks to many months after infection. In maintenance hosts, leptospires also may persist in the genital tract and, less commonly, in the cerebrospinal fluid and ocular vitreous humor.

Localization and persistence of the organism in the uterus of pregnant animals may result in fetal infection, with subsequent abortion, stillbirth, birth of weak neonates, or birth of healthy but infected offspring. An animal usually aborts only once. In maintenance host infections, infection often persists in the male and female genital tract. Leptospires have been demonstrated in bull semen and infection can be transmitted during breeding; artificial insemination is not likely to be a source of infection when semen is treated with antibiotics. Venereal transmission seems to be common in serovar *bratislava* infection of swine and serovar *hardjo* infection of cattle.

CLINICAL SIGNS

Clinical signs associated with leptospirosis vary and depend on the infecting serovar and the host. Many leptospiral infections are subclinical, particularly in nonpregnant and nonlactating animals, and are detected only by the presence of antibodies or lesions of interstitial nephritis at slaughter. Acute or subacute leptospirosis is most commonly associated with incidental host infections and occurs during the leptospiremic phase of infection. Clinical signs associated with chronic infections are usually associated with reproductive loss through abortion and stillbirth. Chronic infection of the female genital tract also may be associated with infertility in swine and cattle.

Cattle

Serovars of major importance are *hardjo* and *pomona* in North America and *hardjo* in Europe. Illness due to other serovars is relatively uncommon. Seroprevalence (agglutinating antibody titers ≥100) among cattle in the United States is estimated to be 29% for serovar *hardjo*; 23% for *pomona*; 19% for *icterohaemorrhagiae*; and 11% for *canicola*. In recent years, infection with serovar *hardjo* has become increasingly recognized along with a decline in importance of serovar *pomona* infections.

Acute Infection

Uncommonly, severe acute disease occurs in calves infected with incidental serovars, particularly serovar *pomona*. Clinical signs include high fever, hemolytic anemia, hemoglobinuria, jaundice, pulmonary congestion, meningitis (occasionally), and death. In lactating cows, incidental infections are often associated with agalactia with small quantities of blood-tinged milk. Recovery is prolonged.

The most common form of acute leptospirosis occurs in dairy cows as a transient pyrexia with a marked drop in milk production lasting for 2 to 10 days. In this acute *milk drop syndrome*, the milk has the consistency of colostrum, with thick clots, yellow staining, and high somatic cell count, and the udder has a uniformly soft texture. This condition occurs most commonly with serovar *hardjo* type *hardjoprajitno* infection but may be caused by other serovars. Leptospiral milk drop syndrome varies

---

Table 1
COMMON *Leptospira* SEROVARS AND THEIR MAINTENANCE HOSTS IN NORTH AMERICA

Genus and Species	Serovar	Maintenance Host(s)
L. interrogans	bratislava	Swine, horses
L. interrogans	canicola	Dogs
L. kirschneri	grippotyphosa	Raccoons, skunks, opossum, squirrels
L. borgpetersenii	hardjo type hardjo-bovis	Cattle
L. interrogans	icterohaemorrhagiae	Rats
L. interrogans	pomona type kennewicki	Skunk, raccoon, opossum, swine

from an epizootic infection in a previously unexposed herd, involving more than half the herd over a period of 1 or 2 months, to a more common endemic infection affecting cows in their first or second lactation. Recovery is usually in 10 days without treatment, although cows in late lactation may dry up. A subclinical form of this milk drop syndrome may occur in *hardjo*-infected lactating cows in the absence of other clinical evidence of infection.

Chronic Infection

The chronic form of disease, most commonly associated with serovars *hardjo* and *pomona*, is associated with fetal infection in pregnant cows presenting as abortion, stillbirth, or birth of premature and weak infected calves. Infected but apparently healthy calves also may be born. Retention of fetal membranes may follow *hardjo*-induced abortion. Abortion or stillbirth is commonly the only manifestation of infection, but it may sometimes be related to an episode of illness up to 6 weeks (serovar *pomona*) or 12 weeks (serovar *hardjo*) earlier. Serovar *hardjo* type *hardjoprajitno* appears to be more virulent than type *hardjo-bovis*.

Accurate data for the frequency of abortion due to *hardjo* and *pomona* serovars are not readily available in North America. Abortion due to serovar *pomona* has decreased in importance over the last decades, probably because of vaccination. Abortion and stillbirth due to serovar *hardjo* are recognized more commonly. Serovar *hardjo* is more important than is *pomona* because it causes endemic rather than more sporadic infection. In Northern Ireland, where the more virulent type *hardjoprajitno* occurs, *hardjo* was recognized as being responsible for nearly half of all bovine abortions in one study. Type *hardjoprajitno* was isolated from the majority of aborted fetuses, whereas type *hardjo-bovis* was isolated mainly from the kidney and genital tract of carrier cows. In one large study in Ontario, where type *hardjo-bovis* is prevalent, serovar *hardjo* caused about 6% of abortions; abortions from *pomona* infection were not recognized.

The pattern of *hardjo* infection in a herd varies with the husbandry conditions and with the type of *hardjo* present. In addition, to the major types of serovar *hardjo*, *hardjo-bovis* and *hardjoprajitno*, genetic differences and differences in tissue localization and immune response to infection have been identified in serovar *hardjo* isolates from different parts of the world. Data from Britain, where the more virulent *hardjoprajitno* is present, may not be fully applicable to North America. In Britain, where heifers are often reared separately from the main herd, abortion and stillbirth commonly occur in a proportion of these susceptible animals after their introduction into an endemically infected herd. In such herds, between 3% and 10% of cows in the herd may abort or produce stillborn or weak calves. Four patterns of *hardjo* infection were identified in cattle in Britain, based on herd serologic findings and clinical history: (1) endemic infection, described in the preceding; (2) active infection in yearlings, in which subsequent abortion was rare; (3) frequent and high titers in cows of all ages, indicating recent infection in a susceptible herd; and (4) a *fading herd infection*, in which titers were confined largely to older cows, but their clinical significance was unclear. In Ontario, *hardjo* infection and abortion was largely a problem in beef rather than in dairy cattle, and the serologic pattern conformed most to the pattern of fading herd infection.

Infertility, which has apparently responded to vaccination and treatment, has been described in *hardjo*-infected herds. Such infertility, which has not been well documented, may follow localization of leptospires in the uterus and oviduct of *hardjo*-infected cattle.

Swine

Whereas any leptospire may infect and cause disease in swine, until recently, the most common and important serovar recognized in swine in North America was *pomona* (type *kennewicki*). In Australia and some European countries, serovar *tarassovi* (formerly *hyos*), another swine-adapted pathogen, causes losses as serious as those of *pomona*. Serovars such as *canicola* and *grippotyphosa* can be locally important. Antibodies to *icterohaemorrhagiae* are widespread, but the serovar is of little disease significance. Understanding of leptospirosis in swine is changing rapidly with the recognition of the widespread and dominant prevalence of antibodies to the *australis* serogroup (serovars *bratislava* and *muenchen*) and the isolation of *bratislava* and *muenchen* from aborted and stillborn pigs. In contrast to other serovars, the role and importance of serovars *bratislava* and *muenchen* in swine is not fully understood, in part because of the difficulty of isolating these bacteria.

Acute Infection

Only a small proportion of infected animals develop clinical illness, which is characterized by transient and mild pyrexia, anorexia, and depression. Hemoglobinuria and jaundice occur rarely in piglets.

Chronic Infection

Abortion in the last trimester of pregnancy and the birth of stillborn or of weak and unthrifty piglets are the result of chronic infection with serovars other than *bratislava* and *muenchen*. In nonpregnant swine, variable lesions of interstitial nephritis are commonly observed grossly at slaughter. Infection with *pomona* or *tarassovi* may result in abortion storms when first introduced into a susceptible herd, but abortions diminish once herd immunity develops, and gilts are most affected.

Evidence for the role of serovars *bratislava* and/or *muenchen* in abortion includes their recovery from aborted and stillborn swine in Northern Ireland, their isolation from the kidneys and genital tracts of recently aborting sows, the improvement in fertility and number of piglets born to sows vaccinated with *bratislava* as reported in Italy and the United States, and serologic studies showing a significant relationship between titers and infertility in sows.

In Northern Ireland, late-term reproductive losses caused by serovars *bratislava* and *muenchen* have been characterized by the birth of live, dying, and dead piglets. Infection in herds in Ireland often had a 2-year cyclicity. Marked annual variation has occurred in incidence in Northern Ireland, from 6% to 40% in different years.

Infertility is also associated with *bratislava* and *muenchen* infections and is characterized as a repeat breeder syndrome, described as endemic in most breeding herds in Northern Ireland. Disease is most noticeable in sows in certain age groups, particularly those bred for the first time to infected boars. Disease is at its worst when susceptible animals are introduced into an endemically infected herd, for example, when sows from specific-pathogen free (SPF) herds are brought into the herd. Serovars *bratislava* and *muenchen* have been commonly isolated from the genital tracts of sows and boars in infected herds; venereal transmission is thought to be a major means of transmission.

In Britain, *bratislava* type *B2b* is almost exclusively isolated from swine and from aborted fetuses; type *B2a* is widespread in several hosts, including swine, but it is rarely isolated from aborted piglets. This pattern is not apparent in the United States, where *B2a* and *B2b*, and an additional type *B1*, have been isolated from cases of reproductive failure as well as from the kidneys of swine at slaughter. All three types have even been isolated from piglets in the same litter.

Serovar *bratislava* has been isolated from stillborn and weak pigs in Iowa and is less commonly associated with abortion. Serovar *bratislava* was isolated from 12% of swine sampled at one slaughter facility in the United States, which indicates the importance of this infection.

Sheep and Goats

Sheep appear less susceptible than cattle to clinical leptospirosis. Sheep are maintenance hosts for serovar *hardjo*, and the infection is maintained in populations of sheep independent of their contact with cattle. Other serovars may also cause disease. Acute disease in lambs is characterized by fever, hemolytic anemia, hemoglobinuria, and jaundice. Serovar *hardjo* infection of ewes may cause late-term abortion, stillbirth, weak lambs, and agalactia in recently lambed ewes. Other serovars occasionally cause abortion. Leptospirosis in goats has attracted little attention, but goats are susceptible to a wide range of leptospiral serovars and may develop acute and chronic leptospirosis.

PATHOLOGY AND NECROPSY FINDINGS

In acute infection, calves and piglets show pathologic changes of subserosal and submucosal hemorrhage, hemolytic anemia, hemoglobinuria, and jaundice, with histologic changes of interstitial nephritis and centrilobular hepatic necrosis.

In chronic infection, pathologic findings in most aborted bovine fetuses are negligible. Mild focal tubular necrosis and interstitial nephritis may be present. Jaundice is rarely recognized. In swine, nonmummified fetuses often show excess serosal effusions and, quite commonly, scattered 1- to 4-mm necrotic foci in the liver. Adult swine and cattle commonly show 1- to 3-mm gray foci of chronic lymphocytic interstitial nephritis at slaughter.

DIAGNOSIS

Diagnosis of leptospirosis is dependent on a good clinical and vaccination history and the availability of diagnostic testing at a laboratory with experience in the diagnosis of leptospirosis. Diagnostic tests for leptospirosis can be separated into those designed to detect antibodies against the organism and those designed to detect the organism or its DNA in tissues or body fluids of animals. Each of the diagnostic procedures, for detection of the organism or for antibodies directed against the organism, has a number of advantages and disadvantages. Some of the assays suffer from a lack of sensitivity and others are prone to specificity problems. Therefore, no single technique can be recommended for use in each clinical situation. Use of a combination of tests allows maximum sensitivity and specificity in establishing the diagnosis. Serologic testing is recommended in each case, combined with one or more techniques to identify the organism in tissue or body fluids.

Serologic Tests

Serology is the most commonly used technique for diagnosing leptospirosis in animals. The microscopic agglutination test and various enzyme immunoassays are the serologic tests most frequently used. Serology is inexpensive, reasonably sensitive, and widely available.

The microscopic agglutination test is available worldwide and involves mixing appropriate dilutions of serum with live leptospires of serovars prevalent within the region. The presence of antibodies is indicated by the agglutination of the leptospires. Enzyme immunoassays have been developed using a number of different antigen preparations and assay protocols. An assay that measures anti-leptospiral IgM may be useful for detecting recent infection in livestock. Use of these assays is complicated in areas of the world in which vaccination is common, because some vaccinated animals develop IgM titers as well as IgG titers, thus giving positive results in the enzyme immunoassays. In general, animals develop relatively low agglutinating antibody titers (100 to 400) in response to vaccination, and these titers persist for 1 to 3 months after vaccination. However, some animals develop high titers after vaccination, and although these high vaccination titers decrease with time, they may persist for 6 months or more after vaccination.

Detection of high titers of antibody in animals with a disease consistent with leptospirosis may be sufficient to establish the diagnosis. This is particularly true in the investigation of abortions caused by incidental host infections in which the dam's agglutinating antibody titer is 1600 or greater. However, in maintenance host infections, particularly *hardjo* in cattle and *bratislava* in swine, infected animals often have a poor agglutinating antibody response to infection. Often, at the time of abortion, antibody titers are quite low or negative in the maintenance host. In these cases, the herd serologic response to infection is often more helpful than is the individual's response in establishing the diagnosis. In abortion or stillbirth, it is often useful to do serologic testing on fetal serum, but dilutions should start at 1:10, in contrast to adult studies in which the usual starting dilution is 1:100.

Interpretation of leptospiral serologic results is complicated by a number of factors: cross-reactivity of antibodies, antibody titers induced by vaccination, and lack of consensus about what antibody titers are indicative of active infection. Antibodies produced in an animal in response to infection with a given serovar of *Leptospira* often cross-react with other serovars of leptospires. Therefore, a pig infected with a single serovar is likely to have antibodies against more than one serovar in an agglutination test. In some cases, these patterns of cross-reactivity are predictable based on the antigenic relatedness of the various serovars of *Leptospira*. Unfortunately, patterns of cross-reactivity of antibodies vary widely between species of animals and between individuals within a species. However, in general, the infecting serovar is assumed to be the serovar to which that animal develops the highest titer. Paradoxical reactions may occur with the agglutination test early in the course of an acute infection, with a marked agglutinating antibody response to a serovar other than the infecting serovar.

Interpretation of leptospiral serologic titers is variable; an agglutinating antibody titer of 100 or greater is considered significant by many. However, this cutoff level may be exceeded in vaccinated animals and may not be reached in maintenance host infections. Therefore, diagnosis of leptospirosis based on a single serum sample must be made with caution and with full consideration of the clinical picture and vaccination history of the animal. In cases of acute leptospirosis, a fourfold rise in antibody titer is often observed in paired serum samples. However, in cases in which appropriate antibiotic therapy is instituted promptly after the onset of clinical signs, titers may not rise in paired serum samples, or, indeed, a significant titer may never develop. Maintenance hosts are commonly actively infected and shedding leptospires with antibody titers of 100 or less. Therefore, a low antibody titer does not necessarily rule out a diagnosis of leptospirosis. Antibody titers can persist for months following infection and recovery, although the antibody titer usually declines gradually with time.

Detection of Leptospires

Other techniques available for the diagnosis of leptospirosis in livestock involve procedures to detect leptospires or leptospiral DNA in tissues or body fluids. These techniques include dark-field microscopy, immunofluorescence, culture, histopathology with special stains, and polymerase chain reaction assays. Each of these assays is useful in the diagnosis of leptospirosis and each presents special advantages and disadvantages for routine use.

Dark-field microscopy has been used as a rapid screening tool to identify leptospires in the urine of animals. The advantage of dark-field microscopy is speed; disadvantages include low specificity and sensitivity. Direct visualization of the organisms is problematic, and artifacts present in body fluids are difficult to distinguish from leptospires, even by experienced observers. The sensitivity of dark-field microscopy is low; approximately 10^5 leptospires per milliliter of urine must be present to be detected. It is also important to remember that leptospires are present in the urine to varying degrees with different serovars and are not usually present in urine in the early stages of acute disease. In general, dark-field microscopy can be useful to make a preliminary positive diagnosis of leptospirosis, but it should not be relied on to make a definitive diagnosis.

Immunofluorescence can be used to identify leptospires in tissues, blood, or urine sediment. The availability of this test is increasing, and the test is rapid, has good sensitivity, and can be used on frozen samples. The fluorescent antibody conjugate currently available for general use is not serovar-specific; serologic examination of the animal is still required to identify the infecting serovar. Serovar-specific fluorescent antibody conjugates have been prepared and are in use in Canada and in some research laboratories in other countries.

Bacteriologic culture of blood, urine, or tissue specimens is the definitive method for the diagnosis of leptospirosis. Leptospiremia occurs early in the clinical course of leptospirosis and is usually of short duration and low level. Therefore, blood is only useful for culture in the first few days of clinical illness and prior to antibiotic therapy. Leptospires are usually present in the urine of animals 10 days or more after the onset of clinical signs. Urine for culture should be collected after injection of furosemide. Furosemide increases the glomerular filtration rate and "flushes" more leptospires into the urine and produces dilute urine, which enhances survival of the leptospires. Urine, blood, and tissue samples for culture should be diluted in 1% bovine serum albumin transport medium as soon as possible after collection. Culture of leptospires is difficult and time-consuming and it requires specialized culture medium. However, isolation of the organism from the animal allows definitive identification of the infecting serovar.

The use of special stains in histopathology can be effective for identification of leptospires in animal tissues. This common diagnostic technique is the only one that can be routinely used on formalin-fixed tissues. Application of silver stains or immunohistochemical stains to tissue sections will allow detection of leptospires or leptospiral antigens in the renal tubules and interstitium of the kidney, liver, lung, or placenta. Low sensitivity is a disadvantage of this diagnostic technique. Leptospires are often present in small numbers in affected tissues, particularly in chronic leptospirosis. The infecting serovar cannot be determined by histopathology; serologic studies also should be conducted.

Techniques have been developed that allow detection of leptospiral DNA in clinical samples. These tests include DNA probe tests, which detect leptospiral DNA directly, and tests that rely on the polymerase chain reaction amplification of DNA in tissues or body fluids. In general, DNA probes are not used because of a lack of sensitivity and technical difficulties in their use. Polymerase chain reaction tests, however, are being used for the diagnosis of leptospirosis in animals. A number of polymerase chain reaction procedures are available. In general, polymerase chain reaction testing of urine is more reliable than testing of tissues. Processing of tissue samples is more difficult, and tissues often contain inhibitors to the amplification reaction and therefore may cause false-negative results. Most polymerase chain reaction assays are able to detect the presence of leptospires but are not able to determine the infecting serovar. Polymerase chain reaction assays can be sensitive and specific techniques for the diagnosis of leptospirosis. Unfortunately, the process is complex and exquisitely sensitive to contamination with exogenous leptospiral DNA.

Cattle

Paired samples in an individual animal are particularly useful for acute and subacute infections. Titers in these animals are often considerably greater than 100. In abortion caused by incidental serovars, agglutinating antibody titers against *pomona* and other incidental serovars are high, often 3000 or greater.

Paired serum samples are of no value in chronic infections because abortion occurs weeks after infection, so that titers are static or declining. For chronic *hardjo* infections, a recently aborting cow with a titer of 300 or greater has about a 60% chance of fetal infection; 1000 or greater, an 80% chance; and 3000 or greater, a 90% chance. If several aborting cows in a herd show high titers (≥300), this is usually sufficient evidence for a diagnosis of leptospirosis in unvaccinated herds. However, 25% or more of the cows with *hardjo*-infected fetuses may have no detectable agglutinating antibody titer.[12]

Because of these serodiagnostic difficulties in chronic disease, herd rather than individual serologic testing may be useful for determining the presence of active infection, especially due to *hardjo*. The herd should be divided for sampling into different management and age groups for representative testing. For *hardjo* infection, titers of 300 or greater indicate active infection, and for incidental serovars, titers are often higher (≥1000 to 3000). The herd serologic profiles will show seasonal and individual variation over time. Diagnosis of chronic infections is thus best made by combination of direct detection of leptospires with the individual animal and herd serologic findings.

Swine

Several fetuses in each litter must be examined for leptospires (e.g., by pooling kidneys and lungs from four piglets for immunofluorescence). Serosal effusions or the vitreous humor of the eye may show viable leptospires, especially in *pomona* or *tarassovi* infection, which can be identified by dark-field microscopy or immunofluorescence. Serologic testing on several piglets (aborted, stillborn, or weak piglets that have not sucked) in the litter is particularly useful to identify *bratislava* or *muenchen* infection. Titers may be as low as 10, and are rarely more than 100, and cross-reactions with other serovars may occur, but these usually have a lower titer than that to *bratislava*. Several litters should be examined before it is concluded that Australis serogroup leptospires are not involved.

Sows that have recently aborted because of *pomona*, *tarassovi*, or other incidental serovars often have high agglutinating antibody titers (1000 to 30,000). Because individual sows may have low titers, testing a dozen herdmates is often valuable. Agglutinating antibody titers in sows aborting because of *bratislava* or *muenchen* infection are unhelpful because many will have low titers (100 to 400) and many will be negative. Seroconversion may occasionally be demonstrated. Antibody titers in herds vaccinated for *bratislava* will often be much higher than those associated with infection, regardless of the infection status of the herd. Therefore, in these herds, diagnostic methods must be used to identify the organism in tissues or fluids.

TREATMENT AND CONTROL

Animals with acute leptospirosis can be treated with streptomycin (12.5 mg/kg twice daily for 3 days) or tetracycline (10 to 15 mg/kg twice daily for 3 to 5 days). Streptomycin treatment can be combined with ampicillin or large doses of penicillin G. Leptospires also are highly susceptible to erythromycin, tiamulin, and tylosin, although these antibiotics cannot be relied on to remove the renal carrier state. A single dose of streptomycin (25 mg/kg) will usually remove the chronic renal carrier state caused by *pomona* or other serovars; chronic *hardjo* type *hardjoprajitno* infections may resist this treatment regimen. Streptomycin is no longer available for use in the United States. Injectable, long-acting oxytetracycline at a dose of 20 mk/kg may be substituted for streptomycin to treat chronic infections.

Control is based on prevention, vaccination, and treatment. In all cases, there should be limitation of direct and indirect transmission by carriers of incidental infections (e.g., by rodent control around buildings, fencing of swampy ground or streams). Immunity is serovar specific. Polyvalent vaccines containing common serovars endemic to the host and region are generally available. These may contain unnecessary serovars (e.g., *canicola* and *icterohaemorrhagiae*). Different vaccines vary in efficacy, and vaccine failures may occur.

There are two basic approaches to control: eradication by a combination of progressive identification of carriers and antibiotic treatment, or control by annual herd vaccination and judicious use of antibiotics. The decision as to which approach to use depends on the purpose of the herd, the herd history, and the seroprevalence of leptospirosis; most people favor control over eradication.

Cattle

Annual vaccination of all cattle in a closed herd with appropriate vaccines, or twice yearly vaccination in an open herd, is the most effective approach to control. Newly introduced cattle should be treated with dihydrostreptomycin (25 mg/kg, given intramuscularly [IM], in two doses 10 days apart) or long-acting oxytetracycline (20 mg/kg, IM, two doses 10 days apart) for elimination of most chronic renal infection and vaccinated before they enter the herd. Streptomycin or oxytetracycline treatment will not remove all carriers of *hardjo* (particularly *hardjo-prajitno* carriers), but it is usually effective for *pomona*. Vaccination can be combined with antibiotic treatment in the face of an outbreak. Calves should be 6 months or older before vaccination and should be vaccinated twice, with 3 to 4 weeks between vaccinations; younger animals respond poorly. Vaccination thereafter is with a single dose annually. Because of the short-lasting, low-titer agglutinating antibody response, annual vaccination with most available vaccines will progressively reduce and eventually abolish the herd seroprevalence of leptospirosis. In an infected animal, vaccination will not reduce urinary shedding, but it often considerably increases the antibody titer. Persistent low-titer reactions, which may last for years, may prevent bulls from entering studs or cattle from being exported. Treatment often does not abolish these titers. Because of the low sensitivity of the agglutination test for detecting *hardjo* carriers, international recommendations for importation of livestock (Internal Zoo-Sanitary Code, Office International des Epizooties) suggest reliance on antibiotic treatment before any movement, rather than on serologic testing. Regulations generally should be changed for bull studs or export requirements to allow control by the combination of vaccination and antibiotic treatment rather than by the use of serologic tests to detect carriers.

Vaccination with incidental serovars usually gives excellent protection against challenge. Field evidence has shown that *hardjo* vaccination reduces reproductive losses due to *hardjo* infection as well as leptospiruria. However, some studies have shown that *hardjo* vaccination does not prevent renal infection, urinary shedding, or fetal infection with type *hardjo-bovis*. The efficacy of serovar *hardjo* vaccines may vary as a result of vaccine composition, husbandry conditions, and type and pathogenicity of serovar *hardjo* strains prevalent in the region.

Swine

A single streptomycin injection (25 mg/kg IM) stops leptospiruria in the majority of swine infected with *pomona*, although administration for 3 days may be slightly more effective. Oxytetracycline (20 to 40 mg/kg IM, once daily for 3 to 5 days), although cumbersome, is a useful alternative where streptomycin is no longer available. The value of streptomycin in the treatment of *bratislava* and *muenchen* infections has not been investigated but would be likely to be less effective than for *pomona*. Penicillin is ineffective against the carrier state. Administration of tetracycline in feed (800 to 1000 g/ton) has in some, but not all, cases eliminated renal infections with *pomona*. Herd administration of tetracycline at 4000 g/ton on a month-on, month-off pattern has been used to control *bratislava* and *muenchen* infection, but infection usually recurs within 4 or 5 months of cessation of treatment.

Vaccines will markedly reduce abortion and stillbirth rates, and will reduce (but may not fully eliminate) renal colonization and leptospiruria. They have, however, been used to eradicate infection in combination with hygienic measures. Double vaccination of gilts just before mating and of vaccinated sows at each weaning is a useful approach to control on endemically affected farms. Field studies of *bratislava* vaccines have shown that their use has been followed by increased litter sizes and farrowing rates. Eradication of *pomona* and *tarassovi* has been accomplished by a combination of serologic testing, isolation, vaccination, and treatment of seropositive animals. Control can be achieved by a combination of twice-yearly vaccination, with antibiotic treatment and double vaccination of all introduced pigs. Careful design of effluent channels and pen and pig separation can reduce transmission.

BIBLIOGRAPHY

Alt DP, Bolin CA: Preliminary evaluation of antimicrobial agents for treatment of *Leptospira interrogans* serovar *pomona* infection in hamsters and swine. Am J Vet Res 57:59, 1996.

Bolin CA: *Leptospira interrogans* serovar *bratislava* infection in swine. Swine Consultant, Fall 1993, p 3.

Bolin CA, Cassells JA: Isolation of *Leptospira interrogans* serovars *bratislava* and *hardjo* from swine at slaughter. J Vet Diagn Invest 4:87, 1992.

Bolin CA, Cassells JA: Isolation of *Leptospira interrogans* serovar *bratislava* from stillborn and weak pigs in Iowa. J Am Vet Med Assoc 196:1601, 1990.

Bolin CA, Cassells JA, Hill HT, et al: Reproductive failure associated with *Leptospira interrogans* serovar *bratislava* infection of swine. J Vet Diagn Invest 3:152, 1991.

Bolin CA, Thiermann AB, Handsaker AL, et al: Effect of vaccination with a pentavalent leptospiral vaccine on *Leptospira interrogans* serovar *hardjo* type *hardjo-bovis* infection of pregnant cattle. Am J Vet Res 50:161, 1989.

Dhaliwal GS, Murray RD, Ellis WA: Reproductive performance of dairy herds infected with *Leptospira interrogans* serovar *hardjo* relative to the year of diagnosis. Vet Rec 138:272, 1996.

Ellis WA: Effects of leptospirosis on bovine reproduction. *In* Morrow DA (ed): Current Therapy in Theriogenology, ed 2. Philadelphia, WB Saunders, 1986, pp 267–271.

Ellis WA: *Leptospira australis* infection in pigs. Pig Vet J 22:83, 1989.

Ellis WA: The diagnosis of leptospirosis in farm animals. *In* Ellis WA, Little TWA (eds): The Present State of Leptospirosis Diagnosis and Control. Dordrecht, The Netherlands, Martinus Nijhoff, 1986, pp 13–24.

Ellis WA, Michna SW: Bovine leptospirosis: Infection by the *hebdomadis* serogroup and abortion—a herd study. Vet Rec 99:409, 1976.

Hathaway SC, Little TW, Pritchard DG: Problems associated with the serological diagnosis of *Leptospira interrogans* serovar *hardjo* infection in bovine populations. Vet Rec 119:84, 1986.

Miller DA, Wilson MA, Beran GW: Survey to estimate prevalence of *Leptospira interrogans* infection in mature cattle in the United States. Am J Vet Res 52:1761, 1991.

Prescott JF, Miller RB, Nicholson VM, et al: Seroprevalence and association with abortions of leptospirosis in cattle in Ontario. Can J Vet Res 52:210, 1988.

■ The *Haemophilus somnus* Complex

Thomas J. Inzana, Ph.D.

Haemophilus somnus was first identified in 1960 as a cause of central nervous system disease in cattle, currently referred to as thrombotic meningoencephalitis (TME). Since its initial identification, *H. somnus* has also been confirmed to be an important cause of bovine diseases such as pneumonia, septicemia, myelitis, arthritis, abortion, infertility due to endometritis, orchitis, vaginitis, retinal hemorrhage, conjunctivitis, laryngitis, otitis, myocarditis, and other local infections. TME, abortion, and pneumonia have been reproduced under experimental conditions.

ETIOLOGY

H. somnus is a small, gram-negative coccobacillus, similar in microscopic appearance to other *Haemophilus* spp. It is highly pleomorphic and under some conditions may form long filaments. Its growth requirements are complex; it does not require X (hemin) or V factor (NAD), but it does require nicotinamide and blood for growth. Carbon dioxide (5% to 10%) is required for growth on agar media, and the amount of CO_2 provided by a candle extinction jar is usually sufficient. When grown in a broth medium, additional CO_2 is not required. Following in vitro passage, strains adapt to growth in ambient air. Colonies at 24 hours are small (about 0.2 to 0.6 mm) and clear, and enlarge to 2 to 3 mm by 48 to 72 hours on a blood-based enrichment medium. Colonies are raised, circular, smooth, and off-yellow on blood agar. Hemolysis on blood agar occurs within 48 hours due to an exotoxin produced by most disease isolates. *H. somnus* is not encapsulated.

A detailed taxonomic study of *H. somnus* has not been done. This bacterium has been classified as incertae sedis by *Bergey's Manual of Systematic Bacteriology*, and has been proposed to be transferred to a new genus, possibly *Histophilus*.

OCCURRENCE

TME was first reported in Colorado in 1956, and *H. somnus* was confirmed to be the etiologic agent of this disease in 1960. Since then, diseases caused by *H. somnus* have been identified in regions throughout the world, including North America, South America, Europe, Australia, New Zealand, Russia, and Japan. Diseases caused by *H. somnus* are primarily problematic in feedlots where there is a large concentration of animals, which facilitates stress and transmission. However, infections in pasture animals, dairy cattle, and adults of beef breeds in cow-calf operations have also been reported. In the United States and Canada, *H. somnus* has been commonly isolated in the West and the Midwest, but rarely in the Northeast or Southeast. The incidence of *H. somnus* fibrinous pneumonia in calves in Canadian feedlots increased almost 50% between 1988 and 1991 over the period 1985 to 1987.

PREVALENCE

In the United States it has been difficult to evaluate the impact of *H. somnus* on morbidity and mortality of cattle because greater than 58% of the deaths in feedlots do not undergo a postmortem examination. In Canada, *H. somnus* is considered a substantial pathogen and a major contributor to respiratory disease. *H. somnus* is recognized as one of the three primary bacterial pathogens in respiratory shipping fever, along with *Pasteurella haemolytica* and *Pasteurella multocida*. The rate of isolation of *H. somnus* from the genital tract has been reported to be as high as 28.6% in Australian cows and as low as 6.0% in German cows. *H. somnus* has been isolated from the vagina of 15% of cows in the United States and of 8% in Canada. In one Canadian study, *H. somnus* was reportedly responsible for greater than 40% of the mortality of feedlot calves per year. The exact incidence of diseases caused by *H. somnus* is not known. However, when all syndromes that may be caused by *H. somnus* are taken together, *H. somnus* may be the most economically significant bovine pathogen in feedlots.

PATHOGENESIS

The first step in pathogenesis is usually adherence of the bacterium to host cells. Adherence of *H. somnus* to a variety of host cell types has been documented, particularly endothelial cells and vaginal epithelial cells. Degeneration of the endothelial cells and vasculitis are key features of *H. somnus* infection, and attachment to these cells may be a prerequisite for the ensuing disease. *H. somnus* can survive within macrophages and polymorphonuclear leukocytes (PMNs). This survival may be due to toxicity by *H. somnus* within bovine phagocytic cells. Hence, virulent *H. somnus* strains are not killed by phagocytic cells because of degeneration of the phagocytes or suppression of phagocytic function. Purine and pyrimidine bases, ribonucleotides, and a ribonucleoside have been identified as the bacterium-associated factors responsible for inefficient killing by PMNs, not the hemolysin. Exposure of PMNs to *H. somnus* reduces the oxidative respiratory burst by these cells. Furthermore, although catalase-negative, viable *H. somnus* can eliminate hydrogen peroxide from its environment and significantly decrease bovine macrophage superoxide production.

Virulent and nonvirulent strains of *H. somnus* have been identified. Isolates from bovine disease can clearly be distinguished from commensal isolates from the normal prepuce or vagina. While essentially all disease isolates are resistant to complement-mediated killing by normal serum, 25% of preputial isolates are serum-sensitive and most vaginal isolates have a delayed susceptibility to killing. Two linked genes have been identified that encode 120-kDa and 76-kDa proteins that are present in serum-resistant disease isolates, but are not present in serum-sensitive preputial isolates. Pathogenic isolates of *H. somnus* demonstrate antigenic phase variation in their lipooligosaccharide (LOS) following in vivo infection or in vitro passage, but this does not occur in nonpathogenic isolates. In addition to phase variation, *H. somnus* is also capable of adding *N*-acetyl-neuraminic acid to the terminal galactose residue of its LOS. The result of this sialylation is decreased binding of some antibodies to LOS and enhanced serum resistance. Again, preputial isolates do not seem capable of sialylating their LOS. Furthermore, preputial isolates cannot cause disease in established *H. somnus* mouse models.

The LOS of *H. somnus*, like the lipopolysaccharide component of enteric bacteria, is also an endotoxin. It is likely that *H. somnus* LOS is a key factor in the inflammation and vasculitis that are characteristic of infections caused by this organism. *H. somnus* also contains Fc receptors that bind to bovine immunoglobulins (IgBPs). These IgBPs may influence virulence by nonspecifically binding immunoglobulin, which then protects the organism from host defenses. Additionally, IgBPs may enhance serum resistance.

Most systemic infections probably occur following dissemination due to septicemia. Factors stated above that promote serum resistance in disease isolates may enable these strains to disseminate and form infectious foci in various organs, such as the myocardium, placenta, lungs, brain, joints, and other organs. The cytotoxicity of *H. somnus* for epithelial, phagocytic, and other cells may result from the direct effect of cytotoxicity by extracellular toxin and inflammation due to endotoxin.

CLINICAL SIGNS

Infections caused by *H. somnus* may occur in animals of all ages, although certain infections are more prominent in certain age groups. The *H. somnus* complex of diseases occurs most often in feedlot calves, where a high concentration of animals and stress (e.g., weather and shipping) probably contribute to transmission of, and susceptibility to, the bacterium. Infections in very young animals are rare, probably because of passive maternal immunity. When infections in young calves do occur, they usually manifest as conjunctivitis or pneumonia. Most systemic infections occur in calves or young animals 6 months to 2 years of age. Infections may be peracute, acute, or chronic. Peracute infections usually involve the respiratory tract or the central nervous system (TME). Clinical signs include fever, prostration, sudden stiffness, and death. Affected cattle will often appear normal one day and severely morbid or dead the following day. Acute infections may present with symptoms in any organ or system, such as the respiratory tract, central nervous system, myocardium, liver, kidneys, and female reproductive tract (abortion). Cattle with these infections may have fever, depression, somnolence, aggression, dyspnea, nasal discharge, excessive lacrimation, stiffness, and/or high morbidity. Chronic infections affect many internal organs subsequent to septicemia, such as the liver, kidneys, and joints. Respiratory tract infections may also be chronic. Rarely, orchitis with swollen testes and infertility may occur in males, but chronic carriage of *H. somnus* in the male reproductive tract is usually asymptomatic. Vaginitis or cervicitis may occur in cows and can result in infertility.

Cattle with joint infections will often appear lame with swollen joints. Paresis in the hind or all four limbs may occur due to myelitis. Retinal hemorrhage is often present due to septicemia, but is usually not diagnosed until necropsy. Myocarditis may result in acute or congestive heart failure. Laryngitis may cause a nonproductive cough. Otitis may result in facial nerve paralysis, nystagmus, ear drooping, or a foul discharge due to rupture of the eardrum. Many of these symptoms are nonspecific and may be caused by a wide variety of other infectious agents, including *Pasteurella* spp., *Actinomyces pyogenes*, *Listeria monocytogenes*, *Mycoplasma* or *Chlamydia* spp., and viruses. There-

fore, chronic, nonspecific symptoms require a broad diagnostic workup.

PATHOLOGY AND NECROPSY FINDINGS

The type of lesions observed at necropsy will usually be reflected by the acuteness of the disease. There may be no gross pathologic findings following peracute death, but microscopic lesions will be present throughout the vasculature. Acute septicemia with subsequent infection of organ systems will result in thrombosis and lesions of the vascular endothelium. The type and extent of the lesions, however, are extremely variable depending on the organ system.

Respiratory tract lesions may be variable, in part because concomitant infections with other bacteria and viruses are common. Common lung lesions include fibrinous pneumonia or pleuritis, suppurative bronchopneumonia, diffuse hemorrhagic interstitial pneumonia, thrombosis, necrotizing bronchiolitis, and diffuse congestion. Vasculitis is also usually present. Myocarditis is often accompanied by fibrinous pleuritis. The myocardium itself may have hemorrhage and necrosis with fibrin exudates on the surface, and miliary or larger abscesses on the ventricular walls and papillary muscles (Fig. 1).

Brain lesions consisting of parenchymal necrosis and multifocal hemorrhage are almost pathognomonic for *H. somnus* infection. These lesions are usually 1 to 5 mm in size with foci up to 2 cm in the cortex (Fig. 2). The presence of thrombi in the lesions accounts for the clinical name TME. The cerebrospinal fluid may be cloudy, and clot, with large numbers of PMNs present. Animals with TME usually have serofibrinous polyarthritis as well. The joints most commonly affected are the stifle or atlanto-occipital, but many joints of the legs and spinal column may be involved. In more chronic infections the arthritic exudate becomes more fibrinous.

Following abortion, edema and necrosis of cotyledons are typical placental lesions resulting from fibrinoid necrosis of arteries in the placenta. Metritis may occur and be severe enough to cause death of the cow. The fetus and fetal membranes may also be infected, resulting in petechial hemorrhages in fetal tissues.

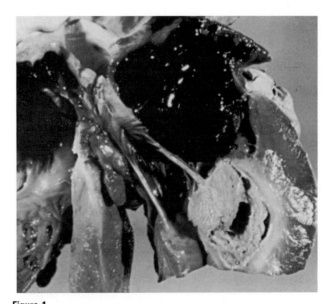

Figure 1

H. somnus myocardial abscess in the papillary muscle of a 700-lb feedlot steer. (Courtesy of M. Savic, D.V.M., D.V.Sc, Guelph, Ontario.)

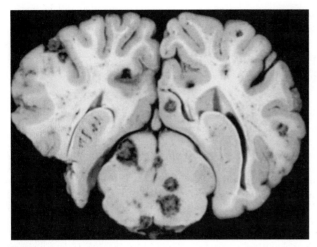

Figure 2
Feedlot steer with multiple focal septic infarcts in the parietal cortex caused by *H. somnus* thrombotic meningoencephalitis (TME).

Chronic infections may be difficult to attribute to *H. somnus* because other bacteria are usually present. Chronic inflammation of the affected site (e.g., vaginitis) would be expected. Lesions in the gastrointestinal tract may also occur. These lesions occur as solid blebs in the submucosa of the esophagus which are 2 to 5 mm in size. Histopathologically, the lesions consist of vasculitis, inflammation, necrosis, and hemorrhage. Laryngeal necrosis is a common necropsy finding, but may be indirectly caused by septic thrombosis of laryngeal vessels.

DIAGNOSIS

Infection by *H. somnus* should be considered in any cattle with neurologic signs, respiratory disease, stiffness, or in cases of reproductive failure. Since *H. somnus* is a normal commensal of the mucous membranes of cattle, care must be taken in determining the clinical significance of recovering *H. somnus*. Isolation of this bacterium from normally sterile sites (e.g., the brain, joints, internal organs) is diagnostic even at necropsy because *H. somnus* is too labile and slow-growing to compete with enteric and gram-positive bacteria in colonizing tissues following death. To be considered a significant etiologic agent, *H. somnus* should be isolated in pure culture or in predominance from the respiratory or urogenital tract, or identified in tissues by histopathology. Immunoperoxidase techniques have been used to identify *H. somnus* in the respiratory tract, where they have been identified free in the alveoli and in degenerating alveolar macrophages.

H. somnus has a relatively long generation time (greater than 60 minutes), and can easily be missed on culture due to overgrowth of commensal bacteria from contaminated specimens. Selective media have been described, but it is not clear if all strains of *H. somnus* will grow on these media. Specimens should be collected as soon as possible, particularly from necropsy, and inoculated onto an enriched medium, such as brain-heart infusion or Columbia base agar containing 10% blood or chocolatized blood. Agar plates must be incubated in an atmosphere containing 5% to 10% CO_2, although a candle extinction jar is usually sufficient. Adequate growth may require incubation of the plates for 36 to 48 hours at 35 to 37°C. If samples cannot be inoculated immediately on agar media they should be refrigerated and cultured within 48 hours. Tissues that are quickly frozen at low temperatures will preserve the bacteria indefinitely. If tissue samples are to be shipped to a diagnostic laboratory,

recovery of *H. somnus* will be most successful if the specimens are frozen and shipped on dry ice. Fluids, such as cerebrospinal fluid from suspected cases of TME or synovial fluid from an affected joint, should be collected aseptically in a sterile syringe and submitted cold directly to the laboratory. If swabs are used, one of the commercial transport systems is recommended. Isolation of *H. somnus* from animals treated with antibiotics may be difficult. Isolation of a slow-growing, yellow, gram-negative coccobacillus that requires blood and CO_2 for growth, and is catalase-negative and oxidase-positive, provides a presumptive diagnosis of *H. somnus* infection.

Serologic tests for *H. somnus* antibodies are available at some major state diagnostic laboratories. However, healthy animals may have high titers because of the high rate of carriage of this bacterium in cattle. Furthermore, the antigens used for the test must be species-specific because cross-reactions with other species can occur using crude antigens or whole cells. The use of specific membrane antigens or measuring only the IgG2 response improves specificity. Current tests include complement fixation, microagglutination, and an enzyme-linked immunosorbent assay. If serologic testing is warranted, such as for monitoring a herd for potential infection and treatment, paired sera should be obtained at least 2 weeks apart. A fourfold or greater rise in titer would help identify animals with active *H. somnus* infection from animals that are only colonized. A serologic typing scheme for *H. somnus* is not yet available.

PROGNOSIS

Cattle with advanced neurologic symptoms due to TME are not likely to recover. Cattle in the early stages of TME may respond better following intracisternal inoculation of antibiotic. Infections that result in extensive necrosis of the vasculature, even if not life-threatening, may be slow to resolve owing to poor blood supply to the affected area. A chronic cough or lameness may persist beyond the standard treatment time owing to vascular damage in the trachea or joints, respectively. However, *H. somnus* is very sensitive to a wide variety of antibiotics and appropriate early treatment usually results in prompt recovery.

PREVENTION AND THERAPY

Septicemic disease is difficult to prevent because of uncertainties about its pathogenesis. Respiratory disease is probably transmitted via aerosol between animals. Therefore, sick animals should be isolated and exposed animals treated prophylactically. As stress and overcrowding are important cofactors in the development of *H. somnus* disease, management practices should be used to minimize these conditions.

Postarrival prophylaxis of feedlot calves with long-acting oxytetracycline has not reduced mortality in *H. somnus* disease. It is not clear if prophylactic antibiotics have any effect on morbidity. In endemic regions it may be useful to combine postarrival antibiotic prophylaxis with vaccination. This may reduce the establishment of *H. somnus* disease in animals before protective antibodies develop. In combination with antibiotic therapy, treatment may also include corticosteroid treatment to reduce inflammation and intravenous fluids to counter fluid loss due to endotoxic shock.

Commercial bacterins are available for vaccination of animals against *H. somnus* disease. Although antibodies to *H. somnus* are induced in vaccinated animals, the efficacy of current vaccines is incomplete. Studies that have examined vaccine efficacy on TME and pneumonia vary considerably depending on the study design and methodology. Two immunizations at least 14 days apart are required to obtain any protective effect. Prevention of reproductive disease by vaccination has not been examined. A semipurified outer membrane antigen free of LOS from *H. somnus* used as a vaccine against calf pneumonia significantly reduced lung lesions. However, when LOS was added to the outer membrane fraction in the vaccine, the protective effects were eliminated. In fact, immunized animals had more severe lesions than control animals. It is possible that phase variation of the LOS may result in selection of more virulent phase variants that are not cleared by vaccination-induced LOS antibodies to the vaccine strain. Efforts to design more efficacious vaccines to prevent *H. somnus* disease are continuing.

ANTIBIOTIC TREATMENT

Antibiotic treatment should be based on the most efficacious, cost-effective drug appropriate for the infected site. The choice of antibiotic therapy should be guided by standardized susceptibility testing. The National Committee for Clinical Laboratory Standards (NCCLS) has recently released a tentative standard for antimicrobial susceptibility testing of veterinary bacterial pathogens, including *H. somnus*. A new medium, veterinary fastidious medium (VFM), was developed that will reliably grow all isolates of *H. somnus* for testing by minimal inhibitory concentration or disk diffusion. At this time susceptibility testing of *H. somnus* should be done using VFM and following NCCLS recommendations. Although *H. somnus* is typically sensitive to a wide variety of antibiotics, a variable response to antimicrobial therapy has been noted. In general, *H. somnus* is most susceptible to the penicillins, second- and third-generation cephalosporins, tetracyclines, chloramphenicol (not approved for food animal use), trimethoprim-sulfamethoxazole, aminoglycosides, novobiocin, and the new quinolones. Isolates are often or always resistant to lincomycin, spectinomycin, neomycin, spiramycin, and sulfonamides.

BIBLIOGRAPHY

Corbeil LB, Gogolewski RP, Stephens LR, et al: *Haemophilus somnus:* Antigen analysis and immune responses. *In* Donachie W, et al (eds): *Haemophilus, Actinobacillus,* and *Pasteurella.* New York, Plenum Press, 1995, pp 63–73.

Gogolewski RP, Leathers CW, Liggitt HD, et al: Experimental *Haemophilus somnus* pneumonia in calves and immunoperoxidase localization of bacteria. Vet Pathol 24:250–256, 1987.

Humphrey JD, Stephens LR: *Haemophilus somnus:* A review. Vet Bull 53:987–1004, 1983.

Inzana TJ, Hensley J, McQuiston J, et al: Phase variation and conservation of lipooligosaccharide epitopes in *Haemophilus somnus.* Infect Immun 65:4675–4681, 1997.

Keister DM: *Haemophilus somnus* infections in cattle. Compendium Continuing Educ Pract Vet 3:S260–S267, 1981.

Kilian M, Biberstein EL: Genus 11 *Haemophilus. In* Krieg NR, et al (eds): *Bergey's Manual of Systematic Bacteriology,* vol 1. Baltimore, Williams & Wilkins, 1984, pp 558–569.

Miller RB, Lein DH, McEntee KE, et al: *Haemophilus somnus* infection of the reproductive tract of cattle: A review. J Am Vet Med Assoc 182:1390–1392, 1983.

Moisan PG: I. Clinical manifestations of *H. somnus* infection. Top Vet Med 6:7–16, 1995.

Primal SV, Silva S, Little PB: The protective effect of vaccination against experimental pneumonia in cattle with *Haemophilus somnus* outer membrane antigens and interference by lipopolysaccharide. Can J Vet Res 54:326–330, 1990.

Van Donkersgoed J, Janzen ED, Potter AA, et al: The occurrence of *Haemophilus somnus* in feedlot calves and its control by postarrival prophylactic mass medication. Can Vet J 35:573–580, 1994.

■ Porcine Contagious Pleuropneumonia

Brad Fenwick, D.V.M., M.S., Ph.D., Diplomate, A.C.V.M.
Steve Henry, D.V.M.

Contagious porcine pleuropneumonia is caused by *Actinobacillus pleuropneumoniae* (App). App is a gram-negative pleomorphic rod which colonizes and causes disease in pigs. The organism is found in all regions of the world where pigs are produced. In some areas it is one of the most common disease reasons for depopulation of swine herds. In its more virulent form, App has the potential to cause significant economic losses through deaths, treatment costs, and increases in the costs of production (reduced growth and feed conversion rates).

In contrast to the widespread epizootics that occurred during the late 1970s in North America, clinical disease is now most common as an endemic problem in individual herds which suffer from repeated disease outbreaks. This should not be interpreted as evidence that the number of infected herds has declined, but rather that management procedures have been developed which reduce the risk of clinical disease outbreaks.

There is strong serologic evidence that most commercial herds in North America are infected with App, yet in only a relatively small proportion of these herds is clinical disease recognized.[1] Clinically apparent disease outbreaks are often related to minor changes in production methods or occur seasonally because of rapid changes in environmental conditions (temperature and humidity). In addition, disease outbreaks continue to occur following the mixing of clinically healthy pigs that are colonized with App with pigs immunologically susceptible to infection. In a similar fashion, management systems that alter the immunologic stability of the various age-related subpopulations of pigs within an endemically infected herd increase the risk of a clinical disease outbreak.

Recent research has provided a better understanding of a number of important aspects of the epidemiology and pathogenesis of porcine pleuropneumonia. The development and application of improved serologic tests as well as DNA fingerprinting of App isolates have been instrumental in unraveling the natural history and epidemiology of the disease. Detailed studies of the toxins, capsule, and outer membrane proteins of App have added a new dimension to our understanding of the pathogenesis of the disease. This new information, plus a clearer understanding of the principles of infectious disease control in various pork production systems, has provided new, more effective ways to reduce the risk of clinical disease; the ability, in some circumstances, to eradicate the organism from selected populations of pigs; and reliable procedures for preventing transmission of App between herds.[2]

PATHOGENESIS

App is environmentally fragile and apparently can survive outside the pig for only a limited time. The pig is the only known animal host. As such, the major means of transmission is via healthy, yet persistently infected carrier pigs which may subsequently transmit App to susceptible pigs. Transmission by healthy carrier pigs not only occurs between herds, but is also an important means of transmission between subpopulations of pigs within the same herd. This is particularly relevant when continuous-flow production methods are used. Other, less common means by which App is thought to be transmitted over short distances are via contaminated clothing, machinery, and insects (particularly flies).

It is critical to understand that like many bacterial diseases, App only rarely results in severe clinical disease. In most cases, infection with App results in mild to clinically unrecognizable disease. This is particularly the case if infection occurs (as it often does) while the piglet is protected by colostral immunity. At some point, colostral immunity is sufficient to prevent overt disease but not colonization. The difference between those pigs that following exposure become colonized but do not develop clinically overt disease and those that die acutely or require aggressive antibacterial treatment is related to three factors: (1) the App serotype involved (virulence), (2) the number of organisms to which the pig is exposed (exposure dose), and (3) the pig's immunologic status (susceptibility).

There are 12 recognized capsular serotypes of App. Structural and antigen variability within a serotype occur. Country-to-country as well as regional differences in the distribution of serotypes are recognized. Knowledge as to the serotypes which are most common within a specific area helps to focus diagnostic and prevention strategies. Nevertheless, the changing nature of the pork production industry which now often involves transporting pigs over long distances, including between continents, has caused the emergence of serotypes in areas where they were not recognized previously.

While all App serotypes have the potential to cause significant clinical disease under the right circumstances, the relative virulence of the 12 serotypes can be divided into those that are highly virulent (serotype 1), those that are moderately virulent (serotypes 2, 5, 9, 10, 11), and those that are least virulent (serotypes 3, 6, 7, 12). There are a number of serotypes that are seen so infrequently as to create uncertainty as to their relative ability to cause disease. In addition, there may be regional differences in the virulence of strains of the same serotype.

Following exposure, App colonizes the respiratory epithelium and tonsils, and the inhalation of organisms results in pneumonia. Given how rapidly clinical signs develop in the peracute form of the disease, initial colonization of the upper respiratory system occurs rapidly or is not required. Presumably, in these cases the number of organisms in the environment is sufficiently large to allow the organism to colonize the lung directly. At lower exposure doses, the likelihood of clinical disease is reduced even though colonization and seroconversion occur. The management and environmental factors which promote high levels of exposure are continuous-flow production, high stocking densities, poor ventilation, and high humidity. In addition to influencing the number of organisms in the environment, these factors can alter the susceptibility of the pigs, and thus lower the threshold number of organisms necessary to cause disease.

In sharp contrast to many bacteria that colonize the respiratory system and cause disease only following some insult to the respiratory system by some other organism (e.g., viral or mycoplasma infections), App is a primary pathogen in that it can cause disease in otherwise healthy pigs under optimal environmental conditions. On the other hand, it is clear that prior or concurrent infection with a number of other respiratory pathogens can increase the frequency and severity of the clinical disease which follows exposure to App. It should be noted that management and environmental conditions which increase risk of disease due to other respiratory pathogens are, of themselves, also risk factors for App. Prominent among these contributing infections are mycoplasmas, salmonellae, and pseudorabies virus. Current research and some clinical evidence suggest that porcine reproductive and respiratory syndrome (PRRS) virus does not enhance the virulence potential of App.

A number of interdependent virulence factors have been described for App. These include capsule, lipopolysaccharides (endotoxin), outer membrane proteins, iron acquisition systems, and cytotoxins. The relative importance of any one of these factors in isolation from the others is difficult to assess. The capsule provides resistance from complement and cell-mediated host defenses. Capsular antigens are the basis for the serotyping classification system, are important antigens in serologic tests, and are the basis for the serotype-specific protective immunity provided by vaccines. The lipopolysaccharides of App can be used in serologic tests and endotoxin is thought to play a contributing role in the peracute form of the disease. Outer membrane proteins, particularly those involved in iron acquisition, allow the organism to survive in the face of host defenses and are hypothesized to contribute to App being a porcine-specific pathogen.

At least three functionally and genetically related cytotoxins are produced by App.[3] The combination of cytotoxins that are produced is related to serotype. The cytotoxins of App belong to a family of bacterial toxins (RTX toxins), which kill or interfere with host cells' function by forming pores in their membranes.[4] The toxins can be hemolytic, cytotoxic, or both. Those App serotypes which produce the most functionally active toxins are also more virulent. Neutralizing antibodies to these toxins are an important component of protective immunity which follows recovery from a natural infection. Unfortunately, current vaccines do not reliably induce cytotoxin-neutralizing antibodies.

CLINICAL SIGNS

Clinical signs associated with an App infection are highly variable and can be confused with a number of other respiratory diseases. Although clinical disease is most commonly seen in finishing pigs, pigs of all ages are susceptible and outbreaks with deaths in sows and boars as well as piglets prior to weaning occur occasionally. Herds that are endemically infected with App but have uniformly high levels of immunity may be free of recognizable clinical disease or may have infrequent, clinically mild respiratory disease. In the same fashion, infected herds that do not have other diseases, have good facilities and environmental controls, have progressive management systems, or are infected with a low-virulence strain of App may not have overt clinical disease even though a high percentage of the pigs are serologically positive.

Clinical signs may develop following the introduction of carrier pigs into a susceptible population of pigs (different herd or different age group in the same herd), changes in management that alter the immunologic stability of the herd or allow a higher App exposure dose, outbreaks of other diseases, as well as following sudden changes in environmental temperature or humidity.

Subclinical infections are recognized only by serologic testing, while in the peracute form of the disease death may occur within hours after exposure. During the early stages of a disease outbreak the clinical signs of anorexia, shifting leg lameness, reluctance to move, and elevated temperature ($\geq 41°C$) are often overlooked. In some of these pigs, the disease progresses rapidly. The respiratory rate may increase dramatically with efforts to minimize thoracic wall movement resulting in exaggerated abdominal effort. Nonproductive coughing and gagging is common. As the disease progresses blood-tinged foam may flow from the nose. Ultimately, death is due to respiratory insufficiency and shock. Pigs found dead are often noted to have evidence of bleeding from the nose and marked ventral cutaneous congestion. Chronic disease is characterized by marked reduction in growth and a nonproductive deep cough. Clinical signs related to pneumonia within a given group of pigs will diminish over a period of 1 to 2 weeks. In affected and recovering pigs, reduced feed efficiencies and reduced gain may result in a delay of 4 to 6 weeks in the time it takes pigs to reach market weight.[5]

NECROPSY DIAGNOSIS

Lesions associated with App infection are restricted to the lung and pleura. The highly variable nature of the lung lesions induced by App is not well appreciated. While the classic lesions of App are easily recognized, App lesions can be mistaken for those induced by *Salmonella*, *Actinobacillus suis*, *Haemophilus parasuis*, and concurrent infections of mycoplasma and *Pasteurella multocida*. Infections with *A. suis* in high-health-status herds has become a particularly important differential diagnosis because the lesions are very similar to those caused by App.

Characteristically, the lesions of App involve one or more focal areas in the diaphragmatic lung lobes which are markedly congested, swollen, and associated with focal fibrinous pleuritis. The lesions can range from a few centimeters in diameter to large areas that involve nearly the entire lung. On cut surface, the involved lung is grossly replaced by a well-delineated, firm mass of necrotic tissue and clotted blood. In addition, bronchi contain moderate to large amounts of blood-tinged foam to frank blood, pulmonary septa are thickened with edema, and mediastinal lymph nodes are congested and edematous.

The focal lung lesions heal rapidly so that in a few weeks all that remains is a small (often less than 1.0 cm), firm fibrotic nodule surrounded by a grossly normal lung parenchyma. Pleural adhesions may or may not be associated with these areas. As such, the use of slaughter checks to determine if a herd is infected with App are reliable only if the infection occurs within a few weeks of slaughter.[6]

LABORATORY DIAGNOSIS

It is important to isolate the strain of App that is causing disease. Under the right circumstances, a number of other organisms can produce clinical disease and lung lesions that mimic those of App. These include *A. suis*, *P. multocida*, *Streptococcus suis*, *H. parasuis*, and *Salmonella*. Only by isolating App can the etiologic diagnosis be confirmed with absolute certainty. In addition, the isolation of App allows for the selection of the most appropriate antibiotic; determination of the serotype, which is important if the use of vaccines is to be considered; and DNA fingerprinting, which provides epidemiologic information important in determining the source of the specific App strain which is causing disease (an endemic or newly introduced strain). Given the difficulty in distinguishing biotype 2 strains of App (strains that do not require NAD) from *A. suis* using standard microbiologic techniques, molecular biology–based techniques are now used.[7]

Isolation is most often successful when pneumonic lesions from acute cases are cultured. Lung lesions from subacute and chronic cases are often heavily contaminated with other organisms, particularly *P. multocida*. Chilled tissue samples should be submitted directly to a laboratory experienced in the isolation and identification of App. The use of culture swabs and transport media should be avoided as App will not survive under these conditions and is easily overgrown by contaminants. The best site for isolating App from healthy carrier pigs is the cut surface of the tonsil.

The use of serologic tests designed to detect serum antibodies specific to App has become an important component in the diagnosis and control of the disease. Serologic tests are used to evaluate the success of disease control and eradication programs and to compare the health status of herds before purchase or commingling of pigs. A number of serologic tests have been developed which use a variety of antigens. The most commonly used tests include complement fixation (CF) assays using whole organisms as antigens, enzyme-linked immunosorbent assays (ELISA) using purified capsular or lipopolysaccharide as antigens, and assays which measure the ability of serum to neutralize the function of the cytotoxins produced by App. As a group, the CF assays have very low numbers of false-positive results, but a very high rate of false-negative results, particularly if the test is run a few months post infection. The ELISA and toxin neutralization tests have low numbers of both false-positive and false-negative results.[8]

TREATMENT

Effective treatment for the acute disease in the individual pig requires the use of injectable antibiotics to which the causative App is sensitive. In general, the response is rapid and even pigs with severe clinical signs can be saved. A 3-day course of antibiotics is recommended.

If necessary, the involved pig should be isolated and orally hydrated. While injectable penicillin remains the antibiotic of choice, multiple antibiotic-resistant strains have developed in several regions and are becoming a problem in others. In these cases, tiamulin and ceftiofur are generally effective. Recently approved, the in-feed antibiotic Pulmotil offers a new, potentially valuable means of controlling App. In general, however, the use of other sources of water or feed medications are not reliable treatments, as effective antibiotic concentrations are not established in the tissues. Pretreating pigs with oral antibiotics prior to exposure to App may reduce the severity of clinical disease but does not prevent colonization.

Individual animal treatment is not an effective means of controlling disease outbreaks in intensively managed herds. To reliably limit the severity of a disease outbreak, all pigs in the air space should be treated with the appropriate injectable antibiotic. In large part, this is because the rapid course of the disease does not allow sufficient time to effectively treat pigs individually. In addition, as the disease outbreak progresses, the number of organisms in the environment increases rapidly. This causes the disease to spread more quickly and because of the higher exposure dose the mortality rate may increase.

PREVENTION

The most reliable means of preventing outbreaks of App is to avoid its introduction into the herd in the first place. This is best accomplished when the herd is initially formed or repopulated.

The medical history and health assessment of the source herd should be thoroughly investigated and the serologic status of the herd determined. In existing herds, the introduction of new pigs and the commingling of pigs from several sources should be done only after comprehensive efforts have been made to assure that the pigs have the same App status.[2] This is best done by reviewing the medical history of the herds, including slaughter checks, vaccine programs, treatment records, and because of the subclinical nature of most App infections, the serologic profiles.

Pigs that recover from an App infection are solidly immune to clinical disease from all other serotypes of App. In contrast, current App vaccines do not reliably prevent colonization or clinical disease but may reduce the mortality rate. To be effective, vaccines must contain the same serotype of App which is causing disease. Autogenous vaccines are occasionally more effective than commercial vaccines. Two, and sometimes three or four, immunizations are necessary to provide optimal levels of protection. Only rarely is vaccination a long-term solution to controlling App.

At the center of any program to reliably prevent App is an effective health management program. In herds with a history of clinical disease, special efforts should be made to minimize fluctuations in temperature and humidity, to control concurrent diseases (particularly mycoplasmosis), and to avoid overstocking. All-in–all-out and multiple-site production by grouping subpopulations of pigs by age and consequently by health status are very effective methods for reducing the App infection rate as well as the frequency of disease outbreaks.

In herds where clinical disease occurs at a predictable stage of production, the use of oral or water antibiotics during these periods (strategic medication) may be beneficial. The goal is to reduce the severity of disease, but since infection still occurs the pigs develop protective immunity. Another strategy is to medicate the pigs for a few days followed by a few days without antibiotics (pulse medication). Again, the concept is that the infection is allowed to occur in a more controlled fashion.

One of the notable success stories of segregated early weaning (SEW) is the ability to control and eradicate App.[9] On the other hand, SEW programs that are not appropriately designed or instituted can actually increase the risk of clinical disease. By weaning piglets at an age prior to the time they become infected with App via the sow, isolating them from other pigs, and taking steps to prevent lateral introduction of App from other sources, it is possible to produce App-free pigs from endemically infected sow herds. The correct weaning age to reliably prevent transmission of App varies from herd to herd and must be determined experimentally by evaluating the serologic status of piglets after colostral immunity has been lost and again when the pigs are marketed. Treating the sow or piglets, or both, with antibiotics does not substantially influence the success of these programs.

In large part, the weaning age necessary to prevent piglets from becoming colonized with App depends on the collective immunologic status of the sow herd and gilts. As the level of sow herd immunity declines and becomes more variable, the weaning age must decline. The addition of gilts with little or no immunity to App reduces sow herd immunity and contributes increased variability. As such, efforts to stabilize sow herd immunity and to limit variation between sows and gilts reduces the risk that App will be transmitted to the piglet and that a clinical disease outbreak will occur at a later stage of production. In the case of App, this can best be done by introducing replacement gilts at a young age so that they can develop immunity prior to farrowing.

App will continue to be a challenge to clinicians, whether the challenge be management of an infected herd or prevention. Through serology the interaction of the organism with the herd can be appreciated. While options for controlling App are clearly limited, exercising positive controls over pig flow, strategic therapy, weaning age, herd introductions, and environment can successfully limit the economic consequences of this organism.

REFERENCES

1. Devenish J, Rosendal S, Bosse JT, et al: Prevalence of seroreactors to the 104-kilodalton hemolysin of *Actinobacillus pleuropneumoniae* in swine herds. J Clin Microbiol 28:789–791, 1990.
2. Fenwick B, Henry S: Porcine pleuropneumonia. J Am Vet Med Assoc 204:1334–1340, 1994.
3. Frey J: Virulence in *Actinobacillus pleuropneumoniae* and RTX toxins. Trends Microbiol 3:257–261, 1995.
4. Menestrina G, Moser C, Pellet S, et al: Pore-formation by *Escherichia coli* hemolysin (HlyA) and other members of the RTX toxin family. Toxicology 87:249–267, 1994.
5. Straw BE, Shin SJ, Yeager AE: Effect of pneumonia on growth rate and feed efficiency of minimal disease pigs exposed to *Actinobacillus pleuropneumoniae* and *Mycoplasma hyopneumoniae*. Prev Vet Med 9:287–294, 1990.
6. Noyes EP, Feeney DA, Pijoan C: Comparison of the effect of pneumonia detected during lifetime with pneumonia detected at slaughter on growth in swine. J Am Vet Med Assoc 197:1025–1029, 1990.
7. Frank RK, Chengappa MM, Oberst RD, et al: Pleuropneumonia caused by *Actinobacillus pleuropneumoniae* biotype 2 in growing and finishing pigs. J Vet Diagn Invest 4:270–278, 1992.
8. Montaraz J, Fenwick B, Hill H, et al: Evaluation of antibody class specific ELISA, complement fixation, and Apx-1 hemolysin neutralization test to detect serum antibody in pigs known to be infected with *Actinobacillus pleuropneumoniae* serotype 1. Swine Health Prod 4:79–83, 1996.
9. Harris DL: New approaches for the elimination of infectious diseases from swine. *In* Proceedings of the Annual Meeting of the Animal Health Association, 1989, pp 416–426.

■ Brucellosis

Paul Nicoletti, D.V.M., M.S.

Brucellosis in food-producing animals is caused by four of the six members of the genus *Brucella*. Infections in cattle are caused primarily by *Brucella abortus*, in swine by *B. suis*, in goats and sheep by *B. melitensis*, and also in sheep by *B. ovis*. Cross-species infections are uncommon, and clinical symptoms occur rarely.

HISTORY

In 1886, a micrococcus was isolated from the spleen of human patients, and the associated disease was named *undulant fever* in 1897. In 1904 a young British physician, Bruce, was commissioned to determine the cause of the human malady on the Isle of Malta. In the meantime a Danish veterinarian, Bang, isolated a microorganism from an aborting heifer that was later named *B. abortus*. Traum, in California in 1914, isolated *B. suis* from a sow. In 1953 Buddle and Boyes, in Australia and New Zealand, identified *B. ovis* as a cause of epididymitis in sheep.

Brucellosis is the term now used for infections by any member of the genus *Brucella*. In humans it is occasionally referred to as *undulant* or *Malta fever* and in cattle as *Bang's disease*. All species infect humans except *B. ovis* and *B. neotomae*. Sporadic cases occur in goats and humans when introduced from and contracted in other countries, respectively.

The incidence of cattle brucellosis in the United States was reduced from 5% in 1957 to less than 0.1% in 1996 according to U.S. Department of Agriculture (USDA) statistics. Thirty-six states were classified brucellosis-free and the number of infected herds was less than 50. The annual losses caused by the disease are low and are from abortions, decreased milk yield (especially because of early calving), and sale and replacement of diseased cattle. Estimates of losses are not available for human, swine, or sheep. The incidence of swine brucellosis has declined to less than 0.01% among marketed swine. More than 40 states are validated as being swine-brucellosis–free.

ETIOLOGY

Brucellae are gram-negative coccobacilli that are nonmotile and nonencapsulated. They are aerobic, but some species require added carbon dioxide for cultivation. The colonies appear in approximately 4 to 5 days, are round and convex, and display a somewhat characteristic bluish color when examined with light transmitted at a 45-degree angle. Differentiation of species and biovars in the genus *Brucella* is based on various growth requirements, sensitivity to dyes in media, oxidation of metabolic substrates, serologic reactions, and bacteriophage susceptibility (Table 1).

Table 1
SOME GENERAL CHARACTERISTICS OF FOUR SPECIES OF *Brucella**

Species	No. of Biovars	Growth Requirements			
		CO_2	H_2S	Basic Fuchsin	Thionin
Brucella melitensis	3	−	−	+	+
B. abortus	8	+	+	+	−
B. suis	4	−	+	−	+
B. ovis	1	+	−	+	+

*Variations occur among some biovars.

CLINICAL SIGNS

Cattle

After the ingestion of brucellae, there is a temporary septicemia with phagocytosis by the neutrophils and fixed macrophages of local lymph nodes. Sites of predilection are the endometrium and fetal placenta in pregnant cows and the supramammary lymph nodes and the udder. Uterine infection may be related to the presence of a natural compound, erythritol, which stimulates the growth of *B. abortus*. The severity of uterine infection varies, but the numbers of organisms are greatest at the time of abortion or parturition. Genital infection usually disappears within 30 days after calving but may recur during subsequent pregnancies. Inflammation of the allantochorion may interfere with circulation to the fetus and cause subsequent fetal death and expulsion. Abortions frequently occur after the fifth month of pregnancy, and a retained placenta may follow. Not all infections result in abortion, and few cattle have abortions more than once. A small percentage of cattle spontaneously recover. A high percentage of cattle have permanent udder infection with shedding or organisms in the milk.

In bulls, *B. abortus* may produce orchitis with abscesses, epididymitis (Fig. 1), and inflammation of accessory reproductive organs. Orchitis is usually unilateral and results in reduced libido and impaired fertility. Brucellae may be discharged into the semen, but there is little evidence that transmission to cows is by natural breeding.

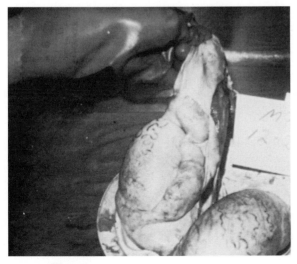

Figure 1
Epididymitis in a bull with *B. abortus* infection.

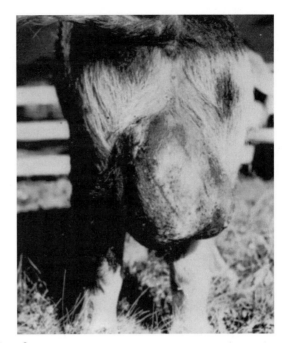

Figure 2
Unilateral orchitis from *B. suis*. (Courtesy of Dr. B. Deyoe, Nevada, Iowa.)

Swine

Clinical evidence of *B. suis* infection varies and is influenced by many factors. The typical syndrome is that of abortion or birth of stillborn or weak pigs, infertility, orchitis (Fig. 2), and sometimes posterior paralysis or lameness as a result of spondylitis. Genital infection is more permanent in boars than in sows. The semen usually contains large numbers of organisms, and sows may become infected during breeding.

Sheep and Goats

B. melitensis infections occur in both sheep and goats and produce abortions in late pregnancy (Fig. 3). The abortion rate varies considerably, and susceptibility also varies among breeds of sheep. In general, milking breeds of sheep are more susceptible to *B. melitensis*. Infected ewes and goats excrete organisms in the milk and in vaginal discharge. Sheep may recover from the disease.

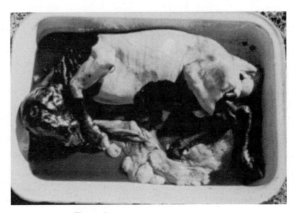

Figure 3
Abortus from sheep with brucellosis.

B. ovis infections in sheep usually cause epididymitis and orchitis. Abortions may occur even though the ewe appears to be more resistant than the ram, and the disease may not persist. Lesions of scrotal edema, fibrosis, and adhesions are observed. Aspermia and abnormalities in the motility or morphology of spermatozoa may be seen. Although uncommon, transmission from ram to ram during preputial or rectal contact and from ram to ewe during mating do occur.

DIAGNOSIS

A correct diagnosis depends on the herd or flock history along with information concerning the individual, in addition to serologic, bacteriologic, or pathologic examination. Antibodies to *Brucella* are found in a number of fluids, but most tests are performed on serum or milk. Herd surveillance methods include milk ring and blood tests on marketed cattle. The milk ring test is much more efficient because it surveys nearly all the population at one time. Identification of infected herds is also through blood tests for cattle marketed for breeding or slaughter. This method depends on the sale of an animal with positive results, and it may be slow to identify infected herds.

SEROLOGY

Positive results from serologic tests indicate present or past exposure to an antigenic stimulus and cannot always be equated with infection. These tests also do not measure immunity. The only international standard for the diagnosis of brucellosis in individual cattle is the tube agglutination test (Fig. 4), which measures antibodies in international units. The test methods and interpretation of results vary in both veterinary and human medicine and from country to country. In the United States, tests on nonvaccinated cattle are considered positive if the serum reacts in a 1:100 or greater dilution and is positive for vaccinated cattle at a 1:200 or greater dilution. Test results from cattle with lower titers are classified as suspect or negative, depending on the vaccination status. The tube agglutination test is influenced by many factors, and there are many false-positive and false-negative results. Causes of false results are early or chronic infections, vaccination, and heterospecific antigens. Difficulties in performing the test and in interpreting the results have led

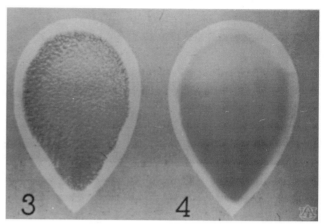

Figure 5
Card test showing agglutination *(left)*.

to the development and use of several other procedures. The tube agglutination test is usually performed in the United States and several other countries only when required for international commerce of cattle.

Plate Agglutination Test

The plate agglutination test is comparable to the tube agglutination test in sensitivity and is subject to most of the same factors that influence the results. Other tests have largely replaced the plate agglutination test. These other tests are procedures that use acidification of the antigen solution to reduce agglutination caused by IgM antibodies, which are largely due to previous vaccination.

Card Test or Rose Bengal Test

The card test (Fig. 5) is performed on a card or a white tile. It is simple and can be completed at the farm, ranch, market facility, or laboratory. The test is a good screening procedure (there are few false-negative results) but should generally be supported by other tests (there may be many false-positive results, especially in vaccinated populations) and information on herd and individual history.

Rivanol Precipitation Test

The Rivanol (ethacridine lactate) precipitation test depends on the precipitation of high-molecular-weight agglutinins and examination of the supernatant with a special antigen. It is less sensitive than the tube or plate agglutination test or the card test and is simpler than the complement fixation test.

Complement Fixation Test

Many studies have shown the superiority of the complement fixation test in specificity and sensitivity, especially for chronically infected or vaccinated cattle, when compared with the aforementioned tests.

Other Tests

The particle concentration fluorescence immunoassay has been developed by a commercial company (IDEXX Corp, Port-

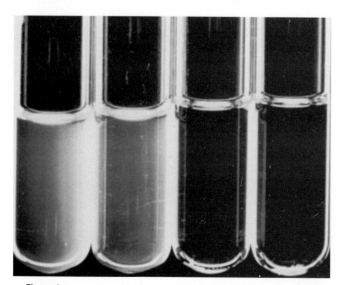

Figure 4
Tube agglutination test with negative *(left)* and positive *(right)* results.

land, Me) and uses submicron polystyrene particles to which soluble antigens and a fluorescence marker are attached. The system is automated and used as a screening test. Other test methods that have been used are enzyme-linked immunosorbent assay, heat inactivation, mercaptoethanol, Coombs' antiglobulin, hemagglutination, milk ring (individual) and whey tests, and vaginal mucus and semen plasma agglutination.

Regardless of the test used, the results should be properly evaluated. Emphasis should be placed on kinds of antibodies (qualitative) instead of numbers of antibodies (quantitative) and on bacteriologic studies of appropriate specimens.

BACTERIOLOGY

The milk and other udder secretions are good specimens for culture of organisms. The supramammary lymph nodes are the preferred site at necropsy, but other lymph nodes are also useful. Abomasal fluid should be cultured from the fetus.

Swine

It is agreed that individual animal test results are less accurate in swine than in cattle. False-negative or false-positive results may occur. A herd test result profile is best. The card test is very useful, and supplemental procedures can be used. Sites for cultures include the lymph nodes, especially those in the cervical region, and the seminal vesicles.

Sheep and Goats

No international standard has been established for the selection of a test or interpretation of results for the diagnosis of *B. melitensis* infection. The tube agglutination test or the rose bengal test is generally used, but complement fixation and dermal hypersensitivity tests are preferred by some diagnosticians. Bacteriologic examinations can be made on vaginal discharges, milk, lymph nodes, placentas, and aborted fetuses.

The diagnosis of *B. ovis* infection requires clinical examination, semen evaluation, and interpretation of results of the complement fixation test on blood sera and cultures if indicated. A gel diffusion test has also given good results. Recent research studies have found that an indirect enzyme-linked immunosorbent assay is superior in sensitivity to other procedures.

EPIDEMIOLOGY

Infected cows are the source of most infections through discharges and products associated with parturition (Fig. 6). Cows are not generally infectious to other cattle by 2 to 4 weeks after parturition. Hygienic measures are important but may not be effective in controlling the disease owing to seronegative infected cattle that abort or calve normally. The variable incubation period of a few weeks to several months is related to the gestation period and severity of exposure.

Brucellae are intracellular parasites and, in this environment, are not antigenic and are thus protected from host defenses and chemotherapy.

Calves born to infected cows and those ingesting contaminated milk are temporarily infected. The permanency of this infection has been disputed; however, it is now certain that latent infections occur, but the frequency and contributing factors are unknown. An additional problem is that the heifer becomes seronegative during most of prepuberty and prior to calving. Many reports have been published of latent infection that has resulted in new herd infections or in reinfections of herds considered free of brucellosis.

Under normal conditions the bull appears to play a minor role in the transmission of brucellosis. However, contaminated semen used in artificial insemination may result in infection.

Brucellosis in wildlife species has rarely proved to be a source of transmission to domesticated livestock. The disease exists in certain bison and elk populations in the United States and in caribou and reindeer populations in the Arctic. The presence of *B. abortus* in bison and elk populations of the Yellowstone National Park region has caused much controversy about possible control methods and the risk of transmission to cattle herds in the area.

Brucella organisms may survive within protected environments for several weeks, but sunlight kills them within a few hours. The virulence of strains varies, but no satisfactory in vitro method for virulence measurement has been developed.

TREATMENT

Development of a satisfactory treatment for brucellosis in domestic animals has been difficult. Spontaneous recoveries may

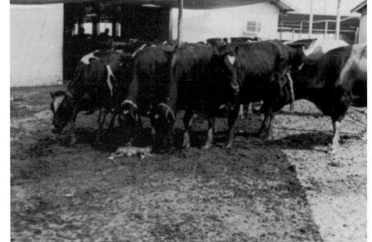

Figure 6

Ingestion of contaminated fluids from an aborted fetus is the most common source of *Brucella* infection.

occur in all species. Treatment of *B. ovis* infections in sheep and *B. abortus* in cattle with tetracyclines and streptomycin has been successful, but use of these regimens has been limited owing to cost and the regulatory aspects of cattle brucellosis.

PUBLIC HEALTH CONSIDERATIONS

Brucellosis is a true zoonosis, and control in humans is directly related to its prevalence among animals. Occupationally related infections predominate, with slaughterhouse workers being the group at highest risk. Approximately 100 human cases in the United States are reported each year to the Centers for Disease Control and Prevention.

B. melitensis is considered the most virulent species for humans, followed by *B. suis* and *B. abortus* in that order. Direct contact with contaminated fluid and tissue is the chief source of infection. Outbreaks in slaughterhouses from the inhalation of *B. suis* have been reported. Accidental inoculation of strain 19 has caused infection in veterinarians and laboratory workers. Ingestion of contaminated and unpasteurized dairy products is a very serious public health problem when *B. melitensis* is prevalent.

Symptoms in humans vary in severity from acute to chronic, and many infections are undiagnosed. The classic symptoms are headache, undulating fever, joint pain, chills, and weakness. Relapses after apparently successful treatment are not uncommon. The serum agglutination test is most often used to aid in diagnosis, but methods of performing the test and interpretation of results may vary. The card test is very useful for acute infections. Intradermic tests should be avoided.

CONTROL

The control of brucellosis in livestock is a responsibility of the herd owner and regulatory agencies. The major phases are identification and slaughter of diseased livestock, vaccination, herd management, and control of livestock movements.

Strains 19 and RB51 of *B. abortus* are vaccines approved in the United States to prevent *B. abortus* infection in cattle. RB51 is a laboratory-derived lipopolysaccharide O antigen–deficient mutant of the virulent strain 2308. It does not cause the production of antibodies that react in serologic tests used to diagnose cattle brucellosis. Other vaccines such as 45/20 and H38 have been studied by many investigators, often with conflicting findings, and they are rarely used. An attenuated strain of *B. melitensis*, Rev 1, which is used in other countries for control of *B. melitensis* and sometimes *B. ovis*, is very effective.

Currently, strains 19 and RB51 are recommended for the vaccination of calves 4 to 12 months of age. They are also used for adult cattle in a lower dose and under restricted conditions. High rates of vaccination in herds are important to reduce infection rates.

The immunity produced by *Brucella* vaccines is cell mediated and related to the dose and virulence of the challenge strain. The effectiveness of vaccination is best when a high percentage of the herd is immunized so that exposure potential is minimized. Individual effectiveness is often quoted to be about 65% to 70%, but herd effectiveness is much greater. Vaccinated animals are much more likely to resist the disease or have less severe disease, so fewer organisms are excreted.

Herd size is very important in brucellosis control, especially if there is close confinement. Introduction of replacement animals increases the risk of herd infection. The status of the herd of origin is very important. Negative test results on purchased animals are not a sole satisfactory means of preventing the introduction of cattle that are incubating the disease. Isolation and retests are recommended.

A cooperative program for control and eradication of bovine brucellosis began in 1934 largely as a drought relief effort. It received special emphasis in the early 1950s, and the current federal budget in the United States is about $65 million annually. The Uniform Methods and Rules are administered by the USDA. Strain 19 vaccination has been an integral part of the program, with peak usage in 1988, when approximately 10 million calves were vaccinated. The program emphasizes surveillance, prompt herd tests, slaughter of seropositive animals, vaccinations, and owner cooperation.

Swine

Purchase of swine from *Brucella*-free herds or rearing replacements is the best prevention. If brucellosis exists, it is best to depopulate the herd. A second proposal is to retain young pigs and test them prior to breeding and farrowing. A third, but inferior approach is to test and remove reactors until the last two herd tests reveal no more infected swine. The criteria for validating herds and areas are given in the Uniform Methods and Rules.

Sheep and Goats

Where *B. melitensis* exists, consideration is given to slaughter of the entire flock or herd. The use of Rev 1 vaccine, with or without identification, along with slaughter of infected animals is another form of control. Rev 1 vaccine has been recommended for young female sheep and goats. Studies have found successful and more practical control with the use of a reduced dose of Rev 1 in sexually mature animals.

Control of *B. ovis* is accomplished by maintaining young rams separate from mature rams. In addition, mature male sheep are examined, and those with clinical and serologic evidence of infection are slaughtered. In some countries Rev 1 vaccine is also used.

BIBLIOGRAPHY

Alton GG, Jones LM, Angus RD, et al: Techniques for the Brucellosis Laboratory. Paris, Institut National de la Recherche Agronomique, 1988.

Deyoe BL: Brucellosis. *In* Leman AD, Straw B, Glock RO, et al (eds): Diseases of Swine, ed 6. Ames, Iowa, Iowa State University Press, 1986, pp 599–607.

Kimberling CV: Jensen and Swift's Diseases of Sheep, ed 3. Philadelphia, Lea & Febiger, 1988.

Nicoletti P: The epidemiology of bovine brucellosis. Adv Vet Sci Comp Med 24:69–98, 1980.

Nielson K, Duncan JR (eds): Animal Brucellosis. Boca Raton, Fla, CRC Press, 1990.

Schurig GG, Roop RM, Bagchi T, et al: Biological properties of RB51, a stable rough strain of *Brucella abortus*. Vet Microbiol 28:171, 1991.

■ Pasteurellosis in Cattle

Anthony W. Confer, D.V.M., Ph.D., Diplomate, A.C.V.P.

Cyril R. Clarke, B.V.Sc., Ph.D., Diplomate, A.C.V.C.P.

In cattle, *Pasteurella multocida* and *P. haemolytica* are primarily associated with hemorrhagic septicemia and pneumonia. *P. multocida* causes hemorrhagic septicemia, a disease of major importance in cattle and water buffalo in Africa and Asia. *P. haemolytica* and *P. multocida* are both involved in severe fibrinous pleuropneumonia (bovine pneumonic pasteurellosis) in dairy and beef cattle worldwide. In addition, *Pasteurella* spp. have been sporadically isolated from bovine diseases such as meningitis, localized infections, abortions, and mastitis. *P. haemolytica* and *P. multocida* are ubiquitous in the cattle population as commensals in the nasopharynx. Therefore, mechanisms of immunity to them have been difficult to determine, efficacious vaccines have been a challenge to develop, and vaccine efficacy has been hard to evaluate.

P. haemolytica can be typed into 16 serotypes (1 to 16) and 2 biotypes (A or T). Recently, *P. haemolytica* biotype T (a cause of septicemia in lambs) has been reclassified as *P. trehalosi*. *P. multocida* is classified into five serogroups (A, B, D, E, and F) based on capsular antigens and 16 serotypes (1 to 16) based on somatic antigens. *P. haemolytica* A:1 and *P. multocida* A:3 are the most common serotypes isolated from bovine respiratory disease. *P. multocida* B:2 and E:2 are the main antigenic types associated with hemorrhagic septicemia.

P. haemolytica– and *P. multocida*–induced diseases of cattle are of worldwide economic importance. Severe respiratory disease is the major cause of clinical disease and death loss in stocker and feedlot cattle and second only to diarrhea as a major disease syndrome in dairy calves. In North America alone, bovine respiratory disease results in economic losses to producers estimated at $800 million annually. Quantitative estimates of economic losses resulting from hemorrhagic septicemia are lacking; however, losses are particularly severe in Southeast Asia and are related both to epidemics affecting young and old animals and to constant endemic disease of young animals.

SEPTICEMIA

Hemorrhagic septicemia, an acute disease affecting cattle and water buffalo primarily in Southeast Asia and Africa, is caused by *P. multocida*, serotypes B:2 and E:2. The epidemiology of the disease is dependent on the presence of both immune and active carrier animals. Immune carriers most often become active carriers (shedders) in response to stressful situations. The disease is particularly associated with the wet humid weather of the rainy season in Southeast Asia.

Infection occurs through the inhalation or ingestion of *P. multocida*. The bacteria replicate in the tonsillar region, and if host immunity is overcome, bacteria gain access to the circulation and septicemia results. Endotoxin appears to be the major virulence factor responsible for clinical signs and death. In animals in which host defenses prevail, the bacteria persist, and the animals become immune carriers.

Clinical signs can occur within 48 hours after exposure to the virulent bacteria. The clinical course is usually short, with the first sign often being sudden death. Affected animals that are found alive are febrile (41 to 42°C) and anorectic. Profuse salivation and respiratory distress develop and lead to recumbency and death within 24 hours. Petechiation on mucosal surfaces may occur, and subcutaneous edema may develop in the throat, neck, brisket, and perineum.

At necropsy, there is generalized petechiation on serosal surfaces and within the lymph nodes. The lungs are diffusely edematous, and there may be acute bronchopneumonia. *P. multocida* can be readily isolated from the spleen and heart blood.

Treatment

The acute course of hemorrhagic septicemia requires urgent antibacterial therapy and attention to the possible development of septic or endotoxic shock. It is imperative that bactericidal concentrations of an antibacterial agent be attained in the blood as soon as possible and that initial serum concentrations be high enough to cause adequate distribution of drug into peripheral tissues, where localized infections may become established. Therefore, initial intravenous administration of antibacterial agents followed by intramuscular or subcutaneous dosing is recommended. Prophylactic use of antibacterial agents in all in-contact animals should be employed in case of an outbreak.

Prevention

The immunogens in *P. multocida* B:2 and E:2 that are responsible for protection are not known. Recent studies have concentrated on the potential role of *P. multocida* outer membrane proteins in stimulating immunity in hemorrhagic septicemia.

In countries where hemorrhagic septicemia is endemic, control is achieved through the use of plain-broth, alum-precipitated, aluminum hydroxide gel, or oil adjuvant bacterins. Use of the plain-broth bacterin is discouraged because of short-lived immunity (6 to 8 weeks) and a potential for induction of anaphylactic shock. Alum-precipitated bacterins stimulate immunity for 4 to 6 months, whereas oil adjuvant bacterins stimulate immunity for 6 to 9 months after initial vaccination. Vaccination of cattle and buffalo with oil adjuvant bacterins at 4 to 6 months of age, followed by a booster 3 months later and annual vaccination, effectively controls the disease. In some countries, the alum-precipitated bacterin is preferred, and annual booster injections are recommended prior to the rainy season.

RESPIRATORY DISEASE

P. haemolytica A:1 is the most commonly isolated bacterium in fibrinous pleuropneumonia associated with shipping fever (prevalence, 65% to 75%). *P. multocida* A:3 is the second most common bacterium isolated from fibrinous pneumonia in beef cattle (prevalence, 21% to 34%) and the major cause of fibrinous bronchopneumonia in dairy calves (prevalence, >65%). The latter condition is part of the enzootic pneumonia complex of dairy calves.

The pathogenesis of pneumonic pasteurellosis involves several bacteria-host interactions: nasopharyngeal colonization, inhalation of aerosolized droplets containing bacteria, pulmonary alveolar colonization, host response to colonization, and bacterial evasion of host defenses. Both *P. haemolytica* and *P. multocida* are carried in the nasopharynx and tonsils of cattle in low, often undetectable numbers. In the case of *P. haemolytica*, isolates from the nasal cavity of normal cattle often yield serotypes other than A:1, especially A:2. Viral infections, inclement weather, overcrowding, poor ventilation, transportation, and other causes of stress result in the proliferation of *P. haemolytica* A:1 or *P. multocida* A:3 with subsequent inhalation of bacteria into the lung.

More is known about the host—*P. haemolytica* interactions occurring in the lungs of cattle than about host—*P. multocida* interactions. Therefore, the following discussion of pathogenesis will concentrate on *P. haemolytica*. Once *P. haemolytica* gains access to the pulmonary alveoli, local host defenses, including pulmonary surfactant, alveolar macrophages, the cough reflex, and mucociliary protection, must be overcome for pneumonia to result. These local mechanisms, together with cellular and humoral systemic defenses, usually destroy bacteria before pulmonary damage is severe. However, when those responses are insufficient or overwhelmed, several bacterial and host factors (particularly leukocyte products) induce localized tissue damage and incite systemic responses associated with the acute inflammatory process.

P. haemolytica produces a thick polysaccharide capsule that protects the organism from phagocytosis and complement-mediated killing. Endotoxin, which is associated with the outer membrane of *P. haemolytica*, causes alveolar capillary endothelial damage. Endothelial damage results in fluid exudation and neutrophil infiltration into alveoli, activation of the coagulation cascade, and stimulation of platelet aggregation with subsequent thrombosis. In addition, endotoxin stimulates bovine alveolar macrophages to release inflammatory mediators. Leukotoxin causes damage and activation of neutrophils and macrophages; this results in the release of proteolytic enzymes that damage alveoli and inflammatory mediators, which further enhances the inflammatory response in the alveoli.

Clinical signs of pneumonic pasteurellosis usually become evident 3 to 10 days after cattle are stressed. Occasionally, cattle are found dead with minimal warning of disease, but most affected cattle become depressed and are first observed standing alone with their heads dropped. Severely affected animals may be found in dorsal recumbency. Respirations are usually shallow and rapid and accompanied by a slight productive cough, especially when cattle are moved. A mucopurulent nasal discharge is common. Most cattle lose their appetite but continue to drink water. Affected cattle are febrile (40 to 41°C or higher), and bronchial tones, wheezes, and pleuritic friction sounds may be auscultated. The clinical course usually lasts 2 to 4 days. If treated early, clinical responses may be noted within 24 to 36 hours. Treatment failures result in death or chronic pneumonia with continued anorexia, weight loss, and lack of vigor.

The lesion attributed to *P. haemolytica* A1 infection is a severe fibrinous pleuropneumonia. Variable amounts of fibrin-rich fluid are present in the pleural cavity, with abundant fibrin strands adherent to pleural surfaces. The cranioventral lung lobes are dark reddish black to grayish brown and firm with marked distention of interlobular septa by gelatinous yellow fluid and sharply demarcated areas of coagulation necrosis. Microscopically, intra-alveolar fibrin, neutrophils, oat-shaped macrophages, necrotic areas that usually have numerous bacteria at their margins, thrombus- and fibrin-filled interlobular septa, and fibrin-filled lymphatics can be seen. In animals that survive, the pleural fibrin organizes and fibrous adhesions develop between the lung and thoracic wall. Necrotic lung tissue usually undergoes liquefaction, and *Actinomyces pyogenes*–associated abscesses may develop.

The lesion caused by *P. multocida* A:3 in either beef or dairy calves is usually a cranioventral fibrinous bronchopneumonia that is less fulminating and more chronic than the lesion caused by *P. haemolytica*. The pleural surfaces contain adherent fibrin, and the cranioventral portion of the lungs is consolidated and dark red to reddish gray with minimal distention of the interlobular septa. On a cut surface, the consolidated areas contain uniformly spaced grayish foci (bronchioles) from which yellow-gray fibrinopurulent exudate can be expressed. Small foci of necrosis or abscesses may be present. Microscopically, bronchiolar epithelial changes vary from necrotic to hyperplastic, and bronchiolar lumina are filled with neutrophils and fibrinonecrotic debris. Alveoli are likewise distended with neutrophils and fibrinonecrotic debris, and these changes are most intense in peribronchiolar alveoli.

Treatment

Antibacterial therapy must be initiated as soon as possible because animals in which severe pneumonia is allowed to develop are less likely to respond favorably. Even if initial treatment is successful, animals in which advanced pneumonia is allowed to develop are more likely to suffer permanent lung damage leading to a decreased growth rate and subsequent relapse. Body temperature provides the useful quantitative determinant of when treatment should be initiated. The precise temperature used to determine whether antibacterial treatment is needed depends on an assessment of the relative cost and benefits of therapy and the effects of ambient temperature and physical exertion. Generally, a critical temperature of 104°F is used. When considering whether the response to therapy has been satisfactory, both body temperature and clinical signs should be assessed.

Selection of an appropriate antibacterial agent should be guided by consideration of the in vitro sensitivity of the etiologic bacterium, the pharmacokinetic disposition of the drug, and the potential for adverse effects. An antibacterial agent selected for use against bovine respiratory disease should achieve effective concentrations in infected lung. Assessment of in vitro sensitivity can be accomplished by using the agar disk diffusion technique or by direct determination of minimum inhibitory concentrations. Although the use of such data provides a more quantitative approach that is more likely to result in satisfactory treatment responses, in vitro susceptibility assays are conducted in the absence of host defenses and therefore may not always be predictive of in vivo efficacy.

Managerial and economic constraints, coupled with the necessity of treating pneumonic animals as soon as possible, preclude culture and sensitivity testing in many cases. Instead, large numbers of animals in which respiratory disease has been diagnosed but not yet treated with antibacterial agents should be sampled periodically. These samples may be collected from the nasal cavity or the laryngotracheal region with swabs or from the lung by lavage. Culture and sensitivity data from these animals can then be used to guide the selection of antibacterial agents for initial therapy. Subsequent testing of isolates from treatment failures will provide information relevant to the selection of alternative agents for use in animals that have not responded satisfactorily to initial therapy. In the absence of appropriate culture and sensitivity information, selection of antibacterial agents must be based on past experience and published efficacy data. Approved antibacterial agents to which isolates of *P. haemolytica* are least likely to be resistant are ceftiofur, tilmicosin, and florfenicol. These agents can be considered first-choice agents to be used at the onset of an outbreak of respiratory disease when more definitive in vitro sensitivity data are not available. Caution should be exercised when using agents to which animals have previously been exposed because of the possibility of antibacterial resistance developing.

In acute cases of pneumonic pasteurellosis, prior to the development of consolidated lesions, concentrations of drugs in pulmonary interstitium will be similar to corresponding serum concentrations. Antibacterial concentrations in chronically infected lung tissue are more difficult to estimate, and it is recommended that the antibacterial agent selected achieve a concentration in the lung that exceeds the minimum inhibitory concentration. Maximum lung concentrations achieved by the administration of approved doses of antibacterial agents can be predicted by estimating the degree to which each drug penetrates tissue (Table 1).

In vitro susceptibility studies have indicated that the number of isolates of *P. haemolytica* sensitive to antibacterial therapy may be increased by combining antibacterial agents. Furthermore, combinations of antibacterial agents may be necessary to treat

Table 1
VALUES LIKELY TO BE ACHIEVED AFTER ADMINISTRATION OF SINGLE APPROVED OR RECOMMENDED DOSES OF ANTIBACTERIAL AGENTS TO ANIMALS WITH SUBACUTE OR CHRONIC INFECTION

Drug	Approved/Recommended Dosage (Interval)	C_{max}* (μg/mL)	C_{min}* (μg/mL)	% Penetration	L_{max} (μg/mL)
Ceftiofur	1–2 mg/kg IM (24 hr)	4.58	0.05	30	1.37
Erythromycin	15 mg/kg IM (24 hr)†	2.4	0.15	250	6.00
Oxytetracycline	6.6–11 mg/kg IV, IM, SC (24 hr)				
Hydrochloride		4.37	1.17	65	2.84
Base		2.93	1.30	65	1.91
Florfenicol	20 mg/kg IM (48 hr)	3.07	0.57	100	3.07
Spectinomycin	20 mg/kg IM (12 hr)†	52.54	0.05	30	15.76
Sulfachlorpyridazine	40 mg/kg IV (12 hr)	166.71	0.13	—	—
Sulfadimethoxine	55 mg/kg IV, then 27.5 mg/kg IV (24 hr)	297.30	34.25	50	148.65
Sulfadiazine	17.6 mg/kg IV (24 hr)†, ‡	20.65§	0.12	—	—
Tilmicosin	10 mg/kg SC (1 dose only)	0.64	—	1450	9.28
Trimethoprim	3.5 mg/kg IV (24 hr)†	1.78	0.01	300	5.34

C_{max}, maximum serum concentration; C_{min}, minimum serum concentration at the end of the dosage interval; % Penetration, degree of penetration into consolidated lung tissue; L_{max}, estimated peak lung concentration; IM, intramuscularly; IV, intravenously; SC, subcutaneously.
*Using the highest approved/recommended dose and dosage interval.
†Not approved for use in cattle or as an extra-label dose.
‡Combined with trimethoprim.
§Zero-time plasma concentration.

pneumonia caused by multiple organisms, including chlamydiae and mycoplasmas. However, most of the antibacterial agents recently approved for use against bovine respiratory disease already have a fairly wide spectrum of activity, and despite the theoretical advantages of combination therapy, field trials have not demonstrated substantial benefits of combination therapy in comparison with treatment using a single antibacterial agent. A combination of antibacterial agents with other pharmacologic agents such as nonsteroidal anti-inflammatory agents, corticosteroids, antihistamines, and immunomodulators has had limited success, and the use of these agents is not recommended.

Treatment of sufficient duration can be achieved only if the response to treatment is carefully monitored. Therapy must be continued for at least 48 hours after clinical signs have abated; if there is no improvement by 48 hours after initiation of therapy, an alternative treatment should be selected and then continued until 48 hours after the abatement of clinical signs. Failure to treat animals for a sufficient duration will promote the development of bacterial resistance and result in high relapse rates.

The cost-effectiveness of therapeutic strategies on a herd basis depends on the user's appropriate selection of antibacterial agents, early treatment, use of an adequate dosage and treatment duration, condition of the animals, and the season of the year when they are first introduced into the feedlot or stocker operation. Treatment response rates are usually lower in the fall, during inclement weather, and when shipping stress has been excessive. Response rates may also be influenced by the management and care of diseased animals. Pneumonic animals should be sheltered from extreme temperatures, good-quality grass hay should be provided, and overcrowding should be avoided. All these factors need to be considered when assessing the success of treatment strategies. Generally, targets of greater than 85% for the response rate and less than 5% for the case fatality rate are recommended.

Prevention

The current method of raising, processing, and marketing beef cattle in North America results in severe stress and trans-

mission of numerous respiratory pathogens among cattle. As long as this situation exists, complete prevention of pneumonic pasteurellosis is probably not feasible. However, prophylactic treatment and vaccination can reduce morbidity and mortality.

Prophylactic use of antibacterial agents has become increasingly popular. Administration of long-acting oxytetracycline (20 mg/kg intramuscularly) or tilmicosin (10 mg/kg subcutaneously) is effective in controlling outbreaks of bovine respiratory disease or may be used on arrival at the feedlot when morbidity exceeds a critical level, such as 10%. Parenteral administration of antibacterial agents at this time is a superior alternative to mass medication of food and water. However, the long-term implications of prophylactic use of antibacterial agents have yet to be determined; in particular, the prophylactic use of agents that are frequently used for therapy may promote the establishment of bacterial populations resistant to these agents.

The specific *P. multocida* immunogens that are important for stimulating immunity in cattle against respiratory disease have not been identified. Of potential interest as immunogens are purified *P. multocida* capsule, lipopolysaccharide, outer membrane proteins, and iron-regulated outer membrane proteins. Preliminary experimental evidence favors outer membrane proteins as the major immunogens against *P. multocida*–induced pneumonic pasteurellosis. Two types of *P. multocida* vaccines are currently available for use against pneumonic pasteurellosis: bacterins and a live streptomycin-dependent mutant vaccine. The efficacy of these vaccines has yet to be well documented.

The specific *P. haemolytica* immunogens that are important for stimulating immunity in cattle are leukotoxin, surface antigens (including capsular polysaccharide, lipopolysaccharide, outer membrane proteins, and iron-regulated outer membrane proteins), and possibly the sialoglycoproteinase that is present in culture supernatants. Experimental data indicate that the most important *P. haemolytica* surface antigens are proteins and that these are most likely outer membrane in origin.

Various commercial formulations of *P. haemolytica* vaccines are currently available (Table 2). Their efficacies have been demonstrated primarily with experimental challenge methods; however, demonstration of efficacy against experimental challenge may not necessarily indicate that the vaccine will be efficacious against natural disease. Determination of which

Table 2
TYPES OF COMMERCIAL *PASTEURELLA* VACCINES AVAILABLE FOR USE AGAINST PNEUMONIC PASTEURELLOSIS

Types of *Pasteurella* Vaccines Available	Examples of Commercial *Pasteurella* Vaccines
Bacterins	Pneumosyn-H, Pasturpro, Shipguard
Bacterins/toxoid	One Shot
Cell-free extracts	Presponse
Bacterin extract	Septimune PH-K
Modified live	Once PMH

Pasteurella vaccine to use is difficult. In general, traditional *Pasteurella* bacterins have not been shown to be efficacious. Experimental and field studies with several of the "new-generation" vaccines such as One Shot, Presponse, and Once PMH demonstrated efficacy in many of the trials. These vaccines stimulate antibodies to *P. haemolytica* leukotoxin, surface proteins, and in some cases other antigens present in culture supernatants. Only Once PMH contains *P. multocida*. One of these newer vaccines should be considered as part of a bovine respiratory disease prophylaxis program. However, because Once PMH consists of live bacteria, concurrent use of prophylactic antibiotics might lower antibody responses to the bacteria.

The use of one dose of *P. haemolytica* vaccine has become the industry standard. Experimental studies have demonstrated that one injection of experimental *P. haemolytica* vaccine stimulates significant protection against challenge and that protection was no different from that induced by two doses of vaccine administered 1 week apart. By the time that levels of maternal antibodies decline, *P. haemolytica*—specific antibodies have developed in most cattle from aerosol exposure to nasopharyngeal bacteria. Therefore, although those titers may not be long-lived, the first vaccination with a *P. haemolytica* vaccine stimulates essentially an anamnestic response.

Timing of vaccination is a critical issue in the management of respiratory disease in feedlot and stocker cattle. There is evidence that cattle entering a feedlot with preexisting serum antibody titers to *P. haemolytica* have less respiratory disease and fewer deaths than those without serum antibodies. Therefore, cattle should be vaccinated against *Pasteurella* spp. while on the farm of origin, approximately 2 to 3 weeks prior to shipment. Studies have indicated that one injection of a commercial *P. haemolytica* vaccine stimulates maximum serum antibody titers 2 to 3 weeks after vaccination. Those titers, however, rapidly decline to baseline by 6 weeks after vaccination. Vaccination of cattle against pneumonic pasteurellosis on arrival at the feedlot does not allow enough time for the development of immunity prior to the period of highest morbidity; however, results in several field trials indicate that this practice can afford some protection against the disease.

BIBLIOGRAPHY

Clarke CR: Bovine Respiratory Disease: Sourcebook for the Veterinary Professional. Trenton, NJ, Veterinary Learning Systems, 1996, pp 40–48.

Clarke CR, Burrows GE, Ames TR: Therapy of bovine bacterial pneumonia. Vet Clin North Am Food Anim Pract 7:669–694, 1991.

Confer AW: Immunogens of *Pasteurella*. Vet Microbiol 37:353–368, 1993.

Confer AW, Fulton RW: Evaluation of *Pasteurella* and *Haemophilus* vaccines. Bovine Proc 27:136–141, 1995.

de Alwis MCL: Haemorrhagic septicemia (*Pasteurella multocida* serotype B: and E:2 infection) in cattle and buffaloes. *In* Donachie W, Lainson FA, Hodgson JC (eds): *Haemophilus, Actinobacillus* and *Pasteurella*. London, Plenum, 1995, pp 9–24.

Perino LJ, Hunsaker BD: A review of bovine respiratory disease vaccine field efficacy. Bovine Pract 31:59–66, 1997.

Shewen PE: Host response to infection with HAP: Implications for vaccine development. *In* Donachie W, Lainson FA, Hodgson JC (eds): *Haemophilus, Actinobacillus,* and *Pasteurella*. London, Plenum, 1995, pp 165–171.

Smith RA: Bovine Respiratory Disease: Sourcebook for the Veterinary Professional. Trenton, NJ, Veterinary Learning Systems, 1996, pp 49–56.

■ Pasteurellosis in Swine

Lorraine J. Hoffman, Ph.D.

Pasteurella multocida, a frequent commensal in the nasopharynx and tonsils of pigs, is present in a high percentage of swine herds throughout the world. It is the primary cause of progressive atrophic rhinitis (AR), and it is a frequent and significant secondary bacterial pathogen in cases of enzootic (*Mycoplasma*-induced) pneumonia and porcine respiratory disease complex (PRDC) common in growing-finishing swine. *P. multocida* is one of the milieu of respiratory pathogens that results in millions of dollars of lost income within the pork industry each year.

P. multocida is a small gram-negative rod or coccobacillus that grows optimally on blood agar at 37°C in an aerobic environment. The colonies are nonhemolytic and often mucoid in appearance, with most strains producing a distinctive sweet, musty odor. *P. multocida* will not grow on MacConkey or tergitol-7 agar. A series of biochemical tests is commonly used to aid in the definitive identification of this organism, including oxidase (+), catalase (+), indole (+), urease (−), and several carbohydrate fermentations. Five serogroups or types of *P. multocida* are differentiated according to capsular polysaccharides (types A, B, D, E, and F). Types A and D are the most common types found in swine. Type A strains are frequently associated with bronchopneumonia, pleuritis, or abscess formation, and they may be toxigenic or nontoxigenic. These strains usually produce large, mucoid colonies because of the hyaluronic acid in their capsule. The type D strains, which are often toxigenic and associated with AR, are less mucoid because of a different capsular composition.

A large number of type D and type A strains produce a heat-labile exotoxin that is a primary virulence factor responsible for atrophy of the turbinate bones, growth depression, and damage to parenchymal organs such as the kidney and liver. Toxigenic and nontoxigenic *P. multocida* organisms have been recovered from numerous other species such as sheep, goats, rabbits, and cattle. Numerous instances may occur in which individuals of these species act as carriers with no overt clinical signs. The carriage of pathogenic strains by humans and animals that are in close proximity to swine creates epidemiologic possibilities for transmission routes and sources of infection within and between swine herds.

PNEUMONIA

Most swine pneumonias are complex. They pose a serious problem for swine producers because of a reduction in feed efficiency, disruption in pig flow, and increase in days to market weight. *P. multocida* is a common secondary bacterial invader in cases of pneumonia. In 6- to 12-week-old pigs, *P. multocida* is frequently associated with enzootic or mycoplasmal pneumonia. This syndrome generally begins with the invasion of *Mycoplasma hyopneumoniae* potentiated by stressors such as dust, extreme temperatures, or poor ventilation, followed by invasion and colonization of the lung by *P. multocida* and other opportunistic bacterial pathogens.

Severe outbreaks of PRDC, which cause growth stall-outs in 18- to 20-week-old pigs, are becoming more frequent in large units. The most common pathogens recovered from pigs with this syndrome are porcine reproductive and respiratory syndrome virus, swine influenza virus, and *M. hyopneumoniae*. *P. multocida* is cited as one of the common opportunistic bacteria associated with PRDC. Treatment focused on *P. multocida* and other bacterial invaders decreases the severity of PRDC.

P. haemolytica and unclassified *Pasteurella/Actinobacillus*-like bacteria are sometimes isolated from pneumonic swine lungs. The exact role of these agents is not well defined. There are also infrequent occurrences of *P. multocida*–induced septicemia in young pigs.

Epidemiology

An in-depth understanding of the epidemiology of pneumonic pasteurellosis is difficult because each outbreak is complex and highly influenced by a multiplicity of other predisposing and potentiating infectious and environmental factors. *P. multocida* type A can be found in the nasal cavities and/or tonsils of healthy pigs and appears to be transmitted most frequently by oral or nasal droplets. Aerosol transmission does occur, but with low frequency. Vertical transmission from sow to piglet is not as common as lateral transmission from pig to pig later in life. The organism may also be spread by fomites contaminated with respiratory secretions. Nonclinical carrier animals in addition to swine may also play an important role in maintenance and spread of this agent on a given production site.

Pathogenesis and Virulence Factors

A normal pig lung is capable of tolerating massive numbers of *P. multocida* when introduced intranasally or intratracheally. Clearance of the organism undoubtedly occurs very quickly because mild, transient lesions resolve in a few days without treatment. The only successful experimental models are those in which the animals are first compromised by other respiratory pathogens or large volumes of infected fluids are instilled directly into the lung. These investigations corroborate the observed pathogenesis of naturally occurring *P. multocida*–related pneumonias in which superinfections occur after primary pathogens and/or environmental influences diminish the pulmonary defense mechanisms. Because type A and D strains of *P. multocida* (toxigenic and nontoxigenic) consistently colonize the nasal passages and tonsillar tissue of pigs, this provides two locations from which the agent can easily access the lower respiratory tract.

Virulence factors play a major role in the development of pneumonic pasteurellosis, but total understanding of these factors has yet to be elucidated. Type A strains, which are predominant in pneumonic lungs, possess a thick polysaccharide capsule that interferes with phagocytosis by alveolar macrophages. Pneumonic type A strains also adhere to lung cells with greater affinity than do type D strains, thus indicating differences in cell attachment receptors and tissue tropism.

The contribution of dermonecrotic toxin to the pathogenesis of *P. multocida*–complicated pneumonias remains largely unanswered. Even though numerous investigators have recovered A and D toxigenic and nontoxigenic strains from pig lungs, it remains unclear whether the toxin is associated with enhanced virulence. Other cellular components that need further investigation to determine their contribution to pathogenesis include endotoxin, outer membrane proteins, and enzymes.

Clinical Signs and Pathology

The clinical features of *P. multocida* vary in severity depending on virulence of the organism, immune status of the pig, and time of treatment intervention. Intensification of preexisting pneumonic lesions by colonization of *P. multocida* results in acute bronchopneumonia manifested by a dry nonproductive cough with dyspnea. As the disease progresses, a more productive, moist cough is noted. Acute situations commonly result in pigs with elevated body temperature, depression, and inappetence. Although acute disease may persist for several days, if treatment is prompt, the mortality is generally low. Some strains of *P. multocida* cause pleuritis in growing-finishing to market-weight hogs which results in emaciation and loss of productivity. It is important to distinguish *P. multocida*–induced pleuritis from similar infections caused by *Actinobacillus pleuropneumoniae* or *A. suis*.

The chronic form of pneumonia is the most common and may persist for several weeks. This usually occurs in nursery or early–growth stage pigs and also in the late-finish (18 to 20 weeks) stage of confinement-reared swine. Pigs are in poor condition with impaired feed conversion and rate of gain. Clinical signs can be inconsistent and confusing because of the presence of other organisms; therefore, respiratory outbreaks frequently present diagnostic challenges for the veterinarian and producer.

Gross lesions associated with *P. multocida* are those common to purulent bronchopneumonia, often superimposed on pulmonary lesions induced by the primary invader. A typical finding would be anteroventral consolidation with a definite line of demarcation separating healthy and diseased lung. The affected tissue is often firm and red to gray. There may be cases in which abscessation and pleuritis are present in varying degrees. It is frequently difficult to differentiate lung lesions associated with *P. multocida* from those caused by *M. hyopneumoniae* and other secondary bacterial pathogens because the gross and microscopic lesions are similar.

Diagnosis

A definitive diagnosis of *P. multocida* pneumonia is based on isolation and identification of the organism, in association with bronchopneumonia or pleuritis. Lung, trachea, bronchial exudate, and tonsils are the preferred specimens for isolation of *P. multocida*. Additional tissues that may yield growth of *P. multocida* are thoracic fluid, pericardial fluid, and heart blood. If tissues and fluids are collected in the field, they should be cooled and delivered expediently to the laboratory. Swabs are not recommended unless nasal or tonsil specimens are collected from live pigs when rhinitis and pneumonia are occurring simultaneously.

P. multocida is easy to isolate unless samples are not collected aseptically or the tissues are autolyzed. In either situation, there may be excessive contamination that conceals low numbers of colonies or interferes with good colony separation. A number of methods have been used to circumvent this situation, the most frequent of which is the use of a selective medium containing antibiotics. Immunohistochemical and polymerase chain reaction tests are not currently available for the diagnosis of *P. multocida*–complicated pneumonias.

Lung isolates of *P. multocida* are not commonly serotyped or toxin-tested in the laboratory. Antibiotic susceptibility testing is routinely conducted because resistant strains of *P. multocida* are now commonplace and need to be identified, especially in situations where empirical treatment has not been effective.

Treatment, Prevention, and Control

Early and accurate diagnosis followed by appropriate treatment and sound managerial and environmental modifications provides the best results in altering the course of swine respiratory disease. Pigs exhibiting acute signs of pneumonia should be treated parenterally with appropriate antimicrobials. Selection of antibiotics should be based on antibiograms of *P. multocida* isolates from the particular herd involved. Nonclinical pigs in the pen and/or building should be mass-medicated in their water or feed. Antibiotics commonly used for treatment and prevention include ampicillin, penicillin, ceftiofur, tetracyclines, sulfonamides, tiamulin, quinolones, tilmicosin (feed additive used only in swine), and tylosin.

Killed vaccines for *Pasteurella*-induced pneumonias are commercially available, but their effectiveness remains largely undetermined. Field immunoprophylaxis has been disappointing; thus the cost-effectiveness of vaccine usage to protect against *Pasteurella*-complicated pneumonias is highly questionable.

P. multocida is only one of several secondary bacterial agents that may be involved in swine respiratory disease; therefore, treatment and prevention programs must be focused on resolving or reducing the major pathogens as well as maintaining the conditions necessary for raising highly productive hogs. Reduction of disease depends on sound husbandry and management practices, appropriate medications (based on accurate susceptibility testing whenever possible), and effective immunization programs to control primary pathogens. Management decisions that must be considered are all-in/all-out movement of pigs, closed herds to minimize exposure to pathogens, reduction of building and pen size to decrease animal density, and air quality upgrades to control dust, humidity, and temperature. Segregated early weaning programs and multiple-site reproduction should also be considered when respiratory diseases pose a serious challenge to efficient production.

PROGRESSIVE ATROPHIC RHINITIS

Atrophic rhinitis is a contagious disease of pigs that is of importance to hog producers throughout the world. A 1991 report indicated that only 10% of the producers surveyed thought that their herds were completely free of AR and 42% indicated that they were vaccinating growing pigs for the causative agents of AR. The progressive form of AR is due to a concurrent infection with toxigenic *P. multocida* and *Bordetella bronchiseptica*. It has been agreed that management, environment, nutrition, and disease status of the herd contribute significantly to the development and severity of AR. Clinical aspects of progressive AR include shortening and deformation of the snout, sneezing, mucopurulent nasal discharge, nasal bleeding, and, frequently, growth retardation.

Etiology/Extrinsic Factors

Certain strains of *P. multocida* elaborate a potent dermonecrotic toxin associated with irreversible or progressive turbinate atrophy. Some toxigenic strains of *B. bronchiseptica* cause transient turbinate atrophy in young pigs and also facilitate the colonization of *P. multocida* through either mucosal irritation or the release of soluble substances. Combined invasion by toxigenic *P. multocida* and *B. bronchiseptica* results in the most severe forms of epithelial and bony atrophy, sometimes causing complete disappearance of the turbinates within 10 to 14 days. The central role that *P. multocida* toxin plays in progressive AR is well established inasmuch as both turbinate atrophy and growth retardation occur in piglets exposed to purified toxin by various injection routes. Systemic effects of the toxin may also occur that result in kidney and liver dysfunction as well as inhibition of growth plates. This finding suggests that turbinate lesions themselves are only partially responsible for the decreased growth rate in pigs with progressive AR. Viruses such as porcine reproductive and respiratory syndrome virus, swine influenza virus, porcine respiratory coronavirus, porcine cytomegalovirus, and pseudorabies virus may also damage turbinate epithelium and allow enhanced colonization by *P. multocida*, *B. bronchiseptica*, and other bacteria.

Despite the major role of infectious agents, other factors contribute to the clinical manifestations of progressive AR and are often difficult to evaluate and quantify. High population density or overcrowding will increase the transmission of primary agents. Excessive mixing of pigs, reduced or inadequate ventilation, and high levels of dust or noxious gas can contribute significantly to the seriousness and expression of this syndrome. It is likely that genetics play a role in a pig's susceptibility to a particular agent, and nutritional factors can influence the severity of disease. Herds may be infected with toxigenic strains of *P. multocida* and not display clinical signs, especially if extrinsic factors and other disease agents are well controlled.

Epidemiology

Toxigenic *P. multocida* and *B. bronchiseptica* are common organisms, not only in swine, but also in several other domestic and wild species, that represent potential vectors for carrying these organisms into swine herds. *B. bronchiseptica* can be found in ciliated respiratory mucosa, tonsils, and the intestines of pigs, whereas *P. multocida* resides in the tonsils and nasal passages. Animal-to-animal infection through direct contact is the most common mode of transmission, although aerosolization and fecal-oral exchange may also occur. Breeding females may harbor and thus maintain both organisms on the farm. Piglets can acquire *P. multocida* within 1 week of birth, and pig-to-pig transmission can occur at any time. Dissemination of *B. bronchiseptica* is common at 2 to 3 weeks of age and immediately following weaning.

The development of AR lesions is influenced by the type and amount of immunity (passive or active) and also by the timing of infection with the primary infectious agents. The addition of carrier animals can infect a naive herd. In some herds toxigenic *P. multocida* is present without overt signs of progressive AR because other potentiating bacteria and environmental irritants are controlled. Cases of clinical AR may also occur from which it is difficult to isolate toxigenic *P. multocida*.

Pathogenesis and Virulence Factors

The most significant virulence properties of *P. multocida* are toxin production and colonizing ability. Fimbrial structures or adhesins are found on toxigenic strains of *P. multocida* recovered from pigs with progressive AR. These structures contribute to colonization of the nasal mucosa following damage induced by *B. bronchiseptica* and environmental stressors. Release of the toxin causes irreversible turbinate atrophy, growth retardation, and lesions in tissues such as growth plates, spleen, liver, and testicles. Because the tonsil is a colonizing site for *P. multocida*, it is assumed that intranasal lesions can result from toxin released by organisms at that location also.

Clinical Signs and Pathology

Sneezing and nasal discharge may be noted in suckling piglets, and clinical signs progress as the pigs move through the nursery and growing-finishing stage. Characteristic clinical signs include sneezing, mucopurulent nasal exudate, and staining of the medial canthus of the eye as lacrimation increases and drainage decreases. In severe cases, affected animals may bleed from the nose and exhibit shortening ("bullnose") and twisting or deviation of the snout. Diminished weight gain and loss of feed efficiency as a result of rhinitis are the most economically apparent signs.

Gross lesions are generally restricted to the nasal cavity and adjacent structures of the skull. Ventral scrolls may be slightly shrunken to moderately atrophied in mild cases. Complete atrophy of the ventral and dorsal turbinates accompanied by septal deviation and deformity of the face is present in more severe cases. Nasal structures are frequently evaluated for damage during necropsy in the laboratory or at the packing plant. Snouts are sectioned vertically between the first and second premolar teeth, and the degree of nasal structure loss is quantified. These evaluations are helpful in assessing the disease level in a herd, particularly when overt physical signs are minimal or absent.

Diagnosis

The diagnosis of progressive AR can be made on the basis of clinical signs, morphologic changes in turbinates, and recovery of toxigenic *P. multocida* and *B. bronchiseptica*. Swabs of turbinates and tonsils along with tonsillar biopsy specimens can be obtained from live pigs or at necropsy and cultured for bacterial pathogens. When nasal swab specimens are collected from live pigs, it is imperative to restrain the pigs properly and clean the external nares with 70% alcohol. A sterile, cotton swab is then inserted into both sides of the nasal cavity and rotated gently to avoid excessive trauma. Swabs should be placed in a nonnutrient transport medium, cooled, and transported to the laboratory within 24 hours of collection. Because *P. multocida* colonizes the tonsils, the tonsils should also be cultured if the animals are to undergo necropsy. It may be impractical to swab or perform a biopsy on the tonsils of live pigs.

P. multocida is easily recovered on blood agar, but various selective media containing antibiotics have been used to help reduce contaminants and provide improved recovery of pasteurellae, which are often present in low numbers. MacConkey's agar is routinely used for the isolation of *B. bronchiseptica*. Another method that has been successful in the recovery of *P. multocida* is intraperitoneal mouse inoculation with nasal swab contents diluted in saline. However, this method is not commonly used because of high cost, labor intensiveness, and humanitarian concerns.

Capsular serotyping of *P. multocida* strains is conventionally done by an indirect hemagglutination test, but this is not a routine procedure in diagnostic laboratories. A simple test to differentiate types A and D is the hyaluronidase test, but some porcine strains cannot be typed with this method.

Toxin detection can be achieved by several different methods, including observation of dermonecrotic lesions in guinea pigs, mouse lethality, and cytopathic effect on Vero cells. These procedures have been essentially replaced with in vitro methods such as enzyme-linked immunosorbent assay, colony blot assay using monoclonal antibodies, and DNA hybridization.

Isolation of *B. bronchiseptica* and *P. multocida* is not always indicative of a problem because they are part of the normal microflora of pigs; however, recovery of toxigenic strains of *P. multocida* type D is significant. Severe lesions have been observed in pigs from which there is no isolation of toxigenic *P.*

multocida from nasal swabs. This suggests that other agents are capable of causing AR or that toxigenic strains reside principally in the tonsil and thus toxin is causing turbinate atrophy without the presence of toxigenic strains in the nasal cavity.

Treatment, Control, and Prevention

Selected combinations of chemotherapy, vaccination, management, and environmental changes are imperative for lowering the prevalence and severity of AR within a herd. Improving the overall environment for swine by all-in/all-out pig flow in the nursery, providing optimal ventilation, and controlling temperature shifts and overcrowding will contribute to control of this disease. Intensification in large units results in spread by aerosolization. *P. multocida* loses viability quickly when aerosolized, but under conditions of high humidity, it remains infectious much longer. Poor survival in other liquids suggests that routes of transmission other than direct exposure are unlikely.

No drugs have been specifically cleared to prevent or treat AR. Antibiotics that have been effective are potentiated sulfonamides, tetracyclines, tylosin, and ceftiofur. These may be used in sows prior to farrowing, in newborn piglets, and in newly weaned pigs. Mass antibiotic medication in water or feed is commonly used in weaned pigs.

Variable success in preventing AR has been achieved with vaccination programs. Some of the vaccines contain only *B. bronchiseptica*, whereas others contain both *B. bronchiseptica* and *P. multocida* with or without *Pasteurella* toxoid. Bacterins alone may not affect growth reduction or colonization of the pathogens. Varying degrees of success have been noted with vaccines containing the toxoid component. The multivalent vaccines are most often recommended and have been effective when combined with production changes such as decreased weaning age and all-in/all-out pig flow. Gilts are typically vaccinated twice, the second dose being 1 to 2 weeks prior to farrowing, and sows should be revaccinated each year 2 weeks prior to farrowing. Vaccination of pigs at 7 to 14 days (weaning) then again 2 to 3 weeks later is a common practice unless high colostral protection is present in the herd.

Producers who maintain AR-free swine herds must pay strict attention to avoid purchases of breeding stock infected with toxigenic *P. multocida* and *B. bronchiseptica*. There should be absolutely no acquisitions from known positive herds or those of questionable status. Segregated and medicated early weaning methods, as well as adoption of a specific pathogen-free system, are ways in which stock can be raised free of the pathogens common to AR. Veterinarians and producers must remain cognizant that reduction or eradication of AR requires constant dedication to good management and health procedures.

BIBLIOGRAPHY

Ackerman MR, Debey MC, Register KB, et al: Tonsil and turbinate colonization by *Pasteurella multocida*. J Vet Diagn Invest 6:375, 1994.

Ackermann MR, Register KB: Update on atrophic rhinitis control. *In* Proceedings of the First Annual Swine Disease Conference of Swine Practitioners. Ames, Iowa, 1995, p 27.

Ackermann MR, Register KB, Stabel JR: Effect of *Pasteurella multocida* toxin on physeal growth in young pigs. Am J Vet Res 57:848, 1996.

Baekbo P: Pathogenic properties of *Pasteurella multocida* in the lungs of pigs. *In* Proceedings of the 10th International Pig Veterinary Society, Rio de Janeiro, 1988, p 58.

Chanter N, Rutter JM: Pasteurellosis in pigs and the determinants of virulence of toxigenic *Pasteurella multocida*. *In* Adlam C, Rutter JM (eds): Pasteurella and Pasteurellosis. London, Academic Press, 1989, pp 161.

Ciprian A, Pijoan C, Cruz T, et al: *Mycoplasma hyopneumoniae* increases the susceptibility of pigs to experimental *Pasteurella multocida* pneumonia. Can J Vet Res 52:434, 1988.

De Jong MF: (Progressive) atrophic rhinitis. *In* Diseases of Swine, ed 7. Ames, Iowa State University Press, 1992, pp 414–435.

Desrosiers R: Diagnosis and control of swine respiratory diseases. *In* Proceedings of the 28th Meeting of the American Association of Swine Practitioners. Quebec City, 1997, p 333.

Fuentes M, Pijoan C: Phagocytosis and killing of *Pasteurella multocida* by pig alveolar macrophages after infection with pseudorabies virus. Vet Immunol Immunopathol 13:165, 1986.

Halbur PG: Defining the causes of PRDC. Swine Consultant/Pfizer, vol 4, Fall 1996, pp 4–15.

Hall W, Bane D, Kilroy C, et al: A model for the induction of pneumonia caused by *Pasteurella multocida* type A. *In* Proceedings of the 10th International Pig Veterinary Society, Rio de Janeiro, 1988, p 59.

McCaw MB: Management techniques for atrophic rhinitis control. Compend Contin Educ Pract Vet 16:1615–1618, 1994.

Morbidity/Mortality and Health Management of Swine in the United States. National Animal Health Monitoring System, U.S. Department of Agriculture, Animal and Plant and Health Inspection Service, Vet Services, National Swine Survey, Fort Collins, Colo, 1991, p 20.

Pijoan C: Pneumonic pasteurellosis. *In* Leman AD, Straw BE, Mengeling WL, et al (eds): Diseases of Swine, ed 7. Ames, Iowa, Iowa State University Press, 1992, pp 552–559.

Quinn PJ, Carter ME, Markey BK, et al: Clinical Veterinary Microbiology. London, Wolfe Publishing, 1994, pp 254–258.

Stevenson GW: Bacterial contributors to porcine respiratory disease complex (PRDC). *In* Proceedings of the 24th Meeting of the American Association of Swine Practitioners, Kansas City, Mo, 1993, p 351.

Sundberg P: Transmission and immune response studies of toxigenic *Pasteurella multocida* (dissertation). Ames, Iowa, Iowa State University, 1996.

Turnquist SE: Etiology and diagnosis of progressive atrophic rhinitis. Swine Health Production 3:168–170, 1995.

▪ Swine Dysentery

Robert D. Glock, D.V.M., Ph.D.

Swine dysentery (bloody scours) is a common diarrheal disease of swine throughout the world. It is feared by swine producers because it is easily transmitted and tends to cause long-term economic losses. The exact prevalence is unknown because of a lack of reliable methods for determining whether there may be carrier animals in a particular herd. However, studies in 1982 produced an estimate that 40% of the swine herds in the central United States were infected. The infection rate is probably lower currently because of improved control methods.

The term *swine dysentery* refers to a specific disease. The primary causative agent, and the key to transmission of the disease, is an anaerobic spirochete, *Serpulina hyodysenteriae*. Other gram-negative bacteria normally present in swine intestines may play a synergistic role in the pathogenesis.

Mechanisms of pathogenesis in swine dysentery are not clearly defined. *S. hyodysenteriae* organisms are located deep in crypts and often invade the epithelial layer of the large intestine. Colonic malabsorption leads to dehydration and acidosis.

CLINICAL SIGNS

Swine of all ages are susceptible to swine dysentery, but pigs in the postweaning and early fattening periods are most frequently affected. The disease rarely occurs in suckling pigs. Peracute deaths, before the onset of diarrhea, are infrequently encountered. These pigs usually have typical enteric lesions. Clinical signs in most pigs begin as mucoid diarrhea, which often progresses to dysentery with blood, mucus, and fibrin in the feces. Initially, flecks of blood may be scattered in the mucoid feces. If the disease progresses, the blood may be thoroughly mixed in watery feces. Abdominal pain, weight loss, and dehydration cause a gaunt, arched-back appearance. The diarrhea and anorexia result in depletion of serum electrolytes, metabolic acidosis, and some deaths. However, the majority of economic losses are the result of reduced performance, the cost of continuous medication, and the loss of breeding-stock markets.

DIAGNOSIS

There are many causes of diarrhea or dysentery. A diagnosis of swine dysentery should include an appropriate history such as the recent movement of swine into a clean herd. Previously infected pigs may have no clinical signs until after the stress of movement, environmental change, or altered feeding routine. The incubation period for swine dysentery may range from 2 or 3 days to a number of months, depending on the amount of exposure and host resistance. Some swine carry the organism without showing clinical signs. However, clinical signs often appear within 1 or 2 weeks after exposure.

Clinical dysentery with blood in the feces may be caused by other diseases such as salmonellosis, trichuriasis, and proliferative enteritis (ileitis). Gastric ulcers can also cause gastrointestinal bleeding, although the feces are much darker and firmer than those of pigs with swine dysentery.

Necropsy of an acutely affected pig may aid in diagnosis. Specific lesions of swine dysentery are limited to the large intestine, which is usually hyperemic and edematous. The mucosa is diffusely inflamed, swollen, superficially eroded, and covered by variable combinations of mucus, fibrin, blood, and cellular debris, depending on the stage of the disease. Salmonellosis differs because lesions are usually also found in other parts of the intestine or in other organs. Trichuriasis is best diagnosed by carefully inspecting the cecal and colonic mucosa for the parasites. The lesions in proliferative enteritis are located primarily in the small intestine.

Presumptive diagnosis of swine dysentery may include examination of mucosal scrapings (or dysenteric feces) by dark-field or phase microscopy to identify numerous large, motile spirochetes with tapered ends. Organisms can also be identified in smears stained with crystal violet or Victoria blue 4-R, and they can be seen in silver-stained histologic sections of the large intestine. The reliability of these presumptive diagnostic aids is jeopardized by the fact that very similar nonpathogenic spirochetes, *Serpulina innocens*, may be present in large numbers in pigs without swine dysentery.

Milder forms of colitis, sometimes referred to as intestinal spirochetosis, have been related to weakly β-hemolytic intestinal spirochetes. One of this group is *S. pilosicoli*, which has been associated with transient colitis in growing pigs. This group of organisms can be differentiated from *S. hyodysenteriae* through a variety of laboratory procedures.

Definitive diagnosis of swine dysentery is based on isolation and identification of *S. hyodysenteriae* from colonic mucosal or rectal swabs. Trypticase soy agar with 5% bovine blood and selective inhibitory antibiotics such as spectinomycin (400 μg/mL) may be streaked, incubated anaerobically at 42°C, and examined for the presence of typical complete hemolysis. Specimens submitted for culture should be kept cool and moist but not frozen. It is also important to culture for *Salmonella* spp. Combinations of swine dysentery, salmonellosis, proliferative enteritis, or trichuriasis are common, so the mere presence of one organism does not exclude the presence of others.

Detection of individual carrier animals is very difficult, but rectal swab cultures and serologic tests on specimens from numerous animals have some promise as methods of determining whether carrier animals are present within a given herd.

CONTROL

After establishing a diagnosis of swine dysentery, medication in the feed or water is recommended. In a very acute outbreak, medication of water is preferred because of reduced feed consumption by sick pigs. Parenteral treatment with drugs such as tylosin or lincomycin is also useful in some cases. Initial medication can be followed by the use of therapeutic or control levels of medication as feed additives. The disease is likely to persist in infected premises, so it is frequently necessary to medicate continuously or at least repeatedly. Table 1 lists some drugs commonly used for the treatment of swine dysentery.

It is imperative that pig comfort and sanitation be given primary attention in any control program. There is a direct correlation between levels of contamination and severity of disease. Combinations of sanitation, medication, and isolation have been used to eliminate the infection from some herds. Success depends on a good cooperative effort between a determined herd manager and an experienced veterinarian. Possible approaches to eradication are described by Walter and Kinyon and by Fujioka and colleagues (see Bibliography).

PREVENTION

The most important consideration for prevention of swine dysentery is to maintain a closed herd. Any new stock should be purchased from a reliable supplier who can provide a history free of swine dysentery. Any new arrivals should be isolated and observed for several weeks before entry into the main herd. If diarrhea should occur, feces should be analyzed by culture to determine whether *S. hyodysenteriae* is present. It is also imperative that animals be transported in a truck that has been thoroughly cleaned.

S. hyodysenteriae can survive for at least a few days in moist, cool feces, so infection can be easily transmitted by fomites such as truck tires and boots. Because mice can be long-term carriers of infection, rodent control is an important part of control programs.

It may be wise to use preventive levels of medications in situations in which animals of unknown origin are combined with the herd or previously contaminated facilities are used. Survival times of *S. hyodysenteriae* range from a few hours or less on clean, dry surfaces to a number of weeks in cool, moist feces. Survival time in anaerobically stored waste may be quite long.

Table 1
SOME DRUGS USED FOR TREATMENT OF SWINE DYSENTERY*

Compound	Water	Feed
Bacitracin	+	+
Carbadox	−	+
Dimetridazole†	+	+
Gentamicin	+	−
Ipronidazole†	+	+
Lincomycin	+	+
Sodium arsanilate	+	+
Tiamulin	+	+
Tylosin	+	+
Virginiamycin	+	+

*Always follow label direction for dosage and withdrawal before slaughter.
†Use of these compounds is prohibited in the United States.

BIBLIOGRAPHY

Egan IT, Harris DL, Hill HT: Prevalence of swine dysentery, transmissible gastroenteritis, and pseudorabies in Iowa, Illinois, and Missouri swine. *In* Proceedings of the U.S. Animal Health Association, Nashville, pp 497–502.

Fellstrom C, Pettersson B, Johansson K, et al: Prevalence of *Serpulina* species in relation to diarrhea and feed medication in pig-rearing herds in Sweden. Am J Vet Res 57:807–811, 1996.

Fujioka K, Nakamoto S, Nishida H, et al: A trial of Lincomix 44 Premix for the eradication of swine dysentery. *In* Proceedings of the 11th Congress of the International Pig Veterinary Society, Lausanne, Switzerland, July 1–5, 1990, p 132.

Harris DL, Lysone RJ: Swine dysentery. *In* Leman AD, Straw BE, Mengeling WL, et al (eds): Diseases of Swine, ed 7. Ames, Iowa, Iowa State University Press, 1992, pp 599–616.

Kinyon JM, Harris DL, Glock RD: Enteropathogenicity of various isolates of *Treponema hyodysenteriae*. Infect Immunol 15:638–616, 1977.

Songer JG, Kinyon JM, Harris DL: Selective medium for isolation of *Treponema hyodysenteriae*. J Clin Microbiol 4:57–60, 1976.

Walter DH, Kinyon JM: Recent MIC determinations of six antimicrobials for *Treponema hyodysenteriae* in the United States: Use of tiamulin to eliminate swine dysentery from two farrow to finish herds. *In* Proceedings of the 11th Congress of the International Pig Veterinary Society, Lausanne, Switzerland, July 1–5, 1990, p 129.

■ Salmonellosis

Jerome C. Nietfeld, D.V.M., Ph.D., Diplomate, A.C.V.P.
George A. Kennedy, D.V.M., Ph.D., Diplomate, A.C.V.P.

Salmonellosis is a ubiquitous disease caused by members of the genus *Salmonella*, family Enterobacteriaceae, that affects nearly all species of vertebrates. *Salmonella* spp. are gram-negative bacilli, generally motile, facultative anaerobes, that invade tissue and induce inflammation and tissue damage. The precise classification of salmonellae is confusing and controversial. Salmonellae are serotyped according to somatic or O antigens and flagellar or H antigens and, in the case of only a few serotypes, virulence or Vi antigens. Some serotypes are further divided into biovars, for example, *Salmonella choleraesuis* biovar *kunzendorf*. More than 2300 serotypes have been identified. Before 1983, each *Salmonella* serotype was recognized as a separate species. Then it was proposed that all *Salmonella* serotypes be placed into three species: *S. typhi*, the cause of typhoid fever in humans; *S. choleraesuis*, the principal cause of salmonellosis in pigs; and *S. enteritidis*, which would include all the remaining serotypes, referred to as serovars of *S. enteritidis*. For example, *Salmonella typhimurium* would be referred to as *S. enteritidis* serovar *typhimurium*. Since then, two additional classification schemes have been proposed. In one system, all serotypes are classified as a single species, *S. choleraesuis*, and this species would be subdivided into seven subgroups based on DNA similarity and host range. In another scheme, all pathogenic salmonellae would be included in a single species, *S. enterica*. With the latter two systems, each serotype would be referred to as a serovar of either *S. choleraesuis* or *S. enterica*, for example, *S. choleraesuis* serovar *typhimurium* biovar *copenhagen* or *S. enterica* serovar *typhimurium* biovar *copenhagen*. However, none of the newer classification systems have gained much acceptance, and almost everyone continues to refer to each serotype as a separate species. In this discussion we have chosen to use the older species designations. Knowledge of the serovar can be important in that it may influence the way an outbreak will be managed, provide information on the zoonotic potential, and be a starting point for epidemiologic studies.

Clinically, salmonellosis may be systemic, enteric, or inapparent and may be acute or chronic. The disease tends to occur in the young, debilitated, and very old, although all ages can be affected. Subclinical carriers, some of which shed the organisms intermittently, occur in all species, which makes salmonellosis difficult to control. Stressors such as crowding, chilling, starvation, transportation, concomitant disease, and others predispose animals to clinical disease and increased fecal shedding. Salmonellae survive in stagnant water, soil, and dried manure for months or years. Freezing decreases the number of viable bacteria, but it does not entirely eliminate salmonellae inasmuch as both *S. choleraesuis* and *S. typhimurium* were still culturable after being buried in an Indiana pasture for 450 days. Salmonellae are inactivated by heat and direct sunlight. Contaminated feed, water, pasture, dirt lots, buildings, liquid manure slurries, lagoon water, effluent from human sewage treatment plants, sick animals, and healthy carriers are all possible sources.

Salmonella infections are considered to be transmitted by the fecal-oral route, but there has been considerable speculation that *S. choleraesuis* can be transmitted by aerosol. Experimentally, greater than 10^6 organisms are usually required to induce clinical disease, and attack rates, severity of infection, and length of shedding increase with increasing inoculating dose. However, epidemiologic studies of human outbreaks have demonstrated that a few individuals become sick after ingesting only 10^2 to 10^3 salmonellae. Domestic animals are probably similar, with low numbers of organisms inducing illness in a few animals. Diarrhea develops in these animals, and they shed large numbers of bacteria into the environment. Concentration of large numbers of animals has the effect of increasing the number of salmonellae in the environment and thus increasing the incidence of salmonellosis. Stomach acidity is an important barrier to infection because salmonellae are killed at normal gastric pH. Ingestion with agents that buffer gastric acidity or pass through the stomach quickly increases susceptibility. The normal bacterial flora of the intestine inhibits salmonellae, as evidenced by the significant decrease in intestinal colonization by *Salmonella* spp. in young chicks fed bacterial cultures from the cecum of normal adult chickens. Reduction in the normal flora is probably the reason that *Salmonella* outbreaks sometimes occur following antibiotic therapy.

The pathogenesis of salmonellosis has been intensively studied but is still incompletely understood. Salmonellae must pass through the intestinal epithelium and invade to cause diarrhea. The amount of diarrhea and intestinal damage is related to the magnitude of intestinal invasion and inflammation, and much of the diarrhea and tissue damage is undoubtedly caused by neutrophil degranulation with release of cytotoxic enzymes and inflammatory responses to endotoxin. Enterotoxins and cytotoxins that are active in vitro have been described for several serotypes, but their importance remains unknown. Given the large number of *Salmonella* serotypes, the differences in virulence, and the different syndromes caused by salmonellae, it is likely that one or more toxins, other than endotoxin, play a role in disease. The most virulent serotypes, such as *S. choleraesuis*, *S. typhimurium*, and *S. dublin*, have virulence plasmids that are necessary for the full development of clinical signs. The exact role of these plasmids remains uncertain. The plasmids are not necessary for intestinal invasion, but they are necessary for progressive growth in extraintestinal tissue such as the liver and spleen. Recent research indicates that virulence plasmids enable salmonellae to lyse macrophages after being ingested and modify the host's immune response to promote increased bacterial growth. Salmonellae are generally regarded as facultative intracellular pathogens that invade and proliferate in cells, especially macrophages. This concept is largely based on the finding that strains of *Salmonella* that are resistant to in vitro killing by macrophages are the most virulent in vivo. However, some researchers believe that the ability of salmonellae to evade phagocytosis and multiply extracellularly is the key to their virulence.

CLINICAL SIGNS
Pigs

In most surveys, *S. choleraesuis* accounts for greater than 70% and sometimes greater than 90% of all *Salmonella* serotypes isolated from clinically ill pigs. There is a definite age susceptibility to clinical disease. Weaned pigs less than 4 months of age are primarily affected. Market-weight and adult swine are occasionally affected, and suckling pigs are rarely affected. Morbidity may range from a single animal to greater than 50%. In a survey of 702 outbreaks, the average morbidity was 16% and the average mortality, 4%.

Two different syndromes consisting of acute septicemia and enterocolitis are associated with *S. choleraesuis*. Acute septicemia is the more common and frequently follows some form of stress. Often owners find pigs acutely dead with no observed illness. More commonly, dyspnea, high fever, anorexia, depression, and cyanosis of the ears, tail, and ventral portion of the abdomen are present. Occasionally, affected swine display posterior weakness, restlessness, and other signs of neurologic involvement. In pigs that survive this phase, gangrene of the ears and tail may develop and, on the third or fourth day, yellow diarrhea, which often contains flakes of fibrin. Pregnant sows may abort. Enterocolitis may develop secondary to septicemia, but it is usually insidious in onset. Affected pigs may continue to eat and drink even though several in the herd have profuse yellow diarrhea that contains fibrin. Many animals recover, but their weight gain is subnormal, and they remain unprofitable.

Salmonella typhimurium, the second most common serotype that affects pigs, is usually manifested as acute or chronic enterocolitis. Septicemia can occur, but it is uncommon. Outbreaks usually occur in feeder pigs and are characterized by fever, weakness, anorexia, and yellow, watery diarrhea that often contains fibrin, shreds of mucosa, and sometimes mucus and blood. Morbidity is high and although mortality is usually low, it can be quite high, especially if septicemia is present. Many survivors will be unthrifty to maintain and have intermittent diarrhea. Rectal strictures may be a sequela of chronic colitis.

S. typhisuis infection is uncommon and characterized by intermittent diarrhea, emaciation, and frequently, enlargement of the cervical lymph nodes and parotid salivary glands and abscessation of the tonsils. It is possible that some cases of *S. typhisuis* may be missed because the organism is difficult to isolate in the laboratory.

A large number of other serotypes are commonly isolated from pigs, and enterocolitis and even rectal strictures are occasionally associated with serotypes such as *S. agona* and *S. derby*. However, serotypes other than *S. choleraesuis*, *S. typhimurium*, and *S. typhisuis* are generally considered to be of low pathogenicity for pigs, and their major importance is as potential human pathogens.

The differential diagnosis for septicemic salmonellosis includes erysipelas, streptococcal septicemia, edema disease, *Actinobacillus pleuropneumoniae* infection, pseudorabies, hog cholera, and African swine fever. For the enteric form, swine dysentery, the proliferative enteropathies caused by *Lawsonia intracellularis*, whipworms, and postweaning *Escherichia coli* infection must be considered.

Cattle

Salmonellosis affects both dairy and beef cattle. It is more difficult to categorize the disease in cattle as strictly systemic or enteric because in any given case one form may merge into the other, particularly in calves. Prevalence of the various serovars changes with different geographic localities, but *S. typhimurium* tends to be common worldwide. *S. dublin*, *S. newport*, and *S. anatum* are among the important serovars in cattle but tend to have a more patchy geographic distribution. *S. dublin*, once confined to the Pacific northwest in the United States, is becoming more widespread geographically, and severe outbreaks have occurred throughout the United States.

Acute salmonellosis is more common in dairy than beef cattle. It usually does not occur in calves less than 2 weeks old. However, it has occurred in beef calves on pasture and in calves less than 1 week old. A common history includes a moderately high incidence of intractable diarrhea with some deaths, with the disease continuing to develop in calves over an extended period. The initial fever may or may not have subsided by the time the calf is examined. The temperature commonly drops upon initiation of diarrhea, and extreme weakness is often a prominent sign. The most characteristic feature is brownish, watery diarrhea with shreds of sloughed mucosa, flakes of fibrin, and streaks of fresh blood. Meningitis, polyarthritis, and pneumonia may occur in septicemic cases. Even in the enteric form most calves will be terminally septicemic, and those that survive may remain unthrifty.

Clinical signs in adult cattle are acute illness with depression, fever, cessation of milk flow, and severe diarrhea. Parturition can be a precipitating factor. The feces tend to be fetid and watery and contain mucus, fibrinous casts, and sometimes considerable quantities of fresh blood. Persistent diarrhea and unthriftiness characterize the more chronic syndrome. Pregnant cows may abort. Although abortion is more commonly associated with *S. dublin*, it may occur with a variety of serovars. Cows may or may not be sick at the time of abortion.

Salmonellosis in the feedlot may occur anytime during the fattening period, but it generally appears soon after cattle arrive owing to the stresses and infections encountered in shipping. Morbidity and mortality can vary from a few sporadic cases to significant numbers within a pen or group. A sudden onset of semifluid to mucohemorrhagic diarrhea accompanied by depression, fever, and weakness is characteristic, but the acute septicemic form may predominate in some cases. The diarrhea may mimic bovine virus diarrhea or coccidiosis. *Salmonella* has frequently been found as a co-pathogen in cases of bovine virus diarrhea.

The differential diagnosis includes colibacillosis, rotavirus, coronavirus, and cryptosporidiosis in calves and bovine virus diarrhea, Johne's disease, coccidiosis, parasitism, and certain poisonings such as arsenic in older calves and adults.

Blood study results may include either neutrophilia or neutropenia, lymphopenia early in the course of disease, and increased fibrinogen, but there are no diagnostic clinical pathologic changes. Hyponatremia, hypokalemia, and hypoalbuminemia can occur and may be worth monitoring for treatment purposes in valuable animals.

Sheep and Goats

Salmonellosis is most frequent and economically most important in feeder lambs. It generally affects lambs soon after arrival at the lot. Affected lambs have watery diarrhea that often contains mucus and streaks of blood. Fever and depression are less specific features. Morbidity may exceed 25%, and mortality can be high. Salmonellosis in feedlot lambs must be differentiated from coccidiosis and enterotoxemia. Coccidiosis is more common, tends to appear 1 to 3 weeks after arrival, and commonly causes more blood in the feces.

Several serovars of *Salmonella* may cause abortion in ewes.

The ewe is usually sick at the time of abortion with *S. typhimurium* and *S. dublin* infections, whereas *S. arizonae* and *S. montevideo* may cause abortion in healthy-appearing ewes. *S. abortus ovis*, a host-adapted serovar causing pregnancy termination in sheep and goats, appears to be restricted to parts of Europe.

Salmonellosis in goats is reported to be generally similar to the disease in cattle. It occurs in neonatal goats, older nursing kids, and adults. The enteric form is most common, with a watery or hemorrhagic diarrhea. Coccidiosis, parasitism, and enterotoxemia should be included in the differential diagnosis.

NECROPSY FINDINGS

Pigs dying of the septicemic form of *S. choleraesuis* have a purplish discoloration of the extremities and ventral portion of the abdomen. The peripheral and visceral lymph nodes are swollen, edematous, congested, and often hemorrhagic. There may be petechial hemorrhage on the epiglottis, bladder, kidneys, and intestinal tract. The spleen is consistently blue-black and swollen. Miliary whitish foci of necrosis are occasionally macroscopically visible, and foci of necrosis are consistently visible microscopically in the liver and are a valuable diagnostic aid. The lungs do not collapse because of edema and interstitial pneumonia. The mucosal surface of the greater curvature of the stomach is typically dark red to purple, and in animals that survive for several days, the mucosal epithelium may slough. Usually there are no intestinal lesions with the septicemic form.

Ruminants with *Salmonella* septicemia may also have interstitial pneumonia, generalized lymphadenopathy, splenomegaly, widespread serosal hemorrhage, and hyperemia of the abomasal mucosa. Enteric lesions are more likely to be present in septicemic ruminants. The presence of clotted bile in the gallbladder is said to be highly suggestive of septicemic salmonellosis, especially that caused by *S. dublin*.

In both swine and ruminants with the enteric form, intestinal changes are primarily confined to the distal end of the jejunum, ileum, cecum, and colon. The mucosal surface can vary from normal to angry red to grayish yellow with adherent flakes of fibrin and ingesta. A diphtheritic pseudomembrane may cover large areas of the mucosal surface, and sloughed mucosa and fibrin may form casts in the lumen. In these cases the intestinal wall is thick and rigid. Circular *button ulcers* may be seen in pigs with enteritis caused by *S. choleraesuis* and *S. typhisuis*, but they are uncommon with *S. typhimurium*. Mesenteric lymph nodes are consistently enlarged, wet, and reddened.

Isolation of *Salmonella* from animals with typical clinical signs and lesions confirms the diagnosis. The samples of choice include the lung, liver, and spleen for the septicemic form and the large intestine, ileum, and mesenteric lymph nodes for cases of enteritis. *S. typhisuis* is very fastidious in its growth requirements, so special techniques are required for isolation.

PREVENTION

Salmonellae are widespread in the environment, and clinically normal carriers occur; thus, prevention is not easy and requires considerable labor and dedication on the part of the owner and veterinarian, and then there are no guarantees that infection will not be introduced by a source that cannot be controlled. Knowledge of the serotype can be useful. *S. choleraesuis* and *S. typhisuis* are host-adapted to pigs, and *S. dublin* to cattle. These host-adapted serotypes are rarely isolated from other species, feed, fomites, or environments other than those containing infected pigs or cattle. Long-term and possible lifetime carriers occur with the host-adapted serotypes, whereas the carrier state is much shorter for non–host-adapted serotypes. Thus *S. choler-*

aesuis, *S. typhisuis*, and *S. dublin* are almost always, if not always, introduced by a carrier animal, whereas other serotypes can enter a herd via feed, water, fomites, rodents, or birds.

Closed herds are best, and buying replacement stock from herds that have no history of salmonellosis is helpful but does not guarantee success. Identification of carriers by culture is unreliable inasmuch as multiple samples cultured over a long period are sometimes required to detect intermittent shedders. Serologic testing is more sensitive and can detect animals that have been exposed and, if multiple samples are evaluated over time, can detect active infections. Cattle that maintain a stable titer for 5 months or more should be considered to be chronic carriers, even if they are culture negative. In the past, serologic examination has been unreliable, but recently several investigators have experimented with enzyme-linked immunosorbent assays, which appear to be reliable and sensitive and will probably be used more in the future.

It is advisable to purchase feedstuff from reputable manufacturers and dealers. Dried milk, meat scraps, bone meal, and other animal or fish products are potential sources of salmonellae. These products are required to be heat-treated, which should kill all salmonellae, but if they are not handled properly, they may be contaminated after processing. Grain is less of a problem, but it can become contaminated by bird or rodent excreta. For example, *Salmonella* organisms were isolated from 2.8% of 1264 samples of feed and feed ingredients from 30 pig farms, and 14 (46.7%) of the sampled farms had at least one positive sample. Most likely much of the contamination occurs on the farm because *Salmonella* spp. were significantly more likely to be isolated on pig farms without bird proofing. Buildings that are easily cleaned and disinfected help reduce salmonellosis; for example, pigs raised on the same farm were significantly more likely to be culture positive if finished in a building with a solid floor than in one with partially slotted floors. All-in, all-out production, segregation of young from older animals, and rigorous cleaning and disinfection between groups are helpful in preventing salmonellosis in all species. The common phenolic-, chlorine-, and iodine-based disinfectants are all effective. Raw milk is a potential source of salmonellae. *S. dublin* carriers intermittently shed the organism in the milk, and other serovars have been found to intermittently contaminate the milk in some dairies with a *Salmonella* problem. Water from livestock lagoons and from streams that contain effluent from livestock farms and human sewage treatment units should be considered to be contaminated. When disposing of infected carcasses, owners must remember that they are sources of contamination for other unexposed groups of animals. Also, trucks from rendering plants are potentially contaminated, so they should not be allowed to enter pens to pick up dead animals. Carcasses should be taken to a site at the edge of the farm where there is no danger of exposing livestock to the truck.

The effectiveness of *Salmonella* bacterins is somewhat controversial. There is little doubt that they are not fully protective, and the authors have seen outbreaks of salmonellosis in animals vaccinated with both autogenous and commercial bacterins. Experimentally, bacterins stimulate high levels of serum antibodies and increase the numbers of salmonellae required to cause clinical disease. Therefore, it seems likely that if coupled with sanitation measures to decrease the exposure level, bacterins would be beneficial, and many veterinarians do have the clinical impression that they are helpful. Several commercial *S. choleraesuis*, *S. typhimurium*, and *S. dublin* vaccines are available. Two modified live *S. choleraesuis* vaccines are also available. One is labeled for use in pigs 3 to 8 weeks old and is given by subcutaneous injection, and the other may be given intranasally or in the drinking water at 1 day or 3 weeks of age. Both seem to be effective. There are two commercially produced vaccines composed of core antigens that are common to all gram-nega-

tive bacteria. In a field study with 1000 calves, vaccination at 3 and 10 days of age with a core antigen vaccine significantly reduced mortality from salmonellosis after the calves were older than 1 month.

TREATMENT AND CONTROL

Treatment, especially treatment of the septicemic form, is often not very rewarding; therefore the focus of *Salmonella* control must be on prevention rather than treatment. The role of antibiotics in treatment of the enteric form is controversial, but antibiotics are indicated in cases of septicemia. The use of antibiotics for the treatment of enteric salmonellosis is considered by some to be contraindicated because in humans with enteric salmonellosis, antibiotic therapy does not decrease the severity or duration of diarrhea but it does increase the duration of *Salmonella* shedding. Documentation of either beneficial or deleterious effects of antibiotic therapy in natural cases of animal salmonellosis is lacking. Most studies have shown that if present in the feed when experimentally infected, antibiotics reduce diarrhea, weight loss, and the duration of shedding, but if added after experimental infection, the beneficial effects of antibiotics are reduced or absent. However, a few studies found that antibiotics in the feed increased the severity of clinical signs. Probably the most important effect of antibiotics in the treatment of enteric salmonellosis is that they appear to help reduce the spread and help prevent clinical disease in unaffected animals exposed to diarrheic animals. Because of the deleterious effects of endotoxin, parental use of glucocorticoids or nonsteroidal anti-inflammatory drugs for 1 to 2 days is sometimes advocated for the treatment of septicemic salmonellosis and appears to increase survival. Correction of acidosis and electrolyte loss can be helpful in animals valuable enough to be treated individually. In ruminants, switching to an easily digestible, high-roughage ration can be beneficial.

In 1995 to 1996, more than 90% of all swine *Salmonella* isolates at the Kansas State University Veterinary Diagnostic Laboratory were sensitive to ceftiofur, neomycin, apramycin, gentamicin, and enrofloxacin, and 80% to 90% of the isolates were sensitive to trimethoprim-sulfamethoxazole. Of 681 isolates of *S. choleraesuis* from Missouri, Nebraska, Indiana, and Kansas tested at the University of Missouri Diagnostic Laboratory, more than 90% of the isolates were sensitive to apramycin, neomycin, ceftiofur, gentamicin, trimethoprim-sulfamethoxazole, and enrofloxacin. Resistance to ampicillin, spectinomycin, sulfonamides, and oxytetracycline was evident. Although in vitro resistance to oxytetracycline is common, the combination of neomycin and oxytetracycline is reported to be more effective than either alone. Carbadox is also said to have good activity against salmonellae but has the disadvantage of a long withdrawal time. At Kansas State University, more than 90% of the bovine isolates were sensitive to apramycin, ceftiofur, enrofloxacin, and amikacin, and more than 70% of the isolates were sensitive to gentamicin and trimethoprim-sulfamethoxazole. Neomycin, apramycin, carbadox, and gentamicin are approved for use in the feed or drinking water of pigs, and the likelihood of susceptibility is high. Only neomycin is approved for oral use in cattle, but fewer than half of the Kansas State University isolates were sensitive. Ceftiofur is labeled for parental use in both species and should have a high likelihood of efficacy. Because of long withdrawal times, none of the aminoglycosides are approved in the United States for parental use in food-producing animals, and their use is discouraged by regulatory agencies and veterinary and producer groups. Currently, the extra-label usage of fluoroquinolones in food-producing animals is prohibited by the U.S. Food and Drug Administration, so the use of enrofloxacin or other fluoroquinolones in pigs and ruminants is illegal in the United States. In countries where their use is allowed or if in the future they are approved for use in the United States, fluoroquinolones should have good activity against salmonellae.

For successful control, the focus must be on limiting the outbreak and preventing future outbreaks. Salmonellosis is a multifactor disease with interplay between the agent, the animal, and the environment. Reduction of exposure to salmonellae and reduction of stressors are important. There is a direct relationship between the number of ingested salmonellae and the attack rate and severity of infection. Animals with active diarrhea shed the highest number of organisms; thus it is important to separate clinically ill animals. Buildings, feeders, and waterers should be cleaned and disinfected to reduce the number of organisms in the environment. A warm, dry, draft-free environment with clean water and high-quality feed should be provided and everything within reason done to reduce environmental stressors.

PUBLIC HEALTH CONCERNS

Salmonellosis is an important animal-borne disease of humans, and almost all serotypes are considered to be pathogenic for humans. Ingestion of contaminated food of animal origin is the most important method of transmission, but some outbreaks occur by direct contact with infected animals. The authors have seen several cases involving individuals caring for calves with salmonellosis and one case in a newborn infant born to a mother with *S. typhimurium* enterocolitis acquired from calves. Animal owners, caretakers, and veterinarians need to recognize the potential danger and take appropriate precautions to prevent animal-to-human spread.

Recent U.S. Department of Agriculture (USDA) surveys found that 18% of the hogs and 1% of the beef carcasses sampled at slaughter houses and 12% of the ground pork and 4% of the ground beef sampled at processing plants were culture positive for *Salmonella* spp. Another USDA survey found evidence of fecal shedding on 58 of 153 (38.2%) swine farms. This figure probably underestimates the prevalence of *Salmonella* spp. on farms because several studies have shown that the stress of shipping increases shedding and pigs and cattle that were culture negative on the farm will be culture positive after shipment to a slaughter house. Elimination or reduction of salmonellae in livestock is important to reduce the number of *Salmonella*-infected animals at abattoirs and help reduce the prevalence of contamination in food products. This is very important because with modern food processing procedures, huge quantities of food products are prepared and distributed widely, thus making it possible to infect thousands of people over large geographic areas, especially if the products are inadequately cooked or not cooked at all before ingestion. For example, dairy products are rarely infected with salmonellae because pasteurization kills the organism, but some of the largest outbreaks that affected several thousands of individuals have involved milk and ice cream that were contaminated after pasteurization. Proper food handling and hygiene are important for preventing cross-contamination of other food, and adequate cooking of all ground meat products is important to ensure their safety.

BIBLIOGRAPHY

Barber IK, Van Dreumel AA, Palmer N: Salmonellosis. *In* Jubb KV, Kennedy PC, Palmer N (eds): Pathology of Domestic Animals, vol 2, ed 4. San Diego, Academic Press, 1993, pp 213–227.
Bulgin MS, Anderson BC: Salmonellosis in goats. J Am Vet Med Assoc 178:720–723, 1981.
Harris IT, Fedorka-Cray PJ, Gray JT, et al: Prevalence of *Salmonella* organisms in swine feed. J Am Vet Med Assoc 210:382–385, 1997.
House JK, Smith BP, Dilling GW, et al: Enzyme-linked immunosorbent assay for serologic detection of *Salmonella dublin* carriers on a large dairy. Am J Vet Res 54:1391–1399, 1993.
Losinger WC, Wells SJ, Garber LP, et al: Management factors related to *Salmonella* shedding by dairy heifers. J Dairy Sci 78:2464–2472, 1995.
Pelzer KD: Salmonellosis (zoonosis update). J Am Vet Med Assoc 195:456–463, 1989.
Schwartz KJ: Salmonellosis in swine: Review/update. *In* Proceedings of the George A. Young Swine Conference and Annual Nebraska SPF Swine Conference. Lincoln, Neb, Aug 1–2, 1994, pp 6–11.
Scott P: Management of a salmonellosis outbreak in a cattle herd. In Practice 16:17–20, 1994.
Selim SA, Cullor JS, Smith BP, et al: The effect of *Escherichia coli* J5 and modified live *Salmonella dublin* vaccines in artificially reared neonatal calves. Vaccine 13:381–390, 1995.
Wray C, Sojka WJ: Reviews of the progress of dairy science: Bovine salmonellosis. J Dairy Res 44:383–425, 1977.

■ Anthrax

Derek A. Mosier, D.V.M., Ph.D.
M. M. Chengappa, D.V.M., Ph.D.

Anthrax is a highly fatal infectious disease caused by *Bacillus anthracis*. The disease occurs worldwide and affects many species of domestic and wild animals as well as humans. Of the food production animals, ruminants and pigs are most commonly affected.

ETIOLOGY AND EPIDEMIOLOGY

B. anthracis is a large, gram-positive, spore-forming rod. Spores are very resistant and can remain viable within soil for more than 15 years. The organism has limited capacity for growth in the environment but can grow in alkaline soil containing large amounts of organic matter. Growth is often facilitated by alternating periods of drought and rain and temperatures above 16°C. Although naturally contaminated soil is the primary reservoir of infection, outbreaks can also arise from fodder grown on contaminated soil, contaminated products of animal origin (e.g., bone meal), or contaminated water.

Outbreaks originating from soil-borne spores tend to follow periods of environmental change, such as heavy rainfall, flooding, or drought. During periods of drought, spores that have settled to the bottom of waterholes may become more accessible to animals drinking the contaminated water. Initial cases are usually caused by ingestion of spores in the environment or in contaminated feed. Subsequently, anthrax may be spread by contact with discharges from infected animals or by ingestion of contaminated carcasses. Pulmonary infection may sometimes occur as a result of inhalation of spore-laden dust, and cutaneous infection occasionally occurs in sheep. Biting insects can transmit spores mechanically, but this is not likely to be an important mode of infection.

Worldwide, serious outbreaks and persistence of spores are most common in tropical and subtropical areas. Within the United States anthrax has a regional distribution, with outbreaks having occurred in virtually every state. Outbreaks are most common in the late summer and fall, and are sometimes associated with sparse pasture and close grazing of coarse plants. Even in areas of endemic disease, anthrax occurs infrequently. Many years may elapse between sporadic cases and epizootics in high-risk areas. Multiple, small sporadic outbreaks are reported each year in the United States, but epizootics are uncommon.

The morbidity in an outbreak is variable, but mortality often exceeds 90%. Compared with cattle, sheep and goats are highly susceptible to infection, whereas swine are much more resistant.

Relative risk also varies with age (lambs and calves are seldom affected) and sex (bulls are more susceptible to infection than cows).

PATHOGENESIS

Spores at the initial site of infection pass through mucosal or epithelial barriers and enter the local lymphatics and lymph nodes. Lymphangitis and lymphadenitis occur, with vegetation and proliferation of the organisms in the lymph nodes. Subsequently, there is septicemia, which progresses from the lymphatics to the blood with deposition of the organisms throughout the body. Bacilli at primary and secondary sites of infection produce a complex of plasmid-encoded toxins that includes edema factor (EF or factor I), protective antigen (PA or factor II), and lethal factor (LF or factor III). Although these toxins have minimal effects individually, collectively they result in damage to phagocytes, increased vascular permeability, and inhibition of coagulation and complement activity. Additionally, the capsule of *B. anthracis* is antiphagocytic. Death generally results from shock, renal failure, and terminal anoxia.

CLINICAL SIGNS

In ruminants, sudden death is sometimes the first evidence of disease. Peracute death may occur within 1 to 2 hours of the onset of signs which include depression, listlessness, an abrupt onset of fever (42°C), increased heart and respiratory rates, respiratory distress, congested to cyanotic mucosa, and collapse and terminal convulsions. Animals surviving longer than 24 hours may also develop blood-tinged diarrhea and abdominal pain, and hematuria; pregnant animals may abort, milk production drops dramatically, and milk may be blood-tinged; and there can be edema of the perineum, throat, and abdominal wall. Affected cattle may rarely recover without treatment, but in sheep and goats infection is invariably fatal.

In swine the disease is similar to that in ruminants, except edematous swelling of the head and neck are much more common. The swelling may interfere with breathing and swallowing. Death can occur within 12 to 36 hours after the onset of clinical signs. However, some cases may persist for several days. Chronic infection localized to the tonsils and cervical lymph nodes is common. Subclinical infection may occur with localization of infection in pharyngeal and mesenteric lymph nodes.

PATHOLOGY

The carcasses of animals that die of anthrax putrify rapidly, become gas-distended, have minimal rigor mortis, and exude blood from natural orifices. The blood is dark, clots poorly, and flows freely from cut surfaces.

In cattle the spleen contains the most significant and consistent lesion, and in some cases it is the only recognizable lesion. The spleen is frequently greatly enlarged, dark, and soft, and exudes thick, black-red blood when incised. In some cases the spleen may rupture spontaneously. Other lesions may occur at the site of initial infection, including hemorrhagic to ulcerative enteritis, and less often, abomasitis and colitis. Infection that originates in the oropharynx can be associated with localized lymphadenitis and submandibular edema. Gelatinous edema is often present in the mesentery as a result of lymphangitis. Subserosal, intermuscular, and subcutaneous edema may also be present. Lymph nodes throughout the body can be edematous and hemorrhagic; this is most prominent in the lymph nodes at the initial site of infection (often the mesenteric lymph nodes).

Variably sized hemorrhages are common on the abdominal and thoracic serosa, as well as on the epicardium and endocardium. Serous to blood-tinged fluid is usually present in body cavities. Parenchymatous organs are congested and swollen.

In sheep and goats the course of disease is more rapidly progressive than in cattle and there are rarely local lesions. Splenic lesions are not as prominent as they are in cattle.

Lesions in pigs are most prominent at the initial site of infection. There can be pharyngitis with edematous swelling of the pharyngeal region and neck. The tonsils and cervical lymph nodes are large, red, and inflamed. Diphtheritic membranes or ulcers may develop over the surface of the tonsils. Hemorrhagic enteritis with regional lymphangitis and lymphadenitis can also occur. The organism does not often become septicemic in pigs, and splenic lesions are not extensive.

DIAGNOSIS

Anthrax may be confused with a wide range of diseases causing sudden death, including lightning strike, blackleg and other clostridial diseases, acute leptospirosis, peracute lead toxicity, and hypomagnesemia. If anthrax is suspected, complete necropsy of affected animals should be avoided to reduce environmental contamination and health risks to humans and other animals. A small amount of blood collected aseptically from a superficial vessel such as the jugular vein is the preferred diagnostic specimen. For shipment to the laboratory, the blood can be left in the syringe, which in turn should be enclosed in a leak-proof container. The blood can also be submitted to the laboratory as a dried specimen on a sterile swab or small piece of sterile cotton umbilical tape, or as thin smears on microscopic slides. In swine with localized disease, a small piece of affected lymphatic tissue that has been collected aseptically should be submitted. Tissue specimens other than dried blood should be shipped refrigerated or frozen. Blood smears should be obtained just before or soon after death for demonstration of organisms. Additionally, the organism is rapidly destroyed by putrefaction within a carcass, so tissue samples should be obtained as soon after death as possible.

Examination of blood smears from recently dead animals can provide a rapid, inexpensive tentative diagnosis. On Wright- or Giemsa-stained blood smears, *B. anthracis* appears as single- to short-chained bacilli with square ends. A bacterial capsule that stains pink with Giemsa or polychrome methylene blue stain is a distinguishing feature of the anthrax organism. More definitive diagnosis can be obtained by fluorescent antibody staining using anticapsular antibodies. Aerobic cultures of blood or infected tissues can be used to isolate and separate *B. anthracis* from other closely related organisms.

TREATMENT

Severely ill animals are unlikely to recover, but in the early stages of disease the infection responds well to antibiotic therapy. *B. anthracis* is highly susceptible to a number of antimicrobial agents, including penicillin, amoxicillin, erythromycin, chloramphenicol, gentamicin, streptomycin, and ciprofloxacin. Under field conditions penicillin and oxytetracycline have been reported most consistently as being therapeutically effective. The common recommended daily dose of penicillin for swine, sheep, and goats is 20,000 IU/kg daily; the daily dose for cattle is 5 to 10 million units. Therapy should be continued for at least 5 days, and the daily dose should be administered in two equal parts at 12-hour intervals for the first 2 days. In severely ill animals, the initial dose should be administered intravenously. The daily oxytetracycline dose, administered intravenously or intramuscularly, is 5 mg/kg for all species. The daily dose should be divided into two equal parts for the initial period of therapy, as with penicillin. Hyperimmune anthrax serum has been recommended for use in conjunction with antibiotic therapy in the face of outbreaks.

PREVENTION

Hygiene is the most important factor in preventing spread of the disease. Carcasses of animals that die of anthrax should be either burned completely or buried deeply (2 m of soil) to reduce environmental contamination. Putrefaction within the carcass destroys the bacteria, so if the carcass is unopened, environmental contamination is minimal. Covering the carcasses with a layer of quicklime (calcium oxide) at burial is often recommended, but the benefit of this procedure is unknown. Bedding and other contaminated material should also be burned or buried.

Vaccination can be an effective means of control in endemic areas. Most livestock vaccines used worldwide today for anthrax prevention are derived from the live toxigenic, nonencapsulated spore vaccine developed by Sterne in 1937. Annual vaccination of livestock in areas of endemic anthrax is recommended just prior to the season when outbreaks are expected. Immunity is considered to be due predominantly to the development of antibodies to the PA of *B. anthracis*, but cell-mediated immune responses are also believed to be important. Animals should not be vaccinated within 60 days of anticipated slaughter. Antibiotics should not be administered within 7 days of vaccination since the commonly used vaccines are live and depend on in vivo growth for their effectiveness.

Localized subcutaneous edema commonly develops within 24 hours at injection sites, may last for several days, and is sometimes severe. Localized anthrax at the site of injection with Sterne strain vaccine has been reported in llama calves. Progressive edema at the site of inoculation may occur in goats. Recent vaccine research using different adjuvants and antigen delivery systems may help to alleviate some of these side effects in future vaccines. Additionally, systems for oral delivery of vaccines have been investigated that could be beneficial for the prevention of anthrax in wild animal populations.

All outbreaks should be reported to local regulatory and public health officials. Quarantine should be placed on affected premises to prevent infected animals from being marketed. All susceptible livestock on affected and surrounding premises should be vaccinated. Prior to vaccination of dairy cattle at the time of an outbreak, the procedure required by state health authorities should be determined. If the outbreak is associated with a discrete source, such as contaminated bone meal, antibiotic treatment of exposed animals and removal of the source may be more effective than vaccination in reducing losses.

BIBLIOGRAPHY

Forshaw D, Higgs AR, Moir DC, et al: Anthrax in cattle in southern Western Australia. Aust Vet J 74:391–393, 1996.
Hunter L, Corbett W, Grindem C: Anthrax. J Am Vet Med Assoc 194:1028–1031, 1989.
Iacono-Connors LC, Welkos SL, Ivins BE, et al: Protection against anthrax with recombinant virus–expressed protective antigen in experimental animals. Infect Immun 59:1961–1965, 1991.
Ivins BE, Fellows P, Pitt L, et al: Experimental anthrax vaccines: Efficacy of adjuvants combined with protective antigen against an aerosol *Bacillus anthracis* spore challenge in guinea pigs. Vaccine 13:1779–1784, 1995.
Jubb KVF, PC Kennedy, N Palmer: Anthrax. *In* Pathology of Domestic Animals, ed 4, vol. 3. San Diego, Academic Press, 1993, pp 240–243.
Tuchili LM, Pandey GS, Sinyangwe PG, et al: Anthrax in cattle, wildlife and humans in Zambia. Vet Rec 132:487, 1993.
Turnbull PCB: Anthrax vaccines: Past, present and future. Vaccine 9:533–539, 1991.
Van Ness GB: Ecology of anthrax. Science 172:1303–1307, 1971.

■ Tetanus, Botulism, and Blackleg

Henry Staempfli, D.V.M., Diplomate, A.C.V.I.M. (Large Animals)
Olimpo Oliver, D.V.M., D.V.Sc., M.Sc.

Diseases caused by *Clostridium* spp. are still of considerable economic importance in farm animals. The ubiquitous presence of the organisms in soil and ingesta of animals makes eradication of diseases impossible. In almost all instances diseases caused by *Clostridium* may be prevented by vaccination. Polyvalent vaccines with up to seven key antigens are commercially available and highly effective.

TETANUS

In food animals, tetanus causes a generalized, or occasionally localized, hypertonia of the skeletal muscles, frequently accompanied by clonic paroxysmal muscular spasms. The disease occurs throughout the world but is more prevalent in tropical countries. The incidence and severity decrease, in the following order, from cattle and buffalo to camels, sheep, goats, and pigs. This variation is due to differences in species susceptibility and to a lesser extent to the ecology of *Clostridium tetani*. The organisms are commonly present in feces and are continuously shed into the environment, where they sporulate and persist for long periods. Tetanus usually occurs in sporadic, individual cases, but occasionally outbreaks occur in cattle, young pigs, and lambs. Mortality is high in younger ruminants. Adult cattle have a higher recovery rate, possibly due to higher circulating, naturally acquired antitoxin antibodies. In adult dairy cattle tetanus occurs most commonly as a postparturient complication following placental retention.

Etiology and Pathogenesis

C. tetani is a strictly anaerobic gram-positive bacterium. Infection most often results from contamination of a wound. Upon entrance into devitalized tissue with an anaerobic environment, *C. tetani* will convert to the vegetative form and produce toxin within 4 to 8 hours. The tetanus bacteria remain localized and do not commonly invade surrounding tissue. Tetanus toxin (tetanospasmin) is locally produced, diffuses to surrounding tissue, enters the lymphatics and blood (toxemia), and ascends retrogradely along axons to the spinal cord. It acts by irreversibly blocking the inhibitory synapses of the spinal cord motor neuron, resulting in overactivity of extensor muscles (clinical signs of extensor rigidity) and in uncontrolled stimulation of voluntary muscles. Death most often occurs by asphyxiation. In outbreaks, the tetanus bacteria may proliferate in the forestomachs of normal cattle to produce sufficient concentrations of toxin to produce clinical signs. The toxin may also be ingested in the feed and enter via wounds in the mouth.

Clinical Signs

The first signs usually occur after an incubation period of 1 to 3 weeks and include stiff gait, prolapse of the third eyelid, and trismus (lockjaw). The prolapse of the third eyelid can be accentuated by sudden lifting of the muzzle. With progression of signs, the stiffness becomes more obvious and involves the head, neck, all four extremities, and the tail. Other signs observed include an exaggerated response to external stimuli, erect ear carriage, and drooling of saliva. Regurgitation of food and water may be present due to laryngeal and pharyngeal spasm preventing normal deglutition. Secondary aspiration pneumonia is a potential sequela. At a later stage, the animals become dehydrated due to decreased water intake, hypersalivation, and profuse sweating. Temperature and heart rate are normal early in the course of the disease but rise when muscular tone is increased. Cattle may be mildly bloated as an early sign (esophagus: striated muscle) but maintain normal rumen motility (rumen: smooth muscle). As disease progresses there is great difficulty in walking and the animal may adopt the "sawhorse" posture. Tetanic convulsions, accompanied by opisthotonos, often occur following external stimuli.

Clinical Pathology and Necropsy

Serum muscle enzymes—aspartate aminotransferase (AST), creatine kinase (CK), and lactate dehydrogenase (LDH)—are likely to be elevated. Stress hyperglycemia may occur. Dehydrated cattle may become acidotic (loss of saliva) and may have elevated serum urea and creatinine (prerenal azotemia). No gross or histologic lesions are present in uncomplicated cases. Aspiration pneumonia, prolonged recumbency, and severe dehydration may lead to lesions in lungs, extremities, and kidneys.

Diagnosis

Clinical signs in well-advanced disease are related to spasms of voluntary muscles and are not usually confused with other diseases. Early cases should be differentiated from hypomagnesemic tetany, polioencephalomalacia, rabies, other cerebrospinal meningitides, lead poisoning, and enterotoxemia in lambs. In cattle the stiff gait in polyarthritis may be confused with tetanus. In enzootic muscular dystrophy there is usually no tetany. Attempts at measuring blood levels of tetanospasmin for confirmation of tetanus are often unsatisfactory. Tetanus can be confirmed bacteriologically by demonstrating *C. tetani* in an infected wound, if present.

Treatment

The goals of therapy include elimination of the local infection (wound debridement); parenteral and local procaine penicillin G 25,000 IU/kg b.i.d. for 3 to 5 days, then s.i.d. for another 5 days, or long-acting penicillin; neutralization of circulating toxin (1500 IU tetanus antitoxin subcutaneously [SC] s.i.d. for 3 to 5 days); and relaxation of muscle tetany (acetylpromazine 0.05 mg/kg intramuscularly [IM] b.i.d.; xylazine 0.1 to 0.33 mg/kg IM or 0.02 to 0.05 mg/kg intravenously [IV] b.i.d.) until severe signs subside (10 to 12 days). Supportive treatment is important by keeping the animals in a dark, quiet, and well-bedded stall. If recurrent bloat occurs a rumen fistula may be indicated. This allows temporary feeding and watering of the animal through the fistula. Recovery is a slow process (weeks to months).

Prevention

Proper skin and instrument disinfection at the time of castration, docking, and shearing could prevent many tetanus cases. Passive immunization with 1500 to 2000 IU tetanus antitoxin

in calves and 200 IU in lambs has reduced the incidence of disease after these procedures on tetanus-prone farms. The protection lasts only 10 to 14 days, and the toxoid, an aluminum-precipitated formalin-treated toxin, given IM at the same time but at a different site, gives immunity after 2 weeks, lasting at least 12 months. Prevention of tetanus in lambs is achieved by vaccinating ewes in the last 2 to 3 weeks of gestation and the lambs at 2 to 3 months of age. Vaccination of cattle is usually not indicated unless an outbreak of disease has occurred.

BOTULISM

Botulism is a disease characterized by fatal progressive flaccid paralysis of all voluntary muscles caused by the ingestion of botulinum toxin in contaminated food or water. Cattle, sheep, goats, and horses are more susceptible than pigs, dogs, and cats. The organism is a common inhabitant of the gastrointestinal tract of herbivores and other animals and may persist in the environment in its sporulated form for long periods. The source of toxin for animals is usually a dead animal (carrion), which may include decaying rodents; birds, including dead chickens in poultry manure; or other animals. Proliferation of *Clostridium botulinum* is also possible in decaying plant material (rotten hay and silage). Sporadic epizootics have been reported from many countries and in recent years have been associated with the feeding of poultry litter or its use on pasture, as well as silage bales. The disease is seasonal in range animals, occurring mainly during drought periods, when feed is sparse and animals have a depraved appetite due to phosphorus deficiency. Mortality in cattle is usually 90% to 95%.

Etiology and Pathogenesis

C. botulinum is a spore-forming anaerobic gram-positive rod, mainly proliferating in decaying animal and plant material. It is commonly found in soil samples and aquatic sediments. Different types (A–G) have been identified and different types predominate in different soils. The derivative toxins produced by the different serologic types are physically and chemically very similar to each other and are almost identical to tetanospasmin. Following ingestion, clinical signs appear after 24 to 48 hours. The toxin is absorbed as a protoxin and converted by endogenous gastrointestinal proteases into the active form. The paralysis follows a three-step event: (1) recognition of a receptor on the nerve ending and irreversible binding at that site; (2) internalization of a portion of the molecule into the nerve cell; and (3) the action of this internalized fragment to prevent acetylcholine release at the motor-neuronal junction. Only peripheral cholinergic synapses are affected. The animals die of respiratory paralysis.

Clinical Signs

The incubation period varies with the amount of ingested toxin and with individual susceptibility, and may last from days to weeks. Peracute cases may die without prior clinical signs. In most cases the disease is subacute and death ensues within 2 to 6 days.

Cattle

The first clinical signs are decreased tongue tone and problems with deglutition and prehension of food, followed by progressive muscular weakness until animals become recumbent in a parturient paresis-like posture. The tongue may protrude. Early weakness is usually manifested by ataxia and a stumbling gait affecting the hind legs first. Oral examination can be performed without resistance (decreased jaw tone), and there is ptosis and occasionally a delayed pupillary light reflex. Skin sensation is retained. In some cases there is no obvious impairment of deglutition and animals continue to eat until they die.

Sheep

Flaccid paralysis does not occur in sheep until late in the disease. There is stiffness in the gait. Salivation and serous nasal discharge are common.

Clinical Pathology and Necropsy

Marked indicanuria, glycosuria, and albuminuria have been observed in cattle but are not consistent findings. In peracute cases, toxin can be demonstrated in serum by mouse inoculation. Toxin is often not detected in the serum of subacute cases. Nonspecific changes in the serum biochemical profile may be seen in dehydrated recumbent animals. There are no specific changes at necropsy. Cattle that die often have a very dry omasum and a mild enteritis with congestion of intestinal mucosa. There may be nonspecific hemorrhages in the subendocardium and subepicardium. Perivascular hemorrhages have been reported in the corpus striatum and cerebrocortex.

Diagnosis

Diagnosis by demonstration of toxin is often impossible and therefore relies on the clinical manifestation and epidemiologic pattern of the cases. The veterinarian should look for a potential source of toxin, such as the presence of a carrion contaminating hay, silage, or water. Filtrates of the stomach and intestinal contents can be tested for the presence of toxins but are frequently negative. In epizootics, suspected feed material may be fed to susceptible animals to establish a diagnosis. Recumbent animals and findings at necropsy resemble cows with parturient paresis. Other differential diagnoses should include diseases of the central nervous system (CNS) and spinal cord such as the paralytic form of rabies; Aujeszky's disease; sporadic bovine encephalomyelitis (Buss's disease); listeriosis; polioencephalomalacia; lead poisoning; miscellaneous plant poisonings; and bovine spongiform encephalopathy (BSE, mad cow disease). In sheep, louping ill and some cases of scrapie and plant poisoning may be misdiagnosed as botulism.

Treatment

Treatment should only be attempted in subacute cases. Therapy is mainly symptomatic and should include fluid and nutritional support and general nursing care. Feeding potentially contaminated feeds should cease until the source of the toxin is established, the type of toxin identified, and the rest of the herd is vaccinated. Ruminal lavage, administration of lactic acid (50 to 80 mL lactic acid in 5 to 10 L of water per stomach tube in adult cattle), or purgatives have been suggested to remove or inactivate toxin in the intestinal tract. Polyvalent serum containing antibotulinum toxin antibodies (anti-C and -D mostly) may be tried in very early cases and in animals believed to be at risk, but once toxin is bound at the synapses it cannot be neutralized. Anticholinesterases such as neostigmine have been used with contradictory results. The type of toxoid for vaccina-

tion depends on results of mouse protection testing or the historical experience with a specific type in an endemic area.

Prevention

Control measures consist mainly of good husbandry: proper disposal of carcasses (especially in range cattle areas); avoiding the use of contaminated and spoiled feed (hay, silage); and supplementing phosphorus in deficient regions to prevent pica. In areas with enzootic disease, vaccination with a type-specific or bivalent vaccine (cattle: types C and D toxoid) is recommended. A single dose of vaccine gives good immunity after 2 weeks and lasts for about 24 months.

BLACKLEG

Blackleg is a peracute, noncontagious, highly fatal infection of skeletal muscle by *Clostridium chauvoei* (*C. feseri*) characterized by gaseous edema of muscles and severe toxemia. Causes of similar lesions include *C. septicum*, *C. novyi*, and *C. sordellii*. Blackleg is common in cattle and rarely seen in sheep. The infection is soil-borne but the portal of entrance into the body is still in dispute. The disease affects mainly young cattle (6 months to 2 years) on pastures in blackleg-prone regions. Most cases occur during the hot months of the year. Blackleg may cause considerable economic loss in endemic areas, with mortality approaching 100%, especially where there is frequent flooding.

Etiology and Pathogenesis

C. chauvoei and other agents of blackleg are anaerobic, motile, spore-forming organisms. The spores may survive for many years in the soil. Mixed infections are common. It is assumed that the portal of entry is the mucosa of the alimentary tract. The bacteria can be found in the spleen, liver, and alimentary tract of normal animals. The stimulus causing postulated "latent" spores to proliferate in muscle tissues is often unknown, but muscle trauma associated with transporting, herding, and handling has been incriminated to create suitable conditions in the muscle to allow bacterial multiplication and myonecrosis. Several toxic compounds (cytolysins, necrotizing enzymes) are produced by *C. chauvoei*, causing severe local damage and widespread organ dysfunction.

Clinical Signs
Cattle

Peracute affected animals are often found dead. The incubation period is 1 to 3 days. Prior to local signs there is depression, anorexia, rumen stasis, high fever (41 to 42°C), and tachycardia (>100 beats per minute). These early signs are usually followed by marked lameness with pronounced muscle swelling of the upper part of the affected leg. Lesions can also occasionally be found on the base of the tongue, brisket, and the udder. There is regional lymphadenopathy. The developing edema shows crepitus on palpation and tympanic sounds on percussion. The skin is often discolored in affected areas. On cut section a serosanguineous rancid fluid appears, and gas escapes.

Sheep

Subcutaneous edema is uncommon and crepitation is often absent. There is high fever, anorexia, and depression, followed by rapid death. The first clinical signs observed are lameness, often involving multiple limbs.

Clinical Pathology and Necropsy

Culture, cytology, and Gram's stain may be attempted on fine-needle aspirates of affected tissues. Large numbers of gram-positive spore-forming rods are seen. Serum enzymes derived from skeletal muscle (CK, AST, LDH) are significantly elevated. Terminally sick animals have secondary complications like toxemia and hypovolemia. Clotting of blood occurs rapidly. For necropsy, cadavers must be fresh to avoid the rapid local infiltration of other clostridial organisms which might confuse the bacteriologic diagnosis. On necropsy, affected areas (connective tissues and muscles) are filled with rancid serosanguineous fluid and gas pockets which crepitate when squeezed. The affected muscles appear dry, showing red and black areas with islands of necrosis. Toward the periphery of the lesion the muscle is dark red in color and moist with edema fluid. There is lymphadenopathy. Spleen and liver often look normal but may show gaseous distention. Secondary findings include pulmonary edema, degenerated heart muscle, and some degree of degeneration in the other solid organs. To detect localized lesions it is important to examine all skeletal muscles of the carcass, including the tongue and diaphragm.

Diagnosis

Isolation and identification of *C. chauvoei* and related clostridia is quite demanding, whereas detection by immunofluorescence is relatively simple using commercially available conjugated antisera. Clinically, and on gross necropsy, malignant edema should be ruled out. The epidemiology (local incidence, season, age group, pasture environment) and bacterial confirmation are therefore crucial. Anthrax and lightning strike do not show the typical gaseous edemas. Necropsy findings in bacillary hemoglobinuria are very similar.

Treatment

Treatment is often too late. Large doses of penicillin (20,000 IU/kg b.i.d.) are given to animals that are not moribund. Local antibiotic treatment in affected areas has been attempted. Drainage and slashing of affected tissue to allow oxygen into the tissue may be tried to save individual animals. Supportive treatment (parenteral fluids, analgesics, etc.) is crucial.

Prevention

On farms and in regions where the disease is endemic, annual vaccination of cattle between 6 months and 2 years should be performed shortly before expected epizootics (spring, summer). The formalin-killed, aluminum-precipitated bacterin from a local strain of *C. chauvoei* is the best. Early vaccination (age 3 weeks) with subsequent revaccination has been recommended on disease-prone farms. Immunity develops after 2 weeks, but morbidity and mortality may continue for some time in outbreak situations. The incidence may be reduced by prophylactic antibiotic treatments (penicillin 10,000 IU/kg IM s.i.d.) for up to 2 weeks. Movement from affected pastures is recommended. In sheep less than 1 year old, good immunity does not develop postvaccination, and it is suggested that young first-lambing ewes be vaccinated 3 weeks before parturition. This will provide permanent protection for the adult animals and passive protection of lambs up to 3 weeks. In sheep multivalent clostridial vaccines are preferred. Carcasses of animals should be destroyed by burning or deep burial in safe nonpasture areas to limit soil contamination.

BIBLIOGRAPHY

Hariharan H, Mitchell WR: Type C botulism: The agent host spectrum and environment. Vet Bull 47:95–100, 1977.
Rings DM: Bacterial meningitis and diseases caused by bacterial toxins. Vet Clin North Am Food Anim Pract 3:85–98, 1987.
Stogdale L, Booth AJ: Bacillary hemoglobinuria in cattle. Compend Contin Educ Pract Vet 6:S284–S290, 1984.
Wallis AS: Some observations of the epidemiology of tetanus in cattle. Vet Rec 75:188–191, 1963.

▪ Bacillary Hemoglobinuria, Braxy, and Black Disease

Olimpo Oliver, D.V.M., D.V.Sc., M.Sc.
Henry Staempfli, D.V.M., Diplomate, A.C.V.I.M.

BACILLARY HEMOGLOBINURIA

Bacillary hemoglobinuria (BHU) is an acute, toxemic, and highly fatal clostridial disease with the liver being the main target organ. The disease occurs worldwide, is sporadic, and most commonly affects cattle, and occasionally sheep and pigs. In North America it is seen more commonly during the summer and early fall. BHU occurs more frequently in areas where fascioliasis is a problem and is spread from infected areas to noninfected areas by flooding, natural drainage, contaminated feed, or carrier animals. In the United States BHU occurs predominantly in poorly drained pastures, particularly where the soil is alkaline (pH 8.0 or higher). Bacillary hemoglobinuria is rare in calves less than 1 year old and in cattle with poor body condition. On endemic farms the mortality averages 5% but mortality rates up to 25% have been observed in outbreaks among feedlot cattle.

Etiology and Pathogenesis

BHU is caused by *Clostridium hemolyticum*. It is a soil-borne anaerobe. The organism has been successfully isolated from the bone of dead animals up to 1 year after death. *C. hemolyticum* produces several exotoxins, with β-toxin being mainly responsible for the tissue damage. The infection results from ingestion, and in some instances from inhalation, of the clostridial spores, which are then absorbed and transported via blood to the liver. Once in the liver, the spores may remain latent for an indefinite time and may be isolated from healthy cattle. It has been difficult to determine the natural incubation period of the disease, but from experimental and observational evidence, it seems that local hepatic injury is necessary to trigger the onset. It has been suggested that telangiectasis, necrobacillosis, fascioliasis, or *Cysticercus tenuicollis* is the triggering factor causing local anaerobic conditions for germination of dormant spores. Once spore germination occurs there is local production of exotoxins, causing severe hepatic necrosis and local thrombosis. With the increasing concentrations of exotoxin in the blood, erythrolysis ensues, producing acute hemolytic anemia and hemoglobinuria. β-Toxin also causes endothelial damage of arterioles throughout the body with extravasation of blood in the tissue and body cavities.

Clinical Signs

Animals with peracute disease die before any signs have been noted. In acute cases, the animals stand separated from the rest of the herd and appear very ill. The back is arched, and the abdomen is "tucked up." Appetite, lactation, rumination, and defecation suddenly cease. Animals are reluctant to move and have to be forced to walk. Grunting occurs when walking. Tachycardia, tachypnea, and weak pulse are present. Fever (40 to 41°C) is prominent throughout the clinical disease with subnormal temperature being observed terminally. Initially there is frequent passage of small amounts of bile-stained feces, often later progressing to diarrhea. The urine is dark red with no erythrocytes present, jaundice may be observed, and anemia may be severe. The duration of the clinical syndrome is 18 to 36 hours. Death occurs as a consequence of the severe hemolytic anemia and toxemia. Mortality in untreated animals reaches 95%.

Clinical Pathology and Necropsy

Anemia with a hematocrit as low as 0.10 L/L (10%) is frequently observed and the erythrocyte count is low and may reach values as low as 1 million cells per microliter. Hemoglobin can also drop to 35 g/L. The white blood cell count is highly variable; the urine is red in color and contains hemoglobin. Blood culture may be positive. Necropsy findings are characterized by subcutaneous edema, petechiae, and diffuse hemorrhages throughout the body. The pleural and peritoneal cavities contain large quantities of hemoglobin-stained transudate. Hemorrhagic abomasitis and enteritis may be present. Red urine is found in the bladder, the lungs are edematous, and bronchi are filled with a blood-tinged foam. Large hepatic infarcts are always present and are pathognomonic. They vary from 5 to 25 cm in diameter and are pale and conical in shape on cut surface and often surrounded by a reddish zone of congestion. Histologically, the necrotic liver tissue is sharply demarcated from the unaffected tissue by a wide band of bacteria and a mild leukocytic infiltrate. *C. hemolyticum* can be consistently isolated from heart blood, the liver infarct, and sometimes from other organs of fresh carcasses. Postmortem invaders may obscure its presence.

Diagnosis

Clinical diagnosis of BHU is mainly obtained by excluding other causes of hemoglobinuria. Peracute disease is difficult to diagnose. Appropriate specimens from dead animals should be collected, especially those tissues showing pathologic lesions. BHU can be confused with acute leptospirosis, postparturient hemoglobinuria, and hemolytic anemia caused by cruciferous plants, including rape or kale. The plant-induced hemoglobinurias are not usually accompanied by severe febrile reactions.

Babesiosis and anaplasmosis are geographically limited and protozoal parasites can be detected in peripheral blood smears. Pyelonephritis, enzootic hematuria, and cystitis have intact red blood cells in urine. Chronic copper poisoning, especially in sheep, is differentiated postmortem by the absence of liver infarcts.

Causes of sudden death in cattle and sheep, as in anthrax, blackleg, and infectious necrotic hepatitis, have to be differentiated from BHU, especially when terminal hematuria occurs.

Treatment

If treatment is attempted, 500 to 1000 mL of *C. hemolyticum* antitoxin should be administered along with specific antibiotics:

procaine penicillin (20,000 IU/kg IM, b.i.d.) or tetracycline (10 mg/kg IV or IM s.i.d.). The response to antibiotic treatment without the antitoxin is poor. Supportive treatments with blood transfusions, parenteral fluid, and electrolytes may help to control the hemolytic anemia and dehydration. Animals should be kept in a quiet environment to avoid additional stress. Bulls should not be used for service up to 3 weeks after recovery because of the danger of liver rupture and hemorrhage. Vitamins and iron should be administered to recovering animals.

Prevention

BHU can be prevented by the use of vaccination. The vaccine can be administered at any age, but it is recommended that it be used at 6 months of age and again within 3 to 4 weeks, with annual boosters in low-exposure areas and boosters every 6 months in high-exposure areas. Multiway clostridial vaccines include *C. hemolyticum* and are efficacious. In low-prevalence areas, vaccination may not be economically reasonable.

BRAXY

Braxy is a rare acute hemorrhagic abomasitis of sheep caused by *Clostridium septicum* and is associated with toxemia and high mortality (about 50%). The disease is mostly seen in the winter in animals eating frozen silage or hay. The age groups most commonly affected are weaned to yearling sheep. The disease occurs worldwide but appears to be rare in North America. A similar syndrome has been reported in one beef calf.

Etiology and Pathogenesis

C. septicum, a soil-borne organism and probably a normal commensal in the gastrointestinal tract of sheep, invades the abomasal wall under favorable conditions, causing severe abomasitis and toxemia.

Clinical Signs

The course of braxy is peracute. There is sudden onset of depression, segregation from the group, and high fever, with death ensuing within hours. There may be signs of colic and abdominal distention.

Clinical Pathology and Necropsy

Antemortem laboratory tests are of little value. Major changes are observed in the abomasal wall and include congestion of mucosa with areas of necrosis, gas accumulation, and ulceration. Histologically there is acute severe transmural abomasitis. Besides changes associated with toxemia, there are no other histologic lesions present.

Diagnosis

Because of the acute nature of the disease, clinical diagnosis is very difficult. Grain overload may produce similar signs but there are no lesions in the abomasum at necropsy. The syndrome resembles infectious necrotic hepatitis but lacks the liver lesions. Diagnosis is established by direct isolation of *C. septicum* from abomasal tissue or by demonstrating the organism by immunofluorescence on frozen abomasal sections of smears.

Treatment

No treatment of value has been reported.

Prevention

In areas where the problem is prevalent, prophylactic vaccination with formalin-killed whole culture of *C. septicum* given 2 weeks apart has proved to be very effective.

BLACK DISEASE

Black disease (infectious necrotic hepatitis) is a peracute, highly fatal clostridial disease occurring in sheep and cattle, and occasionally in pigs. Horses and goats may also be affected. Black disease has a worldwide distribution. A close association between black disease and fascioliasis has been established. There is a marked seasonal occurrence in the summer and the disease occurs in well-nourished adult sheep between 2 and 4 years of age. Fecal contamination of pasture, infected carcasses, and flooding are the main sources of infection. The infection is also spread by birds and wild animals. In sheep, the morbidity is about 5% with up to 50% being reported.

Etiology and Pathogenesis

Black disease is caused by *Clostridium novyi* type B and a concurrent hepatic insult, most commonly due to *Fasciola hepatica*. The disease has been reproduced in sheep by administration of spores to animals previously infected with fluke metacercariae. *Cysticercus tenuicollis* has also been implicated as another possible factor in precipitating hepatic insult. The spores of *C. novyi* are ingested and transported to the liver where they may remain dormant or proliferate in injured anoxic liver tissue. *C. novyi* type B usually produces α- and β-exotoxin, causing hepatic necrosis, toxemia (mostly α-toxin), and often death.

Clinical Signs

Sheep or cattle with black disease are frequently found dead without preceding signs of disease. Clinically affected animals tend to separate from the flock, are unwilling to move, and may fall if driven. Early in the disease body temperature is increased (40 to 42°C) but tends to fall to normal or subnormal levels in moribund animals. There is tachypnea, and sheep usually remain in sternal recumbency and may even die in this posture. The course of the clinical disease is very short (hours). The clinical findings in cattle are similar to those in sheep, but the course is usually longer (1 to 2 days). New cases may occur up to 9 weeks after removal from fluke-infested pastures or up to 14 days after vaccination is initiated.

Clinical Pathology and Necropsy

Antemortem laboratory tests are rarely possible because of the peracute course. The carcass undergoes very rapid putrefaction. Subcutaneous blood vessels are engorged and cause the carcass to blacken (hence black disease). Varying amounts of fluid are present in the pericardial sac and pleural and peritoneal cavity. Hemorrhages of the endocardium are a consistent finding. There is a generalized engorgement of the liver with areas of necrosis 1 to 2 cm in diameter, surrounded by a zone of hyper-emia. Hepatic necrosis is most frequently subcapsular in the diaphragmatic lobe and consists of a central zone of necrosis surrounded by leukocytes and large numbers of clostridia.

Diagnosis

The diagnosis is based on the history and postmortem findings. The lesions are often unremarkable and, if there is considerable damage by *Fasciola* spp, the diagnosis may be very difficult. Definitive diagnosis is reached by demonstration of the organism in the lesion or preformed mouse lethal toxin. Bacteria are easily identified in smears of hepatic tissue by immunofluorescence. Other causes of sudden death, such as clostridial infections (enterotoxemia, bacillary hemoglobinuria, and blackleg) and anthrax, should be considered. In sheep, acute facioliasis can cause heavy mortalities with a postmortem finding similar to that in black disease. Therefore laboratory diagnosis is necessary for a definite diagnosis.

Treatment

There is no effective treatment available. The longer course in cattle may allow the use of broad-spectrum antibiotics or penicillin.

Prevention

Based on the epidemiology of black disease, control can be effected by eliminating fascioliasis. Vaccination with aluminum-precipitated toxoid is highly effective even in the face of an outbreak. It is recommended that the initial vaccination be repeated 3 to 4 weeks later with annual boosters on problem farms.

BIBLIOGRAPHY

Bagadi HO: Infectious necrotic hepatitis (black disease) of sheep. Vet Bull 44:385–388, 1974.

■ Clostridial Enterotoxemia (*Clostridium perfringens*)

J. Glenn Songer, Ph.D.

Clostridium perfringens is ubiquitous in the environment and can be isolated from the alimentary tract of most healthy animals. Disease results when the organism proliferates and produces one or more toxins.

The species is divided into five types by assessment of the ability to produce four major toxins. Type A produces α-toxin; type B produces α-, β-, and ε -toxins; type C produces α- and β-toxins; type D produces α- and ε-toxins; and type E produces α- and ι-toxins. Types A, C, and D are common causes of enterotoxemia in the United States and elsewhere. Type E is uncommon in the United States, and type B is almost nonexistent.

TYPE A ENTEROTOXEMIA

Strains of type A are common causes of wound contamination, anaerobic cellulitis, and gas gangrene, but they also cause enteric disease. Lamb enterotoxemia (*yellow lamb disease*) occurs primarily in the spring in the western United States. Clinical signs include dyspnea, depression, anemia, and hemoglobinuria, but icterus, evident on all mucous membranes, is the predominant feature. Diarrhea is uncommon, and most animals die of an acute hemolytic crisis following a clinical course of 6 to 12 hours. Morbidity rates may reach 30% or more, and the case fatality rate may be close to 100%. The kidneys are darkened and the spleen is edematous; the liver is enlarged, pale, and friable. Fluid accumulates in the pericardial and peritoneal cavities, and large numbers of *C. perfringens* organisms are often present in intestinal contents.

In calves, the disease may be similar to, although much less severe than, that in lambs. It usually occurs sporadically, but the incidence may be as high as 50%. In calves, an acute abdominal syndrome may develop, the hallmark of which is tympany, often with colic, abomasitis, and abomasal ulceration and occurring with or without diarrhea and sudden death. Gram-positive bacilli are often present on the mucosa and in the submucosa, and isolates of *C. perfringens* from some of these cases produce enterotoxin.

Suckling and feeder pigs can have mild necrotizing enterocolitis and villous atrophy, with type A as a proposed etiologic agent. The small intestine is usually most severely affected, and cultures yield luxuriant growth of *C. perfringens*. A role for a toxin in the pathogenesis of enteric lesions has been proposed, but evidence supporting this contention is equivocal.

TYPE B ENTEROTOXEMIA

C. perfringens type B is the etiologic agent of dysentery in newborn lambs. Isolates of type B are relatively rare in North America, but disease is common in the border country between England and Scotland and in Wales, South Africa, and the Middle East.

Lamb dysentery typically occurs during the first few days of life, although involvement of older lambs is not uncommon. Chronic disease (called *pine*) in older lambs is manifested as chronic abdominal pain without diarrhea, and the disease in calves is similar but less severe, with a clinical course of 2 to 4 days. In typical lamb dysentery, the organism is acquired from the dam or the environment and increases in number in the gut, especially in lambs suckling heavily lactating ewes. Enterotoxemia follows, accompanied by hemorrhage and ulceration of the mucosa of the small intestine. Cessation of feeding, depression, abdominal pain, bloody diarrhea, recumbency, coma, and death less than 24 hours after onset are common. The incidence is often as high as 30%, with case fatality rates approaching 100%.

The most prominent lesion is extensive hemorrhagic enteritis, with ulceration and necrosis of the mucosa. The peritoneal cavity often contains hemorrhagic fluid, the liver is usually enlarged and friable, and the mediastinal lymph nodes are generally enlarged.

TYPE C ENTEROTOXEMIA

Infections by *C. perfringens* type C have been reported in humans and most domestic animals worldwide. Newborn animals are most susceptible, perhaps because of ready colonization of the gut by *C. perfringens* in the absence of well-established normal intestinal flora. Alteration of the flora by sudden dietary changes may provoke type C infection.

Peracute disease is common in piglets 1 to 2 days of age. Depression is followed by diarrhea and dysentery, with blood and necrotic debris in the feces. The intestinal surface is often dark red, with gas in the tissue, hemorrhagic exudate in the lumen, and hemorrhagic necrosis of the mucosa, submucosa, and muscularis mucosa. As many as 10^9 colony-forming units of *C. perfringens* type C can be isolated from each gram of intestinal contents. Morbidity rates may be 30% to 50%, with case fatality rates of 50% to 100%, often with a clinical course lasting less than 24 hours. Piglets affected at 1 to 2 weeks of age usually have a longer clinical course, with nonbloody, yellowish diarrhea and necrosis of the jejunal mucosa. Sows are probably a source of the infection for newborn pigs, but numbers of type C organisms in sow feces may be too low to be detected by culture.

Similar disease occurs in neonatal calves, lambs, and goats. Hemorrhagic, necrotic enteritis and enterotoxemia, often accompanied by abdominal pain, develop in vigorous, healthy calves usually less than 10 days old. In lambs the disease resembles lamb dysentery and is often accompanied by nervous signs such as tetany and opisthotonos. Death may be peracute, but it may also follow a clinical course of several days. Morbidity rates are 15% to 20%, with case fatality rates approaching 100%.

Hemorrhagic inflammation of the jejunum and ileum is the most striking feature of the disease in young animals. The peritoneal cavity often contains serohemorrhagic fluid, and petechial hemorrhages are common on serosal surfaces and in the spleen, thymus, heart, meninges, and brain.

Adult sheep can be affected by type C enterotoxemia, colorfully named *struck* after the rapid death associated with the condition, which often leaves the impression that the animal has been struck by lightning. Damage to the gastrointestinal mucosa, frequently caused by poor-quality feed, is followed by multiplication of type C in the abomasum and small intestine. Subsequently there is mucosal necrosis, usually without dysentery or diarrhea. The peritoneum may contain a large volume of serous fluid; peritoneal vessels are congested and peritoneal hemorrhage may occur. The small intestine may contain areas of mucosal necrosis, and jejunal ulceration is common. Pleural and pericardial transudates provide additional evidence of acute toxemia.

β-Toxin plays a central role in the pathogenesis of type C infections. In pigs, type C organisms adhere to jejunal mucosa, eventually resulting in widespread mucosal necrosis. Mucosal necrosis is progressive, with epithelial cell death and desquamation followed by further bacterial invasion, multiplication, and more toxin production. β-Toxin acts initially in the jejunum under conditions of curtailed proteolytic activity. Pancreatic secretion deficiency shortly after birth or ingestion of protease inhibitors, which compromises the detoxification process, may be responsible. Intestinal lesions can be impressive in extent and severity, but death is probably ultimately due to β-toxemia. Similarities of *cpb*, the gene for β-toxin, to the genes for staphylococcal α- and γ-toxins and leukocidin strengthen suggestions that β-toxin may affect the central nervous system.

TYPE D ENTEROTOXEMIA

Type D strains cause enterotoxemia (sudden death, overeating, or pulpy kidney disease) in sheep of all ages beyond the neonatal period. Although most prevalent in 3- to 10-week-old lambs suckling heavily lactating ewes, enterotoxemia is also a significant cause of death in weaned animals up to 10 months of age, usually those fed rich grain rations in feedlots. Disease often follows upsets in the gut flora resulting from sudden changes in diet or continuous feeding of high levels of feed concentrates. Rapid multiplication of type D organisms and production of ε-toxin is favored by the presence of excess dietary starch in the small intestine; ε-toxin facilitates its own absorption.

Petechial and ecchymotic hemorrhages are present on the

serosal surfaces of the rumen, abomasum, and duodenum and in the diaphragm and abdominal muscles. Excess pericardial fluid and hemorrhage of the epicardium and endocardium are common. The term *pulpy kidney* is derived from the postmortem autolysis that occurs rapidly in hyperemic kidney tissue damaged by ε-toxin. Hyperglycemia and glycosuria are considered by some to be pathognomonic for type D enterotoxemia.

A primary target of toxin is the central nervous system, where it produces foci of liquefactive necrosis, perivascular edema, and hemorrhage, especially in the meninges. The extent of neurologic signs, including incoordination, convulsions, and sudden death, is directly related to the severity of the lesions. Focal encephalomalacia is probably a chronic manifestation of enterotoxemia. Affected sheep are often blind and demonstrate head pressing and an inability to eat.

Type D enterotoxemia is also important in calves and goats and occasionally occurs in adult cattle, deer, domesticated camels, and horses. In goats, catarrhal, fibrinous, or hemorrhagic enterocolitis is a consistent lesion, and the classic pulpy kidney is absent.

TYPE E ENTEROTOXEMIA

Type E may cause about 1% of all cases of enterotoxemia in calves, and disease has also been reported in lambs and rabbits. Calves die acutely, and necropsy reveals hemorrhagic enteritis.

DIAGNOSIS OF ENTEROTOXEMIA

Key components in the diagnosis of enterotoxemia are evaluation of clinical signs and gross and microscopic lesions, bacteriologic culture of appropriate specimens, and detection of toxins in pathologic specimens and in supernatant fluids of pure cultures. Demonstration of toxins by in vivo assays has become less common because of the expense, variability of results, and undesirability, on humanitarian grounds, of the traditional mouse and guinea pig assays. There are recent reports of immunoassays for enterotoxemia-associated toxins of *C. perfringens*, but these methods are not in widespread use. The use of gene probes or polymerase chain reaction assays for the detection of toxigenic *C. perfringens* in affected animals is gaining acceptance as an adjunct to diagnosis. Polymerase chain reaction allows rapid genotyping of isolates, and the correlation of genotype with phenotype is nearly 100%.

TREATMENT AND PREVENTION

Prophylaxis in swine by the use of bacitracin has been effective, and in individual animals, therapy with hyperimmune antiserum may be of value for up to 3 weeks. However, the course of enterotoxemia is usually rapid, so immunoprophylaxis is of greatest importance. Commercial multivalent toxoids or bacterin/toxoids are typically administered semiannually. Immunization of sows during gestation is ordinarily followed in about 2 weeks by protective levels of antibodies in colostrum and can yield more than 10-fold reductions in the mortality of piglets. Ewes may be vaccinated against infection by types B, C, or D, depending on the locale. Serum antibodies against ε-toxin prevent the death of goats from toxemia but provide little protection against enterocolitis. No biologics currently licensed in the United States make a label claim for protection against enterotoxemias caused by type A.

BIBLIOGRAPHY

Daube G, Simon P, Limbourg B, et al: Hybridization of 2,659 *Clostridium perfringens* isolates with gene probes for seven toxins (alpha, beta, epsilon, iota, theta, mu, and enterotoxin) and for sialidase. Am J Vet Res 57:496–501, 1996.

Songer JG: Clostridial enteric diseases of domestic animals: A review. Clin Microbiol Rev 9:216–234, 1996.

■ Streptococcal Disease

John F. Timoney, D.Sc., Ph.D., M.V.B.
E. Denis Erickson, D.V.M., Ph.D.

Streptococcal infections are major sources of economic loss to the dairy cattle and swine industries. Sporadic infections of sheep and goats also occur but are generally of minor significance. Recent advances in taxonomy have resulted in changes in the nomenclature of some members of the Lancefield group C and G streptococci that cause disease in these hosts, and these will be mentioned in the appropriate sections of the text. Although polymerase chain reaction based on 16S rRNA and other gene sequences is the most accurate and rapid means of identifying streptococci, serologic grouping and biochemical typing continue to be the commonly available identification methods. The emphasis in this chapter will be on those streptococcal diseases of food animals that are common and economically important.

DISEASE OF RUMINANTS

Streptococcal infections of sheep and goats occur sporadically and are associated with mastitis in adults and with septicemia, meningoencephalitis, septic arthritis, and otitis media in the young. Bovine streptococcal infections other than mastitis are also of relatively minor importance. Incidental and opportunistic infections of various organ systems may occur but do not represent well-defined syndromes with a consistent primary streptococcal etiology. Respiratory and genital infections as well as abscesses in a variety of locations have been described. Streptococcal species, including *Streptococcus dysgalactiae* subsp. *dysgalactiae*, *S. zooepidemicus*, *S. pneumoniae*, and various α-hemolytic and nonhemolytic streptococci, may be involved. Streptococcal infections of the udder are a very significant veterinary problem and source of economic loss.

Mastitis of Cattle

Streptococcal infections of the udder are either contagious (*S. agalactiae*) and transmitted from cow to cow by fomites, including the milker's hands, milking machines, and the mouths of sucking calves, or are opportunistic (non-*agalactiae*) and derived from the cow's surroundings or its skin. It therefore follows that the streptococcal species involved in an outbreak of mastitis has a profound influence on the strategy and outcomes of control programs.

Etiology

Bovine mastitis may be caused by several species of streptococci, *S. agalactiae*, *S. dysgalactiae* (Lancefield groups B and C), and *S. uberis* being the most common. Other streptococci, including *S. pyogenes*, *S. zooepidemicus*, *S. pneumoniae*, and *S. parauberis*, have been implicated in sporadic cases. Various α-hemolytic streptococci are readily isolated from the skin and teat canal of cows, but their pathogenicity is uncertain.

S. agalactiae, despite its susceptibility to several common antibiotics, still exists in herds in which mastitis control procedures have not been adopted. The infected udder is the usual reservoir for transmission of infections to healthy animals. Heifer calves may become infected by ingesting mastitic milk and may then transfer infection by cross-suckling other calves with which they are housed. *S. agalactiae* can be carried by some adult human beings and may cause serious disease in infants. Although human isolates can produce bovine mastitis under experimental conditions, cows are not regarded as a source of human infection.

Mastitis results when organisms reach sufficient numbers at the teat end, cross the teat canal, adhere to host epithelial cells, and multiply in the gland. Once the infection reaches the acinar level of the ductular system, bacteria penetrate below the secretory epithelium and cause an acute exudative neutrophilic reaction. In later stages a mononuclear cell infiltration develops in areas of chronic inflammation. Fibrosis and scar tissue develop and, along with cellular debris, cause obstruction of the ductular system and progressive loss in production, particularly for *S. agalactiae* infections.

Clinical Signs

Infections by *S. agalactiae* are usually mild, subclinical, and slowly progressive and cause fibrosis and atrophy of glandular tissue. Opportunistic, environmentally derived infections by other streptococci tend to produce acute local inflammation with pain, swelling, abnormal milk, and a systemic reaction, but they may also cause chronic mastitis. Chronic subclinical mastitis may be detectable by cowside tests that detect inflammatory cells (California mastitis test), by changes in the electrical conductivity of foremilk, or by laboratory analysis.

Diagnosis

Although mastitis must be viewed as a herd problem, careful clinical examination of individual animals is necessary. In addition to the obvious signs of acute mammary inflammation and abnormal milk, examination of the udder may reveal damaged teat ends associated with improper milking equipment, freezing, or trauma. Resolution of the mastitis outbreak will occur only after correction of these predisposing problems or risk factors.

The herd evaluation should include a thorough laboratory analysis of the milk, including a determination of the herd somatic cell count and microbiologic analysis of bulk tank milk. Further analysis should include regular testing of all lactating quarters with the California mastitis test or a similar system for detection of elevated leukocyte numbers. Although microbiologic analysis of all quarters is ideal, much information on the infections within a herd can be obtained by sampling a proportion of the quarters that score greater than trace on the California mastitis test.

Treatment

Treatment of mastitis should include good nursing care of the cow and udder, provision of locally and parenterally administered antibiotics and other supportive treatment, and prevention of reinfection or superinfection. Subclinical mastitis is best treated at drying off by using a slow-release formulation to maintain high levels of antibiotic for extended periods of time. Even though many dairy workers abhor the chore, nursing care, particularly frequent stripping of affected quarters, is a first step to recovery. The goal for *S. agalactiae*–infected herds is eradication of the infection. *S. dysgalactiae* and *S. uberis* are present on the skin or in the environment and are less amenable to eradication from the herd. Although *S. agalactiae* is usually sensitive to penicillin, the susceptibility patterns of other streptococcal udder pathogens are much less predictable; therefore it is valuable to monitor these patterns by antibiotic susceptibility testing. For intramammary infusion, only sterile, properly formulated products prepared by licensed commercial drug manufacturers should be used. Too often, hand-mixed preparations in multidose containers are found in dairies. These preparations and the method in which they are used are often the source of new udder infections. Intramammary infusions deliver high concentrations of antibiotic into the ductular system. Depending on lipid solubility, the degree of ionization, and protein binding, parenterally administered antibiotics may achieve high levels in both tissues and milk. Dosages must be those indicated by the manufacturer, with the upper limits being used for parenteral administration.

Prevention

Preventive measures for the control of bovine streptococcal mastitis have been described and reviewed in the veterinary and dairy science literature. The cornerstone of most programs includes a properly functioning milking system, single-use towels to clean and dry the udder before attaching milkers, and teat dipping using an approved germicide after each milking. Early detection and treatment of clinical cases, as well as infusion of appropriate antibiotics at the time of drying off, are important. The objective is to reduce both the duration and the number of infections. Opportunistic (environmental) infections caused by *S. uberis*, *S. dysgalactiae*, and other non-*agalactiae* streptococci may be reduced by providing a clean, dry holding facility for the cows, minimizing soiling and trauma of the udder, and controlling fly populations in the summer.

DISEASES OF SWINE

Streptococci are associated with several important and specific disease syndromes of pigs. The most important of these are meningitis, arthritis, bronchopneumonia, and septicemia associated with *S. suis* and cervical lymphadenitis caused by *S. porcinus*. A variety of other group C and L streptococci, including *S. dysgalactiae* subsp. *dysgalactiae* (*S.* "*equisimilis*"), cause sporadic purulent infections of the joints, meninges, lungs, skin, and other body organs.

Streptococcus suis Infections

Etiology

S. suis is a Lancefield group D, R, and S *Streptococcus* that occurs in at least 35 serotypes based on capsular antigens. Some relationship exists between serotype and clinical disease syndrome. Serotypes 1, 2, 1/2, 3, and 8 appear to be the most prevalent, but patterns of occurrence vary geographically. *S. suis* has its greatest impact on large, intensively managed herds in which other major diseases are controlled. Overcrowding and poor air quality are predisposing factors. Disease episodes have been reported from virtually all swine-raising areas of the world. Pigs of all ages may be affected, but the typical case of septicemia and meningitis occurs in nursing pigs and in weaned pigs, particularly in 8- to 12-week-olds. The incidence varies greatly within an infected herd and among herds under differing environmental and management conditions.

S. suis has been isolated from other animals, including cattle and horses. Infection in human beings, particularly meningitis, is well documented. People associated with swine production and the handling of pork are at greatest risk.

In pigs the organism gains entry by the mouth and nose and colonizes the palatine tonsils. Following colonization, there is a bacteremic phase when *S. suis* can be transported to distant sites, including the central nervous system, by using mononuclear cells as vehicles. As many as 100% of a herd may harbor *S. suis* in their tonsils, and these pigs are a constant source of infection for susceptible penmates.

Clinical Signs

Sudden death is a common sequela to overwhelming infection by *S. suis*. Often, signs of meningitis will be evident, including fever, anorexia, depression, blindness, incoordination, paddling, opisthotonos, tremors, and paralysis. As the disease becomes chronic, residual central nervous system signs may persist together with lameness associated with polyarthritis. In weaned pigs, bronchopneumonia may develop and involve other secondary bacterial invaders such as *Actinobacillus pleuropneumoniae*, *Pasteurella multocida*, or *Salmonella* spp. *S. suis* has also been recovered from aborted fetuses and the postpartum genital tract.

Pathology

No gross lesions are seen in pigs dying peracutely; in those that survive longer, the common lesion is fibrinopurulent exudative polyserositis. Different strains and serotypes of the organism vary in pathogenicity and tissue tropism. Meningitis is a common finding but may not be noticed except on histopathologic examination. Polyarthritis, meningitis, bronchopneumonia, and polyserositis may occur individually or concurrently. Less common lesions of young pigs include pericarditis, myocarditis, and valvular endocarditis.

Diagnosis

Confirmation of *S. suis* infection must rely on postmortem and microbiologic examination. The spectrum of clinical signs allows this infection to be confused with other viremic and bacteremic diseases associated with meningitis, polyserositis, pneumonia, and arthritis. *S. dysgalactiae*, *Haemophilus parasuis*, *A. pleuropneumoniae*, and pseudorabies virus are possible alternative or concurrent diagnoses. Because *S. suis* may be confused with closely related streptococci, accurate identification should include serologic, morphologic, and biochemical studies.

Tissue secretions from a variety of organs, including the brain and meninges, tonsils, lungs, parenchymatous organs, and synovial membranes, should be fixed in buffered formalin for histopathologic examination. Large blocks of the same tissues should be transported to the laboratory at 4°C for microbiologic analysis.

Treatment

Treatment includes good nursing care and specific antibiotic therapy. Weaned pigs with clinical signs should be moved to a hospital pen with clean, dry bedding and adequate heat and ventilation. Severely affected pigs should be given more intensive nursing, including hand feeding, or be euthanized for necropsy.

Although most reports indicate that *S. suis* isolates are susceptible to penicillin and ampicillin, their susceptibility to other antibiotics is much more variable. In one study, 43% of 122 *S. suis* isolates were only moderately sensitive (minimum inhibitory concentration, 0.25 to 2.0 μg/mL) and 6% were resistant (minimum inhibitory concentration, 4.0 μg/mL) to penicillin. It is therefore important to have susceptibility data to guide appropriate antibiotic selection. Because *S. suis* is widely distributed in various tissues, the higher end of the dosage range should be used. Procaine penicillin at 10,000 to 20,000 IU/kg intramuscularly (IM) once or twice per day or ampicillin at 10 mg/kg of body weight IM three times per day has been used. Isolates often have a high level of resistance to trimethoprim-sulfamethoxazole, lincomycin, neomycin, and spiramycin.

Prevention

Management practices that reduce stress and exposure to *S. suis* are very important in prevention and control. Overcrowding must be corrected and air quality improved to reduce stress and the burden of challenge. Pigs from different age groups or sources should not be mixed, and an all-in, all-out management system should be used. *S. suis* is readily killed by most commercial disinfectants but may survive for days or weeks in feces and dust at cool temperatures.

Feed-mixed antimicrobials have been used as a means of controlling infection during peak risk times, such as the moving and commingling of pigs, or to control the spread of an enzootic. Once again, selection of antimicrobials must be based on susceptibility testing. Neither antibiotics nor immunization can be expected to eliminate the infection in carrier pigs.

Commercial and autogenous vaccines are widely used. Because protection is in part serotype specific, vaccines should ideally contain the antigens of strains epidemic on the farm where the vaccine will be used. The self-limiting nature of disease caused by *S. suis* in isolated groups of pigs strongly implicates the emergence of an acquired convalescent protective immune response resulting in serum antibodies. Thus hyperimmune or convalescent serum may be of value in treatment or prophylaxis. The addition of recombinant bovine interleukin-1β greatly improves the efficacy of commercial vaccines. Formalin-killed vaccines do not stimulate levels of protection equivalent to those produced as a result of natural infection.

Eradication of the infection on a premises may be attempted by depopulation and thorough cleaning and disinfection followed by a rest period of at least 6 weeks. It may, however, be difficult to obtain new stock free of *S. suis* infection for repopulation.

Streptococcus porcinus Infection

S. porcinus, a Lancefield group E *Streptococcus*, is the cause of a contagious purulent lymphadenitis of the head and neck of feeder swine. The disease is known as jowl abscess, cervical lymphadenitis, feeder boils, and swine strangles and has been a major cause of carcass trim or condemnation in North American packing plants. Transmission is by nasal contact and drinking water. The disease is not of economic importance in countries other than the United States, although a similar organism is present in swine herds in those areas. *S. porcinus* is occasionally isolated from a variety of lesions such as arthritis, pericarditis, and encephalitis. The development of jowl abscesses may be accompanied by pyrexia, inappetence, and neutrophilia, but the systemic effects are minimal. Palpable thick-walled abscesses develop in the throat region and may rupture. Aspirates are inoculated on colistin–nalidixic acid (CNA)–blood agar and isolates identified by biochemical and serologic procedures.

Antibiotic therapy may have no effect on well-formed abscesses, and resolution requires spontaneous or surgical drainage. Supplementation of starter feed with antibiotics such as tetracycline has been very effective in disease prevention. An avirulent oral vaccine was protective in more than 90% of postweaned pigs but has not been much used because of the convenience and efficacy of antibiotic supplementation of starter feed.

Other Streptococcal Infections

S. dysgalactiae subsp. *dysgalactiae*, formerly described as *S. "equisimilis,"* and other group C streptococci are commonly associated with a wide variety of pyogenic infections of young pigs, including meningitis, otitis, pneumonia, arthritis, endocarditis, abscesses, bacteremia, and pyoderma. Endometritis, mastitis, and abortion in cows may also be caused by these streptococci.

Antibiotics, particularly penicillin or ampicillin, are used in treatment as previously described. Multivalent bacterins containing *S. dysgalactiae* (*S. equisimilis*) are available but provide only limited protection.

S. durans has been associated with enteritis in pigs. The organism is isolated in essentially pure culture from the intestine of affected animals. In these infections numerous gram-positive cocci are seen closely adherent to the brush border of villous enterocytes on histologic examination. The significance and prevalence of this infection are unknown.

BIBLIOGRAPHY

Chanter N, Jones PW, Alexander TJ: Meningitis in pigs caused by *Streptococcus suis*: A speculative review. Vet Microbiol 36:39–55, 1993.

Clifton-Hadley FA: The epidemiology, diagnosis, treatment and control of *Streptococcus suis* type 2 infection. *In* Proceedings of the Annual Meeting of the American Association of Swine Practitioners. 1986, pp 471–491.

Higgins R, Gottschalk M: An update on *Streptococcus suis* identification. J Vet Diagn Invest 2:249–252, 1990.

Prieto C, Garcia FJ, Suarez P, et al: Biochemical traits and antimicrobial susceptibility of *Streptococcus suis* isolated from slaughtered pigs. Zentralbl Veterinarmed 41:608–617, 1994.

Sischo WM, Heider LE, Miller GY, Moore DA: Prevalence of contagious pathogens of bovine mastitis and use of mastitis control practices. J Am Vet Med Assoc 202:595–600, 1993.

Soback S: Mastitis therapy—past, present and future. *In* International Symposium on Bovine Mastitis, Indianapolis. Arlington, Va, National Mastitis Council, 1990, pp 244–251.

Yancey RJ Jr: Recent advances in bovine vaccine technology. J Dairy Sci 76:2418–2436, 1993.

■ Staphylococcal Disease

George C. Stewart, Ph.D.

Staphylococci are gram-positive, facultatively anaerobic cocci which colonize the skin and mucous membranes of a wide variety of animal species. There are currently 32 recognized species of the genus *Staphylococcus*. These species can be divided into two categories—the primary pathogens and the commensals—by virtue of production of the enzyme coagulase. The primary pathogens, which produce coagulase, are *Staphylococcus aureus*, *Staphylococcus intermedius* (primarily associated with canines), and *Staphylococcus hyicus* (coagulase production is reported to be a variable trait in this species). Infections caused by primary staphylococcal pathogens are of two basic types: (1) cutaneous or mucosal infections, and (2) septicemia, which is generally associated with abscess formation at a variety of tissue sites; osteomyelitis; endocarditis; or arthritis. The coagulase-negative staphylococci comprise a number of species which are commensals on the skin and mucous membranes of animals and are occasionally associated with minor infections, including foreign body–associated abscesses and intramammary infections. The prototype coagulase-negative staphylococcus is *Staphylococcus epidermidis*, which is a commensal bacterium of humans and other animals. Because of the ubiquitous nature of these skin commensals, the coagulase-negative staphylococci are frequently contaminants of clinical samples. Because they can on occasion be the disease-causing agent, the significance of their presence in a clinical sample must be interpreted with caution.

VIRULENCE FACTORS AND PATHOGENESIS

The most significant pathogen, and the best studied of the coagulase-positive staphylococci, is *S. aureus*. The virulence factors associated with this organism are complex and not well understood. The bacterium produces a number of secreted toxins and tissue-degrading enzymes which theoretically contribute to the virulence of the organism (Table 1). However, no single virulence factor has yet been shown to be critical for the disease-causing process. Thus the virulence properties of *S. aureus* are considered to be multifactorial, with many staphylococcal proteins contributing to the ability of the organism to cause disease. The production of coagulase is a good example of the complicated nature of the pathogenesis of this organism. Because of the more virulent nature of the coagulase-positive staphylococci, it has been assumed that this enzyme is an important virulence trait, perhaps by allowing the organism to form a fibrin wall to protect itself from the phagocytic cells in the early stages of abscess formation. However, mutants of *S. aureus* that do not produce coagulase remain virulent. Coagulase production, although not absolutely required for virulence, is still the best predictor of the disease-causing potential of the organism and current animal models are inadequate to fully appreciate its role.

Staphylococcal virulence factors can be divided into two categories: cell surface proteins that are involved in attachment and subsequent colonization, and secreted proteins that are involved with evasion of host defenses and spread of the organism from the initial site of infection. These virulence factors are required at specific stages of the infectious process. Initially, it is important for the bacterium to produce colonization factors to allow the organism to adhere and begin replication. Later, mechanisms to ward off the recruited inflammatory cells are necessary to maintain the infection. Lastly, enzymes to degrade host tissues and allow the organism to spread to new sites are required. *S. aureus* possesses a two-component regulatory system to coordinately regulate these virulence determinants. When the bacterial cell numbers are low, as is the case at the initiation of the infection, the system regulates gene expression such that the cell surface components (proteins necessary for adherence to tissues) are maximally expressed and the exoprotein genes are only expressed at very low levels. The bacteria then adhere and begin to replicate at the initial sites of the infection. When the bacterial cell numbers reach a critical mass, the regulatory system causes decreased expression of the cell surface genes and increased expression of the virulence exoproteins. These proteins help the bacteria to resist the host inflammatory response and phagocytosis and to promote bacterial cell detachment and spread to establish new foci of infection at other sites in the infected animal. Thus the exoproteins are needed at this time and the adherence factors are of lesser importance.

CLINICAL SIGNS AND PATHOGENESIS

Staphylococcal Mastitis

With the effectiveness of control regimens against bovine streptococcal intramammary infections (IMIs) and the remark-

Table 1
VIRULENCE FACTORS OF *Staphylococcus aureus*

Virulence Factor	Function	Proposed Role in Virulence
Cell surface proteins†		
Collagen binding protein	Binds collagen	Attachment/colonization
Clumping factor	Binds fibrinogen	Attachment/colonization
Fibrinogen binding protein (bound coagulase)	Binds fibrinogen	Coats self with host protein to avoid the immune system
Fibronectin binding protein A	Binds fibronectin	Attachment/colonization
Fibronectin binding protein B	Binds fibronectin	Attachment/colonization
Microcapsule	Masks cell wall components	Antiphagocytic
Protein A	Binds Fc portion of antibody	Inhibits opsonization
Extracellular proteins		
α-toxin	Forms pores in membranes	Kills phagocytic cells
β-toxin	Sphingomyelinase	Kills phagocytic cells
γ-toxin	Membrane-damaging hemolysin	Unknown
δ-toxin	Membrane-damaging hemolysin	Unknown
Coagulase	Fibrin clot formation	Abscess formation (?)
DNase	Degrades DNA	Unknown
Enterotoxins	Polyclonal T cell activators (superantigens)	Food poisoning; toxic shock syndrome
Exfoliative toxins	Cleavage of desmosomes at level of the stratum granulosum	Exfoliation of epidermis
Fatty acid metabolizing enzyme (FAME)	Breakdown of fatty acids	Detoxifies fatty acids; skin colonization
Hyaluronidase	Breakdown of hyaluronic acid	Spreading factor (?)
Lipase	Glycerol ester hydrolase	Skin colonization
Panton-Valentine leukocidin	Kills leukocytes	Antiphagocytic
Phospholipase C	Membrane-damaging	Unknown
Proteases	Breakdown of protein	Inactivation of antibodies and antimicrobial peptides (defensins) (?); tissue damage
Staphylokinase	Breakdown of fibrin	Spreading factor
Toxic shock syndrome toxin	Superantigen	Hypotension; shock; disruption of immune function

*For details, see Projan and Novick.
†Binding activities have also been described for bone sialoprotein, elastin, laminin, thrombospondin, and vitronectin, but specific surface proteins have not yet been identified for these activities.

able ineffectiveness of similar programs against staphylococcal infections, *S. aureus* has surpassed *Streptococcus agalactiae* as the major cause of bovine contagious mastitis. Contagious mastitis is defined simply as an IMI transmitted from cow to cow. Estimates of the prevalence of *S. aureus* infections range from 7% to 40% of all dairy cows, a fivefold higher prevalence than that assigned to *Str. agalactiae*. The skin of the udder and teats serves as the reservoir for the infection and the population of the organism can be high if the quarter is also shedding the organism. The bacteria may also be deposited on the teat end by contaminated washcloths or sponges used in the premilking cleaning procedure. Cow-to-cow transmission thus occurs primarily during the milking process. Infection is due to entry by the bacteria through the teat canal into the mammary gland. Colonization of the teat canal appears to be requisite for subsequent infection of the mammary gland. Adherence prevents the bacteria from being flushed out of the gland during milking. After *S. aureus* has gained access to the teat canal, the predominant outcome is a chronic subclinical infection. One quarter of the udder is generally infected independently of the other three. In the less acute forms of the disease, there is ulceration and erosion of lactiferous sinus and ductular epithelia. An infiltration of macrophages and polymorphonuclear neutrophil leukocytes (PMNs), which cross the mammary epithelium into lactiferous ducts and glandular alveoli, occurs. This leads to damage to the alveolar secretory cells. Shrinkage of alveoli, proliferation of connective tissue, and accumulation of cellular debris ensue. Pathogen-induced necrosis and immune cell–induced damage result in reduced milk secretion and the presence of bacteria and inflammatory cells in the milk.

The most severe form of staphylococcal mastitis is the gangrenous form, which is usually associated with calving and affects a variable amount of the udder. Symptoms of acute inflammation with heat, redness, swelling, and pain occur and there is progression to necrosis with its associated coldness of the affected area, blue-black color, fluid exudation, and crepitation. The cow may die of toxemia or the quarter may slough. The α-toxin produced by *S. aureus* appears to play a major role in the gangrenous form of the disease.

The outcome of the infection is primarily determined by the ability of the PMNs to control bacterial multiplication. Chronic subclinical mastitis can be converted to the gangrenous form by the induction of neutropenia. On the other hand, experimental induction of IMI failed in quarters with milk somatic cell counts in excess of 6×10^5 cells per milliliter (see Postle and colleagues). This effect of the phagocytic cell count explains the observation that a single bacterial strain may produce gangrenous mastitis on some occasions, and only mild disease on other occasions.

IMIs can also result from infection by *S. hyicus* or by coagulase-negative staphylococcal species. Less tissue damage results from these infections, which may be self-curing. IMI by coagulase-negative staphylococci may result in an elevated somatic cell count sufficient to prevent subsequent establishment of an infection by *S. aureus*.

Exudative Epidermitis of Pigs

Exudative epidermitis (greasy pig disease) is an acute generalized disease of suckling and weaned pigs caused by *S. hyicus*. The clinical signs of this condition are characterized by exfoliation of the skin, excessive sebaceous secretion, and the formation of a brownish coat of exudate. The lesions are prone to superinfection by other bacterial species, which complicates the clinical picture. Exudative epidermitis occurs worldwide, is highly contagious, and mortality rates may reach 90%. The reservoirs for *S. hyicus* include the skin of pigs, the skin and nares of poultry, and occasionally the skin and milk of cattle.

The disease resembles scalded skin syndrome which occurs in human infants. The latter results from infection by *S. aureus* producing one of two forms of exfoliative toxin. The porcine disease appears to be caused by a similar mechanism. An exfoliative toxin purified from *S. hyicus* caused exfoliation in piglets after intradermal or subcutaneous injection. Histopathologically, the skin revealed an intraepidermal cleavage plane between the stratum corneum and stratum granulosum and at the stratum granulosum. A lipase has also been characterized from *S. hyicus* and may be important for successful colonization of the skin.

TREATMENT AND CONTROL

Staphylococcal infections are notoriously difficult to treat. In cases of mastitis, ductal occlusion and microabscesses may impede antibiotic diffusion. Antibiotic therapy may cause the infection to subside clinically, but microabscesses may later rupture and allow *S. aureus* to spread. The presently available antibiotic preparations used during lactation cure less than 50% of *S. aureus* IMI. In addition, antibiotic resistance occurs readily in the staphylococci. The majority of *S. aureus* strains produce β-lactamase and are thus resistant to penicillin.

Control of bovine IMI by vaccination has been a goal for a number of years. Protection against new infections with toxoids or bacterins, however, has not been reproducible. This may be a result of a lack of relevant antigens in the vaccines, insufficient knowledge regarding appropriate immunization schedules, and a paucity of information regarding immune mechanisms operative in the bovine mammary gland. Recent research on *S. aureus* infections has provided some hope that an effective vaccine may be achievable. There are at least eight immunologically distinct polysaccharides which make up the microcapsule of this bacterium which are capable of inducing serotype-specific opsonic antibodies. Conjugate vaccines consisting of the most common capsular polysaccharide types and *Pseudomonas aeruginosa* exoprotein A have provided protection in experimental challenge in mice. The capsular polysaccharides are poorly produced in vitro except on specific low-phosphate culture media. Therefore, their relative absence on cultured bacteria may explain the variable response seen with bacterin immunization. The microcapsule antigen studies were carried out with capsular polysaccharide isolated from strains of serotypes 5 and 8, which constitute approximately 80% of human infections, greater than 70% of bovine IMI isolates, and which are the prevalent serotypes isolated from ovine and caprine IMI (see Sutra and Poutrel). Therefore, the vaccines developed against these two capsular serotypes may ultimately prove useful as IMI vaccines.

Control of staphylococcal mastitis is currently dependent upon hygiene at milking, including premilking washing and postmilking drying of udders with individual cloths, dipping of teats with antiseptic solutions after milking, and observing strict milking machine sanitation practices. Systematic antibiotic treatment by intramammary infusions in dry cows should be carried out to cure chronic subclinical IMI established during lactation.

Antibiotic resistance, frequently plasmid-mediated, is common with exudative epidermitis-causing strains of *S. hyicus*. Treatment failure occurs often. Antibiotic sensitivity testing is critical with this pathogen. The site of the infection and the nature of the lesions also make it difficult to maintain effective local concentrations of the antibiotic, thus rendering antibiotics which are effective in vitro, but much less so in vivo.

BIBLIOGRAPHY

Fattom AI, Sarwar J, Ortiz A, Naso R: A *Staphylococcus aureus* capsular polysaccharide (CP) vaccine and CP-specific antibodies protect mice against bacterial challenge. Infect Immun 64:1659, 1996.
Fox LK, Gay JM: Contagious mastitis. Vet Clin North Am Food Anim Pract 9:475, 1993.
Matthews KR, Harmon RJ, Smith BA: Protective effect of *Staphylococcus chromogenes* infection against *Staphylococcus aureus* infection in the lactating bovine mammary gland. J Dairy Sci 73:3457, 1990.
Penny RHC, Muirhead MR: Exudative epidermitis (greasy pig disease, "marmite" disease). *In* Leman AD, Straw B, Glock RD, et al (eds): Diseases of Swine, ed 6. Ames, Iowa State University Press, 1986, pp 87–88.
Postle DS, Roguinsky M, Poutrel B: Induced staphylococcal infections in the bovine mammary gland. Am J Vet Res 39:29, 1978.
Projan SJ, Novick RP: The molecular basis of pathogenicity. *In* Crossley KB, Archer GL (eds): The Staphylococci in Human Disease. New York, Churchill Livingstone, 1997, pp 55–81.
Sato H, Tanabe T, Kuramoto M, et al.: Isolation of exfoliative toxin from *Staphylococcus hyicus* subsp. *hyicus* and its exfoliative activity in the piglet. Vet Microbiol 27:263, 1991.
Sutra L, Poutrel B: Virulence factors involved in the pathogenesis of bovine intramammary infections due to *Staphylococcus aureus*. J Med Microbiol 40:79, 1994.
Vestweber JG, Leipold HW: *Staphylococcus aureus* mastitis. Part I. Virulence, defense mechanisms, and establishment of infection. Compend Contin Educ Pract Vet 15:1561, 1993.

■ Swine Erysipelas
Jerry P. Kunesh, D.V.M., M.S., Ph.D.

Erysipelas of swine is a contagious disease caused by *Erysipelothrix rhusiopathiae*, a bacterium that also infects many other species, which may act as sources of infection for swine. The most common of these are mice, pigeons, sparrows, and blackbirds. Turkeys, cattle, sheep, goats, horses, and many others may also be infected. Distribution of the disease is worldwide, but regional differences are recognized. The factors that predispose swine to infection are not well understood.

CLINICAL SIGNS

Acute erysipelas is characterized by depression and an elevated temperature of 41°C or higher. When disturbed, affected animals are irritable and noticeably lame. Abortions may occur. Occasionally, individual pigs may be found dead without observed illness. Generally, inappetence and other symptoms of illness will be seen. As the disease progresses, raised rhomboid erythematous skin lesions may occur.

Subacute forms of disease present the same clinical signs in a milder form, whereas chronic forms are characterized by lameness and varying degrees of arthritis.

PATHOLOGY

Rhomboid skin lesions are generally considered to be pathognomonic, but similar lesions can occur in pigs with septicemia caused by *Actinobacillus suis*. All other lesions, including an enlarged spleen, hemostasis, and hemorrhagic lymph nodes, are associated with septicemia and are not specific for swine erysipelas. In the chronic forms, vegetative endocarditis and lesions of arthritis are suggestive of swine erysipelas.

DIAGNOSIS

The arthritic form of the disease must be differentiated from streptococcal, staphylococcal, and mycoplasmal infections. In rare cases, *Actinomyces pyogenes* or *Brucella suis* may present a similar clinical picture. In the absence of rhomboid skin lesions, bacterial cultures are necessary to differentiate erysipelas from other septicemic conditions. Although possibly rare, *A. suis* should be considered, even in the presence of typical skin lesions.

TREATMENT

Penicillin is considered to be the drug of choice. The recommended dosage is 6000 to 12,000 IU/kg of body weight given by intramuscular injection once daily. Other antibiotics that are effective if given once daily by intramuscular injection are ceftiofur, 3.0 to 5.0 mg/kg; lincomycin, 22 mg/kg; and oxytetracycline, 6.6 to 11 mg/kg. Tylosin given at 9.8 mg/kg twice daily is also effective. Antibiotics should be administered so that therapeutic levels are sustained for 4 to 5 days. Any of the tetracyclines or lincomycin may be used for herd treatment by incorporation into the feed or water, in accordance with label directions, as an adjunct to individual treatment. In all cases, the preslaughter withdrawal period must be observed to avoid tissue residue.

Antiserum is available and may be used for herd treatment. More commonly, antiserum use is restricted to suckling or recently weaned piglets and is administered according to label directions in conjunction with injectable penicillin.

PREVENTION AND CONTROL

Prevention of erysipelas on farms or in areas where the disease is endemic is best accomplished by using either bacterins or attenuated live vaccines. Occasional cases of vaccine failure occur, apparently because of incomplete cross-protection among serotypes of *Erysipelothrix*. Breeding stock should be immunized twice annually. Market animals immunized before 4 weeks of age should be revaccinated after 6 weeks of age if protection is to last until the animals are marketed.

Erysipelas can be avoided by following a systematic immunization program, purchasing replacement stock from herds where the disease has not occurred, using good sanitation and disinfection procedures, and protecting feed supplies from contamination by soil or feces.

BIBLIOGRAPHY

Wood RL: Erysipelas. *In* Leman AD, Straw BE, Glock RD, et al (eds): Diseases of Swine, ed 7. Ames, Iowa State University Press, 1992, pp 475–486.

■ Listeriosis (Circling Disease, Silage Sickness)

Melissa R. Finley, D.V.M.
Stanley M. Dennis, B.V.Sc., Ph.D., F.R.C.V.S., F.R.C.Path.

Listeriosis is an infectious disease caused by *Listeria monocytogenes*. In ruminants, listeriosis is characterized by encephalitis or abortion in adults and by septicemia in fetuses and neonates. Infrequently, it can be associated with mastitis, conjunctivitis, or ophthalmitis. In monogastric animals it is usually characterized by septicemia with focal hepatic necrosis. Listeriosis is worldwide in distribution and affects a wide variety of mammalian and avian species, including humans. Recently, listeriosis has emerged as a public health concern. Listeric infection in humans can cause septicemia, meningitis, and abortions.

ETIOLOGY

Six species and 16 serovars of the genus *Listeria* are recognized. *Listeria monocytogenes* is the principal pathogen for both animals and humans, whereas *L. ivanovii* can be pathogenic for sheep and infrequently for humans. The species *L. innocua, L. grayi, L. seeligeri,* and *L. welshmeri* are not generally considered virulent.

Listeria serovars are based on somatic and flagellar antigens, with serovars 1/2a, 1/2b, and 4b most commonly associated with disease.

Hemolysis is an important virulence factor because of the production of a hemolysin, listeriolysin O. Listeriolysin O is the enzyme that enables the organism to disrupt the phagolysosomal membrane and thereby survive and multiply within the cell. *L. monocytogenes, L. ivanovii,* and *L. seeligeri* produce listeriolysin O. Although *L. seeligeri* is capable of producing listeriolysin O, it is not known to cause disease.

L. monocytogenes is a ubiquitous facultative intracellular pathogen. It is a small, gram-positive bacillus that is motile by means of a few peritrichous flagella. *L. monocytogenes* grows well on the usual bacterial media. Primary isolation of *Listeria* is improved under microaerophilic conditions. *Listeria* organisms grow under a wide temperature range, with the optimum temperature being between 30 and 37°C. Its ability to grow at 4°C is important diagnostically and is the basis for the "cold enrichment" method for primary isolation of *Listeria* from suspected cases of listeric encephalitis and contaminated foods.

EPIZOOTIOLOGY

The natural habitat of *L. monocytogenes* is soil and the mammalian intestinal tract. Vegetation and silage become contaminated with soil and/or feces. Grazing animals ingest *Listeria* and further contaminate soil and vegetation, thereby establishing an ecological listeric cycle. The most important environmental sources are silage, grass, surface water, and dust. Animal-to-animal transmission by the fecal-to-oral route occurs. Animal-to-human transmission may occur directly or indirectly via milk, cheese, meat, eggs, or vegetables.

L. monocytogenes has been isolated from the feces of healthy animals and humans. The majority of listeric infections are too mild to be recognized clinically and are inapparent or latent; therefore, asymptomatic intestinal carriers are common. Shedding of *L. monocytogenes* in the feces is very common after clinical listeriosis. Listeriosis is primarily a winter-spring disease, and the fecal excretion of *Listeria* in cattle is highest in the winter months.

Sporadic cases of listeric encephalitis are common. Over a period of months, up to 5% of a cattle herd or 10% of a sheep flock may become infected. Confined sheep and cattle, especially those being fed silage, have a higher incidence than range animals do.

Recovery of *Listeria* from the milk of both mastitic and normal cows emphasizes the potential danger of milk-borne listeriosis in animals and humans. *Listeria* organisms have also been isolated from the milk of sheep, goats, and women. Excretion of *Listeria* in the milk of cattle is usually intermittent but may persist for periods exceeding a single lactation. Typically, *Listeria* is inactivated by pasteurization, but under unusual circumstances the organism may persist. Shedding of the organism into milk was increased in dairy cattle previously infected with *L. monocytogenes* after they were treated with an immunosuppressive dose of dexamethasone for 3 consecutive days. The administration of corticosteroids in this study may have mimicked the environmental stresses placed on production animals.

The distal portion of the intestinal tract is regarded as a reservoir from which *Listeria* invades tissues when the body's defenses are impaired. The most important single source of both clinical and asymptomatic listeric infections is gross environmental contamination. *Listeria* can multiply in soil at 18 to 20°C and can be present on many types of grass, hay, and other crops. In a cool, damp environment, *Listeria* can survive in organic matter for years. Its survival is good in grass, soil, and silage of near-neutral pH but poor in acid soil and good silage.

Outbreaks of listeriosis in sheep and cattle have frequently been attributed to silage. Poor-quality or poorly cured silage (pH 5.4 or greater) provides a favorable substrate for *Listeria*. Pit silage appears to be involved more than silage in tower-type silos, possibly because of greater soil and fecal matter being introduced by tractors during filling and packing. The frequency of listeriosis tends to increase as the lower and damper layers of silage are consumed, shortly before animals are turned out to graze in the spring. It is postulated that *Listeria*-contaminated silage results in a large number of latent infections, often approaching 100% of the herd or flock, but clinical listeriosis develops in only a few animals.

L. monocytogenes has high infectivity but low pathogenicity, and clinical *Listeria* infection is usually not manifested unless the host's resistance is reduced by various stress factors, concurrent disease, or pregnancy. Asymptomatic intestinal carriers disseminate listeric infection to uninfected herds or flocks on their introduction.

PATHOGENESIS

Susceptible animals are exposed to *Listeria* by means of contaminated soil, vegetation, or silage. The organism gains entry through wounds in the buccal mucosa, inhalation, conjunctival contamination, or the gastrointestinal tract. Infection by *L. monocytogenes* is manifested as encephalitis, septicemia, or abortion. Occasionally, mastitis, conjunctivitis, ophthalmitis, and myelitis may occur.

Listerial encephalitis is a local infection involving the medulla, pons, and adjacent areas of the brain. The organism reaches the brain stem by migrating along branches of cranial nerves innervating the oral and nasal mucosa or rarely through hematogenous routes. Small wounds in the oral or nasal mucosa may provide a port of entry for the organism into axons of cranial nerves. However, the exact mechanism by which *L. monocytogenes* gains entry into these nerves remains to be elucidated. In vitro, fetal nervous tissue is capable of taking up *L. monocytogenes*; however, the number of organisms identified within nerve axons was small when compared with macrophages. It has been postulated that uptake of the pathogen into nonphagocytic parenchy-

mal cells may be mediated through interaction with host cell receptors and activation of host cell signal transduction mechanisms that initiate uptake of the organism into a phagosomal vacuole. Intracellular survival and replication of *L. monocytogenes* are dependent on the production of listeriolysin O, which enables the organism to disrupt the phagosomal membrane and enter the cytoplasm. In vitro, *L. monocytogenes* is capable of cell-to-cell transmission between human enterocytes, mediated through interaction with the F-actin of the host cell microfilaments. This may account for the organism's ability to ascend the trigeminal and other peripheral nerves and migrate through neural tissue. Focal lesions of the brain parenchyma are established, and only occasionally do lesions extend into the meninges and ventricular system. The clinical signs vary and are dependent on the site of infection. The selective localization of *L. monocytogenes* in the brain stem is often unilateral and accounts for the signs of facial paralysis and circling. Listerial myelitis has been reported in sheep, but affected animals did not have signs consistent with listerial encephalitis. The pathogenesis of listerial myelitis is unknown.

Septicemic or visceral listeriosis usually results from the ingestion of *L. monocytogenes*. The intestinal epithelium and the specialized epithelial cells covering Peyer's patches are thought to be the primary sites of entry. The production of listeriolysin O enables the organism to survive and grow within the enterocyte, as well as allows for extraintestinal dissemination. Because *L. monocytogenes* is capable of cell-to-cell transmission in vitro, *Listeria* may move between cells and evade the immune system. Following intragastric inoculation, *L. monocytogenes* has been recovered from the liver and spleen of mice. Infection by this route is usually inapparent, although in some cases bacteremia with localization in various organs or fatal septicemia may develop. Infected animals may shed the organism in the feces, which is presumably a result of biliary excretion following hepatic colonization. *Listeria* may also be excreted into the external environment in milk, tears, nasal secretions, urine, and uterine discharge.

The placenta of all pregnant domestic animals is highly susceptible to listeric infection, and placental infection results in placentitis, fetal death, abortion, stillbirths, neonatal deaths, and possibly viable carriers. The uterus is extensively involved only when fetal and placental tissues are retained. Although listerial metritis is constant, it has little or no lasting effect on reproductive function, but *Listeria* may be shed for a month or more. Sporadic abortions resulting from some stress during pregnancy and from the development of listeric congenital infection in individual animals are more likely than a herd or flock pathogen spreading horizontally and causing abortion epizootics. Listerial encephalitis and listerial abortion rarely occur together.

Mastitis caused by *L. monocytogenes* infection is rare. *L. monocytogenes* does not appear to readily invade the bovine udder and probably does so only when hygiene is poor.

Ophthalmitis associated with *L. monocytogenes* infection has been reported in cattle and sheep. It has been associated with the feeding of silage to winter-housed cattle and in ewes fed baled silage. It is believed that the infection is associated with corneal contamination by the organism. Exposure keratitis may occur in association with listerial encephalitis as a result of facial nerve dysfunction.

CLINICAL SIGNS

Clinical listeriosis infection is generally associated with characteristic syndromes in various groups of susceptible animals. Encephalitis is the most common manifestation of *Listeria* infection in adult ruminants. Septicemia usually occurs in swine and neonatal ruminants, and abortion and perinatal mortality occur in all species. Infection is more common in ruminants fed silage.

Ruminants

Encephalitis, the most frequently recognized form of listeriosis, affects sheep, cattle, goats, and pigs. The incubation period is unknown, probably 2 to 3 weeks, and infection generally occurs in winter and early spring. Although both sexes and all ages are affected, it is more common during the first 3 years of life. The morbidity rate is low, but mortality is high.

In the early stages, ruminants with listerial encephalitis are usually depressed and anorectic and separate themselves from the rest of the flock or herd. They may be moderately febrile, tachycardiac, and tachypneic. Many affected animals are dehydrated with electrolyte and acid-base abnormalities. Metabolic acidosis and low serum bicarbonate levels are common in cattle with listeriosis because of salivary fluid losses.

The neurologic signs are usually associated with disease of the midbrain, pons, and medulla and are often asymmetrical. Affected ruminants may demonstrate dysfunction of multiple cranial nerves, including the trigeminal (V), abducent (VI), facial (VII), vestibular (VIII), glossopharyngeal (IX), vagal (X), and hypoglossal (XII) nerves. Lesions of the trigeminal motor nucleus or the mandibular nerve result in weakness of the muscles of mastication and are manifested as poor jaw tone or an inability to masticate feed. Lesions of the sensory portion of the trigeminal nucleus or the trigeminal nerve cause reduced facial sensation, especially the nasal mucosa. Affected animals will fail to respond when the nasal mucosa is stimulated on the ipsilateral side. In sheep with listerial encephalitis, the sensory portion of the trigeminal nucleus is affected more often than the motor portion. A medial strabismus may occur in animals with lesions of the abducent nucleus. Unilateral facial paresis is apparent with lesions of the facial nucleus. Damage to this area results in a dropped ear, a lowered eyelid, a dilated nostril, and flaccid lips on the ipsilateral side. The filtrum of small ruminants may deviate away from the side of the lesion. Exposure keratitis and corneal ulceration are common in animals with poor eyelid function as a result of facial nerve paralysis. Occasionally, facial nerve inflammation may cause eyelid spasticity when the animal is stimulated. Ataxia, circling, and a head tilt toward the affected side are indicative of vestibular nuclei lesions and are common clinical signs in animals with listerial encephalitis. Nystagmus may be present at rest or become apparent when the head is manipulated into extension, and the fast phase is often away from the side of the lesion. Affected animals may also lean or circle toward the side of the lesion. If the affected animal is recumbent, it may lie exclusively on the affected side and resent manipulation to the other side. Lesions involving the glossopharyngeal and vagal nuclei are manifested as dysphagia and drooling. Reduced lip function (facial nucleus) and weak muscles of mastication (trigeminal nucleus) can also contribute to signs of dysphagia. Lesions of the vagal nuclei may also lead to vomiting of ruminal contents. Tongue paralysis and protrusion can occur if the hypoglossal nucleus is affected.

Depression, head tremors, ataxia, and hemiparesis also occur in ruminants with listerial encephalitis. Depression is caused by inflammation of the ascending reticular activating system or, less likely, as a result of meningitis. Head tremors may occur in animals with lesions of the cerebellum. Occasionally, animals circle away from the side of facial paralysis. These signs are usually the result of a vestibular nucleus lesion on the opposite side of the brain stem or a lesion of the cerebellar peduncles on the same side (paradoxical vestibular disease). Hemiparesis may result if ipsilateral lesions exist in the motor neurons of the brain stem and general proprioceptive pathways in the medulla

or cerebellar peduncles. In the terminal stages the animal falls and is unable to rise without assistance. Prostration followed by coma and death may develop rapidly.

Listeric encephalitis in sheep and goats is acute, with death occurring as early as 4 to 48 hours after the onset of clinical signs, and recovery is rare. In cattle the disease is more chronic, with most surviving for 4 to 14 days. Spontaneous recovery is frequent, but recovered animals often have long-lasting brain damage. Listerial encephalitis is rare in neonatal lambs and calves.

The clinical signs associated with listerial myelitis are ataxia, paresis, and paralysis. Affected animals do not have signs associated with cranial nerve dysfunction. The lesions are restricted to the spinal cord.

Primary listerial septicemia in adult ruminants (usually sheep) is reported in Europe but is relatively rare in the United States. The affected animals have general weakness, inappetence, and respiratory distress. The mortality is not as high as that resulting from listerial encephalitis. In neonatal lambs and calves, listeric infection is manifested by septicemia, similar to that in monogastric animals.

Ophthalmitis associated with *L. monocytogenes* infection occurs in both sheep and cattle. Affected animals may have epiphora, blepharospasms, and photophobia. Examination of the eye may reveal hypopyon, iridocyclitis, uveitis, and keratitis. The lesions are usually unilateral with moderate corneal involvement. Listeric ophthalmitis and listeric encephalitis rarely occur together.

Swine

Listeria infection in swine is uncommon. It results in septicemia, encephalitis, localized internal abscesses, and poxlike skin lesions. Mixed infections with hog cholera, erysipelas, and influenza have been reported.

Listeriosis in swine is usually septicemic, with sudden anorexia, coughing, and respiratory distress. In piglets the main signs are depression, fever, prostration, and sudden death. Encephalitis has been reported in older pigs. Signs of central nervous system disturbances include trembling, incoordination, caudal paralysis, stilted gait of the forelegs, and progressive weakness followed by death. Infection during pregnancy may be followed by abortion.

Listeriosis in swine, either septicemic or encephalitic, usually has a rapid and fatal course of 3 to 4 days. The majority of swine listeric infections, however, apparently do not manifest clinical signs, and outbreaks are usually self-limiting.

Pregnant Animals

Regardless of the animal species, stage of gestation, or route of infection, the uterine contents quickly become infected with *L. monocytogenes*. Most listeric abortions occur in the last trimester, but they may occur at any stage of gestation. Near term, the fetus may be stillborn, born alive and die in a few hours or days, or survive. No premonitory signs of abortion are observed, and most dams exhibit few or no signs of general infection and spontaneously recover. The abortion rate in sheep is reported to range from 1% to 20%, with the average being about 10%. Abortion in sheep occurs within 3 to 11 days after exposure, depending on the route of infection.

NECROPSY FINDINGS

Usually no gross lesions are seen in animals dying of listerial encephalitis, apart from some congestion of meningeal vessels and an increase in the amount of cerebrospinal fluid (CSF). Microscopic lesions are confined primarily to the pons, medulla, and anterior spinal cord. Marked perivascular cuffing of mononuclear cells and varying degrees of focal necrosis are present. In sheep and goats, neutrophils predominate in the necrotic foci and cause microabscesses. Edema, hemorrhage, neuron degeneration, neuronophagia, congestion, and some thrombi may be present. In cattle, the perivascular cuffs are smaller, and the focal lesions are usually limited to edema and small accumulations of microglial cells and lymphocytes. Rarely are lesions as extensive as those in sheep—an observation in keeping with the more chronic nature of bovine encephalitis. In septicemic listeriosis, small necrotic foci may be found in any viscus, especially the liver and spleen. Fetuses aborting from listeric placentitis may be slightly to markedly autolytic. There is excess fluid in the serous cavities, clear to blood tinged; some fibrin in the abdominal cavity; and numerous small necrotic foci, up to 2 mm in diameter, in the liver, especially the right half. These lesions are usually not masked by autolysis, grossly or microscopically. Necrotic foci may also be found in other organs such as the lungs and spleen. Shallow erosions 1 to 3 mm in diameter may be present in the abomasal mucosa. Gram-stained smears of abomasal contents reveal numerous gram-positive, pleomorphic coccobacilli.

DIAGNOSIS

A presumptive diagnosis of listerial encephalitis may be made from the history, clinical signs, and laboratory data. Silage-fed animals demonstrating signs compatible with brain stem lesions such as cranial nerve abnormalities are highly suspect. The CSF of ruminants with listeriosis usually contains an increased number of white blood cells and an increase in CSF protein content. The predominant cell type in the CSF of affected animals is the monocyte. Hematology and serum biochemical analysis generally do not contribute to the diagnosis of listeriosis. Isolation of *L. monocytogenes* from the CSF is usually unrewarding because the organism only occasionally gains access to the meningoventricular system. A polymerase chain reaction assay has been developed for the detection of *L. monocytogenes* in the CSF of humans with listerial encephalitis. This test is useful in humans who have previously been treated with antimicrobials, which renders isolation of the organism very difficult. Detection of *L. monocytogenes* in the CSF of affected ruminants is possible with use of the polymerase chain reaction assay, but absence of the organism in the CSF limits the usefulness of this test. *Listeria* can be quickly identified in silage samples by using the polymerase chain reaction assay.

Listerial encephalitis must be differentiated from other diseases. In cattle, the differential diagnosis includes rabies, otitis media and interna, lead poisoning, ketosis, acute gastroenteritis, Aujeszky's disease, and viral encephalitis. In sheep, the differential diagnosis should include rabies, otitis media and interna, *Parelaphostrongylus tenuis* infection, brain abscess, polioencephalomalacia, and pregnancy toxemia. Rabies, Aujeszky's disease, hog cholera, erysipelas, influenza, and certain toxins should be considered in swine.

A definitive diagnosis of listerial encephalitis can be made by histopathologic and bacteriologic studies; prompt examination should be made for both listeriosis and rabies. Anti-*Listeria* immunohistochemical staining, Gram's staining, and bacterial culture are used to identify *Listeria* in the brain parenchyma. These techniques are generally more successful in ovine cases than bovine cases. In sheep, listeric encephalitis is confirmed by finding the characteristic microabscesses in the midbrain.

Listeria infection is confirmed by isolating and identifying *L. monocytogenes*. Difficulties are often encountered in isolating

Listeria from fresh tissue, especially brain. Direct stained smears, especially of fetal or placental tissue, may reveal large numbers of pleomorphic, gram-positive, small rods suggestive of *Listeria*. Fluorescent antibody techniques are effective for rapidly diagnosing and identifying *L. monocytogenes* in smears from animals dead or aborted from listeriosis and from milk and meat.

Serologic procedures are being used more for diagnosing listeriosis, but their value in animals has not been established. A dot-blot assay and an enzyme-linked immunosorbent assay have been used experimentally in cattle to detect anti–listeriolysin O antibodies.

TREATMENT

Listeria organisms are sensitive to many antimicrobials, especially ampicillin, tetracycline, and erythromycin. However, several *Listeria* isolates from human patients in Europe were resistant to tetracycline. Ampicillin reaches therapeutic concentrations in the CSF and has few side effects. Penicillin in high doses is the most economical antimicrobial used for the treatment of listeriosis in food animals.

Early treatment of listerial encephalitis before the onset of severe central nervous system signs is important. A high dose of procaine penicillin G (44,000 U/kg twice daily) administered intramuscularly or subcutaneously for 7 to 14 days, followed by an additional 7 to 14 days at a lower dose (22,000 U/kg twice daily), is an effective treatment protocol for both cattle and sheep with encephalitis. Initially, potassium penicillin (44,000 U/kg) can be given intravenously to rapidly attain high plasma concentrations. Oxytetracycline hydrochloride (10 mg/kg twice daily) is also used in the treatment of listerial encephalitis; treatment should be continued for at least 1 week. The prognosis for listerial encephalitis depends on the duration and severity of clinical signs prior to treatment; if the animal is recumbent, treatment is of little use. However, the prognosis for both sheep and cattle that are ambulatory upon examination is good.

Anorectic or dysphagic animals are often dehydrated and have electrolyte abnormalities. If salivary fluid loss is high, affected animals may have metabolic acidosis because of the high salivary content of bicarbonate. Oral or intravenous fluid therapy is usually required to treat dehydrated animals, especially if they are dysphagic. Bicarbonate replacement and supplementation may be necessary if affected animals are losing saliva. Fluid therapy should be continued until the animal is able to swallow. Transfaunation of ruminal contents may re-establish rumen flora and motility in an anorectic ruminant. Additional supportive therapy to maintain musculoskeletal function may be necessary. A well-bedded stall with nonslip surfaces will reduce the risk of injury in a recumbent or weak patient. Anti-inflammatory drugs and vitamin E–selenium are used to treat muscular trauma associated with recumbency.

Penicillin may be used to treat septicemic listeriosis. Prophylactic administration of penicillin may also reduce the risk of abortion in susceptible animals.

IMMUNITY

Immunologic protection against listeriosis is primarily cell mediated, and *Listeria* organisms producing listeriolysin O initiate a T-cell–mediated response. However, it has been suggested that humoral immunity may play a role in the clinical course of infection in goats and in the elimination of *Listeria* from the gastrointestinal tract of goats. Listeriolysin O appears to be an important target for specific antibody production.

Formol and heat-killed *Listeria* vaccines give poor protection. Good results with live attenuated vaccines in sheep have been reported from Bulgaria, Germany, Norway, and Russia. The live vaccine used in certain areas contains attenuated strains of *L. monocytogenes*, serovars 1/2a, 1/2b, and 4b. Healthy sheep older than 3 months, including pregnant ewes, are vaccinated subcutaneously, and protective immunity results within 2 weeks and lasts for at least 10 months. Annual revaccination is recommended in those countries where vaccine is cost-effective.

CONTROL

Institution of general principles for controlling infectious diseases and good hygiene are the only current control measures available in North America. When listeriosis has broken out, affected animals should be isolated and treated and dead animals disposed of as quickly as possible by a rendering plant or preferably by burning or burying deeply under quicklime. Affected buildings and housing for in-contact animals should be thoroughly cleaned and disinfected, and all contaminated or suspected bedding and feed should be burned.

Silage feeding should be reduced and feeding spoiled silage should be avoided. In affected feedlots, constant feeding of low-level tetracyclines may be beneficial.

Animals with nonfatal *Listeria* infection or those recovering after antibiotic therapy may be carriers for long periods and should therefore be eliminated or isolated. Some lactating cows with listeriosis may excrete *Listeria* in their milk for long periods and are a public health hazard.

BIBLIOGRAPHY

Gray ML, Killinger AH: *Listeria monocytogenes* and *Listeria* infection. Bacteriol Rev 30:309–382, 1966.

Husu JR: Epidemiological studies on the occurrence of *Listeria monocytogenes* in the feces of dairy cattle. J Vet Med 37:276–282, 1990.

Jaton K, Sahli R, Bille J: Development of polymerase chain reaction assays for detection of *Listeria monocytogenes* in clinical cerebrospinal fluid samples. J Clin Microbiol 30:1931–1936, 1992.

Low JC, Wright F, McLauchlin J: Serotyping and distribution of *Listeria* isolates from cases of ovine listeriosis. Vet Rec 133:165–166, 1993.

Marco AJ, Prats N, Ramos JA: A microbiological, histopathological and immunohistological study of the intragastric inoculation of *Listeria monocytogenes* in mice. J Comp Pathol 107:1–9, 1992.

Miettinen ARI, Husu J, Tuomi J: Serum antibody response to *Listeria monocytogenes*, listerial excretion, and clinical characteristics in experimentally infected goats. J Clin Microbiol 28:340–343, 1990.

Rebhun WC: Listeriosis. Vet Clin North Am 3:75–83, 1987.

Rebhun WC, deLahunta A: Diagnosis and treatment of bovine listeriosis. J Am Vet Med Assoc 180:395–398, 1982.

Rocourt J, Berche P: Third Forum in Microbiology Virulence; *Listeria monocytogenes*. Ann Inst Pasteur Microbiol 138:241–284, 1987.

Scarratt KW: Ovine listeric encephalitis. Compend Contin Educ Food Anim 9:F28–F33, 1987.

Seeliger HPR, Jones D: Genus *Listeria. In* Bergey's Manual of Systematic Bacteriology. Baltimore, Williams & Wilkins, 1986, pp 1235–1245.

Wiedmann M, Czajka J, Bsat N: Diagnosis and epidemiological association of *Listeria monocytogenes* strains in two outbreaks of listerial encephalitis in small ruminants. J Clin Microbiol 32:991–996, 1994.

■ Necrobacillosis Associated With *Fusobacterium necrophorum*

T. G. Nagaraja, M.V.Sc., Ph.D.

Necrobacillosis in animals associated with *Fusobacterium necrophorum* generally encompasses diseases typified by necrosis and abscess formation (Table 1). The genus *Fusobacterium*, particularly the species *F. necrophorum*, is a frequent anaerobic isolate from clinical specimens. Necrobacillosis has been reported in cattle, sheep, goats, rabbits, and wild animals. Among *F. necrophorum* infections, hepatic necrobacillosis (liver abscesses), necrotic laryngitis (calf diphtheria), and interdigital necrobacillosis (foot rot) in cattle have the most severe economic impact. The economic losses are generally due to loss of productivity; the infections seldom cause mortality.

CHARACTERISTICS OF *Fusobacterium necrophorum*

F. necrophorum, formerly called *Sphaerophorus necrophorus*, is a gram-negative, strictly anaerobic, non–spore-forming pleomorphic bacterium. It can be differentiated from other *Fusobacterium* species by indole production and the ability to convert lactate to propionate. The organism is a normal inhabitant of the gastrointestinal tract (particularly the rumen), oral cavity, respiratory tract, and genitourinary tract of animals. Although anaerobic, the organism can survive in the soil of feedlot pens and pastures.

Historically, *F. necrophorum* is classified into four biotypes/biovars: A, B, AB, and C. Biotypes A and B, the most frequent types encountered in infections, have been assigned subspecies status: *necrophorum* and *funduliforme*, respectively. Biotype AB has characteristics intermediate to those of biotypes A and B, and its taxonomic status is unclear. It is rarely involved in liver abscesses in feedlot cattle but is isolated more frequently from foot abscesses of cattle and sheep. Biotype C, an avirulent type, has been reclassified as a new species, *F. pseudonecrophorum*.

The two major biotypes or subspecies differ in morphology, growth characteristics, and biochemical and biologic characteristics. Among the biologic characteristics, toxin production and virulence are most relevant to the pathogenesis of infection.

Table 1
NECROBACILLOSIS CAUSED BY *Fusobacterium necrophorum*

Disease	Host	Subspecies/ Biotype	Other Bacteria Commonly Associated
Hepatic abscess	Cattle	*necrophorum, funduliforme*	*Actinomyces pyogenes, Bacteroides* spp.
Foot abscess	Cattle	*necrophorum, funduliforme*	*Actinomyces pyogenes, Prevotella melaninogenicus*
	Sheep	Biotype AB	*Dichelobacter nodosus, Bacteroides* spp.
Calf diphtheria	Calves	*necrophorum, funduliforme*	*Actinomyces pyogenes*
Mastitis	Cattle	ND	*Actinomyces pyogenes, Peptostreptococcus indolicus*

ND, not determined.

The subspecies *necrophorum* (biotype A) is more toxigenic, more virulent, and therefore more frequently isolated from infections than the subspecies *funduliforme* (biotype B).

VIRULENCE FACTORS

Virulence factors implicated in the pathogenesis of *F. necrophorum* include leukotoxin, endotoxic lipopolysaccharide, hemolysin, hemagglutinin, capsule, adhesins or pili, platelet aggregation factor, dermonecrotic toxin, and several extracellular enzymes, including proteases and deoxyribonucleases. Among these factors, leukotoxin and endotoxic lipopolysaccharide have been investigated extensively and are believed to be the major virulence factors.

PATHOGENIC MECHANISMS

The pathogenesis of *F. necrophorum* infections possibly involves the following series of events:

1. Entry into the epithelium, mucosa (rumen and larynx), or epidermis (feet)—facilitated by breaks in the surface from trauma and/or the actions of proteases, dermonecrotic toxin, and adhesins of the organism.

2. Proliferation and colonization of the epithelium, mucosa, or epidermis—facilitated by leukotoxin (prevents phagocytosis) and endotoxin or platelet factor (to create an anaerobic microenvironment) elaborated by the bacterium.

3. Necrosis of local tissues—induced by the cytotoxic effects of bacterial toxins (leukotoxin, hemolysin, and lipopolysaccharide), by enzymatic activities (proteases and DNAses) of the organism, and indirectly by the action of cytolytic products released from damaged tissue.

Generally, *Fusobacterium* infections tend to remain localized, but occasionally the organism may enter the circulation and result in systemic infection.

LIVER ABSCESSES

Liver abscesses occur at all ages and in all types of cattle, but the abscesses of significant economic impact occur in feedlot cattle. Abscesses found in the liver at the time of slaughter or necropsy are often well encapsulated with thick fibrotic walls. Histologically, a typical abscess is pyogranulomatous, necrotic in the center, encapsulated, and often surrounded by an inflammatory zone.

Incidence

Abscessed livers in slaughtered feedlot cattle are generally recognized as part of aggressive feeding programs. The incidence in most feedlots averages 12% to 32% and is influenced by a number of factors, most notably the diet. Generally, the incidence increases as the roughage level in the grain diet decreases. Grains that are categorized as rapidly fermentable (e.g., wheat, barley, high-moisture corn, or steam-flaked corn) promote a higher incidence. In addition, certain feeding practices such as rapid step-up and poor bunk management that result in fluctuations in feed intake may lead to a higher incidence.

Almost all studies involving bacteriologic analyses of liver abscesses have concluded that *F. necrophorum* is the primary etiologic agent. The organism is often associated with other anaerobic and facultative bacteria, including *Actinomyces* (formerly called *Corynebacterium*) *pyogenes*, *Bacteroides* spp., *Clostrid-*

ium spp., *Pasteurella* spp., *Peptostreptococcus* spp., *Prevotella* spp., *Porphyromonas* spp., *Staphylococcus* spp., and *Streptococcus* spp. *Actinomyces pyogenes* is the second most frequent pathogen isolated from bovine liver abscesses.

Economic Importance

Liver abscesses are significant liabilities to the producer and the packer. Abscesses are the major causes of liver condemnation in the United States. Besides loss of the liver, carcass trimming is often necessary. However, the greatest economic impact of liver abscesses is from reduced animal performance. A number of studies involving comparisons of cattle with and without abscesses have documented that cattle with abscessed livers have reduced feed intake, reduced weight gain, decreased feed efficiency, and decreased carcass yield.

Pathogenesis

Liver abscesses are secondary to the primary foci of infection on the ruminal wall. Because of the close correlation between the incidence of ruminal pathology and liver abscesses in cattle, the term *rumenitis–liver abscess complex* is commonly used. Although the precise mechanism is not recognized, it is accepted that rapid fermentation of grain by ruminal microbes and the subsequent accumulation of organic acids (volatile fatty acids and lactate) result in ruminal acidosis. Acid-induced rumenitis and damage to the protective surface, often aggravated by foreign objects (e.g., sharp feed particles, hair), predispose the ruminal wall to invasion and colonization by *F. necrophorum*. Once colonization has occurred, *F. necrophorum* can gain entry into the blood or cause ruminal wall abscesses and subsequently shed bacterial emboli into the portal circulation. Filtration of bacteria from the portal circulation by the liver results in infection and abscess formation.

Diagnosis

Liver abscesses are detected only at the time of slaughter because cattle, even those that carry multiple abscesses, seldom show clinical signs. Occasionally, rupture of a superficial abscess leads to extensive spread, massive infection of other organs, and eventual death. Hematologic analysis and liver function tests are not useful indicators of liver abscesses. Ultrasonography has been tested as a technique for liver abscess detection. The technique is helpful in monitoring the onset and progression of experimentally induced abscesses, but its application in feedlot cattle with naturally developed abscesses is limited.

Prevention

Control of liver abscesses in feedlot cattle has typically depended on the use of antimicrobial feed additives. Five antibiotics (bacitracin, chlortetracycline, oxytetracycline, tylosin, and virginiamycin) have approval claims for use in feedlot cattle. These antibiotics vary in their effectiveness, with bacitracin being the least effective and tylosin being the most effective and widely used compound (Table 2).

An immunoprophylactic approach would be highly desirable in the feedlot industry. However, the results of attempts to induce protective immunity by using various antigenic components of *F. necrophorum* have varied from having no effect to providing significant protection. Recently, a leukotoxoid-based

Table 2
FDA APPROVED FEED ADDITIVES FOR THE CONTROL OF LIVER ABSCESSES IN FEEDLOT CATTLE

Antibiotic	Chemistry	Mode of Action of Bacterial Inhibition	Absorption From the Gut	Recommended Dosage	Reported Reduction in Liver Abscess Incidence
Bacitracin (methylene disalicylate)	Polypeptide	Cell wall synthesis	No	70 mg/head/day	None to ?
Chlortetracycline	Tetracycline	Protein synthesis	Yes	70 mg/head/day	Up to 21%
Oxytetracycline	Tetracycline	Protein synthesis	Yes	75 mg/head/day	Up to 55%
Tylosin	Macrolide	Protein synthesis	Yes	8–10 g/ton of feed to provide 90 mg/head/day	Up to 75%
Virginiamycin	Peptolide and macrocyclic lactone	Protein synthesis	None to minimal	13.5–16.0 g/ton of feed	Up to 38%

vaccine has shown promise in protecting against experimentally induced liver abscesses in steers.

NECROTIC LARYNGITIS

Necrotic laryngitis is more often referred to as "calf diphtheria," which is a misnomer because the disease occurs in cattle up to 3 years of age. The disease is characterized by necrosis of the mucous membrane and underlying tissues of the larynx and adjacent structures. The infection can be acute or chronic and is generally considered to be noncontagious. In severe cases, cattle can die of aspiration pneumonia.

F. necrophorum is the most frequent pathogen isolated from necrotic inflammation of the larynx, either alone or in association with *A. pyogenes.* Because *F. necrophorum* is a poor invader of healthy mucosa, a breach in the mucosal barrier, possibly caused by viruses, allergens, irritants, or other bacteria, is believed to be required for tissue invasion and colonization. Clinically, initial fever is followed by dyspnea that causes a roaring noise on inspiration and, in severe cases, painful swallowing and cough on inspiration and expiration. Necropsy lesions include necrosis of the larynx and vocal cords and mucosa covered by inflammatory exudate. Occasionally, bronchopneumonia may be present.

Treatment for diphtheria is generally based on systemic administration of sulfonamides and antibiotics (tetracyclines) alone or in combination.

INTERDIGITAL NECROBACILLOSIS

Interdigital necrobacillosis (foot rot, foot abscesses, or foul-in-the-foot) is characterized by acute or subacute necrotizing infection involving the skin and adjacent underlying soft tissues of the feet. The infection is the major cause of lameness in dairy and beef cattle in the United States. The economic impact involves loss in productivity (milk production and weight gain). *Fusobacterium necrophorum* is the most frequent isolate. It is always present in large numbers in necrotic material from foot lesions. Another anaerobe, *Prevotella (Bacteroides) melaninogenicus,* is often isolated from the lesions. *A. pyogenes* is also a frequent isolate. Foot rot in sheep is a mixed bacterial infection of the interdigital skin, with *Dichelobacter* (formerly *Bacteroides) nodosus,* an anaerobe, being the primary causative agent.

Predisposing factors involved in the pathogenesis of foot rot are damp soil and injury to the skin of the interdigital area.

Cattle with long overgrown toes are at higher risk of succumbing to infection. Fecal excretion of *F. necrophorum* is believed to provide the primary source of infection in foot rot and abscesses. However, the presence of *F. necrophorum* in cattle feces is rare, which suggests that the organism is not normally shed. Apparently, disturbances of normal gut flora induced by the oral administration of certain antimicrobial agents encourage the proliferation of *F. necrophorum* in the gut and subsequent fecal excretion.

The lesions are characterized initially by mild cellulitis and swelling between the digits. Within a few days, fissure formation with a scabby exudate that eventually becomes pus in the margin of the fissure is observed. Fever and lameness are common clinical signs. Healing is usually rapid once the abscess has discharged.

Diagnosis is based on recognition of the characteristic interdigital lesion accompanied by a foul discharge.

In mild cases detected early, topical application of antimicrobial agents is helpful. Debriding the necrotic area before application of the agent is generally a good practice. Systemic administration of sulfa drugs or antibiotics (penicillin, chlortetracycline, oxytetracycline, tylosin, and erythromycin) is recommended. Ethylenediamine dihydroiodide (10 to 50 mg/head/day) has been used as a feed additive to prevent foot rot in feedlot cattle; however, it is not approved for use in dairy cattle.

Good management practices such as removal of sharp objects, rocks, or coarse stubble from corrals and pastures, well-drained feedlot pens, and prophylactic use of foot baths are beneficial in reducing the incidence of foot rot.

BIBLIOGRAPHY

Mackey DR: Calf diphtheria. J Am Vet Med Assoc 152:822–823, 1968.

Nagaraja TG, Laudert SB, Parrott JC: Liver abscesses in feedlot cattle: I. Causes, pathogenesis, pathology and diagnosis. Compend Contin Educ Pract Vet 18:5230–5241, 1996.

Nagaraja TG, Laudert JB, Parrott JC: Liver abscesses in feedlot cattle: II. Incidence, economic importance and prevention. Compend Contin Educ Pract Vet 18:5264–5273, 1996.

Rebhun WC, Pearson EG: Clinical management of bovine foot problems. J Am Vet Med Assoc 181:437–577. 1982.

Saginala S, Nagaraja TG, Tan ZL, et al: Serum neutralizing antibody response and protection against experimentally induced liver abscesses in steers vaccinated with *Fusobacterium necrophorum.* Am J Vet Res 57:483–488, 1997.

Tan ZL, Nagaraja TG, Chengappa MM: *Fusobacterium necrophorum* infections: Virulence factors, pathogenic mechanism and control measures. Vet Res Commun 20:113–140, 1996.

Protozoal Diseases

Consulting Editor
Robert A. Smith, D.V.M., M.S., Diplomate, A.B.V.P.

■ **Bovine Anaplasmosis***

E. J. Richey, D.V.M.

Anaplasmosis is an infectious, noncontagious, transmissible hemoparasitic disease of cattle caused by *Anaplasma marginale*,[1] a member of the order Rickettsiales. In the United States, anaplasmosis is enzootic in the South Atlantic States, the Gulf States, and the lower plains and western states, but is reported as sporadic in the northern states.[2–4]

TRANSMISSION

The principal means of *A. marginale* transmission are the transfer of parasitized red blood cells (RBCs) (mechanical transmission) and the transfer of the tick stage of *A. marginale* during certain tick feeding (biologic transmission). Mechanical transmission occurs by direct inoculation of infected RBCs into susceptible cattle on blood-contaminated hypodermic needles, surgical or dehorning instruments, or on the mouthparts of biting flies. Horse flies[5] deer flies, stable flies, and less importantly, mosquitoes, and *Dermacentor andersoni* and *Dermacentor occidentalis* ticks, can all spread anaplasmosis and have been implicated as the major means of transmission in enzootic areas of the southern United States.[6–9] These natural mechanical and biologic vectors are usually seasonal and most outbreaks of anaplasmosis coincide with or immediately follow the vector seasons.

---

*© State of Florida.

Contaminated surgical instruments, dehorners, and hypodermic needles are known mechanical vectors used by man. This type of mechanical transmission takes place only when the disease organism is exchanged immediately—within minutes. When this type of transmission occurs, a large number of cattle in the herd show signs of anaplasmosis at nearly the same time, without a few earlier cases having appeared.[10]

CLINICAL SIGNS

All ages of cattle may become infected with anaplasmosis. However, the severity of illness and the percentage of deaths increase with age. Calves under 6 months of age become infected and remain carriers when challenged with *A. marginale*; however, they seldom exhibit any clinical signs of anaplasmosis[11] (Fig. 1). Cattle aged 6 months to 3 years become increasingly ill and more deaths occur with advancing age (Fig. 2). After 3 years of age, a 30% to 50% mortality rate occurs in cattle exhibiting clinical anaplasmosis.[11, 12] (Fig. 3).

The clinical signs found in bovine anaplasmosis are predominantly signs related to acute anemia. However, a febrile response is noted coinciding with the beginning of a detectable parasitemia in the blood system. The fever usually persists through the period of increasing parasitemia and may reach 41°C (106°F); however, subnormal temperatures are noted prior to death.

The acute anemia results in pallor of the mucosa, muscular weakness, depression, dehydration, anorexia, increased heart

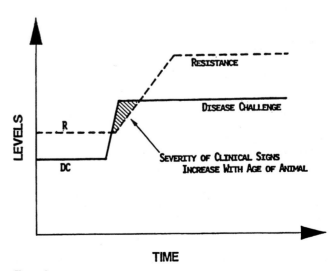

Figure 1
Calf response to *A. marginale* challenge.

Figure 2
Response in cattle, 6 months to 3 years of age, to *A. marginale* challenge.

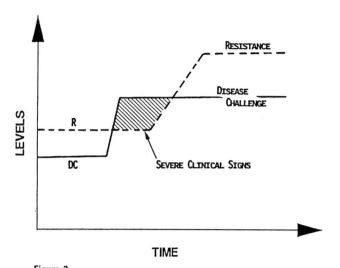

Figure 3
Response in cattle older than 3 years to *A. marginale* challenge.

Table 1	
TYPICAL CLINICAL LABORATORY FINDINGS IN ACUTE ANAPLASMOSIS	
Parasitized RBCs (%)	10–75
Packed cell volume (%)	5–15
Total RBCs ($\times$ 10⁶ cells/µL)	1.5–4.0
Total billirubin (mg/100 mL)	2.0–7.0
Direct bilirubin (mg/100 mL)	0.25–7.0
RBCs, red blood cells.	

rate and, upon exertion, respiratory distress.[13] The animal may be belligerent if inadequate tissue oxygenation has affected the brain. Examination of the blood shows it to be grossly thin and watery. Since the disease is characteristically a hemolytic disease in which the parasitized RBCs are destroyed in the reticuloendothelial system without release of free hemoglobin, hemoglobinuria is not seen in anaplasmosis.[14]

PATHOGENESIS

Anaplasmosis can be divided into four stages: incubation,[10] developmental, convalescent, and carrier. The *incubation stage* is that time from introduction of the *Anaplasma* organism into a susceptible animal until the time 1% of the RBCs are infected. The length of this stage appears to vary directly with the number of organisms introduced into the animal. Under natural conditions, the time may be from 3 to 8 weeks, although shorter and longer times have been recorded. No clinical signs can be seen during this stage. The end of the period coincides with the first rise in body temperature.

The *developmental stage* refers to that time when the characteristic anemia is developing. It begins at the time of 1% infected RBCs and ends when the reticulocytes appear in the peripheral circulation. The length of this stage varies from 4 to 9 days. During this period, most of the signs characteristic of anaplasmosis appear. The infected animal usually shows the first clinical signs about midway, or about the third or fourth day, of the developmental stage. This is the time when owners who observe their cattle carefully each day will notice the animal is ill.

Laboratory values during this stage reflect a severe hemolytic anemia. The percentage of parasitized erythrocytes can range from 10% to greater than 75% in acute infections and the cell count is characterized by numerous basophilic punctate bodies 0.5 to 1.0-µm in diameter in the margin of Wright's- or Giemsa-stained RBCs[1] (Table 1).

The *convalescent stage* extends from the appearance of reticulocytes to the return to normal of the various blood values. The length of this stage varies greatly and may extend from a few weeks to a few months. The differentiation between developmental and convalescent stages is evidence of increased erythropoiesis on stained blood smears. The signs of increased erythropoiesis in the peripheral blood, which identifies the convalescent stage, are reticulocytes, polychromatophils, basophilic stippled

cells, normoblasts, increased hemoglobin, and an increase in the total white blood cells.

Death losses due to anaplasmosis usually occur during the late developmental stage or early convalescent stage (Fig. 4). Postmortem findings are principally attributable to the severe hemolytic anemia. All tissues are pale and the blood is thin and watery; icterus may be present if the animal dies in the later states of acute infection. The spleen is frequently enlarged and a deep red-brown. An enlarged liver and a gallbladder distended with dark bile are common.[1] On a thin blood smear, stained with Giemsa or Wright's stain, the *A. marginale* bodies appear as spherical granules 0.2 to 0.5 µm in diameter located near the periphery of the RBC. The *Anaplasma* bodies are most easily detected during the developmental and convalescent stages.

The *carrier stage* is usually thought of as that time extending from the disappearance of discernible *Anaplasma* bodies sometime during the convalescent stage to the end of the animal's life. Clinically recovered animals remain carriers with a nondetectable parasitemia and thus act as a reservoir of the disease.

SEROLOGY

The complement fixation test and the rapid card test (agglutination) are the most common serologic tests used for the detection of *Anaplasma* titers. Infected animals begin to exhibit positive reactions at about the same time that *Anaplasma* bodies can first be seen in the RBCs. The test reactions are, therefore,

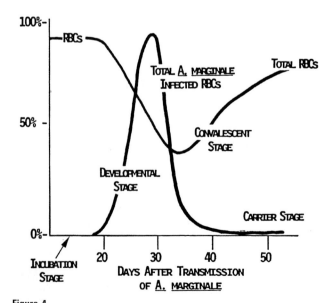

Figure 4
A. marginale infestation of RBCs and change in total RBCs during the different stages of anaplasmosis.

negative throughout the incubation period and positive during the developmental, convalescent, and carrier stages. Because the serologic tests will not differentiate the latter three stages, the use of serologic reactions is of little use when a definitive diagnosis of anaplasmosis is required.

DIAGNOSIS

A tentative diagnosis of anaplasmosis may rely upon suspicion of transmission, characteristic clinical signs, necropsy findings, serologic testing, or clinical laboratory values. However, definitive diagnosis requires the identification of *A. marginale*–parasitized RBCs during the developmental or convalescent stages.

A brief summary of the presence of parasitemia, serologic reactions, and clinical signs in relationship to the stage of disease is presented in Table 2.

TREATMENT OF ACUTE ANAPLASMOSIS

A *single parenteral injection* of oxytetracycline (OTC) can be very effective in reducing the severity of the disease when administered while the percentage of infected cells is less than 15% (about midway through the developmental stage). Animals treated parenterally with OTC at this time have better than average chance for recovery. The OTC will stop the increase in infected RBCs and since it is mainly those cells that are destroyed to produce the anemia, the RBC count hopefully will not drop below a critical level.[15]

When percentages of infected cells above 15% are encountered, the effectiveness of OTC is reduced and recovery of the animal will be due to the natural ability of the bone marrow to produce RBCs in sufficient numbers to compensate for loss of the infected cells[15] (Fig. 5).

Toward the end of the developmental stage and the beginning of the convalescent stage, frequently the best treatment is no treatment. There are two reasons for considering not to treat at this time. First, the animal may suddenly die from anoxia if it is forced to move or becomes excited. Second, OTC treatments do little or nothing to change the outcome of the disease when given at this time. OTC acts only to reduce the number of infected RBCs; the number of infected RBCs has already peaked and they are being rapidly destroyed by the reticuloendothelial system. Hematinic drugs do not have enough time to stimulate erythropoiesis, and a blood transfusion in sufficient amount to be beneficial may overload the anoxia-weakened heart.[15]

MANAGEMENT OF ANAPLASMOSIS

Anaplasmosis outbreaks are related to having no control program, having both anaplasmosis carriers and susceptible animals

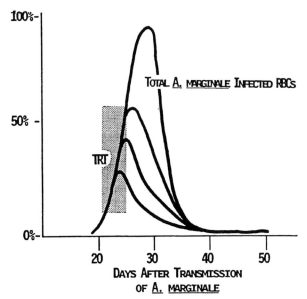

Figure 5
Effect of oxytetracycline on *A. marginale* infestation of RBCs.

present in the herd, and having vector transmission.[15] As with any disease situation, an animal remains healthy or unaffected as long as the animal's "resistance" level remains above the "disease challenge" level (Fig. 6). Relying solely on natural resistance or lack of disease exposure to keep the resistance level above the disease challenge level is not a very comfortable position for a herd to be in. Any rise in the disease challenge level would result in clinical anaplasmosis. Certain tools have been identified that can assist the herd owner to control anaplasmosis by preventing outbreaks and halting outbreaks when they occur. Those tools either raise the resistance or reduce the disease challenge. It is to the herd owner's advantage to create a greater spread between the resistance and disease challenge levels. A wider spread provides a more comfortable situation (Fig. 7).

In general, utilizing both tools (increasing resistance and reducing challenge) simultaneously can be very expensive; therefore, simultaneous use is primarily limited to stopping outbreaks of anaplasmosis, whereas control programs to prevent clinical

Table 2			
FINDINGS DURING DIFFERENT STAGES OF ANAPLASMOSIS			
Stage of Disease	***Anaplasma marginale* on Blood Smear**	**Reaction to Serologic Testing**	**Clinical Signs**
Unexposed	No	Negative	None
Incubation	No	Negative	None
Developmental	Yes	Positive	Present
Convalescent	Yes*	Positive	Present
Carrier	No	Positive	None

*Immature red blood cells also present.

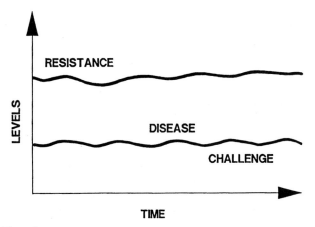

Figure 6
A healthy herd exists when the resistance level is maintained above the level of disease challenge.

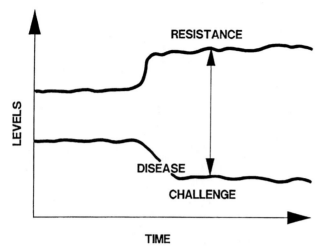

Figure 7

A comfortable spread between the resistance level and the level of disease challenge.

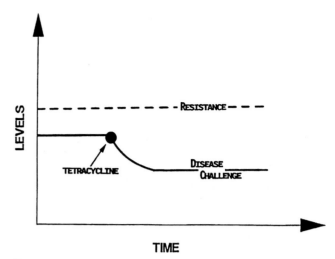

Figure 9

Test and eliminate the carrier state as a control program for anaplasmosis.

anaplasmosis in a herd usually utilize only one tool type at a time.

Prevention Programs

Testing and Removal of Carriers

This program necessitates bleeding each animal, identifying carriers, and removing them.[15] An alternative to disposing of carriers is to separate the carrier animals from the "clean" animals and to maintain two herds, an anaplasmosis-infected herd and an anaplasmosis-clean herd; there are no susceptible animals in a 100% carrier herd. New additions must be protected, however, and there are regulations governing interstate movement of carrier animals (Fig. 8).

Testing and Clearing the Carriers

Anaplasmosis carriers may be cured of the infection by treatment with certain tetracycline antibiotics[16] (Fig. 9). Carrier state

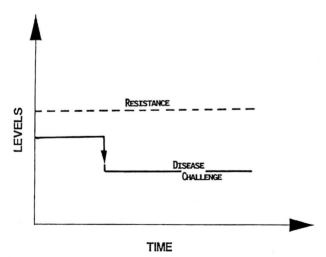

Figure 8

Test and removal of carrier animals as a control program for preventing anaplasmosis.

elimination programs must include postmedication serologic testing. The animal can test positive for months after treatment but may be free of infection. When testing 6 months after stopping treatment, positive reactors should be considered as treatment failures.[10] Failures should be re-treated or separated from the rest of the herd. Animals cleared of the carrier state are susceptible to reinfection, but are known to exhibit resistance to clinical anaplasmosis for up to 30 months after treatment.[17]

Elimination of the carrier state should be conducted after the vector season has ended. The effect of a continuous field challenge exposure while attempting a carrier elimination program has not been fully investigated.

1. OTC 50 to 100 mg/mL to eliminate carrier stages: Treat each animal with OTC at 22 mg/kg (10 mg/lb) of body weight daily for 5 days,[18] or 11 mg/kg (5 mg/lb) of body weight daily for 10 days.[19] Inject not over 10 mL per site intramuscularly (IM). If intravenous, dilute with physiologic saline.

2. OTC 200 mg/mL to eliminate carrier stages: Treat each animal four times with OTC 200 at 3-day intervals at 20 mg/kg (9 mg/lb) of body weight. Each dose should be divided between two sites and given by deep IM injection.[20]

3. Chlortetracycline (CTC) to eliminate carrier stages: It is recommended that CTC be fed at a level of 11 mg/kg (5 mg/lb) body weight daily for 60 days.[21] When fed daily at this level, CTC will eliminate the carrier stage. Oral administration permits treatment on a herd basis and the use of economical antibiotic premixes. This oral dose on rare occasions may cause diarrhea, anorexia, and weight loss during the first week, but the cattle return to normal rapidly after that time. The medicated feed should nevertheless be kept before them during this time. Fed at the rate of 1.1 mg/kg (0.5 mg/lb) of body weight daily for 120 days, CTC eliminates the carrier state.[22] This low dosage fed for 120 days makes the clearing of the carrier state very simple while winter-feeding range cattle.

Continuous Oxytetracycline Medication During the Vector Season

An injection of OTC administered every 28 days, beginning with the start of the vector season and ending 30 to 60 days after the vector season ends, will prevent clinical anaplasmosis from developing.[23] The recommended dose is 6.6 to 11 mg/kg (3 to 5 mg/lb) of body weight when using 50 to 100 mg/mL

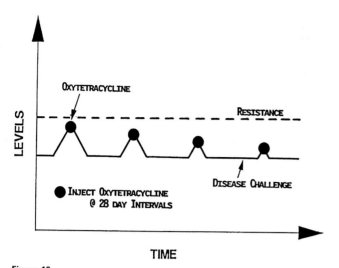

Figure 10
Inject oxytetracycline at 28-day intervals throughout the vector season as a control program for anaplasmosis.

OTC, or 20 mg/kg (9 mg/lb) of body weight when using OTC 200 (Fig. 10).

Continuous Chlortetracycline Medication During the Vector Season

CTC consumed at the rate of 1.1 mg/kg (0.5 mg/lb) body weight daily during the vector season will prevent the transmission of anaplasmosis to susceptible animals. CTC at this dose may be administered by use of medicated feed fed daily, medicated salt-mineral mixes offered free choice, and medicated feed blocks. Consumption data should be available from feed or salt-mineral manufacturers[24] (Fig. 11).

Continuous Chlortetracycline Medication Year-Round

CTC administered in daily doses of 0.22 to 0.55 mg/kg (0.1 to 0.25 mg/lb) of body weight will prevent clinical anaplasmosis.

However, transmission of the *A. marginale* organism has been reported when using this low dose. If the CTC is withdrawn shortly after transmission occurs, you can expect clinical anaplasmosis to appear in the herd after a delayed incubation stage. For this reason, CTC at this dose must be administered year-round. CTC added to salt-mineral mixes is a convenient way to administer this low dose (Fig. 12).[24]

Using salt-mineral mixes or feed blocks as the vehicle for administering CTC requires placing the mix or blocks near water holes, providing sufficient protection from the sun and rain, and replenishing the mix at frequent intervals. It is advisable to routinely check to ensure that the cattle are consuming the medicated mix.

Bulls apparently do not consume adequate CTC and require additional protection, such as vaccination.

Anaplasmosis Vaccine

The initial vaccination schedule, which consists of two doses given 4 weeks apart, is scheduled so that the second dose is given at least 2 weeks before the vector season begins.[25] Each year thereafter a booster should be given 2 weeks or more before the vector season begins.[26] A vaccinated animal is still capable of becoming infected with *A. marginale* and subsequently can become a carrier. The vaccine does not prevent infection, but aids in prevention or reduction in the severity of clinical anaplasmosis[25] (Fig. 13).

Current immunization in the United States is limited to the use of a killed whole organism vaccine (Plazvax, Schering-Plough Animal Health, Kenilworth, NJ). A modified live vaccine has been licensed for use in California.[27] Neither infection nor clinical disease is prevented by the vaccines, but the severity of the anemia, parasitemia, and weight loss is less than that exhibited in nonvaccinated cattle.[28] Although vaccination is recommended when shipping susceptible mature cattle to enzootic areas, vaccination does not guarantee protection and is not feasible for use in developing a disease-free herd.

The use of modified live vaccines for preimmunization will also induce resistance to severe manifestation of clinical disease.[27, 29] The preimmunizing infection can cause a mild to severe case of clinical disease and may require treatment with tetracyclines to control the initial infection. Although its use in enzootically stable areas is effective, it has limited use in routine

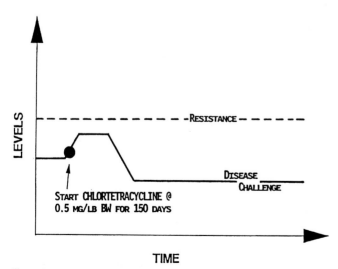

Figure 11
Chlortetracycline administered during the vector season as a control for anaplasmosis.

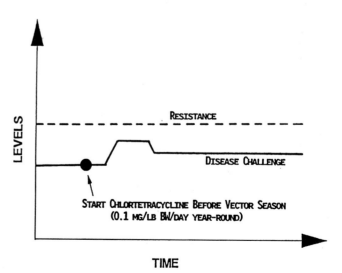

Figure 12
Chlortetracycline administered year-round as a control program for anaplasmosis.

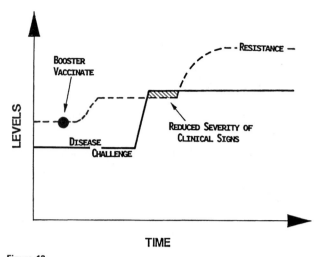

Figure 13

Vaccination to reduce the severity of clinical disease as a control program for anaplasmosis.

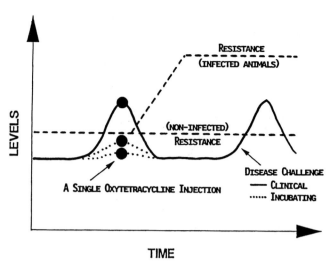

Figure 15

Response of *A. marginale* infection to one oxytetracycline injection.

immunization of mature susceptible cattle. The risk of transmitting other infective agents with the blood-based vaccine (including bovine leukemia virus) will likely limit its approval to intrastate use in the United States.

Clearly, the current vaccine is not effective for routine use to maintain *A. marginale*–free cattle herds or for complete protection when moving susceptible cattle into enzootic areas.

Preimmunization of Calves

Before the development of the tools to prevent anaplasmosis, calves were deliberately inoculated with *A. marginale* to provide lifetime protection. Citrated whole blood, 1 mL, freshly collected from a known *A. marginale*–infected animal, was injected subcutaneously into calves under 6 months of age. The inoculated calves became infected and remained carriers without exhibiting clinical anaplasmosis. Too high a volume into too old an animal can result in clinical disease. The injection of 5 mL

of *A. marginale*–infected blood into yearling heifers has resulted in severe clinical anaplasmosis and death[10–12] (Fig. 14).

Reduction of Vector Transmission

Applications of insecticides that reduce the biting insect population will substantially reduce the number of clinical cases occurring in a herd. Periodic spraying and dipping, as well as forced use of dust bags and back rubbers, are the common methods of insecticide application.

Since man often transmits the disease by carrying the organism from a carrier animal to a susceptible animal via blood-contaminated instruments, a quick rinse of the contaminated instruments in clean water or disinfectant between animals will prevent transmission.

Stopping an Outbreak

Regardless of the availability of adequate control programs, many cattle producers either choose not to use a program or

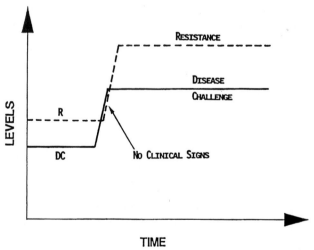

Figure 14

Calf response to a challenge by *A. marginale*.

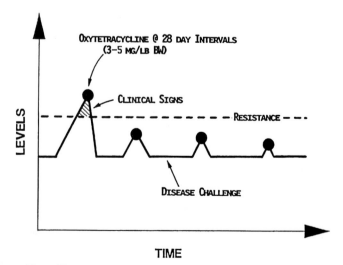

Figure 16

Oxytetracycline injections used to stop an outbreak of anaplasmosis.

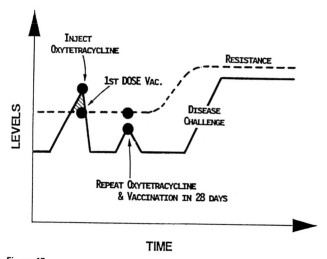

Figure 17
Oxytetracycline plus vaccination used to stop an outbreak of anaplasmosis.

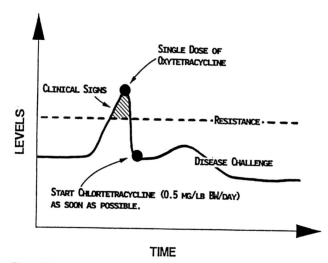

Figure 19
Oxytetracycline and chlortetracycline used to stop an outbreak of anaplasmosis.

have no reason to do so. In either event, it is necessary to describe to a veterinarian and producer the methods available for halting an anaplasmosis outbreak in a herd. The proper handling of an outbreak should include the treatment of clinically ill animals and provide adequate protection for the remainder of the herd. The clinically ill animal may only be the first of many that will become ill or exposed to anaplasmosis.

In addition to treating the clinically ill animals, the remainder of the herd must be adequately protected. Since no clinical symptoms are being exhibited by the animals in the remainder of the herd it is assumed that they could be categorized as being unexposed, in the incubation stage, in the convalescent stage, or in the carrier stage. The unexposed animals and the animals in the incubation stage must be provided with temporary protection until prolonged protection can be established.

The tools used to prevent an anaplasmosis outbreak in a herd can also be used to stop an outbreak. They can be used to provide both temporary and prolonged protection to the herd.

Temporary protection is accomplished by administering par-

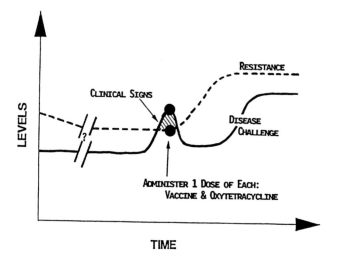

Figure 18
Using vaccine boosters and oxytetracycline to stop an outbreak of anaplasmosis in a previously vaccinated herd.

enteral injections of OTC. Parenteral injection of OTC prior to exposure has no effect on the course of a later infection, but animals injected with a single parenteral dose of OTC during the incubation stage exhibit a prolongation of the incubation stage for 2 to 3 weeks, and a single dose of OTC administered to animals early in the developmental stage will suppress clinical disease for 3 to 4 weeks. In both cases, clinical anaplasmosis is delayed for approximately 28 days (Fig. 15).

1. Use of injectable OTC to stop an outbreak: At the first indication of anaplasmosis, gather all susceptible animals and administer a single dose of OTC at the rate of 6.6 to 11 mg/kg (3 to 5 mg/lb) of body weight for temporary protection. For prolonged protection this treatment must be repeated at 28-day intervals throughout the vector season. After withdrawal of the OTC medication, close observation should continue for symptoms of anaplasmosis that may have been only delayed, not aborted, in some cattle (Fig. 16).

2. Use of OTC and vaccination to stop an outbreak (Fig. 17): At the first indication of anaplasmosis, gather all susceptible animals and administer a single dose of OTC at the rate of 6.6 to 11 mg/kg (3 to 5 mg/lb) of body weight for temporary protection. For prolonged protection give each animal the first dose of anaplasmosis vaccine. Twenty-eight days later, give the second dose of vaccine and another dose of OTC.[30]

3. Use of OTC and vaccination to stop an outbreak in a previously vaccinated herd: If anaplasmosis occurs because a vaccine booster was skipped, administer a single dose of OTC at the rate of 6.6 to 11 mg/kg (3 to 5 mg/lb) of body weight and one dose of vaccine to each susceptible animal. Any previously nonvaccinated animals should receive a second dose of both vaccine and OTC in 28 days[31] (Fig. 18).

4. OTC and CTC to stop an outbreak: At the first indication of anaplasmosis, gather all susceptible animals and administer a single dose of OTC at the rate of 6.6 to 11 mg/kg (3 to 5 mg/lb) of body weight for temporary protection. For prolonged protection, immediately offer CTC free choice at the rate of 1.1 mg/kg (0.5 mg/lb) of body weight in a medicated salt-mineral mix or feed blocks. CTC-medicated mixes or blocks should be offered for at least 60 days[32] (Fig. 19).

Tetracycline treatment regimens for anaplasmosis control, elimination of the carrier stage, and handling outbreaks are provided in Table 3.

Table 3
TETRACYCLINE TREATMENT REGIMENS FOR ANAPLASMOSIS MANAGEMENT*

Use and Drug	Route	Dose (mg/kg of BW)	Frequency of Treatment
Prevention			
Chlortetracycline	Oral	0.22–0.55	Daily year-round
Chlortetracycline	Oral	1.1	Daily during vector season
Oxytetracycline (50–100 mg/mL)	IV or IM	6.6–11	Every 28 days during vector season
Oxytetracycline (200 mg/mL)	IM	20	Every 28 days during vector season
Carrier Elimination			
Chlortetracycline	Oral	1.1	Daily for 120 days
Chlortetracycline	Oral	11	Daily for 60 days
Oxytetracycline (50–100 mg/mL)	IV or IM	11	Daily for 10 days
Oxytetracycline (50–100 mg/mL)	IV or IM	22	Daily for 5 days
Oxytetracycline (200 mg/mL)	IM	20	Four treatments at 3-day intervals
Treatment of Sick			
Oxytetracycline (50–100 mg/mL)	IM	11	Usually one treatment
Oxytetracycline (200 mg/mL)	IM	20	One treatment
Temporary Protection During Outbreaks			
Oxytetracycline (50–100 mg/mL)	IM	11	One treatment
Oxytetracycline (200 mg/mL)	IM	20	One treatment
Prolonged Protection During Outbreaks			
Oxytetracycline (50–100 mg/mL)	IM	11	Every 28 days during vector season
Oxytetracycline (200 mg/mL)	IM	20	Every 28 days during vector season
Chlortetracycline	Oral	1.1	Daily for 60 days

BW, body weight; IV, intravenous; IM, intramuscular.
*Vaccine is used to stimulate prolonged resistance; however, until resistance is established, oxytetracycline injections should be used simultaneously with each dose of vaccine to temporarily reduce the *A. marginale* challenge.

REFERENCES

1. Theiler A: *Anaplasma marginale*: The points in the blood of cattle suffering from a specific disease. In Theiler A (ed): Report of the Government Veterinary Bacteriologist (1908–1909). Transvaal Department of Agriculture, Republic of South Africa, 1910, pp 7–64.
2. National Research Council: Priorities in biotechnology research for international development. In Proceedings of a Workshop. Directed by Development, Office of International Affairs. Washington, DC National Academy Press, 1982, pp 1–9.
3. McCallon BR: Prevalence and economic aspects of anaplasmosis. In Jones EW (ed): Proceedings of the Sixth National Anaplasmosis Conference. Stillwater, Okla, Heritage Press, 1973, pp 1–3.
4. Alderink FJ, Dietrich R: Anaplasmosis in Texas: Epidemiologic and economic data from a questionnaire survey. In Hidalgo RJ, Jones EW (eds): Proceedings of the Seventh National Anaplasmosis Conference. Starkville, Mississippi State University, 1981, pp 27–44.
5. Hawkins JA, Love JN, Hidalgo RJ: Mechanical transmission of anaplasmosis by tabanoids (Diptera: Tabanidae). Am J Vet Res 43:732–734, 1982.
6. Ewing SA: Transmission of *Anaplasma marginale* by arthropods. In Hidalgo RJ, Jones EW (eds): Proceedings of the Seventh National Anaplasmosis Conference. Starkville, Mississippi State University, 1981, pp 395–424.
7. Kocan KM, Hair JA, Ewing SA: Ultrastructure of *Anaplasma marginale* Theiler in *Dermacentor andersoni* Stiles and *Dermacentor variablis* (Say). Am J Vet Res 41:1966–1976, 1980.
8. Kocan KM Hair JA, Ewing SA: Demonstration of *Anaplasma marginale* Theiler in *Dermacentor variablis* (Say) by ferritin-conjugated antibody technique. Am J Vet Res 41:1977–1981, 1980.
9. Oberst RD, Kocan KM, Hair JA, et al: Staining characteristics of colonies of *Anaplasma marginale* Theiler in *Dermacentor andersoni* Stiles. Am J Vet Res 42:3006–3009, 1981.
10. Richey EJ: Bovine anaplasmosis. In Howard J (ed): Current Veterinary Therapy: Food Animal Practice. Philadelphia, WB Saunders, 1981, pp 767–772.
11. Ruby TO, Gates DW, Mott LO: The comparative susceptibility of calves and adult cattle to bovine anaplasmosis. Am J Vet Res 22:982–985, 1979.
12. Jones EW, Kliewer IO, Norman BB, et al: *Anaplasma marginale* infection in young and aged cattle. Am J Vet Res 29:525–544, 1976.
13. Ajaxi SA, Wilson AJ, Campbell RSF: Experimental bovine anaplasmosis: Clinico-pathological and nutritional studies. Res Vet Sci 25:76–81, 1978.
14. Allen PC, Kuttler KL, Amerault TE: Clinical chemistry of anaplasmosis: Blood chemical changes in infected mature cows. Am J Vet Res 42:322–325, 1981.
15. Richey EJ: Discussion on treatment and control. In Hidalgo RJ, Jones EW (eds): Proceedings of the Seventh National Anaplasmosis Conference, Starkville, Mississippi State University, 1981, p 649.
16. Brock WE, Pearson CC, Kliewer IO: Anaplasmosis control by list and subsequent treatment with chlortetracycline. In Proceedings of the 62nd Annual Meeting of the USLSA, 1958, pp 66–70.
17. Renshaw HW, Magonigle RA, Eckbald WT, et al: Immunity to bovine anaplasmosis after elimination of the carrier status with oxytetracycline hydrochloride. In Proceedings of the 80th Annual Meeting of the US Animal Health Association, 1976, pp 79–88.
18. Magonigle RA, Renshaw HW, Vaugh HW, et al: Effect of five daily intravenous treatments with oxytetracycline hydrochloride on the carrier status of bovine anaplasmosis. J Am Vet Med Assoc 167:1080–1083, 1975.
19. Pearson CC, Brock WE, Kliewer IO: A study of tetracycline dosage in cattle which are anaplasmosis carriers. J Am Vet Med Assoc 130:390–292, 1957.
20. Magonigle RA, Newby TJ: Elimination of naturally acquired chronic *Anaplasma marginale* infection with a long acting oxytetracycline. Am J Vet Res 43:2170–2172, 1982.
21. Franklin TE, Huff JW, Grumbles LC: Chlortetracycline for elimination of anaplasmosis in carrier cattle. J Am Vet Med Assoc 147:353–356, 1965.
22. Richey EJ, Brock WE, Kliewer IO, et al: Low levels of chlortetracycline for anaplasmosis. Am J Vet Res 38:171–172, 1977.
23. Miller JG: Protective measures against anaplasmosis in Jamaica for imported animals. In Proceedings of the Fourth National Anaplasmosis Conference, 1962, pp 49–50.
24. Richey EJ, Kliewer IO.: Efficacy of chlortetracycline against bovine anaplasmosis when administered free choice to cattle in medicated feed block and salt-mineral mix. In Hidalgo RJ, Jones EW (eds): Proceedings of the Seventh National Anaplasmosis Conference, Starkville, Mississippi State University, 1981, pp 635–647.
25. Brock WE, Kliewer IO, Pearson CC: A vaccine for anaplasmosis. J Am Vet Med Assoc 147:948–951, 1965.
26. Richey EJ, Kliewer IO: Boosters are required in anaplasmosis control programs utilizing killed *Anaplasma marginale* vaccine. In Hidalgo NJ, Jones EW (eds): Proceedings of the Seventh National Anaplasmosis Conference. Starkville, Mississippi State University, 1981, pp 505–514.
27. Ristic M, Sibinovic S, Welter CJ: An attenuated *Anaplasma marginale* vaccine. In Proceedings of the 72nd Annual Meeting of the USLSA, 1969, pp 56–69.
28. Vizcaino O, Corrier DE, Terry MK, et al: Comparison of three methods of immunization against bovine anaplasmosis: Evaluation of protection afforded against field challenge exposure. Am J Vet Res 41:1066–1069, 1980.
29. Ristic M, Carson CA: Methods of immunoprophylaxis against bovine anaplasmosis with emphasis on the use of the attenuated *Anaplasma marginale* vaccine. In Miller LH, Pino JA, McKelvey JJ

(eds): Immunity to Blood Parasites of Animals and Man. New York, Academic Press, 1977, pp 151–188.

30. Bedell DM, Slater M: The use of a combination of the therapeutic and immunological regiment in an anaplasmosis epizootic. Biochem Rev 33:2, 1966.

31. Richey EJ, Kliewer IO: Boosters are required in anaplasmosis control programs utilizing killed *Anaplasma marginale* vaccine. In Hidalgo NJ, Jones EW (eds): Proceedings of the Seventh National Anaplasmosis Conference, Starkville, Mississippi State University, 1981, pp 505–514.

32. Richey EJ, Kliewer IO: Controlling an acute outbreak of bovine anaplasmosis with oxytetracycline and chlortetracycline. In Hidalgo RJ, Jones EW (eds): Proceedings of the Seventh National Anaplasmosis Conference. Starkville, Mississippi State University, 1981, pp 615–627.

■ Coccidiosis

C.A. Speer, B.Sc., M.Sc., Ph.D.

Coccidiosis is one of the most economically important diseases of livestock, costing the industries in the United States several hundred million dollars annually. Bovine coccidiosis is considered to be the fifth most important disease in the U.S. cattle industry. Although there are no data on the economic effects of coccidiosis on the sheep and swine industries, it is generally known that this disease can have extremely devastating effects. Coccidiosis is an acute or chronic disease associated with hemorrhagic diarrhea, emaciation, growth retardation, and sometimes death. Clinical signs of coccidiosis occur most frequently in young animals, but they may also occur in older animals that are in poor general condition. Compared to clinical coccidiosis, inapparent coccidial infections are probably more important economically because nearly all animals are infected or have experienced infections with coccidia, and many do not thrive or gain weight properly. Coccidiosis is a disease often associated with crowded conditions and intensive animal husbandry, but the disease can also occur in free-ranging animals.

The agents that cause coccidiosis are protozoan parasites belonging to the phylum Apicomplexa. Members of this phylum are obligatory intracellular parasites that have complex life cycles in which they reproduce sexually as well as asexually, and contain motile stages (called *sporozoites* or *merozoites*) that use their apical complexes to penetrate cells of the host (Fig. 1). The apical complex consists of ultrastructural features that are unique to the Apicomplexa, including apical rings, polar rings, a pellicle consisting of a plasmalemma and an inner membrane complex, subpellicular microtubules, rhoptries, micronemes, and a conoid (may be absent, as in malaria parasites). Coccidia use their apical complexes to actively penetrate into cells of the host, where they undergo asexual reproduction (called *schizogony* or *merogony*) followed by sexual reproduction (called *gametogony*), which results in the formation of environmentally resistant oocysts.

The coccidia that cause disease in cattle, sheep, and swine occur chiefly in the genera *Eimeria* and *Isospora* and belong to the same general group as the parasites causing malaria in man. One of the unusual characteristics of the coccidia infecting livestock and poultry is their generally high degree of host specificity in which certain species will infect only a single host or a few closely related hosts. Some of the cattle coccidia, for example, will also infect elk, zebu, water buffalo, and the American bison, but others will infect only cattle.[4, 6] The coccidia of chickens will infect only a single host and will not infect other hosts, including cattle or even other species of poultry. In general, the coccidia also demonstrate an extremely high degree of host cell specificity. For example, first-generation schizonts of *Eimeria bovis* develop only in endothelial cells of the central

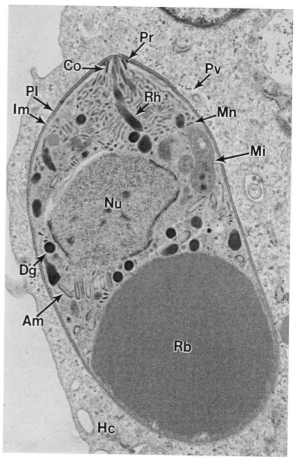

Figure 1

Transmission electron micrograph of a sporozoite of *E. bovis* in a cultured bovine pulmonary artery endothelial cell showing the apical complex and various organelles and inclusion bodies (magnification × 15,000). Am, amylopectin granule; Co, conoid; Dg, dense granule; Hc, host cell cytoplasm; Im, inner membrane complex of sporozoite pellicle; Mi, mitochondrion; Mn, microneme; Nu, nucleus of sporozoite; Pl, plasmalemma of sporozoite; Pr, polar ring; Pv, parasitophorous vacuole; Rb, refractile body; Rh, rhoptry.

lacteal of the small intestine, localizing mainly in the distal ileum.

Older animals are carriers of coccidiosis and continually contaminate pastures, feedlots, and pens by shedding oocysts in their feces (Figs. 2 and 3). Although oocysts are susceptible to the harmful effects of radiation, freezing, and desiccation, they are extremely resistant to disinfectants and can remain viable in moist, shady conditions for several years. Oocysts of *Eimeria* spp. have four sporocysts, each with two sporozoites, whereas those of *Isospora* spp. have two sporocysts, each with four sporozoites (see Figs. 2 and 3). Coccidian parasites can usually be identified by the structural characteristics of their oocysts, especially sporulated oocysts. Important structural features include oocyst shape and size and presence of micropyle or micropylar cap; texture of the oocyst wall; number of layers in the oocyst wall; size, shape, and arrangement of sporocysts; and the presence or absence and size and appearance of oocyst or sporocyst residua. Some coccidian species have oocysts that appear structurally identical. In these situations, species identification is usually based on differences in development stages occurring in the host, length of prepatent period (time from ingestion of oocysts until newly formed oocysts appear in the feces), or some other biologic differences.

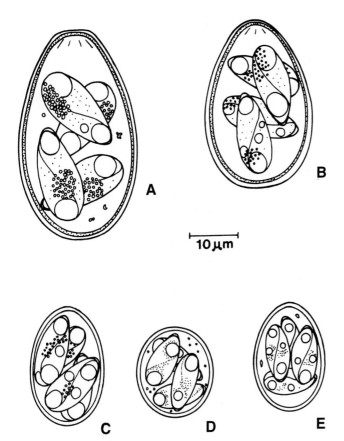

Figure 2

Schematic representations of the oocysts of *Eimeria* species that are commonly found in cattle. *A, E, auburnensis. B, E. bovis. C, E. ellipsoidalis. D and E,* Two forms of *E. zuernii.*

LIFE CYCLE

Coccidia have complex life cycles, with several asexual generations and one sexual generation included in a single cycle (Fig. 4). Confusion sometimes exists among producers and practitioners concerning the endogenous life cycles of *Eimeria* that infect ruminants. It is often assumed that the endogenous developmental cycles are essentially identical to those of *Eimeria* spp. in poultry. Many of the lowly pathogenic *Eimeria* in ruminants have endogenous cycles similar to those of poultry *Eimeria* species, but pathogenic ruminant *Eimeria* differ considerably by having giant first-generation schizonts that are located in the intestinal lamina propria (not in intestinal enterocytes) and substantially longer prepatent periods. For example, first-generation schizogony in *E. bovis* and *E. zuernii* in cattle, *E. ovina* in sheep and *E. ninakohlyakimovae* in goats requires approximately 2 weeks to complete, which results in the formation of more than 100,000 merozoites. In the poultry coccidia, the entire endogenous cycle is completed in about 1 week, and the schizonts contain only a few dozen merozoites.

When discharged in the feces from the host, the oocysts are generally noninfectious, consisting of a condensed protoplasm, called a *sporont*, that is surrounded by an oocyst wall (Fig. 5*A*). Before they are infectious to another animal, the oocysts must undergo a developmental process called sporulation (see Figs. 4 and 5*B*), which requires moist conditions, atmospheric oxygen, and approximately 3 to 10 days to complete. On ingestion by the host, sporulated oocysts are exposed to elevated levels of carbon dioxide, which causes them to become fragile and to rupture, usually at the micropylar end (see Fig. 5*B*). The micro-

pyle is a thin area in the oocyst wall, usually located at one pole of the oocyst. Sporocysts of *Eimeria* spp. and certain *Isospora* spp. have sporocysts with a plug at one pole, called a *Stieda body*. During excystation, which occurs as the oocyst enters the small intestine, trypsin and bile enter the oocyst through the ruptured micropyle and cause the Stieda body to undergo dissolution, creating a gap through which the sporozoites escape. The sporocysts of some *Isospora* spp. have walls that lack Stieda bodies but contain four curved plates held together by sutures.[8] During excystation, the plates in the sporocyst wall separate at the sutures, causing the sporocyst to collapse and release the sporozoites. After excystation, sporozoites penetrate into the intestinal wall, enter a specific type of host cell, and begin to grow as schizonts (Figs. 5*C–E* and 6*A* and *B*). During schizogony, several to many nuclear divisions occur without cytoplasmic division (see Figs. 5*C–E*). Coincidentally with the last nuclear division, merozoite buds develop at the surface of the schizont immediately above each nucleus (Figs. 6*A* and 7). On completion of schizogony, completely formed merozoites (Figs. 6*C* and 8) are released by rupture of the host cell. New host cells are invaded and the process is repeated one or more times (see Figs. 6*D–F*).

After a set number of schizogonous generations, merozoites enter the sexual phase of the life cycle by penetrating new host cells and forming either male or female gamonts, called *microgamonts* and *macrogamonts*, respectively (Fig. 9*A–D*). Microgamonts undergo a process similar to schizogony, which ultimately results in the budding of numerous microgametes at the gamont's surface. Each microgamete contains a nucleus, a mitochondrion, several microtubules, and a pointed anterior

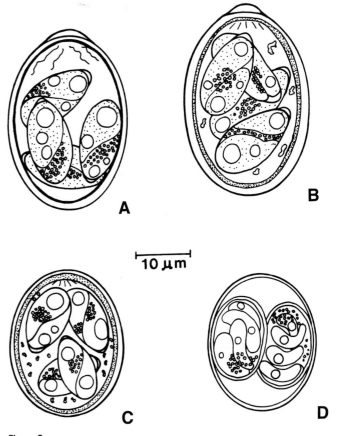

Figure 3

Schematic representations of the oocysts of some of the *Eimeria* species infecting sheep and goats and *Isospora suis* infecting pigs. *A, E. ahsata* from sheep. *B, E. arloingi* from goats. *C, E. ninakohylyakimovae* from goats. *D, I. suis* from pigs.

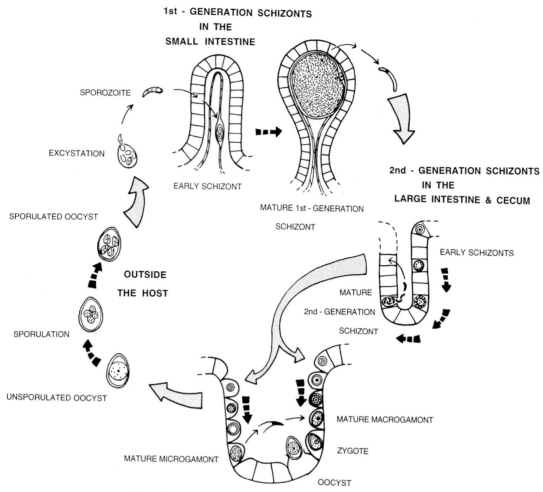

**1st - GENERATION SCHIZONTS
IN THE
SMALL INTESTINE**

SPOROZOITE

EXCYSTATION

EARLY SCHIZONT

SPORULATED OOCYST

**2nd - GENERATION SCHIZONTS
IN THE
LARGE INTESTINE & CECUM**

MATURE 1st - GENERATION
SCHIZONT

EARLY SCHIZONTS

**OUTSIDE
THE HOST**

MATURE
2nd - GENERATION
SCHIZONT

SPORULATION

MATURE MACROGAMONT

UNSPORULATED OOCYST

ZYGOTE

OOCYST

MATURE MICROGAMONT

Figure 4

Schematic representation of the life cycle of *E. bovis* in cattle.

end, called a *perforatorium*, from which two long flagella arise from two basal bodies. Microgametes use their flagella for motility to fertilize macrogamonts (see Fig. 9D). In contrast to microgamonts, macrogamonts do not undergo nuclear division but increase in size, have a large nucleus with a prominent nucleolus, and form numerous wall-forming bodies in their cytoplasm (see Figs. 9B and C). After fertilization of a macrogamont by a microgamete, the wall-forming bodies lay down a resistant oocyst wall at the surface of the zygote (see Fig. 9E).

Parasites resulting from the sexual phase of the cycle are quite numerous at this point and are generally more injurious to their host cells, causing bleeding and partial destruction of the mucous lining of the intestinal tract. The signs of coccidiosis usually occur simultaneously with the discharge of oocysts in the feces. In clinical coccidiosis, the feces may contain blood, shreds of necrotic intestinal mucosa, and oocysts. In general, coccidiosis differs from bacterial and from certain protozoal diseases (e.g., malaria) because the severity of the infection is dependent on the number of organisms that initiate the infection (i.e., the number of oocysts ingested). Because *Eimeria* and most *Isospora* spp. have a set number of asexual generations and a single sexual cycle, the infections they cause are generally referred to as *self-limiting*.

Cattle

Thirteen species of *Eimeria* are known to infect cattle (Table 1), and all species probably contribute to disease. *E. bovis* and *E.*

zuernii are considered to be highly pathogenic; *E. auburnensis* and *E. alabamensis* are moderately pathogenic; and *E. ellipsoidalis* is lowly pathogenic. In outbreaks of coccidiosis, the most frequently seen coccidian oocysts are usually those of *E. bovis* and *E. zuernii* followed by *E. auburnensis* and *E. ellipsoidalis* (see Fig. 2). There are also differences in geographic distribution of *Eimeria* species infecting cattle, with certain species being more prevalent in certain regions of the United States than others.

More is known about infections caused by *E. bovis* than about any of the other species infecting ruminants. The oocysts of *E. bovis* are variable in shape—being ovoid, short ovoid, or subellipsoidal—and they measure 26 to 32 × 18 to 21 μm (see Figs. 2 and 5A and B). After ingestion of sporulated oocysts, sporozoites of *E. bovis* excyst from oocysts and penetrate through the intestinal epithelium, where they localize intracellularly in endothelial cells of the central lacteal of the intestinal villi, especially toward the tips of villi in the distal ileum just anterior to the ileocecal valve. Here, the parasite undergoes schizogony to form giant first-generation schizonts (see Figs. 4, 5C–E, and 6A), which are so large (nearly 0.3 mm in diameter) they can be seen without the aid of a microscope (see Fig. 6B). First-generation schizonts require approximately 2 weeks to reach maturity, and each schizont contains about 120,000 merozoites (see Figs. 6C and 8). First-generation merozoites travel to the large intestine and cecum, where they penetrate glandular enterocytes and develop in 1.5 to 2 days into small second-generation schizonts with 30 to 36 merozoites (see Fig. 6D–F). Second-generation merozoites stay in the same area and penetrate other

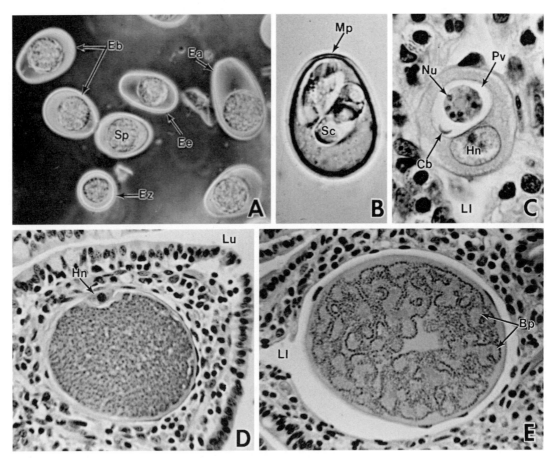

Figure 5

Photomicrographs of *Eimeria* species from cattle. *A*, Unsporulated oocysts (magnification × 750). Ea, *E. auburnensis;* Eb, *E. bovis; Ee, E. ellipsoidalis;* Ez, *E. zuernii;* Sp, sporont. *B*, Sporulated oocyst of *E. bovis* (magnification × 1500). Mp, micropyle. *C*, Young first-generation schizont of *E. bovis* in an endothelial cell of the central lacteal in the ileum (magnification × 1400). Cb, crescent body; Hn, host cell nucleus; Ll, lumen of central lacteal; Nu, nucleus of schizont; Pv, parasitophorous vacuole. *D*, Intermediate first-generation schizont of *E. bovis* in an endothelial cell of the central lacteal. Schizont nuclei appear as black dots within the schizont (magnification × 780). Hn, host cell nucleus with a prominent nucleolus; Lu, lumen of intestine. *E*, More advanced first generation schizont of *E. bovis* showing blastophores (Bp) from which merozoites will bud; blastophores are formed by indentations of the parasite plasmalemma; schizont nuclei appear as black dots at the margins of blastophores (magnification × 780). Ll, lumen of central lacteal.

glandular enterocytes and develop into microgamonts and macrogamonts, which requires about 3 days (see Fig. 9*A–D*). Approximately 80% of the second-generation merozoites develop into macrogamonts, and 20% develop into microgamonts. Microgametogenesis results in the formation of microgamonts containing numerous biflagellate microgametes (see Fig. 9*D*). Fertilization of macrogamonts by microgametes results in the formation of zygotes, which develop into oocysts (see Fig. 9*E*). The final, sexual generation matures in approximately 3 days. Oocysts destroy their host cells and are released into the intestinal lumen and voided with the feces. Thus, the life cycle of *E. bovis* is completed in a minimum of about 18 days, with the peak oocyst discharge occurring at 19 to 22 days after ingestion of oocysts. Few or no oocysts will be seen in the feces after about 26 days.

One of the most impressive aspects of *E. bovis*, as well as other species of *Eimeria* that contain giant first-generation schizonts in their life cycles, is their tremendous biotic potential to produce offspring. For example, a single oocyst contains 8 sporozoites, each of which will form 120,000 first-generation merozoites, and each of these will form 36 second-generation merozoites, 80% of which will form macrogamonts and, therefore, oocysts. Thus, a single oocyst of *E. bovis* will produce 27,648,000 oocysts, which destroy an equal number of host glandular enterocytes.

Less is known about the details of the life cycle of *E. zuernii*,

the other pathogenic species in cattle, because experimental infections are inordinately difficult. Oocysts of *E. zuernii* are variable in shape, being subspherical, subovoid, or elliptical; they measure 15 to 22 × 13 to 18 μm and lack a micropyle (see Figs. 2*D* and *E* and 5*A*). *E. zuernii* also has giant first-generation schizonts with more than 100,000 merozoites, which develop in endothelial cells of the lacteals in the lamina propria; but unlike *E. bovis*, first-generation schizonts of *E. zuernii* also develop in the large intestine and cecum. Mature second-generation schizonts contain 24 to 36 merozoites and develop in glandular enterocytes in the lower small intestine, large intestine, and cecum. Gamonts and oocysts are also formed at these locations. Oocysts appear in the feces at 19 days after ingestion of oocysts. *E. zuernii* appears to cause coccidiosis more frequently in older animals than does *E. bovis* and is generally more commonly seen in the disease known as "winter coccidiosis," which occurs during or following cold or stormy weather in the winter months.

Oocysts of *E. auburnensis* are usually elongated ovoids; they measure 35 to 44 × 19 to 26 μm and appear yellowish brown (see Figs. 2*A* and 5*A*). *E. auburnensis* has giant first-generation schizonts similar to those of *E. bovis* except that they are located more deeply in the small intestinal villi. The second-generation schizonts are small, with approximately 24 merozoites. The gamonts, however, are unusual because they parasitize cells in

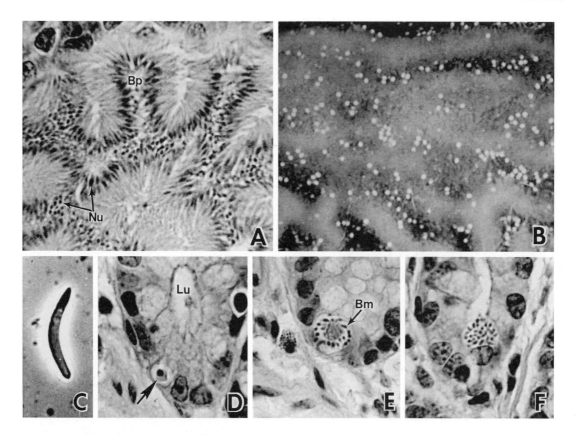

Figure 6

Photomicrographs of *E. bovis* in cattle. *A,* Margin of mature first-generation schizont showing merozoites arranged in rosettes arising from blastophores (Bp) (magnification × 1400). Nu, nucleus of merozoites. *B,* First generation schizonts appear as white spheres on the mucosal surface of the ileum just anterior to the ileocecal valve; 13 days after inoculation of oocysts (magnification × 10). *C,* First-generation merozoite (magnification × 2200). *D,* Uninucleate second-generation schizont *(arrow)* in glandular enterocyte in the cecum; 15 days postinoculation of oocysts (magnification × 1400). Lu, lumen of gland. *E,* Second-generation schizont with budding merozoites (Bm) in glandular enterocyte; 15 days postinoculation (magnification × 1400). *F,* Mature second-generation schizont; 15 days postinoculation (magnification × 1400).

the lamina propria of the small intestine, and the microgamonts are unusually large, containing thousands of microgametes. The epithelium must break or slough off of the epithelial layer for the oocysts to be discharged into the lumen of the intestine. The endogenous life cycle of *E. auburnensis* is completed in approximately 18 days.

E. ellipsoidalis has oocysts that are usually ellipsoid, but they are sometimes ovoid or cylindrical, and they measure 18 to 26 × 13 to 18 μm. *E. ellipsoidalis* develops exclusively in the small intestine, with all stages occurring in the glandular enterocytes. Schizonts are small, containing 24 to 36 merozoites, and oocysts appear in the feces at about 10 days after ingestion of sporulated oocysts. *E. alabamensis* is unusual in that the parasites appear to be intranuclear because they lie within indentations of the nucleus of the host cell. *E. alabamensis* and *E. ellipsoidalis* are normally nonpathogenic, except in unusually heavy infections.

Sheep

It is very common to find sheep infected simultaneously with several species of *Eimeria* (see Table 1). The two most pathogenic species are *E. ahsata* and *E. ovinoidalis*. *E. ovina* is one of the most common eimerians found in sheep, but it is not very pathogenic. The oocysts of *E. ahsata* and *E. ovina* are similar structurally, being ellipsoid to ovoid with a prominent micropyle and micropylar cap (see Fig. 3*A*). The two species differ in size; *E. ovina* measures approximately 23 to 36 × 16 to 24 μm, whereas those of *E. ahsata* are 29 to 37 × 17 to 28 μm.[7] Giant

schizonts of *E. ahsata* occur in the mucosa along the entire length of the small intestine, but they prefer the jejunum. Schizonts appear to develop in the lacteals, with some localizing deep in the mucosa close to the muscularis mucosae. Gamonts are found mostly in glandular enterocytes. The prepatent period is 18 to 20 days. *E. ovinoidalis* is markedly pathogenic and localizes especially in the posterior small intestine as well as the cecum and colon. The oocysts measure 16 to 28 × 14 to 23 μm, are subspherical to ovoid or ellipsoid, and have neither a micropyle nor a micropylar cap.

Goats

Although several species of *Eimeria* occur in goats, *E. ninakohlyakimovae*, *E. arloingi*, and *E. christenseni* are probably the most pathogenic (see Table 1). Developmental stages of *E. ninakohlyakimovae* and *E. arloingi* occur in the small intestine and upper colon, forming giant first-generation schizonts within endothelial cells of lacteals in the small intestine and gamonts in the glandular and villar enterocytes.[7] The oocysts of *E. arloingi* are ellipsoid to slightly ovoid, measure 13 to 27 × 17 to 42 μm, have a 1 μm–thick wall, and have a prominent micropylar cap (see Fig. 3*B*). The prepatent period is 20 days.

The oocysts of *E. ninakohlyakimovae* are ovoid, measure 14 to 21 × 19 to 25 μm, and have a micropyle but no micropylar cap (see Fig. 3*C*). The prepatent period is 11 to 14 days. The oocysts of *E. christenseni* measure 38 × 25 μm, are ovoid and sometimes ellipsoidal, and are occasionally flattened at the mi-

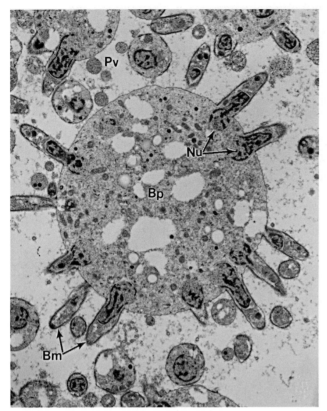

Figure 7

Transmission electron micrograph of a blastophore (Bp) showing budding merozoites (Bm) (magnification × 5610). Nu, nuclei of budding merozoites; Pv, parasitophorous vacuole.

cropylar end, which is covered by a prominent micropylar cap. *E. christenseni* can be fatal to Angora kids.[1]

Swine

Although swine harbor several species of *Eimeria* (see Table 1), members of this genus are not normally associated with disease. *Eimeria scabra* occasionally causes disease in older pigs, but the lesions and symptoms appear to be resolved rapidly. The major coccidian disease in the swine industry is neonatal porcine coccidiosis (also called *isosporiasis*) induced by *Isospora suis*.[10] This disease is ubiquitous in piglets farrowed in confinement and is responsible for 15% to 20% of the cases of piglet diarrhea in the United States and Canada. Clinical disease occurs in piglets younger than 2 weeks and is relatively rare in piglets older than 2 weeks. The oocysts of *I. suis* are ovoid, measure 20 to 24 × 18 to 21 μm, and contain two sporocysts without Stieda bodies (see Fig. 3D).[7] The parasite develops within villar enterocytes throughout the small intestine, with the peak of schizogony occurring at 4 days and gamonts appearing at 5 days after ingestion of oocysts.[5] The prepatent period of *I. suis* is 5 days; the patent period is 5 to 8 days.

PATHOGENESIS

Severity of coccidiosis depends on the number of oocysts ingested. If only a few are ingested, no signs of disease may occur, and repeated infections may produce immunity without disease. If a moderate number of oocysts is ingested, the disease

may be mild and immunity may result. Ingestion of a large number of oocysts usually results in severe disease and, occasionally, death. In severe cases of coccidiosis, gross examination of the intestinal mucosa usually reveals the presence of hemorrhagic and necrotic lesions. Histologically, the villous epithelium may be disrupted and atrophied, which causes a reduction in the absorptive mechanisms for uptake of water and nutrients and the loss of serum proteins and other nutrients into the intestinal lumen.

Bovine coccidiosis is easily recognized by its characteristic signs of bloody diarrhea, rectal tenesmus and anal paralysis, loss of appetite, slight fever, and debility. In severe infections, the rectum may prolapse. In severe bovine coccidiosis, the animal may produce an explosive stream of bloody, watery diarrhea that jettisons 3 to 4 feet.

Clinical neonatal porcine coccidiosis is characterized by a pasty diarrhea that progresses to a watery diarrhea after 2 to 3 days. Mortality and morbidity are variable and the illness does

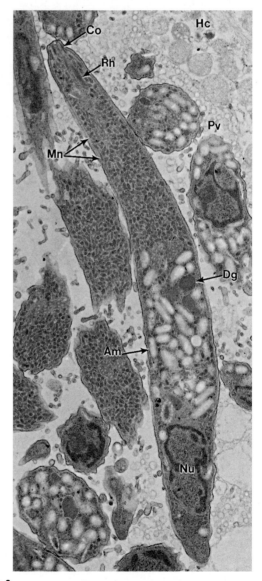

Figure 8

Transmission electron micrograph of a first-generation merozoite of *E. bovis* (magnification × 15,000). Am, amylopectin granule; Co, conoid; Dg, dense granule; Hc, host cell cytoplasm; Mn, microneme; Nu, nucleus of merozoite; Pv, parasitophorous vacuole; Rh, rhoptry.

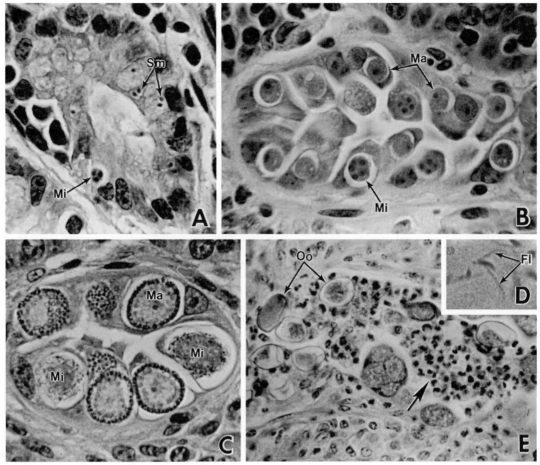

Figure 9

Bright-field (*A* through *C* and *E*) and phase-contrast *(D)* photomicrographs of *E. bovis* in the cecum of an infected calf. *A,* Second-generation merozoites (Sm) and an early microgamont (Mi) in glandular enterocytes (magnification × 1400). *B,* Macrogamonts (Ma) and microgamonts (Mi) in intermediate stages of development in glandular enterocytes; macrogamonts have a single nucleus, microgamonts have several nuclei (magnification × 1400). *C,* Glandular enterocytes infected with several mature macrogamonts (Ma) and two microgamonts (Mi); microgametes appear as commas at the margins of the microgamonts; wall-forming bodies are visible at the margins of the macrogamonts (magnification × 1400). *D,* Microgamete showing its two flagella (Fl) (magnification × 3000). *E,* Cecal gland infected with gamonts and oocysts (Oo) and infiltrated with mononuclear and polymorphonuclear leucocytes *(arrow)* (magnification × 700).

not respond to antibacterial therapy. The diarrhea is yellow to gray and blood is absent. Piglets become covered with diarrhea; they are damp and lethargic and smell of sour milk, but they continue to nurse. Microscopically, the small intestine exhibits severe fibrinonecrotic enteritis, villous atrophy, villar fusion, and epithelial erosion. Because the parasite infects the tips of the villi and does not localize in the crypts, if the piglet can survive the initial onslaught, it recovers rapidly.

IMMUNITY

Animals that recover from coccidiosis are frequently resistant to reinfection, but the degree of immunity to different species of coccidia is not constant. Infections with a given species may soon disappear completely, leaving the host fully protected, whereas resistance to another species may build up only gradually through successive reinfections over a long period and be maintained by the continual development of small numbers of organisms. Immunity is species-specific in that immunity to one species does not confer immunity to another. Immunity to coccidial infection is rarely absolute. Although animals may be resistant to the disease produced by pathogenic species, they

often support parasites in numbers sufficient to produce a few oocysts in the feces. A greater degree of immunity occurs with those species that penetrate deeply and tend to be retained in the tissues of the host, whereas immunity develops slowly with species that superficially infect the host by localizing in the intestinal epithelium. In cattle, infection with *E. bovis* induces immunity, which develops rapidly within a couple of weeks after oocysts appear in the feces and may persist for 3 to 6 months or even a year or longer. In contrast to *E. bovis*, *E. alabamensis* induces little immunity; reinfections can occur as many as four times before evidence of resistance is obtained. Little information is available on the actual mechanisms of immunity to ruminant coccidia. In *E. bovis*, cell-mediated immune responses appear to be more important in resistance to reinfection than humoral immunity.[3, 9]

Older sheep and goats almost continuously discharge moderate amounts of eimerian oocysts in their feces, indicating that a certain, but not complete, degree of immunity is bestowed by various coccidial infections encountered during earlier periods of life. During spontaneous outbreaks of coccidiosis it is almost always only the lambs or kids that fall sick, whereas the older animals remain clinically healthy.

Little is known regarding immune responses in swine to *I.*

Table 1
LIST OF *Eimeria* AND *Isospora* SPECIES INFECTING PRODUCTION ANIMALS

Cattle	Goats
Eimeria alabamensis	E. alijevi
E. auburnensis	E. absheronae
E. bovis	E. arloingi
E. brasiliensis	E. caprina
E. bukidnonensis	E. caprovina
E. canadensis	E. christenseni
E. cylindrica	E. gilruthi
E. ellipsoidalis	E. hirci
E. illinoisensis	E. jolchijevi
E. pellita	E. kocharii
E. subspherica	E. ninakohlyakimovae
E. wyomingensis	E. pallida
E. zuernii	E. punctata
Sheep	**Pigs**
E. ahsata	E. betica
E. crandallis	E. debliecki
E. faurei	E. guevarai
E. gonzalezi	E. neodebliecki
E. intricata	E. polita
E. marsica	E. porci
E. ovina	E. residualis
E. ovinoidalis	E. scabra
E. pallida	E. spinosa
E. parva	E. suis
E. punctata	Isospora suis
E. weybridgensis	
E. gilruthi	

Data from Levine ND: The Protozoan Phylum Apicomplexa, vol 1. Boca Raton, Fla, CRC Press, 1988.

can also cause signs during the schizont phase of its life cycle. In heavy coccidial infections, microscopic examination of the feces may reveal the presence of merozoites, gamonts, blood cells, and sloughed intestinal mucosal cells in addition to oocysts. Occasionally, severe infections may cause so much destruction to the intestinal mucosa that no coccidian oocysts appear in the feces. In these cases, diagnosis depends on finding coccidian stages in the intestinal tract by microscopic examination.

A saturated sugar solution for flotation to concentrate coccidian oocysts is preferable to most salt solutions (except zinc sulfate) because it does not crystallize as readily and causes less distortion of oocysts. A saturated sugar solution can be made by mixing 500 g of sucrose (ordinary cane or beet sugar) in 320 mL of water. The number of oocysts per gram of feces can be determined by the following technique. Briefly, place 3 g of feces in a 15 mL centrifuge tube, add approximately 13 mL of 70% aqueous saturated sugar solution, mix thoroughly, and centrifuge at 200g for 10 minutes. Aspirate 1 mL from the top of the solution and load a three-chambered McMaster slide (Olympic Equine Products, Issaquah, Wash). The oocysts are easily visible microscopically because they rise to the top of the solution, away from other fecal debris. Because the rectangular area counted on the McMaster chamber spans a volume of 0.3 mL, the number of oocysts counted will be the number of oocysts per gram of feces. In general, a few oocysts per gram of feces indicate only a low-grade infection; 50 to 100 oocysts per gram, a moderate infection; and 100 to 1,000 or more oocysts per gram, a high-grade coccidial infection and disease. If the feces contain large pieces of debris, then mix the feces with water and pass this through two layers of cheesecloth before mixing with the 70% sugar solution.

TREATMENT

Table 2 provides information concerning recommended label use, dosage, dosage form, and withdrawal period for the most common and effective drugs used in cattle, sheep, goats, and swine. Treatment of clinical coccidiosis is difficult because the signs of the disease do not become noticeable until it is far advanced. In coccidiosis caused by *E. bovis*, the first signs of disease usually occur at 17 to 18 days after ingestion of oocysts. At this time, most of the life cycle within the host has been nearly or entirely completed, with some damage to the intestinal mucosa having already occurred. Thus, treatment given at this time can, at best, result in lessening of the signs of coccidiosis. However, if drugs are given at an earlier stage of disease, the clinical signs of infection can be largely or entirely prevented. Coccidiostatic drugs are preferred to coccidiocidal ones, because inhibition of the development of coccidian parasites might also inhibit the development of immunity to subsequent infections.

When animals in a pen show signs of coccidiosis, they should be removed from the pen; other animals remaining in the pen should be treated because they have potentially been exposed, and they may harbor parasites in intermediate stages of development that are susceptible to drug treatment.

Drugs Used in Cattle

Amprolium

Amprolium and various sulfonamides are still the most commonly used drugs for treatment of clinical coccidiosis in ruminants. The approved regimen for prevention of coccidiosis is 5 mg of amprolium per kilogram of body weight (226.8 mg per

suis. Swine either develop age resistance or a solid immunity to isosporiasis, because several surveys have failed to show *I. suis* oocysts in older animals.

DIAGNOSIS

Diagnosis of coccidiosis depends on demonstrating the presence of coccidia in clinically affected animals. Because some species of coccidia are nonpathogenic and animals may be partially immune to coccidia, the presence of coccidia does not necessarily indicate clinical coccidiosis.

When coccidiosis is suspected, an examination of fecal samples by a salt or sugar flotation technique is a useful preliminary to a more comprehensive investigation. Many laboratories designate a certain number of oocysts per gram of feces as being indicative of an infection sufficient to cause disease. Diagnosis can be more accurately made if animals are available for postmortem examination. In this way, the exact site of lesions caused by the developmental stages of coccidia can be determined and the severity of infection more accurately assessed. Lesions caused by coccidia are attributable either to the maturation of the asexual phase of the life cycle or the development of the sexual phase, and sometimes both.

Microscopic examination of the feces from animals suffering from coccidiosis usually shows the presence of several species of *Eimeria*. When *E. bovis* is involved, the oocysts are usually demonstrable in the feces because the pathogenicity of this species is at its peak during gametogenesis and oocyst formation. The feces may also contain oocysts of *E. zuernii*, but this species

Table 2
RECOMMENDED USE, DOSAGE, DOSAGE FORM, AND WITHDRAWAL PERIOD OF ANTICOCCIDIAL DRUGS USED IN CATTLE, GOATS, SHEEP, AND SWINE*

Drug	Trade Names	Use	Animal	Dosage	Dosage Form	Withdrawal Time (Days)
Amprolium	Corid	Therapeutic	Cattle	10 mg/kg/day for 5 days	20% soluble powder 9.6% oral solution 1.25% crumbles	1
			Swine‡	25–65 mg/kg 1 or 2 × daily for 3–4 days		Unknown
		Prophylactic	Cattle	5 mg/kg/day for 21 days		1
			Swine	25 mg/kg in piglets for first 3–4 days of life		Unknown
Sulfonamides†						
Sulfamethazine	Sulfasure, Sulfatec	Therapeutic	Cattle	Label	Soluble powder, solution, or bolus	15
Sulfaquinoxaline					Bolus	10
Ionophores						
Monensin	Rumensin	Prophylactic	Cattle and goats	1 mg/kg/day, 10–30 g/ton	Feed additive	
Lasalocid	Bovatec	Prophylactic	Cattle and sheep	1 mg/kg/day, 20–30 g/ton	Feed additive	
Decoquinate	Deccox	Prophylactic	Cattle, sheep, and goats	0.5 mg/kg in feed for at least 28 days (22.7 mg/100 lb)	6% Premix for addition to feed	0

*Always read and follow label instructions.
†Several trade names.
‡Not approved by the FDA for use in swine in the United States.

100 lb) per day in the feed or water for 21 days. Clinically ill animals can be treated with 10 mg/kg/day of amprolium for 5 days (454 mg per 100 lb). Treatment of calves with amprolium for 19 or more days has been shown to be effective in controlling coccidiosis, whereas treatment for 14 days or less provided little or no protection against disease. In some cases, the beneficial effects of amprolium treatment in clinically ill calves have been almost immediately visible, which has caused some practitioners using this drug to report "miraculous" cures of extremely ill animals.

Decoquinate

In the United States, decoquinate is approved for prevention of coccidiosis in cattle at the dosage of 0.5 mg/kg/day, or 22.7 mg per 100 lb. *Eimeria* species in chickens rapidly develop drug resistance against decoquinate, but resistance does not seem to be a problem in cattle. It should be given for at least 28 days during periods of exposure.

Lasalocid

Lasalocid is approved in the United States for use in the feed to improve gain in pasture cattle, gain and feed efficiency in confinement feedlot cattle, and to control coccidiosis. Rations should be formulated to provide lasalocid at 1 mg/kg of body weight up to a maximum of 360 mg/head/day, to control coccidiosis.

Monensin

Monensin is approved in the United States for improvement of feed efficiency at 5 to 30 g/ton. It is also approved for use

against coccidiosis. When given at 30 g/ton (33 ppm) in the feed, which is approximately 1 mg/kg/day, monensin is highly effective against infections with *E. bovis* and *E. zuernii*. Label dosage for control of coccidiosis in cattle is from 100 to 360 mg/head/day.

Laidlomycin

Laidlomycin is approved in the United States for improved feed efficiency and increased rate of gain in cattle fed in confinement for slaughter. Data regarding its potential as a coccidiostat are scanty at this time.

Drugs Used in Sheep

Drug treatment is usually given to clinically ill animals, and in some cases it is given prophylactically to animals at high risk of infection, such as young lambs confined to feedlots.

Amprolium

Amprolium is highly effective in preventing coccidiosis in sheep when administered in the water at 100 to 200 ppm or 10 mg/kg/day for 5 days. Amprolium is not approved for use in sheep in the United States.

Monensin

Monensin is not approved for use in sheep in the United States.

Lasalocid

Lasalocid is approved for use in sheep to prevent coccidiosis. When placed in the feed at 20 to 30 g/ton, it is to be fed continuously to provide not less than 15 mg nor more than 70 mg/head/day of lasalocid, depending on body weight.

Decoquinate

Decoquinate, at a dosage of 0.5 mg/kg (22.7 mg per 100 lb), is approved for use in sheep and should be fed for at least 28 days during periods of exposure.

Drugs Used in Goats

Decoquinate

Decoquinate, at a dosage of 0.5 mg/kg (22.7 mg per 100 lb), is approved for use in goats in the United States. It should be fed for at least 28 days during periods of exposure.

Monensin

Monensin is approved for use in goat rations at a level of 20 g/ton to prevent coccidiosis.

Drugs Used in Swine

I. suis is the main cause of coccidian-induced dysentery and mortality in neonatal piglets raised in large farrowing facilities. Drugs that are effective against *Eimeria* spp. have little or no effect against *I. suis* infections in pigs. At this time, sanitation is probably more effective than any drug treatment.

CONTROL

Because there is still no effective vaccine against coccidiosis in ruminants and swine, good animal husbandry practices and the proper use of anticoccidial drugs are the only effective means of controlling the disease. Coccidiosis occurs primarily in young animals and in stressed older animals, with the severity of disease depending on the number of sporulated oocysts ingested and the immune status of the animal. Older animals are asymptomatic carriers of coccidia and continuously discharge oocysts, which may accumulate over a given pasture and give rise to explosive outbreaks of coccidiosis. Good animal management strategies are to isolate older animals from growing animals and to change the grazing area or bedding as frequently as possible. Pens should be kept clean and dry, with the fecal material being removed daily. Feed troughs should be elevated and constructed so that animals cannot get onto them and contaminate them with their feces. Farrowing pens should be cleaned thoroughly with high-pressure water, scrubbed with a phenol-containing solution, and then steam-cleaned. Moving from one farrowing pen directly to another without cleaning and disinfecting footwear and clothing should be avoided.

The epidemiology of neonatal porcine coccidiosis is puzzling because surveys have failed to find *I. suis* oocysts in sows on farms where this disease is a problem. *I. suis* has not been found in the milk or in the placentas of sows on farms with neonatal coccidiosis. Thus, it seems that once *I. suis* is established on a farm it is transmitted by piglets, which are infected from the contaminated farrowing crate. Controlled studies have shown that amprolium, monensin, and furazolidone have little or no effect. Improved sanitation appears to be the best means of controlling the disease.[2]

Stress and coccidiosis go hand in hand. For example, bovine coccidiosis frequently occurs in cattle during the fall months, when animals are being weaned, culled, and shipped to feedlots. Overcrowding of animals causes stress and higher levels of oocyst contamination. It is good practice to use anticoccidial drugs prophylactically before and during stressful periods. Adequate shelter and high-energy feed should be provided during times of stress. The gradual withdrawal of anticoccidial drugs will allow susceptible animals an opportunity to gradually develop an immunity to clinical disease.

REFERENCES

1. Craig TM: Epidemiology and control of coccidia in goats. Vet Clin North Am Food Anim Pract 2:289, 1986.
2. Ernst JV, Lindsay DS, Current WL: Control of *Isospora suis*–induced coccidiosis on a swine farm. Am J Vet Res 46:643, 1985.
3. Hughes HPA, Whitmire WM, Speer CA: Immunity patterns during acute infection by *Eimeria bovis*. J Parasitol 75:86, 1989.
4. Kogut MH: Host specificity of the coccidia. *In* Long PL (ed): Coccidiosis of Man and Domestic Animals. Boca Raton, Fla, CRC Press, 1990, pp 44–62.
5. Lindsay DS, Stuart BP, Wheat BE, et al: Endogenous development of the swine coccidium, *Isospora suis* Biester 1934. J Parasitol 66:771, 1980.
6. Penzhorn BL, Knapp SE, Speer CA: Enteric coccidia in free-ranging American bison *(Bison bison)* in Montana. J Wildl Dis 30:267, 1994.
7. Pellerdy LP: Coccidia and Coccidiosis. Berlin, Verlag Paul Parey, 1974.
8. Speer CA, Hammond DM, Mahrt JL, et al: Structure of the oocyst and sporocyst walls and excystation of sporozoites of *Isospora canis*. J Parasitol 59:35, 1973.
9. Speer CA, Reduker DW, Burgess DE, et al: Lymphokine-induced inhibition of growth of *Eimeria bovis* and *Eimeria papillata* (Apicomplexa) in cultured bovine monocytes. Infect Immun 50:566, 1985.
10. Stuart BP, Gosser HS, Allen CB, et al: Coccidiosis in swine: Dose and age response to *Isospora suis*. Can J Comp Med 46:317, 1982.

■ Bovine Trichomoniasis

William G. Kvasnicka, D.V.M.
Mark R. Hall, Ph.D.
Donald R. Hanks, D.V.M.

DEFINITION

Bovine trichomoniasis, which is caused by the protozoan *Tritrichomonas foetus*, is a contagious venereal disease of beef and dairy herds.[1,2] Losses occur due to early embryonic death and transient infertility leading to reduced calving rates and an extended calving season.[3] Losses are also associated with abortion and pyometra. The disease is reported worldwide. In some regions of North America, South America, and Australia, where open-range beef operations are common, as many as 50% of the herds can be infected.[4] The disease is widespread in the range areas of the western United States and Florida.[5–6] In some beef herds, bovine trichomoniasis has been diagnosed as a significant cause of infertility for more than 50 years.[7]

T. foetus is a flagellate protozoan assigned to the order Polymasticida and family Trichomonadidae. Trichomonads are pyriform, with a rounded anterior end and a somewhat pointed posterior end.[8] A single nucleus is located in the anterior part of the body. Anterior to the nucleus is a blepharoplast, which is associated with a number of basal granules. Arising from the blepharoplast are the anterior flagella and a posterior flagellum. The posterior flagellum runs along the edge of an undulating membrane and often extends posteriorly from the body. A costa extends along the base of the undulating membrane and an especially characteristic rod-like axostyle emerges from the posterior end (Fig. 1). Several genera occur in this family, and speciation is dependent on the number of anterior flagella. Those with three anterior flagella belong to the genus *Tritrichomonas*. Trichomonadidae are widely distributed and infect nearly every mammal associated with humans as well as humans themselves.

Awareness of bovine trichomoniasis has increased in the past few years because of the economic impact, required testing in some areas, and more frequent diagnosis.[9] The economic impact of *T. foetus* infection can be profound. The calf crop in beef herds, and even in dairies, can be reduced by 14% to 50%, depending on the percentage of bulls infected and the susceptibility of the cows in the herd. In addition to the obvious losses due to the reduced number of calves born, the reduction in weaning weights as a result of an extended calving season affects the profitability of the ranching enterprise. These combined losses can result in a 5% to 35% decrease in the economic return per cow in herds infected with *T. foetus*.[10]

A production management program drafted to control and prevent bovine trichomoniasis requires a thorough understanding of the pathogenesis of the disease and of the immunologic response initiated by natural infection and vaccination.

CLINICAL SIGNS

Trichomoniasis usually has an insidious onset and is well established by the time a veterinarian is consulted. A rancher will notice that cattle exhibit estrus after 60 days into a long breeding season, that the number of pregnant cows at pregnancy

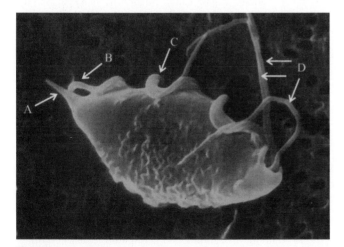

Figure 1

Scanning electron micrograph showing the morphology of *Tritrichomonas foetus*. *A*, Axostyle. *B*, Posterior flagellum. *C*, Undulating membrane. *D*, The three anterior flagella.

examination time is reduced by 20% to 40%, the calving season is spread out, and weaning weights vary.[11]

The infected bull rarely exhibits any signs of the trichomoniasis.[12] The cow may develop vaginitis, cervicitis, and endometritis, which may be accompanied by a mucopurulent discharge. Occasionally a cow has pyometra, which is detected at pregnancy examination.[13] The most common occurrence is the early embryonic death that occurs 50 or more days following conception. A few infected cows will abort a fetus at 5 months or later.[3]

DIAGNOSIS

Because no consistent signs are observed in bulls or cows infected with *T. foetus*, veterinarians must rely on laboratory diagnostic procedures. Lesions in an aborted fetus may lead to a presumptive diagnosis,[14] but confirmation of the diagnosis requires demonstration of the organism in fetal tissue or, most frequently, in samples collected from the bull or cow.

Two cultivation techniques have been successfully employed with consistent results. One uses in vitro Diamond's medium prepared for culture of *T. foetus*.[15] Currently, the most widely used procedure is a commercially available plastic pouch (In-Pouch TF culture system, BioMed Diagnostics), which allows convenient use in the field and contains a proprietary medium with a 12- to 15-month shelf life.[16] These culture methods have repeated sensitivities of 81% to 97%. One test may be adequate to make a herd diagnosis if one or more bulls are infected; however, for an individual bull, three negative tests are necessary to ensure that the bull is not infected.[13–17]

Other diagnostic techniques, including serologic methods and DNA probes, have lacked the sensitivity and specificity needed for effective diagnosis.[18] Michael and co-workers[19] have reported on a promising specific DNA probe and polymerase chain reaction amplification that could be a useful alternative method for the diagnosis of bovine trichomoniasis.

Reliability of the culture techniques depends on proper collection and handling of the specimen. Samples are obtained with a dry infusion pipette attached to a 20 mL syringe. In bulls, the pipette is directed to the distal penis in the sheath. The specimen is collected by scraping the mucosa of the distal penis and the fornix area while applying suction with the syringe. In the cow, the same technique is used in the anterior vagina. A transport medium is not used; rather, the specimen is deposited directly into the selected culture medium in the field. It is incubated at 37°C with the pouch in a vertical position to concentrate the organisms at the bottom.[20] Cultures are usually examined microscopically after 24, 48, and 72 hours of incubation. The specimen should be viewed at a magnification of ×100. Trichomonads are recognized by their jerky movements and characteristic morphology.[20]

PREVALENCE

Bovine trichomoniasis is prevalent in beef herds in which natural breeding is practiced.[5, 6] Most geographic prevalence reports are not derived from randomly selected herds and likely contain sampling biases. Johnson[7] reported in 1964 that 26% of beef herds and 7.6% of all bulls examined in the western United States were infected. Slaughterhouse surveys in Florida and Oklahoma revealed an infection prevalence of 7.3% and 7.8%, respectively.[6, 21] A survey in Nevada, from data collected at the veterinary diagnostic laboratory, found 27% to 44% of ranches to have at least one infected bull.[5]

A recent report from Missouri, where beef production management differs from typical western extensive range-grazing practices, describes *T. foetus* infection in a herd of cattle.[22] In a well-designed random survey in California, BonDurant and colleagues[23] found that 16% of herds contained one or more infected bulls, and 4.1% of the bulls tested one time were positive for *T. foetus*. The California report concludes that trichomoniasis is common in California beef herds.[24]

In an attempt to control trichomoniasis in beef herds, a mandatory bull testing program was initiated by the Idaho Cattlemen's Association with the cooperation of the Idaho Veterinary Association. Program administration and enforcement are directed by the Bureau of Animal Health (BAH), Idaho Department of Agriculture.[9] The results indicate that a program designed to identify only the carrier bulls will lower the prevalence of trichomoniasis but will not eliminate the disease from the population. No data have been collected on the effect of vaccination on the herd prevalence of trichomoniasis in Idaho.

Recent studies by the Idaho Bureau of Animal Health and U.S. Department of Agriculture Animal and Plant Health Inspection Service, Veterinary Services, indicate several factors that may explain the continuing occurrence of trichomoniasis. These factors include the use of aged bulls, a possible lack of compliance with testing requirements, imperfect test sensitivity, retaining open and late-calving cows in the herd, and the carrier cow syndrome. A recent case-control study showed that the risk of trichomoniasis infection increases with an increased number of commingled herds on public grazing lands.

Thus, although trichomoniasis in cattle is an insidious disease without obvious overt clinical signs, the high incidence and transient infertility results in considerable economic loss.[24] The Idaho experience indicates that economic losses can be reduced by strict management.

PATHOGENESIS

Trichomoniasis is a true venereal disease. Transmission of *T. foetus* is from infected bull to susceptible cow or from infected cow to susceptible bull during breeding.[17]

In bulls, *T. foetus* is found only on the penis and the preputial membranes, localizing in the secretions of the epithelial lining of the penis, prepuce, and the distal portion of the urethra.[12] No signs of diagnostic significance are produced. Thus, the infected bull serves only as a carrier of the agent. Older bulls tend to become permanent carriers, possibly because of the increased number and depth of crypts in the epithelial lining in older bulls.[25] Younger bulls are less likely to become permanent carriers, but they may still transmit the organism to susceptible females. Investigators and practitioners have found yearling bulls and even so-called virgin bulls to have positive culture results for *T. foetus*.[17]

It is believed that infection can become established with as few as 100 to 200 motile cells in the anterior vagina in cows and heifers that have had no previous contact with *T. foetus*.[17] *T. foetus* colonizes the vagina, uterus, and oviduct but does not prevent conception. The secretions from these organs contain the organism. A mild inflammation of the vagina and uterus does develop but is usually not observed. The inflammatory response of the uterus occurs 6 to 8 weeks after infection and is most likely responsible for death of the embryo.[3]

Cows infected with *T. foetus* usually harbor organisms for several heat cycles after infection or pregnancy loss. The parasite is then eliminated from the bovine reproductive tract within a few months as a result of an active specific immune response induced by infection. Immunity, however, is not permanent and the cow is subject to reinfection in subsequent breeding periods.[13]

A carrier cow is defined as a *T. foetus*–infected cow that

remains infected through the entire gestation period and into the postpartum period.[26-28] Morgan[26] studied 167 infected cows and found 1 cow infected at the time of parturition and again 3 weeks later. In a second cow, *T. foetus* was cultured once, 6 weeks after calving. Mancebo and co-workers[27] reported on 12 of 120 heifers that were positive for *T. foetus*. In 10 of these heifers, the parasites were observed once: 60 days post breeding in 1 heifer, 160 days after breeding in 7 heifers, and 240 days after breeding in 2 heifers. In the remaining 2 infected heifers, an irregular pattern of isolation persisted for 300 days after breeding. Skirrow[28] found that 2 of 40 infected cows from two herds carried the infection through the entire gestation and for up to 9 weeks postpartum.

The finding of *T. foetus* in heifers 3 weeks[26] and 10 months[27] after exposure is a clear indication that a production management strategy of giving open cows sexual rest or of retaining open cows in the herd is not sufficient to control infection. Thus, the carrier cow presents a problem in controlling the disease and offers a partial explanation for the persistence of infected animals when control measures have concentrated on eliminating the carrier bulls.[20]

The exact disease-causing mechanism induced by *T. foetus* is not fully understood. The pathogenic process results in insidious signs of inflammation in the bull and a mild vaginitis, cervicitis, and endometritis in the cow.[3, 12] *T. foetus* has been considered a noninvasive organism. This concept seems to explain the lack of inflammation induced in the bull.[12] Recent reports describe evidence that *T. foetus* does have the ability to penetrate fetal mucosal epithelium and invade subjacent connective tissue and lymphatics.[29] Such studies should provide a better understanding of the pathogenesis of trichomoniasis.

IMMUNOLOGY

Few reports describe the immune response to *Trichomonas* infection in the bull. Infection in the bull seems to provoke neither disease nor an immune response.[12] As noted earlier, young bulls are less likely to be infected, but the correlation between prevalence and age is not related to immunity; rather, it is related to the microscopic structure of the mucosal coverings of the penis and prepuce.[25]

Cows do mount an effective immune response to *T. foetus*. The parasites incite a mild inflammatory response associated with the termination of pregnancy. Inflammation is mediated by immune mechanisms that usually bring an end to infection.[3] The immune mechanisms apparently fail in the case of the carrier cow, and this failure is important in the maintenance of infection in cattle herds.[27]

The typical local antibody immune response that occurs in the bovine female following *T. foetus* infection consists of immune globulins of the IgG and IgA class in cervical vaginal mucus secreted by the uterus.[30] Gault and co-workers[31] reported specific anti-trichomonal antibodies present in bovine cervical vaginal mucus after initial infection and also after systemic immunization. Other reports define the mechanisms of action of trichomonal antibodies.[32-34] Monoclonal antibodies cause agglutination, promote complement-mediated lysis, prevent adherence of organisms to epithelial cells, and facilitate phagocytosis by bovine monocytes. Aydintug and colleagues[35] reported that specific trichomonal antibody, in combination with complement, enhance killing of *T. foetus* by polymorphonuclear leukocytes. In addition, the IgG fraction is responsible for preventing adherence of *T. foetus* to bovine vaginal epithelial cells.[34]

The vaccines commonly in use against bovine trichomoniasis (Trichguard and Trichguard V5L, Fort Dodge Laboratories; Reprotec-T and Reprotec-TVL5, Franklin Laboratories) are administered by subcutaneous injection. Two injections 3 weeks apart about 1 month before the breeding season and an annual booster 1 month before the breeding season are recommended. Intensive trials involving beef heifers, all bred to infected bulls, report significant improvement in calving rates.[36–38] Data on retention of conceptus were collected monthly, and the final data were determined at the end of the calving season. Neither vaccination and challenge nor challenge alone affected conception rates. Hall and others[37] reported a 56.32% reduction of abortion (calving rate: vaccinees, 82.76%; controls, 60.53%) and Kvasnicka and co-workers[38] reported a 97.1% increase in term pregnancy (calving rates: vaccinees, 62.1%; controls, 31.5%; P = 0.00045). Control heifers remained infected for a mean of 10.6 weeks (range, 0 to 18 weeks), whereas the vaccinated heifers remained infected for 3.2 to 5.0 weeks (Fig. 2).

Immunologic studies showed that total cervical vaginal mucus concentration of IgM, IgA, IgG_1, and IgG_2 did not change after vaccination or challenge exposure. However, enzyme-linked immunosorbent assay (ELISA) titers of total trichomonal antibodies increased up to 1:10,000 in serum following vaccination (Fig. 3). More important, the titers of the cervical vaginal mucus increased 10-fold over those of noninfected animals and thus were elevated before challenge. In control heifers, the local trichomonal antibody response increased 3- to 5-fold after infection but was not elevated until 60 to 75 days following infection (Fig. 4).[31] These data indicate that vaccination with a killed *T. foetus* vaccine induced a significant local antibody response. This response limited the duration of infection in pregnant cows to an early phase of gestation, a period at which fetal losses are minimal. The result was a significant improvement in calving rates reported.[31]

The effect of vaccination on the status of the carrier cow has not been studied. However, the data reported here tend to support a hypotheses that vaccination should reduce or eliminate the carrier cow as a factor in perpetuation of the disease in infected herds.

TREATMENT

Therapeutic agents for the treatment of bovine trichomoniasis are not available. In the past, ipronidazole was used under the

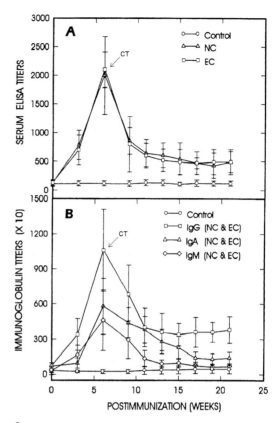

Figure 3

The ELISA titer of total *Tritrichomonas foetus* antibodies *(A)* and *T. foetus* antibody subclasses *(B)* in the serum of control and vaccinated heifers. The arrows marked CT (challenge exposure time) at 6 weeks after initial vaccination indicate the date of challenge exposure by breeding or breeding plus experimentally induced infection. Data plotted as means of the reciprocals of the highest dilution producing a positive ELISA color reaction for each sample collection time, with bars representing the SEM.

provisions of the extra-label requirements of the Food and Drug Administration.[17] Ipronidazole has been declared off-label and is no longer available. Other related compounds are likewise not approved for use in cattle. Although the possibility exists for new therapeutic agents, control of trichomoniasis must be achieved by other means at present.[20]

CONTROL AND PREVENTION

With knowledge of the pathogenesis of trichomoniasis and of the immunologic response following infection or vaccination, a veterinarian can devise a production management program for individual herd situations. The prognosis for reducing the economic impact of the disease is excellent. The basic principles recommended incorporate the general disease prevention recommendations outlined by Richey,[39] the foundation of which program is based on four simple factors.

1. Recognize the disease challenge (diagnosis and surveillance)
2. Know when and why a challenge will occur (pathogenesis)
3. Lower (or eradicate) the challenge (management)
4. Raise the resistance to the specific disease challenge (immunity)

Veterinarians and producers need to consider incorporating the newly introduced production management techniques described in Richey's article. In summary, there has been an in-

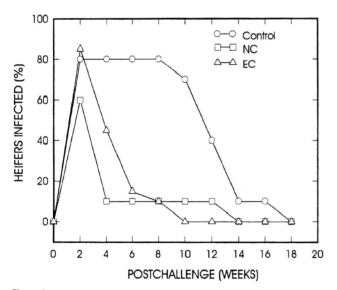

Figure 2

Percentage of *Tritrichomonas foetus* culture-positive cervicovaginal mucus samples obtained at biweekly intervals from 10 control (nonvaccinated, natural challenge exposure) heifers, 10 natural challenge exposure (NC) vaccinated heifers, and from experimental challenge exposure (EC) vaccinated heifers. The samples were cultured in Diamond's media and observed microscopically for growth of *T. foetus*.

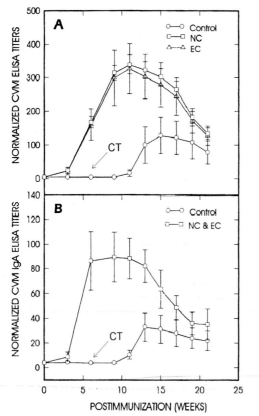

Figure 4

Normalized ELISA titers of total *Tritrichomonas foetus* antibodies *(A)* and *T. foetus* IgA subclass *(B)* in the cervicovaginal mucus of control and vaccinated heifers. The data plotted are the means of the ELISA optical density reading, above background, multiplied by 100 for each sample time, with bars representing the SEM.

creased emphasis on culturing and culling positive bulls,[9] a reliable field culture system is available,[16] and a commercial vaccine with proven efficacy is available.[36, 37, 38]

The following proposals are for naturally bred herds in range locations. However, the same ideas apply to other management situations.

- Replace old bulls with young bulls, keeping the average bull age as young as possible.[12]
- Culture all newly purchased bulls, regardless of age.[11]
- Avoid borrowing or leasing bulls.[11]

Culture bulls 2 weeks after the breeding season and cull those that test positive. Veterinarians should be experienced with the diagnostic collection procedure and have confidence in their ability to isolate and identify *T. foetus*. Culturing of bulls can also be accomplished at the time of breeding soundness examination.[17]

- Use artificial insemination if it can be effectively managed. Check the source of the semen to ensure that bulls at the source facility are tested for trichomoniasis.[17]
- Cull open cows at pregnancy check time.[13] Veterinarians can also identify late-calving cows, cows with pyometra, and any cow with an abnormality suggestive of an impending abortion. It is advisable to sell those cows that calve near the end of an extended calving season. In known infected herds, veterinarians often recommend sorting the late-calving cows for re-palpation in 30 to 60 days.[27, 28] These recommendations should reduce the challenge imposed by the carrier cows.

- Avoid purchase of bred or open cows from herds in the western range regions of the United States.[9, 23, 28]
- Limit the breeding season to 90 days or less. In the event of an outbreak, it will be obvious that there is a problem with some reproductive disease. Trichomoniasis is difficult to prevent or eradicate if the breeding season is extended or year-round.[20]
- Avoid grazing public lands in common with other herds. If common grazing lands are used, keep bulls out of these areas, if possible. Keep fences repaired. Make a note of any commingling of the herd with neighboring herds.[20]
- Vaccinate cows and heifers against *T. foetus* if a disease challenge has been diagnosed or is suspected as well as when the threat of exposure is imminent.[40] Commercial vaccines containing killed *T. foetus* and a proprietary adjuvant are available for use in a control program. Controlled trials have shown the vaccine to significantly reduce the abortion losses when cows are challenged. The vaccines do not prevent infection of the cow; however, they limit the duration of the infection and thus prevent the pathologic effect of the organism by allowing elimination of infection from the cow's system before damage is done to the fetus.[24, 37, 38] Timing of vaccination is important to ensure that adequate resistance is achieved before the challenge occurs.[39] As stated in this article, it is reasonable to assume that vaccination should reduce or eliminate the carrier cow from the herd. Vaccination of bulls is reported to be of limited value in most situations.[41]

Various authors have questioned the efficacy of the currently available vaccines.[42, 43] Resistance and immunity to natural *T. foetus* infection are similar to other pathogenic organisms (e.g., campylobacteriosis) that cause local infection of the reproductive system.[30] When veterinarians evaluate the efficacy of *T. foetus* vaccines, they should review the efficacy of current vaccines that are routinely used to control campylobacteriosis. In 1965, Hoerlein and co-workers[44] reported that when the immunity induced in heifers was severely challenged by natural breeding to infected bulls, pregnancy rates in all groups of vaccinated cattle were substantially better than those in nonvaccinated control cattle. Sixty-three days following breeding and challenge, 60% of the vaccinees were pregnant and only 35% of the controls were pregnant. These data are similar to those reported for the commercial *T. foetus* vaccines.[37, 38]

- The final production management procedure recommended is to control other reproductive diseases such as campylobacteriosis, infectious bovine rhinotracheitis, bovine viral diarrhea, and leptospirosis, with a program to raise the resistance and lower the challenge for these diseases.[39]

Prevention and control of bovine trichomoniasis requires management decisions based on the pathogenesis and immunology of the infection. Management is critical to control disease. Vaccination results in more rapid elimination of infection and reduces early abortions, which are associated with the disease.

REFERENCES

1. Bartlett DE: *Trichomonas foetus* infection and bovine reproduction. Am J Vet Res 8:343, 1947.
2. Goodger WJ, Skirrow SZ: Epidemiologic and economic analyses of an unusually long epizootic of trichomoniasis in a large California dairy herd. J Am Vet Med Assoc 189:772, 1986.
3. Parsonson IM, Clark BL, Dufty JH: Early pathogenesis and pathology of *Tritrichomonas foetus* infection in virgin heifers. J Comp Pathol 86:59, 1976.
4. Dennett DP: Observations on the incidence and distribution of

serotypes of *Tritrichomonas foetus* in beef cattle in North-Eastern Australia. Aust Vet J 50:427, 1974.

5. Kvasnicka WG, Taylor REL, Huang J-C, et al: Investigations of the incidence of bovine trichomoniasis in Nevada and of the efficacy of immunizing cattle with vaccines containing *Tritrichomonas foetus.* Theriogenology 31:963, 1989.

6. Abbitt B, Meyerholz GW: *Trichomonas foetus* infection of range bulls in south Florida. Veterinary Medicine Small Animal Clinician 74:1339, 1979.

7. Johnson AE: Incidence and diagnosis of trichomoniasis in western beef bulls. J Am Vet Med Assoc 145:1007, 1964.

8. Soulsey EJL: Helminths, arthropods and protozoa of domesticated animals, ed 6. Philadelphia, Lea & Febiger, 1977.

9. Idaho Animal Health Regulation 187: Trichomoniasis. By provision of title 25, chapter 2, Idaho Department of Agriculture, Bureau of Animal Health, Boise.

10. Rae DO: Impact of trichomoniasis on the cow-calf producers profitability. J Am Vet Med Assoc 194:771, 1989.

11. Berry SL, Norman BB: Trichomoniasis in beef cattle. Angus, pp 14, 18, and 21, Feb. 1990.

12. Parsonson IM, Clark BL, Dufty JH: Early pathogenesis and pathology of *Tritrichomonas foetus* infection in the bull. Aust Vet J 50:421, 1974.

13. Ball LR: Trichomoniasis: Diagnosis, pathogenesis, treatment and control. Proc Am Assoc Bovine Pract 16:163, 1984.

14. Rhyan JC, Stackhouse LL, Quinn WJ: Fetal and placental lesions in bovine abortion due to *Tritrichomoniasis foetus.* Vet Pathol 25:350, 1988.

15. Kimsey PB: Bovine trichomoniasis. *In* Morrow DA (ed): Current Veterinary Therapy in Theriogenology, ed 2. Philadelphia, WB Saunders, 1986, pp 275–279.

16. Thomas MW, Harmon WM, White C: An improved method for the detection of *Tritrichomonas foetus* infection by culture in bulls. Agri Pract 11:13, 1990.

17. BonDurant RH: Diagnosis, treatment and control of bovine trichomoniasis. Compend Cont Ed Pract Vet 7:S179, 1974.

18. Appel LH, Mickelsen WD, Thomas MW: A comparison of techniques used for the diagnosis of *Tritrichomonas foetus* infections in bulls. Agri Pract 14:2, 1993.

19. Ho MSY, Conrad PA, Conrad PJ, et al: Detection of bovine trichomoniasis with a specific DNA probe and PCR amplification system. J Clin Microbiol 32:98, 1994.

20. Thomas MW, Harmon WM: Bovine trichomoniasis: General information, diagnosis and control. Res Bull Calif Agri Tech Inst, publ No. 940301, March 1994.

21. Wilson SK, Kocan AA, Baudy ET, et al: The prevalence of trichomoniasis in Oklahoma beef bulls. Bovine Pract 14:616, 1979.

22. Peter DA, Fales WH, Miller RB, et al: *Tritrichomonas foetus* infection in a herd of Missouri cattle. J Vet Diagn Invest 7:278, 1995.

23. BonDurant RH, Anderson ML, Blanchard P, et al: Prevalence of trichomoniasis among California beef herds. J Am Vet Med Assoc 196:1590, 1990.

24. Corbeil LB: Vaccination strategies against *Tritrichomonas foetus.* Parasitol Today 10:103, 1994.

25. Ladds PW, Dennet DP, Glazebrook JS: A survey of the genitalia of bulls in Northern Australia. Aust Vet J 49:335, 1973.

26. Morgan BB: Studies on the trichomonad carrier-cow problem. J Anim Sci 3:437, 1944.

27. Mancebo OA, Russo AM, Carabajal LL, et al: Persistence of *Tritrichomonas foetus* in naturally infected cows and heifers in Argentina. Veterinary Parasitology 59:7, 1995.

28. Skirrow SZ: Identification of trichomonad carrier cows. J Am Vet Med Assoc 191:553, 1987.

29. Rhyan JC, Blanchard PC, Kvasnicka WG, et al: Tissue-invasive *Tritrichomonas foetus* in four aborted bovine fetuses. J Vet Diagn Invest 7:409, 1995.

30. Skirrow SZ, BonDurant RH: Immunoglobulin isotype of specific antibodies in reproductive tract secretions and sera in *Tritrichomonas foetus* infected heifers. Am J Vet Res 51:645, 1990.

31. Gault RA, Kvasnicka WG, Hanks D, et al: Specific antibodies in serum and vaginal mucus of heifers inoculated with a vaccine containing *Tritrichomonas foetus.* Am J Vet Res 56:454, 1995.

32. Hodgson JL, Jones DW, Widders PR, et al: Characterization of *Tritrichomonas foetus* antigens by use of monoclonal antibodies. Infect Immunol 58:3078, 1989.

33. Burgess DE: *Tritrichomonas foetus*: Preparation of monoclonal antibodies with effector function. Exp Parasitol 62:266, 1986.

34. Corbeil LB, Hodgson JL, Jones DW, et al: Adherence of *Tritrichomonas foetus* to bovine vaginal epithelial cells. Infect Immunol 57:2158, 1989.

35. Aydintug MK: Bovine polymorphonuclear leukocyte killing *of Tritrichomonas foetus.* Infect Immunol 61:2995, 1993.

36. Schnackel JA, Wallace BL, Kvasnicka WG, et al: *Trichomonas foetus* vaccine immunogenicity trial. Agri Pract 10:11, 1993.

37. Hall MR, Kvasnicka WG, Hanks D, et al: Improved control of trichomoniasis with *Tritrichomonas foetus* vaccine. Agri Pract 14:29, 1993.

38. Kvasnicka WG, Hanks D, Hall MR, et al: Clinical evaluation of the efficacy of inoculating cattle with a vaccine containing *Tritrichomoniasis foetus.* Am J Vet Res 53:2023, 1992.

39. Richey EJ: Facilitating veterinary and producer communication. Large Anim Vet, March–April, p 5, May–June, p 8, 1991.

40. Hjerpe CA: Bovine vaccines and herd vaccination programs. Vet Clin North Am Food Anim Pract 6:171, 1990.

41. Clark BL, Dufty JH, Parsonson IM: Immunization of bulls against trichomoniasis. Aust Vet J 60:178, 1983.

42. Perino LJ, Rupp GP: Beef cow immunity and its influence on fetal neonatal calf health. Proceedings of American Association of Bovine Practitioners 28th Annual Convention, 1995, p 145.

43. Ikeda JS, BonDurant RH, Campero CM, et al: Conservation of a protective surface antigen of *Tritrichomonas foetus.* J Clin Microbiol 31:32289, 1993.

44. Horelein AB, Carroll EJ, Kramer T, et al: Bovine vibriosis immunization. J Am Vet Med Assoc 146:828, 1965.

▪ *Neospora caninum* Infection and Abortion in Cattle

Mark C. Thurmond, D.V.M., Ph.D.
Sharon K. Hietala, Ph.D.

Neospora caninum is a common coccidian parasite of cattle that typically causes asymptomatic infection, and is associated with abortion, reduced milk production, and premature culling. Infected cattle have been found worldwide, with prevalence in some herds approaching 100%. Infection is lifelong and readily transmitted congenitally from an infected dam to her fetuses, thereby perpetuating infection from generation to generation and effectively maintaining infection in a herd. Cows need not acquire infection during pregnancy to abort, and can abort repeatedly. The close relationship between *N. caninum* and *Toxoplasma gondii* suggests the two parasites may have similar life cycles and that postnatal transmission of *N. caninum* may involve a carnivorous definitive host, similar to *T. gondii.*

N. caninum infection was first characterized in 1984 in dogs,[1] and first suggested as a cause of bovine abortion in the late 1980s when a *Neospora*-like infection was identified in connection with an abortion epidemic in a New Mexico dairy.[2] Although the disease in cattle has been recognized only since 1989, the extensive worldwide distribution of infection[3] and stable annual rates of infected aborted fetuses[4] indicate the disease probably has been present in some cattle populations for many years or centuries. Analysis of ribosomal RNA gene sequences estimated that *N. caninum* and *T. gondii* diverged 80 million years ago, about the time of mammalian divergence, indicating that *N. caninum* has been present for at least as long as cattle.[5] Efficient transplacental transmission of *N. caninum* and the relatively low risk of endemic abortion suggest an evolution that has ensured the parasite's successful symbiotic existence with cattle.[6–8]

THE PARASITE

Current knowledge of the parasitology of *N. caninum* is available in recent reviews.[3, 9] Studies comparing isolates from dogs and from aborted bovine fetuses have concluded that they are the same.[10] Although the parasite has been placed in its own genus, *Neospora*, studies demonstrating a close relationship with *T. gondii* suggest that *N. caninum* should be placed in the family Sarcocystidae and in the same genus as *T. gondii*.[5, 11, 12]

Life Cycle

The tissue cyst and tachyzoite forms are the only known stages of *N. caninum* in cattle. Tachyzoites, the intracellular stage of the parasite, are found in several organs, including brain, heart, adrenal, skeletal muscle, kidney, and placenta. Tissue cysts enclose bradyzoites and are found typically in brain and other neural tissue.

Life cycles of other well-studied parasites in the Sarcocystidae family, such as *T. gondii* and *Sarcocystis* spp. involve both a carnivorous definitive host and a ruminant intermediate host,[13] strongly suggesting a similar life cycle for *N. caninum*. In *T. gondii* transmission, a carnivorous definitive host becomes infected following ingestion of cysts in placental or fetal tissues of the intermediate host (e.g., cow). After undergoing development in the intestinal epithelium of a definitive host, *T. gondii* oocysts are shed in the feces for a limited time. It is important to note that recently weaned carnivores, such as kittens, are more likely to have *T. gondii* oocysts in their feces, compared with adults that may not shed oocysts for years after becoming infected. The life cycle is completed when the intermediate host is infected by consumption of feces containing oocysts. Though speculated and extensively sought among domestic and nondomestic dogs, cats, and birds, definitive hosts for *N. caninum* have not been identified. In cattle, *N. caninum* cysts are most frequently described in brains of infected fetuses; however, adult cattle have not been sufficiently studied to determine if cysts can be found in neural tissue to serve as a source of infection in carnivorous hosts.

A wide range of potential definitive and intermediate hosts may exist for *N. caninum*, including those with evidence of natural infection (sheep, goats, deer, dogs, horses, raccoons, coyotes), or for which experimental transmission has been demonstrated (cats, pigs, gerbils, rabbits, and foxes).[3] The possibility of a carnivorous definitive host for *N. caninum* remains viable based on several observations and findings, including the point-source pattern of bovine abortion epidemics,[2, 14, 15] the resistance of bradyzoites in tissue cysts to hydrochloric acid,[16] evidence of natural infection in dogs and coyotes and experimental infection in cats, pigs, and foxes,[3] and the observed correlation between a large number of cats and high seroprevalence in some herds.

The role rodents and birds play in establishment and maintenance of herd infection also is unknown. Studies of crows, hawks, owls, and vultures suggest that carnivorous birds may not be effective definitive hosts.[17] The successful experimental infection of mice suggests that, in addition to cattle, mice may be an intermediate host that could help maintain the life cycle. If mice are indeed an intermediate host, the role of cats as a definitive host of *N. caninum* becomes even more plausible.

Congenital transmission has been shown to be the major means of transmission. Similar to the maintenance of *T. gondii* infection in mice and wild rats,[18, 19] transmission via a definitive, carnivorous host is not necessary to maintain *N. caninum* infection in cattle. Other means of transmission of *N. caninum* that should not yet be excluded are infection directly by tachyzoites through ocular or oral exposure, as for *T. gondii* in sheep, or through direct exposure to tissue cysts.[20] Exposure to tachyzoites or tissue cysts might occur when cattle rub on or eat an infected fetus or placenta. If mice, rats, and other rodents can be an intermediate host for *N. caninum*, as they are for *T. gondii*, then one also might expect exposure of cattle following accidental consumption of infected rodent tissue, as in silage or total mixed rations. *N. caninum* infection can enter a herd through additions of infected female cattle, or theoretically through additions of infected definitive hosts.

CLINICAL PRESENTATION

Clinically, *N. caninum* infection can present as abortion or, rarely, as central nervous system (CNS) signs in a neonatal calf.[21, 22] Aborted fetuses are frequently autolyzed, and may range in age from 3 to 7 months, depending on the parity of the dam and on the epidemiologic pattern of abortion in the herd.[23] Although mummies have been observed in infected cows, the role of *N. caninum* in causing mummification, if any, has not been reported. Information is not available on diagnostic changes in hematologic or clinical chemistry values for *N. caninum*–infected cattle. Generally, morbidity and mortality of infected calves can be expected to be no different from that of noninfected calves. In some herds, infected calves may experience less diarrhea and improved survivorship during the preweaning period, presumably due to immunologic cross-protection against related parasites, including cryptosporidia and coccidia.[6]

Subclinically, congenitally acquired *N. caninum* infection has been found to manifest as reduced milk production in first-lactation dairy heifers;[24] the effect of infection on production in subsequent lactations is not known. No changes in milk production have been reported, however, for epidemics of abortion believed to be due to *N. caninum*.

EPIDEMIOLOGY

Abortion

N. caninum–associated herd abortion problems appear in two distinct epidemiologic patterns. Endemic abortion is the most common pattern in which a herd consistently experiences an elevated abortion rate greater than 5% year after year. Abortion may be attributable to cows that acquired *N. caninum* congenitally and can be a function of the prevalence of infection in the herd. In herds with this endemic-congenital pattern of *N. caninum* abortion, infected cows can be expected to experience, on average, a two- to threefold higher rate of abortion, compared with noninfected cows.[23, 25–27]

The abortion risk for cows congenitally infected with *N. caninum* varies with fetal age and parity. Fetal age for *N. caninum*–associated abortions during the first pregnancy of congenitally infected heifers can range from 3 to 7 months, but can narrow to the 4- to 5-month period in subsequent pregnancies. In the first pregnancy, the risk of abortion in infected heifers was seven times that of noninfected heifers, but declined for subsequent pregnancies, and by the second lactation was no different from that of noninfected cows.[23] Such a decline in prevalence with subsequent pregnancies suggests that the perceived contribution of *N. caninum* to an overall herd abortion problem may depend on the proportion of the herd that is heifers. As demonstrated by abortion in congenitally infected cows, acquisition of *N. caninum* infection during pregnancy is not required for abortion to occur.[26, 27]

In addition to the increased risk of abortion associated with *N. caninum* per se, infected cows that abort can be expected to experience a higher risk of subsequent abortion than infected cows that do not abort.[23] The role *N. caninum* plays in a herd abortion problem can depend on the culling philosophy applied to the herd. *N. caninum* would be expected to contribute to a greater proportion of abortions of infected cows in herds for which aborting cows were retained and rebred, compared to a herd in which aborted cows were culled aggressively.

The other less common but more dramatic epidemiologic pattern is the epidemic occurrence of abortion, where a high proportion of pregnant cows abort during a 2- to 4-week period. In contrast to the endemic pattern, the risk of abortion for infected cows can be as much as 40-fold higher than for noninfected cows.[25] Although one study found that most of the cows that aborted during an epidemic probably were infected postnatally,[25] preabortion serology typically is unavailable to determine if cows were infected before or during the aborted pregnancy or whether congenitally infected cows also could experience an epidemic of *N. caninum* abortion. The point-source type of epidemic pattern suggests cows were exposed to a common source of an abortifacient, which could be a common source of *N. caninum* or a common source of a predisposing factor that might trigger abortion of *N. caninum*–infected fetuses. The latter hypothesis has developed from clinical observations of *N. caninum*–associated epidemics with a history of exposure to bovine virus diarrhea virus (BVDV) or of moldy feed consumption 2 to 3 weeks before onset of the epidemic.[28] Little is known about possible risk factors associated with abortion in cows infected postnatally, or to what extent the epidemiology resembles abortion following congenitally acquired infection.

Experimental and clinical evidence has accumulated to suggest a possible link between *N. caninum* abortion and BVDV infection,[29, 30] although no reports have specifically addressed an interaction between the two. Until further research clarifies the role of BVDV in *N. caninum* abortion, BVDV should be considered in diagnostic investigations of suspected *N. caninum* abortion.

Congenital Infection

Studies of the epidemiology of congenital transmission have not identified a relationship between congenital infection in a fetus and dam age, lactation number, history of abortion, or sex of the fetus.[6] The dam's *N. caninum* antibodies during pregnancy, however, have been found to predict whether or not a calf would be infected congenitally. Cows with increasing antibodies between 90 and 240 days of gestation and high antibody level at 240 days of gestation were significantly more likely to give birth to a precolostrally seropositive calf than were cows with low values.[26, 27] These findings suggest that some as yet unknown factors of pregnancy might stimulate tachyzoite proliferation or promote transmission of tachyzoites to the fetus, or that the dam may develop an enhanced humoral response as the fetus becomes infected. Congenital transmission to the fetus can be expected in 95% or more of infected cows, indicating that *N. caninum* probably is the main means by which infection is perpetuated through multiple generations of a herd, in the absence of postnatal transmission.[6–8] Congenital infection also is possible for potential carnivorous hosts, such as the dog, and intermediate hosts other than the cow, such as mice.[3]

Postnatal Infection

Little information is available on postnatal transmission of *N. caninum*, and most of the epidemiology is speculation, based on assumptions that transmission resembles that for *T. gondii* in sheep. Persistence of postnatally acquired infection and its effect on risk of repeated fetal infection and abortion has not been reported. In a limited study of two dairies with 30% to 50% of cows infected, the annual rate of postnatal infection was estimated to be only about 2% to 4% to the first freshening,[31] and only 1% per year in cows.[32] Calves born to noninfected cows

did not develop infection after consuming colostrum or milk from infected cows, suggesting that milk or colostrum-borne transmission was unlikely. The limited postnatal infection, first appearing in cattle more than 6 to 8 months of age, coincided with initial feeding of total mixed rations.

Beef herds tend to have low herd prevalences of infection, ranging from 0% to 10%, and few, if any, reported epidemics of *N. caninum*–associated abortion.[33] The low prevalence in beef herds, compared with dairy herds, has suggested that the epidemiology of postnatal transmission may relate to features of dairy herd management that generally are not present in beef herds. Based on clinical observations of abortion epidemics in dairies, several features of management and the environment may be prerequisite to an epidemic of infection or abortion caused by a common-source exposure to *N. caninum* oocysts. Possible examples include *Neospora*-contaminated feed that could permit dissemination of the organism to a large number of cattle, concentration of fecal material from a potential carnivorous host shedding oocysts in locations readily accessible to cows, or an environment conducive to the life cycle of *N. caninum*. Unfavorable conditions would include very cold conditions, or conditions that favor desiccation of oocysts shed into the environment.

ECONOMICS

In the early years following discovery of *N. caninum* in cattle, the economic impact of *N. caninum* was perceived to be related to abortion epidemics, which tend to be rare for a given herd. More recently, however, other direct and indirect costs of the disease have been identified that suggest the disease can have a major impact on profitability of cattle production. In addition to abortion epidemics, *N. caninum* endemic abortion may contribute to sustained and costly reproductive inefficiency in a herd.[25] For an assumed loss of $1000 per abortion, a typically observed abortion rate of 20% for infected cows, a 40% herd seroprevalence, and a 40% attributable abortion rate in seropositive cows,[23] the annual cost of endemic *N. caninum* abortion in a herd with 500 pregnant cows per year would be roughly $16,000 ($0.4 \times 500 \times 0.2 \times 0.4 \times 1000$). In addition, milk production during the first lactation may be 2.5 to 3.0 lb/day less in infected cows,[24] and infected cows may be culled prematurely by as much as 6 months.[32]

Other less tangible and more indirect costs relate to the effect of the disease on marketability. The value of infected replacement heifers may be expected to decline, as buyers stipulate in purchase contracts that cattle must be free of *Neospora*. Internationally, it is not yet known whether countries will attempt control through programs that prevent sale or movement of infected cattle, which could have considerable impact on selected cattle markets.

DIAGNOSIS

Aborted Fetuses

Historically, the diagnosis of *N. caninum* abortion for an individual cow or a herd has been based on evidence of *N. caninum* infection in an aborted fetus, as indicated by positive fetal serology, presence of compatible histopathologic lesions, or a positive immunoperoxidase (IPX) stain of a tissue cyst or tachyzoites. Problems associated with use of aborted fetuses to diagnose herd abortion problems relate to the sampling bias inherent in examination of aborted fetuses[34] and to the low predictive values anticipated for histopathologic or IPX assessment of fetal tissues.[35] Diagnostic findings for aborted fetuses typically will be biased by submission of large, mid- to late-gestation fetuses, which are more likely to be recovered for diagnostic submission. Herd abortion problems related to deaths in fetuses less than 4 months of age are frequently overlooked or misdiagnosed.[36]

In addition to the bias inherent in sampling large fetuses, use of fetal infection as a criterion for abortion is inappropriate given the knowledge that most calves of *N. caninum*–infected cows are born with the infection and that histopathologic lesions or IPX staining can be found in nonaborted fetuses and calves. If the sensitivity of such a criterion were perfect, assuming all fetuses aborted due to *N. caninum* had evidence of infection, the low specificity associated with congenital infection could account for a false-positive rate as high as 82%.

Serology

N. caninum antibody is detectable relatively early in gestation, typically by midgestation in infected fetuses, and persists for life in congenitally infected cattle. Specific antibodies produced against *N. caninum* in response to postnatal vs. congenital infection, and their role in protecting the cow have not been well characterized. Antibody levels or titers have not been directly associated with protection from abortion or congenital infection; however, there is some evidence that the specific level of antibody during certain stages of gestation influences pregnancy outcome, predicting either congenital infection or abortion from *N. caninum*–infected dams.[6] Because there are currently no vaccines, detection of *N. caninum* antibody is an indication of natural exposure to the organism, making serology an extremely effective tool for diagnosing the infection and for studying the epidemiology and economic impacts of the agent in cattle.

The serologic tests described for *N. caninum* include the indirect fluorescent antibody (IFA) test and enzyme-linked immunosorbent assays (ELISAs). For the IFA method, cell culture–propagated *N. caninum* tachyzoites are used as antigen and bovine sera are tested in serial dilutions. Cross-reaction with other members of the Apicomplexa parasites, including *Eimeria* sp., *Cryptosporidia* sp., *Sarcocystis* sp., *Hammondia* sp., and *Toxoplasma* sp., can be readily distinguished by trained laboratory technicians who recognize the specific pattern of tachyzoite fluorescence.[37–39] Various cutoffs have been used for interpretation of a positive reaction (Table 1).

Several ELISAs, utilizing *N. caninum* tachyzoites but differing in the preparation of the antigen or in test format, have been described. The ELISA techniques described include kinetic,[37] competitive,[40] recombinant,[41] formalin-fixed antigen,[42] iscomantigen,[43] and sonicated antigen ELISA.[44] In addition, a modification for testing milk from individual cows showed a 95% agreement between serum and milk ELISA results.[45] All tests measure antibodies directed at one or more *Neospora* surface antigens, including the IFA test. Some of the ELISAs additionally recognize internal *N. caninum* antigens. The sensitivity and specificity of the different test systems are reported as similar, though most have not yet been validated by testing sera from confirmed infected and noninfected cows. Table 1 provides sensitivity and specificity estimates based on a panel of 70 and 85 sera from *Neospora*-infected and noninfected cows, respectively, for IFA and the kinetic ELISA.[37]

Serology for *N. caninum* is a useful addition to existing bovine abortion serology screens. A negative serologic test for an aborted cow can be used to exclude *N. caninum* as the cause of abortion in individual cows. Because not all seropositive cows abort, a positive antibody test confirms infection, but not abortion. Similarly, positive fetal serology can be used to indicate infection, but should be interpreted as evidence of infection and not necessarily definitive for the cause of the abortion. There is not a high correlation between fetal histopathologic lesions and serologic findings in either the aborted dam or fetus, most probably because of the high rates of vertical transmission resulting in apparently healthy calves.[46] *N. caninum*–positive fetal serology has been reported in fetuses in which abortion was attributed to other causes.[47, 48] The increased risk of fetal loss due to interaction of *Neospora* and other abortifacients is not yet understood.

Seroconversion, from seronegative to seropositive or seropositive to seronegative in paired samples following abortion, is not typically observed with natural infection, though it has been reported in experimental infections[38, 44] and occasionally in association with an abortion epidemic.[15] In cases of congenital neosporosis, serologic status persists for the life of the cow. Passively derived antibody (colostral antibody) persists for about 4 to 5 months in uninfected calves. The serologic status of cows with natural postnatal infection has not been sufficiently documented.

Diagnosing *Neospora caninum* as the Cause of Abortion on a Herd Basis

Because of the inherent problems in using fetal necropsy information to diagnose herd abortion problems, diagnostic epidemiologic methods have been developed to determine the extent to which *N. caninum* is associated with a herd abortion problem.[25, 28] The general approach is to compare the proportion of aborted, seropositive cows with the proportion of nonaborted seropositive cows in a representative sample of the herd.

The method is illustrated using data obtained from a 1200-cow dairy herd that experienced an abortion epidemic involving about 120 cows aborting over a 4-week period (Table 2). A sample of aborting cows was bled within the first 2 weeks of the epidemic, and nonaborted cows that were in the same stage of pregnancy in the same corrals were selected for bleeding after the epidemic had subsided. A 2 × 2 table was used to calculate the χ^2 statistic, which indicates whether or not the association between seropositivity and abortion is real (significant), where a P-value <0.05 or 0.10 indicates significance. The relative risk (RR) is the estimate of the strength of the association between seropositivity and abortion in an epidemic. In this case, the seropositive cows were 16.9 times more likely to have aborted than seronegative cows. The proportion of abortion due to *N. caninum* is estimated by the attributable proportion (AP), which is calculated as (RR − 1)/RR. In this case, 94% of the abortions

Table 1
SENSITIVITY AND SPECIFICITY, AND OVERALL CORRECT CLASSIFICATION OF THE INDIRECT FLUORESCENT ANTIBODY (IFA) AND KINETIC ENZYME-LINKED IMMUNOSORBENT ASSAY *Neospora caninum* (ELISA)

	Sensitivity	Specificity	Overall Correct Classification
IFA at a dilution of 1:320	90%	82%	86%
IFA at a dilution of 1:640	87%	92%	90%
Kinetic ELISA	89%	97%	93%

Data from Paré J, Hietala SK, Thurmond MC: An enzyme-linked immunosorbent assay (ELISA) for serological diagnosis of *Neospora* sp. infection in cattle. J Vet Diagn Invest 7:352,1995; and Paré J, Hietala SK, Thurmond MC: Interpretation of an indirect fluorescent antibody test for diagnosis of *Neospora* sp. infection in cattle. J Vet Diagn Invest 7:273,1995.

Table 2

RELATIVE RISK (RR) OF ABORTION IN *Neospora caninum*-SEROPOSITIVE COWS DURING AN EPIDEMIC OF ABORTION ON A DAIRY MILKING 1200 COWS

| *N. caninum* Serologic Status | No. of Cows Sampled (N = 167) | | Proportion Aborting |
	Aborted (n = 45)	*Nonaborted (n = 122)*	
Positive	43	51	0.457
Negative	2	71	0.027

RR = 0.457/0.027 = 16.9
Attributable proportion = 15.9/16.9 = 0.94
P-value < .0001

Table 4

ODDS RATIO (OR) OF SEROPOSITIVITY FOR DAUGHTERS BORN TO SEROPOSITIVE AND SERONEGATIVE DAMS ON A DAIRY MILKING 1200 COWS AND EXPERIENCING AN ABORTION EPIDEMIC ASSOCIATED WITH *Neospora caninum* IN 1997

| *N. caninum* Serologic Status of the Dam | Daughter *N. caninum* Status (N = 28) | | Proportion of Positive Daughters |
	Positive (n = 5)	*Negative (n = 23)*	
Positive	5	51	0.25
Negative	0	8	0.00

Proportion seropositive   5/5 = 1.0   15/23 = 0.65
Proportion of positive daughters = 5/28 = 0.18
Proportion of positive dams = 20/28 = 0.71
OR = (5)(8)/(0)(15) = 2.67 (after substituting 1 for 0)
95% confidence interval of OR = 0.23, 141
P = .16

in seropositive cows were estimated to have been attributable to *N. caninum*.

The association between *N. caninum* seropositivity and endemic abortion can be assessed retrospectively, using a similar approach. In this case the odds ratio (OR), which provides a rough approximation to the RR, is estimated instead of the RR. The attributable proportion (AP) can be estimated in a similar manner as AP = (OR − 1)/OR. For the herd investigated in Table 3, the association between *N. caninum* was significant (*P* = .004), but the OR was considerably less (OR = 2.54) than the RR for the herd with the epidemic pattern of *N. caninum* abortion illustrated in Table 2. An OR of 2 to 4 has been interpreted to indicate an endemic abortion problem with *N. caninum*, which has been observed to be typical of herds in which infection is maintained mainly through congenital transmission.

If the diagnostic results and analysis indicate that a significant amount of abortion in a herd was attributable to *N. caninum*, additional diagnostic assessment can be made to characterize the extent to which herd infection was due to congenital or to postnatal transmission.[25] Information on the nature of transmission is important in planning control strategies and in assessing the likelihood of future success.

An estimate of the extent to which infection is attributable to congenital transmission can be made by applying serology and knowledge that most, if not all, infected cows will give birth to an infected calf. The proportion of seropositive daughters of seropositive cows can be compared with the respective propor-

tion of daughters of seronegative cows. If all of the transmission in a herd took place congenitally, all daughters born to seronegative cows would be seronegative and all born to seropositive dams would be seropositive. Table 4 illustrates how such data can be analyzed in a 2 × 2 table. If χ^2 analysis found no significant association (*P* > .10), then one would conclude that little, if any, of the herd infection was transmitted congenitally, and that all or most were therefore transmitted postnatally. If a significant association (*P*-value ≤ .10) was found, then the OR can be calculated to assess the strength of the association, and the AP of infection associated with congenital transmission can be approximated (AP ∼ (OR − 1)/OR). In the example provided in Table 4, no association was found (*P* = .16), indicating most of the transmission took place after the cow gave birth to the daughter that was tested. For the herd illustrated in Table 5, however, a significant association was found in which positive cows were 9.9 times more likely to have a positive daughter, compared with negative cows. The estimated AP is interpreted to mean that 90% of infections in positive cows that had a positive daughter were due to congenital transmission.

Table 3

ODDS RATIO (OR, ESTIMATED RELATIVE RISK) OF ABORTION DURING THE PREVIOUS PREGNANCY FOR SEROPOSITIVE COWS ON A DAIRY MILKING 800 COWS AND EXPERIENCING ENDEMIC *Neospora caninum* ABORTION

| *N. caninum* Serologic Status | No. of Cows Sampled (N = 199) | |
	Aborted (n = 65)	*Nonaborted (n = 145)*
Positive	36	44
Negative	29	90

OR = (36)(90)/(29)(44) = 2.54
(95% confidence interval of OR = 1.32, 4.88)
Attributable proportion ∼ 1.54/2.54 = 0.61
P = .004

Table 5

ODDS RATIO (OR) OF SEROPOSITIVITY FOR DAUGHTERS BORN TO SEROPOSITIVE AND SERONEGATIVE DAMS ON A DAIRY MILKING 2000 COWS AND WITH ENDEMIC *Neospora caninum* ABORTION IN 1996

| *N. caninum* Serologic Status of the Dam | Daughter *N. caninum* Status (N = 244) | | Total | Proportion or Positive Daughters |
	Positive (n = 123)	*Negative (n = 121)*		
Positive	78	18	96	0.81
Negative	45	103	148	0.30
Proportion seropositive	78/123 = 0.63	18/121 = 0.15		

Proportion of positive daughters = 123/244 = 0.50
Proportion of positive dams = 96/148 = 0.65
OR = (78)(103)/(45)(18) = 9.9 (95% confidence interval = 5.1, 19.5)
P < .0001
Attributable proportion ≈ (OR − 1)/OR = 8.9/9.9 = 0.90

CONTROL AND PREVENTION

Congenital Infection

Currently, no treatment or immunoprophylaxis is available to prevent congenital *N. caninum* infection of a fetus. Results of limited in vitro studies suggest that several anticoccidial drugs may inhibit development of *N. caninum*,[49, 50] but no data from clinical trials are available to determine efficacy in preventing either congenital or postnatal transmission, or in preventing abortion due to *N. caninum*. An incidental finding in one study showed that heifers infected with *N. caninum* and fed monensin 200 mg per head per day during their first pregnancy had a sevenfold higher risk of abortion than noninfected heifers.[23] Although no control group was examined, the observation suggests monensin may not be effective in preventing *N. caninum* congenital infection or abortion.

Congenital transmission of *N. caninum* can be prevented in embryo transfer fetuses by use of recipients not infected with the parasite. Currently, control and prevention of herd infection attributable to congenital transmission requires culling and replacement with noninfected heifers. The cost-effectiveness of a program aimed at reducing or eliminating the prevalence of infection in a herd would depend on such factors as initial herd prevalence, costs of testing, availability and cost of replacement heifers, cost of abortion, milk production loss, and premature culling attributable to *N. caninum*. For herds with a high prevalence of infection, culling infected cows and replacing them with noninfected heifers may not be economically justified.

Postnatal Infection

Recommendations for control of postnatal transmission are based on the assumption that the life cycle of *N. caninum* resembles that of *T. gondii*. A general control strategy would be aimed at breaking the theoretical life cycle by minimizing exposure to oocytes in feces of definitive hosts and to exposure to tachyzoites and cysts in carcass or placental tissues of cattle or other intermediate hosts. Practices employed to minimize postnatal transmission would be those used to enhance general sanitation, which would also control other infectious diseases. Exposure to oocysts would be reduced as follows: minimizing the number of carnivores cohabitating with the herd, reducing access of carnivores to cattle carcasses and placentas and other tissues that may contain *N. caninum* cysts; minimizing exposure of carnivores to other theoretical intermediate hosts, such as mice and rats, through live-trapping, poisoning, or rodent control methods other than use of cats; minimizing exposure of cattle to potential carnivore feces in feed and water; and limiting reproduction of potential definitive hosts, thereby minimizing congenital transmission from generation to generation of carnivores.

Presuming that carnivores play a role in the life cycle of *N. caninum*, congenital infection in carnivorous hosts may be minimized by controlling reproduction of domestic carnivores, including use of castrated or spayed cats and dogs to control rodents and work cattle, respectively. Litters of kittens or pups should be relocated to an environment with no access to cattle. Exposure of carnivores and cattle to *N. caninum* would be controlled by limiting access to carcasses, placentas, and tissues from the premises. Use of individual calving pens or segregation of seropositive and seronegative cows at calving would reduce exposure of noninfected cows to tissues and fluids of infected cows during calving. Preferred sites of defecation for carnivores should be identified and feces routinely removed. Domestic animals should be encouraged to defecate in areas inaccessible to cattle or to cattle feed or water. Commodities and stored feed should be examined routinely to assess whether fecal contamination is taking place.

Vaccination

Currently, no vaccine is available to immunize cattle against *N. caninum*. Although the prospects for an effective vaccine have not been considered favorable,[9] vaccines with claims of efficacy are likely to appear on the market. In determining the appropriateness and effectiveness of a vaccine directed against *N. caninum*, the following issues should be considered: (1) effectiveness of a vaccine in preventing abortion or infection due to natural (as opposed to experimental) exposure, (2) effectiveness in preventing congenital infection of the fetus, (3) effectiveness in preventing postnatal infection, (4) serologic differentiation of vaccine-induced antibody from that produced in natural infection (interference with interpretation of serologic tests), which would allow for vaccination to mask infection, and (6) cost-effectiveness, including expected reduction in congenital and postnatal transmission and in abortion.

REFERENCES

1. Bjerkas I, Mohn SF, Presthus J: Unidentified cyst-forming sporozoon causing encephalomyelitis and myositis in dogs. Z Parasitenkd 70:271, 1984.
2. Thilsted JP, Dubey JP: Neosporosis-like abortions in a herd of dairy cattle. J Vet Diagn Invest 1:205, 1989.
3. Dubey JP, Lindsay DS: A review of *Neospora caninum* and neosporosis. Vet Parasitol 67:1, 1996.
4. Thurmond MC, Anderson ML, Blanchard PC: Secular and seasonal trends of *Neospora* abortion in California dairy cows. J Parasitol 81:364, 1995.
5. Ellis J, Luton K, Baverstock PR, et al: The phylogeny of *Neospora caninum*. Mol Biochem Parasitol 64:303, 1994.
6. Paré J, Thurmond MC, Hietala SK: Congenital *Neospora caninum* infection in dairy cattle and associated calfhood mortality. Can J Vet Res 60:133, 1996.
7. Björkman C, Johansson O, Stenlund S, et al: *Neospora* species infection in a herd of dairy cattle. J Am Vet Med Assoc 188:1441, 1996.
8. Anderson ML, Reynolds JP, Rowe JD, et al.: Evidence of vertical transmission of *Neospora* sp infection in dairy cattle. J Am Vet Med Assoc 210:1169, 1997.
9. Anderson ML, Barr B, Conrad PA: Protozoal causes of reproductive failure in domestic ruminants. Vet Clin North Am Food Anim Pract 10:439, 1994.
10. Barber JS, Holmdahl OJM, Owen RM, et al: Characterization of the first European isolate of *Neospora caninum* (Dubey, Carpenter, Speer, Topper and Uggla). Parasitology 111:563, 1995.
11. Holmdahl OJM, Mattsson JG, Uggla A, et al: The phylogeny of *Neospora caninum* and *Toxoplasma gondii* based on ribosomal RNA sequences. FEMS Microbiol Lett 119:187, 1994.
12. Gua Z-G, Johnson AM: Genetic comparison of *Neospora caninum* with *Toxoplasma* and *Sarcocystis* by random amplified polymorphic DNA-polymerase chain reaction. Parasitol Res 81:365, 1995.
13. Dubey JP: *Toxoplasma, Neospora, Sarcocystis*, and other tissue cyst-forming coccidia of humans and animals. *In* Kreier JP (ed): Parasitic Protozoa, ed 2. San Diego, Academic Press, 1993, pp 1–158.
14. Nietfeld JC, Dubey JP, Anderson ML, et al.: *Neospora*-like protozoan infection as a cause of abortion in dairy cattle. J Vet Diagn Invest 4:223, 1992.
15. McAllister MM, Huffman EM, Hietala SK, et al: Evidence suggesting a point in an outbreak of bovine abortion due to neosporosis. J Vet Diagn Invest 8:355, 1996.
16. Lindsay DS, Dubey JP: Infections in mice with tachyzoites and bradyzoites of *Neospora caninum* (Protozoa, Apicomplexa). J Parasitol 76:177, 1990.
17. Baker DG, Morishita TY, Brooks DL, et al: Experimental oral inoculations in birds to evaluate potential definitive hosts of *Neospora caninum*. J Parasitol 81:783, 1995.

18. Beverley JKA: Congenital transmission of toxoplasmosis through successive generations of mice. Nature 183:1348, 1959.
19. Webster JP: Prevalence and transmission of *Toxoplasma gondii* in wild brown rats, *Rattus norvegicus*. Parasitology 108:407, 1994.
20. Jacobs L, Hartley WJ: Ovine toxoplasmosis: parasitaemia, tissue infection, and congenital transmission in ewes infected by various routes. Br Vet J 120:347, 1964.
21. Dubey JP, Janovitz EB, Skowronek AJ: Clinical neosporosis in a 4-week-old Hereford calf. Vet Parasitol 78:532, 1992.
22. Barr BC, Conrad PA, Dubey JP, et al: *Neospora*-like encephalomyelitis in a calf: Pathology, ultrastructure, and immunoreactivity. J Vet Diagn Invest 3:39, 1992.
23. Thurmond MC, Hietala SK: Effect of congenitally-acquired *Neospora caninum* infection on risk of abortion and repeat abortion in dairy heifers and cows. Am J Vet Res 58:1381, 1997.
24. Thurmond MC, Hietala SK: Effect of *Neospora caninum* infection on milk production in first-lactation dairy cows. J Am Vet Med Assoc 210:672, 1997.
25. Thurmond MC, Hietala SK, Blanchard PC: 1997, Herd-based diagnosis of *Neospora caninum*–induced endemic and epidemic abortion in cows and evidence for congenital and postnatal transmission. J Diagn Lab Invest 9:44, 1997.
26. Paré J, Thurmond MC, Hietala SK: *Neospora caninum* antibodies in cows during pregnancy as a predictor of congenital infection and abortion. J Parasitol 83:82, 1997.
27. Paré J: Epidemiology of *Neospora caninum* infection in cattle. PhD dissertation, University of California, Davis, 1996, p 110.
28. Thurmond M, Hietala S: Strategies to control *Neospora* infection in cattle. Bovine Pract 29:60, 1995.
29. Dubey JP, Miller S, Lindsay DS, et al: *Neospora caninum* associated myocarditis and encephalitis in an aborted calf. J Vet Diagn Invest 2:66, 1990.
30. Barr BC, Rowe JD, Sverlow KW, et al: Experimental reproduction of bovine fetal *Neospora* infection and death with a bovine neospora isolate. J Vet Diagn Invest 6:207, 1994.
31. Thurmond M, Hietala S: Postnatal transmission of *Neospora caninum* before first calving in dairy heifers. *In* Proceedings 38th Annual Meeting of the American Association of Veterinary Laboratory Diagnosticians, Sparks Nev 1995, p. 70.
32. Thurmond MC, Hietala SK: Culling associated with *Neospora caninum* infection in dairy cows. Am J Vet Res 57:1559, 1996.
33. Hietala S: Unpublished data from the California Veterinary Diagnostic Laboratory System. School of Veterinary Medicine, University of California, Davis.
34. Thurmond MC, Blanchard PC, Anderson ML: An example of selection bias in submissions of aborted bovine fetuses to a diagnostic laboratory. J Vet Diagn Invest 6:269, 1994.
35. Thurmond MC, Blanchard PC, Hietala SK: Predictive values of fetal histopathology and immunoperoxidase staining in diagnosing *Neospora caninum* abortion. *In* Proceedings 40th Annual Meeting of the American Association of Veterinary Laboratory Diagnosticians, Louisville, Ky, 1997.
36. Forar AL, Gay JM, Hancock DD, et al: Fetal loss frequency in ten Holstein dairy herds. Theriogenology 45:1505, 1996.
37. Paré J, Hietala SK, Thurmond MC: An enzyme-linked immunosorbent assay (ELISA) for serological diagnosis of *Neospora* sp. infection in cattle. J Vet Diagn Invest 7:352, 1995.
38. Conrad PA, Sverlow KW, Anderson M, et al: Detection of serum antibody responses in cattle with natural or experimental *Neospora* infections. J Vet Diagn Invest 5:572, 1993.
39. Paré J, Hietala SK, Thurmond MC: Interpretation of an indirect fluorescent antibody test for diagnosis of *Neospora* sp. infection in cattle. J Vet Diagn Invest 7:273, 1995.
40. Baszler TV, Kowles DP, Dubey JP, et al: Serological diagnosis of bovine neosporosis by *Neospora caninum* monoclonal antibody–based competitive inhibition ELISA. J Clin Microbiol 34:1423, 1996.
41. Lally NC, Jenkins MC, Dubey JP: Evaluation of two *Neospora caninum* recombinant antigens for use in an ELISA for the diagnosis of bovine neosporosis. Clin Diagn Lab Immunol 3:275, 1996.
42. Williams DJL, McGary J, Guy F, et al: A novel ELISA for detection of *Neospora*-specific antibodies in cattle. Vet Rec 140:328, 1997.
43. Björkman C, Lundén A, Holmdahl OJM, et al: *Neospora caninum* in dogs: Detection of antibodies by ELISA using an iscom antigen. Parasite Immunol 16:643, 1994.
44. Dubey JP, Lindsay DS, Adams DS, et al: Serologic responses of cattle and other animals infected with *Neospora caninum*. Am J Vet Res 57:329, 1996.
45. Björkman C, Holmdahl J, Uggla A: An indirect enzyme-linked immunoassay (ELISA) for demonstration of antibodies to *Neospora caninum* in serum and milk of cattle. Vet Parasitol 68:251, 1997.
46. Reichel MP, Drake JM: The diagnosis of *Neospora* abortions in cattle. N Z Vet J 44:151, 1996.
47. Barr BC, Anderson ML, Sverlow KW, et al: Diagnosis of bovine fetal *Neospora* infection with an indirect fluorescent antibody test. Vet Rec 137:611, 1995.
48. Blanchard PC, Hietala SK, Thurmond MC: Diagnostic interpretation of *Neospora* serology. *In* Proceedings 38th Annual Meeting of the American Association of Veterinary Laboratory Diagnosticians, Sparks, Nev, 1995, p 40.
49. Lindsay DS, Dubey JP: Evaluation of anti-coccidial drugs' inhibition of *Neospora caninum* development in cell cultures. J Parasitol 75:990, 1989.
50. Lindsay DS, Butler JM, Blagburn BL: Efficacy of decoquinate against *Neospora caninum* tachyzoites in cell cultures. Vet Parasitol 68:35, 1997.

■ Toxoplasmosis*

J. P. Dubey, M.V.Sc., Ph.D.

ETIOLOGIC AGENT

Toxoplasmosis is caused by the protozoan parasite *Toxoplasma gondii*. It is an intracellular coccidian parasite that is classified in the phylum Apicocomplexa, class Sporozoasida, order Eucocciiorida, suborder Eimeriorina, and family Toxoplasmatidae. Felids, including the domestic cat (*Felis catus*) and wild Felidae, are definitive hosts, and various warm-blooded animals are intermediate hosts (Fig. 1).

Like all coccidian parasites, oocysts are excreted only by the definitive hosts, cats. Unsporulated, noninfective oocysts (10 × 11 μm) are shed in feces of infected cats. Oocysts sporulate outside in cat feces within 1 or more days, depending on environmental conditions. Sporulated oocysts can survive in soil and elsewhere in the environment for many months, and they are resistant to freezing and drying. Each sporulated oocyst contains two sporocysts, each of which contains four banana-shaped sporozoites (8 × 2 μm). Sporulated oocysts are infectious to virtually all warm-blooded hosts, including humans.

Intermediate hosts can become infected by ingesting sporulated oocysts in food or water. Sporozoites are released from oocysts in the gut lumen and become tachyzoites (Greek *tachy*, "speed"; *zoite*, "organism") within 12 hours of penetration into host cells. Tachyzoites (6 × 2 μm) multiply in virtually all cells of the body by division into two zoites. Within 3 to 4 days, tachyzoites may become encysted in tissues and are called bradyzoites (*brady*, "slow"). Bradyzoites (7 × 2 μm) are enclosed in a thin, elastic wall, and the entire structure is called a tissue cyst. Tissue cysts are formed in many locations, but particularly in the central nervous system and both striated and smooth muscle. They are often elongated (up to 100 μm) in muscles and round (up to 70 μm) in the central nervous system. Tissue cysts may persist for the life of the host.

All hosts, including the definitive felid hosts, can become infected by ingesting tissue cysts. In the intermediate host, bradyzoites become tachyzoites within 18 hours of infection, and the tachyzoite-bradyzoite cycle is repeated. However, in the definitive host, the cat, bradyzoites give rise to a conventional coccidian cycle in the small intestinal epithelium. This coccidian cycle consists of an asexual cycle (schizonts) followed by a sexual cycle (gamonts). Fertilization of the female parasite (macrogamont) by the male parasite (microgamete) gives rise to an oocyst. Both the asexual and sexual cycles can be completed in the feline intestine within 3 days of the ingestion of tissue cysts.

---

*All of the material in this article is in the public domain.

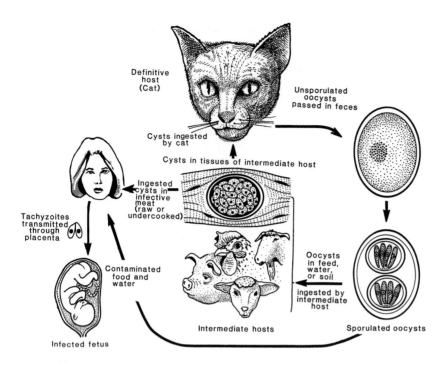

Figure 1
Life cycle of *Toxoplasma gondii.*

The extraintestinal cycle of *T. gondii* in the cat is like that in the intermediate hosts.

The ingestion of tissue cysts or oocysts can cause parasitemia in the mother and lead to infection of the fetus. Congenital *T. gondii* infections are frequent in human beings, sheep, and goats.

CLINICAL SIGNS AND LESIONS

Clinical signs and symptoms vary with the host, mode of infection, immune status, and the organ parasitized. Congenitally acquired toxoplasmosis is generally more severe than postnatally acquired toxoplasmosis.

Chorioretinitis, hydrocephalus, mental retardation, and jaundice may all be seen together in severely affected infants, but chorioretinitis is the most common sequela of congenital infection in children. Toxoplasmosis does not result in hydrocephalus in sheep, goats, or other animals.

In ewes infected during pregnancy, lambs may be mummified, macerated, aborted, or stillborn or may be born weak and die within a week of birth. Lambs that survive the first week generally grow normally to adulthood and produce *T. gondii*–free lambs. Although infected adult sheep have no clinical signs, toxoplasmosis can be fatal in adult goats. Severe congenital toxoplasmosis has been reported in cats, dogs, and pigs but not in cattle or horses.

Clinical toxoplasmosis in dogs is generally seen concurrently with canine distemper virus infection and often involves the lungs, liver, and central nervous system. Pneumonia is the most common entity associated with clinical toxoplasmosis in cats. Clinical toxoplasmosis has not been documented in cattle or horses.

Most infections in immunocompetent human beings are asymptomatic; however, toxoplasmosis can be fatal in immunocompromised hosts, such as individuals with AIDS or patients receiving immunotherapy for tumors or in connection with organ transplants. Whereas lymphadenopathy is the most common symptom in immunocompetent humans, encephalitis predominates in immunosuppressed patients.

T. gondii causes necrosis by active multiplication in cells; it does not produce a toxin. The extent of lesions and associated clinical signs varies depending on the organ parasitized. For example, even small lesions in eyes are debilitating. Early in the infection, *T. gondii* produces enteritis and mesenteric lymph node necrosis before lesions develop in other organs. Some hosts may die of enteritis. Pneumonia and nonsuppurative encephalitis are other important lesions. In sheep and goats, *T. gondii* causes small (1 to 5 mm), chalky white areas of necrosis in cotyledonary villi of the placenta.

Clinical signs of toxoplasmosis are nonspecific and unreliable for a definitive diagnosis. Diagnosis is aided by biologic, serologic, or histologic methods or by combinations of them. *T. gondii* can be isolated from patients by inoculation of laboratory animals (generally mice) and tissue cultures with appropriate material. Secretions, excretions, body fluids, and tissues taken antemortem or tissues taken at necropsy are all possible specimens from which to attempt to isolate *T. gondii*. However, these procedures are too complicated for routine use in most diagnostic laboratories and are performed only in specialized laboratories.

Finding *T. gondii* antibodies aids in the diagnosis. Numerous serologic tests are available for detecting humoral antibodies, and details can be found in Dubey and Beattie (1988). A number of agglutination tests and an enzyme-linked immunosorbent assay that have been modified to detect both IgG and IgM antibodies are commercially available. The IgM antibodies appear and disappear sooner than do the IgG antibodies, and the difference in IgM and IgG antibody titers is helpful in determining the time since infection occurred. IgG antibody titers may persist for life; therefore their presence establishes only that a host has been exposed to *T. gondii*. A 16-fold higher antibody titer in a serum sample taken 2 to 4 weeks after the first sample was collected more accurately indicates an acute acquired infection. In veterinary practice, this rise in antibody titer is difficult to document because acute and convalescent samples must be run at the same time. Moreover, antibodies may have already peaked by the time patients are seen in the clinic. For example, by the time goats and sheep abort pregnancies because of toxoplasmosis, the antibodies have already peaked and waned and are therefore of marginal value in diagnosis. However, finding antibodies in goat, sheep, and pig fetuses is indicative of congenital toxoplasmosis in the fetus because there is no maternal transplacental transfer of antibodies in ruminants and pigs.

The diagnosis of toxoplasmosis can be made by finding *T. gondii* in host tissue removed by biopsy or at necropsy. A rapid diagnosis may be made by making impression smears of lesions on glass slides. After drying for 10 to 30 minutes, smears should be fixed in methyl alcohol and stained with Giemsa or any of several other stains routinely used to stain blood smears. *T. gondii* tachyzoites are crescent shaped, are about 6×2 µm, have a well-defined nucleus, and are often found in macrophages.

TREATMENT

Little is known regarding the efficacy of various drugs for treating naturally occurring toxoplasmosis in animals because antemortem diagnosis is rare. Sulfadiazine and pyrimethamine (Daraprim) are two drugs widely used for the treatment of human toxoplasmosis. Monensin (15 mg/day per ewe) has been advocated in some countries for use in sheep as a prophylactic to prevent abortion. However, the drug is not approved for this use in the United States.

PUBLIC HEALTH SIGNIFICANCE

Cats are the key hosts in the epidemiology of toxoplasmosis. They can excrete millions of oocysts in a gram of feces. Cats generally become infected by eating tissue cysts of *T. gondii* from birds and mammals. Cats excrete oocysts for only 1- to 2-week periods in their lives.

Food animals become infected with *T. gondii* by ingesting food and water contaminated with sporulated oocysts. Tissue cysts can persist in tissues of live animals for many months (probably for life). *T. gondii* infections are more common in sheep, goats, and pigs than in horses and cattle. Therefore, ingestion of beef is of little importance in the epidemiology of toxoplasmosis. Human beings become infected by ingesting tissue cysts in undercooked meat or oocysts in food and water contaminated with cat feces. Approximately 40% of the adult human beings in the United States have antibodies to *T. gondii*, and it is estimated that twice that level of prevalence occurs in Central and South America and in France. Approximately 1 in 1000 children is born infected with *T. gondii* in the United States. Therefore it is essential to prevent infections in human beings during pregnancy.

PREVENTION AND CONTROL

To prevent human infection, hands should be washed thoroughly with soap and water after handling meat. All cutting boards, sink tops, knives, and other materials that come in contact with uncooked meat should be washed with soap and water because the stages of *T. gondii* that occur in meat are killed by water. The meat of any animal should be cooked to 70°C before human or animal consumption, and tasting meat while cooking it or while seasoning homemade sausage should be avoided. Pregnant women should definitely avoid contact with cat feces or litter, soil, and raw meat. Pet cats should be fed only dry, canned, or cooked food. Cat litter should be emptied every day, preferably not by a pregnant woman. Gloves should be worn while gardening. Vegetables should be washed thoroughly before eating because of the risk of contamination with cat feces.

Because most cats become infected by eating infected tissue, cats should never be fed uncooked meat, viscera, or bones, and efforts should be made to keep cats indoors to prevent hunting. Trash cans should be covered to prevent scavenging. Although freezing can kill most *T. gondii* tissue cysts, it cannot be relied on to kill them all. Cats should be spayed to control the feline population on farms. Dead animals should be removed promptly to prevent scavenging by cats. A vaccine for the prevention of toxoplasmosis in human beings is not yet available; however, a vaccine containing live but nonpersistent tachyzoites is available in New Zealand and Europe to prevent abortion in sheep.

BIBLIOGRAPHY

Dubey JP, Beattie CP: Toxoplasmosis of Animals and Man. Boca Raton, Fla, CRC Press, 1988, pp 1–220.

Remington JS, McLeod R, Desmonts G: Toxoplasmosis. *In* Remington JS, Klein JO (eds): Infectious Diseases of the Fetus and Newborn Infant, ed 4. Philadelphia, WB Saunders, 1995, pp 140–267.

Roberts T, Murrell KD, Marks S: Economic losses caused by foodborne parasitic diseases. Parasitol Today 10:419–423, 1994.

■ Sarcocystosis*

J. P. Dubey, M.V.Sc., Ph.D.

ETIOLOGIC AGENT

Sarcocystis spp. are coccidian parasites that belong to the phylum Apicomplexa, class Sporozoasida, subclass Coccidiasina, order Eucoccidiorida, and family Sarcocystidae.

The name *Sarcocystis* (Greek *sarkos*, "flesh"; *kystis*, "bladder") implies parasites in muscle and refers to sarcocysts found in the striated muscle of mammals, birds, and poikilothermic animals.

Sarcocystis has an obligatory prey-predator two-host cycle (Fig. 1). Unlike most other coccidian parasites, the asexual and sexual cycles occur in different hosts. The asexual cycle develops only in the intermediate host, which in nature is often a prey animal. Sexual stages develop only in a carnivorous definitive host. A given host may be parasitized by more than one species of *Sarcocystis*, and intermediate and definitive hosts may vary for each species of *Sarcocystis* (Table 1). The definitive host becomes

---

*All of the material in this article is in the public domain, with the exception of any borrowed figures and tables.

Table 1
INTERMEDIATE AND DEFINITIVE HOSTS FOR SPECIES OF *Sarcocystis* IN CATTLE, SHEEP, GOATS, AND PIGS

Intermediate Host	Species of *Sarcocystis*	Definitive Hosts	Pathogenicity for Intermediate Hosts
Cattle	*Sarcocystis cruzi*	Dog, coyote, fox, wolf, jackal, raccoon	+ +
	S. hirsuta	Cat	±
	S. hominis	Primates, humans	±
Sheep	*S. tenella*	Dog, coyote, fox	+ +
	S. arieticanis	Dog	+
	S. mihoensis	Dog	?
	S. gigantea	Cat	−
	S. medusiformis	Cat	−
Goat	*S. capracanis*	Dog, coyote, fox	+ +
	S. hircicanis	Dog	+
	S. moulei	Cat	−
Pig	*S. miescheriana*	Dog, fox, raccoon, jackal	+
	S. porcifelis	Cat	?
	S. suihominis	Humans, other primates	+

+ +, Highly pathogenic; +, pathogenic; ±, mildly pathogenic; −, nonpathogenic; ?, unknown.

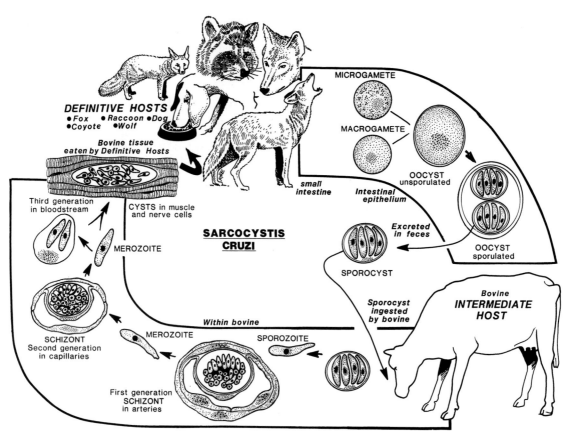

Figure 1

Life cycle of *Sarcocystis cruzi*. (From Dubey JP, Speer CA, Fayer R: Sarcocystosis of Animals and Man. Boca Raton, Fla, CRC Press, 1989, pp 1–215.)

infected by eating sarcocysts containing infective zoites (bradyzoites). The bradyzoites transform into male and female gamonts in the small intestine, and after fertilization oocysts are produced. The oocysts sporulate in the lamina propria and contain two sporocysts, each with four sporozoites. The oocyst wall is thin and often breaks so that both sporocysts and oocysts are excreted in feces, usually 1 week after the ingestion of sarcocysts. The asexual cycle occurs initially in vascular endothelium, later in cells in the bloodstream, and finally in muscles. Two or more asexual cycles (schizonts) are produced in blood vessels. After brief multiplication in leukocytes, merozoites enter muscles and produce sarcocysts.

Sarcocysts mature in about 1 to 2 months and become infectious for the carnivore host. Sarcocysts of some species of *Sarcocystis* may become grossly visible, for example, *Sarcocystis gigantea*, *S. hirsuta*, and *S. moulei*. Many others are microscopic in size.

CLINICAL SIGNS AND LESIONS

Sarcocysts are generally nonpathogenic for the definitive host, and some species of *Sarcocystis* are also nonpathogenic for intermediate hosts (see Table 1). Generally, species transmitted by canids are pathogenic, whereas those transmitted by felids are nonpathogenic. *S. cruzi*, *S. capracanis*, and *S. tenella* are the most pathogenic species for cattle, goats, and sheep, respectively. Clinical signs are generally seen during the second schizogonic cycle in blood vessels (acute phase). Three to 4 weeks after infection with a large dose of sporocysts (50,000 or more), fever, anorexia, anemia, emaciation, and hair loss (particularly on the rump and tail in cattle) develop, and some animals die. Pregnant animals may abort, and growth is slowed or arrested. Animals recover as sarcocysts begin to mature.

Dramatic gross lesions are seen in animals that die during the acute phase. Edema, hemorrhage, and atrophy of fat are commonly seen. The hemorrhages are most evident on the serosa of viscera, in cardiac and skeletal muscle, and in the sclera of the eyes. Hemorrhages vary from petechiae to ecchymoses several centimeters in diameter. Microscopic lesions may be seen in many organs and consist of necrosis, edema, and infiltrations of mononuclear cells. During the chronic phase, lesions are restricted to muscles and consist of nonsuppurative myositis and degeneration of sarcocysts.

DIAGNOSIS

Diagnosis of acute sarcocystosis is difficult. Naturally occurring, clinically acute sarcocystosis has been observed only in cattle. The disease in cattle is generalized in nature with no specific signs. Anemia, hair loss, excessive salivation, abortion, and a history of contamination of feed or water by canine feces should arouse suspicion of acute sarcocystosis. Laboratory examination should include hematologic analysis, serum enzyme chemistry, and serologic examination for anti-*Sarcocystis* antibody. Serum sorbitol dehydrogenase, creatine phosphokinase, and lactate dehydrogenase levels are elevated, packed cell volume is lowered to less than 20%, and levels of anti-*Sarcocystis* antibodies are elevated. Because nearly all cattle and sheep are subclinically infected with *Sarcocystis*, serologic examination alone is not diagnostic.

TREATMENT

Although prophylaxis with certain anticoccidials (monensin, lasalocid, decoquinate, salinomycin, amprolium) can reduce clinical sarcocystosis in animals, treatment is not effective once clinical signs are noted. Because diagnosis is difficult, the efficacy of chemotherapy in natural outbreaks of clinical sarcocystosis is unknown.

Carnivores should be excluded from animal houses and from feed, water, and bedding for livestock. Uncooked meat should never be fed to carnivores. Freezing kills sarcocysts in meat.

Dead livestock should be buried or incinerated. There is no vaccine to protect livestock from acute sarcocystosis.

BIBLIOGRAPHY

Dubey JP: *Toxoplasma, Neospora, Sarcocystis,* and other tissue cyst-forming coccidia of humans and animals. *In* Kreier JP (ed): Parasitic Protozoa, vol 6. New York, Academic Press, 1993, pp 1–158.

Dubey JP, Speer CA, Fayer R: Sarcocystosis of Animals and Man. Boca Raton, Fla, CRC Press, 1989, pp 1–215.

Respiratory Diseases

Consulting Editor

Mike Apley, D.V.M., Ph.D., Diplomate, A.C.V.C.P.

Production medicine begins by defining problems or opportunities through knowledge of the individual animal and the production setting. Solutions then involve control and prevention through management of the environment, management of nutritional influences, vaccination programs, limiting of disease exposure, and therapeutic intervention.

This section emphasizes a production medicine approach to respiratory disease. Each author addressing swine, bovine, or sheep and goat respiratory disease has concentrated on the epidemiology of causal agents, environmental influences, practical preventive measures, and intervention strategies. The article on diagnostic methods details practical knowledge necessary to define a respiratory problem in a production system. The therapeutics article starts with interpretation of susceptibility data, moves through characteristics of selected antimicrobial and ancillary agents, and ends by considering therapeutic populations and drug selection.

Production medicine manages the health of the individual animal by paying attention to all factors influencing health in the production system. This section highlights the areas of emphasis necessary to achieve respiratory health in a production system.

■ Causal Factors in Swine Pneumonia

Barbara Straw, D.V.M., Ph.D.
Oliver Duran, D.V.M., Ph.D., M.R.C.V.S.

GENERAL EPIDEMIOLOGIC CONSIDERATIONS

Pneumonia in swine, especially the chronic forms, must be viewed as a complex. Most cases are caused by infectious agents, but they are strongly influenced by contributing factors. Clinical disease occurs when pigs exposed to a number of microorganisms experience stress and lowered resistance owing to the influence of environmental conditions, genetics, or management factors.

Infectious Agents

Numerous infectious agents can be involved in the pneumonia complex (Table 1). Some are highly pathogenic primary agents capable of causing extensive lung lesions and severe clinical signs. Many other primary pathogens produce only faint lesions without clinical significance. Other organisms are not capable of initiating disease but act as secondary invaders, intensifying damage caused by primary pathogens.

Spread of pneumonia between herds occurs most often through infectious contacts (primarily purchase of pigs and to a lesser extent, transport vehicles, birds, people, etc.) Airborne transmission over several kilometers has been demonstrated for porcine respiratory corona virus (PRCV), *Mycoplasma hyopneumoniae*, and pseudorabies. Aerosol exposure appears to occur for porcine respiratory and reproductive syndrome (PRRS) virus only when there is a dense pig population and a large number of pigs become infected simultaneously, as occurred in the initial outbreaks in Europe. Factors increasing the risk of airborne spread include large herd size, mechanical ventilation, proximity to other herds, direction and velocity of the prevailing winds, cloud cover, minimum turbulence, level topography, and relative humidity over 90%.

The infectious agents responsible for swine pneumonia are extremely common in the swine population. Various surveys have estimated the percentage of midwestern herds positive for *Actinobacillus pleuropneumoniae* as 70% to 80%; for *M. hyopneumoniae* over 90%; and for PRRS, 60% to 80%. Pathogens are found in both healthy and diseased lungs and so culture results must be interpreted in light of expected frequency of isolation. Table 2 gives the frequency of isolation of various lung pathogens from healthy and diseased lungs. *A. pleuropneumoniae* and *M. hyopneumoniae* are common at the herd level but are seldom isolated from healthy individuals. Their presence in the herd is usually associated with clinical, or more often subclinical, disease, particularly during the critical period in young pigs when passive immunity is replaced by active immunity. Although pneumonia organisms are widely distributed throughout herds, the presence of pneumonia agents in the herd is not well correlated with severity or extent of infection.

Interactions Between Infectious Agents

Clinically significant disease is seldom the result of infection with only one pathogen. More typically, several microorganisms are involved. Primary pathogens reduce local and sometimes also systemic defense mechanisms of the host, allowing secondary invaders to colonize the lung. Primary pathogens are usually viruses or mycoplasma, while secondary invaders are bacteria. For example, susceptibility to *A. pleuropneumoniae* is increased

---

Table 1
INFECTIOUS AGENTS ASSOCIATED WITH PNEUMONIA

Bacteria	Mycoplasma	Viruses	Parasites
Actinobacillus pleuropneumoniae *Actinobacillus suis* *Pasteurella multocida* *Salmonella cholerasuis* *Bordetella bronchiseptica* *Haemophilus parasuis* *Streptococcus suis* *Klebsiella pneumoniae* *Actinomyces pyogenes*	*Mycoplasma hyopneumoniae* *Mycoplasma hyorrhinis*	Porcine reproductive and respiratory syndrome virus Swine influenza virus Pseudorabies virus Porcine corona respiratory virus	*Ascaris suum* *Metastrongylus* spp.

---

following infection with *M. hyopneumoniae*, swine influenza, PRRS, or pseudorabies. A common scenario is for pigs to be infected with PRRS virus in the nursery followed by *M. hyopneumoniae* in the finishing phase.

Environment and Management

As more sensitive microbiologic and serologic methods were developed, it became obvious that differences between levels of pneumonia in different herds were not primarily due to type of organism present. Epidemiologic techniques subsequently revealed the major impact of environment and management on clinical disease. Therefore practical control of pneumonia is primarily based on modifying the environment and management when possible and using medication and vaccination when physical limitations prevent modification.

Farm Type and Degree of Integration

Farms producing all their own animals (closed) have less pneumonia than farms that purchase feeder pigs (open). Studies find the prevalence of pneumonia to be nearly twice as great in open vs. closed herds. Typically, farms that purchase feeder pigs buy from multiple sources, so pigs with differing microbiologic and immunologic backgrounds are mixed together. Pigs purchased from only one source do not have a substantially greater risk of pneumonia than the closed herd. Purchase of stock from sales barns confers the greatest risk of pleuropneumonia. Obviously, respiratory problems can be expected if pigs with low health status are introduced into a herd with better health.

However, it is also risky to introduce high-health-status animals into herds with lower health status. High-health animals, insufficiently protected by specific immunity, easily develop clinical disease. As a consequence there is a sudden rise in excretion of pathogens, and the established equilibrium between infection and immunity in the lower-health herd is unbalanced.

Pneumonia control is greatly simplified in farrow-to-feeder and feeder-to-finish herds compared with that in farrow-to-finish herds owing to the "pathogen generator" effect associated with growing pigs. In farrow-to-finish herds periodic transmission of airborne pathogens from growers to the breeding herd is inevitable. In herds with an inadequate separation between pigs of different age groups there remains a continuous transmission of microbials from older to younger pigs with a subsequent continuous replication of pathogens. Dissimilar environmental needs of different age groups may be a contributing factor.

The introduction of purchased replacement gilts has been linked with outbreaks of PRRS, probably due to the gilts having insufficient protective immunity after natural infection or by introducing the virus to a naive sow population or transmitting a new strain of the PRRS virus. A prolonged isolation (60 days) and effective acclimatization procedures for gilt replacements reduce the risk of flares of PRRS.

Movement of Pigs Through Facilities

Numerous studies have demonstrated the benefit of utilizing all-in, all-out movement of pigs into buildings compared with continuous addition and removal of animals. Prevalence of pneumonia in facilities with all-in, all-out flow is generally 20% to 25% less than in continuous-flow facilities.

Mixing and Sorting of Pigs

Frequently, when animals are moved from nursery to grower barn or grower barn to finishing barn, they are regrouped so that all animals in a pen are approximately the same size. Farms with all-in, all-out pig flow have less tendency to mix or regroup animals, but often at least a few animals are sorted out and moved back. By contrast, farms with continuous flow of animals are conspicuous for the amount of mixing and regrouping. Often pneumonia is the reason pigs fail to grow as rapidly as their contemporaries. Thus, when pigs are mixed, healthy younger animals under stress of establishing a new social order are placed in direct contact with older diseased pigs.

Herd Size and Space

Generally, the risk of contracting respiratory disease increases with increasing herd size. However, very large herds frequently

---

Table 2
RELATIVE FREQUENCY OF ISOLATION OF INFECTIOUS AGENTS FROM GROSSLY NORMAL AND PNEUMONIC SWINE LUNGS

Organism	Normal Lungs With Organism (%)	Pneumonic Lungs With Organism (%)	Relative Risk Ratio
P. multocida	6.8	30.9	4.5
M. hyopneumoniae	16.3	29.4	1.8
B. bronchiseptica	2.1	3.8	1.8
M. hyorrhinis	7.9	13.6	1.7
A. pleuropneumoniae	0.2	1.8	10.4
S. cholerasuis	0.2	1.0	5.9
Coliforms	8.8	7.9	0.9
Streptococcus	23.6	13.8	0.6
Staphylococcus	9.4	5.0	0.5

have a lower level of respiratory disease than medium-sized herds. This probably occurs because very large herd facilities are forced to subdivide and move pigs in groups, while for small and medium-sized herds it is not cost-effective to divide facilities for all-in, all-out production. Therefore the health status of medium-sized and small herds is often surpassed by that of large herds.

Barns that contain few pigs have less pneumonia than barns with many animals. While the ideal barn capacity in terms of pneumonia control is 150 to 300 animals, a facility of this size is uneconomical to construct. Isolated finishing facilities operated as all-in, all-out facilities with a high health status of pigs commonly accommodate up to 1000 pigs. The number of pigs housed in the same air space significantly affects the prevalence of pneumonia, even on farms with all-in, all-out production. Densely crowded pigs have higher levels of pneumonia than pigs that are allowed more space. Herds that crowd pigs beyond a recommended level of 0.7 m^2 per pig have increased levels of pneumonia.

Ventilation

Forced air ventilation is required in confinement buildings to remove excess moisture and waste gases. The smaller the air space allotted per pig, the higher the air exchange needed. While air exchange rates of greater than 60 m^3 hour per pig have been associated with reduced frequencies of pneumonia, it is not possible to offset an increase in stocking density with a proportional increase in ventilation rate. For example, if the stocking rate is doubled within a fixed air space, the ventilation rate would have to be increased by 10 times to maintain the same clearance of air contaminants. Ventilation systems often recirculate air, and this mixing of air contributes to the spread of respiratory pathogens in the barn. Pneumonia is less severe in buildings with negative-pressure ventilation where polluted air is removed and exchanged for fresh air.

Within confinement facilities the amount of air space per animal is significantly associated with the risk of pneumonia. Based on the amount of pneumonia observed at slaughter, an air space of at least 3 m^3 per pig in the growing-finishing period has been recommended. This amount of space is especially critical in continuous-flow facilities.

Lack of uniform air flow through a building is associated with increased levels of pneumonia. Pigs raised in buildings with solid pen dividers, which minimize draftiness, have less pneumonia than pigs raised in an open environment.

Temperature

Cold environmental temperatures reduce the young pig's ability to clear bacteria from its lungs. Cold uninsulated floors, which cause heat loss from the pig's body through conduction, are associated with higher levels of pneumonia. With low outside temperatures there is a reduction in the ventilation rate and often an increased stocking density on farms, which indirectly increases the incidence of respiratory disease. Fluctuations in temperature depress the pig's ability to mount an immune defense. Air temperature should not be allowed to vary by more than 3°C in 24 hours.

Ammonia

Ammonia in concentrations of 10 to 100 ppm interferes with respiratory tract function and predisposes the pig to infection. Prolonged exposure to 20 ppm ammonia causes excessive nasal, lacrimal, and oral secretions, increased coughing, and increased number of bacteria in the lung.

Waste Disposal System

Liquid manure handling and slatted floors are associated with higher levels of pneumonia. This is possibly due to a cold environment, drafts, and high ammonia concentration, which frequently accompany slatted flooring.

Dust

While aerial hog-house dust can induce acute or chronic malfunction of the respiratory tract in humans, there is little evidence to incriminate it as a major contributor to swine pneumonia. Several investigations have failed to demonstrate any significant relation between dust and respiratory disease in pigs.

Pneumonia-Associated Diseases

Pigs from herds in which diarrhea occurs either in unweaned or weaned pigs are at greater risk of developing pneumonia. Litters of pigs with rotavirus or transmissible gastroenteritis (TGE) have been shown to have higher rates of respiratory disease than virus-free litters. Outbreaks of pneumonia have been reported in which control could not be achieved until pigs were treated for mange.

Within-farm studies have generally failed to demonstrate an association between the presence of atrophic rhinitis and pneumonia, while between-farm studies have shown that herds with high levels of one disease tend also to have high levels of the other. Shared predisposing factors probably account for herd associations, but atrophic rhinitis does not predispose to pneumonia in individual animals.

Migration of *Ascaris suum* enhances the lesions of pneumonia in swine. Lung consolidation in mycoplasmal pneumonia may be increased 10 times if pigs undergo concomitant ascarid migration.

Age

The maximum prevalence of pneumonia has traditionally occurred in pigs between 16 and 19 weeks of age, which is probably related to loss of maternal immunity and elevated stocking density. Recently, onset of severe pneumonia in nursery pigs has been seen in herds infected with the PRRS virus. Sows carry a lower burden of pathogenic organisms and confer higher levels of maternal antibody via colostrum to the piglets as they become older.

Castration

Slaughter surveillance of market swine shows the prevalence of pneumonia and pleuritis in castrated males to be 10% higher than in females.

Nutrition

Feed or water restriction and low protein content of the diet exacerbate the severity of pneumonia in swine.

Heredity

Respiratory disorders are to some extent influenced by heredity. Antibody production and phagocytic functions of pulmonary alveolar macrophages differ among breeds. Yorkshire pigs have higher levels of pneumonia than Hampshire, Landrace, or Duroc pigs.

DIAGNOSIS OF RESPIRATORY DISEASE

The definitive diagnosis of respiratory disease is based on a combination of history, clinical observation, laboratory tests, necropsy, and slaughter checks. A clinical diagnosis can only be tentative, as respiratory distress may result from dysfunction of other organs. Also, certain disorders of the respiratory system may be without clinical signs or signs typical of respiratory disorders. Often acute pleuropneumonia may be widespread in a herd before the disease is discovered. Clinical signs of "lazy pigs" and decreased appetite in fatteners should trigger investigation of possible causes of pneumonia. Table 3 lists various differentiating features of cough, and dyspnea in swine.

MONITORING PNEUMONIA

Pneumonia levels are monitored to provide feedback for use in determining the appropriateness and efficacy of specific intervention. Action is taken to reduce economic loss or maintain the health status of seed stock. Pneumonia has been estimated to reduce average daily gain by 37 g for every 10% of the lung with lesions (Straw and colleagues, 1990).

Monitoring pneumonia entails collecting data from clinical and production records, laboratory tests, and slaughter examinations.

Examinations in the Herd

Clinical observations include the amount of coughing or dyspnea and unevenness in size. Postmortem examinations of dead or euthanized animals are used to determine the character of lesions and for isolation of infectious agents. Records are reviewed for feed consumption, growth rate, number of treatments, and accumulated mortality. Weight or age of dead pigs should be noted.

Laboratory Tests

Tremendous progress in biotechnology has accelerated the development of new, highly specific laboratory tests for pneumonia. To determine the presence of a pathogen in the herd, typically sera from 30 animals provide 95% confidence in detecting a 5% prevalence of infected animals. Another common use of serology is to sample 10 animals from each age group, for example, growing pigs at 2- to 3-week intervals, to determine the level and duration of maternal immunity and the development of active immunity.

Examinations of Slaughter Swine

Slaughter checks are used to determine the extent and character (reflection of cause) of pneumonia. Commonly used measures include prevalence and severity of lesions such as consoli-

dation, pneumonic abscesses, and pleuritis. Recent infections show up as darker, firm areas of the lung; fissures in lung tissue represent earlier resolved lesions. Details of various examination techniques are described elsewhere (Straw and others, 1986).

Interpretation of slaughter findings are made in light of the dynamic nature of infection and seasonal influences. Acute infection resolves in 6 to 8 weeks, so lesions at slaughter reflect only the last part of the finishing period. Fissures in lung tissue indicate earlier infection. Pneumonia is most prevalent and severe in pigs slaughtered in the spring and fall and is mildest in the summer.

CONTROL AND PREVENTION

Pathogenic microorganisms are involved in all respiratory disorders of importance. While it is possible to eliminate certain organisms from the herd, in practice it is impossible to protect pigs from every pathogenic microorganism, and the development of respiratory disease fundamentally depends on the balance between pressure from pathogenic microorganisms and the pig's ability to resist them. This equilibrium is very fragile and greatly affected by the above-mentioned factors. Therefore control of pneumonia at the herd level is based on two principles: (1) elimination of certain pathogens and (2) strengthening the herd's defense mechanisms and diminishing the infection pressure in the herd.

Elimination of Pathogens

Freedom from certain pathogens (M. hyopneumoniae, A. pleuropneumoniae, the PRRS virus, pseudorabies virus) greatly simplifies pneumonia control. This can be accomplished for the above-named organisms because the agents can be definitively identified, transmission routes can be effectively blocked, and sufficient diagnostic capability is available. The process of elimination and maintenance of pathogen-free status require an extremely motivated owner.

Minimal Disease ("High Health") Herds

Freedom from M. hyopneumoniae and A. pleuropneumoniae has been achieved in herds composed of hysterectomy-derived pigs and their offspring, raised on site or at other isolated farms. The usual contributing factors (crowding; lack of age separation; infection with influenza, PRRS, or pseudorabies; enteric disorders; etc.) are tolerated to a greater extent in minimal disease herds than in conventional herds infected with these two organisms.

Segregated Early Weaning

M. hyopneumoniae, A. pleuropneumoniae, and pseudorabies may be eliminated from the growing-finishing section by weaning piglets before 10 days of age and raising them in a facility far removed from the sow herd. This technique is less effective in eliminating the PRRS virus.

Culling Techniques

Heavy medication in conjunction with repeated serologic testing and removal of positive sows has been used to eradicate A. pleuropneumoniae from smaller herds with a low initial prevalence of infection.

Table 3
CHARACTERISTICS OF DISEASES THAT CAUSE COUGH AND DYSPNEA IN PIGS

Clinical Signs	Associated Agents	Necropsy Findings	Diagnosis
Signs primarily referable to the respiratory tract: dyspnea, cough, anorexia, fever, abdominal respiration, varying severities of clinical signs in a group of pigs	*A. pleuropneumoniae* *M. hyopneumoniae* *A. suis* *M. hyorrhinis* *P. multocida* *S. cholerasuis* *B. bronchiseptica* *H. parasuis* *Streptococcus suis* *Klebsiella pneumoniae* *Actinomyces pyogenes* PRRS virus Swine influenza virus Pseudorabies virus	Usually cranioventral distribution of lesions; firm areas of tissue with variable intralobular edema; fibrinous pleuritis suggests involvement with *A. pleuropneumoniae, H. parasuis, P. multocida, M. hyorrhinis,* or *S. cholerasuis*	Culture of organism; fluorescent antibody (FA) test for mycoplasma; serology or FA for pseudorabies; virus isolation, serology, or immunoperoxidase monolayer assay, immunohistochemistry for PRRS virus
Dyspnea, fever, anorexia, possible cyanotic extremities	PRRS virus	Enlarged tan lymph nodes; edema and extensive interstitial pneumonia	Virus isolation, serology, or immunoperoxidase monolayer assay, immunohistochemistry
Rapid clinical course, high fever, anorexia, depression, severe dyspnea, open-mouth breathing, cyanosis, foamy blood-tinged discharge from nose and mouth	*A. pleuropneumoniae*	Acute hemorrhagic necrosis distributed throughout the lungs, especially dorsally in the diaphragmatic lobes; fibrinous pleurisy; some blood-tinged fluid in the pleural cavity; bloody foam in the trachea	Isolation of organism; serology, pathology
Coughing with minimal other signs	*A. suum*	Areas of atelectasis, hemorrhage, edema, and emphysema in lung; septal and periseptal hemorrhage and necrosis in liver	Fecal examination for eggs (may be negative early); typical necropsy findings; history of access to soil (absolute requirement for *Metastrongylus*)
	Metastrongylus spp.	Bronchitis, bronchiolitis in caudoventral margins of diaphragmatic lobes; areas of atelectasis	
Dyspnea, abdominal respiration, cyanosis, no coughing	Diaphragmatic hernia (possibly related to selenium deficiency, genetics, or trauma)	Tear in diaphragm; abdominal organs in chest	Necropsy
No coughing, but dyspnea and cyanosis, depression, fever, anorexia, reluctance to move, lameness, stiff gait, swollen joints, ataxia, convulsions	*H. parasuis* *M. hyorrhinis* *S. suis*	Fibrinous to serofibrinous pleuritis; pericarditis, arthritis, meningitis	Isolation of organism
Very acute onset, near 100% morbidity, extreme prostration, complete anorexia, labored jerky respiration, hard paroxysmal cough, fever	Swine influenza	Often there is no opportunity to do a necropsy since death due to uncomplicated swine influenza is rare; tenacious mucus in pharynx, larynx, trachea, and bronchi; depressed deep-purple areas in lung	Physical examination, serology; virus isolation from pharyngeal swab
Labored respiration, minor cough	*Eubacterium moniliforme* toxicity	Pulmonary edema and hydrothorax	Necropsy, mycotoxin analysis on feed
Rapid or abdominal respiration, moist nonproductive cough if present, pale mucous membranes	Anemia	Pale musculature, lung edema, dilated heart, excess pericardial fluid, contracted spleen	Packed cell volume 15%–20%; hemoglobin concentration 6–7 g/dL
Rapid, panting respiration, no cough, open-mouth breathing, gasping, high temperature	Porcine stress syndrome; heat prostration; puffer sow syndrome	Areas of pale, soft, or exudative muscle; edema and congestion of lungs; rapid autolysis	Creatine kinase, DNA analysis, physical examination

Long-Term Control Measures

Long-term control of pneumonia often requires more radical and expensive changes in production systems and housing. Long-term strategies should incorporate as many control options as possible. Table 4 lists factors that predispose to pneumonia and their relative importance.

Practical application of disease control principles does not necessarily require expensive construction. Large finishing barns may be partitioned into rooms using sheets of heavy plastic to create walls. Pressure-treated plywood is placed below the floor, extending into the liquid surface of the pit to totally separate ventilation between sections. Barn sections should be designed to hold the number of animals that are introduced (weaned) in a 2-week or, ideally, 1-week period, and then operated on an all-in, all-out basis.

Ventilation and housing should be carefully assessed and deficiencies corrected. Often this requires adding additional insulation, placing solid partitions between pens, and supplying the correct amount of air exchange while maintaining incoming air flow at 600 ft/minute.

Table 4
FACTORS PREDISPOSING HERDS TO PNEUMONIA

Factor	Effect
Production system	
Large herd size	+ + +
High stocking density	+ + +
Conventional health system (not minimal disease production system)	+ + +
Introduction of animals from herds with unknown/low health status	+ + +
Continuous flow of animals through facilities	+ + +
Low average age of sows	+ + +
Average age of piglets at weaning	
Very low	+ +
Medium	+
High	+ +
Housing	
Badly insulated and ventilated facilities (cold or fluctuating temperature, inadequate air exchange, drafts)	+ + +
Poor division of facilities combined with housing of differently aged animals in same air space	+ + +
Pen dividers without solid separations	+ + +
Large grower-finisher apartments (containing > 200–300 pigs)	+ +
Nutrition	
Caloric intake insufficient	+
Improper content of macro- or microelements in feed	+
Presence of Nonrespiratory Pathogens	
Colibacillosis	+ +
Dysentery	+ +
Mange	+
Ascarids	+
Management	
Poor control of climate	+ + +
Poor monitoring of signs of disease	+ +
Lack of or incorrect treatment	+ +
Lack of or incorrect preventive measures (vaccinations, strategic medications)	+ +
Poor care of sick animals (isolation, handling)	+
Poor hygiene	+ +

+, slight effect; + +, moderate effect; + + +, marked effect.
Adapted from Christensen G, Mousing J: Respiratory system. In Leman AD, et al (eds): Diseases of Swine, ed 7. Ames, Iowa, Iowa State University Press, 1992.

Short-Term Measures

Short-term measures against pneumonia include strategic medication procedures, vaccination, immediate treatment of sick animals, climate modification, and isolation or dispersion arrangements.

Medication

Successful control of pneumonia outbreaks requires immediate medication of diseased individuals and penmates. Pigs showing clinical signs should be treated for 2 to 3 days by injection with penicillin, long-acting tetracycline, or ceftiofur, since their consumption of water and feed is significantly reduced. Pigs in contact with diseased pigs should be administered with chlortetracycline, tiamulin, or sulfamethazine in their water or chlortetracycline or tiamulin in their feed for 4 to 7 days. Antibiotic withdrawal periods need to be observed and products containing sulfonamides should be avoided in finishing pigs.

Strategic medication is useful when outbreaks can be anticipated. Common times for the development of clinical pneumonia include about 1 week after pigs are moved to the grower-finisher unit, and at about 50 to 75 kg when passive immunity to *A. pleuropneumoniae* is lost. Feed (tilmicosin, tiamulin or chlortetracycline) or water (chlortetracycline, tiamulin, or sulfamethazine) medication should be given for 4 to 7 days just prior to the time when signs of disease are expected. Medication is designed to prevent the severe consequences of infection, but still allow pigs to receive sufficient exposure to the current infections to develop immunity. Totally preventing exposure through administration of therapeutic levels of antibacterials for a prolonged period only delays the outbreak.

Evaluation of the economics of medication for the control and treatment of pneumonia need to be considered to avoid excessive costs to the producer and to assess the longer-term savings that could be achieved by instituting improvements in facilities and changes in pig transit.

Vaccination

Vaccines against pseudorabies are generally efficacious, as are *M. hyopneumoniae* vaccines when used in PRRS-positive herds. Existing vaccines against *A. pleuropneumoniae*, *H. parasuis*, PRRS, and swine influenza have only limited value.

Dispersion and Partial Depopulation

During an outbreak of pneumonia, new cases can be avoided by dispersing pigs over a large area. If weather conditions permit, pigs may be moved to an outside lot. Dispersion is more common in chronic pneumonia when one room or building is emptied and allowed to remain vacant for several weeks before being restocked with pigs.

Climate Modification

Obvious deficiencies in environment should be corrected. Hovers or plastic partitions can be erected to reduce drafts. Sources of dampness should be removed. Provision of straw bedding raises the effective environmental temperature. Air exchange should not be compromised to increase air temperature.

BIBLIOGRAPHY

Alexander TJL, Harris DL: Methods of disease control. *In* Leman AD, Straw BE, Mengeling WL (eds): Diseases of Swine, ed 7. Ames, Iowa State University Press, 1992.

Christensen G, Mousing J: Respiratory system. *In* Leman AD, Straw BE, Mengeling WL (eds). Diseases of Swine, ed 7. Ames, Iowa State University Press, 1992.

Straw BE: Controlling pneumonia in swine herds. Vet Med, Jan 1992, pp 78–86.

Straw BE, Backstrom L, Leman AD: Evaluation of swine at slaughter. Part I—Sample size, mechanics of examination, scoring systems and seasonal effects. Compendium Continuing Educ Pract Vet 8:541, 1986.

Straw BE, Shin SJ, Yeager AE: Effect of pneumonia on growth rate and feed efficiency of minimal disase pigs exposed to *Actinobacillus pleuropneumoniae* and *M. hyopneumoniae*. Prev Vet Med 9:287–294, 1990.

■ Ovine and Caprine Respiratory Disease: Infectious Agents, Management Factors, and Preventive Strategies

Sherrill Fleming, D.V.M., Diplomate, A.C.V.I.M., A.B.V.P. (Food Animal)

In 1994, respiratory diseases in lambs and breeding sheep were the third highest category of death losses, behind lambing losses and digestive disorders.[1] These death losses represented 0.64% of the national sheep inventory (approximately 61,000 lamb and 39,000 breeding sheep deaths). Pneumonia losses in lambs were highest in the North Central States. Despite documented losses, the 1996 Sheep Health and Productivity Needs Assessment survey did not identify respiratory disease as a high or moderate concern of producers.[2]

A variety of infectious agents, alone or in combination, have been identified from cases of sheep respiratory disease (Table 1) and goat respiratory disease (Table 2).[3, 4] Many of these agents can be isolated from the nasal passages, pharynx, and tonsillar areas of normal, adult sheep. Individually, these agents cause mild respiratory disease when inoculated into susceptible animals. More severe respiratory disease occurs when a combination of agents is sequentially introduced to naive animals.[5]

Parainfluenza 3 virus, adenoviruses, and respiratory syncytial virus are frequently isolated from sheep and goats.[5–10] However, the inoculation of these viruses into susceptible animals usually results in mild catarrhal inflammation of the upper respiratory tract or subclinical respiratory disease. Seroconversion occurs in most animals, and antibodies in the general population are widespread. Introducing *Pasteurella hemolytica* several days after viral exposure results in more severe clinical disease and possible mortality.[5, 11, 12] *P. hemolytica* is often the bacteria isolated from "quick" pneumonia which causes sudden death with few premonitory signs in neonatal lambs. *Mycoplasma* spp. are reported from respiratory outbreaks and chronic pneumonia problems, particularly in areas which confine sheep and goats during winter months.[13–16] Catastrophic outbreaks of *Mycoplasma mycoides* subsp. *mycoides* have been reported in goats, associated with mastitis, arthritis, pneumonia, pleuritis, and abortion.[17]

Retroviral infections are slow viral diseases which can involve the respiratory tract and are of major importance to the economics of sheep and goat production.[18] Ovine progressive pneumonia (OPP) and caprine arthritis and encephalitis (CAE) viruses affect sheep and goats (see Chapter 80) respectively. These diseases limit the productive life of sheep and goats, as well as

decrease the milk production and weaning weights of offspring.[19] The presence of retroviral infection predisposes to chronic bacterial pneumonia.[20] Producers that attempt to control these diseases have a significant investment in testing and culling of infected animals.

Caseous lymphadenitis caused by *Corynebacterium pseudotuberculosis* is another chronic infection which may involve the respiratory tract with abscess formation in the lungs or mediastinal or retropharyngeal lymph nodes. This disease is a major concern of producers, particularly meat goat producers. High rates of condemnation and carcass trimming are caused by the presence of abscesses in internal organs and peripheral lymph nodes. The respiratory tract is an important reservoir for spreading the bacteria to other animals. Abscessation of lungs affects individual production.[21] Both chronic retroviral pneumonia and caseous lymphadenitis represent a drain on the individual animal's resources which makes it more susceptible to other respiratory diseases.

DIAGNOSIS OF RESPIRATORY DISEASE

Physical examination of affected animals should include observation of attitude and appetite. Depression, listlessness, separation from the flock, and decreased to absent appetite are common presentations. The rectal temperature (normal 101.5 to 103.5°F) and respiratory rate are usually elevated. Elevated respiratory rates in sheep and goats can also be caused by handling and high environmental temperature. Auscultation of the lung fields demonstrates an increase in breath sounds and if

Table 1

SUMMARY OF INFECTIOUS CAUSES OF SHEEP RESPIRATORY DISEASES BY CLINICAL SIGNS

Coughing	Serous Nasal Discharge	Mucopurulent Nasal Discharge
Pasteurella spp.*	*Pasteurella* spp.*	*Pasteurella* spp.*
Lungworm infection/ verminous pneumonia	Lungworm infection/ verminous pneumonia	Lungworm infection/ verminous pneumonia
Mycoplasma spp.*	*Mycoplasma* spp.*	*Mycoplasma* spp.*
Ovine progressive pneumonia	Ovine progressive pneumonia	Ovine progressive pneumonia
Ovine adenovirus*	Ovine adenovirus*	—
Reovirus type 3	Reovirus type 3	—
Chlamydia spp.	*Chlamydia* spp.	
Pulmonary adenomatosis, jaagsiekte	Pulmonary adenomatosis, jaagsiekte	Pulmonary adenomatosis, jaagsiekte
—	*Oestrus ovis*, nose bots*	*Oestrus ovis*, nose bots*
—	Early bacterial pneumonia*	Chronic bacterial pneumonia*
—	Bluetongue	Bluetongue
—	Border disease, hairy shaker	
—	—	Postviral bacterial infection of respiratory tract*
—	—	Abscesses/caseous lymphadenitis*
—	—	Ovine nasal granuloma

*Common.

Table 2
SUMMARY OF INFECTIOUS CAUSES OF GOAT RESPIRATORY DISEASES BY CLINICAL SIGNS

Coughing	Serous Nasal Discharge	Mucopurulent Nasal Discharge
Pasteurella spp.*	Pasteurella spp.*	Pasteurella spp.*
Lungworm infection/ verminous pneumonia	Lungworm infection/ verminous pneumonia	Lungworm infection/ verminous pneumonia
Mycoplasma spp.*	Mycoplasma spp.*	Mycoplasma spp.*
Mycoplasma mycoides subsp. mycoides	Mycoplasma mycoides subsp. mycoides	Mycoplasma mycoides subsp. mycoides
Caprine arthritis and encephalitis virus	Caprine arthritis and encephalitis virus	Caprine arthritis and encephalitis virus
Respiratory syncytial virus	Respiratory syncytial virus	—
Caprine herpesvirus	Caprine herpesvirus	Caprine herpesvirus
Chlamydia spp.	Chlamydia spp.	—
Pulmonary adenomatosis, jaagsiekte	Pulmonary adenomatosis, jaagsiekte	Pulmonary adenomatosis, jaagsiekte
—	Oestrus ovis, nose bots*	Oestrus ovis, nose bots*
—	Early bacterial pneumonia*	Chronic bacterial pneumonia*
—	—	Postviral bacterial infection of respiratory tract*
Abscesses/caseous lymphadenitis*	—	Abscesses/caseous lymphadenitis*

*Common.

secondary bacterial infections are present, squeaks and wheezes may be audible in the peripheral lung fields. Radiographs of the thorax may be helpful in assessing the degree of consolidation present and the prognosis. Radiographs can also be diagnostic of abscesses in the lungs. Transtracheal washes for viral or bacterial isolation and cytology may be attempted if the animal is not dyspneic and overly stressed. In the event of a flock outbreak of disease, one or two representative cases should be selected for euthanasia and necropsy. Collection of a serum sample from affected animals on initial presentation for follow-up serology is a wise precaution. Producers should be encouraged to submit, as promptly as possible, animals that die for necropsy examination.

TREATMENT

Few antimicrobials are labeled for use in small ruminants, and veterinarians must rely on extralabel uses. Viral diseases on their own usually do not require treatment other than nursing care (provision of shade, shelter, fresh water, and palatable feed within easy reach). Prophylactic antibiotics are often administered during viral outbreaks in an attempt to prevent secondary bacterial infections.[22] There are a variety of antibiotics which are routinely used, including procaine penicillin G, amoxicillin, ampicillin, oxytetracycline, ceftiofur, tylosin, erythromycin, and tilmicosin (sheep only).[23] *Tilmicosin should not be used in goats,* as a high percentage of goats may have an adverse reaction which results in acute death. Florfenicol is a relatively new antibiotic that is not labeled for use in small ruminants but may be useful in some instances. Oxytetracycline and tylosin are often chosen because of their efficacy against chlamydial and mycoplasmal agents. Care must be taken to recommend appropriate withdrawal periods for slaughter in small ruminants that are treated

with extralabel antibiotics. Supportive therapy includes the use of nonsteroidal anti-inflammatory drugs. Flunixin meglumine and ketoprofen in the acute stages can be useful in combating the toxic effects of bacterial pneumonia and making animals more comfortable. Monitoring of temperature, pulse, respiration, appetite, and attitude during therapy is important. Treatment with antibiotics should continue for at least 48 hours after the animal returns to normal.

MANAGEMENT OF RESPIRATORY DISEASE

During an acute outbreak within a flock or group of small ruminants, isolation of affected individuals should be attempted. Rectal temperatures of all in-contact sheep or goats can be used to identify those animals that are in the early stages of infection. The ability to do this will depend on the facilities of the producer and the number of animals involved. In flocks that have tendencies for annual respiratory outbreaks, inclusion of chlortetracycline in the feed prior to problem time periods has been successful in reducing morbidity and mortality in many herds. The immediate postweaning period seems to be when most respiratory problems are seen in sheep.

Producers are often anxious to attempt vaccination programs if they have had repeated problems with respiratory disease. Currently there are no licensed vaccines for commonly encountered pathogens in ovine or caprine respiratory disease.[24] The use of modified live intranasal parainfluenza 3 vaccines, which also include infectious bovine rhinotracheitis (IBR), virus, have been popular among producers.[25] Cattle *Pasteurella* vaccines have been used in sheep but there are questions about their ability to cross-protect against different serotypes. Other than anecdotal testimonials, there is little documentation that these products are effective in reducing morbidity and mortality from respiratory disease. The ability to produce ovine adenoviral vaccines is available but has not been attempted by vaccine companies because of limited markets.[26] Several commercial vaccines for caseous lymphadenitis have been produced.[27, 28] Currently, Colorado Serum Company, Denver, markets a vaccine for use in sheep which is reasonably effective. There have been reports of adverse reactions in goats that have received this vaccine.[29]

RISK FACTORS

Respiratory disease in ruminants is a multifactorial process that is affected by the interplay of individual animals, flock, infectious agents, and environmental conditions. The immunity of the individual to infectious agents is determined by previous exposure or passive immunity, nutritional status, vitamin and mineral deficiencies, environmental stressors, level of exposure, and possibly genetic factors. Younger animals are at higher risk as they are initially dependent on colostral immunity and have had limited opportunities to develop immunity. Young animals are also limited in their resources to withstand extremes in environmental conditions.

There are a wide range of environmental conditions across the United States resulting in major regional differences in farm management. In the Northeast, sheep are in smaller flocks, with more confinement and more dependence on stored feeds. Confinement during cold weather may result in decreased ventilation and increased humidity and ammonia levels, which predispose to respiratory disease. The Southeast is greatly dependent on grazing, and provides minimal housing. Flock size is small and gastrointestinal parasitism is a major problem. Hot, humid conditions are experienced during the summer, which results in animals crowding into shaded areas. The mountainous areas have very large flocks that must be grazed in extensive pastures high on the mountains during the summer and moved to more sheltered areas during the winter. Housing is virtually nonexistent for these large flocks. However, inclement weather can result in severe stress of lambs and adults. Lamb feedlots are located in the western part of the country and often have difficulty with dry and dusty environments. Grain supplements in all types of production tend to contain cracked or ground grain which can be very dusty unless pelletized or dried molasses is added.

Times of particular stress for sheep and goats are at lambing or kidding, weaning, processing (castration, shearing, etc.), prolonged transportation or moving between ranges, overcrowding, and extremely hot, cold, wet, or humid weather. Provision of shade and fans during hot and humid weather, windbreaks, or open-sided sheds during cold weather can help decrease the adverse effects of the weather. Adequate ventilation and protection from drafts during winter housing is crucial. Limiting the time that groups are held in overcrowded conditions is accomplished by planning in advance. Attention to proper nutrition and consideration of prophylactic antibiotic treatment (chlortetracycline in feed) will help to minimize the incidence of respiratory disease under adverse conditions.

Biosecurity is a subject which does not appear to be well-known by many producers. The axiom "buyer beware" is commonly encountered when purchases of breeding animals are made. Producers should be aware of diseases that can be introduced into their flocks by purchased additions. Testing programs for CAE and OPP are relatively common so that seronegative sheep and goats can be purchased. There are serology tests for caseous lymphadenitis, but they may be difficult to interpret depending on the vaccination history of individuals.[30, 31] Johne's disease and the purchase of animals carrying anthelmintic-resistant nematodes are also potential dangers. Outbreaks of sore mouth or orf and upper respiratory disease are common sequelae after commingling purchased additions to a farm. A receiving protocol should be instituted on farms for any new arrivals and for reintroducing individuals that have participated in shows. These protocols should include an isolation area that has no contact with sheep or goats on the farm. Inspection for presence of footrot and external abscesses should be made before arrival on the farm. Deworming on arrival, with follow-up fecal examinations a week following deworming, should be performed.[32] After 30 days on the farm with no observed disease, several sentinel sheep or goats from the farm may be introduced to the purchased group. If no illnesses are noted in either group after 2 weeks, the flock additions may be commingled with the main flock.

REFERENCES

1. Sheep—1994 Death losses due to health-related problems. Fort Collins, Colo., Centers for Epidemiology and Animal Health, January 1996.
2. 1996 Sheep Health and Productivity Needs Assessment. Fort Collins, Colo., Centers for Epidemiology and Animal Health, 1996.
3. Wilson WD, Lofstedt J: Alterations in respiratory function. *In* Smith BP (ed): Large Animal Internal Medicine, ed 2. St. Louis, Mosby–Year Book, 1996, pp 46–64.
4. Smith MC, Sherman, DM. Goat Medicine. Philadelphia, Lea & Febiger, 1994, pp 247–274.
5. Lehmkuhl HD, Contreras JA, Cutlip RC, et al: Clinical and microbiologic findings in lambs inoculated with *Pasteurella haemolytica* after infection with ovine adenovirus type 6. Am J Vet Res 50:671, 1989.
6. Lamontagne L, Descoteaux JP, Roy R: Epizootiological survey of parainfluenza-3, reovirus-3, respiratory syncytial and infectious bovine rhinotracheitis viral antibodies in sheep and goat flocks in Quebec. Can J Comp Med 49:424, 1985.
7. Lemkuhl HD, Cutlip RC, Brogden KA: Seroepidemiologic survey for adenovirus infection in lambs. Am J Vet Res 54:1277, 1993.
8. LeaMaster BR, Evermann JF, Lehmkuhl HD: Identification of ovine adenovirus types five and six in an epizootic of respiratory tract disease in recently weaned lambs. J Am Vet Med Assoc 190:1545, 1987.
9. Pommer J, Schamber G: Isolation of adenovirus from lambs with upper respiratory syndrome. J Vet Diagn Invest 3:204, 1991.
10. Whetstone CA, Evermann JF: Characterization of bovine herpesviruses isolated from six sheep and four goats by restriction endonuclease analysis and radioimmunoprecipitation. Am J Vet Res 49:781, 1988.
11. Trigo FJ, Breeze RG, Liggitt HD, et al: Interaction of bovine respiratory syncytial virus and *Pasteurella haemolytica* in the ovine lung. Am J Vet Res 45:1671, 1984.
12. Davies DH, Long DL, McCarthy AR et al: The effect of parainfluenza virus type 3 on the phagocytic cell response of the ovine lung to *Pasteurella haemolytica*. Vet Microbiol 11:125, 1985.
13. Brogden KA, Rose D, Cutlip RC, et al: Isolation and identification of mycoplasmas from the nasal cavity of sheep. Am J Vet Res 49:1669, 1988.
14. Jones GE, Gilmour JS, Rae AG: Investigations into the possible role of *Mycoplasma arginini* in ovine respiratory disease. Res Vet Sci 38:368, 1985.
15. Bölske G, Msami H, Humlesjö NE, et al: Mycoplasma capricolum in an outbreak of polyarthritis and pneumonia in goats. Acta Vet Scand 29:331, 1988.
16. Brandâo E. Isolation and identification of *Mycoplasma mycoides* subspecies *mycoides* SC strains in sheep and goats. Vet Rec 136:98, 1995.
17. DaMassa AJ, Brooks DL, Holmberg CA, et al: Caprine mycoplasmosis: An outbreak of mastitis and arthritis requiring the destruction of 700 goats. Vet Rec 120:409, 1987.
18. Madewell BR, Gill DB, Evermann JF: Seroprevalence of ovine progressive pneumonia virus and other selected pathogens in California cull sheep. Prev Vet Med 10:31, 1990.
19. Pekelder JJ, Veenink GJ, Akkermans JPWM, et al: Ovine lentivirus induced indurative lymphocytic mastitis and its effect on the growth of lambs. Vet Rec 134:348, 1994.
20. Myer MS, Huchzermeyer HFAK, York DF, et al: The possible involvement of immunosuppression caused by a lentivirus in the aetiology of jaagsiekte and pasteurellosis in sheep. Onderstepoort J Vet Res 55:127, 1988.
21. Paton MW, Rose IR, Hart RA, et al: New infection with *Corynebacterium pseudotuberculosis* reduces wool production. Aust Vet J 71:47, 1994.
22. Appleyard WT, Gilmour NJL: Use of long-acting oxytetracycline against pasteurellosis in lambs. Vet Rec 126:231, 1990.
23. Diker KS, Akan M, Haziroglu R: Antimicrobial susceptibility of *Pasteurella haemolytica* and *Pasteurella multocida* isolated from pneumonic ovine lungs. Vet Rec 134:597, 1994.
24. Council Report: Vaccination guidelines for small ruminants (sheep, goats, llamas, domestic deer, and wapiti). J Am Vet Med Assoc 205:1539, 1994.
25. Salsbury DL: Assessing the effectiveness of bovine respiratory vaccines for treating sheep with rhinitis. Vet Med 79:1520, 1984.
26. Lehmkuhl HD. Personal communication, 1996.
27. Eggleton DG, Middleton HD, Doidge CV, et al: Immunization against ovine caseous lymphadenitis: Comparison of *Corynebacterium pseudotuberculosis* vaccines with and without bacterial cells. Aust Vet J 68:317, 1991.
28. Menzies PI, Muckle CA, Brogden KA, et al: A field trial to evaluate a whole cell vaccine for the prevention of caseous lymphadenitis in sheep and goat flocks. Can J Vet Res 55:362, 1991.
29. Bretzlaff KN. Personal communications, 1996.
30. Menzies PI, Muckle CA, Hwang YT, et al: Evaluation of an enzyme-linked immunosorbent assay using an *Escherichia coli* recombinant phospholipase D antigen for the diagnosis of *Corynebacterium pseudotuberculosis* infection. Small Ruminant Res 13:193, 1994.
31. ter Laak EA, Bosch J, Bijl GC, et al: Double-antibody sandwich enzyme-linked immunosorbent assay and immunoblot analysis used for control of caseous lymphadenitis in goats and sheep. Am J Vet Res 53:1125, 1992.
32. Herd R: Slowing the spread of anthelmintic resistant worms of sheep. Shepherd 16(4):28, 1995.

■ Bovine Respiratory Disease

Louis J. Perino, D.V.M., Ph.D.
Mike Apley, D.V.M., Ph.D., Diplomate,
A.C.V.C.P.

DISEASES OF THE UPPER RESPIRATORY TRACT

Rhinitis

Excessive nasal discharge, rubbing, sneezing or snorting, and erythema of the nares are clinical signs of rhinitis. Causes include fungal infections, viral infections, and environmental irritants. The irritants may include allergens ("summer snuffles"), exhaust fumes during shipment, feedlot dust, or inadequate ventilation in buildings with manure pits. Viral causes such as infectious bovine rhinotracheitis virus (IBRV) are discussed later.

Sinusitis

A common cause of sinusitis in cattle is postdehorning infection. The diagnosis is usually obvious as a result of the clinical history combined with drainage. Indication of bone involvement suggests *Actinomyces* infection and an associated poor prognosis along with a requirement for extended antimicrobial therapy.

A chronic sinusitis resulting from dehorning or ascension from an infectious rhinitis may require trephining a dependent region of the affected sinus. The physical examination should include examination of the oral cavity for teeth-related causes.

Conditions of the Larynx and Pharynx

Traumatic pharyngitis should be suspected in cases of pharyngeal trauma in cattle that have been treated with oral instruments. Balling guns, used to administer boluses, and stomach tubes can cause extensive damage to soft tissues and laryngeal cartilage when excessive force is used. This condition is one of many good reasons to completely remove the tongue and upper respiratory tract during every necropsy to monitor for these lesions. Crew medication technique may need to be continuously monitored.

Necrotic laryngitis, resulting from, at least in part, *Fusobacterium necrophorum*, may occur in neonates through cattle in the feedyard. This pathogen can invade areas of ulcer formation on the laryngeal cartilage of heavy feeder cattle. The clinical presentation often involves inspiratory stridor, extension of the head during breathing, and open-mouth breathing in severe cases. It is noteworthy that cattle are quick to breath through their mouth if the obstruction or air exchange problem is at the level of the larynx or lower in the respiratory tract, yet cattle must be almost totally unable to pass air through the nasal passages before resorting to mouth breathing. Suspected necrotic laryngitis requires ruling out traumatic laryngitis, tumors, abscesses, and laryngeal edema. Some of these conditions warrant early slaughter of animals that do not have significantly elevated rectal temperatures rather than attempting therapy. Widely differing epidemiologic patterns of necrotic laryngitis can occur, probably because of differences in the particular predisposing factors or differences in the susceptibility of the animal population to the specific predisposing factors. Occurrence is often sporadic, but clustered, high-morbidity outbreaks occur.[1] In high-morbidity pens, the actual morbidity may be considerably greater than clinical morbidity would indicate. One report suggests that animals with lesions have lower slaughter weights.[1]

Tracheal Edema

The honker syndrome in the feedlot occurs when the dorsal membrane of the trachea swells to partially obstruct the lumen. Various infectious causes have been proposed, as well as environmental irritation combined with a heavy animal trying to keep cool in hot weather. A characteristic "goose honk" accompanied by open-mouth, extended-head dyspnea in heavy, overheated cattle indicates the need for immediate anti-inflammatory therapy with minimal agitation of the animal.

DISEASES OF THE LOWER RESPIRATORY TRACT

Interstitial Pneumonia

The primary interstitial pneumonia of feedlot cattle is atypical interstitial pneumonia (AIP), which is often accompanied by edema and emphysema. Affected cattle are usually found in varying stages of acute respiratory distress. Rapid incubation of this syndrome (18 to 24 hours) is suggested by cases being detected within several hours of the pen being examined for diseased cattle. Attempts to reproduce this syndrome with bovine respiratory syncytial virus (BRSV) have been unsuccessful. It is not uncommon to find the ventral portion of a bovine lung involved in fibrinous bronchopneumonia, whereas the dorsal portion is consistent with AIP. Current speculation and research emphasis on causes of feedlot AIP include examination of diet-related causes.

Etiologic agents that have been shown to cause acute pulmonary edema and emphysema include the D,L-tryptophan fermentation product 3-methylindole ("fog fever"), paraquat, stinkwood and perila mint toxicity, and the mold *Fusarum solani* associated with moldy sweet potatoes. An in-depth review of acute bovine pulmonary edema and emphysema is contained in the third edition of this book (pp. 643–646).

Hematogenous Pneumonia

Hematogenous pneumonia results from blood-borne pathogens lodging in the lungs. The insult may be a result of generalized septicemia or a pyemia resulting from a localized infection such as an abdominal or liver abscess. The primary isolate from hematogenous pneumonia in ruminating calves is *Haemophilus somnus*. *Salmonella* spp., *Escherchia coli*, and *Streptococcus* spp. are commonly isolated from hematogenous pneumonia in neonates.

Venal caval thrombosis results in large-scale showering of the lungs with emboli. Case presentations range from acute death to chronic respiratory disease signs lasting for weeks. Hemoptysis following pulmonary arterial rupture is a clinical sign differentiating this syndrome from bronchopneumonia. Venal caval thrombosis is extensively described in the third edition of this book (pp. 647–652).

Bronchopneumonia—The Bovine Respiratory Disease Complex

Bovine respiratory disease complex (BRDC), also known as shipping fever, is aptly called a "complex" because of the involvement of environmental, viral, and bacterial factors. These causative factors may occur in various combinations to produce clinical presentations ranging from subclinical infections to acute bronchopneumonia or fibrinous pneumonia.

Epidemiology

Pneumonia typically starts to appear soon after significant environmental, physiologic, or psychological stress or exposure to new disease organisms. Production examples include weaning, commingling at points-of-sale followed by shipping, increasing dietary energy–density in the feedlot, parturition and lactation in dairy cattle, and heat or cold stress in pasture cattle.

Each bovine production system has a typical time for respiratory disease to develop in the population. In feedlot cattle, the morbidity pattern differs with source and management history. High-quality, low-stress (low-risk) yearling cattle would typically be expected to have a BRDC morbidity of less than 5%. Low-risk calves with proper management may have BRDC morbidity rates of less than 10%. In contrast, high risk (marginal-quality or very high-stress) yearlings and calves may have BRDC morbidity rates exceeding 50% in severe outbreaks. BRDC case fatality rates (dead/treated) are typically 5% to 10% when considering true BRDC cases.

In a vaccine study, cattle that were preconditioned before transport to the feedyard were 19.5 times less likely to experience feedlot morbidity than cattle purchased from auctions and then transported to the feedyard. Cattle shipped directly from the ranch to the feedyard were 5.7 times less likely to experience feedlot morbidity than cattle purchased from auctions and then transported to the feedyard. Cattle that were preconditioned before being shipped directly from the ranch to the feedyard were 3.4 times less likely to experience feedlot morbidity than cattle shipped directly from the ranch to the feedyard.[2]

An example of a distressor associated with BRDC is transport. A positive association between increased transport shrink in cattle hauled to Oklahoma and increased feedlot morbidity and mortality has been reported.[3] However, in a more recent report of cattle hauled to Alberta, there was a positive association between increased distance hauled and transport shrink, but not between distance hauled and risk of fatal fibrinous pneumonia.[4] However, the authors noted a relationship between the degree of mixing of calves from various sources and the risk of fatal fibrinous pneumonia among truckloads of cattle.[5]

A Colorado-based study evaluating BRDC risk factors in feedlot cattle found that lower respiratory tract disease peaked before 20 days on feed, with 58% of total morbidity occurring before 40 days on feed.[6] The number of animals put into a group on separate days had the greatest effect on respiratory disease morbidity. A review of the literature concerning morbidity in calves found that overall (all diseases) morbidity ranged from 0% to 69% with most in the range of 15% to 45%.[7] The morbidity peak was in the first 3 weeks after arrival. Respiratory infection was the most common clinical and necropsy diagnosis. Data from 59 feedyards for the period January 1990 to May 1993 (over 38 million cattle) indicated that respiratory death loss accounted for 44.1% of total death loss.[8] Death loss peaked in November and December. It is not uncommon for respiratory disease to account for 75% of morbidity in feedlots.

The amount of time that cattle spend in the marketing system can influence our perception of morbidity and mortality. If cattle have spent 5 to 10 days in the marketing system, the incubation periods will seem to be unusually quick. In fact, the incubation period is unchanged; we have simply moved our arbitrary day 0 (arrival at the feedyard) well into the incubation period. This can also have practical implications for intervention strategies. The farther along in the incubation period that cattle are, the less likely they are to benefit from arrival immunizations. Conversely, fresh, naive cattle that will begin incubation periods after arrival at the feedlot are unlikely to benefit from arrival metaphylaxis because their peak morbidity will likely not occur for several days.

In neonates, a study of 410 dairy heifers in 18 dairy herds found a pneumonia morbidity of 25.6%, with a likely case fatality risk of 2.2% before 3 months of age.[9] Other studies report morbidities in similar periods of 0.8% to 39%.

The morbidity patterns of BRDC are well described for most production systems. Unfortunately, many of the risk factors are associated with production practices that are currently refractory to change.

Detection

One of the primary signs of respiratory disease drawing the attention of caretakers is depression. Affected animals stand apart from penmates and attempt to keep other animals between themselves and the observer. The movement of affected animals has been characterized as "walking in concrete." Animals in moderate to advanced stages may have significantly diminished flight zones and refrain from moving away from the observer unless absolutely necessary. More advanced cases may develop weakness sufficient to cause "knuckling" of the rear fetlocks during locomotion, often accompanied by swaying of the hips and staggering.

Different observers rely on varying key indicators. Some pay particular attention to the eyes, watching for a "glazed" look resulting from pain and discomfort. Nasal and ocular discharge, along with elevated respiratory rate, are unreliable indicators by themselves when present in the absence of depression. Respiratory character (outstretched head or labored breathing) is a better indication of BRDC than rate. These signs should be evaluated with allowance for normal appearance of the animals in the current environmental conditions (i.e., dust, glare, heat).

Rumen fill is an indicator of feed intake. Description of gaunt animals would usually include at least a sunken right paralumbar fossa. Severe anorexia usually is accompanied by a dramatically sunken left paralumbar fossa. A common misconception is that ill animals will not eat. Some feedlot personnel do not closely examine cattle when they are at the feed bunk, associating this pen location with good health. However, sick cattle can fool us by nosing their way into the bunk to avoid pen checkers, thereby giving the appearance of eating. Moreover, many calves in the early stages of pneumonia, when therapeutic response is best, will continue to eat. Sunken flanks should draw attention to an animal for further evaluation. A full rumen is not a valid reason to skip further examination of an animal that is displaying other signs of BRDC. Given these considerations, it is a good idea to closely check cattle at the bunk and congregating around water tanks.

Further evaluation of clinical BRDC cases starts with the rectal temperature. Readings as high as 42°C (108°F) can occur. Practices vary, but approximately 40°C (104°F) is used as the start of the temperature range that "indicates" BRDC. We must be careful not to interpret increased rectal temperature as an absolute indicator of BRDC. We have observed highly agitated, newly received cattle with rectal temperatures of approximately 41.5°C (107°F) which were brought to the treatment facility on a hot afternoon because of depression and inappetence, not treated for BRDC by the crew, and then returned to the pen with no further BRDC occurrences during the feeding period.

Our ability to appreciate the impact of management factors on pulmonary disease rates is greatly affected by our ability to measure the clinically relevant outcomes such as respiratory morbidity rate, respiratory mortality rate, and weight changes. The ability to assess weight changes quickly and accurately has improved tremendously with the advent of reasonably priced, rapid scales that can be integrated into handling chutes, along with computers to process the information. In addition to visual inspection, changes in body weight may serve as a useful prognostic indicator. Cattle gaining 0.5% or greater than 5.0% of body weight during hospital stay were 2.7 or 11 times less likely to relapse, respectively, than cattle losing body weight.[10] Mortality resulting from respiratory disease, as determined by postmortem examination, is a specific and useful outcome. More clinicians are working proactively to increase the proportion of animals receiving at least a gross postmortem examination. There is still room for improvement. Failure to obtain a gross postmortem examination can result in a 10% to 30% misclassification bias in the mortality database, compromising the value of this information.[11] A limitation of using mortality to evaluate pulmonic immunity is that it usually occurs at a low rate, giving it poor statistical power to find real differences resulting from the effects of management decisions. Morbidity rate is probably the indicator most often used to determine the success or failure of decisions made to manage respiratory immunity.

The methods we use to detect calves with pulmonic disease may be seriously flawed. In many feedyards, 25% to 50% of respiratory deaths occur in the pen, before treatment can be initiated.[11, 12] Recent studies indicate that pulmonic disease is widespread in populations of feedlot cattle—even in cattle that seem normal throughout the feeding period. In surveys of cattle in packing plants, well over half the cattle that were not detected as clinically ill during the feeding period display pulmonary lesions.[13] Cattle having these lesions gain approximately 0.1 lb/day less than cattle that do not have pulmonary lesions, suggesting that these lesions are clinically relevant.

The converse of this dilemma, the treatment of cattle that do not have pulmonic disease, is much more difficult to assess. Among calves removed from the pen and treated for pneumonia, 22% did not display any evidence of pneumonia at slaughter. It is possible that the pulmonary lesions in these cattle were never present, had completely resolved, or were to small or in a place that prevented detection.

Accurately identifying cattle with pneumonia based on clinical signs can be further confounded by genetics. The genetics of individual cattle may affect the degree to which they show clinical signs of disease.[14] Clearly, these problems with clinical outcome assessment point to opportunities to improve and refine our detection systems for clinical disease. They also lead to the conclusion that subjectively determined clinical illness may be a very imprecise indicator of the success or failure of our management decisions.

Clinical evaluation of possible BRDC cases is an inexact science. In any kind of cattle, we must rely on our best judgment of a combination of depression, appetite, respiratory character, various discharges, and rectal temperature to arrive at a therapy decision. This judgment must be constantly refined based on therapy results.

Agent-Specific Pathogenesis and Disease Development

Pasteurella haemolytica, biotype A, serotype 1 (A1) is the primary bacterial pathogen in bovine respiratory disease in the United States. A survey involving 435 lung samples from feedlots in Kansas, Oklahoma, Texas, and New Mexico over a 1-year-period found *P. haemolytica* in 49.7% of the cases.[15] *Mycoplasma* spp. were found in 33.3% (409 cultured), *Pasteurella multocida* in 14.7%, *Actinomyces pyogenes* in 5.7%, *H. somnus* in 5.5%, and *Salmonella* spp. in 3.2%. The *Mycoplasma* isolates were all found in conjunction with one of the other pathogens. Other bacterial isolates in bovine respiratory disease (usually from chronic lesions) include *Staphylococcus aureus*, *Neisseria* spp., and *Bacteroides melaninogenicus*. *Escherichia coli* may also be found in neonatal pneumonia resulting from septicemia.

P. haemolytica is found in the nasopharynx of healthy cattle,

and is pathogenic only in ruminants, presumably because of the ability of a heat-labile leukotoxin that is active only against ruminant leukocytes. *P. haemolytica* A2 seems to be the primary serotype colonizing the nasopharynx in cattle on the farm, whereas *P. haemolytica* A1 proliferates during shipping and becomes the primary isolate in feedlots.[16, 17] Infection with bovine respiratory viruses has been shown to enhance nasopharynx colonization by *P. haemolytica* A1, even in the face of active immunity.[18, 19] Sudden changes in climate have also been shown to contribute to colonization.[20] Colonization of the nasopharynx allows inspiration of *Pasteurella* organisms, which are cleared from the lungs if a competent immune system is present. High-stress environments, viral immunosuppression, or inadequate nutrition in the form of energy, protein, and trace elements may allow inspired *Pasteurella* to colonize the lungs.

Once *P. haemolytica* gains access to the lungs, tissue damage is heightened by leukotoxin-mediated toxicity to leukocytes resulting in lysosomal enzyme release and excessive stimulation of eicosanoids. Addition of *P. haemolytica* leukotoxin to cell cultures has been shown to significantly accelerate alveolar macrophage deterioration without apparent effects on pulmonary parenchymal cells.[21] The encapsulated nature of *P. haemolytica* makes phagocytosis by neutrophils and macrophages more difficult.

P. multocida is viewed as secondary in importance to *P. haemolytica* in bovine pneumonia except in veal and dairy calves, where the prevalence of *P. multocida* infection may be higher than *P. haemolytica*. A study of 14 epizootics of pneumonia in dairy calves found *P. multocida* involved in 12 of the 14, whereas *P. haemolytica* was detected in only four.[22] *P. multocida* is also thought of as a less acute pneumonia, with isolates often recovered from chronic pneumonia cases or in cattle with more time in the feedlot. *P. multocida* differs from *P. haemolytica* in that a potent leukotoxin has not been identified for *P. multocida*. It is, however, thought to be capable of significant contributions to lung disease when present. Susceptibility to antimicrobials may vary between *P. multocida* and *P. haemolytica*, making extrapolation of efficacy from one genus to another tenuous at best without susceptibility testing or supporting literature.

H. somnus has been reported as a major cause of respiratory disease in fall-weaned calves shipped to feedlots in Canada. A 1990–1992 study in a commercial feedlot in Saskatchewan found that *H. somnus* accounted for greater than 40% of mortality in calves each year.[23] It has received less attention as a primary pathogen in the United States, but is still reported in respiratory disease outbreaks. Unlike *Pasteurella*, *H. somnus* is also frequently isolated from other disease conditions in cattle such as thromboembolic meningoencephalitis (TEME), arthritis, myocarditis, metritis, and abortions. It is not uncommon to observe myocarditis, TEME, and arthritis cases occurring in a group of cattle beginning 2 to 3 weeks after a respiratory disease outbreak from which *H. somnus* was isolated. Another Canadian feedlot study found the median fatal disease onset for *Haemophilus* pneumonia was 12 days on feed (DOF) compared with 18 DOF for polyarthritis, 22 DOF for myocarditis and pleuritis, and 29 DOF for TEME.[24]

Virulence factors for *H. somnus* include endotoxin (lipooligosaccharide) and immunoglobulin binding proteins. *H. somnus* is also thought to be able to function as a facultative intracellular parasite, with the ability to inhibit the oxidative burst in bovine neutrophils.

Mycoplasma organisms are currently considered to play a secondary role in bovine respiratory disease. Mycoplasma contribution to pathogenesis is uncertain, and attempts at establishing artificial infection models have met with little or no success. Increased reports of *Mycoplasma* involvement in bovine respiratory disease may be a result of improved and more routinely used culturing techniques rather than an absolute increase in occurrence. *Mycoplasma bovis*, as well as *A. pyogenes*, staphylococci, and streptococci, are isolated from focal and disseminated abscesses in advanced cases.

Viral isolates from bovine respiratory disease cases include IBRV, bovine viral diarrhea virus (BVDV), BRSV, parainfluenza 3 (PI-3) virus, malignant catarrhal fever virus, reovirus, calicivirus, and bovine adenovirus, parvovirus, herpesvirus 4, rhinovirus, reovirus, enterovirus, and respiratory coronavirus. Of these, IBRV, BVDV, and BRSV have been shown to be of major importance in field cases of bovine respiratory disease in the United States.

IBRV is a DNA herpesvirus (bovine herpesvirus 1, or BHV-1) responsible for numerous disease entities in cattle, including keratoconjunctivitis, abortion, infectious pustular vulvovaginitis, and meningoencephalitis, as well as respiratory disease. BHV-1 is further subdivided into three subtypes, with subtypes 1 and 2 responsible for respiratory disease.

The affinity of IBRV for mucous membranes results in visible clinical signs involving the upper respiratory and ocular membranes. IBRV alone causes severe hyperemia of the muzzle ("red nose") and upper airways, with lesions extending as far down as the larger bronchi. Pustules and a diphtheritic membrane in the nares may be observed, along with extreme pyrexia and depression. Severity of clinical symptoms following IBRV infection has been linked to genotypic traits in cattle.[14] Specific alleles were identified as associated with severe or mild clinical disease expression after inoculation of 98 unrelated cattle with IBRV.

The adverse effects of IBRV on the immune system include predisposition to BRDC by impairing the function of neutrophils, macrophages, and lymphocytes. IBVR is commonly recognized as being a predisposing agent for *P. haemolytica*. The epidemiology of IBRV is linked to the ability to establish latent infections in the trigeminal ganglion and recrudesce under future stressful conditions, such as those described as promoting colonization of the nasopharynx with *P. haemolytica* A1. IBRV is spread through nasal secretions and aerosols. Feedlot outbreaks typically occur in the first few weeks on feed, with later outbreaks indicating a problem in vaccination response.

BVDV is an RNA pestivirus that is involved in several disease entities of cattle. Diarrhea and mucosal disease, abortion and fetal mummification, and congenital defects are commonly reported in addition to involvement with respiratory disease. Like IBRV, the role of BVDV in respiratory disease is mainly as an immunosuppressive agent. Synergism has been shown between BVDV and IBRV,[25] BVDV and *P. haemolytica*,[26] and BVDV and BRSV.[27] One study found that BVDV was the most common isolate from multiple viral respiratory tract infections in calves.[28] Acute BVDV infections may incite bacterial respiratory disease without clinical signs suggestive of BVDV. Absence of mucosal lesions at necropsy does not rule out the involvement of BVDV in a respiratory disease outbreak.

The epidemiology of BVDV is extremely complex. It is spread through direct contact and is very prevalent in the bovine population. BVDV has a very high mutation rate for antigenic changes. Recent advances in diagnostic techniques have identified types I and II BVDV, with each containing the previously recognized cytopathic and noncytopathic forms. Cattle infected in utero with a noncytopathic form before approximately 130 days' gestation become persistent carriers, shedding the virus to herdmates throughout the production cycle. These cattle develop mucosal disease only when exposed to a cytopathic form of "their" virus through exposure to another animal, mutation of the persistent infection virus to a cytopathic form, or through vaccination.

BRSV is a paramyxovirus affecting cattle. A respiratory syncytial virus also affects sheep and goats. BRSV may be present as a primary pathogen or in combination with bacterial pathogens. BRSV has been shown to work in concert with *P. haemolytica*.[29, 30] BRSV may interact with *P. haemolytica* in calves by causing functional deficits in neutrophils and alveolar macrophages. The epidemiology of BRSV most likely involves adults acting as reservoirs for immature animals.

As opposed to IBRV, BRSV is a very significant factor in pneumonia in dairy calves. A study of 14 epizootics of pneumonia in dairy calves found BRSV to be involved in 10 of the 14.[31]

Host Factors

Stress is an important factor in determining an animal's ability to fight infection and respond to vaccines. Stress comes from a variety of sources, including transport, nutritional changes, weaning, handling, and adjustment to new social groups. Stress is associated with increased cortisol levels, decreased immune function indicators, and increased disease occurrence.

We should make efforts to minimize as many stressors as possible to prevent compromised host defense systems. The concept of additive stressors is especially relevant when discussing the immunologic sequelae of stress. Usually it is not a single stressor that debilitates the immune system. More often, the cumulative effects of a series of mild and moderate stressors experienced over a period of hours to days depress immune function below a threshold that prevents an effective immune response from occurring. Not only does each animal have a unique immunologic history but each animal varies in response to stressors, resulting in the wide spectrum of morbidity and response to vaccination frequently seen in cattle.

Genetic predisposition to disease occurs in other species and is speculated to occur in cattle. An example in cattle is the recently described bovine leukocyte adhesion deficiency.[32] Also, calves with certain interferon genotypes display more severe clinical signs than calves having other interferon genotypes, following the same experimental exposure to IBRV; this suggests that genetics partially determines the degree of clinical signs that calves display.[14]

Passive transfer of maternal antibodies present in colostrum is an important event in preventing disease, including respiratory disease, early in a calf's life.[33] However, the impact of health and growth performance continues past weaning.[34] Calves classified as having failure of passive transfer as indicated by inadequate IgG or plasma protein (PP) concentrations at 24 hours post partum were not only at greater risk of mortality from birth to weaning (odds ratio [OR] = 3.2) but were also at greater risk of feedlot respiratory morbidity (OR = 3.1). The lowest calf weaning weights were observed among calves classified as having inadequate IgG or PP concentration at 24 hours. However, multivariable modeling indicated that the effect of passive transfer on weaning weight was indirect through its effect on neonatal morbidity. Morbidity during the first 28 days of life resulted in a 35 lb lower expected weaning weight. Similar to weaning weight, passive immune status at 24 hours was not directly associated with feedlot growth rate; rather, feedlot growth rate was associated through the effect of PP concentration at 24 hours on feedlot morbidity. Adjusted mean daily gain for calves with respiratory morbidity while in the feedlot was 0.09 lb less than that for nonmorbid calves.

Age is another important host factor. The bovine immune system begins to develop during gestation.[35] Even though the bovine fetus is capable of recognizing and responding to antigens before birth, the immune system does not reach its peak function until around puberty. During old age, immunocompetence wanes.

A calf's previous nutritional status and parasite burden can affect its overall physiology and immune responsiveness. Parasites produce immunosuppressive substances as they progress through larval molts.[36] Because the immune system is a part of the larger organism—the calf—nutritional deficiencies in energy and protein will likely compromise overall physiology and immune function. Paradoxically, high levels of energy or protein in diets have been associated with increased morbidity. It is not known if this is truly a result of infectious disease or some other phenomenon that causes calves to "look sick." Trace minerals and vitamins play an important role in maintaining optimal immune function, although this is incompletely understood, and the practical implications are even more obscure.

Management

As previously mentioned, increased respiratory morbidity and mortality are associated with weaning, marketing, transport, arrival, and acclimatization to the feedyard environment. It must be remembered that association is not necessarily causation. Although it is likely that some combination of these events is at least partially responsible for increased bovine respiratory disease rates, specific combinations have not been well characterized. Despite the recent surge in integration and alliances, the great majority of cattle will continue to be marketed in much the same way, at least in the near future. In order to reduce the BRDC rate associated with weaning and marketing, we must continue to determine which specific factors, or combination of factors, are associated with increased BRDC risk. However, we must use epidemiologic techniques that allow us to simultaneously evaluate and control for multiple risk factors.

Some producers will elect to avoid high-risk calves or work proactively to reduce respiratory morbidity by ensuring that calves are immunologically and behaviorally prepared to move to the feedyard—moving them quickly, cleanly, and with minimal sorting—and making sure their transition into the feedlot is a smooth, organized event. However, when high-risk calves are offered for sale, someone is going to buy them. Thus, we must ensure that the producer understands the liability associated with the calves and has realistic expectations of their health and growth performance. Our greatest contributions in this scenario are the ability to accurately predict performance and to intervene to minimize disease.

A positive management intervention point for health managers is identifying and minimizing preventable stressors. Many stresses that cattle encounter result from the marketing and management systems peculiar to the cattle industry in the United States. We often can have little impact on such stresses. However, if we examine our management strategies objectively, we will see that we tolerate many controllable stressors in the interest of economics or convenience.

An obvious and important way to help the immune system is to prevent exposure. Examples of management strategies that can accomplish this are closed herds or screened replacements, sanitation, and herd immunization.

With a closed herd, opportunity for exposure to pathogens is reduced. However, this management strategy often is not practical. One alternative is to isolate and screen new animals for disease before introduction into the herd. Neither of these measures is practical in feedlots, making other means of reducing exposure, such as sanitation, even more important.

Sanitation is an often underemphasized management tool. Pathogens are everywhere in the environment, so we can never hope to eliminate them, but we can reduce their numbers. The number of pathogens an animal encounters is a critical determinant of whether infection and disease will result.

Space and sunlight can be useful tools for reducing exposure. Decreasing animal density can decrease transmission events by reducing animal contacts; sunlight kills many pathogens. Other strategies include keeping receiving pens and hospital areas as clean as possible.

Another way to prevent exposure of susceptible animals to disease agents is through herd immunity. Herd immunity is based on the fact that transmission of communicable disease requires contact between infectious and susceptible individuals. Raising resistance in a herd by natural exposure or vaccination reduces the number of susceptible animals and the number of infected animals during an outbreak, thereby reducing the number of contacts between susceptible and infected animals. This indirectly protects all susceptible animals, especially in outbreaks of highly contagious disease.

Our goal in herd immunization is to raise the level of immunity in a sufficient number of animals to prevent disease outbreaks. This reduces, but does not eliminate, the occurrence of diseases with high morbidity or mortality. Paradoxically, individual animals can still become ill when the vaccine is successfully stimulating an effective level of herd immunity.

Although an animal is frequently exposed, infection and disease do not commonly occur. The agent must infect the animal to cause disease. A calf's ability to defend its respiratory system against infectious agents results from several complex, interrelated defense mechanisms. These include innate defenses, such as intact epithelium, mucus, ciliated epithelial cells, complement, interferon, natural killer cells, and phagocytes, as well as acquired defenses, such as antibodies and cytotoxic T lymphocytes. During weaning, marketing, transport, and arrival in, and acclimatization to the feedyard environment, the function of these defense mechanisms is compromised. An important concept to remember is that many of the host defense mechanisms listed above are influenced only by husbandry, not by vaccines.

Vaccine-induced immunity is one of several management tools available to the veterinarian to help livestock achieve optimal productivity through disease prevention, control, and eradication. Sound husbandry and good management are key to maintaining immunocompetence. Management decisions can be passive or active and can be a choice to do something good for the calf's immune system or avoid something that would be bad for the immune system. Biologic and pharmacologic products are valuable aids, but they cannot replace sound animal care practices.

Disease surveillance is critical to determining need and to evaluating the effectiveness of immunization. This surveillance requires accurately monitoring clinically affected animals and postmortem examination of all dead calves.

Two key components required for each successful immunization are an efficacious vaccine and an immunocompetent animal. Despite its simplicity, these, along with challenge dose considerations, are the basis of all vaccination successes. Vaccine failures arise from inattention to details in these critical areas.

If we consider the biology of the immune system, it is obvious that in order for a vaccine to work, the immune response that it elicits must occur before challenge. If a vaccine is used during or after exposure, reduced efficacy can result.

Market forces often affect management decisions more than does understanding the biology of the immune system. Over the past several years, there have been myriad of efforts to integrate different segments of the beef cattle production system. These have sparked renewed interest in monitoring the downstream effects of different management decisions that might affect pulmonary immunity.

One aspect of this renewed interest is the "rediscovery" of the biologically rational use of vaccines, in other words, using vaccines in cattle a sufficient time before disease challenge to allow the immune system to mount a response. Attempts to standardize and document management interventions to prepare calves for weaning and movement into confined feeding facilities, termed *preconditioning*, have been going on since the 1960s. Preconditioning, which includes preexposure vaccination, has proved beneficial, but is not a panacea. In a review of controlled studies of the effect of preconditioning on feedlot health performance, morbidity was reduced from 26.5% to 20.4% and mortality was reduced from 1.44% to 0.74%.[37] The same author reviewed survey reports and cited a reduction of 20% to 30% in morbidity and of 0% to 1.7% in mortality. Recently, several demonstration studies have shown similar effects.[38] Additionally, these demonstration studies have attempted to quantify the growth performance effects and monetary value of the management interventions. Although the effects cannot be ascribed to one specific intervention and may be the result of genetics, nutrition, vaccines, preweaning acclimatization to feed bunks, environment, or some combination of these, this does not obviate the fact that there seems to be large, important monetary advantages in managing cattle "correctly."

What we know about the immune system, as well as the data described above, support the concept that preexposure immunization reduces morbidity and mortality. There are several important details to note. Preconditioning does not eliminate disease. Morbidity and mortality rates in preconditioned calves will rarely be zero. Thus, without a valid control group it can be difficult to know the true value of preconditioning. Similarly, if no disease occurs in a given group, it will not be possible to show a benefit. A final consideration is cost-effectiveness. Even if we accept that reduced morbidity and mortality rates by preexposure immunization are usually statistically significant, this does not necessarily equate to cost-effectiveness. Economic variables such as cost of vaccine and cost of additional handling must be considered.

Vaccines

We use both live and killed vaccines. The advantages of one are usually the disadvantages of the other. Modified live vaccine attributes include a strong, long-lasting immune response achieved with fewer doses; less reliance on adjuvants; possible stimulation of interferon production; stimulation of the effector component of cell-mediated immunity (cytotoxic T lymphocytes); and the bacteria or virus may look and behave more like the pathogenic form of the organism. Some advantages of killed vaccines are that they are more stable in storage and they are unlikely to cause disease as a result of residual virulence or reversion. Numerous brands of vaccines provide a variety of combinations of live and killed antigens. These include IBRV, BVDV, P-I3 virus, BRSV, *Pasteurella* spp., and *H. somnus.*

IBRV vaccines are available in modified live virus form for intramuscular, subcutaneous, or intranasal use, as well as killed and chemically altered virus for intramuscular use. Intramuscular modified live virus vaccines are thought to quickly induce immunity following proper administration of a single dose. Intranasal modified live virus vaccines induce immunity at the mucosal surface through stimulation of acquired mucosal immunity and production of interferon. They may be used safely in calves suckling pregnant cows and induce immunity in the face of residual maternal antibody titers. They are, however, more difficult to administer. Killed virus vaccines require two doses, administered at 14- to 28-day intervals, to induce immunity. This, along with higher cost and concerns about shorter duration of immunity, make them less practical to use in a typical feedlot setting.

In a review of IBRV vaccine clinical efficacy studies, results were positive or neutral; however, none were negative.[39] The studies date to 1958 and 1974 and may not apply to current cattle feeding management practices in North America. In a field trial using modified live IBRV vaccine on arrival, the incidence of upper respiratory disease was reduced from 17.2% in 3371 unvaccinated calves to 1% in 3345 vaccinees (relative risk [RR] = 16; $P < .0000$).[40] A well-designed trial using modified live IBRV given on arrival failed to show benefits in health

performance.[41] Another report that failed to show IBRV vaccine efficacy involved additional antigens and is discussed later. The current consensus is to include IBRV in preconditioning and arrival vaccine regimens.

BVDV vaccines are available in modified live and killed viral forms, and they are one of the most controversial vaccines used in U.S. cattle. Lack of large-scale efficacy trials, widespread infection in the U.S. cattle population, the presence of persistently infected cattle that subsequently develop mucosal disease, and the emerging role of heterologous and novel strains of the virus all combine to create confusion and controversy. There is no clear consensus concerning use. Measurements of certain immunologic values suggest that immunosuppression following use of modified live virus may be a concern;[42] however, the lack of complications following their use in large numbers of cattle suggest these may not be of practical concern.[43] They may be of greater concern in highly stressed cattle, but well-controlled studies evaluating this are not available. Like BHV-1, dosage and timing requirements of killed BVDV vaccines are a severe limitation in most feedlot settings.

There are no reliable peer-reviewed reports of field trials examining the clinical effects of BVDV vaccines in North American beef cattle that are based on research that uses scientifically valid methods with clinically relevant outcomes.[39] Use is based on extrapolation from challenge or licensing data and personal preference.

BRSV vaccines are available in modified live and inactivated virus forms. Because recovery from natural infection with BRSV does not engender protective immunity in most species, it is unlikely that vaccination will prevent subsequent infection. However, it may still be possible for vaccination to attenuate clinical signs of subsequent infections and reduce time to recovery. One experimental challenge of a small number of calves showed that passive antibodies reduce the pathologic changes associated with BRSV.[44] Moreover, there are reports of improvement in gain and feed efficiency.[45] Mixed results are reported from studies investigating the clinical efficacy of BRSV vaccination of calves upon arrival. A statistically significant benefit of BRSV vaccination was shown in auction market–purchased and transported calves with vaccinated calves two times less likely to be treated for BRDC (OR = 2.0, $P < .00001$). Freshly weaned and transported calves were 1.4 times less likely to be treated for BRDC (OR = 1.4; $P < .001$). A statistically significant benefit of BRSV vaccination was not shown in the two classes of calves with low morbidity rates. These included preconditioned calves ($P = .11$) and freshly weaned calves that were not transported ($P = .75$).[2] In a Canadian study, results of five separate trials designed to assess BRSV vaccine efficacy were equivocal for calves vaccinated before weaning; however, reduction of the treatment rate was reported in calves vaccinated once upon arrival. No benefit was found for vaccination upon arrival of yearling cattle.[46] Two additional trials involving calves[47, 48] and one trial involving stocker cattle[49] failed to demonstrate a benefit of BRSV vaccination on arrival. Although there is evidence to support BRSV vaccine usage in naive and mismanaged calves, inclusion in vaccine regimens is not universal.

Studies show the PI-3 virus compromises innate defenses of the respiratory tract.[50, 51] Because many older cattle arriving at feedlots are likely immune, the value of PI-3 virus vaccination in yearling cattle is questionable. Vaccination may be valuable in preweaning or arrival programs for less immunologically experienced calves. There are no reliable peer-reviewed reports of field trials examining the clinical effects of PI-3 virus vaccines in North American beef cattle, based on research that uses scientifically valid methods with clinically relevant outcomes.[39] As a practical matter, it is difficult to select a multivirus bovine respiratory vaccine that does not include PI-3 virus, making its inclusion less of an issue.

Findings reported in the literature are equivocal on the use of more recently available *Pasteurella* sp. vaccines before and at feedlot arrival. The largest body of *Pasteurella* vaccine data exist for *P. haemolytica* toxoid. Three studies have shown statistically significant reduction in morbidity and mortality in calves administered a *P. haemolytica* toxoid on arrival.[52–54] However, two clinical trials showed no significant effects when the same vaccine was given on arrival[55] or 3 weeks before shipment or arrival.[56] In no reports was health performance in vaccinees negatively affected.

There are individual reports on various other commercial or experimental *Pasteurella* sp. vaccines. These include reports of significant efficacy in field studies of a streptomycin-dependent live *Pasteurella* sp. vaccine[57] and an intradermally administered live *P. haemolytica* vaccine.[58] Alternatively, a field study of a *P. haemolytica* capsular antigen vaccine failed to show significant health effects,[59] as did a study using a tissue culture–derived *P. haemolytica* bacterin.[60]

For some currently available *Pasteurella* sp. vaccines there are no reliable peer-reviewed reports of field trials examining clinical effects in North American beef cattle that are based on research that uses scientifically valid methods with clinically relevant outcomes. There are reports of lack of field efficacy with earlier *Pasteurella* sp. bacterins.[61, 62] There is also a report of increased health problems following vaccination with earlier *Pasteurella* sp. bacterins.[63] However, this study did not mention whether treatment assignment was random and the experimental unit is unclear, making the validity of the data analysis suspect. Because of dosage and timing requirements for optimal immunity (7 to 10 days following a 14- to 21-day booster dose) their value should be compromised when used only in a feedlot arrival program. Paradoxically, the available data support the use of *P. haemolytica* toxoid on arrival. Current consensus is that it is best to administer at least the priming dose and sometimes the booster dose before weaning.

As with other vaccine antigens of bovine respiratory disease prophylaxis, results of field trials evaluating the efficacy of *H. somnus* bacterins have been conflicting. One group of investigators has reported negative effects of a single vaccination with a commercial *H. somnus* bacterin, in that significantly more animals in groups of calves vaccinated once were treated for respiratory disease compared with groups of unvaccinated control calves or groups of calves vaccinated twice after a 21-day interval.[64] However, these findings conflicted with earlier reports by these authors that no significant difference in the number of animals treated was found between groups of calves immunized once with a commercial *H. somnus* bacterin and groups of unimmunized control calves.[62] Conversely, these investigators had reported earlier that morbidity (number of animals treated for respiratory disease) was significantly reduced in groups of calves vaccinated with a commercial *H. somnus* bacterin upon arrival at the feedlot and revaccinated 21 days later compared with groups vaccinated twice with a bivalent *P. haemolytica* or *P. multocida* bacterin or unvaccinated controls.[61]

Ability of *H. somnus* vaccine to reduce bovine respiratory disease in U.S. feedlots may be limited by the low incidence and sporadic nature of the disease.[65] While studies demonstrate vaccine efficacy, most have shown vaccine efficacy using septicemic challenge.[66] Some have shown efficacy in experimental respiratory challenge.[67, 68] To date, however, efficacy has not been unequivocally demonstrated in well-controlled trials in a U.S. field setting. It is logical to assume that these vaccines are subject to the same dose and timing limitations as *Pasteurella* vaccines. There is no clear consensus on usage.

Field trials have been carried out with vaccinees receiving multiple antigens, making it impossible to determine the effects of individual antigens. These can be subdivided into two broad groups—vaccine administered at or near the time of feedlot arrival and vaccine administered several weeks before feedlot arrival. Assuming valid design, execution, and analysis, interpretation of the first group is fairly straightforward. Some studies of arrival vaccination suggest it does not affect or may even compromise health performance. A well-designed study using modified-live IBRV and PI-3 virus vaccine along with a *P. haemolytica* toxoid failed to show health performance benefits.[69] This is supported by findings in a multiyear observational study in Ontario, Canada, which reported that administration of respiratory vaccines (IBRV or IBRV-PI-3 virus or IBRV-PI-3 virus-*Pasteurella*) to calves vaccinated within 2 weeks of arrival was associated with increased risk of mortality (RR = 2.4).[70] In contrast, subcutaneous vaccination with a *P. haemolytica* and *H. somnus* vaccine on arrival reduced BRDC morbidity from 41% to 29%.[71]

The second type of mixed-antigen study is when vaccines are administered several weeks before feedlot arrival. These are often part of a preconditioning or preweaning study. Because an unvaccinated, but similarly managed group is rarely included in these studies, the effects of management interventions such as preweaning and bunk acclimation are totally confounded with vaccine effect. Hence, it is impossible to know which accounts for improvements in health performance.

Optimizing Vaccination

As stated initially, vaccine injection only ensures that the animal has been exposed to the antigens contained in that vaccine, not that a protective immune response will ensue. The two key components required for a successful immunization are an efficacious vaccine and an immunocompetent animal.

Achieving a protective immune response to every pathogen in every animal in a population is probably impossible for several reasons. Even if it were possible, the cost would likely be prohibitive. Based on their pathogenesis, some pathogens require each individual in a population to be immune for the vaccine to be efficacious. One example is an infectious, but noncommunicable, disease such as tetanus. For other pathogens, especially those that are highly contagious, reducing the number of susceptible animals below a critical threshold may be sufficient for the vaccine to be efficacious by preventing a disease outbreak—the concept of herd immunity.

A vaccine may seem ineffective if it does not contain antigens that induce protective immunity to the disease-causing agent currently challenging the calf. There are respiratory pathogens that can influence calf health for which no vaccines are available, such as *Chlamydia* sp.[72] There are situations where antigenic differences among strains and species of pathogens or changes in antigens the organism displays may compromise vaccine efficacy. One example of this is the genetic and antigenic instability of BVDV.[73] This instability was thought to contribute to the failure of repeated annual doses of inactivated virus vaccine to protect animals from infection.[74] For many infectious agents of cattle, immunologically important antigens are relatively stable.

A more likely cause of vaccine ineffectiveness is improper storage or handling. We must store and administer vaccines according to recommendations or risk reducing their efficacy.

Once we have done everything to properly care for the vaccine and the equipment, we must carefully administer the vaccine. Training sessions should be conducted to ensure that personnel are knowledgeable about the proper locations and techniques for vaccine administration.[75] Intramuscular injections should not be made behind the calf's front leg. The subcutaneous route should be used whenever label instructions allow. As a general rule, the smallest needle through which the product is easily delivered should be used. For thin, watery products, an 18-gauge needle works well. Strict attention to proper restraint and changing needles to keep them sharp is critical when using 18-gauge needles. Needle length should be adjusted for calf size and injection route. Give intramuscular injections with a 1½-in. needle, except in the case of small calves, where a 1-in. needle should be used. Make subcutaneous injections with a needle less than 1 in. Change needles whenever they become dull, barbed, or bent. Use a clean needle when refilling syringes to avoid contaminating the vaccine bottle. Good handling facilities help minimize injection site reactions by ensuring that cattle are adequately restrained, thereby preventing movement should a calf struggle during an injection.

Sanitation is an important component of any vaccination plan and helps minimize injection site reactions and abscesses. Contamination of a multidose container can result in vaccine inactivation and injection site problems. Disinfectants inactivate modified live vaccines, so we must properly clean and rinse all equipment that comes in contact with vaccine.

Timing of vaccine administration can also influence our perception of vaccine effectiveness. If an animal is incubating a disease, or if it is exposed to the disease-causing agent soon following vaccination, it may get sick and the vaccine will seem ineffective. It takes several days for an animal's immune system to respond to a vaccine and for the animal to be protected, especially if the calf is immunologically naive.

Experimentally, if we give enough of the disease-causing organism, we can cause disease even in immune animals. When cattle are assembled in close quarters, the amount of disease agent to which they are exposed may be quite large, resulting in disease even in immune animals.

In summary, specific vaccine recommendations should be made by the veterinarian familiar with the management of the operation, including the type of cattle handled and disease problems typically experienced. There are few cookbook solutions. Fine-tuning the program by including or excluding certain vaccines requires identification of the specific disease entities present in an operation. This requires good records, complete postmortem examinations, and a good diagnostic support system. Effective management to optimize immunocompetence and timing of vaccine administration is as important as selecting the correct antigens and type of vaccines used.

Environment

The environment into which we thrust the calf can make or break both our prevention and treatment programs. This is especially true in critical areas such as feedlot receiving and hospital pens. Although this makes intuitive sense, data that quantify the individual contributions of environmental components to the healthfulness of the calf are not available. These components include pen space, pen surface, bunk space, water space, pen layout, windbreaks, sanitation, pen size, and shades.

Specific recommendations are difficult to provide because of the huge variation in climates in which cattle are raised and the seasonal variations within a geographic region. Pen space recommendations vary in the literature from a minimum of 18 sq. ft per calf for slotted-floor, covered confinement feeding to a maximum of 800 sq ft per animal for high-rainfall regions with outdoor, flat pens (<2% slope).

General guidelines and common sense are our best tools. A handy number to remember is that, in general, a calf needs 20 sq ft of space. Look at a hospital pen. Does it provide 20 sq ft of dry, comfortable pen space per animal? In regions where ambient temperatures exceed 100°F for more than 14 days/year, shades might be considered. Again, approximately 20 sq ft per animal should suffice. In moderate- to high-rainfall areas, mounds are indicated. They should be sized to provide 20 sq ft

per animal; this same area is also a good guide for hospital shelters if the environment warrants them.

Although 20 sq ft of dry pen surface per calf is a useful guide, the number of total square feet required in the pen will vary. Visual evaluation of pen conditions and cattle is vital. Assess their level of comfort by observing their behavior, such as cud chewing. If pens are too small, they will be wet, dirty, and uncomfortable. If pens are too large, cattle will unnecessarily expend energy wandering around the pen and valuable land will be wasted. Keeping receiving pens and hospitals clean is often a challenge. These pens are frequently small and sometimes difficult or impossible to access with cleaning equipment. Pens should be constructed so as to make cleaning easy, as well as to facilitate moving cattle into and out of the pen.

Bunk space is another highly variable number. Aggressive cattle that have had previous experience with bunk feeding might only need 7 in. of linear bunk space per animal. Cattle that are timid, inexperienced with bunks, sick, or tired from transport may require two to three times more linear bunk space per animal. In areas where tired or sick cattle are placed, such as receiving or hospital pens, 24 in. of linear bunk space per calf is desirable, with 18 in. a minimum. Waterers need to provide 10 (cold environment) to 20 (hot environment) gal per animal per day and a minimum of 0.75 in. per animal of linear waterer space.

In receiving pens, arrange fresh feed to attract cattle (hay with the starting ration layered on top). Evaluate the freshness of the feed and the condition and cleanliness of the waterers. If logistics and labor allow, bunks or hay feeders can be placed at right angles to the fence so that cattle will encounter them as they circle the pen. In hospital and receiving pens, hay should be fed in feeders or bunks, not on the ground.

Putting these recommendations into practice is a challenge. The key is to evaluate facilities before the operation is in the middle of a heavy workload. Evaluate each hospital and receiving pen in terms of pen space, bunk space, waterer space, and, when appropriate, barn or shade space. Unless the pen is perfectly designed, one of these will be a limiting factor. Determine the routine and maximum occupancy that will be allowed for each pen, then compare these figures with the historical and expected cattle receipts and morbidity rates. This will help to identify potential shortfalls before it is too late to respond.

Nutrition

Water is the least expensive, and perhaps most important nutrient for an animal recovering from respiratory disease. Intake by normal feedlot cattle may vary from 300% of dry matter feed consumption at 4°C (~40°F) to around 800% at 32°C (~90°F). It might perhaps be better stated that cattle will only have a dry matter consumption of approximately 33% of water intake (2.5 lb of dry matter per gallon of water) in cold conditions ranging down to approximately 12.5% (1 lb dry matter per gallon of water) in a hot environment. If you want cattle to eat, they must drink. A target feed intake of 2% of body weight per day on a dry matter basis in newly received 250-kg calves during late fall would require around 15 kg (15 L, ~4 gal of water per day). Stimulation of water intake is best accomplished by providing fresh water in routinely cleaned tanks. Once-a-day cleaning of hospital tanks is not excessive. The water tank in pens used to house newly received feeder calves should be at the periphery of the pen where cattle walking the fence will find it. Adding vertical tubes to the float valves in automatic waterers creates a water sound that may attract calves familiar with range conditions. Some managers choose to limit water availability for the first few hours after arrival to "encourage feed intake." This may be a mistake since a calf that has just lost 4% to 10% of its body weight during shipment is likely to eat only minimal amounts before rehydration.

Feed intake during the first 30 days in a feedyard can easily turn into too much of a good thing. Limiting feeding calves to a moderate-energy diet for the first month decreases the stress of production and dietary adaptation, which may translate to reduced morbidity. Calves fed a receiving ration containing 75% concentrate had higher gains and 57% morbidity compared with lower gains and 47% morbidity in calves receiving a 25% concentrate ration during the arrival period.[76]

The presence of fermented feeds (silage, high-moisture corn) in excessive amounts soon after arrival may discourage feed intake by calves during the adaptation period. Likewise, high added fat concentrations may discourage feed intake.

The choice of feed in recovery pens is subject to much debate. Newly received calves may eat a high-quality grass hay or a medium-quality alfalfa much more readily than a prepared bunk ration ("mill feed"). The mill feed, however, will contain more energy and protein than hay. Realizing that a full rumen resulting from hay intake may be misleading as to true energy intake, a system of feeding an approximately 25% to 50% concentrate milled diet over hay is recommended for newly received cattle in the hospital. Cattle on a more concentrated ration should receive a higher-energy diet while away from the home pen to minimize the return transition.

Trace element nutrition in highly stressed calves is extremely important to the health outcome. Suggested dietary contents, as listed in the seventh revised edition of *Nutrient Requirements of Beef Cattle* include 15 ppm copper, 0.1 to 0.2 ppm selenium, 400 to 500 IU/kg ration of vitamin E, and 4000 to 6000 IU/kg of vitamin A.[76]

CONCLUSION

Optimal prevention of pneumonia in feedlot cattle begins with effective management of passive transfer in newborn calves, followed by rational and proper use of vaccines in preconditioning programs. Control continues through maintenance of innate respiratory defenses by minimizing time in market channels, choosing to manage cattle in a manner that eliminates or minimizes as many physical and behavioral stressors as possible, and, to the extent possible, minimizing unnecessary exposure to pathogens.

REFERENCES

1. Panciera RJ, Perino LJ, Baldwin CA, et al: Observations on calf diphtheria in the commercial feedlot. Agri Pract 10:12, 1989.
2. Hansen DE, Syvrud R, Armstrong D: Effectiveness of a bovine respiratory syncytial virus vaccine in reducing the risk of respiratory disease. Agri Pract 13:19, 1992.
3. Griffin DD: Epidemiology—Its use in cattle feeding. *In* Proceedings of the 18th Annual Conference of the American Association of Bovine Practitioners, 1985, p 130.
4. Ribble CS, Meek AH, Shewen PE, et al: Effect of transportation on fatal fibrinous pneumonia and shrinkage in calves arriving at a large feedlot. J Am Vet Med Assoc 207:612, 1995.
5. Ribble CS, Meek AH, Shewew PE, et al: Effect of pretransit mixing on fatal fibrinous pneumonia in calves. J Am Vet Med Assoc 207:616, 1995.
6. Alexander BH, MacVean DW, Salman MD: Risk factors for lower respiratory tract disease in a cohort of feedlot cattle. J Am Vet Med Assoc 195:207, 1989.
7. Kelly AP, Janzen ED: A review of morbidity and mortality rates and disease occurrence in North American feedlot cattle. Can Vet J 27:496–500, 1986.
8. Vogel GJ, Parrott C: Mortality survey in feedyards: The incidence of death from digestive, respiratory, and other causes in feedyards on the great plains. The Compendium—Food Animal, February, 1994, p 227.
9. Virtala AK, Melchor GD, Grohn YT: Epidemiologic and pathologic characteristics of respiratory tract disease in dairy heifers during the first three months of life. J Am Vet Med Assoc 208:2035, 1996.
10. Blood KS, Perino LJ, Dewey CE, et al: Body weight change during respiratory disease treatment as a treatment success indicator in feedlot cattle. Agri Pract 17:6, 1996.
11. DeGroot BD, Dewey CD, Griffin DD: Effect of booster-vaccination with a multivalent clostridial bacterin-toxoid on sudden death syndrome mortality rate among feedlot cattle. J Am Vet Med Assoc 211:749, 1997.
12. Pierson RE, Jensen R, Lauerman LH, et al: Sudden deaths in yearling feedlot cattle. J Am Vet Med Assoc 169:527, 1976.
13. Wittum TE, Woollen NE, Perino LJ, et al: Relationships among treatment for respiratory tract disease, pulmonary lesions at slaughter, and rate of weight gain in feedlot cattle. J Am Vet Med Assoc 209:814, 1996.
14. Ryan AM, Hutcheson DP, Womack JE: Type-I interferon genotypes and severity of clinical disease in cattle inoculated with bovine herpesvirus 1. Am J Vet Res 54:73, 1993.
15. Welsh RD: Bacterial and mycoplasma species isolated from pneumonic bovine lungs. Agri Pract 14:12, 1993.
16. Frank GH, Briggs RE, Loan RW, et al: Serotype-specific inhibition of colonization of the tonsils and nasopharynx of calves after *Pasteurella haemolytica* serotype A1 after vaccination with the organism. Am J Vet Res 55:1107, 1994.
17. Frank GH, Briggs RE, Loan RW, et al: Respiratory tract disease and mucosal colonization by *Pasteurella haemolytica* in transported cattle. Am J Vet Res 57:1317, 1996.
18. Frank GH: Colonization of the nasal passages of calves with *Pasteurella haemolytica* serotype 1 and regeneration of colonization after experimentally induced viral infection of the respiratory tract. Am J Vet Res 47:1704, 1986.
19. Jericho KWF: Bovine herpesvirus-1 and *Pasteurella haemolytica* aerobiology in experimentally infected calves. Am J Vet Res 47:205, 1986.
20. Jones CDR: Proliferation of *Pasteurella haemolytica* in the calf respiratory tract after an abrupt change in climate. Res Vet Sci 42:179, 1987.
21. Wilkie IW, Fallding MH, Shewen PE, et al: The effect of *Pasteurella haemolytica* and the leukotoxin of *Pasteurella haemolytica* on bovine lung explants. Can J Vet Res 54:151, 1990.
22. Baker JC, Werdin RE, Ames TR, et al: Study on the etiologic role of bovine respiratory syncytial virus in pneumonia of dairy calves. J Am Vet Med Assoc 189:66, 1986.
23. Van Donkersgoed J, Janzen ED, Potter AA, et al: The occurrence of *Haemophilus somnus* in feedlot calves and its control by postarrival prophylactic mass medication. Can Vet J 35:573, 1994.
24. Van Donkersgoed J, Janzen ED, Harland RJ: Epidemiological features of calf mortality due to hemophilosis in a large feedlot. Can Vet J 31:821, 1990.
25. Potgieter LND, McCracken MD, Hopkins FM, et al: Effect of bovine viral diarrhea virus infection on distribution of infectious bovine rhinotracheitis in calves. Am J Vet Res 45:687, 1984.
26. Potgieter LND, McCracken MD, Hopkins FM, et al: Experimental production of bovine respiratory tract disease with bovine viral diarrhea virus. Am J Vet Res 45:1582, 1984.
27. Kelling CL, Brodersen BW, Perino LJ, et al: Potentiation of bovine respiratory syncytial virus infection in calves by bovine viral diarrhoea virus. *In* Proceedings of the 19th World Buiatrics Congress, vol 1, 1996, p 20.
28. Richer L, Marois P, Lamontagne L: Association of bovine viral diarrhea virus with multiple infections in bovine respiratory disease outbreaks. Can Vet J 29:713, 1988.
29. Al-Darraji AM, Cutlip RC, Lehmkuhl HD, et al: Experimental infection of lambs with bovine respiratory syncytial virus and *Pasteurella haemolytica*. Am J Vet Res 42:224, 1982.
30. Trigo FJ, Breeze RG, Liggitt HD, et al: Interaction of bovine respiratory syncytial virus and *Pasteurella haemolytica* in bovine lung. Am J Vet Res 48:1663, 1984.
31. Baker JC, Werdin RE, Ames TR, et al: Study on the etiologic role of bovine respiratory syncytial virus in pneumonia of dairy calves. J Am Vet Med Assoc 189:66, 1986.
32. Gilbert RO, Rebhun WC, Kim CA: Clinical manifestations of

leukocyte adhesion deficiency in cattle: 14 cases (1977–1991). J Am Vet Med Assoc 202:445, 1993.

33. Perino LJ, Sutherland RL, Woollen NE: Serum gamma-glutamyl-transferase activity and protein concentration at birth and after suckling in calves with adequate and inadequate passive transfer of immunoglobulin. Am J Vet Res 54:73, 1993.

34. Wittum TE, Perino LJ: Passive immune status at postpartum hour 24 and long-term health and performance of calves. Am J Vet Res 56:1149, 1995.

35. Schultz RD, Dunne HW, Heist CE: Ontogeny of the bovine immune response. J Dairy Sci 54:1321, 1974.

36. Gasbarre LC, Romanowski RD, Douvres FW: Suppression of antigen- and mitogen-induced proliferation of bovine lymphocytes by excretory-secretory products of *Oesphagostumun radiatum.* Infect Immun 48:540, 1985.

37. Cole NA: Preconditioning calves for the feedlot. Vet Clin North Am Food Anim Pract 1:401, 1985.

38. McNeill J: 1994–95 Texas A&M Ranch to Rail North/South Summary Report. College Station, Texas Agricultural Extension Service, Texas A&M University System.

39. Perino LJ, Hunsaker BD: A review of bovine respiratory disease vaccine field efficacy. Bovine Pract 31:59, 1997.

40. York CJ, Schwarz AJF, Zirbel L, et al: Infectious bovine rhinotracheitis vaccine. Vet Med, October 1958, p 522.

41. Curtis RA, Angulo A: A field trial to evaluate an intranasal infectious bovine rhinotracheitis vaccine. Can Vet J 15:327, 1974.

42. Roth JA, Kaeberle ML: Suppression of neutrophil and lymphocyte function induced by a vaccinal strain of bovine viral diarrhea virus with and without the administration of ACTH. Am J Vet Res 44:2366, 1983.

43. Edwards AJ: The effect of stressors like rumen overload and induced abortion on BRD in feedlot cattle. Agri Pract 10:10, 1989.

44. Bleknap EB, Baker JC, Patterson JS, et al: The role of passive immunity in bovine respiratory syncytial virus–infected calves. J Infect Dis 163:470, 1991.

45. Armstrong DA: Conclusion. *In* Proceedings of the Academy of Veterinary Consultants, Aug 27, 1987, p 62.

46. Van Donkersgoed J, Janzen ED, Townsend HG, et al: Five field trials on the efficacy of a bovine respiratory syncytial virus vaccine. Can Vet J 31:93, 1990.

47. Baker JC, Rust SR, Ciszewski DK, et al: A safety trial of a bovine respiratory syncytial virus vaccine in feedlot calves. Bovine Pract 21:70, 1986.

48. Morter RL, Amstutz HE: Effectiveness of vaccination of feedlot cattle with bovine respiratory syncytial virus (BRSV). Bovine Pract 21:67, 1986.

49. Johnson BD, Hays VS, Gill DR: Respiratory syncytial virus vaccine for stressed stocker cattle. Oklahoma Agricultural Experiment Station Animal Science Research Report MP-125, 105, 1988.

50. Reed SE, Boyd A: Organ cultures of respiratory epithelium infected with rhinovirus or parainfluenza virus studied in a scanning electron microscope. Infect Immun 6:68, 1972.

51. Lopez A, Thompson RG, Savan M: Pulmonary clearance of *Pasteurella haemolytica* in calves infected with bovine PI3 virus. Can J Comp Med 40:385, 1976.

52. Jim K, Guichon T, Shaw G: Protecting feedlot calves from pneumonic pasteurellosis. Vet Med 83:1084, 1988.

53. Bechtol DT, Ballinger RT, Sharp AJ: Field trial of a *Pasteurella haemolytica* toxoid administered at spring branding and in the feedlot. Agri Pract 12:6, 1991.

54. Macolm-Callis KJ, Galyean ML, Duff GC: Effects of dietary supplemental protein source and a *Pasteurella haemolytica* toxoid on performance and health of newly received calves. Agri Pract 15:22, 1994.

55. McLean GS, Smith RA, Gill DR, et al: An evaluation of an inactivated, leukotoxin-rich, cell-free *Pasteurella haemolytica* vaccine for prevention of undifferentiated bovine respiratory disease. Oklahoma State University Animal Science Research Report MP-129, 135, 1990.

56. Thorlakson B, Martin W, Peters D: A field trial to evaluate the efficacy of a commercial *Pasteurella haemolytica* bacterial extract in preventing bovine respiratory disease. Can Vet J 31:573, 1990.

57. Kadel WL, Chengappa MM, Herren CE: Field-trial evaluation of a *Pasteurella* vaccine in preconditioned and nonpreconditioned lightweight calves. Am J Vet Res 46:1944, 1985.

58. Smith RA, Gill DR, Hicks RB. Improving the performance of stocker and feedlot calves with a live *Pasteurella haemolytica* vaccine. Vet Med 81:978, 1986.

59. Hill WJ, Kirkpatrick J, Gill DR, et al: The effects of Septimune on health and performance of stressed stocker cattle. Oklahoma State University Animal Science Research Report P-933, 301, 1993.

60. Frank GH, Briggs RE, Loan RW, et al: Respiratory tract disease and mucosal colonization by *Pasteurella haemolytica* in transported calves. Am J Vet Res 57:1317, 1996.

61. Amstutz HE, Horstman LA, Morter RL: Clinical evaluation of the efficacy of *Haemophilus somnus* and *Pasteurella* sp. bacterins. Bovine Pract 16:106, 1981.

62. Morter RL, Amstutz HE, Crandell RA: Clinical evaluation of prophylactic regimens for bovine respiratory disease. Bovine Pract 17:56, 1982.

63. Bennett BW: Efficacy of *Pasteurella* bacterins for yearling feedlot cattle. Bov Pract 3:26, 1982.

64. Morter RL, Amstutz HE: Evaluating the efficacy of a *Haemophilus somnus* bacterin in a controlled field trial. Bovine Pract 18:82, 1983.

65. Hjerpe CA: Clinical management of respiratory disease in feedlot cattle. Vet Clin North Am Large Anim Pract 5:119, 1983.

66. Stephens LR, Little PB, Wilkie BN, et al: Isolation of *Haemophilus somnus* antigens and their use as vaccines for prevention of bovine thromboembolic meningoencephalitis. Am J Vet Res 45:234, 1984.

67. Groom SC, Little PB: Effects of vaccination of calves against induced *Haemophilus somnus* pneumonia. Am J Vet Res 49:793, 1988.

68. Cairns R, Chu HJ, Chaves LJ, et al: Efficacy of an outer membrane complex *Haemophilus somnus* bacterin in preventing symptoms following *Haemophilus somnus* challenge. Agri Pract 14:35, 1993.

69. Bateman KG: Efficacy of a *Pasteurella haemolytica* vaccine/bacterial extract in the prevention of bovine respiratory disease in recently shipped feedlot calves. Can Vet J 29:838, 1988.

70. Martin SW, Meek AH, Davis DG, et al: Factors associated with mortality and treatment costs in feedlot calves: The Bruce County Beef Project, years 1978, 1979, 1980. Can J Comp Med 46:341, 1982.

71. Van Donkersgoed J, Schumann FJ, Harland RJ, et al: The effect of route and dosage of immunization on the serological response to a *Pasteurella haemolytica* and *Haemophilus somnus* vaccine in feedlot calves. Can Vet J 34:731, 1993.

72. Palotay JL, Christensen NR: Bovine respiratory infection I. Psittacosis–lymphogranuloma venereum group of viruses as etiological agents. J Am Vet Med Assoc 134:222, 1959.

73. Corapi WV, Donis RO, Dubovi EJ: Characterization of a panel of monoclonal antibodies and their use in the study of the antigenic diversity of bovine viral diarrhea virus. Am J Vet Res 51:1388, 1990.

74. Kelling CL, Stine LC, Rump KK, et al: Investigation of bovine viral diarrhea virus infections in a range beef cattle herd. J Am Vet Med Assoc 197:589, 1990.

75. Hudson DB, Perino LJ: Proper injection procedures for cattle. University of Nebraska NebGuide G92-1082-A, 1992.

76. Implications of stress, *In* Nutrient Requirements of Beef Cattle, ed 7. Washington, DC, National Academy Press, 1996.

■ Diagnostic Methods for Respiratory Disease

Steven D. Sorden, D.V.M., Ph.D., Diplomate, A.C.V.P.

Disease in any organ system results from alteration of the balance between host defense mechanisms and pathogens in the host's environment. Although inflammatory responses induced by infectious agents are the proximate causes of respiratory disease in food animals, the ultimate causes are those host and environmental factors that make the host more susceptible to the injurious effects of microbes that in most cases are common inhabitants of the host or environment. Diagnostic investigation that is limited to examination of animal hosts can therefore provide only a part of the total diagnostic picture of a respiratory disease problem.[1] Examination and evaluation of the host's environment (air quality, stocking density, etc.) is crucial to solving such problems, and is covered elsewhere. This discussion describes current methods used to obtain maximal diagnostic information through the examination or sampling of diseased animals or their healthy cohorts. Examination of the host enables the clinician to (1) define the nature of the disease, (2) identify the proximate causes of the disease, and (3) evaluate host factors, such as trace mineral deficiencies, that may be contributing to the herd's respiratory disease problem.

GENERAL APPROACH TO RESPIRATORY DISEASE DIAGNOSIS

The ideal approach to the diagnosis of any herd disease problem is to deliver multiple live, untreated animals in various stages of the disease process or phases of the production system to a diagnostic laboratory. This provides the laboratory with the necessary specimens with which to obtain a cross-sectional overview of the herd problem. If the ideal approach is chosen, then the clinician's most important task is to select appropriate animals for submission. *Acutely affected and untreated* animals provide the most information. Acutely affected animals usually have high fevers, clear nasal discharge, and other signs of respiratory disease of less than 24 hours' duration. The most severely affected are often not the most acutely affected.[2] The temptation to allow untrained personnel to select animals for submission should be resisted, as should the temptation to submit runts, chronic poor doers, or other individuals that are not good examples of the herd problem.

Obviously, various economic and disease constraints preclude the ideal approach in many instances. Respiratory disease problems tend to occur as acute outbreaks with high morbidity and variable mortality or, more frequently, as chronic problems of variable morbidity and mortality. *Enzootic respiratory disease* is more suited to the ideal approach. *Acute outbreaks* of respiratory disease can be further divided into predictable and unpredictable outbreaks. *Predictable acute outbreaks* allow for preonset sampling and comparison of serologic and other values in the same animal over time, in contrast to *unpredictable acute outbreaks*. In any situation, the clinician should bear the ideal approach in mind and obtain as many samples from as many different animals as circumstances allow.

EXAMINATION AND SAMPLING

Antemortem Tests

Antemortem tests demonstrate the presence of pathogens and detect immune responses to those pathogens. It is unlikely that practical, economical antemortem diagnostic techniques that approach the accuracy of postmortem examination will ever be developed; this is primarily due to the inability of antemortem tests to definitively correlate the presence of a pathogen with a characteristic lesion. However, antemortem sampling can be extremely useful, and in many cases is the only method by which a reasonable sample size can be obtained.

For the investigation of enzootic respiratory disease problems, as well as predictable acute outbreaks, serum is probably the most useful sample that can be obtained from living animals. Serologic profiling, in which a cohort of uniquely identified animals is repeatedly bled at various time points as they progress through the production system, enables the clinician to identify which pathogens the herd encounters and when in the production system seroconversion occurs. Since seroconversion indicates infection but does not necessarily indicate disease, serologic profiling is best done in conjunction with necropsy of

representative individuals. Serology may be less valuable for unpredicted acute outbreaks, especially if high mortality prevents convalescent sampling. However, particularly in the case of cattle, if individuals are to be restrained for treatment, obtaining blood samples requires little additional effort. Blood should be allowed to clot at room temperature for 1 to 2 hours, and then serum should be removed from the clot and frozen ($-20°C$). Refrigeration is adequate if sera arrive at the laboratory within 24 to 48 hours. Frozen sera can always be discarded at a later time, but it is impossible to obtain "acute" serum from convalescent animals. If possible, hold acute sera frozen until convalescent sera are drawn and submit all samples simultaneously, so that all will be tested in the same run. Formulas exist for determining the appropriate sample sizes for detecting infection in a given population.[3] For large (>100) groups, a sample size of 30 is often adequate to detect infection by most of the important respiratory pathogens. Serum can also be used to assay some trace minerals, but is not as reliable as liver.[4]

Nasal swabs are frequently used to detect respiratory pathogens in live animals. Nasal swabs can be used successfully to detect bacterial or viral causes of rhinitis, and to detect viruses that replicate in both the lung and nasal mucosa. Unfortunately, pneumonia, not rhinitis, is the major cause of morbidity and mortality due to respiratory disease. Not all pulmonary viral pathogens replicate to a great extent in the nasal mucosa, and antimicrobial sensitivity patterns of bacteria isolated from nasal swabs do not correlate well with those of bacteria isolated from lung tissue.[5] Nevertheless, nasal swabs are often the most practical method available. Cotton swabs are adequate for bacterial isolation, but most laboratories prefer Dacron-tipped swabs for virus isolation; clinicians should contact the diagnostic laboratory to which the samples will be submitted for specific instructions. Swabs should be obtained from acutely affected animals and from as deep in the nasal cavity as possible to avoid skin contaminants, and should be kept moist and chilled for transport. Swabs for bacterial culture should be shipped on ice but not frozen. Swabs for virus isolation should be handled as recommended by the particular laboratory; in general, swab aggressively in order to penetrate the mucus and obtain epithelial cells, and transport overnight on ice in an antibiotic-containing cell culture medium or viral transport medium. Freezing may be preferable if transport time is prolonged. Swabs can also be rolled onto glass slides to deposit epithelial cells, then fixed in acetone and submitted for fluorescent antibody testing for the presence of specific viruses.

Given the limitations of nasal swabs, other antemortem diagnostic techniques have been employed, particularly in cattle. Laryngotracheal swabs, using equine uterine culture swabs, allow sampling of exudate that contains microbial agents that are derived from the lung and thus are more representative of the pulmonary disease process. Bronchoalveolar lavage provides an even better sample[6] but is time-consuming and is unlikely to be employed on significant numbers of food animals.

Postmortem Examination

If the best approach is to euthanize and perform necropsies on acutely affected animals, the worst approach is to fail to perform necropsies. As many animals as possible should be examined post mortem on each visit, initially to characterize the problem, and later to monitor the response to therapy. Necropsy of 2 of 10 dead animals may be very misleading if the two animals are not representative of the herd problem. Useful information on the nature of the disease process can often be gleaned from moderately autolyzed carcasses; detection of etiologic agents usually requires minimally decomposed material.

The most important rule of tissue submission is to submit multiple samples obtained from multiple sites and animals. Pathogens are distributed nonhomogeneously within tissues and populations, and can be easily missed if, for example, only one small piece of lung from one animal is submitted to the diagnostic laboratory. As a rule, tissue samples should be submitted both fresh and in 10% neutral buffered formalin. Fresh tissue should be cooled in a refrigerator or on ice, then submitted between ice packs in a Styrofoam container. Fresh tissue should normally not be frozen, since freezing and thawing impair both bacterial culture and virus isolation. Freezing is acceptable if it will be several days before the fresh tissue can be delivered to a laboratory. In addition, tissue submitted for toxicologic examination or trace mineral analysis can usually be stored and submitted frozen. Tissue samples to be placed in formalin should generally be no larger than 2 × 2 cm and no thicker than 1 cm (0.5 cm is best). It is always preferable to submit some tissue in formalin rather than to submit only fresh tissue; tissue in formalin will be less autolyzed and can be processed immediately upon arrival at the diagnostic laboratory, resulting in more accurate and timely histopathologic diagnoses. If fixed tissue must be mailed in extremely cold weather, consider holding tissue overnight in formalin (long enough to fix if pieces are only 0.5 cm thick) and shipping in 70% ethanol, which has a much lower freezing point than neutral buffered formalin.

Lung. Most attention should be given to the lungs. The thoracic cavity should be opened so that at least one lung can be examined in situ. Excessive clear pleural fluid (transudate) should be noted but is rarely worth sampling. Fibrinous or fibrinopurulent exudate should be sampled; submission of fluid is preferable to submission of swabs. Firm, fibrous pleural adhesions in animals dying of acute respiratory disease indicate chronic or resolved pleuritis and are usually incidental findings.

If possible, the larynx, trachea, and thoracic viscera (the pluck) should be removed as a unit. The pleural surface of the excised hemithorax makes a handy field table. Open major bronchi in one lung all the way to the distal portion of the caudal lobe; *Dictyocaulus viviparous* infestation in cattle is easily missed if this is not done. Make transverse incisions into the parenchyma and examine the cut surface. The nature and distribution of lung lesions should be noted to formulate a provisional gross diagnosis and should be indicated on the diagnostic laboratory submission form. In addition to distribution, the most important feature of a lung lesion is its *texture*; firm or consolidated, swollen (cranioventral) lung tissue usually indicates bronchopneumonia and aerogenous bacterial infection, while rubbery, poorly demarcated lesions are more likely to be viral in origin. Diffusely noncollapsed, congested, and edematous lungs (interstitial pneumonia) suggest bacterial septicemia or pneumonia induced by viral infection or toxicosis. If possible, an entire lung (one side), or generous portion (hand-sized) of lesional and adjacent unaffected lung, should be submitted fresh or chilled. If both lungs are similarly affected, tissue for formalin fixation should be obtained from the contralateral lung. Submit at least four, preferably six, 0.5-cm-thick, 2-cm² pieces of lung in formalin. Sample several different areas, including cranial and caudal lobes, and be sure to include obvious lesions and the diseased-normal interface. Many small pieces from widely separated areas are much more helpful than one or two large pieces. Acute lesions most likely to hold active causative agents are usually at the diseased-normal interface. Chronic lesions in dependent tips or lobes may no longer hold primary pathogens.

Other Respiratory Tissues. Tracheobronchial lymph nodes should be submitted fresh; histologic evaluation is generally unrewarding. The larynx and trachea from at least a few animals should be opened to exclude lesions in these organs. Congestion and mild hemorrhage are common nonspecific findings in the tracheal mucosa of dyspneic animals. Mucopus derived from the lung may be coughed up and coat the tracheal mucosa; this material is easily removed and reveals normal underlying mucosa. If the trachea and bronchi are filled with froth, this should be noted, but the cause of the pulmonary edema should be sought by examining and sampling the lung and heart. Tracheal swabs for bacterial culture collected at necropsy are usually not worthwhile, and may detect aspirated normal nasal flora; bacteria isolated from lung lesions are much more significant. Erosions, ulcerations, fibrinonecrotic exudate, or submucosal edema severe enough to noticeably reduce the luminal diameter is significant, and representative 2-cm segments should be submitted both chilled and in formalin; be sure to include lesion margins. In swine, fixed and fresh palatine tonsil should always be collected. Fixed and fresh or chilled samples of turbinate should be collected if there are gross lesions or in cases of suspected acute viral pneumonia. The nasal cavity is best accessed by splitting the head; this has the added advantage of providing access to the brain. Evaluation of swine for lesions of atrophic rhinitis is the major exception to this approach (see below). Nasal swabs for bacterial culture and virus isolation should be performed as discussed above.

New Laboratory Techniques. Many diagnostic laboratories now employ immunohistochemistry (IHC) on formalin-fixed, paraffin-embedded tissues to detect viral and, less often, bacterial antigens. Advantages of this technique are that fresh tissue is not required and that lesions and antigens can be visualized simultaneously, increasing diagnostic accuracy. Turnaround time is usually only slightly longer than that of routine histology. The prime consideration for the submitter is that tissues for IHC should not be kept in formalin for more than a few days; again, overnight delivery is optimal.

Detection of viral nucleic acid by in situ hybridization or polymerase chain reaction (PCR) is more rapid than virus isolation and is not affected by the presence of neutralizing antibody. PCR can detect extremely small amounts of viral nucleic acid in a variety of samples that are unsuitable for virus isolation or viral antigen detection, and holds great promise in the antemortem diagnosis of viral respiratory infections.

SPECIES-SPECIFIC DIAGNOSTIC METHODS

Ruminants

Antemortem Diagnosis. As noted above, bacteria recovered from nasal swabs may not be identical to those causing disease in the lung, making antibiograms of these isolates of questionable validity. Pulmonary lavage fluid is the ideal antemortem specimen, but may not be practical in many situations. Laryngotracheal swabs taken from several acutely affected animals are a reasonable compromise.

Antemortem diagnosis of viral infection is often challenging. Sampling several very acutely affected animals will increase the likelihood of obtaining a positive diagnosis. Direct immunofluorescent antibody (IFA) tests on cytologic preparations (swabs rolled on a glass slide) are more reliable and economical than virus isolation.[7] Dacron-tipped swabs and viral transport media, and cotton-tipped swabs and bacterial transport media should be kept on hand so that they are available when unpredicted outbreaks occur and can be used on the first visit. Infectious bovine rhinotracheitis virus (IBRV), bovine coronavirus,[8] and parainfluenza 3 (PI-3) virus may be detected using nasal swabs, either by virus isolation or direct IFA. Bovine respiratory syncytial virus (BRSV) is best detected in lavage fluid, but may also be demonstrated by the direct FA technique on cells obtained from nasal swabs.[9] BRSV isolation is usually not worth attempting unless lavage fluid can be delivered to the laboratory in less than 1 hour.[2] Liquid nitrogen is ideal for storing specimens for virus isolation, and is available on many dairy and some beef farms; liquid nitrogen storage of swabs immersed in viral transport media should be considered if virus isolation is critical. In some laboratories, BRSV infection can be diagnosed via antigen detection with a human RSV kit.[10]

If bovine viral diarrhea virus (BVDV) or border disease infection is suspected, serum and whole (heparinized) blood should be obtained and submitted chilled for virus isolation attempts. Persistent infection is easily demonstrated by virus isolation from serum. In acutely infected immunocompetent animals, virus may only be present in peripheral blood mononuclear cells (buffy coat).[11] Store half of each serum sample frozen; uniquely identified animals can be resampled 3 to 4 weeks later for paired serology.

Postmortem Examination. Tissue collected as described in the preceding section will be adequate for most cases of respiratory disease in cattle and small ruminants. *Pasteurella haemolytica*, *Pasteurella multocida*, and *Haemophilis somnus* are routinely isolated from lung tissue. The characteristic feature of fibrinous pleuropneumonia induced by *P. haemolytica* is the irregular, dry, pale or hemorrhagic areas of parenchymal necrosis observable on the cut surface of the lung; this feature is more reliable than the presence of fibrin on the pleural surface or within interlobular septa. Within a few days, zones of necrosis develop thin, pale borders representing leukocytic infiltrates. Bronchopneumonia without obvious necrosis, as seen in enzootic pneumonia in calves or lambs, is usually associated with *P. multocida* or *H. somnus* infection; these cannot be reliably distinguished grossly. Other thoracic lesions induced by *H. somnus* in cattle include fibrinous pleuritis without pneumonia, and myocarditis. The myocardium should be incised in multiple sites so that the latter lesion is not missed. *H. somnus* myocarditis is characterized by pale, friable areas that are usually most prominent in the papillary muscles of the left ventricle. If present, fixed and fresh samples of these lesions should be submitted. Multiple abscesses 1 to 5 mm in diameter (bronchiectasis) within cranioventral lung lobes usually indicate infection with *Mycoplasma bovis* or other mycoplasmas, and are frequently seen in conjunction with chronic fibrinous arthritis. *M. bovis* can be detected via culture of lung tissue or joint fluid, or via IHC on formalin-fixed lung or joint capsule.[12]

Direct FA tests or IHC can be performed on lung tissue for IBRV, PI-3 virus, BRSV, BVDV, and coronavirus.[8] IBRV, PI-3 virus, and BVDV are the viruses most likely to be isolated from lung. The characteristic fibrinonecrotic rhinotracheitis induced by IBRV is almost pathognomonic. This lesion may extend into major bronchi. Direct FA tests on fresh trachea or nasal turbinate with erosions or ulcers will confirm the diagnosis. Viral pneumonias are usually complicated by secondary bacterial infection. PI-3 virus infection by itself is almost never fatal. Severe BRSV pneumonia can be fatal, and is characterized by cranioventral red-brown, collapsed lung, and caudodorsal lung that is noncollapsed due to emphysema, edema, and in some cases interstitial pneumonia. Several areas of the cranioventral lung should be submitted fresh, especially from the diseased-normal interface, and both samples of cranial and caudal lung should be submitted in formalin.

Several additional tissues are required to diagnose BVDV infection. Fixed and fresh samples of spleen, liver, kidney, thymus, ileum, and mesenteric lymph node should be included, as well as fixed samples of any mucosal ulcers or erosions from the oral cavity, esophagus, forestomachs, abomasum, or interdigital skin. Virus isolation and IHC are the most reliable methods. The rapid, direct FA technique is prone to give both false-positive and false-negative results.[13] Although not as sensitive as IHC, virus isolation is necessary if determination of viral strain, genotype, or biotype is desired.

Noninfectious interstitial pneumonias are primarily seen in pastured cattle (acute bovine pulmonary edema and emphysema, or fog fever, induced by 3-methylindole), or feedlot cattle (idiopathic). Lungs are noncollapsed, rubbery, and mottled or diffusely red brown. Interlobular edema and emphysema are frequently but not always observed. The two syndromes are differentiated on the basis of the presence or absence of a history of access to lush pasture. There is currently no way to determine whether or not a particular lesion was induced by metabolites of 3-methylindole. Histology and IHC or FA tests should be utilized to differentiate these syndromes from interstitial pneumonia induced by BRSV.

Sampling to Evaluate Factors Contributing to Respiratory Disease. Trace mineral analysis is best done on liver, which can be frozen for this purpose. Frozen liver, kidney (with fat), rumen contents, and brain can be held if a toxicosis is suspected. Lesions of white muscle disease can be detected in formalin-fixed heart, tongue, diaphragm, and hind limb muscle. Evaluation of body condition should be included in any necropsy study; depletion or serous atrophy of fat indicates preexisting malnutrition or prolonged illness. Fresh feces and formalin-fixed samples of abomasum (*Ostertagia*, *Haemonchus*) and small intestine and colon (coccidia) may assist in ruling in underlying parasitism. Brain should be included if nervous signs or sudden death has been observed; section longitudinally and submit one half in formalin and one half fresh or chilled, and be sure to include the brain stem.

Swine

Antemortem Study

Serology is commonly used to detect exposure to porcine respiratory pathogens.[14] The general principles discussed earlier are applicable. Bacterial culture of nasal and tonsillar swabs has been used to detect the presence of toxigenic *P. multocida* type D; direct detection of the dermonecrotic toxin gene via PCR may replace culture in the next few years.[15] Swine influenza virus (SIV) and porcine respiratory corona virus (PRCV) can be isolated from nasal swabs, using the general approach outlined above. Again, swabs from deep in the nasal cavity of multiple acutely affected animals are critical. Clinicians should contact the diagnostic laboratory prior to submitting samples to familiarize themselves with the specific media and specimens, preferred by that laboratory.

Postmortem Examination

Euthanasia and necropsy of clinically affected pigs is often the most cost-effective method by which to diagnose a respiratory problem. In contrast to cattle, individual pigs have a low enough economic value relative to that of the entire herd or unit that submission of several live pigs to a diagnostic laboratory is an affordable investment. Selection of appropriate individuals is discussed above. If necropsies are performed by the clinician, samples should be collected as described below. Serum should always be collected from euthanized pigs; blood is most easily obtained from the axillary artery after a front limb is reflected immediately following euthanasia.

Porcine Reproductive and Respiratory Syndrome (PRRS). The respiratory form of PRRS is characterized by mottled tan, noncollapsed lungs and generalized lymph node enlargement. Collect fixed and fresh lung, tracheobronchial lymph nodes, and tonsil from euthanized pigs. Histology and IHC allow demonstration of typical lesions and viral antigen in the same piece of tissue.[16] Sampling multiple areas of the lung is absolutely critical, since antigen is often widely scattered. If obtaining a viral isolate is important, lung lavage fluid is the best specimen, since lavage harvests macrophages from throughout the lung.[17] Lavage requires an intact lung or lung lobe, depending on the size of the pig, and can be performed with a 20-mL pipette or large catheter-tip syringe using cell culture medium or saline. Insert the tip of the pipette or syringe into the trachea or bronchus and instill enough fluid to moderately distend the lung. Aspirate and reinstill the fluid three times. Final recovery of even 30% to 50% of the original 30- to 60-mL volume is satisfactory. Lavage fluid should be frozen if it will not arrive at the laboratory within 24 to 48 hours. PRRS virus is not stable in autolyzed tissue, and virus isolation attempts from such tissues are unlikely to be successful.

Swine Influenza Virus. Acute SIV infection typically produces lungs with multiple coalescing red to hemorrhagic lobules, predominantly in the cranioventral lung. Secondary bacterial infection is common and makes a presumptive diagnosis of swine influenza on the basis of gross lesions alone very difficult. Direct FA testing is most likely to demonstrate SIV antigen in bronchi near the hilus, especially at the diseased-normal interface. Autolytic sloughing of airway epithelium greatly impairs the sensitivity of this test, so submission of live pigs or tissue from euthanized pigs is optimal. Again, histology and IHC allow demonstration of typical lesions and viral antigen in the same piece of tissue.[18] SIV replicates in the lung for only a few days following infection, and typical microscopic lesions (necrotizing bronchitis and bronchiolitis) are often present in the absence of detectable antigen. Virus isolation can also be performed on lung or nasal turbinate.

Mycoplasma byopneumoniae. Sharply demarcated areas of tan-purple consolidation in the cranioventral lung are suggestive of mycoplasmal pneumonia, but laboratory confirmation is required for definitive diagnosis. Direct FA testing on fresh lung and histopathologic examination are the primary postmortem diagnostic tools. Large airways near the diseased-normal interface are best for direct FA testing; as in the case of SIV, autolysis frequently results in false-negative results. Typical microscopic lesions are highly suggestive but not pathognomonic. Isolation of *M. hyopneumoniae* (Mh) is difficult and expensive, and is generally not attempted. Seroconversion in conjunction with typical lesions provides a presumptive diagnosis; seroconversion occurs 1 to 3 weeks following the onset of coughing, depending on the assay utilized.[19] An IHC test for Mh antigen, enabling demonstration of Mh antigen within typical lesions, is greatly needed.

Pseudorabies. Respiratory disease associated with pseudorabies virus infection is more common in growing-finishing pigs than in neonates, in which the nervous form tends to predominate. Fixed and fresh tonsil and brain should be submitted for histology, direct FA, and virus isolation. Virus isolation provides definitive evidence of infection but may require up to 2 weeks. Direct FA testing is rapid, but false-positives and -negatives are possible; FA results should be correlated with typical microscopic lesions. A variety of serotests for PRV infection are available, and serodiagnosis is often the most reliable method in older pigs.[20]

Porcine Respiratory Corona Virus. PRCV is an uncommon cause of significant respiratory disease, but may be a problem in occasional herds. Nasal swabs or turbinates from acutely affected pigs are required for virus isolation, and isolation is required to distinguish this virus from transmissible gastroenteritis virus (TGEV). Positive direct FA or IHC testing using monoclonal antibodies to TGEV provides presumptive evidence of PRCV infection, as does seroconversion to TGEV in herds without enteric disease.[21]

Actinobacillus pleuropneumoniae. Typical lesions of fibrinohemorrhagic pleuropneumonia are usually caused by *A. pleuro-*

pneumoniae, but *Actinobacillus suis* and, less commonly, *Salmonella choleraesuis* may produce grossly indistinguishable lesions. Histology will confirm the lesion, but bacterial culture of fresh lung is required to diagnose *A. pleuropneumoniae* infection. Coagglutination tests on fresh lung may be helpful in detecting antigen in culture-negative lungs. Recently, isolates that are biochemically intermediate between *Actinobacillus* and *Pasteurella* have become more common; these require genetic analysis for definitive identification.[22]

Other Bacterial Pneumonias. *P. multocida* type A is the most common bacterial secondary invader. *Streptococcus suis* and *Haemophilus parasuis* are also frequent isolates from porcine bronchopneumonias. Since these three organisms are present in the nasal cavities or tonsils of healthy pigs, isolation from diseased lung and microscopic demonstration of compatible lesions is recommended.[23] Isolation of *S. choleraesuis* from lung is always significant. Fixed and fresh liver, spleen, kidney, lymph node, and intestine should be included if septicemic salmonellosis is suspected.

Rhinitis. In pigs less than 30 to 40 lb, heads should be split longitudinally, nasal and tonsillar swabs obtained for bacterial culture, and fixed and fresh samples of turbinate obtained. In growing-finishing pigs, snouts should be sectioned at the level of the first or second premolar to evaluate turbinate atrophy prior to obtaining samples. In severe cases, gross lesions are diagnostic of progressive atrophic rhinitis. In mild cases, histology reveals suppurative rhinitis and fibrous replacement of turbinate bone.[24] Toxigenic *P. multocida* type D is most easily isolated from tonsil. Inclusion body rhinitis (porcine cytomegalovirus) infection is most easily diagnosed histologically.

Sampling to Evaluate Factors Contributing to Respiratory Disease

Gross and microscopic evaluation of heart to rule out mulberry heart disease should be performed if there is pulmonary edema and pericardial effusion. Liver is the best tissue for assessment of vitamin E and selenium status. Heart should also be sampled to detect inflammatory lesions associated with PRSV infection.

In 1997, a disease referred to as postweaning multisystemic wasting syndrome was described in western Canada.[25] This syndrome also occurs sporadically in the United States. Progressive weight loss is the most common clinical sign. At necropsy, most pigs have interstitial pneumonia characterized by noncollapsed, gray, mottled lungs, and severe lymph node enlargement. Porcine circovirus infection has been associated with this syndrome. The diagnosis is based on histologic demonstration of characteristic lesions.[25] Submissions should include fixed brain, tonsil, lung, lymph node, thymus, heart, liver, kidney, pancreas, spleen, stomach, duodenum, ileum, and colon.

REFERENCES

1. Hancock D: Strategic laboratory use: How to use hypothesis-based laboratory testing. Bovine Pract 28:118–125, 1996.
2. Dubovi EJ: Diagnosing BRSV infection: A laboratory perspective. Vet Med 88:888–893, 1993.
3. Thrushfield MV: Veterinary Epidemiology. London, Butterworth, 1986, p 158.
4. Wikse SE, Herd D, Field RW, et al: Diagnosis of copper deficiency in cattle. J Am Vet Med Assoc 200:1625–1629, 1992.
5. Clarke CR: Live animal sampling for antibacterial susceptibility testing. Bovine Pract 27:150–151, 1995.
6. Kimman TG, Zimmer GM, Straver PJ, et al. Diagnosis of bovine respiratory syncytial virus infections improved by virus detection in lung lavage samples. Am J Vet Res 47:143–147, 1986.

7. Kennedy GA: Diagnostic considerations for bovine respiratory disease. Bovine Pract 29:142–146, 1997.
8. Kapil S, Goyal SM: Bovine coronavirus-associated respiratory disease. Compend Contin Educ Pract Vet 17:1179–1181, 1995.
9. Elvander M: Severe respiratory disease in dairy cows caused by infection with bovine respiratory syncytial virus. Vet Rec 138:101–105, 1996.
10. Osorio FA, Anderson GA, Sanders JS, et al: Detection of bovine respiratory syncytial virus antigen using a heterologous antigen-capture enzyme immunoassay. J Vet Diagn Invest 1:210–214, 1989.
11. Dubovi EJ: Laboratory diagnosis of bovine viral diarrhea virus infections. Vet Med 91:867–872, 1996.
12. Adegboye DS, Rasberry U, Halbur PG, et al: Monoclonal antibody-based immunohistochemical technique for the detection of Mycoplasma bovis in formalin-fixed, paraffin-embedded calf lung tissues. J Vet Diagn Invest 7:261–265, 1995.
13. Ellis JA, Martin K, Norman GR, et al: Comparison of detection methods for bovine viral diarrhea virus in abortions and neonatal death. J Vet Diagn Invest 7:433–436, 1995.
14. Hill H: Interpretation of serologic results of some important swine diseases. Compend Contin Educ Pract Vet 10:979–985, 1988.
15. Kamp EM, Bokken GCAM, Vermeulen TMM, et al: A specific and sensitive PCR assay suitable for large-scale detection of toxigenic Pasteurella multocida in nasal and tonsillar swabs specimens of pigs. J Vet Diagn Invest 8:304–309, 1996.
16. Halbur PG, Andrews JJ, Huffman EL, et al: Development of a streptavidin-biotin immunoperoxidase procedure for the detection of porcine reproductive and respiratory syndrome virus antigen in porcine lung. J Vet Diagn Invest 6:254–257, 1994.
17. Mengeling WL, Lager KM, Vorwald AC: Diagnosis of porcine reproductive and respiratory syndrome. J Vet Diagn Invest 7:3–16, 1995.
18. Vincent LL, Janke BH, Paul PS, et al: A monoclonal-antibody-based immunohistochemical method for the detection of swine influenza virus in formalin-fixed, paraffin-embedded tissues. J Vet Diagn Invest 9:191–195, 1997.
19. Bereiter M, Young TF, Joo HS, et al: Evaluation of the ELISA and comparison to the complement fixation test and radial immunodiffusion enzyme assay for detection of antibodies against Mycoplasma hyopneumoniae in swine serum. Vet Microbiol 25:177–192, 1990.
20. Kluge JP, Beran GW, Hill HT, et al: Pseudorabies (Aujeszky's disease). In Leman AD, Straw BE, Mengeling WL (eds): Diseases of Swine, ed 7. Ames, Iowa State University Press, 1992, pp 312–323.
21. Paul PS, Halbur PG, Vaughn EM: Significance of porcine respiratory coronavirus infection. Compend Contin Educ Pract Vet 16:1223–1233, 1994.
22. Fenwick B, Henry S: Porcine pleuropneumonia. J Am Vet Med Assoc 204:1334–1340, 1994.
23. Straw BE, Dewey CE, Erickson ED: Interpreting culture reports from swine lungs. Swine Health Prod 4:200–201, 1996.
24. De Jong MF: (Progressive) atrophic rhinitis. In Leman AD, Straw BE, Mengeling WL (eds): Diseases of Swine, ed 7. Ames, Iowa State University Press, 1992, pp 414–435.
25. Clark EG: Post-weaning multisystemic wasting syndrome. In Proceedings of the American Association of Swine Practitioners, 1997, pp 499–501.

■ Parasites of the Respiratory System

Robert K. Ridley, D.V.M., Ph.D.

Although lungworms are found in cattle, sheep, pigs, and goats, the most important parasite of the respiratory system in food animals worldwide is *Dictyocaulus viviparus*, the only lungworm found in cattle. In the United States, dictyocaulosis has been reported sporadically from different parts of the country, but it is most often associated with cool, moist climates. *Dictyocaulus viviparus* larvae have been reported to survive winters on heavily contaminated pastures as far north as Canada, so extensive movement of cattle may result in clinical disease in areas where formerly it was not considered a problem. *D. filaria*, *Muellerius capillaris*, and *Protostrongylus rufescens* are found in sheep and goats. *D. filaria* has about the same distribution as *D. viviparus*; *Muellerius* occurs infrequently and *Protostrongylus* is thought to be uncommon in domesticated animals in the United States and Canada. However, a disease outbreak associated with *Protostrongylus* in a flock of sheep in Maryland may alert veterinarians to include lungworms in the differential diagnosis of sheep with respiratory tract signs, especially if they do not respond to antibiotic therapy.[1] *Metastrongylus apri* is the common lungworm found in pigs.

Dictyocaulus viviparus

Life Cycle

Female *D. viviparus* in the trachea and bronchi produce embryonated eggs that are coughed up, swallowed, and usually hatch while still in the digestive tract, so L_1 larvae are found in fresh bovine feces. Under favorable conditions, first-stage larvae develop to the infective third stage in less than a week. A coprophilic fungus (*Pilobolus* spp.) greatly facilitates the spread of larvae on pasture. The infective larvae ascend the fungus as it grows on the dung pat and invade the sporangia. When the sporangia rupture, the infective larvae are dispersed with the fungal sores. Cattle are infected when they ingest infective third-stage larvae from contaminated pastures. The third-stage larvae penetrate the intestine and migrate via the lymphatics to the mesenteric lymph nodes, where they molt to the fourth stage and gain access to the blood vascular system. From here they are carried to the lungs and penetrate the alveoli. Adult worms are found in the trachea and bronchi. It takes 3 or 4 weeks for worms to reach maturity and start producing larvae. Mature females are up to 80 mm long; males are smaller with long, heavy spicules. The life cycle of *D. filaria* is essentially the same as that of *D. viviparus*.

The metastrongylid nematodes, unlike *Dictyocaulus*, have indirect life cycles and require intermediate hosts. *Muellerius* and *Protostrongylus* use a mollusk (slugs) and *Metastrongylus* requires an earthworm. Transplacental transmission apparently occurs in *P. rufescens* in sheep because larvae have been found in ovine fetuses and newborn lambs.

Pathogenesis

Larvae migrating through the alveoli and bronchioles produce an inflammatory response that may block small bronchi and bronchioles with inflammatory exudate. The bronchi contain fluid and immature worms; adult worms and the exudate they produce also block the bronchi. Secondary bacterial pneumonia and concurrent viral infection are often complications of dictyocaulosis. Because the larvae migrate through the lymphatics, a good immunologic response is usually seen beginning a week or so after the initial infection, and the disease lasts only 3 to 4 weeks if few larvae are ingested and acute disease does not occur. In the absence of continued exposure to infective larvae, immunity wanes and reinfection will occur if the animals are placed on contaminated pasture the next grazing season. Prior infection with *Ostertagia* spp. and *Cooperia* spp. exacerbates subsequent lungworm infections in cattle, whether or not the worms are in the gut at the time. *D. viviparus* recovered from animals previously infected with those two gastrointestinal worms were more numerous and larger than lungworms recovered from cattle that did not have *Ostertagia* and *Cooperia* infections. Although the mechanism of this is not fully known, it is tempting to speculate that other trichostrongylid nematodes can also influence the course of lungworm infection in cattle.

Clinical Signs

Clinical signs of dictyocaulosis range from none to a mild cough with no deterioration in condition, through a more severe cough, rapid weight loss, and death. Clinical disease is most frequently seen in young animals 4 to 6 months of age running in pasture. Subacute forms of this verminous pneumonia do not result in heavy death losses, but the lungs may be badly affected. Treatment will rid the host of the parasites but does not necessarily result in resolving the lesions. *D. filaria* causes a severe parasitic bronchitis in sheep (husk, verminous pneumonia). *Metastrongylus apri* produces similar signs in pigs.

Diagnosis

Although clinical signs in endemic areas are suggestive of dictyocaulosis, definitive antemortem diagnosis depends on finding the first-stage larvae in fresh feces. (*Dictyocaulus* larvae are the only nematode larvae found in rectal samples of bovine feces.) Larval recovery is usually done with the Baermann technique, although some investigators believe that zinc sulfate flotation is equally or more effective. Practitioners should be aware that it is necessary to set up Baermann examinations shortly after feces are passed because first-stage *Dictyocaulus* larvae become lethargic quickly and are not recovered in Baermann funnels after being subjected to refrigerator temperatures. In our laboratory, just holding fecal samples in obstetric sleeves at room temperature overnight significantly reduced the recovery of L_1 larvae by the Baermann technique. Obtaining rectal samples will obviate the need to distinguish L_1 *Dictyocaulus* larvae from the free-living larvae found as normal inhabitants of soil. It should also be noted that larvae will not be found when the disease is caused by immature worms.

Adults are easily found in the trachea and bronchi at necropsy, but finding immature stages usually necessitates dissecting the pulmonary tissue and either allowing it to sit in physiologic saline or baermannizing the tissue in physiologic saline. Immunodiagnostic tests, including a dipstick immunoassay, have recently been developed but are not yet commercially available.

Like *Dictyocaulus*, antemortem diagnosis of *Muellerius* and *Protostrongylus* depends on finding larvae in the feces. In sheep, it is necessary to differentiate between *D. filaria*, *Muellerius* spp., and *Protostrongylus* spp. *D. filaria* first-stage larvae are 0.5 mm in length and have a distinct "knob" on the anterior end. *Muellerius* and *Protostrongylus* are shorter, about 0.3 mm in length.

Epidemiology

Arrested development (hypobiosis) is a phenomenon usually associated with *Ostertagia ostertagi*. It has also been found that *D. viviparus* can cause arrest in the lungs of animals early in the fifth stage (adult). Animals that harbor arrested stages do not show clinical signs and are "silent carriers." Arrested immature worms are thought to constitute a part of naturally acquired lungworm infections and result in pasture contamination when conditions become favorable for their survival. Because hypobiosis has been demonstrated in *D. viviparus*, one cannot assume that the pastures are safe in spring after a severe winter. One also assumes that "silent carriers" may carry the infection through other times when larvae would be unlikely to survive on pasture, e.g., a hot, dry summer.

Because most animals at pasture carry both *Ostertagia* and *Cooperia* infestations, bringing cattle from areas where lungworms are endemic to areas where lungworms were formally not a problem may result in economic losses because of the synergistic effects of lungworm infection.

Comparatively few larvae, when ingested by susceptible animals, will result in unsafe pastures over the course of a grazing season. Only a few are needed because over time the pasture will become so heavily contaminated with larvae that the infection will be potentially fatal if susceptible calves are introduced and allowed to graze.

Neither of the metastrongylid nematodes (*Muellerius* or *Protostrongylus*) is a major pathogen because unlike *Dictyocaulus* spp., which have direct life cycles, both *Protostrongylus* and *Muellerius* spp. require a mollusk (land snail or slug) as an intermediate host and these are not ingested in large enough numbers to cause serious disease.

Treatment

D. viviparus is one of the few parasites for which an effective vaccine is available, although not in the United States. The vaccine is composed of irradiated larvae that are not killed but survive long enough to reach the mesenteric lymph nodes and elicit an immune response. Most irradiated larvae die before reaching the lungs; however, some do reach the lungs and produce eggs, so the use of this vaccine in areas not known to be contaminated with *Dictyocaulus* is contraindicated.

Anthelmintics approved for treating *D. viviparus* infection in beef and nonlactating dairy cattle include albendazole* (paste, suspension), oxfendazole† (paste, suspension, intraruminal injection), levamisole‡ (drench, bolus, pour-on, injectable solution, feed additive), ivermectin§ (injectable solution, pour-on, sustained-release bolus), and doramectin¶ (injectable solution).[2]

Fenbendazole# (paste, suspension, free-choice mineral, molasses and protein blocks) is the only anthelmintic approved for treating *D. viviparus* in beef and lactating dairy cattle. There is no milk withdrawal time with fenbendazole. Withdrawal times for the aforementioned anthelmintics vary widely, and the label should be consulted before animals are sent to slaughter.[2]

Treatment should be initiated as soon as clinical signs appear and a positive diagnosis is made. Such timely treatment will prevent the disease from progressing and minimize further pasture contamination and consequent continued infection and increasing parasite burden in commingled animals.

Ivomec Sheep Drench is effective against lungworms and nose bots in sheep, and Ivomec for Swine is labeled for *M. apri* in pigs.[2] Levamisole is also very effective in controlling lungworms in pigs. There are no approved anthelmintics for controlling lungworms in goats, but *Muellerius* and *Protostrongylus* infections, because there are few worms involved, usually do not warrant anthelmintic intervention. The choice of anthelmintic will be dictated by whether gastrointestinal nematodes, especially inhibited *Ostertagia*, are present.

OTHER PARASITES

Oestrus ovis

"Nose bots" are larvae of dipteran flies. These flies are active from late spring until autumn during the hot part of the day and larviposit around the nostrils of sheep. The larvae develop

---

*Valbazen, Pfizer Animal Health, Exton, Pa.

†Synanthic, Fort Dodge Laboratories, Fort Dodge, Iowa.

‡Levasol, Tramisol, Totalon; Mallinckrodt Veterinary, Inc., Mundelein, Ill; Agri Laboratories, Ltd., St. Joseph, Mo; Aspen Veterinary Resources, Ltd., Kansas City, Mo.

§Ivomec, Merck AgVet Division, Merck & Co., Rahway, NJ.

¶Dectomax, Pfizer, Inc., North American Region, Animal Health Group, Exton, Pa.

#Panacur, Safe-Guard, Hoechst Roussel Vet, Somerville, NJ.

through the second and third instars in the frontal and maxillary sinuses of the host. Third-instar larvae crawl out of the sinuses and pupate for 10 to 70 days in the ground. The complete life cycle takes from 2 to 10 months, so there is usually only one cycle per year. When the flies are active, sheep will seek shade, keep their noses to the ground, or try to protect their nostrils in the wool of other sheep. The first-instar maggot causes a mucoid to mucopurulent nasal discharge. Because the second- and third-instar larvae have small keratinized oral hooks and ventral spines, these stages can traumatize the nasal mucosa and produce hemorrhage, causing blood in the nasal discharge. If the larvae die in situ, they may become calcified or cause abscesses. Occasionally, *Oestrus* larvae penetrate through the sinuses to the brain and cause death. Clinically, sheep infested with nose bots will sneeze and shake their heads in futile attempts to dislodge the larvae. Except for the aforementioned nasal secretions, sheep infected with nose bots appear in good health.

Ascaris suum

Although ascarids do not occur as adults in the respiratory system of food animals, in pigs, migrating larvae can cause respiratory signs ("thumps") when they reach the lungs. Details of ascariasis in pigs are covered elsewhere in the section on porcine respiratory disease complex.

Cryptosporidium Species

Respiratory cryptosporidiosis has recently been described in a suckling calf simultaneously infected with intestinal cryptosporidia. *Cryptosporidium* organisms were recovered at necropsy from unciliated bronchial epithelial cells.[3]

REFERENCES

1. Mansfield LS, Gamble HR, Baker JS, et al: Lungworm infection in a sheep flock in Maryland. J Am Vet Med Assoc 202:601–606, 1993.
2. Arroija-Dechert A (ed): Compendium of Veterinary Products, ed 4. Port Huron, Mich, Adrian J Bailey, 1997.
3. Mascaro C, Arnedo T, Rosales MJ: Respiratory cryptosporidiosis in a bovine. J Parasitol 80:334–336, 1994.

■ Respiratory Disease Therapeutics

Mike Apley, D.V.M., Ph.D., Diplomate, A.C.V.C.P.

We are fortunate in the veterinary profession to have a large selection of antimicrobial compounds for the therapy of respiratory disease in food animals. While providing us with many therapeutic options, this situation also places a high demand on our ability to select the most appropriate agent for each situation. A balance must be struck between efficacy, cost, and regulatory considerations. Further challenges include the consideration of combination antimicrobial therapy, ancillary therapy, pathogen susceptibility profile interpretation, and the evaluation of antimicrobial selection within the context of other factors affecting response to therapy. Withdrawal information for extralabel drug use may be acquired through the Food Animal Residue Avoidance Databank (FARAD). Unfortunately, at the time of this writing, funding for FARAD has been discontinued and the future of this valuable resource is uncertain.

INTERPRETING SUSCEPTIBILITY PROFILES

The ideal method for determining microbial susceptibility profiles is to do serial dilution minimal inhibitory concentration (MIC) determinations on each isolate. Unfortunately, economics and current techniques prohibit this procedure on a large scale, so we are forced to select "breakpoints." We speculate that if pathogen growth is inhibited in the laboratory by concentrations of an antimicrobial which are achievable in the animal (serum or plasma), then the pathogen will be "susceptible" in vivo. This first concentration is used as the susceptible or moderately susceptible breakpoint.

A higher concentration is also used in the laboratory to check for pathogen growth inhibition if the susceptible concentration did not inhibit growth. This becomes the moderately susceptible or resistant breakpoint. Antimicrobial concentrations above this point are considered clinically unreasonable, and pathogens still growing at this breakpoint concentration would likely be resistant in clinical cases.

Plate dilution systems (Sensititer) typically use two wells, one at each of the breakpoint concentrations. These are the breakpoint concentrations reported in Tables 1, 2, and 3. An example of interpretation using standard oxytetracycline breakpoints is shown in Figure 1. Kirby-Bauer susceptibility tests (zone of inhibition around an antimicrobial disk) also use breakpoints. The breakpoint concentrations are converted to zone diameters. Points to keep in mind when interpreting susceptibility results include the following:

1. The pharmacokinetic values used to arrive at the breakpoints represent estimates of the mean for a population. This applies well to production medicine, but we should expect significant variations within individual animals. Newer antimicrobials have breakpoints determined through animal trials.

2. Even more variation is introduced into the equation when susceptibility summaries, such as in Tables 1 through 3, are used to select therapy for an individual animal or production unit. This is especially true for susceptibility summaries from another area of the country. Repeated sampling within a group of animals will give the best analysis.

3. The laboratory conditions under which susceptibility testing occurs (aerobic, neutral pH, debris-free) are ideal for most antimicrobials. In vivo conditions may adversely affect efficacy. For example, aminoglycosides bind readily to cellular debris, are inactive in anaerobic conditions due to reliance on an oxygen-dependent uptake system into pathogens, and exhibit decreased efficacy in environments with a decreased pH. Extrapolation of sulfonamide susceptibility results to clinical efficacy is also particularly frustrating because of environmental effects.

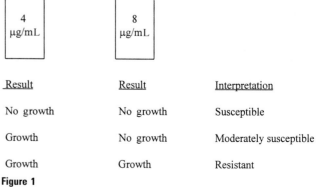

4 µg/mL	8 µg/mL	
Result	Result	Interpretation
No growth	No growth	Susceptible
Growth	No growth	Moderately susceptible
Growth	Growth	Resistant

Figure 1

Susceptibility results using breakpoint concentrations, oxytetracycline example.

Table 1
SUSCEPTIBILITY PROFILES FOR SELECTED BOVINE RESPIRATORY PATHOGENS SUBMITTED TO THE IOWA STATE UNIVERSITY DIAGNOSTIC LABORATORY FOR THE PERIOD APRIL 1996 TO DECEMBER 1996

Antimicrobial	Breakpoints	Pasteurella haemolytica (%) (N = 75)			Pasteurella multocida (%) (N = 67)		
		Sus.	M. Sus.	Res.	Sus.	M. Sus.	Res.
Amikacin	16, 32	97	0	0	94	3	3
Gentamicin	4, 8	97	0	0	97	3	0
Neomycin	8	79	—	19	81	—	19
Spectinomycin	8, 16	3	5	89	13	36	51
Apramycin	8, 16	27	68	3	28	49	22
Penicillin	0.12, 2	33	45	19	96	0	4
Ampicillin	0.25, 2	83	1	13	96	0	4
Ceftiofur	1, 2	97	0	0	97	1	1
Cephalothin	8, 16	96	1	0	97	1	1
Tilmicosin	6.25, 12.5	88	3	24	85	10	4
Erythromycin	0.5, 4	0	87	11	4	79	16
Tylosin tartrate	5, 10	1	1	95	4	6	90
Tetracycline	4, 8	76	5	16	87	9	4
Sulfadimethoxine	20, 40	17	5	75	7	7	85
Sulfachlorpyridazine	20, 40	43	39	16	18	13	69
Trimethoprim-sulfadiazine	1/19, 2/38	97	0	0	96	1	3
Clindamycin	0.5, 4	1	7	89	1	3	96

Sus., susceptible; M. Sus., moderately susceptible; Res., resistant.

4. Realize that breakpoints are economically mandated compromises indicating which of three zones (susceptible, moderately susceptible, or resistant) that an isolate is in. Figure 2 illustrates that a moderately susceptible organism could be almost susceptible or almost resistant.

Suggested Susceptibility Test Interpretation Guidelines for Production Animal Settings

1. Susceptibility patterns from a single case extrapolated to an entire population or production unit can be misleading both as to the pathogen(s) involved and the susceptibility profile of the isolate. Repeated profiles should be coupled with observations of clinical response to evaluate drug therapy. (Would you rely on an unpaired titer for a definitive diagnosis?)

2. Keep track of, and pay close attention to, changes in susceptibility profiles over time, especially in different production units. Changes in laboratories may bring about changes in susceptibility profiles. When changing laboratories, check to see if the new laboratory uses NCCLS standards (National Committee for Clinical Laboratory Standards) to ensure consistency.

3. Place the most weight on susceptibility profiles from un-

Table 2
SUSCEPTIBILITY PROFILES FOR SELECTED PORCINE RESPIRATORY PATHOGENS SUBMITTED TO THE IOWA STATE UNIVERSITY DIAGNOSTIC LABORATORY FOR THE PERIOD APRIL 1996 TO DECEMBER 1996

Antimicrobial	Breakpoints	Actinobacillus suis (%) (N = 49)			Actinobacillus pleuropneumoniae 1 (%) (N = 67)			Actinobacillus pleuropneumoniae 5 (%) (N = 73)			Actinobacillus pleuropneumoniae 7 (%) (N = 55)		
		Sus.	M. Sus.	Res.	Sus.	M. Sus.	Res.	Sus.	M. Sus.	Res.	Sus.	M. Sus.	Res.
Amikacin	16, 32	100	0	0	97	1	1	100	0	0	100	0	0
Gentamicin	4, 8	100	0	0	97	1	1	100	0	0	98	2	0
Neomycin	8	92	—	8	90	—	10	100	—	0	85	—	15
Spectinomycin	8, 16	2	4	94	13	22	64	3	12	85	11	13	76
Apramycin	8, 16	84	20	0	69	27	4	23	69	8	22	76	2
Penicillin	0.12, 2	35	43	22	6	49	45	23	77	0	5	31	64
Ampicillin	0.25, 2	80	4	12	57	1	42	99	1	0	38	2	58
Ceftiofur	1, 2	100	0	0	100	0	0	100	0	0	96	0	4
Cephalothin	8, 16	100	0	0	100	0	0	100	0	0	100	0	0
Tilmicosin	6.25, 12.5	98	2	0	94	6	0	63	34	3	62	38	0
Erythromycin	0.5, 4	0	100	0	0	88	12	0	56	44	0	64	36
Tylosin tartrate	5, 10	4	0	96	1	12	87	1	5	93	4	4	93
Tetracycline	4, 8	41	33	27	24	40	36	58	22	21	24	13	64
Sulfadimethoxine	20, 40	61	4	35	7	0	93	4	4	92	11	5	84
Sulfachlorpyridazine	20, 40	84	12	4	51	15	34	23	21	56	24	36	40
Trimethoprim-sulfadiazine	1/19, 2/38	100	0	0	100	0	0	100	0	0	100	0	0
Clindamycin	0.5, 4	0	57	43	0	97	3	1	81	18	2	89	9
Tiamulin	8, 16	67	2	0	70	25	4	52	42	5	67	25	7

For abbreviations, see footnote to Table 1.

Table 3
SUSCEPTIBILITY PROFILES FOR SELECTED PORCINE RESPIRATORY PATHOGENS SUBMITTED TO THE IOWA STATE UNIVERSITY DIAGNOSTIC LABORATORY FOR THE PERIOD APRIL 1996 TO APRIL 1997

Antimicrobial	Breakpoints	Streptococcus suis (%) (N = 874)			Haemophilus parasuis (%) (N = 385)			Pasteurella multocida (%) (N = 923)		
		Sus.	M. Sus.	Res.	Sus.	M. Sus.	Res.	Sus.	M. Sus.	Res.
Amikacin	16, 32	98	2	1	99	1	0	99	0	0
Gentamicin	4, 8	99	1	0	100	0	0	99	0	0
Neomycin	8	92	—	8	94	—	6	98	—	2
Spectinomycin	8, 16	56	30	14	36	5	59	1	17	82
Apramycin	8, 16	66	31	2	46	49	5	20	73	7
Penicillin	0.12, 2	84	14	1	96	0	3	86	11	2
Ampicillin	0.25, 2	100	0	0	94	2	3	99	0	1
Ceftiofur	1, 2	100	0	0	98	0	1	99	0	0
Cephalothin	8, 16	99	0	1	99	0	1	99	0	0
Tilmicosin	6.25, 12.5	32	1	67	99	0	1	74	21	6
Erythromycin	0.5, 4	30	16	54	9	89	1	1	84	15
Tylosin tartrate	5, 10	30	1	69	35	36	28	1	3	95
Tetracycline	4, 8	5	1	94	93	2	5	80	5	15
Sulfadimethoxine	20, 40	25	3	72	5	2	94	14	9	78
Sulfachlorpyridazine	20, 40	26	3	70	5	7	87	21	8	70
Trimethoprim-sulfadiazine	1/19, 2/38	98	1	1	97	2	1	99	0	0
Clindamycin	0.5, 4	30	3	68	11	85	3	0	1	98
Tiamulin	8, 16	95	2	3	90	6	2	8	39	52

For abbreviations, see footnote to Table 1.

treated animals. Be sure sampled animals are in a representative stage of the disease.

4. "Susceptible" results indicate that a correct antimicrobial regimen at an appropriate time in the disease process has a good chance of success in the majority of cases.

5. "Moderately susceptible" indicates that stressed or immunocompromised animals may require an elevated dose to achieve results, or that satisfactory clinical results may not be obtained. Immunocompetent animals may still respond to the label regimen.

6. "Resistant" suggests that the antimicrobial is not a good choice in most cases.

INDIVIDUAL DRUG GROUPS

Sulfonamides

The sulfonamides are a fairly homogeneous group in relation to potency on a milligram basis. However, radical differences in elimination pharmacokinetics and protein binding require

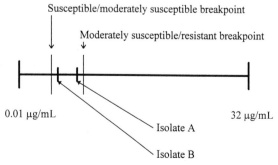

Susceptible/moderately susceptible breakpoint

Moderately susceptible/resistant breakpoint

0.01 μg/mL   32 μg/mL

Isolate A

Isolate B

Figure 2

Illustration of oxytetracycline breakpoint categories in relation to MIC scale. The location of the actual MICs of isolates A and B illustrate that the breakpoint categories are not an exact determination of an isolate's MIC.

differences in dosing regimens and withdrawal times. For example, the elimination half-time of sulfachlorpyridazine in cattle is reported as 1.2 hours, while that of sulfadimethoxine is reported as 12.5 hours.[1,2] In swine, the elimination half-time for sulfathiazole has been reported as 9 hours while that of sulfamethazine has been reported as 9.8 and 16.8 hours.[3,4] These differences underscore the necessity of researching dosing regimens and withdrawal times carefully when using different sulfa drugs, especially when switching brands of long-acting sulfamethazine boluses in cattle, where label slaughter withdrawal times vary between 8 and 28 days.

Resistance to the sulfonamides is a major issue in the therapy of respiratory disease. This resistance develops primarily through plasmid-mediated mechanisms, although chromosomal mutation may also occur. Conditions at the site of infection affect sulfa efficacy. An extremely important consideration is the presence of necrotic debris, which provides high concentrations of folic acid for bacteria, bypassing the sulfa mode of action. In my opinion, a sulfa drug should not be a primary choice as therapy in a severe respiratory outbreak, especially with severely distressed or immunocompromised animals.

The short withdrawal time and intravenous (IV) injection route for injectable sulfadimethoxine in cattle suggests it as a good choice in animals close to market. It is absolutely inappropriate to inject sulfadimethoxine intramuscularly (IM) or subcutaneously (SC) in cattle or swine owing to significant tissue damage by the extremely basic solution. Various sulfas are available as feed additives, water-soluble powders for drinking water, oral boluses, and injectable solutions. Use of sulfa drugs in lactating dairy cows is prohibited by the Center for Veterinary Medicine except for approved uses of sulfadimethoxine, sulfabromomethazine, and sulfaethoxypyridazine.

Potentiated sulfonamides have been used in an extralabel manner in swine and cattle. The administration of trimethoprim (oral or parenteral) to cattle with functional rumens will result in rapid hepatic biotransformation of the trimethoprim, with elimination half-times after IV administration declining to 0.9 hour by 42 days of age.[5] Although the susceptibility results in Table 1 for cattle suggest a possible high clinical efficacy, the trimethoprim likely will not be around long enough to have a significant clinical effect.

Penicillins

The penicillins used in food animals include penicillin G and the aminopenicillins amoxicillin and ampicillin. They are acidic compounds with high bioavailability after IM injection. Suspensions of these compounds contain water-insoluble forms (penicillin G procaine, ampicillin, and amoxicillin trihydrate). These forms should not be administered IV, especially procaine penicillin G, from which the procaine may rapidly dissociate and lead to toxicity. Penicillin G is rapidly degraded by stomach acid.

Penicillins are water-soluble, with good distribution to tissues with the exception of the central nervous system and joints. They should not be counted on for exceptional penetration into consolidated lung tissue with a reduced blood supply. They tend to reach low concentrations in milk. Elimination is rapid and occurs through the kidneys as the unchanged compound. The length of time that the plasma concentration is above the MIC of the pathogen is most closely related to efficacy for the penicillins. Short elimination half-times (usually 2 to 6 hours) may require more than once-daily administration in refractory infections. Toxicity is limited to hypersensitivity reactions. This class of compounds is usually more 'tissue-friendly' after IM injection than most other antimicrobial classes.

The penicillins are bactericidal compounds with noted anaerobic capability. The aminopenicillins have expanded gram-negative spectra and are susceptible to *Staphylococcus* spp. penicillinases to the same degree as penicillin G. Resistance to the penicillins may be either through chromosomal mutation (gram-positive organisms primarily) or through plasmid-mediated properties (primarily gram-negative organisms).

Bovine labels for respiratory disease include injectable penicillin G procaine, amoxicillin, ampicillin, and benzathine penicillin G in combination with penicillin G procaine. Only penicillin G procaine is approved for use in swine. The other compounds are not specifically approved for swine, but may be used under the Animal Medicinal Drug Use Clarification Act (AMDUCA) guidelines for extralabel therapy. Penicillin G is available as a feed additive in swine for growth promotion and in combination with chlortetracycline and sulfathizole or sulfamethazine for maintenance of weight gain in the presence of atrophic rhinitis.

The label dose for penicillin G is inadequate for therapy of respiratory disease. In cattle, an elevated dose of 30,000 IU/kg gives peak plasma concentrations of 1.5 to 2.2 μg/mL.[6, 7] These concentrations well represent the breakpoint concentrations used in Tables 1 to 3, but require the assignment of an extended withdrawal time. Benzathine penicillin G–penicillin G procaine combinations have difficulty obtaining the same therapeutic concentrations without giving extremely high doses. Administration of a benzathine penicillin G–penicillin G procaine combination at 24,000 IU/kg IM resulted in a peak plasma concentration of 1.06 μg/mL with an elimination half-time of 58 hours.[8] The majority of the plasma concentration in the first 48 hours is due to the penicillin G procaine. The subsequent plasma concentrations are due to the benzathine fraction, but these concentrations are well below therapeutic concentrations. "Long-acting penicillin" has little place in the therapy of bovine respiratory disease (BRD).

Penicillin G is probably most commonly used in combination with another antimicrobial for the therapy of respiratory disease in cattle. A common reason is "covering the gram-positive side." Concern with gram-positive agents (*Staphylococcus*, *Streptococcus*, *Actinomyces pyogenes*) early in the course of therapy indicates the possibility of other major causes contributing to case fatality (i.e., intervening too late in the disease process). *Pasteurella multocida* may be an indication for the use of penicillin G in respiratory disease in cattle. The use of penicillin G in the therapy of BRD requires an accurate assessment of the population being treated and an extended slaughter withdrawal time to accommodate a clinically effective dose.

There are aminopenicillins available (amoxicillin, ampicillin) with improved gram-negative spectra that may be used if a penicillin group member is desired in the therapy of respiratory disease. These compounds are considerably more expensive than penicillin G. However, the commercially available ampicillin preparation has the advantage in cattle of a meat withdrawal of 6 days and a milk withdrawal of 48 hours when used according to the label.

Tetracyclines

The tetracyclines are bacteriostatic at clinically prudent doses, although bactericidal activity against some pathogens may occur at significantly elevated doses. Significant activity exists for both gram-negative and gram-positive organisms in aerobic and anaerobic environments. Resistance development, which is largely plasmid-mediated, calls for scrutiny of the classic tetracycline spectrum before using this spectrum as a basis for clinical use.

The tetracyclines are essentially equipotent on a milligram basis. Differences in clinical efficacy between tetracycline compounds may be attributable to pharmacokinetic differences in lipid solubility or bioavailability. The tetracyclines are well distributed to tissues. Elimination is primarily through the kidney, although a significant portion is eliminated through the bile. Enterohepatic recirculation occurs, contributing to elimination half-times in the 6- to 10-hour range. The kidney is the primary organ of toxicity, especially at high parenteral doses.

Tetracycline and chlortetracycline are available as in-feed additives alone and in combination with other antimicrobial compounds. Oxytetracycline is available as an IM injection. Tetracycline and chlortetracycline are also available as oral water-soluble powders. Long-acting oxytetracycline products (Liquamycin LA-200, Pfizer Animal Health, and related generic products) are labeled for respiratory disease in cattle and swine. Two of these products (Liquamycin LA-200 and Bio-Mycin 200, Delmarva) are labeled for SC as well as IM and IV use in cattle. A conventional formulation of oxytetracycline was also recently labeled for subcutaneous use in beef cattle with a 48-hour slaughter withdrawal (Status SQ, Boehringer-Ingelheim). The SC use of oxytetracycline is preferred over IM injection to avoid possible adverse injection site reactions.

Oxytetracycline continues to be used in feedlot animals for respiratory disease. Extralabel doses are commonly used. IV administration at doses above 22 mg/kg (10 mg/lb) should be discouraged because of the possibility of toxicity.[9-11] IM injections of oxytetracycline should be confined to the neck and excluded from high-value areas of the carcass such as the top-butt and the round. IV injection of a long-acting product *does not* result in prolonged serum concentrations as compared to a conventional product injected IV. Recent approval of oxytetracycline and chlortetracycline doses of 10 mg/lb/day in the feed raises the possibility of delivering meaningful concentrations through the feed in respiratory outbreaks.

Evaluating plasma concentrations of oxytetracycline after administration of a long-acting product in relation to reported pathogen MIC values would appear to predict poor therapeutic response. However, I have observed acceptable treatment responses in yearling cattle and low-stress calves with the use of long-acting oxytetracycline at the label dose. As for other antimicrobials, the rational selection of patient populations is an absolute necessity.

I suggest moving severely ill, nonresponding cattle to a new antimicrobial at 48 hours after injection of a long-acting oxytetracycline. Some very severe cases may warrant moving to a second therapy at 24 hours postinjection. A long-acting oxytetracycline is probably not the right choice for first treatment if more than 5% to 10% of the cattle require additional therapy at 24 hours. A decision either to retreat the animal or classify it as "cured" should absolutely be made at 72 hours post-treatment. Using ampicillin, amoxicillin, penicillin G, or ceftiofur (β-lactams) as a second therapy 24 or 48 hours after long-acting oxytetracycline therapy is not the most logical choice, as the oxytetracycline may slow growth of the pathogen enough to impede the activity of a cell wall–active bactericidal agent. Logical choices for continued therapy in cattle would include tilmicosin or florfenicol. Using β-lactams at the same time as oxytetracycline is not a good choice for the same reason.

Cephalosporins

The only cephalosporin labeled for use in food animals is ceftiofur, which was first introduced as ceftiofur sodium (Naxcel, Pharmacia & Upjohn) in 1988. Ceftiofur sodium is labeled for respiratory disease and footrot in cattle (including lactating dairy cattle) and respiratory disease in swine. Ceftiofur is also available as ceftiofur hydrochloride sterile suspension (Excenel, Pharmacia & Upjohn), labeled for respiratory disease in swine. Ceftiofur is a bactericidal antimicrobial which inhibits cell wall formation by binding with strategic proteins in the cell wall of dividing bacteria.

Ceftiofur is a weak acid which is acid-stable and water-soluble. The thioester bond of ceftiofur sodium is cleaved within 15 minutes after IM administration, yielding furoic acid and desfuroylceftiofur, the active metabolite in plasma. The pharmacokinetics of both ceftiofur forms in swine are essentially the same.[12] Absorption after IM injection is rapid with peak concentrations obtained by 2 hours. Cephalosporins are eliminated through the kidneys. The time that ceftiofur plasma concentrations remain above the pathogen MIC is correlated with therapeutic efficacy. The long elimination half-life of ceftiofur sodium and desfuroyl-related metabolites in cattle (9 to 10 hours) should be noted as being extended beyond the 2 to 4 hours often seen for the penicillins in food animals. Although labeled only for IM administration, SC administration of ceftiofur sodium in cattle results in a plasma profile virtually identical to IM administration.[13]

The label should be consulted for reconstitution and storage instructions. A recent label change allows the storage of Naxcel at room temperature (59 to 86° F) prior to reconstitution. The labels for both Naxcel and Excenel are excellent sources of pharmacokinetic and pathogen MIC range information. Considering the gram-negative component of the ceftiofur spectrum, it is difficult to understand the rationale behind substituting a human-label, first-generation cephalosporin such as cephalexin (oral) or cefazolin (injectable) for a ceftiofur product in the therapy of respiratory disease of cattle or swine. Regardless of spectrum considerations, the regulations promulgated to enact the AMDUCA are clear in that the compounds labeled for food animal application must be found to be ineffective when used as labeled, or in an extralabel manner, before a human-labeled compound may be used.[14] Cost is clearly not a valid reason for extralabel use under the AMDUCA and accompanying regulations.

Ceftiofur toxicity potential is minimal. Injection site reaction from IM injection of ceftiofur is similar to that from injecting sterile saline.[15] One of the advantages of ceftiofur sodium is a zero-day withdrawal for meat in both cattle and swine, and for milk in lactating dairy cows when administered according to label directions. Ceftiofur hydrochloride sterile suspension also

has a zero-day slaughter withdrawal in swine when used according to label directions.

Macrolides

Macrolides used in food animals include tylosin, erythromycin, and tilmicosin, which was introduced in 1992. They are highly lipid-soluble, basic compounds, which are well absorbed after oral administration. Erythromycin and tylosin are extensively distributed to tissue with the exception of variable distribution to the central nervous system. The macrolides tend to distribute into milk in high concentrations. Administration of tilmicosin according to label directions will result in prolonged milk residues in lactating dairy cattle ranging from 19 to 31 days.[16] Elimination of the macrolides is primarily through the liver with some renal excretion. IM injection of the macrolides is extremely irritating and may result in prolonged injection site reactions.

The macrolides are bacteriostatic for the majority of pathogens at therapeutically reachable concentrations. They may act in a bactericidal, concentration-dependent fashion with some pathogens. Tilmicosin has been shown to preferentially concentrate in macrophages and may contribute to an anti-inflammatory action by reducing release of neutrophil contents after cell death.[17, 18] Their spectrum is considered primarily gram-positive with some gram-negative activity. Tylosin has superior *Mycoplasma* activity compared to erythromycin. An in vitro postantibiotic effect of tilmicosin has been demonstrated for *Pasteurella haemolytica* and *P. multocida*.[19] Resistance to the macrolides is thought to be primarily through chromosomal mutation, although this resistance may be unstable. Plasmid-mediated resistance may also occur.

Tylosin is available as a feed additive for cattle for prevention of liver abscesses, and for swine to prevent swine dysentery, maintain weight gains in the presence of atrophic rhinitis, and increase rate of gain and feed efficiency. Tylosin is also available as an injectable product labeled for respiratory disease and other indications in cattle and swine, as well as a poultry-labeled water additive product. Erythromycin is available as an injectable product for respiratory disease and other indications in sheep, cattle, and swine. Tilmicosin is available as a feed additive for respiratory disease in swine and as an injectable product for respiratory disease in cattle.

It is difficult for me to recommend tylosin or erythromycin for respiratory disease therapy in cattle in view of a combination of reported in vitro resistance and concerns over injection site reactions. IV injection of tylosin and erythromycin in an extralabel manner is possible, although the reaction of cattle to this injection route is best termed as "rough." Unless the intent is to create a multiple-macrolide treatment rotation, it is questionable to choose either of these compounds instead of tilmicosin. Also, in my opinion, "veining" another compound at the time of tilmicosin administration to achieve more rapid lung concentrations is not necessary because of the time frame of lung tilmicosin accumulation.

Adverse reactions may include edema and erythema of the rectal mucosa, anal protrusion, diarrhea and pruritus reported with tylosin use in swine. The tilmicosin phosphate label carries warnings relating to accidental injection of humans, which may be fatal. Elanco has received reports of 1462 accidental human exposures for the period May 1992 to December 1996.[20] No serious sequelae were reported after follow-up of these exposures, which included 718 exposures by puncture or scratch, 214 by injection of less than 1 mL, 209 dermal contacts, 201 exposures by ingestion, and 120 cases of exposure by a combination of skin, eye, and ingestion contact. These data should not be interpreted as not advocating caution in the handling of tilmicosin. It is important that tilmicosin be used in accordance with label directions.

IV tilmicosin has been fatal to cattle at 5 mg/kg. There were no adverse systemic effects at doses up to 150 mg/kg SC, and three times the label dose has been given SC three times, 3 days apart, with no adverse effects. Tilmicosin is fatal to swine when given at 20 mg/kg IM.[21]

Florfenicol

Florfenicol (Nuflor injectable solution, Schering-Plough) was new to the U.S. animal health market in 1996. It is a synthetic, lipid-soluble antimicrobial, structurally derived from chloramphenicol. Significant molecular changes lower bacterial resistance to some pathogens as well as potential toxicity to humans. It is labeled for treatment of BRD associated with *P. haemolytica*, *P. multocida*, and *Haemophilus somnus* in cattle. Chloramphenicol is considered a bacteriostatic, protein synthesis inhibitor. However, a comparison of MICs and minimal bactericidal concentrations (MBCs) of florfenicol for *P. haemolytica* and *P. multocida* suggests that florfenicol more closely fits the definition of a bactericidal antimicrobial (MBC two to four times the MIC) for these pathogens. A swine label is being developed. Diagnostic laboratories are just becoming equipped to run routine florfenicol susceptibility testing, so Tables 1 to 3 do not include florfenicol data.

Intracellular penetration of phagocytes in high concentrations and maintenance of activity within these cells have been demonstrated for chloramphenicol.[22] It is reasonable to assume that florfenicol shares these characteristics to some degree.

Residue warnings from the product label state the following: (1) Do not use in female dairy cattle 20 months of age or older. Use of florfenicol in this class of cattle may cause milk residues. (2) Do not use in veal calves, calves under 1 month of age, or calves being fed an all-milk diet. Use in these classes of calves may cause violative tissue residues to remain beyond the withdrawal time. The product label lists inappetence, decreased water consumption, and diarrhea as adverse effects that may occur transiently following treatment.

Aminoglycosides

The aminoglycosides include gentamicin, neomycin, and amikacin. They are polar bases which are very water-soluble but insoluble in lipids. Distribution in tissues is more limited than lipid-soluble compounds such as the macrolides. Bioavailability after oral administration is usually much less than 10%. Elimination is through the kidneys.

The aminoglycosides are bactericidal compounds with a mainly gram-negative spectrum, although some gram-positive bacteria such as *Staphylococcus* spp. are susceptible. Aminoglycosides are taken up into pathogens by an oxygen-dependent mechanism, preventing activity against anaerobic pathogens or facultative anaerobes in an anaerobic environment. Tissue debris (binding) and low pH may also inhibit the in vivo activity of aminoglycosides. Laboratory susceptibility results for aminoglycosides may be overly optimistic when actual in vivo activity is considered. The primary resistance mechanism is a plasmid-mediated production of enzymes which inactivate the aminoglycosides. Cross-resistance among the veterinary aminoglycosides is common, with less cross-resistance involving amikacin.

Gentamicin is available as an injectable solution for piglets less than 3 days of age and as an oral solution for swine dysentery therapy. Neomycin is available in combination with tetracycline as an in-feed medication for swine and as a feed medication and oral solution for scours therapy in cattle.

The aminoglycosides require extensive withdrawal times, as well as having the potential for nephrotoxicity when used in an extralabel manner. Gentamicin is not available in any form labeled for cattle, so no residue tolerance has been developed. Any gentamicin residue which is detected in cattle is violative. No published clinical trials are available to evaluate the efficacy of aminoglycosides compared with labeled compounds for respiratory disease therapy in cattle. In response to these issues, the Academy of Veterinary Consultants and the American Association of Bovine Practitioners have adopted statements discouraging the extralabel use of aminoglycosides in cattle. In addition, the National Cattlemen's Beef Association has adopted a resolution endorsing the Academy of Veterinary Consultants' position statement. Before using the aminoglycosides for extralabel use in respiratory disease, all labeled compounds (used in a label or extralabel manner) must first be judged ineffective as required under the AMDUCA and its regulations.[14]

Aminocyclitols

Spectinomycin is available as an injectable product labeled for turkey poults and newly hatched chicks, as an oral solution for *Escherichia coli* scours in pigs less than 4 weeks of age, and as a water-soluble powder for use in broilers. Spectinomycin remains active in the gut after oral administration, with any that is absorbed excreted by glomerular filtration. A label is currently being developed for BRD.

There has been extralabel use of spectinomycin for respiratory disease in cattle and swine. The compounding of a swine or cattle injectable formulation from the water-soluble powder has been used by the Center for Veterinary Medicine in the Compliance Policy Guideline as an example of an adverse reaction in compounding in food animals.[23] As for the aminoglycosides, a practitioner must be prepared to defend the extralabel use of spectinomycin for respiratory disease by supporting the statement that all labeled compounds are less effective as described in the regulations under the AMDUCA.[14]

Lincosamides

Lincomycin is a basic, lipid-soluble compound which is incompletely absorbed following oral administration in swine. The majority of the absorbed drug is eliminated through the liver with a smaller portion excreted unchanged through the kidneys. The basic status, coupled with a pK_b of 7.6, indicates significant ion trapping leading to high levels in acidic fluids such as milk. It is a bacteriostatic compound with activity against gram-positive and anaerobic bacteria as well as *Mycoplasma*.

Resistance may be either chromosomal or plasmid-mediated. There is frequently cross-resistance with the macrolides. Combining lincosamides and macrolides in therapeutic regimens is possibly antagonistic. Lincomycin is available as a swine feed additive and as an oral, water-soluble powder for the control of swine dysentery and mycoplasmal pneumonia, and as an IM injection for arthritis and mycoplasmal pneumonia in swine. The susceptibility results for clindamycin (another lincosamide) in Tables 1 to 3 suggest that extralabel use for other respiratory indications would be of questionable value.

A combination water-soluble product (with spectinomycin) labeled for poultry has been compounded for extralabel use in the therapy of respiratory disease in cattle and swine. Given the questions about lincomycin effects on the rumen and AMDUCA requirements for extralabel use discussed earlier, I find little support for this compounding.

Diterpines

Tiamulin is a lipid-soluble, basic compound, available as a feed additive for swine dysentery and in a water-soluble form for use against swine dysentery and pneumonia caused by *Haemophilus pleuropneumoniae*. Oral absorption is almost complete and distribution to tissues is extensive, including milk. It is extensively metabolized, with the majority of the numerous metabolites excreted through the liver, although a small percentage is excreted renally.

Resistance to tiamulin occurs by chromosomal mutation, with variable cross-resistance with macrolide or lincosamide antimicrobials. Acute fatalities may occur if tiamulin is administered in combination with polyether antibiotics. Tiamulin is available as an in-feed additive and as an oral water-soluble powder. Other areas of reported activity include *Actinobacillus pleuropneumoniae*, *Pasteurella*, and *Haemophilus* spp.

Fluoroquinolones

At the time of this writing, enrofloxacin is approved for use in dogs, cats, and poultry and is in the final stages of approval in the United States for the therapy of BRD. The extralabel use of fluoroquinolones is currently banned in food animals in the United States. Sarafloxacin is approved for use in poultry.

The spectrum of enrofloxacin, like most fluoroquinolones, encompasses a broad range of gram-negative aerobes, a more limited number of gram-positive aerobes, as well as *Mycoplasma* spp. Activity against anaerobes is much more limited. However, activity may not be based on the presence or absence of oxygen, as activity has been demonstrated against *E. coli* in anaerobic conditions.[24]

EXTRALABEL DRUG USE

Valid reasons for extralabel antimicrobial use are clearly limited to situations where approved new animal drugs are not available or are clinically ineffective.[14] Cost is not included as a valid reason for extralabel drug use in the AMDUCA, nor in the regulations promulgated to implement the act. A provision allowing extralabel use for production purposes was not included in the AMDUCA or the regulations. Extralabel use of human drugs or an animal drug approved only for use in animals and not intended for human consumption requires that additional steps be taken as regards the extralabel use of drugs labeled for use in food animals. Extralabel use of an approved human drug in a food-producing animal is not permitted under the regulations if an animal drug approved for use in food-producing animals can be used in an extralabel manner for the particular use. The regulations are clear that consideration of label and extralabel use of compounds labeled for respiratory disease is required prior to the use of compounded antimicrobials.[23]

It is important for practitioners to realize that the AMDUCA and the accompanying regulations do not give free rein to extralabel drug use. In fact, the intent of Congress was stated during floor debate as being that of codifying existing compliance policy guidelines (such as 7125.06, Extra-Label Use of New Animal Drugs in Food Producing Animals).*

---

*A source for pertinent documents relating to extralabel drug use is: on the World Wide Web, http://www.cvm.fda.gov/; by mail, Communications Staff, FDA-CVM, 7500 Standish Place, HFV-12, Rockville, MD 20855; by telephone, (301) 594-1755. Questions regarding individual practices may be addressed to the Office of Surveillance and Compliance, (301) 594-1761.

COMBINATION ANTIMICROBIAL THERAPY

In my opinion, combining antimicrobials for therapy of BRD, in most cases, needlessly drives up the cost of therapy, results in additional, unnecessary injection sites or stress on the animal, and in some combinations may compromise the activity of one or both of the antimicrobials. Reasons for selection of combination therapy for BRD may include one or more of the following: (1) the search for synergism, (2) to suppress resistance, (3) to extend the spectrum, and (4) "one of them should work."

One study examining in vitro interactions suggested that erythromycin and spectinomycin was a clinically useful combination while erythromycin and oxytetracycline were of marginal benefit when combined in vitro against *P. haemolytica* and clinically practical concentrations were considered.[25] However, there was significant variation in results due to the isolate tested and also due to varying the accepted clinically relevant antimicrobial concentrations. This variation would likely be magnified in a clinical setting where additional factors besides drug-pathogen interaction determine the outcome of therapy.

Antagonism is also a possible result of combining antimicrobials. It is logical that introducing a compound which works by slowing bacterial growth at clinically achievable concentrations (bacteriostatic) would impede the activity of a bactericidal antimicrobial that works by inducing cell wall lysis in rapidly growing bacteria (a β-lactam). Other antagonism may come about by antimicrobials competing for the same site of action. The line between synergism and antagonism may depend on dose. When searching for synergism, remember that toxicity may be additive too.

Suppression of resistance through combination therapy is based on the premise that pathogens resistant to antimicrobial A are susceptible to antimicrobial B. The amount of "resistance overlap" is impossible to predict in the case of empirical therapy. The study cited above utilized many resistant *P. haemolytica* isolates. The inconsistent results support the concept that suppression of resistance is as variable as synergism and additive effects. Combining two less expensive antimicrobials to address the issue of resistance in BRD therapy brings the cost much closer to, if not higher than, the cost of a single, more effective antimicrobial. If resistance to an antimicrobial is a concern, why include it in a regimen if another antimicrobial with minimal resistance is available?

Combining antimicrobials to give broad-spectrum coverage makes sense in empirical therapy of diseases with unpredictable pathogen involvement. However, in cattle, respiratory disease pathogen possibilities are fairly predictable. We expect early involvement of *P. haemolytica*, *P. multocida*, and possibly *H. somnus*. Pathogens cultured from more advanced cases include *Staphylococcus* spp., *Streptococcus* spp., *A. pyogenes*, and *Mycoplasma* spp. With this in mind, it is of questionable value to add antimicrobials to "extend the spectrum" to the gram-positive, opportunistic pathogens during therapy of cattle in the early stages of respiratory disease. The role of *Mycoplasma* in BRD has yet to be conclusively defined. A constant finding of gram-positive organisms at necropsy of cases with short therapy records indicates case selection problems, not the need for an expanded first-therapy spectrum.

Suggested rules for combination antimicrobial therapy of BRD are listed below. These are not guaranteed to prevent adverse reactions or antagonism. They may also rule out combinations which could show in vivo additive or synergistic properties. These qualifications underscore the fact that we really do not know what we are doing in the area of combination BRD therapy.

1. Avoid combining a bacteriostatic antimicrobial (macro-

lides, tetracyclines) with a β-lactam antimicrobial (penicillin G, amoxicillin, ampicillin, or ceftiofur).

2. Select bacteriostatic combinations that have different sites or mechanisms of action. Macrolides (erythromycin, tylosin, tilmicosin) and florfenicol primarily function at the 50S ribosomal subunit of bacteria. The tetracyclines primarily function at the 30S ribosomal subunit. Sulfa drugs interfere with the production of folic acid for purine synthesis.

3. There is no such situation as "adding it can't hurt." Recent work in cattle has shown that even the injection of sterile saline in the top-butt has adverse effects on the degree and consistency of tenderness of the meat approximately 190 days after injection.[15] At the very least, combination therapy of BRD increases the cost of treatment.

METAPHYLAXIS AND PROPHYLAXIS

Administration of antimicrobials to all animals in a group is utilized in outbreak situations in both swine and cattle production settings. The treatment may be prophylactic when the antimicrobial is given immediately prior to an outbreak predicted by previous experience in a production setting (i.e., after weaning, before shipment). The treatment may also be metaphylactic, when previous experience and current clinical signs indicate that the majority of animals in a group are in the incubatory stages of a disease. Administration may be through the water, feed, or by individual injection. Regulations limit feed administration to label uses only, while parenteral or water administration may be extralabel if required.

An in-depth review of techniques and procedures for prophylaxis and metaphylaxis is beyond the scope of this discussion. An extensive review of the bovine literature (review article of 107 field trials) indicated that mass medication with long-acting oxytetracycline or tilmicosin consistently reduced morbidity, but effects on mortality and performance were inconsistent.[26] Another review article cited several studies where morbidity and case fatality were reduced and performance was enhanced during 30- and 60-day trials.[27] The challenge in administering antimicrobials in a prophylactic or metaphylactic manner is selecting the optimal groups. Questions to answer when considering prophylactic or metaphylactic use of antimicrobials include the following:

1. Do historical groups and the condition of the present group indicate that a disease outbreak is likely or is in an early stage? What is the probability in this case?

2. Have all management factors which may affect the probability or severity of the outbreak been addressed (i.e., nutrition, environment)?

3. Would an alternative method suffice to reduce morbidity and mortality (vaccination)?

4. Is the considered compound labeled for the indication? If extralabel, is it appropriate?

5. What potential toxicity or penalty in slaughter withdrawal time might occur?

6. What are the comparative economics of administering antimicrobials, using alternative management methods, and treating affected cases with no preventive intervention?

ANCILLARY THERAPY FOR RESPIRATORY DISEASE

The goal of ancillary therapy for respiratory disease is to improve the clinical efficacy of antimicrobials. Attempting to ameliorate the harmful effects of inflammation, blocking the activity of histamine, and improving immune function are at-

tractive targets for ancillary therapy. Other areas of interest are improving pulmonary function, regulating the febrile response, and stimulating feed intake. When ancillary therapy is evaluated in light of production medicine principles, it is often difficult to justify the use of ancillary compounds on a cost vs. efficacy basis. Anti-inflammatory agents and antihistamines are useful as examples.

Anti-inflammatory Agents

The theoretical aspects of nonsteroidal anti-inflammatory drugs (NSAIDs) and glucocorticosteroids would seem to indicate that this class should dramatically affect the outcome of BRD therapy, if only by making the animal feel better. However, there is no published clinical evidence to support this conclusion for phenylbutazone or aspirin. The duration of a meaningful serum concentration for aspirin indicates it is not a rational choice for ancillary therapy of respiratory disease in cattle unless administration every 6 to 8 hours is possible. The published evidence available for the use of glucocorticosteroids indicates mixed clinical effects with ample evidence for real immunosuppression with indiscriminate use.

Steroids may have a place in the therapy of inflammatory respiratory diseases such as diphtheria and tracheal edema provided they are used reasonably. It is unlikely that a one-time administration of a glucocorticosteroid at a reasonable dose will have clinically significant effects on the immune system. However, a very large dose of dexamethasone (2.8 mg/kg IV) given once in a rabbit latency model for bovine herpesvirus 1 (BHV-1) resulted in all of the rabbits again shedding BHV-1 in ocular fluid by 72 hours postinjection.[28] The authors cited additional results to support the argument that reactivation of BHV-1 from trigeminal ganglia is due to a nonimmunologic method of action on the part of glucocorticosteroids. This work calls into question the high, one-time doses of glucocorticosteroids sometimes administered during BRD therapy as possibly contributing to BHV-1 reactivation even if a significant adverse immunologic effect does not occur.

Cattle appear to be much more susceptible to the immunosuppressive effects of dexamethasone than swine. Dexamethasone 2 mg/kg administered to swine does not have the immunosuppressive effects of 0.04 mg/kg administered to cattle.[29] Dexamethasone administered at 0.04 mg/kg (0.9 mL/100 lb of a 2 mg/mL solution) daily for 3 days is used as an immunosuppression model in cattle.[30, 31]

There are positive model data published for flunixin meglumine, but the clinical data found by me could not be classified as conclusive.[32–34] This seems to be fairly consistent across the NSAIDs.

Antihistamines

The H$_1$ blockers discussed here are competitive antagonists of histamine at the H$_1$ receptor. Pyrilamine maleate and tripelennamine hydrochloride are two ethylenediamine H$_1$ blockers used in veterinary medicine. There has apparently been very little work done in the form of clinical trials to validate the efficacy of these drugs in the treatment of BRD. Their primary application may be respiratory syndromes where a hyperimmune component is suspected, as in atypical interstitial pneumonia. However, there are no clinical data to support this use. In regard to airway constriction, it is interesting to note that antihistamines are ineffective in the treatment of human asthma, as are cyclo-oxygenase inhibitors. It is believed that leukotrienes are predominantly responsible for allergic bronchoconstriction, as evidenced by protection provided by lipoxygenase inhibitors.[35]

CONSIDERATION OF THERAPEUTIC POPULATIONS

The lack of an accurate, consistent case definition of respiratory disease in most field situations makes evaluation of treatment response and case fatality difficult. Helping a client develop an accurate case definition for instituting therapy may be more important than selecting among the high-efficacy antimicrobials available today. Start by evaluating what the client is currently treating as respiratory cases. Animals being treated for respiratory disease may be split into three categories: (1) those that do not require therapy and are being treated for signs due to a noninfectious condition which would resolve without antimicrobials, (2) those that need antimicrobials to recover, and (3) those that are receiving therapy too late for a significant impact on recovery.

Individual producers will often lean toward excessive amounts of category (1) or (3). Clients treating a high proportion of category (1) animals will have extremely impressive case fatality rates (i.e., less than 1% in BRD) with high drug use and related costs. In contrast, respiratory disease case fatality rates greater than 10% suggest that the antimicrobial is ineffective, or (more likely) that the animals are being treated too late. Veterinarians are sometimes too quick to switch therapy without examining the case definition. Correcting problems involves working with clients as they select animals for therapy and evaluating records.

This section is not intended to promote an attitude of ignoring differences in drug efficacy and the potential benefit of adjusting the therapeutic regimen. There *are* differences in drug efficacy. However, ignoring the client's respiratory disease case definition when evaluating poor treatment response is a major error.

SELECTION OF A DRUG ROTATION, OR, WHERE DO I PUT THE MOST EFFECTIVE ANTIMICROBIAL?

Should you take the chance of placing a less expensive, less effective antimicrobial in the first-treatment position and hope to catch nonresponders with a more expensive, more effective agent? This strategy works if the right animals are put with the right client and crew. Candidates include low-risk cattle such as most yearlings and fresh, short-haul calves. In short, any source of animals with a history of good treatment response coupled with a client and crew that have demonstrated an ability to accurately detect cases of respiratory disease might be considered for this approach. Consistent treatment of a high percentage of animals described in category (1) above also indicates this approach as an option. An absolute requirement is intense monitoring of posttreatment animals and aggressive rotation to additional therapy as needed.

I do not recommend using a lower-efficacy antimicrobial as first treatment for any animal that would be designated as "high risk." This includes long-haul, sale-barn, and highly distressed cattle. Any animal in which prophylactic or metaphylactic therapy was justified also fits in this category. A high percentage of animals in category (3) require the most effective initial therapy regimen possible. Attempting to differentially assign first-treatment antimicrobials based on degree of rectal temperature elevation is a doubtful practice. This approach assumes a smooth, textbook temperature response indicating severity and stage of disease. It also prohibits accurately evaluating drug response over the whole population.

THERAPY FOR FIRST-TREATMENT NONRESPONDERS

One of the biggest obstacles to turning around refractory cases is maintaining a constant therapeutic pressure on the pathogen(s). Timing of continued therapy is likely as, or more, important than the selection of the second antimicrobial. A breakdown in the system happens all too easily in crowded production environments or when animals are returned to or left in the pen after initial therapy.

Part of the treatment regimen also involves knowing when to stop. In my opinion, continuing therapy for bovine respiratory disease beyond three antimicrobials over 9 to 10 consecutive days does little for the animal and may actually impede recovery (we can make chronic cases out of animals that are slow to recover). Another rule of thumb is that it is time to quit when you start to search for injection sites. These animals need to be left alone in the best environment your client can offer.

SUGGESTED APPROACH TO A PERCEIVED LACK OF TREATMENT RESPONSE

It is easy to become disoriented in the middle of a "wreck." I suggest the following progression of emphasis when treatment response is less than expected:
1. Is the problem one of morbidity or treatment response?
2. What is the case definition—too many category (1) or (3)?
3. If a lack of treatment response in cattle in the early stages of BRD is determined,
   a. Is the agreed upon regimen being followed?
   b. Are first-treatment nonresponders being aggressively moved to the next regimen?
   c. Is drug quality being protected?
   d. Is the hospital environment conducive to recovery?

REFERENCES

1. Nielson P, Rasmussen F: Half-life, apparent volume of distribution, and protein-binding for some sulphonamides in cows. Res Vet Sci 22:205–208, 1977.
2. Boxenbaum HG, Fellig J, Hansen LJ, et al: Pharmacokinetics of sulphadimethoxine in cattle. Res Vet Sci 23:24–28, 1977.
3. Van Poucke LSG, Van Peteghem CH: Pharmacokinetic and tissue residues of sulfathiazole and sulfamethazine in pigs. J Food Protect 57:796–801, 1994.
4. Sweeney RW, Bordalaye PC, Smith CM, et al: Pharmacokinetic model for predicting sulfamethazine disposition in pigs. Am J Vet Res 54:750–754, 1993.
5. Shoaf SE, Schwark WS, Guard CL: Pharmacokinetics of sulfadiazine/trimethoprim in neonatal male calves: Effect of age and penetration into cerebrospinal fluid. Am J Vet Res 50:396–403, 1989.
6. Luthman J, Jacobsson SO: Distribution of penicillin G in serum and tissue cage fluid in cattle. Acta Vet Scand 27:313–325, 1986.
7. Bengtsson B, Granklin A, Luthman J, et al: Concentrations of sulphadimidine, oxytetracycline and penicillin G in serum, synovial fluid and tissue cage fluid after parenteral administration to calves. J Vet Pharmacol Ther 12:37–45, 1989.
8. Papich MG, Korsrud GO, Boison JO, et al: Disposition of penicillin G after administration of benzathine penicillin G, or a combination of benzathine penicillin G and procaine penicillin G in cattle. Am J Vet Res 55:825–829, 1994.
9. Griffin DD, Amstutz HE, Morter RL: Oxytetracycline toxicity associated with bovine respiratory disease therapy. Bovine Pract 14:29–35, 1979.
10. Griffin DD, Morter RL: Experimental oxytetracycline toxicity in feedlot heifers. Bovine Pract 14:37–40, 1979.

11. Lairmore MD, Alexander AF, Powers BE, et al: Oxytetracycline-associated nephrotoxicosis in feedlot calves. J Am Vet Med Assoc 185:793–795, 1984.

12. Excenel package insert, Kalamazoo, MI: Pharmacia & Upjohn.

13. Brown SA: Personal communication. Kalamazoo, MI: Pharmacia & Upjohn, 1994.

14. Extralabel drug use in animals: Final rule. Federal Register 1996 61(217)(Nov 7):57731–57746.

15. George MH, Ames RA, et al: Incidence, severity, amount of tissue affected and effect on histology, chemistry, and tenderness of injection-site lesions in beef cuts from calves administered a control compound or one of seven chemical compounds. Final Report to the National Cattlemen's Beef Association, 1996.

16. Helton-Groce SL, Thomson TD, Readnour RS, et al: A study of tilmicosin residues in milk following subcutaneous administration to lactating dairy cows. Can Vet J 34:619–621, 1993.

17. Buret A, Morck DW, Merrill JK, et al: Neutrophil apoptosis in the infected lung: Anti-inflammatory benefits of tilmicosin (abstract H99). Biochem Soc Trans 24:617S, 1996.

18. Thomson TD, Laudert SB, Chamberland S, et al: Micotil—Pharmacokinetics of tilmicosin, a semi-synthetic macrolide antibiotic, in acutely pneumonic cattle and primary bovine alveolar macrophages. *In* Proceedings, Sixth International Congress, European Association for Veterinary Pharmacology and Toxicology, Edinburgh, 1994.

19. Diarra MS, Malouin F. Postantibiotic effects of tilmicosin and of other antibacterial agents at MICs and sub-MICs on swine and bovine pathogens (abstract A-81). Presented at American Society of Medicine General Meeting, 1994.

20. Elanco Animal Health: Personal communication. Indianapolis: Elanco, 1997.

21. Micotil package insert. Indianapolis: Elanco Animal Health, NADA No. 140–929.

22. Adams PE, Varma KJ, Powers TE, et al: Tissue concentrations and pharmacokinetics of florfenicol in male veal calves given repeated doses. Am J Vet Res 48:1725–1732j, 1987.

23. Compounding of Drugs for Use in Animals. Compliance Policy Guide, Chapter 6, Subchapter 600, Section 608-400. Center for Veterinary Medicine.

24. Wetzstein HG, Schmeer N: Bactericidal activity of enrofloxacin against *Escherichia coli* growing under strictly anaerobic conditions. *In* Proceedings General Meeting of the American Society of Microbiology, Washington, DC, 1995, p 150.

25. Burrows GE: In vitro assessment of the efficacy of erythromycin in combination with oxytetracycline or spectinomycin against *Pasteurella haemolytica*. J Vet Diagn Invest 1:299–304, 1989.

26. Donkersgoed JV: Meta-analysis of field trials of antimicrobial mass medication for prophylaxis of bovine respiratory disease in feedlot cattle. Can Vet J 33:786–7795.

27. Young C: Antimicrobial metaphylaxis for undifferentiated bovine respiratory disease. Compend Food Anim January 133–142, 1995.

28. Rock D, Lokensgard TL, Kutish G: Characterization of dexamethasone-induced reactivation of latent bovine herpesvirus 1. J Virol 66:2484–2490, 1992.

29. Roth JA, Flaming KP: Model systems to study immunomodulation in domestic food animals. Adv Vet Sci Comp Med, 35:26–27, 1990.

30. Roth JA, Kaeberle ML: In vivo effect of ascorbic acid on neutrophil function in healthy and dexamethasone-treated cattle. Am J Vet Res 46:2434–2436, 1985.

31. Roth JA, Kaeberle ML: Effect of levamisole on lymphocyte blastogenesis and neutrophil function in dexamethasone-treated cattle. Am J Vet Res 45:1781–1784, 1984.

32. Scott PR: Field study of undifferentiated respiratory disease in housed beef calves. Vet Rec 134:325–327, 1994.

33. Selman IE, Allan EM, Dalgleish RG, et al: Evaluation of the efficacy of flunixin meglumine using four different experimentally induced bovine respiratory disorders. *In* Proceedings, International Symposium on Nonsteroidal Anti-inflammatory Agents. 1986, pp 23–32.

34. Selman IE, Allan EM, Gibbs HA, et al: The effect of antiprostaglandin therapy in an acute respiratory distress syndrome induced in experimental cattle by the oral administration of 3-methylindole. Bovine Pract 22:124–126, 1985.

35. Campbell WB: Lipid-derived autacoids: Eicosanoids and platelet-activating factor. *In* Gilman AG, Rall JW, Nies AS, et al (eds): Goodman and Gilman's the Pharmacological Basis of Therapeutics, ed 8. New York: Pergamon Press, 1990, pp 600–615.2.

Circulatory Diseases

Consulting Editor

Robert N. Streeter, D.V.M., M.S., Diplomate, A.C.V.I.M.

■ Diagnostic Methods in Food Animal Cardiology

Bimbo Welker, D.V.M., M.S.

The definitive diagnosis of cardiac disease in food animals can be hampered by the relative infrequency of occurrence and the lack of equipment usable in a field setting. Most affected animals, however, can be identified as having a diseased cardiovascular system, and a tentative diagnosis can usually be made by available field techniques. Specialized techniques are typically available at referral hospitals or universities for confirmation or differentiation of the disease process.

The first step in diagnosing diseases of the cardiac system involves recognition of the signs, clinical findings, and historical information suggestive of dysfunction.

SIGNS OF CARDIOVASCULAR DISEASE

Most signs are not specific for heart disease but rather can result from other disease processes. These should serve as a signal for further investigation of the cardiovascular system. Such signs include edema, ascites, lethargy, wasting, diarrhea, coughing, syncope, and sudden death. A thorough physical examination and basic blood work will help to determine if these signs are cardiogenic or noncardiogenic in nature.

CLINICAL FINDINGS

Murmurs, muffled heart sounds, arrhythmias, and abnormal jugular pulses are all highly suggestive of cardiac disease. Murmurs and arrhythmias are first detected by auscultation and, if necessary, can be more clearly defined by specialized tests.

AUSCULTATION

Proper auscultation requires a good-quality stethoscope, quiet environment, and adequate restraint of the patient to allow uninterrupted listening. Knowledge of auscultation sites is also important. The points of maximal intensity (PMI) for the various valves are as follows:

Pulmonic valve: Left, third intercostal space, approximately 5 cm below the level of the shoulder.
Aortic valve: Left, fourth intercostal space, above the level of the pulmonic valve.
Mitral valve: Left, fifth intercostal space, at or just dorsal to the level of the elbow.

Tricuspid valve: Right, at the third or fourth intercostal space, between the shoulder and elbow.

The most common mistake in auscultation of large animals is listening at improper locations. The locations for auscultation of the pulmonic, aortic, and tricuspid valves require that the stethoscope be pushed cranially into the axillary area.

Abnormalities noted with auscultation can be in the form of disturbances in blood flow (murmurs), changes in audibility of sounds, or alterations in rhythm.

Disturbances in Blood Flow or Murmurs

Normal heart sounds are produced by vibration of the cardiogenic structures as a result of energy imparted to them in the processes of the normal cardiac cycle. Anything that disturbs the usual flow of blood in the heart creates turbulence and can result in an audible murmur. Murmurs are characterized as either physiologic or pathologic. Physiologic (also termed *functional*) murmurs are not associated with cardiac dysfunction but must be differentiated from those that are. Physiologic murmurs are typically of low to medium intensity, peak in early or midsystole, end before the second heart sound, do not radiate, and are variable in intensity from one auscultation to the next. They are usually found over the semilunar valves. The most common causes of physiologic murmurs include fever, excitement, and anemia.

Pathologic murmurs are those associated with cardiac dysfunction. When a murmur is detected, it should be characterized to better define it. The characteristics to be evaluated include the PMI (side, intercostal space, and level); loudness or intensity (scale of 1 to 6); location in the cycle (systolic [from S_1 to S_2], diastolic [from S_2 to S_1], or continuous); and timing in the cycle (early, mid, late, or throughout). This information will allow the auscultator to approximate the structures involved and speculate on the type of lesion present. If valves are involved in the pathologic condition, the murmur can be classified as an ejection or regurgitant type. Ejection murmurs occur when blood is forced through a narrowed opening during systole. The PMI is usually over the semilunar valves and can occur during any stage of systole. Differential diagnoses include physiologic murmur, stenosis of semilunar valves, or congenital defects allowing blood to move across the septum. Regurgitant murmurs can occur during systole or diastole. Systolic regurgitant murmurs are evident with atrioventricular valve incompetence, whereas diastolic regurgitant murmurs are suggestive of semilunar valve incompetence.

Changes in Audibility of Sounds

With proper auscultation techniques, the cardiac sounds can be heard in any large animal. Conditions such as obesity, thick chest walls, and poor technique should be ruled out when muffled sounds are encountered. If the sounds are decreased in amplitude, the conditions considered should include fluid around the heart (hydropericardium) or in the chest (pleural effusion), masses positioned between the body wall and heart (abscesses or neoplasms), fluid within the lungs (pulmonary edema or pneumonia), and emphysema. In addition, electrolyte imbalances, such as hypocalcemia, can cause decreased strength of contraction and, therefore, an apparent muffling of sound.

Confirmation or clarification of the conditions that result in murmurs or muffled sound may require additional tests. Thoracocentesis/pericardiocentesis, echocardiography, and/or thoracic radiographs are helpful.

Alterations in Rhythm

Rhythm disturbances occur as a result of abnormalities in impulse generation and/or conduction. The most common types of dysrhythmias in food animals include bradycardia associated with high vagal tone and decreased feed intake; ventricular premature contractions (VPCs) associated with conditions resulting in myocardial irritation (e.g., myocarditis, pericarditis); atrial premature contractions (APCs) associated with abnormalities in electrolyte or acid-base status, high vagal tone, or possibly irritation or disruption of the atrial musculature; and atrial fibrillation. Atrial fibrillation is classically associated with gastrointestinal disease and thought to result from acid-base, electrolyte, or autonomic nervous system abnormalities. Differentiation of the type of dysrhythmia present is best accomplished by performing an electrocardiogram.

Abnormal Jugular Pulses or Distention

Pulsation of the jugular vein can be demonstrated in the normal animal. The pulsations generally extend no higher than the midcervical region when the head is held level. These pulsations are a reflection of events occurring in the right atrium and ventricle. Abnormal pulsation, evidenced by extension farther up the neck and/or erratic configuration, occurs as a result of resistance to right heart filling. Resistance to filling may be due to abnormal electrical activity (dysrhythmias), obstruction to flow (heart base tumors or abscesses, pericardial effusion), or myocardial failure. Distention of the jugular veins may be another indication of filling problems. The normal jugular vein is thin walled and easily compressed. It should fill rapidly when held off at the thoracic inlet and empty rapidly when released. Persistence of jugular distention should be differentiated from an inflamed jugular vein (phlebitis) secondary to previously administered intravenous drugs. The most common causes of jugular distention or pulsation in ruminants include traumatic reticulopericarditis, lymphosarcoma of the right atrium, tricuspid insufficiency resulting from endocarditis, jugular phlebitis, and dysrhythmias (APCs, VPCs, and atrial fibrillation in particular). Differentiation of these conditions may require an electrocardiogram (ECG), ultrasound, and/or pericardiocentesis.

SPECIALIZED TESTS

Electrocardiography

The ECG may or may not be considered a specialized test, depending on availability of equipment. It can still be considered a "cowside" test, however, and can be used whenever dysrhythmias are suspected.

Because of the type of conduction system present in the heart of large animal species, the ECG is useful for evaluation of conduction disturbances and little else. A basic lead configuration that demonstrates all the components of the electrical cycle is adequate. A simple base-apex lead in the following configuration will suffice: the left arm lead is attached to the left axillary area adjacent to the point of the elbow; the right arm lead is attached in the right jugular furrow in the midcervical region; and the chest lead is attached anywhere on the animal as a ground lead. When this setup is run on lead I, a positive P wave, a positive QRS deflection, and a positive T wave will be recorded in a normal animal.

Common dysrhythmias will appear as follows:

APCs: Random P-QRS-T complexes will occur throughout the strip. Note that a P is associated with each configuration.

VPCs: Random QRS-T complexes occur throughout the strip. Note that a P *is not* associated with each configuration, and the configurations are shaped differently.

Atrial fibrillation: No P waves, a variation in the R-R interval, a variation in the amplitude of the QRS complexes, and the presence of F waves.

Any of a number of other types of dysrhythmias are possible in food animals as in other species. If the veterinarian at least has a rhythm strip in hand, it can be studied and compared or sent for a second opinion.

Pericardiocentesis

Another test that should be included in a list of field diagnostic methods is thoracocentesis/pericardiocentesis. This diagnostic test is indicated any time abnormal fluid is suspected in the pleural space or pericardium. The most common cause of pericardial effusion is traumatic pericarditis. The technique for pericardiocentesis is as follows: in the standing cow, the skin just behind the elbow is clipped and surgically prepared. A 6- to 8-in. 18-gauge needle is inserted aseptically through the skin at the fifth or sixth intercostal space, approximately level with the elbow. The needle is advanced *slowly* until pericardial fluid is obtained.

Complications can occur with pericardiocentesis, but the incidence is low. Complications include laceration of a coronary artery or the myocardium, ventricular premature beats, or ventricular fibrillation. Death may also occur as a result of cardiac tamponade. Once again, the incidence is low and pericardiocentesis is indicated in any case in which effusion is suspected.

Echocardiography

The greatest diagnostic advance in large animal cardiology has occurred with ultrasound, which allows visualization of the cardiac structures for evaluation of individual components and their function. It should be prescribed for evaluation of murmurs, suspected congenital defects, valvular dysfunction, muffled sounds, or unexplained dysrhythmias. It is an excellent noninvasive method of evaluation. The disadvantages include the cost of the equipment and the specialized training required to perform the examination and interpret the data.

Radiography

Radiographic evaluation of the heart is limited to small ruminants and neonates of large animals. The information derived from radiographs, even in these cases, is at best supplemental to the ultrasound data. Radiographs are more likely to provide information regarding the status of the pulmonary tree relative to cardiac function or to reveal evidence of thoracic effusion and possibly gross cardiac enlargement. Detailed information is rarely derived. Contrast studies in the smaller species or young may provide useful information when defective circulation is suspected (congenital defects).

Proper use of field methods should allow the practitioner to identify cardiac dysfunctions and generate a tentative differential diagnosis list. Because of food animal economics, this may be all that is necessary to instigate treatment and arrive at a prognosis.

BIBLIOGRAPHY

Bonagura JD, Herring DS, Welker F: Echocardiography. Vet Clin North Am Equine Pract 1:311–334, 1985.
Ducharme NG, Dill SG, Rendano VT: Reticulography of the cow in dorsal recumbency: An aid in the diagnosis and treatment of traumatic reticuloperitonitis. J Am Vet Med Assoc 182:585–588, 1983.
Fregin GF: Electrocardiology. Vet Clin North Am Equine Pract 1:419–432, 1985.
Levine SA, Harvey WP: Clinical Auscultation of the Heart, ed 2. Philadelphia, WB Saunders, 1959.
Raphel CF, Fregin GF: Clinical examination of the cardiovascular system in cattle. Compend Contin Ed Pract Vet 2:S259–S264, 1980.

■ Circulatory Shock

Robert N. Streeter, D.V.M., M.S., Diplomate, A.C.V.I.M.
Charles McCauley, D.V.M.

Circulatory shock is a state of acute cardiovascular dysfunction characterized by widespread inadequacy of tissue perfusion resulting in cellular hypoxia. Untreated, the hypoxia can induce cellular injury, and eventually result in organ dysfunction and death of the animal. Circulatory shock develops subsequent to many common disease processes and its successful treatment depends on early recognition and aggressive therapy.

CIRCULATORY CONTROL MECHANISMS

Knowledge of the pathogenesis, signs, and treatment of circulatory shock is enhanced by an understanding of the body's circulatory control mechanisms and how they are altered in various shock states. Regulation of blood pressure, volume, and distribution is dependent on neural, local, and humoral mechanisms.

A reduction of arterial blood pressure or reduced cardiac output stimulates increased sympathetic vasomotor tone and release of vasoactive hormones (angiotensin, vasopressin). The resultant arteriolar and venular constriction occurs most strongly in the gastrointestinal tract, skin, and kidneys. Peripheral vasoconstriction increases venous return and cardiac output, preserving perfusion of vital organs (brain and heart). Arteriolar vasoconstriction reduces capillary hydrostatic pressure, facilitating the movement of fluid into the intravascular space, expanding blood volume. Increased sympathetic activity increases the heart rate and contractility, thus increasing cardiac output.

Blood flow is also controlled locally. A myogenic reflex occurs within vessel walls wherein reduced blood flow results in muscle relaxation and vasodilation, improving tissue perfusion. Decreased local concentration of oxygen or increased metabolic byproducts stimulate arteriolar dilation, increasing blood flow.

Humoral factors (angiotensin, vasopressin, aldosterone), released in response to reduced arterial pressure, function to increase renal sodium and water retention, thus increasing blood volume.

With mild circulatory insults, the compensatory mechanisms may be capable of maintaining arterial pressure and tissue perfusion with only subtle external evidence of cardiovascular derangement. With more severe insults, the mechanisms may be overwhelmed and a state of decompensated shock ensues. Alternatively, disease processes may interfere with the compensatory mechanisms and predispose to the development of shock.

PATHOPHYSIOLOGY

Circulatory shock can be organized into four pathogenic processes: (1) reduction of circulating blood volume, (2) sequestration of blood volume in capacitance vessels, (3) vascular obstruction, and (4) intrinsic cardiac dysfunction.

The basal insult in all forms of shock is prolonged tissue hypoxia. Without oxygen, cellular energy stores are rapidly depleted and energy-dependent activities, such as transmembrane pumps, are impaired. This results in altered intracellular electrolyte content, cellular edema, loss of lysosomal integrity, and eventually cell lysis.

Hypoxic tissues generate lactic acid. Metabolic acidosis may develop, which, if severe, inhibits cellular metabolism, myocardial contractility, and the vasopressor response. An array of vasoactive, inflammatory, and procoagulant compounds (cytokines, eicosanoids, oxygen free radicals, lysosomal enzymes, etc.) are released from injured and lysed cells. In large amounts, these compounds can cause tissue damage, both locally and systemically. Eventually, the cellular dysfunction is of sufficient magnitude to result in organ dysfunction.

Organ dysfunction initially develops in the least vital (and perfused) organs, progressing to the most vital organs. Persistent gastrointestinal hypoxia leads to mucosal necrosis, which allows invasion by enteric microorganisms and absorption of toxins. Transudation of large quantities of fluid may occur across the damaged mucosa, reducing circulatory volume. Hepatic hypoxia hinders reticuloendothelial function, allowing portal bacteria or toxins to traverse the liver and enter the vasculature.

Reduced renal blood flow may result in renal tubular cell necrosis and renal failure. Pulmonary injury is prominent in some forms of shock (septic), resulting in hypoxemia. Eventually, cerebral and coronary perfusion are critically reduced, compensatory mechanisms fail, and cardiopulmonary arrest occurs. The above changes are common to all types of shock. Unique features of separate causes of shock are described below.

Hypovolemic Shock

Hypovolemia refers to a absolute reduction in circulating blood volume. Acute loss of more than 25% of the blood volume can result in shock. Hypovolemia may be due to hemorrhage, or loss of intravascular fluid via diarrhea, intestinal obstruction, polyuria, body cavity transudation, or simple dehydration.

Vascular Obstructive Shock

Obstruction to the flow of blood through areas of the vascular tree may interfere with cardiac output by increasing afterload or reducing preload. If severe, the reduction in cardiac output can lead to hypoperfusion and shock. Conditions resulting in vascular obstructive shock include pericardial tamponade, tension pneumothorax, hydrothorax, and bloat.

Cardiogenic Shock

Disorders of the myocardium, valves, or conduction system may interfere with cardiac pump function and lead to cardiogenic shock. The more common of these conditions in food animals are described in this section in the article "Acquired Diseases of the Heart".

Distributive Shock

Approximately 70% of the blood volume resides within the venous circulation. Thus, an abrupt increase in venous capacity due to widespread vasodilation results in a relative hypovolemia. The abnormal distribution of the blood volume leads to reduced venous return and cardiac output, and can induce a state of shock. Examples of distributive shock include anaphylactic, neurogenic, and septic shock.

Anaphylactic shock is a generalized immunologic response wherein the mediators released cause pronounced systemic vasodilation and increased capillary permeability. Neurogenic shock develops subsequent to an abrupt reduction in sympathetic vasomotor tone as may occur with profound general anesthesia, head trauma, or spinal anesthetic overdose.

Septic shock is a complex syndrome perpetuated by an overwhelming and destructive host response to microbial infection. Several microbial substances produced by invading microorganisms can have profound circulatory effects. The most significant such mediator in large animal medicine is endotoxin, the lipopolysaccharide component of gram-negative bacterial cell walls. Disruption of the microbial cell wall through death or division releases endotoxin. Conditions commonly associated with endotoxemia include neonatal septicemia, coliform mastitis, puerperal metritis, pasteurellosis, salmonellosis, peritonitis, and intestinal accidents.

Circulating endotoxin activates macrophages, endothelium, and other cells, causing the release of a variety of vasoactive, proinflammatory, and procoagulant host mediators including cytokines, eicosanoids, complement components, and platelet activating factor. Inflammatory mediators induce increased capillary permeability, resulting in edema and reduced blood volume. Vasoactive mediators alter vasomotor tone. A maldistribution of blood flow can develop due to a local disorganization of vasoconstrictive and vasodilative events, resulting in arteriovenous shunting of blood. Procoagulant mediators lead to platelet and neutrophil aggregation. This can impair local blood flow, concentrate the release of toxic cellular components, and potentiate the development of disseminated intravascular coagulation. Ruminants are particularly susceptible to endotoxin-induced pulmonary injury due to a large population of pulmonary intravascular macrophages. Pulmonary hypertension, increased microvascular permeability, and ventilation-perfusion mismatching occur, resulting in pulmonary edema and hypoxia.

The hemodynamic effects of endotoxemia are dependent on the dose and duration of the toxemia. Acute and severe endotoxemia results in a hypodynamic cardiovascular state, characterized by severe pulmonary hypertension, reduced cardiac output, and systemic hypotension. Pulmonary edema and hypoxia develop. Death may occur subsequent to right heart or respiratory failure.

Recurrent or chronic endotoxemia results in a hyperdynamic cardiovascular state characterized by increased cardiac output, decreased systemic vascular resistance, hypotension, and a less pronounced pulmonary response. This syndrome is termed the "warm" phase of septic shock. Tissue hypoxia occurs despite the hyperdynamic cardiovascular state. The oxygen debt may be due to arteriovenous shunting or altered cellular metabolism, which interferes with oxygen utilization. If prolonged, the hypoxia ultimately leads to multiple organ failure and death.

CLINICAL SIGNS AND RECOGNITION

In the early stages of shock, compensatory mechanisms result in minimal external clinical signs. Elevated heart rate and reduced pulse pressure may be the only clinical abnormalities. The presence of shock should be considered when tachycardia occurs in the absence of identifiable chronotropic stimuli such as excitement, anemia, or pain. In more advanced cases, evidence of peripheral vascular collapse becomes evident with pale mucous membranes, prolonged capillary refill time, cool extremities, and reduced urine output. Depression and muscular weakness may be noted. Tachycardia becomes more extreme, pulse pressures decline, and heart sounds weaken as the condition progresses. Tachypnea may occur due to lactic acidosis or pulmonary edema.

Exception to the above scenario occurs in the hyperdynamic stage of septic shock, wherein clinical findings may include increased heart sounds, strong pulse pressure, and hyperemic mucous membranes with shortened capillary refill time. Ruminal stasis and low-volume diarrhea are often present in endotoxemic ruminants. Animals will usually be febrile during this stage, but the temperature will decline in advanced stages of shock, such that an animal with severe sepsis may be normo- or hypothermic.

Signs indicative of cardiogenic shock may include venous distention, murmurs, arrhythmias, and abnormal jugular pulses. Severe tachypnea and dyspnea occur with acute left heart failure, and this must be distinguished from primary pneumonia. Animals in left heart failure are typically less febrile and depressed than are animals with infectious pneumonia and lung sounds characterized as crackles are present rather than wheezes or friction rubs.

The diagnosis of shock is usually based on the history and physical findings. Hemodynamic monitoring and blood gas analysis can be valuable tools in the differentiation and management of various shock states, but are not often employed because of practical constraints.

THERAPY

The primary therapeutic objective in all forms of shock not associated with cardiac failure is restoration of an effective circulating blood volume. Other considerations include maximizing blood oxygen content, correction of acid-base abnormalities, antibiotic therapy, cardiovascular support, and counteracting the effects of harmful mediators (Table 1). Therapy of cardiac failure is discussed in this section in the article "Therapeutic Management of Cardiovascular Diseases."

Blood volume expansion should be accomplished by intravenous or intraosseous (neonates, swine) fluid administration. Fluids given by subcutaneous or oral routes are unlikely to be absorbed rapidly enough in shock states to warrant their sole use. The most appropriate type of fluid to be administered is dependent on the underlying pathogenesis, economics, and temporal restraints.

Isotonic sodium-rich electrolyte solutions are the standard fluid type recommended for the treatment of shock. Large volumes are required because two thirds of the infused volume is distributed to the extravascular compartment shortly after administration. Approximately 60 mL/kg of body weight (BW) should be infused acutely. Rapid administration should proceed until evidence of increased peripheral perfusion is noted in the

Table 1
THERAPY FOR CIRCULATORY SHOCK

Treatment Objective	Therapy/Dose	Target Response
Restore blood volume	Isotonic crystalloids (0.9% NaCl, lactated Ringer's) 60–90 mL/kg rapidly; then as needed Hypertonic saline (7% NaCl) 4 mL/kg over 5–10 min; may repeat once followed by IV or oral replacement fluids	Absence of clinical dehydration Capillary refill time < 2 sec Urine output > 1 mL/kg/hr Central venous pressure 5–10 cm H_2O
Blood oxygen content	Oxygen insufflation 2–4 L/min/100 kg Blood transfusion 10–40 mL/kg given over 1–4 hr	Pink mucous membranes Hematocrit > 25 mL/dL Arterial oxygen tension (Pa_{O_2}) > 70 mm Hg
Correct acidosis	Sodium bicarbonate 3–5 mEq/kg over 15–30 min IV drip	Maintain blood pH > 7.25
Eliminate/prevent infection	Intravenous antibiotics Local debridement or drainage	Reduced fever Improved leukogram
Cardiovascular support	Inotropic agent Dopamine: 2–10 μg/kg/min IV drip Vasopressor Dopamine: 5–10 μg/kg/min IV drip	Strong palpable pulse Mean arterial pressure > 80 mm Hg
Mediator inhibition	Dexamethasone sodium phosphate: 1–2 mg/kg IV Flunixin meglumine: 0.3–1.0 mg/kg IV Polymixin B: 6000 IU/kg	

form of improved pulse pressures, mucous membrane color, and capillary refill. The rate can be slowed thereafter in accordance with the animal's condition. While a medical standard, this method of fluid administration is impractical in field settings for large animals.

Small volumes of hypertonic saline are transportable and can be administered rapidly, offering a practical alternative. The hypertonic solution draws body water into the vascular space, rapidly expanding the blood volume at the expense of tissue hydration. Hypertonic saline (7.5% NaCl) is infused at 4 mL/kg of BW over 5 to 10 minutes. The effect is transient, lasting about 1 hour, and should be followed immediately by other fluid administration. Ideally, this would be in the form of intravenous isotonic electrolytes, but a more practical alternative is oral administration of water or a hypotonic electrolyte solution. Contraindications to the use of hypertonic saline include hypernatremia, hypokalemia, severe dehydration, or uncontrolled hemorrhage. Synthetic colloids can be added to hypertonic saline to prolong its hemodynamic effect, but their use is cost-prohibitive for most food animal patients.

Maximizing blood oxygen content involves oxygen supplementation and correction of significant anemia. If available, oxygen should be supplemented via facemask, transtracheal catheter, nasal insufflation, or endotracheal intubation. With acute hemorrhagic shock, volume expansion should be employed while blood is collected for transfusion. If hemorrhage has been severe or the packed cell volume falls below 20% with fluid administration, at least 10 to 20 mL/kg BW of whole blood should be administered.

Correction of metabolic acidosis and electrolyte abnormalities should be undertaken cautiously unless laboratory analysis is performed. Empirically, a bicarbonate dose of 3 to 5 mEq/kg of BW can be estimated for moderate to severe shock.

Antibiotics should be administered to animals in septic shock. The choice of antibiotic should be predicated on knowledge of the likely pathogens in an identified focus of infection. If a source of infection is not identified, broad-spectrum, intravenous, and nontoxic drugs should be chosen. Focal sources of infection should be removed by drainage or debridement. Antibiotics may be of benefit in other types of severe shock as translocation of bacteria may occur across the hypoperfused

intestinal tract. In such cases, antibiotics should be chosen for efficacy against gram-negative and anaerobic bacteria.

Hemodynamic support may be indicated in the form of positive ionotropic agents and vasopressors or vasodilators in individual cases. Most of these drugs should be given by constant-rate infusion and under hemodynamic monitoring; thus their use is typically impractical in clinical food animal practice.

A variety of drugs have been utilized to block some of the deleterious effects of biologic mediators released during shock. These include corticosteroids, nonsteroidal anti-inflammatory drugs (NSAIDs), hyperimmune serum, and polymyxin B. The therapeutic value of these agents in the treatment of shock is controversial and some can have significant adverse effects; thus their utility should be assessed based on the circumstances in individual cases.

If corticosteroids are to be beneficial in shock therapy, they must be given early, in aqueous formulations, and in large doses. Corticosteroids can induce peripheral vasodilation, worsening a hypotensive state, and should be given only after volume expansion has been initiated. Certain NSAIDs are capable of reducing the adverse effects of endotoxemia. Flunixin meglumine and ketoprofen (approved for use in horses) are probably the most effective for this purpose. These NSAIDs carry the risk of renal and gastrointestinal toxicity and should be used cautiously in hypoperfused patients. Subanti-inflammatory doses (one-third to one-fourth of the full dose) of NSAIDs have proved effective in treatment of experimental endotoxemia and the reduced dose may lessen the risk of adverse effects. Polymyxin B is a cationic antibiotic that combines with endotoxin and may reduce its biologic effect. In studies performed in foals, a subantibacterial dose of polymyxin B (6000 IU/kg) was found to lessen the severity of clinical signs associated with endotoxemia. Polymyxin B is nephrotoxic and neurotoxic and should be used cautiously in shock states. Conflicting results have been reported on the efficacy of antiendotoxin antibody (hyperimmune serum) in clinical endotoxemia. The high cost of this mode of therapy and its questionable efficacy preclude its use in most cases of septic shock in food animal patients.

When anaphylactic shock is diagnosed, epinephrine should be given immediately (1 mL/100 kg of 1:1000 epinephrine intramuscularly; with cardiopulmonary arrest, give one-half the dose diluted 1:10 with saline intravenously). Additional therapy in the form of corticosteroids, antihistamines, bronchodilators, and intravenous fluids may be indicated if prompt recovery is not evident after epinephrine administration.

BIBLIOGRAPHY

Bottoms GD, Adams HR: Involvement of prostaglandins and leukotrienes in the pathogenesis of endotoxemia and sepsis. J Am Vet Med Assoc 200:1842–1849, 1992.

Cullor JS: Shock attributable to bacteremia and endotoxemia in cattle: Clinical and experimental findings. J Am Vet Med Assoc 200:1894–1902, 1992.

Ferguson DW: Cardiogenic Shock. In Wyngaarden JB (ed): Cecil Textbook of Medicine, ed 20. Philadelphia, WB Saunders, 1996, pp 477–496.

Holbrook TC, Moore JN: Anti-inflammatory and immune support in endotoxemia and septicemia. Vet Clin North Am Equine Pract 10:535–547, 1994.

Olson NC, Hellyer PW, Dodam JR: Mediators and vascular effects in response to endotoxin. Br Vet J 151:489–522, 1995.

St Jean G, Constable PD, Yvorchuk K: The clinical use of hypertonic saline in food animals with hemorrhagic and endotoxic shock. Agri Pract 14:6–11, 1993.

Tobias TA, Schertel ER: Shock: concepts and management. In DiBartola SP (ed): Fluid Therapy in Small Animal Practice, Philadelphia, WB Saunders, 1992, pp 436–470.

Traber DL, Flynn JT, Herndon DN, et al: Comparison of the cardiopulmonary responses to single bolus and continuous infusion of endotoxin in an ovine model. Circ Shock 27:123–138, 1989.

■ Acquired Diseases of the Heart

Bimbo Welker, D.V.M., M.S.

The most common acquired cardiac conditions in food animals include traumatic pericarditis, bacterial endocarditis, lymphosarcoma, atrial fibrillation, and nutritional dystrophies. The food animal practitioner should be familiar with diagnosis, treatment, and prognosis of these five conditions, realizing that other less common conditions may also occur.

TRAUMATIC RETICULOPERICARDITIS

Signs, Clinical Findings, and Diagnosis

Nonspecific signs suggestive of cardiac dysfunction and consistent with traumatic reticulopericarditis include lethargy, inappetence, rapid drop in production, and mild pyrexia. The physical examination findings that are suggestive of pericardial involvement include bilateral jugular distention or abnormal pulsation, a muffling of cardiac sounds, or a characteristic "washing machine" murmur. The signs and examination findings vary depending on the volume of fluid accumulation within the pericardium and the stage of the disease. The differential diagnoses for jugular distention or pulsation include any cause of right heart failure, compression of the precava by intrathoracic lesions (abscess, tumor, or fibrosis), jugular thrombophlebitis, or pericardial disease. The muffled heart sounds must be differentiated from masses or fluid in the thorax that decrease the audibility of the sounds. Pleuritis is an important differential diagnosis for pericarditis. Pericarditis can tentatively be differentiated from pleuritis by characteristics found on auscultation.

Pericarditis typically results in a muffling of heart sounds, an absence of lung sounds ventrally, and an increase in the audibility of lung sounds dorsally. In contrast, pleuritis results in a muffling of both heart and lung sounds ventrally, but not of radiation of the heart sounds. In fact, the heart sounds will radiate over a wider than normal area, and they are often accompanied by abnormal breath sounds and/or pleural friction rubs. The characteristic "washing machine" or "splashing" murmur is heard in cases of pericarditis in which the associated bacteria are gas producers. Although this murmur is pathognomonic for septic pericardial disease, its absence does not rule it out.

The definitive diagnosis of pericardial disease must be made using pericardiocentesis and, if it is available, echocardiography. Pericardiocentesis allows evaluation of the effusion. Collected fluid can be used for culture and sensitivity to determine appropriate antibiotic therapy. A false-positive result can occur if the fluid obtained is actually from the thoracic cavity rather than the pericardial sac. Auscultation characteristics and performing the aspiration at alternate locations might help alleviate this problem. Ultrasonography of the thorax provides the best method of establishing the location of the fluid.

A definitive diagnosis of traumatic reticulopericarditis can be made only by identifying penetration of a foreign body from the reticulum into the pericardial sac. This requires evidence of cranial reticulitis at the time of a laparotomy and/or rumenotomy, identification of a foreign body on ultrasound within the pericardial sac, or visualization of a foreign body on thoracic radiographs. In a field setting, and depending on economics, laparotomy/rumenotomy may be the most practical method of diagnosis. Both ultrasound and radiography can be costly and difficult to interpret, even for specialists.

Nontraumatic or primary pericardial effusion may occur and should be considered as a differential diagnosis when a foreign body or reticulitis cannot be identified. Hematogenous pericarditis has been reported in cattle. The characteristics of the fluid obtained from pericardiocentesis may be similar. A single isolate is likely to be found in cases of hematogenous pericarditis as compared to a mixed bacterial population found in traumatic reticulopericarditis. Transudation of fluid into the pericardial sac as a result of congestion, hypoproteinemia, or neoplastic effusion may also occur. The fluid characteristics should be confirmatory.

Etiology

Traumatic reticulopericarditis is the result of penetration of the reticular wall, diaphragm, and pericardial sac by a sharp metal object, from which septic inflammation ensues. The condition occurs most commonly in older cattle. Dairy cows and beef cattle in feedlot conditions are at higher risk. Confinement and other management practices increase their exposure and probability of ingesting foreign objects, such as wire and nails.

Ingested metal objects tend to settle into the first compartment or reticulum. During reticular contraction or episodes of increased abdominal pressure, such as parturition, the sharp object may be pushed through the wall. Because of the close anatomic relationship between the pericardium and the reticulum, an object penetrating the cranial wall may be directed into the pericardial sac. Penetration into the pericardial sac may inoculate the area with ruminal bacteria. If the offending structure persists long enough to allow significant inoculation, and the body defenses cannot overcome the insult, the bacteria proliferate. The result may be acute, subacute, or chronic fibrinopurulent pericarditis. Absorption of bacterial toxins results in systemic signs of fever and malaise. Accumulation of fluid within the pericardial sac or thickening of the pericardium and epicardium will impair cardiac function and result in the development of right heart failure.

Treatment and Prognosis

An animal with a diagnosis of traumatic reticulopericarditis should never be given anything better than a guarded (30%) prognosis. The chronicity of the condition is a major factor in determining the possible outcome. Chronicity, however, may be difficult to ascertain. Acute cases may respond to prolonged antibiotic therapy and removal of the foreign object, if it is still present, via left laparotomy and rumenotomy. Repeated pericardiocentesis or pericardiotomy and/or pericardiostomy for drainage and lavage have been useful in a few cases for short-term salvage. The best treatment is prevention. Management practices to prevent exposure to metal objects combined with prophylactic magnet administration can reduce the incidence of traumatic reticulopericarditis.

Nontraumatic cases of suppurative pericarditis should be given a similar prognosis and treated similarly, except for the rumenotomy. A laparotomy may still be utilized as a diagnostic tool.

BACTERIAL ENDOCARDITIS

Signs, Clinical Findings, and Diagnosis

The clinical signs of bacterial endocarditis vary depending on the stage of the disease. The most common complaints on admission are recurrent fever, anorexia, weight loss, and poor production. Lameness or stiffness may even be the predominant presenting sign. In the early stages of the disease these signs can be present without evidence of cardiac malfunction. Of these nonspecific signs, the identification of recurrent fever should at least suggest the possibility of early bacterial endocarditis. As the disease progresses, some sign of cardiac dysfunction usually develops. Early evidence includes tachycardia (80 to 120 beats/minute), murmurs, loud and pounding heart sounds, arrhythmias, and/or pulse deficits. These signs, although more specific for cardiac disease, are not specific for endocarditis. Finding nonspecific signs, especially recurrent fever, in combination with a murmur is highly suggestive of bacterial endocarditis and warrants specific diagnostic investigation. As the disease process advances, signs of congestive heart failure begin to appear. At this stage, peripheral edema, jugular and mammary vein distention, dyspnea, pulmonary edema, and cachexia may appear.

Diagnosis of bacterial endocarditis in the early stages is difficult. Because clinical signs can occur without evidence of cardiac abnormalities, the practitioner must be sensitized to the very nonspecific signs, especially recurrent fever, and be alerted to conditions that may predispose to the disease, such as chronic infectious processes elsewhere in the body. Identifying bacterial endocarditis at this stage or even at later stages requires a positive blood culture and/or echocardiographic detection of the lesion.

Proper blood culturing technique is critical for a correct diagnosis. Sampling should be done from multiple (a minimum of three) aseptically prepared sites. Arterial and venous sites are acceptable. Sampling from indwelling catheters is not recommended. Blood should generally be drawn during fever spikes to improve efficacy. It is important that two or more of the samples be positive to decrease the possibility of contamination at one site causing a false-positive result. Additionally, multiple negative cultures do not definitively rule out the disease.

Echocardiographic evaluation (if available) is a noninvasive and quick method of diagnosing endocarditis. False-positive and -negative results can occur. In the early stages, the lesions may be very small and may be missed on ultrasound. Failure to identify the lesion is therefore not conclusive.

Etiology

Bacterial endocarditis in cattle is typically a sequela to a chronic infectious process at some distant site and to persistent bacteremia. Common sources of chronic or recurrent bacteremia in cattle include traumatic reticulitis, liver abscesses, metritis, mastitis, omphalophlebitis, and musculoskeletal diseases. Circulating bacteria may colonize the valve leaflets either by direct adherence or by embolism of the valve capillaries. The tricuspid valve is typically the most commonly involved in ruminants, but any valve or combination of valves can be affected. *Actinomyces (Corynebacterium) pyogenes* and α-hemolytic *Streptococcus* are the organisms most commonly isolated from these lesions in cattle.

The lesion produced on the valve leaflets varies depending on chronicity. In acute cases the lesion may develop into a large, cauliflower-like (vegetative) growth on the free edge of the leaflet. As the disease becomes chronic, the lesion becomes smaller and wart-like (verrucose), and the valves are shrunken and distorted.

The consequences of such valvular lesions result from either the interference with normal valve function or the showering of septic emboli. Large vegetative lesions can interfere with normal blood flow and cause cardiac dysfunction. Dysfunction results from regurgitation through an incompetent valve or from the myocardium's having to work harder to expel blood through an obstructed orifice. In addition, the vegetative lesions tend to fragment easily, sending emboli throughout the systemic circulation, which can lodge and create abscesses at distant sites. Typical sites include the lungs, kidneys, and joints. As the lesions become more chronic they are less fragile, and the pathology produced is related primarily to the distortion of the valves (heart failure).

Treatment and Prognosis

Successful treatment of bacterial endocarditis requires early detection and long-term antibiotic therapy (minimum, 4 weeks). Treatment in the early stages, before evidence of cardiac dysfunction develops and when diagnosis is most difficult, results in a fair (50%) to good (70%) prognosis for recovery. As the signs of right heart failure develop (e.g., edema, jugular distention or pulsation), the prognosis progressively drops to poor. Even with successful treatment of the infection, any valvular disfigurement and subsequent murmurs or insufficiencies are likely to persist.

Antibiotic selection should optimally be based on culture and sensitivity results. During the interim period, considering the most common organisms involved, penicillin is a reasonable selection. Procaine penicillin G (minimum 20,000 units/kg, twice daily) is safe and inexpensive for the long-term therapy required. If evidence of congestive heart failure is present, diuretics and a low-salt diet may be beneficial. Recovery is likely to be slow and gradual. Improvement in appetite, weight gain, and cessation of febrile episodes are signs of recovery. However, even with successful treatment of the infection, signs related to valve distortion may persist.

To prevent bacterial endocarditis, the chronic disease processes that result in episodes of chronic bacteremia should be prevented or treated.

ADULT LYMPHOSARCOMA

Signs, Clinical Findings, and Diagnosis

The clinical signs associated with infiltration of the heart by lymphosarcoma vary depending on the structures involved and the size and position of the lesions. Characteristically, cardiac lymphosarcoma begins in the right atrium, but it is by no means limited to this structure. As the tumor infiltrates the musculature of the heart and/or enlarges in size, function of the myocardium becomes impaired. Clinical signs of cardiomyopathy may ensue (e.g., brisket edema, jugular distention or pulsation). Disruption of the sinoatrial node in the right atrium may result in cardiac arrhythmias. These signs are not specific for lymphosarcoma and must be differentiated from other causes of cardiac malfunction.

A diagnosis of lymphosarcoma as the cause of cardiomyopathy or arrhythmia can be very challenging. If lymphosarcoma can be identified elsewhere in the body, a tentative diagnosis can be made. Echocardiographic examination can be useful in identifying masses associated with the cardiac structures. This may allow differentiation of lymphosarcoma from other common causes of cardiac dysfunction, such as pericarditis and bacterial endocarditis. Pericardiocentesis may be performed if hydropericardium is suspected on the basis of ultrasound or from auscultation of muffled heart sounds. Occasionally, abnormal lymphocytes may be identified in the fluid. Leukemia is a characteristic of only one third of clinical cases, but it is very significant if identified. The primary differential diagnosis to consider is persistent lymphocytosis (PL), a benign lymphoproliferative response to bovine leukemia virus (BLV). The definitive diagnosis of lymphosarcoma can be made only by histologic examination of tissues obtained at biopsy or necropsy. Serologic tests for BLV infection are available. Positive titers to the virus indicate infection by the virus; however, this finding cannot be interpreted as a diagnosis of clinical lymphosarcoma. Estimates suggest that anywhere from 10% to 20% of adult cattle across the United States will have titers to BLV. A negative titer in an animal suspected of having adult lymphosarcoma is more valuable in ruling out the diagnosis than is a positive titer, which may only indicate infection, exposure and seroconversion, in confirming the diagnosis. Fewer than 5% of cattle infected with BLV develop lymphosarcoma.

Etiology

Adult bovine lymphosarcoma, also known as enzootic bovine leukosis (EBL), is a fatal systemic neoplasm of the lymphoreticular tissue. The heart is only one of many tissues that can be affected. The diverse types of tissues and organ systems that can be affected result in a potential myriad of presenting clinical signs. Seroepidemiologic studies indicate that BLV is the causative agent of EBL. BLV is a retrovirus.

The spread of BLV is mainly by contact. Transmission can occur by the transfer of infected lymphocytes via hematophagous (bloodsucking) insects or blood-contaminated instruments (e.g., needles, syringes). Although BLV and/or BLV-infected lymphocytes are present in the milk of most infected dams, transmission to the calf via the milk is thought to be infrequent. Maternal antibodies in the colostrum are believed to protect the calf from infection during the nursing period. Prenatal transmission is also uncommon. Fewer than 20% of calves born to BLV-infected dams are infected with BLV in utero (i.e., BLV positive at birth). Recent studies raise the possibility of transmission of BLV in semen. BLV-infected lymphocytes could possibly be present in semen from bulls with inflammatory conditions of the urogenital tract. Transmission of the infection via artificial insemination is considered unlikely.

Bovine lymphosarcoma affects both sexes and all breeds but is most common in adult dairy cattle. The majority of cases occur in the 4- to 8-year-old age group, with most patients being 3 years of age. There also appears to be a tendency for clinical cases to aggregate along familial lines, suggesting a hereditary predisposition to tumor development.

Treatment, Prevention, and Prognosis

No effective treatments for lymphosarcoma have been available to date; therefore the prognosis is grave. The economic losses due to death, loss of productivity, and export restrictions can make this disease very economically significant in certain herds.

Eradication of BLV infection, and therefore EBL, is possible, but the cost effectiveness of an eradication program must be considered on a farm-to-farm basis. Such eradication programs should be based on accurate identification and removal of BLV-positive animals from the herd and institution of management practices to reduce transmission of the infection. A vaccine may be present in the future.

ATRIAL FIBRILLATION

Signs, Clinical Findings, and Diagnosis

Cows with atrial fibrillation (AF) generally do not present with signs specifically related to the cardiovascular system. The most common complaints associated with cows having AF are anorexia and poor production. Obviously these signs are very nonspecific and, in fact, are probably more related to the underlying cause of the arrhythmia than to the AF itself.

Atrial fibrillation can be detected during cardiac auscultation. This conduction disturbance creates an *irregularly irregular* rhythm. During auscultation, absolutely no pattern can be detected in the intervals between beats. The heart rate varies from normal to very rapid with this disturbance. When the rate is very rapid, the irregularity in intervals may not be easily appreciated. Another auscultatory finding is variation in intensity from beat to beat. This sound is referred to as "jungle drum" beats. Either or both of these auscultation findings are highly suggestive of atrial fibrillation in the cow.

The definitive diagnosis of atrial fibrillation requires electrocardiography. The base-apex lead is performed by placing the left arm (LA) lead on the point of the left elbow, the right arm (RA) lead in the right jugular furrow, and the chest (C) lead as a ground lead anywhere on the animal. This arrangement, recorded on lead I, will generate a positive P wave, a positive QRS deflection, and a positive T wave in the normal animal. Criteria used to diagnose atrial fibrillation will include the absence of P waves, the presence of F waves (baseline flutter), an irregular R-R interval, and variation in the amplitude of the QRS complex.

Etiology

Atrial fibrillation is one of the most common arrhythmias detected in cattle. It can and usually does occur without apparent underlying primary heart disease. It is therefore often referred to as a *functional arrhythmia*. The clinical significance of this is that if the underlying cause of the disturbance can be corrected, the arrhythmia may convert back to normal sinus rhythm. The most common underlying causes that tend to predispose to atrial fibrillation are gastrointestinal disorders. It should be noted, however, that atrial fibrillation has been associated with diseases of other systems. The acid-base and electrolyte abnormalities frequently seen with these disturbances have been incriminated as contributing to the development of atrial fibrillation. Therapy is usually directed at these imbalances and at correction of the primary disease process.

Primary heart disease must be considered a differential diagnosis, especially in those that fail to respond to correction of the primary problem and its associated imbalances. Ultrasound may be useful in identifying gross abnormalities in the right atrium (e.g., lymphosarcoma).

Treatment and Prognosis

Treatment of atrial fibrillation is warranted in any cow valuable enough to keep in the herd. Persistence of atrial fibrillation may lead to poor performance and progressive cardiac disease.

Treatment of atrial fibrillation should first be directed at the suspected underlying disease, usually gastrointestinal, and the concomitant acid-base and electrolyte disorders. Once these are corrected, self-conversion to normal sinus rhythm occurs within 5 to 7 days in 40% to 50% of cattle. Failure of spontaneous conversion to occur after resolution of concurrent disorders is a criterion for antiarrhythmic therapeutic intervention. The treatment of choice is quinidine sulfate (44 mg/kg dissolved in 4 L of distilled water, administered in a slow intravenous infusion (approximately 1 L/hour). In most cases conversion will occur in 2 to 4 hours. At whatever time conversion does occur, the drug is stopped immediately. When conversion is achieved using this technique, normal sinus rhythm is generally maintained. Oral administration studies have not proven as effective. Quinidine can be toxic to the heart, and treatment associated fatalities may occur; therefore, treatment should be monitored with an ongoing electrocardiogram. A widening of the QRS complex on ECG is suggestive of toxic effects. Side effects that are noted in all cases include ataxia, blepharospasm, diarrhea, increased frequency of defecation, and increase in rumen contractions. These effects are transient, lasting less than 12 hours. In cases in which heart rates are very high, the conversion may be facilitated by administering digoxin (1 mg/100 kg, given intravenously) prior to quinidine treatment. A failure to respond to treatment suggests either inappropriate treatment or underlying heart disease. A poor prognosis for performance is typical in these cases, and progressive cardiac disease may ensue.

NUTRITIONAL MYODEGENERATION (WHITE MUSCLE DISEASE)

Signs, Clinical Findings, and Diagnosis

Nutritional myodegeneration, or white muscle disease, presents as two distinct syndromes: a cardiac form and a skeletal muscle form. Both forms tend to affect the young, but they have been suspected in yearlings and adults. The cardiac form typically affects neonates in the first week of life. The clinical course is acute, or peracute, and usually results in severe debilitation or sudden death. Because the heart, diaphragm, and intercostal muscles are affected, animals may present with signs predominantly referable to the respiratory system. Cardiac murmurs and irregular heartbeats may be detected. Murmurs at this age require consideration of congenital anomalies as differential diagnoses. If the animal presents without significant signs of cardiac dysfunction but with severe debilitation or sudden death, the differential diagnosis list must include septicemia, pneumonia, diarrhea and dehydration, or toxic effects.

White muscle disease should be considered as a differential diagnosis any time these signs are present in a neonate from a geographic area where the problem is endemic. The antemortem diagnosis of white muscle disease should be based on *whole-blood levels of selenium and plasma levels of vitamin E*. Whole-blood selenium concentrations range from 0.07 to 0.1 ppm in normal animals. The critical levels of vitamin E in *plasma* are 1.1 to 2.0 ppm. Vitamin E in plasma deteriorates rapidly; therefore, samples need to be put on ice immediately and stored at $-21°F$ ($-16°C$) if the analysis is not going to be performed immediately. The blood and plasma levels of selenium and vitamin E, respectively, do not assess body stores. Tissue samples taken by antemortem biopsy or at postmortem can be useful in evaluating body stores. Liver selenium levels of 0.9 to 1.75 µg/g of dry matter (DM) for cattle and 0.9 to 3.5 µg/g of DM for sheep are considered normal. A diagnosis of selenium and/or vitamin E deficiency can also be supported by ration analysis.

The postmortem findings are typical and include white streaks in the muscle bundles, which represent bands of coagulation necrosis; in chronic cases they may represent fibrosis and calcification. In calves, the left ventricular wall and septum are most frequently affected.

Etiology

Deficiencies of selenium and/or vitamin E apparently result in destruction of cell membranes and proteins, leading to a loss of cellular integrity. Cell damage results from the presence of free radicals and peroxides. Normal cellular metabolism produces high levels of reactive forms of oxygen (free radicals) such as hydrogen peroxide, hydroperoxides, superoxides, and various other radicals. Vitamin E in the cell membrane scavenges these free radicals before they can combine with unsaturated fatty acids to form lipid hydroperoxides. Selenium as a component of the enzyme glutathione peroxidase destroys the peroxides that have already formed.

Soils in certain regions of the United States and other countries are inherently low in selenium. The northeastern and eastern seaboard and the northwestern regions of the United States are particularly deficient. Acid soils, soils originating from volcanic rock, and high-sulfur soils or those treated with sulfur-containing fertilizers are likely to be low. In addition, forages may vary in selenium content. Legumes take up less than grasses, and all forages take up less selenium during rapid growth and in times of high rainfall.

Vitamin E deficiencies become a problem when animals are fed poor-quality hay, straw, or root crops. Stored grains lose their vitamin E content with time. Cereal grains, green-growing pastures, and properly prepared hays usually have adequate concentrations of vitamin E.

Selenium and vitamin E tend to have a sparing effect on one another. Adequate levels of vitamin E can decrease the level of selenium required in the diet. In contrast, low levels of vitamin E will increase the selenium requirement.

Treatment and Prognosis

The calf that presents with signs of cardiac dysfunction as a result of vitamin E and/or selenium deficiency must be given a poor prognosis. Most affected animals die within 24 hours. If therapy is to be instituted it must be immediate, before signs advance. Injectable vitamin E/selenium (at 2.5 to 3.0 mg/45 kg), given either intramuscularly or subcutaneously, is recommended.

Prevention of myocardial degeneration from white muscle disease must be aimed at proper supplementation of the dam either by salt mix or by total ration supplementation and, if late in gestation, prepartum injection of vitamin E/selenium.

BIBLIOGRAPHY

Blood DC, Radostits OM: Veterinary Medicine, 7th ed. Baltimore, Williams & Wilkins, 1989.
Ferrer JF: Bovine lymphosarcoma. Compend Contin Educ Pract Vet 2:S235–S241, 1980.
Ferrer JF, Marshak RR, Abt DA, et al: Relationship between lymphosarcoma and persistent lymphocytosis in cattle: A review. J Am Vet Med Assoc 175:705–708, 1979.
Krishnamurthy D, Nigam JM, Peshin PK, et al: Thoracopericardiotomy and pericardiectomy in cattle. J Am Vet Med Assoc 175:714–718, 1979.
Maas JP: Diagnosis and management of selenium-responsible diseases in cattle. Compend Cont Ed Pract Vet 5:S393–S400, 1983.
McGuirk SM, Muir WW, Sams RA: Pharmacokinetic analysis of intravenously and orally administered quinidine in horses. Am J Vet Res 42:938–942, 1981.
McGuirk SM, Muir WW, Sams RA: Pharmacokinetic analysis of intravenously and orally administered quinidine in cows. Am J Vet Res 42:1482–1487, 1981.
Miller JM: Bovine lymphosarcoma. Bovine Proc 20:34–36, 1988.
Power HT, Rebhun WC: Bacterial endocarditis in adult dairy cattle. J Am Vet Med Assoc 182:806–808, 1983.
Smith JA: Bacterial endocarditis in cattle. Bovine Clin 3:8, 1983.
Ströber M: The clinical picture of the enzootic and sporadic forms of bovine leukosis. Bovine Pract 16:119–129, 1981.

■ Hematology of Food Animals

Marlyn S. Whitney, D.V.M., Ph.D., Diplomate, A.C.V.P.

Hematologic evaluation is useful for the assessment of many disease states. Primary alterations in hematologic parameters result from disorders within the hemic system itself. Perhaps more important, secondary hematologic alterations commonly occur as the result of abnormalities in other body systems, so hematologic evaluation can provide important diagnostic clues to many diverse conditions. Because similar hematologic abnormalities may occur in response to widely different processes, determination of hematologic parameters alone rarely provides a definitive diagnosis. However, when hematologic alterations are interpreted in conjunction with other patient information, such as the history, physical examination findings, and other relevant laboratory data, appropriate diagnostic decisions can often be made. This article emphasizes general principles regarding the use and interpretation of hematologic tests. Hematology laboratory methods are described elsewhere.[2, 4, 11]

LABORATORY EVALUATION OF THE HEMIC SYSTEM

Parameters Evaluated

The complete blood count (CBC), the most commonly performed hematologic procedure, serves as a broad screening test for hematologic abnormalities. If the CBC provides incomplete information regarding hematologic abnormalities, additional diagnostic procedures may be warranted.

A CBC aids assessment of any animal that has clinical indications of anemia, infection, inflammation, or bleeding disorders. Additionally, a CBC may provide useful diagnostic clues in animals with vague or nonspecific clinical signs. The CBC usually consists of the following: hematocrit, hemoglobin, red blood cell (RBC) count, total white blood cell (WBC) count, platelet count or estimate, and examination of a stained blood film to determine the WBC differential distribution and to evaluate individual blood cell staining characteristics and morphology. In addition, an estimate of the total plasma protein level is often done by refractometer. An estimate of the plasma fibrinogen level is often included in the CBC for food animal species.

A bone marrow examination may assist in explaining CBC findings that cannot be explained by the patient's history, physical examination findings, or other diagnostic tests. Bone marrow examination is indicated when the CBC identifies any unexplained peripheral blood cytopenia and is used for evaluation of animals with suspected hematopoietic neoplasia.

In addition to a platelet count, the most common laboratory procedures for assessment of the hemostatic mechanism are the activated clotting time (ACT) and the activated partial thromboplastin time (PTT) for assessment of the intrinsic and common coagulation cascades, and the prothrombin time (PT) for assessment of the extrinsic and common coagulation cascades. If a thrombotic disorder, such as diffuse intravascular coagulation, is suspected, the PTT and PT may be supplemented with determinations of antithrombin III (ATIII) and plasma fibrinogen levels and a test to detect the presence in serum of excessive fibrin degradation products (FDP). Other tests used to evaluate hemostasis, such as determinations of specific coagulation factor levels, von Willebrand factor assays, and platelet function tests, are rarely requested for food animal patients, and the availability of these tests for these species is restricted to a few hemostasis research laboratories.

For animals suspected of having iron deficiency or disordered iron metabolism, determination of serum iron and transferrin levels is helpful. The serum transferrin level is usually determined as the serum total iron binding capacity (TIBC). Body iron stores can be estimated by microscopic examination of Prussian blue–stained bone marrow specimens.

The Office Hematology Laboratory

The types of laboratory procedures performed in house in an individual practice are determined by the caseload of the practice, economic considerations, and the accessibility of reliable outside laboratories. It is within the capability of most veterinary practices to perform in-house CBCs. Some practitioners may elect to perform additional hematologic procedures in their practice laboratories.

Cell counts can be performed either manually with a hemocytometer or with an automated blood cell counter. Sample preparation for manual cell counting is most easily done using Unopette* blood dilution chambers. Dilution chambers are available for performing reasonably accurate WBC and platelet counts. Manual RBC counts are less accurate. The hematocrit can be determined via centrifugation of microhematocrit tubes, or it can be calculated from the RBC count and mean red cell volume (MCV) as measured by an automated blood cell counter. A hand-held temperature-compensated clinical refractometer is used to estimate the total plasma protein level. If a heated water bath is available, the plasma fibrinogen level can be estimated refractometrically by the heat precipitation method. This

_____
*Available from Becton Dickinson & Co., Rutherford, NJ.

method is suitable for detecting the elevated fibrinogen levels characteristic of inflammatory processes but is not sensitive or accurate enough to be reliable for detecting the decreased fibrinogen levels characteristic of consumptive coagulopathies. Various hemoglobinometers intended for office or field use are available. Polychrome stains, such as Wright's or Wright-Giemsa stain, are routinely used for staining blood and bone marrow aspirate smears. Commercially available quick stains such as Diff-Quik* are easy to use and give excellent results. New methylene blue stain is used for reticulocyte counts. The ACT is a useful office screening test for detecting disorders in the intrinsic and common coagulation pathways.

Sample Collection and Handling

Samples for routine CBCs should be collected into tubes containing ethylenediamine-tetraacetate (EDTA). Blood collection tubes should be filled to capacity. If tubes are filled to less than half of their capacity, EDTA will be excessive in relation to the blood volume. This results in artifactual spiculation of erythrocytes due to cell shrinkage, which falsely reduces the hematocrit and alters RBC morphology on blood smears. Underfilling of EDTA tubes may also cause a falsely high refractometric protein estimation because EDTA has a high refractive index.

If the CBC is not performed immediately in the office laboratory, a few blood smears should be made and allowed to air dry, and the remainder of the specimen should be kept at refrigerator temperature until the cell counts are done or it is shipped to an outside laboratory. Platelet counts must be done within 2 hours of sample collection. If this cannot be done, platelet numbers can be estimated using the stained blood smear. Although reasonably accurate WBC and RBC counts can be obtained on properly cooled specimens held for several days, accurate determination of the WBC differential distribution, estimation of platelet numbers, and assessment of blood cell morphology require that blood smears be made as soon as possible after sample collection. Staining can be delayed for several days if necessary. Once made, smears that are not stained immediately should be protected from water, dust, and flies. Bone marrow aspirate smears should be handled in the same manner as blood smears. Bone marrow core biopsies are routinely fixed in formalin in the same manner as other tissue biopsies. (Caution: exposure of blood and bone marrow smears to formalin vapors may impair staining. Slides should be put in slide holders and then sealed in plastic bags to protect them, or they should be shipped separately from formalin-fixed tissues.)

Samples for coagulation tests should be collected by careful venipuncture and handled per the instructions of the laboratory that is performing the analysis. Plastic syringes and plastic or silicon-coated collection and storage tubes should be used. Sodium citrate is the anticoagulant used for PTT and PT determinations. The blood-to-anticoagulant (3.8% sodium citrate solution) volume ratio must be correct: 9:1. Samples for FDP analysis are collected into special tubes intended specifically for that purpose. Specimens for most coagulation tests must be analyzed as quickly as possible after sample collection, or the plasma must be harvested and frozen at $-20°C$ until the analyses can be performed.

Samples for other laboratory tests that may be required should be collected and handled per the instructions of the laboratory performing the analysis.

---

*Available from VWR Scientific Products, Suwanee, Ga.

Hematologic Reference Ranges

Reference ranges for selected hematologic parameters of adult cattle, sheep, goats, and swine are presented in Table 1. Animals younger than 6 months tend to have somewhat lower hematocrits, RBC counts, hemoglobin levels, and plasma protein levels and somewhat higher total WBC counts. Neonates generally have a high hematocrit that decreases rapidly owing to colostrum ingestion. The hematocrit continues to decrease during phases of rapid growth, when body size is increasing faster than blood volume. Although fewer than 1% of the circulating erythrocytes are reticulocytes in healthy adult swine, suckling pigs have moderate to marked reticulocytosis and metarubricytosis owing to intense erythrogenesis related to rapid body growth and attendant increase in blood volume. In all species, lymphocyte counts tend to decrease with advancing age. Lactating animals, especially high-yield dairy cows, may have decreased hematocrits, RBC counts, and hemoglobin levels. Animals grazing at high altitude tend to have increased hematocrits, RBC counts, and hemoglobin levels. Whenever possible, reference ranges derived by the laboratory performing the hematologic tests should be used.

GENERAL PRINCIPLES OF HEMATOPOIESIS

General Information

With the exception of lymphocytes, blood cell formation in the normal healthy adult animal occurs only in the bone marrow. In normal adults, much of the marrow space is hematopoietically inactive and filled with fat. Active bone marrow remains in the flat bones and in the ends of the long bones. If the marrow hematopoietic tissue itself is healthy and has a proper nutrient supply, it can expand again into the fat-filled areas in response to increased peripheral use, loss, or destruction of blood cells. The capacity to respond to increased need for blood cells varies with the species and is generally less in food animal species than in companion animals. If the marrow is unable to respond adequately, extramedullary hematopoiesis may occur in the spleen and/or liver.

The Effects of Disease on Hematopoiesis

The hematopoietic tissue is liable to the same pathologic processes as other tissues: hyperplasia, hypoplasia, neoplasia (primary or metastatic), fibrosis, inflammation, and infarction. Hyperplasia, hypoplasia, and hematopoietic neoplasms may affect single or multiple components of the bone marrow. For example, following an episode of hemorrhage, an animal may develop hyperplasia of the erythroid compartment of the bone marrow, with the myeloid and megakaryocytic compartments remaining relatively normal. In this case there is an increased stimulus for erythrocyte production but less for leukocytes and platelets. In the case of toxins that damage the marrow stem cells that have not yet differentiated into specific cell lines, all three marrow compartments may become hypoplastic or aplastic simultaneously.

Lesions in the bone marrow may have either a diffuse or a focal distribution. Diffuse lesions will almost surely affect hematopoiesis and cause alterations in CBC findings, whereas focal lesions may have little or no effect on overall hematopoiesis. Hyperplastic and hypoplastic responses, primary hematopoietic neoplasms, and myelofibrosis usually have a diffuse distribution throughout the bone marrow. Osteomyelitis and bone

Table 1
HEMATOLOGIC REFERENCE RANGES

Parameter	Cattle	Sheep	Goats	Swine
Hematocrit (%)	24–46	27–45	23–38	32–50
Hemoglobin (g/dL)	8–15	9–15	8–12	9–16
RBC count ($\times 10^6/\mu$L)	5.0–10.0	9.0–15.0	8.0–18.0	5.0–8.0
Reticulocytes (% of RBC)	0	0	0	0–1
MCV (fL)	40–60	28–40	16–25	50–68
MCHC (g/dL)	30–36	31–34	30–36	29–34
Platelet count ($\times 10^5/\mu$L)	1.0–8.0	2.5–7.5	3.0–6.0	2.0–7.2
WBC count (cells/μL)	4000–12,000	4000–12,000	4000–13,000	11,000–22,000
Band neutrophils (cells/μL)	0–120	Rare	Rare	0–800
Segmented neutrophils (cells/μL)	600–4000	700–6000	1200–7200	2000–15,000
Lymphocytes (cells/μL)	2500–7500	2000–9000	2000–9000	3800–16,500
Monocytes (cells/μL)	25–850	0–750	0–550	0–1000
Eosinophils (cells/μL)	0–2400	0–1000	50–650	0–1500
Basophils (cells/μL)	0–200	0–300	0–120	0–500
Total plasma protein (g/dL)	6.0–8.5	6.0–7.5	6.0–7.5	6.0–8.0
Fibrinogen (g/dL)	1–7	1–5	1–4	1–5
Serum iron (μg/dL)	57–162	162–222		91–199
TIBC (μg/dL)	120–348	293–373		191–461
ATIII (% of normal canine pool)	130–153			
PT (seconds)	22–55			11–12
PTT (seconds)	44–64			34–39
FDP (μg/mL)	<10	<10	<10	<10
ACT	90–120			

Data from Duncan JR, Prasse KW: Veterinary Laboratory Medicine: Clinical Pathology, 2nd ed. Ames, Iowa, Iowa State University Press, 1986; Jain NC: Schalm's Veterinary Hematology, 4th ed. Philadelphia, Lea & Febiger, 1986; and the Clinical Pathology Laboratory of the Veterinary Teaching Hospital, Texas A&M University, College Station, Texas. See text for expected variations due to age, elevation, etc.

marrow infarction are usually focal lesions, but osteomyelitis may become multifocal and widespread in the case of bacterial infections that have spread hematogenously.

Neoplasms that metastasize to the bone marrow from other tissues may be focal, localized lesions that do not cause any widespread effects on blood cell production, or they may become so widespread in later stages as to have a diffuse distribution that essentially replaces the bone marrow. The latter situation may occur in the case of bovine lymphosarcoma, which may arise in the lymph nodes or other extramedullary tissue and subsequently metastasize to the bone marrow.

Lesions in virtually any tissue may have secondary effects on the hematopoietic tissues, affecting the results of a CBC. It is common for multiple processes to be simultaneously operant on the hematopoietic tissue.

DISORDERS OF THE ERYTHRON

Evaluation of the erythroid portion of the CBC is directed toward the detection and classification of anemia or polycythemia and toward the detection of any abnormalities in erythrocyte size, staining affinity, or morphology.

Anemia

Anemia is a common condition with diverse etiologies; it is a component of many diseases. The erythroid portion of the CBC is used to confirm the presence of anemia and, together with the remainder of the CBC data and the information obtained from the patient's history and physical examination findings, it often provides the necessary clues for determining the cause of anemia. A flow chart for the assessment of anemia is presented in Figure 1. The anemia is first classified as regenerative or nonregenerative. Especially in the case of nonregenerative ane-

mias, it is helpful to further classify the anemia with respect to RBC size (normocytic vs macrocytic or microcytic) and color (normochromic vs hypochromic). Classification of the anemia in this manner greatly shortens the list of etiologic possibilities.

Regenerative anemias are those in which marrow production and release of reticulocytes have increased to compensate for the increased loss of erythrocytes via blood loss or hemolysis. In contrast, nonregenerative anemias result from a decreased ability of the bone marrow to produce and release erythrocytes in response to peripheral needs. They can result from an intrinsic problem in the hematopoietic tissue, such as the lack of an essential nutrient or the presence of a toxin, or from an abnormality in the humoral signaling mechanisms that normally elicit an adequate level of erythropoiesis.

The reticulocyte count is used to determine if an anemia is regenerative or nonregenerative. With Wright's stain, reticulocytes appear as polychromatophils—erythrocytes that take up some blue stain as well as pink. Therefore, Wright's-stained blood smears from animals with highly regenerative anemias show marked polychromasia. More accurate identification and enumeration of reticulocytes is accomplished via the use of new methylene blue–stained smears. The reticulocyte count is expressed as the percentage of erythrocytes that display the blue reticulum characteristic of reticulocytes stained with new methylene blue. For accurate assessment of the adequacy of a regenerative response, the reticulocyte count must be adjusted for the severity of the anemia. To adjust the reticulocyte count, divide the patient's hematocrit by the mean normal hematocrit for the species and multiply the result by the patient's reticulocyte count expressed as a percentage. For example, a cow with a hematocrit of 18 and a reticulocyte count of 10% would have an adjusted reticulocyte count $(18 \div 35) \times 10 = 5.1$. An adjusted reticulocyte count of greater than 2.0 indicates a regenerative response, whereas a value less than 0.5 indicates a nonregenerative response. Values between 0.5 and 2.0 may occur early in a regenerative response (before the marrow has had time to

- Obtain clinical history and perform physical examination
- Identify or confirm anemia with Hct or hemoglobin determination

If the cause of anemia is not evident from the above:
- Do a complete CBC
- Do a reticulocyte count and adjust it for the severity of the anemia to determine if the anemia is regenerative or nonregenerative
- Determine the MCV and MCHC
- Further narrow the list of etiologic possibilities using the diagnostic clues indicated below each type of anemia (1a–2b)

1 Regenerative Anemia*
- Adjusted reticulocyte count >2.0
- Normal to slightly increased MCV
- Normal to slightly decreased MCHC
- Basophilic stippling common in ruminants

2 Nonregenerative Anemia*
- Adjusted reticulocyte count <0.5
- MCV and MCHC variable (see below)
- Bone marrow evaluation may be necessary to differentiate between 2a and 2b

1a Blood Loss
- Total protein decreased
- ± Hypovolemia (severe acute hemorrhage)
- ± Trauma
- ± Hemorrhagic effusion
- ± Hematuria
- ± Melena or fecal occult blood
- ± Evidence of endo- or ecto-parasites
- ± Evidence of hemostatic disorder
- See Table 3 for causes

1b Hemolysis
- Total protein normal or increased
- ± Hyperbilirubinemia†
- ± Bilirubinuria†
- ± Hemoglobinemia†
- ± Hemoglobinuria†
- ± Abnormal RBC morphology (e.g., schistocytes,† spherocytes,‡ RBC ghosts,† agglutination)
- ± RBC parasites
- ± Spleno/hepatomegaly‡
- See Table 3 for causes

2a Ineffective Erythropoiesis
- Nuclear maturation arrest often causes increased MCV
- Cytoplasmic maturation arrest often causes decreased MCV and/or decreased MCHC
- MCV and MCHC may be normal
- Erythroid compartment of marrow hyperplastic, but maturation sequence not complete
- See Table 4 for causes§

2b Erythroid Hypoplasia
- MCV and MCHC usually normal
- Erythroid compartment of marrow hypoplastic or aplastic
- See Table 4 for causes§

*If the corrected reticulocyte count is >0.5 but <2.0, the anemia may be a hemolytic or blood loss anemia that has not yet had sufficient time (4 to 6 days) to become regenerative.
†These findings suggest intravascular hemolysis.
‡These findings suggest extravascular hemolysis.
§Diagnosis of the anemia may be facilitated by a search for physical or laboratory evidence of the conditions listed in Table 4.
Hct = hematocrit; CBC = complete blood count; MCV = mean corpuscular volume; MCHC = mean corpuscular hemoglobin concentration; RBC = red blood cell.

Figure 1
Procedures for the assessment of anemia.

respond maximally) or as the result of secondary factors that impair a regenerative response. In cattle, and to a lesser degree in sheep and goats, regenerative responses are often characterized by prominent basophilic stippling of erythrocytes as well as by reticulocytosis. Basophilic stippling is readily observable with Wright's stain. Nucleated red blood cells (nRBCs) may be present in the circulation of animals with regenerative anemias, but they will be outnumbered by reticulocytes. Since nRBCs may be present in the circulating blood in some nonregenerative anemias, their presence alone cannot be used to differentiate regenerative from nonregenerative anemias.

Calculated parameters that are used to further classify anemias are the mean red cell volume (MCV) and the mean red cell hemoglobin concentration (MCHC), calculated as follows:

$$MCV = (Hct/RBC\ ct) \times 10$$

$$MCHC = (Hgb/Hct) \times 100$$

where Hct is the hematocrit (%), RBC ct is the erythrocyte count (10^6 cells/µL), and Hgb is the hemoglobin level (g/dL). The MCV is given in femtoliters, and the MCHC is expressed as grams per deciliter.

An increased MCV (macrocytosis) may be a feature of a regenerative anemia, because reticulocytes are somewhat larger than mature erythrocytes. If a nonregenerative anemia is due to ineffective erythropoiesis, the MCV and/or the MCHC is often (but not always) abnormal. An increased MCV in the absence of a regenerative response is indicative of ineffective erythropoiesis due to interference with mitosis of the developing erythrocytes. A decreased MCV (microcytosis) suggests interference with hemoglobin production, as does a decreased MCHC (hypochromasia). If a nonregenerative anemia is due to erythroid hypoplasia, the MCV and MCHC are usually normal. See Table 4 for causes of ineffective erythropoiesis and erythroid hypoplasia.

True increases in MCHC do not occur. If the calculated MCHC is above the normal range, an error in determination of one of the parameters used in the calculation is likely. Hemolysis causes a falsely elevated MCHC because only intact erythrocytes are included in the hematocrit reading, and all the hemoglobin in the specimen is included in the hemoglobin measurement.

Abnormalities in erythrocyte size, morphology, and staining affinity should be noted when the blood smear is evaluated, as these often provide important diagnostic clues. If anemia is present, the RBCs should be examined for parasites such as *Anaplasma*. The MCV and MCHC should always be checked for accuracy by examination of the stained blood smear. For example, if the MCV is decreased, the erythrocytes should appear microcytic on the blood smear. If a discrepancy occurs between measured or calculated values and what is seen on a blood smear, interpretation should be based on what is seen on the smear. See Table 2 for a list of selected morphologic abnormalities of erythrocytes and their diagnostic significance.

Table 2
POSSIBLE SIGNIFICANCE OF ALTERATIONS IN ERYTHROCYTE SIZE, STAINING, AND MORPHOLOGY

Size changes

Increased MCV	May be a feature of regenerative anemias; often present in ineffective erythropoiesis due to nuclear maturation defects
Decreased MCV	Often a feature of ineffective erythropoiesis due to disorders of hemoglobin synthesis (iron deficiency is most common cause)

Altered Staining Affinity*

Polychromasia	Signifies increased release of immature RBCs (reticulocytes) into the circulation; therefore a feature of regenerative anemias
Hypochromasia	Often a feature of ineffective erythropoiesis due to disorders of hemoglobin synthesis (iron deficiency is most common cause)
Basophilic stippling	Commonly seen in regenerative anemias in ruminant species; in absence of regenerative anemia, may signify lead toxicity

Morphologic Abnormalities

Nucleated RBCs	May be present in highly regenerative anemias (reticulocytes should outnumber nRBCs in this situation); in absence of regenerative anemia, consider bone marrow stromal damage (endotoxemia; heavy metal toxicity, such as lead poisoning; neoplastic infiltration), extramedullary hematopoiesis
Acanthocytes	Liver disease; disordered lipid metabolism; sometimes seen in calves with pneumonia
Spherocytes	Immune-mediated hemolytic anemias; Heinz body hemolytic anemias
Schistocytes	Thrombotic disorders (including localized and diffuse intravascular coagulation); vasculitis, chronic renal disease, vascular tumors (hemangiosarcoma)
Ovalocytes	Characteristic of the family Camellidae; sometimes associated with myelophthisic syndromes
Heinz bodies	Hemolysis due to oxidant toxins (cruciferous plants, castor beans, rye grass, onions, copper); sometimes seen in cattle with postparturient hemoglobinuria (possibly associated with increased susceptibility to oxidants)

*Wright's-type stains.

Regenerative Anemias

Regenerative anemias are due to excessive loss of erythrocytes via blood loss or hemolysis. Table 3 lists causes of hemorrhage and hemolysis. If the bone marrow is healthy, erythroid hyperplasia occurs to compensate for peripheral erythrocyte losses. Because it takes 3 to 6 days for the bone marrow to increase circulating reticulocyte numbers significantly, a CBC performed early in the course of a hemorrhagic or a hemolytic anemia may give the false impression of a poorly regenerative or nonregenerative anemia. Regenerative anemias are often characterized by the presence of diagnostic clues that help to shorten the list of potential etiologies.

Blood loss anemias are characterized by a decrease in the plasma protein level because all components of blood, not just the cells, are lost via hemorrhage. A site of hemorrhage may be evident, or other clinical or laboratory evidence may suggest occult loss of blood. Severe acute bleeding episodes result in hypovolemia as well as hypoxia owing to a decreased erythrocyte mass. Affected animals may present with hypovolemic shock to compound the hypoxia owing to the anemia. The hematocrit of animals with acute hemorrhage will not fully reflect the severity of the anemia until approximately 48 hours after bleeding has ceased. Compensatory shifts of body water from extravascular compartments to restore blood volume (thus diluting the remaining erythrocyte mass) take time.

Chronic blood loss, as from chronic infestation with bloodsucking parasites or a chronically bleeding ulcer, progresses slowly. If chronic blood loss gradually depletes the body iron stores, the anemia may change from a regenerative anemia to a nonregenerative iron deficiency anemia.

Hemolysis generally results in a stronger and somewhat quicker regenerative response than does hemorrhage because the components of the erythrocytes (iron and proteins) are not lost from the body and can be readily recycled. The plasma protein level is usually normal or increased.

Hemolysis can be either an intravascular or an extravascular phenomenon. The clinical and laboratory findings vary according to which type of hemolysis predominates in a particular case. In extravascular hemolysis, erythrocytes are phagocytized at an increased rate by macrophages in the spleen, liver, and perhaps other tissues. In intravascular hemolysis, the erythrocytes rupture in the circulating bloodstream, releasing their hemoglobin into the plasma. Therefore splenomegaly and hepatosplenomegaly are most consistent with extravascular hemolysis, whereas hemoglobinemia and hemoglobinuria indicate intravascular hemolysis. Hyperbilirubinemia may occur with any hemolytic process, but it is more frequent in intravascular than

Table 3
CAUSES OF REGENERATIVE ANEMIA IN FOOD ANIMALS

Hemorrhage*
Trauma
Surgery
Hemostatic disorders
Gastrointestinal ulcers
Parasitism: infestation with endoparasites or ectoparasites that feed on the blood supply
Hematuria
Vascular neoplasia (e.g., hemangiosarcoma)
Hemolysis
Intravascular
  Bacteria (e.g., *Leptospira* spp., *Clostridium perfringens* type A, *C. hemolyticum*)
  RBC parasites (*Babesia*)
  Toxins (e.g., onions, rye grass, cruciferous plants, castor bean plants, copper)
  Immune-mediated hemolysis (e.g., neonatal isoerythrolysis occurring in calves of dams given bovine-origin vaccines against anaplasmosis, drug-induced immune-mediated hemolysis, autoimmune hemolytic anemia)
  Postparturient hemoglobinuria of cattle
  Intrinsic erythrocyte defects (e.g., bovine congenital erythropoietic porphyria)
Extravascular
  RBC parasites (e.g., *Anaplasma, Eperythrozoon*)
  Toxins (e.g., onions, rye grass, cruciferous plants, castor bean plants, copper)
  Immune mediated (e.g., drug-induced immune-mediated hemolysis, autoimmune hemolytic anemia)
  Intrinsic erythrocyte defects

*Chronic blood loss may lead to iron deficiency, causing the anemia to change from regenerative to nonregenerative.

extravascular hemolysis. Early in the course of hemolysis, hyper-bilirubinemia is due to increased unconjugated (indirect-reacting) bilirubin. As the process progresses, conjugated bilirubin may also increase. The blood smears of patients with intravascular hemolysis may contain fragmented erythrocytes (schistocytes) or the membranes of ruptured cells (erythrocyte "ghosts"). Heinz bodies may be seen on the erythrocytes of animals with intravascular or extravascular hemolysis owing to oxidant toxins. Blood smears of patients with extravascular hemolysis may contain spherocytes, but these are difficult to identify in food animals because their erythrocytes are normally small and lack a distinct central pallor.

Intravascular hemolytic episodes tend to cause a rapid decrease in the hematocrit, allowing the animal no time to compensate for the resultant anemia. In general, these anemias tend to present with clearly evident clinical signs of anemia and its attendant hypoxia, and signs of a regenerative response may not yet be present in the peripheral blood. In contrast, anemias due primarily to extravascular hemolysis may progress more slowly. As increased destruction of erythrocytes decreases the hematocrit, the bone marrow undergoes erythroid hyperplasia to compensate for the lost erythrocytes. Because the marrow usually cannot fully compensate, the net effect is a progressive anemia. The animal has time to compensate for the anemia with cardiac hypertrophy and adaptive alterations of erythrocyte metabolism. By the time medical attention is sought, the hematocrit may be quite low, and a regenerative response is often evident.

Nonregenerative Anemias

These anemias are due to decreased production of erythrocytes either because of defects in the maturation of erythrocyte precursors (referred to as maturation arrest anemias, or ineffective erythropoiesis) or because of hypoplasia or aplasia of the erythroid compartment of the bone marrow. Because nonregenerative anemias are primarily the result of decreased erythrocyte production, and because erythrocytes have long life spans, nonregenerative anemias generally develop slowly. Slow development of anemia allows time for compensatory cardiovascular changes and alterations of erythrocyte metabolism, which help counteract the anemia by increasing the efficiency of oxygen delivery to the tissues. For this reason, nonregenerative anemias can become quite severe before clinical signs, such as exercise intolerance, become evident.

Causes of nonregenerative anemias are listed in Table 4. Sometimes etiologic clues can be identified by the CBC (alterations of the MCV and MCHC), but bone marrow examination may be necessary for the complete evaluation of a nonregenerative anemia. In those nonregenerative anemias due to ineffective erythropoiesis, the erythroid compartment of the marrow is hyperplastic. However, the maturation sequence is interrupted, causing an increase in early precursors relative to more mature cells. In nonregenerative anemias due erythroid hypoplasia or aplasia, marrow erythroid cells of all stages of development are decreased. The most common hypoplastic anemia is the anemia of chronic inflammation. This type of anemia can occur secondary to chronic neoplastic as well as chronic inflammatory disorders. The anemia is usually mild, and bone marrow findings typically include myeloid hyperplasia, increased iron stores, and plasmacytosis, in addition to mild erythroid hypoplasia.

Polycythemia

Polycythemia is an increased erythrocyte mass per volume of blood. There are two kinds of polycythemia: relative and absolute. In relative polycythemia, the hematocrit is increased be-

---

Table 4
CAUSES OF NONREGENERATIVE ANEMIA IN FOOD ANIMALS

Ineffective Erythropoiesis (Maturation Arrest Anemias)
Nuclear maturation arrests (disorders of nucleic acid synthesis)
   Vitamin B_{12} deficiency
   Cobalt deficiency*
   Folic acid deficiency
Cytoplasmic maturation arrests (disorders of hemoglobin synthesis)
   Iron deficiency
   Pyridoxine deficiency
   Copper deficiency
   Molybdenum toxicity
   Lead toxicity
Erythroid Hypoplasia/Aplasia
Anemia of chronic disease
   Chronic inflammation
   Chronic neoplasia
Inadequate erythropoietin production
   Chronic renal disease
   Hypothyroidism†
Cytotoxic bone marrow damage‡
   Radiation
   Bracken fern
Immune mediated
   Pure red cell aplasia
Myelophthisic syndromes
   Leukemia
   Metastatic neoplasia
   Myelofibrosis
Infections
   Trichostrongyles (non–blood-sucking)

*Because rumen microflora can synthesize vitamin B_{12}, vitamin B_{12} deficiency does not occur in ruminants unless they are grazing on cobalt-deficient soils (cobalt is required for vitamin B_{12} synthesis).
†Has been seen in cattle with hypothyroidism secondary to fluorosis.
‡Usually accompanied by leukopenia and thrombocytopenia.

---

cause the aqueous portion of the blood has decreased due to dehydration or shock, or splenic contraction has forced increased numbers of erythrocytes into circulation. Absolute polycythemia is due to an actual increase in the total erythrocyte mass in the body. This can be the result of an appropriate response of the bone marrow to increased erythropoietin levels generated in response to tissue hypoxia. Examples of this type of polycythemia include those cases occurring due to high altitude or chronic severe pulmonary disease. Polycythemia can also be the result of a response to a tumor, usually of renal origin, that is producing erythropoietin or an erythropoietin-like substance. Some cases of absolute polycythemia are the result of inappropriate production of erythrocytes (not in response to increased erythropoietin levels). This situation is usually idiopathic and is sometimes a prelude to the development of a hematopoietic malignancy. Hereditary polycythemia has been seen in inbred Jersey cattle. Affected animals have hematocrits of 60% to 80%, with no reticulocytosis and no lesions to explain secondary polycythemia. They are weak, lethargic, and dyspneic and often die by 6 months of age. Survivors usually have a remission of clinical signs by the time they reach maturity.

DISORDERS OF THE LEUKON

The leukocytic portion of the CBC is used to detect leukocytosis or leukopenia and to determine which specific types of leukocytes are altered in number. Table 5 lists the causes of shifts in the absolute numbers of leukocytes. The morphology of the leukocytes should also be assessed. As is the case with the

<table>

Table 5
CAUSES OF SHIFTS IN LEUKOCYTE NUMBERS

Neutrophilia
Epinephrine release (physiologic leukocytosis)*
Corticosteroid effects (stress leukogram)†
Inflammation
Infection (especially bacterial; also fungal, viral, parasitic)
Myelogenous leukemia
Neutropenia
Acute inflammation
Severe, overwhelming infection/inflammation (common with coliform
    infections, endotoxemia)
Bone marrow cytotoxicity (irradiation, bracken fern)
Myelophthisic syndromes
Lymphocytosis
Chronic viral infections
Epinephrine release (physiologic leukocytosis)*
Lymphoid leukemia
Persistent lymphocytosis of cattle (see text)
Lymphocytopenia
Acute viral infections
Mycoplasma infections
Septicemia
Corticosteroid effects†
Loss of lymph (ruptured thoracic duct, alimentary lymphosarcoma,
    enteric neoplasia, granulomatous enteritis, Johne's disease, protein-
    losing enteropathy)
Lymphosarcoma
Hereditary thymic aplasia (T-cell deficiency) of Black-Pied Danish
    cattle
Monocytosis
Resolving inflammation
Chronic persistent inflammation
Acute inflammation
Tissue necrosis
Corticosteroid effects†
Eosinophilia/Basophilia
Endogenous or exogenous parasites that cause tissue reactions
Allergic reactions

</table>

*Associated with fear, excitement, strenuous exercise. Lymphocytosis may be a feature of physiologic leukocytosis in pigs. This response has been seen 3 to 5 hours after feeding in healthy pigs.
†Can be due to increased endogenous corticosteroid release or to administration of exogenous corticosteroids. Associated with pain and temperature extremes. In cattle also seen with displaced abomasum, milk fever, ketosis, dystocia, feed overload, and indigestion. In pigs also seen with parturition, strenuous exercise, and immediately after transport.

erythroid portion of the CBC, detection of abnormalities in the leukocytic compartment may not provide a specific etiologic diagnosis but usually provides diagnostically and prognostically useful information, especially when used in conjunction with other patient data.

Although differential leukocyte counts are often reported as the percentages of each type of cell present (relative numbers), interpretations should always be based on the absolute numbers of each cell type (derived by multiplying the percentages by the total WBC count). A relative neutrophilia can be due to either absolute neutrophilia or absolute lymphocytopenia or a combination of the two. If the total number of leukocytes is sufficiently decreased, it is possible to have a relative neutrophilia although there is absolute neutropenia. In health, the food animal species have a higher proportion of lymphocytes than of neutrophils in circulation, so when a relative neutrophilia occurs it is sometimes called a "lymph-seg reversal." "Lymph-seg reversal," like "relative neutrophilia," is an ambiguous term that has no diagnostic usefulness until translated into terms of what the absolute numbers of the neutrophils and lymphocytes are. Throughout this article, terms such as neutrophilia, neutro-

penia, and lymphocytosis, refer to absolute numbers of leukocytes.

Morphologic abnormalities of leukocytes include the presence of increased numbers of immature neutrophils (a "left shift"), toxic changes in neutrophils, and reactive changes in lymphocytes. In addition, cells with morphology consistent with neoplastic transformation are sometimes seen in the circulating blood of animals with leukemia.

Disorders of the leukocytic portion of the hemic system may occur alone or in conjunction with abnormalities in the erythron and/or thrombon. Various combinations of increases and decreases in the circulating numbers of the different leukocytes occur, with some general patterns being associated with inflammation, epinephrine effects, and corticosteroid effects. Two or more factors may simultaneously affect the leukogram.

Inflammation

Inflammation can cause neutrophilia or neutropenia or can leave neutrophil numbers in the normal range, depending on the type, stage, and severity of the inflammatory process. During the acute phase of inflammation, neutrophil numbers may be normal or decreased and there may be a left shift. As a suppurative inflammatory process progresses, an adequate bone marrow response resolves any left shift and may lead to neutrophilia as the bone marrow reaches a higher steady state of neutrophil production. As inflammation subsides, neutrophil production decreases to normal again. In general, localized suppurative inflammatory processes, such as abscesses and metritis, cause higher neutrophil counts than more diffuse inflammatory processes.

The magnitude of the left shift and the likelihood of the development of neutropenia in the acute phase of inflammation depends on the size of the bone marrow storage pool of mature neutrophils at the onset of inflammation, the severity of the inflammation, and the ability of the bone marrow to increase its production of neutrophils in the face of increased peripheral demands. In ruminants, severe acute inflammation may cause a period of neutropenia, and a left shift may develop and persist for several days. Ruminants do not have a large bone marrow storage pool of mature neutrophils to draw on, and they do not mount as strong a neutrophilic response to suppurative inflammatory processes as occurs in many other animals. However, by 3 to 5 days after the onset of inflammation, neutrophil production should increase sufficiently to begin to correct a left shift. A left shift that persists for more than 4 to 5 days, especially in combination with neutropenia, indicates an inadequate bone marrow response.

With severe inflammation, the marrow may be unable to respond adequately to tissue demands for neutrophils, and neutropenia will persist or worsen as the inflammatory process progresses. This is especially likely to happen in infections by gram-negative bacteria, which may produce systemic toxemia, damaging developing neutrophils in the marrow and impairing adequate production. Morphologic alterations of circulating neutrophils associated with such toxicity include Döhle body formation, foamy cytoplasmic basophilia, and enlargement of neutrophils. Persistent or worsening neutropenia accompanied by neutrophil toxicity and/or a left shift warrants a poor prognosis.

Because ruminants may not develop a pronounced neutrophilic response during inflammation, fibrinogen determination is a useful adjunct to the leukogram for the detection of inflammation in ruminants. Hyperfibrinogenemia occurs during inflammation, but it also occurs with dehydration. The plasma protein-to-fibrinogen ratio is used to differentiate the two. All plasma proteins are proportionately elevated in dehydration, but fibrinogen is disproportionately elevated in inflammation. A protein-to-fibrinogen ratio of less than 10 indicates inflammation, whereas a value of greater than 15 is consistent with normalcy or dehydration. In addition to fibrinogen, others of the so-called acute-phase proteins have been evaluated as potential markers of active inflammation in ruminants. Of these, haptoglobin has been the most extensively studied. Haptoglobin elevations slightly precede fibrinogen elevations, usually occurring within 36 hours of onset of inflammation. Although fibrinogen levels may remain elevated in chronic inflammation, haptoglobin usually returns to normal. Glucocorticoids may also elevate serum haptoglobin. The combination of fibrinogen and haptoglobin may prove useful for assessing and staging inflammation in ruminants.

Monocytosis and lymphocytosis are frequent features of chronic inflammatory leukograms. Monocytosis can also occur during the acute and subacute phases of inflammation. Reactive lymphocytes are often seen during inflammation; the reactive changes signify antigenic stimulation and are seen in many infectious processes. Inflammatory responses involving hypersensitivity reactions often result in eosinophilia, sometimes in conjunction with basophilia. Parasitic diseases in which a stage of the parasite invades or migrates through tissues are likely to incite eosinophilia.

Corticosteroid Effects (The Stress Leukogram)

Classic findings associated with corticosteroid release or administration are mild to moderate neutrophilia, lymphocytopenia, and eosinopenia. These findings are commonly referred to as a "stress leukogram," because endogenous steroid release occurs in response to stress. Lymphocytopenia is the most consistent characteristic. The neutrophilia is due to decreased margination of neutrophils on vascular walls, decreased migration of neutrophils into tissue, and increased release into circulation of neutrophils from the marrow storage pool. The neutrophilia is usually mature (no left shift), but there may be a left shift if the corticosteroid response occurs in conjunction with inflammation. The total WBC count of cattle typically reaches 8000 to 18,000/μL in response to steroids. Leukogram alterations are usually most pronounced 4 to 8 hours after steroid administration, and are usually gone by approximately 24 hours after a single therapeutic dose or within 72 hours after a longer treatment regimen.

Epinephrine Effects (Physiologic Leukocytosis)

Epinephrine release, which is usually the result of an animal's being excited or fearful at the time of sample collection, causes a mature neutrophilia. In pigs, lymphocytosis may occur as well. The effect is primarily the result of increased blood pressure and muscular activity, which cause the portion of the neutrophils that are normally marginated on the vascular walls to be dislodged into the flowing blood, and which may cause increased ejection of lymphocytes from the thoracic duct into the bloodstream. Epinephrine has no effect on the bone marrow. Epinephrine effects are usually short-lived, disappearing soon after the animal becomes quiet.

Hematopoietic Neoplasia

Leukograms of animals with hematopoietic neoplasia are variable. The proliferation of neoplastic cell lines in the bone mar-

row may crowd out the normal hematopoietic cells and cause anemia or other cytopenias. Neoplastic cells may be released from the bone marrow into the blood; their numbers in the blood can range from very low to extremely high. The most common hematopoietic neoplasms in food animals are those of lymphoid origin, and these are most common in cattle. Myeloproliferative diseases are rare in food animals.

Lymphoid leukemias in cattle are most often the result of the adult form of lymphosarcoma caused by bovine leukemia virus (BLV). The neoplasm often arises in the peripheral lymphoid tissue (e.g., lymph nodes) but may metastasize to the bone marrow. Neoplastic cells are found in the circulation in approximately 30% of cases. Because the clinical course of the disease is usually rapid and the erythrocytes of cattle have long life spans (up to 160 days), severe anemia is usually not a sequela of lymphoid leukemia in cattle.

Bovine Persistent Lymphocytosis

BLV infection is also associated with a condition called *persistent lymphocytosis* (PL). PL is defined as an increase in the absolute lymphocyte count beyond the normal level for the patient's age for at least 3 months. Only a small percentage of cattle with PL develop lymphosarcoma, but about 65% of cattle with BLV-associated lymphosarcoma previously had PL.

Functional Disorders of Leukocytes

Functional disorders of leukocytes may be either hereditary or acquired. Few hereditary disorders have been described in food animals. Some experimental work has been done in food animals (mostly cattle) to determine the effects of various infectious agents on the functions of leukocytes.

Chédiak-Higashi syndrome is a hereditary abnormality found in cattle of the Hereford and Angus breeds. It is a generalized cellular disorder characterized by abnormal fusion of cytoplasmic granules of leukocytes. The basic abnormality underlying the syndrome is unknown. Because the granules of melanocytes are also abnormally fused, affected animals have coat color dilution. Giant granules can usually be seen in the neutrophils and eosinophils on Wright's-stained blood smears from affected cattle. Leukocyte function is abnormal, so affected animals have increased susceptibility to infection. Platelet function is also abnormal, causing mild bleeding abnormalities. Affected animals may be neutropenic and thrombocytopenic. There is a propensity for lymphohistiocytic proliferation in the bone marrow, liver, and spleen of animals with Chédiak-Higashi syndrome, which contributes to pancytopenia and increased susceptibility to infection.

Bovine leukocyte adhesion deficiency (BLAD) is an autosomal recessive hereditary disorder of Holstein cattle in which leukocytes lack surface glycoproteins, known as β_2 integrins, which are important for normal cell adhesion. Neutrophil chemotaxis and phagocytosis are also abnormal. Affected animals have recurrent bacterial infections, progressive periodontitis, oral ulcers, delayed wound healing, and stunted growth, and they usually die before adulthood. A persistent marked neutrophilia, usually without a left shift, is present. The myeloid compartment of the bone marrow is expanded.

DISORDERS OF THE THROMBON AND HEMOSTATIC MECHANISMS

Disorders of the thrombon and hemostatic mechanisms may be either hereditary or acquired. A few hereditary disorders have been identified in food animals. Acquired disorders may be the result of bone marrow dysfunction in the case of thrombocytopenia or thrombocytosis, of increased platelet destruction or consumption in the case of thrombocytopenia, or of decreased synthesis, increased utilization, or increased loss in the case of deficiencies of coagulation factors and other proteins involved in the coagulation cascades. Platelet function defects may occur secondary to various disease states.

Thrombocytopenia

Thrombocytopenia may result from decreased production, increased consumption, increased destruction, or sequestration of platelets. Decreased platelet production may result from bone marrow toxicity that affects the megakaryocytes or their progenitors. Increased platelet consumption is most commonly associated with thrombotic disorders, including diffuse intravascular coagulation (DIC). DIC is a potential sequela of many diseases. Increased platelet destruction due to an immune response directed against platelets is seen in some species of animals. Endotoxemia may cause splenic sequestration of platelets. Viruses may cause thrombocytopenia. Certain strains of noncytopathic bovine viral diarrhea virus are known to induce thrombocytopenia in calves and adult cattle, and this manifests as hemorrhage in some affected animals.

Thrombocytosis

Thrombocytosis is sometimes a feature of iron deficiency anemia. In iron deficiency anemia, circulating levels of erythropoietin are increased and erythropoietin has some thrombopoietic effect. Thrombocytosis may also be a feature of some forms of hematopoietic malignancy.

Thrombocytopathies

A familial thrombocytopathy has been seen in Simmental cattle. Affected animals have prolonged bleeding times, and mild to severe hemorrhage may occur, especially following trauma or surgery. As stated previously, cattle with Chédiak-Higashi syndrome have abnormal platelet function and may have prolonged bleeding times. A hereditary platelet function defect due to abnormalities in the platelet granules has been seen in pigs. Acquired platelet function defects may occur secondary to various disease states, but these have not been studied extensively in food animals. Platelet function defects secondary to renal uremia may occur in food animals.

Disorders of Hemostasis

Both congenital and acquired deficiencies of the proteins involved in the hemostatic mechanism occur and may cause a bleeding diathesis. Acquired deficiencies may result from hepatic failure, toxic responses, or the development of DIC.

The coagulation factor deficiency of hepatic failure is due to decreased protein synthesis by the liver and may result in prolongation of the PTT and PT. Poisoning with coumarins (found in many rodenticides and in moldy sweet clover hay) or with other rodenticides that are vitamin K antagonists may result in deficiencies of the vitamin K–dependent coagulation factors and prolong the PTT and PT. Diffuse intravascular coagulation is typically characterized by prolongation of the PT and PTT, thrombocytopenia, hypofibrinogenemia, decreased ATIII level, and increased fibrin degradation products.

Congenital disorders of hemostasis are seen in food animals. Hereditary deficiency of coagulation factor VIII has been seen in Hereford cattle, and factor XI deficiency has been seen in Holstein cattle. These disorders are characterized by an increased PTT; specific coagulation factor assays are used to identify and confirm the specific factor deficiency present. Some Poland-China cross and Yorkshire-Hampshire cross pigs have a hereditary deficiency of von Willebrand factor, resulting in a disease that is analogous to autosomal recessive type III von Willebrand disease of humans. Homozygotes have a moderate to severe bleeding tendency. Routine coagulation test results are often normal, but occasional animals have a slightly increased PTT. Von Willebrand factor assays are used to confirm the diagnosis. Heterozygotes are detectable by laboratory tests (von Willebrand factor assays) but are asymptomatic. A hereditary afibrinogenemia has been reported in Saanen goats. Affected newborn and young kids have a severe hemorrhagic diathesis characterized by hemarthroses and bleeding from the umbilicus into the subcutaneous tissues and from the mucous membranes. The disorder is inherited as an incomplete dominant trait, with homozygous goats having no detectable fibrinogen and heterozygotes having decreased levels.

REFERENCES

1. Alsemgeest SPM, Kalsbeek HC, Wensing T, et al: Concentrations of serum amyloid-A (SAA) and haptoglobin (HP) as parameters of inflammatory diseases in cattle. Vet Q 16:21–23, 1994.
2. Benjamin MM: Outline of Veterinary Clinical Pathology, 3rd ed. Ames, Iowa, Iowa State University Press, 1978.
3. Bezek DM, Grohn YT, Dubovi EJ: Effect of acute infection with noncytopathic or cytopathic bovine viral diarrhea virus isolates on bovine platelets. Am J Vet Res 55:1115–1119, 1994.
4. Coles EH: Veterinary Clinical Pathology, 3rd ed. Philadelphia, WB Saunders, 1980.
5. Corapi WV, Elliott RD, French TW, et al: Thrombocytopenia and hemorrhages in veal calves infected with bovine viral diarrhea virus. J Am Vet Med Assoc 196:590–596, 1990.
6. Dodds WJ: Hemostasis. In Kaneko JJ (ed): Clinical Biochemistry of Domestic Animals, 4th ed. New York, Academic Press, 1989, pp 274–315.
7. Duncan JR, Prasse KW: Veterinary Laboratory Medicine: Clinical Pathology, 3rd ed. Ames, Iowa, Iowa State University Press, 1994.
8. Gilbert RO, Rebhun WC, Kim CA, et al: Clincial manifestations of leukocyte adhesion deficiency in cattle: Fourteen cases (1977–1991). J Am Vet Med Assoc 202:445–449, 1993.
9. Higuchi H, Katoh N, Miyamoto T, et al: Dexamethasone-induced haptoglobin release by calf liver parenchymal cells. Am J Vet Res 55:1080–1085, 1994.
10. Jain NC: Essentials of Veterinary Hematology. Philadelphia, Lea & Febiger, 1993.
11. Jain NC: Schalm's Veterinary Hematology, 4th ed. Philadelphia, Lea & Febiger, 1986.
12. Nagahata H, Nochi H, Tamoto K, et al: Characterization of functions of neutrophils from bone marrow of cattle with leukocyte adhesion deficiency. Am J Vet Res 56:167–171, 1995.
13. Skinner JG, Brown RAL, Roberts L: Bovine haptoglobin response in clinically defined field conditions. Vet Rec 128:147–149, 1991.
14. Skinner JG, Roberts L: Haptoglobin as an indicator of infection in sheep. Vet Rec 134:33–36, 1994.
15. Wittum TE, Young CR, Stanker LH, et al: Haptoglobin response to clinical respiratory tract disease in feedlot cattle. Am J Vet Res 57:646–649, 1996.

Therapeutic Management of Cardiovascular Diseases

Peter D. Constable, B.V.Sc., M.S., Ph.D., Diplomate, A.C.V.I.M.

The aim of this article is to provide an overview of current therapeutic agents and techniques used in treating diseases of the cardiovascular system of food animals. The emphasis is placed on the treatment of specific conditions in cattle because therapy is more frequently attempted and documented in this species. However, many of the principles outlined herein can be directly extrapolated for use in other ruminant species.

ANEMIA

The numerous causes of anemia and their differentiation are discussed in greater depth elsewhere in this volume. The clinician needs to be cognizant that characterization of the anemia should be attempted before blood transfusions are administered because the immunologic response to the infused blood may alter many of the tests used to reach a diagnosis.

From a therapeutic perspective, anemia can be conveniently attributed to (1) acute blood loss, (2) chronic blood loss, or (3) chronic inflammation.

Acute Blood Loss

Acute hemorrhage is often life threatening. Immediate treatment is required to minimize further blood loss and rapidly increase venous return. It is important to realize that the cause of death after acute hemorrhage is usually hypovolemia rather than inadequate oxygen-carrying capability. The immediate focus of treatment after severe hemorrhage should therefore be rapid restoration of perfusion pressure and plasma volume. This is best achieved by the rapid administration of balanced electrolyte solutions and/or hypertonic saline solutions once hemorrhage is controlled.

Hypertonic saline (2400 mOsm/L of sodium chloride [7.2%], 4 to 5 mL/kg given intravenously over 2 to 10 minutes) has been used successfully to resuscitate a variety of species from hemorrhagic and/or hypovolemic shock.[1, 2] Hypertonic saline is believed to exert its beneficial effects primarily through rapid plasma volume expansion and associated increases in systemic arterial pressure, cardiac output, and urine production. Hypertonic saline also constricts venous capacitance beds and redistributes the cardiac output away from muscular and cutaneous vascular beds, facilitating perfusion of vital organ systems.[3] The advantages of hypertonic saline in the setting of hemorrhagic shock include the following:

- Accomplishes rapid and economical resuscitation of animals
- Has a long shelf life owing to its hypertonicity
- Can be stored and transported conveniently
- Is easily and rapidly infused
- Rapidly restores cardiac output
- Minimizes increased pulmonary vascular resistance and edema observed with rapid administration of isotonic crystalloid fluids

Hypertonic saline is thus an attractive choice for the initial resuscitation of food animals in acute hemorrhagic shock.

Contraindications to hypertonic saline administration include hypernatremia, hypokalemia, severe acidosis, and inability to control hemorrhage. Profound hypotension can result from extremely rapid infusions of hypertonic saline. It should be empha-

sized that this treatment is applicable only to the *initial* management of hemorrhagic shock, allowing sufficient time for the clinician to control hemorrhage definitively or to obtain blood for transfusion. The dose rate of hypertonic saline can usually be repeated once after 30 minutes if necessary, but additional treatments should not be contemplated because of the risk of hypernatremia.

Volume expansion with isotonic crystalloid fluids (such as normal saline) can improve oxygen delivery in animals with mild hemorrhagic shock. The volume of isotonic saline administered should be approximately three times the volume of blood lost. Infusion of an adequate volume of isotonic fluid cannot usually be performed rapidly enough in large animals, and hypertonic saline administration or blood transfusion should be considered as a more practical alternative.

Indications for blood transfusion following acute hemorrhage include (1) inability to control hemorrhage (such as bleeding from an abomasal ulcer), (2) lethargy and weakness, (3) inappetence, (4) elevated heart rate, and (5) late pregnancy, when hypoxia may result in fetal death. A good clinical examination is usually the best method of evaluating the severity of an acute bleeding episode and the necessity for blood transfusion. Laboratory determination of the hematocrit and plasma protein level is not an accurate guide to the extent of acute hemorrhage because these parameters do not change for some hours after the bleeding episode. The most accurate laboratory indicator of the need for blood transfusion is the oxygen tension in mixed venous blood, which is well approximated by jugular venous oxygen tension. Venous oxygen tensions less than 30 mm Hg indicate inadequate oxygen delivery to the tissues, regardless of tissue oxygen demands. Volume expansion with hypertonic saline or isotonic fluid can improve oxygen delivery through increasing cardiac output; however, blood transfusions may be more beneficial in selected cases because they increase venous return *and* the oxygen-carrying capacity of blood.

Iron supplementation is not required after one episode of acute blood loss because body iron stores are usually adequate and grazing ruminants ingest sufficient quantities of iron on a daily basis. Additional iron may be required by the animal when bleeding episodes have been recurrent, as outlined below, or when anorexia is present.

Chronic Blood Loss

Chronic blood loss is a common occurrence in food animals and frequently results from internal or external parasitism. The anemia is usually microcytic and hypochromic. Because blood loss occurs over a prolonged period, the animal can successfully adapt to very low hematocrit values. Ruminants can frequently stand and graze with a hematocrit as low as 5%, provided that the rate of blood loss is slow enough to allow compensatory mechanisms to be evoked.

Therapy should be directed primarily at removal of the cause of the chronic blood loss. Blood transfusions are generally not indicated in animals with chronic anemia because transfused red blood cells are short-lived (3 to 4 days). Additionally, transfused red blood cells interfere with the animal's normal bone marrow response to anemia. A possible benefit of transfusion is the provision of rapidly utilizable hemoglobin because these animals may have total depletion of their iron stores. Administration of iron may be of benefit in rapidly replenishing body iron stores.

Chronic Inflammation

Anemia of inflammatory disease is usually normocytic, normochromic, and mild in nature. It is characterized by low serum iron concentration, normal or decreased total iron-binding capacity, and increased bone marrow iron stores.[4] The anemia results from sequestration of iron by the mononuclear phagocytic cell system as a defensive measure. Blood transfusions and iron supplementation are contraindicated in the treatment of this disorder because excess iron may enhance the pathogenicity of the invading bacteria. There is no depletion of body iron stores, making iron supplementation superfluous.

Blood Transfusions

The objective of blood transfusion is to supply the animal with one of four factors: (1) RBCs, (2) clotting factors, (3) immunoglobulin, or (4) protein. Clotting factors can be deactivated when blood is collected in glass; thus, plastic containers should be used in treatment of coagulation disorders.

Blood is readily obtained from the jugular vein of a cow through a 10-gauge bleeding trocar. Placement of a choke rope will facilitate venous distention and hasten blood flow. Up to 15% of the blood volume, corresponding to approximately 1.2 L of blood/100 kg, can be removed safely over 15 to 20 minutes from the donor. Blood is most easily collected in an open-mouth glass jar containing 4 g of sodium citrate per liter of blood to be collected. The blood is gently swirled during collection to ensure adequate mixing of the anticoagulant. Excess sodium citrate should not be added because hypocalcemia can be induced if the blood is administered rapidly. The blood should be administered immediately or refrigerated at 4°C for up to 24 hours prior to use. Filters are not required for transfusion if fresh blood is used and anticoagulation has been adequate. To prevent transmission of infective agents, the blood donor should be free of anaplasmosis, bovine leukemia virus, and persistent infection with bovine viral diarrhea virus.

Blood is usually administered intravenously, although in exceptional circumstances the intraperitoneal route may be used. Cross-matching of blood is unnecessary for the first transfusion but may be advisable for subsequent transfusions, particularly if separated by an interval greater than 1 week. The most practical way of ensuring compatibility of blood types is to monitor the recipient's response during the first 20 minutes of blood administration. The transfusion should be stopped if trembling, tachypnea, weakness, and salivation are observed. These responses are more common in neonates, in which they may result from a rapid rate of administration rather than an anaphylactic reaction. Treatment of transfusion reactions primarily consists of discontinuing blood administration. Epinephrine and antihistamine given intramuscularly are of benefit in severe cases. Recommencement of blood transfusion, preferably from another donor, should be done under close supervision and using slow infusion rates.

Iron Administration

Oral administration of iron is most economical and safe. Ferrous salts are absorbed the most efficiently. Suggested daily oral dose rates of ferrous sulfate are as follows: cattle, 8 to 15 g; sheep, goats, and swine, 0.5 to 2 g. Treatment can be continued for up to 2 weeks.[5] Dark feces, reflecting the presence of unabsorbed iron, may be observed after oral dosing. Heavy oral dosing is not recommended because iron toxicity has been induced in piglets administered large doses (0.6 g/kg) of ferrous iron.[6]

Parenteral iron injections can be prohibitively expensive when administered to adult cattle, and anaphylactic reactions and cellulitis have occasionally been observed following iron injection. Caution should be exercised if multiple treatments are administered because iron cannot be rapidly excreted from the body and iron toxicity may result. Iron must be injected as a slow-release compound, usually as iron dextran (100 mg/mL). Injection of quick-release salts containing iron, or intravenous injection of iron dextran, will result in rapid death, as the excess iron causes the rapid precipitation of blood proteins.

Parenteral iron administration should be considered in animals with documented iron deficiency (microcytic, hypochromic anemia; low serum iron level; and low ferritin concentrations with normal iron-binding capacity) and abnormal gastrointestinal function. Dose rates for ruminants are empirical, and additional treatments with iron should be given when indicated by the mean corpuscular hemoglobin concentration and total hemoglobin concentration. Neonatal pigs routinely require iron injections within the first week of life, because they are born with minimal iron stores, and the sow's milk is low in iron. Parenteral iron administration is not routinely required in other neonates.

Vitamin B$_{12}$

There are very few indications for the use of vitamin B$_{12}$ in the treatment of anemia in food animals. Vitamin B$_{12}$ is synthesized in adequate quantities by ruminal bacteria. The adult ruminant liver usually has stores of vitamin B$_{12}$ that can maintain normal blood levels for at least 6 months. Supplementation of anemic animals with vitamin B$_{12}$ is indicated only in ruminants with cobalt deficiency (causing absorbed vitamin B$_{12}$ to be inactive) or inadequate liver stores (suckling ruminants, extremely prolonged anorexia). Vitamin B$_{12}$ deficiency should be considered in ruminants with a macrocytic anemia that is not attributable to a regenerative response. Suggested intramuscular doses of cyanocobalamin are as follows: cows, 2500 μg; calves, 1000 to 1500 μg; sheep, goats, and swine, 1000 μg. The dosage can be repeated in 7 days if necessary.

Anabolic Steroids

These agents are potentially useful adjunctive treatments for anemia. The mechanism of action of anabolic steroids is through erythropoietin-mediated stimulation of red cell production and nonspecific stimulation of bone marrow. Anabolic steroids are most effective when therapeutic endeavors have been instituted against the etiologic agent, and the erythron is showing some regeneration. The erythron's response to androgen therapy may be variable and should not be relied on as the sole means of treatment. Appropriate dose rates have not been developed; however, the following intramuscular dosages are suggested: testosterone propionate in oil (three times per week), cow, 100 to 300 mg; sheep and goat, 25 mg; nandrolone phenpropionate (every 7 to 10 days), cow, 100 to 200 mg; sheep, goat, and pig, 50 to 100 mg; stanozolol (repeated weekly up to four doses), cow, 250 to 350 mg; sheep, goat, and pig, 25 to 50 mg; boldenone undecylenate (may repeat treatment in 3 weeks), cow, 500 to 700 mg; sheep, goat, and pig, 50 to 100 mg. None of these anabolic steroids are approved for such use in animals intended for food; thus, their use should be restricted accordingly. Androgenic compounds containing nandrolone are most widely used for the treatment of anemia in human patients.

ANTIARRHYTHMIC AGENTS

Cardiac arrhythmias are relatively common in sick ruminants. Most arrhythmias are not associated with structural heart disease and do not constitute a significant threat to the animal's well-being. Whenever cardiac arrhythmias are identified, the clinician should closely evaluate the animal for evidence of heart failure or cardiac murmurs (suggestive of organic heart disease) or gastrointestinal and metabolic abnormalities (suggestive of functional arrhythmias resulting from dysautonomia or electrolyte and acid-base abnormalities). The vast majority of arrhythmias in cattle respond to resolution of dysautonomia and electrolyte or gastrointestinal abnormalities, and therapy should therefore be directed primarily toward these areas.

Only four pharmaceutical agents (quinidine, lidocaine, digoxin, and atropine) are routinely used to treat cardiac arrhythmias in food animals. These drugs should be administered only when the arrhythmia is producing serious hemodynamic effects. Therapy should be closely monitored because marked variations in plasma concentrations occur following dosage. Both quinidine and digoxin are excreted in milk, and adequate withdrawal times should be used if treated animals are slaughtered or their milk is sold for consumption.

Quinidine

Quinidine is a class Ia antiarrhythmic agent possessing membrane-stabilizing ability. It slows cardiac conduction, prolongs the effective refractory period, and decreases the excitability of myocardial tissue. Quinidine is considered the treatment of choice for sustained atrial fibrillation in cattle with normal or only partially compromised ventricular function. Because of the potential toxic effects of quinidine, treatment should ideally be confined to cattle that have normal gastrointestinal motility, acid-base status, and serum electrolyte concentrations or whose clinical signs (lethargy, anorexia, poor milk production) are thought to be a result of atrial fibrillation. Because the majority of cattle with atrial fibrillation spontaneously convert to normal sinus rhythm, and fatalities can occur with intravenous quinidine infusions, quinidine should not be administered for at least 3 weeks after resolution of any concurrent disorders.

The therapeutic range of quinidine in animals is thought to be 2 to 3 μg/mL of plasma,[7] and appropriate dosage schedules are presented in Table 1. Extremely large doses of quinidine are required for oral administration, necessitating slow intravenous infusion for effective and economical treatment. Quinidine should be administered intravenously under continuous ECG monitoring with frequent recordings performed at a paper speed of 50 mm/second. Widening of the QRS complex and heart rate corrected QT interval is considered a normal therapeutic response to quinidine. Another normal response to quinidine infusion is an increase in the frequency of the ventricular response rate, which can progress to transient, supraventricular tachycardia. Infusion should be stopped or slowed in this eventuality. Treatment should be discontinued if the QRS duration is prolonged more than 25% during administration, indicating that toxic levels of quinidine may be present. Blepharospasm, diarrhea, increased rumen motility, weakness, ataxia, and depression have been observed during quinidine infusion in cattle.[8] Sodium bicarbonate (1 mEq/kg, given intravenously) should be administered if toxic signs are severe because it increases quinidine binding to albumin and lowers the plasma potassium concentration, decreasing the effect of quinidine on cardiac tissue.

Lidocaine

Lidocaine is a class Ib antiarrhythmic agent possessing membrane stabilizing activity. Lidocaine decreases automaticity and conduction velocity of cardiac tissue with only minimal alterations of the refractory period. Its electrophysiologic effects are dependent on an adequate potassium concentration; therefore it is less effective in the presence of hypokalemia. Lidocaine is considered the drug of choice for the treatment of ventricular arrhythmias and is usually administered as a bolus intravenous dose (over 10 seconds) of 1 to 2 mg/kg followed by continuous intravenous infusion (0.025 to 0.060 mg/kg/minute). If continuous intravenous infusion is not done, a second bolus of lidocaine can be given 30 to 120 minutes after the first dose. Higher doses should be administered with caution because toxic effects can occur with intravenous doses of 4 mg/kg. Absorption from intramuscular injections is too erratic for therapeutic purposes.

Table 1
PHARMACOKINETIC DATA AND DOSE RATES FOR SELECTED ANTIARRHYTHMIC AGENTS IN CATTLE AND SHEEP

Antiarrhythmic Agent	Dose	$T_{1/2}$ (hr)	V_d (L/kg)	Cl_t (mL/m/kg)	Reference
Cattle					
Quinidine sulfate	49 mg/kg IV in 4 L water over 4 hr 42 mg/kg IV q 6 hr maintenance 209 mg/kg oral loading dose 180 mg/kg oral q 6 hr maintenance	2.3	3.8	19	7
Digoxin	0.022 mg/kg IV loading dose, then 0.0034 mg/kg IV q 4 hr maintenance, or 0.0086 mg/kg/hr continuous IV infusion	7.8	6.4	9.5	10
Sheep					
Digoxin					
Ewes	0.025 mg/kg IV q 8 hr × 3 loading dose 0.005–0.015 mg/kg q 12 hr maintenance	15.2	27.6	17	17
Lambs	0.04 mg/kg IV (q 8 hr × 3 loading dose) 0.008–0.025 mg/kg q 12 hr maintenance	13.7	35.5	22	17
Lidocaine	1–2 mg/kg IV over 60 sec 0.3–0.4 mg/kg/min IV infusion for 15 min followed by 0.1–0.2 mg/kg/min IV for 45 min	1.0	1.3	38	18

$T_{1/2}$, Half-life; V_d, volume of distribution; Cl_t, total clearance; NA, not applicable.

The therapeutic blood concentration of lidocaine is 1.5 to 5 μg/mL.[9]

Lidocaine toxicity is manifested by neurologic and cardiopulmonary abnormalities. Signs of toxicity include muscle tremors, dullness, opisthotonos, blindness, extensor rigidity, and convulsions. Lidocaine is rapidly metabolized and excreted; therefore the duration of toxicity should be short, provided that hepatic and renal blood flow is adequate. At least 5 mg/kg of lidocaine can be administered subcutaneously to cattle before toxic signs are observed.

Digoxin

Digoxin exerts its antiarrhythmic effect indirectly through alterations in autonomic tone and cardiac contractility. Digoxin slows the sinus rate, depresses atrioventricular conduction, and prolongs the atrial effective refractory period. It is the antiarrhythmic agent of choice in food animals when heart failure is present. The therapeutic plasma concentration of digoxin is thought to be 0.8 to 2.0 ng/mL, with toxic effects usually occurring at concentrations exceeding 2.5 ng/mL. Signs of toxicity include development of third-degree atrioventricular (AV) block and ventricular premature complexes. Sheep may require lower plasma concentrations for successful therapy, and neonates require higher doses of digoxin on a body-weight basis than do adults.

Digoxin must be administered intravenously in ruminants because ruminal bacteria degrade orally administered digoxin, and intramuscular injections of digoxin produce severe muscle necrosis. The half-life of digoxin in ruminants is much shorter than that observed in other species, necessitating frequent dosing. Appropriate dosages are outlined in Table 1. The constant intravenous infusion dose is the preferred method of digoxin administration in cattle because it is associated with reduced risk of reaching toxic levels.[10] The doses stated differ significantly from those previously proposed, which appear to be inaccurate.

The requirement for frequent intravenous administration of digoxin makes long-term treatment impractical and uneconomical. An alternative method of digoxin administration is oral drenching immediately following induced closure of the esophageal groove. This allows digoxin to bypass the rumen and escape degradation. Esophageal groove closure is best accomplished by pharyngeal administration of 100 to 250 mL of 10% sodium bicarbonate solution in cattle or 5 mL of 10% copper sulfate solution in sheep[11] and intravenous injection of 0.5 IU/kg of lysine-vasopressin injection in goats.[12] Esophageal groove closure remains for up to 2 minutes following these treatments. This technique has successfully been used in the treatment of heart failure in sheep, as demonstrated by the presence of therapeutic blood levels of digoxin in conjunction with clinical improvement.

Atropine

Atropine is a muscarinic receptor antagonist that is used in ruminants to inhibit bradycardic states resulting from administration of agents with vagomimetic activity, such as xylazine and calcium borogluconate. In cattle, atropine usually reverses second-degree AV block produced by excessive administration of calcium ions, converting the rhythm to sinus tachycardia.[13] Atropine is not routinely used in ruminants because prolonged inhibition of gastrointestinal motility predisposes the animal to free gas bloat. Suggested dose rates of atropine (as atropine sulfate) are 0.04 mg/kg, given intramuscularly (preferably), or 0.02 mg/kg, given intravenously. It should be administered only when cardiac output is thought to be inadequate as a result of bradycardia or second-degree AV block.

HEART FAILURE

Inotropic agents may be indicated on a short-term basis in food animals undergoing surgical procedures or in animals with heart failure in late gestation, when the birth of a viable fetus is desired. In contrast, long-term treatment of heart failure is rarely attempted because it usually indicates severe, irreversible cardiac pathology that is incompatible with an economical, productive life. Despite these reservations, the treatment of selected cases of heart failure may be undertaken.

The most cost-effective treatment of heart failure in food animals involves stall rest, restriction of sodium intake, and furosemide administration. Minimizing exertion decreases cardiac work. Unrestricted access to salt blocks or consumption of high-salt forages can exacerbate the clinical signs of heart failure in cattle; however, it is usually impractical to formulate a low-sodium diet for affected animals. Furosemide is inexpensive and is administered orally (2 to 5 mg/kg every 12 to 24 hours) or by intravenous or intramuscular injection (1 to 2 mg/kg every 12 to 24 hours). Dramatic clinical improvements have been observed in ruminants with heart failure within 1 day of instituting furosemide therapy. Prolonged therapy can lead to hypokalemia, necessitating periodic monitoring of serum potassium concentrations. This is particularly important when cardiac glycosides are administered because hypokalemia potentiates digoxin toxicity.

Specific inotropic agents (Ca^{2+}, digoxin, dopamine, and dobutamine) should be administered in selected cases. The serum calcium concentration should be closely monitored in ruminants with heart failure because lactating, anorexic animals are often hypocalcemic. Calcium is most economically administered as calcium gluconate. Digoxin can be given intravenously but is prohibitively expensive if prolonged treatment is anticipated (see above). Dopamine and dobutamine infusions (1 to 4 μg/kg/minute, given intravenously) are widely used as inotropic agents during general anesthesia; however, they are impractical for long-term use. Cattle with heart failure arising from mountain sickness (high-altitude disease) should be treated initially by movement to a lower altitude. Unresponsive animals may respond to furosemide, inotropic agents, and intranasal oxygen administration.

Nonspecific agents that could be used in the treatment of heart failure are aminophylline, nitroprusside, and nitroglycerin. Aminophylline is principally used as a bronchodilator; however, it also possesses weak inotropic and diuretic activity. Therapeutic blood levels have been achieved following oral administration of theophylline (20 mg/kg every 12 hours), although blood levels need to be monitored.[14] Vasodilators (such as nitroglycerin and nitroprusside) have been used in selected cases of heart failure without obvious success. The impression gained from using these agents is often one of delaying the inevitable.

ENZOOTIC BOVINE LEUKOSIS

The most common proliferative hemolymphatic disorder in cattle is enzootic bovine leukosis. Chemotherapy and immunotherapy of cattle with enzootic bovine leukosis have been reported.[15, 16] The results suggest that short-term remission can be obtained in cattle with enzootic bovine leukosis, although optimal treatment regimens have yet to be developed, and the agents used are quite expensive or not readily available. Treatment may therefore be considered a short-term measure in the treatment of valuable breeding animals with lymphosarcoma when the defined goal is embryo transfer or semen collection. However, before chemotherapy is initiated, the possibility that affected cattle are genetically susceptible to development of lymphosarcoma should be considered. Propagation of this genotype may therefore be undesirable.

REFERENCES

1. Nakayama S, Sibley L, Gunther RA, et al: Small volume resuscitation with hypertonic saline (2,400 mOsm/L) during hemorrhagic shock. Circ Shock 13:149–159, 1984.
2. Schmall LM, Muir WW, Robertson JT: Hemodynamic effects of small volume hypertonic saline in experimentally induced hemolytic shock. Equine Vet J 22:273–277, 1990.
3. Constable PD, Schmall LM, Muir WW, et al: Small volume hypertonic saline (2400 mOsm/L) treatment of calves in endotoxic shock: Hemodynamic changes. Am J Vet Res 52:981–989, 1991.
4. McGillivray SR, Searcy GP, Hirsch VM: Serum iron, total iron binding capacity, plasma copper, and hemoglobin types in anemic and poikilocytic calves. Can J Comp Med 49:286–290, 1985.
5. Szabuniewicz M, McGrady JD: Anemia and hematinic drugs. *In* LM Jones, NH Booth, LE McDonald (eds): Veterinary Pharmacology and Therapeutics, 4th ed. Ames, Iowa, Iowa State University Press, 1977, p 481.
6. Campbell EA: Iron poisoning in the young pig. Aust Vet J 37:78–83, 1961.
7. McGuirk SM, Muir WW, Sams RA: Pharmacokinetic analysis of intravenously and orally administered quinidine in cows. Am J Vet Res 42:1482–1487, 1981.
8. McGuirk SM, Muir WW, Sams RA, et al: Atrial fibrillation in cows: Clinical findings and therapeutic considerations. J Am Vet Med Assoc 182:1380–1386, 1983.
9. Morishima HO, Gutsche BG, Stark RI, et al: Relationship of fetal bradycardia to maternal administration of lidocaine in sheep. Am J Obstet Gynecol 134:289–296, 1979.
10. Koritz GD, Anderson KL, Neff-Davis CA, et al: Pharmacokinetics of digoxin in cattle. J Vet Pharmacol Ther 6:141–148, 1983.
11. Constable PD, Hoffsis GF, Rings DM: The reticulorumen: Normal and abnormal motor function: II. Secondary contraction cycles, rumination, and esophageal groove closure. Compend Cont Ed Pract Vet 12:1169–1174, 1990.
12. Mikhail M, Brugere H, Le Bars H, et al: Stimulated esophageal groove closure in adult goats. Am J Vet Res 49:1713–1715, 1988.
13. Littledike T, Glazier D, Cook HM: Electrocardiographic changes after induced hypercalcemia and hypocalcemia in cattle: Reversal of the induced arrhythmia with atropine. Am J Vet Res 37:383–388, 1976.
14. Langston VC, Koritz GD, Davis LE, et al: Pharmacokinetic properties of theophylline given intravenously and orally to ruminating calves. Am J Vet Res 50:493–497, 1989.
15. Masterson MA, Hull BL, Vollmer LA: Treatment of bovine lymphosarcoma with L-asparaginase. J Am Vet Med Assoc 192:1301–1302, 1988.
16. Onuma M, Yasutomi Y, Yamamoto M: Chemotherapy and immunotherapy of bovine leukosis. Vet Immunol Immunopathol 22:245–254, 1989.
17. Berman W, Musselman J, Shortencarrier R: The pharmacokinetic of digoxin in newborn and adult sheep. J Pharmacokinet Biopharm 10:173–186, 1982.
18. Bloedow DC, Ralston DH, Hargrove JC: Lidocaine pharmacokinetics in pregnant and nonpregnant sheep. J Pharm Sci 69:32–37, 1980.

Digestive Diseases

Consulting Editor
D. Michael Rings, D.V.M., M.S., Diplomate, A.C.V.I.M.

■ Actinobacillosis (Wooden Tongue, Woody Tongue, Big Head)

Karl W. Kersting, D.V.M., M.S.
James R. Thompson, D.V.M., M.S.

Actinobacillosis is a disease that occurs worldwide. The classic site affected is the bovine tongue in which a hard diffuse nodular swelling is found, leading to the term "wooden tongue." The organism responsible for this condition is *Actinobacillus lignieresii*, a gram-negative rod that is a normal inhabitant of the rumen and mouth of cattle, sheep, and goats. The bacteria affect all ages of animals and enter the body through mucosal lesions. A local lesion then develops which can spread to regional lymph nodes. Saliva and exudate from infected animals can lead to a more contaminated environment, with the possibility of more cases developing. The condition is usually sporadic but herd outbreaks have been reported.[1] Atypical lesions involving the lips, nose, and lymph nodes of the head and neck are especially seen in sheep but can involve other sites in the body as well.[2-4]

CLINICAL SIGNS

Initial signs in an animal with actinobacillosis may be excessive salivation progressing to an inability to prehend food. Since actinobacillosis is a disease of the soft tissues; often intermandibular swelling is seen and eventually an enlarged tongue may protrude from the mouth. An oral examination should always be performed in cases suspected of being wooden tongue. The base of the tongue is usually hard and painful with nodular ulcerations occurring frequently. These lesions may be filled with plant material. Granulomas resulting from actinobacillosis have been reported in the esophagus, pharynx, palate, flank, and internal iliac lymph nodes as well as peripheral lymph nodes.[3-6] Lesions have also been found subcutaneously and in the testes.[5]

The differential diagnosis in a bovine includes conditions affecting the oral cavity. Cases of actinomycosis, dental disease, oral foreign bodies, pharyngeal trauma, abscesses caused by other pyogenic bacteria, neoplasms, and tuberculosis are conditions that should be included in the differential diagnosis.

In sheep, the tongue appears to be less commonly affected than the lips and face or the parotid and submaxillary regions. The nasal cavity and internal organs have also reportedly been affected in sheep.[2] In sheep, the differential diagnosis should include contagious ecthyma and caseous lymphadenitis.

CLINICAL PATHOLOGY

Hematology and chemistries are usually not helpful in diagnosing actinobacillosis. Results are usually normal or perhaps indicative of a chronic infection. No serology is available. Biopsy or needle aspirate and culture would lead to a definitive diagnosis. Sulfur granules may be identified in the exudate by either crushing the exudate between two glass slides or palpating it between the fingers. Similar granules may be present in cases of actinomycosis and occasionally with staphylococcal infections.

NECROPSY

Postmortem examination will reveal firm, pale, gritty, granulomatous abscesses that are yellowish and granular in appearance.

TREATMENT

When only the tongue is involved, the response to treatment is usually very good. The classic treatment continues to be sodium iodide given intravenously at the rate of 70 mg/kg as a 10% to 20% solution. At least two treatments are usually required at an interval of 7 to 10 days. If or when signs of iodism occur, treatment should be discontinued. Signs of iodism include excessive tearing, coughing, inappetence, diarrhea, and dandruff. Sodium iodide is labeled with a contraindication for pregnant cattle. However, reports of it causing abortion are very rare.[7] Oral organic iodines have been used as a treatment at a dose of 60 mg/kg/day.[6] Often, affected animals may respond to treatment in 48 hours. The mode of action of the iodides is unclear but apparently anti-inflammatory effects on the granulomatous inflammation are more significant than any direct antibacterial effects.[8] Some practitioners include antibiotics or sulfa drugs in the treatment. *A. lignieresii* is usually sensitive to sulfa drugs, tetracycline, and aminoglycosides. Choosing an antibacterial agent can be done on the basis of culture and sensitivity. Occasionally, surgical debulking of lesions is necessary, especially when air flow is obstructed, but, hemorrhage can be a problem during surgery.

PREVENTION AND CONTROL

Since the organism usually gains entrance through lesions caused by feedstuffs, sharp, stemmy, coarse feeds should be avoided. If several cases are seen in a herd, perhaps a change to a softer feed would be beneficial.

REFERENCES

1. Campbell SG, Whitlock RH, Timothy JF, et al: An unusual epizootic of actinobacillosis in dairy heifers. J Am Vet Med Assoc 166:604–606, 1975.
2. Sproat JB: Cud-dropping in sheep. Vet Rec 123:582, 1988.

3. Fubini SL, Campbell SC: External lumps on sheep and goats. Vet Clin North Am 5:457–476, 1983.
4. Swarbrink O: Atypical actinobacillosis in three cows. Br Vet J 123:70–75, 1970.
5. Palotay JL: Actinobacillosis in cattle. Vet Med 2:52–54, 1951.
6. Rebhun WC, King JM, Hillman RB: Atypical actinobacillosis granulomas in cattle. Cornell Vet 78:125–130, 1988.
7. Miller HV, Drost M: Failure to cause abortion in cows with intravenous sodium iodide treatment. J Am Vet Med Assoc 172:466–467, 1978.
8. Smith HW: A laboratory consideration of the treatment of *Actinobacillus lignieresii*. Vet Rec 63:674–675, 1951.

■ Actinomycosis (Lumpy Jaw)

Karl W. Kersting, D.V.M., M.S.
James R. Thompson, D.V.M., M.S.

Lumpy jaw is a condition in cattle, rarely in sheep and goats, usually involving the bony structures of the face, mainly the mandible and less commonly the maxilla.[1, 2] Occasionally, lesions can be found in the soft tissues of the head, esophagus, forestomachs,[3] and trachea.[4, 5] The condition is caused by *Actinomyces bovis*, a gram-positive, nonencapsulated, branching, filamentous bacterium and a normal inhabitant of the ruminant mouth and upper respiratory tract. The organism gains entrance through openings in the oral cavity caused by punctures from plant awns or other dry, coarse, stemmy feeds. Foxtails, thorns, and other feed with stickers have been incriminated. Dental disease may also furnish a route of entry for bacteria.

CLINICAL SIGNS

Animals affected with lumpy jaw usually are identified by the detection of a hard immovable nonpainful bony mass, usually on the horizontal ramus of the mandible. As the condition progresses, fistulous tracts may develop. Animals may appear to be in pain when chewing, and weight loss eventually develops. Examination of the mouth should be performed. Loose teeth, gingivitis, and plant awns may be found. Oral examination will also help rule out the possibility of pathologic fractures, tooth root abscesses, tumors, or osteomyelitis caused by other organisms.

CLINICAL PATHOLOGY AND DIAGNOSIS

Clinical laboratory tests, including hematology, chemistries, and pathologic studies, are not usually very helpful in diagnosing lumpy jaw since results are usually normal or perhaps indicative of a chronic inflammatory response. Radiographs can be very helpful both in diagnosing the condition and in determining the extent of involvement for determining prognosis. Radiographs can identify dental involvement or the presence of pathologic fractures, resulting in a poorer prognosis. Usually a central radiolucent area of osteomyelitis is found surrounded by periosteal new bone formation. Contrast studies of fistulous tracts can be performed to evaluate their extent. A Gram stain of exudate can be performed. Sulfur granules are usually identified in this exudate.

NECROPSY AND BIOPSY

Postmortem examination will reveal a granulomatous abscess condition in bony tissue. Basophilic clumps of bacteria are found surrounded by eosinophilic clublike projections on histopathologic examination.

TREATMENT AND PROGNOSIS

Treatment of lumpy jaw is usually successful only in arresting the lesion. Seldom does the size of the hard bony mass decrease. If the condition is treated before fistulous tracts or loose teeth develop, medical therapy alone may be sufficient to arrest the lesion. If fistulous tracts are present, the lesions should be curetted and flushed with organic iodine. Often curetting leaves a large cavity that can be flushed and packed with iodine-soaked gauze. Usually these lesions have a very good blood supply and hemorrhage control may be difficult. If teeth are affected, they should be removed. The empty alveolus can be packed with iodine-soaked gauze to keep feed material out. When more radical curettage is performed, avoid fracturing the mandible. Medical therapy consists of sodium iodide and antimicrobial drugs to which the organism is sensitive. Sodium iodide can be given at the rate of 70 mg/kg intravenously every 7 to 10 days until signs of iodism occur. These signs would be lacrimation, coughing, inappetence, diarrhea, and the development of dandruff. Sodium iodide is contraindicated for pregnant cattle. However, reports of it causing abortion are very rare.[6] Oral organic iodides at a dose of 60 mg/kg/day for 3 weeks have been used. The effect of the iodide seems to be through decreasing the granulomatous inflammation rather than directly affecting the bacteria.[7] Penicillin is the antibiotic most commonly given in conjunction with sodium iodide. A dose of 10,000 IU/kg intramuscularly twice a day for 7 to 14 days is usually recommended. In the past, isoniazid has been given orally at a dose of 10 mg/kg/day for 1 month as a treatment for lumpy jaw. Although radiation therapy has been used, it is not very practical because of the special equipment and facilities that are needed.

PREVENTION

Since actinomyces is a normal inhabitant of the ruminant mouth, prevention is aimed at avoiding coarse, sharp, stemmy feeds that may cause oral lesions.

REFERENCES

1. Watts TC, Olson SM, Rhodes CS: Treatment of bovine actinomycosis with isoniazid. Can Vet J 14:223–224, 1973.
2. Patgiri GP, Bashar H: Actinomycosis in the bovine-case reports. Livestock Adviser Bangalore 10:35–36, 1985.
3. Bruere AN: Actinomycosis of the digestive tract in cattle. NZ Vet J 3:121–122, 1955.
4. Bertone AL, Rebhun WC: Tracheal actinomycosis in a cow. J Am Vet Med Assoc 185:221–222, 1984.
5. Stevenson RG, Taylor RG: Actinomycosis of the trachea in a mature cow. Can Vet J 18:278–280, 1977.
6. Miller HV, Drost M: Failure to cause abortion in cows with intravenous sodium iodide treatment. J Am Vet Med Assoc 172:466–467, 1978.
7. Smith HW: A laboratory consideration of the treatment of *Actinobacillus lignieresii* infection. Vet Rec 63:674–675, 1951.

generally fruitless and afflicted animals can be expected to remain respiratory cripples.

Preventive strategies for necrotic stomatitis and laryngitis have traditionally hinged on avoidance or control of predisposing factors. Reduction of oropharyngeal trauma, sanitation of feeding and medication implements for calves, biologic control of upper respiratory pathogens, and environmental management of upper respiratory irritants like dust and ammonia may all contribute to reducing the incidence of disease. An *F. necrophorum* bacterin is available as an aid in the control of bovine footrot; however, its efficacy in preventing necrotic stomatitis and laryngitis has been insufficiently investigated to provide a label indication for these diseases.

REFERENCES

1. Jensen R, Lauerman LH, Braddy PM, et al: Laryngeal contact ulcers in feedlot cattle. Vet Pathol 17:667–671, 1980.
2. Beeman KB: *Haemophilus somnus* of cattle: An overview. Compend Contin Educ Pract Vet 7:S259–S263, 1985.
3. Keister DM: *Haemophilus somnus* infections in cattle. Compend Contin Educ Pract Vet 3:S260–S267, 1981.
4. Stephens LR, Little PB, Wilkie BN, Barnum DA: Infectious thromboembolic meningoencephalitis in cattle: A review. J Am Vet Med Assoc 178:378–384, 1981.
5. DeMoor A, Verschooten F: Surgical treatment of laryngeal roaring in calves. Vet Rec 83:262–264, 1968.

■ Esophageal Obstruction (Choke)

D. Michael Rings, D.V.M., M.S., Diplomate, A.C.V.I.M.

DEFINITION

Esophageal obstruction (choke) can be defined as a partial to complete obstruction of the esophagus resulting in the onset of clinical signs in the affected animal. In domestic ruminants, esophageal obstructions are more likely to occur in cattle than in sheep or goats owing to the more haphazard eating habits of cattle.

PATHOGENESIS

Cattle tend to ingest objects and feedstuffs indiscriminately. Among the more common foreign bodies found obstructing the esophagus of adult cattle are hedge apples, ear corn, apples, sugar beets, and potatoes. Esophageal chokes can occur in young calves associated with bolus administration. A case of esophageal obstruction has been reported in a cow due to regurgitation of a trichobezoar.[1] Additionally, problems in innervation can lead to local dilation of the esophagus, in which event even normal feedstuffs such as hay and concentrate may obstruct. The more common sites along the esophagus for obstructions to lodge include the pharyngeal-esophagus junction, the thoracic inlet, the base of the heart, or immediately in front of the cardia.

CLINICAL SIGNS

The clinical signs vary somewhat depending on whether the obstruction is partial or complete. In either instance the affected animal will stand with the head and neck extended and attempt to regurgitate the obstruction. Animals appear anxious and uncomfortable. Most salivate profusely. Dehydration is more likely to develop in cattle with partial obstructions owing to their more chronic nature, while complete obstructions tend to be a more life-threatening situation because of the animal's inability to eructate rumen gas. This results in ruminal tympany. Severe tympany will put pressure on the diaphragm and cause acute respiratory dyspnea. Occasionally choked animals are observed to regurgitate saliva, water, or feed ingested after the obstruction has occurred (trapped proximally). Volumes will be small with no evidence of digestion.

In partial obstruction cases, the condition may go undetected for several days. Pressure necrosis of the esophagus can occur with resultant rupture. This usually is seen as a focal midcervical swelling.

DIAGNOSIS

The presence of excessive salivation and inability to swallow suggest the possibility of esophageal obstruction. A history of exposure to commonly offending feedstuffs is additional support for the diagnosis (i.e., cattle grazing harvested corn fields). Because the differential diagnosis includes rabies, any attempt at oral examination should be done with appropriate precautionary measures. Obstructions in the proximal esophagus can often be palpated externally as the esophagus runs down the left side of the neck. When no obstruction is found externally, the passage of a stomach tube will indicate the location of the obstruction. Care must be taken when applying pressure to the obstructing object to avoid laceration or perforation of the esophagus. Endoscopy can be used to visualize obstructions in the proximal esophagus, but, most endoscopes are only 1 m long and are not useful in obstructions distal to the midcervical region.

Contrast radiographs may be of diagnostic benefit in cattle with a history of vomiting or recurring esophageal obstructions. Focal dilations and achalasias may be outlined using contrast and may show areas of ulceration or perforation in chronic choke cases.

The differential diagnosis for esophageal obstruction based on dysphagia and excessive salivation includes (1) rabies, (2) pharyngeal lacerations, (3) retropharyngeal abscesses, (4) esophageal or pharyngeal ulcerations associated with bovine virus diarrhea or other viral causes of stomatitis, (5) actinobacillosis, (6) tetanus, or even (7) oral foreign bodies, for example, a stick wedged across the dental arcade, cactus spines in the tongue.[2] Compressive lesions around the esophagus such as thymic lymphosarcoma or other intrathoracic masses may cause bloat, as can the reaction to dying *Hypoderma lineatum* during their larval migration around the esophagus.

TREATMENT

The bloated animal presents as a medical emergency. Trocarization of the rumen or creation of a temporary rumen fistula may be necessary to save the animal's life. Once this is done, the dislodging of the foreign body can be undertaken. The veterinarian should remember at this point that it is more important to be careful than quick. Attempts to dislodge the obstruction by stomach tube should be done judiciously because of the risk of esophageal perforation. Large-bore stomach tubes (Kingman tube) may be more beneficial than small-diameter tubes because they engage a larger portion of the obstruction and are less likely to slip off the obstruction and be jammed through the wall. If the mass fails to pass with reasonable pressure, pumping fluid proximally may facilitate passage. Again, great care must be taken to prevent reflux and aspiration. A two-tube method has been advocated in which a cuffed tube is first passed into the esophagus and a smaller-bore tube is then passed through the center of the first tube to the obstruction. Fluids

■ Necrotic Stomatitis and Laryngitis (Oropharyngeal Necrobacillosis, Calf Diphtheria)

Karl W. Kersting, D.V.M., M.S.
James R. Thompson, D.V.M., M.S.

Necrotic stomatitis and necrotic laryngitis are often addressed as separate clinical entities, yet they represent a disease continuum involving the colonization of the oropharyngeal or laryngeal mucosa by *Fusobacterium necrophorum*. Local inflammation and necrosis result in varying degrees of dysphagia and dyspnea in conjunction with systemic illness from bacterial toxins.

PATHOGENESIS

F. necrophorum is a common resident of the bovine oral cavity; however, its inability to breach healthy mucosa makes the organism harmless under normal circumstances. Mucosal injury allows bacterial colonization of the damaged tissues. Local coagulation necrosis and diphtheritic exudate are characteristic of the disease. Adjacent tissues, such as the arytenoid cartilages of the larynx, may become involved. The gram-negative bacillus produces a potent endotoxin and toxemia is a common feature of the disease.

Predisposing factors are generally related to oral and laryngeal mucosal damage. Physical trauma to the oral cavity may result from injurious feeds, rough oral medication techniques, and sharp cheek teeth. Laryngeal necrobacillosis is believed, in part, to be secondary to laryngeal contact ulcers.[1] These ulcers presumably develop due to repetitive laryngeal closure associated with prolonged, harsh coughing. The coughing episodes themselves may be due to upper respiratory tract infections, cold air, irritating aerosols, or hot, dusty conditions. Respiratory pathogens such as infectious bovine rhinotracheitis virus may also directly contribute to laryngeal mucosal damage. An alternative pathogenesis is laryngeal mucosal necrosis following laryngeal vasculitis induced by *Haemophilus somnus* infection.[2–4] Holstein calves with bovine leukocyte adhesion deficiency (BLAD) seem particularly prone to necrotic stomatitis due to poor oral mucosal integrity coupled with neutrophil dysfunction.

CLINICAL SIGNS AND DIAGNOSIS

Necrotic stomatitis is usually a disease of young calves in the first 2 to 3 months of life. An increased incidence of disease may be observed in calves weaned onto excessively coarse feed. Anorexia, fever, ptyalism, dysphagia, and foul breath are typical signs. The calves develop a characteristic chipmunk-like swelling of the cheeks. Oral examination will reveal an accumulation of diphtheritic exudate and feed between the cheek teeth and buccal mucosa. Removal of the material will allow visualization of deep buccal mucosal ulcers. Occasionally, lesions will be observed on the tongue, palate or sublingual mucosa. Phlegmon of adjacent facial structures may occur. Untreated calves may succumb to toxemia or bacteremia.

Necrotic laryngitis is most often observed in older calves and yearlings. The disease is a particular problem in feedlot cattle owing to their frequent exposure to predisposing factors of laryngeal mucosal damage. Some clinical signs overlap with necrotic stomatitis, including anorexia, salivation, dysphagia, foul breath, and fever. Loud coughing, stridor, and inspiratory dyspnea are observed with necrotic laryngitis. Inspiratory dyspnea is indicative of an upper respiratory obstructive pr[...] Auscultation of the upper respiratory tree can aid in localiz[...] of the obstruction. The larynx will be the site of the [...] intense sounds of turbulence. Pharyngeal swelling is [...] noted, and even moderate pressure applied to the pharynx [...] completely obstruct air flow.

Cattle afflicted with necrotic laryngitis may die acutely [...] asphyxia. Severe cases may be so hypoxic that they die sudde[...] during examination or treatment. Alternatively, fatalities m[...] result from toxemia or inhalation pneumonia. Partially reco[...] ered animals may suffer from chronic inspiratory dyspnea d[...] to laryngeal stricture or arytenoid abscesses.

The diagnosis of necrotic laryngitis can be confirmed b[...] visualization of the characteristic diphtheritic necrosis of th[...] laryngeal mucosa. The lesion can often be observed through an illuminated common oral speculum inserted over the base of the tongue. Endoscopy via the nasal passage can be a valuable adjunct diagnostic aid, particularly for the evaluation of chronic laryngeal strictures.

Necrobacillosis of the oral cavity and larynx is distinctive and seldom represents an overwhelming diagnostic dilemma. The presence of *F. necrophorum* in characteristic lesions can be demonstrated by conventional anaerobic bacterial culture. The differential diagnosis in necrotic stomatitis includes infectious diseases that result in oral necrosis, such as bovine virus diarrhea, and papular and mycotic stomatitis. Conditions that cause facial swelling, such as mandibular or maxillary fractures and dental abscesses, may also be considered. The primary differential diagnosis in necrotic laryngitis is other diseases that result in acute upper respiratory tract obstruction, including traumatic pharyngitis and retropharyngeal phlegmon, pharyngeal or laryngeal foreign bodies, necrotic tracheitis, and acute tracheal edema or honker syndrome.

TREATMENT AND PREVENTION

The primary focus in resolving necrotic stomatitis or laryngitis is antimicrobial therapy. Penicillin G procaine 15,000 units/lb intramuscularly (IM) or subcutaneously once a day (s.i.d.) for a minimum of 1 week is a reasonable drug of choice. Daily antimicrobial alternatives include sulfonamides, oxytetracycline, tylosin, erythromycin, ampicillin, and amoxicillin. Long-acting oxytetracycline and tilmicosin provide the possibility of extended therapy when logistics prohibit daily medication; however, the sustained-release products often require repeat dosages. Anti-inflammatory drugs are common adjuncts to therapy. Immunosuppressive effects notwithstanding, corticosteroids may be used judiciously as a single dose to rapidly reduce laryngeal swelling and prevent asphyxia in cases of acute necrotic laryngitis. More commonly, flunixin 0.5 mg/lb IM s.i.d. can be used to reduce swelling and pain associated with stomatitis or laryngitis. To prevent further tissue damage, it is not recommended that oral anti-inflammatory drugs such as aspirin or phenylbutazone be administered into a highly irritated oropharynx.

Debridement of necrotic material from the mouths of calves with stomatitis seems to speed recovery. The efficacy of oral mucosal cauterization with strong disinfectants, such as Lugol's iodine, is a matter of conjecture. Temporary tracheostomy may be lifesaving for some calves with necrotic laryngitis. A conventional midcervical tracheostomy and insertion of a tracheostomy tube for several days can allow for ventilation while laryngeal swelling is controlled medically. Cattle produce copious amounts of respiratory mucus and tracheostomy tubes require frequent cleaning to remain patent. Cranial cervical tracheostomy and arytenoidectomy for the treatment of calves with chronic laryngeal stricture has been described.[5] Medical therapy of chronic laryngeal stricture due to arytenoid chondritis is are then pumped, under pressure, through the smaller tube. If the obstruction does not move, the fluid exits out the larger tube. The passage of a cuffed endotracheal tube into the trachea will prevent refluxed fluids from entering the lungs but requires that the patient be anesthetized.

Esophagotomy can be used to remove cervical foreign bodies that cannot be retrieved manually from the oral cavity or pushed into the rumen. This is a procedure of last resort because of complications associated with esophageal surgeries (poor wound healing, fistula formation).

With intrathoracic obstructions, a rumenotomy can be performed and a stiff wire loop passed through the cardia with the intention of snaring the obstruction and pulling it into the rumen. Simultaneous passage of an oral stomach tube will permit additional pressure to be applied to the obstruction and facilitate its passage.

With long-standing obstructions (>48 hours), the possibility of esophageal necrosis should always be considered. Salvage is an acceptable option in these cases or in cattle having recurring obstructions associated with neurogenic dilations.

REFERENCES

1. Patel JH, Brace DM: Esophageal obstruction due to a trichobezoar in a cow. Can Vet J 36:774–775, 1995.
2. Migaki G, Hinson LE, Imes GD Jr, et al: Cactus spines in the tongues of slaughtered cattle. J Am Vet Med Assoc 155(9):1489–1492, 1969.

■ Pharyngeal Lacerations and Retropharyngeal Abscesses in Cattle

D. Michael Rings, D.V.M., M.S., Diplomate, A.C.V.I.M.

Injuries of the oropharynx are most often associated with trauma caused by balling guns, Frick specula, drench syringes, oral calcium gel tubes, or the boluses themselves.[1] Often the operator has no idea that an injury has occurred until several days later when the cow's inappetence or throat swelling has become apparent. Although many lacerations are small and heal spontaneously with minimal clinical signs, identifiable pharyngeal lacerations cause much distress to affected cattle resulting in significant weight loss or death. A review of case records of cattle with pharyngeal laceration and retropharyngeal abscess[2] showed the presenting complaints to be dyspnea (65%), excessive salivation (40%), high cervical swelling (40%), anorexia (40%), bloat (6%), and malodorous breath (6%). The respiratory signs in these animals were primarily upper respiratory, although pneumonia was also detected in several animals. The degree of respiratory embarrassment in greater than 10% of the cattle was severe enough to warrant tracheostomy.

DIAGNOSIS

Visual assessment of the oropharynx is important in diagnosing and prognosing animals with pharyngeal lacerations. Endoscopy has the distinct advantage over the flashlight-speculum method by allowing the veterinarian to determine not only the width of the injury but also its depth. Digital palpation of the pharyngeal area, using a McPherson mouth speculum, will often allow removal of offending boluses and magnets. With retropharyngeal abscesses, no opening into the pharynx may be apparent, but compression or displacement of the larynx may be seen.

The size of the laceration does not always correlate well with clinical outcome, although as a rule cattle with large openings do worse than cattle with smaller lesions. The development of retropharyngeal abscesses may actually be greater in cattle with openings less than 1 in. than in larger lacerations. Smaller laceration openings may interfere with drainage of the area.

One of the most significant and grave prognostic signs is the presence of swelling extending ventrally and caudally down the neck. These swellings are evident immediately behind the mandibles and give the affected animal's neck a full appearance. This swelling often indicates the development of dissecting tracts along the fascial planes of the cervical muscles. It is difficult to accurately assess the degree of adjacent soft tissue involvement for several days following the institution of treatment. For this reason, repeated endoscopic examinations are advantageous in determining how well the cow is walling off the infection. Radiographs of the throat and neck area are also useful if endoscopy is not available. Infected tracts show up as a result of air or gas accumulation along the muscle planes. Radiograph machines with high capacity are needed for good resolution.

TREATMENT

Treatment of pharyngeal lacerations causing clinical signs can be both tedious and costly. In cattle with dysphagia, emaciation and dehydration can progress rapidly. Measures should be taken as early as possible to remedy these situations. Suturing a nasogastric tube in the external nares will enable the owner or veterinarian to pump fluids to maintain hydration without causing excessive trauma. A rumen fistula will accomplish this as well and has the advantages of allowing supplementation of feeds in addition to fluids, preventing gaseous bloat in cattle having eructation problems, and permitting easier fluid administration (takes less restraint). The major disadvantages are related to making the fistula and spillage of rumen contents over the cow's side.

In making a rumen fistula, only the 2-in.-diameter circle of skin is actually removed. The muscular layers and peritoneum can be separated by blunt dissection (grid incision). A towel clamp or vulsellum forceps can be used to grasp the rumen and pull it above the level of the skin (1 to 2 in.). A modified right-angle Cushing suture or horizontal mattress pattern using nonabsorbable suture is performed, tacking the rumen wall directly to the skin. Particular attention should be paid to the most ventral portion of the fistula to make sure the seal is tight enough to prevent leakage into the abdomen. If at all possible, the rumen cap should not be opened for 24 hours to allow formation of a fibrinous seal. Once the rumen is opened, anyone administering fluids through the fistula must be careful not to tear the rumen wall away from the skin edge.

Despite placement of a rumen fistula, the nutritional requirements of the cow will not be met but may minimize weight lost. Healing of both pharyngeal lacerations and fistulas can be a slow process. Owners and veterinarians should realize that treatment may extend several weeks.

In cattle with large pharyngeal lacerations, all hay and grain should be withheld once the retropharyngeal pocket has been cleared so the space is not immediately refilled. The fact that many cows do not feel well enough to ruminate or eructate is beneficial in keeping the throat area clear. If animals exhibit a strong desire to eat, removal of all bedding for several days is desirable so the space can start to heal.

Surgical drainage of retropharyngeal abscesses is essential to successful resolution. Ultrasonic imaging can be used to determine the exact location and capsule thickness prior to drainage. In most instances, stab incisions and blunt dissection to and through the abscess wall are done externally using only local anesthesia. The preferential incision site is the ventral cervical area because it maintains ventral drainage. This area is highly vascular and attention must be paid to avoid excessive hemorrhage. Systemic antibiotics are indicated to help limit spread from the primary site.

Ancillary treatments such as local hydrotherapy (hot packs) or direct irrigation of the wound may be beneficial. Direct irrigation can be used in already drained retropharyngeal abscesses but should be carefully considered before being used in a closed space because of the potential to push the infection further down the neck, possibly to the chest. For this reason, direct flushing of the wound is not done until the swelling has localized and is no longer descending the neck. Hot packing can be useful in localizing swellings and bringing abscesses to a head. It is, however, time-consuming and tedious with the benefits not being readily apparent.

Tracheostomy can be a lifesaving procedure in animals with severe inspiratory dyspnea, as is occasionally seen with retropharyngeal abscesses. The tracheostomy need only be maintained until the abscess can be lanced and the trachea decompressed. Very few animals have required maintenance of the tracheostomy beyond 24 hours.

REFERENCES

1. Davidson HP, Rebhun WC, Habel RE Pharyngeal trauma in cattle Cornell Vet 71:15–25, 1981.
2. Medical Records, College of Veterinary Medicine, Ohio State University, Columbus.

■ The Ruminant Forestomach

Peter D. Constable, B.V.Sc., M.S., Ph.D., Diplomate, A.C.V.I.M.

The forestomach is a specialized fermentation vat consisting of two primary structures, the reticulorumen and the omasum, which are functionally separated by a sphincter, the reticulo-omasal orifice. Fermentation is controlled by the ruminant through forage selection, addition of a buffer (saliva), and constant mixing through specialized contractions of the forestomach. Reticuloruminal motility ensures a constant flow of partially digested material into the abomasum for further digestion. This constant flow of digesta into the abomasum differs markedly from the intermittent flow observed in monogastric animals.

RETICULORUMINAL MOTILITY

Four specialized contraction patterns can be clinically identified in the reticulorumen[1-5]:

1. Primary or mixing cycle
2. Secondary or eructation cycle
3. Rumination (associated with cud chewing)
4. Esophageal groove closure (associated with suckling milk)

The motility pattern and function of the four specialized contraction patterns should be understood, since specific disorders such as vagal indigestion, rumen bloat, lactic acidosis, and ruminal drinking produce characteristic alterations in forestomach motility.

Primary Contractions

Primary cyclic activity results in the mixing and circulation of the digesta in an organized manner. The contraction cycle be-

gins with a biphasic reticular contraction, followed by contraction of the dorsal and then the ventral ruminal sac. This contraction sequence is initiated, monitored, and controlled by the gastric center in the medulla oblongata and mediated by the vagus nerve.[1, 4] Numerous excitatory and inhibitory inputs are summated in the gastric center to determine both the rate and strength of contraction. Ruminants are clinically categorized as having either normal forestomach motility, forestomach atony, hypomotility, or hypermotility.

Forestomach *atony* is defined as the complete absence of reticuloruminal motility. Atony can result from the absence of excitatory inputs or an increase in inhibitory inputs to the gastric center, direct depression of the gastric center (associated with generalized depression and severe illness), or failure of vagal motor pathways.

Forestomach *hypomotility* refers to a reduction in the frequency *or* strength of primary contractions, and is caused by either a reduction in the excitatory drive to the gastric center or an increase in inhibitory inputs. The distinction between primary contraction frequency and strength is clinically important, particularly with reference to the therapy of reticuloruminal hypomotility. The *frequency* of primary contractions indicates the overall health of the ruminant. In the cow the primary contraction frequency averages one cycle per minute. The rate increases transiently during feeding and decreases during rumination and recumbency.[3] Because of this variability, auscultation should proceed for at least 2 minutes when determining the frequency of contractions. The *strength* and *duration* of each contraction is determined primarily by the nature of the forestomach contents, although alterations in serum electrolyte concentrations (particularly hypocalcemia) can also decrease contraction strength. The strength of contraction is subjectively determined by observing the movement of the left paralumbar fossa and assessing the loudness of sounds associated with rumen contraction.

Forestomach *hypermotility* refers to an increase in the frequency of primary contractions, and is caused by an increase in the excitatory drive to the gastric center (typically mild reticuloruminal distention).

Secondary Contractions

Secondary contraction cycles occur independently of primary contraction cycles and at a slower frequency (usually one every 2 minutes). They are concerned primarily with the eructation of gas, the rate being determined by the gas or fluid pressure in the dorsal ruminal sac.[2, 3] Rumen contractions are essential to eructation.[3] Tension receptors in the medial wall of the dorsal ruminal sac initiate the reflex via the dorsal vagus nerve. Contractions start in the dorsal and caudodorsal ruminal sacs and then spread forward to move the gas cap anteriorly to the cardia region, which subsequently opens.[6] The cardia remains firmly shut if foam (frothy bloat) or fluid (laterally recumbent animals) contacts the cardia. Free gas bloat is often observed in ruminants in lateral recumbency. Eructation occurs in these animals after they become sternally recumbent, when fluid moves away from the cardia. Bloat can also result when peritonitis, abscesses, or masses distort the normal forestomach anatomy, preventing active removal of fluid from the cardia region. Esophageal obstructions, associated with intraluminal, intramural, or extraluminal masses, are also a common cause of free gas bloat. Passage of a stomach tube usually identifies these abnormalities and forestomach motility is unimpaired unless the vagal nerve is damaged. Bloat is also observed in cattle with tetanus, the bloat arising from spasm of the esophageal musculature.

A persistent mild bloat is often observed in ruminants that have ruminal atony or hypomotility secondary to systemic disease. The bloat usually requires no treatment and disappears with the return of normal motility. Although the fermentation rate is lower than normal in these cases, rumen contractions are not strong enough to remove all of the gas produced.[5]

Auscultation of the left paralumbar fossa (which detects rumen motility) cannot differentiate secondary contraction cycles from primary contraction cycles, unless synchronous eructation is heard. However, when palpation of the left paralumbar fossa is coupled with reticular auscultation (by placing the bell of the stethoscope at the left costochondral junction between the seventh and eighth ribs), the two contraction cycles can be distinguished.[7] Reticular contractions (indicating a primary contraction) can usually be heard a few seconds before the dorsal ruminal sac contraction is seen or palpated. The reticular contraction is not easy to identify and this technique requires practice. The absence of a reticular contraction before dorsal ruminal sac motility indicates a secondary contraction.

Rumination

Rumination is a complex process involving regurgitation, remastication, insalivation, and deglutition.[3] It is initiated by the "rumination area," located close to the gastric center in the medulla oblongata. Rumination allows further physical breakdown of food with the addition of large quantities of saliva (buffer) and is an integral part of ruminant activity. Rumination has been associated with a sleeplike state and appears to be an enjoyable experience.[5] The time spent ruminating each day appears to be determined by the coarseness of the rumen contents and the nature of the diet.[8] Rumination usually commences 30 to 90 minutes after feeding and proceeds for 10 to 60 minutes at a time, resulting in 6 to 9 hours per day (maximum of 10) spent in the activity.

Epithelial receptors located in the reticulum, esophageal groove area, reticuloruminal fold, and ruminal pillars detect coarse ingesta and initiate rumination.[2, 8] These epithelial receptors are unspecialized sensory nerve endings and therefore respond to a number of different stimuli.[4, 5] They can be activated by increases in ruminal volatile fatty acid concentration or severe stretch (resulting in alterations in primary or secondary cycle activity) or mild mechanical "rubbing," (inciting rumination).[8] The epithelial receptors are ideally located to contact coarse ingesta, which usually floats on top of the more fluid ventral ruminal contents. An intact dorsal *or* ventral vagus nerve is necessary for regurgitation to proceed.[3] Regurgitation follows an extra contraction of the reticulum before the normal biphasic contraction of the primary cycle.[2, 3] The glottis is closed and an inspiratory movement lowers the intrathoracic pressure, causing the distal esophagus to fill with rumen contents when the cardia relaxes. Reverse peristalsis carries the bolus up to the mouth where it undergoes further mastication.[3] The extra reticular contraction is not essential for regurgitation as fixation or removal of the reticulum does not prevent cattle from ruminating.

It is often difficult to quantify the time spent ruminating; therefore, only the absence or presence of rumination is normally noted. Rumination is often absent in sick ruminants. In these animals, the reappearance of rumination is considered a good prognostic sign, since it often heralds an improvement in the clinical condition of the animal. Additional causes for a reduction or absence of rumination include reticuloruminal hypomotility or atony, central nervous system depression, excitement, pain, liquid rumen contents (no coarse fiber present to stimulate the epithelial receptors), mechanical damage to the reticulum (peritonitis), and a high rumen fluid osmotic pressure (>350 mOsm/L).[9] More unusual causes of the absence of rumination are chronic emphysema (difficulty in creating a negative thoracic pressure) and massive damage to the epithelial recep-

tors which incite the reflex (seen in rumenitis). The effect of osmotic pressure on ruminal function is significant and should not be disregarded. In particular, electrolyte solutions administered orally to sick ruminants should be isotonic, since hypertonic solutions will exacerbate dehydration unless adequate water is available for immediate consumption.

Esophageal Groove Closure

The esophageal groove reflex allows milk in the suckling preruminant to bypass the forestomach, directing milk from the esophagus along the reticular groove and omasal canal into the abomasum. Milk initiates the reflex by chemical stimulation of receptors in the buccal cavity, pharynx, and cranial esophagus.[10] Once the reflex is established in neonates, sensory stimuli can cause esophageal groove closure without milk contacting the chemoreceptors. Esophageal groove closure is therefore normal in calves given water in manner identical to that by which the calf previously received milk or in calves abruptly changed from nipple to bucket feeding.[11] Reflex closure continues to operate during and after the development of a functional rumen, provided that the animal continues to receive milk. Esophageal groove closure has been observed in cattle up to 2 years of age, and can probably be induced pharmacologically in older cattle.[12]

Esophageal groove closure can be induced by the oral administration of particular salt solutions. In adult sheep, 5 mL of a 10% solution of copper sulfate consistently causes esophageal groove closure. This lasts for at least 15 seconds, during which time a second orally administered liquid will pass directly into the abomasum. Watery rumen contents favor the establishment of this reflex.[13] Repeated administration of $CuSO_4$ should be avoided because of the high risk of copper toxicity. Closure of the esophageal groove in cattle less than 2 years of age can be induced by oral drenching with solutions of sodium bicarbonate, sodium chloride, or sugar.[12] A 10% solution of sodium bicarbonate 100 to 250 mL induces esophageal groove closure in 93% of cattle.[12, 14] Closure is immediate and usually lasts for 1 to 2 minutes. Oral solutions administered during this time are directed into the abomasum, avoiding dilution in the rumen. In goats, closure is best induced by injection of vasopressin 1 IU/kg.[15] Reflex closure can be useful in the treatment of abomasal ulcers in younger animals, since magnesium hydroxide or Kaopectate can be given orally shortly after the sodium bicarbonate solution.

The esophageal groove reflex is inhibited by abomasal distention, causing milk to enter the rumen instead of the abomasum. Liquid administered to calves via an esophageal feeder will not induce groove closure; this should be remembered when administering colostrum to newborn calves and oral fluids to diarrheal calves. In calves less than 3 weeks of age, overflow of fluid from the reticulorumen into the abomasum begins when 400 mL is administered. This means that the fluid volume administered by an esophageal feeder should exceed 400 mL if rapid absorption is required.[16]

Reticuloruminal contractions decrease or cease during suckling via a dopaminergic pathway.[17] Esophageal groove closure is also inhibited by dopamine administration. Because incomplete closure of the esophageal groove is thought to be involved in primary digestive disturbances in milk-fed calves, metoclopramide (an antidopaminergic agent) may therefore be of benefit in the treatment of digestive disturbances in suckling ruminants. The clinical effectiveness of this therapy is yet to be determined.

OMASAL MOTILITY

The omasum is a compact spherical organ, comprising the omasal canal and omasal body. Motility of the omasal canal is coordinated with that of the reticulorumen, while omasal body contractions occur independently of and at a slower rate than reticuloruminal contractions. The function of the omasum is incompletely understood. However, it plays an important role in (1) the transport of appropriately sized feed particles from the reticulorumen to the abomasum, (2) esophageal groove closure, (3) fermentation of ingesta, and (4) absorption of water, volatile fatty acids, and minerals. Sheep and goats have a relatively small omasum compared to cattle.

The omasum is situated centrally in the anterior abdomen, preventing examination through techniques such as abdominal palpation and percussion. Auscultation of omasal activity has been described.[18] The technique requires placement of the stethoscope on the right lateral thorax between the 7th and 10th ribs at the level of the shoulder joint. Flowing liquid sounds, indicating flow of ingesta along the omasal canal into the abomasal fundus, are heard approximately 12 seconds after the second reticular contraction. This is an extremely difficult technique that requires practice, since it is hard to be certain that omasal motility was directly responsible for the generated sound.

Definitive evidence of an omasal disorder requires exploratory celiotomy or rumenotomy. Clinical diseases affecting the omasum occur rarely but include omasal impaction, omasal canal obstruction, and omasal erosions. Omasal canal obstructions usually result from ingestion of baling twine or plastic, and are easily diagnosed during rumenotomy. Omasal erosions may be severe enough to lead to perforation of one or more omasal leaves. These erosions are commonly seen in healthy cattle and their pathogenesis is unknown, although inflammation resulting from *Fusobacterium necrophorum* infection is a likely cause.[19] Omasal lesions are also observed in cattle dying of diseases such as bovine virus diarrhea, infectious bovine rhinotracheitis, and rinderpest.

Omasal impaction is a clinical disease of controversial significance, primarily because the normal bovine omasum varies markedly in size and consistency. The disorder is characterized by anorexia, an extremely firm and enlarged omasum which may be painful on palpation, the absence of other pathologic abdominal conditions, and clinical improvement following softening of the omasum. Treatment consists of intraoperative kneading of the omasum until the contents become pliable. Four liters of mineral oil should be administered intraruminally for 3 to 5 days postoperatively to facilitate softening. Omasotomy is indicated in nonresponsive cases. The omasum is exteriorized through a midline abdominal incision, opened along the greater curvature, and flushed with water until it becomes soft and pliable. The omasum is closed with a two-layer inverting pattern and the abdomen is closed routinely.[20]

CLINICAL ASSESSMENT OF FORESTOMACH FUNCTION

Assessment of the primary contraction cycle should be part of the routine clinical examination of ruminant animals. Secondary contraction cycles, esophageal groove closure, and rumination need only be examined when problems associated with the gastrointestinal tract have been identified. Careful assessment of forestomach motility will help the clinician identify the nature of any dysfunction and provide a rational course of treatment.

When assessing forestomach function, the clinician must determine:

1. The rate and strength of rumen contractions
2. The rumen volume
3. The nature of rumen contents
4. The nature of feces

This is best approached using the following two-stage sequential technique for the cow:

Physical Examination of the Forestomach

1. Visual examination. The abdominal profile is examined critically to determine if any distention is present, and the organ most likely to cause the distention. In addition, the left paralumbar fossa is inspected for periodic distention, and the frequency and strength of ruminal contractions are determined.

2. External ruminal palpation. The physical nature of ruminal contents is assessed by ballottement and succussion of the left paralumbar fossa and flank region. Normal primary cyclic motility leads to a stratification of ruminal contents, with firmer fibrous material floating on top of a more fluid layer. The normal rumen therefore feels doughy in the dorsal sac and more fluid ventrally. Abnormal ruminal stratification, or an excessively firm or watery rumen, suggests that a forestomach disorder is present. Very watery rumen contents that splash and fluctuate on ballottement are suggestive of lactic acidosis, vagal indigestion, ileus, or prolonged anorexia. Firm rumen contents are observed with restricted water intake.

3. Auscultation. Identification of rumen contractions requires both auscultation and observation of the left paralumbar fossa. Sound is produced when fibrous material rubs against the rumen wall during contraction. Very little sound is produced when the rumen contains small quantities of fibrous material (i.e., watery rumen). In this case observation of the left paralumbar fossa for periodic distention is needed to detect rumen motility. Rumen hypomotility or hypermotility is usually associated with a change in the type of sound heard during auscultation, with a distant bubbling replacing the normal close crescendo-decrescendo crackling sound. Auscultation should proceed for at least 2 minutes in two locations: (1) the left paralumbar fossa; (2) the seventh to eighth intercostal space at the costochondral junction. Auscultation of the left paralumbar fossa does not differentiate primary from secondary contraction cycles unless synchronous eructation is heard, while auscultation at the left costochondral junction does allow differentiation of the two basic cycles. Less than three contractions per 2 minutes indicates hypomotility, while greater than five contractions per 2 minutes indicates hypermotility.

4. Internal (rectal) ruminal palpation. The rumen (specifically the dorsal and caudodorsal ruminal sacs) should be palpated during rectal examination and the volume and consistency determined. The results should then be compared with those obtained during external ruminal palpation. A portion of the ventral ruminal sac may be palpated on some cows by lifting the ventral abdomen dorsally with a horizontal bar placed at the level of the umbilicus.

5. Examination of fecal material. The size of digested plant fragments in ruminant feces provides an indirect measure of forestomach function, since solid matter normally stays in the rumen until the particle size is sufficiently small to pass through the reticulo-omasal orifice.[21] Excessively large fibers (>0.5 cm) or fine plant particles in the feces indicate rapid or prolonged rumen turnover time, respectively. The nature of the feces can also provide information on the diet; numerous corn kernels may provide evidence of excessive grain consumption.

Laboratory Examination of Rumen Fluid

Collection of Rumen Fluid

Rumen fluid can be obtained by two methods: passage of a stomach tube or rumenocentesis. Analysis is best performed on freshly collected samples. A detailed description of rumen fluid analysis is available.[22]

Ororuminal Collection

This involves ororuminal passage of a tube to collect rumen fluid. Although this technique is safe and practical, the major difficulty is avoiding saliva contamination of the rumen sample, thereby necessitating collection of fluid from the ventral ruminal sac. Specialized stomach tubes have been developed that minimize saliva contamination, such as weighted stomach tubes and Dirksen's guidable probe, although neither tube predictably collects fluid from the ventral ruminal sac. The best method to be developed utilizes a magnet attached to the weighted head of the collecting tube.[23] The tube is passed ororuminally until an obstruction is felt, at which time the surface of the left ventral abdominal area is scanned with a compass to confirm that the sample is being collected from the ventral ruminal sac. This technique is initially successful in 72% of attempts. If the compass indicates that the tube is not located in the ventral ruminal sac, the tube is removed and the procedure is repeated. Using this technique, 500 mL of ruminal fluid can be rapidly and easily removed from the ventral ruminal sac.[23]

Rumenocentesis

This involves percutaneous aspiration of rumen contents from the ventral ruminal sac. An area on the lower left ventrolateral abdominal quadrant, horizontal with the patella and 8 in. caudal to the last rib, is clipped and surgically scrubbed. The cow is then restrained by tail elevation and hobbling the hind feet or by mild xylazine sedation 0.04 mg/kg intravenously, and a 5-in. 16-gauge needle attached to a 12-mL syringe is thrust firmly and quickly perpendicular to the skin into the rumen. Rumen contents are then aspirated and the pH is measured immediately using a portable pH meter. If the needle becomes blocked with ingesta, 3 mL of air is pushed through the needle in an attempt to clear the blockage.[24, 25]

Problems associated with rumenocentesis include subcutaneous abscesses (at least 1% of cattle sampled),[24, 25] localized peritonitis (observed by me in four of six cattle within 2 days of sampling), penetration of the uterus in late gestation or the abomasum in cows with left displaced abomasum, and a small sample volume (<10 mL). Until the safety of rumenocentesis has been adequately documented in large numbers of cattle, the method should remain confined to research animals.

Analysis of Rumen Fluid

Color. This is dependent upon the diet; corn silage and straw diets produce yellow-brown rumen contents, concentrates produce an olive-brown color, and pasture produces a green color. A black-green color usually indicates ruminal stasis while a milky gray–brown color is often observed in lactic acidosis.

Odor. Rumen fluid normally has a slightly aromatic, unobjectionable odor. An acidic or sour smell is suggestive of lactic acidosis. Rumen putrefaction produces a rotting odor.

Consistency. Rumen contents are normally slightly viscous. Excessive viscosity indicates significant saliva contamination and the sample should be discarded since it is not a valid representation of rumen fluid. A watery sample with little particulate matter indicates anorexia, and is usually associated with reduced protozoal and bacterial numbers. Rumen fluid that has numerous stable bubbles that do not coalesce is indicative of frothy bloat.

pH. Rumen pH is best measured 2 to 4 hours after feeding a concentrate meal or 4 to 8 hours after offering a fresh total mixed ration. Rumen pH is most practically determined using pH papers, although use of a portable pH meter is advocated when using herd rumen pH as a screening method for diagnosing subacute rumen acidosis. The normal pH of grass-fed ruminants is 6 to 7. A pH value of 5.5 to 6.0 is seen in cattle on high grain diets or pasture-fed cattle with very early lactic acidosis. pH values less than 5.5 are virtually pathognomonic for lactic acidosis, although feedlot cattle well adapted to very high grain diets can have rumen pH values approaching 5.0. A reduced feed intake of 2 or more days' duration often increases rumen pH up to 7 or 8. Rumen pH values exceeding 8 are due to (1) saliva contamination, in which case the sample should be discarded, (2) severe putrefaction of ingested protein associated with prolonged rumen stasis, or (3) urea toxicity.

Methylene Blue Reduction. This test measures the reducing ability of anaerobic ruminal bacteria. Ten milliliters of fresh rumen fluid is added to a test tube containing 0.5 mL of a 0.03% solution of methylene blue and the time taken for the solution to clear is measured. In cattle, the clearance time is normally between 2 and 6 minutes, the faster rate being observed in cattle on high grain diets. Clearance times greater than 10 minutes indicate inadequate anaerobic bacterial numbers and rumen transfaunation is required. The clearance time is much faster in sheep (usually 1 to 4 minutes). This test is invalid at a rumen pH less than 5.5.

Protozoa. One drop of fresh rumen contents is placed on a slide and examined under low power ($\times$ 40). Normal rumen fluid contains greater than 40 protozoa per low-power field, with actively moving protozoa that can be broadly characterized into three sizes (small, medium, big). Low protozoal numbers (less than eight per low power field), nonmotile protozoa, or loss of population heterogeneity all indicate an abnormal intraruminal environment. Transfaunation is indicated if these abnormalities are identified, particularly if the methylene blue reduction time is prolonged. It is not usually necessary to identify the protozoal species present, but occasionally it is valuable to differentiate isotrichids (formerly holotrichs), which are usually the larger protozoa, from oligotrichs (entodiniomorphs), which are smaller and more resistant to pH values of less then 6. Protozoal energy stores can be assessed by adding one drop of Lugols' iodine to one drop of rumen fluid on a slide. Healthy protozoa are almost uniformly stained by iodine, while protozoa that have been starved have diminished starch stores, evidenced by decreasing numbers of starch granules.

Chloride Concentration. The rumen fluid should be centrifuged and the supernatant submitted for determination of the chloride concentration, which is normally 10 to 25 mEq/L in cattle and less than 15 mEq/L in sheep. Elevated rumen chloride concentrations result from abomasal reflux (internal vomition), ileus, or high salt intake. Rumen chloride concentrations are extremely useful in localizing the site of gastrointestinal obstruction in ruminants with rumen distention, since high values indicate obstruction at or distal to the pylorus, while low values indicate obstruction at the level of the omasum or reticuloomasal orifice. The physical examination may provide evidence as to whether this obstruction is functional or pathologic.

Rumen Osmolality. The rumen osmotic pressure is actively controlled by the ruminant and closely approximates serum osmotic pressure. A constant osmotic pressure ensures homeostatic conditions for ruminal microbes, which are susceptible to lysis or swelling if large and rapid variations in rumen osmolality occur.[9]

Gram Stain. Rumen fluid normally contains a large heterogeneous population of bacteria which are predominantly gram-negative. Lactic acidosis produces a more uniform bacterial population which is predominantly gram-positive.

Other Tests. A number of other laboratory tests, such as sedimentation time, cellulose digestion test, and total titratable acidity, have also been used in the examination of rumen fluid. These tests seldom add additional information to that obtained above, and their routine use is not recommended.

SIMPLE INDIGESTION

Definition

Simple indigestion is a common disease primarily affecting nongrazing ruminants. The disorder is relatively easy to diagnose when a large number of ruminants become inappetant immediately after a change in feeding practices. It is much more difficult, however, to diagnose simple indigestion when only one animal is affected and the diet has been unchanged. In this case, simple indigestion is diagnosed by exclusion.

Pathogenesis

The cause of simple indigestion is presumed to be an altered ruminal microbial population, secondary to a rapid change in the intraruminal environment. The ruminal microbial population is normally in a continual state of flux, the population characteristics being determined by feeding frequency, nature of diet, and water intake. Diurnal variations in the rumen microbial population therefore occur. Since these variations are more pronounced in ruminants fed once or twice daily than in animals grazing pasture or fed a total mixed ration, indigestion is more likely to occur in intermittently fed ruminants.

Clinical Signs

The first indication of simple indigestion is a reduction in appetite, accompanied by a moderate decrease in milk production in lactating animals. The fecal consistency is usually altered, and typically a malodorous loose stool is voided within 12 to 24 hours of the onset of clinical signs. Reticuloruminal motility is decreased or absent, and rumination ceases. The rumen contents are more fluid on external palpation. Systemic signs of illness are not observed.

Diagnosis

Three criteria must be fulfilled before a diagnosis of simple indigestion can be made: (1) forestomach hypomotility or atony, (2) abnormal rumen contents, and (3) exclusion of all known diseases affecting the forestomach and gastrointestinal tract. Rumen fluid is required to confirm a diagnosis of simple indigestion. Strong supportive evidence for a diagnosis is a recent change in feed substrate, feeding frequency, or quantity of feed available, and more than one animal being affected.

Differential diagnoses that must be strongly considered when only one animal is affected are traumatic reticulitis, left displaced abomasum (LDA), and acetonemia. Traumatic reticulitis is usually accompanied by an abrupt and marked decrease in appetite and milk production, and abdominal pain and pyrexia are often present. Forestomach motility may appear decreased in cattle with LDA, but the characteristic ping of the LDA is usually identified during simultaneous auscultation and percussion. Acetonemia occurs most frequently in the first 6 weeks following parturition and is diagnosed by assessment of urine and milk acetoacetate concentration.

Treatment

The primary goal of treatment is rapid attainment of a normal intraruminal environment. This is most easily achieved through rumen transfaunation, which provides a balanced, buffered, nutrient-dense solution that also includes essential microorganisms. At least 3 L of freshly strained rumen juice are needed to transfaunate an adult dairy cow; 8 to 16 L is considered ideal. Rumen contents can be collected at the local abattoir or from cattle on the farm by passing a stomach tube and backsiphoning rumen juice. The latter is a time-consuming process and a number of cattle and special stomach tubes are required since the volume obtained varies from animal to animal. Stealing cuds from ruminating cattle has also been proposed as a means of obtaining rumen juice, but this method is impractical for routine use and is incapable of producing adequate volumes. Probiotic agents may be of additional benefit to rumen transfaunation if imbalances in the small intestinal microbial population are suspected. Probiotic preparations contain certain bacterial species (*Lactobacillus, Streptococcus*) that "implant" in the small intestine, potentially preventing or reducing establishment of a pathogenic bacterial species in the intestinal tract. Further work is required to determine the optimal way to use probiotic agents. Good-quality grass hay and straw should be available to the anorexic animal, since sick ruminants often prefer these feeds over alfalfa or concentrates. Oral administration of specific alkalinizing or acidifying agents should not be routinely undertaken in cases of indigestion. Magnesium hydroxide or magnesium oxide (450 g per adult cow) should only be administered to cattle with a confirmed diagnosis of lactic acidosis. These compounds can cause a severe alkalemia and hypermagnesemia when administered to cattle with a normal or high rumen pH, the latter being frequently encountered in cattle with simple indigestion. Acetic acid (vinegar, 4 to 10 L) can be administered to cattle with putrefaction of the rumen, associated with a high rumen pH.

Ruminatorics, such as nux vomica, ginger, tarter, and parasympathomimetics, have a very limited application in the present-day treatment of forestomach dysfunction. Parasympathomimetic agents, such as neostigmine or carbamylcholine, should not be used when rumen atony is present. Neostigmine requires vagal activity to be effective and therefore cannot incite normal primary contractions in atonic animals. Neostigmine may be of some benefit in hypomotile states since it increases the strength of the primary contraction without upsetting rhythm or coordination. Carbamylcholine causes uncoordinated, spastic, and functionless forestomach contractions, and therefore has no place in the treatment of forestomach dysfunction.

Simple indigestion can be prevented by increasing the feeding frequency, adding buffers to the feed (such as crude fiber or sodium bicarbonate), and avoiding rapid changes in feeding practices and substrate.

REFERENCES

1. Leek BF: Reticulo-ruminal function and dysfunction. Vet Rec 84:238–243, 1969.
2. Kay R: Rumen function and physiology. Vet Rec 113:6–9, 1983.
3. Sellers AF, Stevens CE: Motor functions of the ruminant forestomach. Physiol Rev 46:634–659, 1966.
4. Leek BF, Harding RH: Sensory nervous receptors in the ruminant stomach and the reflex control of reticulo-ruminal motility. *In* McDonald IW, Warner ACI (eds). Digestion and Metabolism in the Ruminant. Armadale, Australia, New England Publishing, 1975, pp 60–76.
5. Leek BF: Clinical diseases of the rumen: A physiologist's view. Vet Rec 113:10–14, 1983.

6. Dougherty RW, Habel RE, Bond HE: Esophageal innervation and the eructation reflex in sheep. Am J Vet Res 19:115–128, 1958.
7. Williams EI: A study of reticulo-ruminal motility in adult cattle in relation to bloat and traumatic reticulitis with and account of the latter condition as seen in general practice. Vet Rec 67:907–911, 1955.
8. Ash RW, Kay RNB: Stimulation and inhibition of reticulum contractions, rumination and parotid secretion from the forestomach of conscious sheep. J Physiol 149:43–57, 1959.
9. Welch JG: Rumination, particle size, and passage from the rumen. J Anim Sci 54:885–894, 1982.
10. Ruckebusch Y: Pharmacology of reticulo-ruminal motor function. J Vet Pharmacol Therap 6:245–272, 1983.
11. Abe M, Iriki T, Kondoh K, Shibui H: Effects of nipple or bucket feeding of milk-substitute on rumen by-pass and on rate of passage in calves. Br J Nutr 41:175–180, 1979.
12. Riek RF: The influence of sodium salts on the closure of the esophageal groove in calves. Aust Vet J 30:29–37, 1954.
13. Monnig HO, Quin JI: Studies on the alimentary tract of the merino sheep in South Africa, II. Investigations on the physiology of deglutition, II. Onderstepoort J Vet Sci 5:485–499, 1935.
14. Wester J: The rumination reflex in the ox. Vet J 86:410–410, 1930.
15. Mikhail M, Brugere H, Le Bars H, et al: Stimulated esophageal groove closure in adult goats. Am J Vet Res 49:1713–1715, 1988.
16. Chapman HW, Butler DG, Newell M: The route of liquids administered to calves by esophageal feeder. Can J Vet Res 50:84–87, 1986.
17. Beuno L, Sorraing JM, Fioramonti J: Influence of dopamine on rumino-reticular motility and rumination in sheep. J Vet Pharmacol Ther 6:93–98, 1983.
18. Asai T: Transfer of ingesta in the omasum of calves. Jpn J Vet Sci 37:609–13, 1975.
19. Brownlee A, Elliot J: Studies on the normal and abnormal structure and function of the omasum of domestic cattle. Br Vet J 116:467–473, 1960.
20. McDonald JS, Witzel DA: Three cases of chronic omasal impaction in the dairy cow. J Am Vet Med Assoc 152:638–640, 1968.
21. Ulyatt MJ, Dellow DW, John CSW et al: Contribution of chewing during eating and rumination and the clearance of digesta from the ruminoreticulum. In Milligan LP, Grovum WL, Dobson A (eds): Control and Digestion and Metabolism in Ruminants. Englewood Cliffs, NJ, Prentice-Hall 1986, pp 498–517.
22. Alonso AN: Diagnostic analysis of rumen fluid. Vet Clin North Am Food Anim Pract 1:363–376, 1979.
23. Geishauser T: A probe for collection of ruminal fluid in juvenile cattle and cows. Bovine Pract 28:113–116, 1994.
24. Nordlund KV, Garrett EF: Rumenocentesis: A technique for collecting rumen fluid for the diagnosis of subacute rumen acidosis in dairy herds. Bovine Pract 28:109–112, 1994.
25. Nordlund K. Questions and answers regarding rumenocentesis and the diagnosis of herd-based subacute rumen acidosis. Bovine Pract 28:75–81, 1996.

BIBLIOGRAPHY

Constable PD, Hoffsis GF, Rings DM: The reticulorumen: Normal and abnormal motor function. Part I. Primary contraction cycle; Part II. Secondary contraction cycles, rumination, and esophageal groove closure. Compend Contin Educ Pract Vet 12:1008–1015, 1169–1174, 1990.
Constable PD: Introduction to the ruminant forestomach. In Howard JL (ed): Current Veterinary Therapy 3. Food Animal Practice. 1993, pp 706–712.
Ruckebusch Y: Gastrointestinal motor functions in ruminants. In Wood J (ed): Handbook of Physiology. The Gastrointestinal System, Bethesda, Md, American Physiologic Society, 1990, pp 1225–1282.

DISEASES OF THE RUMINANT FORESTOMACH

■ Lactic Acidosis (Rumen Overload, Rumen Acidosis, Grain Overload, Engorgement Toxemia, Rumenitis)

Karl W. Kersting, D.V.M., M.S.
James R. Thompson, D.V.M., M.S.

DEFINITION

Several distinct syndromes are recognized. Ingestion of excessive quantities of highly fermentable carbohydrate feed leads to lactic acidosis with systemic dehydration and severe depression. It is by far the most common of the acute syndromes.

Ration ingredients characteristically involved include any of the common feed grains fed in quantities larger than those to which the animal has been accustomed. Finely ground grains are more likely to cause severe problems, but grinding is by no means a prerequisite. Other products known to have caused lactic acidosis in cattle include brewers' grains or distillery by-products such as corn gluten. Green corn, sweet corn, bakery bread, and apples and similar fruits have also been involved.

The propensity of a given feed to induce lactic acidosis is dependent on its content of precursors of lactic acid. Carbohydrates that can lead to accumulation of lactic acid are starch, maltose, sucrose, lactose, cellobiose, fructose, and glucose.[1] Ingestion of large quantities of highly fermentable proteinaceous material causes excess ammonium ion production, leading to alkalosis with excitement and hyperesthesia. (Consumption of soybeans and soybean derivatives is the most common cause in the midwestern region of the United States.) Either or both syndromes are commonly observed wherever intensive livestock management is practiced.

A syndrome of chronic rumen acidosis has been described in which lactic acidosis may not be a prominent feature, the lactic acid generated having been metabolized by other microorganisms. This disorder occurs in beef or dairy cattle fed for high production and results from feeding high proportions of concentrate at the expense of appropriate quantities of fibrous roughage or from too rapid introduction to such high-energy rations. Associated findings in affected animals include low milk fat, reduced rate of gain, liver abscesses, chronic laminitis, ketosis, rumenitis or rumen parakeratosis, bloat, and obesity.

PATHOGENESIS

The normal ruminant forestomach can be correctly visualized as a continuous culture fermentation receptacle. The normal microflora constitutes the culture; the ration being fed constitutes the medium or substrate on which the culture grows. The fermentation end products are normally acetic, propionic, and butyric acid, short-chain volatile fatty acids that are absorbed from the rumen as the animal's primary energy source. Bacterial cell protein is also produced and is digested farther down the tract as an amino acid source. Water-soluble vitamins are additional byproducts.

When the ration is abruptly changed to larger than normal quantities of highly fermentable carbohydrate, normal fermentation patterns change. Gram-positive streptococci and lactobacillus organisms become predominant, and lactic acid (both D- and L-isomers) becomes a principal fermentation end product. Lactic acid production increases osmotic pressure within the rumen so that fluid is drawn into the rumen from the circulatory system and thus from other tissues as well. The rumen pH drops, resulting in rumen stasis, and a large percentage of the normal rumen microflora is destroyed. Most of the gram-negative microorganisms and protozoa disappear. Symptoms become severe when the pH reaches 4 to 5.

The D- and L-lactic acids are converted to sodium lactate. In the rumen, they contribute to hypertonicity. Some are absorbed into the circulation (mainly D-lactate because of its slower metabolism) and contribute to a depression of the blood pH. There is some absorption of lactate from the omasum and abomasum and some as a result of continuing fermentation in the intestinal tract. An osmotic gradient is also established within the intestine, drawing fluid into the lumen and contributing to the profuse diarrhea. Chemical damage to the surface epithelium of the rumen mucosa occurs and later results in adherence of debris and penetration by particulate matter from the rumen ingesta, such as hair and sharp pieces of plant material. Bacterial and mycotic organisms begin to invade the rumen wall, and absorption patterns are changed.

The urine volume will usually be greatly decreased as a result of the dehydration, and secreted urine will be high in D-lactate and will be acidic.

The initial syndrome of acidosis is often followed by bacterial or mycotic rumenitis. Other possible sequelae are liver abscesses and peritonitis. Bloat may result from the decreased rumen motility and altered fermentation patterns. The development of acute, and later chronic, laminitis observed in some animals is thought to be related to the relative levels of histamine produced during the acute phases of the process. Thiaminase production by acidophilic microflora may lead to an increased incidence of polioencephalomalacia.

Pregnant animals frequently abort some days or weeks after the acute phases of illness. Secondary rumenitis may cause an increased incidence of bloat, and this is thought to be a major cause of unexplained deaths in feedlots, commonly diagnosed as "sudden death syndrome."

The entire disease process is complex and variable. A suggested additional component is likely endotoxic shock from toxins released during the destruction of large numbers of gram-negative microorganisms from the rumen ingesta.[2, 3]

CLINICAL SIGNS

The rapidity of onset of clinical signs varies and depends on the nature and quantity of the feed consumed and the adaptation of the animal to that feed. Unadapted animals may die from quantities of feed that are readily consumed by animals conditioned to the feed. On the other hand, even animals on "full feed" will overeat and develop acute lactic acidosis under some circumstances.

Usually, clinical signs will become apparent in 12 to 36 hours after engorgement on grain or similar material. Incoordination and ataxia are first noticed, followed by profound weakness and depression. Anorexia will be apparent, and affected animals appear blind. Rumen stasis is complete, with abdominal pain evidenced by occasional grunting and grinding of the teeth. Abdominal fullness and fluid distention of the rumen are observed. Significant dehydration will become apparent within 24 to 48 hours. Fetid diarrhea develops but may not be observed in animals that die early. Profuse diarrhea may be considered a sign of improvement if the animals are not seriously depressed.

In severe cases, the animals may become recumbent in 24 to 48 hours because of weakness and toxemia. The respiratory rate will most likely be increased because of acidosis. Body temperature may be subnormal by the time other signs are observed. The pulse is usually weak and thready. Recumbent animals will lie quietly, often with the head tucked to the side, as in parturient paresis. Crusty mucus will be present on the muzzle because the animal fails to clean its nostrils.

When a herd problem is observed, it is common to see several animals with profound depression and acute lactic acidosis. Animals with less severe cases will also be present and are likely to show only mild depression and diarrhea. Some animals may have acute laminitis with a characteristic lameness.

Acute deaths usually occur in 24 to 48 hours, but many animals have apparent recovery with later deterioration and death due to secondary complications. It is not unusual for losses to continue for 3 to 4 weeks in severely affected herds.

Some animals will partially recover but perform poorly in the feedlot because of chronic rumenitis, liver damage, or laminitis.

CLINICAL PATHOLOGY AND NECROPSY

Affected animals have hemoconcentration and acidic rumen content. The pH of ingesta aspirated from the rumen may be 4 or lower, and the urine pH may be as low as 5. Blood pH changes within a narrow range and requires more precise conditions and sophisticated equipment for measurement. Samples should be collected in heparinized tubes containing a layer of mineral oil, or the tubes should be completely filled, sealed, and then refrigerated (4° C) until measured. Accurate assessment of the blood pH requires that bicarbonate or total carbon dioxide be measured. Values below 7.2 generally indicate severe acidosis and a poor prognosis. Hypocalcemia may be superimposed on the metabolic acidosis.

If soybeans or other high-protein feeds have been consumed, rumen pH may be alkaline due to ammonia production. This will be reflected in the blood and urine pH as well.

Necropsy of acute cases demonstrates that the rumen is distended and filled with fluid content. The offending material is likely to be evident but postmortem measurements of pH levels are not likely to be valid because of rapid changes in the dead animal.

Rumen engorgement of slightly longer duration is characterized by rumenitis. However, postmortem autolysis occurs rapidly in the rumen so observations on the rumen mucosa must be interpreted carefully.

DIAGNOSIS

Diagnosis is usually based on history and clinical examination. The history alone is often sufficient but often it may be misleading if the pattern of feed consumption is not known. Laboratory evaluations, especially of the rumen ingesta, plasma, and urine pH, are particularly helpful.

The condition must be differentiated from polioencephalomalacia, urolithiasis, fulminating peritonitis, parturient hypocalcemia, and other diseases that cause profound depression.

TREATMENT

Animals with mild cases may recover without treatment; but in more severe forms the damage to the animal may be so extensive that even with intensive therapy only limited success will be achieved. Emptying of the rumen by oral lavage or rumenotomy is indicated if circumstances permit. The oral administration of antacids, such as magnesium carbonate or magnesium hydroxide, is indicated. These should be mixed in 2 to 3 gal (8 to 12 L) of warm water and given by stomach tube to ensure dispersion throughout the rumen. Initial doses of up to 1 g/kg body weight (454 g for an adult bovine) should be followed by smaller doses repeated at 6- to 12-hour intervals. If the rumen has been evacuated, the initial dose should not exceed 0.5 lb (225 g).

It is important that dehydration and acidosis be corrected as well. Balanced electrolyte and sodium bicarbonate solutions should be given intravenously. A 450-kg animal with 10% dehydration may require as much as 50 L of fluid over a 24-hour period. Sodium bicarbonate should be given at the rate of 0.5 mEq/kg body weight initially and repeated in 24 hours if necessary (1 g of sodium bicarbonate will supply 12 mEq of bicarbonate ion). Correction of blood pH to within the normal range is vital for survival of the animal even if the offending rumen ingesta are removed.

Oral administration of activated charcoal at the rate 2 g/kg body weight is said to enhance clinical recovery from acute lactic acidosis. This effect may be achieved by inactivating endotoxin thought to be released by the destruction of gram-negative rumen microorganisms.[4] Administration of antihistamines is considered to be of value by some. Recent field experience indicates that oral administration of thiabendazole in normal anthelmintic doses helps in controlling secondary mycotic rumenitis.

PREVENTION

Avoiding sudden and drastic changes in the ration is paramount in preventing rumen acidosis. Bunk-fed cattle need regular quantities of ration at regular intervals, and adequate bunk space must be available so that all animals have an opportunity to feed normally. The ration must include adequate roughage (generally ≥10%) regularly. Animals on self-feeder programs are particularly vulnerable to excessive consumption, especially early in the feeding program. Every precaution must be taken to ensure that roughage is available (mixed in the feed if possible) and that animals are brought onto full feed slowly. Feeders must be checked regularly and not permitted to run low or stand empty so that excessive intake by hungry animals is avoided after the feeders have been refilled. Feeder management must be particularly astute following sudden adverse weather conditions that temporarily force cattle away from the diet.

Progress has been made in the prevention of rumen lactic acidosis by pharmacologic means. The ionophore antibiotics, including monensin, lasalocid, and salinomycin, appear to be particularly useful in maintaining higher rumen pH and lower rumen lactate concentrations, as well as in improving feed efficiency in treated as compared with control animals.[5]

RUMENITIS (RUMINAL PARAKERATOSIS, CHRONIC RUMEN ACIDOSIS)

Definition

The term *rumenitis* refers to a series of inflammatory changes that develop in the rumen mucosa and underlying tissues in cattle fed high-energy rations with inadequate roughage. Clinically, the syndrome includes the associated lesions of liver abscess and laminitis. The incidence may be as high as 100% in cattle fed all-concentrate rations for prolonged periods or those that have not been carefully adapted to such rations. Rumenitis also occurs as a secondary stage of acute rumen engorgement with acidosis.

Pathogenesis

The association between liver abscess formation and ruminal lesions was first reported by Smith[6] and later by Jensen and colleagues.[7] A definite relationship between rumen adaptation to high-energy rations and the development of rumen lesions is now generally understood.

The exact pathogenesis of the rumen lesions has not been elucidated, but it is commonly accepted that the end products of rumen fermentation accumulate and change in relative quantity, causing an increase in hydrogen ion concentration and leading to inflammation of the rumen mucosa. Lactic acidosis is often not a prominent feature of this disorder, and affected animals may not go through an acute phase of illness. Some animals may perform very well, showing acceptable weight gains or producing high volumes of milk in the case of dairy cows. The rumen fluid may be moderately acidic, but in the absence of lactic acid that is probably metabolized by other microorganisms, the effects are mostly chronic and insidious.[8]

The sequence of events would appear to be (1) inflammation of the rumen mucosa, (2) adherence of debris to the mucosa, (3) ulceration and infection of deeper layers in the rumen wall, and (4) focal abscess formation in the rumen wall. Suppurative rumenitis may initiate liver abscesses via portal vein emboli. Similarly, liver abscesses may lead to caudal vena cava phlebitis, endocarditis, and pulmonary abscesses and hemorrhage.

Chronic laminitis is a later sequela. Its relationship is uncertain and appears less well correlated with the preceding events. Other independent factors may be involved in the development of chronic laminitis. Laminitis is frequently observed in cattle fed high-energy rations for 60 to 90 days and the incidence appears to be higher among females. Laminitis sometimes occurs in the absence of rumen and liver lesions. Likewise, there is nothing specific about the lesions in the rumen or the liver; the lesions in either could arise from other causes.

CLINICAL SIGNS

Cattle do not necessarily become clinically ill during the early stages of rumenitis and liver abscess formation. Feed consumption is usually good, and weight gains on all-concentrate rations for periods over 100 days are very acceptable. The addition of good-quality hay or silage for at least 10% to 20% of the ration will often result in increased feed consumption and average daily gain. Dairy cattle may suffer losses in milk production related to undulating or diminished dry matter intake. Butterfat content of milk is often negatively affected.

Animals with advanced rumen and liver lesions may show reduced appetite and weight gains, usually late in the feeding period. Affected individuals show an apparent lack of fill, as evidenced by gauntness of the abdomen. Other clinical signs, possibly relating to peritonitis or septicemia, may be seen. There will be elongation and flatness of the hooves with a very apparent alteration in gait if there is a chronic laminitis.

NECROPSY

Lesions are usually observed only at slaughter and result in the condemnations of livers and rumens. The rumen mucosa will have edema and clumping papillae in mild cases. More advanced causes demonstrate matting and necrosis of papillae with diffuse ulcerations. Hair and debris will adhere to the mucosa. Extensive thickening of the rumen wall with abscessation is also observed. There is increased thickness of the cornified portion of the rumen epithelium and increased numbers of vacuoles on histologic examination. The lesion is characteristic of an acid burn.

Abscesses will be observed on cut sections of the liver and are apparent as light-colored spots on the uncut surface in severe cases.

DIAGNOSIS

Chronic laminitis may be the first visible sign, but in many instances its appearance accompanies or precedes a noticeable reduction in feed consumption and rate of gain. Negative changes in herd milk production and increased culling rates of mature cattle may be observed.

The condition can be suspected in any group of cattle being fed for maximal gains on high-energy or all-concentrate rations, or in dairy animals consuming a total ration containing inadequate amounts of coarse fiber.

A diagnosis of chronic acidosis may be arrived at despite vague clinical signs. Documentation of the condition requires rumen fluid evaluation. Numerous methods of rumen liquor assay and collection have been described.[9] The critical determination for diagnosis of acidosis is pH. Percutaneous aspiration of rumen fluid from the lower left flank has been cited as the least cumbersome collection method for sampling a number of animals for a herd investigation.[10] This method also avoids salivary contamination associated with oral probe sampling which may artificially raise the pH. The fluid can be tested with a pH meter or pH paper and a pH below 5.5 is considered abnormal.

TREATMENT

Treatment and prevention depend on the inclusion of adequate good-quality roughage in the ration. Stemmy hay is preferred as a roughage source and should equal at least 10% of the dry matter in the ration. Chopped or finely ground hay is less effective in preventing rumenitis. Total mixed rations should include 10% coarse fiber particles measuring 1.5 in. or more. Ensilage can be used, but greater quantities are necessary. Ground corncobs are commonly used as roughage but should be supplemented with some hay.

Several antibiotics are approved as feed additives for the reduction of liver abscess incidence; however, tylosin appears to be the most effective.[11] *Fusobacterium necrophorum* vaccines may offer an additional measure of control.[12]

Individual animals that survive acute rumen engorgement develop secondary rumenitis, often with severe mycotic involvement. Thiabendazole (25 mg/kg body weight) given daily may be helpful in reducing the severity.

REFERENCES

1. Cullen AJ, Harmon DL, Nagoraja TG: In vitro fermentation of sugars, grains and by-product feeds in relation to initiation of ruminal lactate production. J Dairy Sci 69:2616–2621, 1986.
2. Dougherty RW, Coburn KS, Cook HM, et al: Preliminary study of appearance of endotoxin in circulatory system of sheep and cattle after induced grain engorgement. Am J Vet Res 36:831–832, 1975.
3. Mullenox CH, Keller RR, Allison MJ: Physiologic responses of ruminants to toxic factors extracted from rumen bacteria and rumen fluid. Am J Vet Res 27:857–868, 1966.
4. Buck WB: Activated charcoal: Preventing unnecessary death by poisoning. Vet Med 81:73–77, 1986.
5. Nogaraja TG, Avery TB, Galitzer SJ, et al: Prevention of lactic acidosis in cattle by lasalocid or monensin. J Anim Sci 53:206–216, 1981.
6. Smith H: Ulcerative lesions of bovine rumen and their possible relation to hepatic abscesses. Am J Vet Res 5:234–242, 1944.
7. Jensen R, Deane HM, Cooper LF, et al: The rumenitis-liver abscess complex in beef cattle. Am J Vet Res 15:55, 1954.
8. Garry FB: Diagnosing and treating indigestion caused by fermentative disorders. Vet Med 85:660–670, 1990.
9. Rings DM, Rings MB: Rumen fluid analysis. Agri Pract 14:26–29, 1993.
10. Nordlund KV, Garrett EF: Rumenocentesis: A technique for collecting rumen fluid for the diagnosis of subacute rumen accidosis in dairy herds. Bovine Pract 28:109–112, 1994.
11. Nagaraja TG, Laudert SB, Parrott JC: Liver abscesses in feedlot cattle II. Incidence, economic importance and prevention. Compend Contin Educ Pract Vet 18:S264–273, 1996.
12. Saginala S, Nagaraja TG, Tan Z, et al: Serum neutralizing antibody response and protection against experimentally induced liver abscesses in steers vaccinated with *Fusobacterium necrophorum*. Am J Vet Res 483–488, 1996.

▪ Rumen Putrefaction (Esophageal Groove Dysfunction, Rumen Drinkers)

Franklyn B. Garry, D.V.M., M.S., Diplomate, A.C.V.I.M.

DEFINITION

In rumen putrefaction a putrefactive decomposition of forestomach contents replaces the normal fermentation processes of rumen microbial digestion. The disease can occur in calves or adult cattle, but it is very uncommon in adults fed typical ruminant rations. It is more frequently seen in calves prior to weaning, before conversion to a ruminant diet and the attainment of full rumen digestive function. The existence of an established, active forestomach microbial population is usually effective in inhibiting the abnormal decomposition of ingesta that causes this disease. The disease has a chronic course, and typically occurs in individual animals, even though herdmates are exposed to similar management and a similar diet.

Putrefactive indigestion is associated with abnormal feeds or with continued deposition of milk in the rumen of the preweaned calf. The disease in calves has been associated with poor function of the esophageal groove. In milk-fed calves, this results in ongoing exposure of milk to bacterial degradation in the forestomach, with consequent abnormal fermentation and disease development. Affected calves have been called "rumen drinkers," and are characterized by chronic poor growth, a potbellied appearance, free gas bloat, poor hair coat or hair loss, abnormal feces, and sometimes a depraved appetite and licking of the hair coat.

PATHOGENESIS

Properties of ingested feed and the forestomach microbial population are primary determinants of the type of digestive processes that occur in the forestomach. High protein diets favor a proliferation of proteolytic organisms. The resulting high rumen fluid pH, paired with repeated inoculation of abnormal bacteria, can promote the development of putrefactive decomposition. In adult cattle, spoiled fermented forages or concentrates, and fecal contamination of feed or water can provide the abnormal microbial inoculum. These conditions are not common, and a well-established rumen microflora inhibits the development of such aberrant digestive patterns, so the disease is uncommon.

The young calf without well-developed rumen fermentation is apparently more susceptible to this form of indigestion. Repeated deposition of milk in the developing rumen stimulates abnormal digestion. Milk can gain access to the rumen by several means. These include failure of esophageal groove closure, prolonged maintenance of calves as preruminants (>3 to 4 months), and abomasal reflux. The latter can result from fluid feeding beyond the capacity of the abomasum (approximately 5% of body weight), fluids that delay abomasal emptying or inhibit curd formation, and abomasal inflammation. The high fat and protein content and relatively low carbohydrate content of milk predispose to a microflora in the rumen that decomposes these constituents, producing spoiled and rancid rumen ingesta. Development of problems is further encouraged by feeding contaminated or spoiled fluids.

CLINICAL SIGNS

Cattle affected by rumen putrefaction have reduced appetite and productivity, decreased rumen activity, recurrent bloat, and intermittent diarrhea. Occasionally frothy rumen contents are found. Overt systemic signs of disease are usually absent.

Calves with this type of indigestion typically display poor growth and evidence of malnutrition. These likely result from abnormal digestive end products, and herdmates on a similar feeding regimen may be performing adequately. Affected calves typically develop a poor hair coat, and sometimes a depraved appetite with excessive licking of the hair coat. The abdomen is mildly distended (potbellied) and flaccid, and the rumen is distended with fluid. Ballottement during auscultation reveals tinkling fluid sounds or pings of rumen origin. Rumen motility is poor and recurrent bloat is common. Feces are commonly pasty or fluid in consistency. The disease develops gradually, so the animal's poor condition may be well advanced before it is noticed.

This disease can occur in association with neonatal enteritis in calves 1 to 2 weeks old. In these cases the evaluation of the calf is usually focused on the intestinal tract and body fluid balance, while the rumen is overlooked and not evaluated. Calves with esophageal groove dysfunction may have prolonged diarrhea and poor response to the usual therapeutic procedures. Although the rumen is not well developed, auscultation with ballottement and percussion of the left flank usually reveals splashing and tinkling fluid sounds and pings. Auscultation during drinking can be especially revealing. Other clinical signs include prolonged mild depression and poor appetite compared with calves that have diarrhea without esophageal groove dysfunction.

DIAGNOSIS

Diagnosis requires evaluation of rumen fluid characteristics. Typically the history is unrevealing until after the diagnosis is achieved, since the animal is maintained similarly to other, normal, herdmates. After diagnosing the condition, a further investigation may reveal predisposing factors.

In adult cattle the rumen fluid color is typically dark green to black, solid and liquid components are mixed and sometimes frothy, the odor is foul, pH ranges between 7.5 and 8.5, and the number of protozoa is greatly reduced.

Milk-fed calves with this problem are also identified based on rumen fluid analysis. Rumen fluid pH in older calves (2 to 4 months) is often alkaline as a result of the proteolytic formation of ammonia. The rumen fluid pH is usually acidic in young calves (1 to 2 weeks) with esophageal groove failure and neonatal enteritis, apparently resulting from lactic acid or butyric acid generation. These pH findings contrast with a normal rumen fluid pH between 6 and 7 in young calves. Color is typically milky to beige, and milk clots and curdling may be apparent. The odor is rancid to sour to stale. These findings, combined with the physical findings described above, define the disease, but usually fail to define the cause in an individual, and further workup may be required to evaluate abomasal health and possible causal involvement. Rumen fluid chloride concentration is high in normal milk-fed calves (40 to 95 mEq/L), and its measurement is therefore not particularly helpful in achieving this diagnosis, nor in identifying abomasal disease as the cause. Typically a specific cause is not determined, and further diagnostic efforts may be unwarranted unless response to treatment, including dietary changes, fails to produce satisfactory improvement.

Treatment

The primary goal, as in other fermentative indigestions, is restoration of a normal forestomach environment and microbial digestion pattern. There are three general steps to accomplish this goal: (1) correct the current fluid abnormalities, (2) reinoculate the rumen with microbes appropriate for normal carbohydrate fermentation, and (3) change the feeding pattern and the rumen ingesta available for fermentation.

The rumen fluid pH abnormality can be corrected by administration of alkalinizing (magnesium hydroxide at 1 g/kg) or acidifying (acetic acid or vinegar at 2 mL/kg) agents via stomach tube. Intraruminal administration of antibiotics, such as oxytetracycline or erythromycin, has been used to decrease undesirable populations of rumen microbes.

In my view, the best approach is removal of the accumulated ingesta. Especially in young calves that have little dry matter content in the rumen, the fluid can be drained off by siphoning via stomach tube. Emptying the contents via rumenotomy may be more expedient and more effective than siphoning when the ingesta has a significant fiber component. The rumen may be lavaged with warm fluids to enhance thorough emptying.

Following the correction of rumen fluid abnormality, rumen transfaunation is used to inoculate the rumen. This procedure is described in the discussion of simple indigestion. Transfaunating several days in a row is desirable, and has the additional benefit of providing a nutrient-dense supplement to the affected animal. Probiotic preparations are not a substitute for rumen fluid administration. Administration of alfalfa pellets mixed into a gruel will provide substrate for fermentative activity, and can be especially helpful in younger animals that have limited experience consuming solid feed.

The final treatment objective, changing the feed pattern, can include provision of good-quality grass hay or other coarse feed such as dry oats or calf starter pellets. Pasture grazing of fresh green grass remains an ideal means of stimulating normal forestomach digestion. If the calf is more than 1 month old it is preferable to wean it and encourage conversion to full rumen function. Very young calves will require continued milk feeding, but establishing an active forestomach flora and intake of solid feed will enhance the plane of nutrition, reduce the need for full milk feeding, and is effective in preventing recurrence of the abnormal rumen digestion.

Both the animal and the rumen microflora have trace mineral requirements that will not have been met during the period of abnormal rumen activity. Oral supplementation of minerals and parenteral administration of B vitamins may be helpful until normal rumen function is reestablished.

BIBLIOGRAPHY

Breukink HJ, Wensing T, Weeren-Keverling-Buisman A: Consequences of failure of the reticular groove reflex in veal calves fed milk replacer. Vet Q 10:126–135, 1988.

Dirksen G: The digestive system. In Rosenberger G (ed): Clinical Examination of Cattle. Berlin, Verlag Paul Parey, 1979, pp 184–242.

Dirksen G, Dirr L: Oesophageal groove dysfunction as a complication of neonatal diarrhea in the calf. Bovine Pract 24:53–60, 1989.

Dirksen G, Garry F: Diseases of the forestomachs of calves. Part I and part II. Compendium Continuing Educ Pract Vet 9:F140–F147, F173–F179, 1987.

Garry F: Indigestion in ruminants. In Smith BP (ed): Large Animal Internal Medicine, ed 2. St Louis, Mosby–Year Book, 1996, pp 824–857.

van Bruinesses-Kapsenberg EG, Wensing T, Breukink HJ: Indigestionen der Mastkälber infolge fehlenden Schlundrinnenreflexes. Tierarztliche Umschau 7:515–517, 1982.

■ Bloat, or Rumen Tympany

Robert N. Streeter, D.V.M., M.S., Diplomate, A.C.V.I.M.

Maria E. Prado, M.V.

DEFINITION

Bloat is an excessive accumulation of fermentation gases within the reticulorumen. This disorder can develop rapidly and become life-threatening. The complete absence of eructation in intensively fed ruminants is a medical emergency. Bloat may occur in an individual or in numerous animals in a herd or flock. Economic losses due to bloat can represent a significant burden to producers in the form of deaths, reduced gains, cost of preventive strategies, and inability to maximally utilize certain forages.

ETIOLOGY AND PATHOGENESIS

The capacity for eructation in a healthy ruminant exceeds the maximal rate of gas production, even at the highest rates of microbial fermentation.[1] Therefore, bloat is not a consequence of excessive gas production, but rather a failure of eructation. This failure may be due to a mechanical or functional disturbance anywhere along the path of the eructation mechanism (reticulorumen, esophagus, pharynx, nervous system) and result in free gas bloat. Alternatively, the failure may be in the form of the gas (foam mixed with digesta), wherein relaxation of the cardia will not occur due to reflex inhibition, resulting in a frothy bloat. A complete description of rumen motility and eructation is presented earlier in this section.

Free gas bloat is not a disease in itself, but rather a manifestation of an underlying primary disorder. Free gas bloat occurs sporadically, usually affecting a single animal without an associated change in the diet. Numerous conditions and disturbances can lead to free gas bloat as summarized in Table 1 and discussed elsewhere in this book.

Frothy bloat is a primary disease wherein the ruminal gases are trapped in small bubbles within abnormally viscous digesta. The development of a stable foam in the rumen fluid is an incompletely understood process, but is known to be dependent on interactions between the diet, ruminal microflora, and animal. Frothy bloat occurs in animals consuming a variety of

Table 1
CONDITIONS LEADING TO FREE GAS BLOAT

Esophageal Dysfunction
Intraluminal: foreign body (choke)
Intramural: papilloma, granuloma, tetanus
Extramural: mediastinal lymphadenopathy
Positional: lateral recumbency, hypocalcemia, surgery
Ruminal Motility Dysfunction
Muscular inactivity: hypocalcemia, xylazine, atropine
Reticular adhesions: hardware, abomasal ulcers
Vagal nerve injury: many
Abnormal rumen environment:
    Grain engorgement (lactic acidosis)
    Rumen impaction with microbial inactivity
    Rumen putrefaction
Severe abomasal distention:
    Left displaced abomasum (particularly in calves)
    Milk engorgement/overeating

different feedstuffs. Offending diets include many legumes, lush wheat or ryegrass, and high-concentrate rations. The bloat that develops is referred to as legume bloat, wheat pasture bloat, and grain bloat, respectively. There are several factors contributing to the pathogenesis of all causes of primary frothy bloat, the most important of which are (1) small particles in the rumen content, (2) rapidly digested feedstuff (3) rumen microorganisms (4) foam-promoting compounds, and (5) foam-retarding compounds.[2]

Ruminal bacteria adhere to small feed particles (fine kernel elements or plant membrane fragments) in the digesta. The small particle size allows for a large population of adherent bacteria for subsequent fermentation. A rapidly digested feedstuff then provides adequate nutrients for explosive microbial proliferation. The multiplying bacteria release large amounts of a mucopolysaccharide, termed *slime*, which is highly viscous. Small gas bubbles released during fermentation become trapped in a particle-slime-gas complex (froth or foam).[2] The stability of the foam is enhanced by factors such as low ruminal pH and surface-active foaming agents in certain plants. Salivary mucoproteins have foam-retardant properties, so reduced saliva production enhances foam stability.

There are significant differences in the bloat-inducing potential of pasture forages, as summarized in Table 2. An important forage characteristic promoting the development of frothy bloat is a high rate of digestion, which is influenced by the plant's leaf structure, mesophyll cell wall characteristics, and maturity.[2] Other factors include the concentration of foaming agents (soluble leaf proteins, pectins), soluble nitrogen, and antifoaming agents (tannins) in the plant. Environmental influences on the bloat potential of forages are complex, and are probably related to digestibility of the forage, grazing patterns of the animals, and saliva production.

Processing of grain to produce small particle size appears to be the primary feed-related factor controlling the development of frothy bloat. Coarsely processed rations are less bloat-pro-

Table 2
BLOAT POTENTIAL OF FORAGES

High Risk	Moderate Risk	Low Risk
Alfalfa	Arrowleaf clover	Lespedeza
Sweet clover	Spring wheat	Birdsfoot trefoil
Red clover	Oats	Sainfoin
Winter wheat	Perennial ryegrass	Most perennial grasses

voking. The foam-producing compounds in grain bloat are derived from the ruminal microflora (mucopolysaccharide slime). The regulation and modulation of bacterial slime production is an area of research interest.

Individual cattle vary in their susceptibility to frothy bloat. Bloat-susceptible cattle have slower clearance of particulate matter from the rumen and larger rumen volume than bloat-resistant cattle. Differences in the rate of eructation, saliva production, and salivary composition may also affect an animal's susceptibility to bloat. Some degree of the susceptibility to bloat appears to be inherited, but information on this subject is limited.[3]

Omasal transport failure, a type of vagal indigestion, can cause frothy bloat. This rumen outflow disturbance results in increased rumen contents, which reflexly initiates hypermotility. The excessive mixing of digesta generates a stable foam and recurrent frothy bloat.

CLINICAL SIGNS

Bloat results in an asymmetrical abdominal distention, most pronounced in the left paralumbar fossa. Mild bloat is often subclinical but may be associated with reduced feed intake and production. As the condition progresses, animals display signs of abdominal discomfort manifested by restlessness, kicking at the abdomen, and rolling. Rumen motility is increased in the early stages, but later is inhibited by extreme distention. As distention becomes severe, the diaphragm and lungs are compressed, interfering with ventilation and venous return to the heart. The respiratory and heart rates progressively increase. Animals may exhibit open-mouth breathing with protrusion of the tongue, and eventually die of asphyxia. Acute bloat is of short duration with death occurring within 30 minutes to 4 hours after onset of mild signs, depending on the specific cause and previous diet.

DIAGNOSIS

The primary diagnostic information for a case of rumen tympany is gained while passing an orogastric tube (Fig. 1). Diagnosis of the cause of free gas bloat not associated with esophageal obstruction can be challenging. Close inspection of the rumen and its motility patterns is warranted. Helpful ancillary diagnostic techniques include rumen fluid examination, esophageal endoscopy, reticular ultrasonography, and exploratory laparotomy or rumenotomy.[4]

The differential diagnosis of abdominal distention that could be confused with bloat includes ruptured bladder, hydroallantois, left displaced abomasum in calves, abomasal volvulus, and mesenteric volvulus. Careful evaluation of the abdominal contour, physical examination, and rectal palpation should allow differentiation.

Postmortem diagnosis of bloat is complicated by the fact that some gas accumulates in the rumen after death from any cause. In primary bloat, the rumen may be markedly distended by foamy contents, but the viscosity of the digesta will decline with increasing postmortem interval. Other findings include congestion of the head, neck, and forelimbs contrasted with compression and pallor of the abdominal viscera and pelvic limbs. A line of demarcation (bloat line) between the congested extrathoracic esophagus and the blanched thoracic esophagus is strong evidence for antemortem bloat.[5]

TREATMENT

Bloated animals that are dyspneic and recumbent require emergency ruminal decompression via trocarization (free gas)

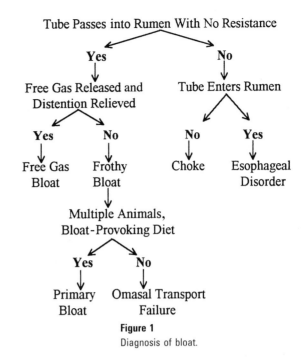

Figure 1
Diagnosis of bloat.

or emergency rumenotomy (frothy). For less severely affected animals, an orogastric tube is passed to facilitate gas removal. Highly frothy digesta will not escape through a tube and antifoaming agents should be administered. Available compounds include poloxalene (2 oz/1000 lb), mineral or vegetable oils (1 to 2 pt/1000 lb), and docusate sodium (2 oz/1000 lb). The antifoaming agent should be deposited near the cardia and be provided in enough volume or diluent to allow dissemination throughout the rumen contents. Poloxalene is more effective in cases of forage bloat than in grain bloat. Animals should be monitored closely for response to therapy over the next hour. In outbreaks of severe frothy bloat, all animals should be removed from the offending diet. Affected animals should be encouraged to walk and should be monitored for the need of individual treatment for the following few hours.

Free gas bloat requires treatment for the primary eructation disorder. Chronic cases may be symptomatically treated by a temporary rumenostomy for long-term bloat relief. Animals with recurrent bloat of any type that fails to respond to conventional measures should be considered for culling.

CONTROL AND PREVENTION

Grazing management is important for the control of bloat on pastures. Cattle should not be exposed to bloat-causing forages when hungry. A full feeding of coarse roughage should precede the first exposure and may be indicated following periods of reduced feed intake (transport, processing, inclement weather). Animals should be turned onto pastures after the dew evaporates. Continued supplementation with coarse roughage or grains may reduce the incidence of bloat by reducing the intake of the pasture. On severely bloat-prone pastures, the above measures may afford incomplete protection, and the provision of specific antifoaming agents is necessary.

The surfactant poloxalene is highly effective in reducing losses from wheat pasture and legume bloat. All animals at risk must receive the compound daily for maximal protection. Poloxalene is available as a top-dressing for grain, in molasses blocks, and in liquid supplements. The ionophore antibiotics monensin and lasalocid have been shown to reduce the incidence of both legume and wheat pasture bloat, but are not as effective as poloxalene.[6] The ionophores have the additional advantage of improving feed efficiency.

Grain bloat is best prevented by allowing adequate adaptation to high-concentrate diets, ensuring that the particle size of the ration is sufficiently large, and providing at least 10% of the diet as coarse roughage. Roughage and concentrate should be fed mixed together. Ionophores in the ration reduce the incidence of grain bloat and have other economic benefits in grain-fed cattle.[7] Other feed additives which have been used to reduce the severity of grain bloat include mineral oil, tallow, salt, and poloxalene, but their utility is reduced by constraints of cost, processing requirements, or reduced gains.

REFERENCES

1. Leek BF: Clinical diseases of the rumen: A physiologist's view. Vet Rec 113:10–14, 1983.
2. Howarth RE, Chaplin RK, Cheng KT, et al: Bloat in Cattle. Agriculture Canada Publication 1858/E. Ottawa, Communications Branch, Agriculture Canada, 1991, pp 6–32.
3. Hall JW, Majak W: Plant and animal factors in legume bloat. *In* Cheek PR (ed): Toxicants of Plant Origin. Boca Raton, Fla, CRC Press, 1989, pp 93–106.
4. Garry F: Managing bloat in cattle. Vet Med 85:643–650, 1990.
5. Mills JHL, Christian RG: Lesions of bovine ruminal tympany. J Am Vet Med Assoc 157:947–952, 1970.
6. Majak W, et al: Pasture management strategies for reducing the risk of legume bloat in cattle. J Anim Sci 73:1493–1498, 1995.
7. Corah LR: Polyether ionophores—Effect on rumen function in feedlot cattle. Vet Clin North Am Food Anim Pract 7:127–132, 1991.

■ Traumatic Reticuloperitonitis and Its Sequelae

Robert N. Streeter, D.V.M., M.S., Diplomate, A.C.V.I.M.

Traumatic reticuloperitonitis (TRP) is a sporadic disease of ruminants caused by perforation of the reticulum by ingested foreign material with resultant contamination of body cavities or organs. Cattle are principally affected owing to their indiscriminant feeding behavior. The disorder occurs rarely in other ruminant species (sheep, goats, and llamas). A variety of clinical syndromes can result, but they all have a common underlying pathogenesis. The following discussion focuses on the disease in cattle.

ETIOLOGY AND EPIDEMIOLOGY

Traumatic reticuloperitonitis is most often caused by linear metallic foreign bodies such as wires and nails. Nonferromagnetic objects are occasionally responsible. Metallic debris is encountered more commonly in processed feeds and forages than on pastures; hence the condition is seen more in confined cattle. Cattle can also acquire linear foreign material when they graze near construction sites, deteriorating buildings, and downed fences. Most cases occur in adult animals, probably due to differences in feeding practices between adult and young stock and to increased exposure occurring over time. Dairy cattle are more commonly affected than beef cattle, which likewise reflects a difference in husbandry practices. Foreign material is frequently found in the reticulum of cattle, often without consequence. Scars within the reticulum or evidence of adhe-

sions associated with TRP have been noted in up to 70% of adult dairy cattle at postmortem inspection.[1]

PATHOPHYSIOLOGY

Ingested particles enter the rumen after deglutition and, with ensuing ruminal contractions, come to rest within the reticulum. Linear objects may lodge within the "honeycombed" internal surface of the reticulum, and with continued reticular contractions, can be forced to penetrate the wall.

Foreign body perforation is usually in the cranioventral aspect of the reticulum and less commonly in a medial or lateral direction. Lesions with intramural penetration without disruption of the serosal surface are probably subclinical or result in a mild self-limiting disease. Once the foreign material penetrates the serosa, the accompanying reticular microflora initiates a local peritonitis, and clinical signs develop. Progression of the disease beyond this stage is variable. The possible outcomes include acute local peritonitis, chronic local peritonitis, diffuse peritonitis, perireticular abscess formation, liver puncture and abscessation, vagal neuritis and vagal indigestion, traumatic splenitis, and transdiaphragmatic migration with resultant pericarditis, mediastinitis, pleuritis, or pulmonary abscessation.

Characteristics of the perforating foreign body may influence its migration. In an experimental model of TRP in which wires and nails were given simultaneously, wires were more frequently found both within the reticulum and to be perforating the wall.[2] Abdominal compression due to an enlarged rumen or advanced pregnancy has been postulated to predispose to transdiaphragmatic migration of foreign objects.[3]

CLINICAL SIGNS

Acute Localized Peritonitis

Acute localized peritonitis is common to all cases of TRP. The most consistent clinical and historical findings are an elevated temperature and heart rate, evidence of abdominal pain, decreased or absent reticuloruminal motility, and rapid decline in appetite and milk production.

Pyrexia is usually moderate (39.5 to 40.5°C); in uncomplicated cases the temperature returns to normal within a few days. Likewise, the heart rate is moderately (80 to 100 beats per minute [bpm]) and transiently elevated. Alterations in respiratory parameters are variable and mild unless significant lung abscessation or pleuritis occurs. An increased rate and shallow depth of respiration may occur due to pyrexia and pain.

Manifestations of abdominal pain may be subtle or quite obvious. In severe cases, animals may resist movement, have a short stilted gait, stand with elbows abducted, have a markedly arched posture, or audibly grunt with respiratory efforts or while walking. Other signs include extended head and neck, tensed facial and abdominal muscles, fasiculations of forelimb muscles, and odontoprisis. Maneuvers used to detect pain include pinching the withers, percussion over the area of the reticulum, and lifting of the cranioventral abdomen with the knee or a pole. Such manipulations may evoke an audible and visual response in severe cases, whereas in milder cases or those of some chronicity, the response can be detected only by simultaneous auscultation over the trachea. Signs of abdominal pain may regress to the point that they are difficult to detect after a few days.

Evidence of abdominal pain is not specific for TRP and may be found in other disorders of the cranial abdomen such as abomasal ulcers, liver abscesses, rumenitis, and abomasal lymphoma. Discriminant palpation and percussion of the right and left abdomen may assist in ruling out potential causes by identification of a most painful locus over a particular organ or viscus. Also, thoracic pain can mimic that originating in the abdomen. Pain elicited on deep intercostal palpation and abnormal thoracic auscultation should alert the clinician to a thoracic disease.

Ruminal abnormalities are a constant feature of acute TRP. Reticuloruminal motility is invariably affected early in the course of the disease with absence or marked suppression of ruminal contractions. As motility returns, evidence of pain may coincide with contraction of the reticulum. Mild free gas bloat with distention of the left paralumbar fossa may occur due to less frequent eructation. Occasionally, animals may be noted to vomit or drop their cud. Rumen contents may be firmer than normal due to dehydration and decreased motility. Feces are frequently scant and dry in the early stages of the disease. Defecation may be more frequent, small in volume, and accompanied by grunting or other evidence of abdominal pain. Diarrhea early in the course of the disease, especially when accompanied by symptoms of toxemia, should alert the clinician to the possibility of acute diffuse peritonitis or a diagnosis other than TRP.

A precipitous drop in milk production and appetite are characteristic of TRP. These historical findings can be helpful in distinguishing subacute TRP from a variety of diseases with similar vague signs of gastrointestinal atony such as left displaced abomasum, simple indigestion, and ketosis. The drop in milk yield is usually greater than 50% to 75% during the first 24 hours in TRP in contrast to the more gradual and modest decline noted in these other conditions.[4]

The course of the disease with acute localized peritonitis is typically short. Most uncomplicated cases will show progressive improvement over 3 to 5 days. If signs persist after this time, the development of chronic active peritonitis or other complications should be considered.

Chronic Localized Peritonitis

Chronic peritonitis may occur due to persistence of the foreign body or its tract and the associated bacteria. Clinical findings are similar to those seen with acute local peritonitis but are less extreme. There is less evidence of abdominal pain and its detection can be difficult. Body temperature and heart rate may return to normal or be slightly elevated. Appetite and milk production usually remain subnormal. Feces continue to be scant but their character may range from firm to loose depending on the animal's hydration status and degree of toxemia. Poorly digested plant material may be found in the feces, suggestive of forestomach dysfunction.

Diffuse Peritonitis

Diffuse peritonitis is an uncommon result of TRP because of the inherent ability of the bovine to form adhesions in response to peritoneal injury. When it does occur, it is often a fulminant and highly fatal disease. Generalized peritonitis usually develops as a primary event directly after foreign body perforation, although cases may develop some time (weeks) after onset of typical TRP signs. The disease course is usually short with animals progressing to prostration, recumbency, and death within 24 to 36 hours. Features distinguishing this from routine cases of TRP include very high heart rate (100 to 120+), high fever (40 to 41°C) with rapid progression to hypothermia, severe dehydration, diarrhea, profound depression, and recumbency. The prognosis for such cases is poor despite aggressive therapy.

Thoracic Sequelae: Pericarditis

Transdiaphragmatic migration of the foreign body occurs in a significant proportion of cases and the result is often catastrophic. Diaphragmatic involvement is reported to occur in 28% to 60% of TRP cases and pericarditis in 6% to 8%.[5, 6] The actual incidence may be significantly less since many mild cases of TRP may not be included in such surveys. Pulmonary or mediastinal abscessation and pleuritis may occur separately or in conjunction with pericarditis. Recognition of intrathoracic involvement in cases of TRP is important as it worsens the prognosis significantly and additional therapeutic measures should be considered in those animals undergoing treatment. The time span between reticular perforation and involvement of the pericardium is variable, ranging from a few days to weeks or months.

Clinical signs referable to traumatic pericarditis are due to a combination of pain, toxemia, and the development of congestive heart failure. The heart rate of affected cattle is continually elevated, typically over 100 bpm. Pyrexia is present in cases suffering from toxemia, but may be absent in subacute cases wherein congestive heart failure predominates. The auscultatory findings depend on the duration of the condition and the presence or absence of gas within the pericardial space. Gas may be present within the pericardium owing to its production by multiplying microorganisms, but it is not present in all cases. Initially, a pericardial friction rub is heard which may be confused with a pleural friction rub if an inflamed portion of the pleura is in contact with the pericardium. With time, exudation into the pericardial sac occurs, producing muffled heart sounds. If gas and fluid are present concurrently, pathognomonic splashing sounds will be heard on cardiac auscultation.

As exudate accumulates within the pericardial space, cardiac tamponade develops. The clinical signs generated are primarily due to right heart failure because of its thinner wall and lower systolic pressure. Signs include venous distention, abnormal jugular pulses, and brisket edema. In severe cases hepatic and portal congestion may lead to profuse diarrhea, ascites, and a palpable liver under the right costal arch. Peracute death can occur due to laceration of a coronary vessel with resultant hemopericardium and cardiac tamponade. Occasionally, subcutaneous emphysema may be detected over the lateral and dorsal thorax as gas produced within the mediastinum escapes to the subcutis.

Other Sequelae

A syndrome of omasal transport failure may occur in association with perireticular and liver abscesses subsequent to TRP.[7] Other forms of vagal indigestion are also potential sequelae to TRP; a variety of clinical manifestations are described[3] (see Vagal Indigestion, which is the next article in this section).

Involvement of the spleen in TRP is rare. Traumatic splenitis may be clinically silent, result in chronic low-grade sepsis and pyrexia, or lead to diffuse peritonitis (if a large abscess is subsequently ruptured). Rarely, sepsis associated with TRP can serve as the precursor to the development of diseases such as endocarditis, septic arthritis, embolic pneumonia or nephritis, and amyloidosis.[8, 9] TRP is also reported to be a predisposing factor in the development of acquired diaphragmatic herniation in the bovine.[10]

DIAGNOSTIC AIDS

Thorough clinical examination is often sufficient to make a tentative diagnosis of acute TRP. Subacute and chronic cases are more difficult to diagnose and ancillary diagnostic techniques are sometimes necessary. Techniques useful in the evaluation of an animal suspected of having TRP include hematologic tests, abdominocentesis, ultrasonography, and radiography.

Changes in the leukogram in cases of TRP are dependent on the duration of the disease and the sequelae present. The classic response is a neutrophilic leukocytosis. However, many cases will have a normal total leukocyte count and the differential count must be relied upon to reflect the presence of a neutrophilia (>4000 cells per microliter) and thus an inflammatory process. The leukogram in uncomplicated cases returns toward normal within 3 to 5 days. In cases of diffuse peritonitis the leukogram may reveal a leukopenia and degenerative left shift. Traumatic pericarditis and pleuritis tend to generate higher total leukocyte counts (14,000 to 20,000/μL) than cases of acute or chronic localized peritonitis. Overall, leukograms are variable in TRP.

Elevation of plasma fibrinogen concentration is a fairly constant feature of inflammatory diseases in cattle.[11] Owing to the influence of dehydration on this parameter, it is suggested that a ratio of plasma protein to fibrinogen of less than 10:1 be used as a finding consistent with TRP.[12] Elevation of total plasma protein (TPP) has been examined as an index for suspicion of TRP. High levels of TPP (>10 g/dL) had a high positive predictive value (76%) in determining the presence of TRP.[13]

Examination of peritoneal fluid is a sensitive means of detecting peritoneal inflammation. The differential cell count appears to be a more reliable indicator of abdominal inflammation than does the total nucleated cell count and protein level. Laboratory values indicative of peritonitis in cattle include the presence of greater than 40% neutrophils and less than 10% eosinophils, cell counts greater than 6000/μL, and protein levels greater than 3.0 g/dL.[14, 15] Gram staining or bacterial culture of the sample also provides useful information regarding subsequent antimicrobial therapy.

Ultrasonographic evaluation of the cranioventral abdomen is useful in the detection of TRP. Ultrasonography allows for the identification of reticular motility and mobility, the position and contour of the reticulum, the presence of perireticular fibrin deposition and abscesses, and the presence of localized or generalized abdominal effusion.[16] The contents of the reticulum (magnets and foreign bodies) cannot be visualized ultrasonographically due to the impedence of the reticular ingesta to sound waves.

Radiography is a useful diagnostic tool in the identification of traumatic reticuloperitonitis, pericarditis, and perireticular abscesses.[17, 18] Owing to the size of the animal, only a lateral view is obtainable; therefore, the absolute location of the foreign body is difficult to determine. The procedure may be performed standing or with the patient in dorsal recumbency. Standing reticulography requires powerful equipment not available to most practitioners. Placement of the animal in dorsal recumbency provides the advantages of being able to use a portable unit on most cows. Dorsal recumbency allows gas to accumulate in the reticulum which increases contrast and visualization of foreign material and allows nonpenetrating foreign bodies to fall out of the reticulum. Dorsal reticulography is not without risk, however, especially in acute cases (in which the procedure can lead to disruption of fibrinous adhesions and dissemination of the infection) and in animals with compromised cardiovascular function (i.e., pericarditis).

Radiographic findings suggestive of foreign body perforation include (1) the foreign body extending through or within the reticular wall, (2) the foreign body not on the floor of the reticulum or with an angle of greater than 30 degrees to the floor, (3) abnormal contour of the cranioventral reticulum, and (4) abnormal gas shadows or gas-fluid interface adjacent to the reticulum.[19] Gas within the abomasum may be confused with an abscess caudal to the reticulum. These criteria must be evaluated collectively because foreign bodies will not be detected radiographically in all animals with TRP.

Additional diagnostic aids applicable to suspected cases of pericarditis include electrocardiography, pericardiocentesis, and thoracic ultrasonography.

TREATMENT

The appropriate treatment for TRP will depend on the stage of the disease, the sequelae present, the value of the animal, and the diagnostic and surgical facilities available to the clinician. Medical management alone gives favorable results in a high percentage of cases. Surgery (rumenotomy) is typically reserved for those cases not showing significant and continuing improvement after 3 to 4 days of medical therapy. Surgery may also be indicated in valuable animals, especially if the offending foreign body is detected radiographically within the diaphragm or is not in contact with a reticular magnet.

Medical management of TRP includes administration of parenteral antibiotics, provision of a reticular magnet, and strict confinement to a small area. The choice of antibiotics should ideally be predicated on an abdominocentesis culture. Empirically, the decision is based on the knowledge that this is a polymicrobial infection; agents commonly encountered include *Actinomyces pyogenes*, coliforms, and anaerobes. Consideration should be given to using a drug with a short slaughter withdrawal time such that salvage may remain an option should therapy be unsuccessful. Commonly utilized antibiotics include ceftiofur, oxytetracycline, and penicillins. Reticular magnets are utilized to stabilize incompletely penetrating foreign bodies and prevent their migration. Magnets give therapeutically may remain within the rumen for several days due to the lack of reticuloruminal motility. Also, only foreign bodies in the ventral aspect of the reticulum are likely to be affected by a magnet. Thus, strict confinement of the animal is advisable to allow adhesions to develop around the perforation, hence limiting the spread of the peritonitis. Elevation of the animal's forequarters in a tie-stall may also help to retard forward migration of a foreign body.

Surgical management involves a left-sided exploratory laparotomy, and rumenotomy.[20] Abdominal exploration should preceed the rumenotomy. Adhesions between the reticulum and surrounding structures supports a diagnosis of TRP. Fibrinous adhesions should not be broken down and retrieval of the foreign body should only be performed during the rumenotomy. With the rumen opened and evacuated, the reticulum is examined for areas of adhesion by grasping and lifting up the wall. Adherent areas are palpated closely for a perforating foreign body, which should be removed. In subacute cases, the offending foreign body may have returned to the lumen and be attached to a magnet. The cranial abdomen is then explored by palpating through the reticular wall. If a perireticular abscess is found, determine if it is firmly adherent to the wall of the reticulum. Needle aspiration confirms the diagnosis and the abscess can be drained by lancing it through the reticular wall at a point of firm attachment. This provides chronic active drainage of the area and recurrence does not appear to be a significant problem.[6] If an abscess is not tightly adherent to a portion of the forestomachs, a second surgery and drainage through a ventral approach is indicated.

Cases of diffuse peritonitis require intensive therapy consisting of intravenous fluids, antibiotics, and anti-inflammatory agents, but the mortality is high despite aggressive and expensive therapy. If large quantities of exudate have accumulated within the peritoneal cavity, its drainage via a catheter placed in the ventral abdomen may be beneficial. Peritoneal drainage and lavage are difficult to accomplish in cattle owing to the size of the animal, the extensive omentum, and large amounts of fibrin and subsequent adhesions.

Therapy for traumatic pericarditis is frequently unsuccessful and usually reserved for valuable individuals. Antibiotic considerations are similar to cases of TRP, except that a longer course (2 to 4 weeks) is indicated. Rumenotomy should be performed early in the disease to increase the probability of retrieving the foreign body. Drainage of the pericardial sac can be accomplished via pericardiocentesis, pericardial catheterization, or pericardiotomy.

Pericardiocentesis provides short-term benefit. Placement of a pericardial catheter is more difficult but enables repeated drainage and lavage. Fibrin clots present in the exudate may occlude the catheter, and adhesions often develop within the pericardial sac leading to compartmentalization and ineffective drainage. Use of proteolytic enzymes in the lavage solution may lessen these occurrences. The catheter is left in place until the fluid retrieved is no longer septic.

Pericardiotomy via a fifth rib resection allows for more complete drainage of the pericardium and removal of foreign bodies inaccessible by rumenotomy. The procedure can be performed under local anesthesia and is followed by marsupialization of the pericardium or insertion of an indwelling drain with closure.[21] Intra- and postoperative complications and mortality are high, but successful recovery is possible.

PREVENTION AND CONTROL

The use of magnets on feed-processing equipment can significantly reduce the incidence of TRP. General cleanliness and discontinued use of baling wire may also be advantageous on problem farms. The prophylactic use of reticular magnets has been demonstrated to be highly effective in preventing the occurrence of TRP.[22] Reticular magnets are probably warranted in individual valuable cattle and all animals in herds known to have a significant problem with this disease.

REFERENCES

1. Maddy KT: Incidence of perforation of the bovine reticulum. J Am Vet Med Assoc 124:113–115, 1954.
2. Kingrey BW: Experimental bovine traumatic gastritis. J Am Vet Med Assoc 127:477–481, 1955.
3. Rebhun WC, Lesser FR: Vagus indigestion in cattle: Clinical features, causes, treatments, and long-term follow-up of 112 cases. Compendium Continuing Educ Pract Vet 10:387–392, 1988.
4. Blood DC, Hutchins DR: Traumatic reticular perforation of cattle. Aust Vet J 31:113–123, 1955.
5. Traumatic gastritis and "tramp iron" (editorial). J Am Vet Med Assoc 125:331–332, 1954.
6. Blood DC, Hutchins DR: Traumatic pericarditis of cattle. Aust Vet J 31:229–232, 1955.
7. Fubini SL et al: Failure of omasal transport attibutable to perireticular abscess formation in cattle: 29 cases (1980–1986). J Am Vet Med Assoc 194:811–814, 1989.
8. Power HT, Rebhun WC: Bacterial endocarditis in adult dairy cattle. J Am Vet Med Assoc 182:806–808, 1983.
9. Johnson R, Jamison K: Amyloidosis in six dairy cows. J Am Vet Med Assoc 185:1538–1543, 1984.
10. Bristol DG: Diaphragmatic hernias in horses and cattle. Compend Contin Educ Pract Vet 8:S407–412, 1986.
11. McSherry BJ, et al: Plasma fibrinogen levels in normal and sick cows. Can J Comp Med 34:191–197, 1970.
12. Schalm OW, Jain NC, Carroll EJ: Plasma proteins, dysproteinemias, and immune deficiency disorders. In Jain NC (ed): Veterinary Hematology. Philadelphia, Lea & Febiger, 1986, p 960.
13. Dubensky RA, White ME: The sensitivity, specificity, and predictive value of total plasma protein in the diagnosis of traumatic reticuloperitonitis. Can J Comp Med 47:241–244, 1983.
14. Wilson AD, et al: Abdominocentesis in cattle: Technique and criteria for diagnosis of peritonitis. Can Vet J 26:74–80, 1985.
15. Hirsch VM, Townsend HGG: Peritoneal fluid analysis in the diagnosis of abdominal disorders in cattle: A retrospective study. Can Vet J 23:348–354, 1982.
16. Braun U, et al: Ultrasonographic findings in cows with traumatic reticuloperitonitis. Vet Rec 133:416–422, 1993.
17. Fubini SL, et al: Accuracy of radiography of the reticulum for predicting surgical findings in adult dairy cattle with traumatic reticuloperitonitis: 123 cases (1981–1987). J Am Vet Med Assoc 197:1060–1064, 1990.
18. Ducharme NG, et al: Reticulography of the cow in dorsal recumbency: An aid in the diagnosis and treatment of traumatic reticuloperitonitis. J Am Vet Med Assoc 182:585–588, 1983.
19. Braun U, et al: Radiography as an aid in the diagnosis of traumatic reticuloperitonitis in cattle. Vet Rec 132:103–109, 1993.
20. Ducharme NG: Surgery of the bovine forestomach compartments. Vet Clin North Am Food Anim Pract 6:371–397, 1990.
21. Ducharme NG, et al: Thoracotomy in adult dairy cattle: 14 cases (1979–1991). J Am Vet Med Assoc 200:86–90, 1992.
22. Poulsen JSD: Prevention of traumatic indigestion in cattle. Vet Rec 98:149–151, 1976.

■ Vagal Indigestion

Robert H. Whitlock, D.V.M., Ph.D., Diplomate, A.C.V.I.M.

DEFINITION

The term "vagus indigestion" was introduced in 1940 to describe functional disturbances of the ruminant forestomachs.[1] Although affected cattle characteristically present with abdominal distention, primary vagal nerve injury is rarely the cause of the syndrome. Cattle with chronic or vagal indigestion have gradual abdominal enlargement due to ruminal distention with fluid or gas, or both. Vagal indigestion is not one specific disease entity, but a syndrome resulting in ruminal distention.[2] The site of functional disturbance within the forestomach compartments allows classification into four distinct types: type I, failure of eructation, or free-gas bloat; type II, failure of omasal transport; type III, abomasal impaction; and type IV, partial obstruction of the forestomach compartments.[3]

HISTORY AND CLINICAL SIGNS

Intermittent bouts of indigestion, anorexia, reduced milk production with characteristic abdominal distention, and weight loss typify the history. Occasionally, this syndrome affects cattle in late gestation. The enlarging fetus may mask initial signs of weight loss, but the continuing loss of muscle mass becomes apparent as the abdomen increases in size. Intermittent vomiting or regurgitation may, on occasion, be the chief complaint. When several animals in a herd are vomiting, spoiled forage should be suspected. Other causes of vomiting in individual cows include (1) frothy bloat, (2) reticulitis, and (3) ingestion of toxic plants such as rhododendron and mountain laurel.

PATHOPHYSIOLOGY

The pathophysiology of vagal indigestion represents a collage of several diseases, all characterized by reduced digesta transit through the stomachs. The lesion site will determine the clinical signs. Commonly, vagal indigestion is a sequela to traumatic reticuloperitonitis.[1, 2] Evidence is accumulating to suggest that vagal neuritis or injury is only one factor in the development of clinical vagal indigestion. Other factors include space-occupying lesions, that is, tumors and abscesses; foreign bodies in the omasal canal or pylorus (hairballs); and adhesions. Some abscesses may cause nerve dysfunction by neuropraxia,[4] while adhesions or abscesses in the cranial part of the abdomen may disrupt normal tension receptor activity of the reticulum, inhibiting normal reticuloruminal motility.[5]

TYPE I: FREE-GAS BLOAT, FAILURE OF ERUCTATION

Free-gas bloat (type I vagal indigestion) may rarely be caused by partial esophageal obstruction due to foreign bodies such as potatoes, tubers, apples, or pears, and less commonly by extraesophageal compression such as by lymphosarcoma, thyroid tumors, or rarely, a chronic mediastinal inflammatory process, tuberculosis, or lung abscesses.

Intermittent free-gas bloat is rarely life-threatening, but may cause mild abdominal distress and require emergency treatment, if only to alleviate the producer's apprehensions about the animal's problem. Following alleviation of gaseous distention, some animals eat vigorously, but as the rumen distends, the feeding ceases because of the recurrence of gaseous distention.[6] Affected cattle often drink water normally or even excessively, further contributing to the rumen distention.

Simple failure of eructation is most often caused by an inflammatory lesion adjacent to the vagus nerve (i.e., chronic pneumonia) or localized peritonitis or abscessation in the left ventral wall of the reticulum and adjacent diaphragm. Normally, eructation occurs during the secondary ruminal contraction; if the cardia is partially flooded with fluid, eructation proceeds more slowly and chronic free-gas bloat may develop.

TYPE II: FAILURE OF OMASAL TRANSPORT

Failure of omasal transport (type II vagal indigestion) may result from a process that impairs the transport of ingesta from the reticulum through the omasal canal into the abomasum. "Reticulo-omasal stenosis" has been advanced as a term to describe failure of omasal transport,[7] but stenosis is believed to rarely occur. Since the major function of the omasum is to pump ingesta from the reticulorumen into the abomasum,[8, 9] any disease process that interferes with the pump should be referred to as "failure of omasal transport." For example, a postparturient cow may eat the placenta which may obstruct the omasal canal. Abscesses can usually be palpated across the reticulum during a rumenotomy. An atonic, easily distensible reticulo-omasal orifice found on digital examination indicates omasal canal atony and failure of omasal transport.

Space-occupying lesions such as lymphosarcoma, papilloma, squamous cell carcinoma, a large infarct, and most commonly, adhesions between the reticulum and diaphragm cranial to the omasum may lead to failure of omasal transport. The abscesses or adhesions are typically located in the right lateral wall of the reticulum and may arise from liver abscesses.[10] Liver abscesses arising from the left lobe of the liver seem to exert pressure on the ventral vagus nerve and not adhere directly to the reticulum or rumen to cause failure of omasal transport.

TYPE III: ABOMASAL IMPACTION OR PYLORIC STENOSIS

Abomasal impaction (type III vagal indigestion) may be subdivided into two major subtypes. Primary abomasal impaction is associated with restricted access to water when cattle are fed very dry, coarse roughage such as wheat or oat straw. It may occur on a herd basis, especially in western Canada or in regions of the United States where beef cattle are pastured on straw stalks or other crop aftermath and the water supply is frozen due to cold weather.[11] The lack of adequate water and coarse roughage may cause high mortality rates in beef cattle. Feeding excessive almond shells led to a herd outbreak of abomasal impaction with death of 15 pregnant dairy replacement heifers.[12]

Secondary abomasal impactions (resembling pyloric obstruction) occur as a result of decreased abomasal emptying and are often a sequela to traumatic reticuloperitonitis. The abscess or local adhesion interferes with normal abomasal emptying, resulting in an impaction.[13] The site of the adhesions or abscess formation is consistently in the right lateral wall of the reticulum, often with minimal involvement of the diaphragm. The pylorus may appear to restrict abomasal outflow, but pyloric stenosis is rarely documented in cattle. Foreign bodies, such as hairballs or placenta, may obstruct the pylorus in adult cattle and result in abomasal impaction. Use of toggle-pin fixation for left abomasal displacement may cause pyloric obstruction resulting in signs of acute abomasal impaction. This syndrome should be suspected if the cow has recently had surgery to correct the displaced abomasum.[14]

Vagal neuritis as a cause of failure of omasal transport or abomasal impaction is still unclear, but evidence is accumulating that vagal nerve injury is not always involved. In my opinion failure of omasal transport and abomasal impaction are associated with mechanically interfered motility due to adhesions or abscesses, which are often sequelae to chronic traumatic reticuloperitonitis. When the contents of the abscess are removed, cows with failure of omasal transport often recover, suggesting local pressure to be an important factor and not an inflammatory lesion in the vagus nerve.

Abomasal impaction has been reported in adult sheep with parasitic lesions about the vagus nerve. Although the abomasum was firmly distended with fibrous digesta, in some cases no lesions were found to account for the impaction.[15, 16] Suffolk sheep have been reported to have an unusual abomasal emptying defect with lesions in the abomasal wall and vagus nerve. Metabolic alkalosis was absent, but increased rumen chloride levels may be helpful diagnostically.[17, 18] The prognosis is poor despite intensive medical and surgical intervention.

TYPE IV: INDIGESTION OF ADVANCED PREGNANCY OR PARTIAL OBSTRUCTION

Type IV vagal indigestion, or partial obstruction of the forestomach compartments, is the most difficult type of define. It occurs more commonly in dairy cattle in advanced pregnancy. As the gravid uterus enlarges, the abomasum is forced further forward, interfering with normal abomasal motility. If abomasal motility has already diminished, then a partial impaction may result. Cattle with this form of vagal indigestion may represent a combination of omasal transport failure and abomasal impaction in the early stages. However, if prolonged and progressive, it often develops into one type or the other. Some cases, even with advanced ruminal distention, may have marginally low plasma chlorides (80 to 95 mEq/L), which makes definitive classification difficult.

The apparent increase in rumen motility in some cases of vagal indigestion may be due to increased secondary ruminal contractions with a possible decrease in primary contractions. Experimentally, if the rumen is insufflated with gas, the frequency of secondary contractions is independent of the primary contractions and the effective stimulus for the former is increased ruminal tension. As many cows with vagal indigestion have a mild chronic free-gas bloat, this is the most logical explanation for the observed increased rumen contraction rate.

Afferent vagal and splanchnic nerve input may also reflexly inhibit reticuloruminal movements by marked distention of the reticulorumen. The marked distention excites high-threshold tension receptors in contrast to the stimulation of low-threshold tension receptors which stimulate contractions.[19, 20]

A rise in the intraruminal pressure triggers the reflex opening of the cardia and other events involved in eructation. However, if the cardia is flooded with fluid or foam, the reflex cardial opening does not occur. Thus, if cattle are unable to clear the cardia because of frothy bloat, extensive reticular adhesions, or malpositions (recumbency), then more gas would accumulate to the point of respiratory embarrassment or death. Large increases in ruminal pressure stimulate the high-tension inhibitory receptors impairing rumen motility, which occurs in cases of severe bloat and is rarely seen in advanced vagal indigestion.

PHYSICAL EXAMINATION

The clinical signs are usually gradual in onset, with a steady decrease in milk production (if lactating), gradual abdominal distention despite a poor appetite, and decreased fecal output. The nature and character of the feces typifies vagal indigestion: scant volume and pasty consistency which upon close inspection often contain 2- to 4-cm-long pieces of hay suggesting poor digestion. The omasal canal determines the hay particle size transported to the abomasum, and if not properly functioning, allows longer hay particles into the lower tract which can be evaluated by close inspection of the feces.

The single most important clinical sign characterizing vagal indigestion is a distended abdomen, with or without bloat; anorectic cattle without vagal indigestion are typically gaunt or "tucked up." In cases of vagal indigestion the rumen is distended with fluid or gas or both. Mild free gas and occasionally frothy bloat occurs in 40% to 60% of cases of types II, III, and IV vagal indigestion and in 100% of type I. As the disease progresses the animal may develop a "papple" shape, resembling an apple on the left and a pear on the right. The apple shape is the result of bloat or excess rumen gas. The pear shape is due to heaviness or distention of the lower right quadrant associated with fullness of the abomasum or rumen with ingesta.

The heart rate may be normal or bradycardic (<60 beats per minute [bpm]) depending on the stage of the disease. The heart rate is decreased (bradycardia) to 40 or 50 bpm in about 20% to 30% of the affected cattle.[21] The normal pulse rate for dairy cattle is 60 to 80 bpm. Bradycardia has been shown to be associated with fasting; therefore, it is not specific for vagal indigestion.[22] However, since bradycardia is an uncommon clinical sign, one should consider vagal indigestion when bradycardia is detected.[23]

Auscultation of the rumen typically reveals increased rumen contractions (three to four per minute). In rare cases no contractions will be detected. Extreme care must be used to assess rumen motility in those cattle with a distended rumen in which the fluid rumen contents produce little sound during a ruminal contraction. Palpation of the rumen may be a better technique for detecting rumen motility in these cases. The absence of rumen motility often signifies a poor prognosis, as it is usually associated with more extensive reticular adhesions to the point of diffuse peritonitis. Simultaneous auscultation-percussion of the rumen will occasionally elicit a ping or tinkle sound typical of a left abomasal displacement (LDA). However, if the size of the gas-filled viscus is critically evaluated, it will be too large for an LDA and the size and shape will be more compatible with a rumen ping. A rumen ping in cases of vagal indigestion

occurs most often in association with excessive fluid in the rumen or with minimal distention due to gas. Obvious cases of bloat are rarely associated with a ping or tinkle sound.

Determination of rumen consistency is a key point in the physical examination of a patient suspected of vagal indigestion. Palpation of the rumen in the upper left paralumbar fossa may reveal a mild to moderate accumulation of gas. The free-gas bloat is easily removed by the passage of a stomach tube, but recurs within several hours. Ballottement of the upper left paralumbar fossa is an important aid in the evaluation of any cow suspected of vagal indigestion. Anorexia typically leads to a firm or doughy rumen as the contents become stratified following anorexia. In vagal indigestion, however, obstruction to the flow of ingesta results in the accumulation of saliva, ingesta, and water, which gives the impression of a fluid or "splashy" consistency when ballottement of the rumen is performed. Determination of rumen consistency and the assessment of rumen size will also assist in the estimation of the acid-base and electrolyte status. Cattle with marked increase in rumen fluid due to abomasal reflux from abomasal impaction are likely to have a hypochloremic, hypokalemic metabolic alkalosis proportional to the extent of reflux.

Rectal examination is an important adjunct to any physical examination and will give further evidence concerning the severity of ruminal distention in animals with suspected vagal indigestion. The ventral sac of the rumen becomes disproportionately distended compared to the dorsal sac, and forms an **L** shape in chronic cases of vagal indigestion. The ventral sac may occupy 75% of the abdominal cavity in advanced vagal indigestion. In rare cases gas may accumulate in the right side of the ventral sac to produce a ping sound upon simultaneous auscultation-percussion of the right abdominal wall.

In cases of advanced pregnancy, rectal examination is of less value since the enlarged uterus precludes accurate assessment of the rumen size. Only rarely can the distended impacted abomasum be palpated during a rectal examination, but if detected it will confirm the diagnosis of type III vagal indigestion. If the omasum is palpated during rectal examination, then liver disease, such as hepatic abscess or fibrosis, should be suspected. The enlarged liver displaces the omasum caudally in the abdomen, and enables it to be felt. Evidence of abdominal pain in cases of vagal indigestion is often difficult to assess as the cow may be depressed. A carefully done Williams reticular grunt test may occasionally give evidence of localized pain in the xiphoid region. The withers pinch test may also indicate pain in the cranial abdomen, but rarely is either test strongly positive.

DIAGNOSIS

Early cases of vagal indigestion may be confused with abomasal displacement or traumatic reticulitis. Unless the cow has been sick for several days (subacute to chronic), then vagal indigestion should not be considered.

The diagnostic rule-outs for abdominal distention include frothy bloat, uterine enlargement (hydrallantois or hydramnios), ascites due to right heart failure, venal caval thrombosis, or abdominal neoplasia such as lymphosarcoma or mesothelioma. A ruptured bladder will also present as abdominal enlargement, but occurs much more commonly in feedlot steers than in dairy cattle. Occasionally, diffuse peritonitis will cause abdominal distention, but the clinical course is usually of shorter duration.

Intestinal obstruction such as a small intestinal intussusception, cecal volvulus, abomasal volvulus, inguinal hernia, or fat necrosis may cause intestinal distention, but with only a mild increase in abdominal size. Other physical findings (rectal examination and percussion) easily differentiate these syndromes from vagal indigestion. Bradycardia, if present, may be an important diagnostic aid suggesting vagal indigestion. Bradycardia is an unusual clinical sign (it may also occur with botulism, milk fever, addisonian crisis, diaphragmatic hernia, or pituitary abscess). One should consider vagal indigestion in cases of abdominal distention.

LABORATORY EVALUATION

The single most rewarding laboratory determination is the serum or plasma chloride determination. Cattle with a distended rumen and normal plasma chloride do not have abomasal reflux, which infers the lesion is in the omasal canal or reticulum; whereas hypochloremia (<85 mEq/L) is evidence of abomasal reflux from an abomasal impaction or stasis of the forestomach compartments.[7] Profound hypochloremia (<90 mEq/L) and hypokalemia (<3.0 mEq/L) are typically found in cattle with type III vagal indigestion.[24] Cattle with abomasal impaction will occasionally have a severe metabolic alkalosis with a plasma chloride of 50 mEq/L or less. Although very low plasma chloride values (<50 mEq/L) suggest a grave prognosis, cattle may survive if treated vigorously.

An assessment of abomasal reflux can also be established by determining the rumen chloride concentration, as reflux causes the rumen chloride concentration to increase above 30 mEq/L. A moderate hypocalcemia (6 to 8 mg/dL) often accompanies any type of indigestion. It may occasionally be sufficiently low to result in recumbency resembling periparturient hypocalcemia.

Dehydration often results in prerenal azotemia with increased concentrations of blood urea nitrogen (BUN) and creatinine. The BUN rarely exceeds 80 mg/dL and the creatinine rarely exceeds 8 or 9 mg/dL in prerenal azotemia. Similarly, the packed cell volume (PCV) and total plasma proteins (TPP) are elevated as a reflection of dehydration. If vagal indigestion is associated with a chronic inflammatory process, such as an abscess, the TPP may be disproportionately elevated as a reflection of chronic antigenic stimulation and hypergammaglobulinemia. The PCV may be decreased (<30%) as a reflection of bone marrow depression and anemia of chronic disease.

The leukogram in cattle with vagal indigestion will reflect the lesions causing the problem. Lymphocytosis suggests lymphosarcoma, reversal of the neutrophil-lymphocyte ratio suggests chronic inflammation, leukocytosis suggests a subacute response to inflammation, and leukopenia may indicate the development of an overwhelming peritonitis.

TREATMENT OF FREE-GAS BLOAT

The treatment of chronic free-gas bloat (type I vagal indigestion) is relatively simple: establishment of a rumen fistula. A rumenostomy can be performed by suturing the rumen to the body wall or by the use of a commercially available rumen trocar (Buff's screw trocar). With a small 1- to 3-cm rumen fistula, the gases produced by fermentation can be expelled. The appetite returns and as the omasal function is normal, digesta will pass down the tract unimpeded, allowing return of the animal to the herd as a productive unit. In time (2 to 6 months), the fistula will spontaneously close with granulation tissue. Most cattle regain the ability to eructate. Failure of eructation, be it due to adhesions of the reticulum or to an inflammatory lesion associated with a vagus nerve, is potentially reversible. If the lesion heals, the cow regains the ability to eructate normally in some cases. Contrary to popular opinion, purported antifermentatives such as turpentine or other noxious liquids containing turpentine are of no value in the prevention or treatment of free-gas bloat. The concentration of these materials necessary to inhibit gas formation by the rumen microflora is large and

would cause death of most microfloras before decreasing rumen gas production. Therefore, their use should not be encouraged in free-gas bloat but reserved for frothy bloat where they are effective as surface tension–reducing agents.

TREATMENT OF OMASAL TRANSPORT FAILURE

The initial therapy in early cases of failure of omasal transport, abomasal impaction, or partial obstruction include ruminatorics and cathartics to promote gastrointestinal tract evacuation, calcium gluconate subcutaneously to maintain normocalcemia, and fluids to correct dehydration. It is recognized that many so-called ruminatorics or parasympathomimetics do little to promote effective rumen contractions, but do promote catharsis, which is a desired effect. Few cattle respond to symptomatic therapy; most require surgical intervention. Those cattle in advanced pregnancy will often benefit from a therapeutic abortion. Economics will dictate in what manner the cow will be treated, if at all. Normal water supply, feed, and exercise are especially important.

The treatment of failure of omasal transport is primarily surgical and usually includes a rumenotomy to remove any foreign bodies and to localize any foreign object that may be occluding the omasal canal, such as a placenta or papilloma.[25] If a neoplasm is present, a needle biopsy may be obtained to make a definitive diagnosis and, if confirmed, then euthanasia may be recommended. If a mass palpated between the reticulum and diaphragm is ascertained to be an abscess, it should be drained. The abscess can be drained via a needle suction apparatus wherein the pus is removed via a long tube through the rumenotomy incision. If the reticular wall is firmly adherent to the abscess, an incision can be made through the reticular wall directly into the abscess allowing purulent material to drain into the rumen via the reticulum. A certain degree of courage is needed to make the incision for fear of causing a diffuse peritonitis. It is occasionally advantageous to insert a 20- to 30-cm-long, 8-gauge needle percutaneously through the body wall directly into the abscess and obtain drainage in this manner.[10] On occasion, the abscess can be surgically extirpated via a paramedian incision if it is loosely attached to surrounding tissues.

Other supportive therapy considered of value in failure of omasal transport includes passing a stomach tube through the nasal passages, down the esophageal groove, and directly into the abomasum. In this way, gruel can be pumped through the nasogastric tube several times daily. As the abomasum and small intestine function normally, the gruel can be digested and help meet the metabolic requirements. If the tube is placed in the rumen, it would cause more ruminal distention and bloat, adding to the severity of the problem. Other supportive therapy includes systemic antibiotics to control the localized peritonitis.

TREATMENT OF ABOMASAL IMPACTION

Abomasal impaction requires vigorous therapy if it is to be treated at all.[13] The owner should be made aware of the poor prognosis associated with this form of the disease. If the cow is not valuable, salvage is recommended. If the cow is valuable and worthy of therapy despite the poor prognosis, oral cathartics such as magnesium hydroxide and other commercially available laxatives are indicated in dosages ranging from 0.5 to 1.0 kg/day. However, magnesium oxide may exacerbate a preexisting metabolic alkalosis.[26] Metaclopramide, a dopamine antagonist, has the potential for restoration of forestomach motility, but few studies have been conducted. Subcutaneously administered doses of 0.1, 0.3, and 0.5 mg/kg decreased the strength of ruminal contraction but had no effect on the rumen contraction rate in normal calves.[27] Intravenous administration may result in severe hypotension. Subcutaneous calcium gluconate to correct the mild hypocalcemia will help to increase abomasal motility. Intravenous fluids are also very important in correcting the metabolic alkalosis and hypokalemia that is usually present. Once the acid-base and electrolyte status is corrected, a rumenotomy may be indicated. If the abomasum is only partially impacted, docusate sodium or magnesium sulfate may be infused directly into the abomasum. The abomasum is then massaged through the ruminal wall. In mild cases, this form of therapy seems to be effective. If an abscess is present between the rumen, reticulum, and diaphragm, and firmly adherent to the reticulum, it may be incised and the purulent contents drained into the reticulorumen. If not, it may be advantageous to drain the abscess percutaneously.

Abomasotomy is only used as a last alternative. Abomasotomy is usually not beneficial to the patient, in that most surgery will promote further adhesions in the fundic area and further diminish abomasal motility. It is best to enhance motility by extra-abomasal means, rather than directly removing the contents from the abomasum itself. It is possible to remove substantial abomasal contents through the omasal orifice during rumenotomy and not produce further adhesions.

Only rarely is there any evidence of a foreign body obstructing the pylorus.[28] The use of pyloromyotomy or pyloroplasty procedures to correct pyloric stenosis in cattle is usually ineffective.

TREATMENT OF INDIGESTION OF ADVANCED PREGNANCY

Therapeutic principles for treatment of type IV vagal indigestion follow those for the other types: fluids to correct dehydration, hypokalemia, hypocalcemia, and alkalosis if present. Once it is determined the cow is pregnant and has ruminal distention, the owner needs to decide which is more valuable, the cow or the calf, or both, since therapeutic abortion of the fetus often helps resolve impaired motility of the forestomachs. If within 4 to 6 weeks of parturition, symptomatic treatment may allow both the dam and fetus to be salvaged. The longer the time to parturition, the less likely both will survive. Rumenotomy to explore the abdomen to determine the nature of the lesion is the first priority. Once the lesion is located, then options will become clear.

PROGNOSIS

The owner should be made aware that a rumen fistula will allow foul gas to escape from the rumen into the environment where cows are being milked and may cause "off-flavored" milk. Occasionally, spillage of rumen contents from the fistula may predispose to localized peritonitis. However, adequate surgical technique carries a minimal risk of peritonitis. Overall, the success rate of rumenostomy for correction of simple failure of eructation is excellent (95%). In feedlot cattle the prognosis is less favorable if a chronic respiratory disorder is the predisposing problem. Even with correction of the bloat, the animal may fail to thrive. Prognosis for survival with failure of omasal transport is fair to good. A more definitive prognosis can be made at the time of surgical intervention. A neoplasm such as lymphosarcoma warrants a hopeless prognosis, whereas a pedunculated papilloma (wart) offers a good prognosis. An abscess between the omasum and diaphragm warrants a fair to good prognosis, as does a liver abscess,[4, 29] but a placenta causing the obstruction offers an excellent prognosis. In cases of abscesses or adhesions between the omasum, diaphragm, and reticulum, the prognosis is approximately 80% for survival depending on the size, the extent of adhesions to the reticulum and, most important, whether its contents can be drained without causing diffuse peritonitis.[29] The prognosis for life in this situation depends on the stage of gestation. The closer to parturition, the better the prognosis. Removal of the fetus should allow improvement in abomasal motility and may improve the prognosis.

REFERENCES

1. Hoflund S.: Investigations of functional defects of the ruminant stomachs caused by damage to the vagus nerve. Svenck Vet Tidskr (Suppl) 45, 1940.
2. Hutchins DR, Blood DC, Hyne R: Residual defects in stomach motility after traumatic reticuloperitonitis of cattle. Pyloric obstruction, diaphragmatic hernia and indigestion due to reticular adhesions. Aust Vet J 33:77–82, 1957.
3. Ferrante PL, Whitlock RH: Chronic (vagus) indigestion in cattle. Compend Contin Educ Pract Vet 3:S231–S238, 1981.
4. Fubini SL, Ducharme NG, Murphy JP, et al: Vagus indigestion syndrome resulting from a liver abscess in dairy cows. J Am Vet Med Assoc 186:1297–1300, 1985.
5. Leek BF: Vagus indigestion in cattle. Vet Rec 82:498, 1968.
6. Rebhun, WC, Fubini SL, Miller TK: Vagus indigestion in cattle: Clinical features, causes, treatments, and long-term follow-up of 112 cases. Compend Contin Educ Pract Vet 10:382–392, 1988.
7. Kuiper R, Breukink HJ: Reticulo-omasal stenosis in the cow: Differential diagnosis with respect to pyloric stenosis. Vet Rec 119:169–171, 1986.
8. Bueno L, Ruckebusch Y: The cyclic motility of the omasum and its control in sheep. J Physiol 238:295–312, 1974.
9. Stevens CE, Sellers AF, Spurrell FA: Function of the bovine omasum in ingesta transfer. Am J Physiol 198:449–455, 1960.
10. Fubini SL, Smith DF: Failure of omasal transport due to traumatic reticuloperitonitis and intraabdominal abscess. Compend Contin Educ Pract Vet 4:S492–S494, 1982.
11. Ashcroft RA: Abomasal impaction of cattle in Saskatchewan. Can Vet J 24:375–380, 1983.
12. Mitchell KL: Dietary abomasal impaction in a herd of dairy replacement heifers. J Am Vet Med Assoc 198:1408, 1991.
13. Rebhun WC: Vagus indigestion in cattle. J Am Vet Med Assoc 176:506–510, 1980.
14. Kelton DF, Fubini SL: Pyloric obstruction after toggle-pin fixation of a left displaced abomasum in a cow. J Am Vet Med Assoc 194:677, 1989.
15. Naeland G, Helle O: Functional pyloric stenosis in sheep. Vet Rec 74:85–90, 1962.
16. Kline EE, Meyer JR, Nelson DR, et al: Abomasal impaction in sheep. Vet Rec 113:177–179, 1983.
17. Rings DM, Welker FH, Hull BL, et al: Abomasal emptying defect in Suffolk sheep. J Am Vet Med Assoc 185:1520–1522, 1984.
18. Kopcha M: Abomasal dilatation and emptying defect in a ewe. J Am Vet Med Assoc 192:783–784, 1988.
19. Leek BF: Reticulo-ruminal function and dysfunction. Vet Rec 84:238–243, 1969.
20. Ruckebusch Y: Pharmacology of reticulo-ruminal motor function. J Vet Pharmacol Ther 6:245–272, 1983.
21. Braun U, Hausmann K, Oertle C: Vagus indigestion in 20 cows as a result of failure of omasal transport. Berl Munch Tierartzl Wochenschr 103:192, 1990.
22. McGuirk SM, Bednarski RM: Bradycardia associated with fasting in cattle. ACVIM Proc 82:29–32, 1986.
23. Smith DF, Becht JL, Whitlock RH: Anorexia and abdominal distention in cattle. In Anderson NV (ed): Veterinary Gastroenterology, ed 2. Philadelphia, Lea & Febiger, 1992, chap 30.
24. Takuchi K: Relationship between degree of dehydration and serum electrolytes and acid-base status in cows with various abomasal disorders. J Vet Med Sci 57:257, 1995.

25. Whitlock RH: Failure of omasal transport: Fact or fiction? Proc ACVIM 14:482, 1996.
26. Ogilvie JH, Butler DG, Gartley CJ, et al: Magnesium oxide induced metabolic alkalosis in cattle. Can J Compr Med 47:108–111, 1983.
27. Guard C, Schwark W, Kelton D, et al: Effects of metoclopramide, clenbuterol and butorphanol on ruminoreticular motility of calves. Cornell Vet 78:89–98, 1988.
28. Kuiper R, Breukink HJ: Secondary indigestion as a cause of functional pyloric stenosis in the cow. Vet Rec 119:404–406, 1986.
29. Fubini SL, Ducharme NG, Erb HN, et al: Failure of omasal transport attributable to perireticular abscess formation in cattle: 29 cases (1980–1986). JAVMA 194:811–814, 1989.

■ Abomasal Physiology, and Dilation, Displacement, and Volvulus

Gilles Fecteau, D.M.V., Diplomate, A.C.V.I.M.
Nicolas Sattler, D.M.V.
D. Michael Rings, D.V.M., M.S., Diplomate, A.C.V.I.M.

ABOMASAL ANATOMY AND PHYSIOLOGY

The abomasum is the fourth compartment of the ruminant stomach. It is analogous to the stomach of the monogastric species. Macroscopically it consists of fundic, body, and pyloric regions. It normally lies ventrally on the midline, but its position may be influenced by pregnancy.[1] It is possible in normal, nongravid adult cattle to localize the abomasum slightly to the left of the midline, directly under the ruminal recess with the pylorus projecting toward the right. A natural stricture, the pylorus, separates the abomasum from the first part of the duodenum. The pylorus of the cow, however, does not function as a total obstruction to flow. A firm muscular structure, the torus pyloricus, can be felt immediately cranial to the pylorus, projecting into the abomasal lumen. The abomasum is lined by glandular mucosa. The mucosal surface is greatly increased by the presence of large abomasal folds. The mucosa of the fundic and body regions contain true peptic glands (secreting hydrochloric acid). The pyloric regions secrete mucus.

Cranially, the abomasum is attached to the omasum and to the reticulum through a band of smooth muscle.[2] This attachment limits its mobility. Figure 1 presents a schematic view of the attachment of the lesser omentum. The superimposed U indicates approximately the attachments. However, the caudal attachment to the greater omentum provides greater mobility, allowing displacement of the abomasum in different directions.

The abomasum is highly vascular, receiving its arterial supply from the left gastric and gastroepiploic arteries. These arteries eventually unite with the right gastric and gastroepiploic arteries. Venous drainage follows the path of the arteries and eventually joins the hepatic portal vein.[2] The dorsal and ventral vagal trunks innervate the abomasum (parasympathetic) while the celiac and cranial mesenteric ganglia and plexuses serve as a site for the synapse of preganglionic sympathetic neurons.[1] Vessels and nerves can be damaged along their course through the omenta when an abomasal volvulus occurs.

After the forestomachs prepare the ingesta, it moves aborad through the abomasum continuously but at a variable rate. Preabomasal preparation consists of (1) digestion and reduction in size of the particles by the rumen flora and (2) reduction of water content by the omasum.

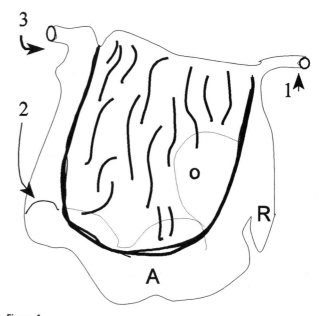

Figure 1

Schematic view of the attachment of the lesser omentum. The thick black line (U) approximately indicates the attachments. A, abomasum; R, reticulum; O, omasum; 1, esophagus; 2, pylorus; 3, duodenum.

Abomasal function consists of further digestion of partially degraded substrate from the rumen, reticulum, and omasum. The abomasum is a pepsinogen- and hydrochloric acid–secreting organ. The abomasal pH will be maintained at approximately 3 under normal conditions.

Abomasal motility can be decreased in many ways. There are normally periods of abomasal inactivity lasting several hours in adult cattle.[3] Overdistention of the rumen, reticulum, or omasum can inhibit motility of the abomasum,[4] as can ulcers and ostertagiasis.[5] Additional factors associated with abomasal content makeup may also be inhibitors of motility: (1) low pH,[6, 7] (2) particle size and fiber content of the ration,[8, 9] (3) the amino acid, peptide, and fat content of duodenal fluid,[4] (4) high volatile fatty acid concentration,[10, 11] and (5) high ruminal histamine synthesis.[12] Other systemic factors reported to negatively influence abomasal motility are (1) endotoxemia,[13] (2) hyperinsulinemia,[14] (3) hypokalemia,[15] (4) epinephrine release (stress),[16, 17] (5) histamine release during inflammation,[18] (6) metabolic alkalosis,[19] (7) hypocalcemia,[20] (8) prostaglandins,[18, 21, 22] (9) lack of exercise,[11, 23] (10) high blood gastrin concentrations,[13, 24] and (11) acetonemia.[25]

ABOMASAL DISPLACEMENT, DILATION, AND VOLVULUS

Abomasal problems are frequent clinical occurrences in bovine practice. Displacements, dilations, and volvulus are now recognized as the most commonly encountered surgical disorders of the gastrointestinal tract in modern dairy practice.[2] These are defined as malposition and dilation of the last gastric compartment. The displacement can be on the left side (left displaced abomasum, LDA) or the right side (right displaced abomasum, RDA). LDA and RDA serve as physiologic impairments to flow while abomasal volvulus (AV) actually can produce mechanical obstruction of this organ. Palpation of a firm twist between the abomasum and the other forestomachs indicates an AV. Depending on the location of the twist, a diagnosis of AV, omaso-abomasal volvulus (OAV), or reticulo-omaso-abomasal volvulus (ROAV) can be made. Wensvoort and van der Welden[26] stated that the term *volvulus* is more appropriate than torsion because the twist is not on the longitudinal axis of the organ. Several review articles are excellent sources of information on abomasal conditions and should be consulted for greater detail.[2, 18, 27–29]

Prevalence and Incidence

Displacement is probably a worldwide problem. One survey of the prevalence of this problem in dairy herds found that 24% of herds had at least one LDA during a 3-year period.[8] The prevalence of abomasal displacement among dairy herds is variable depending on geographic location, management practices, and climate, as well as other factors. Left displacement is the most common of the abomasal twists, constituting 85% to 95.8% of the cases.[2] Although treatment remains an important aspect of this problem, veterinarians should investigate herd health management in order to reduce the incidence of abomasal problems.

Etiology

There is general agreement in the literature that abomasal displacement is a multifactorial syndrome and that abomasal atony is an absolute prerequisite to this condition (see above for causes). Distention of the abomasum with gas produced by microbial fermentation will precipitate the displacement. It has been hypothesized that the orientation of the displacement (left or right) will depend on the size of the rumen, that is, small rumen—left, large rumen—right.[10] Other factors influencing the incidence of displacement include total size of the abdominal cavity, stage of gestation, and perhaps external factors such as transportation, exercise, prior surgery, and stress.[11] Figure 2 shows the relationship between these factors and displacement. Predisposing factors regarding LDA have been studied and reviewed.[30] The heritability of this condition has been estimated to be approximately 28%.[31]

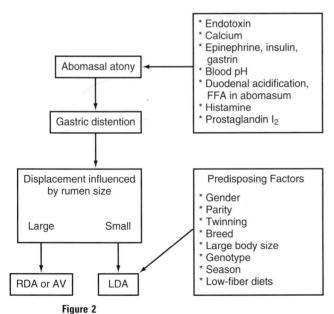

Figure 2
Relationship between factors and displacements.

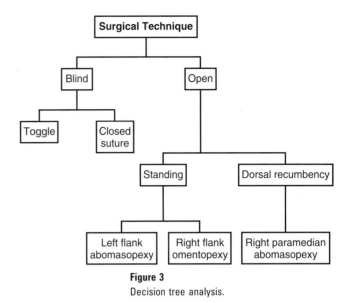

Figure 3
Decision tree analysis.

Treatment

Goals

Treatment of RDA, LDA, and AV is aimed at (1) returning the abomasum to its original position or a close approximation, (2) creating a permanent attachment in that position, (3) correcting the electrolyte, acid-base, and hydration deficits of the patient, and (4) providing appropriate therapy for concurrent disease problems. Goals should be achieved with consideration of the cost of the procedure, the negative impact on current milk production, and the likelihood of the animal returning to normal function.

While a conservative approach (i.e., rolling) has been used for many years, it does not always achieve the goals described above. Since no permanent attachment is created, recurrence of the displacement is likely. Moreover, in most conservatively handled cases, the recovery period will be longer, leading to a greater negative impact on milk production. For these reasons, surgical correction appears to be the most beneficial approach (Fig. 3).

Surgical Therapy

Numerous surgical techniques are used and have been described.[2] Their advantages and disadvantages have also been studied.[29] The permanent attachment is usually created by either suturing the abomasum (abomasopexy) or the greater omentum (omentopexy) to the abdominal wall. Fixation techniques are shown in the decision tree of Figure 3. The decision to treat by either open or closed techniques is usually based on economic factors.[32] If surgical fixation is selected, the surgeon commonly selects the procedure which he or she is most comfortable performing.

In the blind technique, the cow is placed in dorsal recumbency and the abomasum is identified by auscultation and percussion. Tacking sutures are placed through the body wall and into the abomasum using a large 1/2 curved needle. The toggle pin technique is done similarly except that two self-retaining plastic toggles are placed into the lumen of the abomasum through a trocar needle and then tied together, holding the abomasum in place. Neither technique allows for identification of the exact placement of the fixation and both leave the possibility of leakage from the abomasal lumen into the abdomen, the abdominal wall, and the subcutaneous tissues. These "roll-and-tack" procedures should be limited to animals with LDAs only. Other possible complications of these techniques include tacking other structures, for example, the intestine or rumen, fixing the abomasum in an abnormal position, or obstructing outflow by tacking at the pylorus.

When considering a surgical technique for correction of an LDA, the preference of the surgeon is most important because all techniques have approximately the same success and recurrence rates. The paramedian approaches provide an excellent attachment (abomasopexy) with minimal invasion of the abdomen. The ability to explore extensively in the abdomen, however, is severely restricted. Ventral approaches also have the potential to compromise the cow's ventilation. This approach leaves a ventral wound open to potential development of infection and/or herniation.

The left flank abomasopexy is used to visualize a portion of the abomasum in the standing patient. It is a good approach in cows with suspected abomasal adhesions and in cows in late gestation (later than 7 months). This approach cannot be used prophylactically and does require more than one person to complete the procedure. Placement of the sutures through the right paramedian area must be done carefully to avoid trapping omentum or bowel under the suture.

The right flank omentopexy is a well-accepted technique but relies heavily on the strength of the omentum to hold the abomasum in place. Therefore, cows suspected of having fatty omentum should probably be corrected by a method that does not rely on omental strength for fixation. Additionally, variation in placement of the omentopexy can provide sufficient slack to allow RDA to occur. This is a one-person technique and can be done on cows previously diagnosed with LDA but which is not displaced at the time of surgery. The right flank approach does allow the surgeon the most complete exploration of the abdomen.

Supportive Care

Most cattle with either an abomasal displacement or volvulus have some degree of electrolyte imbalance. Potassium and calcium are important for maintenance of muscular function and should be kept within normal limits. It can be anticipated that some degree of hypochloremia and metabolic alkalosis will be present. Fluid composition can be adjusted depending on the biochemistry profile or based on the veterinarian's experience. Isotonic saline and Ringer's solution are commonly used and excellent choices. Additional calcium and potassium salts can be supplemented as needed. Potassium should be administered at a maximum rate of 0.5 mEq/kg/hour when given intravenously.[33] The volume of fluids to be given will depend on the degree of dehydration. Oral rehydration therapy can be used following displacement or volvulus surgery but is not suitable by itself in cattle more than 8% dehydrated. Combinations of NaCl and KCl can be offered in oral fluids free-choice following correction of displacement and volvulus.

Antibiotic therapy can be beneficial but should not be used in all cases without consideration of the three T's: *t*ime (duration of the procedure), *t*rash (surgical sepsis), and *t*rauma (irritation from manipulation). Additional considerations for antibiotic usage should include the viability of the abomasum (as in AV) and whether concurrent disease problems are present (metritis, mastitis). The choice of antibiotics should take into account cost, withdrawal time, ability to reach infection sites, and route of administration.

Prevention

Because abomasal displacement is a multifactorial syndrome, prevention will involve controlling, when possible, the known predisposing factors. Nutritional management is among the most influential factors. Transition to production diets should be gradual to reduce chances of indigestion (lead feeding). The factors influencing hypocalcemia around the time of parturition should be reviewed and corrected as needed. High-concentrate rations need to be correctly adjusted and managed. Any inflammatory disease of the periparturient cow (i.e., metritis, mastitis) should be appropriately treated.

LEFT DISPLACED ABOMASUM

Clinical Signs

LDA occurs most commonly in the period around parturition (2 weeks pre- to 8 weeks postpartum). Cattle with LDA usually show a reduction in appetite accompanied by a progressive decrease in milk production. Often cattle show a preferential loss of appetite for grain while still consuming forages. Ketosis may develop as a secondary problem. Feces are often softer than normal. Rectal temperature should be normal, as should the pulse and respiratory rates. If tachyarrhythmia is noted, atrial fibrillation should be suspected. An electrocardiogram (ECG) will confirm the diagnosis. In a majority of cases, correction of the LDA combined with supportive care (balancing electrolytes) will result in correction of the arrhythmia.

Diagnosis

Simultaneous auscultation and percussion of the left flank should be done in suspected cases to elicit the characteristic metallic "ping" or tinkle. Most displacements can be found on or above an imaginary line drawn from the left tuber coxae to the left elbow. The size and location of the ping can vary depending on the amount of gas trapped, the amount of compression of the abomasum by the rumen, and even, perhaps, the size of the animal itself. The ping can be as far forward as the ninth rib and can extend caudally into the paralumbar fossa. In some cattle the last few ribs may appear elevated in large displacements. If, during auscultation and percussion, the pitch of the ping changes as if moving up or down a music scale, the examiner can be confident that the ping originates within the abomasum. The pitch change is due to pressure variations within the abomasum as contractions move through. Rumen pings do not change that much in pitch because the size of the organ and the pressure generated by contractions do not change that much.

The differential diagnosis of LDA includes other causes of left-sided pings, such as ruminal tympany and pneumoperitoneum. The location and intensity of the ping can be useful in differentiating these. Pneumoperitoneum pings are located dorsally under the transverse vertebral apophysis. The ping will be less musical, of a lower pitch, and should extend to the right side as well. A rumen ping can cover a large area and a rumen ping can sometimes be heard when percussion of the shaft of the ilium or the transverse apophysis is performed. Passage of a stomach tube and blowing into the tube while someone listens in the left flank can serve to differentiate between rumen and abomasal pings. If doubt persists, a percutaneous aspiration of fluid from the gas-filled viscus and measurement of the pH should differentiate between rumen (pH 6 to 7) and abomasum (pH 2 to 3).

Clinical Pathology

The hallmarks of high intestinal impairments to flow—hypochloremia, hypokalemia, and metabolic alkalosis—can be found in varying degrees in cattle with LDA. These changes are due to sequestration of abomasal hydrochloric acid secretions in the abomasum, and possibly the forestomachs. Hypokalemia and hypocalcemia likely result from the reduced intake caused by anorexia and the presence of alkalosis. If acetonemia is present, the blood glucose may be low. Stress, however, may create a transient hyperglycemia.

RIGHT DISPLACED ABOMASUM AND ABOMASAL VOLVULUS

Clinical Signs

The clinical signs of RDA resemble those of LDA, but the ping is heard on the right side. The ping is usually located under the last few ribs and should extend no further craniad than the 10th rib.

Cattle with AV are more likely to appear systemically affected than those with RDA or LDA. Clinical signs referable to shock, hypovolemia, and pain may be present associated with distention and necrosis of the abomasum, or severe electrolyte and acid-base imbalances, or both.

AV causes total anorexia and an abrupt decline in milk production. Feces are scant and often dark and diarrheal. Abdominal pain may be evident (bruxism, tachycardia, tender abdomen). In some cases of abdominal pain, the only signs may be a reluctance to move or recumbency. Clinical dehydration is easily recognized by the retracted position of the eye in the orbit and lack of skin turgor. The rectal temperature is often subnormal. The heart rate is usually increased and may be indicative of the severity of the volvulus (greater than 100 beats per minute [bpm]). Rumen contractions are decreased or absent. Auscultation and percussion of the right flank reveal the characteristic ping. The location of the ping may extend from the last rib cranially as far forward as the diaphragm. In severe cases, the ping may also extend posteriorly to the wing of the ilium. Simultaneous succussion and auscultation can help evaluate the amount of fluid in the volvulus. Abdominal distention is evident and the animal may have a rounded appearance. Rectal examination will allow palpation of the greater curvature in more than 50% of the cases. The clinical distinction between an early AV and RDA may be very difficult (Table 1).

Pathophysiology and Clinical Pathology

A hemogram and biochemistry profile will reveal more dramatic changes with AV than with RDA or LDA. Clinical and clinicopathologic findings include hypovolemia, dehydration, hemoconcentration, metabolic alkalosis, hypochloremia, hypokalemia, and, often, paradoxical aciduria. Hyperglycemia, hypocalcemia, and hyponatremia can be observed in some cases. Later, a superimposed metabolic acidosis may be present. The anion gap gradually increases with severity of the disease. Systemic shock eventually causes death.

Reduced fluid intake and sequestration of large quantities of chloride-rich fluid in the abomasum, as occurs in AV (third space problem), lead to dehydration and hypovolemia. Reflux of abomasal fluid, termed "internal vomiting," may occur. The triad of proximal gastrointestinal obstruction—hypochloremia, hypokalemia, and metabolic alkalosis—is more severe with AV than with LDA and RDA. Dehydration, accompanied by prolonged or severe hypochloremia and hypokalemia, may result in paradoxical aciduria. Low chloride concentrations limit the resorption of Na^+ in the proximal renal tubule because an anion must accompany reabsorbed sodium to maintain electroneutrality. Sodium resorption in the distal renal tubule is coupled with secretion of H^+. Correcting the hypochloremia and hypokalemia results in reversal of the aciduria.

Metabolic acidosis develops in cattle with long-standing volvulus. Decreased tissue perfusion, secondary to dehydration, promotes anaerobic generation of lactate and other organic acid anions, producing a metabolic acidosis. The longer the duration of the volvulus, the greater the release of phosphates and sulfates from tissue catabolism. This further contributes to the development of the acidosis. Calculation of the anion gap $(Na^+ + K^+) - (Cl^- + HCO_3^-)$, can be performed to evaluate accumulation of acid products. Normally, the anion gap ranges from 13.9 to 20.3 mEq/L. With the accumulation of unmeasured anions, the anion gap rises.

Hyperglycemia is often observed, likely resulting from glucocorticoid release. Hypocalcemia is observed and probably associated with reduced feed consumption. In the final stage, hyponatremia can develop and is believed to be the result of the third space problem.

AV can result in obstruction of blood flow through the abomasum. This will lead to congestion, edema, and, eventually, necrosis of the abomasal wall. AV may also directly damage the vagus nerve. Lesions can vary from nerve inflammation and swelling to complete avulsion of the nerve.[34]

Diagnosis

Any condition causing right-sided ping may be included in the differential diagnosis of RDA and AV. Among those of clinical importance, cecal dilation or torsion is probably the most common and difficult to differentiate. In most cases of cecal volvulus, rectal palpation will reveal the presence of the distended viscus caudally in the upper right quadrant. Less important causes of right-sided pings include gas in the duodenum or colon, physometria, pneumoperitoneum, and pneumorectum. The location and intensity of the ping will help in the differentiation. The entire clinical picture must be considered. Disease causing abdominal pain and colic should be included in the differential. Essentially, the diagnosis of AV is based on clinical findings, that is, the presence of a right-sided ping in a severely affected animal with compatible rectal findings.

Clinically, RDA can be difficult to differentiate from an early AV. In fact, the degree of rotation necessary to confirm an AV probably varies from one veterinarian to another. Prior experience of the surgeon and knowledge of the normal topographic anatomy aid in making the diagnosis.

Treatment

Cattle with AV should be monitored closely because they are more prone to severe systemic signs such as profound dehydra-

---

Table 1
DIFFERENTIATING RIGHT DISPLACED ABOMASUM (RDA) FROM ABOMASAL VOLVULUS (AV)

	Tentative Diagnosis	
	RDA	*AV*
Heart rate	Normal (60–80 bpm)	>100 bpm
Dehydration	<8%	>10%
Rumen motility	Normal	Absent
Feces	Present	Absent
Ping size and location	10–25 cm Centered around 11th–13th rib	>20–40 cm from 8th–13th rib
Rectal finding	Nonpalpable	Usually palpable
Blood gas analysis	Normal/mild alkalosis	Metabolic alkalosis (early) Metabolic acidosis (late)

tion, electrolyte disturbances, and poor peripheral perfusion. Surgical correction should be attempted as soon as possible. Spontaneous recovery is unlikely to occur and conservative treatment such as rolling will not return the abomasum to a correct anatomic position. Because of the systemic effects of AV, the ventral surgical approach may not be the technique of choice. A standing approach is less likely to affect respiration and ventilation.

Following a standard right flank celiotomy, the abomasum can be palpated in the dorsocranial right abdomen. The liver will be displaced from the body wall by the AV. Palpation along the greater curvature will allow identification of the location of the twist. This should allow differentiation between RDA, AV, OAV, and ROAV. To correct the volvulus, the abomasum should first be decompressed. Following deflation, the left hand of the surgeon is placed dorsally on the greater curvature. The abomasum is pushed cranioventrally to a point against the ventral body wall. When this is accomplished, the abomasum is pushed to the left, allowing the abomasum to untwist. The pylorus can then be pulled to the incision and an omentopexy performed. If the abomasum continues to pop up, this usually indicates that the omasum is also involved and has not been corrected. The omasum can be derotated in a clockwise motion separate from the abomasum and the motion to correct the AV repeated.

Therapy pre- and postoperatively should include intravenous administration of isotonic fluids such as normal saline and Ringer's solution. Large volumes will likely be necessary because of the cow's body weight. Volumes in excess of 60 L may be required during the first 24 hours.

Anti-inflammatory drugs (nonsteroidal or glucocorticoids) may benefit cattle with signs of shock. Administration of these drugs should precede correction of the AV since manipulation may release toxins and inflammatory mediators trapped in the vasculature or lumen of the abomasum.

Prognosis

Establishing an accurate prognosis is the goal of the veterinarian because treatment will involve expense and the chance of the cow recovering sufficiently to pay back this cost must be considered. There are two times when economic decisions must be made: prior to surgery and in the postoperative period. The first decision will be whether to operate or salvage immediately. The second critical time is following surgery in cows not recovering appropriately. The decision will be whether to continue to treat (cost) or salvage, if possible.

Some veterinarians recommend salvaging most cattle with AV prior to any treatment. Presurgical assessment of the postoperative outcome (death, salvage, productivity) is useful since surgery is a major expense and likely to affect salvage value. Preoperative assessment is difficult. In our experience, assessment should not be done on the basis of a single clinical observation or biochemistry value. The best published studies looked at two different classifications of outcome: death vs. survival and productivity vs. nonproductivity. A logistic regression model,[35] looking at heart rate, base excess, and serum chloride level, was developed as a preoperative predictor of death or survival. The study by Constable et al,[36] found that four variables (hydration, heart rate, duration of inappetence, and alkaline phosphatase level) could be used to best predict cattle as productive or nonproductive prior to surgery.

Surgical assessment of outcome has been investigated. The overall success rate of surgery varies between 61.5% and 86.3%.[37–40] The number of forestomachs involved in the twist has been found to adversely affect survival and productivity. Wallace[40] found only 20% success in cattle with reticulo-omasal-

abomasal volvulus. Another study[41] reported success in 55% of cattle with omasal-abomasal volvulus and 87% success in cattle with only an AV. The appearance of the abomasum at surgery has also been correlated with outcome. Edema of the abomasum carries a guarded to poor prognosis.[40, 42, 43] Edema around the proximal duodenum was associated with a poor outcome in Pearson's study[42] but Fubini et al[44] found no association with outcome. Purple discoloration of the abomasal serosa tends to bode poorly for long-term outcome, as does total distention of this organ, abomasal necrosis, and thrombosis of the gastric veins.[35, 40] When it has been necessary to drain the abomasum of fluid to correct the twist, the animals have usually not done well.[38] The measurement of intraluminal pressures of greater than 16 cm Hg also carries a poor prognosis because of mucosal damage.[45] A logistic regression model using some of the surgical findings did not predict outcome any better than with the preoperative model.[35]

Following correction, cattle with AV should be expected to have a diarrheal stool for 24 hours. The stool should then firm up to normal consistency. Clinical signs associated with a poor prognosis include melena, anorexia, persistent tachycardia, and dehydration.[38, 43, 46, 47] It is our experience that even if appetite and general attitude are initially good, persistence of a loose, low-volume stool 72 hours after surgery may indicate vagus indigestion. Cattle developing vagus indigestion will develop abdominal distention and dehydration along with smaller fecal quantities, usually within the first week postoperatively. This happens in 14% to 21% of the AV cattle surviving surgery.[15, 27, 37, 40, 48] Once vagal signs develop, the survival rate is only 11.5% to 20%.[40, 49] Prolonged treatment seems irrelevant because neither surgical treatment (pyloroplasty, abomasal or ruminal fistula) nor medical treatment (prokinetic drugs or laxatives) has been effective.[18, 38, 50] Thus, the best decision when vagal signs appear following surgery seems to be salvage. Although the prognosis for these cattle remains poor, improvement had been observed in cattle as long as 15 days post surgery.[27]

REFERENCES

1. DeLahunta A, Habel RE: Applied Veterinary Anatomy. Philadelphia, WB Saunders, 1986.
2. Trent AM: Surgery of the bovine abomasum. Vet Clin North Am Food Anim Pract 6:399–448, 1990.
3. Kuiper R: Abomasal diseases. Bovine Pract 26:111–117, 1991.
4. Argenzio RA: Gastrointestinal motility. In Swenson MJ, Reece WO (eds): Duke's Physiology of Domestic Animals, ed 11. Philadelphia, WB Saunders, 1993.
5. Leek BF: Digestion in the ruminant stomach. In Swenson MJ, Reece WO (eds): Duke's Physiology of Domestic Animals, ed 11. Philadelphia, WB Saunders, 1993.
6. Singleton AG: The effect of duodenal contents on abomasal motility in goats. J Physiol 115:336–340, 1951.
7. Bell FR, Green AR, Waas JAH, et al: Intestinal control of gastric function in the calf: The relationship of neural and endocrine factors. J Physiol 321:603–610, 1981.
8. Coppock CE, Noller CH, Wolfe SA, et al: Effect of forage-concentrate ration in complete feeds fed ad libitum on feed intake prepartum and occurrence of abomasal displacement in dairy cows. J Dairy Sci 55:783–789, 1972.
9. Grymer J, Willeberg P, Hesselholt M: Feed composition and left abomasal displacement in dairy cattle. A control study. Nord Vet 33:306–309, 1981.
10. Svendsen P: Etiology and pathogenesis of abomasal displacement in cattle. Nord Vet 21(suppl. 1):1–60, 1969.
11. Breukink HJ: Abomasal displacement: Etiology, pathogenesis, treatment and prevention. Bovine Pract 26:148–153, 1991.
12. Brikas P: Motor-modifying properties of 5-HT3 and 5-HT4 receptor agonists on ovine abomasum. Zentralbl Vetmed A 41:150–158, 1994.
13. Vlaminck K, van Meirhaeghe H, van der Hende C, et al: Einfluss

von Endotoxinen auf die Labmagenentleerung beim Rind. Dtsch Tierztliche Wochenschr 92:392–395, 1985.

14. Van Meirhaeghe H, Desperz P, van der Hende C, et al: The influence of insulin on abomasal emptying in cattle. J Vet Med Ser A 35:213–220, 1988.

15. Poulsen JSD: Right sided abomasal displacement in dairy cattle: Pre- and post-operative clinical chemical findings. Nord Vet 26:65–69, 1974.

16. Cunningham JG: Endocrine glands and their functions. *In* Cunningham JG (ed): Textbook of Veterinary Physiology. Philadelphia, WB Saunders, 1992, p 415.

17. Duncan DL: Responses of gastric musculature of the sheep to humoral agents and related substances. J Physiol 125:475–487, 1954.

18. Constable PD, Miller GY, Hoffsis GF, et al: Risk factors for abomasal volvulus and left abomasal displacement in cattle. Am J Vet Res 53:1184–1192, 1992.

19. Poulsen JSD: The influence of metabolic alkalosis and other factors on the abomasal emptying rates in goats and cows. Nord Vet 26:22–30, 1974.

20. Madison JR, Troutt HE: Effects of hypocalcemia on abomasal motility. Res Vet Sci 44:264–266, 1988.

21. Vandeplassche G, Korteweg M, Verdonk G, et al: The influence of prostaglandins on in-vitro motility of the antrum pyloricum of the bovine abomasum. Arch Int Pharmacodyn 256:324–326, 1982.

22. Vandeplassche G, Oyaert W, Houvenaghel A: The influence of prostaglandins on in-vitro motility of the fundus and pyloric sphincter of the bovine abomasum. Arch Int Pharmacodyn 260:306–308, 1982.

23. Horney FD, Wallace CE: Surgery of the bovine digestive tract. *In* Jennings PB (ed): The Practice of Large Animal Surgery. Philadelphia, WB Saunders, 1984, pp 493–554.

24. Bell FR, Titchen DA, Watson DJ: The effect of gastrin analogue, pentagastrine, on gastric electromyogram and abomasal emptying in the calf. Res Vet Sci 23:165–170, 1977.

25. Boosman R, Nemeth F, Gruys E: Bovine laminitis: Clinical aspects, pathology and pathogenesis with reference to acute equine laminitis. Vet Q 13:163–171, 1991.

26. Wensvoort P, van der Velden MA: Torsion of the abomasum in ruminants: Diagrammatic representation of rotary movements based on post mortem findings. Tijdschr Diergeneeskd 105(suppl 3):125–135, 1980.

27. Kumper H: Right displacement of the abomasum and abomasal volvulus in cattle. Part I: Pathogenesis, clinical symptoms and prognosis. Tierartzliche Praxis 23:351–359, 1995.

28. Geishauser T: Abomasal displacement in the bovine—a review on character, occurrence, aetiology and pathogenesis. J Vet Med Ser A 42:229–251, 1995.

29. St-Jean G, Hull BL, Hoffsis GF, et al: Comparison of the different surgical techniques for correction of abomasal problems. Compend Contin Educ Pract Vet 9(1):F377–F382, 1987.

30. Radiostits OM, Blood DC, Gay CC: Left abomasal displacement, right abomasal displacement, abomasal volvulus. *In* Radostits OM, Blood DC, Gay CC (eds): Veterinary Medicine: A Textbook of Diseases of Cattle, Sheep, Pigs, Goats and Horses, ed 8. London, Bailliere Tindall, 1994, pp 292–301.

31. Uribe HA, Kennedy BW, Martin SW, et al: Genetic parameters for common health disorders of Holstein cows. J Dairy Sci 78:421–430, 1995.

32. St-Jean G: Decision making in bovine abdominal surgery. Vet Clin North Am Food Anim Pract 6:335–358, 1990.

33. Guard C: Abomasal displacement and volvulus. *In* Smith BP (ed): Large Animal Internal Medicine, ed 2. St Louis, Mosby–Year Book, 1996, pp 868–874.

34. Habel RE, Smith DF: Volvulus of the bovine abomasum and omasum. J Am Vet Med Assoc 179:447–455, 1981.

35. Grohn YT, Fubini SL, Smith DF: Use of a multiple logistic regression model to determine prognosis of dairy cows with right displacement of the abomasum or abomasal volvulus. Am J Vet Res 51:1895–1899, 1990.

36. Constable PD, St-Jean G, Hull BL, et al: Prognostic value of surgical and postoperative findings in cattle with abomasal volvulus. J Am Vet Med Assoc 199:892–898, 1991.

37. Menard L, St-Pierre H, Lamothe P: Les affections de la caillette chez la vache laitière au Quebec. II. Étude rétrospective de 1000 cas. Can Vet J 19:143–149, 1978.

38. Smith DF: Right-side torsion of the abomasum in dairy cows: Classification of severity and evaluation of outcome. J Am Vet Med Assoc 173:108–111, 1978.

39. Garry FB, Hull BL, Rings DM, et al: Comparison of naturally occuring proximal duodenal obstruction and abomasal volvulus in dairy cattle. Vet Surg 17:226–233, 1988.

40. Wallace CE: Reticulo, omasal, abomasal volvulus in dairy cows. Bovine Pract 24:74–76, 1989.

41. Constable PD, St-Jean G, Hull BL, et al: Preoperative prognostic indicators in cattle with abomasal volvulus. J Am Vet Med Assoc A 198:2077–2085, 1991.

42. Pearson H: The treatment of surgical disorders of the bovine abdomen. Vet Rec 92:245–254, 1973.

43. Esperson G: Dilatation and displacement of the abomasum to the right flank and dilatation and dislocation of the caecum. Vet Rec 76:1423–1432, 1964.

44. Fubini SL, Grohn YT, Smith DF: Right displacement of the abomasum and abomasal volvulus in dairy cows: 458 cases (1980–1987). J Am Vet Med Assoc 198:460–464, 1991.

45. Constable PD, St-Jean G, Koenig GR, et al: Abomasal luminal pressure in cattle with abomasal volvulus or left displaced abomasum. J Am Vet Med Assoc 199:892–898, 1991.

46. Hjortkjaer RK, Svendsen CK: Right abomasal displacement in dairy cows: Clinical, clinical chemistry and hemodynamic findings with special reference to prognosis and circulatory disturbance. Nord Vet 31(suppl 2):1–28, 1979.

47. Hoffsis GF, McGuirk SM: Diseases of the abomasum and intestinal tract. *In* Howard JL (ed): Current Veterinary Therapy 3: Food Animal Practice. Philadelphia, WB Saunders, 1993, pp 723–735.

48. Garry FB, Hull BL, Rings DM, et al: Prognostic value of anion gap calculation in cattle with abomasal volvulus: 58 cases (1980–1985). J Am Vet Med Assoc 192:1107–1112, 1988.

49. Rebhun WC, Fubini SL, Miller TK: Vagus indigestion in cattle: Clinical features, causes, treatments and long-term follow-up of 112 cases. Compend Contin Educ Pract Vet 10:387–391, 1988.

50. Smith DF: Abomasal volvulus. Bovine Pract 22:162–164, 1987.

DISEASES OF THE ABDOMEN

■ Abomasal Ulcers

Robert H. Whitlock, D.V.M., Ph.D., Diplomate, A.C.V.I.M.

Abomasal ulcers may be classified into two major types: (1) those that bleed but do not perforate and thus do not result in abdominal distention secondary to peritonitis and (2) those that perforate and result in localized or diffuse peritonitis. Both nonperforating and perforating abomasal ulcers will be discussed here because the pathophysiology for each type is similar.

The clinical signs resulting from an abomasal ulcer are highly variable and depend on the type and location of the ulcer. The initial erosion or early ulcer lesion may not elicit any clinical signs, yet such lesions are commonly detected in abattoir surveys.[1] Ulceration that progresses to hemorrhage or perforation of the abomasal wall results in quite different signs.

Clinically, abomasal ulcers with significant bleeding rarely perforate, and ulcers that perforate rarely bleed. One practical classification of abomasal ulcers based on clinical signs is listed in Table 1. Bleeding abomasal ulcers are commonly subdivided into types I and II or III, which refer, respectively, to simple

Table 1
CLASSIFICATION OF ABOMASAL ULCERS

Nonperforating ulcers

Type I — Incomplete penetration of the abomasal mucosa resulting in minimal intraluminal hemorrhage, focal abomasal thickening, or local serositis.

Type II — Ulceration causing severe blood loss and penetration of the wall of a major abomasal blood vessel, usually in the submucosa, resulting in severe intraluminal hemorrhage. Type II ulcers commonly occur during the early postpartum period and in cattle less than 5 years of age.

Type III — Ulceration causing blood loss and penetration of the wall of a major abomasal blood vessel, usually in the submucosa, resulting in intraluminal hemorrhage and associated with abomasal lymphosarcoma. These ulcers occur at any stage of lactation or gestation. Affected cattle are typically over 5 years of age and clinical signs develop more gradually than with type II ulcers.

Perforating ulcers

Type IV — Perforating ulcer with acute, localized peritonitis. Penetration of the full thickness of the abomasal wall results in leakage of abomasal contents. The resultant peritonitis is localized to the region of the perforation by adhesion of the involved portion of the abomasum to adjacent viscera, omentum, or the peritoneal surface.

Type V — Perforating ulcer with diffuse peritonitis. Penetration of the full thickness of the abomasal wall resulting in leakage of abomasal contents. The resulting peritonitis is not localized to the region of the perforation. The ingesta is spread diffusely throughout the peritoneal cavity.

Adapted from Smith DF, Becht JL, Whitlock RH: Anorexia and abdominal distention in cattle with or without pain. *In* Anderson NV (ed): Veterinary Gastroenterology. Philadelphia, Lea & Febiger, 1980, pp 425–428.

erosions/ulcers and bleeding ulcers. Bleeding ulcers are further classified as benign (type II) or lymphosarcoma-associated ulcers (type III). Abomasal ulcers that perforate are further subdivided into those that result in local circumscribed peritonitis (type IV) or diffuse peritonitis (type V).

Surveys report the prevalence of abomasal ulceration in cattle to be approximately 3% in feedlot cattle, 9% with fatal bleeding ulcers among 141 cows sent to emergency slaughter, 1% in asymptomatic dairy cows at slaughter, and as high as 97% in dairy calves at slaughter.[1–3] The latter study found a lower prevalence of ulcers in calves raised in wooden crates than in calves loose-housed on straw or wood shavings. Nearly all reports indicated that the lesions occur most frequently in the pyloric region, yet duodenal ulceration is rare. Abomasal ulcers in feedlot cattle occur more commonly when the cattle are first placed on feed during the winter months.[2] Clinically important abomasal ulcers were detected in 69 of 6385 cattle admitted to a referral hospital. Of those 69 cases, 24 were bleeding ulcers, 12 were benign, and 12 were associated with lymphosarcoma.[4] The prevalence of abomasal ulcers in beef calves has been increasing, with reports of up 50% of calves being affected in some calf crops.[5] Despite several investigations of abomasal ulcers in beef calves, the cause remains elusive.

PATHOPHYSIOLOGY

As with gastric ulcers in other animals and humans, abomasal ulcers are multifactorial in origin. They occur as a result of an imbalance in defensive factors to protect the gastric mucosa, which include local blood flow, mucus cover, mucosal cell resistance, and duodenal influence on gastric acid secretion. Aggressive factors that promote ulceration include excess pepsin, trauma, hyperacidity, hormonal factors, and stress.

The precise mechanism or mechanisms underlying mucosal resistance to the corrosive effects of acid-pepsin have not been fully defined. Gastric mucus, secreted by mucous cells of gastric glands, is a gelatinous material that coats the mucosal surface of the stomach. The mucus coating serves as an unstirred layer through which the diffusion of acid-pepsin is reduced. Normally the gastric luminal epithelial cell surfaces and intercellular tight junctions provide a nearly impermeable barrier to backdiffusion of hydrogen ions from the lumen. Such backdiffusion to intracellular and intercellular sites may result in cellular injury, release of histamine from mast cells, further stimulation of acid secretion, damage to small blood vessels, mucosal hemorrhage, and superficial ulceration. Group E prostaglandins are of foremost importance in the preservation of mucosal integrity. Prostaglandin functions include increasing mucus secretion and microcirculation and reduction of the secretion of hydrochloric acid.[6] Decreased mucosal blood flow accompanied by backdiffusion of hydrogen ions also appears to contribute to damage to the gastric mucosa. Both short-chain fatty acids, which have a detergent action, and bile acids, which may reach the abomasum by abomasal reflux, may destroy the mucous coating.[7] Drugs that inhibit prostaglandin E (such as acetylsalicylic acid) predispose to ulcers.[6]

The so-called stress factors may play a role in ulcerogenesis in cattle. A higher stocking rate of dairy cattle per acre was associated with a significantly higher prevalence of ulcers.[3] This Dutch study reported bleeding ulcers to be most common during the summer months (May to October) and to be highly associated with heavy nitrogen fertilization of pastures, especially new pastures. Ulcers occurred more commonly in higher-producing cows but were not associated with recent parturition. North American studies report a higher prevalence during the stabling period (January to April), with a close association with recent parturition.[4, 8] Clearly, different predisposing factors must exist. Other stress factors occurring during the time when the peak occurrence of abomasal ulceration is diagnosed include parturition; other concurrent early postpartum diseases such as retained placenta, mastitis, metritis, and hypocalcemia; and attainment of peak lactation. Perhaps increased abomasal volatile fatty acids following feeding of high-concentrate diets may induce a hyperacidity within the abomasum that predisposes to ulceration when compounded by the presence of concurrent disease. In one case report, five cases of perforated fatal ulcers occurred in a herd of 40 Jersey cattle within a period of 1 month. The rapid change from pasture to a high-moisture corn and silage ration was thought to predispose to the unusual number of cases.[9]

Helicobacter pylori was successfully cultured from human gastric ulcers.[10] In subsequent reports of therapeutic trials,[11, 12] epidemiologic studies,[13] and animal models,[14] *H. pylori* was shown to be an important agent for human gastritis, gastroduodenal ulceration, and gastric carcinoma.[15] At least two reports suggest that the *Campylobacter*-like organisms observed in histologic sections of ulcerated bovine abomasums may be *H. pylori*.[16] A prospective study of beef calves failed to provide any histologic or microbiologic evidence that *H. pylori* was associated with perforating or bleeding abomasal ulcers.[17] This report is compatible with reports in humans in which perforated duodenal ulcers were not associated with *H. pylori* but were commonly associated with chronic gastric and duodenal ulceration.[18] Only rarely do cattle have chronic nonperforating abomasal ulcers. Most commonly, the lesions are either acute perforating or bleeding ulcers.

Other bacteria, including *Campylobacter*[19] and streptococci,[2] as well as fungi,[20] have been associated with abomasal ulceration. Most investigators believe that mycotic or fungal agents invade the ulcer after its formation and are not causal. Only *Clostridium perfringens* continues to be considered a risk factor for abomasal ulcers in cattle. Earlier reports have suggested an association between acute abomasal ulcers and *C. perfringens*, especially in beef cattle.[19, 21–23] Experimental intraruminal inoculation of *C. perfringens* type A caused depression, diarrhea, abdominal bloat, abomasitis, and abomasal ulceration.[23] The ulcers produced were frequently multiple, never perforating, and associated with petechial and ecchymotic hemorrhage. By contrast, naturally occurring ulcers are typically singular, frequently perforating, rarely hemorrhagic, and often localized in the fundic portion of the abomasum. The same prospective study found *C. perfringens* type A in 78.6% of the calves with ulcers and 75% of the control calves.[17] Thus, at this time no specific bacterial agent has consistently been associated with perforating or bleeding ulcers in cattle, although copper deficiency and abomasal hairballs have also been suspected.[24] For a comprehensive review on abomasal ulcers in calves see Dirksen.[25]

A retrospective study was made of 296 cattle with signs of gastrointestinal dysfunction, including 26 animals with confirmed abomasal ulcers. Fecal occult blood, abdominal pain, and packed-cell volume (PCV) were evaluated for sensitivity, specificity, and positive or negative predictive value for abomasal ulcers.[26] The fecal occult blood test had a sensitivity of 77% for all types of abomasal ulcers, whereas if all three tests were negative or normal, there was only an 11.5% chance that ulcer disease was present. It was noteworthy that 6 of 17 cows with bleeding ulcers had evidence of abdominal pain and 7 of 9 cows with perforating ulcers had a positive fecal occult blood test. False-positive tests occurred most commonly in cattle with traumatic reticulitis, abomasal displacement, liver disease, cecal volvulus, and pneumonia or pleuritis.[26]

NONPERFORATING ABOMASAL ULCERS

Diagnosis of Type I Abomasal Ulcers

Most cases of type I abomasal erosion and ulceration in cows occur early in the postpartum period and are typically associated with left displacement of the abomasum (LDA), coliform mastitis, or septic metritis.[8, 27] The characteristic clinical features of type I ulceration are darkened, soft to fluid feces and minimal anemia. The clinical signs are attributable to the primary disease and not the abomasal ulcers. Feces may be positive for occult blood, and some cows exhibit a painful response to xiphoid pressure.[26] The abnormal dark feces resolve as the primary disease responds to therapy. Most type I ulcers are detected at slaughter or necropsy and are typically multiple and superficial. Type I abomasal ulcers were found in 20.5% of 912 abomasums examined at slaughter.[28] Other ulcer types were not found in any of these cattle; however, 32% were anemic with a PCV less than 28% and 11% of the cattle were hyperfibrinogenemic (>700 mg/dL).

Diagnosis of Type II Abomasal Ulcers

The hallmark of bleeding abomasal ulceration is black, tarry feces and anemia.[4, 8, 26] Rarely, the affected cow may die peracutely from exsanguination into the abomasal lumen. This type of ulceration typically involves one large ulcer that erodes through the wall of the gastroepiploic artery in the greater curvature of the abomasal fundus. These ulcers tend to occur in cows younger than 5 years.[4] Because most type II ulcers are singular, they are not considered to be a progression of type I ulcers.

Typically, cattle with this type of ulcer have clinical signs referable to anemia. The history often includes a sharp drop in milk production, depression, and a capricious appetite. Concurrent disease problems such as a displaced abomasum, ketosis, metritis, mastitis, and retained placenta are often present.[4] Rumen motility is usually decreased both in strength and in rate of contraction.

Anemia is clinically manifested by pale mucous membranes, tachycardia, muscle weakness, and melena, although occasionally an affected cow may die before melena becomes evident. Laboratory findings usually support the presence of profound anemia (PCV less than 15%) and mild leukocytosis. With loss of whole blood, total plasma protein is also lowered, usually less than 6.0 g/dL. The guaiac test for occult blood is more sensitive and reproducible, as Payton and Glickman showed when comparing it with two commercial tablet tests.[29] As little as 75 mL/day of blood loss could be detected in the feces. For further clinical and laboratory findings, the reader is referred to a paper by Braun and co-workers.[30]

Diagnosis of Type III Abomasal Ulcers

Bleeding abomasal ulcers associated with lymphosarcoma occur most often in cattle 5 years and older and at any stage of gestation and lactation. Benign bleeding ulcers occur more frequently in cows less than 5 years of age, often with concurrent diseases such as metritis or mastitis.[4] Lymphosarcoma-associated bleeding ulcers tend to have more gradual blood loss and other clinical signs of lymphosarcoma, such as detectable tumor masses and weight loss. Approximately 50% of the cattle with type III ulcers have enlarged peripheral lymph nodes and/or masses detectable on rectal examination. The absence of a bovine leukemia virus (BLV) titer would rule out lymphosarcoma-associated tumor, whereas the presence of a BLV titer would only indicate that the cow had been exposed to the virus, not that clinical lymphosarcoma was present, inasmuch as 20% of the cattle in the United States have a titer to BLV.[31] Although approximately 75% of the cattle with type II bleeding ulcers survive with supportive treatment,[4] the prognosis for recovery is nil for lymphosarcoma-associated ulcers. It is therefore important for the clinician to be able to differentiate benign bleeding ulcers from lymphosarcoma-associated ulcers.

Other causes of blood loss into the digestive tract include duodenal ulcers or abomasal lymphosarcoma-associated ulcers, which may be the underlying cause for the type II ulceration, or hemoptysis secondary to embolic pneumonia associated with caudal vena caval thrombosis. Cows with salmonellosis, coccidiosis, and rectal lacerations often have bright red blood in the feces and are thus easily differentiated from cows with abomasal ulceration (Table 2). Because lymphosarcoma may be the cause of the ulceration, this possibility should be thoroughly investigated in any cow with type II abomasal ulceration. A negative BLV titer in an adult cow with type II abomasal ulceration would rule out lymphosarcoma as the cause because nearly all cows with the adult form of lymphosarcoma have a BLV titer. Both peripheral and internal lymph nodes should be examined. Cows 6 years or older with evidence of a bleeding ulcer have ulcers predominantly associated with lymphosarcoma. Benign ulcers typically occur in cows younger than 5 years, early in the postpartum period, and frequently in cows with concurrent disease.[4]

Table 2
DIFFERENTIAL DIAGNOSIS FOR ABOMASAL ULCERS
Bleeding abomasal ulcers
Salmonellosis
Coccidiosis
Rectal lacerations
Duodenal ulceration
Benign bleeding abomasal ulcers
Lymphosarcoma-associated bleeding ulcers
Bovine virus diarrhea with thrombocytopenia
Duodenal or jejunal bleeding syndrome
Perforating abomasal ulcers
Ruptured uterus
Ruptured abdominal abscess
Perforated rectum

Treatment of Nonperforating Abomasal Ulcers

Type I abomasal ulcers resolve as the primary disease process is corrected. Although the ulcers may heal with a superficial mucosal scar, secondary complications are uncommon. Management of a cow with type II abomasal ulceration is directed at restoring blood volume with either hypertonic saline (1 L) or whole blood if the anemia becomes severe (PCV less than 15%). The most reliable indication for blood transfusion is assessment of the general condition of the patient. Marked weakness with dyspnea, tachycardia (more than 100 beats per minute), and pale membranes is evidence for blood transfusion. If whole blood is to be given, a minimum of 4 L is recommended. Cross-matching the donor's red cells with the recipient's plasma is not necessary because cattle have so many different blood groups.[32] Analgesics such as flunixin meglumine (250 to 500 mg/1000 lb) are often indicated for the alleviation of discomfort. Other supportive measures include dietary change to a more fibrous diet, including high-quality hay. Although type 2 histamine receptors occur in the abomasum, preliminary studies to alter abomasal acidity with type 2 antagonists (cimetidine, famotidine, and ranitidine) have been only partially successful.[33] Ranitidine (6.6 mg/kg) has been shown to reduce abomasal pH.[33] Metoclopramide has been advocated as a means of promoting abomasal emptying by its gastrokinetic effects. Surgical intervention with extirpation of the ulcer is difficult and not commonly attempted. Correction of LDA in cattle with concurrent abomasal displacement and type II ulcers usually results in resolution of the bleeding ulcer.

The prognosis for bleeding abomasal ulcers not associated with LDA is guarded inasmuch as many are associated with lymphosarcoma. Some cows respond transiently to supportive care only to die of exsanguination at a later date.

PERFORATING ABOMASAL ULCERS: TYPE IV AND V

History and Clinical Signs

Abomasal ulcers may perforate the abomasal wall without involving large vessels and cause either localized (type IV) or diffuse (type V) peritonitis. Abdominal distention in association with type V ulcers is not an early sign but can occur. Thus affected cattle are anorectic but usually do not have abdominal distention and are therefore considered in this section. Most cases of type IV and V ulcers occur during the early postpartum period. An investigation of 209 cases of fatal abomasal ulceration in Canadian beef calves found that more than 93% were perforating, with 85% occurring in calves less than 2 months of age and a range of 5 days to 6 months of age.[34] Abomasal hairballs were thought to be related to the occurrence of ulcers in beef calves,[35] but an investigation of 56 calves with perforated ulcers showed a similar frequency of hairballs (>60%) in control calves.[36] The majority (89%) of perforating ulcers in calves occurred along the greater curvature.

The history and clinical signs attributed to perforating abomasal ulcers (type IV) with local peritonitis are similar to the signs of traumatic reticuloperitonitis.[8, 26] The primary difference is the site of localized pain. In cows with traumatic reticuloperitonitis, the pain is to the left side of the xiphoid or on the midline, whereas with abomasal perforation the pain is typically on the right side of the midline, often near the costal arch. However, occasionally cows with LDA have concurrent abomasal ulceration with localized pain, which may confound the diagnosis somewhat.

Cattle with localized peritonitis secondary to type IV ulcers tend to have variable clinical signs of abomasal displacement without evidence of peritonitis, chronic indigestion typified by intermittent anorexia, fever, mild bloat, rumen stasis, or more complete gastrointestinal stasis resembling vagal indigestion.[27]

Cows with type IV ulcers are often seen as medical emergencies with abruptly decreased milk production, rumen stasis, and evidence of abdominal pain. Concurrent disease conditions, in particular, abomasal displacement, are present in nearly 75% of cattle with perforating ulcers.[8, 27] The rectal temperature and heart rate tend to be minimally elevated (75 to 90 beats per minute). Epigastric pain can often be detected by the cow's reluctance to ventroflex the spine. The feces, although scant, are of normal color without evidence of melena. Cattle with perforating ulcers rarely bleed, and cows with bleeding ulcers rarely have perforation. Statistically, the events are nearly mutually exclusive.[27] Approximately 50% of perforating ulcers in adult cows occur within the first month postpartum.[8]

Cattle with perforating abomasal ulcers leading to diffuse peritonitis (type V) have more severe clinical signs, including prominent tachycardia (more than 120 beats per minute), cessation of milk production, complete rumen stasis, profound depression, progressive severe dehydration, and in advanced stages, recumbency and cold extremities suggestive of shock. Many affected cows have low-volume diarrhea, but in rare instances a cow will be constipated.[27] Owners of affected cows recognize the disorder as severe and life-threatening and request medical assistance to salvage the animal during this medical emergency.

Diagnosis of Perforated Abomasal Ulcers: Type IV and V

The diagnosis of abomasal ulcers with perforation requires a comprehensive examination by an astute diagnostician. Local or diffuse peritonitis may be confirmed by intracellular bacteria and toxic changes in the cells on cytologic examination of fluid obtained by peritoneocentesis. Both disorders are usually associated with leukopenia or leukocytosis, lymphopenia, and mild dehydration with an elevated PCV (>35%). Cows with diffuse peritonitis usually have a normal or low plasma protein (total plasma protein, <6.0 g/dL) concentration with profound hemoconcentration (PCV, >40%). The disparate values of elevated PCV and low total plasma protein concentrations signal the possibility of diffuse peritonitis, one cause of which is a perforating abomasal ulcer.[27]

Occasionally, perforating ulcers are first detected during the process of surgical correction of a displaced abomasum. Depending on the surgical approach used, the ulcers may be oversewn or surgically resected and then the displacement corrected, or a second approach can be made. When the surgical findings include an early perforating ulcer or a complete-thickness ulcer, the prognosis for survival is fair to good.[26]

Most abomasal perforations (85%) are confined to the omental bursa along the lesser curvature of the abomasum and result in local peritonitis. Diffuse peritonitis and contamination of the peritoneal cavity proper into the omental bursa occur more commonly with ulceration along the greater curvature according to Hemmingsen.[37]

Treatment of Perforating Abomasal Ulcers

The objectives for treatment of a perforating abomasal ulcer with circumscribed peritonitis are similar to those for traumatic reticuloperitonitis (i.e., antimicrobials to control the infection, restricted exercise to allow a firm adhesion to develop, and perhaps, elevation of the front quarters). For cows with concurrent abomasal displacement, a paramedian celiotomy to locate and oversew the ulcerated lesion is recommended. Tulleners and Hamilton[38] reported successful surgical resection in 4 of 10 suckling calves despite abdominal contamination. The paramedian approach offers the best exposure of the abomasal surface and, once the ulcerated lesion is oversewn or extirpated, offers an excellent method for permanent correction of the displacement. Some surgeons prefer the left paralumbar fossa approach for the repair of abomasal ulcers in cows with concurrent LDA.

Prognosis and Complications

Type I abomasal ulcers heal as the affected animal recovers from the primary disease. In animals that die of the primary disease, multiple abomasal ulcers will be found in the abomasal mucosa. Only rarely will the blood loss associated with these ulcers ever cause clinical anemia.

Cattle with type IV ulcers generally have a fair to good prognosis for survival.[8] Occasionally, adhesions develop and interfere with forestomach motility, which may lead to vagal indigestion syndrome. Type V ulcers with resultant diffuse contamination of the peritoneal cavity carry a uniformly grave prognosis.

REFERENCES

1. Welchman D, Baust GN: A survey of abomasal ulceration in veal calves. Vet Rec 121:586–590, 1987.
2. Jensen R, Pierson RE, Braddy PM, et al: Fatal abomasal ulcers in yearling feedlot cattle. J Am Vet Med Assoc 169:524–526, 1976.
3. Aukema JJ, Breukink HJ: Abomasal ulcers in cattle with fatal hemorrhage. Cornell Vet 64:303–317, 1974.
4. Palmer JE, Whitlock RH: Bleeding abomasal ulcers in adult dairy cattle. J Am Vet Med Assoc 183:448–451, 1983.
5. Jelinski MD, Jansen ED, Hoar B, et al: A field investigation of fatal abomasal ulcers in western Canadian beef calves. J Agri Pract 16:16–18, 1995.
6. Highland RL, Upson DW: Simplified role of prostaglandins in the gastrointestinal tract. Compend Contin Educ Pract Vet 8:188–194, 1986.
7. Braun U, Hausmann K, Forrer R: Reflux of bile acids from the duodenum into the rumen of cows with reduced intestinal passage. Vet Rec 124:373–376, 1989.
8. Smith DF, Munson L, Erb HN: Abomasal ulcer disease in adult dairy cattle. Cornell Vet 73:213–224, 1983.
9. Sanford SE, Josephson GKA: Perforated abomasal ulcers in postparturient Jersey cows. Can Vet J 29:392, 1988.
10. Marshall BJ: Unidentified curved bacilli on gastric epithelium in active chronic gastritis. Lancet 1:1273–1275, 1983.
11. Mantzaris GJ, Hatzis A, Tamvakologos G, et al: Prospective randomized, investigator-blind trial of Helicobacter pylori infection treatment in patients with refractory duodenal ulcers. Dig Dis Sci 38:1132–1136, 1993.
12. Morris A, Nicholson G: Ingestion of Campylobacter pyloridis causes gastritis and raised fasting pH. Am J Gastroenterol 82:192–199, 1987.
13. Blaser M: Epidemiology and pathophysiology of Campylobacter pylori infections. Rev Infect Dis 1(suppl):99–106, 1990.
14. Lee A, Fox JG, Murphy J: A small animal model of human Helicobacter pylori active chronic gastritis. Gastroenterology 99:1315–1323, 1990.
15. Graham DY, Go MF: Helicobacter pylori: Current status. Gastroenterology 105:279–282, 1993.
16. Haringsma PC, Mouwen JMVM: Mogelijke betekenis van spirilvormige bacterien bij het ontstaan van lebmaagzweren bij het volwassen rund. [Possible role of spiral-shaped bacteria in the pathogenesis of abomasal ulcers in adult cattle.] Tijdschr Diergeneeskd 117:485–486, 1992.
17. Jelinski MD, Ribble CS, Chirino-Trejo M, et al: The relationship between the presence of Helicobacter pylori, Clostridium perfringens type A, Campylobacter spp, or fungi and fatal abomasal ulcers in unweaned beef calves. Can Vet J 36:379–382, 1995.
18. Reinbach DH, Cruickshank G, McColl KEL: Acute perforated duodenal ulcer is not associated with Helicobacter pylori infection. Gut 34:1344–1347, 1993.
19. Mills KW, Johnson JL, Jensen RL, et al: Laboratory findings associated with abomasal ulcers/tympany in range calves. J Vet Diagn Invest 2:208–212, 1990.
20. Gitter M, Austwick PKC: The presence of fungi in abomasal ulcers of young calves: A report of seven cases. Vet Rec 69:924–927, 1957.
21. Berkhoff GA, Braun RK, Buergelt CD, et al: Clostridium perfringens type A associated with sudden death of replacement and feeder calves. In Proceedings of the 23rd Annual Meeting of the American Association of Veterinary Laboratory Diagnosticians, St Louis, 1980, pp 45–52.
22. Johnson JL, Hudson DB, Bohlender RE: Perforating abomasal ulcers and abomasal tympany in range calves. In Proceedings of the 24th Annual Meeting of the American Association of Veterinary Laboratory Diagnosticians, St Louis, 1981, pp 203–210.
23. Roeder BL, Chengappa MM, Nagaraja TG, et al: Experimental induction of abdominal tympany, abomasitis, and abomasal ulceration by intraruminal inoculation of Clostridium perfringens type A in neonatal calves. Am J Vet Res 49:201–207, 1988.
24. Johnson JL, Schneider NR, Slanker MR: Trace element concentrations in perinatal beef calves from West Central Nebraska. Vet Hum Toxicol 31:521–524, 1989.
25. Dirksen GU: Ulceration, dilatation and incarceration of the abomasum in calves: Clinical investigations and experiences. Bovine Practitioner 28:127–135, 1994.
26. Smith DF, Munson L, Erb HN: Predictive values for clinical signs of abomasal ulcer disease in adult dairy cattle. Prev Vet Med 3:573–580, 1986.
27. Palmer JE, Whitlock RH: Perforated abomasal ulcers in adult dairy cows. J Am Vet Med Assoc 184:171–174, 1984.
28. Braun U, Eicher R, Ehrensperger F: Type 1 abomasal ulcers in dairy cattle. J Vet Med A 38:357–366, 1991.
29. Payton AJ, Glickman LT: Fecal occult blood tests in cattle. Am J Vet Res 41:918–921, 1980.
30. Braun U, Bretscher R, Gerber D: Bleeding abomasal ulcers in dairy cows. Vet Rec 129:279–284, 1991.
31. Ferrer JF: Bovine leukosis: Natural transmission and principles of control. J Am Vet Med Assoc 175:1281–1286, 1979.
32. Kallfelz FA, Whitlock RH: Survival of ^{59}Fe-labeled erythrocytes in cross-transfused bovine blood. Am J Vet Res 34:1041–1044, 1973.
33. Wallace LLM, Reecy J, Williams JE: The effect of ranitidine hydrochloride on abomasal fluid pH in young steers. J Agri Pract 15:34–38, 1994.
34. Jelinski MD, Ribble CS, Campbell JR, Janzen ED: Descriptive epidemiology of fatal abomasal ulcers in Canadian beef calves. Prev Vet Med 26:9–15, 1996.
35. Katchuik R: Abomasal disease in young beef calves: Surgical findings and management factors. Can Vet J 33:459–461, 1992.
36. Jelinski MD, Ribble CS, Campbell JR, et al: Investigating the relationship between abomasal hairballs and perforating abomasal ulcers in unweaned beef calves. Can Vet J 37:23–26, 1996.

37. Hemmingsen I: Ulcus perforans abomasi bovis. Nord Vet Med 19:17–30, 1967.
38. Tulleners EP, Hamilton GF: Surgical resection of perforated abomasal ulcers in calves. Can Vet J 21:262–264, 1980.

■ Abomasal Impactions in Cattle

Guy St. Jean, D.M.V., M.S., Diplomate, A.C.V.S.
David E. Anderson, D.V.M., M.S., Diplomate, A.C.V.S.

Abomasal impaction is defined as the accumulation of ingesta within the abomasum with failure of aboral transport.[1] Abomasal impaction is uncommon in cattle and results from a mechanical or functional obstruction of abomasal outflow of ingesta. Functional obstruction results from the ingestion of a large quantity of poor-quality roughage and inadequate water intake, vagal indigestion (forestomach dysfunction), or dysfunction of the abomasum secondary to abomasal volvulus (type III vagal indigestion). Mechanical obstruction of the abomasum results from the presence of intraluminal foreign bodies or extramural or mural lesions in the area of the pylorus.[2]

Primary functional abomasal impaction is usually seen during the winter months in beef cows fed poor-quality, coarse roughage with minimal or no water available. Cows fed straw, late-cut hay, and corn stover are particularly predisposed to this condition.[1] Abomasal impaction with sand (malnourished cattle fed hay on top of sandy soil) and with almond shells (3.6 kg per head per day) has also been reported.[3, 4] These feeds accumulate in the abomasum and secondarily fill the reticulum and rumen. Cows consume the offending feed until the physical capacity of the rumen limits further intake. Because nutrients are not absorbed, these cows are in a state of starvation. Cows in mid to late gestation appear to be affected more frequently. Calves may suffer from impaction of the abomasum by eating bedding or other rough forage when receiving poor-quality milk replacer.[1] An anomaly of the vagal nerve has been suggested as a possible cause of abomasal impaction.[5] Impaction has been seen following traumatic reticuloperitonitis (possibly caused by vagal neuritis) and after correction of abomasal volvulus (possibly caused by stretching of the vagal nerve).[5, 6] Functional impaction following abomasal volvulus may also be due to vascular thrombosis or muscular damage in the abomasal wall from overdistention.[6]

Placenta, bailing twine, phytobezoars, and trichobezoars are capable of obstructing the pylorus and causing an abomasal impaction.[2, 5] The most commonly recognized mural lesion around the pylorus is lymphosarcoma, which can result in partial or complete outflow obstruction.[5] Extramural lesions include abscesses, fat necrosis, adhesions, improper placement of an omentopexy or pyloropexy suture, inadvertent fixation of the pylorus with a toggle pin during an attempt to correct left displacement of the abomasum,[2] and extramural compression of the pylorus by a near-term gravid uterus.[7]

DIAGNOSIS

Abomasal impaction results in an animal with bilateral ventral abdominal enlargement and bulging of the left paralumbar fossa. Cattle often have a round, fat appearance from a distance, but on close examination they are very thin and often dehydrated. Anorexia is usually present, and rumen contractions are often increased early in the disease process but are decreased or absent in late stages of the disease. Feces are absent or very scant and hard. It may be possible to perform ballottement on an enlarged, firm abomasum caudal to the rib cage in the ventral right flank area. In calves, the abomasum may fill the majority of the abdomen and be firm on external palpation. In a small nongravid cow or in a steer it may be possible to rectally palpate the caudal aspect of an enlarged abomasum.[5] With type III vagal indigestion, the abomasal contents are of normal consistency.[6]

Respiration may be labored because of abdominal distention. The heart rate is usually normal or low during most of the course of the disease, but tachycardia may be seen in the terminal stage of the disease because of hypovolemic shock.[1] Also in the terminal stage of abomasal impaction, cattle may be recumbent and groan with each respiration.

Transabdominal ultrasonography can be used to identify the size and content of the abomasum and differentiate it from the rumen. Affected cattle are typically dehydrated and have hypokalemic hypochloremic metabolic alkalosis caused by the sequestration of abomasal secretions.[8] Analysis of rumen fluid usually reveals an increased concentration of chloride (>26 mEq/L). A definitive diagnosis of abomasal impaction is often made during exploratory celiotomy.

TREATMENT

Options for treatment depend on the severity and chronicity of the impaction and the value of the animal. Options include slaughter, medical therapy, rumenotomy, and abomasotomy. In chronic cases, salvage by slaughter is often the most economical recommendation. In acute cases of abomasal impaction, medical therapy can be effective.[2] The rumen should be decompressed with a large-bore stomach tube. Fluid and electrolyte abnormalities should be corrected by intravenous administration. Saline cathartics (magnesium sulfate, 2 kg/day orally) can initiate and facilitate evacuation of the abomasum. Orally administered laxatives and lubricants such as mineral oil (8 mL/kg/day) and dioctyl sodium sulfosuccinate (50 mg/kg/day) can soften impacted ingesta. Easily digestible feeds should be offered. Cattle affected with sand impaction responded to a mixture of molasses, mineral oil, Epsom salts, and water.[4] Cattle with almond shell impaction had variable response to the oral administration of laxatives and mineral oil.[3] Pregnancy can be terminated by induction of parturition with corticosteroids (dexamethasone, 20 mg) or prostaglandins, which leads to decreased extramural pressure on the abomasum, more abdominal space, improved comfort, and less energy requirements. If medical treatment is not effective or in more advanced cases, surgery may be offered as a treatment option. Rumenotomy can be used to decompress the rumen, and then medication can be infused into the abomasum through the reticulomasal orifice.[1, 9] A tube can also be inserted from the nose to the reticulo-omasal orifice to allow infusion of fluids into the abomasum after surgery. If pyloric obstruction is suspected, a right flank celiotomy is indicated.[10] From this approach the abomasum cannot be emptied, but fluids can be infused into the abomasum. An abomasotomy can be performed from a right paramedian or a right paracostal approach. Abomasotomy allows exposure of the pyloric portion of the abomasum and ensures initial relief of the impaction.[10] The authors prefer the exposure afforded by the right paramedian approach.[10] However, dorsal recumbency in an adult with abomasal impaction causes significant stress on the cardiovascular and respiratory systems, especially if the animal is in the last trimester of pregnancy.[10] Decompression of the rumen with a large tube orally should be done before positioning the animal for an abomasotomy. The abomasum should be isolated with towels to avoid contamination of the abdomen.[2] Following removal of the contents, foreign body, or mass, a two-layer inverting-pattern suture should be placed in the abomasum. If the pyloric region is severely affected and normal outflow cannot be restored through the pylorus, an abomasoduodenal bypass may be necessary to avoid the obstruction. The impaction may recur if the original cause persists or if previous distortion has resulted in permanent abomasal damage.

The prognosis for abomasal impaction depends on the cause, chronicity of the impaction, and the method of treatment. Calves have a better prognosis because the abomasum is easier to access surgically.[5, 10] In adult cattle with chronic cases of abomasal impaction, the prognosis is usually poor. However, in the authors' opinion, functional impaction from indigestible feed and limited water intake without permanent neuromuscular damage (early cases) can be treated successfully. Type III vagal indigestion carries a poor prognosis.[6]

PREVENTION

Prevention of abomasal impaction is extremely important, especially prevention of functional obstruction caused by the ingestion of a large quantity of poor-quality roughage because other cattle in the herd may be affected.[1] Proper dietary management of cattle in cold weather needs to be implemented because their energy requirements are high. Coarse roughage should be limited, high-quality hay should be made available, in lots with sandy soil roughage should not be placed on the ground, and concentrates should be given. Body condition should be monitored, and thin cows should be given supplemental feed. With calves, the milk replacer should be of high quality and the bedding removed.[1] Foreign material should be removed from the area where the cattle are kept to prevent mechanical obstruction. Cattle suffering from abomasal volvulus need early surgical correction to prevent dysfunction of the abomasum (type III vagal indigestion).[6]

REFERENCES

1. Hoffsis GF, McGuirk SM: Abomasal impaction. Diseases of the abomasum and the intestinal tract. *In* Howard JL (ed): Current Veterinary Therapy, Food Animal Practice, vol 2. Philadelphia, WB Saunders, 1986, pp 732–733.
2. Blikslager AT, Bristol DG, Hunt EL: Abomasal impaction in cattle. Compend Contin Educ Pract Vet 15:1571–1575, 1993.
3. Mitchell KJ: Dietary abomasal impaction in a herd of dairy replacement heifers. J Am Vet Med Assoc 198:1408–1409, 1991.
4. Hunter R: Sand impaction in a herd of beef cattle. J Am Vet Med Assoc 166:1179, 1975.
5. Trent AM: Surgery of the bovine abomasum. Vet Clin North Am Food Anim Pract 6:412–415, 1990.
6. Constable PD, St Jean G, Hull BL, et al: Preoperative prognostic indicators in cattle with abomasal volvulus. A prospective study in 80 animals. J Am Vet Med Assoc 198:2077–2085, 1991.
7. Van Meter DC, Fecteau G, House JK, et al: Indigestion of late pregnancy in a cow. J Am Vet Med Assoc 206:625–628, 1995.
8. Taguchi K: Relationship between degree of dehydration and serum electrolytes and acid-base status in cows with various abomasal disorders. J Vet Med Sci 57:257–260, 1995.
9. Baker JS: Abomasal impaction and related obstructions of the forestomachs in cattle. J Am Vet Med Assoc 175:1250–1253, 1979.
10. St Jean G, Hull BL, Hoffsis G, et al: Comparison of the different surgical techniques for correction of abomasal problems. Compend Contin Educ Pract Vet 9:377–382, 1987.

▪ Abomasal Emptying Defect in Sheep

D. Michael Rings, D.V.M., M.S., Diplomate, A.C.V.I.M.

DEFINITION

Abomasal emptying defect (AED) is a syndrome of chronic weight loss in sheep which is associated with abomasal distention. The breed most frequently affected is the Suffolk[1]; however, other sheep have been diagnosed with this condition, including Hampshire, Columbia, Corriedale, and Dorset.

ETIOLOGY AND PATHOGENESIS

The mechanism responsible for this condition has not been defined. The high proportion of clinical cases occurring in Suffolk sheep suggests a hereditary aspect. Supporting this is the increased number of AED-affected animals identified within a particular Suffolk family line. However, a previous study[2] investigating an outbreak of this condition in a large flock was unable to show any heritability. In Great Britain, a similar condition was found in sheep infected with scrapie.[3] No evidence of scrapie has been detected in AED-affected sheep in the United States.

The problem appears to be neither seasonal nor sex-linked in its incidence and both pregnant and nonpregnant ewes have been affected. Clinical cases have occurred in sheep managed under range conditions as well as those under intensive husbandry. There does not appear to be any geographic area with an increased incidence. Clinical signs have been observed primarily in sheep between 1 and 5 years of age.

One distinctive feature of this problem differing from abomasal impaction in cattle is that the distention of the abomasum is almost exclusively in the body of the organ (normal atrium and pyloric portion). Because the pylorus is open, some abomasal secretions and ingesta continue to pass into the small intestine. The classic clinicopathologic findings in abomasal obstructive disease (hypochloremia, hypokalemia, metabolic alkalosis) are not usually seen in AED sheep. The distention of the abomasum is often slow to develop. The persistent neural feedback to the brain's satiety center in the hypothalamus caused by abomasal distention leads to loss of appetite. The animal starves with a full stomach. Volumes of greater than 18 L have been removed from the abomasum of AED-affected sheep (normal volume <2 L).

CLINICAL SIGNS

Most animals have a history of gradual weight loss varying from weeks to months, but, weight loss in sheep with heavy fleeces may not be apparent until shearing when the loss may seem dramatic. Although affected sheep lack a good appetite, the gregarious nature of the species causes owners to believe they are eating because they stay with the flock during feeding and may be observed taking an occasional mouthful. AED sheep often continue to pass relatively normal amounts of pelleted stool, but diminished fecal production is also seen. Heart rates are usually elevated (>90 beats per minute) while body temperature and respiratory rates are within normal limits. Ruminations are variable, with some sheep having exaggerated rumen movements while others may have no motility evident. Ventral abdominal distention can be detected in about 50% of the animals by visual observation. Ballottement of the right ventral abdomen can often identify a distended, firm viscus in this quadrant.[4] Although the clinical course may be slow, the untreated condition will be fatal.

DIAGNOSIS

The clinical history of chronic weight loss in a Suffolk sheep in which no other cause is apparent should suggest the possibility of AED. Physical examination findings of tachycardia, weight loss, ventral abdominal distention, and the presence of a firm viscus in the right ventral quadrant are strongly suggestive of AED. Confirmation of the diagnosis can be made using ultrasonography to image the right ventral abdomen or via laparotomy. Laboratory evaluation of electrolytes (K^+, Cl^-) and blood gases will be normal, but measurement of rumen fluid chloride content will often be elevated (>15 mEq/L) due to reflux of hydrochloric acid.

TREATMENT

AED remains a disease with a poor prognosis using treatment regimens previously reported. Sheep diagnosed early in the course of the problem (before the abomasum becomes overdistended) can be treated medically using a combination of gastric motility drugs such as metoclopramide (0.1 mg/kg b.i.d.) and 2 to 4 oz of mineral oil orally for 10 to 21 days. Successful treatment is usually apparent within 7 days of the initiation of treatment. Abomasums which become distended to greater than 6 L respond poorly to medical treatment alone. Abomasotomy and evacuation of the contents, with or without imbrication of the abomasum, can be attempted; however, the recovery rate for these animals is even lower because of chronic abomasal atony.

REFERENCES

1. Rings DM, Welker FH, Hull BF, et al: Abomasal emptying defect in Suffolk sheep. J Am Vet Med Assoc 185:1520–1522, 1984.
2. Ruegg PL, George LW, East NE: Abomasal dilitation and emptying defect in a flock of Suffolk ewes. J Am Vet Med Assoc 193:1534–1536, 1988.
3. Sharp MW, Collins DF: Ovine abomasal enlargement and scrapie (letter). Vet Rec 120:215, 1987.
4. Rings DM: Abomasal emptying defect in Suffolk sheep. In Proceedings of the American College of Veterinary Internal Medicine, 1987, pp 759–762.

■ Intestinal Volvulus in Cattle

David E. Anderson, D.V.M., M.S., Diplomate, A.C.V.S.
Guy St. Jean, D.M.V., M.S., Diplomate, A.C.V.S.

DEFINITION

Volvulus refers to the rotation of viscera about its mesenteric attachment. Torsion refers to the rotation of viscera about its own (or long) axis. Although torsion of the abomasum and of the uterus are found in cattle, torsion of the small intestine is rare. Small intestinal volvulus may occur in different forms.[1–3] The most severe form of intestinal volvulus is volvulus of the root of the mesentery and involves the entirety of the small intestine and mesenteries. Volvulus of the root of the mesentery causes obstruction of venous outflow and arterial blood supply to the intestines. Ischemic necrosis of the intestine proceeds rapidly, which causes metabolic acidosis, shock, and death. Volvulus of the jejunoileal flange refers to volvulus of the mid- to distal jejunum and proximal ileum where the mesentery is long. This long mesentery and associated bowel has been termed the "flange" and may rotate about its mesentery without involving the remaining small intestine. Often, arterial occlusion is not found with volvulus of the jejunoileal flange, possibly because extensive fat deposits within the mesentery may prevent compression of the muscular wall of the arteries until the volvulus becomes severe. However, obstruction of outflow of venous blood may be equally detrimental because of mural edema,

shunting of blood away from the mucosa, and progressive ischemia.

Cattle of any breed, age, or sex may be affected by intestinal volvulus at any time during the year. In a review of 190 cattle having intestinal volvulus, dairy breeds were at a higher risk of developing volvulus compared with beef breeds.[1] This difference was believed to be associated with differences in management. Neither lactation nor gestation were identified as risk factors, and calves were not found to be at an increased risk compared with adult cattle. In a separate study of 100 cattle having intestinal volvulus, 86 were calves between 1 week and 6 months old.[4]

CLINICAL SIGNS

Cattle having volvulus of the root of the mesentery may be found dead with severe abdominal distention. Early in the course of the disease, affected cattle demonstrate acute, severe abdominal pain (kicking at the abdomen, rolling, lying down and getting up frequently, grunting) and have marked elevation in heart rate (>120 beats per minute [bpm]) and respiratory rate (>80 breaths per minute). The rapid progression of the disease precludes development of significant dehydration, but cardiovascular shock is usually present.

Cattle having volvulus of the jejunoileal flange may present similarly to cattle having volvulus at the root of the mesentery. However, these cattle often demonstrate clinical signs consistent with acute intestinal obstruction rather than cardiovascular shock. Cattle show signs of abdominal pain, are tachycardic (80 to 120 bpm), and pass minimal feces. Cattle may be dehydrated at the time of examination.

CLINICAL PATHOLOGY

Because of the rapid onset and progress, cattle having intestinal volvulus may not demonstrate changes in serum biochemistry or hematologic valves. The changes expected with intestinal volvulus are consistent with intestinal obstruction, stress, and dehydration: azotemia, hypocalcemia, hyperglycemia, and a leukocytosis with a mild left shift.[1] In the early stages of the disease, cattle develop alkalemia with normal serum potassium concentration. As cardiovascular compromise and intestinal ischemia proceed, cattle develop metabolic acidosis and hyperkalemia. Cattle having the shift to acidosis and hyperkalemia have a poor prognosis for survival.[1]

DIAGNOSIS

Diagnosis of intestinal volvulus is by exploratory laparotomy. Rectal palpation reveals multiple loops of distended intestine filling the caudal abdomen and excessive tension on the intestinal mesentery. Simultaneous auscultation and percussion of the abdomen yields multifocal pings of variable pitch and location. Findings of scant feces, abdominal pain, sudden onset of abdominal distention, and multiple loops of distended intestine on rectal palpation in cattle are highly suggestive of intestinal volvulus. The differential diagnosis includes intussusception, cecal volvulus, abomasal volvulus, intraluminal obstruction, and severe indigestion.

TREATMENT

Immediate surgical correction is the treatment of choice. Intravenous fluids should be administered to treat cardiovascular shock, but preparation for surgery should not be delayed. The volvulus must be corrected before irreversible ischemic injury or thrombosis of the mesenteric arteries has occurred. A right paralumbar fossa laparotomy with the cow standing is the approach of choice. Restoration of the normal anatomic position of the intestines is more easily done with the patient standing. Cattle that are thought to be at great risk of becoming recumbent during surgery should be placed under general anesthesia, in left lateral recumbency, and the laparotomy performed through the right paralumbar fossa. The presence of the volvulus and the direction of the twist is assessed by palpating the root of the mesentery and, in the case of jejunoileal flange volvulus, following this ventrally to the location of the twist. The intestinal mass is gently derotated, being careful not to cause rupture of the viscera. This procedure may require exteriorization of various portions of the intestinal mass. After correction of the volvulus, the intestinal tract should be examined for evidence of nonviable bowel. If compromise of the intestine is found (arterial thrombosis, blackened serosa, friable wall of the affected segment, mural edema), then intestinal resection and anastomosis is indicated (see Intussusception in this section). Also, exploration of the abdomen should be done to rule out the presence of a second lesion (abomasal displacement, fecalith, intussusception, anomalous fibrovascular bands, peritonitis, etc.).

Postoperative management is directed toward maintaining optimal hydration, and electrolyte and acid-base status. Antibiotics and anti-inflammatory drugs are indicated. Ileus may be seen during the first 48 hours after surgery, but the use of prokinetic drugs should be weighed against the risk of leakage at the site of the anastomosis if intestinal resection was performed. Passage of large volumes of diarrhea within 24 hours after surgery is considered to be a favorable prognostic indicator.

PROGNOSIS

Prognosis varies with the severity and duration of the lesion. Prognosis for survival of cattle having volvulus of the root of the mesentery (44%) is less than for volvulus of the jejunoileal flange (86%).[1] Overall, dairy cattle had a better prognosis for survival (63%) than beef cattle (22%). This difference was presumed to be because dairy cattle are observed more frequently and, therefore, treatment is sought earlier in the progression of the disease. Of 92 cattle in which surgical correction of intestinal volvulus was attempted, 13 were euthanized during surgery, 25 died within 24 hours after surgery, 13 died between 2 and 7 days, and 41 (45%) survived.[4]

PREVENTION

Specific recommendations for strategies to prevent intestinal volvulus are not possible because no risk factor has been identified. Some authors have suggested that turning out to graze lush pastures is a risk factor for intestinal volvulus.[5] This has not been our experience. Feeding of concentrates, frequent dietary changes, confinement housing, and selection for high productivity may place dairy cattle at higher risk compared with beef cattle. These management techniques are also used in feedlot operations, but these cattle may not be presented for treatment to teaching hospitals because of their lower perceived economic value. Therefore, recommendations should be aimed to optimize cattle health by gradual changes in diet and environment.

REFERENCES

1. Anderson DE, Constable PD, St-Jean G, et al: Small-intestinal volvulus in cattle: 35 cases (1967–1992). J Am Vet Med Assoc 203:1178–1183, 1993.
2. Fubini SL, Smith DF, Tithof PK, et al: Volvulus of the distal part of the jejunoileum in four cows. Vet Surg 15:150–152, 1986.
3. Tulleners EP: Surgical correction of volvulus of the root of the mesentery in calves. J Am Vet Med Assoc 179:998–999, 1981.
4. Rademacher G: Diagnosis, therapy, and prognosis of the intestinal mesenteric torsion in cattle. *In* Proceedings, 17th World Buiatrics Congress and 25th American Association of Bovine Practitioners Conference, St Paul, Minn, vol 1, 1992, pp 137–142.
5. Willet MDJ. Intestinal torsion in cattle. N Z Vet J 18:42–43, 1970.

■ Intraluminal Intestinal Obstruction: Trichobezoars, Phytobezoars, and Enteroliths

David E. Anderson, D.V.M, M.S., Diplomate, A.C.V.S.
Guy St. Jean, D.M.V., M.S., Diplomate, A.C.V.S.

DEFINITION

Intraluminal obstruction of the intestinal tract of cattle, sheep, and goats is most commonly caused by a trichobezoar, phytobezoar, or enterolith.[1, 2] These foreign bodies form in the rumen or abomasum and may pass into the intestinal tract where they become lodged within the small intestine or spiral colon. Hairballs (trichobezoars) are caused by frequent ingestion of hair (Figs. 1 and 2). This is seen most commonly in cattle infested with lice or mange, or during the spring when shedding of the winter hair coat occurs. Phytobezoars and enteroliths form around undigested materials (e.g., nylon fibers, cotton fabric). In a necropsy survey of 166 dead calves less than 90 days old in western Canada, 56 calves died because of perforation of an abomasal ulcer.[3] Calves having an abomasal ulcer were 2.74 times more likely to have an abomasal hairball. Calves less than 31 days old and having an abomasal ulcer were 3.81 times more likely to have an abomasal hairball. However, the authors were unable to establish a causative relationship between the presence of abomasal hairballs and a perforating ulcer. During a study of confined cattle being fed a roughage-limited diet, cows began biting hair from each others' hair coats and developed multiple ruminal hairballs (range of 2 to 10 hairballs weighing 0.2 to 3.8 kg each).[4] The investigators speculated that the cows began

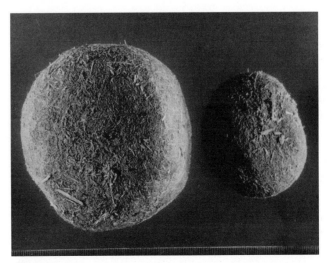

Figure 1
Two trichobezoars removed from the jejunum of a Polled Hereford bull.

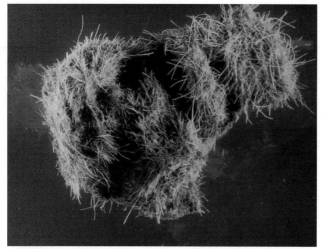

Figure 2
Trichobezoar disrupted to demonstrate formation by compacted hair and ingesta.

"grazing" hair because of the lack of roughage in the diet and high stocking density. One report describes clinical findings in two sheep having 107 individual hairballs.[5] The authors speculated that pruritus or some unknown dietary deficiency was the cause of excessive ingestion of the wool.

CLINICAL SIGNS

Animals affected with ruminal or abomasal bezoars may be observed to have decreased appetite, weight loss, decreased fecal production, lethargy, and apparent depression. Multiple bezoars present in the rumen or abomasum of calves, sheep, and goats may be found during transabdominal palpation or on abdominal radiographs. When an obstruction of the small intestine or spiral colon occurs, affected animals initially show clinical signs of abdominal pain (restlessness, kicking at the abdomen, lying down and getting up frequently, arching the back, stretching out the legs while standing) and progress to recumbency and apparent depression. Progressive bloat or abdominal distention and lack of fecal production are noted.

CLINICAL PATHOLOGY

Serum biochemistry analysis reveals hypokalemic, hypochloremic metabolic alkalosis, the severity of which depends on the duration and location of the lesion. These changes are most severe with proximal intestinal obstruction and become more severe with increasing duration. If ischemic necrosis of the intestinal wall has occurred, an inflammatory leukogram with increased numbers of immature neutrophils may be seen. As peritonitis develops and organic acids are released into the bloodstream, the serum biochemistry changes to a metabolic acidosis with relative hyperkalemia. These changes are consistent with a poor prognosis. Perforation of an abomasal ulcer or rupture of the intestine and contamination of the abdomen with ingesta carries a poor to grave prognosis.

DIAGNOSIS

In affected cattle, serum biochemistry changes are consistent with intestinal obstruction. Rumen chloride concentration may

be elevated (>30 mEq/L). The cause of intraluminal obstruction is rarely palpable per rectum, but small intestinal distention may be palpable. Ultrasonographic examination of the abdomen may be useful in calves and small ruminants. Intraluminal intestinal obstruction should be suspected in cattle with recurrent rumen tympanites which is transiently responsive to decompression and is associated with minimal fecal production. The differential diagnosis includes intussusception, vagus indigestion syndrome, intestinal lymphosarcoma, fat necrosis, intestinal entrapment around anomalous fibrovascular bands, and volvulus of the jejunoileal flange.

TREATMENT

Trichobezoars, phytobezoars, or enteroliths located within the rumen are unlikely to cause clinical signs unless the number and magnitude of the foreign bodies are severe (e.g., two sheep in which hairballs accounted for $>10\%$ of the animals' body weight[5]). A cow suffered esophageal obstruction after suspected attempted regurgitation of a rumen trichobezoar.[6] Ruminal foreign bodies are removed via a left paralumbar fossa celiotomy and rumenotomy (see Traumatic Reticuloperitonitis earlier in this section).

Abomasal hairballs may cause pyloric obstruction which leads to rapid onset of abdominal distention. We prefer to perform a right paramedian or ventral paracostal laparotomy to exteriorize the abomasum. An abomasotomy is performed along the greater curvature of the abomasum, the foreign bodies are removed, and the abomasum is closed with absorbable monofilament suture material (e.g., 0 polydioxanone) using two layers of an inverting suture pattern.

When obstruction of the duodenum, jejunum, or spiral colon is suspected, a right paralumbar fossa celiotomy and exploration of the abdomen should be performed. The foreign body is found by exteriorizing a segment of normal or distended intestine and tracing this segment orad, or aborad, respectively, until the obstruction is found. This segment of intestine is exteriorized from the abdomen and isolated using moistened surgical towels. Manual breakdown of some enteroliths through the intestinal wall may be possible. When this cannot be accomplished, an enterotomy is performed. After removal of the foreign body, the enterotomy is closed with absorbable suture material (e.g., 2-0 polydioxanone, polyglactin 910) using two lines of an inverting suture pattern. The enterotomy may be closed transversely to maximize the lumen of the affected segment of intestine and minimize the tension endured by the suture line during contraction of the intestinal wall. When the perceived economic value of the affected cattle is high, surgery may be performed with the patient under general anesthesia. This will minimize the risk of ingesta contamination of the abdomen during surgery.

Intravenous (IV) fluid therapy is based on the clinical estimate of dehydration, severity of intestinal lesions identified at surgery, and severity of serum biochemistry changes. In general, cattle should receive 20 to 60 L of isotonic saline IV over 12 hours. We routinely add calcium (1 mL of 23% calcium gluconate per kilogram body weight) and dextrose (to create a 1.25% solution) to the IV fluids. Nonsteroidal anti-inflammatory drugs (flunixin meglamine, 1 mg/kg body weight, IV, q. 12 h. for 3 days) and antibiotics (for 3 to 5 days) also are administered.

PROGNOSIS

The prognosis for return to productive use is based on the animal's body condition, severity of changes in serum biochemistry variables,[7] presence of visceral perforation or peritonitis, and ability to perform surgical removal of the foreign body without contaminating the abdomen. Cattle that are less than 10% dehydrated and have mild to moderate hypochloremia (e.g., >80 mEq/L) and metabolic alkalosis (e.g., bicarbonate >32 mEq/L) have a fair to good prognosis for recovery. Cattle that are more than 10% dehydrated, have severe hypochloremia (e.g., <80 mEq/L) and metabolic acidosis (e.g., bicarbonate <20 mEq/L), or have visceral perforation have a poor prognosis for survival. Therefore, immediate surgical intervention is required for alleviation of clinical signs caused by intraluminal foreign bodies.

PREVENTION

Intraluminal obstruction of the intestine occurs infrequently in cattle. The sporadic nature of the problem limits recommendations for prevention. Adequate dietary roughage should be made available to cattle at all times. Lice control strategies, particularly during the winter months, will prevent pruritus-associated ingestion of hair.

REFERENCES

1. Pearson H, Pinsent PJN: Intestinal obstruction in cattle. Vet Rec 101:162–166, 1977.
2. Pearson H: The treatment of surgical disorders of the bovine abdomen. Vet Rec 92:245–254, 1973.
3. Jelinski MD, Ribble CS, Campbell JR, et al: Investigating the relationship between abomasal hairballs and perforating abomasal ulcers in unweaned beef calves. Can Vet J 37:23–26, 1996.
4. Cockrill JM, Beasley JN, Selph RA: Trichobezoars in four Angus cows. Vet Med Small Anim Clin 73:1441–1442, 1978.
5. Ramadan RO: Massive formation of trichobezoars in sheep. Agri Pract 16:26–28, 1995.
6. Patel JH, Brace DM: Esophageal obstruction due to a trichobezoar in a cow. Can Vet J 36:774–775, 1995.
7. Anderson DE, Constable PD, St-Jean G, et al: Small-intestinal volvulus in cattle: 35 cases (1967–1992). J Am Vet Med Assoc 203:1178–1183, 1993.

■ Intussusception

David E. Anderson, D.V.M., M.S., Diplomate, A.C.V.S.
Guy St. Jean, D.M.V., M.S., Diplomate, A.C.V.S.

DEFINITION

Intussusception is the invagination of one segment of intestine within another. The invaginated portion of intestine is termed the *intussusceptum*, and the outer, or receiving, segment of intestine is termed the *intussuscipiens*. Intussusception occurs sporadically in cattle of all ages, breeds, and sex and may be seen at any time during the year.[1, 2] However, in a case-control epidemiologic study of 336 cattle, intussusception occurred most commonly in calves less than 2 months old, Brown Swiss cattle appeared to be overrepresented, and Hereford cattle appeared to be underrepresented compared with Holstein cattle.[1] Although the inciting cause is rarely identified, intussusception may occur secondary to enteritis, intestinal parasitism, sudden changes in diet, mural granuloma or abscess, intestinal neoplasia (especially adenocarcinoma), mural hematoma, and administration of drugs that affect intestinal motility. Any focal disturbance of intestinal motility may facilitate the invagination of an orad segment into an aborad segment of intestine. Intussusception occurs most commonly in the distal portion of the jejunum, but intussusception has been found affecting the proximal jejunum, ileum, cecum, and spiral colon.[1-7] In a review of 336 intussusceptions in cattle, 281 affected the small intestine, 7 were ileocolic, 12 cecocolic, and 36 colocolic.[1]

CLINICAL SIGNS

Cattle affected with intussusception demonstrate clinical signs of abdominal pain (restlessness, kicking at the abdomen, lying down and getting up frequently, assuming abnormal posture) for up to 24 hours after the onset of disease. Cattle are frequently anorectic, lethargic, and reluctant to walk. After the initial signs of abdominal pain subside, affected cattle become progressively lethargic, recumbent, and show apparent depression. Abdominal distention becomes apparent after 24 to 48 hours' duration. This is caused by gas and fluid distention of the forestomach and intestines, and sequestration of ingesta within the gastrointestinal tract results in progressive dehydration and electrolyte depletion. The heart rate will increase proportionally to abdominal pain, intestinal necrosis, and dehydration. Fecal production may be normal for up to 12 hours after the occurrence of the intussusception, but minimal fecal production is noted after 24 hours' duration. Passage of blood and mucus from the rectum is common at this time.

CLINICAL PATHOLOGY

Hemoconcentration is usually present (increased packed cell volume and total protein), and the leukogram may indicate inflammation if ischemic necrosis of the intussusceptum has occurred. Often, changes in the white blood cell count and differential are minimal and changes in peritoneal fluid constituents are not seen because the intussusceptum is isolated by the intussuscipiens. Hypochloremic metabolic alkalosis is found with serum biochemistry analysis. Hyponatremia, hypokalemia, hypocalcemia, azotemia, and hyperglycemia also may be found. The magnitude of these changes is dependent on the location and duration of the lesion. Proximal jejunal intussusception causes rapid and severe dehydration, electrolyte sequestration, and metabolic alkalosis. Most lesions occur in the distal jejunum and may require more than 48 hours to develop these changes. Elevation of rumen chloride concentration (>30 mEq/L) may be found if fluid distention of the rumen is present.

DIAGNOSIS

Diagnosis of intussusception is usually made during exploratory laparotomy. Occasionally the intussusception can be felt during rectal palpation, but distention of multiple loops of small intestine is most commonly identified. In our experience, an intussusception may be present for 48 hours or more in adult cattle without being able to find intestinal distention during rectal palpation. In calves and small ruminants, percutaneous palpation and ultrasonographic examination of the abdomen may be used to identify intestinal distention and, possibly, the intussusception. Intussusception should be suspected in cattle with a history of abdominal pain and having abdominal distention, minimal feces consisting of blood and mucus, and palpable distention of the intestine. The differential diagnosis includes primary indigestion, functional ileus, trichobezoar, foreign bodies, intestinal incarceration or strangulation, vagal syndrome, intestinal neoplasia, fat necrosis, and jejunoileal flange volvulus.

TREATMENT

Affected cattle must be stabilized before surgical intervention. Fluid therapy should be aimed at replacing fluid and electrolyte deficits. Surgical correction may proceed after the patient has been assessed as a suitable candidate. Right paralumbar fossa exploratory laparotomy is the surgical approach of choice for treatment of intussusception. The majority of the small intestine of cattle has a short mesentery, preventing adequate exteriorization of the intussusception through a ventral midline incision. Also, the attachments of the greater omentum limit exposure with this approach. The presence of the rumen in the left hemiabdomen prevents adequate exteriorization of the intussusception through a left paralumbar incision. Most often diagnostic exploratory laparotomy is performed with the cow standing after regional anesthesia. Tension on the mesentery of the small intestine results in pain and cattle may attempt to lie down during the procedure. Preoperative planning should anticipate this possibility. When intussusception is suspected and the animal is of high perceived economic value, right paralumbar fossa celiotomy may be performed with the patient under general anesthesia and in left lateral recumbency. The intussusception may be more difficult to elevate through the incision in recumbent cattle because the fluid-filled bowel gravitates away from the surgical site, but isolation and resection of the intussusception can be done without risk of the animal lying down during the procedure and with minimal risk of contamination of the abdomen.

Surgical removal by resection and anastomosis is the treatment of choice for intussusception. Manual reduction of the intussusception is not recommended because of the risk of rupture of the intestine during manipulation, probable ischemic necrosis of the intestine after surgery, possible reoccurrence of the intussusception, and prolonged ileus caused by motility disturbance and swelling in the affected segment of bowel. The margins for excision are selected in healthy-appearing intestine. In general, the distal margin may be 10 cm aboral to the lesion, but the proximal margin should be a minimum of 30 cm orad to the lesion. The larger proximal segment is chosen because chronic distention, inflammation, microvascular thrombosis, relative ischemia, and noxious ingesta accumulated in this segment may cause severe and prolonged postoperative ileus. The mesenteric vessels (arteries and veins) are ligated using "mass ligation" with absorbable suture material, being sure not to compromise the blood supply to the intestine to be preserved. Mass ligation is required because cattle do not have an arcuate vascular anatomy, as do horses. The sutures are placed in an overlapping pattern such that double ligation of the vessels is accomplished. In our experience, stapling instrumentation is highly unreliable for occlusion of mesenteric vessels because of the large amount of fat normally found in the intestinal mesentery of cattle. After completion of mesentery ligation and transection, Doyen intestinal forceps are used to occlude the lumen of the normal and abnormal bowel. The intussusception and associated bowel is then resected and discarded. The proximal segment of bowel is carefully exteriorized to its maximum length and the Doyen forceps is removed. Ingesta contained within the intestine orad to the lesion is "milked" out through the enterectomy site, being careful not to contaminate the incision or abdomen with ingesta. This procedure will lessen the severity of postoperative ileus and shorten convalescence. The two segments of intestine are reunited by end-to-end or side-to-side anastomosis with an absorbable suture material, using a simple continuous suture pattern. The anastomosis is performed in three overlapping suture lines, each placed in one third of the circumference, or in four overlapping suture lines, each placed in one fourth of the circumference, so that a "purse-string" effect is not created. The initial suture line should be placed at the mesenteric attachment because this is the most likely site of leakage. A second row of sutures is placed to prevent leakage using interrupted segments of inverting suture patterns (e.g., Cushing or Lembert). The affected intestine is thoroughly washed with sterile isotonic fluids, checked for the presence of leakage, and replaced into the abdomen. We prefer to place a solution of antibiotic 5 million units penicillin G potassium, or 1 of sodium ceftiofur, heparin (20 units/kg body weight), and saline (1000 mL) into the abdomen before closing the abdominal wall in routine fashion.

Postoperative management should be directed at preventing dehydration, maintaining optimal blood electrolyte concentration, controlling for infection and inflammation, and stimulating appetite. Intravenous (IV) fluids are beneficial during the first 24 hours after surgery. Rumen transfaunation, 12 to 24 hours after surgery, may stimulate forestomach motility and appetite. Withholding food after surgery should not be done. Administration of butorphanol tartrate (0.02 to 0.04 mg/kg, IV) may help with the pain induced by ileus by providing mild visceral analgesia without direct adverse effects on intestinal motility.

PROGNOSIS

The prognosis for return to productivity after surgical correction of intussusception is variable and somewhat dependent on the duration of the lesion. Cattle generally respond favorably to surgery if operated on within 48 hours of the onset of the disease. Cattle presenting with severe dehydration (>12%), tachycardia (heart rate > 120 beats per minute), severe decrease in serum chloride concentration (<80 mEq/L), and severe abdominal distention are considered to have a poor prognosis for survival. Calves appear to respond more favorably to surgery than adult cattle. If viscera rupture is present at the time of surgery, the prognosis is grave. Of cattle in which surgical correction was attempted, 85 of 143 cattle with small intestinal intussusception, 0 of 4 with ileocolic, 10 of 11 with cecocolic, and 10 of 20 with colocolic intussusception were discharged from the hospital.[1]

PREVENTION

Recommendations for prevention of intussusception are difficult because the cause is seldom identified and a seasonal predilection has not been demonstrated. Changes in dietary management should be made gradually, and good hygiene and control strategies should be practiced to minimize transmission of enteric diseases or internal parasites.

REFERENCES

1. Constable PD, St-Jean G, Hull BL, et al: Intussusception in cattle: 336 cases (1964–1993). J Am Vet Med Assoc 210:531–536, 1997.
2. Pearson H: Intussusception in cattle. Vet Rec 89:426–437, 1971.
3. Smart ME, Fretz PB, Gudmundson J, et al: Intussusception in a Charolais bull. Can Vet J 18:244–246, 1977.
4. Archer RM, Cooley AJ, Hinchcliff KW, et al: Jejunojejunal intussusception associated with a transmural adenocarcinoma in an aged cow. J Am Vet Med Assoc 192:209–211, 1988.
5. Horne MM: Colonic intussusception in a Holstein calf. Can Vet J 32:493–495, 1991.
6. Hamilton GF, Tulleners EP: Intussusception involving the spiral colon in a calf. Can Vet J 21:32, 1980.
7. Strand E, Welker B, Modransky P: Spiral colon intussusception in a three-year-old bull. J Am Vet Med Assoc 202:971–972, 1993.

Intraluminal-Intramural Hemorrhage of the Small Intestine in Cattle

Guy St. Jean, D.M.V., M.S., Diplomate, A.C.V.S.
David E. Anderson, D.V.M., M.S., Diplomate,
A.C.V.S.

Intramural hemorrhage of the digestive tract occurs when localized collections of blood extravasate into the interstitial tissues or into the subserosal, intramuscular, or submucosal layers. There may be so much destruction of the tissues that exact localization of the affected tissue layer may be impossible. In humans, especially children, the duodenum is most frequently occluded by the hematoma and occasionally obstructs the pancreatic and common bile ducts.[1] In humans with intramural hematoma and obstruction, the clinical features have been described as severe upper abdominal pain, discomfort, and vomiting. The diagnosis is usually made using an upper gastrointestinal radiographic series.[1] Treatment consists of evacuation of the blood. The mucosa and submucosa are usually intact. In the absence of complete obstruction, the hematoma may resolve with medical treatment. Most duodenal intramural hematomas result from blunt trauma. Intraluminal hemorrhage occurs following ulceration or mucosal vascular rupture subsequent to an intramural hemorrhage. In cattle, intraluminal hemorrhage is most commonly caused by an abomasal ulcer. Abomasal ulceration type II involves rupture of a major abomasal vessel, with intraluminal abomasal bleeding, anemia, melena, and tachycardia often observed clinically.[2]

In our experience, intraluminal-intramural hemorrhage of the small intestine in cattle has been associated with various clinical signs including abdominal pain, inappetence, weakness, decreased milk production, dehydration, scant feces, abdominal distention, and sudden death.[3] Multiple loops of gas-distended small intestine are found on rectal palpation. Laboratory results are usually consistent with an intestinal obstruction.[4] Packed cell volume and total protein are increased because of dehydration. A leukocytosis may be present in chronic cases because of intestinal ischemia and necrosis. The electrolyte and acid-base status will vary and reflect the segment or segments of intestine being obstructed. If the hematoma and blockage are located in the duodenum or proximal to the midjejunum, hypochloremic, hypokalemic metabolic alkalosis is observed. If the obstruction is located in the caudal jejunum and ileum, normal acid-base and electrolyte status may be found for up to 2 days following obstruction. In the terminal stages of the disease process, the animal may be acidemic because of hypovolemic and endotoxic shock.

Intraluminal-intramural hemorrhage of the small intestine must be differentiated from other causes of intestinal obstruction.[4] In our experience, it is very difficult to differentiate this condition clinically from an intussusception.[4] The final diagnosis is usually made at surgery. Surgery is considered to be the treatment of choice for intraluminal-intramural hemorrhage of the small intestine. Appropriate fluid and electrolyte replacement is critical to recovery. We recommend a right flank celiotomy with the animal standing. This permits an adequate exploration of the abdomen. Single or multiple darkened loops of small intestine are observed during the celiotomy. The small intestine oral to the lesion is distended with fluid and gas. A single or multiple hematoma can be found. We have seen intestinal contents ranging from thick blood clots to bloody fluid creating an obstruction. At surgery, it is often difficult to differentiate an intraluminal from an intramural hemorrhage. In our experience, the length of the obstruction is extremely variable.

Intestinal viability is usually compromised and requires a resection and intestinal anastomosis. An end-to-end anastomosis is preferred by us. We have seen animals with multiple hematomas involving a large portion of the small intestine. In these animals intestinal resection was judged to be too extensive and euthanasia was performed. Culture of the hemorrhagic intestine most commonly yields *Escherichia coli*, but we also have cultured *Clostridium perfringens* and *Salmonella* sp. in a limited number of cows.

The prognosis is guarded to grave despite a combination of surgical and medical management. We have attempted medical treatment alone, without success. A combination of hypovolemic and endotoxic shock is often present and multiple resection of the intestine may be needed. Since the exact cause of this condition is not known, recurrence is possible and prevention only speculative. In animals in which the condition is suspected, we recommend immediate surgical exploration.

REFERENCES

1. Bailey WC, Akers DR: Traumatic intramural hematoma of the duodenum in children. A report of fives. J Surg 110:695–703, 1965.
2. Ruggles AJ, Sweeney RW, Freeman DE, et al: Intraluminal hemorrhage from small intestinal ulceration in 2 cows. Cornell Vet 82:181–186, 1992.
3. West HJ, Baker JR: Duodenal ulceration in a cow associated with left displacement of the abomasum. Vet Rec 129:196–197, 1991.
4. Constable PD, St Jean G, Hull BL, et al: Intussusception in cattle: 336 cases (1964–1993). J Am Vet Med Assoc 210:531–536, 1997.

Cecocolic Dilation and Volvulus

Peter D. Constable, B.V.Sc., M.S., Ph.D.,
Diplomate, A.C.V.I.M.

The ruminant large intestine comprises the cecum, ascending colon (which contains the proximal loop, the centripetal and centrifugal coils of the spiral loop, and the distal loop), transverse colon, descending colon, and rectum. The cecum and proximal loop of the ascending colon function as a single fermentative unit (the cecocolic unit) that further degrades the digesta through microbial fermentation.[1] Normal cecocolic motility consists of regular coordinated peristaltic and antiperistaltic contractions of the cecum and proximal loop of the ascending colon (frequency approximately one per minute in the cow) that result in thorough mixing of digesta. A number of pacemaker sites exist for these regular cecocolic contractions, but two important locations appear to be the ileocecal junction and the blind end of the cecum. Superimposed on this basic mixing pattern is the periodic discharge of ileal contents into the cecum, as well as complete evacuation of cecocolic contents into the spiral loop (approximately every 4 hours).[1, 2] Cecocolic gas also passes on to the spiral loop in association with periodic cecocolic contractions.[1]

CECOCOLIC DILATION

Definition

Cecocolic dilation is defined as an enlarged gas-filled cecum and proximal loop of the ascending colon, without vascular compromise or obstruction to the flow of digesta. The condition is most commonly diagnosed in lactating dairy cows,[3–12] although cecocolic dilation has also been reported in sheep and the goat.[13]

Pathogenesis

Cecocolic hypomotility or atony is considered a prerequisite for cecocolic dilation, with accumulation of gas and fluid preceding dilation. Cecocolic motility is decreased in ileus and hypocalcemia. The regular peristaltic and antiperistaltic contractions of the cecum and proximal colon are also markedly inhibited by a decrease in cecal digesta pH, associated with an increase in cecal volatile fatty acid concentration.[5] The feeding of grain or lush alfalfa is therefore considered a causative factor in cecocolic dilation, since it is accompanied by an increase in cecocolic fermentation.

In vitro studies demonstrate that α_1- and β-adrenergic receptors relax longitudinal and circular muscle of the bovine large intestine.[14] This means that sympathetic activation (such as that induced by abdominal pain) decreases large intestinal motility in cattle. Xylazine 0.05 mg/kg intravenously (IV) also decreases cecocolic motility in the cow.[15, 16]

Clinical Signs and Diagnosis

Cecocolic dilation is often secondary to diseases such as mastitis, metritis, left displaced abomasum, and other gastrointestinal disorders, so the presence of a dilated and dislocated cecum does not necessarily indicate a pathologic condition of the large intestine. The clinical signs of cecocolic dilation are nonspecific and result from the concurrent disease process. A tympanic resonance is often detected in the right paralumbar fossa caudal to the 10th rib, but the sound is usually not high-pitched and varies in quality over time. Rectal examination reveals a moderately distended large viscus (or more than one) in the posterior right abdominal quadrant or pelvic inlet and the presence of a normal or slightly reduced quantity of fecal material in the rectum. The most common clinicopathologic abnormality is hypocalcemia.[11]

The major differential diagnoses are cecocolic volvulus or cecal torsion (see below). These conditions are differentiated from cecocolic dilation on the basis of heart rate, hydration status, resonant ping size, presence of abdominal pain, fecal characteristics, and extent of large intestinal distention determined during rectal palpation.

Treatment

Cecocolic dilation does not require surgical correction. Treatment should be directed toward resolution of concurrent disease and correction of any blood gas, pH, or serum electrolyte abnormalities. The cow should be periodically monitored to ensure that cecocolic volvulus or cecal torsion does not develop. Dilation of the cecum and ascending colon can persist for months without any deleterious effect on milk production or appetite.[6]

If additional treatment is required, bethanechol 0.07 mg/kg subcutaneously (SC), a direct-acting cholinomimetic drug, is the best pharmacologic agent for increasing cecocolic motility and tone, with neostigmine 0.02 mg/kg SC or cisapride 0.08 mg/kg IV having lesser utility as a potential treatment.[4, 16] Bethanechol will also induced urination when administered at this dose rate. Metoclopramide 0.15 mg/kg intramuscularly (IM) and naloxone 0.05 mg/kg IV are probably ineffective treatments for cecocolic dilation.[4, 16] Treatment with these pharmacologic agents constitutes extra-label drug use, and appropriate withholding times should be observed.

CECOCOLIC VOLVULUS (CECAL VOLVULUS) AND CECAL TORSION

Definition

Dilation and displacement of the cecum and proximal loop of the ascending colon can result in severe distention, vascular compromise, and obstruction to flow of digesta. This condition is defined as *cecocolic volvulus*. The term *cecocolic volvulus* is preferred to cecal volvulus, since the cecum and proximal loop of the ascending colon twist about an axis through the mesenteric attachment of the colon.[3, 7–9] The term also conveys the integral role that dilation and translocation of the proximal loop of the ascending colon plays in the pathogenesis.

Cecal torsion is defined as rotation of the cecum along its longitudinal axis. The colon is not involved in the twist.[3, 17] Since the ileum enters at the junction of the cecum and proximal loop of the ascending colon, cecal torsion can be readily differentiated from cecocolic volvulus at surgery by observing the site of the twist in relation to the ileocecal valve.

Cecocolic volvulus and cecal torsion occur most frequently in cattle,[18, 19] although cases have also been described in sheep.[3] Cecal torsion appears to occur much less frequently than cecocolic volvulus.[3, 7, 19] Although the incidence of both conditions has increased markedly in cattle over the last 30 years, they do not occur as commonly as left displaced abomasum or abomasal volvulus.

Pathogenesis

Cecocolic volvulus is assumed to result from dilation and displacement of the cecum and proximal loop of the ascending colon,[3, 7] although direct evidence is lacking. The same factors that produce cecocolic dilation are therefore thought to produce cecocolic volvulus and cecal torsion. The twist is located in the proximal loop of the ascending colon because this region is relatively fixed in position, being attached by the greater omentum and common intestinal mesentery dorsal to the descending duodenum.[9] The common mesentery will occasionally be so displaced by the cecocolic volvulus that volvulus of the entire intestinal tract ensues.[3] This is a rapidly fatal condition.

Cecal torsion results from dilation and rotation of the cecum at its apical end, since the distal third of the cecum is unattached and therefore free to move. Once a volvulus or torsion has been created, the pathophysiologic changes are identical to those observed with strangulating obstruction elsewhere in the intestinal tract.

Clinical Signs

The two conditions can only be differentiated during surgical correction. Cecocolic volvulus and cecal torsion occur most commonly in lactating dairy cows, particularly during winter and early spring. The majority of cases occur within 2 months of parturition. There does not appear to be any breed predilection among dairy cattle.[18, 19]

Most affected cattle exhibit signs of abdominal pain, associated with a precipitous drop in milk production and appetite. Tachycardia and rumen hypomotility or atony are often present. A large gas-filled viscus is usually detected on simultaneous auscultation and percussion of the right paralumbar fossa, and fluid splashes are often heard following succussion of the right flank. The ping normally fills the entire paralumbar fossa but does not extend as far proximal as the ninth rib. A tentative diagnosis is confirmed by rectal examination. Fecal material is usually absent, or much reduced in quantity. One or more large (>10 cm diameter) loops of distended large bowel are detected on careful palpation per rectum, with the distended colon or blind end of the cecum often filling the pelvic inlet. The small intestine may also be distended with fluid. The presence of more then one distended large viscus is suggestive of cecocolic volvulus.

The acid-base and electrolyte status is normal in acute cases. This is expected, since experimental occlusion of the ascending colon for 4 days has no effect on the acid-base or electrolyte status.[20] A mild hypocalcemia and hypochloremic, hypokalemic metabolic alkalosis is present with more prolonged volvulus duration,[19] as a result of small intestinal distention and obstruction. Severe acid-base and electrolyte alterations are observed with advanced cases associated with the onset of circulatory shock.

Diagnosis

The diagnosis of cecocolic volvulus and cecal torsion is usually straightforward. The major differential diagnoses are cecocolic dilation and colonic obstruction. Cattle with cecocolic dilation usually have a concurrent disease, the distended cecum or proximal loop of ascending colon is not tense on palpation, feces are present in the rectum, signs of abdominal pain are not evident, and the heart rate is usually normal. Colonic obstruction can mimic cecocolic volvulus or cecal torsion, depending upon the location of the obstruction, and exploratory celiotomy may be required to make a definitive diagnosis. Severe abomasal volvulus can be confused with these large intestinal disorders, but the resonant right-sided ping is usually located in a more anterior location and only one large distended viscus can be palpated rectally.

Treatment

The overall survival rate to normal production levels with surgical intervention is 75% to 85%.[18, 19] Surgical correction is best achieved through a standing right flank celiotomy, since this approach facilitates cecal emptying. Flunixin meglumine 1 mg/kg IV may be administered preoperatively to provide analgesia since pain from surgical manipulation of distended and ischemic bowel can cause cattle to become recumbent during the procedure. Treatment with flunixin meglumine constitutes extralabel drug use, and appropriate withholding times should be observed. Severe distention of the large bowel is immediately observed after opening the abdominal cavity, and the greater omentum is difficult to identify. Gas decompression of the large intestine is normally required before a thorough exploration of the abdomen can be performed. After decompression, the surgeon should determine whether the twist is primarily located in the proximal loop of the ascending colon (cecocolic volvulus) or cecum (cecal torsion). The direction of the twist is either clockwise or counterclockwise when viewed from the right-hand side.[18] The blind end of the cecum is gently exteriorized and a typhlotomy is performed at the most ventral portion. Up to 20 L of a green-brown malodorous liquid can be removed. The proximal colonic contents are also evacuated by gently advancing the digesta to the typhlotomy site. The typhlotomy site is closed with a two-layer inverting suture pattern and the cecum is thoroughly rinsed with isotonic saline. The cecum is then returned to the abdominal cavity, and the twist is corrected. The cecum and ascending colon should then be carefully inspected to assess the nature and extent of the damage. A partial typhlectomy should be performed if the cecum appears necrotic. The twist is usually located distal to the ileocecocolic junction, mak-

ing direct visualization difficult in some cases. The ascending colon is usually the site of the most severe vascular damage, and resection of necrotic colon, although technically difficult, has been accomplished.[21] Severe damage to this area is more easily handled by infolding the necrotic portion if it is focal, bypassing the area with a side-to-side colo-colic anastomosis, placing an omental patch over the necrotic area, or simply leaving the necrotic area in situ. Parenteral antibiotics and IV fluid therapy should be administered, as required.

A profuse, watery diarrhea should be present within 12 hours of surgical correction. Failure to pass feces within 24 hours of surgery suggests that the volvulus has not been completely corrected, and a second surgery is indicated. A recurrence rate of at least 10% has been reported,[18, 19] in which case partial typhlectomy should be performed at the second surgery. Recurrence may reflect a preexisting anatomic abnormality, since marked abnormalities in the omental attachments to the large intestine have been observed in a bull with recurrent cecocolic volvulus.[22] Resection of the blind end of the cecum is not routinely performed at the initial surgery, since typhlectomy prolongs surgery time and increases the degree of contamination.[19] In addition, typhlectomy has not been proved to successfully prevent further episodes of cecal dilation and subsequent volvulus. Partial typhlectomy could potentially predispose the cow to further episodes of cecocolic dilation and displacement, by altering normal cecocolic motility.

REFERENCES

1. Ruckebusch Y: Gastrointestinal motor functions in ruminants. In Wood JL (ed): Handbook of Physiology, Gastrointestinal Tract II. Bethesda, Md, American Physiological Society, 1990 pp 1225–1281.
2. Steiner A, Roussel AJ, Brumbaugh GW, et al: Myoelectric activity of the cecum and proximal loop of the ascending colon in cows. Am J Vet Res 55:1037–1043, 1994.
3. Pearson H: Dilatation and torsion of the bovine cecum and colon. Vet Rec 75:961–964, 1963.
4. Steiner A, Roussel AJ, Martig J: Effect of bethanechol, neostigmine, metoclopramide, and propranolol on myoelectric activity of the ileocecocolic area in cows. Am J Vet Res 56:1081–1086, 1995.
5. Svendsen P, Kristensen B: Cecal dilatation in cattle. Nord Vet Med 22:578–583, 1970.
6. Duelke BE, Whitlock RH: Persistent cecal dilatation in a lactating dairy cow. Cornell Vet 66:301–308, 1976.
7. Dirksen G: Dilatatio et torsio caeci et ansae proximalis coli in cattle. Dtsch Tierärztliche Wochenschr 15:409–416, 1962.
8. Espersen G: Dilatation and displacement of the abomasum to the right flank, and dilatation and dislocation of the cecum. Vet Rec 76:1423–1432, 1964.
9. Smith DF, Kolb D, Wilsman N, et al: Clinical and anatomic description of dilatation and dilatation with volvulus of the cecum and proximal loop of the ascending colon in adult cattle. In Proceedings of the Second International Congress on Diseases of Cattle, 1988, p 1571.
10. Braun U, Eicher R, Hausammann K: Clinical findings in cattle with dilatation and torsion of the caecum. Vet Rec 125:265–267, 1989.
11. Braun U, Hermann M, Pabst B: Haematological and biochemical findings in cattle with dilatation and torsion of the caecum. Vet Rec 125:396–398, 1989.
12. Braun U, Steiner A, Bearth G: Therapy and clinical progress of cattle with dilatation and torsion of the caecum. Vet Rec 125:430–433, 1989.
13. Waldeland H: Caecal dilatation and displacement in sheep. Vet Rec 111:455–456, 1982.
14. Steiner A, Denac M, Ballinari U: Effects of adrenaline, dopamine, serotonin, and different cholinergic agents on smooth muscle preparations from the ansa proximalis coli in cattle: Studies in vitro. J Vet Med Assoc 39:541–547, 1992.
15. Steiner A, Roussel AJ, Ellis WC: Colic motor complex of the cecum and proximal loop of the ascending colon observed in an

experimental cow with large intestinal obstruction. J Vet Med Assoc 41:53–61, 1994.

16. Steiner A, Roussel AJ, Iselin U: Effect of xylazine, cisapride, and naloxone on myoelectric activity of the ilececocolic area in cows. Am J Vet Res 56:623–628, 1995.

17. Oehme FW: Torsion of the cecum in a cow. J Am Vet Med Assoc 150:171, 1967.

18. Whitlock RH: Cecal volvulus in dairy cattle. *In* Proceedings of the First International Congress of Diseases of Cattle, 1976, pp 60–63.

19. Fubini SL, Erb HN, Rebhun WC, et al: Cecal dilatation and volvulus in dairy cows; 84 cases (1977–1983). J Am Vet Med Assoc 189:96–99, 1986.

20. Hammond PB, Dziuk HE, Usenik EA, et al: Experimental intestinal obstruction in calves. J Comp Pathol 74:210–221, 1964.

21. Pankowski RL, Fubini SL, Stehman S: Cecal volvulus in a dairy cow: Partial resection of the proximal portion of the ascending colon. J Am Vet Med Assoc 191:435–436, 1987.

22. Wynn Jones E, Johnson L, Moore CC: Torsion of the bovine cecum. J Am Vet Med Assoc 130:167–170, 1957.

■ Atresia Coli

Peter D. Constable, B.V.Sc., Ph.D., Diplomate, A.C.V.I.M.

D. Michael Rings, D.V.M., M.S., Diplomate, A.C.V.I.M.

DEFINITION

Atresia coli is defined as the absence of a colonic segment. The condition most commonly affects the spiral loop of the ascending colon in calves; however, atresia coli has also been identified in sheep and swine.

PATHOGENESIS

Atresia coli occurs most commonly in Holstein calves; however, cases have been observed in Angus, Ayrshire, Belgium Blue, Hereford, Maine-Anjou, Shorthorn, Simmental, and crossbred calves.[1–3] Atresia coli is believed to develop early in embryonic life as a result of vascular insufficiency to the developing spiral colon. An association between atresia coli and early pregnancy diagnosis (between days 36 and 42 of gestation) by amniotic palpation has been observed, which suggests that in utero trauma might damage the colonic blood supply.[4] The sporadic nature, the multiple breed involvement, the association with rectal palpation, the development in only one calf of a set of identical twins,[5] and the absence of atresia coli in 14 progeny of affected cattle all suggest a nonhereditary cause. However, a study[6] has indicated that the condition is likely a homozygous recessive trait, at least in Holstein calves. The overrepresentation of Holsteins in two reported case series supports this premise.[1, 2] Holstein cattle are predisposed to atresia coli, probably because their developing colon grows at a faster rate or to a greater extent than is the case in other breeds of cattle.

CLINICAL SIGNS AND DIAGNOSIS

The absence of feces from birth, coupled with progressive abdominal distention, depression, and inappetence during the first 2 to 4 days of life, should alert the clinician to the possibility of atresia coli. Some calves exhibit a high-stepping gait, which is suggestive of abdominal pain. Passage of a well-lubricated flexible tube per rectum is occasionally helpful in establishing the diagnosis; however, great caution must be taken because the distal colon is quite fragile and easily torn. Atresia is indicated by resistance at 10 to 20 cm of insertion associated with the absence of feces. Cytologic examination of rectal contents for the absence of squamous epithelial cells has been used as a presumptive test for atresia coli. This test requires lavage of the rectum with isotonic solution, centrifugation, and staining of the sediment with new methylene blue.[7] The test is difficult to interpret. Barium contrast enemas are also of limited value in aiding diagnosis. They are often nondiagnostic and may result in rectal rupture, as well as increasing the cost of treatment.[1] Definitive diagnosis of atresia coli is made during right flank exploratory celiotomy. Surgical intervention is considered urgent because continued distention of the large intestine leads to ischemic necrosis, peritonitis, and perforation.

The differential diagnosis includes acute intestinal accident, abomasal volvulus, neonatal septicemia, acute diffuse peritonitis, and atresia ani. Feces are present or have been present at some time previously in the first four conditions, whereas atresia ani is easily identified on close inspection of the perineum. Meconium impaction is not considered a primary differential diagnosis because there do not appear to be any reports of this condition in calves.[1]

TREATMENT

Atresia coli is fatal unless surgically corrected. Despite poor initial success rates, advances in the surgical and medical management of affected calves have increased the long-term success rate to approximately 35%.[1, 2] Calves that are able to stand, appear bright and alert, and have a normal temperature and immunoglobulin status are considered the best candidates for surgery. Failure of passive transfer is present in at least one third of affected calves, and plasma should be administered when needed.[1]

Surgery is best attempted under general anesthesia via a right flank celiotomy. The distended cecum is elevated out of the abdomen and the meconium removed through a stab incision. After closure of the typhlotomy site with a two-layer inverting pattern, the colon is traced and the proximal atretic segment is identified. The descending colon is identified by retrograde passage of a soft flexible tube through the anus. A portion of the proximal blind end of the colon is then resected and an end-to-side colocolic anastomosis is performed. This technique minimizes postoperative motility disturbances and stenosis at the anastomotic site.[1, 2] An alternative technique that may be useful in sick calves is colonic depression, followed by cecostomy. This surgery can be performed quickly under local anesthesia. Success rates using this approach have not been favorable, however.[3]

Postoperative treatment should consist of administration of broad-spectrum antibiotics, frequent feedings of milk, and general supportive care. Calves can become severely dehydrated after infection by enteric pathogens because the spiral colon is often absent, limiting the capability of the large intestine to reabsorb water. A postoperative sequela in some calves will be gradual abdominal distention due to impaction of the colon associated with impaired nerve supply to the proximal colon segment.

REFERENCES

1. Constable PD, Rings DM, Hull BL, et al: Atresia coli in calves: 26 cases (1977–1987). J Am Vet Med Assoc 195:118–123, 1989.

2. Ducharme NG, Arighi M, Horney D, et al: Colonic atresia in cattle: A prospective study of 43 cases. Can Vet J 29:818–824, 1988.

3. Martens A, Gasthuyts F, Steenhaut M, et al: Surgical aspects of intestinal atresia in 58 calves. Vet Rec 136:141–144, 1995.

4. Hess M, Leipold G, Muller W: Zur Genese des angeborenen Darmverschlusses des Kalbes. Monatsschr Vet Med 37:89–92, 1982.
5. Hoffsis GF, Brunner RR: Atresia coli in a twin calf. J Am Vet Med Assoc 171:433–434, 1975.
6. Syed M, Shanks RD: Atresia coli inherited in Holstein cattle. J Dairy Sci 75:1105–1111, 1992.
7. Constable PD, Shanks RD, Huhn J, et al: Evaluation of breed as a risk factor for atresia coli in cattle. J Theriogenol 48:775–790, 1997.

■ Rectal Prolapse in Food Animals

Marylou B. Rings, D.V.M.

Rectal prolapse involves the protrusion of rectal mucosa and associated structures through the anus. It occurs in all domestic animals, with the highest incidence in cattle, sheep, and swine.[1] The greatest incidence of rectal prolapse occurs in sheep at 6 to 12 months of age, in cattle at 6 to 24 months of age, and in swine at 6 to 12 weeks of age.[1] A 1% to 5% incidence has been reported in lambs during the feeding period.[2] Animals are predisposed to developing this problem when tenesmus occurs or if there is a marked increase in abdominal pressure. Tenesmus may result from enteritis, constipation, coccidiosis, vaginitis or vaginal prolapse, dystocia, post rectal examination irritation, false copulation, or urolithiasis. An increase in abdominal pressure may result from constant overfilling of the rumen, heavy deposits of fat within the abdomen, pregnancy, prolonged recumbency, chronic coughing from pneumonia, parasites, or adverse environmental conditions.

Rectal prolapse has been associated in lambs with short docks (0.5 in. or less), perhaps resulting from damage to the supporting muscle structure and the nerves innervating the perineal area.[2] The muscles surrounding the anal sphincter have points of insertions on the caudal coccygeal vertebrae.[3] The removal of all or some of these vertebrae during the docking procedure may lead to anal sphincter relaxation and loose attachments of supporting structures of the rectum.[2, 4]

Plant estrogen intake by sheep can increase the prevalence of rectal and vaginal prolapse.[2] The use of estrogens as growth promoters and exposure to estrogenic mycotoxins have also been implicated as a causal factor in rectal and vaginal prolapse in lambs.[4] RALGRO (Mallinckrodt), the approved growth implant for feedlot lambs, contains the active ingredient zeranol, which has anabolic activity similar to the estrogenic compound diethylstilbestrol, but very little uterotropic estrogenic activity.[2] No direct association between the use of zeranol feedlot implants and rectal prolapse has been documented.[2]

A prolapsed rectum may be a sign of pyrrolizidine alkaloid toxicity associated with diarrhea and tenesmus.[1] Tenesmus followed by rectal prolapse has been seen in some cattle with liver disease.[1] It may be associated with diarrhea or be part of hepatic encephalopathy or may be aggravated by edema of the bowel from portal hypertension.[1]

Other factors associated with increased incidence of prolapsed rectums are high protein diets causing enteritis; antibiotic feeding causing anal irritation (pruritus); frigid weather, especially with pigs; and overcrowding in confinement areas or stressing animals through narrow passageways.[5]

The types of rectal prolapse have been divided into four categories: (1) mucosal prolapse (2) complete prolapse (3) complete prolapse with invagination of colon, and (4) intussusception of the peritoneal rectum or colon through the anus.[6] Types 1 and 2 are more common that types 3 and 4.[8] The first three types are continuous with the mucocutaneous junction of the anus, while the fourth type is a protrusion with a palpable trench inside the rectum.[7]

Small prolapses (1 to 2 in. or less), which are evident when the animal is lying down, may self-replace when the animal rises. More extensive prolapses will not self-correct and will become longer and larger as pressure from the anal sphincter causes failure of venous return leading to edema.[8] Exposure of the prolapsed tissue results in drying, inflammation, and necrosis. The resulting anal constriction leads to partial or complete obstruction to passage of feces.[8] The combination of these events leads to continual straining and the continued abdominal pressure pushes the intestines and cecum against the rectal floor causing circulatory changes which weaken tissue and may result in a tear of the rectal wall.[4] Viscera may then be forced through this tear into the lumen of the rectum where, with continued straining, evisceration occurs.[4] Loops of intestine may also be forced into the pouch of peritoneum created within the prolapsed layers of rectum, complicating repair techniques.[4]

TREATMENT

An effort should always be made to correct the underlying cause and prevent the occurrence of prolapses in other herd or flock members as well as to lessen the inciting factors in the prolapsed animal. Surgical correction in some food animals, such as feedlot lambs, is thought to be economically prohibitive. Affected lambs should be slaughtered as soon as possible after the prolapse develops. For show animals, registered stock, or animals of greater economic value, treatment options consist of amputation techniques or replacement of the prolapse.

Various anesthetic techniques may be employed to aid in the correction of the prolapsed rectum. A caudal epidural lidocaine block may be used in cattle and sheep.[5] If difficulty is encountered with the caudal epidural technique, perianal local infusion of 2% lidocaine, especially around the subsacral area, may be used.[5] A lumbosacral epidural block may be used in sheep, administering 0.5 to 1.0 mL of 2% lidocaine to provide up to 2 hours of perineal anesthesia.[9] In adult swine, a subsacral paravertebral lidocaine block may be used. In smaller pigs, under 50 lbs, lumbosacral epidural anesthesia may be used.[5]

Techniques of Replacement

The following techniques may be used if the rectal mucosa is not necrotic, torn, or too dried out or edematous to be replaced.

Purse-String Suture

After replacement of the prolapsed tissue, a purse-string suture is placed deep into the tissues just outside the anal sphincter (0.5 in. from the mucocutaneous junction), drawn down to the diameter of a thumb, and tied in a bowknot. The material used should be broad (⅛ or ¼ in. umbilical tape) to prevent sawing or tearing of the tissue. Often this procedure may be followed by reprolapse of the rectum after the removal of the purse-string suture.

Pararectal Injections

This procedure is used to promote fibrosis of the terminal rectum in the pelvic cavity, providing a more permanent fixation technique. This technique is often used by the author in show lambs. An irritating substance, such as 2% Lugol's solution combined with mineral oil or iodine crystals dissolved in mineral oil, is injected into the rectal serosa, resulting in fibrous adhesions between the rectum and pelvic structures. Injections are made at the 9-, 12-, and 3-o'clock positions around the anus using an 18-gauge 3-in. needle. A volume of 1 mL of the

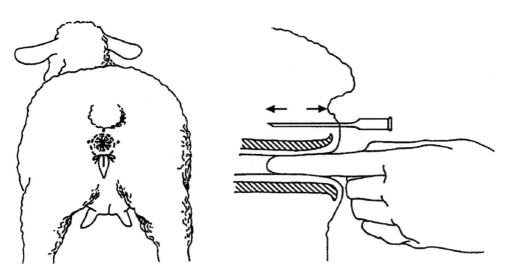

Figure 1
Fibrosis should develop around the sphincter and at a depth as great as the finger can reach along the rectal serosa.

sclerosing solution is injected at each of the three sites. One-half (0.5) milliliter is injected at the depth of the needle advancement and the remaining 0.5 mL is injected as the needle is withdrawn. A forefinger should be placed inside the rectum to direct the needle as it is advanced to make sure the sclerosing solution is placed along the rectal serosa and not in the rectal wall itself. Injection into the rectal wall could result in stricture or abscess formation. Fibrosis should develop around the sphincter and at a depth as great as the finger can reach along the rectal serosa (Fig. 1). A purse-string suture should be placed around the rectum for 5 days. The prognosis is good and an 80% cure rate is expected, assuming the underlying cause is removed.

In both the purse-string and pararectal injection technique, the amount of straining following the procedure may be reduced by the application of a mild antibiotic ointment to the rectal tissue if inflamed or irritated.

Amputation Techniques

Amputation of the Prolapsed Segment Using Prolapse Rings

These rings consist of rigid-walled cannulas with a suture-retaining constriction in the outer wall. The prolapse ring is inserted into the lumen of the prolapsed segment so that the constriction matches the anorectal line. The prolapse ring is anchored with a circumferential ligature (umbilical tape or elastrator bands), effectively cutting off the blood supply to the distal tissue. The avascular tissue will require several days to slough off and allow the prolapse ring to drop out. This procedure is not thought to lead to anal stricture. It is used most commonly in pigs but could be used in other food animals.

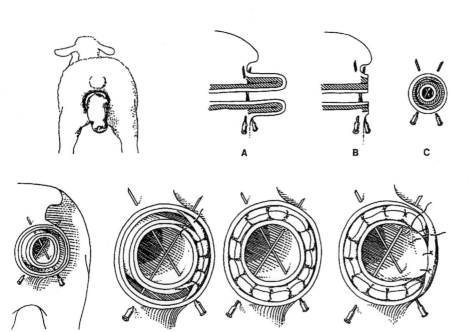

A   B   C

Figure 2
Full surgical amputation.

Mucosal Layer Resection

This procedure is recommended for mucosal or marginally complete prolapses when mucosa lacks viability or is moderately lacerated. This procedure can be used for the first three types of prolapses, although the third type may require a celiotomy.[8] A circumferential incision is made at the proximal portion of the prolapse. The mucosal layer only is incised. A second circumferential incision is made at the distal portion of the prolapse (is at the junction of normal and abnormal tissue). A dorsal longitudinal incision is used to join the two incisions. The mucosa is peeled away and the large blood vessels are ligated. Using absorbable suture in a simple interrupted pattern, viable mucosal edges are brought into apposition (it may be unnecessary to suture in young pigs). A purse-string suture around the anal opening is used in ruminants. The purse-string suture may not be needed in young pigs.[5] The advantages of this procedure are (1) less risk of peritonitis because the adventitia is not exposed, (2) the rectal arteries are not involved, (3) less postoperative straining, (4) the rectal lumen is less constricted, (5) no loss of healthy tissue, and (6) healing is rapid.[10]

Emasculatome

An emasculatome may be used for simple mucosal prolapses. Properly used, this constitutes mucosal resection. It should not be used in complete prolapses.[5]

Full Surgical Amputation

This procedure can be used on extensive prolapses or severely lacerated or necrotic prolapses. Retention needles are placed in the prolapsed segment (Fig. 2) to prevent retraction following amputation. The prolapsed segment is amputated 0.5 in. posterior to the crossed needles. Seroserous and mucosa-to-mucosa sutures are placed using a simple interrupted suture pattern. Another technique describes placement of the retention needles followed by amputation of one third of the prolapsed segment. Full-thickness sutures are then placed through the outer and inner segments and continued around the circumference of the prolapse prior to amputation of the prolapsed segment.[8]

When using either replacement or amputation methods, it is a good idea to administer 100 to 200 mL of mineral oil orally and withhold feed for 24 hours, followed by a reduced portion of a bland diet for 3 to 4 days.

REFERENCES

1. Smith BP: Large Animal Internal Medicine, ed 2. St Louis, Mosby–Year Book, 1996, pp 915–928.
2. Thornsberry RM: Rectal prolapse in feeder lambs: A clinical evaluation. Compend Contin Educ Pract Vet 15:1433, 1993.
3. Sisson S: The Anatomy of Domestic Animals, ed 5. Philadelphia, WB Saunders, 1975, pp 400–401.
4. Kimberling CV: Jensen and Swift's Diseases of Sheep, ed 3. Philadelphia, Lea & Febiger, 1988, pp 169–171.
5. Noordsy JL: Food Animal Surgery. Trenton, NJ, Veterinary Learning Systems, 1994, pp 149–154.
6. O'Conner JJ: Dollar's Veterinary Surgery, ed 4. London, Bailliere Tindall, 1958, pp 699–702.
7. Turner TA, Fessler JF: Rectal prolapse in the horse. J Am Vet Med Assoc 177:1028–1032, 1980.
8. Fubini SL: Surgery of the bovine large intestine. Vet Clin North Am Food Anim Pract 6:2:468, 1990.
9. Constable PD: Diseases of the large intestine. In Howard JL (ed): Current Veterinary Therapy 3: Food Animal Practice. Philadelphia, WB Saunders, 1993, pp 741–742.
10. Johnson HW: Submucosal resection, surgical correction of prolapse of the rectum. J Am Vet Med Assoc 102:113, 1943.

■ Helminth Parasites of the Gastrointestinal Tract
NEMATODE INFECTIONS IN CATTLE, SHEEP, GOATS, AND SWINE

R.P. Herd, M.V.Sc., Ph.D.
A.M. Zajac, D.V.M., Ph.D.

CATTLE

Major Parasites

Although gastrointestinal parasitism in cattle may involve several species, the abomasal nematode *Ostertagia ostertagi* is the most pathogenic and economically important in temperate regions of the world, including most areas of the United States. It is consequently important to understand the life cycle, epidemiology, and pathogenesis of this parasite and to plan control strategies with *Ostertagia* as a major target. Although *O. ostertagi* has been incriminated in most outbreaks of ostertagiasis, *Ostertagia leptospicularis* and *Ostertagia bisonis* may also cause disease. Control strategies effective against *Ostertagia* will also be effective against most other strongylid worms. While these other species, including *Haemonchus, Cooperia, Trichostrongylus,* and *Bunostomum* may contribute to production losses caused by *Ostertagia*, they are much less likely to be a primary cause of disease in North America.

Life Cycle

Ostertagia spp. have a direct life cycle. Eggs passed in the feces hatch first-stage larvae (L1), which develop and molt to become second-stage larvae (L2), which in turn develop and molt to become third-stage infective larvae (L3). This development may occur within a week under optimal conditions, and L3 may then migrate from the dung pat to herbage if there is adequate moisture. Following ingestion of infective L3 by cattle, the parasitic cycle involves development through the L3-L4-L5 stages within the gastric glands. This usually takes 18 to 21 days, by which time the young adult emerges from the glands into the lumen of the abomasum. Under certain conditions to be discussed later, the parasite undergoes hypobiosis (arrested development, inhibited development) and does not develop to the adult stage for several months.

Epidemiology

Seasonal Development of Infective Larvae

In Britain, western Europe, and the northern United States, contamination of pastures with worm eggs starts early in the grazing season, but it is not until summer that conditions are ideal for rapid development of eggs to L3. Hence there is an explosive increase in potentially dangerous L3 in summer resulting from eggs passed over a period of several months. New populations of L3 accumulate in the fecal pats through July, August, and September in northern temperate regions and become available to grazing cattle provided there is sufficient rainfall to assist the migration of L3 from feces to herbage. This pattern may be modified in a dry summer when L3 become trapped within the fecal mass and do not escape to herbage until fall rains occur, resulting in a big increase in pasture infectivity in the fall when L3 are likely to become conditioned for arrest. Young, nonimmune cattle are often exposed to light infection in the first half of the grazing season and heavy infection in the second half.

Marked seasonal patterns of pasture infectivity also occur in the southern hemisphere and southern United States. In many regions the hot dry summers or the alternating wet and dry weather in summer is adverse to larval survival. Even with irrigation systems, the alternating wet and dry conditions each day are lethal to larvae. In most regions with a mild winter there is a progressive increase in pasture contamination and infectivity from fall through spring because of the combination of high worm egg output and favorable environmental conditions. In summer, there is likely to be high mortality of pasture larvae and little transmission of infection.

Dairy cattle in confinement or beef cattle in feedlots are not exposed to significant numbers of infective larvae, although type II ostertagiasis can occur if cattle were harboring massive numbers of hypobiotic larvae when moved from pasture to confinement or feedlot. Although eggs may be passed in the feces of animals removed from pasture, it seems that conditions in confinement are inimical to development of eggs to infective larvae. It is possible that the high concentration of urine has an inhibitory effect in these situations. Infection with coccidia is often a bigger problem in confinement housing and feedlots.

Longevity of Infective Larvae

Although contamination of pastures with worm eggs may be continuous throughout the year, development to infective L3, migration of L3 from dung pats, and the subsequent survival of L3 on herbage differ markedly throughout the year in response to prevailing weather conditions. The fecal pat with its high moisture content acts as an important reservoir of infection and provides a safe haven for L3 during dry periods. The migration of L3 from dung pats to herbage is intermittent and dependent on sufficient moisture to provide a continuous film of water. Once a dung pat has dried out, rainfall of 50 to 100 mm over 2 or more days is needed to induce migration. When rainfall is intermittent, migration tends to occur in waves. The L3 rarely migrate more than a meter from the dung pat, but larvae may be spread over a wider area by temporary localized flooding after heavy rainfall, or by hooves, farm equipment, and insects. Preferred locations for L3 are close to the ground on the undersides of legume leaves and in leaf axils of grasses that spread laterally.

In northern temperate regions, numbers of L3 on pasture tend to be highest in summer and autumn following development from eggs passed in spring and summer. The L3 survive until the following spring when rising temperatures trigger enhanced activity and death following exhaustion of food reserves. Infective L3 of many trichostrongylid species survive well under winter snow and are then available to infect cattle turned out to pasture in early spring. The decrease in numbers of L3 as they die in the spring is accentuated by the diluting effect of accelerated herbage growth. In southern temperate regions numbers of L3 on pasture escalate in fall, winter, and spring if there is adequate warmth and precipitation, but die off rapidly under hot conditions in summer.

Hypobiosis (Arrested Development, Inhibited Development)

Hypobiosis is a temporary cessation of development of a parasite at a precise point in its early life; in the case of *O. ostertagi*, this occurs at the early L4 stage. It has been reported in a large range of nematode parasites (at least 30 species). It has important practical implications because it enables the parasite to survive in a dormant state during adverse periods, when it would otherwise be eliminated by host immunity or when its progeny would be destroyed by adverse seasonal conditions. This hypobiosis mainly occurs during the adverse conditions of winter in northern states and during the adverse conditions of summer in southern states. Many arrested larvae later resume normal development when the internal or external environment has become more favorable. They then seed pastures with eggs, often at a time when pasture infectivity may be quite low, for example, spring in the North, fall in the South. A massive synchronous maturation of arrested larvae will cause clinical disease, such as type II ostertagiasis.

The patterns of worm transmission tend to be reversed in the northern and southern temperate zones. Major accumulations of pasture L3 occur in summer in the North, whereas major mortality of L3 occurs at that time in the South. Major accumulations of pasture L3 occur in spring in the South, whereas major mortality occurs at that time in the North. Type I ostertagiasis mainly occurs in the first half of the year in the South and in the second half of the year in the North. Pre–type II ostertagiasis, the phase of arrested development, occurs in winter in the North and in summer in the South. Type II ostertagiasis, the clinical syndrome associated with the maturation of arrested larvae, occurs mainly in early spring in the North and in early fall in the South.

Host Immunity

Calves are most susceptible to worms during their first season at pasture, but generally acquire a strong immunity during their second grazing season. Cattle exposed to *Ostertagia* infections normally have a strong immunity by the end of their second grazing season. Hence the disease is mainly a problem of dairy replacement heifers at pasture or beef calves grazing contaminated pasture during the postweaning period. Adult cattle are little affected because of their acquired immunity. Nevertheless problems can develop in cattle that have received minimal exposure to parasites as calves or in cattle suffering immunosuppression from a variety of causes, such as malnutrition, concurrent disease, or chemotherapy. Cattle raised indoors or on drylots will have little exposure to nematodes and may not develop strong immunity. In general, dairy calves develop immunity faster than beef calves because of their greater exposure to parasites. Consequently, clinical parasitism is even less common in adult dairy cattle than in adult beef cattle.

Pathogenesis

The major lesions, biochemical changes, and clinical signs associated with ostertagiasis usually occur immediately after emergence of young adults from the gastric glands. Initially, cellular changes are confined to the parasitized glands, but when young adults begin to emerge, the hyperplasia and loss of cellular differentiation become more generalized, giving the abomasal wall a morocco leather appearance. Destruction of parietal hydrogen chloride–producing cells often elevates the abomasal fluid pH from 2 to 7. This results in a failure to denature protein, failure to activate pepsinogen to pepsin, and loss of a bacteriostatic effect, leading to the onset of diarrhea.

The hyperplastic and undifferentiated mucosa also becomes more permeable to macromolecules, leading to elevated plasma pepsinogen levels (>3000 IU tyrosine) as nonactivated pepsinogen diffuses into the circulation. Plasma proteins also leak in the opposite direction, from the circulation to the abomasal lumen. Necrosis and sloughing of surface epithelial cells may follow emergence of large numbers of worms, and congestion or edema of the abomasal folds may be encountered. The clinical consequences of all these changes are diarrhea and ill-thrift. In addition, a significant result of infection is appetite suppression. Although the mechanism of appetite suppression is not fully understood, it is now recognized that it plays an important role in both subclinical and clinical production losses caused by parasitism.

Clinical Disease

There are two main clinical forms of ostertagiasis: type I and type II.

Type I. This clinical entity results from the rapid acquisition of large numbers of L3 that complete their development to the adult stage in 3 to 4 weeks. It occurs mainly in young cattle up to 18 months of age during their first season at pasture. It is most common from July to October in northern temperate regions and from January to April in southern temperature zones. Clinical signs coincide with the emergence of young adults from the gastric glands 3 weeks or more after cattle are exposed to heavily infected pastures. The main signs are anorexia, weight loss, diarrhea, and mortality. It is common for a large percentage of the group to be affected, in contrast to type II disease in which only a small percentage show signs.

Pre–Type II. In this form, clinical signs are absent or mild in character, and the vast majority of *Ostertagia* worms (often >80%) are arrested in their development at the early L4 stage, slightly over 1 mm in length. Pre–type II ostertagiasis occurs in winter following acquisition of arrested-prone L3 in late fall in northern regions. In southern regions, pre–type II ostertagiasis occurs in late spring and summer after acquisition of arrested-prone L3 in spring. It appears that hypobiosis of *Ostertagia* is largely a seasonal phenomenon triggered by falling temperatures in northern regions and other, unknown stimuli in southern regions. Host immunity is thought to play a relatively minor role in this instance.

Type II. This clinical phase results from the emergence and maturation of large numbers of arrested larvae in the early spring in northern regions and in early fall in southern regions. Clinical cases have been observed in grazing cattle, housed cattle, and feedlot cattle, most commonly 2 to 4 years of age. Diarrhea may be intermittent, coinciding with the emergence of successive waves of developing larvae. Anorexia, weight loss, hypoalbuminemia, moderate anemia, and submandibular edema (bottle jaw) may also occur. Clinical signs are usually seen in only a small percentage (<10%) of animals coincident with massive emergence of larvae or loss of immunity.

Type II ostertagiasis can be differentiated from type I by the different seasonal occurrence, grazing history, older age of animals, small number affected, more protracted course, poorer prognosis, and insusceptibility to most anthelmintics. Although beef and dairy cattle both exhibit type II ostertagiasis, a higher proportion of hypobiosis has been reported in beef cattle production systems. On many dairy farms the year-round pasture contamination by calves ensures continual transmission of worms, and there is probably less selection pressure for the parasite to undergo hypobiosis to ensure survival.

Subclinical Disease

The reduction in feed intake and altered gastrointestinal function produced by *Ostertagia* can also produce significant effects on production in the absence of clinical disease. In many parts of North America, especially northern regions, *Ostertagia* infections are frequently associated with subclinical losses rather than overt clinical disease. Reduced weight gains in untreated stocker cattle and replacement heifers have been documented in a number of studies from a variety of locations and emphasize the importance of active parasite control in these susceptible animals. In contrast to the importance of subclinical parasitism in young stock, it has not been possible to demonstrate consistent, statistically significant, and economically important effects of subclinical infection in adult animals. While a number of studies have shown some beneficial effects of deworming on calf weaning weights and conception rates in beef cattle, and increases in milk production in dairy cattle, many of the studies lack adequate replication and statistical significance. Additionally, other studies have been unable to replicate the positive effect of deworming. The very inconsistency of these experimental results emphasizes the hazards of attempting to use blanket recommendations for adult animals. The potential benefits of deworming will be affected by regional climatic factors and management practices on each farm, and individual decisions regarding use of anthelmintics need to be formulated based on the considerations described under Control Strategies below.

Diagnosis

A detailed history is helpful in arriving at a correct diagnosis, as there is a lack of specificity in clinical signs and a poor correlation between fecal egg counts and worm burdens. Knowledge of seasonal conditions, grazing history, likely levels of pasture infectivity, nutritional and reproductive status, managerial practices, anthelmintic treatments, and the expected degree of immunity to worms is helpful in making a decision. For example, type I disease is most likely to be a herd problem in calves during their first grazing season, whereas type II disease affects only a small percentage of animals at the time when there is emergence and maturation of hypobiotic worms, that is, early spring (northern regions) and early fall (southern regions).

Clinical signs of anorexia, weight loss, diarrhea, rough coat, and submandibular edema are suggestive but not specific for ostertagiasis. Fecal egg counts may remain low in some animals in clinical outbreaks of disease and give no indication of the number of immature worms, inhibited worms, or adult worms in which egg laying has been suppressed by anthelmintic treatment or host immunity. Furthermore, it is difficult to differentiate eggs of *Ostertagia* from those of most other trichostrongylid species (*Haemonchus, Cooperia, Trichostrongylus*) or hookworms (*Bunostomum*). Plasma pepsinogen concentrations are sometimes better correlated with *Ostertagia* burdens than fecal egg counts, but false-positives and false-negatives may occur.

The most positive way to make a diagnosis is by necropsy examination and total worm counts. The distinctive abomasal lesions can be observed and aliquots of abomasal contents and abomasal wall digests counted for worms. Adult *Ostertagia* are fine hairlike worms only 1 cm in length and are easily missed on macroscopic examination, even when many thousands are present. A moribund animal or one that is profusely scouring sometimes expels many of its worms in the feces, so that the worm count is artificially low at necropsy. Whereas moderate worm burdens are pathogenic in young cattle, heavy worm burdens may be required to cause clinical disease in adult cattle.

Table 1
TREATMENT PRIORITIES FOR DAIRY CATTLE

Class of Cattle	Immune Status	Worm Exposure	Action
Bulls	Sex-related susceptibility	Variable	Treat
Cows at pasture	High	Low	No treatment
	Low	High	Treat
Cows on concrete or drylot	Variable	Low	No treatment
Replacement heifers 1st year at pasture	Low	High	Treat
Replacement heifers 2nd year at pasture	Variable	Variable	± Treat

Control Strategies

The question arises as to which herds or animals should be dewormed and which should not. This question must be answered on an individual herd basis and can be answered correctly only by the veterinary practitioner who is familiar with the farm and its livestock. There is no cut-and-dried recommendation that applies to every farm, and each one must be considered separately on its merits or lack of merits. The practitioner must make the decisions, drawing on his or her considerable knowledge of the farm, to provide a custom-made worm control program for each farm, instead of a blanket recommendation for all herds. Consideration should be given to each class of cattle separately, and provided for different control programs for bulls, dairy cows, replacement heifers, cow and calf herds, beef stockers or replacements, and feedlot cattle. It is also essential that practitioners appreciate local and regional climatic effects on prevalence and transmission of parasites which determine the most effective treatment times.

Treatment priorities for dairy cattle and beef cattle are summarized in Tables 1 and 2, respectively. When making decisions about treatment, two key questions should be asked:

1. What is the likely immune status of each group of cattle?
2. What is the likely degree of pasture infectivity and exposure to worms?

The answer to these two questions can be derived from the practitioner's general knowledge of the farm, its grazing history, and seasonal conditions, aided by the use of quantitative fecal egg counts. Laboratory tests may be misleading if considered in isolation, but can be of much value if the most appropriate technique is selected, and if the results are interpreted in relation to the history and management of the herd. Fecal egg counts are useful as a guide to the degree of immunity to worms and the severity of pasture contamination, but they do not measure the severity of infection. This subject is discussed later.

Table 2
TREATMENT PRIORITIES FOR BEEF CATTLE

Class of Cattle	Immune Status	Worm Exposure	Action
Bulls	Sex-related susceptibility	Variable	Treat
Cows at pasture	High	Low	No treatment
	Low	High	Treat
Suckling calves	Low	Variable	± Treat
Weanlings	Low	High	Treat
Feedlot	Variable	Low	Treat on arrival

Immune Status
The following basic facts will be helpful in decision making:

- Well-fed beef or dairy cows usually have a high degree of acquired immunity to worms, resulting in few worms (<3000) and low fecal egg counts (<10 eggs per gram of feces [epg]).
- If adult cattle have fecal egg counts in the hundreds, it generally means that they have lost, or never achieved, immunity. Thus, fecal egg counts are sometimes useful in assessing the immune status.
- Unlike lambing ewes, beef or dairy cows exhibit only a slight periparturient relaxation of immunity to worms. Hence, fecal egg counts may rise only slightly, from a mean of about 5 epg to about 20 epg after calving. This is epidemiologically insignificant.
- Young cattle under 2 years of age may have little immunity to worms, large worm burdens (>100,000), high egg counts (>100 epg), and suffer severe production losses and mortality.
- There is a sex-related susceptibility to worms so that young bulls are more susceptible than steers, which in turn are more susceptible than heifers. Thus, production losses and mortality are likely to be greatest in young bulls.

Pasture Infectivity
The following facts are relevant to any decision taken:

- Pastures perpetuate parasites, so the greatest risk occurs in nonimmune cattle grazing pasture.
- Cattle housed continually in confinement, stalls, loafing pens, drylots, or feedlots are rarely exposed to parasitic larvae, except for *Nematodirus* spp. and *Strongyloides*.
- The degree of pasture infectivity is strongly influenced by the previous grazing of a pasture. Young, untreated, nonimmune animals (especially young bulls) will cause the greatest pasture contamination with worm eggs.
- The degree of pasture infectivity is also strongly influenced by seasonal conditions. Warm, wet conditions favor hatching, development, and migration of infective larvae from feces to pasture. Drought conditions enhance larval mortality.
- Once a pasture becomes highly infective, the larvae survive long periods and pose a threat to all grazing animals. In the northern United States, larvae from one year commonly survive until late spring of the next year. In the southern United States, larvae survive well through fall, winter, and spring, but succumb to high summer temperatures.

Each Farm Is Different
Some examples of different farm scenarios are given below. Each farm needs to be considered as an individual entity and fecal egg counts done to fully evaluate the degree of immunity and pasture contamination.

- If a farm is well managed and the cattle well fed, most adult cattle will have developed a strong protective immunity to worms and there may be no economic benefit to deworming. In the case of beef cows, they should not be considered a serious source of pasture contamination for their suckling calves. This can be checked by fecal egg counts. Low counts will indicate strong immunity and low pasture contamination; high counts will indicate that something is wrong.
- In some herds, problems may occur in only a few individuals that have failed to develop a strong immunity because of genetic or other factors. These few animals with high egg counts can be treated or culled.
- Occasionally, a whole group may fail to develop adequate immunity to worms through lack of exposure because they were raised in confinement, or in arid regions, or in drought conditions where infective larvae failed to survive on pastures. They would later be susceptible to worms if moved to a contaminated pasture, exhibit high egg counts, and respond to treatment.
- Animals that were once strongly immune may lose immunity to worms through malnutrition, disease, or lack of exposure. Winter-starved adult cattle may lose immunity to worms and exhibit high fecal egg counts. In this situation, the adult cattle could be a serious source of pasture contamination of their nonimmune calves, and treatment of both cows and calves would be justified. Check fecal egg counts if in doubt.
- In a well-managed cow and calf operation, the suckling calves are nonimmune, but initially they will be exposed to little pasture infection because of low egg counts in their immune dams and limited reliance on pasture. Suckling calves also gain some protection from the milk diet, which alters ecologic conditions in the gastrointestinal tract to cause reduced establishment of worms and stunting of worm growth. In this situation, both cows and calves are likely to show low fecal egg counts. However, a preweaning treatment of calves weighing more than several hundred pounds may be beneficial in situations where substantial parasite exposure occurs.
- By weaning time, treatment of beef calves is usually warranted. Their fecal egg count, together with their history, will immediately reveal valuable information about their immune status and the degree of pasture contamination. A control program is usually of vital importance in the immediate postweaning period. This is generally a period of high susceptibility combined with high pasture contamination and infectivity.
- Dairy replacement heifers in their first year of grazing are usually very susceptible to worms and likely to be exposed to serious pasture contamination in grazing pastures previously grazed by similar batches of calves. A preventive control program is usually essential and its success can be monitored by fecal egg counts to check pasture contamination.

It is desirable that the veterinarian take control of the situation, consider each group of cattle separately, monitor fecal egg counts, and give the owner a comprehensive worm control program. Decisions should be based on what he or she sees on each farm, rather than on what is seen in advertisements, magazine articles, or nonrefereed journals. Such information can be inaccurate or misleading, often failing to give the whole story.

It is now widely accepted that young beef or dairy cattle are the most susceptible to nematode infections. Dairy replacement heifers are especially at risk during their first season at pasture, and beef calves are often exposed to high pasture infectivity in the immediate postweaning period. Control options for these

---

Table 3
CONTROL OPTIONS FOR DAIRY REPLACEMENT HEIFERS

1. Single rumen retention device at turnout to pasture
2. Two to three treatments at 3-wk intervals after pasture turnout (regional variation will affect optimal time for initial treatment)
3. Two treatments at 5- to 6-wk intervals after turnout with an avermectin product
4. Single "treat and move" to safe pasture
5. Alternate grazing with other species

---

two groups are summarized in Tables 3 and 4 respectively. These control strategies have been tested worldwide and have resulted in substantial economic gains, sometimes in excess of $100 per animal. With regard to mature female cattle, there is no scientific justification for a blanket recommendation to deworm all beef and dairy cows. There is no guarantee of an economic benefit to the producer or any certainty of increased milk production, conception rates, or calf weaning weights. Each farm should be considered individually and there is no blanket recommendation that applies to all farms.

Fecal Egg Counts

Fecal egg counts may be of great value in assessing both the immune status and the degree of pasture contamination if used and interpreted correctly. Samples should be monitored at key periods by quantitative egg counts of fresh fecal samples from a representative number of animals from each age group. Samples from five or six animals per group are often adequate, but a wide variation in counts of the sampled animals would indicate the need to sample a larger group. Samples should be kept refrigerated at 4°C to prevent hatching of eggs before the egg counts are done. Fecal egg counts considered in relation to the history and management of the farm provide an ongoing evaluation of the success of the program, the efficacy of the drugs used, and the need for any changes to ensure low pasture contamination. If pasture contamination is kept low, susceptible cattle will never be exposed to infection levels that cause clinical or subclinical disease.

It is useful to take fecal samples at key times. These may include the day of treatment, to check if the previous treatment was successful in suppressing fecal egg counts for the full interval between treatments. If cattle have high counts in the hundreds or thousands, it is not much use suppressing egg counts for a brief period, and then allowing egg counts and pasture contamination to return to pretreatment levels. Another key time is when cattle are moved to a new pasture. If it is found that they have high counts, they should be treated to ensure that little contamination is carried into the new pasture. In this way, clean cattle going into a safe pasture may be protected for months instead of a few days only. Adult cattle need fewer egg

---

Table 4
CONTROL OPTIONS FOR BEEF WEANLINGS

1. Single rumen retention device at weaning time or pasture turnout
2. Treatment at weaning time or pasture turnout, and repeat at 3-wk intervals with nonivermectin wormers depending on time of year, etc.
3. Treatment at weaning time or pasture turnout, and repeat at 5- to 6-wk intervals with an avermectin depending on time of year, etc.
4. Single "treat and move" to safe pasture
5. Alternate grazing with other species

count checks than young cattle because of their immunity to worms, but a suspected loss of immunity may be detected by a rise in egg counts. Fecal egg counts of young cattle are especially valuable in the postweaning period when it is usually vital to give strategic treatment to keep pasture contamination low.

Quantitative Techniques

A quantitative fecal flotation technique, such as the readily available modified McMaster (Paracount-EPG) technique or the homemade Cornell-McMaster technique, is needed in large animal practice. These techniques are simple, fast, and easy to use. They should be a part of every large animal practice, and are not for "research only!" The modified McMaster slide is commonly used to measure fecal egg counts as low as 25 epg, which is all that is needed for private practice, as any counts below this are epidemiologically insignificant. It should be remembered that only a small percentage of the eggs passed in feces successfully complete development to the infective stage. If a higher sensitivity is needed to detect low egg counts for adult cattle or for research projects, the more laborious Wisconsin double centrifugal-flotation technique can be used.

Fecal egg counts are of major value in measuring pasture contamination and the risk of serious infection, but of limited value in estimating the number of worms in the animal. Fecal egg counts are of little diagnostic value in cattle except when they deviate from the expected pattern. Thus, adult cattle usually have very low fecal egg counts (<10 epg) and contribute little to pasture contamination because of a strong acquired immunity to worms. However, high counts in the hundreds could indicate an absence of immunity and the need for treatment and changes in management. The lack of correlation between worm numbers and fecal egg counts occurs for a variety of reasons, including host immunity, worm fecundity, ratio of male to female worms, age of worms, diurnal and seasonal variations in egg laying, and the presence of hypobiotic or migrating larval stages, which have yet to reach the egg-laying stage.

In one study of 59 calves infected with *Ostertagia*, *Trichostrongylus*, and *Cooperia* spp. in Colorado, the ratio of worms to eggs per gram of feces ranged from four worms per egg to 2796 worms per egg. Striking differences may also occur in worm fecundity between species. Thus, a female *Haemonchus* may lay about 10,000 eggs per day compared with only 100 to 200/day for low producers like *Ostertagia* and *Trichostrongylus*, or 50 per day for *Nematodirus*. As many as 1 million hypobiotic *Ostertagia* larvae have been recovered from the abomasum of cattle with pre–type II ostertagiasis. These larvae have the potential to cause severe damage and death when they emerge from the gastric glands, but do not betray their presence by worm eggs.

Anthelmintics

Anthelmintics approved for cattle are shown in Table 5. Most modern drugs have high efficacy against the important gastrointestinal nematodes of cattle, and several of them (levamisole, ivermectin, doramectin, albendazole, fenbendazole, oxfendazole) are also effective against lungworms. Ivermectin and doramectin are the most efficient drugs against hypobiotic (arrested) larvae. The newer benzimidazole drugs (albendazole, fenbendazole, oxfendazole) also have some activity against hypobiotic larvae, but this is variable. The efficacy appears to depend upon the degree of hypobiosis. It has been shown that oxfendazole (4.5 mg/kg) has high efficiency against hypobiotic larvae in the South during periods of hypobiotic induction (February through April) and emergence (August and September), but efficacy is low during periods of peak arrest (May through July). The variable efficacy of oxfendazole was correlated with expected changes in larval metabolic activity. The newer benzimidazole drugs are also effective against tapeworms, and one of them, albendazole, is effective against mature flukes.

A variety of new delivery systems have been developed in recent years to simplify bovine parasite control. These devices are summarized in Table 6. The individual animal devices have the advantage that every animal gets the correct dosage. This is important to ensure maximum worm kill and reduction in pasture contamination. It also avoids selection for drug resistance due to suboptimal anthelmintic dosage. The group dosing systems have considerable appeal because labor is minimal and they sometimes allow a worm control program to be initiated where it was previously impossible. There is, however, a variable intake of drug, especially in heavily parasitized animals with reduced appetite or thirst. One cannot be certain that every animal gets the correct dosage, and there is a risk that suboptimal dosages will speed up selection for drug resistance.

Serious concerns have been raised in recent years about the ecotoxicity of avermectins. These drugs are almost totally excreted in the feces, where they have a prolonged half-life and high potency against both arthropods and nematodes, at ex-

---

Table 5
ANTHELMINTICS APPROVED FOR CATTLE

Anthelmintic	Trade Name	Spectrum	Dosage (mg/kg)	Safety Index
Albendazole	Valbazen	Nematodes, cestodes, trematodes	10	10
Coumaphos*	Baymix	*Trichostrongylus* spp.	2 (6×)	4
Doramectin	Dectomax	Nematodes, arthropods	0.2	25
Fenbendazole*	Panacur, Safe-Guard	Nematodes, cestodes	5, 10	20
Ivermectin	Ivomec	Nematodes, arthropods	0.2	30
Ivermectin-clorsulon	Ivomec-F	Nematodes, arthropods, trematodes	0.2/7	5
Ivermectin†	Ivomec SR Bolus	Nematodes, arthropods	RRD	
Levamisole	Levasole, Tramisol	Nematodes	8	3
Morantel tartrate*	Nematel, Rumatel	Nematodes	10	30
Oxfendazole	Synanthic	Nematodes, cestodes	4.5	50
Phenothiazine	Various	Nematodes	220	1
Thiabendazole*	TBZ, Omnizole	Nematodes	44	10

*Approved for lactating dairy cattle.
†Rumen retention device (RRD) releases 12 mg/day for approximately 135 days.

Table 6
NEW DELIVERY SYSTEMS FOR BOVINE PARASITE CONTROL

System	Anthelmintic (Trade Name)
A. Individual Animal Administration—Correct Dosage	
1. Rumen retention device	Ivermectin (Ivomec SR Bolus)
2. Pour-ons	Levamisole (Totalon), ivermectin (Ivomec)
3. Rumen injector	Oxfendazole (Synanthic)
B. Group Administration—Variable Dosage	
1. Medicated feed block, mineral, feed additive	Fenbendazole (En-pro-al, Safe-Guard), morantel (Rumatel), levamisole (Tramisol)
2. Medicated drinking water	Various drugs (e.g., Dosetroff)

---

tremely low concentrations. Ivermectin has been shown to have adverse effects on a vast number of beneficial and nonpestiferous arthropod species that are essential to the ecosystem. Most of the 250 invertebrate species found in cattle feces are useful and nonpestiferous, and aid in dung degradation, soil aeration, humus content, water percolation, recycling of soil nutrients, and pasture productivity. Several workers have observed significant changes in the dung-degrading fauna and delayed dung degradation of feces from ivermectin-treated animals, resulting in a reduction in grazing area. More research is required to determine if strategic treatments can be given at safe periods to reduce these adverse ecologic effects. Ivermectin contamination of water may also pose to a threat to wildlife. Ivermectin has been shown to be toxic at extremely low concentrations; the LC_{50} (median lethal concentration) for rainbow trout is only 0.003 ppm.

SHEEP

Sheep in temperate nonarid regions frequently suffer severe clinical disease and production losses from worm infection. Generally, ewes and lambs are most susceptible to helminth infection, whereas dry ewes and wethers are more resistant. Consequently, ewes and lambs (before- and after-weaning) should be given the highest priority in parasite control programs and safe grazing strategies. High concentrations of sheep at pasture and high fecal egg counts often lead to dangerous levels of pasture infectivity. The periparturient rise (PPR) in fecal egg counts is particularly important in lambing ewes, reaching much higher levels than in cattle. Sheep are less able than cattle to withstand the pathogenic effects of many thousands of worms, and serious outbreaks of helminthiasis are common in sheep. A disastrous situation may occur if parasitized sheep are kept on a low plane of nutrition.

Parasite control is most satisfactorily achieved by reducing the exposure of sheep to infection by the integration of strategic anthelmintic treatments and judicious pasture management. This is dependent on a knowledge of the epidemiology of each region. This is lacking in many areas of the United States, and there is an urgent need for more research of this type.

Major Parasites

The trichostrongylid worms constitute the most important group of sheep worms in the temperate regions of the world. Three genera, *Haemonchus*, *Ostertagia*, and *Trichostrongylus*, are the most abundant and most harmful in the Northern and Southern Hemispheres. They are responsible for severe production loss, clinical disease, and mortality. *Haemonchus contortus*, a voracious bloodsucker, is the most damaging species in warm and wet regions, becoming less important in the colder zones where *Ostertagia* and *Trichostrongylus* spp. predominate. Nevertheless *H. contortus* is a major problem for sheep in the nonarid regions of both the northern and southern United States.

Life Cycle and Turnover

The trichostrongylid worms of sheep have a simple and direct life cycle. Eggs passed in feces hatch and develop through free-living L1-L2-L3 stages within a week under optimal conditions. *Nematodirus* is an exception in that free-living development takes place entirely within the egg shell and hatching may be delayed until the following year. The trichostrongylid L3 is the infective stage, and parasitic development from L3 to egg-laying adult normally takes 2 to 4 weeks. Under certain conditions, development of *Haemonchus*, *Ostertagia*, and *Nematodirus* spp. in the gastrointestinal tract may be arrested at the early L4 stage for several months and then resume development later when conditions are more favorable. As with the cattle nematodes, hypobiosis has important implications for epidemiology and control.

It appears that *Ostertagia* and *Haemonchus* spp. have a short adult life span of only about 1 month and a rapid population turnover. Because of this short life span the number of worms present in the animal depends on the current intake of infective larvae from pasture. If the intake of L3 is decreased, as when sheep are moved indoors or to drylot, their worm burdens will rapidly drop. However, anthelmintic treatment of animals that continue to be exposed to new infection at pasture will be of little value. It merely removes an adult population soon to be lost, and the lost worms are quickly replaced by new infection. Anthelmintic treatment gives better protection against long-lived species such as *Trichostrongylus*. Thus, a single anthelmintic treatment may remove a large adult population of *Trichostrongylus* spp. that has accumulated over a long period, and it would be only partly replaced when treated animals were returned to contaminated pasture.

Epidemiology

Seasonal Development of Infective Larvae

The sheep nematodes, like those of cattle, exhibit marked seasonal patterns of infectivity with only one or two disease-producing generations of worms per year. In Britain, western Europe, and the northern United States, most eggs passed in spring and early summer complete their development to infective L3 in midsummer, resulting in an explosive increase of pasture infectivity at that time. In a dry summer, this may be delayed until fall rains occur. Pasture infectivity then persists at high levels until the following spring, when L3 start to die because of rising temperatures. Although L3 on pasture successfully persist through the winter, any contamination of pasture after September rarely results in significant new infections. In the Southern Hemisphere and southern United States, accumulations of L3 on pasture occur from fall through spring but may decline rapidly in summer if the weather becomes dry.

The Periparturient Rise

The PPR appears to be of considerable importance in sheep and swine but is absent or moderate in horses and cattle. The

PPR in goats also appears to be more limited than in sheep. It has serious practical implications for sheep nematode control. It occurs any time from 2 weeks before lambing until 12 weeks after lambing, irrespective of the season of lambing. At this time there is a general reduction in the immune response to worms, so that resistance to incoming larvae, controls on worm fecundity, and the capacity to expel worms are all diminished. It is suspected that lactogenic hormones are indirectly involved in bringing about these changes. The epidemiologic significance of the PPR is that it ensures heavy pasture contamination with worm eggs at the time of birth of the new host generation and transmission of worms from one host generation to the next. Although conditions may not be immediately suitable for the development of eggs to L3, there may be a dangerous accumulation of L3 later when lambs are relying less on milk and more on pasture.

Hypobiosis (Arrested Development)

Hypobiosis has important practical implications because it enables the parasite to survive in a dormant state in the host during adverse periods when there is a hostile immunologic environment or when its progeny would not survive in the outside environment. In contrast to the turnover of normally developing worms, arrested larvae tend to accumulate and may reach very large numbers, apparently unaffected by host immune responses. If a sudden resumption of development to adult worms occurs, it may produce a dramatic increase in pasture contamination and large worm burdens in the host at a time when pasture infectivity may be quite low. Hypobiotic larvae are also of practical importance because they are unaffected by some anthelmintics.

A marked degree of winter hypobiosis has been observed in sheep in the northern United States, with almost the entire worm burden of *H. contortus* (98% to 100%), *Ostertagia circumcincta* (89% to 98%), and *Nematodirus filicollis* (77% to 90%) affected. At this time the adult worm population is limited almost exclusively to *Trichostrongylus* spp. It appears that *Trichostrongylus* spp. have a long adult life span, which allows transmission from year to year, whereas *O. circumcincta* and *H. contortus* have short life spans, and a greater reliance on survival from year to year in the hypobiotic state. Hypobiosis is especially important to *H. contortus*, whose free-living stages survive poorly on pasture during winter. There is little information available on the occurrence of hypobiosis in sheep in the southern states.

Host Immunity

Immunocompetence against gastrointestinal helminth infection is slow to develop in sheep and may not be fully expressed until about 9 months of age. Thus, young sheep on infected pastures generally acquire heavy infections and exacerbate the situation by shedding large numbers of eggs in the feces. Although sheep eventually develop a strong resistance to *Nematodirus* spp. and moderate resistance to *Trichostrongylus* spp., resistance to *Haemonchus* and *Ostertagia* spp. is more labile, and outbreaks can occur in sheep of all ages. Immunologic unresponsiveness has been observed in the neonate, the periparturient ewe, and the nutritionally deprived animal. A genetic approach based on selection for responsiveness in young animals may offer the best approach to improving the immunologic responsiveness of young animals to parasite antigens.

Pathogenesis

Infection with *H. contortus* results in anemia and hypoproteinemia owing to the voracious bloodsucking activities of adults

and fourth-stage larvae (L4). Sudden death may occur as a result of severe blood loss. In addition, the migration of larvae into the pits of the gastric glands and the attachment of adult worms to the mucosa cause abomasitis. There is a significant rise in abomasal pH and plasma pepsinogen levels soon after infection, but not to the same levels as those seen in ostertagiasis. The activities of the parasite are believed to interfere with the digestibility and absorption of protein, calcium, and phosphorus. In chronic cases, death may result from exhaustion of protein and iron stores.

The other trichostrongylid worms have a variety of effects. The pathogenesis of ostertagiasis types I and II is similar to that described for cattle. *Trichostrongylus axei* causes abomasitis, whereas *Trichostrongylus* and *Nematodirus* spp. in the small intestine cause villous atrophy and plasma leakage into the intestine. Anorexia is an important feature and exacerbates the hypoproteinemia resulting from the protein-losing enteropathy. Deficiencies in digestion and absorption may be partly due to the loss of enzymes normally found on the microvilli, which results when villous atrophy occurs. Most sheep acquire multiple infections, and there is evidence of a synergistic effect between *O. circumcincta* and *Trichostrongylus colubriformis*, so that the combined effects are more pathogenic than one would expect from the sum of the effects of the two parasites acting separately.

Clinical Disease

Sheep infected with *H. contortus* may die suddenly without showing clinical signs, especially if driven. The main signs are marked anemia with pale skin and mucous membranes, anorexia, submandibular edema, and weakness. When driven, affected sheep may lag behind, stagger, go down, then rise and walk a little farther after resting. In most cases there is no diarrhea; the feces are drier and harder than normal and greatly reduced in quantity. In chronic cases there is extreme weight loss and the fleece may be lost. Sheep infected with other trichostrongylid worms show anorexia, ill-thrift, weight loss, diarrhea, dehydration, staggering, weakness, recumbency, and death. In some cases there is a black scour. Lamb and yearling flocks are most seriously affected, and once mortality starts, a few animals may die each day.

Diagnosis

Gastrointestinal parasites are the most likely cause of anemia, ill-thrift, and diarrhea in sheep in many parts of North America and should always be considered, especially in sheep suffering malnutrition. Diarrhea without ill-thrift or loss of condition is not often due to worms. A detailed history, including age, sex, reproductive status, likely immune status, managerial practices, and anthelmintic treatments, is helpful in arriving at an accurate diagnosis.

Fecal egg counts are a useful aid to diagnosis in sheep under 12 months of age, but it is dangerous to make a diagnosis on the basis of a fecal egg count alone. A total worm count at necropsy should be done wherever possible. *H. contortus* is the largest of the abomasal trichostrongyles, and the inch-long red-and-white–striped worms can be seen on gross visual examination of the abomasum in heavy infections. The other trichostrongylid worms are fine, hairlike worms that can be easily missed by a cursory inspection, even when many thousands are present. In addition to examining aliquots of abomasal and intestinal contents under the microscope, it is desirable to examine digests of the abomasal wall for larval stages. The interpretation of the total worm count must take into consideration the fact that different species are pathogenic at different levels.

Thus 1000 *H. contortus* may be just as pathogenic as 10,000 *O. circumcincta*.

Control Strategies

Many control programs are guided by guesswork, convenience, or desperation after mortality occurs, and they ignore reinfection, the PPR, hypobiosis, and selection for drug resistance. Many control programs give sheep a few days without worms before the process of reinfection returns their worm burdens to pretreatment levels. By the time that apparent clinical disease occurs, over 95% of the total worm population is likely to be in the environment so that treatment removes less than 5% of all worms, and sheep are subject to immediate reinfection. These haphazard treatments may stop some deaths, but they do not stop production losses. To reduce worm burdens on a more permanent basis, it is necessary either to give repeated anthelmintic treatments at short intervals (e.g., every 2 weeks) or to reduce the rate of infection by some form of integrated control combining the prophylactic use of anthelmintics with appropriate grazing management. The latter approach is preferable because it involves less drug cost, less labor cost, and less selection pressure for the evolution of drug resistance.

The modern epidemiologic strategies are summarized hereafter.

Prelambing Treatments

This is a key strategy for lambing ewes to prevent the potentially damaging PPR and clinical or subclinical disease in both ewes and lambs. When given to ewes in winter in northern regions, it is essential to use an anthelmintic (e.g., levamisole, ivermectin) that is effective against hypobiotic larvae, thus preventing maturation to adults and participation in the PPR. This treatment can be given at the time of winter housing or at any convenient period before the ewes go out to spring pasture. The object is to prevent them from contaminating spring pasture with worm eggs. Late-lambing ewes will require a second treatment just before or at lambing if they have already grazed spring pasture contaminated with overwintered larvae. In the case of both early- and late-lambing ewes, good results will be obtained only if ewes are kept indoors or in drylots or are moved to safe pastures following treatment to avoid immediate reinfection. These strategies do not work well if ewes are maintained on contaminated pastures. The "safe pasture" concept is discussed next.

Turnout of Lambs to Safe Pasture With No Treatment

Lambs raised indoors in a relatively parasite-free environment can be turned out to a safe pasture without the need for any anthelmintic treatment. A safe pasture is not necessarily "clean" or free of infective larvae, but is one where infectivity is sufficiently low that the worm burdens of susceptible stock moved to it increase slowly. Regrowth after mechanical harvesting of hay, silage, or small grain crops can generally be considered safe. The use of electric fencing may facilitate maximum exploitation of safe pastures on many farms. Pastures previously grazed by cattle or other species are generally safe because of the small amount of cross-infection between species. Nevertheless, calves less than 6 months of age are susceptible to *H. contortus*. Rotational grazing is usually not effective for parasite control because of the prolonged survival of infective larvae on contaminated pastures.

Prophylactic Treatment in Spring in Northern Regions

The advantage of prophylactic treatment in the spring is that it prevents the occurrence of the summer buildup of pasture infectivity and resulting clinical and subclinical disease. When market lambs or ewe lamb replacements are turned out to spring pasture, they are immediately exposed to L3 that have survived over the winter on pasture. Suckling lambs acquire infection from progeny of hypobiotic worms carried by ewes in winter as well as from overwintered L3. By midsummer, they may be exposed to a massive buildup of second-generation worms and clinical helminthiasis.

Studies in Ohio showed that four treatments at 3-week intervals, starting 3 weeks after spring turnout, were just as effective as eight treatments at 3-week intervals for the entire grazing season. It was obvious that the early-season treatments were highly beneficial, whereas the late-season treatments were a waste of time and money. Studies in Ohio also demonstrated the value of prophylactic treatments in the spring for horses and dairy replacement heifers. In all three host-parasite systems, this strategy prevents the escalation of second-generation (disease-producing) worms.

A program of prophylactic spring treatments is less successful in controlling parasite populations in the southern and southeastern United States. The milder winters and longer grazing seasons found in these regions often lead to a massive buildup of *H. contortus* larvae which cannot be effectively limited by strategic spring treatments. When strategic spring treatment programs are attempted in the southern United States, it is important to provide careful monitoring of sheep to prevent losses from haemonchosis.

Treat-and-Move Strategies

The rationale of this strategy is to extend the effectiveness of a single treatment by moving animals to a safe pasture to limit reinfection. Thus, if sheep are treated by July 1 and moved to a safe pasture in northern regions, they are unlikely to be exposed to the summer explosion in pasture infectivity. If they are treated and left on the same pasture, they will be exposed to heavy reinfection and derive little benefit from treatment. Thus, the move to a safe pasture is the key factor in this strategy. If a flock is moved to a safe pasture after treatment, it will enjoy several months of low worm burdens rather than only 2 or 3 worm-free days as the result of treatment alone. Infected sheep should not be allowed to graze a safe pasture; they must be treated before being allowed to graze. The treatment serves two purposes: it removes a potentially harmful worm burden from the sheep, and it protects a safe pasture from new contamination.

In the Ohio studies, this strategy initially worked well, but a marked rise in pasture infectivity was observed in early October. It appeared that there had been a buildup of *H. contortus* larvae aided by the high fecundity of this parasite and late-season rains favorable to development and survival of the free-living stages. It was concluded that a single treat-and-move strategy would provide safe pasture for a sufficiently long period for lambs that were to be marketed early, but a double treat-and-move system would be needed for lambs at pasture for longer periods of time. The latter would involve two anthelmintic treatments administered about 6 to 8 weeks apart and the use of two pastures ungrazed by sheep that year. Evidence from studies in Virginia also suggests that at least two moves are required during the grazing season to protect sheep from damaging parasite burdens. There is a need to study the selection pressure for drug resistance with this system because it can be argued that the safe pasture may eventually become populated with the progeny of resistant survivors.

Anthelmintics

There are only four anthelmintics approved for use in sheep in the United States (ivermectin, levamisole, phenothiazine, thiabendazole) and four for goats (morantel, fenbendazole, phenothiazine, thiabendazole). Sheep and goat nematodes have probably now developed resistance to all of these drugs in the United States. Widespread benzimidazole and phenothiazine resistance over many years led to excessive reliance on ivermectin and levamisole, with eventual selection for resistance to these drugs as well. The situation can only get worse in the future, especially as there are no new drugs with different modes of action in the research pipeline. Side-resistance (among drugs in the same group) and cross-resistance (between drugs of different groups) are also present. Side-resistance occurs between all benzimidazole and pro-benzimidazole drugs (albendazole, febantel, fenbendazole, mebendazole, oxfendazole, thiabendazole). Cross-resistance occurs between levamisole and morantel, and cross-resistance between phenothiazine and benzimidazole drugs may explain why benzimidazole resistance occurred so quickly after thiabendazole superseded the use of phenothiazine in the early 1960s.

The future outlook for worm control of sheep and goats is bleak, unless action is taken to abandon traditional approaches and develop new chemical and nonchemical strategies with less selection for drug resistance. The first need on any farm is to determine whether anthelmintic resistance has already occurred and to how many dewormers. The simplest way for the practitioner to do this is to carry out a fecal egg reduction test. This procedure can be done simply, using the McMaster slide kit described in the cattle section. Basically, fresh fecal samples from a representative sample of each test group (at least five animals per group) are counted for worm eggs at the time of treatment and 10 to 14 days later. If the interval is less than 10 days, the suppressive effects of drugs on worm egg production (without killing worms) may result in an overestimation of drug efficacy. If the interval is greater than 14 days, there is time for sheep to become reinfected and shed eggs from new worms. When the product being tested for efficacy is levamisole, the period between the pre- and posttreatment samples should be reduced to 3 to 5 days. Egg counts reach pretreatment levels more rapidly following levamisole treatment because of rapid maturation of larval stages not affected by the drug. Modern broad-spectrum anthelmintics should cause a fecal egg reduction of at least 90% if they are working effectively. This test gives the practitioner a good indication of resistance, but larval cultures, in vitro tests, and total worm counts at necropsy are needed for a complete evaluation. It is also important for the practitioner to ensure that the dose of dewormer given to the animals has been accurately calculated and delivered.

The following strategies will help conserve anthelmintic efficacy and limit the drug resistance problem:

1. *Avoid anthelmintic overkill at all times.* Suppressive treatment programs dosing sheep every 2 to 4 weeks will eliminate susceptible worms, but leave only resistant worms to contaminate pastures.

2. *Develop strategic treatment programs as outlined above.* Fewer treatments, epidemiologically based, will be just as effective for worm control, more economical than continuous treatments, and have reduced selection for drug resistance.

3. *Take care in selecting the anthelmintic.* It is a waste of time and money to use a drug if worms have already developed resistance to it. This is where the fecal egg reduction test is useful. Remember, there may also be side-resistance to a string of related drugs, or cross-resistance to unrelated drugs that share a common mode of action.

4. *Use full anthelmintic dosage.* It is better to set the dosage for the heaviest animal rather than for the average animal of the group, in order to avoid underdosing of some animals. Reduced dosages are likely to allow survival of worms with partial resistance (heterozygotes). They may then mate with similar worms, producing offspring that are highly resistant (homozygotes).

5. *Treat all introductions.* Sheep from an outside farm with a resistance problem may introduce resistant worms to a clean farm. Double dosages or a combination of two anthelmintics may be a useful safeguard.

6. *Avoid prolonged drug encounter.* This can occur with licks, blocks, or low-dose sustained-release retention devices that have a gradual tailing off of drug concentration. It may also occur with injectable ivermectin because of its persistence at low concentrations for several weeks after treatment.

7. *Rotation of anthelmintics.* An annual rotation of drugs of different chemical families (e.g., ivermectin, levamisole, benzimidazoles) is recommended because frequent rotation of anthelmintic types has led to the selection of multiple drug resistance in the past. Do not include any drugs in the rotation to which worms have already developed resistance, or any drugs that are side- or cross-resistant.

8. *Synergism of anthelmintics.* Combinations of drugs sometimes result in synergistic increases in efficacy. For example, administration of both levamisole and a benzimidazole compound resulted in improved efficacy against benzimidazole-resistant worms in both sheep and goats. Simultaneous administration of ivermectin and either levamsiole or fenbendazole was also effective against an *Ostertagia* strain with multiple drug resistance in New Zealand. Chemical modification of existing drugs and novel delivery systems may also be used to enhance drug efficacy in the future.

9. *Improved drug absorption.* Research from Australia has shown that when benzimidazole-resistant parasites are present, the efficacy of benzimidazole treatment can be improved by administering two single-dose treatments separated by a 12-hour interval. This regimen is more effective than giving a single double-dose treatment. Efficacy of both ivermectin and benzimidazole drenches can also be improved by offering little or no feed (while continuing to provide adequate water) to sheep 24 hours before treatment. Limiting food will slow the movement of intestinal contents and extend the period of drug uptake. Following drenching, sheep should be held for an additional 6 hours off feed. Food should not be withheld from sheep which are stressed, in poor condition, or heavily pregnant.

Finally, care should be taken when drenching sheep to ensure that the drug reaches the rumen. If placed in the front of the mouth, the esophageal groove may be activated, which will cause the product to bypass the rumen and go directly into the abomasum, reducing the effectiveness of the drug.

10. *Breeding genetically resistant hosts.* In Australia and New Zealand, successful selection of lines of sheep with enhanced resistance to parasites has been carried out in recent years. New techniques of embryo splitting and transfer introduce the possibility of accelerating the selection of genetically resistant flocks to parasites. Heritability of resistance to worms appears to be high and associations have been found between acquired resistance and certain lymphocyte antigen markers.

11. *Worm vaccines for sheep.* Several antigens of *H. contortus* and *T. colubriformis* have been identified as host-protective and are being genetically engineered prior to their assessment in vaccination trials.

12. *Biological controls of nematodes.* Studies of both dung beetles

and nematode-killing fungi have given promising results and warrant further examination.

13. *Management strategies.* Lambing ewes, suckling lambs, and weanlings are the most susceptible to worms, while dry ewes and wethers are more resistant. It is therefore desirable to design management systems that save the safest pastures for the most susceptible groups. Movement of sheep to safe pastures, the drylot, or indoors after pastures become highly infective is of more value than anthelmintic treatments. Alternate grazing with cattle should induce the same parasitologic benefits as leaving pastures ungrazed for long periods, but without the economic or agronomic disadvantages. Dry ewes and wethers, more resistant to worms, can also help reduce levels of pasture contamination. Rotational grazing with a single species is of little or no value since movement of animals occurs too rapidly to allow substantial reductions in the numbers of infective larvae.

GOATS

The major nematode pathogens of sheep are also the major pathogens of goats, and recommendations for parasite control in goats are frequently based on data obtained in sheep. This approach is not always the most effective, because it ignores differences in management, grazing habits, epidemiology, and the pharmacokinetics of anthelmintics. Parasites are a minor problem where goats browse bushy herbage and avoid grazing close to the ground. Haemonchosis is the primary problem where goats graze pasture in warm, humid areas, particularly in the South and Southeast, but it occurs throughout the United States. *Ostertagia* is more important in the northern and central states, while *Trichostrongylus* spp. contribute to helminthiasis in both northern and southern regions. Signs of helminthiasis include anorexia, anemia, ill-thrift, weight loss, diarrhea, rough coat, and mortality. Evidence suggests that goats may be even more susceptible than sheep to the pathogenic effects of *Haemonchus* and related nematodes.

Suppressive anthelmintic treatments with a variety of dewormers is often relied upon during the peak transmission season but may lead to multiple drug resistance. It would be more logical to initiate some of the prophylactic strategies described in the previous section for sheep, to obtain better parasite control and production gains with less selection for drug resistance. These strategies include preparturient treatments, prophylactic treatments in spring in northern regions, and treat-and-move strategies with movement to safe pastures. This ensures protection for several months instead of several days. Safe pastures, such as regrowth after harvesting, provide safe grazing. This is not the case with rotational grazing, where parasite populations may even be increased. However, improved nutritional status due to rotational grazing may help offset the deleterious effects of increased parasite numbers. Exposure to most nematodes is minimal with goats in confinement, but coccidiosis and *Strongyloides* infection are likely to be problems in nonimmune kids.

Anthelmintics

At the current time there are four anthelmintics approved for goats in the United States: thiabendazole, phenothiazine, morantel, and fenbendazole. Thiabendazole and phenothiazine are associated with considerable drug resistance and are no longer extensively used. Because of side-resistance with the benzimidazole group of anthelmintics, the efficacy of fenbendazole is limited when thiabendazole-resistant worms are present. Resistance to benzimidazole anthelmintics has been increased in goats by underdosing this group of drugs in the past. Recent

research has shown that goats metabolize benzimidazoles and levamisoles more rapidly than do sheep and consequently require higher doses. For years, goats have routinely been treated with ovine anthelmintic doses. This chronic underdosing of goats with the benzimidazole anthelmintics has undoubtedly increased the rate of development of drug-resistant *Haemonchus* in the United States. Treatment of goats with benzimidazole products should include two treatments over a 12-hour period. As suggested for sheep, the efficacy of the drugs can also be increased by withholding food prior to and during the treatment period.

Ivermectin resistance in *Haemonchus*-infected goats has been documented in the United States. Morantel (Rumatel) was approved for use in goats quite recently and can be used in lactating dairy goats. However, because of cross-resistance with levamisole, which has been intensively used in small ruminants, it is likely that morantel-resistant parasites will be encountered.

Other recommendations for effective anthelmintic use described in the sheep section should also be applied to goats. There is clearly a need for more research into the pharmacokinetics of anthelmintics in goats, as well as the development of alternative parasite control strategies based on nonchemical methods.

SWINE

Nematode parasites remain a serious limiting factor to successful swine production, although the prevalence and intensity of infection vary with the region, type of housing, and management system. An increasing trend for total confinement of pigs has been associated with a decline in the incidence of stomach worms (*Hyostrongylus*, *Ascarops*, *Physocephalus*), as well as the thorny-headed worm (*Macracanthorhorhynchus hirudinaceus*) and lungworm (*Metastrongylus* spp.). However, the prevalence of some parasites in confined swine is as high as that in pastured swine. Problems often persist because of the incorrect choice of anthelmintics, inappropriate timing of treatment, and lack of fecal monitoring. In some regions, an increased incidence of *Strongyloides* has been associated with a change to permanent farrowing houses and liberal use of bedding.

Ascaris suum, *Oesophagostomum* spp., and *Trichuris suis* remain as serious pathogens in swine, both in confinement and at pasture. Newborn pigs in some areas suffer high mortality from *Strongyloides ransomi* transmitted via the colostrum. Liver condemnations due to *A. suum* and *Stephanurus dentatus* have increased in some regions, and the stigma of trichinosis still persists on the swine industry in the United States.

Life Cycle and Epidemiology

Pigs become infected with ascarids (*A. suum*) by ingestion of infective eggs. After hatching, L3 penetrate the gut wall and commence the typical ascarid hepatic-tracheal migration. They reach the liver via the portal vein within 24 hours of infection, then pass via the bloodstream to the heart and lungs. Larvae reach the lungs about a week after infection, break out of the capillaries into the alveoli, molt to L4, and migrate up the bronchioles, bronchi, and trachea. They are coughed up and swallowed, molt to L5 in the small intestine, develop to maturity, and pass eggs in the feces 6 to 8 weeks post infection. Female *A. suum* produce enormous numbers of eggs, up to half a million eggs per worm per day. The eggs become infective in 10 to 30 days under optimal conditions and are very resistant to external conditions, remaining viable for up to 5 years if protected from desiccation.

Pigs become infected with the nodular worm (*Oesophagosto-*

mum spp.) by ingestion of infective larvae (L3). These invade the intestinal wall and are found in the mucosa and submucosa of the large intestine as early as 20 hours after infection. The third molt occurs in the gut wall; L4 return to the gut lumen, molt to L5, develop to maturity, and pass strongyle-type eggs in the feces 7 to 8 weeks post infection. There is little host reaction to primary infection, but nodule formation may be marked in subsequent infections of sensitized animals. Sows commonly exhibit a PPR in fecal egg counts, reaching a peak 6 to 7 weeks post farrowing. Newborn pigs may be exposed to serious infection, as eggs can develop to infective L3 within a week under optimal conditions.

The whipworm (*T. suis*) life cycle is unusual in that eggs carry an infective L1 (not L3) when ingested by swine and all larval molts occur within the host. Larvae spend 2 to 3 weeks migrating within the cecal and colonic mucosa before reaching the surface epithelium and maturing to egg-laying adults 6 to 7 weeks after infection. The long filamentous anterior end of the adult worm remains imbedded in the mucosa, forming subepithelial tunnels. The characteristic barrel-shaped, double-operculated eggs become infective 3 weeks after being passed and can survive for up to 6 years in protected environments.

The threadworm (*S. ransomi*) can alternate between a free-living and a parasitic existence. Pigs may be infected prenatally, via colostrum, by ingestion of L3 or by skin penetration of L3. Transcolostral infection appears to be of considerable importance, with the greatest number of L3 passed on the first day of lactation. Counts of up to 50 L3 per milliliter of colostrum have been recorded. Sows apparently harbor arrested L3 in their fat depots until farrowing time when the larvae migrate to the milk cisterns of the mammae. Sufficient larvae may be stored in the fat deposits of the sow to infect four consecutive litters. The prepatent period is only 4 days following prenatal or transcolostral infection and 7 to 10 days following other routes of infection. Embryonated eggs or L1 are passed in the feces, and the parasite persists indefinitely in muddy areas.

Pathogenesis

Penetration of the intestinal mucosa by nematode larvae (*Ascaris, Oesophagostomum, Trichuris, Strongyloides*) or tunneling by adults (*Trichuris*) provides a portal of entry for bacteria, spirochetes, and viruses. Further migration within the gut wall may cause extensive destruction of tissue (*Trichuris, Strongyloides*) or a host nodular reaction, caseation, and calcification (*Oesophagostomum*) leading to interference with digestion and motility. Local peritonitis and adhesions sometimes result in intussusception or necrosis. Emergence of whipworm (*Trichuris*) larvae may produce dysentery 3 weeks after infection, well before eggs are passed in the feces, and be misdiagnosed as swine dysentery or proliferative enteritis. These parasitic cases do not respond to antibiotic therapy. Outbreaks of necrotic enteritis may be activated in pigs carrying *Salmonella* infections.

Migration of larvae through the liver (*Ascaris*) may result in interstitial hepatitis or "milk spots" and cause large-scale condemnation of livers at abattoirs. Larvae of gastrointestinal nematodes migrating through the lungs (*Ascaris, Strongyloides*) cause alveolar injury with edema and consolidation. Pigs become more susceptible to other diseases such as enzootic pneumonia and swine influenza. Severe gastric ulcers with fatal bleeding have been associated with both experimental and natural infection of *A. suum*, although the underlying mechanisms are not clear. Anemia sometimes occurs in pigs heavily infected with *Trichuris* as a result of bloodsucking and tissue destruction. Hypoproteinemia may be associated with any parasite when there is marked anorexia or a protein-losing enteropathy. Death

of young pigs sometimes results from invasion of the myocardium by skin-penetrating *Strongyloides*.

Recent studies have shown that *T. suis* infection facilitated invasion of the colon by opportunistic enteric bacteria causing mucohemorrhagic colitis in young swine. Anthelminthic treatment after the onset of signs reversed all disease and pathologic changes. These results indicate that treatment for enteric parasites such as whipworm can prevent disease due to enteric bacteria.

Clinical Disease

Ascariasis may be manifest in young pigs by ill-thrift, stunted growth, potbelly, and diarrhea. Adult worms may be vomited. Occasional cases of obstructive jaundice or intestinal obstruction and rupture occur. Larvae migrating through the lungs may cause "thumps" and elicit a soft cough. Nodular worms may cause weight loss and diarrhea in pigs of all ages, but rarely death. The diarrhea is often khaki in color and contains undigested food. There may be a blood-stained mucoid diarrhea if massive numbers of larvae penetrate the gut wall. The bloody diarrhea of whipworm infection, starting 3 weeks after infection, may be confused with swine dysentery or proliferative enteritis. Affected pigs may also show anorexia, weight loss, straining, rectal prolapse, and a high mortality rate. Newborn pigs with a heavy threadworm infection may show stunted growth, potbelly, bloody diarrhea, and a high mortality rate.

Diagnosis

The history, clinical signs, fecal examinations, and response to treatment are likely to be of value in making a correct diagnosis. The age of the affected pigs and their likely exposure to infective eggs or larvae are important considerations. Ascariasis is a disease of young pigs, and older animals rarely show clinical signs, although they may be an important source of contamination. Strongyloidiosis is mainly confined to baby pigs and may result from prenatal or transcolostral infection, as well as from L3 in the environment. The major nematode species (*Ascaris, Oesophagostomum, Trichuris*) have a prepatent period of 6 to 8 weeks, and it is possible for clinical signs to develop before the characteristic thick-shelled eggs (*Ascaris*), strongyle-type eggs (*Oesophagostomum*), or double-operculated eggs (*Trichuris*) are passed in feces. By contrast, the smaller embryonated eggs of *Strongyloides* may be passed as early as 4 days post infection.

Fecal examinations are of value in determining which parasites are a major problem, but there is a poor correlation between fecal egg counts and worm burden. A small number of *Ascaris* females may produce millions of eggs, whereas *Trichuris* females are not prolific egg layers and a low or modest egg count may be associated with severe disease. The most positive way to make a diagnosis is by necropsy examination so that the intensity of the worm infection and the degree of tissue destruction can be accurately assessed.

Control Strategies

The North Carolina Swine Parasite Control Program or its modifications can be used effectively in many regions. In this program sows and gilts are given a broad-spectrum anthelmintic 5 to 10 days before breeding and again 5 to 10 days before farrowing to remove parasites from their digestive system, which serve as a source of the PPR and infection in the farrowing house. Boars are treated twice a year. Young pigs are treated at

Table 7
MODERN ANTHELMINTICS APPROVED FOR SWINE

Parasite	Anthelmintic
Large roundworm (Ascaris)	Dichlorvos
	Fenbendazole*
	Hygromycin B
	Ivermectin
	Levamisole
	Pyrantel
Nodular worm	Dichlorvos
(Oesophagostomum)	Fenbendazole
	Hygromycin B
	Ivermectin
	Pyrantel
	Levamisole
Whipworm (Trichuris)	Dichlorvos
	Fenbendazole*
	Hygromycin B
Lungworm (Metastrongylus)	Fenbendazole
	Ivermectin
	Levamisole
Threadworm (Strongyloides)	Ivermectin†
	Thiabendazole
	Levamisole
Kidney worm (Stephanurus)	Fenbendazole (adult and larvae)
	Ivermectin (adult and larvae)
	Levamisole (adult only)

*Fenbendazole is effective against migrating ascarid larvae in the liver and lungs, and migrating whipworm larvae in the cecal and colonic mucosa.

†Ivermectin is effective against somatic Strongyloides L3 so that treatment of sows 3 to 16 days before parturition prevents transfer of larvae from dam to piglets via the colostrum.

5 to 6 weeks of age and treatment is repeated 30 days later. Anthelmintics to consider include dichlorvos, levamisole, or ivermectin as single treatments, fenbendazole for 3 to 12 days, and pyrantel tartrate or hygromycin B as continuous additives to the feed during the period of greatest risk. Swine should be kept on well-drained open lots, on temporary pastures, or on clean concrete or slats. Treatment is normally not needed for pigs in a clean operation on raised decks, but treatment of breeders once yearly offers a safeguard against accidental infection.

A major control problem is the great survival capacity of ascarid and whipworm eggs. Sometimes the only solution is to move range pigs to fresh ground and cultivate the old ground for at least 3 years before reintroducing swine. In housing, thorough cleansing with hot detergents or high-pressure water can be used to prepare surfaces for disinfection with agents such as hot lye (95% sodium hydroxide). The disinfectant should be applied to walls and left for 2 to 3 days and then hosed away before pigs are returned. It is advisable to scrub sows thoroughly with hot detergent and water to remove eggs before moving them into a farrowing pen that has been cleaned and disinfected. Sows should also be treated a few days before they enter the farrowing pen so that feces containing viable eggs and expelled worms will not be introduced. Likewise, if young pigs are to be returned to pasture after treatment, it is preferable to confine them on concrete for 1 to 2 days, and to destroy all feces and expelled worms before the pigs are returned to pasture.

Feeder pigs can receive single treatments or continuous-feed medication with pyrantel tartrate or hygromycin B. Where pigs are run on dirt and subject to continuous reinfection, it is more effective to provide a continuous-feed additive. Baby pigs should be treated with thiabendazole, levamisole, or ivermectin at 5 and 10 days of age if threadworm (Strongyloides) is a problem. It

is imperative to keep breeding stock on dry, well-drained surfaces, because Strongyloides is capable of reproducing in a free-living cycle and will persist indefinitely in muddy areas. If the swine kidney worm (Stephanurus dentatus) is a problem, both adult and larval stages can be killed by fenbendazole and adults by levamisole. The "gilt only" farrowing system may also be considered, but it has the disadvantage of producing smaller litters.

Anthelmintics

Modern swine anthelmintics have high efficiency, high safety, and easy administration. Most are available for administration in the feed, but ivermectin is also available in injectable form and levamisole can be given in the drinking water. Swine anthelmintics have high efficacy against the major parasites (Table 7). A high safety index is essential when swine are treated on a herd basis and there is variation in individual drug consumption rates. The safety of dichlorvos, the only organophosphate approved for swine, has been enhanced by incorporation of the drug into slow-release resin pellets. Cataracts and deafness may occur in swine fed hygromycin B for prolonged periods. At three times the recommended dosage, transient salivation and vomiting may occur in pigs given levamisole. Coughing and vomiting may also occur as pigs infected with lungworms expel the parasites. Fenbendazole and ivermectin are both safe in swine.

TREMATODE INFECTIONS IN CATTLE, SHEEP, AND GOATS
R.P. Herd, M.V.Sc., Ph.D.

Fasciola hepatica is the most important trematode of livestock throughout the world. It is an increasing problem as new dams, irrigation projects, and improved water facilities provide new habitats for the lymnaeid snail intermediate hosts. Acute fluke disease causes high mortality in sheep, while chronic fluke disease causes substantial production losses in both cattle and sheep. Several studies suggest that effective control can result in increased mature cow body weights, conception rates, milk production, and calf weaning weights. Feedlot studies have demonstrated increased weight gains and feed conversion rates, with reduced liver rejection rates at abattoirs.

In the United States, *F. hepatica* occurs primarily in the Gulf States and western states, whereas *Fasciola gigantica* occurs in Hawaii. *Fascioloides magna* is an additional problem in the Gulf States, the Great Lakes region, and in the northwestern states where cattle, sheep, or goats share pastures with deer, elk, and moose natural hosts. *Dicrocoelium dendriticum*, the small black lanceolate fluke, is restricted to foci in New York State. The paramphistomes, or rumen flukes, appear to be of minor economic significance in the United States, although heavy infections can cause severe enteritis and mortality in cattle and occasionally in sheep and goats elsewhere. *Paramphistomum microbothrioides* (syn. *Cotylophoron cotylophorum*) is the most common species in the United States.

LIFE CYCLE

Trematodes have an indirect life cycle with a snail intermediate host. *F. hepatica*, *F. gigantica*, *Fasc. magna*, and *P. microbothrioides* all have aquatic snail intermediate hosts. *D. dendriticum* has a land snail as its first intermediate host and a brown ant as its second intermediate host. One fluke egg passed by the cattle, sheep, or goat final host can give rise to thousands of infective cercariae or metacercariae. This has great epidemiologic importance and is in marked contrast to the situation with nematodes, in which one egg produces only one infective larva. Eggs of *Fasciola*, *Fascioloides*, and *Paramphistomum* spp. hatch in water to miracidia, which develop through sporocyst, redia, and cercaria stages after miracidia actively penetrate the appropriate snail intermediate host. Cercariae later emerge from the snail and encyst as metacercariae on herbage to be eaten by the final host. Eggs of *Dicrocoelium* are ingested by land snails, which later expel slime balls containing up to 400 cercariae. Whole colonies of brown ants may become infected by eating slime balls. The final host is infected by ingesting ants attached to herbage.

Most livestock are infected by ingestion of metacercariae from pasture, although prenatal infection with *F. hepatica* has been reported in a small percentage of calves. Metacercariae excyst in the small intestine, and young flukes migrate through the gut wall and peritoneal cavity to reach the liver in 4 to 6 days. They remain in the hepatic parenchyma for 6 to 8 weeks, then enter the bile ducts and mature to egg-laying adults 10 to 12 weeks after infection. The life cycle of *F. gigantica* is similar to that of *F. hepatica*. *Fasc. magna* completes the full life cycle only in deer, elk, or moose natural hosts. Adults are enclosed in thin-walled cysts in the hepatic parenchyma, and eggs escape via fistulas to the bile ducts. In cattle, young flukes become completely encapsulated by a host reaction in the liver and there is no channel for release of eggs to the exterior. Thus diagnosis is not possible by fecal examination. In sheep and goats, young flukes tunnel extensively, causing severe damage to the parenchyma, and ultimately cause host death. Immature paramphistomes develop in the duodenal mucosa but migrate through the abomasum to the rumen and reticulum as they mature. *Dicrocoelium* migrates up the bile ducts from the duodenum and matures in the bile ducts and gallbladder without invading the liver parenchyma.

EPIDEMIOLOGY

The initiation of effective trematode control programs and the proper timing of treatment are dependent on an understanding of the epidemiology of the disease. Livestock most likely to be affected with *F. hepatica* are those grazing in low-lying swampy areas, flood irrigation areas, or anywhere that surface water or small, slowly moving streams favor the propagation of lymnaeid snails. *F. hepatica* can survive for many years in sheep and shed up to 50,000 eggs per day, but cattle develop resistance and expel most flukes within a year. Cattle appear to have a degree of natural resistance to liver flukes, as well as an ability to develop acquired immunity, whereas sheep and goats seem to be lacking in both. Pastures become infective with metacercariae as early as 2 months after being grazed by infected livestock. Metacercariae may survive on pastures for up to 1 year, but die within 2 weeks under hot dry conditions. Housed animals will be protected against the disease unless they are fed hay with sufficient moisture to enable metacercariae to survive. Metacercariae are killed by ensilage.

On the Gulf Coast, warm and wet conditions in mild winters, spring, and early summer are highly favorable to massive proliferation of snails, hatching of fluke eggs, and development of cercariae within snails. Most fluke transmission occurs between the months of February and July. Transmission ceases with death of eggs, snails, and metacercariae in the first sustained drought of summer. By fall, flukes transmitted in the spring are egg-laying adults and fully susceptible to approved flukicides. The extent of production losses is influenced by the level of nutrition and concurrent nematode infections. In the Gulf States, peak fluke burdens, adult *Ostertagia* burdens, and nutritional stress may all coincide in the winter. Whereas warm, wet conditions favor snail and fluke proliferation, cold winter conditions (below 10°C) inhibit their reproduction. In some regions of the Pacific Northwest, peak fluke transmission is delayed because of the death of metacercariae and infected snails during the freezing winter. Although the summers are semiarid, flood irrigation of pastures provides ample moisture for summer-fall transmission. Considerable success has been achieved in predicting high- or low-risk years for fascioliasis from meteorologic data in both Britain and the Gulf Coast regions of the United States.

PATHOGENESIS

Acute fluke disease due to *F. hepatica* is caused by the sudden invasion of the liver by masses of young flukes. Severe destruction of parenchyma results in acute hepatic insufficiency as well as massive hemorrhage into the peritoneal cavity. Chronic fluke disease develops slowly and is caused by the activities of adult flukes in the bile ducts. In addition to cholangitis, biliary obstruction, and fibrosis, they cause anemia by their bloodsucking activities. Hypoproteinemia may result from seepage of plasma proteins from the damaged bile duct epithelium. The pathogenesis of *F. gigantica* is similar to that of *F. hepatica*. Migration of immature flukes through hepatic tissue and production of anaerobic necrotic tracts may trigger germination of latent spores of *Clostridium novyi* and exotoxin production that causes black disease. This occurs much more commonly in sheep than in cattle. Bacillary hemoglobinuria due to exotoxins of *Clostridium haemolyticum* may also be triggered by migrating liver flukes in cattle.

Fasc. magna infection in cattle is usually clinically inapparent because of massive encapsulation of flukes, but their unrestricted tunneling in sheep and goats can be rapidly fatal. It is reported that a single fluke can cause death. In the wildlife natural hosts, there is only minor liver damage as the adults are enclosed in thin-walled cysts. *D. dendriticum* is relatively nonpathogenic because of its small size, smooth cuticle, and failure to invade the liver parenchyma. It may, however, cause cirrhosis of bile ducts and condemnation of livers. Clinical paramphistomiasis is caused by massive numbers of immature flukes in the duodenal mucosa, whereas adult flukes in the rumen and reticulum cause little harm in most circumstances.

CLINICAL DISEASE

Acute liver fluke disease due to *F. hepatica* is seen in sheep and goats, but rarely in cattle because of both natural and acquired immunity. It is caused by massive hemorrhage and tissue destruction following ingestion of large numbers of metacercariae. Acute fluke outbreaks are likely to occur in seasons of very high rainfall. Death is usually sudden or occurs within 48 hours of the onset of symptoms. Clinical signs include anorexia, dullness, weakness, pale membranes, dyspnea, ascites, abdominal pain, and alternating standing up and lying down. It may be possible to palpate an enlarged liver. The feces are dry and not diarrheal. Outbreaks may last only 2 to 3 weeks but involve high mortality, especially if the fluke migration triggers further deaths from black disease. A subacute syndrome may also occur, with affected animals surviving for 2 weeks after the onset of clinical signs.

The chronic disease is a wasting condition caused by the bloodsucking activities of adult *F. hepatica* in the bile ducts. Sheep progressively lose weight over months and develop pale membranes, submandibular edema (bottle jaw), ascites, or rarely jaundice. Shedding of the wool may also occur. Cattle usually suffer the chronic disease only and experience weight loss, anemia, and a reduction of up to 10% in milk yield. Cattle entering feedlots with liver fluke infection show decreased average daily gains. In Britain and the Pacific Northwest of the United States, most fluke infections are acquired by cattle in the fall and early winter, and the effects on lactation and body condition become apparent in midwinter. The poor body condition can contribute to lowered reproductive performance and a higher percentage of barren cows. Subacute disease sometimes occurs in calves exposed to large numbers of metacercariae. Infection with *F. gigantica* causes clinical signs similar to those caused by *F. hepatica*. *Fasc. magna* infection may cause a syndrome similar to chronic *F. hepatica* disease in cattle and acute *F. hepatica* disease in sheep. In tropical regions, paramphistomes may induce a severe enteritis with weight loss and diarrhea and may be clinically indistinguishable from ostertagiasis or Johne's disease. *D. dendriticum* infection is usually asymptomatic.

DIAGNOSIS

Clinical diagnosis of liver fluke disease is often complicated by the concurrent presence of gastrointestinal nematodes, which produce some of the same clinical signs. A common experience on the Gulf Coast is that of giving one or more treatments for nematodes with little effect. When a flukicide is given, a dramatic clinical improvement occurs. A history of access to snail habitats, seasonal conditions favorable to snail reproduction, and an unexpected drop in milk yield are all important indicators in endemic areas. In outbreaks of acute *F. hepatica* disease in sheep and goats there will be no fluke eggs in the feces, and in cases of *Fasc. magna* infection, patency is unlikely to be reached in domestic animals. In subacute disease due to *F. hepatica*, a few flukes may reach adult stage and pass small numbers of eggs in the feces. In chronic *F. hepatica* infection in cattle, sheep, and goats, variable numbers of eggs occur in the feces. The immature paramphistomes that cause clinical signs do not betray their presence by eggs.

It is desirable to use a sedimentation technique for the detection of fluke eggs, as they do not float well in most flotation solutions. *F. hepatica* eggs are large (up to 150 μm), operculated, thin-walled, and yellow-brown. Eggs of *F. gigantica*, *Fasc. magna*, and *P. microbothrioides* all resemble *F. hepatica* eggs but are a little larger, and those of *P. microbothrioides* have a transparent gray-green appearance. Immature rumen flukes are sometimes passed in the feces. They are 3 to 4 mm in size and can be detected by sedimentation and decanting techniques. The eggs of *D. dendriticum* are quite distinctive, being small (up to 45 μm), dark brown, and operculated, and contain a miracidium when passed in the feces.

Researchers in the southern United States have identified several problems in the diagnosis of *F. hepatica* infection in cattle when using the fecal sedimentation method: (1) it is time-consuming, requiring at least 10 samples per cattle group and 15 to 30 minutes per sample; (2) egg counts are low, usually less than 5 epg, even in heavily infected herds; (3) egg counts vary widely between animals in a herd, because most flukes and egg shedding occur in a few highly susceptible animals; (4) herd egg counts peak and wane according to seasonal transmission; (5) immature fluke infections cannot be detected; and (6) lack of standardization of techniques among laboratories prevents meaningful comparisons of data. The researchers reported a new method based on the use of two sieves (Flukefinder, Visual Difference, Inc., Moscow, Idaho). It is twice as fast, less prone to technical variance, and suitable for use by veterinary practitioners. This technique has been used successfully to evaluate fluke burdens in Louisiana cow and calf operations. Currently, no serologic tests are accurate enough to improve on diagnosis by fecal sedimentation in individual animals. Enzyme-linked immunosorbent assay (ELISA) tests are limited by low sensitivity and specificity and by the difficulty of differentiating current infection from previous infection.

In acute *F. hepatica* outbreaks, the main necropsy findings are an enlarged hemorrhagic liver covered with fibrinous strands, a large amount of blood-stained peritoneal fluid, and over 1000 immature flukes in the liver parenchyma. In the subacute disease, the liver is also enlarged and hemorrhagic, but some of the flukes will have reached the adult stage. The chronic disease is characterized by an emaciated carcass, a small, shrunken fibrotic liver, and 200 or more adult flukes in the bile ducts. In cattle infected with *Fasc. magna*, flukes are found within a thick capsule with heavy black pigmentation of the liver, whereas in sheep or goats tunnels are seen in the parenchyma. In paramphistomiasis, immature flukes may cause thickening and hemorrhage of the duodenal wall but are sometimes overlooked because of their small size.

CONTROL STRATEGIES

Control is best achieved by strategic use of flukicides to remove flukes before productivity is affected and to prevent egg shedding before large numbers of susceptible snails are present. In some situations, the use of molluscacides, grazing management strategies, and fencing or drainage of snail habitats may be successfully integrated with strategic treatments. The timing, frequency, and choice of flukicides are best determined after consideration of the epidemiology of fluke disease in each area. The most appropriate timing may not always coincide with the times when livestock owners normally handle their stock for other purposes. However, the returns from improved weight gains, feed conversion, conception rates, milk production, or calf weaning weights may justify a change in management procedure to allow more effective fluke control. There may also be a need to offset winter nutritional stress, since poorly nourished animals are more susceptible to the effects of liver fluke disease.

Studies in Louisiana suggest that an annual fall treatment with a flukicide is adequate for the sustained reduction of fluke burdens in low- and moderate-risk years, as determined by climatic forecasts, but that a late spring or summer treatment may be needed in high-risk years, or on farms with a history of severe liver fluke disease. The fall treatment is especially important in removing adult fluke burdens prior to the winter nutritional stress period, as well as reducing environmental contamination with fluke eggs prior to the massive late-winter to early-summer buildup of the snail population.

A summer treatment on the Gulf Coast may be superior in preventive value for both fluke and gastrointestinal nematodes, compared with spring treatments. Summer treatment with a broad-spectrum flukicide (e.g., albendazole) or combination of a narrow-spectrum flukicide (e.g., clorsulon) and an anthelmintic would remove a high proportion of flukes in the drug-susceptible mature or late immature stages. This treatment would also remove peak numbers of hypobiotic larvae in southern states and prevent problems when they normally emerge in the subsequent fall. Removal of both worms and flukes from cattle would give prolonged protection because environmental transmission is at its lowest level in summer. The Gulf Coast researchers point out that although summer treatment does not coincide with the most convenient times for handling cattle, recent progress in new drug delivery systems (e.g., pulse-release rumen devices, medicated feed blocks) suggest that it may soon be feasible to treat cattle at critical times dictated by local epidemiologic factors. In the Pacific Northwest, a spring treatment at the start of the pasture season will eliminate many adult flukes before they contaminate pasture with eggs and thus reduce the summer-fall transmission potential.

Effective management systems include grazing systems that avoid high-risk areas during periods of high transmission potential and the fencing off or drainage of snail habitats if practical. Molluscacides, such as copper sulfate, may be of value when applied to relatively small snail habitats and integrated with strategic flukicide treatments. Toxicity to nontarget species and phytotoxicity are important constraints to molluscacide use. Copper sulfate has been widely used in the past but has sometimes resulted in copper poisoning of livestock or killing of fish after drainage into nearby streams. Biologic approaches to snail control have also been attempted, including the release of sciomyzid marsh flies, but the results were disappointing.

FLUKICIDES

Flukicides for cattle are shown in Table 8. Albendazole is the only approved broad-spectrum drug in the United States with efficacy against gastrointestinal nematodes, lungworms, tapeworms, and the adult liver fluke. However, it has little efficacy against immature *Fasciola* spp. less than 12 weeks of age. It is consequently most effective in the fall when flukes are adult, but is considerably less effective in the spring or early summer when a mixed, immature and mature population is present.

Clorsulon is effective against *Fasciola* spp. only, but has activity against late immature flukes (8 to 12 weeks). It can also be combined with modern anthelmintics such as benzimidazoles, levamisole, and ivermectin to provide a broad spectrum of activity. Unfortunately, the dosage of clorsulon in combination with ivermectin (Ivomec-F) is only 2 mg/kg (see Table 8), which limits its usefulness to adult flukes only. Greater efficacy against late immature flukes could be obtained by treating cattle with a combination of clorsulon (7 mg/kg) and anthelmintics at recommended dosages.

A new benzimidazole drug, triclabendazole, is so efficient against all stages of *Fasciola* spp., that it introduces the possibility of complete elimination of fascioliasis by treatment at intervals of 8 to 10 weeks (within the prepatent period). It has high efficacy against both larval and adult *F. hepatica*. It is also a very safe drug with a high safety index (see Table 8), but is not currently available in the United States. Most other flukicides are effective only against *F. hepatica*, 8 weeks and older, by which time severe pathologic damage has already occurred.

Most drugs effective against *F. hepatica* are also effective against *F. gigantica*. Higher dose rates are required for efficacy against *Fasc. magna*, and 100% efficacy is needed in sheep and goats because even a single migrating fluke can kill the host. Most benzimidazole drugs have activity against *D. dendriticum* at high dose rates. Drugs recommended for paramphistome therapy (bithionol, brotionide, niclosamide, resorantel) are not approved for food animals in the United States.

Table 8
FLUKICIDES FOR *Fasciola* SPP. IN CATTLE

Flukicide	Trade Name	Dosage (mg/kg)	Safety Index	Minimum Age of Fluke Efficacy >90%
Albendazole	Valbazen	10	10	Adults only
Clorsulon	Curatrem	7	5	8 wks
Clorsulon-ivermectin	Ivomec-F	2/0.2		Adults only
Triclabendazole*	Fasinex	12	20	1 wk

*Not approved in the United States.

CESTODE INFECTIONS IN CATTLE, SHEEP, GOATS, AND SWINE

R.P. Herd, M.V.Sc., Ph.D.

Gastrointestinal cestodes of food animals are of minor importance, but cystic larval stages of human and canid taeniids that occur in food animal intermediate hosts are of both economic and public health significance.

In the United States, *Moniezia* spp of cattle, sheep, and goats are widely distributed owing to the ready availability of the oribatid pasture mite intermediate hosts. Livestock become infected by accidental ingestion of the mites, which are especially numerous on permanent pasture. The "fringed tapeworm" (*Thysanosoma actinioides*) is limited to western states because the appropriate intermediate host (psocid louse) is not so widely disseminated.

A discussion of cysticercosis and hydatidosis is outside the scope of a discussion of digestive system diseases, but it should be noted that *Taenia saginata* has become more common in the United States over the last decade as a result of the influx of migrant workers from enzootic areas, as a consequence of the use of raw sewage for the fertilization of pasture, and because of sewage contamination of irrigation water. There is a similar risk of the introduction of *Taenia solium* by migrant workers from Mexico and other enzootic areas. Cystic hydatidosis persists as a problem in sheep-raising areas in Utah, California, Arizona, and New Mexico, while alveolar hydatidosis is becoming more important in the northern and central states. Cysticercosis of sheep due to larval *Taenia ovis* and *Taenia hydatigena* causes carcass and organ rejection at abattoirs and adversely affects export markets.

LIFE CYCLE AND EPIDEMIOLOGY

Most cestodes of veterinary importance have an indirect life cycle with one intermediate host. There are no free-living larval stages. In the case of *Moniezia* and *Thysanosoma* spp., eggs disseminated from gravid proglottids passed in cattle, sheep, or goat feces are consumed by an arthropod intermediate host. The oncosphere or hexacanth embryo is released and burrows into the body cavity of the arthropod, where it develops to a cysticercoid (a small cyst with a single depressed scolex) within 100 to 200 days depending on the temperature. Each cysticercoid develops into a single tapeworm if the infected intermediate host is eaten by the appropriate final host.

Moniezia tapeworms are relatively short-lived. They start shedding eggs about 6 weeks after infection, then disappear from the host after about 3 months. The eggs have a poor survival capacity and are infective for mites for only about 3 months after being passed. Development of cysticercoids in mites takes several months depending on the temperature, and it appears that cysticercoids can overwinter in mites. The prevalence of *Moniezia* infection in livestock shows a seasonal fluctuation coinciding with the active period of the vectors. At present it is not clear how much the transmission of tapeworm eggs is affected by wind, water, temperature, vectors, and fomites. Coprophagous flies probably play an important role in egg dissemination. Unlike *Moniezia*, *Thysanosoma* is a long-lived worm surviving for several years.

PATHOGENESIS

The intestinal tapeworms of cattle, sheep, and goats are not serious pathogens, although *Moniezia* infection is sometimes associated with poor growth and diarrhea. Adult tapeworms compete with the host for nutrients, interfere with gut motility, and excrete toxic substances. *Monizia expansa* has been associated with enterotoxemia outbreaks in lambs. It has been suggested that it causes sluggish bowel movements and conditions suitable for the production of *Clostridium perfringens* exotoxins. There is evidence that tapeworm-infected sheep may be more subject to fly strike. Young animals are most susceptible to tapeworm infection, and it is possible that older animals develop an acquired immunity. *Thysanosoma actinioides* infection is not of clinical importance, but its presence in the bile ducts can result in the condemnation of livers.

CLINICAL DISEASE

There is some controversy over the importance of tapeworm infection of food animals, with a tendency for farmers to overemphasize its importance and be more concerned about tapeworms than the more pathogenic nematodes and trematodes. At the same time it is probably a mistake to totally ignore tapeworms and regard them as completely nonpathogenic. Most infections do not cause clinical disease, but heavy infections are sometimes associated with poor growth, diarrhea or clostridial infections. Clinical signs are usually not seen in cysticercosis or hydatidosis of food animals unless large cysts disrupt vital organs.

DIAGNOSIS

Diagnosis is usually made by finding proglottids or the characteristic thick-walled eggs in feces. *Moniezia* eggs contain a distinctive hexacanth embryo in a piriform apparatus. The much smaller *Thysanosoma* eggs have no piriform apparatus. *Moniezia* is a large cestode (200 cm), and it is common to recover masses of them at routine necropsy of lambs in the spring. In spite of their spectacular volume, tapeworms are much less pathogenic than the tiny hairlike trichostrongylid nematodes. The smaller *Thysanosoma* tapeworms (20 cm) are usually found in the duodenum or bile ducts at necropsy.

TREATMENT

Because control of the arthropod vectors is impractical, periodic treatment with cestocides is the main method of control.

In the past, lead arsenate (0.5 g for lambs, 1 g for adult sheep, 0.5 to 1.5 g for calves) was the main drug employed. It has now been superseded by more efficient and safer pro-benzimidazole or benzimidazole drugs, including albendazole, fenbendazole, and oxfendazole. Preliminary studies suggest that albendazole and fenbendazole at dosages of 10 mg/kg and oxfendazole at 4.5 mg/kg have excellent activity against gastrointestinal cestodes. There are no highly effective chemotherapeutic agents for the control of larval cestodes in ruminants, but several drugs (e.g., praziquantel, mebendazole) have shown promising results under experimental conditions. At present, the best approach is to use drugs such as niclosamide and praziquantel to eliminate adult cestodes in the human and canid definitive hosts, with the object of reducing the environmental contamination with cestode eggs.

SUPPLEMENTAL READING

Nematode Infections in Cattle, Sheep, Goats, and Swine

Armour J, Ogbourne CP: Bovine Ostertagiasis: A Review and Annotated Bibliography. Miscellaneous Publication No. 7. Farnham Royal, Bucks, England, Commonwealth Institute of Parasitology, Commonwealth Agricultural Bureaux, 1982, pp 1–93.

Gibbs HC, Herd RP, Murrell KD (eds): Parasites: Epidemiology and Control. Vet Clin North Am Food Anim Pract. 2:1986.

Herd RP: Cattle practitioner: Vital role in worm control. Compendium Continuing Educ Pract Vet 13:879–891, 1991.

Radostits OM, Blood DC, Gay CC: Veterinary Medicine, ed 8. London, Baillière Tindall, 1994, pp 1023–1079.

Reinemeyer CR: The effect of anthelmintic treatment of beef cows on parasitologic and performance parameters. Compendium Continuing Educ Pract Vet 14:678–687, 1992.

Reinemeyer CR: Should you deworm your clients' dairy cattle? Vet Med 90:496–502, 1995.

Snyder DE, Klesius PH (eds): *Ostertagia*. Vet Parasitol 46:1–330, 1993.

Zajac AM, Moore GA: Treatment and control of gastrointestinal nematodes of sheep. Compendium Continuing Educ Pract Vet 15:999–1010, 1993.

Trematode Infections in Cattle, Sheep, and Goats

Gibbs HC, Herd RP, Murrell KD (eds): Parasites: Epidemiology and control. Vet Clin North Am Food Anim Pract 2:1986.

Kaplan RM: Liver flukes in cattle: Control based on seasonal transmission dynamics. Compendium Continuing Educ Pract Vet 16:687–693. 1994.

Malone JB, Craig TM: Cattle liver flukes: Risk assessment and control. Compendium Continuing Educ Pract Vet 12:747–754, 1990.

Radostits OM, Blood DC, Gay CC: Veterinary Medicine, ed 8. London, Baillière Tindall, 1994, pp 1223–1279.

Reproductive Diseases

Consulting Editor

Louis F. Archbald, D.V.M., M.S., Ph.D., Diplomate, A.C.T., M.R.C.V.S.

■ Bovine Mastitis

Peter R. Morresey, B.V.Sc., M.A.C.V.Sc.

Mastitis is the most common disease affecting dairy cows worldwide. At any time, up to 50% of the cows may be infected in one or more quarters.[1] In addition to its effects on milk production, mastitis can also cause loss of glandular secretory tissue, systemic illness, and death of the affected cow. Mastitis has many effects on raw milk components and hence on milk-based product quality and yield. There are decreases in the production of lactose, fat, nonfat milk solids, and casein. Whey proteins, sodium, chloride, pH, and free fatty acids are increased.[2, 3]

Total protein may remain stable as increases in albumin and immunoglobulins offset the decrease in casein. Inflammatory cells (known as somatic cells) are increased.

Milk volume is decreased because of the combined effects of decreased lactose, glandular inflammation and destruction, and depressed appetite in the cow if systemically ill. Product yield and quality are decreased, as are product shelf life and consumer acceptance.

An estimate of a total loss in productive capacity of 10% as a result of mastitis has been made.[2] This estimate considers direct effects on the milk, direct costs of treatment, and effects on the herd itself. A 3% increased culling rate has been attributed to mastitis.[1] In addition to the direct effects on production, the effects on the individual and the total population of dairy cows should be considered. Losses of individual productive capacity as a result of morbidity and mortality may lead to desirable genetic traits being lost from the herd. Maintenance costs for the herd are increased because of the higher number of replacements needed to compensate for the losses from mastitis. In a climate of heightened public awareness and scrutiny of general farming practices, mastitis can be seen as a potentially serious welfare issue.

The potential for violative residue in products through the increased prescription of antibiotics and other therapeutic drugs in response to infection is a threat to both human health and the economic well-being of the producer. The use of prophylactic compounds (e.g., disinfectants), if not managed properly, can also contribute to this problem.

CHANGING PREVALENCE

With an increase in production has come an increase in the risk of mastitis.[2] In many parts of the world, some form of the "five-point plan" to combat mastitis in intensive dairying situations has been adopted. This plan consists of treatment of the clinical cases, teat disinfection at every milking, dry cow antibiotic therapy, regular milking machine maintenance, and culling of persistently infected cows from the herd. In well-managed dairies, this practice has led to a profound decrease or elimination of contagious causes of mastitis with a corresponding rise in the prevalence of environmental causes. This confounding occurrence is thought to be due to a decrease in contagious pathogens, which lowers somatic cell counts (SCCs) and immune cells in the milk and results in greater susceptibility to environmental organisms.

DEFENSE MECHANISMS OF THE BOVINE MAMMARY GLAND

Resistance to infection by the bovine udder may be divided into two categories. The nonspecific system provides a first line of defense. If this fails, the tissues of the gland can manufacture a specific defense against a particular infectious agent. This specific immunity can resist another episode of invasion by the same pathogen.

Nonspecific Mechanisms

The first nonspecific barrier to microbial colonization and infection of the mammary gland is mechanical, the teat orifice and teat canal. Physical closure of these structures prevents the leakage of milk, which provides a vehicle for bacterial penetration into the gland. The teat orifice is largely composed of elastic connective tissue. The teat canal is arranged in longitudinal folds lined with keratin that is shed along with any attached organisms during milking. The length of this structure has not been shown to influence susceptibility.

Proximal to the teat canal lies the rosette of Furstenburg, a circular fold of tissue densely packed with neutrophils, lymphocytes, and plasma cells. Free fatty acids present in keratin within the teat canal have antimicrobial properties. Myristic, palmitoleic, and linoleic acids have a prominent role. Proteins from the teat canal have demonstrated an electrostatic charge at physiologic pH sufficient to bind mastitis pathogens.

The very act of milking provides a regular flushing of the distal portions of the teat by a large volume of milk and thus removal from the gland of any noxious organisms, toxins, and inflammatory mediators.

Within the glandular secretions are nonspecific bacterial inhibitors. Complement can be activated by the lipopolysaccharide in a gram-negative cell wall and lyse bacteria by the alternate pathway. Lactoferrin binds iron irreversibly to remove its availability for bacterial usage and also enhances the neutrophil respiratory burst. This process is aided by bicarbonate and inhibited by citrate. The lactoperoxidase/thiocyanate/peroxide system produces bacteriostatic compounds, this process being aided by IgA secreted from within the gland.

Specific Mechanisms

Specific defense mechanisms, as with other body systems, rely on cellular and humoral means. Lymphocytes in milk are competent but not as active as those in serum, possibly because of soluble immune suppressive factors in milk or increased suppressor cell function. Unlike the situation in other species, T cells do not migrate to the mammary gland from other regions of the mucosal immune system to confer immunity.

B cells in the cow have been shown to migrate to the spleen and regional lymph nodes, as evidenced by serum-derived IgG in colostrum and milk.

The predominant immunoglobulin in milk is IgG1 because of selective transfer from the blood. Immunoglobulin G2 and other proteins are transferred during inflammation, and IgM and IgA are produced locally from lymphoblast and plasma cells located close to the glandular epithelium. Inflammation of the mammary gland leads to rapid increases in immunoglobulins and serum proteins, including complement.

The phagocytic activity of neutrophils is the most effective mammary defense. Macrophages and lymphocytes predominate in healthy cows, but neutrophils increase rapidly in response to the presence of bacteria and their products. Endothelial cell gap junctions relax and allow cellular migration and humoral exudation.

CLINICAL SIGNS

The infected mammary gland may display none or all of the cardinal signs of inflammation—heat, redness, swelling, pain, and loss of function, depending on the interplay between host defenses, agent virulence, and the environment. Systemic illness may be present.

Extensive fibrosis and abscessation may occur and block secretory ducts and glandular alveoli, thereby increasing intraglandular pressure, pain, and the buildup of toxins and inflammatory mediators. Tissue destruction in general and the loss of secretory epithelium specifically lead to long-term depression or loss of productive function. Depending on the agent, milk may display few changes, form visible flakes or fibrin clots, or contain blood.

External signs of infection likewise vary among individuals. Direct examination of the gland may detect no signs of the infection. Conversely, the gland may be swollen, hard, painful, and hot, with the cow being pyrectic, inappetent, and depressed. Life-threatening toxemia may result. Endotoxic shock may occur, as may gangrenous changes to the affected gland. Fibrotic areas may be palpated in chronic infections.

DIAGNOSIS

Clinical mastitis, which is most common in the early lactation period, can be diagnosed by examination of the mammary gland and its secretion. In-line filters, foremilk stripping, udder palpation, and electronic sensors may be used to detect clinical disease.

Subclinical mastitis may be detected by cytologic and biochemical changes in the milk.

Milk from a normal mammary gland is sterile, although the sample may be inoculated from the teat canal during collection. Aseptically collected milk will give a positive indication of a mastitis pathogen if present and allow identification and sensitivity analysis.

Cytologic examination will detect the neutrophil infiltration characteristic of intramammary infection. This is the basis of the gelling reaction of the California mastitis test. Individual cow SCCs and bulk milk SCCs indicate individual infection and herd mastitis prevalence, respectively.

Biochemical tests detect alterations in milk composition, namely, increases in sodium and chloride and decreases in potassium. Conductivity meters make use of the increased conductivity of mastitic milk, although the range overlaps with normal values. Enzymatic changes occur and serum components leak into the mammary gland.

Somatic cell counts are affected by the following:

- Mastitis—gland inflammation leads to cellular diapedesis and chemotaxis.
- Stage of lactation—SCCs are initially high and then decrease to a low level before steadily increasing throughout lactation. This is probably due to the concentrating effect of a smaller milk volume.
- Lactation age—subacute inflammation increases with age.
- General stress, estrus.
- Milking interval—shorter intervals lead to higher counts.

The prevalence of clinical and especially subclinical infection is the most important factor affecting bulk milk SCCs. The rapid elimination of gram-negative infections means that the bulk milk SCC is a poor indicator of these infections. Individual SCCs allow a calculation of the proportion of the herd affected, identification of cows for bacteriologic examination or culling, and monitoring of the effectiveness of dry cow therapy (DCT).

PATHOGENESIS OF INFECTION

Establishment of infection is a product of the interaction between pathogenic bacteria and the immune response of the host. For bacteria to become established, udder defenses must break down. Once the teat canal is breached, alveoli are reached within minutes by diffusion, and penetration of the epithelium occurs within hours. Hematogenous spread is also possible.

Inflammatory mediators are released in response to bacterial infection. Cellular recruitment, vascular permeability changes, and exudation of serum proteins occur. Systemic absorption of toxins leads to generalized illness. The release of endotoxin by gram-negative organisms in response to rapid host clearance of infection is responsible for the clinical signs.

Bacteria that resist phagocytosis and the bactericidal effects of milk leukocytes and humoral responses are cleared less rapidly and thus have a greater potential to cause disease. Encapsulated gram-negative bacteria have the ability to grow in the udder and resist complement-mediated lysis. They also have an environmental reservoir. *Staphylococcus aureus* produces toxins that permit invasive growth, the formation of abscesses, and survival in phagocytic cells. *Streptococcus* spp. are poorly antigenic and hence survive by eliciting only a mild immune response.

SPECIFIC AGENTS

Contagious mastitis pathogens are transferred by infected fomites during milking. These pathogens include the invasive gram-positive mastitis agents *Staphylococcus* spp., *Streptococcus agalactiae*, and *Actinomyces pyogenes*.

In environmental mastitis, the cow's environment is the primary reservoir of the mastitis pathogen. Environmental mastitis is usually associated with clinical cases and is the chief mastitis problem in well-managed, low-SCC herds. Gram-negative infections are involved, chiefly *Escherichia coli*, and are noninvasive with the exception of *Pseudomonas* spp. *Str. uberis*, *Str. dysgalactiae*, and other non-*agalactiae* streptococcal species are included in this group because of their environmental prevalence.

Gram-Positive Agents

Staphylococcus Species

Staphylococcus aureus

Sta. aureus causes predominantly subclinical mastitis, but per-acute clinical cases do occur. The main source of infection is the infected udder, although teat lesions can be colonized and act as a reservoir. Significant reductions in milk yield occur, with deaths possible. This organism may be eliminated by culling, milking hygiene, and teat disinfection. *Sta. aureus* can survive within phagocytic and epithelial cells and induces protective pathologic fibrotic udder changes as a result of the action of α-toxin. Infections early in lactation can result in a severe systemic reaction and death. Gangrenous changes may occur because of thrombosis. Chronic incurable disease with cyclic shedding of bacteria results from infections in the dry period or later lactation.

Coagulase-Negative and Other Staphylococcal Species

Sta. epidermidis, *Sta. xylosus*, and other staphylococci have low virulence and are considered opportunistic causes of mastitis, but they can cause microscopic lesions in the mammary gland. Colonization of the teat duct may prevent infection by the more important pathogens. Usually, only a mild increase in SCC is present, and the SCC may pass the threshold for marketable milk.

Streptococcus Species

Streptococcus agalactiae

The main source of infection is the infected udder, although with poor hygiene environmental contamination can be a factor in outbreaks. Subsequent to the initial febrile episode, inflammation persists and repeated infectious crises occur. Long-term yield is depressed and fibrosis occurs. The effectiveness of intramammary antibiotic therapy has allowed *Sta. aureus* to replace *Str. agalactiae* as the major cause of bovine mastitis. Elimination by teat disinfection and routine DCT is possible. Infections may be acute or subclinical and of shorter duration than infections caused by *Sta. aureus*.

Streptococcus uberis

The most common cause of dry period infections, especially in the month before parturition, is *Str. uberis*. Most clinical episodes occur during the first part of lactation; however, susceptibility to infection is greatest at drying off. In infected herds, *Str. uberis* is a common inhabitant of the cow's skin, especially the belly. Some cows become permanent carriers of infection and shed large numbers of organisms in their feces, thereby leading to environmental contamination. Infection with *Str. uberis* is clinically similar to that with *Str. agalactiae*. Dry cow therapy reduces infection rates, and postmilking disinfection does not aid control. The bacteria are widespread on the cow and in her environment; they multiply in straw and attain high numbers. Chronic infections are common and antibiotic therapy is largely ineffective.

Streptococcus dysgalactiae

Disease caused by *Str. dysgalactiae* can be acute and result in systemic illness. Cow-to-cow transfer is important with *Str.* *dysgalactiae*, and an increase in teat lesions is associated with outbreaks. Teat disinfection and herd hygiene are effective controls. Antibiotic treatment is rapidly effective.

Actinomyces pyogenes

Present in suppurative conditions, *A. pyogenes* is part of the "summer mastitis" complex. Infection is usually associated with teat end damage. Prophylactic use of DCT is effective in controlling *A. pyogenes*.

Gram-Negative (Coliform) Agents

Mastitis caused by gram-negative bacteria is usually due to *Escherichia coli*, but *Klebsiella* spp. and *Enterobacter aerogenes* also cause mastitis. Infection occurs as a result of direct contact with the environment between milkings, which makes traditional gram-positive–type control measures ineffective. The udder is most susceptible at the extremes of the dry period. Rarely, peracute mastitis with life-threatening toxemia can occur, most commonly in the periparturient period. Spontaneous self-cure can occur in the subclinical form. Coliform bacteria are considered to be opportunistic agents, with infection being due to contamination of the teats and udder between milkings. Feces act as the major source for *E. coli*, and bedding may allow rapid buildup of high environmental pathogen pressures. A rapid inflammatory response occurs after inoculation, with neutrophil-mediated elimination of infection within hours. The overall outcome of infection is related to the speed and competence of this neutrophil response. Signs of illness/infection are chiefly related to endotoxin production. High-yielding cows in early lactation are most susceptible.

Other Infectious Agents

The organisms just mentioned can be considered *major* pathogens because of their relatively greater importance, as opposed to the following *minor* pathogens.

Mycoplasma Species

Several *Mycoplasma* species are important infectious agents, but *M. bovis* most commonly causes bovine mastitis. Multiple quarters are involved and are refractory to treatment. The onset of mastitis is rapid, and milk production decreases precipitously. Secretion is initially flaky and then becomes thick and purulent. The udder becomes swollen and hard early in the course of infection and then shrinks as fibroplasia ensues. Spread is thought to be due to contamination of the teats during milking. Cows of all ages and at any stage of lactation are susceptible. Control is by elimination of infected animals, teat disinfection, and hygiene when using intramammary infusions.

Pasteurella Species

Mastitis caused by *Pasteurella* spp. is rare in cattle. Severe toxemia and gangrenous changes may occur.

Nocardia Species

Nocardia spp. cause sporadic infections from soil contamination. Nocardial infection leads to a severe systemic reaction and glandular fibrosis.

Listeria monocytogenes

Listeria monocytogenes is important because of its zoonotic potential. Clinical signs of mastitis are mild, but milk production is decreased in the affected gland.

Fungi and Yeast

Infection by fungi and yeast is rare but may be introduced by contaminated intramammary infusions. Antibiotic therapy may stimulate infection. Systemic illness may occur, and fibrosis of the mammary gland is prominent. Many species are implicated, although *Trichosporon* spp., *Cryptococcus neoformans*, and *Candida* spp. are usually responsible.

SUMMER MASTITIS

Summer mastitis, an acute infection of the nonlactating gland, is of multifactorial origin and often not apparent until parturition. It is considered to be most severe in northern Europe but occurs in many dairying regions of the world. Its incidence is greatest in intensive dairy areas, although stock density is only one factor. European cattle, especially the Holstein/Friesian breeds, seem to be the most susceptible.

Summer mastitis is a complex infection. The pathogens associated with this condition may be found in clinically normal mammary glands. In clinical episodes of summer mastitis, *A. pyogenes* predominates and provides toxic factors enabling synergistic growth with anaerobic bacteria. These toxic factors include a hyaluronidase, coagulase, and hemolysin. The activity and quantity of these tissue-destroying compounds are enhanced by the anaerobe *Peptococcus indolicus*. *Fusobacterium necrophorum* and *Bacteroides* spp. may be present. Commonly, *Str. dysgalactiae* is found and is possibly a predisposing agent to *A. pyogenes*.

Disease prevalence in Europe is coincident with distribution of the sheep head fly *Hydrotaea irritans*. These flies have been shown to carry mastitis pathogens, and control of contact of these flies with cattle has reduced the incidence of summer mastitis. These head flies may spread the disease within the herd once it has occurred and can stress the cattle and thereby predispose them to infection.

Infections are often associated with teat end damage, which suggests a direct mode of infection. Lymphatic and hematogenous spread have also been proposed.

MASTITIS IN HEIFERS

Intramammary infections lead to the destruction of secretory and ductular tissue, which may go undetected for prolonged periods in replacement cattle, hence the potential for severe loss of function. Inflammation of the teat cistern and canal (thelitis) can result in "blind quarters" at parturition.

Str. agalactiae has been the predominant pathogen. It has been shown to be transmitted to calf udders by penmates ingesting contaminated milk, thus potentially establishing infection at an early age. As this organism has been eliminated from the milking herd, *Sta. aureus*, coagulase-negative staphylococci, environmental mastitis pathogens, summer mastitis, and mycoplasmal infection have increased in incidence.

OTHER CAUSES OF MASTITIS

Milking Machines

Milking machines may be involved in the spread of mastitis by allowing direct cow-to-cow transfer of infection via cluster contamination or by the transfer of contaminated milk between quarters or clusters during milking. In addition, high vacuum levels may lead to teat orifice eversion and incompetence and allow pathogen entry. Vacuum fluctuations at the teat end may lead to high-velocity droplet impaction on the teat orifice and inoculation of infection into the gland. Overmilking the gland at correct vacuum levels does not appear to increase the incidence of mastitis; however, incomplete milking of the mammary gland does increase the incidence.

Intramammary Infusions

Intramammary infusions may directly inoculate infection into the gland or damage the keratin lining of the teat canal. Absolute hygiene of the teat end during intramammary applications is necessary. Partial insertion is favored over full insertion because it is less damaging to the canal.

Housing

Clean environments decrease bacterial challenge to the teat end and hence lower rates of infection. Sand has been shown to harbor lower bacterial numbers than straw or wood shavings. To reduce the incidence of mastitis, minimizing environmental stress, facilitating effluent drainage and disposal, and avoiding injury, especially to the teat, should be considered in housing design.

Bovine Somatotropin Usage

Increased milk production in general and bovine somatotropin (BST) use in particular have been associated with a higher incidence of intramammary infections and SCCs.[4]

TREATMENT

Regardless of the compounds used, therapy for mastitis should be aimed at assisting host defense mechanisms in eliminating pathogens or reducing the pathophysiologic consequences of infection.

There are established benefits in using antimicrobial agents in the treatment of mastitis. Peracute cases may be salvaged for slaughter and thus reduce economic loss. Irreversible mammary parenchymal damage may be avoided, thereby allowing the cow to continue as an economically viable unit in the herd. Milk quality along with milk quantity may be improved. Microbiologic cures are possible and can eliminate reservoirs of infection for the herd.

When antibiotics are used, it is important to ensure therapeutic efficacy, economic benefit through increased productivity or quality, and the production of residue-free product for consumption.

Principles of Drug Distribution to the Udder

The bovine mammary gland is a highly vascular tissue. In a normal gland, tight endothelial junctions between epithelial cells form a barrier to the passage of compounds between the blood and milk—the "blood-milk" barrier. Lipophilic drugs will generally be concentrated in the milk.

The route of administration affects plasma and hence milk

Table 1

ANTIBACTERIALS AND THEIR DISTRIBUTION IN THE MAMMARY GLAND

Distribution	Route of Administration	
	Parenteral	**Intramammary**
Good	Fluoroquinolones Lincosamides Macrolides Penethamate Tetracyclines Trimethoprim	Aminopenicillins Cephalexin Fluoroquinolones Lincosamides Macrolides Penethamate Trimethoprim
Moderate	Aminopenicillins Cephalosporins (some) Isoxaloylpenicillins Penicillin G Sulfonamides	Aminopenicillins Cephalosporins Isoxaloylpenicillins Penicillin G Sulfonamides Tetracyclines
Poor	Aminoglycosides Cephalosporins (some)	Aminoglycosides

Data from Ziv G: Drug selection and use in mastitis: Systemic versus local therapy. J Am Vet Med Assoc 176:1109, 1980.

concentrations of many drugs (Table 1). Parenterally administered drugs may fail to reach and maintain therapeutic concentrations.

Intramammary infusion produces high levels of active drug in the udder. In a severely inflamed and swollen gland, infused drug may not be able to diffuse to the site of infection.

Obstacles to Treatment Success

Antibiotic treatment of mastitis is an adjunct to and not a replacement for normal host defense mechanisms. Antibiotics previously indicated to be efficacious by laboratory testing for an episode of mastitis may fail to effect a cure, either clinically or bacteriologically. This failure of antibiotic therapy may be due to one or many of the following factors:

1. Inadequate concentration of the drug for a sufficient time at the site of infection. The pharmacokinetic properties of the drug in vivo may render it unable to maintain sufficient levels to combat the organism in spite of favorable sensitivity results. Drug absorption, distribution, and elimination, as well as plasma protein binding, affect peak plasma concentrations. Ionization at physiologic pH may decrease lipid solubility and hence the ability to diffuse across the blood-milk barrier. The increasing pH of a mastitic gland may unfavorably influence "ion trapping" and decrease drug accumulation in the milk.

2. The intracellular nature of some organisms or fibrosis limits the ability of many drugs to reach the site of infection.

3. Innate resistance to antimicrobial drugs by some organisms or the development of resistance postexposure can cause antibiotic therapy to fail. Resistance genes may be transmitted between species of bacteria by plasmids. Mixed infections may allow one organism to be protected by the extracellular secretions of another, e.g., β-lactamases from *E. coli* protecting *S. agalactiae*.

4. Nonmultiplying stages of the bacterial life cycle (bacterial dormancy) are not sensitive to some drugs.

5. L-forms of bacteria lack cell walls and as such are insensitive to β-lactams.

6. Intramammary treatment with antibiotics may be detrimental to host phagocytosis.

7. Reinfection may occur if the host is unable to fully clear the infection in spite of adequate therapy.

Rational Antibiotic Therapy

Rational antibiotic therapy is centered on the correct use of effective drugs for susceptible infections. Identification of the causative organism determines whether antibiotic treatment has a chance of success or whether other options are preferable, e.g., supportive therapy, drying off, culling, or the use of DCT. The goal of improving animal welfare, productivity, and product quality while safeguarding human health must be met.

Supportive Therapy

Oxytocin alone or in conjunction with other therapies has been shown to have positive clinical effects by improving udder drainage during infection, decreasing the buildup of inflammatory mediators, and helping flush out the causative organism.[5] Frequent milking of the affected gland is beneficial for the same reasons.

Endotoxic shock is a result of gram-negative infection, and fluid therapy is central to combating this life-threatening event. Anti-inflammatory drugs both improve systemic well-being and help minimize parenchymal damage.

Immunostimulants have been shown to have no beneficial effect in mastitis treatment. However, immunomodulation with cytokines, including colony-stimulating factor and interferons, has proved to be of use.[6]

PROPHYLAXIS

Management

Environmental stress and gross udder contamination reduce the cow's ability to ward off infection and increase pathogenic bacterial pressure, respectively. Care should be taken in the design of housing to consider these factors. This point is especially important before calving because contamination of the teat orifice at this time can easily lead to intramammary infection.

Teat Dipping

Postmilking teat dipping/spraying is the major means of preventing new intramammary infections in milking cows. Rapid killing of bacteria reaching and colonizing the teat surface prevents penetration of the teat orifice, which may remain open for up to 2 hours after milking.

Premilking dipping/washing decreases the bacterial count of milk and hence the potential for spread of infection. Teats must be dried before milking or the increased moisture will increase the spread of contamination.

Dry Cow Therapy

The infusion of antibiotics into all quarters of all cows at drying off has been shown to reduce the incidence of new infections over the dry period and result in higher cure rates for existing infections. No milk discard is necessary, and the potential for antibiotic residue in milk is reduced if the correct dry period after treatment is observed.

Culling and Segregation

Chronically infected and nonresponding cows should be culled because they are a danger to the herd. Infected cows, once found and if amenable to treatment, should be segregated and clearly identified to avoid infecting other cows. This also reduces the residue potential of the milk.

Milking Management

Teat wash water should be clean or disinfected. Teats should be dried individually with disposable towels. Clusters should be applied and removed while properly minimizing air admission. Suitable teat disinfection regimens should be used and clusters sterilized between cows in an outbreak situation.

Machine Testing

Milking machines should be tested against established parameters regularly. Correct pulsation characteristics and vacuum levels must be maintained. Low-slip liners and correctly fitting liner designs should be used.

Vaccination

The ideal mastitis vaccine would eliminate chronic and prevent new intramammary infections. At the very least, the incidence and severity of new intramammary infections would be greatly reduced. No vaccines to date have been able to meet these goals because of the inconsistent protection afforded and the inability to reverse pathologic gland changes.

A gram-negative mastitis pathogen vaccine must contain a common antigen to be widely effective, this being provided by the common cell wall structure of these bacteria. R-mutant strains have exposed inner cell walls revealing common core antigens.

Staphylococcus aureus vaccines have centered on capsular antigens and exotoxins with variable results. Because infected cattle are reservoirs of infection, vaccines can be seen as an adjunct to control only. *Streptococcus agalactiae* vaccines generate nonprotective humoral responses, and this organism is easily treated. Other *Streptococcus* spp. with environmental reservoirs are amenable to vaccination.

In summary, traditional control and eradication of contagious pathogens are preferable to vaccination. Immunity against virulence factors such as *S. aureus* α-toxin prevent tissue damage. Where contagious pathogens have been eliminated, vaccination against environmental pathogens would be of benefit.

General Health and Nutrition

Inadequate nutrition is known to increase susceptibility to disease. Vitamins and trace elements play roles in both nonspecific and specific defense mechanisms.

Leukocyte function is second only to the teat canal in importance for mastitis resistance. Phagocytic killing is dependent on the superoxide radical. Copper, selenium, vitamin E, and vitamin A and its precursor β-carotene are necessary for antioxidant enzyme activity to protect the cell from autolysis.

Selenium and vitamin E supplementation through the dry period have been shown to decrease the incidence and duration of mastitis infection for the first 8 months of lactation. The increased exposure of selenium-deficient animals to endotoxin during mastitis resulted in higher levels of diarrhea, dehydration, and agalactia and greater residual gland atrophy. However, there is no evidence that supplementation above the National Research Council guidelines will increase mammary resistance to mastitis.

Applications of nutritional methods in mastitis control include correction of selenium-deficient farms and consideration of vitamin A and E alterations depending on forage quality, especially in late winter/early spring. Decreased selenium supplementation over the dry period occurs at a time when the highest rate of new intramammary infections is seen—in the early dry and periparturient period—with the highest rate of clinical infections occurring in the first 30 days of lactation.

Selective Breeding

Resistance to mastitis is based on morphologic, physiologic, and immunologic factors, for example, udder depth, teat length, teat orifice shape, keratinization of the canal, lysozyme, lactoferrin, immunoglobulins, and leukocyte responses. When compared with milk yield and composition, these factors have little genetic influence and strong environmental influence on resistance to mastitis.

REFERENCES

1. Ziv G: Treatment of peracute and acute mastitis. Vet Clin North Am 8:1, 1992.
2. DeGraves FJ, Fetrow J: Economics of mastitis and mastitis control. Vet Clin North Am 9:421, 1993.
3. Heath SE: The pathogenesis of bovine mastitis. *In* Proceedings of the 12th American College of Veterinary Internal Medicine Forum. San Francisco, 1994, p 668.
4. Kronfeld DS: BST: Efficacy and side effects. *In* Proceedings of the 12th American College of Veterinary Internal Medicine Forum. San Francisco, 1994, p 678.
5. Ziv G: Drug selection and use in mastitis: Systemic versus local therapy. J Am Vet Med Assoc 176:1109, 1980.
6. Daley MJ, Coyle PA, Williams TJ, et al: Staphylococcus aureus mastitis: Pathogenesis and treatment with bovine interleukin-1 beta and interleukin-2. J Dairy Sci 74:4413, 1991.

BIBLIOGRAPHY

American Association of Bovine Practitioners: Proceedings of the 26th Conference. Albuquerque, NM, 1993.
American Association of Bovine Practitioners: Proceedings of the 27th Conference. Pittsburgh, Pa, 1994.
American Association of Bovine Practitioners: Proceedings of the 28th Conference. San Antonio, Tex, 1995.
American Association of Bovine Practitioners: Proceedings of the 29th Conference. San Diego, Calif, 1996.
Andrews AH, Blowey RW, Boyd H, et al (eds): Bovine Medicine—The Diseases and Husbandry of Cattle. Boston, Blackwell, 1992.
Holmes CW, Wilson GF: Milk Production From Pasture. Wellington, NZ, Butterworths, 1984.
Radostits OM, Blood DC, Gay CC: Veterinary Medicine, ed 8. London, Baillière Tindall, 1994.
Tizard IR: Veterinary Immunology: An Introduction, ed 5. Philadelphia, WB Saunders, 1996.

◾ Lactation Failure in Swine

Billy I. Smith, B.S., D.V.M., M.S.

Lactation failure, which leads to reduced milk production in sows, should not be confused with agalactia, which is a complete loss of milk production. Lactation failure has been related to a number of different causes, which has resulted in several names for this syndrome, including puerperal mastitis, coliform mastitis, dysgalactia, periparturient hypogalactia syndrome, and mastitis-metritis-agalactia. Mastitis-metritis-agalactia is the most common name associated with this disease syndrome. Because many sows with lactation failure also have a postpartum vulvar discharge, mastitis-metritis-agalactia was the term used to identify these sows. However, it is now accepted that there is not a complete lack of milk production with this syndrome and therefore agalactia should not be included in the name. Lactation failure primarily results in economic loss because of poor piglet growth, piglet mortality, cost of treatment, and potential loss of productive sow units.

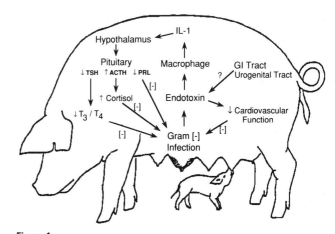

Figure 1

Proposed pathogenesis of lactation failure due to endotoxemia from a gram-negative infection. (From Smith BB, Martineau G, Bisaillon A: Mammary glands and lactation problems. *In* Leman AD, Straw BE, Mengeling WL, et al (eds): Diseases of Swine, ed 7. Ames, Iowa, Iowa State University Press, 1992.)

EPIDEMIOLOGY

Lactation failure frequently occurs within the first 3 days postpartum, with more than 50% of the sows showing clinical signs within 24 hours of farrowing.[1] The disease appears to occur most commonly in sows that farrow indoors in crates. Research has shown that lactation failure is more likely to develop in pluriparous sows than in gilts, with a reported incidence of 4.2% in gilts and 13% in pluriparous sows.[2] The overall incidence, as reported by several studies, is variable.[1, 3] This variation may be due to the complex nature of the disease and the fact that it has been related to a number of different factors. A seasonal variation has been observed, with a higher incidence during the summer than during other months of the year. Generally, lactation failure is not a fatal disease and not a significant cause of sow mortality.[4] The risk factors associated with the disease have not been fully determined; however, contributing elements include infections and nutritional, environmental, and physiologic factors.

ETIOLOGY

There is no one specific cause of lactation failure in sows. It is an extremely complex disease with a number of suggested causes. Noninfectious causes of lactation failure are teat malformation, ergot toxicity, psychogenic agalactia, milk ejection failure, mammary gland edema, ketosis, and hypocalcemia. Many of these causes are infrequent. Management factors, such as poorly maintained farrowing house temperature, improper ventilation, poorly constructed farrowing crates, and poorly maintained farrowing crates, have also been associated with lactation failure.

The most important known cause of lactation failure is infection, and the term *coliform mastitis* has been used to describe this specific cause of lactation failure. Genera of bacteria known to cause this disease include *Escherichia*, *Klebsiella*, *Enterobacter*, and *Citrobacter*. Experimental inoculation of these bacteria into the mammary gland of healthy animals results in clinical cases that mimic the well-described lactational failure syndrome.[5, 6] The resulting clinical signs appear to be caused by lipopolysaccharide endotoxins released from the cell wall of gram-negative bacteria during infection. Proposed sources of endotoxin include the gastrointestinal tract, uterus, and mammary gland. The absorbed endotoxins profoundly affect the immune, cardiovascular, and endocrine systems. Endotoxins alter hypothalamic function by stimulating the release of interleukin-1 and other factors. The altered hypothalamic function results in decreased thyroxine, triiodothyronine, and prolactin, as well as an increase in cortisol concentration. The suppressed prolactin release has been shown to result in a pronounced drop in milk production.[7] The interaction of these changes will alter milk production and is summarized in Figure 1.

Constipation is frequently observed in sows suffering from lactation failure, and changes in the diet of sows during the last week of gestation could result in failure of lactation.[8] However, the occurrence of lactation failure as a result of constipation or gut stasis alone is uncertain. Certain theories associating a change in diet and lactation failure have been developed, one theory being that intense feeding of sows may promote toxin production. A second theory states that the increase in feed consumption may lead to the initiation of lactation and udder engorgement. This could therefore result in increased pressure and leaky teat canals and thus make the sow more susceptible to infection.

The presence of a vulvar discharge in sows experiencing lactation failure led to the assumption that metritis is a cause of this disease. Normal sows will expel a thick, viscous, nonodorous clear discharge during the first 3 days postpartum, which may lead to the incorrect diagnosis of metritis. The presence of a dark brown, foul-smelling vulvar discharge in sows is characteristic of metritis and eventually results in severe toxemia. However, this is not a common finding in sows. Necropsy findings of sows with lactation failure have not been able to consistently link metritis and this disease.[9] Therefore, metritis as a cause of lactation failure has not been confirmed.

Endotoxin concentrations in animals suffering from mastitis are increased. The incidence of mastitis is higher in animals that farrow in crates vs. those that farrow outside, with one study also showing that animals confined to farrowing crates had 300 times greater teat end bacterial counts than did animals with outside access.[8]

DIAGNOSIS AND CLINICAL SIGNS

Failure to nurse piglets is the first clinical sign of this disease. Normally the sow will acknowledge the demands of the piglets and lie in lateral recumbency during nursing. Once in lateral recumbency, the piglets will nose around the mammary glands to find their appropriate feeding sites. This constant nosing behavior from the piglets provides ample stimulation for the complex process of milk letdown by the sow. Normally, once milk letdown occurs, the sow and piglets lie still during feeding. Sows that suffer from lactation failure become disinterested in the piglets and generally lie in sternal recumbency, thus preventing piglets' access to the teats. Sternal recumbency may be assumed in order to avoid the trauma and pain to the teat end associated with the continued nursing efforts of the piglets. If suckling is permitted, it is generally abbreviated and there is continuous movement of the piglets from teat to teat. Because the piglets are unable to obtain a sufficient amount of milk during feeding, they are usually restless and noisy and move frequently to all areas of the farrowing crate in search of food. They often consume urine or water from the floor of the crate, which could lead to diarrhea and other problems.

In the beginning, because of the excessive movement throughout the crate, high mortality from crushing usually occurs. Piglets often fight for teat ends and suffer wounds from biting. Continued movement and jostling for position eventually cause the piglets to lose energy and become weak and quiet. They often move to the warmest places in the farrowing crate. This lack of energy reduces their ability to get out of the way and may also contribute to an increased number of crushed piglets.

Because of the lack of milk necessary for proper growth of the piglets, many of the parameters used to monitor growth can be used to support the diagnosis of this disease. Affected sows may produce poor litters with increased mortality rates, variable weaning weights, and low average weaning weights. These factors can be useful in diagnosing lactation failure in sows.

Sows suffering from lactation failure are generally anorectic and drink only small amounts of water. They are typically depressed and have an elevated body temperature (103 to 105°F). Many sows, including healthy ones, have a slight increase in rectal temperature within the first 2 days postpartum.[10] Therefore it may be difficult to interpret rectal temperature changes in sows during the postpartum period. However, temperatures greater than 104°F are an indication of a severe condition and treatment should be considered.

The appearance of the affected mammary gland ranges from almost normal to grossly abnormal. There may be varying degrees of swelling and inflammation ranging from a normal or firm, warm-to-the-touch mammary gland to an extremely swollen, hot, and blotchy mammary gland.[9] Many sections of the mammary gland may be diffusely involved and lack the normal resiliency of mammary tissue. These have a "meaty" feel when palpated. Large amounts of edema may be present, usually along the outside edge of the glands and extending down their entire length. The skin may be very red and will blanch easily when pressure is applied to the glands, frequently resulting in a mottled appearance.

It is often very difficult to express milk from the teats, and an injection of oxytocin may be necessary to obtain a sample. If milk is obtained, the appearance may vary from a more normal white secretion to a grossly abnormal serous discharge that may contain fibrin or blood.[11] Analysis of the milk sample often leads to confusion. Bacteria are usually present in the milk of sows with lactation failure. However, unless a milk sample is taken from each subsection of the entire mammary gland, culture results may be unrewarding. The pH of the milk from infected sows may range from 7 to 7.8, whereas that of normal milk ranges from 6.4 to 6.5. In addition, somatic cell counts may reveal changes, but when done alone, these counts are extremely variable and unpredictable. However, evaluation of the results of both somatic cell counts and pH can be used to differentiate healthy sows from those with lactation failure.[8]

Other signs suggestive of lactation failure include constipation, vaginal discharge, reduced packed-cell volume, reduced hemoglobin concentration, marked leukopenia, decreased serum calcium, and increased cortisol concentration.

TREATMENT

Because this disease syndrome affects both the sow and the piglet, it is important to consider treatment for both. Removal of the entire litter or part of a litter is dependent on the severity of the disease in the affected sow. Piglets should be removed from sows that have stopped producing milk, and cross-fostering should be done when possible. If cross-fostering is not possible, the piglets must receive supplemental nutrition until the sow recovers and milk production has resumed. The piglets can be fed a solution of electrolytes and 5% glucose for 1 to 2 days. Simple mixtures such as condensed milk diluted with water at a 1:1 ratio can be used. More complicated mixtures such as a mixture of 1 qt cow's milk, 1 oz syrup, and 1 oz corn oil fed to piglets at 10% of the piglet's body weight per day are also effective. In addition, commercial milk replacers are available.

Once treatment is initiated, the sow usually recovers within 3 days. A combination of drugs including antimicrobials, oxytocin, and anti-inflammatory agents is necessary for recovery.[12]

Antimicrobial drugs that are broad-spectrum and effective against *Escherichia coli* and *Klebsiella* bacteria should be used for a minimum of 3 days.

Oxytocin should be administered as soon as possible. A dosage of 5 USP units intramuscularly every hour for at least 6 hours is safe and effective. Any dosage greater than this is excessive and should be avoided. If the sow will allow the piglets to suckle, milk letdown may be enhanced. Warm water massages of the mammary gland in combination with oxytocin every hour may also be beneficial.

Because endotoxins are the primary cause of lactation failure, anti-inflammatory drugs, especially those with antiendotoxic properties, are necessary. Nonsteroidal anti-inflammatory agents such as flunixin meglumine at an extralabel dose of 100 to 250 mg intramuscularly twice daily is effective. Treating sows with 2.2 mg/kg of flunixin meglumine results in a decrease in mammary gland edema, an increase in appetite, and an improvement in piglet weight 7 days after treatment.[8]

Alternatively, corticosteroids can be used in the treatment of lactation failure. They are primarily used to control inflammation, but when used alone, their effects are not noticed. Therefore it is important that they be used in combination with oxytocin and antimicrobial agents. A 20-mg intramuscular dose of dexamethasone given daily for 3 days to sows weighing 150 to 200 kg is recommended. Also, 50 to 100 mg of prednisolone can be used.

Other treatments may include furosemide to control mammary edema and acepromazine to tranquilize the sows to allow the piglets to nurse.

PREVENTION

Because infectious mastitis seems to be the primary cause of lactation failure in swine, it seems that measures used to control bacteria would be helpful in preventing the disease. Therefore, farrowing crates should be thoroughly cleaned and disinfected prior to transferring sows. Sows should be washed prior to being placed into farrowing crates. Crates should be kept as clean as possible, especially immediately before and after farrowing. Stress to the pigs should be minimized. This includes allowing for adequate adjustment to the farrowing crates prior to farrowing (1 week). There should be minimal change in the composition of the diet and the amount fed prior to farrowing. The addition of bran to the diet a couple of days prior to farrowing may reduce the chance of constipation, and the addition of antimicrobial agents may reduce the incidence of this disease complex.

REFERENCES

1. Hermansson I, Einarsson S, Larson K, et al: On the agalactia post partum in the sow: A clinical study. Nord Vet Med 30:465–473, 1978.
2. Backstrom L, Morkoc AC, Connor J, et al: Clinical study of mastitis-metritis-agalactia in sows in Illinois. J Am Vet Med Assoc 183:70–73, 1984.
3. Leman AD, Knudson C, Rodeffer HE, et al: Reproductive performance of swine on 76 Illinois farms. J Am Vet Med Assoc 161:1248–1250, 1972.
4. Chagnon M, D'Allaire S, Drolet R: A prospective study of sow mortality in breeding herds. Can J Vet Res 55:180–184, 1991.
5. Lake SG, Jones JE: Postparturient diseases in sows associated with *Klebsiella* infection. Vet Res 87:484–485, 1970.
6. Ross RF, Harmon RL, Zimmerman BJ, et al: Susceptibility of sows to experimentally induced *Escherichia coli* mastitis. Am J Vet Res 44:949–954, 1983.
7. Smith BB, Wagner WC: Effect of *Escherichia coli* endotoxin and TRH on prolactin in lactating sows. Am J Vet Res 46:175–180, 1985.
8. Smith BB, Martineau G, Bisaillon A: Mammary glands and lactation problems. *In* Leman AD, Straw BF, Mengeling WL, et al (eds): Diseases of Swine, ed 7. Ames, Iowa, Iowa State University Press, 1992, pp 40–61.
9. Jones JET: Reflections on post-parturient diseases associated with lactational failure in sows. Vet Rec 89:72–77, 1971.
10. King GJ, Willoughby RA, Hacker RR: Fluctuations in rectal temperature of swine at parturition. Can Vet J 13:72–74, 1972.
11. Ross RF, Orning AP, Woods RD, et al: Bacteriologic study of sow agalactia. Am J Vet Res 42:949–955, 1981.
12. Radostits OM, Blood DC, Gay CC: Mastitis-metritis-agalactia (MMA) syndrome in sows (toxemic agalactia, farrowing fever, lactation failure). *In* Radostits OM, Blood DC, Gay CC (eds): Veterinary Medicine, ed 8. London, Baillière Tindall, 1994, pp 618–624.

■ Retained Fetal Membranes

Melvyn L. Fahning, D.V.M., Ph.D.

Retained fetal membranes (RFM) is a condition that is very easily diagnosed and yet is complex in terms of its cause, effects, and management. The condition affects cattle and water buffalo more frequently than any of our other food-producing animals. Even sheep and goats, which have a similar type of placentation, have a much lower incidence and few of the associated problems seen in cattle. The abnormal condition of RFM is most often defined as fetal membranes not being expelled by 12 hours after delivery. Some authors extend that period to 24 hours before they consider the retained membranes to be pathologic. This variation in time can affect the incidence of RFM.

INCIDENCE AND ECONOMIC SIGNIFICANCE

The effects of RFM can be varied and manifested in a number of ways. Some of the associated effects include lowered milk production, increased incidence of postpartum metritis and pyometra, and decreased appetite, which can predispose to abomasal displacement. Retained fetal membranes also cause decreased fertility as a result of increased time to first service, reduced first-service conception rate, increased services per conception, and increased days open.

The incidence considered normal for most dairy herds would be in the range of 4% to 12%. The condition is found less frequently in beef cattle.

Economically, RFM represents one of the most significant postpartum abnormalities. Losses occur because of the following factors: longer days open, up to 1% mortality, decreased milk yield and discarded milk because of treatments, higher culling rate, and the cost of veterinary treatment.

ETIOLOGY

Many factors have been implicated in causing RFM, and therefore a single cause has not been elucidated. In general, RFM is attributed to a disturbance of the normal loosening processes in the placentomes, which actually begins days or weeks before parturition. Because we know so little about the normal separation process, it is even more difficult to pinpoint the causes of retention. An increased incidence of RFM has been associated with any abnormal calving or dystocia, twin births, abortions, induced parturition, and premature births or prolonged gestation. Nutritional deficiencies such as vitamin E/selenium and vitamin A deficiency are associated with an increased incidence of RFM. Uterine atony associated with milk fever and hydropic conditions also contributes to the occurrence of RFM, but uterine atony alone, without any other disturbances in the loosening process, is not a major factor in causing RFM. The rate of RFM increases with age and with any infectious cause of placentitis.

Passing of the placenta postpartum involves the loss of fetomaternal adherence and uterine contractions, which physically expel the placenta. Uterine motility is important, but the determining factor for expulsion appears to be disengagement of the fetal and maternal villi.

The process of collagen development in the placental epithelium and maternal crypts begins months before parturition. Contractions of the uterus during the dilation and expulsion phases cause constant changing pressure that results in alternating ischemic and hyperemic conditions. This also results in changes in the shape of the placentomes and surface area of the fetal villi. Attachment of the chorionic epithelium in the maternal crypts becomes impaired, and the first signs of mechanical detachment become evident.

Calving can be induced by the administration of corticosteroids and/or prostaglandins, and RFM is a consistent side effect. Thus the hormonal profile for induced calving is fairly well understood, but its relevance to spontaneous RFM is unclear. Sampling for hormones at parturition is not sufficient because the placenta matures over a period of several days. Consequently, the results of sampling for progesterone and estrogen levels have been inconclusive as they relate to RFM.

Immunologic processes appear to be closely involved in placental release. A reduction in the chemotactic activity of leukocytes was found in cows in which retained placentas eventually developed.[1] Joostens and Hensen[2] found a link between retained placentas and compatibility of the major histocompatibility complex (MHC) of the calf and dam. They suggest that compatibility of the MHC may have an effect on placental maturation.

One can easily conclude that much remains to be learned about normal placental separation and the causes of retention.

TREATMENT

Few topics elicit as much discussion among practitioners and academicians as the subject of how to treat RFM. Veterinarians have diverse opinions about how this condition should be handled and treated. A review by Paisley and co-workers[3] demonstrated the wide variety of treatment alternatives that exist for RFM. One of the earliest and most widely practiced forms of treatment for RFM has been manual removal. One of the main reasons for manual removal is for the benefit of the farmer: to improve milking parlor hygiene. The other reason for removal should be for the benefit of the cow. The first goal can easily be achieved, but the benefit to the cow is much less clear. Most of the scientific literature concludes that manual removal with or without chemotherapy results in reduced rather than enhanced fertility. Considerable trauma to the endometrium occurs even during conservative attempts at manual removal, and manual removal is also associated with inhibition of the uterine defense mechanism. The use of intrauterine antiseptics and other therapeutic agents further inhibits uterine phagocytosis, which is already suppressed. Total removal can only be accomplished if placental separation is complete, which is unlikely. Thus there is a high risk of parts of the placenta remaining in the uterus. Consequently, the overall effect of manual removal is to increase the risk of subsequent metritis. Bolinder and colleagues[4] reported a higher incidence and more severe uterine infections in cows after RFM removal than in untreated cows with RFM. Manual removal also prolonged the occurrence of the first functional corpus luteum by 20 days.

Stevens and associates[5] compared the use of intrauterine infusion of oxytetracycline, subcutaneous injection of fenprostalene, or a combination of both for the treatment of RFM in dairy cows. The conclusions of this study were that the interval from parturition to expulsion of fetal membranes was unaffected by the treatment regimen, as was the frequency of displaced abomasum, ketosis, and mastitis. Reproductive efficiency, as determined on the basis of the interval from parturition to conception, was also unaffected by the treatment protocol.

Drugs that increase uterine motility are frequently used in the treatment of RFM. Estrogen has been used extensively and was thought to have a uterotonic effect. Burton and associates[6] found that it had no such effect. If estrogen has any merit in cases of RFM, it would be due to its stimulation of phagocytic activity and increased uterine blood flow. Other drugs administered to increase uterine motility include oxytocin, ergot derivatives, calcium solutions, and prostaglandin. However, they have been shown to be of limited value. The lack of response should not be surprising in view of the low incidence of uterine atony as a primary cause of RFM.

Eiler and Hopkins[7] reported a different type of treatment for RFM in which the enzyme collagenase is infused into the umbilical arteries. These authors reported that the procedure requires about 25 minutes to complete. A dose of 200,000 IU of collagenase was dissolved in 1 L of saline. It was reported that 85% of the retained membranes were released or loosened in 36 hours. About 15% of the cows do not respond, and repeated or increased doses of collagenase are not effective. The author of this article has not had any experience with this technique. No recent reports of its use have appeared in the literature, which would indicate a lack of widespread acceptance of this technique. Still unanswered is the question of whether there would be a difference in subsequent fertility if this technique were used in a controlled trial as compared with no treatment.

The use of intrauterine therapy does decrease putrefaction and the associated fetid odor of RFM. Although this may be an important consideration aesthetically from the client's viewpoint, it still makes the use of intrauterine therapy questionable economically because of the cost of treatment and withholding of milk for human consumption after treatment. Prostaglandins administered during the immediate postpartum period (within 1 hour) have been advocated by some practitioners as a means of preventing or at least lowering the incidence of RFM; how-

ever, no good evidence exists to support this use of prostaglandin.[5] Burton and co-workers[6] reported that neither prostaglandin $F_{2\alpha}$ nor an analogue of prostaglandin (fenprostalene) was uterotonic during the early postpartum period.

In summary, the results of most studies support the conclusion that no treatment is the best way to manage RFM in the cow. The cow should, however, be closely monitored for signs of systemic involvement so that appropriate supportive therapy can be administered if systemic involvement occurs. Routine postpartum examination starting at about 2 weeks postpartum as part of a routine fertility program should be practiced. Some clients will demand manual removal of RFM, and the practitioner will probably comply with this request; however, one should be conservative in attempts to manually remove the RFM to minimize damage. The practitioner should make use of these opportunities to educate the client.

To prevent or reduce the incidence of RFM, the veterinarian should encourage the client to maintain an effective vaccination program and maintain pregnant animals on a good nutritional program with special emphasis on vitamin E/selenium and vitamin A and proper mineral supplementation. It is also important to have a clean and sanitary calving environment.

Other species of food animals that experience RFM include sheep, goats, and swine, but these species have a much lower incidence of RFM. However, in swine, the membranes may be retained in the apical part of the horn and not be visible externally. Septic metritis often develops in these sows, and mortality can be relatively high. In swine, if RFM is suspected, repeated doses of oxytocin (20 to 30 units every 2 to 3 hours) and broad-spectrum antibiotics should be administered.

REFERENCES

1. Heuweiser W, Grunert E: Significance of chemotactic activity for placental expulsion in cattle. Theriogenology 278:907, 1987.
2. Joostens I, Hensen EJ: Involvement of major histocompatibility complex class I compatibility between dam and calf in the aetiology of bovine retained placenta. Anim Reprod Sci 28:451, 1992.
3. Paisley LP, Mickelson WD, Anderson PB: Mechanisms and therapy for retained fetal membranes and uterine factors in cattle. Theriogenology 278:907, 1987.
4. Bolinder A, Seguin B, Kindahl H, et al: Retained fetal membranes in cow: Manual removal versus nonremoval and the effect on reproductive performance. Theriogenology 30:45, 1988.
5. Stevens RD, Dinsmore RP, Cattell MB: Evaluation of the use of intrauterine infusions of oxytetracycline, subcutaneous injections of fenprostalene, or a combination of both, for the treatment of retained placenta in dairy cows. J Am Vet Med Assoc 207:612, 1995.
6. Burton MJ, Herschler RC, Dziuk HE, et al: Effect of fenprostalene on postpartum myometrial activity in dairy cows with normal or delayed placental expulsion. Br Vet J 143:549, 1987.
7. Eiler H, Hopkins FM: Successful treatment of retained placenta with umbilical cord injection of collagenase in cows. J Am Vet Med Assoc 203:436, 1993.

■ Metritis and Endometritis

Gavin F. Richardson, D.V.M., M.V.Sc.

Metritis and endometritis in cows can result in considerable economic loss to producers. These losses result from reduced reproductive efficiency, loss of production, cost of therapy, increased replacement costs, forced culling, and sometimes the adverse effects of systemic illness. Under appropriate circumstances, veterinarians can reduce these economic losses by promoting good nutrition of breeding stock and encouraging proper sanitary practices at calving and during the early postpartum period.

Puerperal metritis occurs in the early postpartum period. In dairy cows this period has been defined as the period following parturition when the pituitary gland is insensitive to gonadotropin-releasing hormone (the first 7 to 14 days).[1] Conditions that predispose to puerperal metritis include retained fetal membranes, dystocia, trauma to the reproductive tract, an emphysematous fetus, hydrallantois, and unsanitary conditions.

Pathologic uterine infections that persist into the intermediate postpartum period are referred to as *metritis* or *endometritis*. The intermediate period in dairy cows begins when the pituitary gland becomes sensitive to gonadotropin-releasing hormone and lasts until the first ovulation (generally 10 to 30 days postpartum).[1] Endometritis and occasionally metritis can still be present in the postovulatory period (which in normal dairy cows lasts until uterine involution is complete at 40 to 45 days).[1] Endometritis can also result from pyometra or the introduction of pathogens during insemination (e.g., by breeding during the luteal phase).

ETIOLOGIC AGENTS

Actinomyces pyogenes is thought to be the most important aerobic organism involved in metritis or endometritis.[1, 2] Gram-negative anaerobes that act synergistically with *A. pyogenes* to produce these infections include *Fusobacterium necrophorum* and *Bacteroides* spp.[1, 2] Infections with streptococci, staphylococci, *Pasteurella* spp., *Bacillus* spp., *Pseudomonas* spp., and so on rarely persist, cause permanent endometrial damage, or lead to impaired fertility.[1, 2] However, they may be responsible for acute septic metritis in some cows.

Escherichia coli may produce endotoxins. Less commonly, clostridial infections can produce severe or fatal disease. Other organisms that can cause endometritis include mycoplasmas, ureaplasmas, *Haemophilus somnus*, *Campylobacter fetus* subsp. *veneralis*, *Brucella abortus*, *Tritrichomonas foetus*, and certain viruses; these organisms are not discussed in this article.

CLINICAL SIGNS

Cows with acute septic metritis can exhibit signs of toxemia such as anorexia, depression, tachycardia, rumen atony, dehydration, and even weakness and shock. Laminitis may develop in an occasional affected cow. Subinvolution of the uterus usually occurs, which is often fluid-filled and atonic. The vaginal discharge is foul smelling and purulent to reddish brown.

Cows with less severe metritis may have slightly elevated temperatures, be somewhat anorectic, have reduced milk production, or show no systemic signs. There is subinvolution of the uterus and usually a malodorous or purulent vaginal discharge.

Endometritis can be characterized by infertility and a purulent vaginal discharge, which is most often observed during estrus. Affected cows can exhibit shortened or prolonged estrous cycles because of excessive prostaglandin release or embryonic death, respectively. The uterus can be slightly enlarged and may contain a small amount of fluid; however, there may be no palpable abnormalities on transrectal examination.

Perimetritis occurs when uterine infections extend through the uterine wall. A localized or generalized peritonitis can result, and the uterus often forms adhesions to adjacent structures. Because of these adhesions, the reproductive tract can be difficult to palpate or retract. Infertility can result, especially if the ovaries, oviducts, or ovarian bursae are involved or if an abscess drains into the uterine lumen. If the adhesions are extensive, they can compromise the ability of the uterus to expand and result in affected cows becoming chronic aborters. Attempts to break the adhesions down generally result in the formation of more extensive adhesions.

DIAGNOSIS

The characteristics of the vaginal discharge from a postpartum cow must be interpreted carefully to avoid misdiagnosis or incorrect or unnecessary therapy. Manual or speculum examination of the vagina in a sanitary manner is often necessary to inspect this discharge. The discharge of reddish brown, non-odorous fluid that may contain flecks of debris or exudate during the first 10 to 18 days postpartum may be normal lochia and not caused by puerperal metritis. As long as the discharge does not become foul smelling, uterine involution usually proceeds normally.[1] Purulent vaginal discharge in a cycling postpartum cow may not be a sign of metritis or endometritis, but it may be a sign of an active uterine defense mechanism.[2] Evidence suggests that a cloudy, mucous discharge at estrus is not more likely to be infected with pathogenic organisms than is clear mucus.[2]

The diagnosis of postpartum endometritis can be difficult in a clinical setting. Examination of the vagina with a speculum may be the most effective method of diagnosing this condition.[3, 4] This should be combined with an accurate history, visual inspection of the perineum, examination of the tail for evidence of vaginal discharge, and transrectal examination of the reproductive tract. Transrectal ultrasonography of the reproductive tract may be a useful diagnostic technique, particularly when examining the contents of the uterus. Endometrial culture and biopsy can be used, but there are difficulties in interpretation. Furthermore, reduced fertility in cows during the breeding period immediately following postpartum endometrial biopsy has been reported.[3, 5] In most instances, a decision must be made regarding therapy prior to the availability of culture or biopsy results. Nonetheless, culture and biopsy results can be useful in providing retrospective information. A wide variation in the rate of uterine involution can make the results of a single clinical examination of the uterus prior to 21 days postpartum difficult to interpret.

TREATMENT

Cows with metritis that are not affected systemically usually recover satisfactorily without veterinary intervention. Cows with metritis should be examined 30 to 40 days postpartum to make certain that the uterus is involuting normally and that there is no evidence of pyometra, endometritis, or cystic ovarian disease.

Systemic antibiotic therapy is required in septicemic cows or if the oviducts, ovaries, or deeper layers of the uterus are involved. Penicillin (at a dosage of 22,000 units/kg intramuscularly every 12 hours) or broad-spectrum antibiotics at the appropriate dosage can be administered. Once instituted, systemic antibiotic therapy should be continued for a minimum of 5 days.

Cows with severe metritis that are exhibiting signs of toxemia such as dehydration and/or shock will require appropriate fluid and other supportive therapy. Nonsteroidal anti-inflammatory agents such as flunixin meglumine, 0.25 mg/kg every 8 hours, may be beneficial in reducing the effects of toxemia. (Note: One or both of these drugs are not approved for food animal use in some countries.)

Little conclusive evidence exists that intrauterine infusions of antimicrobials are of any benefit in the treatment of metritis or endometritis.[2, 4] In fact, intrauterine antiseptics and many antibiotics are capable of inhibiting phagocytosis for several days after application.[2] This depressed leukocyte activity could be disastrous, especially if the organism involved is resistant to the antibiotic or antiseptic used. Irritating solutions should not be used in the uterus because they will increase the inflammation that is already present. Very few antimicrobial preparations list milk withdrawal times on the label for intrauterine infusion.

Infusing warm water or saline into the early postpartum uterus and then siphoning it off has been suggested as means of removing infected materials and improving the condition of the cow.[6] Although controlled studies to evaluate this form of therapy are lacking, the removal of most or all of the material from an infected uterus should logically be of benefit. Nonetheless, several hazards or difficulties can be associated with this type of therapy. The uterus can be punctured or damaged during the procedure, irrigation fluid might flow into the oviducts and cause salpingitis, placental tissue and debris can block the hose during siphoning, and a large, dependent uterus may be difficult to empty satisfactorily. This procedure can therefore be ineffective and is not without risk. It is contraindicated in situations in which the uterine wall is damaged or friable. If used, initial infusion volumes of 1 L have been recommended until it can be determined whether the fluid can be retrieved. After this, infusion volumes may vary from 1 to 4 L and are continued until the effluent is clear. Transrectal massage of the uterus might assist in expelling the fluid.

Cows with chronic endometritis have been reported to benefit from flushing the uterus with physiologic saline during diestrus by using techniques for the nonsurgical collection of embryos.[7] This can be followed by the administration of prostaglandins and breeding at the induced estrus. For severe endometritis, flushing can be repeated every 48 hours, as indicated.

Cows with retained fetal membranes and/or metritis have been reported to benefit from therapy with prostaglandin $F_{2\alpha}$ or its analogues (PG).[2] There are indications that prostaglandin stimulates ovarian activity in the postpartum period.[8] However, cows with retained fetal membranes or metritis probably already have elevated levels of prostaglandins.[8] There is also evidence that prostaglandin (PG) levels are not important in the dynamics of uterine involution.[8] Furthermore, the prostaglandin preparations currently used do not increase myometrial activity in the early postpartum cow, even when the uterus is primed with estrogen.[9] Oxytocin has been shown to be more effective than prostaglandins in stimulating myometrial activity up to 9 days postpartum,[10, 11] and estrogen priming does not enhance this effect.[12] Oxytocin has also been reported to increase phagocytosis by uterine leukocytes.[2] Thus oxytocin at 20 to 30 units repeated every 2 to 3 hours for several treatments could possibly be of benefit in treating cows with puerperal metritis. Higher dosages of this hormone have been reported to result in spasms of the uterine musculature.[11]

Prostaglandins are indicated in the treatment of endometritis or metritis in the postovulatory period.[1, 2] The optimal time for PG therapy would be after day 7 of the estrous cycle, the time when the corpus luteum is most responsive. This timing is used because successful resolution of endometritis has been associated with the occurrence of estrus. Nonetheless, there may also be a benefit to cows that are not in the luteal phase.[5] Prostaglandins may have a beneficial effect on the postpartum uterus that is independent of their luteolytic effect.[13] The uterine health and fertility of cows experiencing dystocia, retained fetal membranes, and/or metritis may be improved by administering PG at 2 to 3 weeks postpartum and again 2 weeks later.[14]

METRITIS AND ENDOMETRITIS IN OTHER FOOD-PRODUCING ANIMALS

Metritis and endometritis in sheep and goats can resemble these conditions in cows. In sows, urogenital infections can occur as endemic infections or as epidemics.[15] Abnormal vulvar discharge can originate from infections of the urinary tract, vagina, uterus, or a combination of these. Many different bacteria have been isolated from these infections, often in mixed cultures. Viruses or even ureaplasmas could also be involved. The boar may transmit some of the causative organisms venereally. History, clinical signs, and slaughterhouse inspections are commonly used methods of determining the site and nature of these infections. It is important to distinguish between normal vaginal discharge, which usually occurs within 10 days after mating, and abnormal discharge, which usually occurs later.[16] In addition, record analysis will help identify key epidemiologic features of the problem. Uterine infections are commonly associated with reduced conception and farrowing rates and regular return to estrus.[15]

The principles of therapy for uterine infections in cows can be applied to small ruminants and swine. However, PG therapy may not be beneficial in sows. Proper sanitation and hygiene (including at breeding), culling of affected animals, and good management practices will probably reduce the incidence of these infections much more effectively and economically than will therapy, especially in sows.[16, 17] Tetanus prophylaxis should be considered when treating uterine infections in small ruminants.

REFERENCES

1. Olson JD, Bretzlaff KN, Mortimer RG, et al: The metritis-pyometra complex. *In* Morrow DA (ed): Current Therapy in Theriogenology, ed 2. Philadelphia, WB Saunders, 1986, pp 227–236.
2. Paisley LG, Mickelson WD, Anderson PB: Mechanisms and therapy for retained fetal membranes and uterine infections of cows: A review. Theriogenology 25:353, 1986.
3. Miller HV, Kimsey PB, Kendrick JW, et al: Endometritis of dairy cattle: Diagnosis, treatment, and fertility. Bov Pract 15:13, 1980.
4. Gilbert RO: Bovine endometritis: The burden of proof (editorial). Cornell Vet 82:11, 1992.
5. Etherington WG, Martin SW, Bonnett B, et al: Reproductive performance in dairy cows following treatment with cloprostenol 26 and/or 40 days postpartum: A field trial. Theriogenology 29:565, 1988.
6. Montes AJ, Pugh DG: Clinical approach to postpartum metritis. Compend Contin Educ Pract Vet 15:1131, 1993.
7. Johnson WH: Embryo transfer in repeat breeder cows. *In* Morrow DA (ed): Current Therapy in Theriogenology, ed 2. Philadelphia, WB Saunders, 1986, pp 60–62.
8. Thatcher WW: Role of prostaglandins during the periparturient period in the cow. *In* Proceedings of the Annual Meeting of the Society for Theriogenology. Orlando, Fla, 1988, p 55.
9. Ko JCH, McKenna DJ, Whitmore HL, et al: Effects of estradiol cypionate and natural and synthetic prostaglandins on myometrial activity in early postpartum cows. Theriogenology 32:537, 1989.
10. Eiler H, Hopkins FM, Armstrong-Backus CS, et al: Uterotonic effect of prostaglandin $F_{2\alpha}$ and oxytocin on the postpartum cow. Am J Vet Res 45:1011, 1984.
11. Burton MJ, Zuelke KA, Dziuk HE, et al: Postpartum myometrial response to oxytocin in the cow. *In* Proceedings of the 67th Conference of Research Workers in Animal Diseases, Chicago, 1986, p 40.
12. Burton MJ, Dziuk HE, Fahning ML, et al: Effects of oestradiol cypionate on spontaneous and oxytocin-stimulated postpartum myometrial activity in the cow. Br Vet J 146:309, 1990.
13. Bonnett BN, Etherington WG, Martin SW, et al: The effect of prostaglandin administration to Holstein-Friesian cows at day 26 postpartum on clinical findings, and histological and bacteriological results of endometrial biopsies at day 40. Theriogenology 33:877, 1990.
14. Olson JD: Metritis/endometritis: Medically sound treatments. *In* Proceedings of the 29th Annual Convention of the American Association of Bovine Practitioners. San Diego, 1996, p 8.
15. Dial GD, MacLachlan NJ: Urogenital infections of swine: I. Clinical manifestations and pathogenesis. Compend Contin Educ Pract Vet 10:63, 1988.

16. Almond G: Urogenital infections and uterine immunity. *In* Proceedings of the Swine Reproduction Symposium of the American College of Theriogenologists, Society for Theriogenology and American Association of Swine Practitioners. Kansas City, 1996, p 113.

17. Dial GD, MacLachlan NJ: Urogenital infections of swine: II. Pathology and medical management. Compend Contin Educ Pract Vet 10:529, 1988.

■ Bovine Vaginitis

Gavin F. Richardson, D.V.M., M.V.Sc.

NECROTIC VAGINITIS

Necrotic vaginitis can occasionally occur as a result of trauma to the birth canal following dystocia or concurrent with metritis. The condition can be painful, and affected cows may arch their backs, strain, and become anorectic. A necrotic, diphtheritic inflammation of the vestibule and vagina is accompanied by a fetid, watery, reddish discharge. Some degree of vaginal stenosis may result.

Treatment consists of the local application of bland, oily antibiotic preparations two to three times daily. One must be careful not to carry infection forward into the uterus when administering local therapy. Antibiotics should also be administered systemically. In addition, analgesics and nonsteroidal anti-inflammatory agents may be beneficial. If severe pneumovagina is a problem, the dorsal portions of the vulvar lips can be sutured closed (Caslick's operation).

Cows with chronic tenesmus can be treated with a conventional epidural anesthetic. Epidural anesthesia can be prolonged by installing a catheter in the epidural space and capping it between infusions of local anesthetic.[1] Prolonged epidural anesthesia using alcohol preparations in small increments administered to effect (usually 3 to 8 mL is required) has been described; however, this practice can lead to prolonged paralysis of the tail with its associated problems.

VESTIBULOVAGINITIS

Vestibulovaginitis most often occurs when a uterine and/or cervical infection is also present. In addition, it can result from poor vulvar tone and poor perineal conformation. Besides the organisms usually involved in uterine infections, mycoplasmas, ureaplasmas, *Haemophilus somnus*, and an enterovirus have also been associated with this disease. The "Epivag" virus causes infection of the entire tubular genital tract of cows in Africa. The vaginal inflammation may result in a mucopurulent vaginal discharge. However, vaginoscopy is essential to confirm the diagnosis of this condition.

If a uterine infection is also present, therapy would be as described for metritis and endometritis. If poor perineal conformation is the cause, the dorsal portion of the vulva can be sutured closed (Caslick's operation). If indicated, bland, oily antibiotic preparations can be applied locally. Rest from sexual activity will aid healing and help prevent possible spread of the disease. Good sanitation and isolation of affected animals will help prevent the spread of a contagious infection.

GRANULAR VULVITIS

Granular vulvitis is a transient, disseminated lymphoid hyperplasia in the vulvar mucosa that disappears without treatment in 10 to 14 days. The hyperplasia is a characteristic reaction of this area to various infectious organisms and irritants; it should not result in infertility unless pathogenic organisms such as ureaplasmas are involved. Severe infections can result in a mucopurulent discharge from the vulva. The counterpart in the bull is known as granular balanoposthitis.

Treatment of this condition is not usually required. However, in a natural breeding situation, rest from sexual activity for 2 to 4 weeks might be advisable in case a pathogenic organism is involved. If artificial insemination is used, the double-sheath insemination technique should be used to prevent possible transfer of pathogens into the uterus.

INFECTIOUS PUSTULAR VULVOVAGINITIS

Infectious pustular vulvovaginitis is caused by a herpesvirus very similar or identical to the virus that causes infectious bovine rhinotracheitis. Vesicles form in the vagina and become pustules and eventually ulcers. The lesions may become secondarily infected with bacteria and/or coalesce. A mucopurulent vaginal discharge may be present. The counterpart in bulls is known as infectious pustular balanoposthitis. Pain is exhibited and infertility can result from a reluctance to breed. If breeding should occur, there is an unproven potential for reduced conception and/or pregnancy rates. The diagnosis is often based on clinical signs alone but can be confirmed by isolation of the virus.

Rest from sexual activity is recommended for 3 to 4 weeks or more to allow for healing and prevent spread of the disease. Oily antibiotic preparations can be applied locally to combat secondary bacterial infections and reduce the possibility of preputial adhesions in bulls. The use of infectious bovine rhinotracheitis vaccines to prevent the disease is questionable.

REFERENCE

1. Elmore RG: Food-animal regional anesthesia. Bovine blocks: Continuous epidural anesthesia. Vet Med Small Anim Clin 75:1174, 1980.

BIBLIOGRAPHY

Roberts SJ: Veterinary obstetrics and genital diseases. *In* Theriogenology, ed 3. Ann Arbor, Mich, Edward Brothers, 1986.

■ Pyometra in Cattle

Louis F. Archbald, D.V.M., M.S., Ph.D., M.R.C.V.S.

Pyometra is the accumulation of purulent exudate in the uterus. It is an infectious uterine disorder characterized clinically by retention of the corpus luteum and anestrus. Because there are no systemic manifestations of the disease, affected cows do not appear ill. However, these cows are economic liabilities inasmuch as they often experience infertility and, in some instances, sterility. Spontaneous recovery from the disease is uncommon.

Pyometra should not be confused with chronic endometritis, which may be associated with thickening or enlargement of the uterine wall and the presence of a purulent vulvar discharge. In most instances, these cows are cyclic, although there may be irregularities in the length of the estrous cycles.

OCCURRENCE

Pyometra occurs most often during the early postpartum period (15 to 60 days postpartum). Pyometra may be a sequela of dystocia, retained fetal membranes, or acute septic metritis. It can also occur at various intervals after breeding. Such cases are associated with early embryonic death, which may result from an infection introduced at the time of breeding or one already present in the uterus at breeding. Intrauterine insemination of cows during the luteal phase or of pregnant cows will often result in embryonic death and pyometra. The use of bulls infected with the protozoan *Trichomonas foetus* often results in cases of pyometra.

ETIOLOGY

Postpartum pyometra is caused by infection of the uterus by a variety of microorganisms, including hemolytic streptococci, hemolytic staphylococci, coliforms, *Actinomyces pyogenes*, and *Pseudomonas aeruginosa*. Occasionally, animals may be infected with clostridia or different types of fungi. *A. pyogenes* is probably the most common cause of bovine pyometra and can be the cause of pyometra in several cows within a herd.

Postbreeding pyometra, although relatively uncommon, is usually caused by the same microorganisms as those causing postpartum pyometra. However, a more common cause of postbreeding pyometra is the protozoan *T. foetus*.

CLINICAL SIGNS

Affected cows show no general signs of illness, even though the uterus contains a considerable amount of purulent material. Because of failure of the uterine luteolytic mechanism, the corpus luteum persists and true anestrus is commonly observed. In some cases of postpartum pyometra, a purulent vulvar discharge may be observed when the cow lies down. The consistency of the discharge is usually thick and mucoid. However, its color may be yellow, creamy white, grayish white, greenish gray, or reddish brown. In some cows the cervix may be closed and there is no evidence of such a discharge.

On palpation of the uterus per rectum, the uterus is distended with fluid and there is a corpus luteum on one of the ovaries. The size of the uterus can correspond to that characteristic of any stage of pregnancy. Distribution of the fluid in the uterus may be bilaterally symmetrical, or the fluid may predominantly occupy one uterine horn. In cases of unilateral uterine enlargement, the corpus luteum may be observed on the contralateral ovary. It should be noted that pyometra may occasionally exist even if no corpus luteum can be palpated. In addition, it is not uncommon to find that the corpus luteum is smaller than that observed during the luteal phase.

In most cases, vaginal examination will reveal degrees of enlargement of the cervical os and the presence of purulent material in the anterior of the vagina.

DIAGNOSIS

Mucometra, hydrometra, and pregnancy are the three most important conditions that must be differentiated from pyometra. Mucometra or hydrometra occurs most frequently in cases of chronic cystic follicles of the ovaries. However, cases of segmental aplasia of the tubular tract derived from the müllerian duct system should also be considered when mucometra or hydrometra is observed. The most diagnostic feature of pyometra is the absence of any positive signs of pregnancy (amnionic vesicle, fetal membranes, placentomes, and the fetus) in a fluid-filled uterus.

TREATMENT AND PROGNOSIS

Treatment of pyometra is directed toward re-establishment of the estrous cycle through destruction of the corpus luteum (luteolysis). This can be achieved by several different methods.

The most effective and safest method is by the use of exogenously administered prostaglandins and their analogues. The intramuscular administration of 25 mg of dinoprost tromethamine (Lutalyse*) has been shown to be effective in causing luteolysis and evacuation of the uterine contents of cows with pyometra. Estrus is usually observed within 3 to 4 days following treatment, and complete uterine evacuation is observed in most cows at this time. Cloprostenol, a prostaglandin analogue, has also been shown to be effective when administered intramuscularly at the dosage of 0.5 mg.

Recent research[1] has demonstrated that persistence of the corpus luteum in cows with pyometra is not due to an insufficiency in the synthesis of uterine prostaglandin $F_{2\alpha}$ ($PGF_{2\alpha}$) but may be associated with inadequate secretion of luteal oxytocin. Because luteal oxytocin is involved in the release of uterine $PGF_{2\alpha}$ at the time of luteolysis,[2] it may be argued that in cows with pyometra, the release of uterine $PGF_{2\alpha}$ is inadequate to cause luteolysis. Therefore it would appear that multiple dosages of $PGF_{2\alpha}$ may be more effective in causing luteolysis. In fact, it has been demonstrated[3] that more cows exhibit estrus following treatment with two doses of $PGF_{2\alpha}$ (25 mg given intramuscularly) 8 hours apart than cows receiving similar treatment 24 hours apart. In light of these research reports, it is recommended that at the time of diagnosis, cows with pyometra be given two doses of $PGF_{2\alpha}$ (25 mg each, given intramuscularly) 8 hours apart.

Various estrogens can also be used as luteolytic agents in the treatment of pyometra. However, the results are inconsistent, and cystic follicles, ovaritis, ovarian adhesions, and relaxation of the pelvic ligaments are disadvantages of this approach to treatment.

In some cases lysis of the corpus luteum may occur, but rectal palpation of the uterus indicates the continued presence of intrauterine fluid. Partial or complete cervical stenosis, possibly as a result of trauma at calving, should be considered when determining the cause of this apparent lack of response to treatment.

Manual enucleation of the corpus luteum by rectal palpation is an effective but unacceptable method of destroying the corpus luteum. The major disadvantages of this method include excessive hemorrhage and subsequent ovarian adhesions. In some instances it may be difficult to positively identify the corpus luteum by rectal palpation of the ovaries, possibly because the corpus luteum is smaller and more deeply embedded in the ovary of cows with pyometra.

Manual draining of the uterus and intrauterine infusion with antibiotics following evacuation of the uterine contents have not been shown to increase subsequent fertility.

REFERENCES

1. Vighio GH, Liptrap RM, Etherington WG: Oxytocin-prostaglandin interrelationships in the cow with pyometra. Theriogenology 35:1121–1129, 1991.
2. Flint APF, Sheldrick EL: Evidence for a systemic role for ovarian oxytocin in luteal regression in sheep. J Reprod Fertil 67:215–225, 1983.
3. Archbald LF, Risco C, Chavatte P, et al: Estrus and pregnancy rate of dairy cows given one or two doses of prostaglandin $F_{2\alpha}$ 8 or 24 hours apart. Theriogenology 40:873–884, 1993.

*Upjohn Co, Kalamazoo, Mich.

■ Ovarian Follicular Dynamics and Endocrine Profiles in Cows With Ovarian Follicular Cysts

H. Allen Garverick, Ph.D.

Ovarian follicular cysts (cysts) are anovulatory follicular structures that occur in a number of mammalian species. The incidence in dairy herds in the United States probably ranges between 10% and 13%. This is a serious economic problem for producers because cows affected with cysts have extended calving intervals of approximately 50 days. Cows are infertile as long as the condition persists. Several recent publications have reviewed the occurrence, etiology, treatment.[1–3] Cysts have traditionally been defined as follicular structures on the ovary 2.5 cm in diameter or larger that persist for extended periods of time in the absence of a corpus luteum. Recent discoveries have led to a re-examination of the concept of persistent follicular cysts.

OVARIAN FOLLICULAR DYNAMICS

The dynamics of follicular growth in cattle was a subject of debate for many years. The use of real-time ultrasonic examination of the ovaries has provided a much clearer picture of ovarian follicular dynamics in the past 6 to 10 years. Daily examination of ovaries with ultrasound has shown that the estrous cycle of cattle is characterized by the growth of two, three, or four waves of follicular development. In each wave, a cohort of one to five follicles is recruited to continue growth. From this cohort, one follicle is typically selected for continued growth toward dominance and ovulation and the others undergo atresia. If luteolysis occurs while the dominant follicle is in the growing phase, ovulation of the dominant follicle occurs. If luteolysis does not occur during the growth phase, atresia occurs and another wave of follicular growth is initiated.

CYST DYNAMICS

Based on the earlier definition provided, it was assumed that cysts were static structures that persisted for considerable periods of time, which is contrary to our current knowledge of ovarian follicular dynamics in cattle. However, in one early report in which cyst development was monitored by rectal palpation and long-term changes in reproductive hormone secretion it was suggested that cysts were not static structures. Long-term changes in cystic structures and hormone concentrations indicated that cysts were dynamic in nature.[4] Cows with cysts exhibited great variation in circulating hormone concentrations and appeared to be trying to correct the condition but were unable to do so until normal concentrations of hormones were achieved.

Another stumbling block in studying the etiology of cysts was the unpredictable nature of their occurrence. Nearly all of the earlier studies were retrospective studies of cysts taken after their development. However, it was discovered that cysts can be induced with daily exogenous injections of 30 mg of estradiol-17β and 150 mg of progesterone dissolved in alcohol for 7 days. The treatment regimen raises serum concentrations of the injected hormones to levels similar to those observed near the end of gestation. Following completion of the steroid injections, ovaries become static for 25 to 30 days, after which follicular growth begins and results in the development of either a cyst

or an ovulatory follicle. A study using the treatment regimen to induce cysts was then undertaken to determine the turnover rate and fate of cysts.[5] Cysts were induced in 23 dairy cows. After the diagnosis of cysts, ovaries were observed via midventral laparotomy and the cysts were marked around their periphery with subepithelial injections of charcoal. Cysts were then removed 10, 20, or 40 days after marking, and structures on the ovary were recorded along with their position relative to the marked cyst (Table 1). Three different responses were observed. In most cases (20/23), the response was turnover, in which case the cyst decreased in size and was replaced by another follicular structure that either ovulated (7/23) or developed into a new cyst (13/23). In no case did the marked cyst ovulate. The marked cyst did persist at a similar or greater size in 3 of the cows for the duration of the experiment.

However, the actual time of cyst turnover and dynamics was not determined in that study. A second study used real-time ultrasonographic examination of ovaries in cows with induced cysts to study their growth and turnover rate.[6] Similar types and proportions of responses were observed in this study as in the previous study.[5] Cysts persisted for various periods but turned over (decreased in size and were replaced by new follicular

---

Table 1

TURNOVER RATE OF OVARIAN FOLLICULAR CYSTS IN DAIRY CATTLE AT 10, 20, OR 40 DAYS AFTER CHARCOAL MARKINGS OF CYSTS

Group	Days After Marking	Response			
		No.	Ovulation	Turnover	Persistence
1	10	8	1	6	1
2	20	8	4	4	0
3	40	7	2	3	2
Total		23	7*	13*	3*

*Significantly different ($P < .01$).
From Cook DL, Smith CA, Parfet JR, et al: Fate and turnover rate of ovarian follicular cysts in dairy cattle. J Reprod Fertil 90:37, 1990.

Table 2

CHARACTERIZATION OF FOLLICLE OR CYST DEVELOPMENT IN COWS WITH CYSTS AND COWS WITH NORMAL ESTROUS CYCLES

	Cystic Cows*	Control Cows†
Cows (no.)	8	14
Follicular or cystic waves (no.)	28	36
Turnover interval (days)	13.0‡ ± 1.1	8.5 ± 0.5
Range	6 to 26	6 to 14
Follicles or cysts per wave (no.)	3.1 ± 0.3	3.6 ± 0.2
Follicle or cyst size (cm)	2.8‡ ± 0.19	1.6 ± 0.05
Growth rate from detection		
To ovulatory size (days)	7.2 ± 0.3	6.9 ± 0.4
To maximum size (days)	12.7 ± 0.8	

*Cows with spontaneously occurring cysts (n = 3) and cysts induced by steroids (n = 5).
†Cows with ovulatory cycles include controls (n = 6) and those with ovulatory cycles following self-recovery from cysts (n = 8).
‡Significantly different from controls ($P < .05$).
From Hamilton SA, Garverick HA, Keisler DH, et al: Characterization of ovarian follicular cysts and associated endocrine profiles in dairy cows. Biol Reprod 53:890, 1995.

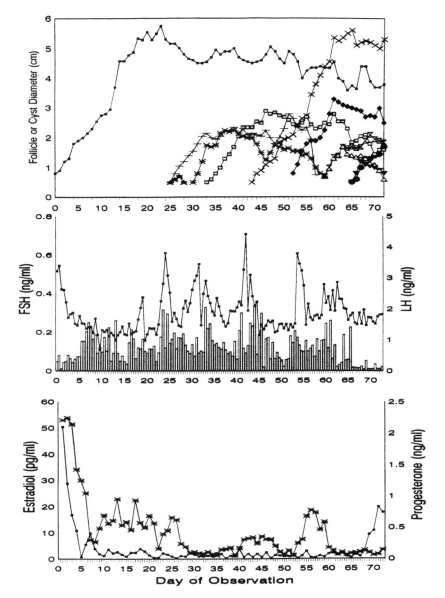

Figure 1

Example of persistence and turnover of follicles or cysts *(top panel)* during the period of observation from a single cow. Changes in size of individual follicles are shown in the top panel. Concentrations of FSH *(line)* and LH *(bars)* relative to the day of observation are displayed in the *middle panel*. Concentration of estradiol-17β *(asterisk)* and progesterone *(black square)* relative to the day of observation are shown in the *bottom panel*. The first follicle/cyst wave (day 0) was detected 10 days after the end of the steroid injections, which were used to induce cysts. (From Hamilton SA, Garverick HA, Keisler DH, et al: Characterization of ovarian follicular cysts and associated endocrine profiles in dairy cows. Biol Reprod 53:890, 1995.)

structures) in most cases. In most cows the new follicular structure developed into a cyst. Development of new cystic structures was characterized by recruitment of a cohort of follicles and selection of a dominant follicle similar to that observed in cows during normal estrous cycles. Following selection of the dominant follicle/cyst in the new wave, the rate of growth to ovulatory size was similar between structures that developed into ovulatory follicles and those that developed into cysts (Table 2). The cysts continued to grow for an additional 5 days. The interval between follicular/cyst waves in cows with cysts was nearly double that observed between follicular waves during normal estrous cycles. Of interest was the growth pattern of follicles/cysts in one cow (Fig. 1). At the beginning of the experimental period, a large cyst was observed that remained dominant for at least 25 days, and little other follicular growth was noted. However, after 25 days, growth of follicular waves was initiated in a periodic manner. However, the cyst remained the largest structure on the ovary for 58 days before another cyst of larger size finally replaced the original cyst. Of importance here is that the usual diagnosis of cysts by a single examination via rectal palpation would have detected only the largest structure, which had lost at least partial dominance after day 25.

Thus this cyst may not have been capable of responding to exogenous treatment with gonadotropin-releasing hormone (GnRH) or human chorionic gonadotropin (hCG).

ASSOCIATED ENDOCRINE PROFILES

Most of the early reports of endocrine changes in cows with cysts were usually retrospective studies of changes that occurred after the cyst had developed. A common finding of studies of endocrine changes in cows with cysts was that mean concentrations and changes in reproductive hormones were quite variable.[1] Based on our current knowledge of ovarian follicular and cyst dynamics, the endocrine parameters observed are explainable by the dynamic nature of cysts. That is, the endocrine milieu was dependent on the stage and steroidogenic capacity of other structures on the ovaries, as well as cysts. However, the ability to provide a model (previously described) whereby cysts could be developed in a predictable manner following exogenous injection of estradiol-17β and progesterone allowed the endocrinology of cysts to be studied.[6, 7] Following steroid treatment, a static period (no follicular growth) occurs for about 30 days, after which a follicular phase is initiated that results in the development of either a cyst or a follicle that ovulates.[7]

During the follicular phase, concentrations of circulating follicle-stimulating hormone were similar between cows that subsequently formed cysts and those that ovulated at similar stages of growth. Conversely, concentrations of circulating luteinizing hormone (LH) were nearly twice as high (mean concentration and pulse amplitude) in cows in which cysts developed when compared with those that ovulated. Similarly, mean LH secretion was nearly twice as high around the time that the follicular wave was detected or the cyst reached the size of a normal ovulatory follicle when compared with similar times in cows that ovulated the dominant follicle of a wave (Fig. 2).[6] However, a preovulatory surge of LH was not detected in any of the cows in which cysts developed in either study whereas the LH surge was detected in controls.[6, 7] Also of interest was the finding that

the content of GnRH was nearly twice as high in the median eminence (site of GnRH release) and about half that in the hypothalamus proper (LH synthesis) in cows in which cysts developed when compared with cows with normal estrous cycles.[7] Thus the higher content of GnRH in the median eminence might explain the higher circulating concentrations of LH in serum. The mechanism(s) behind the lack of a preovulatory surge in cows in which cysts develop is unknown. However, cows with cysts have also been shown to produce higher amounts of estradiol-17β than that observed in cows that ovulate. Cows that have a high estrogen content and are grazing on clover have been shown to have an increased incidence of cysts. Perhaps the higher absolute level of endogenous estradiol-17β or the way it is presented to the hypothalamus and pituitary (rate of increase) might be associated with the lack of an LH surge.

TREATMENT

Evaluation of the success of treatment of cysts is complex because some cysts, particularly those that develop during the postpartum period, spontaneously recover and normal estrous cycles follow; misdiagnoses of cysts occur, and management practices by producers may not be adequate to take advantage of treatment. The success of treatment and re-establishment of pregnancy depend on good overall management by the producer.

If left untreated, approximately 20% of the cows with cysts spontaneously resume ovulatory ovarian cycles (for a review, see Kesler and Garverick[1]). Early treatments used crude pituitary extracts of LH or preparations of hCG. More recently, GnRH analogues have been used. The success rate for these treatments is approximately 80%. Cysts usually respond to LH, hCG, or GnRH treatment by luteinization of the cystic structure. Following treatment, plasma estradiol-17β concentrations often decrease, some dramatically, i.e., within 24 hours. The cystic structure then generally decreases in size and becomes firmer over the subsequent 5- to 15-day period. Circulating progesterone concentrations increase over the next 3 to 9 days and remain elevated until day 15 to 18 after GnRH treatment before declining. Estrus and ovulation then occur, and normal estrous cycles are usually initiated. In some cases, LH, hCG, or GnRH treatments initiate ovulation of the dominant follicles on the ovary with cysts at the time of treatment. Ovulation of the cyst following treatment has not been observed.

Prostaglandin F$_{2\alpha}$ causes lysis of cysts that luteinize spontaneously or luteinize following treatment with GnRH or hCG. The use of PGF$_{2\alpha}$ may reduce the interval from diagnosis and treatment to estrus. However, efficient estrus detection practices are necessary to capitalize on the reduced time to estrus. Prostaglandin F$_{2\alpha}$ appears to be more effective in inducing luteolysis when given 9 to 14 days after GnRH or hCG than when given earlier.

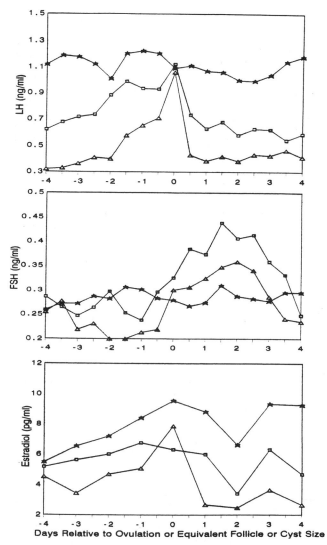

Figure 2

Mean concentrations of LH (*top panel;* SEM ± 0.11), FHS (*middle panel;* SEM ± 0.04), and estradiol-17β (*bottom panel;* SEM ± 1.40) are depicted relative to the time of ovulation or when cysts reached a diameter equal to the mean diameter of follicles that ovulated (1.60 cm). Day 0 denotes the day of ovulation or equivalent cyst size. Symbols for groups are as follows: Control, *open triangle* (n = 6); self-recovery, *open square* (n = 8), and cysts, *asterisk* (n = 8). (From Hamilton SA, Garverick HA, Keisler DH, et al: Characterization of ovarian follicular cysts and associated endocrine profiles in dairy cows. Biol Reprod 53:890, 1995.)

REFERENCES

1. Kesler DJ, Garverick HA: Ovarian cysts in dairy cattle: A review. J Anim Sci 55:1147, 1982.
2. Ax RL, Peralta RU, Elford WG, et al: Studies of cystic ovaries in dairy cows. *In* Baker FA, Miller ME (eds): Dairy Science Handbook, vol 16. Boulder, Colo, Westview Press, 1984, p 205.
3. Garverick HA: Ovarian follicular cysts in dairy cows. J Dairy Sci 80:995, 1997.
4. Kesler DJ, Garverick HA, Caudle AB, et al: Reproductive hormone and ovarian changes in cows with ovarian cysts. J Dairy Sci 63:166, 1980.

5. Cook DL, Smith CA, Parfet JR, et al: Fate and turnover rate of ovarian follicular cysts in dairy cattle. J Reprod Fertil 90:37, 1990.
6. Hamilton SA, Garverick HA, Keisler DH, et al: Characterization of ovarian follicular cysts and associated endocrine profiles in dairy cows. Biol Reprod 53:890, 1995.
7. Cook DL, Parfet JR, Smith CA, et al: Secretory patterns of LH and FSH during development and hypothalamic and hypophysial characteristics following development of steroid-induced ovarian follicular cysts in dairy cattle. J Reprod Fertil 91:19, 1991.

■ Estrus Synchronization

Brad Seguin, D.V.M., Ph.D., Diplomate, A.C.T.

Progesterone, whether natural from the ovarian corpus luteum (CL) or administered, prevents estrus. When the progesterone block is removed, estrus occurs in about 2 to 4 days. In natural reproductive physiology, the nonpregnant uterus sends a signal to the ovary ending the life of the CL, which stops progesterone production and allows or causes the return to estrus. The ability to control or synchronize estrus in domestic animals has been studied extensively over the last 40 years. Reasons for this interest have usually been tied to the desire to increase use of artificial insemination (AI), although potential use of estrus synchronization with natural breeding systems or in individual animal or unique management situations has also been investigated.

NOMENCLATURE

Terms such as estrus *induction* or *induced* estrus should be avoided, at least in cattle, as available products and techniques are generally not able to induce or create a physiologic, fertile estrus in females that are not having normal regular estrus cycles. True anestrus, that is, not having the ovarian activity associated with regular estrus cycle patterns, is most commonly due to females being (1) prepubertal, (2) post partum, (3) under-conditioned, or (4) in their nonbreeding season—for seasonal breeding species. Several indicators are used to measure the reproductive performance of animals in estrus synchronization programs. *Estrus response* is the percent showing estrus of those treated. *Synchronized conception rate* is the percent conceiving of those inseminated, and *synchronized pregnancy rate* is the percent conceiving of those treated. Also, *pregnancy rate is the product of the estrus detection rate and the conception rate.* The pregnancy rate equals the conception rate in systems using appointment AI, because all treated animals are inseminated, but in systems using AI based on estrus detection, the pregnancy rate is almost always lower (if not much lower) than the conception rate.

TWO BASIC APPROACHES TO SYNCHRONIZATION IN CATTLE

Progesterone

One approach to estrus synchronization is to mimic the estrus-blocking effect of progesterone produced by the CL. Exogenous progesterone is used as an injection, implant, feed additive or pessary for a period equal to or slightly longer than the species' normal estrous cycle length. When progesterone is withdrawn, estrus follows in 2 to 4 days. Some synthetic forms of progesterone, known as progestins, are also effective. Synchrony of estrus with progesterone or progestins is more precise when their removal is more precise, for example, after implant removal rather than after the end of injections or ingestion. Progesterone for estrus control works as follows (in cattle):

1. After natural CL regression, exogenous progesterone blocks estrus.
2. Blood progesterone drops when the source of progesterone is removed.
3. Estrogen rises as a follicle develops.
4. Estrus begins in 36 to 48 hours (more variable for progesterone given by injection or orally).
5. Luteinizing hormone (LH) surge occurs at the start of estrus, initiating the ovulation process.
6. Standing estrus lasts 8 to 18 hours.
7. Ovulation occurs 24 to 30 hours after estrus onset.

Prostaglandin

Another approach to estrus synchronization is administration of a substance that will trigger the end of the animal's own CL function. Prostaglandin $F_{2\alpha}$ ($PGF_{2\alpha}$) is the most active example, and commercial products include Lutalyse from Pharmacia & Upjohn, Estrumate from Bayer, and others in other parts of the world. An older but less effective example is injectable estradiol. Of potential interest to organic dairies is a report that bovine colostrum has a luteolytic effect.[1] PGF products act as follows (in cattle):

1. Progesterone output by the CL stops.
2. Blood progesterone decreases in 1 to 2 hours and is nearly undetectable in 24 hours.
3. CL size decreases over 2 to 3 days.
4. Estrogen from the developing follicle rises over 24 to 72 hours.
5. Estrus begins in about 72 hours (range, 60 to 120 hours).
6. LH surge occurs near the onset of estrus, starting the ovulation process.
7. Standing estrus lasts 8 to 18 hours.
8. Ovulation occurs 24 to 30 hours after estrus onset.

No difference was found in the abilities of Estrumate and Lutalyse at standard approved doses to initiate the events listed above.[2] These events can be expected only when a mature, functional CL is present in the cattle being treated; that is, during the diestrous phase (days 7 through 18) of the estrous cycle. There was no response to PGF treatments given to dairy cows between 0 and 5 days after estrus, only a 25% response to treatments on day 6, a 66% response to treatments on day 7, and a greater than 90% response thereafter.[3] So, in order to get desired response rates, PGF treatment for lactating dairy cows needs to be delayed until day 7 or 8 after estrus. The problem is recognition of this time in a clinical situation, given the variations of CL size and shape in individual animals.

Combination Approach

Exogenous progesterone or progestins plus CL termination (by estradiol or PGF injection), can be used to shorten the required duration of progesterone or progestin exposure to 9 or 10 days, which seems to be key to achieving normal fertility at the synchronized estrus.

ESTRUS SYNCHRONIZATION APPLICATIONS FOR CATTLE

Progesterone or Progestins Alone

Progesterone or progestins alone have been used for estrus synchronization in the United States, but are rarely used today except in combination with a luteolytic product (see later). An example is melengestrol acetate (MGA) which is given as a daily feed additive and is sold in the United States by Pharmacia & Upjohn for estrus suppression in feedlot heifers. This method has generally produced very good estrus control, but reduced fertility has been observed at the synchronized estrus, which is a result of the relatively long treatment period (21 to 25 days) required for progesterone products alone to control estrus in groups of cattle.

Prostaglandin Products

PGF can be used in four basic plans to synchronize estrus in groups of cattle. Each has its characteristic advantages and disadvantages, and each has the potential to be used repetitively within the same breeding season or even all year-round, for example, in dairy herds.

1. The classic method is *two PGF injections 11 to 14 days apart*, with *AI after the second PGF injection* based on (a) estrus detection, or (b) timed appointment at 72 to 80 hours for cows and 60 to 68 hours for heifers, or (c) a double-timed appointment at about 72 and 96 hours for cows and 60 and 80 hours for heifers. The response expected of cows at each of the days of the 21-day estrous cycle to this plan is shown in Table 1. Reproductive results with this PGF system, with AI once at 75 to 80 hours (183 cows) or twice at 72 and 96 hours (176 cows) after the second injection, were compared to a control using AI based on conventional estrus detection for 21 days (176 cows) on two farms.[4] Results showed no advantage for the double AI in this system (46% vs. 47% conception rates); similar conception rates between controls and PGF groups (50% vs. 46% and 47%) were seen, and advantage of an increased AI submission rate (61% vs. 100% and 100%) on pregnancy rate (30% vs. 46% and 47%) was demonstrated.

2. A modification of method 1 is to give *one injection to the entire group* with AI in the next 5 days for those observed in estrus, and then *a second injection only for nonresponders in 11 to 14 days* based on estrus detection or timed appointment. This method lowers the doses of PGF required and spreads the AI effort over more time. A 61% conception rate and a 58% pregnancy rate was achieved with this plan in 985 dairy heifers on many farms.[5]

3. Another approach is to *select cows by ovarian palpation or milk progesterone that have a responsive CL for a single PGF injection*, with AI based on estrus detection or by timed appointment. It is best to use double-appointment AI at about 72 and 96 hours for cows or at 60 and 80 hours for heifers when only one injection was used. This method could be used once per group or repeated at intervals of 7 to 14 days to get a greater portion of the group inseminated. When Howard (personal communication, 1977) used this plan on beef cows, the conception rate was 36% (172 cows) with one timed insemination at 72 to 86 hours vs. 49% (185 cows) with two timed inseminations at 72 and 96 hours. In another trial, this plan was compared with conventional heat detection and AI in three dairy herds in stanchion barns using 99 breedable heifers (48 in the PGF system and 51 controls) and 447 cows (219 in the PGF system and 228 controls).[6] In the PGF system, a veterinarian visit occurred the same day each week for palpation of cows and heifers ready for breeding, and PGF was given when a mature CL was found. AI was based on once-daily A.M. heat detection. The program was conducted in three consecutive fall-through-spring breeding seasons. The PGF system decreased the number of days to first AI (by 13 days for heifers and 11 days for cows) and to conception (by 18 days for both heifers and cows) relative to controls. The 267 animals in the PGF system were treated with 313 doses of PGF; and 88% of first inseminations and 82% of all inseminations in the PGF system occurred on days 2 through 5 after the veterinarian's visit and day of PGF treatment; and the conception rate for inseminations 2 to 5 days after PGF was higher than that at all other inseminations in the study (58% vs. 47%).

4. Another popular way to get started with PGF estrus synchronization in a more gradual manner is a *12-day program in which AI based on estrus detection starts for a group of cattle without PGF treatment and then PGF is given on day 7 to all cattle not yet inseminated, and then AI is continued for 5 more days*. This method uses the fewest doses of PGF per animal bred and the first 6 days allows a good monitoring period of the group's cyclicity status (see general guidelines for anestrus later in this section) before PGF is given, but the AI effort is spread over 12 days. In one field trial, this plan was applied to 52 Hereford cows with suckling calves 51 to 87 days old on the first day of breeding.[7] Twenty cows were in estrus and bred prior to PGF and 28 of 32 were in estrus and bred after PGF injection. Day 3 after PGF was the busiest day, with 18 cows (35% of the group of 51 cows) bred. Prior to PGF, the average daily estrus rate was 6.4% (see general guidelines for anestrus), indicating little or no anestrus in this group. The conception rate was 65%, the pregnancy rate was 60%, and number of services per conception was 1.7 (four cows were bred twice). Conception rates before PGF (60%) and after PGF (68%) did not differ.

Progesterone or Progestins plus PGF or Estrogen

Combinations are available for cattle that shorten the treatment period to 9 or 10 days. Syncro-Mate-B (SMB) (Rhone

---

Table 1
MECHANISM OF ACTION BY WHICH THE DOUBLE-PROSTAGLANDIN INJECTION PLAN SYNCHRONIZES ESTRUS IN GROUPS OF CATTLE

Day of Estrous Cycle at 1st PGF →	Status in 3 Days	11 Days Later →	Day of Estrous Cycle at 2nd PGF →	Status in 3 Days	
Day 1	Day 4		Day 15	*Estrus*	
Day 2	Day 5		Day 16	*Estrus*	
Day 3	Day 6		Day 17	*Estrus*	
Day 4	Day 7		Day 18	*Estrus*	
Day 5	Day 8		Day 19	*Estrus*	
Day 6	*Estrus*/day 9		Day 11	*Estrus*	*Estrus rate near 100%*
Days 7→17	*Estrus*	*Estrus rate 55%–60%*	Day 11	*Estrus*	
Day 18	*Estrus*		Day 11	*Estrus*	
Day 19	Day 1		Day 12	*Estrus*	
Day 20	Day 2		Day 13	*Estrus*	
Estrus	Day 3		Day 14	*Estrus*	

Merieux) is the only product of this type in the United States. It has Food and Drug Administration (FDA) approval as an estrus control agent for beef cattle and dairy heifers but not for lactating dairy cows. It consists of placing an implant in the ear (6 mg norgestomet) and giving an intramuscular (IM) injection (3 mg norgestomet and 5 mg estradiol valerate). The ear implant is removed after 9 days and AI is based on observed estrus, usually beginning in about 36 hours, or by appointment 48 to 54 hours after implant removal. In the same field trial cited above,[7] another group of 54 Hereford cows with suckling calves 51 to 87 days old were treated with SMB and then bred based on estrus detection. The conception rate was 65%, the pregnancy rate was 57% and number of services per conception was 1.7 (five cows were bred twice in the 5 days after implant removal). The busiest breeding day was day 2 after implant removal with 42 cows (78% of the group) bred.

In another SMB trial, 79 control heifers were bred by AI based on estrus detection for 25 days vs. 79 SMB-treated heifers bred based on estrus detection vs. 80 SMB-treated heifers bred by timed AI at 48 hours.[8] Respectively, estrus rates were 94%, 84%, and 100%; conception rates were 72%, 73%, and 55%; and pregnancy rates were 67%, 61%, and 55%. The conception rate was influenced by treatment (lower for SMB heifers bred by timed AI), but the pregnancy rate was not different among treatments. Seguin et al.[9] compared the classic PGF system (double-PGF 11 days apart with timed AI at 60 to 62 hours after the second PGF) and the SMB system (timed AI at 48 to 50 hours after implant removal) in seven groups of beef or dairy heifers. Results in five cycling groups were 41 (53%) of 77 heifers pregnant with the PGF system and 34 (45%) of 75 heifers pregnant after the SMB system, but in two groups of anestrus heifers only 6 (18%) of 34 heifers were pregnant after PGF and 7 (21%) of 33 heifers were pregnant after SMB. So these PGF and SMB systems were equally effective for cyclic heifers and equally ineffective for anestrus heifers.

A *controlled intravaginal drug-releasing device (CIDR)* and a *progesterone-releasing intravaginal device (PRID)* are available in other countries to deliver progesterone via a pessary. The injection used with these products is estrogen if given at the beginning of the treatment period, but it is PGF if given at or near the end of treatment. The only option in these programs is deciding whether AI will be based on estrus detection or on timed appointment. The CIDR and PRID have been studied as a way to synchronize second service in cows not pregnant to the first AI by reinserting them 10 days after a first AI and then removing them 9 days later, without PGF or estrogen injection, with all second services based on estrus detection.

Melengestrol acetate (MGA) followed by PGF has been used only in heifers because of its long treatment time (30 to 32 days). MGA 0.5 mg/head/day is fed for 14 days and PGF is given 16 to 18 days after the end of MGA feeding. Although many heifers show estrus after withdrawal of MGA, breeding is delayed until after PGF to maximize synchrony and fertility. This system requires that heifers are fed some concentrate or total mixed ration in which the MGA can be mixed to assure that each heifer gets the required MGA each day. In one trial, this method was compared with conventional SMB with AI based on estrus detection in 310 yearling beef heifers. The method produced higher conception (69% vs. 41%) and pregnancy (57% vs. 37%) rates.[10]

Calving Patterns After Synchronized Breeding

It is commonly asked, when estrus synchronization procedures for groups of cattle are being considered, if cattle conceiving on the same day will calve on the same day. In one group of 100 beef cows that conceived 1 day following estrus synchronization, calvings were spread over a 22-day period with no more than nine calves born on any one day.

Estrus Synchronization for Dairy Herd Reproductive Management

This discussion is restricted to PGF since that is the only estrus synchronization product approved in the United States for use in dairy cows, but in some other countries the CIDR and PRID can be used in lactating dairy cows.

Why Consider Dairy Herd Estrus Control Programs? These systems can provide the following advantages:

1. Elimination of estrus detection and AI from some days of each week or from some weeks of each month. This can change labor needs and improve herd performance by making reproductive management a major task to be performed on fewer but preplanned days, rather than one of many jobs to be done every day.

2. Provision of intermediate indicators of herd reproductive performance before pregnancy examination results are available.

3. Improvement of herd reproductive performance by (a) increasing chances of more than one cow being in estrus at a time, which will create groups of sexually active cows and make estrus detection easier; (b) raising estrus detection rate from the industry average of about 45% to 50%; (c) decreasing average days in milk at first AI and days open without lowering the herd's voluntary waiting interval (see Considerations, later in this article); (d) focusing attention on pregnancy rate per estrus cycle (percent pregnant every 21 days of those ready for breeding) rather than on conception rates.

Monday Morning Program

Seguin and colleagues et al,[6] as described earlier in this section, initially tested a single injection scheme with palpation selection every 7 days for cows with a PGF-responsive CL and saw improved reproductive performance concurrent with evidence of decreased labor inputs for estrus detection. One Wisconsin veterinary practice promoted a variation of this scheme, in which a veterinarian visits the farm every 14 days to perform palpations and, if a CL is found, PGF treatment is given.[11] All first services must be preceded by a PGF treatment, and AI based on standing estrus is stressed. This allows estrus detection efforts to be focused on a 4-day period every 14 days, although 21-day repeats would not fall within this 4-day window. Improved herd reproductive performance, reduced labor, increased income ($76 per cow per year), and higher client satisfaction were reported with this program. This practice expects 60% to 70% of PGF treatments to produce a strong estrus and successful AI. If the estrus response falls below 50% despite a good estrus detection effort, nutritional problems are suspected and feed analysis and ration balancing are recommended. Estrus response rates that are too high (near 100%) may indicate that cows are being inseminated because they were treated, not because strong signs of estrus were seen, which will lower the conception rate.

Target Breeding Program

The *target breeding program* is essentially the 14-day plan discussed above,[11] with two changes: (1) each cow gets a PGF injection before she is ready for AI to "set up" her estrus cycle and increase her chances of being in diestrus 14 days later when she is ready for breeding and given a second PGF treatment; and (2) palpation selection for PGF responsiveness is not usually used.[12] One day in each 2-week interval is selected that will be convenient for PGF injections and for optimal estrus detection 3 to 6 days later. To start, cows in the last 14 days of their voluntary waiting period (not necessarily the same for all cows or all groups of cows; e.g., first-lactation heifers vs. older cows) are given the initial set-up PGF injection. Each cow then gets a second PGF injection 14 days later, followed by a maximized estrus detection effort and AI. At the same time, the next cows ready for breeding (group 2) are given their set-up injection. In another 14 days, group 1 cows not yet inseminated get a third PGF injection, group 2 cows get their first breeding shot, and group 3 cows get their set-up shot. This continues every 14 days thereafter. Appointment AI may be used after the second or third PGF "breeding" injection. One Pennsylvania herd in the target breeding program for 2 years increased cows' pregnancy rate at 120 days post partum from 60% to 80%. More evaluations of the program in controlled research situations are needed, however.

Two possible shortcomings should be understood by potential users. One is that noncycling cows will not respond in this system and to the extent that true ovarian inactivity or anestrus exists as a herd problem at PGF injection times, the program will fail to meet expectations. Another point is that although the first impression may be that this program will allow farms to decrease estrus detection efforts to one 4-day window every 14 days, cows returning to estrus 21 days after a "controlled" breeding will be outside this observation window.

Ovsynch Program

Ovsynch is a new idea in bovine estrus control designed to synchronize ovulation and allow AI without estrus detection in dairy cows.[13] In the Ovsynch program, each cow gets three injections. Injection 1 is gonadotropin-releasing hormone (GnRH), given on day 1 to synchronize growth of a new wave of follicles and to ensure presence of a CL (needed to keep cows from coming into estrus before the next injection and to make them PGF-responsive). Injection 2 is PGF, given on day 8 to regress all CLs (hopefully now present in every cow), which will allow or cause the new dominant follicle to proceed toward maturation. Injection 3 is GnRH, given on day 10, about 48 hours after PGF, to trigger ovulation. AI occurs on day 11, about 16 to 20 hours after GnRH. [Note: Some of the time intervals are still being studied and may change in the future.]

Ovsynch emphasizes the pregnancy rate as the way to improve overall herd reproductive efficiency. This program raises the estrus detection rate (better named the AI submission rate here) to 100% by relying totally on timed breeding, while hoping to maintain reasonable conception rates. To illustrate, note the theoretical calculations in Table 2. It is apparent by this example that some sacrifice in conception rate in exchange for a 100% estrus detection or AI submission rate can be worthwhile when the pregnancy rate is the end point. Pregnancy rates with Ovsynch in lactating dairy cows were equal to those of control cows that were bred based on estrus detection after PGF (38%, n=156 vs. 39%, n=154) but were much lower in Ovsynch-treated dairy heifers than in control heifers that were bred based on estrus detection after PGF (35%, n=77 vs. 74%, n=78).[14] Therefore, this program is not currently recommended for heifers. The program's effect on reproductive end points has been further tested in three herds of 333 dairy cows.[15] Relative to controls, Ovsynch cows had fewer median days to first AI (54 vs. 83) and fewer days open (99 vs. 118), and more Ovsynch cows were pregnant at 60 days (37% vs. 5%) and 100 days (53% vs. 35%) after calving. A Minnesota grazier dairy used Ovsynch

on one group of 54 cows and 36 heifers, with somewhat poorer results—although it happened that the AI day was the hottest day of the summer! The pregnancy rate was 19% in cows and 28% in the heifers treated and bred according to the plan (9 pregnant of 48 cows and 10 pregnant of 36 heifers), but 4 of the remaining 6 Ovsynch cows became pregnant when bred 24 hours early, based on signs of estrus, for an overall pregnancy rate of 26% (23 pregnant of 90 total females). Another farm used Ovsynch on 24 cows, with a pregnancy rate of 25% (6 pregnant of 24 cows). Other anecdotal reports have been made of considerable satisfaction with Ovsynch results.

Users of this protocol must be aware that the second Gn-RH injection has the effect of cutting short full development of behavioral signs of estrus, so AI should be based on appointment timing rather than on detection of estrus. Ovsynch can be modified into an AI system based on estrus detection by using only the first two injections (GnRH on day 1 and PGF on day 8) of the usual three injection Ovsynch scheme.

Basic Methods 1 and 4 Applied to Dairy Herds

In addition to the three dairy herd programs discussed above, basic PGF methods 1 and 4, described earlier in this article, have potential for dairy herds and have been simulation-tested and discussed.[16]

Considerations

Reconsider the Length of the Postpartum Voluntary Waiting Period (VWP). When formulating estrus control plans for entire dairy herds, previously accepted reproductive standards and guidelines should always be open for reevaluation. For example, it may not always be appropriate to continue using a short postpartum VWP, as estrus detection failure will no longer be a factor in determining average days to first AI or days open. Rather it may be better to plan the system, that is, postpartum starting dates, to meet specified goals. For example, it may be best to delay the start of breeding to coincide with the herd's desired average interval to first AI, as some of these programs are guaranteed to produce that figure as the herd's actual result. This change could (1) eliminate the excessively short lactations that occur with first-service conceptions in herds with short postpartum VWPs, (2) allow more cows to overcome postpartum anestrus by the time of the controlled breeding, and (3) increase first-service conception and pregnancy rates by allowing a longer time for postpartum uterine involution.

Table 2

ESTRUS DETECTION RATE, CONCEPTION RATE, AND PREGNANCY RATE INTERACTIONS FOR ACTUAL MINNESOTA DHIA DATA VS. THEORETICAL DATA WITH ESTRUS CONTROL AND APPOINTMENT AI IN DAIRY HERDS

Reproductive Indices	Estrus Detection and AI	Estrus Control and Appointment AI
1. Estrus detection or AI submission rate	43%*	100%
2. Conception rate	52%*	35%
3. Pregnancy rate for one cycle	22%	35%

AI, artificial insemination.
*1994 Minnesota Dairy Herd Improvement Association (DHIA) averages.

Perform Pregnancy Diagnosis as Early as Possible. In all ongoing PGF programs for reproductive management of dairy herds, identifying nonpregnant cows as soon as possible following AI, so they may be placed into the next new injection group and be rebred as soon as possible, is important for overall success. Ultrasonography can have an advantage in this regard.

Choosing an Interval Between Starting New Groups of Cows. Most dairy herds, except graziers, breed throughout the year, so the programs just described must be used repetitively to incorporate new cows, as they complete their VWP, and previously bred cows found to be nonpregnant. Although many farms seem to opt for starting new groups every 14 days, consideration should be given to a 7- or 21-day interval between groups. Because cows have 21-day estrous cycles, either 7- or 21-day intervals between starting groups on these estrus control programs has the advantage that estrus activity from the new round of program treatments will coincide with the time when many of the nonpregnant cows bred on the previous treatment cycle will be returning to estrus. This is not the case if the interval between starting new groups is 14 days. In larger herds, starting new groups at 7-day intervals can have the same advantage over the 14-day interval and will reduce treatment groups to more manageable sizes.

Which Is the Best Program? Each has advantages and disadvantages, so none of them is clearly best for all situations. One of the strengths of estrus control methods in cattle today is the variety of options available. However, some have been put off by this selection opportunity, apparently preferring to accept or reject a single "cookbook recipe" approach. To take full advantage of options, decisions must be made, hopefully from an informed point of view, and most people will need to closely scrutinize the programs to fully understand and utilize them.

Estrus Synchronization for Individual Dairy Cows

Failure to observe estrus within 21 days after the postpartum VWP (preservice anestrus) or after service in cows which have not conceived (postservice anestrus) is the major negative influence on reproductive performance in dairy herds. Zemjanis et al[17] reported that anestrus occurred at 43% of expected estrus periods in dairy cows. However, true anestrus accounted for only 10% of this incidence, with the remaining 90% due to estrus detection failure or failure of cycling cows to adequately exhibit signs of estrus. Thus the authors' title, "Anestrus: The Practitioner's Dilemma," in recognition that man's role in estrus detection is a greater problem than are conditions directly preventing ovarian function and estrus behavior in cows. True anestrus caused by ovarian atrophy can be a problem in individual cows that have complications at calving and on a herd basis where nutritional deficiencies and lack of good body condition exist. Therapy for this problem is rarely successful and the condition is best prevented through management changes.

Since most dairy cows presented to veterinarians for anestrus are having estrous cycles but not being observed in estrus, the condition is more accurately named *unobserved estrus*. Palpation of these cows finds about 55% in diestrus with a functional CL (a smooth plump protruding structure about 2.0 to 2.5 cm in height and diameter that greatly alters the ovary's size and shape), 15% in proestrus 1 to 3 days before estrus, 5% in estrus, and 25% in metestrus 1 to 6 days after estrus. Two basic approaches to these cattle are (1) prediction of estrus based on palpation findings and (2) PGF for estrus control in diestrus cows.

The literature on field results using PGF products in dairy cows shows that, in most cases, only about 65% of clinical cases of unobserved estrus treated with PGF products are observed

in estrus and inseminated as a result of PGF treatment.[2] Why this relatively disappointing result? Three factors are involved: (1) absence of a PGF-responsive CL in treated cows, (2) estrus detection failure after PGF treatment, and (3) perhaps stress related to production, heat, or social interaction among herdmates, depressing behavioral expression of estrus. In one field study,[2] distribution of observed estrus in 280 dairy cows responding to PGF treatment for unobserved estrus was: day 1, 2%; day 2, 8%; day 3, 38%; day 4, 32%; day 5, 14%; and day 6, 6%. This spread can destroy a farm's enthusiasm for the estrus detection efforts needed to maximize PGF results. Even in Minnesota, season can affect PGF results. On one farm, the observed estrus rate was 66% for 32 summer treatments vs. 80% for 40 winter treatments, and resulting conception rates were only 30% in summer vs. 52% in winter for a pregnancy rate as a direct result of PGF of 20% in summer vs. 42% in winter.

Recommendations for Artificial Insemination

Most veterinarians and dairy farmers seem to prefer AI based solely on estrus detection after one-time PGF treatment in dairy cows for unobserved estrus. This is most appropriate in view of the three factors just discussed regarding the apparent estrus response after PGF treatments and the relative costs of PGF and semen. Concerted estrus detection efforts two to three times per day are encouraged at all times but especially during periods of expected estrus response to PGF, and AI should be restricted to those cows showing strong signs of *standing* estrus. As a secondary recommendation (but one that may be most appropriate on some farms), appointment AI may be considered. The advantage and/or disadvantage of appointment AI is that all treated cows get inseminated. Lactating dairy cows should be inseminated about 72 and 96 hours after PGF and heifers about 12 hours earlier, because double-appointment AI has produced a significantly higher pregnancy rate (59%)[18] than is likely with a single-appointment AI in this single-PGF injection situation. This is explained by Table 3, which compares PGF effects in heifers to cows at two times during diestrus.[3] Heifers begin estrus sooner after PGF than cows, and estrus occurs sooner and more predictably when PGF is given on days 7 to 9 of the estrous cycle than if it is given on days 10 to 13. These differences are caused by follicle variables rather than by CL effects. Note also in Table 3 that at day 7 dairy cows are less responsive (72%) than are dairy heifers (89%), indicating that CL growth can be slower in cows than in heifers. Single-

---

Table 3

ESTRUS RESPONSE RATE AND ESTRUS TIME VARIABILITY TO PROSTAGLANDIN TREATMENT AFFECTED BY TYPE OF ANIMAL AND STAGE OF DIESTRUS

	Heifers (Day Treated*)		Cows (Day Treated*)	
	7	10	7	10
No. treated	27	24	25	23
Estrus rate (%)	89	100	72	96
Time to estrus (hr)	49	79	60	100
SD	±4	±19	±9	±39

*Day of the estrous cycle relative to estrus (day of estrus = day 0).
Data from Momont HW: Reproductive response factors of dairy cattle treated with cloprostenol (doctoral thesis). Minneapolis, University of Minnesota, 1985.

appointment AI following a single PGF treatment at an unknown stage of diestrus, as is the case when dairy cows are treated for unobserved estrus, frequently produces an unsatisfactory conception rate of only 20% to 30%.

Another consideration on this point is that when appointment AI is used, veterinarians will feel more pressure for very accurate selection of cows for PGF treatment, because every animal treated gets inseminated. Other disadvantages are that more semen is needed and that some cows (up to 20%) will show estrus after the last-appointment AI, and therefore require a third AI.

Economics

Using computer modeling techniques, AI by detected estrus was more profitable than that with appointment AI at nearly all input assumptions.[19] The exceptions were if the estrus detection rate was poor (<40%), the cost of semen was low (<$5 per dose), or the CL diagnosis was very accurate (>90%).

General Guidelines for Success

All estrus synchronization applications require that cows are having normal estrous cycles to respond successfully. Cows not having normal estrous cycles are said to be in "anestrus." Causes include nutritional deficiency (especially energy or phosphorus), inadequate age (less than normal onset of puberty), inadequate VWP and effect of calf nursing (beef cows with nursing calves seldom resume estrus cyclicity before 50 to 60 days after calving, even with the best management, herd health, and nutrition), and debilitating disease or injury. Guidelines for screening groups of cattle for anestrus are as follows:

1. Before any estrus control treatment has occurred, 4% to 5% of a group should be in estrus each day, and 50% to 60% must have a large CL by rectal palpation at any time.
2. After a first PGF treatment, 50% to 60% should be seen in estrus on days 2 through 5.
3. At the time of a second PGF treatment (11 to 14 days after a first PGF), nearly 100% must have large CL by rectal palpation.

Other management requirements necessary for a successful estrus synchronization and AI effort include:

1. Good facilities so cattle can be sorted and individually handled, injected, palpated, inseminated, and so on.
2. An individual identification (ID) system for each animal that is easily read from a distance.
3. A record system for individual animal reproductive (birthdate, parentage, breeding dates and service sire, calving dates, offspring ID, synchronization treatment dates, etc.) and health (vaccinations, parasite control, etc.) events.
4. Excellent technical services such as ovarian palpation for CL identification (if required in the synchronization program used), semen handling and intrauterine placement, and pregnancy diagnosis.
5. Awareness that the postpartum interval at AI has an effect on fertility. In the beef cow trial above,[7] conception rates were 38% (n = 26), 62% (n = 26), 64% (n = 36), and 71% (n = 17), respectively, for cows 51 to 59, 60 to 69, 70 to 79, and 80 to 87 days post partum at the start of the estrus control program.

Precaution! These estrus synchronization products, especially PGF, will cause pregnant animals to abort, so this possibility must be considered before estrus synchronization is started. The health of females that are more than 100 days' pregnant treated with these products is a special concern in that these animals may not be able to completely expel the aborted calf and therefore develop serious, if not fatal, metritis and septicemia.

ESTRUS SYNCHRONIZATION IN GOATS AND SHEEP

Many of the principles and methods described for estrus synchronization in cattle also apply to goats and sheep, with the following notable qualifiers: (1) ovarian palpation for determination of CL status is not possible in does and ewes, so this technique cannot be used to select responsive or cycling females as is done with cattle; (2) does and ewes are seasonal breeders and therefore unresponsive to estrus synchronization during seasonal anestrus; (3) the AI procedure (semen freezing, timing of insemination, and insemination technique) is still being refined, so that it has been difficult to know where the weak link may be when estrus synchronization and AI results are disappointing; (4) the availability, FDA marketing clearance, and appropriate dosages of these products in does and ewes are uncertain.

During the breeding season, the basic approaches described above of (1) blocking natural estrus by exogenous progesterone or progestins in administration and (2) terminating CL function by PGF or possibly estrogen also apply to ewes and does.

Progesterone or progestins alone have been used, mainly via vaginal pessary administration, for estrus synchronization in goats and sheep, with the same disadvantages seen in cattle. One is the relatively long exposure equal to or slightly greater than the length of the normal estrous cycle (16 to 17 days for ewes and 20 to 21 days for does) required to gain external control of the estrous cycles of all animals in a group. A second is reduced fertility, although synchrony of estrus is usually very good, at the first estrus after progesterone treatment. In both ewes and does, 500 IU of pregnant mare serum gonadotropin (PMSG) is frequently given at the end of progesterone or progestin exposure to improve ovulation rate and synchrony. P.G. 600 (Intervet America, Millsboro, Del), which contains PMSG plus human chorionic gonadotropin (hCG), may be a more readily available alternative to PMSG.

PGF will lyse the mature CL from about days 5 through 14 for ewes and about days 5 through 17 for does, but the basic method 3—pretreatment selection of responsive animals by rectal palpation for mature CL—cannot be used in these small ruminants. The basic double-injection plan is probably the most commonly used method using only PGF, with intervals between PGF injections usually being 9 days for ewes and 11 days for does. PGF doses with Lutalyse are usually 15 to 20 mg for ewes and 8 to 15 mg (but even as low as 1.25 mg) for does.[21]

Combinations of progesterone or progestins and PGF or estrogen have the same advantages observed in cattle, that is, shorter required duration of progesterone or progestin blockage of estrus and improved fertility at the first synchronized estrus. The SMB system for cattle has been used in does and ewes at one-half dosage with apparent success, as have the MGA followed by PGF and the Ovsynch programs described earlier for cattle.

During the nonbreeding season, induction of estrus for breeding is desirable in some goat and sheep management systems. At this time, does and ewes are not cycling and do not have CL function, so estrus synchronization methods based on that physiology, especially PGF, will not work. Artificially shortening daylight will "fool" does and ewes into responding as if the natural breeding season were approaching and thereby induce out-of-season cyclicity. Ram exposure will hasten the onset of cyclicity in does and ewes, especially in the early transition phase between the nonbreeding and breeding seasons. Out-of-season cyclicity and breeding are influenced by breed. Some breeds, which cycle all year long, and their crossbreed offspring are more likely to respond to these stimuli.

Progesterone or progestins given by vaginal pessary for 10 to 14 days, with PMSG given at the end of exposure, will induce estrous cyclicity in many does and ewes.

ESTRUS INDUCTION AND SYNCHRONIZATION IN SWINE

Swine differ in several ways in their response to the general estrus synchronization principles discussed above for cattle: (1) weaning is a very strong stimulus to a fairly well-synchronized estrus, (2) gonadotropins are much more potent stimulants of follicular development, estrus, and ovulation in swine than in cattle, goats, and sheep, and (3) luteolytic agents such as PGF and estrogens are relatively ineffective in swine. In fact, estrogens are actually luteotropic in swine, whereas progesterone still has an estrus-suppression effect.

Induction of Estrus and Ovulation (in Anestrus Females)

Weaning about 21 to 28 days after farrowing induces many sows to be in estrus in 3 to 7 days. This effect is influenced by season, as 82% of sows have estrus within 7 days when weaned from October through June vs. 69% of sows weaned in July through September.[22] Several management systems, increase the percentage of sows exhibiting estrus after weaning or shorten the interval from weaning to estrus. Exogenous hormone treatments can induce follicular growth, estrus, and ovulation in prepubertal gilts and in that portion (10% to 30% on many swine farms) of gilts failing to show estrus within 45 days after puberty. Response is best in gilts that are at least 5 to 6 months old. Gonadotropins such as PMSG or equine chorionic gonadotropin (ECG), human chorionic gonadotropin (HCG), Gn-RH, and estradiol have been used alone or in combinations for this purpose. Only P.G. 600 is marketed for this purpose in the United States. Estrus and ovulation occur in ≥90% of gilts, with greatest estrus activity on days 4 to 6 after treatment. The resulting reproductive performance (pregnancy rate and litter size) is normal. In lactating sows, gonadotropins to induce estrus and ovulation have little effect, unless used after day 30 of lactation or in combination with partial weaning. Boar exposure, group rearrangement, and transport have some stimulatory effect on induction of estrus and ovulation in anestrus gilts ready for breeding, but results are highly variable.

Estrus Synchronization

Of the two general methods of controlling estrus discussed above, that is, controlled termination of progesterone influence via CL lysis and prolonged progesterone blocking of estrus via exogenous progesterone, only the latter is practicably effective in swine. CLs in swine are unresponsive to the luteolytic action of PGF products except for a short period in late diestrus. An interesting but probably impractical alternative is to breed gilts and sows, and then give PGF after day 14, which will produce a synchronized estrus (and abortion) in those that were pregnant.

Progesterone and progestins will delay estrus in swine for as long as they are given, and if given for the duration of an estrus cycle, will produce estrus synchronization when withdrawn. As in other species, adverse effects on fertility and so on of the resulting synchronized estrus have been observed. One compound (methallibure) used for estrus synchronization is terato-

genic if fed for 20 days during the first 49 days of gestation.[23] One of the orally active progestins studied for estrus synchronization in swine is allyl trenbolone, or RU 2267, which is also known as altrenogest or Regu-Mate (Hoechst-Roussel, Somerville, NJ) when marketed for progesterone supplementation in mares. After feeding allyl trenbolone to gilts at the rate of 15 mg/day for 18 days, estrus occurred in 4 to 7 days after withdrawal in nearly all (58 of 60) gilts, with no reduction in farrowing rate or litter size.[24]

The current trend in swine for increased use of AI is likely to stimulate renewed interest in estrus synchronization procedures for this species.

REFERENCES

1. Turner CB, Holdsworth RJ: Effects on the oestrous cycle of dairy cows of the administration of colostrum in the mid-luteal phase. Vet Rec 114:85, 1984.
2. Seguin B, Momont H, Baumann L: Cloprostenol and dinoprost tromethamine in experimental and field trials treating unobserved estrus in dairy cows. Bovine Pract 20:85, 1985.
3. Momont HW: Reproductive Response Factors of Dairy Cattle Treated With Cloprostenol. PhD thesis, University of Minnesota, Minneapolis, 1985.
4. Young IM, Henderson DC: Evaluation of single and double artificial insemination regimes as methods of shortening calving intervals in dairy cows treated with dinoprost. Vet Rec 109:446, 1981.
5. Fogwell RL, Reid WA, Thompson CK, et al: Synchronization of estrus in dairy heifers: A field demonstration. J Dairy Sci 69:1665, 1986.
6. Seguin BE, Tate DJ, Otterby DE: Use of cloprostenol in a reproductive management system for dairy cattle. J Am Ved Med Assoc 183:533, 1983.
7. Fortin MR, Momont HW, Seguin BE: Synchronization of estrus in lactating beef cows: Comparison of prostaglandin with progestin-estradiol therapy. Minn Vet 25:38, 1985.
8. Anderson GW, Banbonis GD, Riesen JW, et al: Control of estrus and pregnancy in dairy heifers treated with Syncro-Mate-B. Theriogenology 17:623, 1982.
9. Seguin BE, Momont HW, Fahmi H, et al: Single appointment insemination for heifers after prostaglandin or progestin synchronization of estrus. Theriogenology 31:1233, 1989.
10. Brown LN, Odde KG, King ME, et al: Comparison of melengestrol acetate–prostaglandin $F_{2\alpha}$ to Syncro-Mate-B for estrus synchronization in beef heifers. Theriogenology 30:1, 1988.
11. Belschner A: A breeding program for dairy cattle. AgriPract 7(5):7, 1986.
12. Hitting the target, *Dialogue*, No. 2, 1993, p 1.
13. Pursley JR, Mee MO, Wiltbank MC: Synchronization of ovulation in dairy cows using $PGF_{2\alpha}$ and GnRH. Theriogenology 44:915, 1995.
14. Pursley JR, Wiltbank MC, Stevenson JS, et al: Pregnancy rates per artificial insemination for cows and heifers inseminated at a synchronized ovulation or synchronized estrus. J Dairy Sci 80:295, 1997.
15. Pursley JR, Kosorok MR, Wiltbank MC, et al: Reproductive management of lactating dairy cows using synchronization of ovulation. J Dairy Sci 80:301, 1997.
16. Seguin BE: Reproductive management programs for dairy cows using prostaglandin products to reduce labor. Comp Contin Educ Pract Vet (special issue), 1984, p 22.
17. Zemjanis R, Fahning ML, Schultz RH: Anestrus: The practitioner's dilemma. Vet Scope 14:14, 1965.
18. Seguin BE, Gustafsson BK, Hurtgen JP, et al: Use of the prostaglandin $F_{2\alpha}$ analog cloprostenol (ICI 80,996) in dairy cattle with unobserved estrus. Theriogenology 10:55, 1978.
19. Fetrow J, Blanchard R: Economic impact of the use of prostaglandin to induce estrus in dairy cows. J Am Vet Med Assoc 190:163, 1987.
20. Hackett AJ, Robertson HA: Effect of dose and time of injection of prostaglandin $F_{2\alpha}$ in cycling ewes. Theriogenology 13:347, 1980.
21. Bretzlaff K: Control of the doe's/ewe's reproductive cycle. Proceedings of the Annual Meeting of the Society for Theriogenology, Austin, 1987, p 322.

22. Hurtgen JP, Leman AD, Crabo B: Seasonal influence on estrous activity in sows and gilts. J Am Vet Med Assoc 176:119, 1980.
23. King GJ: Deformities in piglets following administration of methallibure during specific stages of gestation. J Reprod Fertil 20:551, 1969.
24. Pursel VG, Elliott DO, Newman CW, et al: Synchronization of estrus in gilts with allyl trenbolone: Fecundity after natural service and insemination with frozen semen. J Anim Sci 52:130, 1981.

■ Problems Associated With Artificial Insemination in Cattle

Dale Paccamonti, D.V.M., M.S.

Artificial insemination (AI) has been responsible for tremendous genetic improvement in the dairy industry. The use of frozen semen has allowed the widespread use of bulls of proven genetic value, thereby greatly increasing milk production. However, despite the tremendous advantages of AI, significant problems remain.

SEMEN QUALITY

Semen quality is rarely a problem when the semen has been purchased from a reputable source. Frozen semen prepared and stored according to Certified Semen Services standards can be assumed to be of good quality. For example, the optimum number of spermatozoa per straw varies with the fertility of the individual bull. Thus bulls of low fertility may require more sperm per straw than bulls of high fertility,[1] but this is taken into account during processing. If questions arise about the quality of the frozen semen, a straw from the lot in question should be evaluated according to recommended procedures.[2]

Although the potential for disease transmission in AI exists, semen processed according to Certified Semen Services standards should be free of disease-producing organisms. Concern has been expressed that the widespread use of a particular bull could increase the prevalence of a genetic defect. However, with current testing procedures, most common genetic defects are noted before a bull is used widely by the industry.

SEMEN STORAGE AND HANDLING

Most semen today is stored in 0.25- or 0.50-mL French straws. Studies have failed to show any difference between the two types of straws or any interaction between individual bulls and straw type in subsequent pregnancy rates.[3] When a straw of semen is removed from the liquid nitrogen, the cane containing the semen should be raised no higher than necessary. Exposure to the warmer temperatures in the neck of the tank results in damage to the remaining straws. Semen should be transferred immediately from the tank to the thawing vessel and thawed according to the directions provided by the semen processor. Lacking specific guidelines, a warm water thaw (95°F) for at least 40 seconds is recommended by the National Association of Animal Breeders for 0.5-mL straws. Thawing the straw by means other than a warm water bath will adversely affect the sperm. Semen should be used within 15 minutes of thawing. Thawed sperm cells are susceptible to cold shock, so care should be taken to protect the semen until it is placed in the cow, including warming the AI gun before loading.

HYGIENE

Equipment used for AI should be kept clean and free from contamination. When handling the equipment in preparation for insemination and thawing of semen, cleanliness is very important. The vulva of the cow should be properly cleaned before introducing the AI pipette. Double sheathing the AI pipette will reduce contamination of the uterus from vaginal flora.

ESTRUS DETECTION

Estrus detection is the major problem associated with AI. The effort needed for estrus detection is a primary reason for the low use of AI in the beef industry. Often, poor estrus detection is also the most difficult problem for a veterinarian to alleviate for a herd owner. True anestrus is uncommon in properly fed, healthy dairy cows after 45 days postpartum. Most cows with suspected cases are pregnant or have pathologic conditions such as cystic follicular degeneration or pyometra. In beef herds, anestrus may be a significant problem, especially in herds with *Bos indicus* breeding. Rectal palpation and progesterone levels of suspected anestrous animals will help diagnose the condition. Ultrasonography is a very useful tool to determine the reproductive status of a cow. Questionable ovarian structures can be identified, and the uterine condition can be evaluated as well.

Measures of Efficiency

Estrus detection efficiency can be assessed by examining the herd records. For example, the ratio of normal interestrus intervals to multiples of normal intervals is unaffected by early embryonic death and therefore reflects missed estrous periods. A parameter easily calculated during a herd visit is the percentage of cows presented for pregnancy check that are pregnant. Nonpregnant cows represent missed estrous periods because they will have had at least one estrus between the time they were bred and when they were subjected to pregnancy examination. Although examination of Dairy Herd Improvement Association records is not helpful in assessing estrus detection in a beef herd, an estrus detection trial can be used to check detection efficiency. Nonpregnant cows are observed for 24 days and all estrous periods and services recorded. The number of cows detected in estrus divided by the total number of available cows is an estimate of estrus detection efficiency because normal cycling cows should exhibit one or more estrous periods in this 24-day period. If a low percentage of cows are detected in estrus, rectal palpation or ultrasonography of the internal genitalia can verify that the cows are cycling and not pregnant.

Concentrations of milk or serum progesterone can also be helpful for verifying luteal function and assessing the capabilities of the producer to detect estrus in the herd. An evaluation of progesterone concentrations in a group of cows to be bred can be used to detect the percentage of cows with high progesterone levels that are being serviced (i.e., cows not truly in estrus).

Methods to Increase Efficiency

The best results with AI occur when breeding of cattle is based on observation of standing estrus. The practitioner should be certain that observers can accurately identify animals in estrus. Observation periods of 30 to 45 minutes during the morning and the evening remain the optimum method for detecting estrus. In warm, humid climates it is recommended that a third check be made during the night. In a recent study, movement of the cattle before the observation period combined with observation for more than 15 minutes significantly improved estrus detection.[4]

Many estrus detection aids are available to increase the efficiency of estrus detection. However, sole reliance on detection aids as the means of identifying animals in estrus usually results in a decrease in heat detection efficiency. Aids frequently used include heat detector patches, tail paint or chalk, androgenized steers or heifers, and surgically altered bulls. Using a combination of aids increases heat detection efficiency and accuracy.[5] Heat expectancy charts and breeding wheels can be used to identify animals anticipated to return to estrus. Pedometer systems are available and under some conditions are very efficient in identifying cattle in estrus.[6] In the future, pedometry may be combined with other automated features to help identify animals in estrus.[6]

Prostaglandins can be used to induce luteolysis and subsequent estrus. Two doses of prostaglandin given 8 hours apart resulted in more cows being observed in estrus than was the case with a single dose or to two doses 24 hours apart.[7] Estrus synchronization often results in increased estrous activity among grouped animals, thus making detection easier.

TIMED ARTIFICIAL INSEMINATION

Because of the difficulties surrounding estrus detection, many efforts have been directed at insemination based on factors other than visual observation. Breeding based on frequent milk progesterone tests instead of visual observation was associated with a reduced calving-to-conception interval and a reduced rate of reproductive culls in the United Kingdom.[8] Breeding at a fixed time following estrus induction has been proposed as a means of avoiding the problem of estrus detection. However, results are often disappointing if ovarian activity is not verified before treatment. Palpation, ultrasonography, or progesterone determination can be used to select individuals to be included in an estrus induction program. Unfortunately, even when prostaglandins are administered to cattle with functional corpora lutea, the results of AI at a fixed time after prostaglandin administration are disappointing. This is attributed to variation in the time of ovulation after estrus induction. Recently a protocol was reported in which gonadotropin-releasing hormone (GnRH) was given, followed by prostaglandin 7 days later. A second injection of GnRH was administered 48 hours later, and AI was performed 24 hours after the second GnRH injection.[9] Ovulation occurred within an 8-hour period, 24 to 32 hours after the second GnRH injection, and a 50% conception rate was achieved.[9] More recently, a similar regimen was followed in a much larger group of cows, and AI was performed 16 hours after the second GnRH injection.[10] Conception after fixed-time AI was equal to that achieved by estrus detection and breeding on standing heat.[10] This new regimen, which uses two injections of GnRH along with prostaglandins, seemingly eliminates the need for estrus detection and may provide an effective alternative in some herds.

INSEMINATION

Timing of Insemination

Contrary to producers' beliefs, good results can be achieved from once-a-day AI service.[4] It has been shown that pregnancy rates are equal with breeding once per day vs. twice per day. Animals detected in estrus by the morning should be inseminated that morning and any others observed in estrus later in the day mated the next morning. This recommendation is justified because animals exhibiting estrus early in the morning have probably been in estrus during the previous night and those not exhibiting estrus until later in the day are probably just coming into estrus. A recent report found that the best results were

obtained with once-per-day AI based on observed standing estrus and when performed between 8 and 11 AM.[4]

Site of Deposition

It has long been recommended that semen be placed in the uterine body just inside the internal cervical os. Although this is a sound recommendation in theory, in practice it has probably been responsible for the failure of some inseminators to achieve good results. Placement of semen in the cervix is associated with a decrease in pregnancy rates when compared with placement of the semen in the uterus. Studies have found that many inseminators have difficulty fully penetrating the cervix. Inseminators who underwent retraining to place semen in either the uterine body or the horns were initially equally capable of accurate placement. However, after 6 months, those attempting placement in the body showed a significant reduction in accuracy whereas inseminators placing semen in the horn retained their proficiency.[11] This suggests that the horns provide a more easily identifiable landmark than the cervix, with a higher degree of repeatability. Depositing the semen in the uterus is the key factor, and if this can be achieved more consistently by horn placement than by body placement, that target is preferable.

Unintentional withdrawal of the insemination gun during semen deposition is not unusual. If the gun is placed in the uterine body initially, semen will be deposited in the cervix if it is withdrawn during insemination. However, if the gun is initially placed in the horn, even if the pipette is withdrawn during insemination, the semen will be deposited in the uterus. Semen placement can be evaluated in abattoir specimens with the use of dye or radiographically to determine an inseminator's proficiency. A procedure using ultrasonography to evaluate the site of deposition in live cows has been described and is preferable to the use of abattoir specimens.[12]

Spermatozoa can migrate freely in the reproductive tract in the cow. In heifers inseminated in one horn of the uterus, sperm were present in all parts of the uterus and oviducts, even in the contralateral oviduct distal to a surgical resection within 2 hours.[13] Moreover, of 62 repeat breeder cows inseminated intraperitoneally, 9 became pregnant, a rate not different from that seen with intrauterine insemination.[14] Therefore, assessment of the left-to-right pregnancy ratio is not a useful tool to evaluate inseminator proficiency. It is unclear whether placement of semen into the horn contralateral or ipsilateral to the ovulatory follicle greatly influences pregnancy rates.[15,16] A report examining a large number of cows found that deep cornual insemination ipsilateral to the follicle favored an increased pregnancy rate; however, results were also influenced by the relationship to the previously gravid horn.[16] Although ipsilateral insemination would have limitations for the AI technician, it may be useful for a veterinarian called to breed a repeat breeder cow with no apparent abnormalities.

Usually veterinarians are called to analyze a situation and provide recommendations for improvement. In some cases, a more active role of the veterinarian in estrus detection and AI may be warranted and prove to be economically beneficial.[17]

REFERENCES

1. Kommisrud E, Steine T, Graffer T: Comparison of fertility rates following insemination with different numbers of spermatozoa per insemination dose of frozen bovine semen. Reprod Domest Anim 31:359, 1996.
2. Barth AD: Evaluation of frozen bovine semen. *In* Proceedings of the Annual Meeting of the Society of Theriogenology, 1989, Coeur d'Alene, Idaho, p 92.

3. Johnson MS, Senger PL, Allen CH, et al: Fertility of bull semen packaged in .25- and .5-milliliter French straws. J Anim Sci 73:1914, 1995.

4. Nebel RL, Walker WL, McGilliard ML, et al: Timing of artificial insemination of dairy cows: Fixed time once daily versus morning and afternoon. J Dairy Sci 77:3185, 1994.

5. Pennington JA, Callahan CJ: Use of mount detectors plus chalk as an estrous detection aid for dairy cattle. J Dairy Sci 69:248, 1986.

6. Lehrer AR, Lewis GS, Aizinbud E: Oestrus detection in cattle: Recent developments. In Dieleman SJ, Colenbrander B, Booman P, et al (eds): Clinical Trends and Basic Research in Animal Reproduction. Amsterdam, Elsevier, 1992, p 355.

7. Archbald LF, Risco C, Chavatte P, et al: Estrus and pregnancy rate of dairy-cows given 1 or 2 doses of prostaglandin-$F_{2\alpha}$—8 or 24 hours apart. Theriogenology 40:873, 1993.

8. Williams ME, Esslemont RJ: A decision support system using milk progesterone tests to improve fertility in commercial dairy herds. Vet Rec 132:503, 1993.

9. Pursley JR, Mee MO, Wiltbank MC: Synchronization of ovulation in dairy-cows using $PGF_{2\alpha}$, and GnRH. Theriogenology 44:915, 1995.

10. Burke JM, De La Sota RL, Risco CA, et al: Evaluation of timed insemination using a gonadotropin-releasing hormone agonist in lactating dairy cows. J Dairy Sci 79:1385, 1996.

11. Senger PL, Becker WC, Davidge ST, et al: Influence of cornual insemination on conception in dairy cattle. J Anim Sci 66:3010, 1988.

12. Beal WE, Edwards RB III, Kearnan JM: Use of B-mode, linear array ultrasonography for evaluating the technique of bovine artificial insemination. J Dairy Sci 72:2198, 1989.

13. Larsson B: Transperitoneal migration of spermatozoa in heifers. Zentralbl Vetmed 33:714, 1986.

14. Lopezgatius F: Intraperitoneal insemination in repeat-breeder cows: A preliminary-report. Theriogenology 44:153, 1995.

15. Momont HW, Seguin BE, Singh G, et al: Does intrauterine site of insemination in cattle really matter? Theriogenology 32:19, 1989.

16. Lopezgatius F: Side of gestation in dairy heifers affects subsequent sperm transport and pregnancy rates after deep insemination into one uterine horn. Theriogenology 45:417, 1996.

17. Phatak AP, Whitmore HL: Greater participation by veterinarians in the reproductive management of dairy cattle. J Am Vet Med Assoc 199:74, 1991.

■ Management of the Repeat Breeder Female

Dwight F. Wolfe, D.V.M., M.S.

A female is usually considered to be a repeat breeder if she fails to conceive after three or more regularly spaced services in the absence of detectable abnormalities of the internal reproductive tract. The incidence of the condition ranges from 5.0% to 15.1% in dairy herds, with an apparent average of 10% of dairy cattle affected. Repeat breeder beef cattle or small ruminants appear to be less common, although approximately 20% of sows culled for reproductive failure are culled because of return to estrus following breeding.

NORMAL REPRODUCTIVE EXPECTANCY

In normal healthy cows with estrous cycles, a 63% conception rate is expected after the first service. Similar results are expected on each subsequent service such that 5% of a normal, healthy, cycling cattle population can be expected to be repeat breeders based on the previously mentioned classification of failure of conception after three services (100 × 63% = 63 pregnant, 37 not pregnant after the first service; 37 × 63% =

14 not pregnant after the second service; and 14 × 63% = 5 not pregnant after the third service).

ECONOMICS

Failure to conceive in timely fashion accounts for significant economic loss to the livestock producer. Standardized performance analysis has shown that a producer may lose as much as $75 (U.S.) for each estrous cycle in which a beef cow fails to conceive. Therefore, a repeat breeder may cost the livestock producer several hundred dollars per year just from failure to conceive in an appropriate time. Although failure of conception may be less costly than abortion or the production of inferior offspring, repeat breeder Holstein cattle in the United States produce 144 kg less milk, 0.15 fewer calves, and 8.8% less annual income than cows that are not repeat breeders.

FERTILIZATION FAILURE

Fertilization requires that viable, competent sperm and ova arrive in the uterine tube at the appropriate time. The fertilization rate approaches 100% in healthy first-service heifers as compared with approximately 85% in normal pluriparous cows and only 60% in repeat breeders.

Congenital Anatomic Defects Causing Fertilization Failure

Segmental aplasia of the müllerian ducts is one of the more common abnormalities causing fertilization failure. The developmental defects may involve any portion of the vagina, cervix, uterus, or uterine tubes. Imperforate hymen, imperforate cervix, aplasia of all or part of one or both uterine horns or uterine tubes, and double external or internal cervical ora are manifestations of this condition. Additional forms of the abnormality are didelphia, in which each uterine horn is connected by a separate cervical canal, and uterus unicornis, in which only one uterine horn is present. Any manifestation of these conditions may cause fertilization failure by preventing the union of sperm and ova.

Diagnosis and Treatment

Most of the conditions can be confirmed by physical examination. Varying degrees of vaginal constriction, imperforate hymen, and anomalies of the external cervical os are detectable by speculum, endoscopy, ultrasound, or digital vaginal examination. An accumulation of normal cyclic secretions may occur anterior to an obstruction and produce dilation of a portion of the tubular tract. Careful rectal palpation or ultrasound examination will distinguish this condition from pregnancy. The incidence of congenital anomalies is reported to be less than 1.0%, and surgical repair is not recommended because of the expected heritable nature of the anomalies. However, in cattle, this condition most often results from freemartinism because of the heifer being born twin to a bull.

Defects of Sperm, Ova, or Zygote Causing Conception Failure

Chromosomal abnormalities of sperm or ova may prevent fertilization or cause conception failure by the creation of lethal gene products. Male and female animals heterozygous for a genetically balanced autosomal abnormality are usually phenotypically normal, but they may produce unbalanced products of meiosis that may be lethal to embryos, which die in utero. Chromosomal abnormalities have been reported in all domestic species.

Polyploidy (more than the 2N number of chromosomes) can be caused by two or more sperm penetrating (polyspermy) and fertilizing (polyandry) an ova or by suppression of the second polar body and fertilization of a diploid ova by one sperm (polygyny). The resultant polyploidy is usually lethal. This condition occurs more frequently in aged gametes. Fertilization of aged gametes seldom occurs with natural mating but may occur as a result of improper timing of insemination when artificial insemination is used.

Diagnosis of Chromosomal Abnormalities

Chromosomal analysis of blood leukocytes from a heparinized blood sample by a cytogenetics laboratory will detect the presence of numerical or gross structural autosomal abnormalities. Leukocyte culture may be required to detect balanced autosomal abnormalities. Diagnosis of lethal abnormalities is difficult and depends on cytogenetic studies of the embryo or parents of the embryo. Embryos should be submitted to the cytogenetics laboratory in tissue culture medium containing antibiotics.

Acquired Abnormalities Causing Fertilization Failure

Acquired lesions of the genital tract are probably more common than developmental abnormalities and are usually due to infections or parturient trauma. Often the acquired lesions are detectable by physical examination, perhaps augmented with ultrasound or endoscopic evaluation.

Diseases of the Ovary and Ovarian Bursa

Adhesions, mild to severe, between the ovary and fimbria may prevent ova entrance into the uterine tube. The right ovary appears to be more frequently involved, although the condition may be bilateral. Mild lesions may not affect fertility.

The incidence of the disease is rare in heifers but increases with age. Adhesions may occur in all species but appear to be most common in cattle. Mycoplasmas have been isolated from a high proportion of ovarobursal lesions in cattle, and it has been suggested that there is a relationship between semen-borne mycoplasmas and this disease. Also, the anatomy of the uterotubal junction in the ruminant permits retrograde access to the uterine tube from the uterine lumen. Consequently, overzealous intrauterine therapy may allow contamination of the uterine tube and ovary from the uterine contents. Such therapy could lead to bursal adhesions because of exposure of the fimbria to septic or irritating agents.

Diagnosis and Treatment

Diagnosis of ovarian adhesions is difficult. Careful rectal palpation of the ovaries may detect a small percentage of the fertility-limiting adhesions, and ultrasonography may enhance the accuracy of the diagnosis. Exploratory laparotomy or laparoscopy may be indicated in valuable females. The diagnosis is made even more difficult by the fact that some females with ovarobursal adhesions maintain normal fertility. Therefore the adhesions may not be the source of the infertility. Therapy for fertility-limiting bursal adhesions is disappointing in bilaterally affected cows. If the condition is unilateral, either unilateral ovariectomy or rectal palpation with breeding only when ovulation occurs on the normal ovary may prove successful.

Cows that are infertile because of ovarobursal adhesions may be able to continue to reproduce through assisted reproductive techniques. Ultrasound-guided oocyte aspiration to harvest oocytes for in vitro fertilization may extend the reproductive life of the affected female.

Occlusion or Inflammation of the Uterine Tube

Occlusion or inflammation of the uterine tube (oviduct) may prevent fertilization. These conditions prevent sperm or ova transport or create an environment unsuitable for fertilization. Salpingitis, hydrosalpinx, pyosalpinx, or pachysalpinx may be sequelae to puerperal metritis and not consistently detectable by rectal palpation.

Diagnosis and Treatment

Rectal palpation or ultrasonographic examination may detect occlusive disease of the uterine tube. Other than collection of fertilized ova, there are no reliable tests to assess uterine tube function. Valuable cows that are infertile because of uterine tube disease may be candidates for in vitro fertilization.

Improper Timing of Insemination

Improper timing of insemination is a primary cause of fertilization failure and is almost exclusively associated with the use of artificial insemination. In some herds up to 20% of the inseminated cows are in the luteal phase of the estrous cycle, an indication of inadequate estrus detection programs. If the problem is anticipated, the veterinarian should review the estrus detection program. Client education, palpation of cows by the veterinarian, serum or milk progesterone analysis at the time of insemination, and the use of estrus detection aids such as surgically altered teaser males, heat detection patches, or computer-aided estrus detection devices may improve estrus detection accuracy. Additionally, improper semen handling or placement during artificial insemination may cause fertilization failure.

OVULATORY DISORDERS

Ovulation occurs 10 to 12 hours after the end of behavioral estrus in the cow, 12 to 36 hours after the onset of estrus in the doe, 24 hours after the onset of estrus in the ewe, and 24 to 42 hours after the onset of estrus in the sow.

Ovulatory defects are generally believed to be due to endocrine disturbances. The quantity and timing of luteinizing hormone release from the anterior pituitary gland determines when ovulation occurs. Inappropriate luteinizing hormone release in relation to estrus may lead to anovulation. The preovulatory follicle then becomes cystic. Cows with cystic ovarian disease display irregular estrous cycles and therefore do not qualify as a classic repeat breeder. Insemination during an anovulatory estrus results in fertilization failure.

Delayed ovulation is diagnosed by sequential rectal palpation or ultrasonographic evaluation of the same follicle on the same ovary at more than 24 hours after estrus. Treatment may involve repeat insemination every 12 to 24 hours until ovulation occurs.

Alternatively, gonadotropin-releasing hormone (100 μg intramuscularly) or human chorionic gonadotropin (3000 to 4500 units intravenously) given 6 hours before or at the time of insemination in the ensuing estrus may hasten ovulation.

SEMEN AND FERTILITY

Bulls with high and low conception rates have been identified through artificial insemination records. Fertilization failure or early embryonic death may occur more frequently from bulls with low fertility. This condition presumably occurs in other species.

Careless handling of frozen semen can drastically lower fertilization rates. Infertility in bulls and infertility associated with faulty artificial insemination techniques are discussed elsewhere.

CONCEPTION FAILURE

Conception failure is the result of early embryonic death. In cows, early embryonic death must occur before day 16 to maintain regular estrous cycle length, and numerous studies indicate that most embryonic losses occur before day 15. In ewes and sows, embryonic death must occur by day 12 to maintain regular cycle length.

Physiologic Causes of Early Embryonic Death

Aging of the ovum or sperm may occur in delayed ovulating females or in those that are not inseminated at the appropriate time in relation to ovulation. Generally an aged ovum is fertilizable, but a defective zygote develops and undergoes early embryonic death.

Endocrine Influence on Embryonic Death

Improper balance of estrogen and progesterone during the early postovulatory period can affect ovum transport through the uterine tube. Excessive estrogen delays tubal transport so that the ovum does not enter the uterus at the proper time. Excessive progesterone hastens transport. Either condition prevents the ova from arriving in the uterine lumen at a time when the uterine environment is synchronous with the physiologic needs of the ovum and results in early embryonic death.

The primary source of progesterone during early pregnancy is the corpus luteum. Progesterone or luteal insufficiency has been proposed as a cause of early embryonic failure in many species. Blood progesterone levels greater than 2 ng/dL are necessary for pregnancy maintenance. Numerous empirical treatments have been used for progesterone insufficiency. Injections of human chorionic gonadotropin or gonadotropin-releasing hormone 1 to 10 days after breeding have been recommended to stimulate luteinizing hormone in the cow. Various regimens of exogenous progesterone have been used, ranging from 500 mg of repositol progesterone beginning 10 days after breeding and every 10 days thereafter to the addition of progestins to the diet daily throughout pregnancy.

ENVIRONMENTAL INFLUENCES ON FERTILITY

Reduced conception rates in cows are well documented during the warm months of the year, especially in subtropical and tropical climates. Excessive solar radiation the day of insemination in cattle and high environmental temperature the day following insemination through day 17 have a negative impact on fertilization or embryo viability. Ewes and sows subjected to high ambient temperatures also suffer greater embryonic losses. The elevated uterine temperature may cause fertilization failure by sperm or ova damage, or early embryonic death may occur. Livestock managers should provide relief from thermal stress by supplying adequate water, shade, and forced ventilation.

AGE

Fertility generally declines in all species with advanced age. In cattle, heifers have higher fertilization rates than mature cows but also experience a higher incidence of embryonic death. The number of repeat breeders is lowest in first-calf heifers and increases with age. It is reported that over 13% of cows older than 9 years are repeat breeders.

UTERINE DISEASE

Diseases of the uterus can prevent sperm transport with resultant fertilization failure or may cause early death after a viable embryo arrives in the uterine lumen. Endometritis, metritis, pyometra, and hydrometra are discussed elsewhere in this text.

INFECTIOUS CAUSES OF INFERTILITY

Camplyobacter fetus subsp. *veneralis* and *Trichomonas foetus* are both significant pathogens of cattle that may cause repeat breeders. Infertility is due to fertilization failure or early embryonic death. These diseases are discussed elsewhere in this text.

BIBLIOGRAPHY

Almeida AP, Ayabon N, Faingold D, et al: The relationship between uterine environment and early embryonic mortality (EEM) in normal (NB) and repeat breeder (RB) Friesian cows. *In* Proceedings of the 10th International Congress on Reproduction and Artificial Insemination, Urbana, Ill, 1984, p 438.

Almond GW: Factors affecting reproductive performance of the weaned sow. Vet Clin North Am 8:503–515, 1992.

Bartol FF, Floyd JG: Critical periods, steroid exposure and reproduction. *In* Proceedings of the Society for Theriogenology, Kansas City, 1996, p 101.

Drost M, Thatcher WW: Reducing embryonic death in cattle. *In* Proceedings of the Bovine Shortcourse, Society for Theriogenology, San Antonio, 1995, p 133.

Hawkins HE: Breeding soundness evaluation and fertility in beef bulls. *In* Proceedings of the Society for Theriogenology, Kansas City, 1996, p 58.

Hunter MG: Characteristics and causes of the inadequate corpus luteum. J Reprod Fertil Suppl 43:91, 1991.

Kidder HE, Black WG, Ulborg LE, et al: Fertilization rates and embryonic death rates in cows bred to bulls of different levels of fertility. J Anim Sci 34:312, 1956.

King WA: Chromosome abnormalities and pregnancy failure in domestic animals. Adv Vet Sci Comp Med 34:229, 1990.

Leipold HW: Inherited disorders in large animals. *In* Proceedings of the Society for Theriogenology, Kansas City, 1994, p 15.

McGrann JM: Economic assessment of reproductive management. *In* Proceedings of the Society for Theriogenology, San Antonio, 1992, p 20.

Putney DJ, Drost M, Thatcher WW: Embryonic development in dairy cattle exposed to elevated ambient temperatures between days 1 and 7 post insemination. Theriogenology 30:195, 1988.

Roberts RM, Schalue-Francis J, Francis H, et al: Maternal recognition of pregnancy and embryonic loss. Theriogenology 33:175, 1990.

Sreenan JM, Diskin MG: The extent and timing of embryonic mortality in the cow. *In* Sreenan JM, Diskin MG (eds): Embryonic Mortality in Farm Animals. Dordrecht, The Netherlands, Martinus Nijhoff, 1985, pp 1–11.

Walton JS, Halbert GW, Robinson NA, et al: Effects of progesterone and human chorionic gonadotropin administration five days postinsemination on plasma milk concentrations of progesterone and pregnancy rates of normal and repeat breeder dairy cows. Can J Vet Res 54:305, 1990.

Wolfe DF: Breeding soundness evaluation of bulls. *In* Proceedings of the Annual Meeting of the Alabama Cattleman's Association, Birmingham, 1997.

■ Potential of Embryo Transfer for Infectious Disease Control

M. Daniel Givens, D.V.M.
David A. Stringfellow, D.V.M., M.S.

Technological advances and obvious economic and humane advantages have resulted in an increased demand for the use of embryo transfer to move genetic material between populations of livestock, including cattle, small ruminants, and swine. Research involving specific bovine pathogens has shown that transfer of in vivo–derived embryos can be an effective means for introducing germ plasm into herds while minimizing the introduction of infectious disease–producing agents. Based on an assessment of epidemiologic factors associated with in vivo embryo transfer, it is clear that the movement of these embryos is innately safer than the movement of postnatal animals whenever the transmission of specific pathogens is a concern. Assurance that in vivo–derived embryos are free of pathogens can be provided by screening the health status of donors, by special handling of embryos, or by a combination of these two methods. Affirmation of the disease control potential of embryo transfer is provided in this chapter through an assessment of the epidemiologic factors involved in embryo transfer, a summary of the results of studies concerning the transmission of specific pathogens through embryo transfer, and an outline of effective methods for ensuring that in vivo–derived embryos are pathogen-free.

In vitro embryo production is the newest reproductive technology to be applied commercially in the cattle industry. Information on the association of specific pathogens with in vitro–derived (i.e., in vitro fertilization [IVF]) embryos is limited; however, contemporary evidence suggests a greater potential for producing pathogen-associated IVF embryos because of a higher risk of introducing specific pathogens and differences in the zona pellucida. Therefore, the risks of disease transmission through production and transfer of IVF embryos are assessed separately in this chapter, as are proposed methods for ensuring that these embryos are pathogen-free.

IN VIVO–DERIVED EMBRYOS

Epidemiologic Aspects of Embryo Transfer

For an infectious disease to be transmitted through transfer of in vivo–derived embryos, a series of essential events must occur. Initially, embryos must be exposed to a pathogenic agent, with subsequent adherence of the agent to the embryo, infection of the embryo, or contamination of recovery fluids. Then, sufficient quantities of the pathogen must survive the processes of embryo collection and transfer to result in introduction of an infective dose into a recipient. Each of these events can be

thought of as links in a chain of infection. If a single link is broken, transmission of disease will not occur.

A variety of factors intrinsic to the process of embryo transfer can deter the spread of infectious disease. There is a temporal limit to the potential for exposure of transfer-stage embryos to pathogens because embryos are collected shortly after conception (7 days). Exposure to agents not regularly found in the reproductive tract within a week after estrus is especially unlikely to occur. The immune status of the donor's reproductive tract during the period of conception and early embryonic development also minimizes exposure potential. If exposure does occur, infection of embryos or adherence of pathogens is prevented for many agents by the zona pellucida that surrounds transfer-stage, in vivo–derived embryos. Additionally, a variety of obstacles must be overcome by the agent for transmission to occur. These include the dilution factor of the recovery medium and the effects of antibiotic therapy, cryopreservation and thawing, mechanical washing, and special treatments (e.g., enzymes). The capability of an infectious agent to prevail and be transmitted to a recipient despite each of these obstacles has not been documented in a naturally occurring circumstance in any livestock species.

Embryo-Pathogen Interaction: Specific Research

Early concerns about the potential for transmission of infectious agents through embryo transfer procedures resulted from work in laboratory animals, but there is little evidence for naturally occurring, vertical transmission of pathogens through the embryos of livestock. Numerous studies using zona pellucida–intact (ZP-I), in vivo–derived bovine embryos have resulted in the declaration that these embryos can be transferred with a relative degree of safety. In vivo–derived bovine embryos have been exposed in vitro to Akabane virus, bovine leukemia virus, bluetongue virus (BTV), bovine viral diarrheal virus (BVDV), foot-and-mouth disease virus, infectious bovine rhinotracheitis virus, vesicular stomatitis virus, bovine cytomegalovirus, and *Brucella abortus* and subsequently washed and assayed for infectious agents. Only infectious bovine rhinotracheitis virus, vesicular stomatitis virus, and bovine cytomegalovirus adhered to the zona pellucida of these embryos, and it has been shown that trypsin treatment is effective for the removal of infectious bovine rhinotracheitis virus and bovine cytomegalovirus. In vitro studies with *Haemophilus somnus*, *Ureaplasma diversum*, *Mycoplasma bovis*, and *Mycoplasma bovigenitalium* have shown adherence of these organisms after the recommended washing procedures were used. Of these, *H. somnus* was inactivated by the use of standard levels of antibiotics in embryo wash medium. Treatments to ensure freedom of ZP-I bovine embryos from the other agents have yet to be documented, but neither a significant exposure potential for transfer-stage embryos to these agents nor natural transmission of the agents through embryo transfer has been demonstrated, so the use of such treatments might be unnecessary. In vivo studies are being conducted on the prevention of transmission of bovine spongiform encephalopathy and the equivalent spongiform encephalopathy in sheep (scrapie). Conflicting reports exist concerning the transmission of scrapie by experimentally infected sheep through in vivo–derived embryo transfer.

In livestock other than cattle, embryo-pathogen interactions have been less extensively studied. There is experimental evidence that BTV, *Brucella ovis*, and *B. abortus* adhere to ZP-I ovine embryos after in vitro exposure to these agents, but the infectious agent did not remain when the embryos were washed subsequent to exposure to *Campylobacter fetus* and border disease virus. It is noteworthy that transmission of disease was not demonstrated when ovine embryos were collected and transferred from donor ewes that were known to be infected with BTV, *Chlamydia psittaci* (etiology of enzootic abortion in ewes), and maedi/visna virus. Similarly, transmission of disease could not be demonstrated after the transfer of caprine embryos collected from donors that were serologically positive for BTV or caprine arthritis-encephalitis virus.

Zona pellucida–intact porcine embryos have been exposed in vitro to African swine fever virus, foot-and-mouth disease virus, hog cholera virus, porcine parvovirus, pseudorabies virus (PRV), swine vesicular disease virus, and vesicular stomatitis virus. Washing was not 100% effective in removing any of these viruses, although there appeared to be a substantial beneficial effect for the removal of foot-and-mouth disease virus and PRV. Additional treatment of ZP-I porcine embryos with trypsin after in vitro exposure to hog cholera virus, PRV, and vesicular stomatitis virus was reported to be effective for ensuring that the embryos were free from these viruses. In further attempts to determine the potential for transmission of viral pathogens, embryos were collected from donor swine that were infected with hog cholera virus, PRV, or swine vesicular disease virus and transferred to negative recipients. Seroconversion occurred in recipients receiving embryos from PRV-infected donors, but only in those situations in which the virus was artificially introduced directly into the uterus. Again, it is noteworthy that none of the diseases have been shown to be transmitted with embryos under "natural" circumstances.

Pathogen-Free Embryos

A conservative approach to certifying the pathogen-free status of in vivo–derived embryos for transfer is to ensure that the donor is free of the specific infectious agents of concern. In cattle, for example, it is possible to collect serum samples from the donor on the day of embryo collection or earlier and at some time after collection while the embryos are stored in the frozen state. The measure of safety when using this method is absolute if a reliable test for a specific antibody to the pathogen of concern is available, the transfer media is free of the pathogen, and sufficient time is allowed between the collection of paired sera for the normal incubation period of the disease. This method is also effective for screening the health status of the sire of the embryos because the embryo donor serves as a sentinel animal for agents that might be introduced with the semen at the time of insemination. With the use of this conservative approach, the former in vivo environment of the embryo is certified to be pathogen-free before the frozen embryo is actually thawed and transferred.

Substantial evidence indicates that testing of donors is not necessary if the standard materials and methods described in the *Manual of the International Embryo Transfer Society* are used in handling in vivo–derived embryos. The following methods that conform to the standards are suggested.

Washing of Embryos

Only ZP-I embryos can be effectively washed. To ensure the efficacy of washing, all surfaces of the embryos are examined by using a stereomicroscope set at a minimum magnification of ×50 to ensure that the zonae pellucidae are intact (Fig. 1) and free of adherent material. This visualization is done before and after washing. When adherent material is noted, it must be removed prior to beginning the official washing procedure. Ten 35-mm sterile plastic Petri dishes containing 2 mL of Dulbecco's phosphate-buffered saline plus 2% fetal bovine serum with antibiotics (PSF: 100 units of penicillin [base], 100 μg of streptomy-

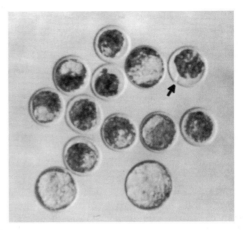

Figure 1

Day 7 bovine embryos enclosed by the zona pellucida (× 50). One embryo had a defective zone *(arrow)* and could not be certified to be pathogen-free after washing.

cin [base], and 0.25 μg of amphotericin B per milliliter of medium) are used for washing of the embryos. A separate, sterile 20-μL micropipette is used to carry groups of embryos between wash dishes. A hand-held micropipetter that provides for easy exchange of pipettes and does not have a plunger that enters the pipette is essential to avoid contamination. The ratio of the volume of medium containing embryos in the micropipette to the volume of medium in each wash dish should be at least 1:100. While embryos are in each wash dish, the dishes are gently rotated in a circular motion alternating between clockwise and counterclockwise to ensure adequate dilution and washing action. Only embryos from a single donor animal are washed together in groups of 10 or fewer.

Trypsin Treatment

Treatment of ZP-I embryos with the enzyme trypsin has been shown to be effective for the removal and/or inactivation of certain viral pathogens that adhere to the zona pellucida. Trypsin treatment should not be regarded as a "general disinfectant" and is only recommended for pathogens adhering to the zona pellucida for which this treatment has proved effective in the laboratory. Trypsin treatment is required for embryos to be imported into certain countries. As in the standard washing technique, before and after treatment the embryos are examined over all surfaces with a stereomicroscope set at a minimum magnification of ×50 to ensure that the zonae pellucidae are intact and free of adherent material. Embryos from only one donor animal at a time are treated in groups of 10 or fewer. Equipment and techniques for pipetting as well as dilution factors are the same as presented for washing of embryos. Trypsin treatment involves the use of 2 mL of medium in twelve 35-mm Petri dishes. Dishes 1 to 5 contain phosphate-buffered saline, 0.4% bovine serum albumin, and PSF; dishes 6 and 7 contain 0.25% trypsin in Hanks' balanced salt solution (pH 7.6 to 7.8); and dishes 8 to 12 contain phosphate-buffered saline plus 2% fetal bovine serum and PSF. It is acceptable to substitute 0.4% bovine serum albumin for the fetal bovine serum in washes 8 to 12. Generally, the embryos are exposed to trypsin for about 2 minutes and all treatments are conducted at ambient temperature (approximately 25°C). It is known that exposure to trypsin for up to 5 minutes does not have a detrimental effect on the developmental capabilities of transfer-stage bovine embryos.

The development of additional treatments for in vivo–derived embryos of livestock has been the subject of research. Specific studies have tested the use of various antibiotics, photosensitive chemical disinfectants, enzymes, and specific antibodies. Although one or more of these new techniques may be adopted in the future to create a variety of options for ensuring the pathogen-free status of embryos, it should not be forgotten that current procedures already provide an extremely high degree of safety.

IN VITRO–DERIVED EMBRYOS

There are differences between embryos produced in the cow and those produced in the laboratory. In general, IVF embryos do not undergo complete compaction and have fewer cells. Critical to a consideration of embryo-pathogen interactions is the difference between the zona pellucida of in vivo– and in vitro–derived bovine embryos. The zonae pellucidae of both types of embryos appear the same when viewed with a stereomicroscope; however, topographic and compositional differences between in vitro– and in vivo–derived embryos have been described. Whether the structural differences affect the in vitro–derived embryo's capability to resist adherence or penetration by infectious agents requires further investigation. It is vitally important to determine whether the zonae pellucidae of IVF embryos provide similar resistance to pathogens and whether pathogen-limiting procedures such as washing are similarly effective.

Epidemiologic Aspects of In Vitro Fertilization–Embryo Transfer

Production of pathogen-associated IVF embryos would in all probability be initiated with introduction of the infectious agent via the gametes (i.e., semen or primary oocytes), somatic cells (e.g., uterine tubal cells, cumulus cells, or continuous cell lines), or media components of animal origin (e.g., serum, bovine serum albumin, or follicle-stimulating hormone). Although it is less likely, environmental contamination could also occur (e.g., fecal or vaginal pathogens introduced during transvaginal ultrasound-guided oocyte collection). After introduction, active replication or tenacious survival of the pathogenic agent would be necessary to produce an infective dose associated with transferred morulae or blastocysts.

As with in vivo embryo production, several factors intrinsic to IVF embryo production are likely to reduce the potential for producing pathogen-associated embryos. For example, some pathogenic viruses will be cytopathic and destroy somatic cells during in vitro maturation of oocytes, IVF, or in vitro culture of embryos. In this circumstance, a clear indication of pathogenic contamination is provided. Also, if an embryocidal pathogen is present, no embryos will be available for transfer.

Other potentially beneficial factors are the use of antibiotics, specific neutralizing antibody, washing at various stages, and specific quality controls designed to prevent environmental contamination and screen materials of animal origin for pathogens. The washing and trypsin treatment recommended by the International Embryo Transfer Society for in vivo–derived embryos may be beneficial, but the efficacy of these treatments has not been thoroughly evaluated for IVF embryos. Indeed, specific research on the epidemiology of IVF embryo transfer has been limited.

In Vitro–Derived Embryo–Pathogen Interaction: Specific Research

Available information indicates a clear potential for the introduction of infectious agents into IVF production systems. Surveillance of ovaries, follicular fluid, cumulus cells, oocytes, sperm, and uterine tubal cells for specific pathogens indicates the potential for the introduction of viruses. Bovine herpesvirus-1 and BVDV can be expected in at least a small proportion of raw materials, and bovine herpesvirus-1 has actually been found in association with embryos produced from such materials. It is clear that essential tissues from cows actively infected with either bovine herpesvirus-1 or BVDV are likely to contain virus and have a high potential for the production of pathogen-associated IVF embryos. Washing, swim-up, Percoll gradients, glass wool separation, and glass bead filtration were all ineffective in removing BVDV virus from the semen of a bull persistently infected with BVDV.

The interactions of pathogens with the zonae pellucidae of IVF embryos are clearly unlike interactions with the in vivo counterparts developed in the cow's uterine tube and uterus. It is clear that washing procedures are not reliable for removing the few agents that have been tested (bovine herpesvirus-1 and BVDV) from in vitro–derived embryos. Research also indicates that trypsin treatment is not effective in removing cytopathic or noncytopathic BVDV from IVF embryos artificially exposed to virus.

Results of limited research on IVF embryo–pathogen interactions indicate a meaningful potential for the introduction of certain pathogens via materials of animal origin that are used for the in vitro production of bovine embryos. Reliable quality control measures to screen these materials are a necessity to ensure the production of specific pathogen-free IVF embryos.

Developing Methods to Ensure Pathogen-Free In Vitro–Derived Embryos

Prevention of disease transmission through transfer of IVF embryos is clearly achievable because of the multiple opportunities for quality control provided by the in vitro system. Additional research is necessary to provide a basis for the establishment of specific sanitary guidelines, and there is a potential that guidelines will vary between different IVF embryo production systems. The following precautionary measures based on current information are suggested:

- Exposing embryos to broad-spectrum antibiotics in media should be effective in controlling many prokaryotic agents. Additional research to test a variety of antibiotics for efficacy as well as toxicity in IVF systems is desirable.
- Washing and trypsin treatments are likely to provide some benefit in reducing the contamination of in vitro–derived embryos.
- Pretesting of the sera and somatic cells used in IVF systems is a necessary quality control measure to verify the absence of pathogens.
- Pretesting of the semen used in IVF is essential to determine that specific pathogens are not present.
- Acquiring animal tissues (e.g., cumulus-oocyte complexes and uterine tubal cells) from sources that are not verified to be pathogen-free (i.e., abattoir origin) may be necessary at times, but the donors should be healthy animals subjected to antemortem and postmortem inspection.
- Testing samples from the IVF system (e.g., media or somatic cells) for the presence of specific pathogens allows additional quality control.
- "Quarantine" of IVF embryos after cryopreservation should occur until it is known that the materials of animal origin used in their production were pathogen-free. The exception would be when all materials were determined to be pathogen-free prior to use.

Although the ability to produce pathogen-free IVF bovine

embryos is certainly attainable, the measures used to provide assurance are likely to differ from those used to ensure that in vivo–derived embryos are free of pathogens. Additional research is necessary to clarify the potential risks of contamination and finalize the most efficient treatment or testing protocols that will ensure that IVF embryos are free of specific pathogens.

CONCLUSION

Transfer of both in vivo– and in vitro–produced embryos has become widely available at a reasonable cost to livestock producers in many parts of the world. Transfer of embryos, where practical, should be the preferred method for introducing germ plasm into herds and flocks because of the potential for prevention of disease transmission.

EQUIPMENT AND SUPPLY LIST

Equipment

Micro-pipettor (#19803/0558), Minitub of America, Rte. 1, Box 3, Cambridge, IA 50046

Twenty-μL micropipettes (#21-175c), Fisher Scientific, 585 Alpha Dr., Pittsburgh, PA 15238

Supplies

Dulbecco's phosphate-buffered saline (#14040-042), Grand Island Biological Co. (GIBCO BRL), Grand Island, NY 14072

Bovine albumin fraction V solution (#A8918), Sigma Chemical Co., St. Louis, MO 63178

Fetal bovine serum (#SH30070.03), HyClone Laboratories, Inc., 1725 S. State Hwy. 89-91, Logan, UT 84321

Penicillin-streptomycin–amphotericin B combination (#15240-062), GIBCO BRL, Grand Island, NY 14072

Trypsin (10× liquid) (#15090-038), GIBCO BRL, Grand Island, NY 14072

Hanks' balanced salt solution (#14170-120), GIBCO BRL, Grand Island, NY 14072

BIBLIOGRAPHY

Guerin B, Nibart M, Marquant-LeGuienne B, et al: Sanitary risks related to embryo transfer in domestic species. Theriogenology 47:33–42, 1997.

Stringfellow DA, Seidel SM (eds): Manual of the International Embryo Transfer Society, ed 3. Champaign, Ill, International Embryo Transfer Society, 1998.

Stringfellow DA, Wrathall AE: Epidemiological implications of the production and transfer of IVF embryos. Theriogenology 43:89–96, 1995.

Wrathall AE: Embryo transfer and disease transmission in livestock: A review of recent research. Theriogenology 43:81–88, 1995.

▪ Abortion Diagnosis in Food Animals

Larry D. Holler, D.V.M., Ph.D.

Abortion in food animal species causes significant economic loss to animal production systems throughout the world. However, the average herd or flock abortion rate reported in the literature is usually quite variable, with much of the variation associated with differences in case definition (what constitutes an abortion), methods of data recording, management styles, geography, and the regional prevalence of significant abortifacients. It is interesting to note that despite an abundance of vaccine products for abortion disease prevention, abortion rates have remain virtually unchanged. Old abortion foes such as brucellosis and pseudorabies have been replaced by new challenging disease agents such as *Neospora caninum*–like protozoa and porcine reproductive and respiratory syndrome virus. The battle for prevention of abortion losses will continue. The first step should always include obtaining an accurate and rapid diagnosis before prevention strategies are formed. Unfortunately, diagnostic success with abortion cases remains consistently low, with rates varying between 23% and 46% in laboratories around the world.[1]

A certain percentage of fetal loss associated with abortion is to be expected in any livestock production system. Because of the sporadic nature of many abortion pathogens, as well as the numerous noninfectious causes of abortion, including genetic factors, toxic plants, hormonal dysfunction, nutrition, and trauma, a 0% abortion rate is not a reality. When one considers the complex mechanisms that must suppress the maternal tendency for immunologic rejection of the conceptus while maintaining and protecting the fragile relationship between the dam and the immunologically naive offspring, it is truly amazing that calves, lambs, or piglets are ever born. If we accept that abortion will occur in a flock or herd at some level, the question for the producer and veterinarian becomes at what level of loss is a diagnostic investigation warranted. This decision will vary between the species of interest, the lost production threshold of the owner, and the owner's desire for specific answers. Veterinarians should be familiar with their diagnostic laboratory's procedures and capabilities when submitting case materials to achieve the greatest success rate for the dollars spent.

ABORTION INVESTIGATION AND SAMPLE SUBMISSION

Submission of case material for abortion diagnosis is usually a straightforward process. However, a high percentage of submissions to diagnostic laboratories every year are incomplete, which reduces the already limited diagnostic success rates. The practitioner should start every abortion investigation by obtaining a complete clinical history, including a description of on-farm management practices and vaccination protocols and an evaluation of recent on-farm events that may have predisposed the dam to abortion disease. Previous disease problems, new purchases, and nutritional programs should be recorded. A complete history is received in probably fewer than 10% of the submitted cases. It is highly recommended that interested practitioners develop a questionnaire that will consistently collect all the information needed for a complete investigation. A partial list of questions is included in Table 1. Realistically, each species may need its own specific list. In abortion outbreaks, all aspects of the operation, including housing, nutrition, feed storage, environmental conditions, and sanitation practices, should be evaluated.

An intact, fresh fetus or fetuses with placenta are most desirable for diagnostic evaluation. If the fetus is large and shipping costs become prohibitive, a complete necropsy should be performed on the farm or at the veterinary clinic. A necropsy is not a difficult task; however, diagnostic success will often hinge on the submission of appropriate samples. Producers should be encouraged to attempt to recover the placenta. Often the placenta is retained and must be retrieved from the cow, or it is left lying on the ground or lost to scavengers. It cannot be overemphasized that the placenta is the most important tissue

---

Table 1

BASIC QUESTIONS TO ASK THE LIVESTOCK OWNER TO ASSIST IN INVESTIGATING ABORTION OUTBREAKS

Number of abortions, traditional abortion rate?
Parity or age of the dam?
Nutritional status?
Change in management procedures, feed programs?
Recent farm events, i.e., transporting, processing, etc?
Feedstuff and water sources?
New additions to the herd or flock?
Vaccination procedures, products used?
Natural service or artificial insemination?
Dams showing clinical illness?
Previous or concurrent disease problems?
Previous abortion diagnoses?

---

for abortion diagnosis, especially in cattle and sheep. Without it the odds of an etiologic diagnosis are significantly reduced.

NECROPSY PROCEDURES

The procedure for a complete necropsy on a fetus is relatively easy and requires no specialized equipment. A sharp knife, pruning shears, meat saw or backsaw, scissors, forceps, Whirl-Paks (leakproof plastic bags; Nasco) and a leakproof container of 10% buffered neutral formalin are required. Pruning shears are excellent for removing the rib cage. A saw is useful for removal of the brain. The secret to success in performing necropsies is repetition and observation. The diagnostic laboratory should be contacted to obtain a list of recommended tissues for submission, and this list should be kept available for use during the necropsy procedure. A list of routine samples to submit for laboratory examination is presented in Table 2. Necropsy observations should be recorded and included on the submission form. Samples should be packaged so that cross-contamination between tissues will be minimized. Fetal stomach contents and thoracic fluid are collected with a sterile 18-gauge needle and syringe and transferred to a sterile tube to avoid the risks associated with sending syringes with attached needles through the mail. Whirl-pak bags that are properly sealed will not leak during transit. An insulated container system is available for purchase from many laboratories and will aid in the shipment of fresh samples to the diagnostic laboratory. The ambient temperature should be taken into consideration when samples are submitted and weekend stays in the post office avoided if possible. Elevated temperatures for a prolonged time tend to adversely affect an already autolyzed fetus. Conversely, histologic examination of frozen fetuses is also less than ideal for diagnostic success.

LABORATORY PROCEDURES

When a case submission is received at a diagnostic laboratory, samples are processed and forwarded to the appropriate laboratories for further investigation. Detailed procedures for specific tests are outlined in Kirkbride's *Laboratory Diagnosis of Livestock Abortion.*[2] For bacterial culture, fetal lung and stomach contents are the tissues of choice. Occasionally, other tissues, including the liver and placenta, will be cultured. Routine samples are cultured on Columbia agar with 5% sheep blood. The plates are incubated at 37°C in an atmosphere containing 10% CO_2 and routinely examined at 24-hour intervals. Stomach contents are often examined by darkfield microscopy for preliminary identification of *Tritrichomonas foetus*, *Campylobacter* spp., and

Leptospira spp. For *Campylobacter* spp., special media with added antibiotics are used for primary isolation. Specific atmospheric conditions are also required. *Campylobacter jejuni* is the most common *Campylobacter* species isolated from bovine and ovine abortions. If *Chlamydia psittaci* is suspected, fluorescent antibody (FA) procedures on fresh frozen sections and culture methods using embryonated chicken eggs or specialized cell lines are used. Yolk sac material or fixed cells are then stained to detect the presence of chlamydial elementary bodies by the FA or Gimenez method. The diagnosis of leptospirosis is also best accomplished by FA analysis on kidney homogenates by using group-specific reagents that will recognize all the relevant serovars that would be encountered. Culture of this organism is not routinely performed.

Mycotic abortion is frequently reported as a cause of bovine abortion, but it is extremely rare in other food animal species. These cases are best diagnosed by examination of affected placentas. Gross examination of the placenta will often lead to a presumptive diagnosis of mycotic abortion based on the characteristic thickening in intercotyledonary spaces. The placenta should be spread out flat and any extra debris removed for a complete examination. A fluorescent dye is routinely used to detect fungal elements in placental scrapings and impression smears. Routine fungal cultures are plated on appropriate media, including Sabouraud's and mycobiotic agar, and incubated at 25°C for 7 days.

Viral causes of abortion are diagnosed by a combination of FA and virus isolation procedures. Infectious bovine rhinotracheitis

---

Table 2

MATERIALS TO BE SUBMITTED TO THE DIAGNOSTIC LABORATORY FOR INVESTIGATION

1. Fetus(es) and placenta
   The entire fetus and placenta, chilled, not frozen, are the preferred specimens when transportation can be arranged
   When the entire fetus cannot be submitted to the laboratory, the following specimens are the minimum if a complete examination is to be done:

Formalin Fixed*	Fresh (Chilled)*
Lung	Lung†
Liver	Liver
Kidney	Kidney
Spleen	Spleen
Heart	Heart
Brain (half)	Brain†
Skeletal muscle (tongue, diaphragm)	Placenta†
Thymus	
Any abnormal tissues	
Placenta (grossly examine for focal lesions)	

2. Also collect
   Stomach contents—1–3 mL in a sterile disposable syringe‡
   Thoracic fluid or heart blood from the fetus—3–5 mL in a sterile disposable syringe‡
   Ocular fluid (nitrate and nitrite analysis)‡
   Maternal blood, with 3–5 mL of serum separated from the clot. Serologic analysis on individual animals is often unrewarding. Samples should be saved for further evaluation in a whole-herd profile at a later date, if not submitted with the initial case

3. Other samples (collect if needed)
   Feedstuff, especially if recent changes in rations
   Water samples

---

*Put the fresh tissues in sterile bags, and chill or freeze if delivery to the laboratory will be prolonged. Put formalin-fixed tissue in an unbreakable, leakproof container. Label samples accordingly. Ship in an insulated container with enough ice packs to maintain refrigerated conditions until arrival at the laboratory.
†Package these tissues in separate Whirl-paks.
‡Transfer to a sterile tube if possible.

virus and bovine viral diarrhea virus in cattle, border disease virus in sheep, and porcine reproductive and respiratory syndrome virus, porcine parvovirus, and pseudorabies virus in swine are readily identified by FA tests. These tests are rapid and produce results within the first 24 hours. Commercial fluorescein-conjugated antibodies are used on fresh frozen sections from selected tissues. Virus isolation procedures are routinely performed on all submitted cases that are considered suitable for examination. This procedure is one of the most reliable tests for the diagnosis of bovine viral diarrhea in individual animals. Fetal tissues, including the lung, spleen, kidney, heart, and liver, are pooled and inoculated onto appropriate susceptible cell lines. Samples of placenta are usually cultured separately. Cultures are evaluated for cytopathic effect daily for 7 days. Cultures free of cytopathic effect are passed to fresh cells and incubated for an additional 7 days. Isolates are identified by FA or immunoperoxidase techniques. Infectious bovine rhinotracheitis virus grows rapidly in cell culture and is usually easy to diagnose by FA analysis. In contrast, bovine viral diarrheal virus is much more difficult to identify because of the presence of noncytopathic strains and may not be isolated until after the first passage. Porcine reproductive and respiratory disease virus is rarely isolated from aborted porcine fetuses, but it may be successfully recovered from serum samples of acutely ill sows during an abortion outbreak.[3]

Tissues for histologic examination are preserved in 10 volumes of 10% buffered neutral formalin. Adequate formalin and thin slices of tissue (<0.5 cm) will ensure adequate fixation of fetal tissue. Formalin-fixed tissues are sectioned at 5 μm, stained with hematoxylin-eosin, and examined microscopically. It should be kept in mind that autolysis of fetal tissue is often advanced if the fetus was retained in utero for a prolonged period. Immunocytochemistry procedures on formalin-fixed tissues are routinely available for many infectious causes of abortion. This technique may prove to be of considerable value for cases in which fresh tissue is unavailable or unsuitable for examination.[4]

Serologic testing is often of little value in individual animal cases; however, serologic profiling for common abortion agents may be of value on a herd basis. Serologic tests are commonly available for many abortion pathogens. The diagnostic laboratory should be consulted for a complete list of available tests and interpretation guidelines.

NEW DIAGNOSTIC METHODS

Laboratory methods for abortion disease diagnosis continue to evolve as new biomedical technologies are developed. It is hoped that the development of polymerase chain reaction technologies in which minute amounts of pathogen-specific nucleic acid can be detected from a variety of samples will reduce the 60% to 70% of abortion cases that go undiagnosed every year. Established technologies such as enzyme-linked immunosorbent assays and immunocytochemistry are becoming routine tools in abortion diagnosis. It is certain that new technologies will be developed that may add to the diagnostic success in food animal abortions. However, the challenge to veterinary diagnosticians will be to provide all these technologies to veterinarians and producers in a useful and *affordable* format.

CONCLUSIONS

Successful abortion disease investigation requires a joint effort of the producer, veterinarian, and diagnostic laboratory. Unfortunately, a significant number of investigations are incomplete and unrewarding for all parties involved. It is critical to remember that many cases of abortion are associated with noninfec-

tious causes and will always be difficult to confirm with a laboratory diagnosis. However, with continued education concerning investigation techniques and sample submission, combined with improved communication between all the participants involved, the possibility for improved success in abortion diagnosis and prevention could be a reality in the future.

REFERENCES

1. Barr BC, Anderson ML: Infectious diseases causing bovine abortion and fetal loss. Vet Clin North Am Food Anim Pract 9:343–368, 1993.
2. Kirkbride CA: Laboratory Diagnosis of Livestock Abortion, ed 3. Ames, Iowa State University, 1990.
3. Holler LD: Diagnosis of swine abortion. Swine Health Production 2:29, 1994.
4. Haines DM, Ellis JA: Special tests for the diagnosis of infectious causes of reproductive failure in ruminants. Vet Clin North Am Food Anim Pract 10:561–585, 1994.

■ Elective Termination of Pregnancy

Dragan Momcilovic, D.V.M., Ph.D.

Maintenance of pregnancy depends on an undisturbed uterine environment and a constant source of progesterone (corpus luteum, placenta, and to a lesser extent, adrenal glands).[1] Pregnancy can be terminated physically either by manual disruption of the conceptus or by intrauterine infusion of chemical agents and hormonally by eliminating the source of progesterone. All treatment methods intended to terminate pregnancy must eliminate the sources of progesterone, and these vary with the stage of gestation.

COW

Elective termination of pregnancy is indicated in feedlot heifers, after incidental breeding (mismating), and in cases of abnormal pregnancy (hydrops of fetal membranes, fetal mummification, fetal maceration, and prolonged gestation). The corpus luteum is the main source of progesterone during the first 150 days of gestation in the cow. The placenta produces enough progesterone to support gestation until 250 days, at which time the corpus luteum is again the main source of this hormone.

Termination of Normal Pregnancy

Pregnancy can be terminated by physical or by hormonal methods (Table 1).

Physical

Intrauterine infusion of 50 to 100 mL of 1% to 2% Lugols' solution, chlorine or potassium permanganate solutions, or other antiseptic solutions will induce abortion if performed between 7 and 60 days of pregnancy.[2] If done later than 60 days, metritis and fetal maceration are common sequelae. The amniotic vesicle can be ruptured manually per rectum between 35 and 66 days of gestation, and the fetus can be decapitated between 66 and 120 days of gestation. Any of these will cause abortion 21 to 27 days later. Decapitation can result in fetal mummification.[1] Manual removal of the corpus luteum per rec-

Table 1
METHODS OF ELECTIVE PREGNANCY TERMINATION IN THE COW

Physical		Hormonal		
Action	*Days*	*Drug*	*Dose**	*Days*
Douching	7–60	Estradiol cypionate	4–8 mg IM	1–2
Enucleation of the corpus luteum	7–150	Oxytocin	100–200 IU IM	2–7
		Prostaglandin F_2	25 mg IM	7–90
Rupture of amnionic vesicles	35–66	Prostaglandin F_2 + dexamethasone	25 mg IM	90–180
		Dexamethasone	25 mg IM	
			25 mg IM	180–250
Decapitation of the fetus	66–120	Prostaglandin F_2	25 mg IM	>250

IM, intramuscularly.
*According to the manufacturer's suggestion and previously reported dosages.

tum will result in abortion 3 to 5 days later.[3] This method, however, is not recommended because of the risk of hemorrhage, which may be fatal, and subsequent formation of adhesions of the ovary and adnexa.

Hormonal

Estrogens given intramuscularly (IM) 24 to 48 hours after service will interfere with migration of the embryo within the uterine tube. Intramuscular injection of 100 to 200 IU of oxytocin between days 2 and 7 of the estrous cycle will interfere with formation of the corpus luteum and disrupt pregnancy. A luteolytic dose (25 mg IM) of prostaglandin F_2 (PGF$_2$) or its analogues (cloprostenol, 500 μg, and fenprostalene, 1 mg) will terminate pregnancy if administered between 6 and 90 days of gestation, and expulsion of the fetus usually occurs 5 to 10 days later. Prostaglandins alone will terminate pregnancies in most cows if administered between 90 and 150 days of pregnancy; however, after 150 days of gestation, dexamethasone should be given in conjunction with prostaglandins to achieve abortion between 2 and 10 days after treatment. After 180 days of gestation, a single dose of dexamethasone will terminate pregnancy in most animals. The corpus luteum is the mandatory source of progesterone after 250 days of gestation, and prostaglandins alone will cause abortion at that time. Undesirable side effects of causing abortion in cows after 120 days are retained fetal membranes and fetal mummification.[1]

Termination of Abnormal Pregnancy

Hydroallantois is characterized by the rapid accumulation of a large volume (up to 150 L) of watery fluid in late gestation because of abnormal function of the placentomes. Hydroamnios, in contrast, is characterized by a gradual increase of fluid in the amnion (up to 80 L) in mid-gestation, usually as a result of a fetal anomaly. A combination of prostaglandin and dexamethasone can be used to induce abortion, which occurs within 48 hours of the treatment. Single or repeated IM injections of 20 to 40 mg of dexamethasone or 10 to 20 mg of flumethasone are also effective. The prognosis for future pregnancy is poor in cows with hydroallantois and fair to good in those with hydroamnios.

Fetal mummification occurs from 90 to 240 days of gestation, whereas maceration may occur at any stage of pregnancy. Mummification is a result of resorption of fluid from the dead fetus in a sterile environment, and maceration results from bacterial infection of the dead fetus. In both conditions the corpus luteum fails to regress. Therefore, prostaglandin is effective in resolving

this condition. The administration of a single dose of PGF$_2$ causes expulsion of the fetus within 2 to 4 days, and a second treatment may be indicated. Diethylstilbestrol (40 to 80 mg) or estradiol cypionate (5 to 10 mg IM) can cause abortion of the mummified fetus within 24 to 72 hours. Because fetal maceration is characterized by permanent damage to the endometrium, slaughter is the recommended treatment for this condition.

EWE

The corpus luteum is the primary source of progesterone during the first 50 days of pregnancy in the ewe. A luteolytic dose of PGF$_2$ (5 to 10 mg IM) will terminate pregnancy in the ewe when given between days 5 and 50. Abortion occurs between 3 and 5 days after treatment. Dexamethasone (10 mg) has no effect on early pregnancy but is lethal to the fetus after 85 days of gestation.[2] Epostane, an inhibitor of the enzyme that converts pregnenolone to progesterone, can induce abortion and parturition when administered between 137 and 156 days of gestation.[3]

DOE

The corpus luteum is the major source of progesterone throughout pregnancy in the doe. The administration of prostaglandins, corticosteroids, and estrogens can successfully terminate pregnancy in the doe. Prostaglandins are frequently used as the first choice because they terminate pregnancy anytime after day 5 of pregnancy. Large variation in the dose of PGF$_2$ (2.5 to 20 mg) for pregnancy termination has been reported. The recommended doses of the prostaglandin analogues cloprostenol and fenprostalene are 150 to 500 μg IM, respectively. Corticosteroids can be used successfully around 141 days of gestation. The administration of 20 to 25 mg dexamethasone IM causes abortion 44 to 48 hours after treatment. Estradiol-17β (16 mg IM) causes premature delivery in the doe similar to corticosteroids. Estradiol benzoate (25 mg) is an effective abortifacient, but subsequent fertility may be affected.[4]

SOW

Accidental or undesirable matings, pseudopregnancy, and fetal mummification are some situations that require abortion in the sow. Prostaglandin F_2 (10 mg) or its analogue cloprostenol (500 μg) will cause abortion in most sows within 24 to 48 hours after treatment. Occasionally a second dose of PGF$_2$ is necessary (10 mg, 12 hours apart).[5]

Induction of parturition is an important procedure in swine reproduction and can be used in sows that are pregnant for at least 110 days. Prostaglandin F_2, as well as its analogue cloprostenol, induced abortion in 65% of all sows between 20 and 36 hours.[5] An effective synchrony of parturition can be achieved by the use of PGF_2 followed in 20 to 24 hours by 5 to 30 IU of oxytocin. Parturition occurs within 6 hours. Carazolol (3 mg IM), a β-adrenergic blocking agent, given 20 hours after prostaglandins initiates parturition within 1.2 to 2.6 hours.[6] Exogenous glucocorticoids such as dexamethasone can effectively induce parturition in the sow, but because large doses (75 to 100 mg) need to be used over a period of 4 days, their use is very limited.

Experimentation with RU 486, a competitive inhibitor of the progesterone receptor, has shown promising results when used in food animal production. It has been tested in the cow, ewe, and sow. Parturition occurred 55 hours after treatment (2 mg/kg of body weight IM) of beef cows, after 31 hours in ewes (4 mg/kg of body weight IM), and after 48 hours in sows (4 mg/kg of body weight IM). The use of RU 486 alone or in combination with relaxin did not cause retention of fetal membranes, and there were no detrimental effects on subsequent reproductive performance. At present, the use of RU 486 is not allowed in this country.

REFERENCES

1. Morrow DA (ed): Current Therapy in Theriogenology, ed 2. Philadelphia, WB Saunders, 1987.
2. Roberts SJ: Veterinary Obstetrics and Genital Diseases, ed 3. Ann Arbor, Mich, Edwards Brothers, 1986.
3. Silver M, Fowden AL: Induction of labour in sheep by inhibition of 3-hydroxysteroid dehydrogenase: Role of the fetal adrenal. J Dev Physiol 15:169, 1991.
4. Smith MC, Sherman DM: Goat Medicine. Philadelphia, Lea & Febiger, 1994, pp 430–431.
5. Pressing AL: Pharmacological control of swine reproduction. Vet Clin North Am 8:707, 1992.
6. Holtz W, Schmidt-Baulain R, Meyer H, Welp C: Control of prostaglandin-induced parturition in sows by injection of the beta-adrenergic blocking agent carazolol or carazolol and oxytocin. J Anim Sci 68:3967, 1990.

■ Diseases of the Testes and Epididymis

Dwight F. Wolfe, D.V.M., M.S.

Developmental abnormalities of the testicles include hypoplasia when one or both testicles are small (<30 cm scrotal circumference in postpubertal bulls) and more obscure defects when a variable portion of one testicle is involved.[1] The condition is probably heritable in the food animal species and should be differentiated if possible from testicular atrophy, usually by history or by long-term observation. In contrast to testicular hypoplasia, testicular atrophy results in the loss of testicular mass over time. Moderate hypoplasia involves subfertility but does not equate with sterility. Thus the condition may be insidious in its effect on breeding performance and male offspring. Affected males will usually cause conception, although bulls with mild to moderate testicular hypoplasia will not function efficiently in a controlled breeding season and calving may be spread over several months. There is no treatment.

Among fertile males and breeds of the various species, there is wide variation in testicular size as related to scrotal circumference, sperm output, age, and body weight. Scrotal circumference measurement affords practical evaluation of testicular size and

has been standardized for bulls by the Society for Theriogenology.[2]

Blind or aberrant efferent ductules cause sperm stasis and extravasation and subsequently sperm granulomas. In time, even after a period of service, granulomas in the epididymal head produce occlusion of the epididymal duct, retrograde pressure on the seminiferous epithelium, and testicular degeneration. The condition appears to be heritable in polled goats. If the head of the epididymis is enlarged and firm, it is usually because of sperm granulomas.[3]

Aplasia of any portion of the epididymis blocks sperm transit, but blockage in the body or tail does not affect testicular function. Thus the testicle may appear normal. Bilateral granulomatous occlusion or epididymal aplasia constitutes irreversible sterility.

TESTICULAR DEGENERATION

Varied insults such as hormonal imbalance, hydrocele, infection, and ambient or local thermal interference with the testicular thermoregulatory system cause the most commonly diagnosed disease of testicles, testicular degeneration.[3] Cryptorchid and ectopic testicles are degenerate. Males experiencing insulation of the scrotum, e.g., scrotal dermatitis, periorchitis, or prolonged recumbency from lameness, rapidly sustain testicular degeneration. The condition may appear after a short febrile episode or during prolonged hot and humid weather. Scrotal frostbite affects many males. Boars may acquire testicular degeneration from prolonged exposure to cold floors or, infrequently, from torsion of a testicle.

At least a portion of the progressive degeneration that attends aging is probably due to multiple insults over time. A larger proportion of old bulls with testicular degeneration have distal fibrosis of the testicle, which is indicative of vascular lesions.

If not reversed, degeneration may progress to spermiostasis, inspissation of sperm, granulomas, fibrosis, and calcification.

Diagnosis

Degeneration often appears as a loss of the normal turgidity and elasticity as the testicle is palpated superficially and gently. The epididymis may feel disproportionately large, and there may be an unusually large gap between the epididymal tail and the testicle.[4] A tonometer has been devised to provide more objective evaluation, but it is not widely used. In chronic cases, deeper (firmer) palpation reveals fibrosis, degeneration is advanced, and the prognosis is worsened. Many of the previously listed local causes are self-evident, but the causes of degeneration often escape detection.

Serial semen evaluations through the course of unchecked degeneration show nonspecific progression from a minor increase in sperm abnormalities to oligospermia, an increase in major head and midpiece abnormalities, and the appearance of primitive germinal cells. In degeneration without obvious cause and with a vague history, evaluation of but a few ejaculates often fails to assist in differentiating the condition from moderate hypoplasia.

Ultrasonography may be useful in diagnosing testicular degeneration.[5, 6]

Thermography uses infrared radiation to measure body surface temperature and is a sensitive indicator of altered testicular thermoregulation and subsequent testicular degeneration.[7] Radiography provides a valuable aid to palpation findings of fibrotic areas or masses and is especially useful in indicating the degree and pattern (isolated or diffuse) of calcification. Diagnostic radiography is not deleterious to spermatogenesis.

Treatment

There is no specific treatment for testicular degeneration. The use of exogenous hormones should be avoided, and known causes should be removed. Young sires with moderate degeneration often recover 60 to 90 days after removal of the insult.

ORCHITIS AND PERIORCHITIS

Treatment and occasional neoplasia aside, the most common cause of inflammation of the testicle and surrounding tunica vaginalis is a myriad of infectious agents, including *Brucella abortus*, *Corynebacterium pyogenes*, *Escherichia coli*, *Pseudomonas*, *Proteus mirabilis*, *Actinobacillus seminis*, *Actinomyces bovis*, *Nocardia farcinica*, *Haemophilus*, and *Salmonella*. Bovine herpesvirus and cytopathogenic enterovirus cause orchitis in bulls. Chlamydial and mycoplasmal agents have also been reported.[1]

Infections are usually hematogenous but may invade punctures and lacerations. Regardless of the mode of entry, the condition is usually unilateral. Acute inflammation of the testicle or tunica causes swelling and pain and may be associated with a stilted gait. Severe enlargement is usually due to fluid and fibrin accumulation within the cavity of the tunic, and suppurative organisms may cause abscesses. Chronic inflammation results in degeneration and its sequelae. Unilateral inflammation may reduce or destroy spermatogenesis in the contralateral testicle.

Diagnosis

If the testicle can be palpated, orchitis may be evident. A firm distended tunic cavity that prevents palpation of the testicle is evidence of periorchitis. An aid to diagnosis is radiography, as described for testicular degeneration. Thermography and thermovision, which detect variations from the normal concentric color bands transformed from infrared surface emissions, are particularly useful in detecting mild inflammation.[7] Also, ultrasound units, such as those commonly used to aid in the rectal diagnosis of pregnancy in mares, provide an excellent means of noninvasive examination of the scrotal contents.[5]

Identifying microbial causes by culture of semen is hampered by contamination during collection but may be helpful. Testicular biopsy for culturing is usually regarded as a last resort.

Treatment

Gentle cold water sprays for 30 minutes twice daily help reduce the damaging inflammatory heat. Although systemic antibiotics may traverse the normally impervious blood-testis barrier, reduced tissue perfusion makes penetration unlikely and probably ineffective.

Early in the course of unilateral inflammation of a testicle, concern should be directed toward the unaffected testicle. Although summary removal of a mildly inflamed testicle and adnexa might constitute overtreatment, careful aseptic hemicastration is indicated when the prognosis for the affected side is poor. Minimal additional inflammatory insult is caused by the surgery. A healthy or completely restorable remaining testicle can be expected to compensate for 60% to 80% of the original sperm output of two testicles.

EPIDIDYMITIS

The tail of the epididymis is vulnerable to infection, especially in rams but also in bulls and bucks. It is less common in boars.

Unilateral caudal epididymitis without testicular involvement is common in bulls. The opportunistic microorganisms of orchitis may be involved, and concomitant infections of the pelvic genitalia are common.

In adult rams, a specific severe epididymitis caused by *Brucella ovis* causes significant loss of flock reproductive efficiency. The organism may exist in the epididymis without palpable enlargement, or there may be extreme swelling and fibrosis even with draining sinus tracts through the scrotum. The testicles may be involved. Transmission is by the genital, oral, and respiratory routes and is enhanced by the animal's sampling of urine of other rams. The condition is often bilateral and causes sterility.[8, 9]

A separate epididymitis affecting ram lambs is attributed to a group of *lamb epididymitis organisms*, mostly Brucellaceae but not including *B. ovis*. The epididymis appears to acquire particular vulnerability in the peripubertal hormonal environment. Both ascending and oral infections from sodomy and filthy environments are suspected. Infertility is the result.

Diagnosis

Palpation of swollen, painful, indurated epididymal tails is the best method of diagnosis. In endemic flocks, palpation several times a year helps identify new cases. Acute inflammation in bulls causes resistance to even gentle palpation.

B. ovis epididymitis in rams usually produces numerous leukocytes in the ejaculate, and the organism is relatively easily cultured from semen. Large numbers of leukocytes accompany detached sperm heads and low motility. Leukocytes in semen are not uniformly characteristic of lamb epididymitis.

Control

No good, widely documented treatment is available for infectious epididymitis. Many bulls appear to recover spontaneously, but unilateral castration is considered in severe cases.

Ram epididymitis requires palpation of the epididymides, separation of clinically affected rams, and culling. Vaccination is of marginal value—it may reduce palpable lesions but usually not the inflammation and leukocyte content of semen. Lamb epididymitis appears to be controlled at times by feeding of tetracycline. No vaccine is available.

REFERENCES

1. McEntee K: Pathology of the testis and epididymis of the bull and stallion. *In* Proceedings of the Society for Theriogenology, Mobile, Ala, 1979, p 80.
2. Chenoweth PJ, Spitzer JC, Hopkins FM: A new breeding soundness evaluation form. *In* Proceedings of the Society for Theriogenology, San Antonio, 1992, pp 63–70.
3. Roberts SJ: Infertility in male animals. *In* Roberts SJ: Veterinary Obstetrics and Genital Disease, ed 3. Woodstock, Vt, Stephen J Roberts, 1986, pp 826–838.
4. Blanchard TL, Varner DD, Bretzlaff KN, et al: The causes and pathologic changes of testicular degeneration in large animals. Vet Med 86:531, 1991.
5. Pechman R, Eilts B: B-mode ultrasonography of the bull testicle. Theriogenology 27:431, 1987.
6. Ahmad N, Noakes DE: Ultrasound imaging in determining the presence of testicular degeneration in two male goats. Br Vet J 151:101, 1995.
7. Purohit R, Hudson R: Thermography of the bovine scrotum. Am J Vet Res 46:2388, 1985.
8. Bulgin MS, Anderson BC, Kirk JH: Ram epididymitis. *In* Proceedings of the Society for Theriogenology, Spokane, Wash, 1981, p 173.

9. Memon MA: Male infertility. Symposium on sheep and goat medicine. Vet Clin North Am 5:619, 1983.

■ Diseases of the Penis and Prepuce

R.L. Carson, D.V.M., M.S., Diplomate, A.C.T.

The frequency and wide variety of significant lesions of the penis and prepuce of food animals dictate careful examination by the veterinarian. This may be done by close observation of the animal during coitus, while serving an artificial vagina, or during stimulation with an electroejaculator. Alternatively, the penis may be extended manually, which may be the preferred method when a lesion is suspected because the aforementioned methods often worsen a preexisting condition. Manual extension is easily done in a standing restrained ram or buck; bulls may require that an assistant place a hand in the rectum to help relax the retractor penis muscles. Once the technique of manual extension is mastered, there is little or no need for tranquilizers, which carry the risk of postexamination penile injury. Boars usually resist manual manipulation and require sedation or anesthesia.

BULL

Balanoposthitis primarily affects young bulls and may be due to infectious bovine rhinotracheitis or to nonspecific abrasions sustained during excessive service. The associated pain may cause bulls to refuse to serve, and the edema and swelling may lead to more serious conditions such as preputial prolapse and laceration. Healing of balanoposthitis is usually spontaneous, and service may be resumed in 2 weeks. This form of infectious bovine rhinotracheitis is venereally transmitted, and affected bulls may shed virus in their semen. Intranasal vaccination may offer some degree of protection from this disorder.

Viral papillomas (warts) are frequently found on the penis but not on the prepuce of young bulls. This condition is more commonly seen in group-housed young bulls that mount each other and obtain penile abrasions. Abrasions admit the virus, and warts grow rapidly and may surround the tip of the penis. Surgical removal is the preferred treatment, the primary concern being preservation of the urethra and the glans penis. Ligating and suturing are preferable but may be difficult because of the broad bases and short stalks of certain papillomas. Thermocautery is a viable option but should be used with caution because excessive heat may cause deep and serious necrosis. Vaccine, even if available, is of marginal value.

Young bulls commonly have a matted ring of hair surrounding the free portion of the penis. The hair comes from the body coat hair of other bulls that have been mounted. The ring should be removed to avoid a deep annular laceration that might create a urethral fistula, a cavernosal fistula, or penile amputation.

Persistent frenulum, a congenital bandlike attachment of the prepuce to the tip of the penis along the median raphe, is usually found in virgin bulls. The frenulum, not to be confused with a persistent prepubertal preputial adhesion, may cause ventral deviation of the erect penis. The impotence thus induced in *Bos taurus* breeds may not affect *Bos indices* breeds that have excessive prepuce. Strong evidence for heritability dictates culling affected bulls from purebred herds. Otherwise, the frenulum is easily ligated at each end and excised.

Persistent preputial adhesions are seen as attachments between the penis and prepuce. These adhesions are frequently seen in yearling bulls and are believed to be due to failure of separation of the prepuce and penile attachments at puberty. The exact cause and possible heritability are unknown. Treatment is simple: manual separation by pulling the prepuce back from the penis.

Deep lacerations of the dorsum of the penis may interrupt the sensory nerve supply, which is essential for intromission and ejaculation. Scars from lacerations should alert the examiner to possible impotence. Sensation may be tested by stimulation of the glans and dorsum of the penis with an electric prod while holding the retractor penis muscles. A positive response is a surprisingly mild contraction of the muscles. A better test is actual mating.

Deep lacerations of the glans and free portion may result in fistulas into the corpus cavernosum, which could cause erection failure or bleeding during erection, the blood being toxic to sperm. Immediate suturing after injury is indicated. Careful longitudinal wedge resection of the fistulas, separate closure of the tunica albuginea and skin, and 3 weeks of rest from sexual activity are usually successful. Fistulas of the glans are especially resistant to closure and require longitudinal resection, curettage of the cavity of the fistula, and deep suturing.

Lacerations or fistulas of the urethra, if more than 5 cm from the terminus, may reduce effective deposition of the ejaculate. Healing of sutured defects is categorically difficult because of the naturally vigorous wavelike movement of urination. A drastic but effective solution is concomitant ischial urethrotomy with an indwelling catheter. After healing of the distal urethra, the ischial urethra is allowed to heal spontaneously.

Spiral and ventral deviations of the penis prevent intromission and are observed during mating. Deviations usually appear in 3- to 4-year-old bulls after a period of satisfactory service. Both types are thought to be defects of the penile apical ligament. Spiral deviations may be repaired by surgically implanting a 2 × 12- to 2 × 15-cm homologous graft of fascia lata between the tunica albuginea and apical ligament through a midline incision on the dorsum of the penis. Repair of ventral deviations may be attempted with the same procedure, but with reduced success.

Rupture of the corpus cavernosum penis (hematoma) is a common and serious breeding accident. It is often caused by innately vigorous sexual behavior and is characterized by circumscribed symmetric swelling surrounding the penis just cranial to the neck of the scrotum. The prepuce is usually dark purple from extravasated blood and will often be prolapsed. The injury will heal spontaneously in many cases when accompanied by systemic antibiotics and 60 days of sexual rest. However, surgical closure of the rent in the tunica albuginea provides less risk of recurrence and reduces the risk of erection failure from corpus cavernosal shunts.

Surgery performed 1 to 2 days after injury allows easier repair. With the bull under general anesthesia or deep sedation in right lateral recumbency with aseptic conditions, an incision in the cranioventral skin is made over the lateral aspect of the bulge of the hematoma. Subcutaneous tissue incision exposes the blood clot, which is removed. The affected portion of the penis is exposed and pulled through the incision in the skin. Multiple layers of peripenile elastic tissue are incised longitudinally and laterally to the penis to expose the tunica albuginea. The usually transverse rent will be found predictably at the dorsal aspect of the distal bend of the sigmoid flexure. Distraction of the torn edges may be 2 cm. The frayed edges are excised and sutured in a boot lace pattern with no. 1 polyglycolic acid suture. The multiple elastic layers are closed with a single simple continuous suture of 3-0 gut. Loose clots in the cavity are rinsed free with sterile saline at 37°C. The wall of the hematoma is sutured with 1-0 gut without closing space, and then the skin incision is closed. Maximal healing requires 60 days of rest from sexual activity.

Because of the violence of the injury and frequent sequelae, the prognosis for rupture of the tunica albuginea is guarded, whether conservatively or surgically managed. Sequelae are peripenile adhesions, hematogenous abscesses, disruption of the sensory nerve supply, and vascular shunts at the rupture site. These shunts, which cause erection failure, may be repaired by the technique for fresh ruptures.

Failure of erection may arise from posthematomal shunts or congenital and uncorrectable multiple shunts in the free portion of the penis. Both types of shunts may be confirmed by serial contrast radiography of the corpus cavernosum. Obstructive cavernositis, intracorporeal thrombosis, and dystrophic calcification are conditions that also cause erection failure. All are difficult to diagnose during life and are irreparable.

Preputial injuries, which are usually sustained in service, appear most frequently in *B. indices* breeds and their crossbreeds, particularly in bulls with excessively pendulous sheaths, long prepuces, and wide preputial orifices. The initial injury is one of contusion and/or laceration. Mild injuries may require little more than 2 weeks of rest but may become major wounds in animals left in service, thus extending breeding time loss as much as 2 months or more with possible complete loss of breeding use. The typical progression of the condition is traumatic edema, preputial prolapse, increased edema, attempted coitus, and laceration (splitting), usually on the ventrum of the prepuce.

Care of prolapse with or without laceration involves cleansing, application of a lanolin-based protectant ointment, and bandaging with a stockinet and adhesive elastic tape. Latex rubber tubing inserted into the preputial lumen and incorporated into the bandage provides urine drainage. The bandage protects the injury, reduces edema, and should be changed every 3 days or as needed. When reduction of edema allows reversion of the prepuce, bandaging without a stockinet continues until the prepuce remains in place spontaneously. Another method of treatment is to make a sling around the bull's abdomen to hold the unbandaged prepuce up to reduce edema and avoid trauma. Cleansing and ointment application would be necessary as with bandaging.

If the prepuce is too long for containment or if a granulating deep laceration prevents the return to normal function, circumcision is indicated. One technique involves (1) full extension of the penis and prepuce, which may require cutting across stenotic areas of prepuce; (2) application of a latex rubber tourniquet at the preputial orifice; (3) resection of sufficient prepuce between the proximal and distal annular incisions to reduce excessive length; (4) removal of fibrotic tissue while still allowing full penile extension; (5) ligation of all severed vessels; (6) removal of the tourniquet and completion of hemostasis; and (7) suturing of superficial elastic tissue and the skin with simple, interrupted stitches using 1-0 gut. A bandage similar to that described for simple prolapse is applied. The bandage should be removed in 3 days and the stitches removed in 10 days. Bulls can usually return to service in 60 days.

Retropreputial abscesses result from deep preputial lacerations and immediate, complete retraction of the prepuce. The condition is common in *B. taurus* breeds. Without prolapse, the injury may not be discovered until function is severely compromised by the formation of peripenile adhesions. Abscesses should be drained through the original laceration in the prepuce and never through the skin of the sheath. The prognosis is poor, but spontaneous recovery occurs in 60 to 90 days in a small proportion of affected bulls. Surgical excision of peripenile adhesions has been unrewarding.

Bulls regularly serving an artificial vagina occasionally sustain an avulsion of the prepuce from its attachment to the free portion of the penis. The prepuce is severely distracted, and contrary to the usual contraindication for suturing fresh but contaminated preputial wounds in range bulls, these avulsions should be repaired immediately.

BOAR

Penile congenital defects in the boar include a persistent frenulum, which may be managed surgically as in the bull. Erection failure may be caused by heritable micropenis and cavernosal venous shunts, which are irreparable. Cavernosal shunts following bite wounds are occasionally seen and cause erection failure.

Failure of penile extension may also be caused by infrequent or habitual "balling," in which the penis is inserted in the preputial diverticulum. Young boars may be corrected by forced dismounting when the action is noted. Repeated mounting often results in correct extension. If the practice persists, culling should be considered because there is some evidence of heritability. Surgical extirpation of the diverticulum is discouraged.

Lacerations of the distal portion of the penis are common in boars and are usually caused by bites from females or other boars during breeding activity. Lacerations heal with 2 weeks of rest from sexual activity and no treatment. Severe wounds may require daily application of topical antibiotic ointments or, rarely, surgical closure. Occasionally a cavernosal or urethral fistula may follow severe lacerations. Preputial injuries are rare in boars.

RAM AND BUCK

Penile and preputial injuries are quite rare in rams and bucks and can usually be managed similarly to those in bulls. Occasionally the urethral process may be grossly traumatized or blocked with urinary calculi. Amputation of the process is simple and appears to have no suppressant effect on fertility.

Posthitis (pizzle rot) is a chronic necrotizing disease of the preputial orifice. Considered to be caused by the interaction of *Corynebacterium renale* infection and the high (4%) urinary urea content of a high-protein diet and reduced water intake, the condition is a serious cause of impotence. Early in the course of the disease the orifice is ulcerated and exudes thick purulent debris. The condition may progress to fill the entire preputial cavity with exudate and necrotic tissue and occlude the prepuce. Early-stage disease may respond to thorough cleansing and regular application of penile ointment. Systemic treatment is ineffective.

BIBLIOGRAPHY

Carson RL, Hudson RS: Diseases of the penis and prepuce. *In* Howard JL (ed): Current Veterinary Therapy: Food Animal Practice, ed 3. Philadelphia, WB Saunders, 1993.
Hudson RS: Diagnosis of disturbances of mating ability in bulls. Auburn Vet 37:81–84, 1981.

■ Diseases of the Male Internal Genitalia

R.L. Carson, D.V.M., M.S., Diplomate, A.C.T.

Disease of any of the internal genitalia of male food animals is rare. The one exception is disease of the vesicular glands of the bull. The incidence of vesiculitis varies from a sporadic 2% to 5% in adult bulls to 5% to 50% in groups of young bulls, which suggests contagion. Most acute cases occur in bulls either younger than 2 years or older than 9 years; however, evidence of inactive infection can be found in many middle-aged bulls. In addition to the direct effect of vesiculitis on reproduction, it is frequently the most obvious manifestation of a serious and complex disease syndrome, including elusive infections in other pelvic genitalia and concomitant or sequential epididymitis, orchitis, and periorchitis.

In bulls, the relative ease of examination of the vesicular glands and the more obvious response to insult may account for vesiculitis being reported more often than infections of other accessory genitalia. Although ampullitis, prostatitis, and bulbourethral adenitis appear frequently with vesiculitis at necropsy, ampullitis is less readily diagnosed clinically and prostatitis is almost never diagnosed. Greater size and firmness of the ampullae may escape detection, and the dense capsule of the bull prostate precludes enlargement. The bulbourethral glands are not palpable.

ETIOLOGY AND PATHOGENESIS

Numerous microorganisms have been associated with vesiculitis, including *Brucella abortus, Actinomyces pyogenes, Escherichia coli, Pseudomonas, Proteus mirabilis, Actinobacillus seminis, Actinomyces bovis, Nocardia farcinica, Haemophilus, Salmonella, Chlamydia,* and certain viruses. The infectious agent often eludes identification. In some cases, especially in outbreaks among young bulls, infectious bovine rhinotracheitis or enteroviruses appear to initiate the insult and predispose the animal to opportunistic bacterial infections. It appears that some bulls have a predilection for vesiculitis because of a congenital malformation of the duct system of the vesicular gland. *Chlamydia psittaci* has been reported to cause seminal vesiculitis in the buck. The predilection of *Brucella* for genital tissue includes the vesicular glands of all the food animal species. The presence of *Brucella suis* in the seminal vesicles of boars without microscopic lesions causes concern in seminal transmission.

The pathogenesis of vesiculitis is not clear. Outbreaks in groups of young bulls may be related to normal homosexual activity with ascending infection or oral and nasal entry of organisms and hematogenous spread. Likewise, extragenital foci of infection, especially in the lungs, appear to be a source of blood-borne infection. Ascending infection in the rare cases of generalized urinary tract disease must be considered. Often there is a concurrent vesiculitis and epididymitis and occasionally orchitis, but it is difficult to determine which came first. In practice, the veterinarian may not be able to determine the origin or route of infection.

Studies point to increased susceptibility of the seminal vesicles associated with discrete unpalpable congenital abnormalities, but bulls with satisfactory service records and no evidence of vesiculitis may have palpable unilateral hypoplastic or aplastic seminal vesicles or ampullae.

DIAGNOSIS

Overt clinical signs rarely arise. Acute vesiculitis may cause signs of localized peritonitis, tenesmus, and obscure rear limb lameness. The condition is usually discovered on routine rectal palpation or after purulent exudate is found in the semen. Acutely affected vesicular glands are initially swollen, possibly painful, and often devoid of the normal lobulation. Advanced disease may cause abscess formation and fibrosis. In cases of inactive vesiculitis, the glands will be fibrotic and lack normal lobulation. Caution is required in that there is normal variation in the size of the vesicles within and among bulls. Also, some diseased organs elude even careful palpation. Old bulls typically have firmer vesicular glands than young bulls.

Culture of fluid massaged from the vesicular glands and collected through a hygienically inserted sterile urethral catheter is preferable to culture of semen, which always contains contaminants. Even so, the vesicular fluid may be adulterated with the products of other organs.

PATHOGENESIS

Acute vesiculitis may regress spontaneously or may progress to a chronic state of bacterial infection. Abscess formation and fibrosis may form adhesions extending to other organs or form tracts extending to the inguinal rings. Cases of long duration usually involve other foci of genital infection.

The effect of solitary vesiculitis on reproduction is difficult to assess. Greater viscosity of vesicular fluid may reduce the gross motility of sperm. Reports of more sperm abnormalities probably reflect concurrent disease in the testes or epididymides. Survival of frozen-thawed semen is reduced.

Concern for transmission of disease through coitus or artificial insemination is logical, but the extent of the risk is unknown. Many bulls with vesiculitis have been used without detectable suppression of herd fertility. In short, bulls with vesiculitis are classified as unsound but may not be infertile. The threat of infection to other genitalia, especially to the testes and epididymides, outweighs the threat of vesiculitis alone.

TREATMENT AND CONTROL

Spontaneous recovery in many young bulls does not permit a good evaluation of treatment. Most young bulls with acute vesiculitis respond favorably to broad-spectrum antibiotic therapy if adequate dosage and duration of treatment are provided. However, many bulls with well-established bacterial infections resist antibiotic therapy. The cases that are nonresponsive to routine treatment may suggest congenital malformation of the duct system. Confirmed and suspected chlamydial infections seem to respond to daily intravenous oxytetracycline, 5 mg/lb for 10 days. Regression of swelling is often dramatic. Surgical removal of the vesicular gland through the ischiorectal fossa is often disappointing. Easily replaceable bulls of marginal quality should be culled. It may be that the recommendation to cull all bulls with the disease based on a possible predisposition from congenital abnormalities merits consideration. The idea, however, is unlikely to gain popularity among producers working in free enterprise systems.

Vaccination against infectious bovine rhinotracheitis prior to close group housing of young bulls and other management practices that help control infectious diseases of other bodily systems are believed to help reduce the prevalence of vesiculitis.

BIBLIOGRAPHY

Arthur GH, Noakes DE, Pearson H: Veterinary Reproduction and Obstetrics. London, Baillière Tindall, 1982.
Carson RL, Hudson RS: Diseases of the male internal genitalia. *In* Howard JL (ed): Current Veterinary Therapy: Food Animal Practice, ed 3. Philadelphia, WB Saunders, 1993.
McCaulay AD: Seminal vesiculitis in bulls. *In* Morrow DA (ed): Current Therapy in Theriogenology. Philadelphia, WB Saunders, 1980.

■ Dairy Herd Reproductive Efficiency

Carlos A. Risco, D.V.M., Diplomate, A.C.T.
Louis F. Archbald, D.V.M., M.S., Ph.D., M.R.C.V.S.

Dairy herd reproductive efficiency is commonly defined in terms of the herd's calving interval. The calving interval influences the time that cows spend in the most profitable period of milk production, which is the first 120 days in milk. In addition, the calving interval affects the pounds of milk produced per day per herd lifetime and the number of cows culled for reproductive failure. Consequently, farm income is affected by the calving-to-conception interval.

FACTORS AFFECTING THE CALVING INTERVAL

The calving interval is determined by the elective voluntary waiting period, the estrus detection rate, the conception rate, and pregnancy maintenance to term.[1] Cows become pregnant from the elective voluntary waiting period as a function of the estrus detection rate and the conception rate. The pregnancy rate is the product of the estrus detection rate and the conception rate and represents the proportion of cows that become pregnant each estrous cycle.[2] The pregnancy rate determines the speed at which cows become pregnant from the elective voluntary waiting period.[2] The interrelationship between the pregnancy rate and the interval from calving to conception is shown in Figure 1. As the pregnancy rate increases from a higher estrus detection rate, a higher conception rate, or both, the interval from calving to conception decreases. Ferguson and Galligan[2] have shown that the pregnancy rate after the first insemination explained 79% of the variation in calving intervals. These authors concluded that maximizing the estrus detection rate and the conception rate for the first insemination is the most important factor influencing the calving interval. It is therefore suggested that dairy herd managers allocate major resources and effort to improving the estrus detection rate and the conception rate to obtain the greatest return from their reproductive program.

The estrus detection rate of a dairy herd should be evaluated in terms of efficiency and accuracy. The efficiency of detection of estrus is defined as the percentage of eligible cows that are actually seen or detected in estrus.[3] The accuracy of estrus detection is defined as the percentage of estruses observed that are physiologic estrus.[3]

Efficiency of Estrus Detection

An estrus detection rate of 70% should be the goal of every dairy manager if reproductive efficiency is to be achieved. The time and quality of time spent in estrus detection are of critical importance. Early morning and late evening (when combined) are the two periods in a 24-hour day that yield a high percentage of detected estrus. To help improve estrus detection efficiency, estrus detection aids (androgenized heifers, pressure-sensitive mount detector, and tail head color markings) are commonly used. Research has shown that when these heat detection aids are used in conjunction with visual observation, efficiency of estrus detection improves.[4] Electronic mount detectors that record legitimate mounts for individual cows have been developed and evaluated.[5] The manager can access the information electronically to determine which cows were mounted at a particular time.

The interval from calving to first ovulation averages about 3 weeks (usually accompanied by undetectable estrus), and the first detected estrus is usually about 5 weeks postpartum. It is generally assumed that complaints by dairy managers that cows are not cyclic most likely represent inadequate estrus detection because of human error and not true anestrus. However, care should be taken with this assumption during the hot summer months because cows may not readily exhibit signs of estrus and, when they do, the duration of estrus is shorter.[6] In addition, severe negative energy balance during the postpartum period and factors that affect cow comfort should also be evaluated. Rectal palpation of the ovaries for the presence of a corpus luteum, determination of milk or plasma progesterone, or both can be used to determine whether cows are actually cyclic and are being missed in estrus. To rule out nutritional causes, periodic assessment of body scores and evaluation of the prepartum and postpartum transition rations should be conducted.

Some factors that can be used to evaluate estrus detection efficiency are listed in Table 1. The 24-day estrus detection rate is an excellent method to use. It can easily be implemented by the dairy manager to determine how efficiently estrous periods are being detected. A list of the cows most likely to exhibit estrus within the next 24 days is obtained. At the end of this period, the number of cows observed in estrus is divided by the total number of cows eligible to cycle. A positive characteristic of this method is that it takes only 24 days to determine the degree of estrus detection efficiency by the dairy manager.

The palpation pregnancy rate (PPR), which is the percentage of cows pregnant at pregnancy examination performed at definite time periods, is also a very good parameter for evaluating estrus detection efficiency.[7] The defined time period is usually 35 to 42, 43 to 50, or more than 50 days from the last insemination. When evaluating the PPR for a particular herd, it is important that the conception rate be considered. It has been

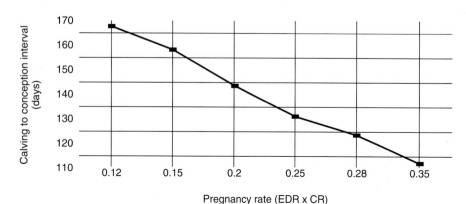

Figure 1

Relationship between calving to conception interval and pregnancy rate. Calculations were based on a voluntary waiting period of 60 days and a range of estrus detection rates (EDR) and conception rates (CR) from .30 to .70 and .40 to .50, respectively. (Adapted from Heersche G, Nebel RL: Measuring efficiency and accuracy of detection of estrus. J Dairy Sci 77:2754, 1994.)

Table 1
PARAMETERS USED TO EVALUATE ESTRUS DETECTION EFFICIENCY

Parameter	Value*
Days in milk to first service	EVWP + 18 days (80% of cows)
24-Day estrus detection rate	80%–85%
Palpation pregnancy rate	80%–85%
Cows detected in estrus by 60 days postpartum (%)	>75%
Cows artificially inseminated by 100 days postpartum (%)	100%

EVWP, elective volunary waiting period.
*The value listed is the desired goal for that parameter.

Table 2
EFFECT OF STANDING TO BE MOUNTED IN COMBINATION WITH OTHER SIGNS OF ESTRUS ON ERROR OF ESTRUS DETECTION BASED ON MILK PROGESTERONE CONCENTRATIONS OF 1 ng/mL OR GREATER

Secondary Sign	Progesterone ≥1 ng/mL Standing Not Recorded	Standing Also Recorded
Rough tail head	7.8*	1.5*
Riding other cows	4.4	1.9
Usually active	7.6	2.1
Mucus on vulva	7.9	2.3
Bawling	6.7	2.5
Fully triggered Kamar device	17.7	3.9
No milk letdown	10.5	5.7
Partly triggered Kamar device	25.8	8.3

*Values are percentages.
From Heersche G, Nebel RL: Measuring efficiency and accuracy of detection of estrus. J Dairy Sci 77:2754, 1994.

demonstrated mathematically that the conception rate influences the PPR.[7] The PPR increases as the conception rate increases. The time period since the last insemination also influences the PPR. If the time frame since the last service is greater than 42 days, the PPR increases because two estrous cycles have occurred since the last service and thus the opportunity to detect an open cow in estrus increases. Therefore, when setting PPR goals to evaluate the herd's estrus detection efficiency, the conception rate and days since last insemination should be considered.[7]

Conception Rate

The conception rate can be directly affected by the following factors: accuracy of estrus detection, competency of the inseminator, fertility of the herd (female), and fertility of the semen sample (bull).

Accuracy of Estrus Detection

As mentioned earlier, the accuracy of estrus detection refers to the percentage of cows exhibiting true physiologic estrus that are detected in estrus.[3] Using natural service, the bull readily detects estrus. However, with artificial insemination the accuracy of estrus detection is vitally important because insemination of cows not in estrus or at the wrong time during estrus results in failure of conception. Research using milk progesterone concentrations to accurately time insemination has shown that many cows (30%) are inseminated when they are not in estrus (Table 2).[3] A major factor affecting estrus detection accuracy is the ability to distinguish primary from secondary signs of estrus. Parameters used to determine estrus detection accuracy are shown in Table 3.

Competency of the Inseminator

The competency of the inseminator is a significanct factor contributing to the conception rate. It has been demonstrated that conception rates can vary as much as 22% among artificial insemination technicians. The technician's major responsibilities are related to proper handling of the semen from the time of removal from the refrigeration tank to correct placement in the uterus of the cow. Other considerations include temperature fluctuations and proper handling of the straw and inseminating gun.

Fertility of the Herd (Female)

A major factor in fertility of the herd is to have as many cyclic cows that are free of reproductive disease when they enter the breeding program as possible. Early resumption of cyclic activity during the first 30 days postpartum has been shown to have a significant and positive effect on fertility.[8] The physiologic and hormonal events associated with estrus restore uterine and ovarian function so that they are conducive to the establishment of pregnancy. A substantial amount of research has demonstrated the relationship of energy balance and resumption of postpartum cyclicity in dairy cattle.[9] In addition, the use of prostaglandin $F_{2\alpha}$ during the elective voluntary waiting period has been shown to improve fertility in dairy cattle, particularly those affected with dystocia, retained fetal membranes, or both at calving.[10]

A major goal of a reproductive herd health program is that cows have the ability to carry their pregnancy to term. To accomplish this, a well-designed vaccination program that maintains the herd's resistance to viral and bacterial challenges causing abortion is of primary importance. The responsibility of the herd veterinarian should be to recommend vaccination protocols and types of vaccine and to ensure proper handling of the products used.

Table 3
PARAMETERS USED TO EVALUATE ESTRUS DETECTION ACCURACY

Parameter	Value* (%)
Interestrus interval (days)	
3–17	<15
18–24	60
25–35	<10
36–48	10
>48	<5
Cows pregnant from previous breeding	<3
High milk progesterone levels at insemination	<10

*The value listed is the desired goal for that parameter.

Fertility of the Semen Sample (Bull)

Two important points should be kept in mind when considering the effect of the semen sample on fertility. First, conception rates after the first insemination can vary as much as 36% among sires that are used for artificial insemination. Second, the quality of the semen sample can rapidly deteriorate after it arrives on the farm because of improper semen storage and handling. Proper care and maintenance of the semen tank should be an integral component of the herd reproductive program.

MONITORING HERD REPRODUCTIVE EFFICIENCY

A number of parameters can be used to monitor the progress that a dairy herd is making toward maximizing reproductive efficiency (Table 4). Of these parameters, days open, days in milk, calving interval, and herd reproductive status index are the more common and traditional ones used to assess reproductive performance by most dairy herd record processing centers. The calving interval and days open are historical parameters, but they consider only cows that conceive, and thus two parturitions are required. Therefore the current reproductive performance of open cows is not known.

The herd reproductive status index is a good measure of the influence open cows impose on meeting the goals of reproductive efficiency. It accounts for all cows that go beyond a specified period of time (e.g., 100 or 120 days postpartum) and have not conceived.[11] This parameter is influenced by the stage of gestation at the time of pregnancy examination, and an index greater than 65 days is acceptable and suggests that only a few cows in the herd are outside the reproductive goals relative to days open.

Because calving is done on a year-round basis in many dairies, calculating the percentage of the herd with diagnosed pregnancies per month is a useful tool. To maintain an equal number of lactating cows, the rate of calving should equal the rate of drying off and should include a small percentage for culling. This means that there should be equal numbers of new pregnancies per month. In other words, 8% to 9% of the cows in the herd should become pregnant every month.

Many of the parameters listed earlier can be used to evaluate the performance of cows that conceived and eventually calved. However, other parameters should be used to evaluate reproductive failures in the herd (Table 5). It should be mentioned that all dairy herds will experience some degree of infertility. However, when the actual figures exceed the ones listed in Table 5, investigation into possible causes should be performed.

To achieve excellent herd reproductive efficiency, managers of dairy herds must focus on the organization and training of personnel. Other factors to consider are grouping of cows for

Table 4
PARAMETERS USED TO EVALUATE REPRODUCTIVE EFFICIENCY IN THE HERD

Parameter	Value*
Calving interval	13 mo
Days open	125 days
Days in milk (for the herd)	160–175 days
Herd reproductive status index	>65 days
Proportion of the herd becoming pregnant per month	8%–9%
Cow open more than 150 days	<10%
Annual culling for infertility	<10%

*The value listed is the desired goal for that parameter.

Table 5
PARAMETERS USED TO EVALUATE REPRODUCTIVE FAILURES

Parameter	Value*
Palpation pregnancy rate†	<70%
Service per pregnancy, all cows	>3.0
Annual culling for infertility	>15%
Days in milk to first service	EVWP + 26 days

EVWP, elective voluntary waiting period.

*The value listed is the level for that parameter at which investigation into possible causes should be performed.

†This value is based on a conception rate greater than 0.30 and a pregnancy examination greater than 42 days since the last service.

intensive reproductive management and the use of accurate records to evaluate reproductive performance. This performance is dependent on the interrelationship between management, environment, and cow factors. The most limiting of these factors is management or human intervention.

REFERENCES

1. DeKruif A: Factors influencing the fertility of a cattle population. J Reprod Fertil 54:507, 1978.
2. Ferguson JD, Galligan DT: Reproductive programs in dairy herds. *In* Proceedings of the First Central Veterinary Conference. Kansas City, Mo, pp 161–178.
3. Heersche G, Nebel RL: Measuring efficiency and accuracy of detection of estrus. J Dairy Sci 77:2754, 1994.
4. Gwasdauskas FC, Nebel RL, Sprecher DJ, et al: Effectiveness of rump-mounted devices and androgenized females for detection of estrus in dairy cattle. J Dairy Sci 73:2965, 1990.
5. Walker WL, Nebel RL, McGilliard ML: Time of ovulation relative to mounting activity in dairy cattle. J Dairy Sci 79:1555, 1996.
6. Thatcher WW, Collier RJ: Effects of climate on reproduction. *In* Morrow DA (ed): Current Therapy in Theriogenology, ed 2. Philadelphia, WB Saunders, 1986, pp 301–309.
7. Barker RP, Risco CA, Donovan GA: Low palpation pregnancy rate resulting from low conception rate in a dairy herd with adequate estrus detection intensity. Compendium 16:801–815, 1994.
8. Thatcher WW, Wilcox CJ: Postpartum estrus as an indicator of reproductive status in the dairy cow. J Dairy Sci 56:608, 1973.
9. Staples CR, Thatcher WW, Clark JH: Relationship between ovarian activity and energy status during early lactation in high producing dairy cows. J Dairy Sci 73:938, 1990.
10. Risco CA, Archbald LF, Elliott J, et al: Effect of hormonal treatment on fertility in dairy cows with dystocia or retained fetal membranes at parturition. J Dairy Sci 77:2562, 1994.
11. Upham GL: Measuring dairy herd reproductive performance. Bovine Pract 26:49, 1991.

■ Evaluation of Beef Cattle Reproductive Performance

D. Owen Rae, D.V.M., M.P.V.M.

The role of reproduction in beef cattle production is critical to the success of the cow-calf enterprise whether it be measured by production or financial success. Financial return to the producer is optimized when economic inputs are balanced against expected outcomes. Financial success is attained when (1) an optimal number of calves are weaned each year, (2) an optimal weaning weight is achieved for the type of cow and production environment, (3) cow maintenance costs (inputs) are kept at an optimal level, and (4) the best contractual sale price is negotiated.

Each of these four factors is either directly or indirectly associated with the cow's reproductive performance. The number of calves weaned relies on a successful conception, the maintenance of gestation to term, the successful delivery of live, vigorous offspring, and the maternal characteristics that support the calf in the neonatal and growing period. The weaning weight of the calf is dependent on the calf's birth weight, its birth time relative to the herd calving season, time of weaning, and maternal sustenance, including lactation. Cow maintenance costs are dependent on expenses for heifer and bull development, feed, breeding, delivery, and neonatal care costs. The contractual sale price is market-driven. Nonetheless, a sale price range exists within which factors such as calf weight, uniformity, and presale processing have an influence. Each of these factors is also influenced by the time of conception of the cow within the breeding season.

Evaluation of reproduction and production variables requires establishment of goals and critical intervention points (Table 1) which can be measured and assessed at regular and timely intervals. To evaluate performance, there must be a goal toward which to work and a critical intervention point at which the producer is aware that action is required.

It should be noted that the individual reproductive performance of a cow is important but even more important is its contribution to the dynamics of the population. In this treatise, some production variables that are closely associated with calf propagation are evaluated with the more traditional reproduction variables.

Assessment by the veterinary practitioner must be on a herd basis. The production unit history and a "physical examination" of the enterprise initially and periodically thereafter add to the cumulative knowledge base. The profile of the enterprise should include cattle inventory by category of cattle (bulls, cows, heifers, calves); the predominant cattle breed type; the breeding season, including the beginning and ending dates and its length; the weaning date, reflecting the calf growing period (Table 2, Fig. 1); when and with what the animals are processed; the age at which replacement heifers are bred; the types of breeding bulls used; and what disease conditions are common to the unit.

Table 2
SAMPLE HERD: PRODUCTION TIME LINE

Breeding season	Begins	4/1/95	
	Ends	6/15/95	
Length			75 days
Pregnancy test date		8/15/95	
Gestational age {	Min.*		61 days
	Max.†		136 days
Calving season	Begins	1/1/96	
	Ends	3/15/96	
Length			74 days
Weaning date	Begins	9/1/96	
	Ends	9/1/96	
Length			0 days
Calf age {	Min.‡		170 days
	Max.§		244 days

*Minimum gestational age at pregnancy examination.
†Maximum gestational age at pregnancy examination.
‡Minimum days of age for calves at weaning.
§Maximum days of age for calves at weaning.

Record-keeping can be accomplished in a variety of ways. Whether by field records, cow cards, or computer, production yardsticks are essential.

PRODUCTION MEASUREMENTS

The individual animal signalment (animal identification, breed, sex, age, and health) is maintained to give a face to a member of the population, the herd. Breeding season measurements might include cow weight, a body condition score, breeding group, breeding sire(s) and dates, pregnancy status, and days pregnant (at pregnancy examination). Calving season data include birth dates, birth weights, calving ease and vigor scores, health, and mothering ability. Weaning information might include the weaning date, calf weaning weight, and cow and calf body condition scores. Heifer and bull development measures should track yearling weights and dates weighed, body condition score, breeding soundness evaluation or a reproductive tract and pelvic area score. Culling reasons should be established for all animal categories.

With this information, reports and summaries germane to the enterprise can be developed for the herd or herds and by animal category for each phase of the production cycle (i.e., breeding, pregnancy, calving, weaning, marketing, replacement stock development). In addition, health data, that is, morbidity and mortality, should be reported.

Financial records, reports, and summaries of herd inventory value by animal category are essential to finding annual maintenance costs of cow units, gross return on calves, and net return per cow (the production unit). These are beyond the scope of this text and will not be addressed in any more detail.

Performance analysis to be meaningful must be consistent, accurate, and repeatable, and it is desirable that it be standardized between herds, ranches, and regions. Performance measures should be specified, provide performance and cost reference points for the beef operation, and use existing data to produce information for management decisions.

Standardization starts with an agreement on definitions. Some are noted.[1, 2] *Calf crop weaned* is that cohort or group of calves weaned during the year being analyzed. *Breeding season* is the beginning and ending dates of the breeding that result in the calves weaned. *Pregnancy test date* is the date(s) of the pregnancy test after the breeding season. *Calving season* is the beginning and ending dates of the calving that resulted in the calves

Table 1
SAMPLE HERD: BEEF PRODUCTION GOALS AND CRITICAL INTERVENTION LEVELS

	Goal	Critical Level
Pregnancy percentage		
Cows (60-day breeding season)	90%–95%	<85%
Heifers (45-day breeding season)	80%–85%	<80%
Abortion percentage (pregnancy loss)	<2%	>5%
Calving percentage	80%–85%	<80%
Calving interval	12 mo	>13 mo
Stillbirth percentage	<2%	>5%
Dystocia percentage—cows	<2%–5%	>5%
Dystocia percentage—heifers (24 mo)	<15%	>15%
Cesarean-section rate	<1%	>2%
Weaned calf crop	>75%	<75%
Weaning weights	500 lb or 40% dam wt	<450 lb / <40%
Weight per day of age	1.60 lb/day	<1.5
Female replacement rate	15%	>20%
Mortality rate (annual)		
Calves, birth to 10 days	<5.0%	>5%
Calves, 11–30 days	<2.0%	>2%
Calves, 31 days to weaning	<1.0%	>1%
Calves, post weaning	<1.0%	>1%
Cows, bulls (breeding stock)	<0.5%	>1%

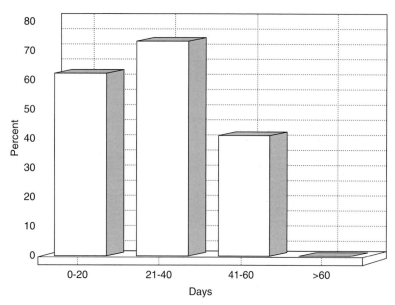

Figure 1
Pregnancy percentage distribution by conception within the breeding season, by 20-day intervals.

weaned. *Births during the calving season* should be categorized in 21-day intervals, if possible. The total number of calves is most important. *Calf deaths* should be recorded as those that die at birth and those that die during the growth phase. *Total calves weaned and their weights* is the most important production measurement. The count should only include calves that are actually weaned and their actual weights at weaning.

The establishment of calf crop or weaning percentage and other more intermediary measures of reproductive performance, that is, pregnancy percentage and calving percentage, require an accurate determination of the denominator, which by definition for each of these measurements is the number of cows exposed to the bull (or cows bred) during the breeding season. The makeup of a cow population is dynamic and may change over the calf production span (an approximately 18-month window, breeding to weaning). The numerator changes with population fluctuations and the denominator must reflect these changes. A tally sheet of "cows exposed to the bull" may be helpful for calculation purposes (Table 3; note that this does not reflect actual cattle inventories on hand).

Some rules apply to cow number adjustments.[1, 2] The beginning breeding inventory is the total number of cows exposed to breeding during the breeding season. This number should include replacement heifers exposed for the first time and mature females acquired and added to the herd. The number must be adjusted for any females exposed but not intended to be kept. This would include females with calves that will be sold when the calves are weaned. After breeding season adjustments, include all transfers-in after the breeding season that have been exposed and have the potential to calve during the calving season. The only adjustment for transfers-out is for pregnant females transferred out. Animals that are open or have undetermined pregnancy status should remain in the herd count. Adjustments after the calving season begins include all females with nursing calves transferred in. Females with nursing calves transferred out should be excluded from this total count. Females transferred out without a nursing calf should remain in the inventory count.

EVALUATION OF BREEDING AND PREGNANCY

Pregnancy percentage portrays the general success rate of the breeding season. It is calculated as the number of females ex-

posed to the bull and diagnosed as pregnant divided by the number of females exposed, multiplied by 100. The raw numbers making up the numerator and denominator are also of importance. Further, information can be gleaned by evaluating pregnancy numbers and percentages for specific production indices, such as cow age, body condition score (at calving or a pregnancy examination), and lactational state (Table 4).

During the pregnancy examination added information can be gathered by staging the gestation of the pregnant cows. With this, a time to conception within the breeding season can be computed based on a breeding season beginning date, representing time zero, a calculation of the maximum days pregnant at the pregnancy examination, and subtraction of the time in days of the per rectum staging of the gestation. Evaluation of these data is best made by categorizing conception time into 10 or 20 (approximately 21-day) intervals to establish a distribution or profile of pregnancy for the herd (Fig. 1). Time to conception in the breeding season can also be evaluated by production

Table 3
SAMPLE HERD: INVENTORY AND ADJUSTMENTS WORKSHEET TO ESTABLISH NUMERATORS AND DENOMINATORS FOR CALCULATIONS THROUGH THE PRODUCTION PHASES

Category	Adj	Count	ExpF
Female inventory at breeding		—	200
Transferred in after breeding	2	—	202
Transferred out after breeding	1	—	201
Total females pregnancy-tested		176	201
Transferred in after test	3	—	204
Transferred out after test	1	—	203
Total females calving		174	203
Total live calves at birth		172	203
Transferred out after calving	1	—	202
Transferred in after calving	1	—	203
Calves died at birth	3	171	203
Calves died during growing phase	3	168	203
Total calves weaned		168	203

Adj, adjustments to inventory values; Count, potential calf count at each point of measurement; ExpF, exposed females—tally through the production cycle.

Table 4
SAMPLE HERD: PREGNANCY EXAMINATION SUMMARY

	n (%)	DTC (days)	Age (yr)	BCS
Females exposed	201 —	23	3.8	5.1
Pregnant	176 (87.6)	23	3.8	5.2
Nonpregnant	25 (12.4)	—	3.6	4.8
Lactating cows	128 (85.9)	26	5.0	5.0
Nonlactating cows	73 (92.0)	17	2.5	5.8

	Conception Interval (days)			
	0–20	*21–40*	*41–60*	*>60*
Pregnancy by period	70	65	37	4
Cumulative pregnancy	70	135	172	176
Cumulative percent	39.8	76.7	97.7	100.0

DTC, average days to conception within the breeding season for each category; BCS, body condition score (1 = thin, 9 = obese).

indices much like pregnancy percentage, that is, by cow age, body condition score, and lactational state.

EVALUATION OF GESTATION AND CALVING PERFORMANCE

Calving percentage is the number of females calving divided by the number of females exposed to the bull, multiplied by 100. Keep in mind that an accurate computation requires adjustments to the number of females actually exposed during the breeding season, that is, cows sold, herd transfers, and so forth. All full-term calves (but not abortions) should be included in the number of calves born, even if they are dead at birth (Table 5).

Calving distribution is the cumulative number of calves born by 21, 42, 63, and greater than 63 days of the calving season. A calving distribution percentage uses this cumulative number by period divided by the total number of calves born, multiplied by 100. The starting date for the first 21-day period is 285 days after the bull turn-in date with the mature cow herd. If this

information is unavailable, start the first 21-day period when the third mature cow (3 years and older) calves. All calves should be included, whether alive or dead.

Pregnancy loss percentage is the number of cows found to be pregnant at pregnancy examination minus the number of cows delivering offspring divided by the number of cows pregnant at pregnancy examination.

Calf death loss can be reported based on cows exposed during the breeding season or by number of calves born, or preferably both. Calf death loss based on cows exposed during the breeding season is the number of calves that died divided by the number of exposed females, multiplied by 100. Calf death loss based on calves born is the number of calves that died divided by the number of calves born, multiplied by 100. Calf death loss should include those calves lost at birth and any that die up to weaning time. Greater reporting detail is possible if mortality is categorized as occurring at birth, birth to 10 days, 11 days to 30 days, and 31 days to weaning. More accurate analysis of calf death loss would include age of the calf at death, age of dam, and cause of death. Abortions before calving should be included in the pregnancy loss percentage.

Calving ease and calf vigor scores are subjective measurements that may identify problems in sire selection, birthing, or maternal traits. Calving ease scores* are given as 1 to 5, where 1 is a natural unassisted delivery, 2 is an easy assisted delivery, 3 is a moderately difficult assisted delivery, 4 is a difficult assisted delivery, and 5 is a caesarean section or a fetotomy. Calf vigor is also scored on a scale of 1 to 5, where 1 is a normal vigorous calf that nurses unassisted, 2 is a calf that nurses but is slow to stand and do so, 3 is a calf requiring assistance to stand and nurse, 4 is a calf that dies shortly after birth, and 5 is a stillborn or dead calf at birth. This information can be used in combination with cow age, calf gender, or calving distribution period to further characterize the calving season.

EVALUATION OF CALF GROWING PHASE (TO WEANING)

Calf crop or weaning percentage is the number of calves weaned divided by the number of females exposed, multiplied

---

*Adapted from the American Hereford Association.

Table 5
SAMPLE HERD: CALVING SEASON SUMMARY

	n (%)	DTP	BWt (lb)	CES
Exposed females calving	174 (85.7)	22	75	1.1
Bull calves	89 (—)	25	79	1.2
Heifer calves	85 (—)	19	72	1.1
Pregnancy loss	2 (1.0)	—	—	—
Calving loss/death	3 (1.5)	40	82	2.3
Calf death 1–10 days	2 (1.0)	45	65	1.4
Calf death 11–30 days	1 (0.5)	25	78	1.0
Calf death >30 days	0 (0.0)	—	—	1.0
Cow death	1 (0.5)	—	—	—

	Calving Interval (days)*			
	0–21	*22–42*	*43–63*	*>63*
Calves born by period	66	71	33	4
Cumulative number	66	137	170	174
Cumulative percent	37.9	78.7	97.7	100.0

DTP, average days to parturition; BWt, calf birth weight by category; CES, calving ease score (1–5).
*Starting date for the 21-day periods is 285 days after the bull turn-in date with the mature cows or when the third mature cow calves.

Table 6
SAMPLE HERD: WEANING SUMMARY

	n (%)	DTW	WWt (lb)	WDA (lb/days)	W/C (lb)
Weaned*	168 (82.8)	216	502	2.3	415
Bulls/steers	86 (—)	219	510	2.3	—
Heifers	82 (—)	218	493	2.3	—
Total wt	— (—)	—	84,322	—	415
Market†	138 (68.0)	216	492	2.3	334
Bulls/steers	86 (—)	219	510	2.3	—
Heifers	52 (—)	211	462	2.2	—
Total wt	— (—)	—	67,879	—	334
Replace‡	30 (14.8)	225	548	2.4	—
Bulls	0 (—)	—	—	—	—
Heifers	30 (14.8)	225	548	2.4	—
Total wt	— (—)	—	16,443	—	—

	Calving Period (days)§				
	0–21	**22–42**	**43–63**	**>63**	**Total**
Calves weaned	66	71	28	3	168
DTW	233	212	191	170	215
WWt	525	500	459	440	502
Total weight	34,650	35,500	12,852	1320	84,322
W/C by interval	171	175	77	8	415
W/C (%)	41.1	42.1	15.2	1.6	100

DTW, average days to weaning; WWt, calf weaning weight by category; WDA, weight per day of age; W/C, weaned pounds of calf per cow exposed to the bull.
*All cows weaned.
†Weaned calves going to market.
‡Weaned calves being kept as breeding replacement animals.
§Calving intervals representing birthing distribution in the calving season; that is, the oldest calves are in category 0–21.

by 100. Remember that an accurate denominator requires adjustments to the number of females actually exposed during the breeding season (Table 6).

Average calf weaning weights (pounds per head) for all weaned calves and for gender classes (steers and bulls, and heifers) can be computed as follows: steer and bull calf weaning weight is the total weight of weaned steer and bull calves divided by the total number of weaned steer and bull calves; heifer calf weaning weight is the total weight of heifer calves weaned divided by the total number of heifer calves weaned; and average weaning weight is total weight of weaned calves divided by the total number of calves weaned. The product of a cow-calf enterprise is a weaned calf measured in terms of pounds or hundredweight. Herd productivity is measured in pounds weaned per exposed female. Pounds weaned per exposed female are the total pounds of calf weaned divided by the total number of females exposed. The number of females exposed must be adjusted for the same factors used in the calf crop percent calculations.

Average calf weaning age identifies the window in which calves are allowed to grow. Average weaning weights are of little meaning if the age at weaning is not known. Production indices can be evaluated by age at weaning in 21-day intervals much like the calving season distribution. Weight per day of age is the weaning weight of all calves or gender classes divided by days of age at weaning.

OTHER IMPORTANT MEASUREMENTS

Measurements of resource utilization include grazing and raised feed calculations as they relate to acres of pasture per exposed female and pounds weaned per acre used by cattle.

Some weaned heifers will be retained as replacement heifers, while previously productive cows will be culled from the herd.

The female replacement rate is the raised replacement heifers exposed for the first time to the bull plus purchased replacement heifers plus purchased breeding cows exposed to the bull divided by the total number of females exposed, multiplied by 100.

CONCLUSION

Systematic, well-defined data collection and analysis allows comparison with target goals and establishes critical control

Table 7
SAMPLE HERD: SUMMARY OF PERFORMANCE

	No. (%)
Exposed females	203
Pregnancy percentage	176 (88.0)
Pregnancy loss percentage	2 (1.0)
Calving percentage	174 (87.0)
Calf death loss based on exposed females	6 (3.0)
Calf crop or weaning percentage	168 (84.0)
Female replacement rate percentage	30 (13.5)
Calf death loss based on calves born	6 (3.4)
Calving distribution	
Calves born during first 21 days	66 (37.9)
Calves born during first 42 days	137 (78.7)
Calves born during first 63 days	170 (97.7)
Calves born after first 63 days	4 (2.8)

Production Performance Measures		
Average age at weaning (days)		218
Weaning weights (lb/head)		
Bulls/steers	86	510
Heifers	82	493
Average weaning weight	168	502
Pounds weaned per exposed female		415

levels that demarcate areas where problems become evident (Table 7). Reproductive (and productive) strengths and weaknesses can be evaluated in each of five calf development phases: (1) the timely establishment of pregnancy, (2) the maintenance of pregnancy throughout gestation, (3) the birthing and delivery of a healthy, vigorous calf, (4) the survival of the neonate and maternal nurturing of same, and (5) the calf's growth and development under maternal care.

REFERENCES

1. Hamilton ED: Standardized performance analysis. Vet Clin North Am Food Anim Pract, 11:199–213, 1995.
2. IRM-SPA Handbook. College Station, Tex, Texas Agricultural Extension Service, 1993.

■ Management of Reproduction of Sheep and Goats

Randall S. Ott, D.V.M., M.S.

Effective management of reproduction is essential to the profitability of livestock enterprises that raise sheep and goats. A population viewpoint (herd approach) is necessary for cost-effective production of these species. Selection of the breed, or crossbreed, that is the best match for the available environmental, nutritional, and management resources is an important first step. For flock replacements, selective preference should be given to the offspring of animals that perform well without requiring therapy or costly management practices. Mating practices, feeding regimens, and vaccination programs must be continually reviewed to ensure that the benefits derived are greater than the costs incurred.

The most important method of increasing the reproductive capacity of a flock is the selection of highly fertile males. Early puberty and enhanced reproductive capacity of males are transferred to female progeny. The male's contribution to the flock's gene pool is manyfold greater than that of a female's even when natural mating is practiced. Estrus synchronization and artificial insemination have the potential to greatly accelerate a male's contribution. Embryo transfer offers minimal impact with increased expense and is not likely to be cost-effective in most sheep and goat production programs.

The most important trait of breeding males is large scrotal circumference for age. Scrotal circumference is an indirect measurement of early puberty and testicular size and is positively related to sperm production. Other important traits include serving capacity (the male's ability to inseminate females) and testicular health. Highly fertile males increase production by causing conception in more females and by fertilizing more ova per female.

Breeding soundness examinations assess the fitness of individual rams and bucks and can help diagnose breeding problems in the flock. Finding that the males are satisfactory breeders causes one to look for other causes such as infections, subfertility of females, or nutritional deficiencies. A breeding soundness examination may confirm a suspected case of male infertility and allow the owner to receive compensation or a replacement animal from the seller if the sire is under warranty. Guidelines for breeding soundness examinations of rams and bucks are available from the Society for Theriogenology.

SHEEP

Most ewes are bred by natural service, although selective or hand mating and artificial insemination are used in certain situations. A suggested mating system for maximum ewe fertility is the use of three rams in each breeding unit. More ewes are detected in estrus when three rams are working together. Breeding pastures should be large enough so that dominant rams do not prevent subordinate rams from mating. A limit of 50 ewes per ram has been recommended. Highly fertile rams with excellent libido can serve more than 100 ewes during a 17-day breeding cycle. Rams are frequently harnessed with tupping crayons so that ewes that have been served by the ram can be identified. The crayon color should be changed every 14 to 15 days. Introduction of the ram to the breeding flock at the beginning of the breeding season can result in partial synchrony of ovulation in the ewes several days later. Sheep tend to ovulate without showing signs of estrus, whereas goats have been reported to exhibit signs of estrus without ovulation at the beginning of the breeding season.

Ewes are serviced 2 to 6 times per estrus. When more than one ram is present, multiple-sire matings occur. Males with good libido may mate 20 to 30 times a day. The duration of estrus in the ewe ranges from 10 to 40 hours, with an average of about 24 hours. The length of the estrous cycle in sheep is 16 to 17 days. Ewes in estrus actively seek the ram. The need to learn how to find and successfully compete for the ram is thought to account for the poor performance of maiden ewes in pasture mating.

A common practice in sheep breeding is to flush the ewes just before and during the breeding season. Flushing ewes is thought to stimulate more ovulations during the early and late breeding season but is probably of little benefit during the middle of the season. Ewes that are fed properly are more likely to have strong lambs and milk well. Most of the growth of fetal lambs occurs in the last 2 months of gestation. Failure to meet energy requirements during gestation may result in pregnancy toxemia (ketosis) in late gestation in ewes or does carrying more than one offspring.

Early born ewe lambs can cycle and conceive in their first breeding season. Bringing ewe lambs into production as early as possible decreases maintenance costs before the start of production and increases lifetime production. To accomplish early breeding, lambs must be large enough (65% of mature weight is suggested) and in good condition. Age at puberty varies greatly among breeds. Female offspring from rams selected for large scrotal circumference for age reach puberty at a younger age.

Care should be taken that animals added to the flock come from herds in which the owners practice disease control. A program of reproductive disease prevention includes sanitation, early diagnosis of disease, and proper vaccination programs. *Brucella ovis* infection causes epididymitis, which greatly reduces the reproductive capacity of affected rams. The presence of grossly palpable epididymal lesions and white blood cells and increased numbers of tailless heads in the semen sample are findings indicative of epididymitis. However, determination of the infection rates of *B. ovis* in flocks is best accomplished by a *B. ovis* enzyme-linked immunosorbent assay on blood serum. Ram epididymitis has been reported as a major cause of reduced fertility in western range flocks; it has affected 95% of Utah range flocks and 35% of the rams in a flock.

Determination of pregnancy in ewe lambs enables the nonpregnant ones to be culled and marketed while they can still command slaughter lamb prices. Real-time ultrasonography has been reported as an accurate and cost-effective method of pregnancy determination in large flocks.

DAIRY GOATS

Selective or hand mating is the usual practice in dairy goat herds. It is not desirable to allow odorous bucks to run free with milking does. The duration of estrus in does is 32 to 40 hours. Does are usually mated at the onset of estrus and at 12-hour intervals until estrus subsides. In artificial insemination programs, the doe is inseminated when she first accepts mounting by a teaser buck and again 12 hours later.

The length of the estrous cycle of dairy goats is 20 days. Abnormally short (5 to 8 days) estrous cycles may occur in does early in the breeding season. A condition called "false pregnancy" occurs in some does. In these does, a large volume of clear fluid is passed at "parturition." Pregnancy diagnosis of does by transabdominal scanning is accurate after 40 days of gestation.

Whether hand mating or artificial insemination is practiced, proper detection of estrus is the most important aspect of goat breeding. Does actively seek the presence of the buck when in estrus. Bucks are sometimes descented at the time of dehorning by burning and destroying the odor glands located posteriorly and medially to the horn buds. This is probably a bad practice because does, when given a choice, will usually prefer a scented buck to a deodorized one. As with sheep, the presence of males can initiate and even synchronize the cyclic activity of females at the beginning of the breeding season. Detection of estrus in does is best accomplished with the use of a buck. An intact buck should be penned in an area where does in estrus can be observed congregating near the pen. Signs of estrus in does are tail wagging, bleating, and urinating near the buck. There may be swelling of the vulva and a mucous discharge from the vulva. The reaction of the buck to the doe being teased is an indication of estrus in does. Some does show few signs of estrus other than limited tail wagging and standing for mounting by the buck, and these signs may be present only after teasing. Does will occasionally stand for mounting by other does; however, the level of homosexual activity in goats is low in reproductively normal females.

A common condition that causes infertility in dairy goats is intersex or hermaphroditism. Female hermaphrodites may have a vulva of normal size but an enlarged clitoris and a short or atretic vagina. A penile clitoris, or ovotestes, can occur in does that otherwise appear phenotypically female. Hermaphroditism and congenital hypoplasia of the reproductive tract are commonly observed in naturally hornless (polled) goats and are more likely to occur when both parents are polled. Despite phenotypic variation, intersex goats are usually genetic females with a normal female chromosome (60,XX) complement.

CONTROL OF REPRODUCTION IN SHEEP AND GOATS*

Sheep and goats are considered "short-day breeders" because they initiate reproductive activity in response to decreasing length of daylight. Both are classified as seasonally polyestrous and become anestrous as a result of either pregnancy or the end of the breeding season. Control of the time of breeding allows control of the time of lambing and kidding and control of milk production in does. Progestogens have been the most widely used agents for ovulation control. Fluorogestone acetate has been administered by the intravaginal route with an impregnated polyurethane sponge. Vaginal pessaries are left in place for 14 days in sheep and for 21 days in goats, and an injection of pregnant mare's serum gonadotropin is given at the time of removal. In goats, an 11-day regimen has proved successful when prostaglandin $F_{2\alpha}$ and pregnant mare's serum gonadotropin were given on day 9. The efficacy of pregnant mare's serum gonadotropin for ovarian stimulation can diminish after repeated use in does.

Prostaglandin $F_{2\alpha}$ or its analogues will induce luteolysis in cyclic ewes or does during the breeding season. A dose of 2.5 mg has been shown to be adequate for induction of estrus in the doe. Doses ranging from 6 to 15 mg have been used for estrus induction of sheep. Fertility after an induced estrus has been reported to be normal in goats; however, some workers have reported reduced fertility in sheep.

Control of the time of parturition in sheep and goats enables closer supervision of lambing and kidding during planned periods when labor could be used more efficiently. In one study, dexamethasone (16 mg) administered to ewes on day 143 of gestation resulted in lambs on days 144 to 146, with the largest litters being delivered earliest. Prostaglandin $F_{2\alpha}$ has been demonstrated to be the drug of choice for induction of parturition in goats. Does receiving either 2.5 mg or 5.0 mg prostaglandin $F_{2\alpha}$ on day 144 gave birth to kids within 28 to 57 hours. Retained fetal membranes have not been reported to be associated with induced parturition in ewes or in does.

A number of factors, including light, temperature, and the presence of the male, influence the onset of the breeding season. However, the photoperiod is believed to be the most important factor. Control of the photoperiod by using artificial lighting has been well researched in sheep. Nevertheless, this method has not had much application in either species. In the United States, the breeding season for sheep and goats generally extends from August to February. Breed differences and the geographic area account for wide variation. Some goat dairies have practiced exposure of breeding animals to total darkness for 17 hours daily after the beginning of June to induce early onset of cyclic activity. There is interest in developing breeds and strains of both species that under proper management might reproduce without seasonal restrictions, thus allowing accelerated lambing in sheep and year-round milk production in goats.

BIBLIOGRAPHY

Bagley CV, Healy MC: Epididymitis in Range and Purebred Rams. Logan, Utah, Utah State University Cooperative Extension Service, EL-228, pp 1–4.
Baril G, Remy B, Vallet JC, et al: Effect of repeated use of progestogen-PMSG treatment for estrus control in dairy goats out of breeding season. Reprod Domest Anim 27:161–168, 1992.
Kimberling CV, Marsh D: Ram breeding soundness evaluations (BSE). *In* Proceedings of Small Ruminant Short Course. Kansas City, American College of Theriogenologists and Society for Theriogenology. 1994, pp 55–71.
Ott RS: Dairy goat reproduction. Compend Contin Educ Pract Vet 4(suppl):164–172, 1982.
Ott RS: Management of noninfectious problems in reproduction of the ewe and female goat. *In* Laing JA, Morgan WJB, Wagner WC (eds): Fertility and Infertility in Veterinary Practice, ed 4. London, Baillière Tindall, 1988, pp 113–119.
Ott RS, Memon MA: Breeding soundness examinations of rams and bucks, a review. Theriogenology 13:155–164, 1980.
Ott RS, Memon MA: Sheep and Goat Manual. Hastings, Neb, Society for Theriogenology, 1980.

■ Management of Reproductive Problems in Swine Herds

Craig A. Smith, D.V.M., Ph.D., Diplomate, A.C.T.

The swine industry is undergoing rapid, massive changes. The industry is evolving, with the end result being that a small number of farms will have a large number of pigs. Reproductive efficiency is a paramount concern that must be addressed for

---

*Some treatment regimens described in this article lack official regulatory approval. Refer to label instructions for proper usage.

Table 1
COMMON REPRODUCTIVE PROBLEMS IN SWINE

Primary Complaint	Factors	Comments and Recommendations
Anestrus (gilts)	Boar exposure	Expose to mature boar daily from 135 to 160 days of age; 15 min of daily exposure sufficient; fence-line contact often most practical
	Estrus detection	Enhanced by use of a mature boar; 15 min of exposure sufficient; continuous exposure not recommended
	Nutrition	Gilts should be fed to achieve goal without overconditioning
	Housing	Recommended stocking rate = 8 sq ft/pig; keeping group size < 50; adequate ventilation
	Ambient temperature	Extremes adversely affect feed intake; supplemental heat recommended in winter, cooling in summer (shade, water cooling system—drip cooling, water backup; air conditioning—zone cooling)
	Season and photoperiod	16–18 hr of daylight required to induce cycling; expose gilts to normal daylength patterns throughout the year
	Endocrine status	Perform serum progesterone analysis for evidence of luteal activity
	Developmental defects	Hermaphrodites, immature and malformed tracts, cystic ovaries; perform slaughter check
	Mycotoxins	Precocious puberty (swollen vulvas common); test feed, perform slaughter check
	Breed	Landrace mature earlier
	Induction of estrus	Natural methods: (1) transportation stress (limited to gilts 190 days and older), (2) regrouping, (3) vasectomized boar
		Hormonal treatments: (1) synthetic progesterone, allyl trenbolone (Regumate, Hoechst-Roussel) fed for 14 days, then withdrawn, will induce estrus in up to 90% of gilts within 4–7 days (not currently approved for use in the United States); (2) injectable PMSG-HCG combination (P.G. 600, Intervet America) will induce estrus in up to 70% of gilts 4–7 days after a single injection (approved for use in the United States)
Postweaning anestrus	Nutrition	High-energy ration (>17 Mcal/sow/day) and sufficient protein (>689 g/sow/day) required throughout lactation (NRC recommendations, 1988)
	Lactation length	Optimum = 18–24 days for intensive operations; for each 10-day reduction in lactation there is a potential 1-day increase in the wean-to-estrus interval; may not be flexible due to facility limitations (often decreased because of a lack of farrowing crates and increased because of poor nursery facilities)
	Parity	Primiparous sows often delayed
	Season	Common during late summer and early fall (especially in primiparous sows)
	Ambient temperature	See Anestrus (gilts)
	Estrus detection	Consider boar exposure, housing (individually housed sows show estrus sooner), and detection procedures
	Metritis	Postmortem, slaughter check
Regular returns	Timing of mating	Breed 12–24 hr after onset of estrus; "in heat in the morning, breed in the afternoon; in heat in the afternoon, breed the following morning"
	Number of matings/estrus	Two or more matings at 12 to 24-hr intervals
	Type of mating	Homospermic (single boar) vs. heterospermic (multiple boars): use of multiple boars during estrus period improves the chance that the effect of a subfertile boar will be canceled by the subsequent use of a fertile boar; natural vs. artificial insemination: comparable results can be achieved with artificial insemination, provided personnel are competent and the technique is correct; hand vs. pen mating: pen mating may yield better results if heat detection is a problem
	Boar usage	≤6 times/week (hand mating), 5–7 sows/boar (pen mating: continuous farrowing), 2–3 sows/boar (pen mating: batch farrowing)
	Quality of mating	Personnel should manage 2 or fewer matings/person at one time (hand mating); observe quality of floor surface
	Infectious disease	Porcine parvovirus, pseudorabies virus
	Endometritis	Postmortem, slaughter check
	Ambient temperature	Temperatures in excess of 90°F adversely affect embryonal survival (embryo is most susceptible during first 30 days) and sperm production (delayed effect); provide shade, water cooling system (drip cooling, water backup), air conditioning (zone cooling)
	Breed	White breeds generally have higher conception rates
Delayed returns	Season	Late summer; usually no change in litter size
	Ambient temperature	Delayed effect of temperature extremes
	Infectious disease	Parvovirus, pseudorabies virus, PRRS virus; leptospirosis (including *Leptospira interrogans* serovar *L. bratislava*) and eperythrozoonosis; isolation (60–90 days) and serologic testing of new introductions (use of antibiotics during this period not recommended)
	Housing	Provide least stressful environment
	Nutrition	Excess energy intake during early gestation may cause embryonal death
	Mycotoxins	See Anestrus (gilts)
Failure to farrow (following positive pregnancy check)	Pregnancy diagnosis	Observe for return to estrus at 18–24 days; use accurate amplitude depth, ultrasound device, or both amplitude depth and Doppler ultrasound devices at 30-day intervals
	Abortion	Failure of personnel to observe abortions
	Mycotoxins	See Anestrus (gilts)
	Infectious disease	Reproductive (especially pseudorabies virus) and systemic disease
	Season	Summer to early fall
	Developmental defects	Cervical hypoplasia in gilts

Table continued on following page

Table 1
COMMON REPRODUCTIVE PROBLEMS IN SWINE *Continued*

Primary Complaint	Factors	Comments and Recommendations
Small litters	Parity	Maximum litter size from parity 3–6; breed gilts on second cycle
	Lactation length	For each 1-day decrease in lactation length <28 days, there is a potential loss of 0.1 pig per litter
	Infectious disease	Reproductive diseases (particularly PPV and enteroviruses)
	Timing of mating	See Regular returns
	Number of matings/estrus	See Regular returns
	Type of mating	See Regular returns
	Boar usage	See Regular returns
	Boar fertility	Semen evaluation or review of records (difficult if heterospermic matings are used)
	Ambient temperature	See Anestrus (gilts)
Abortions	Infectious diseases	Reproductive (particularly leptospirosis, pseudorabies, PRRS, and brucellosis) and systemic disease; laboratory submission of fetal and placental tissue, serology of dam
	Mycotoxins	See Anestrus (gilts)
	Season	Summer to early fall and winter; likely associated with feed intake
	Nutrition	Underfeeding
	Parity	Common in sows beyond parity 6
Stillbirths	Parity	More common in gilts and sows beyond parity 6
	Calcium deficiency	Feed analysis for both calcium and phosphorus
	Infectious disease	Reproductive disease (leptospirosis, PRRS virus, and pseudorabies virus)
	Prolonged labor	Confirm that personnel know when and how to intervene; overconditioned sows or gilts
	Mycotoxins	See Anestrus (gilts)
Mummies	Parity	See Stillbirths
	Infectious disease	Parvovirus, pseudorabies virus, PRRS virus, encephalomyocarditis virus, enteroviruses, influenza virus
	Mycotoxins	See Anestrus (gilts)
Vaginal discharges	Urogenital infection	Sanitation, facility design; vaginal or preputial diverticulum culture may be helpful; medicate breeding herd ration; use an antibiotic preputial wash

PMSG, pregnant mare serum gonadotropin; HCG, human chorionic gonadotropin; NRC, National Research Council; PRRS, porcine reproductive and respiratory syndrome; PPV, porcine parvovirus.

Adapted from Van Der Leek ML, Becker HN: Reproductive management problems in swine. *In* Howard JL (ed): Current Veterinary Therapy 3: Food Animal Practice. Philadelphia, WB Saunders, 1993, p 806.

---

these farms to maintain economic stability and remain viable. Veterinarians must offer their clients optimal service in this business-oriented market. Veterinarians must be cognizant of infectious diseases, but also must provide information on technological advances and modern management techniques.

The challenges facing veterinarians in the swine industry are perhaps most apparent when dealing with reproductive problems. Reproductive problems may be difficult to diagnose because of their insidious, chronic nature. Often, reproductive problems may not be manifest until weeks or months have passed, long after an inciting cause has disappeared. Reproductive problems usually result from the interaction of multiple factors.[1-3] Although infectious agents may be involved, they rarely are the primary cause. Numerous areas of a farm or various portions of a herd may be involved. Thus, veterinarians must attempt to integrate information about infectious diseases, management, and the results of laboratory analyses with their own observations and knowledge of all the areas on each farm to determine the causes of reproductive failure (Table 1).

CAUSES OF REPRODUCTIVE PROBLEMS IN SWINE HERDS

For purposes of simplicity, reproductive problems can be grouped into those caused by infectious agents and those that result from noninfectious causes. A primary goal of the investigation should be to determine whether the problem is one of generalized poor reproductive performance or whether there is a specific cause for the inefficiency.

Infectious Agents Causing Reproductive Failure

Many bacterial[1, 3] and viral[4, 5] causes of reproductive failure have been identified. *Leptospira interrogans*, *Erysipelothrix rhusiopathiae*, *Streptococcus* spp., and *Brucella suis* have long been identified as causes of reproductive failure in sows and gilts. *Salmonella* spp. and *Staphylococcus* spp. are just two of the bacteria that can cause systemic illness in pregnant females, resulting in fetal death and abortion. Similarly, several viruses (porcine parvovirus, porcine enterovirus, pseudorabies virus, and encephalomyocarditis virus) have a long-standing history as causes of reproductive failure. Many of these infectious agents have been almost eliminated through regulatory programs or through the use of vaccines. However, the emergence of porcine reproductive and respiratory syndrome virus as a major cause of infertility, abortions, and stillbirths should remind us that outbreaks of infectious disease can work havoc on the reproductive performance of swine herds.[6-8] Boars also can be affected by infectious agents. Infected males may be subfertile or may act as a source of infection of susceptible females.[9]

Noninfectious Causes of Reproductive Failure

Noninfectious causes of reproductive failure are extremely numerous[10] and probably outnumber the infectious agents. Manifestations of noninfectious reproductive failure include delayed onset of puberty; anestrus in weaned sows; anestrus in nonpregnant, mated females; infertility; irregular return to estrus after mating; abortions; failure to farrow after a positive diagnosis of pregnancy; small litter sizes; excessive numbers of stillbirths or mummies; and vaginal discharges. Genetics,[11] nutrition,[12] housing facilities, season,[13] photoperiod, temperature, toxic substances, and management factors[14] can all contribute to reproductive inefficiency. Again, these factors can affect boars as well as sows and gilts. The effects on the males may be less obvious and may be detectable only when problems become evident in the females (e.g., excessive heat may render boars subfertile, but this may not become apparent until conception or farrowing rates decrease).

DIAGNOSIS OF HERD REPRODUCTIVE PROBLEMS

Accurate diagnosis of the causes of reproductive failure is essential before corrective measures can be instituted. Clinical signs alone may not clearly indicate whether infectious agents are involved. A thorough herd investigation should be conducted.[15-17] A systematic method of assessing reproduction on swine farms, such as those provided by use of algorithms or flow charts (Figs. 1 and 2), will enable veterinarians to explore all facets that are involved in good reproductive performance.

Herd History

Obtaining a history of the herd problem from the workers on the farm is the first and, possibly, most critical step in solving reproductive problems. Discussions with farm personnel should elicit information that will assist in subsequent diagnostic efforts. Information on the time frame (acute vs. chronic onset) for a problem, whether the situation is improving or becoming worse, the nature of previous interventions, and the level of management and managerial expertise should become apparent during this process.

Records Analysis

Information gained from the herd history can yield information about the reliability of records. Reliable records are necessary for evaluation. Often, analysis of the records will indicate the onset of the problem or the severity of the problem, which may differ from the recollections of farm personnel. Monitoring appropriate variables, considering appropriate time frames, and evaluating specific portions of the herd can reveal causes of the problem as well as the economic impact. Records analysis can be used to guide additional areas of management that should be investigated as well as aid in selection of appropriate samples that should be submitted for laboratory testing.

Observation of Herd and Facilities

A walk through the facilities and observation of the herd is helpful in confirming information gathered in the herd history and records analysis. Observation of the animals, their condition, the facilities in which they are housed, and their general environment is essential to determining an accurate diagnosis. Observations of daily activities, especially those of estrus detection and breeding management, are necessary components. It must be borne in mind that the things seen during a visit may not be reflective of the day-to-day operations on the farm, because personnel may be more aware of their responsibilities and more inspired in the performance of their duties when they are being observed by an outsider.

Slaughterhouse Evaluations

Examination of a representative group of animals can assist practitioners with their diagnostic efforts. The ability to observe the reproductive tracts and obtain specimens for additional laboratory analysis can prove invaluable.[18] Furthermore, visual confirmation of the cause of problems can be a strong stimulus for convincing personnel of the accuracy of your diagnosis and the need to implement corrective actions.

Laboratory Analyses

Nutritional factors that could influence reproductive performance should be evaluated. Laboratory confirmation of rations and diets may be necessary. Submission of serologic samples or

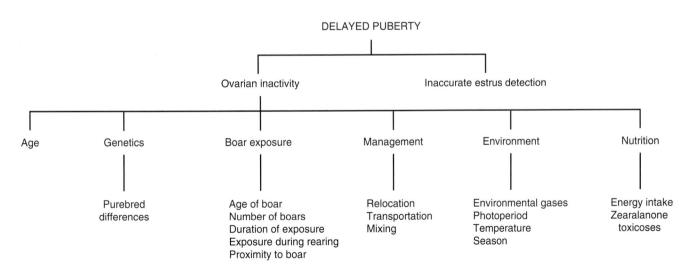

Figure 1

Algorithm depicting interrelationships among factors that affect delayed onset of puberty in gilts. (From Dial GD, Marsh WE, Polson DD, et al: Reproductive failure: Differential diagnosis. *In* Leman AD, Straw BE, Mengeling WL, et al (eds): Diseases of Swine, ed 7. Ames, Iowa, Iowa State University Press, 1992, p 107.)

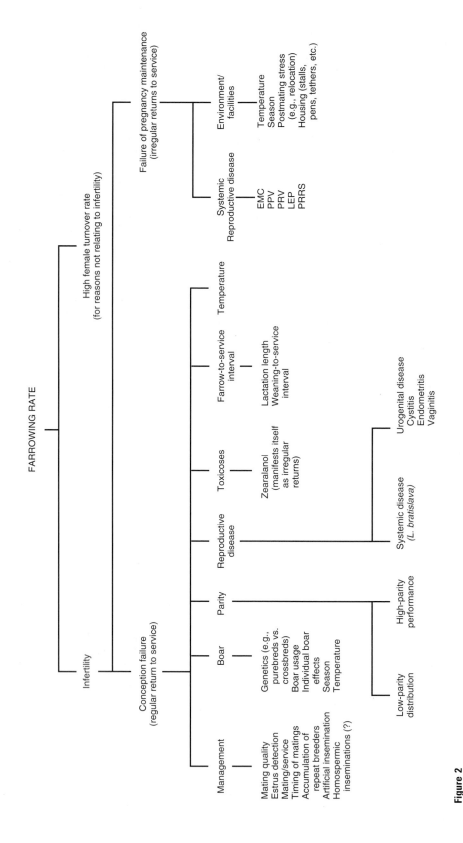

Figure 2

Algorithm depicting interrelationships among factors that affect farrowing rate. EMC, encephalomyocarditis virus; PPV, porcine parvovirus; PRV, pseudorabies virus; LEP, *Leptospira interrogans*; PRRS, porcine reproductive and respiratory syndrome virus. (Adapted from Dial GD, Marsh WE, Polson DD, et al: Reproductive failure: Differential diagnosis. *In* Leman AD, Straw BE, Mengeling WL, et al (eds): Diseases of Swine, ed 7. Ames, Iowa, Iowa State University Press, 1992, p 94.)

tissue specimens to diagnostic laboratories can be used to confirm that an infectious agent is part of the problem. Laboratory testing can also be used to confirm that an infectious agent is not the problem (not detecting the agent in a sufficient number of affected, susceptible animals) or is being adequately controlled (evidence of protective titers in vaccinated animals). Practitioners should consult with laboratory diagnosticians to determine the type and number of samples that should be submitted for analysis.[19, 20]

MANAGEMENT OF REPRODUCTIVE PROBLEMS

Documentation of records analysis, laboratory testing, or personal observations will substantiate and support the final diagnosis. Because of the multifactorial nature of many reproductive problems, it may be necessary for veterinarians to establish those factors that are most contributory to the problem or, alternatively, that have the greatest economic impact, so that implementation of corrective programs can be prioritized.

Infectious agents have historically been handled through use of programs (e.g., cesarean section to derive specific pathogen–free pigs) that prevented the introduction of diseases to farms, programs that resulted in removal of infected animals from farms, or vaccination programs to limit the effects of a disease. Biosecurity and disease prevention and reduction programs will be increasingly important in the future.[21] Artificial insemination can be used to improve reproductive efficiency and simultaneously aid in controlling transmission of diseases; however, use of new technologies may initiate a new set of problems.[22] Veterinarians must thoroughly discuss the benefits and pitfalls of new programs before they are implemented on swine operations. Veterinarians will continue to screen breeding stock for reproductive diseases, but producers also are demanding that prospective breeding stock be screened for diseases that will affect the general health of growing pigs and thereby affect economic returns because of poor feed efficiency.[23]

For noninfectious causes, owners must be committed to implementing programs that will improve reproductive efficiency. Herd performance must be continually monitored to maintain peak reproductive performance and to ensure that the underlying causes are not allowed to recur. Realistic time frames for improvement in reproductive performance as well as the appropriate variables to monitor should be agreed on prior to instituting corrective actions. Management of specific segments of the herd may be necessary to achieve optimal results.[24, 25] For herds in which a definitive diagnosis cannot be achieved, implementation of a program of sound reproductive management coupled with good sanitation and biosecurity measures may remedy the situation. Furthermore, progressive swine producers can institute programs[26] that make use of hormones or other pharmacologic agents to prevent reproductive losses from anestrus, anovulation, or problems encountered at parturition.

REFERENCES

1. Dial GD, Marsh WE, Polson DD, et al: Reproductive failure: Differential diagnosis. *In* Leman AD, Straw BE, Mengeling WL, et al. (eds): Diseases of Swine, ed 7. Ames, Iowa State University Press, 1992, pp 88–137.
2. Cutler R: Diagnosis of reproductive failure in sows manifested as abortion, mummified fetuses, stillbirths and weak neonates. *In* Morrow DA (ed): Current Therapy in Theriogenology, ed 2. Philadelphia, WB Saunders, 1986, pp 957–961.
3. Roberts SJ: Infertility in female swine. *In* Roberts SJ (ed): Veterinary Obstetrics and Genital Diseases (Theriogenology), ed 3. Woodstock, Vt, author, 1986, pp 636–653.
4. Straub OC: The important viral infections of pigs. Swine Health Prod 2:15, 1994.
5. Mengeling WL: Viral reproductive failure. *In* Morrow DA (ed): Current Therapy in Theriogenology, ed 2. Philadelphia, WB Saunders, 1986, pp 949–952.
6. Christianson WT, Joo HS: Porcine reproductive and respiratory syndrome: A review. Swine Health Prod 2:10, 1994.
7. Dee SA, Joo HS: Recurrent reproductive failure associated with porcine reproductive and respiratory syndrome in a swine herd. J Am Vet Med Assoc 205:1017, 1994.
8. Blaha T, Morrison RB, Molitor T, et al.: Update on porcine reproductive and respiratory syndrome (PRRS). Swine Health Prod 3:263, 1995.
9. Prieto C, Suarez P, Bautista JM, et al.: Semen changes in boars after experimental infection with porcine reproductive and respiratory syndrome (PRRS) virus. Theriogenology 45:383, 1996.
10. Hurtgen JP: Noninfectious infertility in swine. *In* Morrow DA (ed): Current Therapy in Theriogenology, ed 2. Philadelphia, WB Saunders, 1986, pp 962–966.
11. Gaughan JB, Cameron RDA, Dryden GM, et al.: Effect of selection for leanness on overall reproductive performance in Large White sows. Anim Sci 61:561, 1995.
12. Tokach MD, Reichert BT, Goodband RD, et al.: Amino acid requirements for lactating sows: New developments. Compendium Continuing Educ Pract Vet 18:S127, 1996.
13. Xue JL, Dial GD, Marsh WE, et al.: Multiple manifestations of season on reproductive performance of commercial swine. J Am Vet Med Assoc 204:1486, 1994.
14. Wilson MR, Dewey CE: The associations between weaning-to-estrus interval and sow efficiency. Swine Health Prod 1:10, 1993.
15. Thacker BJ: Detection and diagnosis of swine reproductive failure. *In* Morrow DA (ed): Current Therapy in Theriogenology, ed 2. Philadelphia, WB Saunders, 1986, pp 996–1001.
16. Tubbs RC: How to evaluate the reproductive efficiency of a swine operation. Vet Med 90:83, 1995.
17. Tubbs RC: Evaluating management causes of swine reproductive failures. Vet Med 90:195, 1995.
18. Almond GW, Richards RG: Evaluating porcine reproductive failure by the use of slaughterchecks. Compendium Continuing Educ Pract Vet 14:542, 1992.
19. Holler LD: Diagnosis of swine abortion. Swine Health Prod 2:29, 1994.
20. Collins J, Dee SA, Halbur P, et al.: Laboratory diagnosis of porcine reproductive and respiratory syndrome (PRRS) virus syndrome. Swine Health Prod 4:33, 1996.
21. Dee, SA, Joo HS, Pijoan C: Controlling the spread of PRRS virus in the breeding herd through management of the gilt pool. Swine Health Prod 3:64, 1995.
22. Ko, JCH, Althouse GC: Toxicity effects of latex gloves on boar spermatozoa. Swine Health Prod 1:24, 1993.
23. Carpenter J, Templeton C: Evaluation of a transmissible gastroenteritis virus eradication program in a breeding stock supply herd. Swine Health Prod 4:239, 1996.
24. Connor JF, Tubbs RC: Management of gestating sows. Compendium Continuing Educ Pract Vet 14:1395, 1992.
25. Doig GS, Friendship RM: Improving gilt performance. Compendium Continuing Educ Pract Vet 15:143, 1993.
26. Huhn U, Jochle W, Brussow KP: Techniques developed for the control of estrus, ovulation, and parturition in the East German pig industry: A review. Theriogenology 46:911, 1196.

Urinary Diseases

Consulting Editor
Richard F. Randle, D.V.M., M.S.

■ Therapeutic Management of Urinary Diseases

Vernon C. Langston, D.V.M., Ph.D., Diplomate, A.C.V.C.P.

As with all diseases, treatment of a urinary disorder is dependent on the pathophysiologic mechanisms involved. Because these mechanisms often overlap, so do the treatments. It is thus necessary to realize what objectives are attainable. Table 1 lists common urinary diseases and the therapies used.

CONTROL OF INFECTION

Although the general principles of rational antimicrobial therapy apply equally to urinary tract infections, there are special considerations that must be taken into account. First, when choosing an antimicrobial it should be remembered that different drugs concentrate in urine to varying degrees. Thus organisms that might normally be resistant to a drug at systemic concentrations can be successfully treated in cystitis or pyelonephritis. For example, ampicillin trihydrate does not normally produce plasma concentrations therapeutic against most *Escherichia coli* infections; however, *E. coli* cystitis can usually be treated by relatively low doses of this formulation. Indeed, cystitis caused by certain *E. coli* can even be treated with high-dose penicillin G, a drug to which similar systemic bacteria would almost certainly be resistant. Care should be taken to ensure that laboratory categorizations of sensitivity are based on urine and not serum concentrations.

Urinary pH also affects the activity of many antimicrobials. Agents such as the penicillins are more active in an acidic environment, and in selected cases such as *Corynebacterium renale* infections, urinary acidification may be of value. Acidification of the urine of food animals is absolutely essential for methenamine use, a urinary antiseptic that has been used anecdotally in veterinary medicine

Urinary tract infections can be notoriously resistant to treatment. It is generally recommended that first-time treatments last at least 10 days. If significant bacteriuria persists after 3 days of therapy, resistance is probable and a change in the antimicrobial might be indicated. In recurrent infections, treatment for 3 to 6 weeks is usually required, and even then the prognosis for cure may be guarded. When dealing with extremely resistant organisms, irrigation of the bladder with drugs that would otherwise be too costly or toxic for systemic administration may be an option. It is important not to overlook contributing factors such as urinary calculi, which may restrict urinary flow from the renal pelvis and thereby aggravate a pyelonephritis (calculi lodged in the ureter) or serve as a nidus

of infection in cystitis. Water and salt should always be provided, and animals that refuse to drink should receive isotonic fluids orally or parenterally to maintain hydration and fluid diuresis. Repeat urinalysis 1 to 2 weeks after ending therapy is prudent for detecting relapses. Care to avoid catheterization-induced reinfection is essential.

When an antimicrobial is selected for long-term use, preference should be given to drugs with minimal toxicity and residue potential. If culture and sensitivity results are lacking, penicillin G is commonly used in combating most gram-positive organisms (e.g., *C. renale*), whereas a cephalosporin such as ceftiofur might be more appropriate when a gram-negative or staphylococcal species is suspected. In the latter instance a potentiated sulfonamide may also have merit, although oral use would be limited to swine and preruminant calves. Even though clinical studies documenting its benefit are lacking, based on its pharmacokinetic profile, florfenicol may be a good alternative for the treatment of many resistant urinary tract infections provided that injection site tissue irritation is not a limiting factor.

Two antibiotic families used in other species could be used successfully to treat urinary tract infections were it not for serious regulatory limitations in food animals. Fluoroquinolones such as enrofloxacin could be an excellent choice; however, at the time of this writing, extralabel use of fluoroquinolones in food animals is banned in the United States because of concerns that increased use might promote fluoroquinolone bacterial resistance. An aminoglycoside could also be used; however, its toxicity and residue potential severely limit its use.

ALTERATION OF URINARY pH

The need to alter the pH of the urine in urinary tract infections has already been addressed. Another indication is urolithiasis, where acidification may help prevent the formation of struvite calculi. Ammonium chloride is given orally at 100 to 200 mg/kg twice daily (or 0.5% to 1% of the ration as dry matter) to prevent urolithiasis in steers and sheep.[1] It should not be used in patients with hepatic failure, renal failure, or metabolic acidosis. In the rare instance in which urinary alkalization is needed, sodium bicarbonate is usually administered.

INDUCTION OF DIURESIS

Fluid diuresis is commonly used for the treatment of urinary tract infections and for the prevention of urolithiasis. The promotion of high urine output will in essence "wash out" bacteria, cellular debris, crystals, and small calculi. Because forced fluid diuresis is not practical for the long-term prevention of urolithiasis, increased water intake (and subsequent urine production) is accomplished by the addition of salt to the diet at 4% (single-

Table 1
COMMON URINARY DISEASES AND THEIR TREATMENTS

Disease	Control Infection	Alter pH*	Induce Diuresis	Induce Micturition	Relax Urethral Tone
Cystitis	+	+	Fluid		
Pyelonephritis	+	+	Fluid		
Urolithiasis					+
Urolithiasis prevention		+	Increase water intake		
Bladder paralysis				+	
Renal failure			+		

+, may be used in treatment; fluid, forced fluid diuresis.
*Dependent on the specific disease entity.

source diet) to 12% (creep-fed calves). It has also been suggested that the increase in chloride ions may decrease the incidence of some forms of urolithiasis. Ammonium chloride has a transient (1- to 3-day) diuretic effect but should be thought of primarily as a urinary acidifier.

In those instances in which rehydration has failed to re-establish urinary flow, e.g., renal shutdown from shock or nephrotoxicity, aggressive diuresis using large doses (e.g., 5 to 10 mg/kg) of intravenous furosemide may be required. Alternatives to furosemide include osmotic diuretics such as mannitol (0.25 to 1 g/kg intravenously over a 5-minute period) or dextrose. The upper limit of the dose should not be exceeded even if administration of an osmotic diuretic fails to induce adequate urine flow, as overhydration and hyperosmolality may result in pulmonary edema. Congestive heart failure is also a contraindication to the use of osmotic diuretics. Dimethyl sulfoxide given intravenously as a 10% to 20% solution at 0.5 to 1.0 g/kg also acts as a potent diuretic, although appreciable hemolysis may occur. Dopamine infusion at 2 to 5 μg/kg/min may also be helpful in oliguria, although it requires continuous intravenous infusion and monitoring. Even though the thiazide diuretics are quite effective in nonrenal diseases such as udder edema or early congestive heart failure, they are not usually capable of inducing urine production in refractory renal cases.

It deserves mention that the commonly used sedative xylazine has a significant diuretic action.[2] In those instances in which bladder rupture is imminent, sedation with an alternative to xylazine may be preferable.

INDUCTION OF MICTURITION

Urinalysis is pivotal to the diagnosis of most urinary diseases, and hence obtaining a urine sample is basic to the diagnostic process. Although perineal stimulation ("feathering") and catheterization are effective means of accomplishing this in the female, obtaining a urine sample from a male is more difficult. Diuretic induction of urine flow with subsequent urination is commonly used, although this prohibits a determination of urine specific gravity and will dilute many constituents. If a more representative urinalysis is desired, bethanechol may be administered subcutaneously at 0.075 mg/kg to directly induce contraction of the detrusor muscle. Usually the animal will urinate within 20 minutes of injection. Bethanechol has been used in humans and small animals for the management of bladder paralysis postobstruction or following spinal lesions and should likewise be useful in large animals for similar conditions. Urinary or gastrointestinal obstruction is a strict contraindication to the use of bethanechol. Intravenous injection can cause pronounced bradycardia and collapse.

RELAXATION OF URETHRAL TONE

Occasionally, relaxation of urethral tone has been advocated as an aid in the treatment of urolithiasis. Aminopromazine was most commonly used for this purpose but is no longer available in the United States. Acepromazine or similar phenothiazine tranquilizers have been advocated in urolithiasis for their ability to relax the internal urinary sphincter, relieve smooth muscle spasms (proximal urethra), and relax the retractor penis muscle to allow for partial extension of the penis.[3] All these benefits are thought to be due to the α-antagonistic effects of acepromazine. The true benefit of such drugs in urolithiasis remains unproven and is probably dependent on the severity of an individual case and the location of the blockage. Relative contraindications against the use of acepromazine include hypotension, anemia (acepromazine causes short-term but significant lowering of the packed-cell volume), animals prone to hypothermia, recent exposure to other cholinesterase inhibitors such as organophosphate or carbamate insecticides, or animals prone to seizures.[4] Although penile paralysis is a rare but serious side effect in stallions, this has not been reported in the bull or boar. In rare instances, some blockages may be cleared by backflushing the urethra. If this is attempted, the use of a local anesthetic as the flushing solution (e.g., 0.5% lidocaine) will relieve urethral spasm.

AVOIDANCE OF DRUG-INDUCED NEPHROTOXICITY

A variety of therapeutic agents are potentially nephrotoxic. Chief among these are the aminoglycoside, sulfonamide, and tetracycline antimicrobials and nonsteroidal anti-inflammatory drugs.

Nephrotoxicity from aminoglycoside antibiotics is well known by most practitioners. Although their use is not banned in the United States, aminoglycoside administration is highly discouraged because of residue concerns, and accordingly, their use has decreased significantly. If aminoglycoside use is considered for the rare multiresistant infection, the reader is referred to the prior edition of this text for methods to minimize the nephrotoxic potential of this group of drugs.

The nephrotoxicity associated with sulfonamides is due to crystalluria. This is primarily a problem with the older sulfonamides such as sulfathiazole when used in species that produce an acidic urine. As long as hydration is well maintained and the newer agents are used, crystalluria is rarely a concern.

The tetracyclines have long been known to be capable of worsening azotemia by their antianabolic properties. Also, a Fanconi-like syndrome is associated with the use of outdated tetracyclines. Most of the tetracycline-induced nephrotoxicities, however, have been seen when high-dose (i.e., 20 mg/kg twice daily) oxytetracycline was administered to animals suffering from *Pasteurella* pneumonia or coliform mastitis. It now appears that the endotoxemia associated with either disease acts synergistically to induce proximal tubular damage.

Nonsteroidal anti-inflammatory drugs are not generally considered to be potent nephrotoxins; however, they can induce severe tubular damage, especially if other nephrotoxins are given concomitantly (e.g., an aminoglycoside) or if hypotension or dehydration is present. Pathologically this is manifested as a renal papillary necrosis or interstitial nephritis.

Other potentially nephrotoxic therapeutic agents used in food animals include monensin, vitamin D, and vitamin K_3.[5]

REFERENCES

1. Bushman DH, Emerick RJ, Embry LB: Effect of various chlorides and calcium carbonate on calcium, phosphorus, sodium, potassium and chloride balance and their relationship to urinary calculi in lambs. J Anim Sci 27:490–496, 1968.
2. Thurmon JC, Nelson DR, Hartsfield SM, et al: Effects of xylazine hydrochloride on urine in cattle. Aust Vet J 54:178–180, 1978.
3. Oehme FW, Tillmann H: Diagnosis and treatment of ruminant urolithiasis. J Am Vet Med Assoc 147:1331–1339, 1965.
4. USP DI, vol 1, Drug Information for the Health Care Professional, Sept update. The United States Pharmacopeia Convention, Rockville, Md, 1997.
5. Rebhun WC, Tennant BC: Vitamin K_3-induced renal toxicosis in the horse. J Am Vet Med Assoc 184:1237–1239, 1982.

■ Urolithiasis in Food Animals (Urinary Calculi, Waterbelly, Calculosis)

James G. Floyd, Jr., D.V.M., M.S.

Urolithiasis in domestic food animals is a disease of significant economic importance that results from urinary tract obstruction by mineral-protein calculi. Urolithiasis produces losses from death and from condemnation of carcasses contaminated by urine. Estimates of losses are 0.6% of the annual production in the U.S. cattle industry[1] and 4% of all deaths in feedyard lambs.[2]

Castrated male ruminants between 5 and 18 months old are primarily affected by urinary calculi and fall into two main classes: (1) feedlot animals with grain as a high percentage of their diets and (2) pastured animals grazing on grasses high in silicates or oxalates.[1, 3, 4] Swine are rarely afflicted with urolithiasis, although the condition is sporadically found in all ages and types of hogs.

PATHOGENESIS

Urolithiasis develops in ruminants as a result of mineral precipitation and binding onto an organic matrix, concretion of the crystallized matrix into urolith(s), and partial or total occlusion of the ureter or urethra by the urolith(s).[5] The proteinaceous matrix that serves as a nidus for mineral crystallization can be desquamated epithelial cells or other urinary tract cellular and organic debris. This debris may collect as a result of infection, inflammation, and factors such as parenteral administration or ingestion of estrogenic substances that promote hypertrophy and keratinization of the accessory sex glands. Higher levels of mucoproteins in the urine associated with rations high in

concentrates and low in roughage may act as a cementing factor and enhance calculus formation.[5]

Male ruminants are predisposed to calculosis because their urethral diameter is smaller than that of females. Urolithiasis occurs in intact bulls and rams[3, 6, 7]; however, males castrated at a young age are at increased risk because their urethral diameter is smaller as a result of their decreased exposure to androgens.[8] Urolithiasis is relatively rare in females, although cases of female calves with ruptured bladders resulting from calculi have been reported.[9] Ureterolithiasis has been reported in a mature cow as a sequela to nephrolithiasis.[10]

Interactions of several dietary and physiologic factors determine the type of urinary calculi formed by ruminants. Urine pH is a major factor determining calculus composition. The range of normal urine pH of ruminants is 7.0 to 9.5.[11, 12] When urine pH exceeds 8.5, calcium carbonate and phosphate crystals begin to precipitate as urine colloids lose their ability to behave as a protective gel.[5, 11, 12] Alkaline urine favors the formation of calcium and magnesium phosphates and carbonates, triple phosphates (calcium, ammonium, and magnesium phosphate calculi), and iron carbonate.[11] Acid urine promotes the formation of oxalate and xanthine calculi. The relationship between the formation of siliceous calculi and urine pH is less clear, although alkali-forming diets have tended to promote silica urolithiasis.[4, 13]

Diet is a main determinant of the type of urinary calculi that may develop. Feedlot cattle and sheep receiving grain-based feedlot rations tend to form phosphate (calcium, ammonium, and magnesium) calculi. Cattle on western U.S. range pastures with grasses high in silica tend to form siliceous calculi.[1] Carbonates (calcium, ammonium, and magnesium) or oxalates tend to be the predominant calculi formed in the urine of grazing animals when grass silica concentrations are not high, such as on clover pastures and with plants high in oxalates.[4, 5, 11] Oxalate calculi in steers receiving feed have been associated with fescue (*Festuca* spp.) seed screenings in the diet.[14] Xanthine calculi have been reported in sheep in New Zealand but are not common in the United States.[5] Elevated dietary magnesium has been experimentally shown to cause urolithiasis in growing male calves.[15, 16]

The gross appearance of calculi differs depending on their predominant chemical composition. Phosphatic calculi tend to be numerous and very small and form a gritty urinary "sludge."[11] These calculi are often noticed as "grit" or "sand" on the preputial hairs of male cattle, sheep, or goats. Phosphatic calculi are smooth and have a softer consistency than silicate calculi.[17] Siliceous calculi tend to be single and form rough, hard white stones of 4 to 7 mm.[11, 17]

Management factors can contribute to the incidence of urolithiasis. Water deprivation from frozen pumps or tanks can cause a relative concentration of urinary mineral solutes and increase the likelihood of their precipitation. Dehydration can also promote urolithiasis by urinary concentration. Vitamin A deficiency, vitamin D excess, and exposure to phytoestrogens such as in subterranean clover have also been implicated.[4, 5] In one study, the estrogenic growth promotant diethylstilbestrol, now banned from use in the United States, was associated with fatal urolithiasis in wethers.[5] There is no known association between urinary calculosis and the estrogenic growth-promoting implants currently approved in the United States.

CLINICAL SIGNS

The course of urolithiasis depends on the location and degree of urinary tract occlusion. Uroliths can be present in the kidney, urine, bladder, or urethral mucosa without necessarily causing obstruction of urinary outflow. Nephroliths do not usually cause clinical signs unless portions of the stone are passed and result in ureteral obstruction and hydronephrosis.[5, 10, 17] Clinical disease occurs when urinary outflow is significantly obstructed, which usually occurs when a calculus lodges in the urethra.[17] Predilective sites of entrapment in the urethra are the ischial arch, the proximal flexure of the penis, and the urethral orifice. In small ruminant males the urethral process is often a site of obstruction. Uroliths are often entrapped in multiple sites.

Clinical signs accompanying partial occlusion of urinary outflow are uneasiness, signs of abdominal pain, stranguria, dribbling urine, and hematuria. Owners or herdsmen may describe an animal afflicted with urolithiasis as being constipated or suffering from gastrointestinal disease. The urethra at the point of calculus obstruction often becomes inflamed and swollen, further decreasing the size of the lumen and exacerbating the occlusion. With total occlusion the animal displays signs of colic, bruxism, rear leg stamping, circling motion of the tail, and decreased feed consumption.[1, 18] Rectal palpation may reveal a pulsating urethra and distention of the bladder.[1]

Within 48 hours after total obstruction of the lower urinary tract a rupture of the bladder or urethra is likely. These animals have a distended abdomen ("waterbelly") with a transmitted fluid wave apparent on ballottement. The differential diagnosis includes bloat, ascites, peritonitis, and pneumonia. Azotemia develops over a period of days, followed by coma and death.[5] If the urethra ruptures, the subcutaneous tissues of the ventral portion of the abdomen become infiltrated with urine, especially in the preputial region. The differential diagnosis includes penile hematoma and preputial abscess.[18] Necrosis and sloughing of the skin over these areas will occur if the animal does not die sooner, with drainage of urine from the deeper tissues resulting in a more prolonged course of disease.[5] Serum urea nitrogen concentrations in cases of bladder or urethral rupture have been reported to be over 200 mg/dL.[17]

Edematous swelling with urinous fluid in the prepuce and ventral abdominal wall has been reported in a lamb with obstructive urolithiasis without bladder or urethral rupture.[19] This report hypothesized that increased urinary pressure forced urine through the accessory glands in the pelvic urethra.

Cystourethrography has been used as a diagnostic tool to differentiate urolithiasis from cystitis in small ruminants and miniature pet pigs.[20, 21] Ultrasonographic measurements of a normal kidney, urinary bladder, and urethra have been made in a group of 20 White Alpine rams as a benchmark for comparison with sheep exhibiting signs of urinary tract disease, although it is unknown how applicable these measurements are across breeds.[22]

Urolithiasis does not always lead to total obstruction of the urinary tract. Chronic partial urethral obstruction by calculi resulting in hydronephrosis, hydroureter, and chronic end-stage renal disease has been reported in a 13-month-old steer.[23]

Although older swine are occasionally found with calculi located in the renal pelvis,[11] urolithiasis is more prevalent in miniature pet pigs than in commercial hogs. Although commercial miniature pig chows are not usually calculogenic, the day-to-day diets of many pet pigs may be calculogenic because of their variability, with table scraps and other treats often being a major portion of the diet.

TREATMENT

Treatment of urolithiasis involves restoration of urinary flow, repair of damaged and contaminated tissues with time, and in many cases, salvage of the animal. Total recovery of normal urinary excretory and reproductive function following treatment for urolithiasis is possible but often not the rule; therefore, slaughter is often the most cost-effective course of action.

A reasonable course of action in feedlot steers or wethers in early stages of clinical urolithiasis is immediate slaughter before bladder or urethral rupture.[4] This salvages the animal and reduces the cost of surgery and treatment, which is prudent in light of the probable recurrence of multiple phosphatic calculi in animals on feedlot diets.[17] Bladder or urethral rupture and infiltration of the ventral abdominal region with urine necessitates that the obstruction be removed to relieve azotemia and acidosis. The animal may then recover and be salvaged for slaughter when the tissues become edible.[17] Linear or stab incisions may be made lateral to the prepuce to drain edematous tissues in cases of urethral rupture, but care must be exercised to avoid the abdominal vasculature.[4] About 30 days is required for tissue damage to resolve prior to slaughter.[24]

Treatment alternatives chosen in cases of urolithiasis depend on the type of animal affected, the type of calculi, and the stage of the disease. Clients will often desire more aggressive treatment of intact males valued as sires or small ruminants valued as pets despite a relatively poor prognosis in more advanced cases. If recovery of an obstructed male to breeding or long-term survival is desired, avoiding trauma to the urethra should be a primary goal. Trauma from repeat catheterization, urethrotomy, or temporary urethrostomy are often followed by the development of a urethral stricture and recurrence of obstructive urolithiasis.

Medical Treatment

Phenothiazine tranquilizers such as acepromazine maleate may promote passage of a urethrolith in a steer or bull if administered shortly after partial obstruction occurs in steers. Medical therapy does not generally succeed in passing uroliths in small ruminants.[25]

Supportive therapy includes intravenous fluids to correct dehydration and electrolyte imbalances. In cases of uroperitoneum, particularly when large volumes of fluid have built up, intravenous fluids may be necessary to prevent shock during drainage.[25] Antibiotic therapy is usually indicated because urolithiasis is often accompanied by urinary tract infection and inflammation. If antibiotics are administered, appropriate withdrawal times should be observed before slaughter. Extended withdrawal times may be required because azotemic animals may have a decreased ability to eliminate drugs. Oral urinary acidifiers such as 3 oz of ammonium chloride per day (in 1-oz capsules or as a feed additive) are essential to dissolve calculi.[26]

Urethral catheterization retrograde from the glans penis is relatively unsuccessful in ruminants and swine because the urethral diverticulum present at the level of the ischial arch precludes the passage of normal catheters past that point.[7, 25] The urethral diverticulum has been successfully avoided by the use of a precurved catheter such as that used for retrograde cystourethrography[20]; however, this equipment is not routinely available. Normograde urethral catheterization is frequently used to flush the urethra during celiotomy and bladder repair.[7]

Surgical Treatment

Published success rates for the surgical treatment of urolithiasis range from 35.3% to 95%.[25, 27] The diversity of outcomes reflects differences in populations of animals, urinary tract damage, surgical procedures, and follow-up evaluation periods. In general, traumatized reproductive tracts with rupture and necrosis create a poorer prognosis for long-term successful surgical treatment.

Urethrotomy over the site of the calculus, determined by palpation and/or catheterization, has been commonly used, particularly when attempting to preserve a male's breeding ability.[25] Stone removal at the proximal sigmoid flexure of the penis can be accomplished through a prescrotal approach in a laterally recumbent animal. In some cases, using a Backhaus towel clamp to crack the stone will allow the pieces to pass. If this fails after one or two attempts, a urethrotomy over the site of obstruction may be performed.[17]

A parapenile urethrotomy approach was used to remove obstructing uroliths in a report of three bulls and five bullocks.[28] With a tourniquet applied to the penis on either side of the obstruction, the urethrotomy was accomplished on the flattened lateral aspect of the penis through the corpus cavernosum penis. The authors stated that this approach eliminated postsurgical strictures, although follow-up was only 10 days.

Urethral process amputation in small ruminants is easily accomplished, and that structure can be sacrificed because it is not required for reproductive success. However, patency is usually restored for only a few hours because of other sites of blockage. Urethral process amputation provided less than 36 hours of relief of obstruction in 14 of 16 cases in one report.[29]

Catheterization following ischial urethrotomy has been successful in bulls and steers.[4, 24] If the urethral obstruction can be relieved, a ruptured bladder will often heal without surgical repair, particularly if the bladder is ruptured on the dorsal aspect.[25] Catheters inserted through ischial urethrotomy incisions have been installed to drain near the urethrotomy site as a salvage procedure for bulls and steers weighing over 700 lb.[24] Alternatively, the catheter may be passed into the bladder with the other end inserted distal along the urethra to emerge and drain at the prepuce.[17] In that case, the catheter can be removed after several days when normal urinary function is restored.

Urethrostomy with penile amputation is appropriate for salvage, with or without urethral fistulization (splitting the dorsal urethra along the midline from the distal aspect of the penile stump to the level of the incision, with mucosal flaps sutured to the skin).[4, 25, 26] A stricture may result if more than 4 weeks elapse before slaughter. A "high urethrostomy" (subischial) can be done with the animal standing. A "low urethrostomy" (postscrotal) is performed at the dorsal aspect of the scrotum with the animal in dorsal or lateral recumbency. Success depends on the degree of concurrent urinary tract trauma and necrosis, with success rates of 38.5% to 95% being reported.[25]

Urethrostomy without penile amputation may preserve breeding status and can be accomplished with the urethral mucosa sutured to the skin.[25] Retrograde flushing can then be used to dislodge calculi and restore urine flow. Strictures or recurrence of urolithiasis has occurred in small ruminants at rates of 45%, 58%, and 78% within a few months after surgery.[25] One report had only a 17% 1-year survival rate,[30] whereas another had a survival rate of 55% at a median follow-up period of 27 months, although 40% of those animals had more than one perineal urethrostomy performed.[29] The lack of long-term success in many small ruminant cases has prompted the recommendation that they not be kept longer than 3 to 4 months.[30, 31]

Cystotomy plus removal of calculi in the bladder, in conjunction with intraoperative normograde and retrograde urethral flushing, was successful in seven of eight small ruminants with obstructive urolithiasis.[29] The six goats and one sheep were healthy at a median follow-up of 23 months, with a range of 5 to 55 months. The authors of this study concluded that cystotomy was more effective than perineal urethrostomy for the management of urolithiasis in small ruminants. Cystotomy may be the procedure of choice in small ruminants in which longevity or maintenance of breeding ability is desired.

Tube cystostomy through a ventral paramedian approach has been successfully used in both small ruminants[2, 32] and cattle[4, 26] as a method of relieving urinary obstruction without incising the urethra. In small ruminants a new Foley catheter is surgically placed in the bladder during celiotomy and bladder repair. The catheter is then sutured into the incision in the ventral aspect of the abdomen to allow for periodic outflow of urine and bladder irrigation with an acetic acid (pH 4.5) solution. This technique is useful in cases of a ruptured bladder or urethra and should be considered when longer-term longevity and salvation of a breeding male are desired.[4] Once urinary outflow has been established and supportive therapies have alleviated inflammation and swelling and dissolved lodged calculi, the catheter can be pulled. Twelve of 15 small ruminants had urethral obstruction successfully relieved by tube cystostomy, with a mean of 11.5 days until free urination was restored and 14.4 days until the tube was removed.[2] The authors concluded that tube cystostomy should be considered as a primary treatment for urethral obstruction in small ruminants with or without rupture of the bladder because of its relative success in comparison to urethrotomy or perineal urethrostomy.

Tube cystostomy has also been reported to be successful in miniature pigs with obstructive urolithiasis.[2] Vietnamese pot-bellied pigs have also been surgically treated with permanent extrapelvic urinary diversion. In one case of obstructive urolithiasis, an extrapelvic urethral anastomosis was performed.[21] In another case of obstructive urolithiasis in a miniature pig that had previously undergone perineal urethrostomy followed by long-term hemorrhage at the surgical site, a permanent urethro-preputial anastomosis was performed.[21]

PREVENTION

Successful prevention of urolithiasis may be accomplished through dietary and water management.

In steers and sheep receiving high-phosphorus diets, increased feeding of calcium can prevent calculosis.[33, 34] Calcium-to-phosphorus ratios of 1.2:1 are normally recommended by the National Research Council, but increasing the ratio up to 2:1 in cattle and up to 2.5:1 in sheep has been advocated as anticalculogenic.[5, 35] On cereal grain diets that are not high in silica, reducing the phosphorus content to less than 0.6% will decrease urolithiasis in sheep.[36] Minerals mixed in sheep feed are more successful than if offered as a free choice.[35]

The occurrence of urolithiasis in feedlot lambs was related to concentrations of magnesium and phosphorus in the diet. At low (0.11%) phosphorus concentrations and magnesium concentrations of 0.63%, urolithiasis did not occur.[16] However, when dietary phosphorus concentrations exceeded 0.30%, the incidence of urolithiasis increased from 8% at a dietary magnesium concentration of 0.35% to an incidence of 100% at a magnesium concentration of 0.65%.

The relationship of silica urolithiasis to calcium-to-phosphorus ratios differs from that in phosphate urolithiasis. In high-silica diets, increasing calcium-to-phosphorus ratios by adding calcium to a level of 0.6% tended to promote the formation of silica uroliths in lambs.[13] Therefore, in the presence of diets or forage likely to cause silica urolith formation, prevention may be enhanced by decreasing the calcium-to-phosphorus ratio to 0.7:1 to 1:1 by adding phosphorus.[4]

Adding up to 4% salt (NaCl) to the feedlot ration has been effective in steers and lambs as a method of increasing urine volume in the presence of adequate drinking water.[5, 35] However, salt can act as an intake limiter, which may decrease gains if excessive salt is added.[4, 36] The urine-diluting effect of salt may also be used as a preventive in cattle grazing on high-silica grasses. It has been recommended that calves be creep-fed with a high-salt supplement during the last 60 days before weaning by starting out with a salt-free supplement and gradually increasing to one with 12% NaCl.[5]

Lowering the urine pH by feeding urine acidifiers such as

ammonium chloride has been effective. Recommendations for daily amounts range from 7.1 to 10 g for sheep and 45 g for steers.[5,35] To prevent silica urolith formation, urine acidification through the addition of 1% ammonium chloride to a wether lamb diet containing 3.3% SiO_2 and a reduction in the dietary Ca to P ratio were effective.[13]

Feeding ammonium or calcium chloride at 1.5% of the diet will reduce urine pH and decrease urolith formation in ruminants ingesting high-phosphorus cereal grain diets.[4,36] The palatability problems that may occur with ammonium chloride can be avoided by substituting ammonium sulfate as a urinary acidifier in the diet of feedlot steers.[4] However, because polioencephalomalacia may be related to increased sulfate intake,[5] caution should be exercised.

Managers should always be aware of the role of a reliable source of palatable water at all times in the prevention of calculosis. Clean water may be consumed preferentially, although individual animal preferences may not always make this hold true. The availability of water is particularly critical in cold weather because of the danger of a freeze.

REFERENCES

1. Jensen R, Mackey DR: Diseases of Feedlot Cattle, ed 3. Philadelphia, Lea & Febiger, 1979, pp 262–267.
2. Rakestraw PC, Fubini SL, Gilbert RO, et al: Tube cystostomy for treatment of obstructive urolithiasis in small ruminants. Vet Surg 24:498–505, 1995.
3. Ogaa JS, Agumbah GJO, Patel JH, et al: Massive obstructive urolithiasis in a bull used for artificial insemination. Vet Rec 117:664–666, 1985.
4. Larson BL: Identifying, treating, and preventing bovine urolithiasis. Vet Med 91:366–377, 1996.
5. Radostits OM, Blood DC, Gay CC: Veterinary Medicine, ed 8. London, Baillière Tindall, 1994, pp 450–455, 1699–1702.
6. Murray MJ: Urolithiasis in a ram. Compend Contin Educ 7(suppl):269–273, 1985.
7. Tulleners EP, Hamilton GF, Farrow CS: Surgical repair of ruptured urinary bladder in a ram. J Am Vet Med Assoc 177:708–709, 1980.
8. Bailey CB: Siliceous urinary calculi in bulls, steers and partial castrates. Can J Anim Sci 55:187–191, 1975.
9. Gera KL, Nigam JM: Urolithiasis in bovines. Indian Vet J 56:417–423, 1979.
10. Divers TJ, Reef VB, Roby KA: Nephrolithiasis resulting in intermittent ureteral obstruction in a cow. Cornell Vet 79:143–149, 1988.
11. Jubb KFV, Kennedy PC: Pathology of Domestic Animals, vol 2, ed 2. New York, Academic Press, 1970, pp 322–326.
12. Sorensen DK: Urinary system. In Amstutz HE (ed): Bovine Medicine and Surgery, ed 2. Santa Barbara, Calif, American Veterinary Publications, 1980, pp 841–846.
13. Stewart SR, Emerick RJ, Pritchard RH: Effects of dietary ammonium chloride and variations in calcium to phosphorus ratio on silica urolithiasis in sheep. J Anim Sci 69:2225–2229, 1991.
14. Waltner-Toews D, Meadows DH: Urolithiasis in a herd of beef cattle associated with oxalate ingestion. Can Vet J 21:61–62, 1980.
15. Kallfelz FA, Ahmed AS, Wallace RJ, et al: Dietary magnesium and urolithiasis in growing calves. Cornell Vet 77:33–45, 1986.
16. Poole DBR: Observations on the role of magnesium and phosphorus in the aetiology of urolithiasis in male sheep. Irish Vet J 42:60–63, 1989.
17. Walker DF: Surgery of the urinary tract. In Walker DF, Vaughan JT (eds): Bovine and Equine Urogenital Surgery. Philadelphia, Lea & Febiger, 1980, pp 59–66.
18. Powe TA: Diseases of the urinary system. In Howard J (ed): Current Veterinary Therapy: Food Animal Practice, ed 2. Philadelphia, WB Saunders, 1986, pp 816–818.
19. King JM: Urethral calculi in a lamb. Vet Med 87:1080, 1992.
20. van Weeren PR, Klein WR, Voorhout G: Urolithiasis in small ruminants II. Cysto-urethrography as a new aid in diagnosis. Vet Q 9:79–83, 1987.
21. Mann FA, Cowart RP, McClure RC, et al: Permanent urinary diversion in two Vietnamese pot-bellied pigs by extrapelvic urethral
or urethropreputial anastomosis. J Am Vet Med Assoc 205:1157–1160, 1994.
22. Braun, U, Schefer U, Fohn J: Urinary tract ultrasonography in normal rams and in rams with obstructive urolithiasis. Can Vet J 33:654–659, 1992.
23. Aldridge BM, Garry FB: Chronic partial obstructive urolithiasis causing hydronephrosis and chronic renal failure in a steer. Cornell Vet 82:311–317, 1992.
24. Winter RB, Hawkins LL, Holtman DE, et al: Catheterization: An effective method of treating bovine urethral calculi. Vet Med 82:1261–1268, 1987.
25. Van Metre DC, House JK, Smith BP, et al: Obstructive urolithiasis in ruminants: Medical treatment and urethral surgery. Compend Contin Educ 18:317–328, 1996.
26. Noordsy JL: Food Animal Surgery, ed 3. Trenton, NJ, Veterinary Learning Systems, 1994, pp 199–208.
27. Gasthuys F, Steenhaut M, De Moor A, et al: Surgical treatment of urethral obstruction due to urolithiasis in male cattle: A review of 85 cases. Vet Rec 133:522–526, 1993.
28. Mouli SP: Parapenile urethral penotomy—a new technique to treat penile urolithiasis in bovines. Indian Vet J 69:1034–1036, 1992.
29. Haven ML, Bowman KF, Engelbert TA, et al: Surgical management of urolithiasis in small ruminants. Cornell Vet 83:47–55, 1993.
30. van Weeren PR, Klein WR, Voorhout G: Urolithiasis in small ruminants I. A retrospective evaluation of urethrostomy. Vet Q 9:76–79, 1987.
31. Oehme FW, Tillmann H: Diagnosis and treatment of ruminant urolithiasis. J Am Vet Med Assoc 147:1331–1339, 1965.
32. Cockcroft PD: Dissolution of obstructive urethral uroliths in a ram. Vet Rec 132:486, 1993.
33. Emerick RJ, Embry LB: Calcium and phosphorus levels related to the development of phosphate urinary calculi in sheep. J Anim Sci 22:510–513, 1963.
34. Huntington GB, Emerick RJ: Oxalate urinary calculi in beef steers. Am J Vet Res 45:180–182, 1984.
35. Pierson RE, Kimberling C: Commercial lamb feedlot management. In Howard J (ed): Current Veterinary Therapy: Food Animal Practice, ed 2. Philadelphia, WB Saunders, 1986, p 179.
36. Hay L: Prevention and treatment of urolithiasis in sheep. In Practice 12:87–91, 1990.

■ Urinary Disorders Associated With the Neonate

Richard F. Randle, D.V.M., M.S.

CONGENITAL DEFECTS

The occurrence of congenital anomalies associated with the urinary system in ruminant species is rare. Often, congenital defects are multiple and associated with more than one body system. A variety of urinary system defects have been recorded and include hydronephrosis, polycystic kidneys, renal dysgenesis, renal agenesis, hypospadias, ectopic ureter, and patent urachus.

Patent Urachus

At birth, the urachus should close rapidly in association with rupture of the umbilical cord. Situations that cause delayed or incomplete closure of the urachus can result in this condition. Congenital patent urachus in ruminants is rare; however, infections of other umbilical structures or the urachus itself may result in incomplete closure and lead to an acquired patent urachus after birth. Aggressive manipulation of the umbilical cord at parturition may predispose to an acquired patent urachus.

Patent urachus is most often diagnosed by direct visualization of urine dripping from the urachus or a persistently wet umbilical stump. Retrograde or intravenous contrast radiography may also be used as an aid in diagnosing a patent urachus.

The usual therapy is surgical removal of the entire urachus. The associated arteries and veins are typically ligated and removed as well. A common sequela of a patent urachus is cystitis secondary to ascending infections; therefore, systemic antimicrobials are indicated. Conservative therapy may be considered and consists of medical management of infection and cauterization of the urachus with such agents as silver nitrate, iodine, or phenol. A potential problem exists with this therapy in that cauterization of the urachus at the umbilical stump may trap organisms higher up in the urachus and lead to infection and urachal abscessation necessitating surgery later.

Polycystic Kidneys

The most commonly reported congenital defect seen in most species is polycystic kidneys. Typically, the condition is unilateral, and no clinical signs appear because of compensation by the other kidney. If the defect is extensive and bilateral, the animal is usually stillborn or dies in the perinatal period. Frequently, other congenital anomalies are found in these animals.

Most often this condition is reported as a finding at necropsy. The affected kidney is enlarged and composed of either a few large cysts or numerous small cysts. A grossly enlarged kidney may be encountered on rectal examination in adult large ruminants. Ultrasonography may aid in the diagnosis of polycystic kidneys.

Renal Oxalosis

Renal oxalosis results from excessive deposition of calcium oxalate crystals in the glomeruli, tubules, and collecting ducts. This condition has been described in aborted fetuses and neonatal calves that have not been exposed to a known oxalate source. Calves with renal oxalosis have a frequent occurrence of cardiac and musculoskeletal defects such as arthrogryposis, osteopetrosis, and chondrodysplasia, which suggests a metabolic disorder involving glycine.

OMPHALITIS

Inflammation of the umbilical arteries, umbilical vein, urachus, or surrounding tissues is termed omphalitis. These structures combine to form the umbilicus, which represents the vestige of the fetal-maternal connection. The umbilical vein, which carries oxygenated blood from the placenta to the fetus via the liver and ductus venosus, becomes the round ligament of the liver. The two umbilical arteries, which carry waste materials from the fetus to the placenta, become the round ligaments of the bladder. The remnant of the urachus becomes incorporated into the apex of the bladder.

Pathogenesis

At parturition, the umbilical arteries retract into the abdomen and close by smooth muscle contraction in response to the increased partial pressure of oxygen in the blood, and the umbilical vein and urachus remain outside the abdomen. The vein closes rapidly by smooth muscle contraction, and the urachus shrinks and dries within a few days.

Of the umbilical structures, the urachus is the most commonly infected in calves, with *Actinomyces pyogenes* being the most frequently identified organism involved. *Escherichia coli*, *Proteus*,

Enterococcus, *Streptococcus*, and *Staphylococcus* species have also been identified as causative agents; therefore, antimicrobial therapy should be based on culture results.

Clinical Signs

Clinical signs associated with omphalitis may be varied. Usually the animal has a history of purulent drainage from the umbilicus at 1 to 2 weeks of age. The umbilicus may be enlarged, firm, hot, and painful on palpation. In approximately 25% of the cases there is an associated umbilical hernia. The animals may have concurrent systemic infections such as bacteremia, septic arthritis, pneumonia, diarrhea, uveitis, or peritonitis. Some animals show no evidence of drainage or inflammation at the umbilicus but are febrile, appear depressed, and are tender in the abdomen on palpation. Other clinical signs include dysuria, pollakiuria, and cystitis as a result of direct communication between the urachus and the bladder or interference with filling and emptying of the bladder.

Diagnosis

Infections of the umbilicus are easily identified in the presence of a draining tract or enlarged umbilicus. For determining the extent of urachal involvement, a metal probe or radiopaque contrast material can be placed in the draining tract and radiographs taken. Radiographic findings include a cranioventrally positioned bladder and a radiopaque structure ventral to the bladder. Deep palpation above the umbilicus with the animal either standing or in lateral recumbency may reveal an abdominal mass or painful areas. Ultrasonography may also be used as an aid in determining involvement of the various umbilical structures. Omphalitis should be considered in neonates with a normal-appearing umbilicus but that are unthrifty or have a fever of unknown origin.

Treatment

The treatment of choice is exploratory laparotomy and surgical excision of the abscesses. Urachal infections extending into the bladder require excision of the apex of the bladder and ligation of the umbilical arteries. In the absence of systemic involvement, the prognosis is good and recovery is usually uneventful.

Prevention

The control of umbilical infections centers on good sanitation and hygiene at parturition. The use of astringents and disinfectants on the umbilicus at birth is widely practiced, but there is limited evidence that this is of significant benefit.

BIBLIOGRAPHY

Baxter GM: Umbilical masses in calves: Diagnosis, treatment, and complications. Compend Contin Educ 11:505–513, 1989.

Dennis SM: Urogenital defects in sheep. Vet Rec 105:344–347, 1979.

Fetcher A: Renal disease in cattle. Part I. Causative agents. Compend Contin Educ 7(suppl):701–708, 1985.

Smith BP: Large Animal Internal Medicine. St Louis, CV Mosby, 1990, pp 370–372.

Trent AM, Smith DE: Surgical management of umbilical masses with associated umbilical cord remnant infections in calves. J Am Vet Med Assoc 185:1531–1534, 1984.

■ Renal Toxicants

Dennis J. Blodgett, D.V.M., Ph.D.

Primary renal toxicoses in food animal veterinary medicine occur relatively infrequently. Oak toxicosis is by far the most common renal toxicosis diagnosed and is discussed in some detail. Other primary renal toxicants are listed in tabular form according to the species that are most likely affected (Tables 1 through 3). Toxicants capable of producing secondary renal lesions are also listed in these tables. Therapeutic drugs associated with renal problems in food animals are discussed in another section.

OAK POISONING

Occurrence

More than 60 species of oak (*Quercus*) are found in North America. Oak species range from shrubs to large trees and are classified as either white or black oak. The acorns of white oak mature in 1 year, whereas black oak species require 2 years for acorn development. Different species of oak do not cause variation in the clinical syndrome. All species of oak should be considered toxic.

Oak toxicoses occur as seasonal problems. In the southwestern United States, shin oak (*Quercus harvardii*) and Gamble's oak (*Quercus gambelii*) cause problems in the spring of the year when new buds and leaves are heavily ingested. Much of the rest of the United States has problems in the fall when animals ingest acorns. More cases occur following summer droughts when forage is scarce or as a result of heavy rains or winds dislodging acorns. Cases in the fall usually cease several weeks after the first hard frost. Immature, green leaves and acorns are more toxic than mature leaves and acorns.

Oak poisoning affects cattle primarily, although sheep and goats are also susceptible. Calves seem more susceptible than adult cattle. Swine are fairly resistant to oak poisoning. Oak poisoning in cattle has a low-moderate morbidity with a moderate-high case mortality of approximately 35% to 85%.

Toxic Principle

Tannin and its metabolites are believed to be the toxic components of oak buds and acorns, and most of the tannin content of acorns resides in the shell. Acorns typically contain 3% to 9% tannin. Tannin is a gallotannin hydrolyzed in the rumen to gallic acid and pyrogallol. A number of polyhydroxyphenolic compounds have been identified in the serum and urine of experimentally poisoned animals, including gallic acid, pyrogallol, resorcinol, pyrocatechol, hydroquinone, phloroglucinol, cresol, and phenol. Lesions similar to those in cattle poisoned by oak developed in rabbits dosed with tannic acid (gallotannin), gallic acid, or pyrogallol. These lesions were not evaluated histologically, however. Lesions produced by tannic acid in rabbits were most like the lesions produced when rabbits were fed oak.

Because the exact toxic principle is unknown, the mechanism of action in oak toxicosis can only be hypothesized. One theory is that phenolic groups of gallotannin or gallic acid bind to proteins in saliva, dietary components, digestive enzymes, or gastrointestinal epithelium. Binding of the phenolic compounds to epithelium has an astringent action. Bound phenolic groups that reach the abomasum may be released by the change in pH. Free phenolic compounds may then be absorbed and cause further destruction of plasma proteins, endothelial cells, and renal tubular epithelium. Endothelial cell damage would promote fluid extravasation and edema. Damage to renal tubular epithelium would cause interstitial edema and increased back-pressure of the glomerular filtrate, with subsequent perirenal edema.

Deer are believed to be resistant to acorn poisoning because of a small glycoprotein in their saliva, which has a high concentration of proline. Browsing animals in general have relatively larger salivary glands and higher concentrations of proline in the saliva than grazers such as cattle and sheep. The tannin-binding glycoprotein in the saliva of browsing animals is not present in the saliva of grazing animals. Tannin bound to the tannin-binding protein is hypothesized to pass through the gastrointestinal track unhydrolyzed. Goats, a partial browsing species, are more resistant than cattle and sheep to oak poisoning.

Clinical Signs

Animals have usually ingested oak buds or acorns for 3 to 14 days (average, 1 week) before clinical signs are apparent. The renal and gastrointestinal systems are predominantly affected. Initially, the animal has anorexia, depression, and weakness. A mucous nasal discharge may be present, although the nose itself may be dry and crusted. The rumen is atonic and initially the animal is constipated with dark brown mucus-covered feces. Later in the course of the disease, black, tarry, fetid diarrhea may develop. Animals are often gaunt and emaciated with an elevated lumbar spine. Ventral edema may be apparent anywhere from the jaw to the perineum. Hydrothorax and ascites are also possible. Hydrothorax may lead to respiratory signs such as tachypnea. Polydipsia, polyuria, and dehydration may occur. Terminally, the animal is recumbent. Epistaxis has also been noted. The course of the disease usually ranges from 2 to 12 days, with 3 to 7 days being average.

Pathology

Anorexia, rumen atony, and renal damage produce many clinical pathologic abnormalities. Azotemia and increased serum creatinine are consistent findings, with the ratio usually being 10:1 or greater. Hypochloremia is also a consistent finding because of trapping of chloride in an atonic gastrointestinal tract. Hyponatremia is commonly associated with renal loss from decreased reabsorptive capability, and hypocalcemia results from decreased ingestion and an inverse relationship with phosphorus. The reason for the hyperphosphatemia is poorly understood because the kidney plays only a minor role in phosphorus excretion in ruminants. Hypermagnesemia may be present from decreased elimination associated with decreased glomerular filtration. Magnesium serum concentrations greater than 3.5 mEq/L are usually prognosticators of death. A general trend toward hypokalemia is present in most animals because of decreased intake and increased salivary potassium excretion with concurrent hyponatremia under the influence of aldosterone. However, hyperkalemia has been noted in some of the more acute oak toxicoses. Alkalosis is more common than acidosis, although acidosis is sometimes found in animals with severe diarrhea. The alkalosis is the result of a functional abomasal atony producing a sequestration of hydrochloric acid in the abomasum and forestomachs. Substitution of bicarbonate ions for chloride ions in the circulation causes the alkalosis. Other possible clinical pathologic abnormalities include neutrophilic leukocytosis, hyperfibrinogenemia, prolonged plasma thromboplastin times, hyperbilirubinemia, and hyperaminotransferasemia. The urine specific gravity is less than 1.020 and is often in the isothenuric range of 1.008 to 1.014. Proteinuria may also be present.

Table 1
BOVINE NEPHROTOXICANTS

Source	Epidemiology	Clinical Signs	Pathology	Comments
Oak (Quercus spp.) Soluble oxalates	See the text See Table 2	See the text See Table 2	See the text See Table 2	See the text See Table 2; many fewer reports in cattle than in sheep because of management differences
Redroot pigweed (Amaranthus retroflexus)	Found throughout US; onset, 3–7 days; drylot or pasture exposure to large quantities of plant in summer to early fall	See Table 3	See Table 3	Unknown toxicant; gross and histologic lesions inseparable from those of oak toxicosis
Cantharidin (blister beetles, Epicauta spp.)	Toxic blister beetles throughout US; primary problems in crimped alfalfa hay from the southwest (i.e., Okla, Tex, Ark, Kan); onset time of a few hours; morbidity and mortality very dependent on dose of blister beetles	Salivation, lacrimation, urination, defecation, anorexia, rumen atony, pollakiuria, colic, shock, hematuria	Increased packed-cell volume, leukocytosis, hypocalcemia, increased serum urea nitrogen and creatinine, hematuria, decreased urine specific gravity; esophageal and GI hyperemia and ulceration, pale swollen kidneys, congested and hemorrhagic ureters and bladder, tubular degeneration/ necrosis	Rare toxicant in cattle; most reports in horses
Ochratoxin	Rare mycotoxin of grain or grain silage (e.g., wheat, barley, sorghum, corn, rye and oats); see Table 3 for onset, morbidity, and mortality	Depression, anorexia, diarrhea, dehydration	Hyperphosphatemia, hypocalcemia, increased serum urea nitrogen; perirenal edema, enteritis; see Table 3 for histopathologic findings	3 cases reported in Iowa and Wyo; silage containing 1–6 ppm ochratoxin A
Lead	Variety of sources involved (e.g., grease, used motor oil, batteries, caulking, linoleum, paint chips, silage contaminated with soil having a high lead concentration); onset times of 2 days to several weeks depending on bioavailability and dose; low-moderate morbidity, moderate-high case mortality	Depression, blindness, anorexia, rumen atony, colic, constipation or diarrhea, bruxism, ataxia, hyperirritability, muscle tremors, convulsions possible	Blood lead >0.35 ppm; lead source sometimes still visible in digestive tract; brain edema, cerebral congestion, laminar cortical necrosis; gastroenteritis, hepatocyte degeneration and necrosis, proximal tubule degeneration and necrosis, thickening and hyalinization of glomerular capsules; possible acidophilic intranuclear inclusions in hepatocytes and tubular epithelium	Common toxicosis in cattle; primary systems affected are CNS and gastrointestinal; blindness is reversible; convulsions are more likely with very bioavailable lead sources (e.g., grease); see CNS toxicant section for treatment
Arsenic (inorganic)	Variety of sources (as found in some herbicides, rodenticides, insecticides, and ashes of salt-treated wood); onset <24 hr; morbidity low-high, case mortality high	Weakness, trembling, ataxia, depression, colic, rumen atony, diarrhea, prostration; course of disease, hours to several days	Hyperemia of abomasum and sometimes duodenum, petechiae of GI serosa; congestion of liver, kidneys, and lungs; edema and necrosis in mucosa and submucosa of abomasum and duodenum; hepatic and proximal tubular degeneration and necrosis	Fairly common bovine toxicosis, primarily a gastrointestinal syndrome; cattle attracted to salty taste of arsenic salts; many cases die before diarrhea is evident; herbicide-treated foliage retains its toxicity
Zinc	Environmental contamination or misformulation of diet; milk replacer implicated previously; chronic toxicosis has onset time of >2 wk; high morbidity, low-moderate case mortality	Pica, anorexia, diarrhea, bloat, polydipsia possible	Possible anemia and hemolysis, ulcers in abomasum, enteritis and congestion of small intestine, possible pale and shrunken kidneys; degeneration and necrosis of pancreatic acinar cells, degeneration and necrosis of proximal tubular epithelium, cast formation possible, hepatocyte necrosis	Infrequent bovine toxicosis, primarily a GI syndrome; dietary concentrations >700 ppm are toxic, especially for young calves
Bracken fern (Pteridium aquilinum)	Found in forested areas throughout US; onset time, 1–3 mo; onset possible several weeks after removal of source; usually low morbidity, high case mortality	Depression, rough coat, anorexia, hemorrhagic diarrhea, elevated temperature (104–109°F), hematuria, epistaxis; course of disease, 1–4 days	Leukopenia, thrombocytopenia, anemia (late); petechiae, ecchymoses, and frank hemorrhage throughout body organs and within body cavities; hypoplasia of bone marrow, possible hyperplasia/ carcinoma of urinary bladder epithelium	Infrequent bovine toxicosis, primarily a bleeding syndrome in cattle; plant is toxic green or dry; toxin in bovine syndromes is ptaquiloside

Table 2
OVINE AND CARPINE NEPHROTOXICANTS

Source	Epidemiology	Clinical Signs	Pathology	Comments
Soluble oxalates Halogeton *(Halogeton glomeratus)* Greasewood *(Sarcobatus vermiculatus)* Curly dock *(Rumex cripsus)* Rhubarb *(Rheum rhaponticum)*	Most problems from sodium oxalate in halogeton found in arid region of western US (i.e., Nev, Utah, Idaho, Wyo, Colo); halogeton is found along roadsides and other disturbed areas; acute toxicosis has onset time of 2–6 hr; high morbidity and case mortality possible	Tachypnea, dyspnea, depression, frothing, ataxia, prostration, rumen atony and bloat, coma, tetany, and convulsions possible; course of disease, 1–48 hr	Hypocalcemia; increase in serum urea nitrogen and aspartate aminotransferase; pale and swollen kidneys, hemorrhagic edematous rumen wall, hyperemia of abomasal and intestinal mucosa, ascites; numerous calcium oxalate crystals in kidney tubules and rumen wall	Parenteral calcium administration will not prevent death; preventive measures include not driving hungry or thirsty animals past dense stands of halogeton and supplementing with dicalcium phosphate
Oak *(Quercus* spp.*)*	See the text	See the text	See the text	See the text
Cantharidin	See Table 1	See Table 1	See Table 1	See Table 1; rare reports in sheep
Ovine toxicants producing secondary renal lesions Copper	Chronic copper accumulation over weeks to months; sporadic occurrences in flock associated with stress (e.g., vaccination, shipping, etc.); morbidity <10%, case mortality >80%	Depression, anorexia, jaundice, prostration, hemoglobinuria, coma; course of disease, 1–2 days	Hemolysis, decreased packed-cell volume, hemoglobinuria, mottled yellow-brown liver, icterus, enlarged spleen, gunmetal-colored kidney; hepatic necrosis, hemoglobin casts in kidney tubules	One of the most common ovine toxicoses, seen when dietary copper-molybdenum ratios >10:1; poor prognosis for chelation therapy with penicillamine

Necropsy lesions also relate primarily to the gastrointestinal tract and the kidneys. The gastrointestinal tract may have congestion, hemorrhage, and ulceration. Ulceration is especially likely in the abomasum and small intestine; however, ulcers are also seen at times in the buccal mucosa, esophagus, rumen, and colon. The subserosal area of the gastrointestinal tract may have petechial to ecchymotic hemorrhages. Acorns or oak foliage may or may not be present because of the delay in onset time. Ventral subcutaneous edema may be severe. Often, ascites and hydrothorax are present. The perirenal area is edematous and often tinged with blood. The kidneys are pale and normal to swollen in size with petechial subcapsular hemorrhages. At times, the liver may appear pale and mottled.

Histopathologic findings include coagulative necrosis of the proximal tubules with the formation of acidophilic granular casts of epithelial and protein debris. Many tubules may be dilated in the cortical and medullary regions. Bowman's capsules may be normal or fluid filled. Sometimes swelling or thickening of the capsular and glomerular epithelium is noted. Chronic cases have mononuclear cell infiltrates and fibrous connective tissue production in the cortex.

Diagnosis

A tentative diagnosis of oak toxicosis is based on the presence of renal failure, compatible clinical signs, and evidence of oak bud or acorn consumption. Renal failure is diagnosed by the presence of azotemia or dehydration in conjunction with low urine specific gravity. Additionally, paper strips impregnated with 2% ferric chloride and dried will turn blue-black when dipped in the phenolic urine of poisoned animals. The prognosis in individual cases correlates with the return of appetite and decreases in creatinine and serum urea nitrogen. The prognosis is guarded at best in view of the fact that two thirds to three fourths of the kidney tubules are affected before increases in

serum urea nitrogen and creatinine and a decreased urine specific gravity are seen.

Treatment

Therapy is aimed at restoration of renal perfusion, extracellular fluid volume, and rumen motility. Renal perfusion and severe dehydration should ideally be corrected by intravenous fluid administration. Deficits of sodium, chloride, and calcium electrolytes are expected. The trend in most cases is toward hypokalemia, although some individual animals have hyperkalemia. In lieu of laboratory electrolyte results, normal saline with added calcium and potassium should be administered. Oral fluid therapy, although less efficacious, may be more practical in certain situations than intravenous administration. Oral fluids should be balanced in electrolytes and preferably low in magnesium.

Rumen motility is often difficult to re-establish. Loss of rumen fermentation necessitates parenteral vitamin B supplementation and transfaunation. High-quality legume forage should be made available for the herd with just a little grain supplement on the side. Animals that remain anorectic may benefit from oral propylene glycol to supplement their energy needs. Even with better-quality feed available, many animals will continue to seek out acorns.

Prevention

Preventive methods are more rewarding than therapeutic attempts. A pelleted ration with 10% calcium hydroxide (slaked lime) will partially prevent oak toxicosis when fed at the rate of 0.9 kg/head/day in calves and 1.8 kg/head/day in adult cattle during problem seasons. The mechanism of action is unknown. An untested method would be to supplement diets with feedstuff high in proline (e.g., corn gluten meal, gelatin, dehulled soybean

Table 3
PORCINE NEPHROTOXICANTS

Source	Epidemiology	Clinical Signs	Pathology	Comments
Redroot pigweed (*Amaranthus retroflexus*)	Found throughout US; onset 3–7 days after ingestion, primarily in confinement-raised pigs turned into unused drylot in summer to early fall; morbidity, 5%–90%; case mortality, ≥75%; isolated reports in cattle and lambs	Initial incoordination, weakness, trembling, and knuckling of hindlegs; sternal recumbency, paresis, and flaccid paralysis; alert, good appetite, and normal temperature early; terminally, coma, ventral edema, and distended abdomen; course of disease, approximately 2 days	Hyperkalemia, increased serum urea nitrogen and creatinine; perirenal edema; pale, normal to small kidneys with subcapsular petechiae; thoracic and abdominal fluid accumulation; proximal tubular nephrosis, necrosis and dilation of distal and convoluted tubules, oxalate crystals in tubules sometimes observed	Unknown toxicant; plant also contains soluble oxalates and nitrate; less common toxicosis than in years past with less access of swine to drylot; chronic cases possible
Vitamin D Cholecalciferol (vitamin D_3) Ergocalciferol (vitamin D_2)	Dose-dependent onset time of 2 days to several weeks; feed formulated >1000× too high; morbidity, 75%–100%; case mortality, ≤25%	Lethargy, emesis, anorexia, rough hair coat, and lameness with more chronic problems; course of disease, 1 day to weeks	Hypercalcemia, hyperphosphatemia, hypermagnesemia, possible increase in serum urea nitrogen; hyperemic gastric mucosa; edematous, firm, and congested lungs; multifocal pinpoint pale spots in renal cortex; chronic cases with fractures of bones (especially femurs and ribs); necrosis and mineralization in kidneys, gastric mucosa, lungs, and heart	Cumulative toxicant, vitamin D_3 more toxic than vitamin D_2; mineralization because of combination of dystrophic and metabolic reasons; fairly uncommon toxicosis
Ochratoxins (especially ochratoxin A)	Rare mycotoxin of grain (e.g., wheat, barley, sorghum, corn, rye, and oats); onset time, 2 days to several weeks; morbidity may approach 100%, case mortality usually less than 35%	Polydipsia, polyuria, decreased weight gain, enteritis, and anorexia (large doses)	Isosthenuria, proteinuria, increased serum urea nitrogen, possible increase in aspartate animotransferase; pale and swollen kidneys, gastric and intestinal hyperemia; proximal tubular necrosis and dilation; chronically, renal interstitial fibrosis and glomerular sclerosis; possible intestinal mucosal, lymphoid, and hepatic necrosis	Feed concentrations >0.2 ppm are toxic; toxin binds strongly to proximal tubules; $T_{1/2}$ in pigs is approximately 3–5 days; few reported cases in US
Porcine toxicants producing secondary renal lesions				
Cocklebur (*Xanthium* spp.)	Found throughout US; onset 1–3 days after ingestion; primarily associated with cotyledon (2-leaf stage) ingestion in field in spring, sometimes associated with seed contamination of feed; low-moderate morbidity, high case mortality	Depression, ataxia, sternal recumbency, jaundice, enteritis, coma, convulsions with paddling; course of disease, 1–3 days	Increased serum liver enzymes and bilirubin, hypoglycemia; mottled and enlarged liver, edematous gallbladder, ascites; centrolobular hepatic necrosis and congestion, possible secondary kidney tubular degeneration and necrosis with granular casts	Carboxyatractyloside is toxin; few confirmed cases in swine; isolated reports also in sheep and cattle

meal) during these times. Certainly, pastures or ranges with fewer oak species should be used in the spring in the southwestern United States and in the fall elsewhere in the country.

BIBLIOGRAPHY

Austin PJ, Suchar LA, Robbins CT, et al: Tannin-binding proteins in saliva of deer and their absence in saliva of sheep and cattle. J Chem Ecol 15:1335–1347, 1989.

Divers TJ, Crowell WA, Duncan JR, Whitlock RH: Acute renal disorders in cattle: A retrospective study of 22 cases. J Am Vet Med Assoc 181:694–699, 1982.

Dollahite JW, Pigeon RF, Camp BJ: The toxicity of gallic acid, pyrogallol, tannic acid, and *Quercus harvardi* in the rabbit. Am J Vet Res 23:1264–1266, 1962.

Fetcher A: Renal disease in cattle. Part II. Clinical signs, diagnosis, and treatment. Compend Contin Educ 8:S338–S345, 1986.

Kasari TR, Pearson EG, Hultgren BD: Oak (*Quercus garryana*) poisoning of range cattle in southern Oregon. Compend Contin Educ 8:F17–F29, 1986.

Kingsbury JM: Poisonous Plants of the United States and Canada. Englewood Cliffs, NJ, Prentice-Hall, 1964, pp 444–446.

Osweiler GD, Carson TL, Buck WB, Van Gelder GA: Clinical and Diagnostic Veterinary Toxicology, ed 3. Dubuque, Iowa, Kendall/Hunt, 1985.

Panciera RJ: Oak poisoning in cattle. In Keeler RF, Van Kampen KR, James LF (eds): Effects of Poisonous Plants on Livestock. New York, Academic Press, 1978, pp 499–506.

Robbins CT, Mole S, Hagerman AE, Hanley TA: Role of tannins in defending plants against ruminants: Reduction in dry matter digestion? Ecology 68:1606–1615, 1987.

Shi ZC: Research on the pathogenesis of oak leaf poisoning in cattle. In James LF, Keeler RF, Bailey EM, et al (eds): Poisonous Plants: Proceedings of the Third International Symposium. Ames, Iowa State University Press, 1992, pp 509–516.

Spier SJ, Smith BP, Seawright AA, et al: Oak toxicosis in cattle in northern California: Clinical and pathologic findings. J Am Vet Med Assoc 191:958–964, 1987.

■ Infectious Pyelonephritis in Cattle

Richard F. Randle, D.V.M., M.S.

Pyelonephritis may occur in a number of ways, including secondary to an ascending infection from the lower urinary tract, by spread from embolic nephritis of hematogenous origin, or as a result of specific infectious processes such as that caused by *Corynebacterium renale* in cattle. The most common route is secondary to ascending infection.

PATHOGENESIS

The primary factors involved in the development of pyelonephritis are the presence of infection in the urinary tract and the stagnation of urine allowing progression of the infection up the tract. Ureteral reflux from the bladder may be involved in the process. The infection ascends from the bladder via the ureters and invades the renal pelvis. Infection of the renal pelvis results in erosion of the papilla, necrotic debris in the renal pelvis, and a suppurative nephritis involving the tubular and interstitial structures of the affected lobes. The infection may be either unilateral or bilateral.

C. renale and *Escherichia coli* are the organisms most commonly responsible. Other organisms involved include *Corynebacterium pilosum*, *Corynebacterium cystitidis*, and a number of gram-negative organisms. The *Corynebacterium* spp. are normal inhabitants of the skin and have shown the ability to adhere to the bovine urinary bladder, vagina, and vulvar epithelium. These organisms are also capable of survival in the environment for long periods of time. Transmission most likely results from direct manipulation of the urogenital tract. Venereal transfer is possible in light of the fact that these organisms have been isolated from the prepuce of healthy bulls.

CLINICAL SIGNS

Cattle affected with pyelonephritis typically exhibit hematuria, pyuria, dysuria, fever, and occasionally colic signs. The presence and severity of these signs can vary considerably early in the course of the disease. As the condition becomes chronic, gross urine abnormalities abate somewhat, and the animal exhibits more generalized signs of chronic disease, including inappetence, loss of condition, and loss of production over a period of weeks.

Rectal examination may reveal thickening of the bladder wall and ureters. Affected kidneys may show enlargement, loss of lobulation, and pain on palpation. These changes are most easily detected in the left kidney. Ultrasonography may be used to detect involvement of the various structures. The right kidney is best imaged from the right paralumbar fossa, whereas the left kidney, ureters, and bladder are best imaged via rectal probe.

DIAGNOSTIC FINDINGS

Urinalysis findings include hematuria, pyuria, and bacteriuria. Culture of urine is necessary for confirming the causative agent. Blood evaluation usually indicates an inflammatory leukogram and elevated fibrinogen levels. Evidence of azotemia or uremia

is usually not present unless there is bilateral involvement or the animal is in the terminal stages of the disease.

NECROPSY FINDINGS

Major necropsy findings are confined to the urinary tract. The affected kidney appears grossly enlarged, and lobulations may appear less evident than normal. Necrotic areas on the surface of the kidney may be present. Abscesses and necrotic debris are evident in the renal pelvis. Affected ureters are thick walled and contain blood, pus, and mucus. The bladder wall is thickened, and the mucosa is hemorrhagic, edematous, and possibly ulcerated.

TREATMENT AND PROGNOSIS

The treatment of choice in cases of *Corynebacterium* infection is penicillin. The prognosis, in most instances, is good provided that therapy is instituted early and extensive structural damage to the urinary tract has not occurred. Infections caused by other organisms are best treated with antimicrobials selected on the basis of urine culture and sensitivity results.

Animals infected with *C. renale* require more agressive therapy, and the prognosis in these animals is guarded. Treatment with procaine penicillin for an extended period of time (2 to 4 weeks) is recommended. The initial response to therapy may be good, but relapse is common and clearing of the infection is difficult. In unilateral infections in valuable animals, nephrectomy may be warranted provided that the functional ability of the other kidney has been established.

Adjunctive therapy should include intravenous fluid therapy in severely affected patients. Animals should be encouraged to drink plenty of fresh water for maintaining or increasing urine output to clear the urinary tract of debris and organisms. The availability of salt will aid in increasing thirst and ensuring adequate water intake. Urinary acidifiers have been used and may be of value in the treatment of pyelonephritis. The adhesive abilities of *Corynebacterium* have been shown to be pH dependent, with less adhesion occurring in an acid pH. Ammonium chloride at 50 to 100 mg/kg twice daily has been recommended.

PREVENTION AND CONTROL

No specific control measures are advocated, but isolation of affected animals, removal of contaminated bedding, and careful hygiene associated with examination of the urogenital tract may reduce environmental contamination and transmission of the disease. Artificial insemination may be considered but, in most instances, is not economically justifiable.

BIBILOGRAPHY

Blood DC, Radostits OM: Veterinary Medicine, ed 7. London, Baillière Tindall, 1989, pp 399–400, 574–575.

Johnson R, Grymer J, Gerloff B, et al: Nephrectomy as treatment for pyelonephritis in a cow. Compend Contin Educ 6:S356–S359, 1984.

Smith BP: Large Animal Internal Medicine. St Louis, CV Mosby, 1990, pp 888–889.

Takai S, Yanagawa R, Kitamura Y: pH-dependent adhesion of piliated *Corynebacterium renale* to bovine bladder epithelial cells. Infect Immun 28:669–674, 1980.

Tulleners EP, Deem DA, Donawick WJ: Indications for unilateral nephrectomy: A report on four cases. J Am Vet Med Assoc 179:696–700, 1981.

Yanagawa R: Causative agents of bovine pyelonephritis: *Corynebacterium renale, C. pilosum, C. cystitidis. In* Pandy R (ed): Progress in Veterinary Microbiology and Immunology. vol 2. Basel, Switzerland, S. Karger, 1986, pp 158–174.

■ Cystitis, Pyelonephritis, and Miscellaneous Diseases of Swine

Roderick C. Tubbs, D.V.M., M.S., M.B.A.

CYSTITIS

Cystitis is an inflammatory condition of the urinary bladder. It appears to occur more frequently in the female than the male, apparently because of the shorter urethra, which predisposes the female to ascending urinary tract infections. Females are also predisposed to trauma of the urethra and anterior vagina at coitus and parturition, with many cases of cystitis in sows occurring after breeding and after farrowing. Solid-floored or solid-backed gestation crates have also been suggested as factors predisposing to cystitis in sows because sows will often sit on the floor or come in contact with the back of the crate, which allows direct access to the lower urinary tract by fecal contaminants and other microorganisms. Other possible predisposing factors include decreased water intake, infrequent micturition, and incomplete emptying of the bladder at micturition. Feet and leg injuries, poor body conformation, poorly designed facilities, and systemic illness may all contribute to an unwillingness by the sow to stand, drink, and urinate frequently. Sows that urinate from the sitting or recumbent positions may fail to empty the bladder completely.

Clinically, cystitis is characterized by pollakiuria, dysuria, oliguria, and depending on the severity of the individual case, variable amounts of hematuria, pyuria, and bacteriuria. Urethritis usually accompanies cystitis and may account for some of the pain, grunting, and straining seen in association with urination. The most consistent diagnostic sign associated with cystitis is the frequent passage of blood-stained, turbid urine.

Most of the organisms associated with cystitis in sows are normal inhabitants or contaminants of the vagina and vestibule. These include *Escherichia coli, Proteus mirabilis, Staphylococcus* spp., *Streptococcus* spp., *Klebsiella*, and enterococci. A specific primary pathogenic organism that causes cystitis and pyelonephritis in swine (*Eubacterium suis,* formerly *Corynebacterium suis*) is discussed separately.

Laboratory tests for confirmation of a clinical diagnosis of cystitis include urinalysis for the presence of protein (a high level in the urine indicates an inflammatory reaction in the urinary tract if collection methods preclude contamination from the lower genital tract) and inflammatory cells, as well as culture of properly collected urine in the presence of microorganisms. One author has suggested that urine pH may be used as a diagnostic and prognostic indicator for urinary tract disease in the sow.[1] A slightly acid pH urine is considered normal. The pH is reported to be higher than 7.5 in problem herds, and in one survey, sows with a urine pH of 8.5 or above frequently lost pregnancies, were culled, or died.

Necropsy lesions of cystitis include the expected components of the inflammatory response in acute cases: swelling, edema, hyperemia, and possibly hemorrhage of the mucosal surface of the bladder. The lesions progress into subacute and chronic cases until the entire bladder wall becomes grossly thickened and the mucosal surface is doughy and coarsely granular.

Treatment of cystitis consists of systemic administration of appropriate antibiotics based on culture and sensitivity testing. Treatment should be continued for 7 to 14 days. In swine, treatment is often initiated with procaine penicillin at 22,000 to 33,000 IU/kg intramuscularly once or twice per day until the results of culture and sensitivity testing are available. It should be noted that this dosage is higher than the label indication for penicillin in swine; therefore, appropriate veterinary-client-patient relationships should exist, and extended withdrawal times for slaughter should be observed. More specific antibiotic therapy may be selected on the basis of laboratory findings. Ampicillin is preferred by some clinicians as initial treatment and should be administered at 11 mg/kg twice per day. This is an extra-label usage in pigs. The prognosis is fair to good if treatment is initiated early in the course of the disease and guarded to poor if the disease has progressed to a more chronic condition before therapy is initiated.

PYELONEPHRITIS

Pyelonephritis is inflammation of the renal pelvis and kidney. It usually occurs secondary to cystitis as the continuation of an ascending urinary tract infection. It may also result from a hematogeneous origin.

Predisposing factors, clinical signs, and the organisms involved are similar to those described for cystitis, with the exception that by the time the infection has ascended to the kidneys, clinical signs may be more severe and, in addition to the hematuria and pyuria observed with cystitis, systemic signs such as depression, fever, inappetence, and weight loss may be a more profound part of the clinical picture. As with cystitis, the frequent passage of blood-stained, turbid urine is the most reliable clinical evidence of pyelonephritis. Renal function tests (e.g., blood urea nitrogen measurement) may be beneficial in determining the extent of kidney damage caused by pyelonephritis but will be elevated only when more than 75% of the nephrons are nonfunctional.[2] At necropsy, mucosal lesions in the ureters and kidneys are similar to those described as occurring in a bladder with cystitis. Treatment for pyelonephritis is very similar to that for cystitis. The prognosis for pyelonephritis is much more guarded than that for cystitis.

Eubacterium suis

Eubacterium suis, a gram-positive anaerobic bacillus, is a specific pathogen affecting the urinary tract[3] and possibly the reproductive tract in female swine. Clinical signs are very similar to those caused by other organisms associated with cystitis and pyelonephritis, except that *E. suis* may cause severe illness with sudden onset and death within hours or days after the clinical signs are first noticed. Other cases may have a more protracted course, such as that seen with cystitis and pyelonephritis caused by commensal or contaminant microorganisms.[3] *E. suis* has also been associated with a chronic course of disease known as the "thin sow" syndrome. This syndrome must be differentiated from the weight loss and emaciation associated with underfeeding, parasites, and other chronic diseases.

A major feature of *E. suis* in pigs is its association with the male.[4] The organism is apparently a normal inhabitant of the male lower urinary tract, particularly the preputial diverticulum. Most boars are asymptomatic, but occasional hematuric episodes may be observed. The high rate of recovery of the organism from asymptomatic males and its association with clinical signs in females have been the basis of the suggestion that the organism is venereally transmitted. Proper handling of specimens (urine, preputial swabs), proper environmental conditions for culture, and the use of selective media are necessary to achieve good culture results.[3–5]

Treatment of *E. suis* infection can be effective if it is applied early in the course of the disease for an appropriate length of time. Procaine penicillin at 22,000 to 33,000 IU/kg once or twice per day for 7 to 14 days is a commonly used antibiotic regimen. Extended slaughter withdrawal times should be used for the extralabel dosage. Ampicillin has also been used with good results and is the preferred treatment of some clinicians but needs to be administered twice per day. Response may be evident as early as 3 to 4 days after the initiation of therapy if treatment is begun early in the course of the disease. As with other causes of cystitis and pyelonephritis, sanitation in the breeding and gestation areas is critical to the control of *E. suis.* Penicillin and ampicillin injections at the time of breeding have been used as prophylactic measures in problem herds with equivocal results. Chlortetracycline at 400 g/ton of feed for 2 weeks followed by 200 g/ton for another 4 to 6 weeks has been used as adjunctive therapy for both treatment and prevention. Although these dosage levels are approved, this is a nonapproved indication, therefore an extended preslaughter withdrawal time may be indicated. Because of the potential for venereal transmission of *E. suis,* flushing the boar's preputial cavity with chlorhexidine, tetracycline, or other antibiotics has been attempted in an effort to prevent cystitis and pyelonephritis in sows. Positive treatment results have been reported in some cases but may in fact be associated with a general increase in attention to sanitation, breeding, and management practices. Selective culling of suspected problem boars may be justified, particularly if individual boars cause excessive trauma with bleeding from the lower urogenital tract of the sow at mating.

MULTIFOCAL INTERSTITIAL NEPHRITIS

Multifocal interstitial nephritis caused by *Leptospira pomona* and perhaps other *Leptospira* serovars is occasionally seen in both sows and finishing pigs at slaughter. The condition is characterized by large white foci in the kidneys and occasional peritonitis resulting in condemnation of kidneys and trimming of the surrounding muscle area. Vaccination for leptospirosis does not appear to prevent the lesions in growing pigs. Leptospiruria is present in most infected animals between 16 and 74 days postexposure. Most infected animals remain clinically normal.

MISCELLANEOUS DISEASES OF THE URINARY SYSTEM OF SWINE

Diseases of the urinary system other than cystitis and pyelonephritis are rarely diagnosed in swine, either because they are masked by the clinical signs of a primary disease or because they do not cause clinical signs unless extensive lesions are present, and even then it is often difficult or impossible to differentiate them from the more common conditions of cystitis and pyelonephritis. Other diseases or conditions that have have been reported or could potentially occur in swine include renal ischemia, glomerulonephritis, nephrosis, interstitial nephritis, embolic nephritis, urolithiasis, and cystic kidneys. A more detailed discussion of these conditions can be found in the second edition of this text and in other standard reference textbooks.

REFERENCES

1. Muirhead M: Sow urine pH mortality key. Int Pigletter 9:43, 1990.
2. Duncan RJ, Prasse KW: Veterinary Laboratory Medicine Clinical Pathology. Ames, Iowa State University Press, 1977, p 115.
3. Walker RL, MacLachlan NJ: Isolation of *Eubacterium suis* from sows with cystitis. J Am Vet Med Assoc 195:1104–1107, 1989.
4. Pijoan C, Lastra A, Leman A: Isolation of *Corynebacterium suis* from the prepuce of boars. J Am Vet Med Assoc 183:428–429, 1983.
5. Dagnall GJR, Jones JET: A selective medium for the isolation of *Corynebacterium suis.* Res Vet Sci 32:389–390, 1982.

BIBLIOGRAPHY

Blood DC, Radostits OM: Veterinary Medicine, ed 7. London, Baillière Tindall, 1989, pp 396–402, 575.

Jones JET: Corynebacterial infections. *In* Leman AD, Straw B, Glock RD, et al (eds): Diseases of Swine, ed 6. Ames, Iowa State University Press, 1986, pp 619–621.

Jones JET: Urinary system. *In* Leman AD, Straw B, Glock RD, et al (eds): Diseases of Swine, ed 6. Ames, Iowa State University Press, 1986, pp 162–167.

Powe TA: Diseases of the urinary system. *In* Howard JL (ed): Current Veterinary Therapy: Food Animal Practice, ed 2. Philadelphia, WB Saunders, 1986, pp 816–817.

Eye Diseases

Consulting Editor
J. Phillip Pickett, D.V.M., Diplomate, A.C.V.O.

■ ## Ophthalmic Examination Techniques for Food Animals

J. Phillip Pickett, D.V.M., Diplomate, A.C.V.O.

A thorough ophthalmic examination is infrequently performed by most food animal veterinarians. Lack of proper equipment, lack of a proper facility for examination, and lack of expertise are all common reasons for not performing an adequate eye/adnexal examination in food animals. Not only is a thorough ophthalmic examination indicated when obvious external ocular disease or apparent vision deficit is present, but also a thorough ophthalmic examination may be useful in conjunction with a physical examination for any apparent systemic disease. Because vision and the eye and its adnexa are integrally involved with cranial nerves II through VIII, the brain stem, the cerebellum, and the cerebral cortex, a thorough ophthalmic examination should be part of any examination for neurologic disease. Prepurchase or soundness evaluations for breeding stock, as well as evaluation of animals afflicted with congenital and/or inherited diseases, are instances where an ophthalmic examination may also be prudent.

The purpose of this article is to acquaint the food animal practitioner with techniques commonly used to examine the eye and its adnexa. It is beyond the scope of this article to cover all the techniques available for ocular examination or describe and/or interpret all the normal and abnormal findings one might see when evaluating a food animal. The practitioner is referred to the bibliography following this article for more specific details concerning advanced ocular examination techniques and detailed interpretation of ophthalmic examination findings.

HISTORY

Prior to actually examining the animal, a thorough history is in order. Information such as age, breed, sex, stage of gestation, and animal use are always useful. Because most food animals are not as closely observed by their herdsman as are horses or small animals, subtle abnormalities or changes may initially go unnoticed by the herdsman, and this should be taken into consideration by the clinician. Clinical signs (including their initial onset and progression), medications used and response to therapy, overall herd involvement, and environmental factors (housing, stress of handling, crowding, temperature extremes, air quality, bedding, and/or potential exposure to toxins) should be elicited from the herdsman.

Questions should be asked in a manner that is understandable to the herdsman and in a manner that does not imply a correct or preferred answer or blame on the herdsman for the problem. In some cases a herdsman may have an idea of what the underlying problem may be, and although it is important to ask the herdsman's opinion, one must not be misled into ignoring other details of the history, no matter how minor, that may be important in diagnosing the problem.

INSTRUMENTS AND SUPPLIES

Besides the usual supplies of various sizes of syringes and needles, cotton balls, and gauze pads, the items listed in Table 1 are recommended for performing a complete ophthalmic examination. Having a kit or special box to carry these instruments to farm calls or having a designated place in the clinic for the instruments makes it easier to always have adequate equipment for a proper examination and thereby ensure that a full ophthalmic examination will be routinely performed. Some of the instruments listed are the author's personal choice, and the use of selected instruments will be discussed in the section involving detailed ocular examination.

RESTRAINT TECHNIQUES

The type of restraint for a close-up and detailed examination of the eyes depends on the species, type, and demeanor of the

---

Table 1
INSTRUMENTS AND SUPPLIES RECOMMENDED FOR OPHTHALMIC EXAMINATION

Instruments
  Ophthalmic/otic diagnostic set with fiber-optic Finnoff transilluminator (No. 41100), direct ophthalmoscope (No. 11720), and otoscope (No. 20260) interchangeable heads with a 3.5-V rechargeable nickel-cadmium battery (Welch Allyn)
  20-D (5×) veterinary viewing lens (Welch Allyn)
  Magnifying head loupe with 1¾× (3 D) to 2½× (5 D) power (Donnegan Optical Co, Kansas City, Mo)
  Dressing forceps with rounded, serrated tips (or a curved Kelly hemostat)
Supplies
  Normal saline or lactated Ringer's solution (as an eyewash solution)
  Fluorescein-impregnated paper strips (Fluor-I-Strips, Ayerst)
  Schirmer tear test strips (Schering-Plough Animal Health)
  Culturette II (Becton-Dickinson)
  3 Fr and 5 Fr open-ended male urinary catheter, red rubber (Sovereign)
  3½ Fr tomcat catheter, polyethylene (Sovereign) or 18-, 20-, and 22-gauge Teflon intravenous catheters (Angiocath, Becton-Dickinson)
  No. 10 Bard-Parker scalpel blade
  Tropicamide, 1% (Mydriacyl, Alcon)
  Proparacaine, 0.5% (Ophthetic, Allergan)
  Lidocaine, 1% or 2% (Butler)

---

animal being examined. The least restraint that will allow for completion of the task at hand and for the safety of the examiner and patient is preferred. A stanchion, chute, or crate and a halter, nose lead, and/or snare may be required. Because eye position tends to follow the long axis of the body, head position can be used to enhance eye position depending on the position desired. Pulling the head up will cause the eye to roll ventrally, and flexion of the head downward will allow for visualization of the ventral aspect of the globe. Pulling the head laterally will expose more of the medial aspect of the globe in the eye away from the direction that the head/neck is bent. Animals in lateral recumbency typically have a ventral strabismus, which makes ophthalmic examination in this position difficult.

The author prefers not to use chemical restraint if at all possible. Xylazine may be used to adequately restrain most food animals, but drug withdrawal times and the risk of apnea, bradycardia, and recumbency following sedation should always be considered. Xylazine will alter the palpebral, corneal, menace, and dazzle reflexes and may cause enophthalmos and third eyelid protrusion, which may hinder a complete ophthalmic examination. It must be remembered that the dosage of xylazine in ruminants is only 10% or less than the recommended equine dose, and if the clinician is going to use xylazine, reversal agents such as tolazoline or yohimbine should be available for reversing the effect of xylazine if necessary.

Blepharospasm can generally be overcome by the local injection of lidocaine around the palpebral branch of the auriculopalpebral nerve (cranial nerve VII). This local block gives partial eyelid akinesia but offers no analgesia and does not affect retraction of the globe or third eyelid movement. In most ruminants the nerve can be palpated subcutaneously as it courses along the zygomatic arch midway between the base of the ear and the lateral canthus. The nerve can be difficult to palpate in heavy fleshed animals (beef cattle and bulls) and in swine. Local infiltration about the nerve (1 to 5 mL of 1% to 2% injectable lidocaine) followed by vigorous massage of the area will usually negate the animal's ability to forcibly close the lids.

Topical anesthesia of the cornea, conjunctiva, and third eyelid may be achieved with commercially available topical anesthetic. For minor procedures (conjunctival scrapings or superficial biopsies), three to five applications of 0.5 to 1.0 mL of a topical anesthetic at 5-minute intervals will provide adequate anesthesia. More extensive procedures (third eyelid excision, deep eyelid resection, or enucleation) will require regional anesthetic blocks.

Unlike the adequately described regional nerve blocks for the lids and adnexa in the horse, species and animal-to-animal variation makes it impossible to describe the exact location of the distribution of the zygomatic, lacrimal, infraorbital, and frontal nerves (sensory branches to the lids and adnexa) in food animals. For palpebral and third eyelid surgery, local infiltration (line blocks) of injectable anesthetic with a small-gauge needle (23 to 25 gauge) will usually provide adequate anesthesia. The Peterson eye block, which allows for placement of local anesthetic behind the globe to provide anesthesia of the orbit and the structures cranial to the orbit, can cause inadvertent injection of anesthetic into the subdural space with resultant death from apnea and cardiac arrest and is not recommended by this author. A four-point nerve block involving the use of a bent 18-gauge spinal needle to deliver retrobulbar anesthetic (the needle is passed through the skin and walked along the orbital bone to a site behind the globe; injections are made at four sites: dorsal, ventral, lateral canthus, and medial canthus) should be used to anesthetize the orbit for extensive surgical procedures (e.g., enucleation or orbital exenteration). The amount of anesthetic agent per site depends on the size of the animal (amounts range from 2 to 6 mL per site for sheep and goats to 10 to 15 mL per site for adult cattle).

NEURO-OPHTHALMIC REFLEXES

The menace response, pupillary light reflex, and dazzle reflex are all well described in the article on neurogenic vision loss later in this section and are not covered here. Other reflexes of importance are the palpebral reflex, corneal reflex, and oculocephalic reflex. The palpebral and corneal reflexes can be elicited by tapping the medial or lateral canthi with the finger and gently touching the cornea with the finger or with the edge of a gauze pad. The normal responses to these stimuli are blinking and retraction of the globe. Application of topical anesthetic, palpebral nerve blocks, and/or sedation may negate or greatly reduce the normal response to these stimuli. The sensory (afferent) branches of these reflexes are the ophthalmic and maxillary branches of the trigeminal nerve (V). The affector (efferent) nerves involved in these reflexes are the abducens nerve (VI—globe retraction) and the facial nerve (VII—blink).

Twisting the head from side to side or up and down results in nystagmus, with the fast phase of the nystagmus being in the direction of head movement. Sensory input for this oculocephalic reflex begins in the semicircular canals of the inner ear and is connected to the brain stem by the vestibular branch of the vestibuloauditory nerve (VIII). Brain stem and cerebellar function are also involved in this reflex. Concerning the efferent nerves, the dorsal, ventral, and medial rectus muscles are innervated by the oculomotor nerve (III), and the lateral rectus muscle is innervated by the abducens nerve (VI).

EXAMINATION OF THE EYE AND ADNEXA

Prior to restraint of the animal, evaluation of the animal free in its environment may be useful for discerning noticeable vision deficits or gross abnormalities. Buckets, hay bales, and other equipment may be used to construct an obstacle course for the animal to negotiate. If unilateral blindness is suspected, alternately patching the eyes with gauze taped over the eye may help with the diagnosis. Head carriage, ear position, and use of the sense of smell should be noted in those animals that may have vision loss. A wide-eyed, head-down, ears-up, sniffing appearance with the head moving side to side may indicate severe vision loss. Gross abnormalities of eyelids or third eyelids, enophthalmos or exophthalmos, periorbital swelling or depression, and ocular discharge should be noted and the right and left sides compared for symmetry.

For safety, close examination of the eyes should be done with adequate restraint. Assessment of pupillary light reflexes and all internal ocular structures should be done in a dimly lit area. Placing a large dark blanket or similarly opaque cloth over the animal's and the examiner's head may be done in the field but is dangerous for the examiner unless the animal and the animal's head are adequately restrained. Once the animal is restrained, re-evaluation of the gross ocular and adnexal structures is indicated. If possible, neuro-ophthalmic reflexes should be assessed without a nose lead, halter, or snare. If culture of the cornea or conjunctiva or a Schirmer tear test is indicated (see later), these tests should be done after gently wiping exudate from the lid margins with cotton balls or dry gauze. Culturing of deep corneal ulcers may be more safely accomplished following a palpebral nerve block.

Detailed examination of the lids, third eyelids, conjunctivae, and corneas is best done with a bright light source (Finnoff transilluminator, light from the direct ophthalmoscope, or an otoscope) illuminating the area obliquely to the examiner's line of sight. A head loupe will allow the examiner to focus at a closer distance with increased magnification (the author prefers a 5 diopter [D] loupe that yields 2½× magnification at a working distance of 20 cm). The surfaces of the eye and adnexa should be viewed from all angles. The initial examination should be performed without touching the face or vibrissae (this will usually result in blepharospasm). If painful, it is almost impossible to open the eyelids of a blepharospastic cow without a palpebral nerve block. To elevate the upper eyelid, the side of the thumb is placed firmly near the lid margin and the thumb rolled upward while pressing against the orbital rim. This puts little or no pressure on the globe. The lower lid may likewise be rolled ventrally. Following gross evaluation, palpation of the orbital rim and digital retropulsion of the globe through the lids with protrusion and examination of the palpebral surface of the third eyelid are indicated. Should the eye be fragile (corneal or scleral laceration or deep corneal ulceration), a palpebral nerve block should be performed prior to any manipulations, and no excessive pressure should be placed on the globe for fear of rupture or expulsion of the ocular contents.

If exudate or foreign material is present on the ocular surface, sterile saline may be flushed across the eye with a syringe to clean the ocular surface. Examination of the cornea, anterior chamber, and iris can be done with a bright light source and loupe as previously described. Deeper structures of the eye (lens, vitreous, and fundus) can best be examined following pupillary dilation. Tropicamide, 1% concentration (applied twice at a 5-minute interval), is the mydriatic of choice because of its rapid action (approximately 30 minutes) and short duration (4 to 12 hours). General evaluation for media opacities (opacities of the cornea, aqueous humor, lens, and vitreous) can be done via the technique of retroillumination. This technique involves placing the light source directly under the examiner's eye, aiming the beam of light into the patient's eye (like sighting down a gun barrel), and looking at the quality of the reflection from the fundus (colored reflection from the tapetum or a red reflex from light reflected off blood vessels). Opacities of the aforementioned structures will appear as dark foci against the fundic reflex because the opacities cast a shadow as light reflects off the fundus back into the examiner's eye. To localize the spot where an opacity may be, a rather crude form of a slit-lamp biomicroscope may be fashioned by using the slit beam from the direct ophthalmoscope and the loupe. As a linear focal light beam passes through the eye, light is refracted at three points: the cornea, anterior lens capsule, and posterior lens capsule (from front to back, respectively). The first two beams (cornea and anterior lens capsule) appear convex (bow outward) when viewed from the side, and the third beam (posterior lens capsule) appears concave (bows inward). Localization of an opacity relative to these three images allows the clinician to determine where in the eye the opacity is located. Examination of the cornea, anterior chamber, lens, and anterior of the vitreous is possible via coaxial illumination of the eye by a direct ophthalmoscope or an otoscope. From a distance of 5 cm, the cornea is in focus with the direct ophthalmoscope at a setting of +20 D, the anterior chamber at +10 D, and the lens at +10 to +7 D. The +10-D objective lens of a veterinary otoscope allows for focusing on the corneal surface at a distance of 10 cm from the instrument to the cornea, focusing on the anterior chamber at a distance of 5 to 10 cm from the eye, and focusing on the lens at 2 to 5 cm from the corneal surface.

The ocular fundus can be examined with a direct ophthalmoscope from a distance of 2 to 5 cm at a setting of −2 to +2 D. Likewise, the fundus can be examined with an otoscope with the objective lens flipped out of the line of sight at a distance of 2 to 5 cm. Both instruments give a right-side-up view (real image) that is greatly magnified. Examination of the periphery of the fundus is difficult with these techniques. Indirect ophthalmoscopy involves the aforementioned technique of retroillumination and a condensing lens. Following establishment of a good fundic reflex at a distance of 40 to 80 cm, a 20-D condensing lens is placed in the line of sight approximately 2 to 6 cm from the ocular surface of the patient. Fine movement of the lens toward or away from the patient allows for fine focus. The image using indirect ophthalmoscopy is virtual (the image is upside down, and the right side of the fundus appears to the left and the left appears to the right), and magnification is much less than with direct ophthalmoscopy, but the periphery of the fundus is readily viewed and the clinician can see a wider panorama of the fundus than is possible with direct ophthalmoscopy.

Additional diagnostic techniques involve evaluation of tear production and drainage, evaluation for corneal ulcerations, examination of the conjunctival fornices and behind the third eyelid, and scrapings of surface ocular tissues for cytologic assessment. Aqueous tear production is very seldom diminished in food animals, but if necessary, the Schirmer tear test can be used to evaluate the amount of aqueous tear production. Following removal of the tear meniscus from the lids with a dry cotton ball, a commercially available strip is bent at the notch and the rounded, short part of the strip placed between the cornea and the lower eyelid centrally with the notched area at the lid margin. Most food animals will wet the entire 30-mm strip in less than 60 seconds. Schirmer tear test readings of less than 15 mm/minute indicate a probable decrease in aqueous tear production. Tear drainage can be evaluated by the passage of fluorescein dye from the eye to the nares. Gently touching a saline-moistened dye strip to the dorsal bulbar conjunctiva or gently dropping saline stained with fluorescein onto the ocular surface will result in the passage of fluorescein from the ipsilateral nares within 1 to 10 minutes. Failure of the dye to pass may be an indication for flushing the nasolacrimal ducts. In most ruminants, the eyelid puncta are paired (one upper, one lower) and are on the lid margin close to the medial canthus at the end of the fibrous tarsal plate. Following the application of topical anesthetic, these puncta may be catheterized with a 3½ Fr open-ended polyethylene tomcat catheter or a Teflon intravenous catheter with the stylet removed. Normograde flushing of the duct may be attempted in this manner. Swine may have only one punctum, on the upper eyelid. Retrograde flushing of the nasolacrimal duct may be achieved by catheterizing the punctum in the nasal vestibule with a red rubber 3 or 5 Fr canine urinary catheter. In the cow, the nasal punctum is laterally positioned under the alar cartilage; in sheep and goats, it is on the medial surface of the alar fold, just off the floor of the nasal vestibule. In swine, the nasal vestibule is usually too small to allow observation or catheterization of the nasal punctum. Fluorescein dye applied to the corneal surface will also delineate areas where corneal epithelium is absent (corneal ulcer). Following dye application, the ocular surface is rinsed with saline. A cobalt blue filter from the direct ophthalmoscope will help delineate areas where the stain cannot be rinsed free. A clear spot in the middle of a deep corneal ulceration usually indicates the presence of Descemet's membrane protruding through the stroma. This is the deepest, most fragile type of ulceration and indicates impending corneal perforation.

To examine the conjunctival fornices and look behind the third eyelid, a palpebral nerve block and topical application of anesthetic are indicated. Nontoothed, serrated dressing forceps or a hemostat may be used to gently grasp the lid margin or third eyelid margin and evert the nictitans to allow examination. The hemostat should not be locked or the tissue grasped too firmly with the dressing forceps because the topical anesthetic will not alleviate the deep pain that occurs when too much pressure is applied to these structures.

Scrapings of the external ocular surface may be evaluated microscopically to diagnose infection or neoplasia. To obtain adequate cells for evaluation, a palpebral nerve block and topical anesthetic are first administered. With the flat, handle end of a scalpel blade, the surface of the lesion is repeatedly scraped gently in the same direction until a pellet of cellular material clings to the blade. This material is gently blotted onto a slide and stained with Diff-Quik or Wright's stain (for cellular morphology) or with Gram's stain (for bacterial identification).

BIBLIOGRAPHY

Barnett KC: Color Atlas of Veterinary Ophthalmology. St Louis, Mosby–Year Book, 1996.

Betts DM: Ophthalmic examination techniques for food and fiber animals. *In* Howard JL (ed): Current Veterinary Therapy: Food Animal Practice, ed 3. Philadelphia, WB Saunders, 1993, pp 829–836.

Gelatt KN: Ophthalmic examination and diagnostic procedures. *In* Gelatt KN (ed): Veterinary Ophthalmology, ed 2. Philadelphia, Lea & Febiger, 1991, pp 195–236.

Severin GA: Examination of the eye. *In* Severin's Veterinary Ophthalmology Notes, ed 3. Fort Collins, Colo, DesignPointe Communications, 1996, pp 1–62.

Whitley RD, Moore CP: Ocular diagnostic and therapeutic techniques in food animals. Vet Clin North Am Large Anim Pract 6:553–575, 1984.

▪ Ophthalmic Therapeutics

David T. Ramsey, D.V.M., Diplomate, A.C.V.O.

Treatment of specific ophthalmic diseases in food animals is frequently initiated after a tentative diagnosis has been made on the basis of clinical impression and experience. Many factors must be considered before a treatment alternative is selected. Treatment of ocular disease is dictated by the type of disease present, the ocular tissue involved, the intrinsic properties and characteristics of the drug used to induce a pharmacologic effect, and the susceptibility of the disease process to medical treatment. Other factors include the temperament of the animal, use of the animal, and the financial and physical willingness or ability of the owner to invest in the treatment protocol. Determining the severity of ocular disease (e.g., irreparable corneoscleral laceration, endophthalmitis) and noting whether eyelid and lacrimal function is normal also influence the selection of a specific treatment alternative.

The treatment objective is the same whether an individual animal or a herd of animals is affected: establishment of an effective and manageable treatment protocol that sustains a therapeutic level of drug in affected ocular tissues to achieve a desired outcome. Treatment strategies differ substantially when many animals in a herd are affected with ocular disease. The ideal treatment protocol that establishes the highest therapeutic concentration of drug in ocular tissues is often unrealistic or impractical in a herd setting. Treatment strategy in a herd setting is directed toward administering an effective therapy that can be achieved with a practical investment of time and capital.

ROUTES OF DRUG ADMINISTRATION

The route of drug administration is as important a consideration as the selection of a drug when attempting to establish therapeutic levels of drug in affected ocular tissues. Factors to consider when selecting the appropriate route of drug administration include (1) the ability of a given drug to achieve an effective therapeutic level in affected ocular tissue (e.g., antibiotic drug to establish a minimum inhibitory concentration), (2) the status of ocular tissue barriers to drug penetration, (3)

drug solubility properties, and (4) the frequency of treatment necessary to induce a therapeutic effect. Most drugs administered parenterally do not establish therapeutic levels in ocular tissues, and effective treatment requires topical or local administration. Penetration of drug into specific ocular tissues is enhanced when the blood-ocular barriers are compromised (e.g., iridocyclitis, chorioretinitis) but may not be possible when the blood-ocular barriers are normal. Drugs administered topically for anterior segment ocular disease must penetrate the lipophilic corneal epithelium and hydrophilic stroma to establish a therapeutic level in the anterior chamber. The frequency of treatment necessary to effect a cure varies necessarily by the route of administration selected. The most practical routes of drug administration include the topical, subconjunctival, and parenteral routes. The subtenon, retrobulbar, intracameral, and intravitreal routes are infrequently used and are seldom necessary.

Topical Application

Conventional practice relies primarily on topical instillation for delivery of most ophthalmic drugs. Topical instillation achieves higher drug levels in the cornea, conjunctiva, aqueous humor, iris, and ciliary body than do other routes of administration. The corneal epithelium is a barrier to the penetration of topically applied drugs. When the corneal epithelium is absent, higher levels of drug can be achieved in the corneal stroma and anterior chamber. Corneal penetration of drug may be facilitated by altering the permeability of the corneal epithelium (addition of wetting agents to the drug preparation); by altering the drug tonicity, pH, particle size, or concentration; or by incorporating lipophilic derivatives of parent drugs (prodrugs) that dissociate to the active fraction after penetrating the corneal epithelium.

Common drug vehicles include solutions, suspensions, ointments, and reservoir devices (collagen shields, soft contact lenses, conjunctival inserts). Solutions and suspensions are difficult to administer to large ruminants without the use of restraint devices to position the head during instillation. The surface ocular contact time of solutions with a low viscosity is short because solutions are rapidly lost through nasolacrimal drainage and drainage onto the face. As a general rule, only a small percentage of a topically instilled dose of aqueous medication (1% to 10%) is absorbed by the corneal stroma or anterior segment of the eye; drugs that drain through the nasolacrimal duct may be absorbed systemically and exert undesired side effects. Surface contact time and subsequent drug absorption are greater for solutions with increased viscosity. Ointments have a longer surface contact time and are not lost as readily by nasolacrimal drainage as is the case with solutions. The frequency of administration is also decreased. Administration of an ointment to the eye of a large ruminant is much easier than administration of a solution. Many ophthalmic ointments are manufactured as a water base and do not delay corneal wound healing. Soft contact lenses are not specifically available for ruminant eyes, but devices manufactured for horses are versatile enough for use in ruminants. Soft contact lenses or dehydrated collagen shields can be presoaked in a drug solution to promote the accumulation of drug in the device. The device acts as a reservoir that releases the drug during initial use. Corneal edema from tissue hypoxia has been reported with the use of hydrophilic contact lenses in cattle. Ocular (conjunctival) inserts are used infrequently in ruminants and are usually cost prohibitive. Drugs manufactured in a powder form for topical ophthalmic use are not recommended because they are extremely irritating to the ocular surface and have low drug bioavailability.

Subconjunctival Injection

Subconjunctival injection of drugs may be used to achieve high local concentrations in anterior ocular tissues. Subconjunctival injection should be used to supplement, not replace, topical treatment. An auriculopalpebral nerve block is usually necessary. Topical anesthetic should be instilled and the head restrained to avoid unintentional intraocular penetration. A maximum volume of 1 mL in large ruminants and 0.5 mL in small ruminants and swine is injected under the bulbar conjunctiva over the dorsolateral quadrant, 5 to 7 mm posterior to the limbus, with a 25-gauge needle and 1-mL syringe. Medications should only be injected under the bulbar conjunctiva; drugs injected into the eyelid or nictitating membrane or under the palpebral conjunctiva are rapidly dissipated and absorbed systemically and offer little advantage over topical instillation. Subconjunctival injection is only recommended for drugs with low solubility and poor corneal penetration. Drugs injected subconjunctivally may bypass the corneal epithelial barrier and enter the corneal stroma or sclera directly, or they may escape back through the conjunctival injection site onto the ocular surface and be absorbed through the corneal epithelium. Unless repository forms of the drug are available, drug concentration and activity are not sustained, and repeated subconjunctival injections are necessary to establish therapeutic levels of drug in ocular tissue. In ruminants, subconjunctival injections are used most frequently as a single dose during the initial treatment of infectious keratoconjunctivitis to establish high levels of antibiotic or corticosteroid drugs or atropine in ocular tissues.

Oral and Parenteral Administration

Frequent application of ophthalmic solutions and ointments or subconjunctival injections necessary to treat ocular diseases is usually impractical in a herd setting. Treatment by the oral or parenteral routes of administration is more feasible, but not all drugs administered systemically achieve therapeutic levels in ocular tissue. The relative distribution of drug administered by the oral or parenteral routes to ocular tissue is determined by the inherent drug properties, the intended ocular tissue that requires a therapeutic level of drug, the stability of the blood-ocular barriers, and the removal of drug from ocular tissue by active transport mechanisms. Some drugs administered orally or parenterally (e.g., oxytetracycline) have an affinity for lacrimal and conjunctival tissues and establish therapeutic levels in these tissues and the tear film. The oral or parenteral routes of administration are ideal for certain diseases of the eyelids, orbit, and sclera. When systemically administered drugs are intended for the treatment of intraocular disease (anterior uvea, vitreous, retina, choroid), the blood-ocular barrier may prevent their penetration into these ocular tissues. Inflammation of intraocular tissue frequently compromises the blood-ocular barriers and makes these tissues readily penetrable by many parenterally or orally administered drugs.

SPECIFIC THERAPY

Most of the common ophthalmic diseases of ruminants affect the ocular tissues of the anterior segment. Treatment is directed toward establishing therapeutic levels of drug in these tissues. When infectious surface ocular disease is suspected, initial treatment should be directed by clinical signs, age at onset, and the results of cytologic studies and Gram staining and confirmed by the results of bacterial culture and susceptibility testing when deemed appropriate. This may not be practical in field settings or when many animals are affected. When economics are an important consideration or when a large number of animals are being treated, convenient and effective treatment strategies must be used.

Antibiotic Drugs

Many different antibiotic drugs have been used to treat infectious keratoconjunctivitis in food animals. Fortunately, most of the infectious agents (*Chlamydia psittaci, Mycoplasma* spp., *Moraxella bovis*) that cause keratoconjunctivitis in food animals have antibiotic susceptibility patterns that allow for the use of a wide range of drugs. Topical ophthalmic preparations containing oxytetracycline are effective in treating most infectious ocular surface diseases of food animals but require frequent instillation (three to four times daily). Initial administration of topical oxytetracycline ointment and concurrent intramuscular injection of long-acting oxytetracycline (cattle, sheep, goats, and swine, 20 mg/kg) can be used to treat infectious keratoconjunctivitis in most food animal species. The administration of oxytetracycline for the treatment of infectious keratoconjunctivitis in sheep, goats, and swine constitutes extra-label drug use. Other antibiotic drugs that have been administered topically or subconjunctivally include gentamicin, bacitracin-neomycin–polymyxin B, gramicidin, erythromycin, benzathine and sodium cloxacillin, furazolidone, nitrofurazone, and some sulfa drugs. Chloramphenicol is not approved for use in food animals in the United States. Subconjunctival administration of the intravenous preparation of gentamicin (50 mg) to cattle with clinical signs of infectious bovine keratoconjunctivitis may be performed, but withdrawal times for milk and slaughter are prolonged.

Mydriatic/Cycloplegic Drugs

Atropine is a parasympatholytic drug that is most frequently used to control intraocular pain attributable to the ciliary muscle and iris sphincter muscle spasm associated with iridocyclitis. Atropine also induces iridoplegia and mydriasis, which decreases the likelihood of posterior synechia formation when the iridocyclitis is severe. Experimental evidence also suggests that atropine may stabilize the blood-aqueous barrier. Atropine (0.25% to 5%) is available in a solution or ointment form and should be instilled four times daily until mydriasis is evident and then instilled as necessary to maintain mydriasis. Initially, injectable atropine solution (0.1 mg, 0.25 mL) can be administered subconjunctivally to effect mydriasis when the iridocyclitis is severe.

Corticosteroid and Nonsteroidal Antiinflammatory Drugs

Topically applied glucocorticoid drugs are used infrequently to treat inflammatory ocular diseases of food animals. Topically and subconjunctivally administered corticosteroids to eyes with ulcerative keratitis may cause stromal collagenolysis by potentiating collagenase activity. Locally administered corticosteroids are contraindicated when corneal ulceration or infection is evident. Ocular immunity is also suppressed after glucocorticoid administration and may result in microbial overgrowth. However, the most common ocular use of glucocorticoid drugs is to reduce the inflammation associated with infectious ocular disease (bovine keratoconjunctivitis), an apparent contradiction in therapeutic logic. Concurrent subconjunctival administration of procaine penicillin G and dexamethasone once daily for 3 days to heifers with corneal ulcers attributable to infectious bovine keratoconjunctivitis does not significantly hasten or delay the clinical course of disease or outcome in heifers with naturally acquired infectious keratoconjunctivitis.[1]

Nonsteroidal anti-inflammatory drugs may be administered topically or systemically to treat inflammatory ocular diseases in food animals. Orally administered aspirin (mature cattle, 240 to 720 grains orally every 12 hours; calves, 240 to 480 grains orally every 12 hours; swine, 10 mg/kg orally every 6 hours) may be used to treat anterior or posterior segment inflammatory ocular diseases but should not be used in lactating dairy animals. Phenylbutazone may also be administered (cattle and swine, 4 to 8 mg/kg orally every 24 hours) to treat inflammatory ocular disease. Flunixin meglumine (2.2 mg/kg intravenously initially and then 1.1 mg/kg intravenously) may be administered to cows but is not indicated for use in cows intended for food. Flunixin meglumine is usually more effective than aspirin or phenylbutazone for ocular inflammatory disease. In the United States, the use of phenylbutazone and flunixin meglumine in food animals constitutes extra-label drug use.

Topical ophthalmic preparations of nonsteroidal anti-inflammatory drugs are expensive and are not commercially available in an ointment vehicle form. Topical ophthalmic nonsteroidal anti-inflammatory preparations should be administered two to four times daily. For these reasons, nonsteroidal anti-inflammatory agents are used infrequently to treat ocular inflammatory diseases in food animals.

Extra-label Drug Use

Withdrawal times have been recommended for many systemically administered drugs. Withdrawal times differ according to the drug formulation, dose, frequency, and route of administration; the species to which the drug is administered; and the weight of the animal. Few studies have evaluated the pharmacokinetics of topically and subconjunctivally administered drugs in food animal species. No studies have investigated drug residues in food animal tissues after topical and subconjunctival injection. Drug residues in milk and meat and standard recommendations for withdrawal times after topical or subconjunctival administration are unknown. When use or withdrawal time recommendations of extra-label drugs are in question, the Food Animal Residue Avoidance Database should be contacted (1-888-US-FARAD [1-888-873-2723]; e-mail address: *farad@ucdavis.edu* [California] or *farad@ncsu.edu* [North Carolina]; World Wide Web sites: *http://ace.orst.edu/info/farad* or *http://cptc.ncsu.edu/farad*) before a drug is used.

REFERENCE

1. Allen LJ, George LW, Willits NH: Effect of penicillin or penicillin and dexamethasone in cattle with infectious bovine keratoconjunctivitis. J Am Vet Med Assoc 206:1200–1203, 1995.

■ Selected Eye Diseases of Food and Fiber-Producing Animals

J. Phillip Pickett, D.V.M., Diplomate, A.C.V.O.

When most food animal practitioners think of ocular disease, infectious keratoconjunctivitis ("pinkeye"), ocular squamous cell carcinoma, and orbital lymphosarcoma are usually the first disease entities that come to mind. Without a doubt, these three entities are responsible for the majority of ocular-based economic losses for food animal producers, especially producers of cattle and small ruminants. There are, however, many ocular disorders seen in food animals that can cause pain and blindness in the animal, with subsequent economic loss to the producer. This article covers ophthalmic diseases that commonly afflict cattle, sheep, goats, and swine. With the exception of systemic diseases in which the ocular signs are a minor component of the overall disease entity, specific therapy is discussed, as well as potential preventive measures for each disorder. In the case of systemic diseases with ophthalmic manifestations, although supportive ocular therapy may be described, the practitioner is referred to other sections within this text for specific therapy for each systemic disease.

ORBIT/GLOBE DISORDERS

Cattle

Congenital anophthalmia (total absence of the eye) and congenital microphthalmos (a small, usually nonfunctional eye) are seen with some frequency in cattle. If the condition is unilateral, clinical signs may include a serous to mucoid to purulent ocular discharge, secondary entropion, or simply the appearance of a small or absent globe in the socket. Bilaterally afflicted animals are usually blind. Any disorder (physical, toxic, or infectious) that can cause in utero maldevelopment could cause microphthalmos. One infectious disease that can cause microphthalmos is in utero infection with the virus causing bovine viral diarrhea/mucosal disease. Infection between days 75 and 150 of gestation can cause cataract formation, retinal and optic nerve degeneration/dysplasia, nystagmus, and microphthalmos, as well as central nervous system disease.

Inherited anophthalmia/microphthalmos is seen in many breeds of cattle. The ocular disease may be seen alone, or there may be multiple congenital anomalies associated with the eye disease. In Herefords, inherited microphthalmos has been described in association with muscular dystrophy and hydrocephalus. Microphthalmos and other ocular defects have been associated with hydrocephalus in Shorthorn cattle. Inherited microphthalmos in Jerseys, Guernseys, and Holsteins may be seen in conjunction with cardiac malformations (high ventricular septal defects), as well as skeletal abnormalities (vertebral defects of the lumbar and/or sacral vertebrae, wrytail, or total absence of a tail). Because the inheritance of these disorders appears to be autosomal recessive, rebreeding the carrier sire and dam together is not recommended and culling of apparent carriers may be in order.

An acquired shrunken eye (phthisis bulbi) may be seen secondary to perforating wounds or ruptured corneal ulcers from infectious bovine keratoconjunctivitis or may be due to intraocular damage from blunt trauma. If there is no secondary entropion or secondary keratoconjunctivitis because of poor eye-to-eyelid conformation, treatment is not needed. Pain and chronic purulent conjunctivitis are both indications for enucleation of the afflicted eye.

Congenital megaloglobus (enlarged eye) secondary to glaucoma is seen in Holsteins in association with malformation of the anterior chamber and lens. Calves with unilateral disease may have one enlarged, blind, nonpainful eye or may have secondary exposure keratitis, corneal ulceration, and pain. Bilaterally afflicted animals are blind. If painful, the globe should be enucleated. Acquired glaucoma in cattle is uncommon and usually secondary to corneal perforation following infectious bovine keratoconjunctivitis or secondary to traumatic or infectious uveitis. Treatment recommendations are the same as for congenital glaucoma.

Convergent strabismus ("crossed eyes," or esotropia) with or without exophthalmos may be congenital or acquired in cattle. In Holsteins, Jerseys, Shorthorns, Ayrshires, and Brown Swiss, strabismus is usually seen at birth. A motor deficiency of the extraocular muscles (lateral rectus and retractor bulbi) innervated by the abducens nerve (VI) causes a nonpainful, non-vision–threatening disorder that appears to be autosomal recessive in inheritance. In the Jersey breed, a recessively inherited, progressive convergent strabismus has also been described and is first noted at 6 to 12 months of age. Divergent strabismus (exotropia) may be seen in cattle and is usually associated with hydrocephalus. Congenital nystagmus has been described in Holsteins (and other breeds) and is seen as a pendular, constant horizontal nystagmus that seems to cause no vision deficit. The disorder is familial, but the mode of inheritance is unknown. Acquired strabismus and/or nystagmus may be seen in cattle as a result of neurologic disorders such as polioencephalomalacia, listeriosis, thromboembolic meningoencephalitis, toxic phenomena, and other nonspecific disorders of the brain stem and cerebellum.

Exophthalmos (normal-sized globe protruding outward from the socket) may be due to retrobulbar neoplasia (see the article Food Animal Ocular Neoplasia in this section), orbital cellulitis, and periorbital sinusitis. Orbital cellulitis is seen as acute swelling of the lids and conjunctiva with third eyelid protrusion, exophthalmos, and potential exposure keratitis. Fever, anorexia, and depression are usually present with orbital cellulitis (which is not always the case with orbital lymphosarcoma unless multiple body systems are involved with the tumor). Puncture wounds through the lids or conjunctiva, maxillary molar root abscessation, and migration of herbaceous material from the mouth into the orbital space are causes of orbital cellulitis. Differentiation of orbital cellulitis from orbital neoplasia may be accomplished by aspiration and cytologic evaluation of material from behind the eye. The material aspirated should include neutrophils, macrophages, and other signs of infection if the exophthalmos is due to orbital cellulitis; if retrobulbar lymphosarcoma is the cause, cell types will include lymphocytes, lymphoblasts, and/or neoplastic cells. Periorbital sinusitis usually involves a more chronic, progressive distortion of the bony periocular tissue than does orbital cellulitis. Maxillary or frontal sinusitis is usually due to infection secondary to trauma (fractures) or dehorning. Infectious agents such as *Actinomyces pyogenes*, *A. bovis*, and *Pasteurella* spp. are common with periorbital sinusitis. Treatment of orbital cellulitis involves protection of the eye (temporary tarsorrhaphy if the animal cannot blink or frequent lubrication with ophthalmic ointments), warm moist compresses to reduce swelling, analgesics (aspirin or phenylbutazone), and antibiotic therapy. If a tract from a foreign body can be found, it should be probed and drainage should be attempted. Unresponsive orbital cellulitis with extensive ocular damage and a blind eye may necessitate orbital exenteration and placement of drains. Treatment of periorbital sinusitis may involve trephination of the sinus to establish drainage, curettage, and broad-spectrum antibiotic therapy.

Sheep and Goats

Inherited microphthalmos is seen in conjunction with multiple ocular anomalies in British, Dutch, and German Trexel sheep. The mode of inheritance appears to be autosomal recessive. Ingestion of the insect chemical sterilant apholate by pregnant ewes can cause congenital microphthalmos and other ocular anomalies, as well as malformation of periorbital bones. Chronic ingestion of plants containing high levels of selenium (over 3 ppm) by pregnant ewes can also cause microphthalmos, ocular cysts, and other ocular malformations. Overzealous selenium supplementation to pregnant ewes by herdsmen can have the same effect.

Consumption of the plant *Veratrum californicum* ("skunk cab-bage") in the high mountain pastures of western North America by ewes and does can cause cyclopia (presence of one central eye) in lambs and kids. Other facial skeletal malformations ("monkey face") and absence of the pituitary gland and other brain malformations can also be seen. The plant must be ingested on day 14 of gestation to result in this facial/ocular malformation. Consumption of the plant later in gestation normally results in embryonal death. Cyclopia has been seen in the eastern United States and Canada in areas where *V. californicum* does not grow. The etiology of the facial/ocular malformation in these areas is unknown.

Glaucoma and megaloglobus are rare in sheep and goats and are usually secondary to ocular puncture wounds or infectious (mycoplasmal septicemia, listeriosis, or neonatal coliform septicemia) uveitis. Similar to the condition in the cow, enucleation is recommended when the enlarged globe has exposure keratitis or is painful. Orbital cellulitis occurs rarely in sheep and goats. Causes include puncture wounds, migration of foreign plant material from the mouth to the orbit, and rarely, caseous lymphadenitis (*Corynebacterium pseudotuberculosis*).

Swine

Congenital microphthalmos is seen in the Yorkshire breed and is believed to be inherited as an autosomal recessive trait. In sows fed a vitamin A–deficient diet (especially during the first month of gestation), microphthalmos (and rarely megaloglobus) is seen in conjunction with other developmental ocular anomalies.

EYELID/THIRD EYELID/ NASOLACRIMAL SYSTEM DISORDERS

Cattle

The two most common congenital adnexal disorders in cattle are dermoids and supernumerary openings of the nasolacrimal ducts. Dermoids are haired, skinlike growths usually of the medial or lateral canthi, the third eyelid (not to be confused with the normal lacrimal caruncle), the bulbar conjunctiva, and/or the limbus and cornea. These choristomas usually cause only minor irritation and epiphora, but severe globe involvement may cause vision loss. The disorder is inherited as an autosomal recessive trait in Herefords, but it can occur in any breed. Accessory openings to the nasolacrimal ducts appear as hairless, depigmented openings on the face inferior to the medial canthi. Tear staining and minor facial dermatitis may occur as a result of this deformity. Brown Swiss and Holsteins seem to be afflicted most commonly.

Acquired lagophthalmos (inability to close the eyelids with secondary conjunctivitis and exposure keratitis) may be seen secondary to palpebral nerve trauma (trauma to the zygomatic arch area caused by blows to the head or as the animal pulls its head from the stanchion) or may be due to central nervous system disease (polioencephalomalacia or listeriosis). Symptomatic therapy includes topical application of ophthalmic ointments or temporary tarsorrhaphies to protect the cornea while waiting to see whether the facial paralysis resolves.

Acute eyelid edema and conjunctival chemosis may be seen as a result of allergic reactions to antibiotics, intravenous fluids, blood transfusions, and/or biologicals. This allergic phenomenon is usually bilateral and may be seen in conjunction with urticaria, skin wheals, generalized facial swelling, and other mucocutaneous junction swelling. Systemic antihistamines, corticosteroids, and/or epinephrine along with cold compresses is the recommended therapy, as well as attempts to identify the offending agent and avoidance of future exposure. Sunburn of the eyelids (especially in color-dilute animals such as Herefords and Holsteins) occurs secondary to photosensitization following phenothiazine administration or the ingestion of toxic plants. Conjunctival necrosis and severe corneal edema (especially ventrally) can be seen with photosensitization. Supportive care includes providing shade for afflicted animals and topical application of antibiotic ointment to the lids, conjunctivae, and corneas to prevent secondary bacterial infection while the area heals.

Treatment of traumatic eyelid lacerations depends on the severity of the lesion. Minor lid margin lacerations may heal following cleansing and the application of antibiotic ointments. If the eyelid is damaged such that lid closure and protection of the globe cannot be achieved, gentle, judicious débridement of necrotic tissue followed by multiple-layer surgical closure of the wound is in order. A palpebral nerve block and local anesthesia are helpful to facilitate meticulous placement of at least two layers of sutures (one deep in the eyelid musculature with absorbable suture while making sure that no suture can come in contact with the corneal surface and one layer in the external skin).

Ocular squamous cell carcinoma, the most common neoplasm involving the lids, the third eyelid, or the globe itself in cattle, is covered in the article Food Animal Ocular Neoplasia in this section. The second most common "mass" involving the lids is fibropapilloma or warts. These virally induced growths are typically seen in the young and are mostly self-limiting. Large warts may be successfully removed by debulking and cryosurgery with liquid nitrogen cryogen.

Occlusion of the nasolacrimal duct is clinically seen as epiphora or a mucoid ocular discharge in animals with minimal other signs of conjunctival or corneal disease. Lack of passage of fluorescein dye through the system from the eye to the nares is diagnostic. Inflammatory debris, food particles, weed seeds, and parasites (*Thelazia* spp.) may occlude the nasolacrimal duct. Treatment involves flushing the nasolacrimal duct (either normograde or retrograde; see the article Diagnostic Examination Techniques) and removal of the inciting cause.

Keratoconjunctivitis sicca (KCS) caused by a lack of aqueous tear production is rarely seen in cattle, but it can be seen after the ingestion of locoweed (*Oxytropis* and *Astragalus*). Supportive therapy includes topical lubricant antibiotic ointment application and/or partial or total temporary tarsorrhaphies to protect the globes. Locoweed-induced KCS may be transient or permanent.

Sheep and Goats

Dermoids occur rarely in sheep and goats but are similar to dermoids in cattle when they do occur. Entropion is the most common congenital eyelid disorder in sheep. Afflicted lambs usually have inrolling of the lower lid, which causes irritant keratoconjunctivitis with pain, ocular discharge, and potential blindness from corneal perforation or scarring. The disorder has a hereditary predisposition but may be augmented by factors such as windy or dusty environmental conditions. Immediate therapy is aimed at reducing the frictional irritation and protecting the cornea. Having the shepherd frequently manually roll the lids out in conjunction with the application of lubricant antibiotic ointment may be too labor-intensive for a large flock. Temporary eversion of the lid margin with skin clips (Michel clips), skin staples, or vertical mattress sutures or injecting penicillin (1 to 2 mL) into the lid to evert the lid margin may break the cycle of irritation followed by blepharospasm, which leads to worsening of the irritation. Most animals will do well with a single temporary eversion technique, but some animals may require a Hotz-Celsus procedure to remove eyelid skin and

permanently repair the defect. This should only be done in older animals (4 to 6 months or older) when temporary techniques have failed. Afflicted animals should not be bred, and sires and dams producing afflicted lambs should be culled.

Numerous infectious and parasitic diseases of the skin may cause blepharitis in sheep. The viral infections that cause cutaneous ecthyma and sheeppox, ulcerative dermatosis, and blue tongue may cause exudative skin lesions about the eyelids. *Dermatophilus congolensis*, *Actinobacillus lignieresii*, and *Trichophyton verrucosum* infections can cause exudative, scablike eyelid lesions. *Clostridium novyi* infection ("big head") can cause eyelid and facial edema. Sarcoptic and demodectic mange, as well as keds, lice, and ticks, can cause blepharitis along with facial dermatitis. Ocular therapy for these disorders is supportive (the eyelids should be kept cleansed and the cornea protected with ophthalmic ointment), and precautions should be taken to prevent the spread of these infections to other animals and/or humans.

As with cattle, photosensitization and KCS can occur in sheep and goats secondary to the ingestion of toxic substances. St. Johnswort, buckwheat, and spineless horsebrush are common plants and phenothiazine is a common drug that causes photosensitization. Locoweed ingestion causes KCS and palpebral nerve paralysis, which can in turn cause severe exposure keratoconjunctivitis.

Swine

Miniature swine and obese Vietnamese pot-bellied pigs may have entropion that might require surgical intervention. Weight loss in Vietnamese pot-bellied pigs in conjunction with temporary eyelid eversion techniques may result in the animal not having to have a permanent correction technique performed.

Phenothiazine toxicity in pigs may cause photosensitization phenomena just as in cattle, sheep, and goats. The treatment is the same. Swinepox may cause pox lesions of the lids, third eyelids, and conjunctivae similar to those seen elsewhere on the body. *Escherichia coli* infections (edema disease and endotoxemia) in pigs may cause severe eyelid edema, conjunctival chemosis and inflammation, and even exophthalmos.

CONJUNCTIVAL DISORDERS

Cattle

The conjunctiva is readily seen and highly vascular, and its appearance may be useful in diagnosing systemic disease. Icterus may first be seen on the bulbar conjunctiva; conjunctival hemorrhage may indicate thrombocytopenia, warfarin toxicity, and/or septicemic states, and pallor may indicate anemia. Subconjunctival hemorrhage in newborns is commonly seen following birthing trauma and usually resolves uneventfully with no specific therapy. Infectious conjunctivitis/keratoconjunctivitis ("pinkeye complex") is discussed in the article on surface ocular microbiology in this section. *Moraxella bovis* and infectious bovine rhinotracheitis virus infections are the most common causes of "pinkeye complex" in cattle. Bovine viral diarrhea infection in adult cattle occasionally causes mild conjunctivitis. Conjunctivitis may also be due to exposure to ocular irritants (ammonia fumes, dust and feed material, plant awns and seeds, and disinfectants). When evaluating one or more animals for ocular discharge and conjunctivitis, it is always important to thoroughly examine the affected eyes, take a good history to rule out some of these other disorders, and not immediately diagnose "pinkeye complex" as the cause of all surface inflammatory eye disease.

Infestation of the conjunctival fornices, recesses around the third eyelid, and the nasolacrimal ducts with the nematode worm *Thelazia* ("eye worms") usually causes little or no surface ocular disease, but keratoconjunctivitis may occur with heavy infestations. The diagnosis of ocular thelaziasis is based on identifying the 1- to 2-cm-long worms in the tear film, behind the lids or the third eyelid, or from nasolacrimal duct flushings. Treatment in severe cases involves the use of oral levamisole or fenbendazole, topical application of ivermectin formulated into an eyedrop (2 μg/mL), or picking the worms out of the eye following topical anesthetic application. Systemic ivermectin at recommended doses is not consistently effective against conjunctival *Thelazia*. Reinfection is likely, especially if measures are not taken to eradicate the biologic vector (face flies).

Sheep and Goats

Infectious keratoconjunctivitis in sheep and goats is covered in the article on surface ocular microbiology in this section. *Mycoplasma* and *Chlamydia* spp. are the two most common causes of infectious keratoconjunctivitis in sheep and goats, but as is the case with cattle, other surface bacteria or fungi should not be overlooked as a cause of conjunctivitis in a single animal.

Thelazia californiensis infection is widespread in North America, but clinical disease is uncommon, as is the case in cattle. Conjunctival or nasolacrimal duct involvement with the nasal botfly *Oestrus ovis* may cause irritant conjunctivitis and epiphora. Systemic organophosphate anthelmintics and ivermectin are effective in killing the parasite. Treatment is best performed in the fall when the larvae are small. Manual extraction of the larvae from the conjunctival cul-de-sacs and flushing the nasolacrimal ducts may also be useful in severe cases.

The filarid nematode *Elaeophora schneideri* commonly afflicts sheep, deer, and elk in the high mountain regions of western North America. Adult worms live in the carotid and internal maxillary arteries, but microfilariae can lodge in the capillary beds of the face and orbit and produce an immunologic reaction with facial swelling, alopecia, encrustations, and ulcerations, as well as severe keratoconjunctivitis. Intraocular disease is discussed later in this article. Adult sheep in the fall and winter months are most likely to be afflicted with "sore head." Therapy may include oral piperazine (50 mg/kg) or diethylcarbamazine (100 mg/kg). The efficacy of ivermectin therapy is unknown. Treatment of heavily parasitized animals may be fatal because of occlusion of the carotid arteries with dead adult worms. Biting flies (*Tabanus* spp.) transmit the microfilariae between animals.

Swine

Chlamydial infection as a cause of infectious conjunctivitis has been reported in swine, but the incidence of the disease in swine is much less than in cattle, sheep, and goats. Two systemic infections that may produce conjunctivitis are pseudorabies (the ocular form itself is usually a very mild, self-limiting keratoconjunctivitis) and hog cholera (early in the disease, profuse conjunctivitis and a mucoid to purulent ocular discharge may be seen).

CORNEAL DISORDERS

As far as congenital corneal disease in cattle is concerned, corneal dermoids have already been mentioned, as well as congenital anterior segment malformation disorders in Holsteins with anteriorly luxated lenses and glaucoma/megaloglobus. A bilateral, congenital, recessively inherited corneal endothelial dystrophy in Holsteins is seen as a nonpainful, diffuse corneal edema that can be severe enough to cause blindness. Animals afflicted with any of the disorders just mentioned should obviously not be used for breeding purposes.

Keratitis (inflammation of the cornea) and corneal ulcerations (loss of the surface epithelial layer of the cornea with extension of necrosis into the corneal stroma) can have many causes in all species. The common causes of infectious bovine keratoconjunctivitis in cattle and infectious keratoconjunctivitis in sheep and goats are described in the article on surface ocular microbiology in this section. Topical application of toxic substances in the form of insecticides, disinfectants, and chemicals may cause corneal epithelial and stromal necrosis. Chlorhexidine is a common disinfectant used in dairies and, when accidentally applied to the corneal surface, can cause epithelial and stromal necrosis in animals and humans. Anhydrous ammonia used as a fertilizer and as a silage additive is equally toxic to the corneal surface. Immediate therapy for any toxic substance on the ocular surface is copious lavage with water followed by symptomatic therapy (see later). Photosensitization secondary to toxic plant or phenothiazine ingestion may cause severe corneal edema and has been described earlier in this article. Severe long-term vitamin A deficiency may cause corneal edema along with retinal and optic nerve disease (described in the article Neurogenic Vision Loss).

Trauma to the corneal surface is a common cause of corneal ulceration. In food animals, hay and straw, weeds and grasses, conjunctival foreign bodies, restraint devices, and even switching tails may disrupt the surface corneal epithelium, which may heal uneventfully or become contaminated by local surface bacteria. Exposure ulcerative keratitis is usually found in a central, horizontally located position on the cornea and may be due to an inability to blink because of exophthalmos or palpebral nerve paralysis. Ulcerative keratitis induced by KCS has this same axial distribution.

Clinical signs of ulcerative keratitis include blepharospasm and ocular discharge (serous to purulent). In food animals, a palpebral nerve block may be necessary to thoroughly examine an ulcerated eye. The definitive diagnosis of a corneal ulcer is based on the retention of fluorescein dye, which indicates an epithelial defect. Additional diagnostic tests include examination of the conjunctival cul-de-sacs and behind the third eyelid for foreign materials that may have caused the ulceration. Corneal scrapings for cytologic evaluation and/or bacterial/fungal culture and sensitivity testing may be indicated in deep, necrotic ulcerations or in the case of ulcerations that are not healing.

The general treatment strategy includes removal of the inciting causes and symptomatic medical therapy. If a conjunctival foreign body is causing the ulceration, removal of the foreign body may allow the cornea to heal uneventfully. Exposure keratitis secondary to lagophthalmos or exophthalmos may necessitate a temporary tarsorrhaphy or a third eyelid flap to protect the cornea until the underlying cause of the lagophthalmos or exophthalmos can be corrected. Symptomatic therapy includes three- or four-times-daily topical administration of broad-spectrum ophthalmic antibiotics (neomycin–polymyxin B–bacitracin, tetracycline, and gentamicin are all good first-choice drugs) and topical 1% atropine ophthalmic ointment (twice daily) to reduce ciliary body and iris sphincter spasm and pain. If culture and sensitivity testing have been done, the sensitivity results may dictate what antibiotic to use topically. Topical or subconjunctival corticosteroids are contraindicated in the treatment of all corneal ulcerations. If the herdsman is unable to treat frequently, topical antibiotics can be augmented by bulbar subconjunctival injection of antibiotics (penicillin, cephalosporins, gentamicin, but not tetracycline), but this will deliver drug to the site for only 12 to 18 hours. Subconjunctival antibiotic injections into the eyelid stroma are rapidly absorbed and are of little use in treating corneal ulcers. Most corneal ulcers in food animals heal uneventfully with medical therapy alone. In the case of valuable animals, referral to a specialist may be in order for the more difficult surgical treatment of deep ulcerations or perforations, which may necessitate general anesthesia and microsurgical techniques. In a field situation, third eyelid flaps will support and protect a deep corneal ulcer and may allow for even small perforations or small full-thickness corneal lacerations to heal with retention of the globe and possibly even vision. Eyes with large corneal perforations or lacerations or eyes with corneal perforations with obvious extension of infection into the eye or prolapse of the intraocular contents should be enucleated.

ANTERIOR UVEAL DISORDERS

The uvea is the vascular portion of the eye and is made up of the iris, ciliary body, and choroid. Commonly used terminology includes anterior uvea for the iris and ciliary body and posterior uvea for the choroid. Because the uveal structures are highly vascular, they have the capacity to become inflamed after local or systemic (blood-borne) stimuli. Congenital defects and malformations (with or without a hereditary predisposition) are rare in food animals and usually important only for recognition purposes so that these animals are not used for breeding. Aniridia (total absence of an iris), iris hypoplasia, persistent pupillary membranes (iris strands bridging across the iris, from the iris to the cornea, or from the iris to the lens), previously described anterior segment dysplasia with glaucoma and megaloglobus, and heterochromia iridis (depigmented or multicolored iris tissue) are commonly occurring congenital/hereditary uveal defects that have been described in food animals.

Inflammation of uveal tissues is the most common and most important uveal disease seen in food animals. Commonly used terms are iritis (inflamed iris), cyclitis (inflamed ciliary body), iridocyclitis or anterior uveitis (inflammation of the iris and ciliary body), choroiditis or posterior uveitis (inflammation of the choroid), chorioretinitis (inflammation of the choroid and adjacent retina), endophthalmitis (inflammation of the uvea and intraocular chambers), and panophthalmitis (inflammation of the internal and external ocular structures and adjacent adnexa and orbit). Common clinical signs of uveitis may include blindness, photophobia, blepharospasm, tearing, episcleral and conjunctival vascular injection, corneal edema, anterior chamber cloudiness as a result of elevated protein levels (aqueous flare), and the presence of settled white blood cells (hypopyon) or red cells (hyphema) in the aqueous humor. Uveitis initially causes a soft eye, but chronic uveitis can cause obstruction of aqueous humor outflow with secondary glaucoma. A swollen iris and a miotic pupil are usually seen with active uveitis. Chronic uveitis can lead to poor lens nutrition and cataract formation.

Because most cases of uveitis in food animals are due to an underlying systemic disease, a thorough physical examination and workup are indicated. Appropriate treatment of the underlying disease is the most important part of a treatment strategy for uveitis. Symptomatic ocular therapy may include topical application of 1% atropine ophthalmic ointment three to four times daily to achieve mydriasis and negate painful ciliary spasm, topical administration of antibiotics similar to those used to treat the systemic infection, and systemic nonsteroidal anti-inflammatory drugs to reduce ocular inflammation and pain. If the cornea is nonulcerated, topical corticosteroids (dexamethasone-neomycin–polymyxin B ointment [Maxitrol, Alcon] four times daily) or bulbar subconjunctival corticosteroids (betamethasone acetate [Celestone Soluspan, Schering], 1 mL) will help relieve the anterior uveitis but will not usually cause systemic immunosuppression.

Blunt trauma to the globe may produce traumatic anterior uveitis. This is usually (but not always) unilateral, and hyphema or subconjunctival hemorrhage is often present. Symptomatic

therapy as described earlier is indicated. Anterior uveitis secondary to surface eye disease (pinkeye complex) is usually mild in comparison to uveitis caused by systemic disease (with the exception of a perforated eye and secondary endophthalmitis). Treatment of the surface eye disease and systemic nonsteroidal anti-inflammatory drugs will usually resolve this form of anterior uveitis. Other systemic diseases causing uveitis are described as follows.

Cattle

Neonatal septicemias caused by navel ill, scours, and pneumonia may cause anterior uveitis in calves. *E. coli*, *Corynebacterium*, *Klebsiella*, *Listeria*, *Salmonella*, *Staphylococcus*, and *Streptococcus* spp. are common etiologic agents. Comatose calves with anterior uveitis many times will also have meningoencephalitis, so the presence of anterior uveitis is an important negative prognostic sign. In adult cattle, anterior uveitis is most commonly seen secondary to metritis, mastitis, peritonitis, and reticulopericarditis.

Tuberculosis may be a cause of granulomatous anterior uveitis and should be ruled out as an underlying disease because of its public health significance. Clinical signs of malignant catarrhal fever in the acute form include bilateral mucoid to mucopurulent ocular discharge with severe episcleral and conjunctival injection, initial peripheral corneal edema and neovascularization that eventually become complete, hypopyon, and miosis. Blindness results from this initial anterior uveitis or from the subsequent panophthalmitis. Listeriosis in young cattle being fed silage may result in anterior uveitis as well as the posterior uveitis and neurologic disease usually seen.

Sheep and Goats

Septicemia secondary to *Mycoplasma agalactiae* infection is a common cause of anterior uveitis or panophthalmitis in sheep and goats. Other neonatal septicemias caused by coliforms, *Staphylococcus* spp., and *Streptococcus* spp. occur less frequently. Listeriosis in 4- to 6-month-old feedlot lambs being fed silage may cause anterior uveitis similar to that seen in calves. In the mountainous regions of western North America, *E. schneideri* infection ("sore head") in sheep may cause keratitis, aqueous flare and hypopyon, cataracts, chorioretinitis, and optic neuritis in conjunction with the previously described lesions of the lids and conjunctiva. Toxoplasmosis is an uncommon cause of anterior uveitis and chorioretinitis in sheep, goats, and cattle.

Swine

Anterior uveitis and chorioretinitis are uncommonly diagnosed in pigs, but they may occur with systemic diseases such as hog cholera, Glasser's disease (*Haemophilus somnus* infection in young piglets), and septicemia secondary to erysipelas.

DISORDERS OF THE LENS

Disorders of the lens are uncommonly reported in food animals, possibly because unless noticeable vision loss is observed, the lenses are not examined (so subtle changes or unilateral abnormalities may go unnoticed). The lenses are seldom evaluated with full pupillary dilation and adequate instrumentation (so subtle changes go unnoticed), and food animals usually do not live long enough for senile lens changes to develop, as is the case in companion animals and horses. The most frequently seen lens disorder is opacification of the lens, or cataract. Cataract is most commonly seen in food animals as a congenital anomaly, but acquired cataract is occasionally noted.

Cattle

Congenital cataracts in calves may be due to inheritance or in utero infection, or they may be due to any toxic, traumatic, or other metabolic disorder that affects development of the eye or lens. There is no way to evaluate a single animal and determine whether the cause of the cataract is inherited, infectious, or toxic in its etiology. If cataracts are found in other age-matched calves from different genetic lines within a herd, a congenital accident or infectious disease may be the cause. When calves of common genetic lines are repeatedly afflicted, inheritance should be suspected. Unless inheritance can be definitively ruled out, bull calves with congenital cataracts should be rejected for use as studs.

In the Jersey, Hereford, Holstein, and Shorthorn breeds, autosomal recessive inheritance of cataracts has been described. In the Jersey breed, congenital cataracts with other anomalies such as lens luxation and microphakia, with or without megaloglobus, have been described. In Hereford and Holstein cattle, a form of congenital cataract that becomes totally mature at 4 to 11 months of age has been noted. There may or may not be other ocular anomalies associated with these cataracts. In Shorthorns, a congenital cataract has been described that may also be seen in conjunction with microphthalmos, hydrocephalus, cerebellar hypoplasia, and myopathy.

Infection in utero between days 75 and 150 of gestation with bovine viral diarrheal virus can cause congenital cortical cataracts in conjunction with microphthalmos, retinal dysplasia and scarring, cerebellar hypoplasia, and brachygnathism. If minimally afflicted, some of these calves may be visual enough to be raised for production purposes.

Anterior uveitis may cause degenerative changes in the anterior segment leading to secondary cataract formation. Young animals with neonatal septicemias, animals with severe infectious bovine keratoconjunctivitis, animals with trauma to the globe or orbit, and adult animals with systemic disease and secondary uveitis may have adhesion of the iris to the anterior lens capsule (posterior synechia), inflammatory debris on the lens capsule, and cataract formation that may lead to vision loss. For this reason, all animals with uveitis should have supportive, symptomatic treatment of the eye in conjunction with definitive systemic treatment for the underlying primary disease.

Sheep and Goats

Cataracts are even less commonly diagnosed in sheep and goats than in cattle. Inherited cataracts have been described in New Zealand Romney sheep. Uveitis-induced cataracts are seen in animals that have uveitis secondary to *E. schneideri* infestation or *M. agalactiae* infection. Uveitis-induced cataracts in sheep and goats appear clinically similar to uveitis-induced cataracts in cattle.

Swine

Cataracts in pigs are very uncommonly seen. Starvation and riboflavin deficiency have been described as causing incomplete cataracts. Hygromycin B has been noted to cause cataracts in adult sows. In Vietnamese pot-bellied pigs, juvenile cataracts are seen with an age of onset of 1 to 4 years. This type of cataract

may be inherited. Uveitis can cause cataracts in pigs just like in sheep, goats, and cattle.

DISORDERS OF THE FUNDUS

As is the case with disorders of the lens, fundic disorders in food animals are often underdiagnosed. However, as is the case with anterior uveitis, examination of the ocular fundus and diagnosis of abnormalities may be useful for systemic diseases (especially those involving the central nervous system), as well as in cases of vision impairment. Fundic disorders may be grouped into congenital disorders, degenerative disorders, and inflammatory diseases. Congenital disorders may be due to inheritance, in utero infection, or deficiencies that lead to abnormal ocular development. Degenerative disorders can be caused by nutritional deficiencies or ingestion of toxic substances that cause retinal or optic nerve death (seen as depigmentation of the nontapetal area, "shiny" hyper-reflectivity of the tapetal zone, and retinal vascular attenuation).

Inflammatory diseases of the fundus are often due to infections involving the vascular choroid and retina. Many inflammatory diseases of the fundus also involve the anterior uvea as well. Aside from vision loss (which may not be seen unless bilateral, end-stage chorioretinal disease is present), clinical signs of active chorioretinal disease include subretinal exudate or hemorrhage that appears as a poorly delineated, dull discoloration of the tapetal and nontapetal zones. Gray exudates are more easily seen when perivascular in location or when in the nontapetal zone than when the tapetal zone is involved. Total separation of the retina from the underlying retinal pigment epithelium and choroid is seen as retinal detachment (a thin, gray "veil" protruding forward from the back of the eye like a "sail in the wind"). Inactive chorioretinal lesions are typically well demarcated, depigmented areas in the nontapetal fundus and shiny, hyper-reflective areas (sometimes surrounding hyperpigmented foci) in the tapetal zone. Active optic neuritis appears as swelling of the optic nerve with indistinct exudate, edema, and/or hemorrhage seen within the nerve head or immediately adjacent to it. Optic nerve atrophy is manifested as a pale, shrunken, sometimes avascular nerve head.

Cattle

In all ruminants, persistence of the hyaloid vasculature is common. In young animals the hyaloid vessels may contain blood, and thin white strands from the optic nerve to the back of the lens may be seen in adult animals. The persistent hyaloid remnant emanating from the optic nerve is called Bergmeister's papilla. Colobomas of the optic nerve and peripapillary choroid are seen in the Hereford and Charolais breeds. Inherited colobomas are typically seen at the 6-o'clock position and are bilateral. Vitamin A deficiency in cows may cause in utero optic nerve hypoplasia and retinal degeneration (vitamin A deficiency–associated optic neuropathy and retinal atrophy are further described in the article Neurogenic Vision Loss in this section). In utero infection with bovine viral diarrhea virus at 75 to 150 days of gestation causes multifocal areas of chorioretinal scarring/dysplasia as a result of virally induced necrosis of the developing retina. Total generalized retinal degeneration leading to total blindness may be seen in some of these calves.

Neonatal septicemias may cause multifocal or generalized chorioretinitis as well as anterior uveitis. Animals that survive may have multifocal chorioretinal scars. Thromboembolic meningoencephalitis caused by *H. somnus* infection in young cattle usually does not cause anterior uveitis, but characteristics of chorioretinal and perivascular exudate ("cotton-wool" spots) and multifocal retinal hemorrhage are often seen. Multifocal scars may be seen if the animal survives. Listeriosis usually causes anterior uveitis, but it can cause multifocal areas of chorioretinitis as well. Other diseases that can cause retinal hemorrhage, chorioretinitis, retinal detachment, and/or optic neuritis are malignant catarrhal fever, tuberculosis, and toxoplasmosis.

Polioencephalomalacia secondary to thiamine deficiency occasionally causes papilledema as well as other neurologic signs (see the article Neurogenic Vision Loss). Ingestion of the male fern *Dryopteris filix-mas* may cause acute papilledema and end-stage changes that can be seen as generalized retinal atrophy. Locoweed toxicity may result in KCS and generalized retinal degeneration along with other central nervous system disorders.

Sheep and Goats

Bluetongue virus exposure during the first half of gestation (either as a viral infection or as a vaccination with modified live virus vaccine) may cause in utero necrosis of the developing retina with subsequent postpartum signs of multifocal retinal scars/retinal dysplasia, vision impairment, and cerebellar hypoplasia and hydrocephalus.

Neonatal septicemias, listeriosis, and toxoplasmosis may cause chorioretinitis, as was the case in cattle. *E. schneideri* infestation may cause chorioretinitis and optic neuritis during acute disease and chorioretinal scars, optic nerve atrophy, and blindness as sequelae to the acute disease. Scrapie virus has a characteristic retinopathy that accompanies the neurologic disease. Multifocal, oval, raised "blister-like" lesions less than 1 disk diameter in size are scattered throughout the tapetal fundus.

Chronic bracken fern (*Pteridium aquilinum*) ingestion causes "bright blindness" in sheep. After many months of grazing, progressive generalized retinal degeneration occurs and results in blindness. In western Australia, "blind grass" (*Stypandra imbricata*) ingestion causes a similar retinal atrophy in sheep. Chronic ingestion of locoweed causes KCS and retinal atrophy in sheep, as was the case in cattle. Hexachlorophene (used in countries outside the United States to treat liver flukes) can cause acute optic nerve-head edema within 24 hours of ingestion of a toxic dose, with subsequent generalized retinal atrophy, optic nerve atrophy, and blindness.

Swine

Optic nerve colobomas (typically bilateral and at the 6-o'clock position) are seen as a presumed inherited defect in miniature swine.

Listeriosis, tuberculosis, toxoplasmosis, and Glasser's disease may cause multifocal areas of chorioretinitis in swine.

Arsanilic acid toxicity can cause optic nerve atrophy in swine (see the article Neurogenic Vision Loss in this section).

BIBLIOGRAPHY

Barnett KC: Color Atlas of Veterinary Ophthalmology. St Louis, Mosby–Year Book, 1996.
Lavach JD: Large Animal Ophthalmology. St Louis, Mosby–Year Book, 1990.
Leipold HW: Congenital ocular defects in food-producing animals. Vet Clin North Am Large Anim Pract 6:577–595, 1984.
Miller TR, Gelatt KN: Food animal ophthalmology. *In* Gelatt KN (ed): Veterinary Ophthalmology, ed 2. Philadelphia, Lea & Febiger, 1991, pp 611–655.
Moore CP, Miller RB: Infectious and parasitic diseases of cattle. *In* Howard JL (ed): Current Veterinary Therapy: Food Animal Practice, ed 3. Philadelphia, WB Saunders, 1993, pp 834–839.
Moore CP, Wallace LM: Selected eye diseases of sheep and goats. *In* Howard JL (ed): Current Veterinary Therapy: Food Animal Practice, ed 3. Philadelphia, WB Saunders, 1993, pp 839–842.
Moore CP, Whitley RD: Ophthalmic diseases of small domestic ruminants. Vet Clin North Am Large Anim Pract 6:641–665, 1984.
Rebhun WC: Diseases of Dairy Cattle. Baltimore, Williams & Wilkins, 1995, pp 443–468.
Rebhun WC: Ocular manifestations of systemic diseases in cattle. Vet Clin North Am Large Anim Pract 6:623–639, 1984.
Severin GA: Severin's Veterinary Ophthalmology Notes, ed 3. Fort Collins, Colo, DesignPointe Communications, 1996.
Smith MC, Sherman DM: Goat Medicine. Philadelphia, Lea & Febiger, 1994, pp 179–192.
Vestre WA: Porcine ophthalmology. Vet Clin North Am Large Anim Pract 6:667–676, 1984.

■ Ophthalmology of South American Camelids: Llamas, Alpacas, Guanacos, and Vicuñas

Juliet Rathbone Gionfriddo, D.V.M., M.S., Diplomate, A.C.V.O.
Deborah S. Friedman, D.V.M., Diplomate, A.C.V.O.

South American camelids have become companion animals of importance to veterinary practice. Llamas and alpacas have considerable economic value in the United States, and in South America these animals are necessary for food, wool, transportation, and fuel. The ocular anatomy of the South American camelid differs greatly from that of other domestic species.

ANATOMY

The large and prominent eyes of camelids are only slightly smaller than equine and bovine eyes despite their considerably smaller body size. They are framed with long lashes and three pairs of vibrissae. The eyelids are tightly adherent to the globe, which makes examination of the conjunctival fornices difficult. Unlike in other domestic animals, no meibomian gland duct openings are present on the eyelid margin. In the camel, a closely related species, meibomian glands are also absent but are replaced by sebaceous glands on the lacrimal caruncle.[1] This is probably the case in the llama as well.

Magnification is helpful in observation of the nasolacrimal puncta, which are 4 to 6 mm inside the medial canthus. The tear drainage system starts with dorsal and ventral canaliculi, which join to form a lacrimal sac. The nasolacrimal duct extends from the lacrimal sac through the lacrimal and maxillary bones and then traverses the nasal cavity. The nasal opening of the nasolacrimal duct is 1.5 to 2 cm proximal to the nares and laterally placed as in sheep and goats. In the adult llama, the duct is 11 to 15 cm long and 2 to 4 mm in diameter.[2]

The prominent appearance of the llama eye is enhanced by the lack of visible sclera within the palpebral fissure. Often the conjunctiva overlying any exposed sclera is pigmented so that no white is evident. The limbus has a dark brown pigment band 2 to 3 mm wide.

The elaborate structure of the iris is a striking feature of the llama eye (Fig. 1). On the dorsal and ventral margins of the pupil, the posterior pigment epithelium of the iris is proliferated and folded vertically. This pupillary ruff is analogous to the corpora nigra of horses but is significantly larger and consists

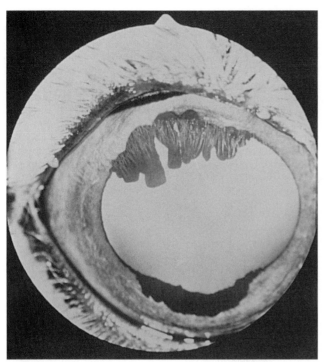

Figure 1

Photograph of a llama iris showing the distinctive pupillary ruff, which represents a protrusion and folding of the posterior pigment epithelium of the iris.

of folded layers rather than globular masses. Iris pigmentation is usually various shades of brown and occasionally blue. Persistent pupillary membranes are common, especially near the pupillary margin. Neonatal llamas occasionally have thin, gray fibrinous strands spanning one or two folds of the pupillary ruff.

The fundus of camelids lacks a tapetum.[1, 3–5] However, it may appear highly reflective because of a prominent Bruch membrane that has been identified histologically.[5] Ophthalmoscopic examination shows the fundus to be either red and brown or blue and brown. The red coloration is due to choroidal vessels being visible through a nonpigmented retinal pigment epithelium.

A study of 29 alpacas demonstrated a relationship between coat color, iris color, and retinal pigmentation.[6] Animals with light coat colors had various combinations of gray, blue, and brown irides and reduced pigmentation of the fundus. Those with dark coat colors had brown irides and pigmented fundi.[6]

The optic disk and retinal vasculature are similar to those of the bovine. A large Bergmeister papilla (hyaloid remnant) may protrude from the disk, and three to five pairs of large retinal vessels emerge from its periphery. Two pairs of vessels leave the optic disk horizontally and are usually accompanied by myelin, which extends several disk diameters peripherally into the fundus (Fig. 2).

The bony orbit of the llama, like that of the horse and ox, is complete and made up of the frontal, lacrimal, zygomatic, maxillary, palatine, temporal, and sphenoid bones. There is a large notch dorsally in the frontal bone that is palpable in living animals. Rostral to the medial aspect of the orbit is a 2-cm-diameter opening into the nasal cavity. This opening is probably associated with a scent gland.

EXAMINATION

A complete evaluation of the camelid eye is important as part of a routine physical examination and when ophthalmic disease

is suspected. In addition, the eyes of all sick camelids should be examined because many systemic diseases have ophthalmic manifestations.[7]

Ocular examination is optimally undertaken with the llama restrained in stocks. Chemical sedation (butorphanol, 0.02 to 0.04 mg/kg) is occasionally necessary to control head movement.[7] Liquids such as tropicamide, topical anesthetic, and fluorescein may be applied to the eye with a "squirt gun" made from a 3-mL syringe and a needle broken at the hub.

A complete ocular examination should include an external eye and anterior segment examination under magnification, reflex responses, a Schirmer tear test, measurements of intraocular pressure, and funduscopy. The menace reflex for testing vision may be elicited by a sudden hand movement across the visual axis. The llama should blink or jump back. Direct and indirect pupillary light reflexes are slow, and movement of the iris is minimal. The mean Schirmer tear test value is 19 mm/minute in a nonanesthetized eye.[8] Fluorescein dye is applied to the eye to help detect corneal ulcers and for the diagnosis of tear drainage problems. Intraocular pressure is most easily measured with an applanation tonometer and averages 14 mm Hg. One application (about 0.25 mL) of 1% tropicamide will cause mydriasis within 20 to 45 minutes.

Dacryocystorhinography may be used for detailed examination of the nasolacrimal drainage system. For this procedure, 5 mL of a sodium and meglumine diatrizoate mixture is injected into the dorsal lacrimal punctum, and lateral and dorsoventral radiographs are then taken.[9]

CAMELID OCULAR DISEASE

Limited information is available concerning the types and frequencies of ocular disease in camelids. Gelatt and colleagues reported on routine ophthalmic examinations of 29 healthy alpacas in South America.[6] In this report, 38% of the alpacas

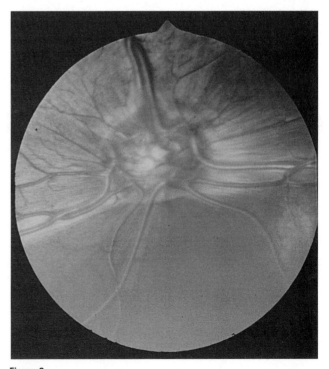

Figure 2

Photograph of the fundus of a llama. Note the large retinal blood vessels and the myelin from the optic disk, which is extending out into the fundus.

had at least one ocular problem, including conjunctivitis, corneal scars, posterior synechiae, cataracts, a subluxated lens, vitreous opacities, and an optic disk coloboma. Most were thought to be secondary to trauma, but some may have been hereditary.[6] A recent retrospective study of the Veterinary Medical Database (VMDB) for a 13-year period found that at least one ocular problem was diagnosed in 6% (194 of 3243) of the llamas seen at veterinary teaching hospitals.[10] Trauma was also considered the primary cause in many of these cases.

Cornea

Corneal disease is the most common ocular abnormality in llamas. Forty-one percent of the llamas with ocular disease reported to the VMDB had corneal disease, and more than half of these were ulcers.[10] Most of them were of unknown cause but were probably traumatic in origin. There is no evidence that llamas or other camelids have primary corneal invasion by bacteria such as *Moraxella bovis*, the main cause of infectious bovine keratoconjunctivitis.[6, 7, 10] Other trauma-associated corneal diseases in llamas include corneal lacerations, foreign bodies, and stromal abscesses.[8, 10] Corneal trauma may be seen in llamas recumbent because of anesthesia, tick paralysis, meningeal worms, or illnesses secondary to a lack of passive transfer.[8, 10]

Treatment of corneal ulcers, lacerations, and infection in camelids is similar to that in other species.[11] Because bacterial pathogens are often present on the normal camelid eye, topical broad-spectrum antibiotics should be used in all cases of corneal ulcers or lacerations.[8] Corneal lacerations may be sutured directly with small-gauge (6-0 to 8-0), absorbable suture material. Deep ulcers in llamas often heal well under the protection of conjunctival grafts as in other species.

Other corneal diseases include dystrophies, degenerations, dermoids, and edema.[10, 12, 13] Bilateral corneal edema was reported in a guanaco and her offspring.[14] The corneal endothelium of camelids appears to be highly sensitive and, if irritated, becomes ineffective in removing excess water from the corneal stroma. Severe corneal edema develops readily after intraocular surgery and corneal trauma.

Conjunctiva

Diseases of the conjunctiva were reported in 19 llamas (10% of the llamas with ocular disease) in a study of the VMDB.[10] Most of these cases were conjunctivitis "due to unknown cause," but there were several conjunctival infections.[10] Numerous bacteria have been isolated from llamas with conjunctivitis.[15] These were suspected to be the primary cause of the disease, although they may have been secondary invaders. *Staphylococcus aureus* was isolated from the inflamed conjunctiva of a llama with keratoconjunctivitis.[16] Clinical signs of bacterial conjunctivitis include hyperemia, serous or mucopurulent ocular discharge, and blepharospasm.

Microbiologic culture (both bacterial and fungal) and sensitivity testing are recommended in most cases of conjunctivitis and keratoconjunctivitis. Most bacterial infections respond well to appropriate topical antibacterial therapy.

Other causes of infectious conjunctivitis include chlamydiae[13] and parasites. *Thelazia californiensis*, a nematode, has been found in the conjunctival sac of many species, including llamas.[17] The pathology of *Thelazia* in llamas ranges from mild conjunctivitis[17] to severe ulcerative keratitis.[8] The initial signs of infection are usually those of nonspecific conjunctivitis. If corneal ulcers are present, however, there may be purulent discharge and photophobia. The nematode is transmitted among animals by face

flies, and *Thelazia* may be seen on the surface of the eye or beneath the third eyelid.[17] Treatment consists of mechanical removal following topical anesthesia, or diethylcarbamazine or ivermectin drops may be instilled into the conjunctival sac to kill the parasite.[17] Many types of flies feed on llama lacrimal secretions and cause conjunctival irritation. Consequently, fly control is important for minimizing this form of conjunctivitis.

Noninfectious conjunctival abnormalities include trauma, foreign bodies, dermoids, and congenital cysts.[8, 10, 18] Large conjunctival wounds should be sutured with small-gauge, absorbable suture material. Small wounds usually heal with medical therapy alone. Congenital cysts have been reported infrequently in crias (neonatal llamas).[19] Schuh and colleagues reported a cystlike structure on the bulbar conjunctiva of a cria.[18] Aspiration of this structure yielded a clear fluid. Because the same eye had other defects, the cyst was thought to be part of a general ocular maldevelopment.[18] A conjunctival cyst, without other ocular lesions, was reported by Johnson.[19] After drainage of the cyst failed to permanently resolve the problem, surgical excision proved curative.

Eyelids and Nasolacrimal System

In the VMDB study only 13 llamas (7%) were reported to have eyelid diseases.[10] Blepharitis was the most common eyelid problem, and several of these llamas had concurrent dermatitis. Blepharitis caused by bacterial infection has been seen and often occurs in conjunction with bacterial conjunctivitis.[13]

Eyelid lacerations in llamas were uncommon in the VMDB study; they were seen in only two animals.[10] Eyelid lacerations can be serious in llamas because of the potential for secondary corneal damage from exposure. Therefore, all full-thickness eyelid lacerations should be sutured.

Nasolacrimal duct disorders seem to be relatively common in camelids. Congenital nasolacrimal duct/punctal atresia was recorded in five crias in the VMDB.[10] Four llamas examined by Severin had congenital punctal atresia.[13] The puncta were successfully opened with a procedure similar to that used in horses.[20] Sapienza and colleagues described a case of severe epiphora caused by bilateral atresia of the nasolacrimal ducts in a cria.[9] The palpebral puncta were patent and the congenital obstruction was at the nasal opening of the duct. Surgical opening of the obstruction was successful.

Lens

Cataracts are the most common abnormalities of the camelid lens. They were reported in 20 animals (10%) in the VMDB.[10] Mature, hypermature, and immature cataracts have been reported.[6, 8, 13, 14, 21, 22] In a South American herd of 29 alpacas, Gelatt and co-workers saw 1 animal with apparently normal vision but with nuclear cataracts.[6] Whether small, immature cataracts in camelids progress to maturity or whether they are inherited is unknown.[14, 17, 21, 22] Some cataracts in camelids severely impair vision.[14, 21, 23] Attempts at cataract removal have had poor outcomes. In a report of cataract surgery in a llama, lens extraction was followed by severe corneal edema, ulcerative keratitis, and phthisis bulbi.[23] Recently, the use of phacoemulsification and viscoelastics for cataract extraction has greatly improved the success rate in dogs. Yet these new techniques do not seem to have improved the success rate for cataract surgery in camelids. Veterinary ophthalmologists report severe, intractable corneal edema in most camelids that have undergone cataract surgery, no matter what surgical techniques are used or which medications are used perioperatively.[15]

Although infrequently seen, other lens diseases in llamas include luxated lenses, traumatic lens rupture, and lens colobomas. A lens coloboma was seen temporally in the left lens of a female guanaco and was associated with nuclear and perinuclear cataracts and corneal edema.[14] A hereditary cause for the defects was suspected.

Uvea

Uveitis (anterior and posterior combined) was the second most commonly diagnosed ocular problem in llamas in the VMDB.[10] Thirty-five llamas (18%) had uveitis. Most were recorded as having "endophthalmitis uveitis" or were "due to unknown cause." Trauma was also a frequent cause of uveitis. Anterior uveitis has been seen in septicemic neonates and crias with juvenile llama immunodeficiency syndrome.[10, 19] Uveitis may also be secondary to deep ulcerative keratitis, trauma, and infectious disease such as equine herpesvirus type 1 (EHV-1).[10, 24]

Posterior Segment: Retina, Optic Nerve

Diseases of the posterior segment are relatively common in camelids. In the VMDB, 11 animals (6%) were reported to have retinal lesions,[10] including retinitis, retinal detachment, retinal dystrophy, and retinal degeneration. Optic nerve disease was reported in 2 llamas: 1 had optic nerve hypoplasia and the other had a coloboma.[10]

Congenital defects of the retina, choroid, and optic nerve of camelids have been reported.[6–8, 18] These defects may be confined to a single structure or, more often, may involve multiple structures. During histopathologic examination of the eyes of neonatal llamas, Dubielzig saw multiple ocular defects including peripapillary colobomas, retinal dysplasia, retinal detachment, and vitreous fibrosis and ossification.[5] A large optic disk coloboma was observed in a young llama during routine ocular examination.[3] Schuh and colleagues described a llama with a large coloboma near the optic disk.[18] Although colobomas are known to be hereditary in cattle,[20] their heritability has not been established in camelids. In general, however, camelids with congenital posterior segment defects should not be bred.[7]

Two infectious diseases have been reported to cause posterior segment disease in camelids: EHV-1 and disseminated aspergillosis, with EHV-1 being the more widely seen. Camelids acquire EHV-1 by contact with members of the family Equidae. Rebhun and associates reported that members of a mixed herd of camelids became blind after exposure to infected zebras.[24] Neurologic signs including head tilt, nystagmus, and paralysis developed in four alpacas. Ophthalmoscopy showed vitritis, retinitis, and optic neuritis. Histopathologic examination of the eyes of two animals showed retinal and subretinal hemorrhage, vasculitis, subretinal exudate, and retinal detachment. Two alpacas also had hypopyon and iritis. All attempted treatments failed to restore vision to any animal. Histologic identification of eosinophilic inclusions in the brain and measurement of high EHV-1 antibody titers in the serum confirmed EHV-1 as the cause.

In 1989 a similar outbreak occurred in a herd of llamas in Illinois.[3] Twenty-eight llamas were exposed to zebras with rhinitis. In 10 to 17 days, neurologic signs including blindness, deafness, head tilt, and circling developed in most of the llamas. Ophthalmic examination showed severe anterior uveitis and chorioretinitis. Equine herpesvirus type 1 was confirmed as the cause of this outbreak.

The extreme pathogenicity of EHV-1 in llamas was shown when three llamas were experimentally infected intranasally with EHV-1.[25] Two of the llamas exhibited severe neurologic signs, including blindness, staggering, head tremors, and depression.

Histopathologic assessment showed severe neuronal changes in the brain and optic nerve. Isolation of EHV-1 was successful in only one (the most clinically ill) of the three infected animals, which suggests that it may be difficult to isolate the virus from infected animals.

Paulsen and colleagues[26] described a llama with chorioretinitis, optic neuritis, and encephalitis. Serologic tests failed to implicate EHV-1, and no intranuclear inclusion bodies were seen histopathologically. The similarity of this animal to the chronically affected alpacas described by Rebhun and co-workers[24] suggests that this may have been a case of chronic EHV-1 in which the virus was not identified.

No effective treatment or method of prevention of EHV-1 infection in camelids is known. Vaccination of llamas for EHV-1 with the equine vaccine has been attempted, but its efficacy has not been evaluated.

Aspergillosis was implicated as a cause of neurologic disease and chorioretinitis in a wild-caught, zoo-housed alpaca.[27] On necropsy, *Aspergillus* was identified in the lung and eye. The fungus was thought to have spread from the lungs to the eye hematogenously.

Toxoplasmosis, a known cause of chorioretinitis in dogs and cats, may also cause blindness in camelids. During an investigation of causes of late-term abortions in llamas, a serologic survey showed an extremely high antibody titer for *Toxoplasma* in a nonaborting blind llama.[19] The llama had lesions of chronic panophthalmitis. Tinsley described a 15-year-old llama with signs of bilateral uveitis.[28] Vitreous humor was collected from one eye at hospital admission and 1 month later. Vitreous toxoplasmosis antibody titers showed a marked rise, although serum antibody titers were negative. These results suggested that an ocular *Toxoplasma gondii* infection may have caused the uveitis.

Miscellaneous Diseases

Although rare, glaucoma has been seen in camelids; two cases were reported in the VMDB.[10] Severin observed increased intraocular pressure in two llamas with normal-appearing eyes.[13] There are no known reports of secondary glaucoma in camelids. Barrie and associates used gonioscopy to examine the drainage angle of a guanaco with corneal edema and normal intraocular pressure.[14] They found the drainage angle to be closed and spanned by uveal tissue. The prevalence of goniodysgenesis and subsequent glaucoma is unknown. Routine tonometry and gonioscopy on diseased and healthy eyes may show a higher prevalence of glaucoma than has been reported.

Visual deficits are being diagnosed with increasing frequency in camelids. Eleven blind neonatal crias with apparently normal fundi were seen at Colorado State University Veterinary Teaching Hospital.[13] Vision gradually returned to all crias; no cause was found. Congenital nystagmus and amblyopia have also been diagnosed in crias.[13] There are numerous reports of permanent blindness with no apparent ocular defects or diseases in adult llamas.[15] These cases may be due to sudden retinal degeneration or a brain disorder. In some cases, electroretinograms and/or visual evoked potentials can be generated in camelids to test the visual pathways and explore the cause of the blindness.

Ocular and periocular neoplasia seems to be rare in llamas. In 14 years only two cases of neoplasia were reported to the VMDB.[10] One was an intraocular medulloepithelioma and the other was an unspecified corneal tumor. No cases of squamous cell carcinoma were reported. This is particularly interesting inasmuch as almost 50% of the cases in the VMDB were from Colorado State University, which serves a region having a relatively high elevation.[10] The increased exposure to ultraviolet light at high altitudes is a predisposing factor to squamous cell carcinoma in cattle and horses.[29] The low tumor incidence in llamas may reflect an adaptation of camelids to exposure to ultraviolet light.

Much remains to be learned about llama eyes. The results of research into the etiology of various ocular diseases, especially the mode of inheritance of suspected hereditary problems (such as cataracts and colobomas), will have practical value for veterinary practitioners advising llama owners about breeding programs and treating camelids with ocular disease.

REFERENCES

1. Duke-Elder S: System of Ophthalmology, vol 1, The Eye in Evolution. St Louis, CV Mosby, 1958, pp 458, 470.
2. Sapienza JS, Isaza R, Johnson RD, Miller TR: Anatomic and radiographic study of the lacrimal apparatus of llamas. Am J Vet Res 53:1007–1009, 1992.
3. Friedman DS: Unpublished data, 1989.
4. Rahi AHS, Sheikh H, Morgan G: Histology of the camel eye. Acta Anat 106:345–350, 1980.
5. Dubielzig RR: Personal communication, 1990, 1997.
6. Gelatt KN, Otzen Martinic GB, Flaneig JL, et al: Results of ophthalmic examinations of 29 alpacas. J Am Vet Med Assoc 206:1204–1207, 1995.
7. Gionfriddo JR: Ophthalmology. Vet Clin North Am Food Anim Pract 16:371–382, 1994.
8. Gionfriddo JR, Friedman DS: Ophthalmology of South American camelids: Llamas, alpacas, guanacos, and vicuñas. In Howard JL (ed): Current Veterinary Therapy: Food Animal Practice, ed 3. Philadelphia, WB Saunders, 1993, pp 842–846.
9. Sapienza JS, Isaza R, Brooks DE, Miller TR: Atresia of the nasolacrimal duct in a llama. J Comp Ophthalmol 6:6–8, 1996.
10. Gionfriddo JR, Gionfriddo JP, Krohne SG: Ocular diseases of llamas: 194 cases (1980–1993). J Am Vet Med Assoc 210:1784–1787, 1997.
11. Severin GA: Severin's Veterinary Ophthalmology Notes, ed 3. Fort Collins, Colo, DesignPointe Communications, 1996.
12. Severin GA: Personal communication, 1993.
13. Severin GA: Unpublished data, 1993.
14. Barrie KP, Jacobson E, Peiffer RL Jr: Unilateral cataract with lens coloboma and bilateral corneal edema in a guanaco. J Am Vet Med Assoc 173:1251–1252, 1978.
15. Gionfriddo JR: Unpublished data, 1990.
16. Brightman AH, McLaughlin SA, Brumley B: Keratoconjunctivitis in a llama. Vet Med Small Anim Clinician 76:1776–1777, 1981.
17. Fowler ME: Medicine and Surgery of South American Camelids. Ames, Iowa, Iowa State University Press, 1989.
18. Schuh JCL, Ferguson JG, Fischer MA: Congenital coloboma in a llama. Can Vet J 32:432–433, 1991.
19. Johnson LW: Personal communication, 1983.
20. Lavach JD: Large Animal Ophthalmology. St Louis, Mosby–Year Book, 1990.
21. Donaldson LL, Holland M, Koch SA: Atracurium as an adjunct to halothane-oxygen anesthesia in a llama undergoing intraocular surgery. Vet Surg 21:76–79, 1992.
22. Boer M, Schoon HA: Untersuchungen zu erblich bedingten Augen- und ZNS-Verdanderungen in einer Zuchtgruppe von Vikunjas (Lama vicugna) im Zoologischen Garten Hanover. Verhandlungsbericht des Internationalen Symposiums über die Erkanungen der Zootier 26:159–164, 1984.
23. Ingram KA, Sigler RL: Cataract removal in a young llama. Proceedings of the annual meeting of the American Association of Zoo Veterinarians. Tampa, Fla, 1993.
24. Rebhun WC, Jenkins, Riis RC, et al: An epizootic of blindness and encephalitis associated with a herpes virus indistinguishable from equine herpesvirus I in a herd of alpacas and llamas. J Am Vet Med Assoc 192:953–956, 1988.
25. House JA, Gregg DA, Lubroth J, et al: Experimental equine herpesvirus-1 infection in llamas (Lama glama). J Vet Diagn Invest 3:137–143, 1991.
26. Paulsen ME, Young S, Smith JA, Severin G: Bilateral chorioretinitis, centripetal optic neuritis, and encephalitis in a llama. J Am Vet Med Assoc 194:1305–1308, 1989.
27. Pickett JP, Moore CP, Beehler BA, et al: Bilateral chorioretinitis secondary to disseminated aspergillosis in an alpaca. J Am Vet Med Assoc 187:1241–1243, 1985.
28. Tinsley D: Unpublished data, 1996.
29. Dugan SJ, Roberts SM, Curtis CR, Severin GA: Prognostic factors and survival of horses with ocular/adnexal squamous cell carcinoma: 147 cases (1978–1988). J Am Vet Med Assoc 198:298–303, 1991.

■ Surface Ocular Microbiology in Food and Fiber-Producing Animals

David T. Ramsey, D.V.M., Diplomate, A.C.V.O.

The microbial population of the ocular surface varies substantially among species. The microbial flora primarily consists of resident and transient bacterial, fungal, mycoplasmal, and chlamydial organisms that exist in a dynamic, homeostatic balance. The resident ocular flora is considered permanent, normal commensal organisms that represent true colonization of the eyelids and conjunctiva. Organisms in the resident flora are always present in large numbers and are obtained consistently on subsequent cultures. In contrast, the transient ocular flora consists of organisms that are present in smaller numbers and are recovered sporadically or inconsistently on subsequent cultures. In concert with surface ocular defense mechanisms, the resident microbial flora aids in maintaining ocular surface health by restricting nutrients to potentially pathogenic microbes. The resident microbial flora produces substances (polypeptide antibiotics) that have antibacterial and antifungal properties that moderate the growth of opportunistic or pathogenic organisms. Microbial population dynamics are frequently altered in diseased ocular states or after the topical use of antimicrobial or corticosteroid drugs. Subsequently, microbial overgrowth by resident flora or alterations in microbial populations by pathogenic organisms may occur.

The relative contribution of specific microbial organisms to the total microbial population of the ocular surface may differ according to geographic location, the season or climate when samples are collected, housing conditions, host nutritional or immune status, sampling technique, and the age of the animal at sample collection. Isolation of a specific organism from the conjunctival sac of an animal with external ocular disease is not definitive evidence of a cause-and-effect association. Knowledge of the normal surface ocular flora is pivotal to interpreting the results of microbial cultures and understanding surface ocular disease dynamics, which constitute a substantial percentage of morbidity in food animal species.

SAMPLE COLLECTION TECHNIQUES

Proper collection methods and handling of samples for microbial culture are imperative and directly correlate with the growth of bacteria in culture. Samples should be collected prior to instillation of topical ophthalmic anesthetic or diagnostic drugs (e.g., 0.5% proparacaine, fluorescein, tropicamide). Topical anesthetic and diagnostic drugs contain preservatives with antibacterial properties that may decrease the in vitro growth of bacteria. Sterile, rayon- or Dacron-tipped swabs should be used to collect samples for microbial culture. The use of cotton-tipped swabs should be avoided because the cottonseed oil coating the cotton fibers also has antibacterial properties. The swab should be premoistened with the transport or nutritional medium prior to sample collection. The swab is then inserted into the conjunctival fornix without touching the swab to the eyelid margin, gently rolled between the thumb and index finger, and then returned to the transport vial. When fungal organisms are suspected, the best growth results are achieved when samples are collected from the cornea or conjunctiva with a sterile, blunt instrument (Kimura platinum spatula) and inoculated directly onto fungal culture medium (Sabouraud's dextrose medium). Before samples are collected, a diagnostic laboratory should be contacted regarding the use of specific transport media.

When bacterial culture and susceptibility testing are not practical, cytologic examination of conjunctival or corneal scrapings may be done. Preparations should be collected with a flat, blunt, round instrument or a dry swab. The cellular material collected should be gently smeared or rolled on a slide and heat- or ethanol-fixed before staining. When bacterial organisms are suspected, slides should be stained with Gram stain. Cellular inclusions that result from viral, mycoplasmal, or chlamydial organisms are poorly defined by Gram staining. Giemsa or Papanicolaou staining allows identification of mycoplasmal, fungal, and chlamydial organisms.

MICROBIAL ISOLATES FROM NORMAL EYES AND EYES WITH EXTERNAL DISEASE

Bovine

Several surveys have evaluated the microbial flora of clinically normal eyes of cows. The predominant bacteria grown in culture from conjunctival swab samples were gram-positive organisms. The most frequently isolated bacterial organisms (and the percentage of recovery) included *Bacillus* spp. (77%), *Staphylococcus epidermidis* (69%), *Streptococcus fecalis* (45%), and *Branhamella catarrhalis* (33%). Growth of *Moraxella bovis*, a gram-negative coccobacillus organism, was evident in 5% of the eyes cultured. Fungal organisms were grown from swab samples in fewer than 1% of the eyes, but no attempt was made to identify fungal species. Isolation of mycoplasmal, chlamydial, or viral organisms and isolation of anaerobic or nutritionally variant bacterial organisms were not attempted in either study. No growth of microbial organisms occurred from 10% of the eyes cultured.

Infectious Bovine Keratoconjunctivitis

The greatest economic losses to cattle producers in the United States are attributable to infectious bovine keratoconjunctivitis (IBK, pinkeye, contagious ophthalmia). In the eyes of cattle with IBK, keratitis, or conjunctivitis, *M. bovis* has been most frequently incriminated as the primary etiologic agent. However, many reports noted failure to recover *M. bovis* from eyes with clinical signs and lesions that typify IBK. This finding suggests that the cause of IBK may be multifactorial (prolonged exposure to ultraviolet light, vector transmission, concurrent ocular or systemic infection, marginal nutritional status) and may have a bearing on singling out *M. bovis* as the etiologic agent. *M. bovis* can exist in a carrier state in the upper respiratory tract of clinically normal cattle. Piliated strains of *M. bovis* are considered pathogenic and are typically recovered from the eyes of affected cattle. Severe clinical signs of ocular disease are attributable to hemolysins produced by piliated strains of *M. bovis*. However, nonpiliated strains that do not produce hemolysins have also been recovered from the eyes of cattle during outbreaks of IBK. Recently, a soluble cell detachment factor produced by *M. bovis* was identified that may be responsible, in part, for the pathogenesis of IBK.[1] Incubation of mammalian cells with *M. bovis* culture filtrate resulted in the detachment of cells from each other and from the substrate. Detached cells remained viable and reattached after removal or destruction of the cell detachment factor.

Calves and *Bos taurus* breeds (specifically, Hereford and Hereford crossbreeds) are at increased risk for clinical IBK disease. Clinical signs of disease are most severe and infection rates are greatest (up to 90%) in calves as compared with mature cattle. Affected cattle have decreased feed consumption and suppression of weight gain and milk production. Initial clinical signs of IBK include excessive lacrimation, photophobia, blepharospasm, and conjunctivitis; the cornea is initially spared gross clinical signs of disease. Subsequently, the axial cornea becomes edematous, and a small, pale white to yellow opacity appears centrally. As the central corneal opacity increases in diameter and depth, corneal ulceration occurs and the character of the ocular discharge becomes mucopurulent. Deep and superficial neovascularization of the cornea becomes evident and iridocyclitis occurs. The corneal ulcer may perforate or may become filled with granulation tissue. Fibrosis of the cornea results in faint opacification (scar) of the central portion of the cornea. Recovery from IBK provides the host moderately protective immunity against severe recurrent ocular disease caused by *M. bovis*.

The diagnosis of IBK is based on clinical signs, seasonal occurrence, and a high incidence of disease in an affected herd. A definitive diagnosis can be made by performing bacterial culture, susceptibility testing, and cytologic examination on samples collected from the cornea or conjunctiva of selected animals in a herd outbreak (see the earlier section Sample Collection Techniques). Collection of samples from all animals in an affected herd is usually impractical and costly.

Medical treatment alternatives include topical, subconjunctival, and oral or parenteral administration of antibiotic drugs and topical treatment with atropine. *M. bovis* is susceptible to many different antibiotic drugs (gentamicin, neomycin-bacitracin–polymyxin B, benzathine and sodium cloxacillin, furazolidone, nitrofurazone, gramicidin, erythromycin, and some sulfa drugs). Resistance of *M. bovis* to sulfa drugs and cloxacillin may make the use of these antimicrobial agents ineffectual. Initial use of oxytetracycline ointment is recommended. Both eyes should be treated topically with antibiotics regardless of whether both eyes are clinically affected. Topical instillation of an antibiotic establishes the highest concentration of antibiotic drug in the tear film but usually requires the application of drug three to four times daily for several days and is impractical for large herds. Intramuscular injection of long-acting oxytetracycline (20 mg/kg) followed by a second injection 72 hours after the initial injection establishes therapeutic levels of drug in surface ocular tissues, decreases the duration of clinical signs and shedding of *M. bovis*, and eliminates the carrier state of *M. bovis* in calves with IBK. A practical treatment protocol includes initial administration of topical oxytetracycline ointment and concurrent intramuscular injection of long-acting oxytetracycline followed by a second intramuscular injection of long-acting oxytetracycline 72 hours after the initial injection. Subconjunctival injection of long-acting oxytetracycline drugs is not recommended because injection results in profound chemosis, blepharoedema, and conjunctival necrosis. Gentamicin (20 mg), penicillin G (500,000 IU), and ampicillin (50 mg) can also be injected subconjunctivally during the initial treatment regimen. Antibiotic drug residues in milk and meat vary according to the drug formulation, dose, frequency, route of administration, and weight of the animal. Therefore, withdrawal times differ substantially among the various antibiotic drugs used subconjunctivally to treat IBK. The Food Animal Residue Avoidance Database should be contacted to determine withdrawal times or whether the use of a particular drug in an extra-label fashion is recommended.

Subconjunctival administration of dexamethasone has been suggested as a means of alleviating severe keratitis in selected cases of IBK. However, subconjunctivally administered procaine penicillin G with or without dexamethasone does not significantly hasten or delay the clinical course of disease or the outcome in heifers with naturally acquired IBK. When iridocyclitis is evident, 1% atropine ointment should be applied topically twice daily to alleviate the intraocular pain associated with ciliary muscle spasm and to induce mydriasis. Alternatively, 0.25 mL of injectable atropine solution (0.1 mg) can be administered subconjunctivally to effect mydriasis and eliminate ciliary muscle spasm. When deep or perforated corneal ulcers are present, mechanical support and protection of the ocular surface in the form of a complete temporary tarsorrhaphy or a nictitans flap is indicated.

Other organisms that have been isolated and identified from the ocular surface of cattle with characteristic clinical signs of IBK include *Mycoplasma bovoculi*, *M. bovirhinus*, *M. verecundum*, *Acholeplasma laidlawii*, *Pasteurella* spp., *Corynebacterium pyogenes*, *Listeria* spp., *Escherichia coli*, *Ureaplasma* spp., *Achromobacter* spp., *Haemophilus* spp., *Micrococcus* spp., and *B. catarrhalis*. These organisms are probably opportunistic resident and transient ocular flora that may decrease ocular defense mechanisms and subsequently predispose the cornea and conjunctiva to *M. bovis* infection; their significance as primary pathogens is speculative and subject to debate.

Infectious Bovine Rhinotracheitis Conjunctivitis

Infectious bovine rhinotracheitis (IBR) conjunctivitis is attributable to bovine herpesvirus. The disposition of herpesvirus to establish latent infection in neurosensory ganglia favors the likelihood of recrudescent or recurrent clinical signs of disease. Young cattle are most susceptible to infection. The eyes may be the only site of infection, or the ocular disease may be a component of upper respiratory or reproductive (infectious pustular vulvovaginitis) disease. Initially, a serous ocular discharge and conjunctival hyperemia are present. As the disease progresses, the character of the ocular discharge becomes mucopurulent, the periphery of the cornea may exhibit deep perilimbal neovascularization and edema, and iridocyclitis may be evident. Corneal ulceration does not occur from IBR infection; the central corneal region remains unaffected, and this is used to clinically distinguish IBR from IBK. However, concurrent infection by bovine herpesvirus and *M. bovis* occurs and may make a definitive diagnosis difficult. Small, white pustules and plaques of the conjunctiva (consisting of lymphocytes and plasma cells) may be observed but are frequently not detected because severe blepharospasm caused by ocular pain makes examination of the conjunctiva difficult.

The diagnosis is based on the appearance of typical clinical signs and the highly contagious nature of the disease. Virus isolation and fluorescent antibody testing from conjunctival or nasal swab samples or serologic titers documenting a fourfold rise in antibody titer are considered definitive evidence of the disease. Because of the propensity for herpesvirus latency, a definitive diagnosis may be difficult to establish. Treatment with antiviral drugs is not recommended because of exorbitant cost and the necessity of frequent application. Supportive treatment is the mainstay recommendation and varies according to the severity of disease. Bacterial overgrowth by opportunistic bacteria is impeded by the administration of topical broad-spectrum antibiotic ointment. Atropine ointment should be administered to maintain mydriasis when iridocyclitis is evident. The clinical course of IBR conjunctivitis is 21 to 28 days. Preventive measures include administering modified live IBR vaccines, isolating affected animals, and minimizing stress in affected herds.

Control and Prevention

Many ocular diseases are not easily preventable because of environmental conditions. Treatment strategies directed toward control or elimination of the vector or infectious agent are advantageous, but there are no foolproof practical methods of completely eliminating many vectors or disease agents from ocular tissues. The use of pyrethrin-impregnated ear tags in both ears to control vector transmission (*Musca autumnalis*, *M. domestica*) has been recommended. Vaccines have been developed to decrease the severity of clinical disease or minimize the carrier state of infectious keratoconjunctivitis in food animals. Vaccines against *Moraxella bovis* to prevent IBK have had a humble debut, and results of vaccination trials indicate limited efficacy.

Caprine

Reports describing the surface ocular flora of normal caprine eyes are sparse. Many early reports documented isolation of microbes from the ocular surface of goats with clinical signs of keratoconjunctivitis, but comparison to the microbial flora of the ocular surface of goats with clinically normal eyes was not done.

Mycoplasma conjunctivae and *Chlamydia psittaci* have been recovered from the ocular surface of goats with clinically normal eyes, but they are the most frequently implicated etiopathologic agents of infectious keratoconjunctivitis in goats in the United States and the United Kingdom. Infectious keratoconjunctivitis in goats may be initiated by exposure of a naive goat to an inapparent carrier of the disease, an environment contaminated by infective ocular secretions, or vector transmission by face flies. *M. conjunctivae* can exist in a carrier state in the conjunctival sac of goats with clinically normal eyes. *M. conjunctivae* may also cause mild clinical signs of concurrent systemic disease. *M. mycoides* subsp. *mycoides* frequently causes keratoconjunctivitis and concurrent polyarthritis, mastitis, and pleuropneumonia in goats. *M. agalactiae* most frequently causes mastitis and septicemia but may cause polyarthritis, keratoconjunctivitis, and iridocyclitis in goats. *M. agalactiae* is infrequently isolated from goats in the United States. *M. capricolum*, *M. arginini*, and *Acholeplasma oculi* usually cause mild keratoconjunctivitis in goats but have also been associated with concurrent mastitis, pneumonia, and polyarthritis.

Two strains of *C. psittaci* may cause naturally occurring or experimentally induced conjunctivitis with or without concurrent arthritis, late-term abortion, and upper respiratory disease in goats. Enzyme-linked immunosorbent assay, complement fixation, culture, immunofluorescent antibody testing, and cytologic examination of conjunctival scrapings may be used to diagnose chlamydial keratoconjunctivitis.

B. ovis has been isolated from the conjunctiva of goats with normal eyes and from goats with clinical signs of keratoconjunctivitis. *Moraxella bovis* does not appear to be a causative etiologic agent in caprine keratoconjunctivitis. Other species of bacteria have also been isolated from the eyes of goats with keratoconjunctivitis but probably represent transient ocular flora and are no longer considered etiologic agents of infectious keratoconjunctivitis in goats. Isolation of anaerobic bacteria or fungal organisms from the ocular surface of goats has not been reported.

Ophthalmic clinical signs caused by *C. psittaci* and *Mycoplasma* spp. are frequently bilateral but asymmetrical and cannot be distinguished solely on the basis of clinical signs. Clinical signs include excessive lacrimation, epiphora, blepharospasm, chemosis, formation of perilimbal conjunctival lymphoid follicles, corneal neovascularization, and fibrosis. Corneal ulceration occurs infrequently. A definitive diagnosis is made by immunofluorescent antibody testing or cytologic examination of samples obtained from the conjunctiva of affected eyes. Topical treatment with oxytetracycline or intramuscular injection of long-acting oxytetracycline (20 mg/kg) is effective if administered early in the course of disease.

Ovine

Reports of microbial isolates from the ocular surface of sheep with clinically normal eyes include *B. ovis*, *Staphylococcus* spp., *Streptococcus* spp., *E. coli*, *Pseudomonas* spp., *Micrococcus* spp., *C. pyogenes*, *Achromobacter* spp., and *Bacillus ovis*. Recovery of low numbers of these organisms from the normal eyes of sheep suggests that they are probably transient ocular flora. There are no reports describing the isolation of anaerobic bacteria or fungal organisms from the ocular surface of sheep.

M. conjunctivae has been recovered from the eyes of sheep with infectious keratoconjunctivitis but not from the clinically normal eyes of healthy sheep. However, some investigators believe that *M. conjunctivae* can infect the conjunctiva of sheep subclinically. Naturally occurring ovine infectious keratoconjunctivitis is most frequently attributable to infection by *M. conjunctivae* and *C. psittaci*. Attempts to induce clinical signs of ovine keratoconjunctivitis in healthy sheep by experimental inoculation of the conjunctival sac with *M. conjunctivae* have been successful for some investigators but unsuccessful for others. *Branhamella ovis* has also been incriminated as an etiologic agent in infectious ovine keratoconjunctivitis, but it may represent a resident opportunistic pathogen that may exacerbate primary infection caused by *M. conjunctivae* or *C. psittaci*. The use of exfoliative cytologic examination on Giemsa-stained slides from conjunctival scrapings may be beneficial in detecting *Mycoplasma* organisms when keratoconjunctivitis is evident.[2]

C. psittaci is a common cause of infectious ovine keratoconjunctivitis. Polyarthritis or late-term abortion may be evident concurrently in affected sheep. Bilateral ocular infection in lambs is more common with *C. psittaci* than with *M. conjunctivae*. Clinical ophthalmic signs of infectious ovine keratoconjunctivitis are similar to signs of infectious caprine keratoconjunctivitis. Clinical signs are more severe in young lambs and morbidity rates of up to 90% are common, which attests to the exceedingly contagious character of the disease. Treatment strategies discussed for caprine keratoconjunctivitis also apply for ovine keratoconjunctivitis. There are no reports that document the growth of chlamydial organisms in culture from sheep with clinically normal eyes.

Porcine

The microbial population of the ocular surface was recently determined in clinically normal eyes of nursing pigs, nursery pigs, feeder pigs, and sows.[3] Bacterial and chlamydial organisms predominated; fungal organisms were isolated infrequently. Eleven aerobic bacterial species were recovered from 98% of the specimens evaluated; culture of anaerobic organisms has not been reported. The most frequently isolated bacterial organisms included α-hemolytic *Streptococcus* spp., *S. epidermidis*, and *Staphylococcus* spp. The greatest number of bacterial isolates was recovered from sows and the least number from feeder pigs. Mycoplasmal organisms were not isolated from any of the specimens. Chlamydial organisms were identified by enzyme-linked immunosorbent assay in all age groups of pigs and in sows but were most prevalent in feeder pigs.

In swine with infectious conjunctivitis and keratoconjunctivitis, the most frequently implicated organisms are *Mycoplasma* and *Chlamydia* spp. Low numbers of mycoplasmal organisms, presumably transient ocular flora, have also been isolated from pigs with clinically normal eyes; their involvement in or association with infectious conjunctivitis and keratoconjunctivitis is questionable. Chlamydial organisms from conjunctival swabs of pigs with conjunctivitis have been reported previously, but the percent recovery rate did not differ from the recovery rate in pigs with clinically normal eyes.[3, 4] It is unlikely that chlamydial organisms initiate conjunctivitis in swine, but chlamydiae may act as opportunistic pathogens when ocular defense mechanisms or ocular immunity is altered.

REFERENCES

1. Halenda RM, Riley LK: Identification and characterization of a cell detachment factor produced by *Moraxella bovis*. Proc Am Coll Vet Ophthalmol 27:71, 1996.
2. Dagnall GJR: Use of exfoliative cytology in the diagnosis of ovine keratoconjunctivitis. Vet Rec 135:127–130, 1994.
3. Davidson HJ, Rogers DP, Yeary TJ, et al: Conjunctival microbial flora of clinically normal pigs. Am J Vet Res 55:949–951, 1994.
4. Rogers DG, Anderson AA, Hogg A, et al: Conjunctivitis and keratoconjunctivitis associated with chlamydiae in swine. J Am Vet Med Assoc 203:1321–1323, 1993.

■ Food Animal Ocular Neoplasia

Carmen M.H. Colitz, D.V.M., Ph.D.
Brian C. Gilger, D.V.M., M.S., Diplomate, A.C.V.O.

The development of neoplasia, benign or malignant, is a multistep process that involves mutations in different genes. These mutations may be caused by spontaneous mutations, the environment, toxins, and viruses. The malignant phenotype is attained when growth of the tumor harms the host because of tissue invasion and metastasis to other sites. Regardless of the initiating cause, cancer is a genetic disease.

Neoplastic disease affecting the eye and periocular structures in cattle results in considerable economic losses every year. Ocular squamous cell carcinoma (OSCC) and orbital lymphosarcoma are the most common tumors affecting cattle. Numerous other neoplasia have been reported to occur in cattle, but little is known about their pathophysiology and subsequent treatment because of the limited number of cases.

OCULAR SQUAMOUS CELL CARCINOMA

Bovine OSCC, also referred to as "cancer eye," is the most economically important neoplasm of cattle. Over the past 50 years, numerous studies have investigated the prevalence of disease in certain breeds, in breeds with a certain periocular pigmentation, and in cattle exposed to a number of risk factors.[1–3] The future of this disease's understanding and treatment will no doubt turn toward a genetic cause.

Bovine OSCC is a disease of high morbidity that results in early culling and carcass condemnation at slaughter (Table 1). Approximately 12.5% of all carcass condemnations in the United States occur because of OSCC.[4] One study showed the association between solar ultraviolet (UV) radiation and the occurrence of OSCC. As radiation levels increased, the average ages of affected cattle decreased. Also important was the presence of periocular pigmentation, which both lessened the susceptibility to lesion development and lessened the probability of

```
┌─────────────────────────────────────────────────────┐
│ Table 1                                             │
│ FEDERAL GUIDELINES FOR CARCASS CONDEMNATION         │
├─────────────────────────────────────────────────────┤
```

Table 1
FEDERAL GUIDELINES FOR CARCASS CONDEMNATION

1. Any animal whose eye has been obscured or destroyed by neoplastic tissue and which is infected, suppurative, and necrotic, usually accompanied by a foul odor, or any animal that is cachectic will be condemned
2. Carcasses with an affected eye or orbit will be condemned if
   a. Extensive infection, suppuration, and necrosis are affecting the osseous structures of the head
   b. Metastasis has occurred from the eye to any lymph node (including the parotid lymph node), internal organ, or any other structure
   c. Cachexia is present to any extent
3. If the carcass is not affected other than the eye, it may be passed for human food after removal and condemnation of the head and tongue
4. Any individual organ or affected part of a carcass with a neoplasm will be condemned. The entire carcass will be condemned if there is evidence of metastasis or if the size, position, or nature of the neoplasm has adversely affected the general condition of the animal
5. Any animal affected with bovine lymphoma will be condemned

Modified from Code of Federal Regulations, Title 9, Chapter 3, parts 309.6, 311.11, and 311.12 (1-1-90 edition).

its development.[5] Squamous cell carcinoma does develop in animals with periocular pigmentation, but less often than in unpigmented animals. In another study, preneoplastic periocular squamous cell carcinoma developed in 75% of the Hereford cattle exposed to solar UV radiation for 16 weeks.[2] Animals living at lower latitudes are exposed to higher intensities of solar UV light and are more prone to the development of OSCC than those at higher latitudes.[2] Therefore, the amount and intensity of exposure to solar UV light are probably the most important risk factors for the development of OSCC, especially in cattle with lightly pigmented periocular structures.

The peak age of incidence of OSCC in cattle is between 7 and 9 years, and OSCC is practically unheard of in cattle younger than 4 years.[1, 6] These data support the environmental component of the disease (i.e., solar UV light) inasmuch as a purely genetic disease would probably be manifested in the younger age group. There is no difference in incidence between males and females. Females seem to be affected more often than males, but this is probably due to the fact that the cows are used for breeding purposes and milk production and are therefore allowed to age. Males are usually slaughtered at a younger age.[4]

Hereford cattle are the most represented of breeds in which OSCC develops. Herefords also outnumber all other breeds of range cattle and cattle at slaughter, so these statistics must be interpreted with care.[3] Ocular squamous cell carcinoma has also been reported in Hereford crossbreeds and Brahman, Charolais, and the dairy breeds.[7]

Factors believed to play a role in the development of squamous cell carcinoma include viruses, nutrition, periocular pigmentation, and solar UV light. As already mentioned, UV light in combination with a lack of periocular pigmentation increases the chances for mutations that can lead to the development of OSCC. The lateral limbus is affected most often (66%), followed by the nasal limbus, the nictitans, the lacrimal caruncle, and the medial canthus.[1, 8, 9]

Pathophysiology

Initially, sun-damaged nonkeratinized stratified squamous epithelial cells of the cornea or conjunctiva become hyperplastic plaques. Plaques may regress spontaneously, they may progress to a papilloma, they may advance to a noninvasive carcinoma (carcinoma in situ), and finally, noninvasive carcinoma may develop into an invasive carcinoma.[9] Noninvasive carcinoma usually remains confined to the epithelium but infrequently can be invasive.[10] Invasive carcinoma varies in clinical appearance with the degree of differentiation, extent of neovascularization, amount of secondary inflammation, and duration.[10] Necrosis, hemorrhage, ulceration, and inflammatory cell invasion characterize an invasive carcinoma.[1] It is not uncommon for these lesions to grow large enough to protrude and cause difficulty in closing the eyelids. Carcinomas affecting the nictitans will consume the structure but usually do not invade the cartilage.[1] Carcinomas that affect the cornea are usually noninvasive.[11] Early lesions in the skin of the eyelid appear as hyperkeratotic plaques or keratoacanthomas and usually occur at mucocutaneous junctions at or near the hairline.[1, 11] These lesions usually regress but will infrequently progress into a papilloma or invasive carcinoma.[4]

Tumors of the eyelid, nictitating membrane, and conjunctival fornix metastasize more readily than those at the limbus and cornea.[12] Metastases from OSCC pass through lymph nodes in the head and neck before arriving at the thoracic duct and the venous circulation to affect the heart, lungs, pleura, liver, kidney, and neighboring lymph nodes.[13]

Diagnosis

The diagnosis of OSCC is often made by gross appearance, although cytologic and histopathologic examination confirms the diagnosis. Cytologically, benign lesions have anucleated superficial squamous cells and vesicular nuclei with coarse chromatin clumping in deeper cells.[8, 11] Lesions of OSCC are typically characterized by enlarged hyperchromatic nuclei with large clumps of chromatin and prominent nucleoli.[8, 9] In 90% of the cases there is agreement between the cytologic diagnosis and the histologic diagnosis.[14] If regional lymph nodes are enlarged, fine-needle aspiration and/or biopsy is indicated.

Treatment

Numerous modalities are available for the treatment of OSCC, but one should first consider the practicality of treatment. That is, the extent of the disease as well as the intended use of the animal and its value should be assessed before investing time and money. If OSCC has invaded the bony orbit or parotid lymph node, the animal should be sent to slaughter because the cost of treatment and probability of its recurrence often preclude any attempt to treat the animal.[14] The smaller the lesion, the better the chance for successful treatment; the bigger the lesion, usually the more expensive the treatment with a lower chance for remission. Smaller lesions are usually more superficial and more amenable to the available treatment options, but larger lesions usually need more than one type of treatment modality.[15]

Complete surgical excision is the treatment of choice for OSCC, although it has been shown that additional lesions may develop within 2 years of surgery.[16] Small lesions with well-defined margins are easily excised and may then be treated with adjunctive cryosurgery or hyperthermia.[15] Lesions involving the nictitans may require amputation of the structure. More extensive lesions or multiple lesions may require either enucleation or exenteration.

Another common treatment modality is cryosurgery. Cryosurgery involves selectively destroying tissue with a cryogen, usually liquid nitrogen. Nitrous oxide is not usually used because it does not attain as suitable a temperature as liquid nitrogen. A double freeze-thaw protocol involves freezing the lesion to between −25 and −40°C, allowing it to thaw slowly, and repeating the cycle; this is the most useful method. When used in lesions smaller than 2.5 cm in diameter, cryosurgery has been shown to have a 97% cure rate.[17] Lesions greater than 5 cm in diameter did not respond well to cryosurgery and had high rates of recurrence. Cryosurgery can also be used in conjunction with surgical excision to destroy the remaining neoplastic cells not removed by excision. It is important to recognize the extent of the disease because even extensive excision and cryosurgery cannot help invasive and metastatic OSCC.[18] Cryosurgery is an easy, rapid, relatively inexpensive procedure that provides analgesia, requires little postoperative care, causes minimal adverse side effects, and can be repeated.[17]

Radiation therapy can also be used to treat OSCC, either alone or in conjunction with surgical excision, depending on the size of the lesion. This modality is usually reserved for extremely valuable animals because of the expense, the need for a radiologist to handle the radioactive isotopes, and public health concerns.[14, 19]

Radiofrequency current hyperthermia involves heating the tumor tissue above normal body temperature (42 to 45°C). Tumor cells are more susceptible to heat damage than are normal cells, so the tumor cells are selectively killed.[8] Heat normally penetrates only 3 to 4 mm into tissues and covers an area of 1 cm²; therefore, larger tumors need to be surgically debulked before hyperthermia can be used effectively.[9, 15] It is recommended that the instrument be applied 3 to 4 mm beyond the tumor margin. A hand-held radiofrequency device is available commercially (Thermoprobe, Hach Co, Loveland, Colo) and consists of electrodes on a surface probe that can heat tissues to 50°C when placed on a lesion for 30 seconds. This increase in temperature results in necrosis of both neoplastic and normal cells and sloughing of the treated tissue.[9] Successful treatment with hyperthermia in small, localized lesions is approximately 90%, and if the tumor should recur, the procedure can be repeated.[15]

Immunotherapy is a treatment option that attempts to stimulate the host's immune system against the tumor. Various antigens, including allogeneic or freeze-dried saline phenol extract of squamous cell carcinoma and emulsified cell walls of *Mycobacterium bovis* (cell walls of the Calmette-Guérin bacillus), have been used in an attempt to initiate active immunity against the tumor. Other agents that have been used to stimulate immunity include levamisole and H_2-receptor blockers. Immunotherapy is not very effective in the treatment of cancer, probably because tumor cells are very capable of evading the immune system either by downregulating major histocompatibility antigens or by tumor-specific immunosuppression.

Herd Management

Careful and proper herd management practices will substantially reduce the economic losses from OSCC. Animals over 2 years of age should be examined for ocular lesions two to three times per year when they are rounded up for routine examination. If suspicious lesions are found, they should be treated immediately by surgical excision, cryotherapy, radiofrequency hyperthermia, and/or immunotherapy.[9, 14] Large noninvasive lesions of the globe or adnexa may require orbital exenteration or culling, depending on the productivity of the animal and market prices. Cattle with invasive and/or metastatic OSCC should be shipped to slaughter immediately.[14] Lines of cattle highly susceptible to OSCC should be culled or bred for pigmented periocular structures, which will decrease the incidence of the disease. Choosing breeds of cattle (Charolais, Angus, and Brahman) that are less predisposed to OSCC will also decrease economic losses.[7]

BOVINE LYMPHOSARCOMA

Enzootic bovine lymphosarcoma is an insidious systemic disease of the reticuloendothelial system that has ocular manifestations. It is responsible for most of the economic losses in dairy cattle and it is the most common orbital neoplasia affecting dairy cattle.[8] Clinically, there is progressive unilateral or bilateral exophthalmos resulting from a retrobulbar neoplastic infiltrate that usually affects the caudal periorbital tissues.[11] Extraocular muscles are often infiltrated by tumor cells. The globe itself is not usually involved.[8] As the disease progresses, exposure keratitis and eventual proptosis occur. The initial complaint may be an acute onset of exophthalmos, although the orbital involvement has probably been present for some time. Subtle signs of exophthalmos are difficult to assess, especially because dairy cattle naturally have slightly exophthalmic eyes. Physical examination will usually reveal other systemic abnormalities.

Definitive diagnosis of bovine leukemia virus infection is by radioimmunoassay. Two negative tests 2 to 3 months apart are necessary to consider cattle bovine leukemia virus–free. Radioimmunoassay uses major internal bovine leukemia virus protein or a virion glycoprotein as an antigen for the most sensitive and specific of serologic tests. Also available is the agar gel immunodiffusion test, but this test is suitable only for screening purposes because of cross-reactivity with bovine viral diarrhea virus.[20] A definitive diagnosis of enzootic bovine lymphosarcoma requires histologic examination of affected lymph nodes or organs.

Treatment is not usually attempted in systemically affected cattle because the prognosis is extremely poor. Cattle will probably be condemned if sent to slaughter. Exenteration of involved eyes provides palliative treatment in cows in late gestation until calving.[11]

REFERENCES

1. Russell WO, Wynne ES, Loquvam GS, et al: Studies on bovine ocular squamous carcinoma ("cancer eye"): I. Pathological anatomy and historical review. Cancer 9:1–52, 1956.
2. Kopecky KE, Pugh GW, Hughes DE, et al: Biological effect of ultraviolet radiation on cattle: Bovine ocular squamous cell carcinoma. Am J Vet Res 40:1783–1788, 1979.
3. Russell WC, Brinks JS, Kainer RA: Incidence and heritability of ocular squamous cell tumors in Hereford cattle. J Anim Sci 43:1156–1162, 1976.
4. Heeney JL, Valli VEO: Bovine ocular squamous cell carcinoma: An epidemiological perspective. Can J Comp Med 49:21–26, 1985.
5. Anderson DE, Skinner PE: Studies on bovine ocular squamous cell carcinoma ("cancer eye"): XI. Effects of sunlight. J Anim Sci 20:474–477, 1961.
6. Blackwell RL, Anderson DE, Knox JH: Age incidence and heritability of cancer eye in Hereford cattle. J Anim Sci 15:943–951, 1956.
7. Bailey CM, Hanks DR, Hanks MA: Circumocular pigmentation and incidence of ocular squamous cell tumors in *Bos taurus* and *Bos indicus* × *Bos taurus* cattle. J Am Vet Med Assoc 196:1605–1608, 1990.
8. Roberts SM: Diseases of the eye. *In* Moore CP (ed): Large Animal Internal Medicine. St Louis, Mosby–Year Book, 1990, pp 1248–1253.
9. Gilger BC, Whitley RD, McLaughlin SA: Bovine ocular squamous cell carcinoma: A review. Vet Ann 31:73–84, 1991.
10. Spencer WH: Conjunctiva. *In* Spencer WH (ed): Ophthalmic Pathology. Philadelphia, WB Saunders, 1996, pp 38–155.
11. Miller TR, Gelatt KN: Food animal ophthalmology. *In* Gelatt KN (ed): Veterinary Ophthalmology, ed 2. Philadelphia, Lea & Febiger, 1991, pp 611–655.

12. Kircher CH, Garner FM, Robinson FR: Tumors of the eye and adnexa. Bull WHO 50:135, 1974.
13. Moulton JE: Tumors in Domestic Animals. Los Angeles, University of California Press, 1961.
14. Kainer RA: Current concepts in the treatment of bovine ocular squamous cell tumors. Vet Clin North Am Large Anim Pract 6:609–622, 1984.
15. Roberts SM, Kainer R: Food animal ocular neoplasia. *In* Howard JL (ed): Current Veterinary Therapy: Food Animal Practice, ed 3. Philadelphia, WB Saunders, 1993, pp 846–857.
16. Lavach JD: Ocular neoplasia. *In* Lavach JD (ed): Large Animal Ophthalmology. St Louis, Mosby–Year Book, 1990, pp 340–345.
17. Farris HE, Fraunfelder FT: Cryosurgical treatment of ocular squamous cell carcinoma of cattle. J Am Vet Med Assoc 168:213–216, 1976.
18. Farris HE: Cryosurgical treatment of bovine ocular squamous cell carcinoma. Vet Clin North Am Large Anim Pract 2:861–867, 1980.
19. Banks WC: Radioactive gold in the treatment of ocular squamous cell carcinoma of cattle. J Am Vet Med Assoc 163:745–748, 1973.
20. Ferrer JF: Bovine lymphosarcoma. Compend Contin Educ 2:235–242, 1980.

■ Neurogenic Vision Loss

Paul E. Miller, D.V.M., Diplomate, A.C.V.O.

Differentiation between the causes of neurogenic vision loss in food animals is often frustrating because many of these entities have a similar range of clinical findings, and it is difficult if not impossible to accurately assess the visual capability of obtunded animals. The purpose of this article is to consider the common causes of neurogenic vision loss in food animals and to discuss methods of distinguishing these disorders from each other from an ophthalmic standpoint. The reader is referred to previous editions of this text and the many textbooks on neurology that review the basic science and neurocircuitry of these disorders.

EXAMINATION

Normal Vision

Any attempt to determine the nature and extent of vision loss first requires an understanding of the normal visual abilities of that species. Unfortunately, this knowledge is relatively limited in domestic ruminants. Their large eyes probably give them a visual acuity (e.g., the ability to see the details of an object separately and unblurred) in the 20/45 to 20/50 range. This is superior to that of dogs and cats and means that they can differentiate the details of an object from 20 ft away that a normal human could do at 45 to 50 ft. The lateral placement of their eyes also gives them a larger, virtually 360-degree visual field of view, with blind spots only anteroventral to the nose and the width of the head posteriorly.

Visual clues are more important to cattle than auditory clues in acquiring feed, and calves have been demonstrated to have a hierarchic attraction for certain colors, with green being preferred over white (incandescent), which is preferred to red. This and other studies have led to a general consensus that cattle have imperfect, although useful color vision. It appears that they can readily distinguish longer light wavelengths such as red, orange, and yellow from gray but have more difficulty in differentiating short-wavelength colors (green, blue, violet) from gray. It has also been suggested that the anatomic differences in the density and biochemical composition of the cone photoreceptors between different cattle breeds may result in breed-related differences in color perception. Pigs also appear to have useful color vision and are able to differentiate between many colors on behavioral testing.

Assessment of Vision

Most clinical tests of animal vision are very crude and only able to discern gross deficiencies in visual function bordering on total vision loss. Because of this, the first indication of vision loss in a herd or flock is often aberrant visually oriented behavior or an increase in self-inflicted injuries resulting from falling into gutters or bumping into objects. More detailed investigation of the visual capabilities of an individual animal usually begins with an assessment of the menace response in which the open hand is rapidly moved parallel to and across the animal's visual field. Care should be exercised to avoid disturbing the vibrissae or periocular hairs because a blink response may be initiated via touch receptors rather than the visual pathway. If the animal lacks a menace response, the ability to blink should be verified by gently tapping with a finger on the skin of the medial canthal region. This stimulation can also be used in uncooperative or somewhat stuporous animals to amplify the response to a subsequent menacing gesture. Because the menace response is a learned response, it may be slow or absent in naive, normal neonatal animals for the first several weeks of life. It should be remembered, however, that a menace response will often be retained in the presence of a visual acuity of 20/1000 or poorer and that it is not particularly reliable for determining the presence or absence of *partial* visual field deficits. Tossing cotton balls across the animal's visual field or maze testing (with or without a pinkeye patch over one eye) may also provide crude estimates of an animal's visual capabilities.

In addition to the menace response, the pupillary light reflex (PLR), swinging flashlight test, and dazzle response should also be assessed, although the presence of these reflexes does not guarantee that vision is normal. Pupillary constriction in response to bright light in large animals is relatively slow in comparison to most carnivores, thus making a bright halogen light source and darkened quarters for examination nearly essential for accurate evaluation of this reflex. Both direct and consensual PLRs should be assessed to adequately localize the lesion(s). A swinging flashlight test may also aid in localizing unilateral lesions by verifying that the deficit is not at the level of cranial nerve III or the iris sphincter muscle. In this test a bright light source is shone into one eye for several seconds, then immediately shifted to the other eye, and then back and forth between the two eyes. Blinding unilateral lesions of the retina or optic nerve will result in an eye in which the pupil constricts when the contralateral eye is stimulated but result in pupillary dilation when the affected eye is illuminated. The dazzle reflex is a subcortical response to bright light and is determined by quickly shining a very bright light into a dark-adapted eye. A positive response is manifested as blinking or withdrawal of the head in response to light. Visual animals will have a positive dazzle reflex, but a positive dazzle reflex may also occur in animals with cerebral cortical disease because the reflex is mediated subcortically.

Once the status of the pertinent neurologic reflexes has been determined, careful examination of the ocular media is warranted. The author prefers to begin by standing approximately at arm's distance from the eye and looking at the tapetal reflex through a direct ophthalmoscope set at "0" D. This technique screens for opacities in the ocular media located between the examiner and the tapetum. Small corneal scars, cataracts, or vitreal debris will appear as black spots within the tapetal reflex. Observation of the animal directly head-on so that the tapetal reflex from both eyes is seen simultaneously may also be used to screen for anisocoria. If the tapetal reflex cannot be readily obtained, it is likely that the cause of vision loss is not neurologic but related to an abnormality of the globe itself. Once the eye is examined at a distance, the clinician may examine the fundus with direct or indirect ophthalmoscopy as described earlier in this section. Indirect ophthalmoscopy is especially useful in animals with horns or dispositions such that it would be unsafe to approach the animal closely.

This rapid screening approach allows the clinician to determine whether neurogenic vision loss is present and to further subdivide the vision loss into two groups, those with and those without a discernible PLR. Although imperfect, the presence or absence of a PLR is often the most reliable clinical parameter because of the difficulty of thoroughly evaluating the visual status of neonatal or depressed animals. The absence of a PLR in a blind eye (with a normal fundus) suggests a lesion of the optic nerve/chiasm. Such eyes also typically fail to exhibit dazzle reflexes (or a menace response) and may or may not have abnormalities of the optic disk discernible by ophthalmoscopy. An intact PLR in a blind eye is typical of lesions of the higher visual pathway. Although these eyes lack a menace response, they may or may not exhibit a positive dazzle reflex. The following is an attempt to use the PLR as a method of differentiating between the most common neurogenic causes of vision loss in food animals—with the realization that in some circumstances overlap in clinical findings in a small percentage of animals may occur.

DISORDERS WITH AN ABSENT PUPILLARY LIGHT REFLEX

Vitamin A Deficiency

Calves born to dams that were vitamin A deficient during gestation may be congenitally blind and exhibit bilateral optic nerve atrophy. Affected animals may also be incoordinated and have thickened carpal joints and hydrocephalus. Acquired vitamin A deficiency most frequently occurs in young (<2 years of age), rapidly growing feedlot steers that are nongrazing and consuming diets high in concentrate with low-quality roughage for a prolonged period of time (>200 days). Heifers appear to be more resistant even if eating the same diet. The development of clinical signs varies with the animal's age, its liver stores of vitamin A, and the duration/severity of the deficiency. Five to 18 months of a deficient diet are usually required before clinical signs readily become apparent, although affected animals are often in poorer condition than normal ones. Early clinical signs include night blindness (usually not recognized until some animals in the herd are completely blind) and papilledema, which results from both increased cerebrospinal fluid (CSF) pressure and bony compression of the optic nerve by a stenotic optic canal. Papilledema occurs before complete vision loss and alterations in the PLR and initially appears as a bilateral, occasionally asymmetric subtle blurring of the optic disk margins. As the deficiency progresses, the disk may enlarge to two to three times normal size and markedly protrude into the vitreous, thus suggesting that the extent of papilledema may indicate the duration of the deficiency. Later in the course of the disease the retinal vasculature may become congested and tortuous, and peripapillary hemorrhage and retinal detachment may occur. The nontapetal region is often focally depigmented, and in advanced stages the optic nerve head becomes atrophic. Some animals may have tonic-clonic seizures, exophthalmos, nystagmus, strabismus, and, uncommonly, corneal edema and conjunctivitis.

The diagnosis is based on clinical signs and determination of vitamin A levels in the serum or liver. Serum levels less than 25 µg/dL and liver values less than 2 µg/g of liver tissue are considered diagnostic. Initial treatment for cattle consists of parenteral vitamin A (440 IU/kg), and long-term control can be achieved by repeated intramuscular injections of 3000 to 6000 IU/kg of vitamin A every 60 days. Alternatively, long-term control may be achieved by the addition of exogenous stabilized vitamin A to the ration or by permitting access to leafy, freshly cured hay, green pasture, or 0.5 to 2 kg of alfalfa meal daily. Night-blind animals typically respond well to treatment, but those with marked retinal degeneration and optic canal stenosis with secondary optic neuropathy should not be expected to regain useful vision.

Orbital Diseases

Inflammatory diseases of the orbit may secondarily involve the optic nerve and cause vision loss (usually unilateral) in individual animals. Unilateral exophthalmos ranging from only a mild resistance to retropulsion of the globe to overt proptosis is almost always present, and many animals also exhibit periorbital or temporomandibular joint pain, anorexia, fever, eyelid swelling, and chemosis. Common causes include periocular puncture wounds, actinobacillosis, plant or other foreign material migrating into the orbit from the oral cavity, and extension of frontal or maxillary sinusitis into the orbit. The diagnosis is based on clinical signs and examination of an aspirate/biopsy of retrobulbar tissue. An elevated white blood cell count and skull radiography/orbital ultrasonography may be supportive of the diagnosis.

Ocular squamous cell carcinoma and lymphosarcoma are the most common orbital neoplasms that can induce neurologic vision loss via secondary optic nerve involvement. In contrast to inflammatory orbital disease, orbital tumors may be manifested as a nonpainful, progressive exophthalmos or as an externally apparent mass invading the orbit. The article Food Animal Ocular Neoplasia in this section discusses these entities in more detail.

Arsanilic Acid

Phenylarsonic derivatives such as arsanilic acid and roxarsone ("3-nitro") have been used as feed additives in the swine industry in the past both as growth promotors and, at higher levels, as therapeutic agents for swine dysentery. Acute symptoms after exposure to high levels of an organic arsenic may occur within 4 to 6 days and include blindness, head tremors, incoordination, euphoria, ataxia, paraparesis, and paraplegia; however, affected animals typically continue to eat and drink. Lower, but still excessive levels of arsanilic acid such as those used for treating swine dysentery may take weeks or months to induce clinical signs and may cause only partial or complete vision loss and possibly paresis. Fundus examination may reveal optic nerve atrophy and thus support the diagnosis. Confirmation of the diagnosis may be difficult because findings of the gross postmortem examination are often unremarkable and the only characteristic histologic feature is demyelination and necrosis of the optic nerves, optic tracts, and some peripheral nerves. Because of rapid excretion, tissue or blood levels of arsenic are rarely diagnostic, and feed levels are more indicative of the true level of exposure. Treatment consists of complete withdrawal of any arsenic-containing compound. The prognosis is fairly good in all but the severely affected, although permanent vision loss or neurologic damage may persist and recovery may require 2 to 4 weeks.

Plant Toxicities

In England, ingestion of the rhizomes of male fern (*Dryopteris filix-mas*) by cattle has been associated with permanent or, more frequently, transient blindness. Blindness may be the primary initial sign, although drowsiness, weakness, malaise, and constipation also occur. Retinal ganglion cells and optic nerve fibers are destroyed, and upon ophthalmoscopy, variable amounts of papilledema and peripapillary hemorrhage are observed initially (thus necessitating differentiation from hypovitaminosis A). In advanced cases, optic nerve head atrophy and retinal vascular attenuation are noted. A similar syndrome has been reported in Australia in sheep and goats after the ingestion of *Stypandra imbricata* ("blind grass") and the flowering phase of *S. glauca* ("nodding blue lily") in the spring.

DISORDERS WITH AN INTACT PUPILLARY LIGHT REFLEX

Polioencephalomalacia

Polioencephalomalacia (PEM) is most common in young feedlot cattle and weaned calves 6 to 12 months old that are receiving a low-fiber, high-concentrate ration. Lambs and kids are typically 2 to 6 months old. Early in the course of the disease, affected animals act blind, walk with the head erect, become anorectic, stagger, and may become detached from the rest of the herd or flock. Diarrhea, hyperesthesia, muscle tremors, and head pressing may also be present. Vision loss is central in origin and may be accompanied by dorsomedial strabismus secondary to trochlear (cranial nerve IV) nuclear dysfunction with variable nystagmus. Dorsomedial strabismus, however, is not diagnostic for PEM by itself. Papilledema and an impaired PLR secondary to increased intracranial pressure have been reported but are uncommon. In some cases, miosis may make interpretation of the PLR difficult. In the latter stages the animal becomes recumbent and tonic-clonic seizures develop.

A tentative diagnosis of PEM is made by observing blindness, muscle tremors, and opisthotonos in cattle 4 to 18 months of age that are being fed high-concentrate rations and by assessing the response to therapy. Thiamine (10 mg/kg intravenously or intramuscularly) every 6 hours for the first day usually results in significant improvement in 24 hours (often within 6 to 8 hours). Therapy should continue at a twice- to four-times-daily schedule for 2 more days, and recovery may take as long as a week. Euthanasia or salvage should be considered in patients not responding to treatment within 3 days. Proper hydration needs to be ensured, and seizures may be controlled with diazepam. Mannitol (1 to 2 g/kg of a 20% solution intravenously) or dexamethasone (1 to 2 mg/kg intravenously) may be useful in reducing cerebral edema. Animals with PEM resulting from high-sulfur diets may not respond to thiamine supplementation, and patients with cortical necrosis may not regain vision. Consideration should also be given to supplementation of high-concentrate diets with thiamine (3 to 10 mg/kg of feed) or allowing access to pasture or good-quality green hay.

Lead Poisoning

Lead is ubiquitous in the environment, and although the risks of ingestion of lead-based paint are well recognized, there are numerous other sources of lead such as grease, used crankcase oil from engines burning leaded fuels, discarded lead-acid batteries, plumbing materials, and possibly other sources discarded onto rural trash piles. Central vision loss (with an intact PLR)

may affect up to 50% of the cattle with lead poisoning. Fixed and dilated pupils, however, have been occasionally reported. Most cattle will exhibit other symptoms such as muscle twitching, hyperirritability, depression, convulsions, ataxia, circling, bruxism, excessive salivation, tucked abdomen, anorexia, or diarrhea. The diagnosis is based on clinical signs, a history or circumstantial evidence of lead poisoning, and excessive lead levels in the blood, liver, kidney or rumen contents. Whole blood lead levels in excess of 0.35 ppm in cattle and probably other ruminants are significant. Unlike listeriosis and thromboembolic meningoencephalitis, lead toxicity typically is not associated with fever, does not have elevated white blood cell counts on a CSF tap, and is unresponsive to antibiotic therapy. In contrast to PEM, lead poisoning frequently affects cattle less than 6 months and over 18 months of age. Thiamine hydrochloride, however, may be beneficial in the treatment of lead toxicity. Treatment is by eliminating the source of lead, inhibiting further absorption (i.e., using gastroprotectants or rumenotomy), and chelation with anhydrous calcium disodium edetate in divided doses two to three times daily and continued for 3 to 5 days. If additional treatment is indicated, a 2-day rest is provided and then followed with another 5-day treatment period. Chelation therapy should be continued despite the apparent lack of clinical improvement because lead first mobilizes from tightly bound tissue depots.

Thromboembolic Meningoencephalitis

Although less common than in the past, the neurologic form of septicemia secondary to *Haemophilus somnus* may cause high fever, unilateral or bilateral blindness, strabismus, nystagmus, anorexia, staggering, paralysis, tonic-clonic seizures, opisthotonos, and paralysis of many cranial nerves in any bovine, but especially calves and feedlot cattle 1 to 12 months of age. Death may occur in a few hours to days. Although vision loss is typically central in origin, approximately 50% of the patients will have fundus lesions consistent with septicemia, which can be a very useful aid in diagnosis. Retinal hemorrhage (secondary to thrombosis of retinal vessels) and small, sometimes coalescing white "cotton-wool" spots with indistinct borders may be seen ophthalmoscopically. Focal areas of retinal detachment and mild papilledema may also be seen. Chronic cases may show only chorioretinal scarring. In contrast to PEM, fever, multifocal cranial nerve deficits, leukocytosis on CSF tap, and a history of respiratory infection in the group are often present. Therapy consists of fluid support and anticonvulsant agents if necessary, as well as systemic tetracycline, ampicillin, penicillin, ceftiofur, or florfenicol. If the animal is still ambulatory, the prognosis is fair to good with intensive therapy. Bacterins are of questionable economic benefit in preventing the relatively sporadic neurologic form of the disease, although they may be useful in other forms of the disease.

Water Deprivation–Sodium Toxicosis

Water deprivation–sodium toxicosis occurs primarily in swine but may also be seen in ruminants consuming a high concentration of sodium with limited access to water. It also occurs in cattle when thirsty animals are given access to saline water or allowed free access to a salt supplement after a period of salt restriction. Generally, as long as water intake is adequate, relatively large intakes of sodium (up to 13% salt) can be tolerated in the diet. Limited water intake may occur as a result of neglect, malfunction of automatic waterers, freezing of water sources, overcrowding, placing the animals in unfamiliar environments, and unpalatable water from the addition of drugs or minerals. Clinical signs are associated with central nervous system edema, and in the initial stages, increased thirst, pruritus, and constipation may be noted. In the later stages (1 to 5 days), vision loss is associated with other neurologic signs such as deafness, circling or running movements, aimless wandering, altered consciousness, walking backward, sialorrhea, and seizures. Seizures in pigs are characterized by sitting on the rear quarters, jerking the head backward and upward, and falling over in a tonic-clonic seizure and opisthotonos. Cattle may exhibit gastrointestinal symptoms, blindness, and convulsions and often characteristically drag their rear feet or even walk on the dorsal surface of the fetlock. The diagnosis is based on a history of limited water intake (which may be difficult to elicit), clinical signs, and the finding of serum sodium levels above 160 mEq/L and cerebral cortex tissue sodium concentrations above 1800 ppm. An increase of 5 mEq or greater in sodium levels in the CSF vs. the serum is also supportive of the diagnosis, especially if water-deprived animals were allowed access to water immediately prior to examination. Additionally, in pigs a characteristic eosinophilic meningoencephalitis is present histologically early in the course of the disease. Treatment is nonspecific and directed at slowly restoring central nervous system and serum sodium and water values to normal levels either by giving small amounts of fresh water frequently (up to 0.5% of body weight every 60 minutes) or by appropriate intravenous fluid support. Approximately 50% of affected animals die regardless of treatment, and recovery may occur within 4 to 5 days.

Listeriosis

Listeria monocytogenes may produce a bacterial encephalitis or meningoencephalitis in adult sheep and sometimes cattle that occasionally results in blindness. Ophthalmic clinical signs vary but may include amaurosis, facial paralysis, optic neuritis (with a diminished PLR), and secondary endophthalmitis. Hypopyon is common, and a unilateral uveitis in the absence of systemic signs may occur. Listeriosis is more commonly manifested as a vestibular syndrome with head tilt, circling, and ataxia or as unilateral facial paralysis, dysphagia, quadriparesis, and depression. It can be distinguished from PEM by the presence of fever, asymmetric cranial nerve deficits, and mononuclear leukocytosis on CSF tap. Cultures of CSF may be useful diagnostically.

Miscellaneous

Virtually any cause of encephalitis or meningitis is capable of being manifested in select circumstances as blindness. Infrequent but potential causes include hydrocephalus, brain tumors, bacterial meningitis, brain abscesses, nervous coccidiosis, *Sarcocystis* infection, *Neospora* infection, the encephalitic form of infectious bovine rhinotracheitis, pseudorabies, rabies, ammoniated forage toxicosis, ethylene glycol ingestion, nitrofurazone toxicosis, and intracarotid drug injection. Vision loss has also been described in sheep with scrapie, *Parelaphostrongylus tenuis* (meningeal worm), the intermediate stages of *Taenia multiceps* (*Coenurus cerebralis*), and inherited ceroid lipofuscinosis.

BIBLIOGRAPHY

Collins BK: Neuro-ophthalmology in food animals. *In* Howard JL (ed): Current Veterinary Therapy: Food Animal Practice, ed 3. Philadelphia, WB Saunders, 1993, pp 851–856.

Holbrook TC, White SL: Assessment of the nervous system. Vet Clin North Am Food Anim Pract 8:285–303, 1992.

Mayhew IG: Large Animal Neurology. Philadelphia, Lea & Febiger, 1989.

McGuirk SM: Polioencephalomalacia. Vet Clin North Am Food Anim Pract 3:107–117, 1987.

Osweiler GD, Carson TL, Buck WB, et al (eds): Clinical and Diagnostic Veterinary Toxicology, ed 3. Dubuque, Iowa, Kendall/Hunt, 1976.

Smith BP: Large Animal Internal Medicine, ed 2. St Louis, Mosby–Year Book, 1996.

Neurologic Diseases

Consulting Editor

Thomas J. Divers, D.V.M., Diplomate, A.C.V.I.M., A.C.V.E.C.C.

The nervous system may be most easily divided into five anatomic divisions: (1) cerebral cortex, (2) brain stem, (3) cerebellum, (4) spinal cord, and (5) peripheral nerves. Dysfunction in each division may produce specific and unique clinical signs in that neuroanatomic area. Bovine neurologic disorders may manifest with localizing signs: polioencephalomalacia and cerebrocortical signs; listeriosis and brain stem signs; midgestation fecal infection with noncytopathic bovine viral diarrhea (BVD); cerebellar signs in a newborn calf; extradural lymphoma causing posterior paresis and cauda equina signs; or recent trauma to a rear limb causing peroneal paresis and inability to extend the fetlock. Conversely, some diseases, such as bacterial meningitis, have a more generalized effect on the nervous system. The recognition of these signs and their association with a specific neuroanatomic location, or a more generalized disorder, can serve as the initial diagnostic step in arriving at a differential diagnosis in bovine neurologic disorders.

■ Diseases of the Nervous System

Thomas J. Divers, D.V.M., Diplomate, A.C.V.I.M., A.C.V.E.C.C.

CEREBRAL DISORDERS

Clinical Signs

Clinical signs suggestive of cerebral or brain stem diseases are commonly seen in cattle. Behavioral changes and central blindness are the characteristic clinical signs of cerebral dysfunction. The behavioral changes may vary from coma or stupor to belligerence and seizures. Cattle with cerebral disease are often found circling (usually toward the side of the lesion) or head pressing. Central blindness can be determined by absence of a menace response with normal pupillary response to light or by observation of the animal as it moves into or around objects. If only one cerebral hemisphere is affected, blindness would appear in the contralateral eye. Ataxia is absent or minimal with cerebral disease alone, although many cattle with cerebral dysfunction walk with a short shuffling gait. Opisthotonus is a common finding with severe cerebral swelling. There are more than 120 diseases that are reported to affect cerebral or brain stem function, resulting in either coma, severe depression, or seizure. Most diseases of the brain in cattle have infectious, toxic, or metabolic causes.

Infectious Causes of Meningitis and Encephalitis

Bacterial meningitis is most common in calves 2 to 14 days of age (mean age of 5 or 6 days). Although inconsistently found, arthritis, omphalophlebitis, or uveitis may be a concurrent clinical problem. *Escherichia coli* is the predominant pathogen causing meningitis in calves. The pathogenic organisms are believed to most often enter via the respiratory or gastrointestinal systems or by way of the umbilicus. Bacteremia ensues, particularly in those calves with inadequate colostral antibody. The least understood step in the pathogenesis of meningitis is the mechanism by which bacteria penetrate the blood-brain barrier and gain entry into the cerebrospinal fluid (CSF). Bacterial piliation appears to be a virulence factor in this step, especially for *E. coli*. Once bacteria reach the CSF, they are likely to survive because of the absence of immunoglobulin and complement in the CSF. Inflammation and tissue destruction rapidly follow, associated with release of bacterial lipopolysaccharide, activation of cytokines, neutrophil adherence to endothelial cells, and release of toxic oxygen metabolites and other inflammatory derivatives. Unless treatment is initiated early in the disease, there is little chance of survival. Antimicrobial and anti-inflammatory therapy, in addition to good nursing care, are the mainstays of therapy. High doses of a cephalosporin (ceftiofur 1 to 3 mg/lb intravenously every 6 to 12 hours) is a reasonable initial treatment. There is evidence that an increasing number of bacteria causing meningitis are resistant to trimethoprim-sulfonamide drugs. Corticosteroid treatment may be beneficial if it is used early in the course of the disease (first 24 hours). Nursing care includes replacement of fluid deficits, plasma treatment, maintaining the head slightly elevated in recumbent calves, proper temperature maintenance, treatment of seizures with phenobarbitol, and intranasal oxygen. Dimethyl sulfoxide (DMSO) has been administered intravenously (IV) as a 5% solution in polyionic crystalloids, but its success in treating any bovine neurologic condition has not been proved.

Prevention of bacterial meningitis or septicemia in calves is of greatest importance and centers around proper colostrum administration to the newborn calf.

Thromboembolic meningoencephalitis (caused by *Haemophilus somnus*) is the most common bacterial meningitis in older calves (usually older than 4 months of age for the encephalitic form). The acute disease is characterized by fibrinopurulent meningitis, multifocal parenchymal necrosis with hemorrhage, and thrombotic vasculitis. Calves that die with a more chronic disease process may have abscessation and cavitation of the brain. The clinical syndrome in dairy replacement heifers may differ slightly from that commonly seen in feedlot animals. The disease is most common in fall and winter and may cause severe clinical signs in a single heifer or small number of replacement heifers. The neurologic signs may or may not be preceded by respiratory signs. The brain, spinal cord, lungs, heart, joints, and larynx may be affected in some calves. The diagnosis can be made from history, clinical signs, postmortem findings, or culturing the organism from the CSF. *H. somnus* is sensitive to most penicillins, cephalosporins, and tetracyclines, but treatment is usually unsuccessful because of the acute and severe inflammation and thrombosis.

Other infectious diseases of the brain include pituitary abscess or septic meningitis associated with sinus infections. Abscesses near the pituitary gland can be seen in calves several months of age or in adult cattle. The organism cultured from the abscess is most often *Actinomyces pyogenes*. In many cases, suppurative foci are found elsewhere in the body and bacteremia may have occurred with the organism(s) localizing in the pituitary region because of the complex vascular network, the rete mirabile, in the bovine. Depression, dropped jaw, exophthalmos, and bradycardia are the most common clinical findings. Antibiotic treatment is not successful.

Increasing numbers of cattle have been affected in the United States with rabies in the past 5 years, which is a result of the epizootic spread of the raccoon, fox, skunk, and bat variant of the virus in several parts of the United States. There are several species-related variants of the virus in the United States, each with different epitopes and nucleotide sequences. The susceptibility to rabies is likely related to the infecting strain, the host's genetic background, the concentration of nicotinic acetylcholine receptors in skeletal muscle, size of the inoculum, degree of innervation at the site of the bite, and proximity to the nervous system. Cattle may manifest either the paralytic, dumb, or furious form of the disease. The variety of form may be related to the distribution of the virus in the nervous tissue. Posterior ataxia, perineal analgesia, bellowing, salivation, hyperesthesia, bizarre behavior, and seizure are some of the most common signs, but no single sign is characteristic. Blindness is rare with rabies. Affected cattle rarely, if ever, purposefully eat or drink. The clinical course of the disease is generally less than 5 days. Confirmation of the disease is by fluorescent antibody testing of the hippocampus and cerebellum. If CSF is collected, it must be handled with great care. An excellent review of rabies by Fishbein and Robinson, including methods of prevention, risks, and treatment recommendations after exposure, has recently been published and veterinarians practicing in rabies endemic areas are encouraged to keep a copy of the article on file.

An encephalitic form of bovine herpesvirus (BHV) may cause encephalitis in young cattle. This neurovirulent strain is BHV-5 which can be distinguished from the respiratory and genital tract isolates of BHV-1 by restriction endonuclease analysis of the viral DNA. It generally causes encephalitic signs and fever in young calves less than 6 weeks of age that are unprotected by passively acquired colostral antibodies against BHV-1 (BHV-1 antibody may be protective against the different subtypes of the virus). Respiratory signs and conjunctivitis may precede the encephalitic signs by 9 to 11 days. The transmission of the virus to the cerebral cortex is thought to be via the trigeminal nerve. The attack rate has been estimated at 15% to 37%, although an isolated case has been documented. Intranuclear inclusion bodies are found in many cases and positive immunoperoxidase staining of the cerebral cortex using antibody against BHV-1 can be used as an aid in confirming the diagnosis. The disease is usually fatal in calves.

Malignant catarrhal fever (MCF) causes nonsuppurative encephalitis, lymphoid necrosis, and vasculitis in cattle. In the United States, the disease is usually seen in cattle that are exposed to sheep (most commonly lambing ewes) and the disease has been called "sheep-associated MCF." There is evidence that the sheep-associated MCF virus is caused by a gammaherpesvirus which is very closely related to the wildebeest-associated MCF herpesvirus. Cattle infected with sheep-associated MCF will seroconvert to this gammaherpesvirus. The clinical disease is usually sporadic in cattle, often causing severe clinical disease in only one animal in the herd. This may be a result of the low infectivity of the virus. There are reports of outbreaks of the disease with some cases having only mild clinical signs. In addition to the neurologic signs (both cerebral and spinal cord signs), purulent nasal and ocular disease is generally present, and diarrhea is variably present. The clinical course of the disease in an affected animal is generally 2 to 5 days.

Bovine spongiform encephalopathy (BSE) has occurred as an epidemic in cattle in Great Britain. The disease is caused by a prior protein transmitted to cattle via ingestion of the scrapie-like agent in feeds containing meat and bone meal. The incubation period is 18 months or longer and the mean age at onset of clinical signs is 60 to 62 months. The neurologic signs most frequently reported include aggressiveness, apprehension, hyperesthesia, persistent licking, and ataxia. These signs are similar to those that might occur with nervous ketosis and a variety of poisons. The potential risk of BSE occurring in the United States has been extensively investigated. The risk or presence of BSE in the United States could not be eliminated. A decline in the number of sheep carcasses used in meat and bone meal, the absence of sheep products in milk replacers, the failure to identify cases in surveillance of cattle imported from Great Britain and Ireland, or in the pathologic review of hundreds of cattle with nervous signs, along with widespread dissemination of information about the disease to appropriate professionals, all suggest that the disease probably does not exist in the United States and the risk of its occurrence is low. Electrophoresis of CSF can be used to identify clinically affected cattle.

Other viral encephalitides in cattle have been sporadically reported, including encephalitis resulting from infection from bovine immunodeficiency virus.

TOXIC AND METABOLIC ENCEPHALOPATHIES

Metabolic causes of cerebral dysfunction include polioencephalomalacia, nervous ketosis, ruminal acidosis, vitamin A deficiency, and uremic or hepatic encephalopathy. Toxic causes are numerous but include lead, salt, organophosphate, and urea poisoning. Until recently, polioencephalomalacia (PEM) has been equated with thiamine deficiency. Recently an association between PEM and increased ruminal sulfide concentrations has been demonstrated. Excessive ruminal production of sulfides may occur from the ingestion of feeds or water with a high sulfate content. Clinical signs most commonly occur 10 to 12 days after beginning a high sulfate, readily fermentable, low fiber diet. Clinical signs include cortical blindness, circling, facial tremors, recumbency, and opisthotonos. Although cattle with PEM experimentally induced by sulfide have had normal blood thiamine concentrations, thiamine, 2.0 mg/kg, should be given every 6 to 12 hours until the animal has recovered. Improvement may be noted within 6 to 12 hours in some cases. Once improvement is noted, full recovery is generally expected, although vision may not return for several days or weeks. If there is no improvement within 2 to 3 days with appropriate therapy, this is a strong indication of cerebrocortical necrosis and recovery is unlikely. Antiedema treatment (DMSO) has been used in some cases, but is unnecessary if treatment with thiamine is initiated early in the disease.

The clinical signs of lead poisoning may be indistinguishable from those of PEM, although extreme nervousness, exaggerated chewing, frequent urination, and facial fasciculations are more common with lead poisoning. Many of the signs may also occur with urea, chlorinated hydrocarbon, organophosphate, or ammoniated forage toxicosis. Thiamine therapy has also been shown to be beneficial in treating and protecting cattle from lead poisoning. In fact, thiamine was more effective than ethylenediaminetetraacetic acid (EDTA) in alleviating the clinical signs in cattle chronically exposed to lead. Treatment with both thiamine and EDTA are recommended for lead poisoning in cattle. There has been a product safety concern that cattle, although clinically recovered from lead poisoning, might continue to produce milk with excessive concentration of lead. Cattle which had exhibited clinical lead poisoning 7 months earlier had increases in blood lead at freshening but lead did not reach detectable levels in the milk. If there are shorter durations between poisoning and milk analysis or if greater or more persistent exposure to lead occurs, there is a possibility of prolonged contamination of the milk.

Hypernatremia (sodium intoxication) seems to be more common now that most oral electrolyte solutions are hypertonic. Toxicity usually occurs from improper mixing of these oral electrolyte solutions and their subsequent administration to calves with neonatal diarrhea. Affected calves usually become extremely depressed, blind, and recumbent. Salt poisoning should be considered in diarrheal calves that become unexplainably depressed and recumbent after being treated by lay personnel with oral electrolytes. Severe hypoglycemia or acidosis can produce identical clinical signs. Serum and CSF sodium concentrations are usually between 170 and 220 mEq/L. Surprisingly, some calves recover if serum sodium is gradually lowered by administering sodium-containing fluids, for example, lactated Ringer's solution with dextrose.

Urea poisoning, vitamin A deficiency, and severe ruminal acidosis are other diseases that may result in blindness and severe depression or seizure in cattle. These are more likely to be found in beef cattle than in dairy cattle. Diagnosis of urea toxicosis is generally based on history and clinical findings. Affected cattle have only a mild increase in blood urea concentrations, but have severe metabolic acidosis, hyperglycemia, and hyperammonemia. Treatment of urea poisoning includes IV fluids to help correct metabolic acidosis and dehydration. Two percent acetic acid, 500 mL/500-kg cow, given orally may be helpful in decreasing the ruminal ammonia concentration. As with most oral toxicants, 0.5 kg of activated charcoal may be helpful. The clinical signs of vitamin A deficiency in cattle may vary according to the animal's age. In calves, the signs include blindness, decreased appetite, poor growth, diarrhea, dermatitis, and pneumonia. In adult cattle, clinical signs are predominantly seizures and blindness. The blindness in hypovitaminosis A is a result of retinal and optic nerve disease, and the pupillary response to light is absent. Absence of pupillary light response is unusual in most other bovine cerebrocortical disorders.

Renal failure may also cause an encephalopathy due to either metabolic or structural changes (Alzheimer type II cells) in the brain. Organophosphate poisoning, especially that caused by terbufos mixed with seed corn, has been commonly seen in dairy cattle. Colic, salivation, depression, frequent urination, and acute death are common findings. Portosystemic shunts have been recently reported in three Holstein heifers. Clinical signs did not occur until the calves were 5 to 8 weeks of age and were being fed increasing amounts of grain and high protein roughage. Seizure, opisthotonus, paddling, and coma may be followed by apparent recovery without treatment, only to recur in a few days. Hepatic failure from hepatic cirrhosis or obstruction of the common bile duct by an abscess may also cause fulminant neurologic signs in cattle. Hepatic enzymes are increased in the serum of cattle with cirrhosis or biliary obstruction, but not in calves with portosystemic shunts.

Ammoniated forages may cause neurologic signs (bonkers) in cattle or in calves nursing cows fed the ammoniated hay. The cause of the syndrome is not proved but it is not the result of high blood ammonia concentration. The clinical signs are hyperactivity, tremors, ear twitching, bellowing, salivation, running in circles, crashing into objects, and terminal seizures with opisthotonus. These signs may be easily confused with those of grass tetany, grass staggers (mycotoxicosis), and nervous ketosis. Once cattle are removed from the forage, no further clinical cases are expected.

Parasitic causes of cerebral dysfunction in cattle include nervous coccidiosis (*Eimeria* sp.), *Sarcocystis* sp., and *Neospora caninum*. The exact pathogenic mechanism of nervous coccidiosis has not been proved. The condition is most common in Canada in feedlots, although it has been observed in most regions of the United States. The neurologic signs (seizure, tremors, ataxia) are generally preceded by diarrhea with mucus and blood and high fecal *Eimeria* oocyst counts. Outbreaks of central nervous system (CNS) signs are not uncommon. There is a high fatality rate in nervous coccidiosis, but IV treatment with polyionic fluids and magnesium and oral sulfamethazine (110 mg/kg every 24 hours) is recommended. Thiamine should be given and is recommended in most CNS diseases of calves. Prevention of severe disease in exposed but clinically inapparent calves should receive adequate attention.

Heavy infestation with *Sarcocystis* in the naive ruminant may result in CNS signs or hemorrhagic myositis. The CNS signs may vary, depending on the pathologic location of the lesions, which are granulomatous meningoencephalomyelitis and malacia. Successful treatment is unlikely and attention should be focused on prevention.

N. caninum is a major cause of abortion and mummified fetuses in cattle in many parts of the United States and the world. Nonfatal infections of the fetus may also occur. Most are clinically normal, but infected newborn calves occasionally will have neurologic signs that could be clinically confused with BVD-induced cerebellar hypoplasia. The pathologic lesions of *N. caninum* include severe cavitation and microscopic nonsuppurative inflammation with encysted protozoa.

TRAUMA AND NEOPLASIA

Injury to the cerebral cortex in cattle may occur from blunt trauma. Affected animals are generally depressed or comatose, and may have blindness, abnormal pupil size, and abnormal respiratory and heart rates. Cerebral edema and hypoxia are the usual sequelae to intracranial injury and should be treated with antiedema drugs (DMSO or corticosteroids) and mild elevation of the head.

If there is a fracture of the skull or hemorrhage into the CSF, antibiotic treatment should be added, but the prognosis with intracerebral hemorrhage is guarded to grave.

Neoplasia of the bovine cerebrum is rare. Non-BLV–associated lymphoma is perhaps the most common neoplasia. It most often causes clinical signs of cerebral cortical disease within the first 2 years of life.

CEREBROSPINAL FLUID COLLECTION AND EVALUATION

The most direct antemortem laboratory method of evaluating the CNS is the examination of CSF. The normal bovine CSF is clear, contains no erythrocytes, less than six white blood cells per microliter (a mixture of lymphocytes and macrophages), and

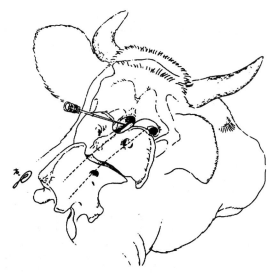

Figure 1
Atlanto-occipital CSF collection from the cow. The cow should be positioned in lateral recumbency for the procedure. The 3½ in. 18-g needle should be introduced at a point exactly between the cranial borders of the atlas.

has a protein content of less than 60 mg/dL. The CSF can be collected from either the atlanto-occipital (Fig. 1) or lumbosacral (LS) sites (Fig. 2). A 3.5-in. needle is usually sufficient for the puncture, even in adult cows. The LS procedure is more difficult in recumbent adults but can be accomplished easily in recumbent calves if the hips are flexed and the pelvic limbs are extended alongside the abdomen. Contamination of the CSF with erythrocytes is also more likely to occur with lumbosacral collection than with atlanto-occipital collection.

The total leukocyte count of the CSF has been shown to be useful in separating septic causes from metabolic or toxic disorders. Cattle with acute bacterial infections of the CNS usually have a neutrophilic pleocytosis. As the infection becomes more chronic, macrophages may predominate, and in brain abscesses, neutrophils may be relatively few. Bacterial meningitis typically causes higher numbers of erythrocytes and greater discoloration of the CSF than with any other disease except acute trauma. Listeriosis generally causes a pleocytosis with the majority of the cells being macrophages, although on occasion the CSF

with *Listeria* may be either normal or have a pleocytosis with macrophages constituting less than 50% of the cells. Polymerase chain reaction (PCR) is effective in detecting *Listeria monocytogenes* in the CSF of nontreated small ruminants, but appears to be less sensitive in cattle.

Viral meningoencephalitis tends to produce a predominantly lymphocytic pleocytosis. Rabies may produce the least cellular response of any septic condition.

Cattle with acute trauma and cerebral cortical signs have increases in CSF protein, erythrocytes, and leukocytes. Erythrophagocytosis is usually present and can be helpful in separating prior hemorrhage from artifactual hemorrhage due to collection. Abnormal number of macrophages may also occur associated with prior hemorrhage and accompanying inflammatory reaction.

Cattle with encephalopathy resulting from metabolic or toxic causes often have normal spinal fluid. CSF protein and leukocytes may be mildly increased.

BIBLIOGRAPHY

Anderson WI, Rebhun WC, de Lahunta A, et al: The ophthalmic and neuro-ophthalmologic effects of vitamin A deficiency in young steers. Vet Med 86:1143–1148, 1991.

Bleem AM, Crom RL, Francy B, et al: Risk factors and surveillance for bovine spongiform encephalopathy in the United States. J Am Vet Med Assoc 204:644–651, 1994.

Boermans HJ, Black WD, Chesney J, et al: Terbufos poisoning in a dairy herd. Can Vet J 25:335–338, 1984.

Brazil TJ, Naylor JM, Janzer ED: Ammoniated forage toxicosis in nursing calves: A herd outbreak. Can Vet J 35:45–47, 1994.

Caldow GL, Wain EB: Urea poisoning in suckler cows. Vet Rec 128:489–491, 1991.

Coppock RW, Wagner WC, Reynolds JD, et al: Evaluation of edetate and thiamine for treatment of experimentally induced environmental lead poisoning in cattle. Am J Vet Res 52:1860–1865, 1991.

Divers TJ: Cerebral and brainstem diseases of cattle: Diagnosis and review of causes. *In* Proceedings of the 27th Annual Convention of the American Association of Bovine Practitioners, Pittsburgh, 1994, pp 75–79.

Divers TJ, Sweeney R, Rebhun WC, et al: Cerebrospinal fluid analysis: A retrospective study in cattle. *In* Espinasse J (ed): Le Recours au Laboratoire en Buiatrie. Societe Francaise de Buiatrie, 1992, pp 207–214.

d'Offay JM, Mock RE, Fulton RW: Isolation and characterization of encephalitis bovine herpesvirus type 1 isolates from cattle in North America. Am J Vet Res 54:534–539, 1993.

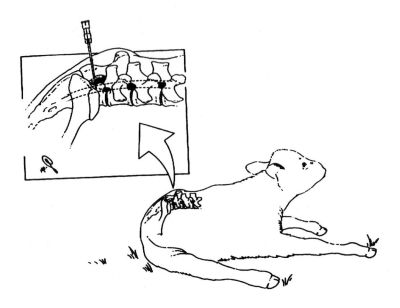

Figure 2
Lumbosacral CSF collection is performed in the recumbent calf by rostrally positioning the rear legs and by introducing the needle on the midline in the palpable lumbosacral space.

Ely RW, d'Offay JM, Ruefer AH, et al: Bovine herpesviral encephalitis: A retrospective study on archival formalin-fixed paraffin-embedded brain tissue. J Vet Diagn Invest 8:487–492, 1996.

Fishbein DB, Robinson LE: Rabies. N Engl J Med 329:1632–1638, 1993.

Fortier LA, Fubini SL, Flanders JA, et al: The diagnosis and surgical correction of congenital portosystemic vascular anomalies in two calves and two foals. Vet Surg 25:154–160, 1996.

Galey FD, Slenny BD, Anderson ML, et al: Lead concentrations in blood and milk from periparturient dairy heifers seven months after an episode of acute lead toxicity. J Vet Diagn Invest 2:222–229, 1990.

Gould DH, McAllister MM, Savage JC, et al: High sulfide concentrations in rumen fluid associated with nutritionally induced polioencephalomalacia in calves. Am J Vet Res 52:1164–1169, 1991.

Green SL, Smith LL: Meningitis in neonatal calves: 32 cases (1983–1990). J Am Vet Med Assoc 201:125–128, 1992.

Hamilton AF: Account of the outbreak of malignant catarrhal fever in cattle in the Republic of Ireland. Vet Rec 127:231–232, 1990.

Hamlen H, Clark E, Janzen E: Polioencephalomalacia in cattle consuming water with elevated sodium sulfate levels: A herd investigation. Can Vet J 34:154–158, 1993.

Hsich G, Kenney K, Gibbs CJ, et al: The 14-3-3 brain protein in cerebrospinal fluid as a marker for transmissible spongiform encephalopathies. N Engl J Med 335:924–930, 1996.

Jones V, Martin TC, Keyes P, et al: Protein markers in cerebrospinal fluid from BSE-affected cattle. Vet Rec 139:360–363, 1996.

Krebs JW, Strine TW, Childs JE: Rabies surveillance in the United States during 1992. J Am Vet Med Assoc 203:1718–1731, 1993.

Mirangi PK, Rossiter PB: Malignant catarrhal fever in cattle experimentally inoculated with a herpesvirus isolated from a case of malignant catarrhal fever in Minnesota. Br Vet J 147:31–41, 1991.

Orr JP: Hemophilus somnus infection: A retrospective analysis of cattle necropsied at the Western College of Veterinary Medicine from 1970–1990. Can Vet J 33:719–722, 1992.

Pringle JK, Berthiaume LMM: Hypernatremia in calves. J Vet Intern Med 2:66–70, 1988.

Schuller W, Cerny-Reiterer S, Silher R: Evidence that the sheep-associated form of malignant catarrhal fever is caused by a herpes virus. J Vet Med B 37:442–447, 1990.

Scott PR, Penney CD: A field study of meningoencephalitis in calves with particular reference to analysis of cerebrospinal fluid. Vet Rec 133:119–121, 1993.

Snider TG, Luther DG, Jenny BF, et al: Encephalitis, lymphoid tissue depletion and secondary diseases associated with bovine immunodeficiency virus in a dairy herd. Comp Immunol Microbiol Infect Dis 19:117–131, 1996.

Sweeney R, Divers TJ, Zeimer E, et al: Intracranial lymphosarcoma in a Holstein bull. J Am Vet Med Assoc 189:555–556, 1986.

Wentink GH, van Oirschot JT, Verhoeff J, et al: Risk of infection with bovine herpes virus 1 (BHV1). Vet Q 15:30–33, 1993.

Wilesmith JW, Ryan JBM: Bovine spongiform encephalopathy: Recent observation of age specific incidences. Vet Rec 130:491–492, 1992.

Wilesmith JW, Ryan JBM: Bovine spongiform encephalopathy: Observations on the incidence during 1992. Vet Rec 132:300–301, 1993.

Yamasaki H, Umemura T, Goryo M, et al: Chronic lesions of thromboembolic meningoencephalomyelitis in calves. J Comp Pathol 105:303–312, 1991.

▪ Brain Stem Diseases of Cattle

Robert H. Whitlock, D.V.M., Ph.D., Diplomate, A.C.V.I.M.

LISTERIOSIS (CIRCLING DISEASE, SILAGE DISEASE)

The encephalitic form of listeriosis most commonly affects adult ruminants (cattle, sheep, and goats, in order of prevalence) during the late winter and spring months of the year. Although the organism may be common in the environment and silage, typically only one or two animals in a herd or flock are affected at any one time. Sheep seem to have more animals affected in a flock than cattle in herds of similar size. *Listeria monocytogenes* can also cause encephalitis, meningitis, ophthalmitis, septicemia, abortion, and mastitis in ruminants.

Etiologic Agent

L. monocytogenes is a gram-positive, motile facultative intracellular, microaerophilic flagellated coccobacillus with an increasingly important zoonotic potential.[1] As an intracellular pathogen, infection is controlled by T lymphocytes and phagocytic cells. A common soil saprophyte that is psychrophilic and widespread in the environment, *L. monocytogenes* easily survives freezing and thawing, and survives in soil and manure for years. *Listeria* may survive longer than *Salmonella* on land sprayed with sewage sludge.[2] The organism is harvested with forage as a soil contaminant, especially silage. With cool temperatures and silage pH greater than 5.5, the organisms proliferate and are more likely to be associated with clinical disease. Some healthy cattle (~10%) and sheep (>20%) carry *Listeria* in their intestinal tract or other body organs and are fecal culture–positive for *Listeria*. The 13 serovars or antigenic types are distinguished by somatic (O) and flagellar (H) antigens.[3] Type 1/2a is the most common pathogenic serovar[4] while serovar 4b is the most common of the three pathogenic serotypes (1/2a, 1/2b, and 4b) in humans.[5] Serotype 4 has been associated with mastitis.

Virulence of *L. monocytogenes* is related to two toxins: hemolysin and cytotoxin. Hemolysin, a cytolysin, is able to lyse tissue and red blood cells. The cytotoxin stimulates cyclic adenosine monophosphate (cAMP) production similar to cholera toxin.[6] Nearly all strains have phosphatase activity, which may play a role in virulence.

Pathogenesis

The lesions of listeriosis include microabscesses and lymphoid perivascular cuffs that are restricted to the brain stem, especially the pontine and trapezoid regions of the medulla. These lesions are nearly pathognomonic for listeriosis. Several authors[7, 8] have provided experimental evidence that the brain stem microabscesses result from an ascending (centripetal) infection of the trigeminal nerve from small wounds in the oral cavity, buccal mucosa, or conjunctiva. Once the organism has gained access to the brain stem, infection is located in the trigeminal nerve nuclei in the pons. Local spread of infection within the brain stem leads to involvement of other adjacent nuclei and resultant meningoencephalitis. Under experimental conditions, clinical neurologic listeriosis resulted about 3 weeks after the inoculation of *Listeria* in the pulp cavity of incisor or premolar teeth in sheep.[7] Goats showed clinical signs 17 to 28 days after experimental infection.[8] Low and Renton[9] recorded the first clinical case 30 days after the introduction of silage in a naturally occurring outbreak.

Epidemiology

The encephalitic form of listeriosis remains the most common form in both cattle and sheep. In a retrospective survey of 75 sheep flocks in Great Britain, listerial encephalitis occurred in 60 flocks with only lambs affected in 10 flocks.[10] The mean attack rate was 2.5% for the encephalic form in adults. Another well-documented outbreak reported the attack rate to be 11.8% with a case fatality rate of 94.3%.[11] The outbreak ceased 2 weeks after removal of the silage that contained the same serovar as isolated from the brains. Listerial meningoencephalitis was detected only in lambs during the postweaning period when lambs were 6 to 12 weeks old.[12] Affected lambs had signs of tooth eruption but no longer had access to silage.

Most clinical cases of listeriosis in ruminants are associated with silage feeding, although not universally.[13] Silage was fed to 59 of the 60 flocks with a mean relative risk of silage feeding of 3.8.[10] Big-bale silage feeding appears more prone to be associated with listeriosis, perhaps due to the increased propensity for spoilage by damage to the bags. Since the organism multiplies at colder temperatures, most cases occur in the late winter and early spring months of the year. When the silage pH is greater than 5.5, organisms proliferate and are more likely to be associated with clinical disease. *L. monocytogenes* survives freezing, and can survive in the soil for at least 2 years and in silage for 10 to 12 years. It has been isolated from feces of apparently healthy animals and humans.[14] A large proportion of healthy sheep may excrete the organism in their feces.[15]

Clinical Signs

A change in mentation (dullness) may be one of the earliest clinical signs, followed by inappetence associated with difficulty in prehension and mastication. Low-grade fever up to 105°F (40.5°C) may be present early but may be normal throughout the disease course of 4 to 10 days.

Unilateral cranial nerve (upper motor neuron paresis) deficits such as facial nerve palsy with a drooped ear; ptosis; hypalgesia of the facial skin, and decreased lip tone on one side of the face, which may allow saliva to drip from the mouth; abnormal nystagmus (fast phase away from the head tilt); loss of a menace response; abducent paralysis (medial strabismus); and vestibular nerve palsy (head tilt) typify the progression of clinical signs.[16]

Lesions of the trigeminal motor nucleus in the brain stem affect the muscles of mastication resulting in poor jaw tone or a "dropped jaw." This is best demonstrated by grasping the upper jaw with one hand and the lower jaw with the other, then moving the jaws laterally. Little resistance is noted in affected animals with lesions of the trigeminal nerve. Circling toward the affected side with evidence of facial nerve palsy occurs in a high percentage of cases. Exposure keratitis, weak tongue, excess salivation, and dysphagia all may present in some cases of listeriosis. Salivation, if profuse, often results in moderate to severe dehydration with metabolic acidosis due to bicarbonate and water loss in the saliva and inability to swallow. A minority of affected cattle may vomit several times early in the course of the disease.

Increased skin tenting and dry mucous membranes reflect the loss of body water. Accordingly the rumen is reduced in size with decreased rumen contractions. The manure often has a more firm consistency and is reduced in volume secondary to dehydration.

Later the tongue may protrude from the mouth and have decreased strength. With development of exposure keratitis, panophthalmitis may result. Many affected cattle have a moderate fever of up to 104°F. Ataxia with tetraparesis occurs with progression of signs. Some cattle develop a propensity to "push" forward against the stanchion with their shoulders. This may persist for weeks, with subsequent development of calluses in front of the shoulders.

Asymmetrical neurologic deficits are nearly always present, which helps to differentiate listeriosis from diffuse cerebral diseases such as thromboembolic meningoencephalitis (TEME), polioencephalomalacia, and lead poisoning. Later stages may include bellowing with central nervous system (CNS) excitement. With progression of clinical signs, the animals become weak, recumbent unable to rise, and die. With recumbency, the prognosis for survival becomes grave despite intensive antimicrobial and supportive therapy.

Necropsy Findings

Gross lesions of listeriosis are typically not found in the brain at necropsy. Histopathologic lesions consist of inflammatory cells in the perivascular spaces, microabscesses with neutrophils and macrophages in the brain stem, and focal necrosis. The peroxidase-antiperoxidase method has been used successfully to detect natural cases of listeriosis in cattle.[17]

Diagnosis

Typical clinical signs (depression with asymmetrical cranial nerve deficits) are usually sufficient to begin antibiotic treatment. Examination of the cerebrospinal fluid (CSF) often provides valuable laboratory data to support a diagnosis of listeriosis. The CSF changes are typical of nonsuppurative encephalitis with mononuclear cell pleocytosis (1 to 300 cells per microliter; normal, <5 cells) and a moderate increase in protein (25 to 140 mg/dL; normal, <40 mg/dL).[18] In recumbent or severely depressed animals, an atlanto-occipital tap is recommended. In stronger standing patients, a lumbosacral tap is used.[19] Visual evoked potentials may be of some value in those animals with central listerial blindness, but most affected animals are not blind, although the menace response may be reduced or absent.[20]

Hematologic changes are of minimal diagnostic value for listeriosis and often reflect stress. An increased packed cell volume (PCV) and total protein (TP) reflect dehydration and serve as guides to fluid therapy. Biochemical changes are of minimal value except for quantitating the severity of the acidosis, if present. Serologic tests including agglutination, dot blot, and enzyme-linked immunosorbent assay (ELISA) tests have been developed to detect antibodies post infection, but are unable to differentiate previous from current infection.[21] These serologic tests also frequently cross-react with antibodies to other bacteria, such as *Staphylococcus aureus*.

The histologic finding of typical brain stem microabscesses provides near-definitive evidence of listeriosis. The finding of *L. monocytogenes* by culture alone is insufficient evidence because some animals may harbor the organisms in their tissues, including brain stem tissues, without clinical signs.[22] The presence of the organism with microabscesses in the brain stem is pathognomonic for listeriosis. Refrigeration of brain stem tissue for 3 to 6 weeks prior to culture will facilitate isolation of the organism, since it is psychrophilic. Immunohistochemistry techniques to identify *Listeria* in the neuropil represent valuable adjunct diagnostic modalities for listeriosis.[23] A direct selective medium for isolation and enumeration of *Listeria* has been described.[11] Recent advances in DNA technology have given rise to new techniques to identify *Listeria* in feed, CSF, and tissue samples.[24]

Treatment

Both tetracycline 10 to 20 mg/kg intravenously (IV) daily and penicillin procaine have been used successfully, but penicillin procaine 44,000 units/kg, b.i.d., is favored by some authors. In valuable cattle, potassium penicillin 10,000 to 20,000 units/kg t.i.d. may be superior to procaine penicillin. Subcutaneously administered procaine penicillin may provide an alternative route whereby larger total doses may be given, but should be given at less than 20 mL per site.[25] This route may be associated with prolonged antibiotic withdrawal times. The treatment should be continued for at least 7 to 10 days and longer in some cases.[16] Cattle and sheep that are recumbent due to listeriosis rarely survive.

Dehydrated and acidotic animals require appropriate bicarbonate-rich fluid therapy, both orally and parenterally, to restore acid-base balance and hydration. In severely acidotic cattle, bicarbonate-rich fluids should be given IV, since orally administered fluids may pool in the atonic rumen. I prefer oral electrolytes for moderately affected cattle since they are easily administered with feed material (alfalfa meal) and rumen contents from another "donor" animal. Analgesics such as phenylbutazone or flunixin meglumine provide anti-inflammatory relief.

Exposure keratitis and corneal ulceration that may result from facial nerve palsy should be treated with atropine ophthalmic ointment to produce mydriasis and with topical ophthalmic antibiotics for the bacterial keratoconjunctivitis. Subpalpebral antibiotics and tarsorrhaphy may be indicated in severe corneal ulceration.

Nursing care, including a well-bedded box stall with a nonslip surface, is important to prevent secondary musculoskeletal injury due to feeble attempts by the patient to rise.

Control and Prevention

Under normal conditions it is virtually impossible to prepare silage free of *Listeria*. *Listeria* grow best at the edge of the silage container where air has access to silage, causing mild growth. In cases of outbreaks, it is recommended that the silage be closely examined and any moldy spoiled silage be discarded. Up to 12,000 organisms per gram of silage have been recovered in some moldy silage in *Listeria* outbreaks.[26] Since alkaline pH silage favors growth of *Listeria*, any measure to favor silage fermentation and acid production will inhibit listeria growth. At the critical pH of 5.5 or less, many fewer *Listeria* organisms are present in silage. Both chlorine-based sanitizers (at 100 ppm) and iodine-containing sanitizers (at 15.5 ppm) were effective against *L. monocytogenes*.

An experimental live vaccine has shown good preliminary results in a field trial in Norway.[27] At this time no U.S. Department of Agriculture (USDA)–approved vaccine is available in the United States.

Zoonotic Potential

Clearly, *L. monocytogenes* has achieved status as a significant zoonotic pathogen which should be of concern to veterinarians. Increased stress (dexamethasone treatment) has been shown to increase listerial shedding in the milk nearly 100-fold compared to pretreatment shedding.[28] One survey of bulk tank milk samples found 4.1% to be contaminated with *L. monocytogenes*.[29] Cattle infected with *L. monocytogenes* in any form may and often do shed the organism in the milk, which is a major zoonotic concern. Raw milk should not be consumed and personnel in close contact with the affected animal should use good hygiene. See Blenden et al.[30] or Pearson and Marth[5] for an excellent review concerning *Listeria* and the food supply.

OTITIS MEDIA

Otitis media remains a major differential diagnosis, especially in early cases of listeriosis. However, strength is preserved in otitis media, whereas *Listeria* cases progress with gradual loss of strength and dullness and depression, all signs of brain stem disease. Ruminants with otitis media often have a sudden onset of head tilt, ear droop, fever, and circling. Some animals may have a suppurative otitis externa with extension to the middle ear. This syndrome may occur more commonly in calves housed in a group pen that allows calves to suck the ears of other calves.

In feedlot calves the disease begins as an acute otitides, most of which resolve. A few persist or recur as chronic suppurative otitis. With adequate therapy the prognosis is favorable for the former and poor to grave for the latter.

Otitis media as a disease of feedlot cattle has been recognized as occurring in two separate age groups: 5- to 7-month-old calves and yearlings 12 to 18 months of age.[31] *Pasteurella* and *Corynebacterium* spp. are the organisms most commonly isolated from infected middle ears. Seventeen (26.6%) of 64 laboratory-confirmed cases in calves were bilateral. Most calves without pneumonia made a clinical recovery.[31]

Cattle with tumors adjacent to the cerebellar-pontine angle may present with clinical signs similar to otitis media. Several case reports document the clinical signs and lesions.[32] Calves with inflammatory lesions of the facial and vestibulocochlear nerves also present with clinical signs resembling otitis media.[33]

REFERENCES

1. Ho JL, Shands KN, Friedland G, et al: An outbreak of type 4B *Listeria monocytogenes* infection involving patients from eight Boston hospitals. Arch Intern Med 146:520, 1986.
2. Watkins J, Sleath KP: Isolation and enumeration of *Listeria monocytogenes* from sewage, sewage sludge and river water. J Appl Bacteriol 50:1, 1981.
3. Jones D: Foodborne listeriosis. Lancet 336:1171, 1990.
4. Low JC, Wright F, McLaughlin J, et al: Serotyping and distribution of *Listeria* isolates from cases of ovine listeriosis. Vet Rec 133:165, 1993.
5. Pearson LJ, Marth EH: *Listeria monocytogenes*—Threat to a safe food supply: A review. J Dairy Sci 73:912, 1990.
6. McCardell BA, Stephens MJ, Madden JM: Production of cyclic AMP stimulating cytotonic toxin by *Listeria monocytogenes*. *In* Proceedings of the Annual Spring Meeting of the Food Research Institute, University of Wisconsin, Madison, May 25–26, 1988.
7. Barlow RM, McGorum B: Ovine listerial encephalitis: Analysis, hypothesis and synthesis. Vet Rec. 116:233, 1985.
8. Asahi O, Hosoda T, Akiyana Y: Studies on the mechanism of infection of the brain with *Listeria monocytogenes*. Am J Vet Res 18:147, 1957.
9. Low JC, Renton CP: Septicemia, encephalitis and abortion in a housed flock of sheep caused by *Listeria monocytogenes* type 1/2. Vet Rec 116:147, 1985.
10. Wilesmith JW, Gitter M: Epidemiology of ovine listeriosis in Great Britain. Vet Rec 119:467, 1986.
11. Vazquez-Boland JA, Dominguez L, Blanco M, et al: Epidemiologic investigation of a silage-associated epizootic of ovine listeric encephalitis, using a new *Listeria*-selective enumeration medium and phage typing. Am J Vet Res 53:368, 1992.
12. Green LE, Morgan KL: Descriptive epidemiology of listerial meningoencephalitis in housed lambs. Prev Vet Med 18:79, 1994.
13. Merideth CD, Scheider DJ: An outbreak of ovine listeriosis associated with poor flock management. J S Afr Vet Assoc 55:55, 1982.
14. Kampelmacher EH, Noorle Jansen LM van: Isolation of *Listeria monocytogenes* from faeces of clinically healthy humans and animals. Zentralbl Bakteriol Parasitol Infect Hyg 211:353, 1969.
15. Grondol H: Listeriosis in sheep. *Listeria monocytogenes* excretion and immunological state in healthy sheep. Acta Vet Scand 20:168, 1979.
16. Rebhun WC, deLahunta A: Diagnosis and treatment of bovine listeriosis. J Am Vet Med Assoc 180:395, 1982.
17. Marco A, Ramos JA, Domingguez M et al: Immunocytochemical detection of *Listeria monocytogenes* in tissue with the peroxidase-antiperoxidase technique. Vet Pathol 25:385, 1988.
18. Scott PR: A field study of ovine listerial meningo-encephalitis with particular reference to cerebrospinal fluid analysis as an aid to diagnosis and prognosis. Br Vet J 149:165, 1993.
19. Divers TJ: Cerebral and brainstem diseases of cattle: Diagnosis and review of causes. *In* Proceedings of the 27th Annual Convention of the American Association of Bovine Practitioners, Pittsburgh, 1995, p 75.
20. Strain GM, Claxon MS, Olcott BM, et al: Visual-evoked response potentials and electroretinograms in ruminants with thiamine-re-

sponsive polioencephalomalacia or suspected listeriosis. Am J Vet Res 51:1513, 1990.

21. Baetz AL, Wesley IV: Detection of anti-listeriolysin O in dairy cattle experimentally infected with *Listeria monocytogenes.* J Vet Diagn Invest 7:82, 1995.

22. Grondol H: Listeriosis in sheep. Isolation of *Listeria monocytogenes* from organs of slaughtered animals and dead animals submitted for post-mortem examination. Acta Vet Scand 21:11, 1980.

23. Johnson GC, Fales WH, Maddox CW, et al: Evaluation of laboratory tests for confirming the diagnosis of encephalitis listeriosis in ruminants. J Vet Diagn Invest 7:223, 1995.

24. Widman M, Czajka J, Bsat N, et al: Diagnosis and epidemiological association of *Listeria monocytogenes* strains in two outbreaks of listerial encephalitis in small ruminants. J Clin Microbiol 32:991, 1994.

25. Divers TJ: Penicillin therapy in bovine practice. Compendium Continuing Educ Pract Vet 18:703, 1996.

26. Fenlon DR: Rapid quantitative assessment of the distribution of *Listeria* in silage implicated in a suspected outbreak of listeriosis in calves. Vet Rec 118:240, 1986.

27. Gudding R, Gronstal H, Larson HJ: Vaccination against listeriosis in sheep. Vet Rec 117:89, 1985.

28. Wesley IV, Bryner JH, Van Der Maaten MJ, et al: Effects of dexamethasone on shedding of *Listeria monocytogenes* in dairy cattle. Am J Vet Res 50:2009, 1989.

29. Rohrbach BW, Draughon FA, Davidson PM, et al: Prevalence of *Listeria monocytogenes, Campylobacter jejuni, Yersinia enterocolitica,* and *Salmonella* in bulk tank milk: Risk factors and risk of human exposure. J Food Protect 55:93, 1992.

30. Blenden DC, Kampelmacher EH, Torres-Anjel MJ: Listeriosis. J Am Vet Med Assoc 191:1546, 1987.

31. Jensen R, Maki LR, Lauerman LH, et al: Cause and pathogenesis of middle ear infection in young feedlot cattle. J Am Vet Med Assoc 182:967, 1983.

32. Roeder BL, Johnson JW, Cash WC: Paradoxic vestibular syndrome in a cow with a metastatic brain tumor. Compendium Continuing Educ Pract Vet 12:1175, 1990.

33. Van Der Lugt JJ, Jordan P: Facial paralysis associated with space occupying lesions of cranial nerves in calves. Vet Rec 134:579, 1994.

■ Cerebellar Disease in Cattle

Cynthia A. Jackson, D.V.M., Diplomate, A.C.V.I.M.

The cerebellum coordinates and refines voluntary movement. It also integrates posture and tone to maintain the normal position of the body at rest or during motion. Cerebellar dysfunction is characterized by truncal ataxia with spasticity and dysmetria, a base-wide stance, and intentional head tremor in an alert responsive animal. Neurologic impairment is usually bilaterally symmetrical. Abnormal nystagmus may occur in animals with severe lesions. Calves affected with a congenital cerebellar disorder may be unable to stand, due to profound ataxia, but they retain voluntary movement with normal strength. Stimulation may induce hyperexcitability and opisthotonus which may be misinterpreted as seizures. A hallmark of cerebellar disease is the absence of a menace (blink) response despite normal vision and intact cranial nerve function. It must be remembered that the menace response is a learned response and may be undeveloped in neonates. Acquired unilateral disease located in a cerebellar peduncle results in vestibular derangement with paradoxical signs, that is, the leaning, circling, and head tilt are all directed away from the side of the lesion.

BOVINE VIRAL DIARRHEA VIRUS

Transplacental infection of calves with bovine viral diarrhea (BVD) virus between 120 and 160 days of gestation frequently results in cerebellar hypoplasia. This is the most common cause of cerebellar disease in cattle in North America. In the bovine species, maximal cerebellar growth occurs between 133 and 162 days of gestation. During this period, the cerebellum is vulnerable to cellular destruction by viruses. The BVD virus disrupts the development of germinal cells of the cerebellum, resulting in Purkinje neuron and granule cell degeneration prior to birth. Destruction of this external germinal layer results in a grossly small, often cavitated, cerebellum. The range of clinical signs with cerebellar hypoplasia ranges from recumbency with opisthotonus to mild hypermetria and ataxia with a slight head tremor. The degree of cerebellar dysfunction appreciated clinically does not always correlate with the damage to the cerebellum. Calves with only mild truncal ataxia may have virtually no remaining cerebellar tissue.

Most acute BVD virus infections in adult cattle are subclinical and frequently dams of affected calves are never noticed to be ill during the period that chronologically corresponds to fetal infection. Review of farm records may document a period of repeat breeding subsequent to the BVD viral infection. Both cytopathic and noncytopathic strains of BVD virus are capable of producing cerebellar hypoplasia and other congenital lesions. The presence of an ophthalmic lesion such as cataracts, microphthalmia, retinopathy with increased pigmentation, and iris defects in a calf with cerebellar signs heightens the index of suspicion of BVD virus–induced disease. Cerebellar hypoplasia is not a progressive condition and mildly to moderately affected calves may seem to improve as they adjust to their impairment. The decision whether to retain a mildly affected heifer calf as a potential herd member will depend not only on the degree of neurologic derangement but more importantly on whether the heifer is persistently infected with BVD virus. Persistent infection is the result of fetal infection with a noncytopathic strain of BVD virus between 40 and 125 days of gestation. The point at which the fetal calf becomes immunocompetent may be as late as 180 days of gestation and therefore the potential for overlap of susceptibility to cerebellar hypoplasia and persistent infection exists. A precolostrum blood sample can be submitted for serology and if antibodies are present, it can be assumed that the fetus was immunocompetent at the time of BVD virus infection. If a precolostrum blood sample cannot be obtained, virus antigen identification can be used to identify virus in the buffy coat of a postcolostrum blood sample.

Appropriate measures should be undertaken if the appearance of calves with cerebellar hypoplasia is the first indication that a BVD problem exists. Vaccination may help to reduce the incidence of cerebellar hypoplasia. Cattle with adequate antibody titers acquired from natural disease or through vaccination did not produce affected calves when challenged with BVD virus at 150 days of gestation.

CEREBELLAR ABIOTROPHY

Cerebellar abiotrophy is the most common late-onset cerebellar disease in a variety of species, including cattle. First reported in 1975, cerebellar abiotrophy is a recessively inherited trait in Holstein cattle which becomes apparent at 3 to 8 months of age. The disease is characterized by a sudden onset of incoordination in a bright alert calf. These calves exhibit classic signs of cerebellar disease such as a spastic dysmetric gait, base-wide stance, loss of menace response, and occasional head tremor. Distinctive features of this condition are the initial rapid progression of signs (affected animals become recumbent within a few days), a dorsomedial strabismus, and extension of the neck. At necropsy the cerebellum appears normal in size with no evidence of cavitation. Histologically, there is degeneration of cerebellar neurons but no evidence of inflammation.

STORAGE DISEASES

Storage diseases can also produce clinical signs indicative of cerebellar dysfunction. These metabolic disorders of the central nervous system are associated with the accumulation and storage of a substrate in the cytoplasm of neurons and other cells resulting from the deficiency of a specific lysosomal enzyme. The storage disease, named for the substrate that accumulates, is inherited as an autosomal recessive trait. GM_1 gangliosidosis and α- and β-mannosidosis are some of the storage diseases reported in cattle.

GM_1 gangliosidosis is described in Friesian cattle due to a 70% to 80% reduction in β-galactosidase activity and accumulation of a glycolipid. Clinical signs appear in the first few weeks of life and include unsteadiness, reluctance to move, and a stiff gait. The disease is often fatal before 1 year of age.

α-Mannosidosis is a recessive trait of Angus and Murray Grey cattle due to a deficiency of α-mannosidase and the resultant storage of an oligosaccharide that contains mannose and glucosamine. Clinical signs are evident at a few weeks to a few months of age and include ataxia, head tremor, aggression, and failure to thrive. Prolonged ingestion of large quantities of plants from the genus *Swainsona* can cause an acquired form of α-mannosidosis in sheep and other livestock due to an alkaloid in the plant that inhibits α-mannosidase.

β-Mannosidosis is an autosomal recessive trait of Saler cattle due to a deficiency in β-mannosidase, resulting in the accumulation of an oligosaccharide in neurons. All 12 calves in a 1991 report were recumbent at birth and unable to stand even with assistance. Calves had a domed calvarium, narrow palpebral fissures, intention tremors, and wide head excursions. Gross lesions included dilated lateral ventricles, loss of cerebral and cerebellar white matter, and bilateral renomegaly.

BIBLIOGRAPHY

Abbit B, Jones MZ, Kasari TR, et al: Beta-mannosidosis in twelve Saler calves. J Am Vet Med Assoc 198:109–113, 1991.

de Lahunta A: Veterinary Neuroanatomy and Clinical Neurology, ed 2. Philadelphia, WB Saunders, 1983.

Leipold HW, Dennis SM: Congenital defects of the bovine central nervous system. Vet Clin North Am Food Anim Pract 3:159–177, 1987.

Mayhew IG: Large Animal Neurology: A Handbook for Veterinary Clinicians. Philadelphia, Lea & Febiger, 1989.

Rebhun WC: Diseases of Dairy Cattle, Media, Pa, Williams & Wilkins, 1985.

Riond JL, Cullen JM, Godfrey VL, et al: Bovine viral diarrhea virus-induced cerebellar disease in a calf. J Am Vet Med Assoc 197:1631–1637, 1990.

Scott FW, Kahrs RF, de Lahunta A, et al: Virus induced congenital anomalies of the bovine fetus. I. Cerebellar degeneration (hypoplasia), ocular lesions and fetal mummification following experimental infection with bovine viral diarrhea-mucosal disease virus. Cornell Vet 63:536–560, 1973.

White ME, Whitlock RH, de Lahunta A: A cerebellar abiotrophy of calves. Cornell Vet 65:476–491, 1975.

Wilson TM, de Lahunta A, Confer L: Cerebellar degeneration in dairy calves: Clinical, pathologic, and serologic features of an epizootic caused by bovine viral diarrhea virus. J Am Vet Med Assoc 183:544–547, 1983.

■ Spinal Cord Diseases

Raymond W. Sweeney, V.M.D.

Bovine patients with spinal cord lesions may present with motor or proprioceptive deficits manifesting as ataxia, paresis or paralysis, abnormal posture, hyporeflexia, or muscle atrophy. The specific clinical signs will depend on the particular segment of spinal cord affected. A complete neurologic examination, as described earlier in this section, should enable the clinician to localize the lesion and determine if a focal, multifocal, or diffuse lesion is suspected. Once the anatomic location of the lesion is discerned, a differential diagnosis can be established and prioritized on the basis of signalment, history, and progression of signs. Because of the poor prognosis associated with most causes of spinal cord disease in cattle, once the determination has been made that a spinal cord lesion exists, often the economic value of the individual patient does not warrant the expense of additional diagnostic testing to establish the etiologic diagnosis. In those cases, postmortem examination should be recommended to ensure that a potential herd problem (e.g., nutritional pathologic fracture) does not exist.

A number of conditions that do not involve spinal cord lesions can be difficult to distinguish from spinal cord disease owing to similarity in clinical signs. For example, cows with rabies will often present initially with clinical signs compatible with a caudal spinal cord lesion, manifested as posterior limb paresis or paralysis, which within a few days progress to signs more typical of encephalitis. Profound weakness caused by neuromuscular paralysis (botulism or hypokalemia), muscle weakness (nutritional myodystrophy), or musculoskeletal injury (coxofemoral luxation, femoral neck fracture) may be quite difficult to distinguish from that caused by spinal cord disease, especially in the recumbent patient. Peripheral nerve injuries may also be difficult to distinguish from spinal cord lesions, especially in cases of bilateral nerve injury, as may occur in calves with femoral nerve palsy following dystocia, or in cases of maternal obstetric paralysis. Signalment, history, and ancillary tests such as radiographs or cerebrospinal fluid (CSF) analysis may assist the clinician in making the distinction between peripheral nerve and spinal cord lesions.

TRAUMA

Spinal cord trauma should always be suspected in cases in which neurologic examination results suggest a focal spinal cord lesion. Typically, there is an acute onset of signs, with minimal exacerbation of signs after 24 hours following the injury. Spinal cord injuries are not common in cattle, but may occur following handling of the animals in a chute, or in heifers that have been mounted by other cattle while in estrus. Spinal cord compression may result from pressure applied by hemorrhage within the spinal canal, or by direct compression from vertebral fracture fragments. Pathologic vertebral fractures, secondary to nutritional osteopenia, should be suspected in calves presented with an acute onset of paralysis. Typically, this occurs in weaned calves less than 1 year of age whose diet is inadequate in calcium or, occasionally, vitamin D. Multiple animals are often affected. Compression fractures of the thoracic or lumbar vertebrae result in paraplegia. Many calves will also have pathologic fractures of long bones or ribs, and palpation of the caudal ribs will reveal greater than normal elasticity, suggestive of osteopenia.

In addition to the neurologic examination, palpation of the vertebrae (externally and per rectum) or overlying soft tissue may reveal evidence of trauma, such as swelling, asymmetry, or pain elicited on palpation. In young stock, radiographs of the spine may be diagnostic, but in adult cattle often only the cervical vertebrae may be imaged well. In cases of pathologic fractures, radiographs may reveal generalized reduced mineralization of bone, and thin cortices of the long bone diaphysis. CSF analysis may reveal a higher than normal red blood cell count, depending on the location of the lesion and the site from which the CSF is collected. The CSF may have a xanthochromic discoloration beginning approximately 24 hours after the injury. In cases of potential pathologic fracture, ration analysis should be performed to determine dietary intake of essential minerals and vitamin D.

The prognosis for cattle with spinal cord trauma is guarded. Those animals with contusions of the spinal cord without vertebral fractures may be expected to recover if they are able to stand. However, cattle that are unable to stand, or those that have spinal cord compression associated with a vertebral fracture, have a poor prognosis. Calves with pathologic vertebral fractures secondary to nutritional osteopenia have a hopeless prognosis.

The aim of treatment is to reduce compression of the spinal cord associated with hemorrhage or edema in the spinal canal. To that end, dexamethasone 0.2 mg/kg of body weight, intravenously (IV) or intramuscularly (IM) once or twice daily, and dimethyl sulfoxide (DMSO), 1 mg/kg diluted in 5% dextrose or 0.9% saline to a 30% DMSO solution, are recommended, although guidelines for extra-label use of these compounds should be followed. Nonsteroidal anti-inflammatory agents may be administered if analgesia is required. Appropriate nursing care for recumbent animals is necessary to prevent secondary problems such as decubitus and muscle ischemic damage.

VERTEBRAL OSTEOMYELITIS

Vertebral body osteomyelitis or spinal cord abscesses usually occur by spread of bacteria to vertebrae hematogenously. Chronic infections, such as pneumonia, in other sites of the body may serve as the source of bacterial organisms, but occasionally no such site can be found in cattle presented with this lesion. Most commonly, *Actinomyces pyogenes* is the bacterium isolated from these lesions. Affected animals are usually young (<3 years old). Signs of spinal cord disease may result from extension of the infection into the spinal canal, leading to meningitis, or from compression of the spinal cord by vertebral fragments following pathologic fracture of the infected vertebra. Onset of signs may be gradual in the case of meningitis, or rapid when fracture results in acute cord compression. Clinical signs are compatible with a focal spinal cord lesion, with the specific deficits depending on the location of the lesion. In my experience, thoracolumbar lesions are most common, resulting in paraplegia. Additionally, animals with vertebral osteomyelitis often exhibit marked stiffness or reluctance to flex the spine, walk, or to lower the head to graze.

In many cases, radiographs of the spine will exhibit findings characteristic of osteomyelitis such as osteolysis, osteoproliferation, and pathologic fracture. Lesions of the lumbar vertebrae in larger cattle may not be apparent. Although nuclear scintigraphy has the potential to be a useful diagnostic aid for this condition, use of radionuclides in cattle may obviate their future use as food-producing animals. Elevation of the plasma fibrinogen concentration above normal is supportive evidence for vertebral osteomyelitis. If infection has extended into the subarachnoid space, results of CSF analysis will show evidence of inflammation such as neutrophilic pleocytosis and high protein concentration. However, often CSF is normal, as the meninges are not penetrated.

Treatment may be attempted with antimicrobials (e.g., penicillin 22,000 IU/kg, IM), but is usually unsuccessful once neurologic signs are manifested. Prolonged treatment (at least 4 weeks) is recommended.

NEOPLASIA

Lymphosarcoma is the most common form of spinal neoplasia found in cattle. Spinal lymphosarcoma is a form of enzootic bovine lymphosarcoma caused by infection with the bovine leukosis virus (BLV). Knowledge of the herd's BLV status may arouse the clinician's suspicion of lymphosarcoma. Tumors are usually extradural within the spinal canal, and are most frequently located in the lumbar or sacral area, resulting in hind limb paresis. As with other forms of lymphosarcoma, older cattle (>4 years of age) are usually affected. Neurofibromas occur rarely in cattle, but may be clinically indistinguishable from lymphosarcoma. These may compress the spinal cord or the peripheral nerve roots.

The onset of neurologic signs is usually gradual over a 1- to 2-week period, but occasionally the onset may be acute. Affected cattle will show clinical signs compatible with a focal spinal cord lesion, usually referable to a lumbar or sacral lesion. Generally, the neurologic signs are indistinguishable from those caused by trauma or vertebral osteomyelitis. However, neurologic signs are usually not progressive in cases of trauma, whereas lymphosarcoma usually results in continued progression of signs after initial detection. Careful physical examination may reveal additional evidence of enzootic lymphosarcoma. Lymphadenopathy is detected in approximately 70% of affected cattle. Other sites of the body (heart, abomasum, uterus) may be infiltrated with tumor, but often cows with spinal cord lymphosarcoma do not have tumors at the other common sites.

Laboratory confirmation of the diagnosis is often not straightforward. Because lymphosarcoma tumor masses are extradural, finding neoplastic lymphocytes on cytologic evaluation of CSF is rare. Occasionally, neoplastic cells may be found if the spinal needle passes directly through the tumor mass when lumbosacral puncture is performed. A positive agar gel immunodiffusion (AGID) test result for antibodies to BLV provides evidence that the cow is infected with the BLV and could have lymphosarcoma, but it does not confirm the diagnosis, as most infected cows never develop lymphosarcoma. Similarly, finding persistent lymphocytosis only provides evidence that the cow is infected with BLV, not that lymphosarcoma is present. Finding other clinical signs compatible with lymphosarcoma, such as lymphadenopathy, pyloric obstruction or abomasal ulceration, heart failure, and so forth would strengthen the diagnosis. If peripheral lymph nodes are involved, cytologic evaluation of a needle aspirate, or histopathologic examination of a biopsy specimen, may confirm the diagnosis. However, even when other supporting evidence is lacking, posterior paralysis in an adult cow older than 4 years of age with no history of trauma is highly suggestive of lymphosarcoma.

Long-term success following treatment of bovine spinal lymphosarcoma has not been reported. Temporary palliation of signs can be achieved in some cases by administration of dexamethasone or, as reported in one case, L-asparaginase. This may permit recovery of genetic potential through superovulation and embryo transfer, or recovery of ova for in vitro fertilization.

PARASITIC DISEASE

Spinal cord disease associated with parasite migration in cattle is caused by larvae of *Hypoderma bovis* (warble flies). Larvae burrow through the skin, migrate to the spinal canal, and lie dormant in the epidural fat for several months. Under normal circumstances, this does not result in neurologic disease. However, if the larvae are killed (e.g., by systemic administration of an organophosphate), the host mounts an inflammatory response to the dead larvae, causing edema and inflammation that results in spinal cord disease.

In North America, the disease is usually seen between July and October, when *H. bovis* typically inhabits the epidural space. The history usually includes an acute onset of neurologic signs 24 to 72 hours after administration of a grub treatment containing organophosphates. Although all four limbs may be affected, more commonly just the hind limbs are affected because of a predilection of the larvae for the lumbosacral region. Clinical signs include ataxia, weakness, and altered reflexes in affected limbs. Clinical signs must be distinguished from those of toxicosis caused by the organophosphate. For example, pour-on chlorpyrifos treatment of bulls has resulted in signs of depression, weakness, and muscle fasciculations 2 to 7 days after treatment that could be mistaken for cerebrospinal nematodiasis.

Treatment with dexamethasone 0.1 to 0.2 mg/kg IV, once or twice daily, may ameliorate the inflammatory response to dying grub larvae. The disease may be prevented by appropriate timing of systemic organophosphate grub treatments to precede the migration of the larvae into the epidural space (i.e., July in North America).

CONGENITAL AND HEREDITARY CONDITIONS

Congenital spinal cord disease is rare in cattle. Occipitoatlantoaxial malformation is a congenital deformation of the cranial cervical spinal column, resulting in progressive tetraplegia in newborn calves. Spina bifida and hemivertebra are vertebral malformations that are usually apparent at birth. Although affected animals may be asymptomatic, often paraplegia or tetraplegia develops. Weaver syndrome is a hereditary progressive degenerative disease of Brown Swiss cattle. Neurologic signs usually develop by 6 months of age, consisting of ataxia, proprioceptive deficits, and eventually recumbency. The prognosis for these and other congenital conditions is poor. When the condition is potentially inherited, as with Weaver syndrome, the diagnosis should be confirmed by postmortem examination.

MISCELLANEOUS CONDITIONS

Cattle are more resistant to the toxin produced by *Clostridium tetani* than horses, but because tetanus prophylaxis is less common in cattle, occasionally cattle will be affected with this disease. Tetanus results when *C. tetani* organisms proliferate in an anaerobic site within the animal and elaborate toxin, which has its effect in the spinal cord. While infection of puncture wounds occurs, tetanus can also occur due to proliferation of organisms in the uterus (in association with postpartum metritis), or the intestinal tract or lesions induced by elastrator bands.

Following inoculation and proliferation under anaerobic conditions, *C. tetani* organisms elaborate at least two toxins. Tetanolysin causes local tissue necrosis and enhances local extension of the infection. Tetanospasmin is transported centripetally (via axons of motor neurons) to the spinal cord. The toxin inhibits the function of Renshaw cells (inhibitory neurons), resulting in uninhibited contraction of motor neurons and spasmodic tetany.

Clinical signs in cattle include bloat due to failure of eructation, rigid extension of the limbs, and tetany of facial muscles resulting in trismus, dysphagia, and retraction of the lips and ears. Signs are exacerbated when the animal is startled or excited. Untreated animals die of respiratory paralysis.

Treatment consists of administration of penicillin and surgical wound debridement to eliminate the *C. tetani* organisms. Administration of tetanus antitoxin 100 IU/kg, subcutaneously, may neutralize unbound toxin and halt progression of the disease. Intrathecal administration of equine-origin antitoxin should not be performed in cattle. Sedation may be required to prevent muscle spasms associated with excitement—promazine 0.5 mg/kg is especially useful for this purpose. Nursing care consists of providing a quiet, darkened stall, and provision for nutritional needs must be made. Water and alfalfa gruel can be force-fed by repeated ororuminal intubation. Alternatively, a temporary rumenostomy can be performed, alleviating bloat and providing access for direct intraruminal feeding.

Tetanus prophylaxis is not usually prescribed in cattle because of the low incidence of the disease. However, inoculation with tetanus toxoid may be recommended if individual farms have had multiple cases. Recovery from clinical tetanus is not associated with active immunity.

Spastic paresis (Elso heel) is a condition of unknown etiology. It affects Holstein, Angus, Hereford, Charolais, and other breeds of cattle. There is disagreement regarding the heritability of this condition. Spastic paresis is characterized by periodic spastic contraction of the gastrocnemius muscle, and usually is observed in young cattle less than 1 year of age. There may be unilateral or bilateral involvement. Typically, signs are seen only when the animal is standing. The hock will be extended in an uncontrolled fashion. The limb is held straight and thus the calf has difficulty advancing the limb when walking. The proximal portion of the tail is often held in an elevated position. Untreated, the disease will usually progress. Surgical interruption of the tibial nerve fibers supplying the gastrocnemius muscle is often successful, although the advisability of introducing these animals to the breeding herd has been questioned in light of the possible heritability of this condition.

Spastic syndrome, or periodic spasticity ("barn cramps"), is seen primarily in adult dairy cattle older than 3 years of age. The syndrome is characterized by episodic muscle spasms of one of the hind limbs. The leg is lifted and held in flexion, accompanied by muscle tremors. Episodes usually last for a few seconds up to 1 minute. Initially the episodes are mild and do not interfere with production, but they may progress over 2 to 3 years to become a dehabilitating condition. Although the onset of the disease is later in life, the condition is inherited as an autosomal recessive trait.

Ankylosing spondylitis is a degenerative intervertebral arthritis of Holstein bulls. Bridging ossification of the ventral ligaments of the lumbar vertebrae results in a stiff or stilted gait. Spinal cord compression does not occur in all cases, but if it occurs will result in progressive hind limb ataxia and paresis. Nonsteroidal anti-inflammatory drugs may alleviate the early clinical signs associated with lumbar pain, but there is no successful treatment available once neurologic signs develop.

BIBLIOGRAPHY

George, LW: Disorders of the nervous system. *In* Smith BP (ed): Large Animal Internal Medicine, ed 2. St Louis, Mosby–Year Book, 1996, pp 1001–1174.

Mayhew IG: Large Animal Neurology: A Handbook for Veterinary Clinicians. Philadelphia, Lea & Febiger, 1989.

Rebhun WC, deLahunta A, Baum KH, et al: Compressive neoplasms of the bovine spinal cord. Compendium Continuing Educ Pract Vet 6:S396–S400, 1984.

Sherman DM, Ames TR: Vertebral abscesses in cattle: A review of five cases. J Am Vet Med Assoc 188:608–611, 1986.

▪ Diseases of the Peripheral Nervous System

Simon Peek, B.V.Sc., M.R.C.V.S., Diplomate, A.C.V.I.M.

The majority of peripheral nerve disorders in ruminants are traumatic in origin, although inflammatory and neoplastic lesions are occasionally encountered. Peripheral nerve dysfunction in cattle may also accompany myopathy secondary to recumbency due to metabolic disease or poor footing. A myriad of potential traumatic causes exist but some of the more common ones are dystocia associated with parturition, mechanical damage during handling, and improper injection techniques. It is important to educate lay personnel with respect to correct injection technique and the risks associated with the overzealous use of force during dystocia if peripheral nerve injuries are to be avoided. Farmers and lay personnel should also be informed of the risks of ill-fitting devices for head restraint, prolonged recumbency on poorly padded tilt tables or concrete flooring, and the overaggressive use of hydraulic chutes in an effort to minimize traumatic injuries causing peripheral nerve damage.

The peripheral nerves of the thoracic and pelvic limbs are individually discussed here alongside a detailed explanation of the specific signs associated with the dysfunction of each nerve.

SUPRASCAPULAR NERVE INJURY

The suprascapular nerve provides motor innervation to the supraspinatus and infraspinatus muscles. The nerve winds distally around the head of the scapula and is most susceptible to trauma at this site. Damage to the suprascapular nerve can occasionally be seen following blunt injury to this region in cattle chutes or following the subcutaneous injection of irritating compounds in the caudal cervical region.

Suprascapular nerve paralysis causes loss of motor innervation to the scapular musculature and leads to limb abduction at rest and circumduction of the affected limb during protraction. Affected cattle will have a shortened stride and an abnormal posture in the acute phase but should the nerve damage be permanent, characteristic neurogenic infraspinatus and supraspinatus muscle atrophy will occur over the following months, giving rise to the condition known as "sweeney."

RADIAL NERVE INJURY

The radial nerve provides motor innervation to the extensor muscles of the forelimb and is particularly susceptible to injury as it courses close to the skin surface over the lateral aspect of the elbow joint. Damage to this nerve is most commonly seen following prolonged lateral recumbency from anesthesia or on tilt tables for foot trimming. Direct trauma to the nerve or damage associated with humeral fractures is also possible.

Radial nerve injury and associated loss of forelimb extensor function typically lead to the animal's being unable to bear weight on the affected limb and the toe being dragged. The toe is knuckled over at rest and the limb cannot be protracted properly. The elbow may be carried lower than in the opposite limb. On the rare occasions when the nerve is damaged distal to the elbow joint, the elbow may not be significantly "dropped" and partial weight bearing may be possible if the distal limb is extended. In chronic cases extensor muscle atrophy and significant soft tissue abrasions on the dorsum of the pastern and fetlock are potential complications.

BRACHIAL PLEXUS INJURY

Brachial plexus injuries are most commonly encountered following excessive traction on the forelimbs of a neonate during parturition. Severe soft tissue shoulder injuries or deep soft tissue lacerations of the axilla may also cause brachial plexus injury in animals of any age.

The clinical signs of brachial plexus injury reflect a complete inability to support weight on the affected limb. The elbow will be dropped to an even lower position than that typically seen with radial nerve paralysis and the animal will be completely unable to protract the affected limb. Affected animals may attempt to compensate for the lack of support in the forequarters by standing with the hind limbs in a more cranial position.

FEMORAL NERVE INJURY

The femoral nerve is most commonly injured following overextension of the coxofemoral or stifle joints. Excessive traction on a posteriorly presented fetus with the stifles in a locked position is probably the most common cause of traumatic femoral nerve injury. The nerve is rarely injured by external blows to the limb, but femoral nerve paralysis can occasionally be seen in down cows that have repeatedly struggled to rise on slippery surfaces or that are suffering from compartment syndrome.

The femoral nerve innervates the principal extensors of the stifle and flexors of the hip such that femoral nerve paralysis is associated with an inability to support weight on the affected limb. In cases of unilateral nerve injury the stifle of the affected limb is flexed, as are all distal limb joints, due to a loss of normal stay apparatus function. However femoral nerve injury does not cause the toe to knuckle over onto the dorsum of the digit, as would be seen with peroneal nerve paralysis. The affected limb is unable to bear weight and cannot be advanced normally. Complete bilateral femoral nerve paralysis results in recumbency and accordingly carries a poor prognosis in both adult cattle and newborn calves. Occasionally, partial bilateral femoral nerve paralysis is seen in down cows. The affected animal will struggle to rise with all the hind limb joints in a continuously flexed position, creating a creeping posture. Femoral nerve paralysis of greater than 2 weeks' duration will be accompanied by significant quadriceps femoris muscle atrophy.

SCIATIC NERVE INJURY

The sciatic nerve and its terminal branches, the tibial and peroneal nerves, are the most commonly injured peripheral nerves of the hind limb. Proximal sciatic nerve damage can occasionally result from pelvic and femoral injuries but is more commonly seen following iatrogenic injury due to poor injection technique or the intramuscular administration of irritating compounds in the gluteal region of calves and small ruminants. Iatrogenic sciatic nerve damage can also result from injections that are directed too laterally into the biceps femoris muscle. Excessive traction of an oversized or malpresented fetus can result in intrapelvic damage to the sciatic nerve and is a significant cause of calving paralysis in postparturient cattle.

The sciatic nerve innervates the extensors of the hip and flexor muscles of the stifle as well as all the distal limb musculature. Sciatic nerve paralysis is therefore associated with a dropped hip, stifle, and hock. The stifle is extended and the fetlock knuckles over dorsally, but the limb is usually able to bear partial weight because of the reciprocal apparatus. Complete sciatic nerve paralysis causes constant knuckling onto the dorsum of the digit but this may not be seen with partial paralysis. Chronic sciatic nerve paralysis is associated with neurogenic atrophy of the caudal thigh and all muscles distal to the stifle.

TIBIAL NERVE INJURY

The sciatic nerve branches into the tibial and peroneal nerves at the level of the distal third of the femur. Injury to the tibial nerve is rarer than injury to the peroneal nerve, but may follow the injection of irritant compounds into the caudal thigh close to the stifle joint. Occasionally tibial nerve deficits are observed in recumbent or downer cattle. Traumatic tibial nerve injury has also been reported in small ruminants following dog attacks.

The tibial nerve supplies motor innervation to the flexors of the digit and extensors of the hock, and paralysis is associated with overflexion of the hock, knuckling of the fetlock, and an asymmetric appearance to the pelvis with the affected side held lower than normal. The limb can usually bear weight and the toe is not knuckled as with peroneal and complete sciatic nerve paralysis. Neurogenic atrophy of the gastrocnemius muscle is a feature of chronic tibial nerve damage. Complete or partial rupture of the gastrocnemius muscle or tendon can produce clinical signs similar to those seen with tibial nerve paralysis. Recumbent cattle that make repeated efforts to stand on slippery surfaces are also at risk of traumatic gastrocnemius muscle injury. Gastrocnemius rupture will also produce an overflexed hock and may be associated with extreme difficulty in rising, particularly if the condition is bilateral. The two conditions can be easily differentiated by palpation of the gastrocnemius muscle and tendon proximal to the point of the hock.

Spastic paresis is a progressive muscular disorder that is associated with periodic spasticity of the gastrocnemius muscle and digital extensors of the hind limbs. Although its cause is uncertain, some cases can be alleviated by tibial neurectomy. Various theories of the etiology and pathogenesis of the condition include demyelination of the red nucleus in the midbrain, reduced neurotransmitter concentrations in the central nervous system (CNS), and overstimulation of spinal gamma motor neurons. The condition is sometimes referred to as Elso heel in Holstein calves. Affected calves usually begin to show signs between 2 and 12 months of age, and the condition is characterized by intermittent extensor tonus of the gastrocnemius muscle in particular. In the early stages of the disease the animal will appear normal while recumbent, but the exaggerated extensor tone becomes evident when the animal stands. The affected limb is held in extension behind the body with only the toes touching the ground. During protraction the extended limb is widely circumducted, giving a pendulum-like appearance to the gait. The condition is progressive and affected animals are usually culled because of increasing discomfort and difficulty in rising. Surgical procedures for the correction of the condition by either tibial neurectomy or a combination of gastrocnemius and superficial digital tenotomy are described.

PERONEAL NERVE INJURY

The peroneal nerve is most susceptible to traumatic injury as it courses superficially over the lateral aspect of the proximal fibula. Peroneal nerve deficits are an unfortunate but common sequela to recumbency in down cattle.

The peroneal nerve innervates the flexors of the hock and extensors of the digit such that damage to this nerve results in hyperextension of the hock and flexion of the fetlock and pastern. The straightened hock will make the limb appear stiff during protraction. Typically the limb is knuckled over onto the dorsum, even at rest. Incomplete paralysis may allow the animal to stand with the foot positioned normally at rest, but the fetlock should characteristically knuckle when the limb is advanced.

OBTURATOR NERVE INJURY

Historically, obturator nerve injury has been incriminated as the major cause of unilateral or bilateral adductor dysfunction in the postparturient cow. However, experimental evidence seems to suggest that this so-called calving paralysis is more commonly the result of combined obturator and intrapelvic

sciatic nerve injury, particularly when the loss of adductor function is accompanied by knuckling of the distal hind limb joints. Anatomic differences in the relative size of the pelvic bones between species makes obturator nerve injury rare except in cattle. The obturator nerve is susceptible to damage as it courses along the medial aspect of the ilium, and paralysis is a potential complication of dystocia, especially in first-calf heifers. The sixth lumbar spinal nerve, which contributes to the sciatic nerve, is also susceptible to injury as it runs ventral to the prominent sacral ridge. Injudicious use of force to deliver an oversized or malpresented fetus is an unfortunate but rather common cause of obturator and intrapelvic sciatic nerve injury in cattle.

Experimentally, it has been shown that given decent footing, cattle may retain their ability to stand and ambulate even if both obturator nerves are severed. The gait is only mildly affected following bilateral injury of this type, with affected animals developing a hopping gait. Adductor function is maintained provided the animal is not placed on a slippery surface. However, combined obturator and sciatic nerve damage results in more severe clinical signs. If the nerve damage is bilateral the cow will be unable to rise and may sit in a froglike position with the hind limbs simultaneously flexed and abducted. Unilateral damage to these nerves results in impaired limb adduction and knuckling of the distal limb joints as described for proximal sciatic nerve paralysis. Cattle may still be able to rise following unilateral injury if good footing and assistance are provided. Unfortunately cattle with obturator and/or sciatic nerve damage are at greater risk of life-threatening musculoskeletal injuries such as femoral neck or shaft fractures, coxofemoral luxations, and severe hind limb myopathy should they repeatedly struggle to rise on slippery surfaces. The potential for secondary compartment syndrome will also increase with the duration of recumbency and the weight of the affected animal.

OTHER PERIPHERAL NERVE INJURIES

Although traumatic forelimb or hind limb peripheral nerve injury is the most common form of peripheral neuropathy encountered in ruminants, veterinarians may occasionally observe neurologic deficits associated with injury to other peripheral nerves.

Peripheral facial nerve injury is occasionally encountered in cattle and small ruminants. Iatrogenic damage from poorly fitted halters, particularly those with metal rings that apply pressure to the facial nerve branches on the caudodorsal aspect of the mandibular ramus, can result in facial nerve paresis. Appropriate padding and loosely fitting halters should be used when animals are restrained on tilt tables or in lateral recumbency for any significant period of time, to prevent facial nerve injury on the down side. The clinical signs of facial nerve paresis include ptosis, lack of menace response on the affected side, ear droop, and an ipsilateral loss of lip tone. In small ruminants the nasal philtrum will be deviated away from the affected side.

Facial nerve deficits can also be seen as a complication of otitis media or interna in calves and small ruminants. Upper respiratory tract infections with organisms such as *Pasteurella* spp., *Haemophilus somnus*, and *Pseudomonas* spp. that extend into the middle ear are particularly common in young calves and feedlot-reared lambs and may be seen to affect individual animals or several animals simultaneously. Facial nerve dysfunction with asymmetric ptosis, drooped ear, and flaccid lips and nostrils is commonly seen. Central vestibular signs with conscious proprioceptive deficits will be absent unless the suppurative process extends into the cranium. Treatment of uncomplicated otitis media or interna with oxytetracycline or penicillin will frequently result in resolution of the facial nerve deficit.

Specific bilateral auriculopalpebral nerve dysfunction has also occasionally been observed in dairy cattle that are restrained in stanchions. If an animal is startled and makes a sudden movement backward, the head can become lodged within the device just caudal to the orbit, thereby applying severe pressure to the auriculopalpebral nerve in the region of the zygomatic arch. The clinical signs of auriculopalpebral nerve injury reflect a loss of motor function to the orbicularis oculae muscles and the muscles of the ear. The palpebral response will be absent, the ears will be drooped, and the animal may be observed to tear excessively. Although it is unlikely that sufficient force will be generated to cause an orbital or zygomatic fracture, cattle may be transiently off their feed due to generalized pain in the area of the temperomandibular joint. Discomfort during palpation and soft tissue swelling in the affected area often assist in making the diagnosis.

PERIPHERAL NERVE INJURY AND THE DOWNER COW

It is of particular importance to consider peripheral nerve injuries as a complication of prolonged recumbency in the downer cow syndrome. Large animal practitioners are only too aware of the frustrations and economic losses that can accompany recumbency of even relatively short duration in adult cattle, and although the continued inability of a downer cow to rise may be due to a number of causes, peripheral nerve dysfunction can undoubtedly contribute to the problem. Experimentally it has been shown that recumbency of even a few hours' duration can be associated with significant myopathy in cattle. Reported values for overall survival rates for downer cows vary widely among authors but there is a consensus that survival rates drop dramatically the longer the animal is down. Although antecedent peripheral nerve damage, particularly following dystocia, may occasionally be directly responsible for a cow being unable to rise, most peripheral nerve deficits in downer cows develop secondary to extensive muscle and soft tissue damage due to prolonged recumbency. Metabolic, endotoxic, and musculoskeletal conditions can result in recumbency and significant secondary muscle and nerve damage. Sciatic and peroneal nerve deficits are particularly common in recumbent cattle, in part because of their anatomic location. Ischemic damage to the caudal and lateral thigh musculature in downer cows can implicate sciatic and peroneal nerve branches and add varying degrees of hind limb paresis to an already challenging clinical picture. There are a number of devices that are available to assist downer cows to stand, but hoisting adult cattle is physically and technically challenging and a time-consuming task. Hip slings, hip clamps, inflatable bags, and mobile flotation tanks are all available, but no single technique is without its drawbacks. Personal preference and the availability of help and the required equipment will dictate which approach is chosen, since there is no categorical research to validate any one technique over another. The value of immersion hydrotherapy for the treatment of severe musculoskeletal and neurologic conditions in other species would intuitively lead one to believe that flotation, if available, would be an excellent choice. Whatever technique is chosen, there is little doubt that early and aggressive assistance in standing and good-quality nursing care are very important if therapy is to stand a reasonable chance of success.

Although strictly speaking a neuromuscular disorder, it is worth considering botulism in the differential diagnosis of weakness and recumbency in adult cattle. In recent years the incidence of *Clostridium botulinum* type B toxicosis has increased in association with the feeding of contaminated silage to cattle, especially in the northeastern United States. Improperly ensiled or baled forages that never attain a pH of less than 4.5 are at particular risk of proliferation of *C. botulinum* type B and the resultant release of the toxin into the feed. Occasional outbreaks of botulism caused by *C. botulinum* type C have been seen in cattle following the incorporation of poultry litter into ensiled feedstuffs or the application of contaminated litter onto pasture. *C. botulinum* type A is more commonly seen in the western United States, and occasional cases of type D toxicosis have been reported in ruminants in association with ingestion of feed that is contaminated with carrion. Following ingestion and absorption the preformed toxin causes selective inhibition of acetylcholine release at peripheral nerve endings. Sensory peripheral nerves and the CNS appear to be spared the effects of the neurotoxin. The clinical signs are therefore those of diffuse neuromuscular weakness which can rapidly progress to recumbency. Dysphagia, tongue protrusion, and excessive salivation are also reported in a high percentage of cases. A definitive diagnosis can be reached by identification of the toxin in feed, serum, or intestinal contents. Treatment is largely supportive and should include specific antisera if permitted by the economic situation of the client. Antibiotics are probably not indicated in the treatment of botulism in ruminants unless the source of the infection is an obvious wound or secondary complications such as aspiration pneumonia develop. Antibiotics that might potentiate neuromuscular weakness, such as procaine penicillin, aminoglycosides, and oxytetracycline, should be avoided.

PERIPHERAL NERVE NEOPLASIA

Clinically relevant peripheral nerve neoplasms are rarely encountered in ruminant practice. It is more common to see peripheral nerve deficits as a complication of other primary or metastatic neoplasms that impinge on peripheral nerve branches. Although more common in a spinal location, lymphosarcoma can occasionally be associated with peripheral nerve deficits that will vary according to the nerve or nerves involved.

The most common primary neoplasm of nervous tissue origin in cattle is the schwannoma and it is usually seen in cattle greater than 5 years of age. This neoplasm can arise in both peripheral and spinal locations. Abbatoir surveys have reported on schwannomas involving the brachial plexus, cardiac nerves, intercostal nerves, cervical spinal nerve rootlets, visceral nerves to the abdomen and thorax, as well as the peripheral nerves to skeletal muscles. However, most accounts of clinically relevant schwannomas in older cattle relate to animals with caudal spinal cord involvement and resultant paraparesis. Current management practices make it unlikely that many beef or dairy animals will live long enough to develop these tumors. A putative hereditary neoplastic disorder involving cells of schwannian descent has also been reported in adult Holstein cattle. Affected cattle had multiple cutaneous nodules involving the skin of the head, neck, brisket, and thorax, but were otherwise clinically normal. The condition resembles cutaneous neurofibromatosis type 1 of humans, an autosomal dominant disorder.

BIBLIOGRAPHY

Ciszewski DK, Ames NK: Diseases of the peripheral nerves. Vet Clin North Am Food Anim Pract 3:193–312, 1987.

Cox VS: Peroneal nerve paralysis in a heifer. J Am Vet Med Assoc 167:142–143, 1975.

Cox VS, Breazile JE: Experimental bovine obturator paralysis. Vet Rec 93:109–110, 1973.

Cox VS, Breazile JE, Hoover TR: Surgical and anatomic study of calving paralysis. Am J Vet Res 36:427–430, 1975.

Cox VS: Understanding the downer cow syndrome. Compendium Continuing Educ Pract Vet 3:5472–5478, 1981.

Cox VS, McGrath CJ, Jorgensen SE: The role of pressure damage in pathogenesis of the downer cow syndrome. Am J Vet Res 43:26–31, 1982.

Cox VS, Marsh WE, Sterernagel GR, et al: Downer cow occurrence in Minnesota dairy herds. Prev Vet Med 4:249, 1982.

Divers TJ, Bartholomew RC, Messick JB, et al: *Clostridium botulinum* type B toxicosis in a herd of cattle and a group of mules. J Am Vet Med Assoc 188:382–386, 1986.

George LW: Peripheral nerve disorders. *In* Smith BP (ed): Large Animal Internal Medicine, ed 2. St. Louis, Mosby–Year Book, 1995.

Hallgren W: Studies of parturient paresis in dairy cows. Nord Vet Med 7:433, 1955.

Rebhun WC: Diseases of Dairy Cattle. Philadelphia, Lea & Febiger, 1995.

Rebhun WC, deLahunta A, Baum KH, et al: Compressive neoplasms affecting the bovine spinal cord. Compend Contin Educ Pract Vet 6:S396–400, 1984.

Sartin EA, Doran SE, Gatz Riddell M, et al: Characterization of naturally occurring cutaneous neurofibromatosis in Holstein cattle. Am J Pathol 145:1168–1174, 1994.

Smith BP, Angelos J, George LW, et al: Down cows and hot tubs. Proceedings of the 12th ACVIM Forum, American College of Veterinary Internal Medicine, San Francisco, 1994, pp 652–655.

Tryphonas L, Hamilton GF, Rhodes CS: Perinatal femoral nerve degeneration and neurogenic atrophy of quadriceps femoris muscle in calves. J Am Vet Med Assoc 164:801–807, 1974.

Vaughan LS: Peripheral nerve injuries: An experimental study in cattle. Vet Rec 76:1293–1301, 1964.

Musculoskeletal Diseases

Consulting Editor
Bruce L. Hull, D.V.M., M.S.

▪ Sole Abscesses

Bruce L. Hull, D.V.M., M.S.

A sole abscess is located between the sensitive laminae and the horny sole of the foot. The purulent exudate in these abscesses varies in color from pinkish-yellow to gray-brown and is usually under considerable pressure. Depending upon duration, a variable amount of the sole is undermined.

ETIOLOGY

Abscesses result from damage to the integrity of the sole. This damage may be caused by foreign bodies, puncture wounds, laminitis, white line separation, and cracks due to overgrown claws. As these breaks in the integrity of the sole are contaminated, they lead to bacterial growth beneath the sole.

CLINICAL SIGNS

The prime sign of a sole abscess is severe pain. This pain is often severe enough to cause the animal to be "three-legged lame." Owing to this lameness and its sudden onset, sole abscesses have often been confused with fractures. With sole abscesses, the animal is reluctant to bear weight on the affected toe. This will lead to a base-wide or base-narrow stance to relieve pressure on the involved toe. Because sole abscesses are most frequent in the lateral toe of the rear foot, the base-wide stance and gait of the animal can easily be confused with that of a stifle injury.

A simple sole abscess is usually not associated with any swelling or inflammation above the coronary band. However, later in the course of the disease a sole abscess may break out and drain at the coronary band. Any time a draining lesion is found at the coronary band, one should evaluate the PII-PIII joint for septic arthritis or osteomyelitis.

Hoof testers may be employed to evaluate pain over a given digit or even an area of a digit. Radiographic evaluation is not indicated and is often unrewarding in the diagnosis of a sole abscess.

Although the signs and symptoms as described may make one suspicious of a sole abscess, the diagnosis is dependent on a foot trim. The foot trim should include following out any black lines or puncture wounds that may be encountered. Although these may appear small and insignificant, they often lead to a large sole abscess.

TREATMENT

While following out the black lines or puncture wounds, dry lines will often become moist shortly before the abscess is opened. Opening the abscess will drain the pus, which is often under considerable pressure and may be accompanied by gas. Often there is a thin layer of new sole deep to the abscess. Because this new sole is thin and soft, care must be taken in removing the undermined sole so that the sensitive laminae are not exposed. All undermined sole should be removed. If undermined sole is left, inadequate drainage may occur due to occlusion by a pack of manure or mud, and the abscess may reform. The undermined sole is usually removed with a hoof knife or a hoof groover.

Although all undermined sole should be removed, the wall of the claw should be left intact to serve as a weight-bearing surface. This wall should be trimmed so that it extends only about 1 cm below the re-forming sole. A long wall promotes the accumulation of manure and mud over the pared-out abscess. After paring off the undermined sole, the foot may be wrapped with an antiseptic ointment. If the wrap becomes soaked with manure and urine, wrapping is undesirable. Consequently, it is probably preferable to leave the abscess open and treat it with a drying agent. It is usually best to clean this abscess area every day or two and apply a topical antifungal drying agent such as Koppertox (Fort Dodge Laboratories) for 7 to 10 days.

Following this treatment, there is usually dramatic relief from the lameness within 12 to 24 hours. The animal is usually back to normal and needs no further treatment after 7 to 10 days. If the lameness persists the diagnosis should be reevaluated or the lameness should be reexamined.

BIBLIOGRAPHY

Greenough PR, Weaver AD: Lameness in Cattle, ed 3, Philadelphia, WB Saunders, 1997.
White ME, Glickman TL, Embree IC, et al: A randomized trial for evaluation of bandaging sole abscesses in cattle. J Am Vet Med Assoc 178:375–377, 1981.

▪ Vertical Wall Cracks

Bruce L. Hull, D.V.M., M.S.

Vertical wall cracks, also called quarter cracks or sand cracks, are usually seen on the cranial aspect of the claws of the front feet. The lateral claw is involved more frequently than the medial claw. These cracks are a loss of continuity of the hoof wall. The cracks start at the coronary band and extend for a variable distance toward the wear surface.

ETIOLOGY

Vertical wall cracks are most common in the front feet of beef bulls. Dry weather and hoof brittleness are definitely involved in the pathogenesis. Excessive weight has also been identified as a causative factor in one study (Goonewardene and Hand). Occasionally, damage to the coronary band caused by an external trauma may initiate a vertical wall crack. Since overly dry or brittle hooves are the prime cause of vertical wall cracks, a higher incidence of the condition can be expected in the late summer or early fall.

CLINICAL SIGNS

Vertical wall cracks range in severity from partial-thickness cracks that are incidental findings, to deep cracks that become infected and lead to septic laminitis. The range in lesion severity is accompanied by a wide range of clinical signs, from a normally moving animal to an abnormally moving or even severely lame animal. In any animal having vertical wall cracks, hoof testers should be used to ascertain if the lameness is indeed caused by the cracks.

TREATMENT

If an animal with vertical wall cracks is not lame, one should not be too vigorous in treatment. Excessive grooving out of the cracks will expose the sensitive laminae and lead to lameness. A good foot trim with special emphasis on shortening the toes is indicated to help relieve abnormal stress on the hoof wall. Also, the hoof wall should be sealed (grease, tar, a drying agent [Koppertox, Fort Dodge Laboratories], or varnish) to help it retain moisture and become more pliable. Resealing is indicated periodically until the crack grows out.

In addition to these procedures, any lame animal should have the crack cleaned out and widened with a hoof groover. Often this treatment will reveal an abscess (septic laminitis). Abscesses are most prevalent distally and in some cases may extend into sole abscesses. If the abscess can be pared out nicely and leave a dry defect in the hoof wall, this defect can be filled with hoof acrylic. However, if the defect has draining tracts it should be kept open. In paring out vertical wall cracks, one should exercise caution. Excessive removal of the wall leads to severe granulation tissue, which protrudes through the defect in the hoof wall. Only remove enough wall to establish drainage.

When fissures extend from the coronary band to the wear surface, a wooden block should be applied to the normal digit with hoof acrylic. This block prevents excessive pull on the hoof wall as the cracks start to heal.

BIBLIOGRAPHY

Amstutz HE: Hoof wall fissures. Mod Vet Pract 59:906–908, 1978.
Goonewardene LA, Hand RK: A study of hoof cracks in grazing cows—Association with age, weight and fatness. Can J Anim Sci 75:25–29, 1995.
Greenough PR, Weaver AD: Lameness in Cattle, ed 3. Philadelphia, WB Saunders, 1997.
Petersen GC, Nelson DR: Foot diseases in cattle. Part 2. Diagnosis and treatment. Compendium Continuing Eds. Pract Vet 6:565–573, 1984.

■ Horizontal Wall Cracks
Bruce L. Hull, D.V.M., M.S.

Horizontal wall cracks have also been called "thimble toe." The loss of continuity of the hoof wall is parallel to the coronary band and extends around the circumference of the toe. The heel area is usually not involved or perhaps grows out before this is recognized as a clinical problem. The lesion usually affects all eight toes of an animal.

ETIOLOGY

Horizontal wall cracks usually follow a severe systemic infection that has been accompanied by an acute febrile response. This febrile episode causes imperfect horn growth at the coronary band that later splits or separates. This imperfect hoof does not usually separate until it nears the wear surface (2 to 3 cm from the coronary band) and begins to have stresses applied to it as the animal walks. Nutritional deficiencies and metabolic diseases are also considered to be a cause by some investigators. Once the split occurs, the distal shell of the hoof is attached only by the sensitive laminae. As the animal walks, this shell moves back and forth, thus pulling on the sensitive laminae and causing pain. In addition to the pulling on the sensitive laminae, dirt and manure may work into the cracks and cause a septic laminitis.

CLINICAL SIGNS

Before the split occurs, clinical signs are minimal. A small horizontal groove may be noted on the hoof, but the animal shows no pain. Once the split occurs, the animal becomes very sore and is often reluctant to move because walking causes the shell of the hoof to move and pull against the sensitive laminae. This stage may be accompanied by weight loss and a sudden drop in milk production.

TREATMENT

The treatment of choice is a foot trim. The trim should be accompanied by removal of any undermined wall to prevent dirt and debris from accumulating. In doing this, care should be taken to avoid injury to the sensitive laminae. Also, the toe should be "dubbed" as short as possible. This helps prevent the shell of the toe from rocking back and forth on the sensitive laminae as the animal walks. Although this treatment will alleviate pain, it usually takes 4 to 6 weeks for the new hoof wall to reach the wear surface and for the outer shell to fall off. Occasionally, another foot trim, as described, will be needed during this time.

BIBLIOGRAPHY

Amstutz HE: Hoofwall fissures. Mod Vet Pract 59:906–908, 1978.
Greenough PR, Weaver AD: Lameness in Cattle, ed 3. Philadelphia, WB Saunders, 1997.

▪ Rusterholz Ulcer

Bruce L. Hull, D.V.M., M.S.

A Rusterholz ulcer is a lesion at the junction of the sole and bulb that starts as a bruise, develops into a devitalized area, and later produces granulation tissue and even osteoarthritis. This lesion is usually located near the axial border of the involved toe and overlies the attachment of the flexor tendons. The ulcerated area is characterized by the presence of a mass of granulation tissue protruding through the sole. This granulation tissue is the result of the piston-like effect of PIII, forcing the sensitive laminae out through the defect in the sole. Rusterholz ulcers are most common in the lateral toes of the rear feet of mature animals, but, when the front foot is involved, it is usually the medial claw.

ETIOLOGY

Although Rusterholz ulcers may occur in pastured animals, they are more frequent in animals confined on concrete. Wet concrete appears to be associated with a higher incidence of Rusterholz ulcers. Chronic bruising is definitely associated with their pathogenesis. Although some workers think genetics or conformation may be involved, the prevailing theory today is that Rusterholz ulcers are secondary to laminitis (see Laminitis).

CLINICAL SIGNS

The lameness associated with Rusterholz ulcers is usually severe and sudden in onset. As this condition often involves the lateral toe of the rear foot, the animal usually walks and stands base-wide to relieve pressure on the lateral digit. Stanchioned animals will often stand back so that only the toe bears weight on the curb of the manure gutter.

Hoof testers will elicit pain when applied over the bulb-sole junction of the affected digit. As with sole abscesses, the final diagnosis must be made in conjunction with a foot trim. The foot trim may reveal granulation tissue, a crack in the sole, or merely a discolored area of the sole. As with a sole abscess, the crack or discolored area must be pared out to reveal the lesion. Although a true sole abscess is possible in this area (axial sole and wall junction), a Rusterholz ulcer characterized by its granulation tissue is usually found.

Untreated Rusterholz ulcers often lead to weakness and necrosis of the flexor tendon near its attachment to PIII. This weakening eventually (3 to 4 weeks) causes a rupture of the tendon attachment. When the tendon ruptures, the toe of the hoof suddenly tips upward owing to the absence of flexion of PIII.

TREATMENT

Treatment of a Rusterholz ulcer is time-consuming and frustrating. After paring out all of the undermined sole, one must gently probe the granulation tissue for fistulous tracts. These tracts, if found, must be explored for evidence of deep abscesses or osteomyelitis. The presence of deep tracts, especially in suspected cases of osteomyelitis, is reason for radiographic evaluation of the foot. If PII-PIII joint involvement is found, digit amputation is the most economical treatment, although drainage and facilitated ankylosis should be considered in valuable animals, as facilitated ankylosis prolongs the animal's useful life.

The granulation tissue that protrudes through the sole must be debrided to the level of the sole and cauterized to prevent excessive hemorrhage. The sole around the ulcer must be "feathered" so as to be thinner and more pliable near the ulcer and thicker away from the ulcer. This thinned sole near the ulcer allows it to give with the piston-like effect of PIII while healing is taking place.

Although bandaging the foot, or drying it, as is done with a sole abscess, may lead to a successful outcome, this is very tedious and time-consuming. It is certainly preferable to apply a wooden, rubber, or plastic block to the normal digit with hoof acrylic (Technovit, Jorgensen Laboratories). Alternatively, a plaster block and cast may be applied to the normal digit. In either case, this relieves pressure on the affected digit. Relief of pressure allows the animal a more pain-free recovery period, but more important, prevents the piston-like effect of PIII, which would lead to new granulation tissue. A block or cast also alleviates stretch on the flexor tendon, which may be weak.

Antiseptic dressings or drying agents such as Koppertox (Fort Dodge Laboratories) should be used in conjunction with elevation of the affected digit. Even with the help of a block, a Rusterholz ulcer will take at least 3 to 6 weeks to heal.

BIBLIOGRAPHY

Greenough PR, Weaver AD: Lameness in Cattle, ed 3. Philadelphia, WB Saunders, 1997.
Petersen GC, Nelson DR: Foot diseases in cattle. Part 2. Diagnosis and treatment. Compendium Continuing Educ Pract Vet 6:565–573, 1984.
Rebhun WC, Pearson EG: Clinical management of bovine foot problems. J Am Vet Med Assoc 181:572–577, 1982.

▪ Aseptic Laminitis of Cattle

Kent Hoblet, D.V.M., M.S., Diplomate, A.C.V.P.M.

The exact cause of aseptic laminitis in cattle is not fully understood. However, it is generally accepted that the active events involve a vascular disturbance in the dermis (corium) of the foot which is mediated by vasoactive substances such as histamine and endotoxin. As a result there is an interruption of nutrient supply and oxygen at the cellular level. The end result is the production of horn of inferior quality in the wall, sole, heel, and white line. In cattle, laminae only extend down the distal half of the hoof. Because there is involvement of the general corium, and not just the laminae, the term *pododermatitis aseptica diffusa* probably more correctly describes the condition than does the term *laminitis*.

FORMS OF ASEPTIC LAMINITIS (PODODERMATITIS ASEPTICA DIFFUSA)

Four broadly defined and generally overlapping forms of aseptic laminitis have been described: In the acute form, the animal exhibits lameness, pain, stiffness, arched back, and occasional recumbency. Redness of the coronary band and increased digital pulse are present. Affected cattle may stand with their front legs crossed or may continually shift their weight from foot to foot. Unlike laminitis in horses, the acute form is not common in cattle. It is most frequently associated with acute acidosis such as might result from grain overload. Occasionally it results from metabolic diseases, mastitis, metritis, or trauma. The subacute form is characterized as a milder form of acute aseptic laminitis. Subclinical laminitis was first described in 1979 by Peterse and subsequently by others. This form is characterized by the absence of overt lameness during the initial episode of vascular disturbance. Hooves must be examined to detect its presence. Even then, lesions in the hoof horn are not observed until several weeks or months after the inflammatory episode occurs in the pododerm. The chronic form develops as a result of the acute, subacute, or subclinical forms of the disease. Hooves typically become elongated, flattened, and widened. There are grooves or ridges in the dorsal hoof wall. If hooves are sufficiently affected to interfere with locomotion, affected cattle may lose condition.

HOOF HORN PRODUCTION

Hoof horn of the wall is produced in the coronary segment at the rate of approximately 5 mm/month varying somewhat with season, claw, and nutritional status. As the hoof wall grows downward it "slides" over the dermal laminae covering the distal one half of the third phalanx. An interruption in growth, such as might occur coincidental with systemic disease or a sudden change in diet, may result in a ridge or transverse groove ("hardship grove") on the hoof wall. By measuring the distance from the coronary segment to the hardship groove one can estimate when the disturbance occurred. The sole of the normal hoof is 8 to 10 mm thick. It is formed by papillae and typically reaches the weight-bearing surface 2 to 3 months after formation. Thus, hemorrhages resulting from an inflammatory episode in the corium will be observed in the surface of the sole 2 to 3 months after the inciting episode. Heel horn is also produced by papillae. In terms of horn hardness in descending order are the wall, sole, and heel. The white line consists of horn formed from three segments of the wall; namely cap horn, terminal horn, and horn leaflets. Horn leaflets are the hardest portion and are produced proximally in the coronary-wall transition region. Cap and terminal horn portions are relatively soft and pliable and constitute a filling substance that occupies the space between horn leaflets in the white line.

LESIONS

Lesions include yellow discoloration of the sole, hemorrhages of the sole, widening and separation of the white line, erosion of the heel, abscess of sole and white line, sole ulceration, sole overgrowth, inflamed coronary band, horizontal grooves in hoof horn, sunken or rotated distal phalanx, overgrowth of claws, and double sole. Hemorrhages range from those barely discernible ("paintbrush" hemorrhages) to ecchymotic hemorrhages of the sole and white line. In a 13-herd field study of first-lactation confined cattle examined during the first 100 days of lactation, it was found that the risk of hemorrhage was significantly greatest in the rear lateral claw. In that same study, 62% of all cattle had detectable hemorrhages of the sole. Hemorrhages of the sole have been observed in the claws of calves 2½ months of age. Separation of the white line in its mildest form has a striated appearance in which the softer, crumbly cap and terminal horn have fallen away with harder horn leaflets remaining as remnants. Separation of the white line permits impaction with debris and possible subsequent abscess formation in the sole and white line. The extent to which aseptic laminitis is involved in heel horn erosion is controversial. Some believe there is direct relationship, while others believe that the relationship is indirect, with poor-quality horn formation resulting in increased susceptibility to erosion by bacteria.

Sole ulcers are observed with greatest frequency in the rear lateral claw near the axial junction of the sole and heel. Often producers and veterinarians attribute sole ulcers primarily to trauma. However, because sole ulcers tend to occur in multiple feet of the same animal and because the highest incidence occurs within 4 months of calving, many believe that the majority of sole ulcers result from aseptic laminitis.

In the hind limb of normal cattle, the lateral claw tends to bear the greater proportion of weight. Laminitis results in overgrowth of the lateral sole of the hind limb with increased height of the lateral relative to the medial claw. The increased height results in the lateral claw bearing an even greater proportion of weight than it does normally and thus becoming even more susceptible to pathologic changes such as sole ulcers.

DIAGNOSIS

Diagnosis of acute and subacute forms may be made based on observation of clinical signs. Clinical lameness, together with characteristic changes in the hooves, forms the basis of diagnosis of the chronic form. In the subclinical form, removing 1 to 2 mm of sole horn is necessary to accurately check for lesions of the sole and white line. Examination of hooves of cattle representing various age categories and stages of lactation within a herd should be helpful in determining if a general herd problem exists.

RISK FACTORS

There is general consensus that causation of aseptic laminitis is multifactorial. Thus, the relative importance of a particular causative factor may be expected to differ from herd to herd. Risk factors considered important include the following:

Parturition. Periparturient stress, including dietary changes, hormonal changes, and the increased risk of acute systemic disease have all been implicated in the pathogenesis of aseptic laminitis. First-lactation cattle seem to be particularly at risk.

Nutrition. Implicated at one time or another have been excess energy, inadequate fiber, excess protein, and deficiency of certain minerals and animo acids.

Feeding Management. Factors which have been considered important have been the forage-to-concentrate ratio, particle length, effective fiber, number of feedings, relative time of feeding forage and concentrate, and whether feeds were fed separately or as part of a total mixed ration.

Environment. Cow comfort is important. The type of housing facilities, bedding materials, stocking density, floor surfaces, and manure management differ greatly among farms and may all be important. Movement of young cattle directly at calving from pasture to concrete without a period of adaptation has been shown to be a risk factor. Excessive standing or inadequate resting has also been implicated. Dry matter content of hooves and erosion of the heel have been shown to be related to cleanliness.

Other Factors. Foot and leg conformation, claw conformation, and claw angle have been mentioned as possible important animal or genetic factors related to the occurrence of aseptic laminitis. Improper foot trimming techniques may result in traumatic laminitis.

TREATMENT

Although data from research in cattle are lacking, judicious extra-label administration of flunixin meglumine 0.5 to 1.0 mg/lb intravenously or intramuscularly s.i.d., phenylbutazone 2 to 4 mg/lb orally every second day, and aspirin 50 mg/lb orally b.i.d. has been recommended during early stages of acute aseptic

laminitis. Moving acutely affected cattle to softer surfaces and "reloading" affected claws (e.g., lateral rear) by applying wood blocks to claws of the less affected side (e.g., medial rear) may be beneficial in early stages. Functional hoof trimming must be used in hooves with chronic changes to restore proper angles of the anterior wall (greater than 45 degrees) and toe length (approximately 75 mm or approximately 3 in. in Holstein cattle). Overgrowth of the lateral claw of the hind limb should be reduced to restore proper weight bearing and transfer weight to the hoof wall and sole adjacent to the wall.

PREVENTION

The relative importance of environment, feeding, and nutrition may be expected to differ from herd to herd. Therefore, although certain basic concepts should be universally adopted by producers, specific intervention strategies—that is, "fine-tuning"—will be expected to vary from herd to herd and should also include evaluation of the replacement heifer program. Reducing stress during the periparturient period, especially in first-calf heifers, is indicated. Special attention should be given to cow comfort and socialization. Clean and dry facilities should be maintained. Avoid acidosis. Research is unclear regarding the severity of acidosis required to trigger an episode of aseptic laminitis or the degree of interaction of nutrition and feeding management with environment or cow comfort. Clearly, there appear to be interactions. Cattle fed similarly but maintained under different environments and management schemes may be affected differently by aseptic laminitis. It must also be noted that most of the reports in the literature relating feeding management and nutrition to aseptic laminitis have resulted from studies conducted in Europe. How different feedstuffs and feeding strategies should be interpreted in light of North American conditions is unclear.

BIBLIOGRAPHY

Budras KD, Mulling C, Horowitz A: Rate of keratinization of the wall segment of the hoof and its relation to width and structure of the zona alba (white line) with respect to claw disease in cattle. Am J Vet Res 57:444–455, 1996.

Smilie RH, Hoblet KH, Weiss WP, et al: Prevalence of lesions associated with subclinical laminitis in first lactation cows from herds with high milk production. J Am Vet Med Assoc 208:1445–1451, 1996.

Toussaint Raven E: The principles of claw trimming. Vet Clin North Am Food Anim Pract 1:93–108, 1985.

■ Interdigital Phlegmon (Interdigital Necrobacillosis)

Aubrey N. Baird, D.V.M., M.S.

Interdigital phlegmon is the appropriate term for the condition commonly referred to as "foot rot." A partial list of synonyms used for interdigital phlegmon includes foot abscess, foot rot, foul-in-the-foot, infectious pododermatitis, interdigital necrobacillosis, and panaritium. The term *blind foul* is used by some to describe lameness typical of interdigital phlegmon without an interdigital skin lesion. Adding to the confusion is the overdiagnosis of interdigital phlegmon. Practitioners, and especially laypeople, tend to call any undiagnosed foot lameness interdigital phlegmon (or foot rot).

Terms defined at the Eighth International Symposium on Disorders of the Ruminant Digit and International Conference on Bovine Lameness in 1994 describe interdigital phlegmon as a highly infectious bacterial condition causing lameness and a necrotic lesion of the interdigital skin, usually with a split in the skin. Interdigital phlegmon is a painful condition that presents as an acute, severe lameness usually affecting one foot. The disease affects animals of any age but is primarily a disease of adults. As many as 25% to 40% of an entire herd may be affected over a period of months, but the incidence is usually lower.

No breed predilection for interdigital phlegmon has been positively identified. *Bos indicus* cattle are believed to be less susceptible to the condition than *Bos taurus*. In Australia, Jersey cows were found to be more resistant than other breeds. The incidence of clinical disease will vary according to age, climate, environmental hazards, grazing periods, housing, season of the year, and weather. The incidence is higher following rainy weather or in conditions of high soil moisture.

The true cost of this disease is difficult to calculate. Other than the obvious expense of veterinary care and drugs, the producers will experience losses from decreased fertility, decreased milk or beef yield, and increased management time to handle affected animals.

Fusobacterium necrophorum and *Bacteroides* are the bacterial organisms most commonly associated with interdigital phlegmon. However, even the organisms involved lead to debate and confusion. Most sources agree that *F. necrophorum* is the predominant organism in this disease, but most cases are found to be mixed infections. Both *Bacteroides melaninogenicus* and *Bacteroides nodosus* have been specifically mentioned in these mixed infections along with various other organisms. Further investigation into these bacterial organisms and their properties has resulted in more detailed identification of subspecies and thus new names. Currently some of the organisms involved will be appropriately referred to as *Dichelobacter nodosus* and *Porphyromones asaccharolytica*.

ETIOLOGY

Cattle are predisposed to infection by *F. necrophorum* and subsequent interdigital phlegmon through compromise of the interdigital skin from mechanical trauma or maceration from wet environmental conditions. Skin lesions associated with other conditions such as interdigital dermatitis may provide an entry site for infection by *F. necrophorum* and other bacteria. Open wounds drain into a favorable environment and "seed" pastures and pens with heavier burdens of causative organisms. The disease is more common during wet, humid weather, especially when the animals are in crowded housing and when the pH of the soil is high. Rocky land, sharp gravel on pathways, and plant stubble in pastures contribute to injury in the interdigital skin. Herd outbreaks are occasionally seen 4 to 8 weeks after rainy weather. Experimentally, skin lesions occur about 5 days after subcutaneous inoculation with *F. necrophorum*.

The *Fusobacterium* exotoxin creates the suppurative necrosis of skin seen in clinical cases. The *Bacteroides* organism produces lytic enzymes that damage subcutaneous tissues and tendons. In addition, secondary infection with *Actinomyces pyogenes* produces factors that consume oxygen in damaged tissues, therefore stimulating growth and proliferation of *F. necrophorum*.

CLINICAL SIGNS

The initial clinical sign of interdigital phlegmon is symmetrical swelling of one limb (usually a rear limb) involving the interdigital skin, occasionally extending proximally to the dewclaws. The animal may be acutely non–weight bearing and mildly febrile. The swelling of the interdigital skin causes the claws to spread apart. Within hours, a fissure may form in the interdigital skin with necrosis of tissue and the presence of suppurative exudate. At this time the characteristic fetid odor associated with this disease will be present. The fissure in the skin of the interdigital cleft exhibits swollen protruding edges. A small volume of purulent exudate and necrotic debris covers the edges of the skin lesion. Swelling as far proximal as the fetlock is often due to cellulitis ascending from the skin lesion. Affected cattle will show a decrease in milk yield, at least temporarily, and possibly infertility related to lameness.

In the United Kingdom where one synonym for foot rot is "foul-in-the-foot," a more severe peracute form of interdigital phlegmon is becoming increasingly important. This condition has accordingly been referred to as "super foul" (see Super Foot Rot).

Animals affected by traditional interdigital phlegmon may recover spontaneously in 10 to 14 days without treatment. However, low-grade lameness may persist for several weeks with negative effects on production and fertility. Untreated cases will more likely result in complications and even debilitation of the animal if joints or tendons become infected.

TREATMENT

Nearly all animals affected by interdigital phlegmon require treatment to adequately control progression of the disease. Most cases of interdigital phlegmon will resolve in 4 to 5 days with systemic antibiotic therapy such as penicillin G procaine 22,000 IU/kg intramuscularly (IM) b.i.d. or oxytetracycline 10 mg/kg intravenously (IV). Many authors suggest higher doses (penicillin G procaine 44,000 IU/kg IM b.i.d.) for nonresponsive cases. Appropriate measures to avoid residues in meat and milk should be followed.

Topical treatment may aid in resolution of clinical signs and help prevent spread of the disease. The benefit is most likely from simply keeping the feet clean. If instituted, topical treatment should consist of thoroughly cleaning necrotic debris from the lesion, possibly followed by topical therapy consisting of antibiotics or an astringent such as copper sulfate. If bandages are used, it is important to change them frequently to allow drainage of necrotic debris. Leaving the digit without a bandage after thorough cleaning may be both effective and efficient when the affected animal can be housed in a clean environment while receiving systemic antibiotic therapy. Most important, prompt treatment is second only to prevention in controlling clinical signs and losses due to decreased production and fertility in affected cattle.

CONTROL AND PREVENTION

The first step in controlling interdigital phlegmon is to isolate affected animals from the rest of the herd as soon as they are noticed. This will decrease contamination of the environment by discharge from skin lesions of affected cattle. Affected animals should also be treated aggressively for optimal results.

Prevention is a management issue of controlling the environment. Vaccines have been investigated and licensed but are not yet the best solution to this problem. Keeping high-traffic areas clean and dry is very important. The busy areas will naturally be the most heavily contaminated. Areas of water sources, gates, and often-traveled paths should be as clean and dry as possible and free of materials (such as stubble or sharp objects) that could traumatize the interdigital skin. Wet, low-lying pastureland may need to be fenced off to deny access to animals during rainy weather.

A foot bath containing copper sulfate or zinc sulfate may help keep the interdigital skin healthy and therefore less susceptible to infection by *F. necrophorum*. Even though most animals affected by interdigital phlegmon have relatively normal-shaped claws, regular foot trimming will lower the incidence of this disease, possibly by simply ensuring that the foot is clean and healthy.

BIBLIOGRAPHY

Bergsten C: Infectious diseases of the digits. *In* Greenough PR, Weaver AD (eds): Lameness in Cattle, ed 3. Philadelphia, WB Saunders, 1997, pp 89–94.

Blowey RW: Interdigital courses of lameness. *In* Proceedings of Eighth International Symposium on Disorders of the Ruminant Digit and International Conference on Bovine Lameness, Banff, Canada, 1994, pp 142–154.

Clark BL: Foot abscess of cattle. *In* Egerten JR, Yong WK, Riffkin GG (eds): Foot Rot and Foot Abscess of Ruminants. Boca Raton, Fla, CRC Press, June 1989, pp 69–79.

Guard C: Recognizing and managing infectious causes of lameness in cattle. *In* Proceedings of the 27th Annual Convention, American Association of Bovine Practitioners, Pittsburgh, January 1995, pp 80–82.

Salman MD, King ME, Odde KG, et al: Annual disease incidence in Colorado cow-calf herds participating in rounds 2 and 3 of the National Animal Health Monitoring System from 1986 to 1988. J Am Vet Med Assoc 198:962–967, 1991.

■ Fescue Foot

Aubrey N. Baird, D.V.M., M.S.

Fescue foot is most commonly seen as a hind limb lameness of cattle grazing tall fescue (*Festuca arundinacea*) infected with the asymptomatic endophytic fungus *Acremonium coenophialum*. Tall fescue is a seed-propagated, cool-season perennial grass that is widely grown in the United States for livestock feed and other purposes. The central and southern regions of the United States contain an estimated 35 million acres of tall fescue. Some reasons that tall fescue is so popular include good forage yield, persistence, wide adaptation, long growing season, and good seed production. Tall fescue is gaining popularity outside the United States, in Argentina, Australia, Belgium, Chile, France, and New Zealand.

The negative side of tall fescue grazing or hay is related to contamination by *A. coenophialum*. The endophyte lives inside the plant without invading the plant cells. It resides primarily in the seed, seed stem, leaf sheaths, and crown. The endophyte remains potentially toxic in fescue hay, as well as in live grass. Endophyte-infected fescue is documented to cause two conditions in cattle other than fescue foot. When summer fescue toxicosis occurs, cattle show signs of stress during elevated ambient temperatures, avoid sunlight, salivate excessively, and have increased respiratory rates and body temperature. Cattle affected by the fat necrosis syndrome develop firm masses of necrotic mesenteric fat. Some sources include agalactia as a fourth endophyte-related syndrome in cattle and cite at least a decreased milk production in cows fed endophyte-infected fescue. However, agalactia has not been experimentally reproduced in cattle and should probably be considered more of an equine problem.

Over a period of 3 years, 54% of seed samples submitted to the Auburn University Fescue Diagnostic Center had endophyte present. The mean contamination rate was 58%. These samples came from 26 different states. While samples from traditionally affected regions had higher infection rates, samples with toxic levels of endophyte were discovered from every region of the United States.

The interaction of the endophyte and tall fescue stimulates the fungus to produce potentially toxic alkaloids, including clavine, ergot, and peramine alkaloids. The fescue plant produces loline alkaloids in response to the endophyte. Ergopeptine and loline alkaloids are associated with the vasoconstriction that leads to necrosis seen in the fescue foot syndrome. Fescue foot is more prevalent on well-fertilized pastures. This is becoming increasingly important as the poultry industry grows in the Southeast and diversified farms dispose of chicken litter by spreading it on fescue pastures for fertilizer.

Fescue foot occurs most often during periods of cooler ambient temperatures and is manifested by vasoconstriction of peripheral vessels, which leads to gangrenous necrosis. The cooler ambient temperatures may indirectly exacerbate the toxicity of the fungus by reducing the need for cooling the body and thus allowing continued consumption of the endophyte, whereas animals exposed to the fungus during warmer summer months will become hyperthermic and stop eating as part of the summer syndrome. The rear feet are most commonly involved, but occasionally the tail and less often the tips of the ears may show avascular lesions.

Severely affected cattle commonly slough the hoof of one digit of the rear limb. Occasionally a necrotic demarcation will occur around the pastern area (or higher up the limb) and the animal will slough skin distal to the demarcation, as well as the hoof, leaving only bone and ligamentous structures intact. The tip of the tail may also slough or lose all the hair of the switch. Ear tips can slough in severe chronic cases after the rear feet and tail show signs of involvement.

DIAGNOSIS

The diagnosis of fescue foot is based on clinical signs and history of exposure to fescue grazing or hay that has been proved to be contaminated with *A. coenophialum*. The fungus is invisible to the naked eye but may be found microscopically in the seed, stem, leaf sheaths, or crown of the fescue plant. Several stems of the plant should be examined to determine the degree of contamination. The pasture is considered endophyte-free if less than 5% of the plants examined contain *A. coenophialum*. Clinical signs of fescue toxicosis may be seen when as little as 20% of the fescue is contaminated. Average daily gain decreases proportionally as the percent contamination increases. It is not uncommon for pastures grazed by affected cattle to be 80% to 100% contaminated. Other than microscopic visualization of the endophyte, an enzyme-linked immunosorbent assay may be used to determine fungal concentration in plants. Dopaminergic activity of ergopeptine alkaloids produced by *A. coenophialum* suppresses prolactin secretion in all species investigated to date. Therefore, measurement of the serum prolactin concentration has become a way to determine the effect of the endophyte.

Cattle may exhibit clinical signs of fescue foot such as hind limb lameness, arched back, and even diarrhea as early as 3 to 5 days after exposure to infected fescue, or they may not develop clinical signs for several months. Animals continually grazing infested pastures may develop clinical signs after a frost or following fertilization of the pasture.

The clinician must remember that other conditions causing similar clinical signs may occur concurrently with *A. coenophialum* toxicity and therefore must rule out those differential diagnoses as contributing to clinical lesions. Those conditions include ergot toxicity, interdigital phlegmon, chronic selenium toxicity, traumatic injury, and frostbite.

PREVENTION

Prevention is based solely on limiting intake of infected fescue. Tilling and replanting the pastures with "clean" fescue seed may be the safest way to prevent *A. coenophialum* toxicity. (I readily acknowledge, however, that the producer must realize benefits that outweigh the time and expense of replanting vs. other prevention methods.) It is often difficult to determine the true cost of *A. coenophialum* toxicosis in the form of decreased rate of weight gain and decreased fertility. The producer should be instructed that the cost of subclinical cases exceeds that of clinical cases. Each producer must ultimately make the decision whether to replant or use other preventive measures.

If replanting is not practical, supplementing concentrate or good-quality hay may be an acceptable way to substantially decrease exposure to *A. coenophialum*. The effect of the endophyte may also be diluted by planting legumes or other grasses in the infected fescue pastures. Planting other grasses is not a permanent solution since the competitive fescue will overtake most other grasses in 1 to 2 years.

Rotating land use between pasture and row crops may be an option for some producers that will help decrease endophyte contamination. Kentucky-31 has historically been the predominant type of fescue. However, varieties are currently available that are more resistant to fungus and should be considered when planting or replanting fescue. The most endophyte-resistant variety is Fawn, followed by Kenmont, Missouri-96, and Kenhy. The producer may also consider limiting grazing of infected fescue pastures by penning cattle intermittently on supplemental feed or pastures free of endophyte.

BIBLIOGRAPHY

Brendemuehl JP: Effects of grazing tall fescue infected with the endophyte *Acremonium coenophialum* on cyclicity, gestation, progestogen production and parturition in the mare and endocrine function in the newborn foal. PhD dissertation, Auburn University, Auburn University, Ala, 1995, pp 1–36.

Garner GB, Cornell CN: Fescue foot in cattle. *In* Wyllie TD, Morehouse LG (eds): Mycotoxicosis of Domestic and Laboratory Animals, Poultry, and Aquatic Invertebrates and Vertebrates. New York, Marcel Dekker, 1978, pp 45–62.

Smart M, Cymbaluk NF: Role of nutritional supplements in bovine lameness—Review of nutritional toxicities. *In* Greenough PR, Weaver AD (eds): Lameness in Cattle, ed 3. Philadelphia, WB Saunders, 1997, pp 158–159.

■ Interdigital Hyperplasia (Interdigital Fibroma, Corn)

Bimbo Welker, D.V.M., M.S.

Interdigital hyperplasia is a common lesion of the interdigital space in cattle, and yet its clinical significance varies from cow to cow. It is characterized as a pedunculated, smooth-surfaced mass arising from the skin of the interdigital cleft. The incidence of these masses can be as high as 4% in dairy cattle and significantly higher in some beef breeds, particularly Herefords, with bulls predominating. Studies show late-lactation dairy cows to have a much higher incidence and that the incidence seems to increase in the winter months and subside in the summer months. Calves as young as 8 to 12 months of age have been observed to have hyperplasia of the interdigital skin.

ETIOLOGY AND PATHOPHYSIOLOGY

Chronic irritation of the skin of the interdigital cleft seems to promote a hyperplastic response of the dermal tissues. The irritation can result from chronic infection (e.g., foot rot), moist environmental conditions that macerate and compromise the integrity of the skin, and trauma. Poor foot care can result in overstretching or pinching of the skin of the interdigital space. Splay toes, an inherited condition of the feet resulting in abnormal separation of the claws at the toes with excessively wide and folded interdigital skin, may be an example of a congenital predisposing factor.

The chronically irritated skin may respond by proliferating, forming a pseudotumorous mass. The mass typically begins at the axial aspect of the lateral digit but can eventually incorporate the entire interdigital space. The protuberance is narrower at the base, pedunculated, and is covered by a smooth covering of epidermis. Histologically, the lesions exhibit hyperkeratosis, parakeratosis, and possibly secondary damage with infection, ulceration, and trauma.

CLINICAL SIGNS

The lameness associated with interdigital hyperplasia ranges from absent to severe, three-legged lameness. The presence of hyperplastic tissue in the interdigital cleft does not constitute a diagnosis of lameness. In my experience most cows demonstrating hyperplastic tissue do not demonstrate an associated lameness. If the protuberance is excessively large, or caudal in the space where it is likely to be pinched, it is more likely to cause problems. If this is the case the examiner can usually demonstrate pain on manipulation. Masses that are traumatized, infected, or ulcerated are more obviously a potential source of the lameness. Recently I observed an increased incidence of corns that would otherwise have been innocuous, with the development of hairy heel warts on their surface.

The typical uninfected corn arises on a pedunculated infundibulum, narrower at the base. Swelling at the base or origination of the corn or swelling above the coronary band is an indication of deep tissue extension or involvement. The degree of lameness at this point will usually be profound.

Because of the classic appearance of the corn, no other disorders should be confused with it. Swelling of the interdigital space due to inflammation, cellulitis, or abscessation from trauma or foot rot does not appear pedunculated. It will cause a bulbous distention of the interdigital cleft that appears to extend down from the deep tissue. Rarely a papilloma will occur in the space, but it is characterized by its wartlike surface.

TREATMENT

It is imperative that the clinical significance of the corn be verified before it is blamed entirely for the lameness. The presence of hyperplastic tissue does not constitute a diagnosis. Areas of hyperplasia may sometimes be resolved by proper foot trimming, treatment of predisposing conditions like foot rot, and environmental management. To surgically remove clinically insignificant hyperplastic tissue may be unnecessary and uneconomical, and may cause more harm than good. Furthermore, if the correct diagnosis has been overlooked, then resolution of the problem is delayed. If the corn is excessively large, caudal in the space, infected, traumatized, or ulcerated, and the animal demonstrates pain on manipulation, then it warrants appropriate treatment. Obviously painful corns are best treated by removal for expedient resolution and return to function. With proper restraint an interdigital block or regional intravenous block is performed. In most cases the interdigital block will suffice. The plexus of nerves that innervate the skin of the interdigital space can be effectively anesthetized by inserting an 18-gauge 1½-in. needle through the skin on the dorsal surface of the foot at the point where the interdigital skin comes to an apex. Approxi-

mately 10 to 20 mL of 2% lidocaine is infused into the area. Using sharp dissection an elliptical incision is made to incorporate the entire tumor. The blade should be angled so as to remove a pie-shaped wedge of interdigital skin. I prefer to leave a thin dermal layer and not to expose the interdigital fat pad. If the fat pad is exposed it should not be removed. The wound is bandaged with medicated ointment using a figure-8 wrap for 10 to 14 days. Preferentially the cow is kept in a clean, dry, well-bedded area until the wrap is removed. It may be advantageous to wire or wrap the toes together to minimize stretching and separation of the claws during healing. Systemic antibiotics are necessary only if there is evidence of deep tissue involvement or swelling above the mass or at the coronary band. Extensive swelling of the foot or localized swelling above the coronary band of one digit portends a poorer prognosis and calls for more extensive diagnostic tests such as radiographs.

Simple, locally irritated or painful corns generally have a good prognosis, while those demonstrating deep tissue involvement warrant a more guarded prognosis.

PREVENTION

The prevention of corns is accomplished primarily by minimizing or removing the sources of chronic irritation. Control or prevention of foot rot, a clean environment with reduced moisture, and proper foot care involving routine, correct trimming are the sine qua non of prevention. Improper trimming can create, rather than prevent, the disease. The feet should be trimmed so that the axial wall is slightly (⅛ to ¼ in.) shorter than the abaxial wall. In addition, the axial wall and sole should be pared to a concave finish to allow more room for the interdigital skin. Overemphasis of wall length differences will exacerbate rather than control the problem.

BIBLIOGRAPHY

Blowey, R: Cattle Lameness and Foot Care. UK., Farming Press, 1993, pp 49–51.
Greenough PR, Weaver DA: Lameness in Cattle, ed 3. Philadelphia, WB Saunders, 1997, pp 119–120.
Peterson GC, Nelson DR: Foot diseases in cattle. Part 2. Diagnosis and treatment. Compendium Continuing Educ Pract Vet 6:5565–5573, 1984.
Rebhun WC, Pearson EG: Clinical management of bovine foot problems. J Am Vet Med Assoc 181:572–577, 1982.
Rowlands GJ, Russell AM, Williams LA: Effects of season, herd size, management system and veterinary practice on the lameness incidence in dairy cattle. Vet Rec 113:441–445, 1983.

■ Ovine Contagious Foot Rot

D. Michael Rings, D.V.M., M.S., Diplomate, A.C.V.I.M.

Ovine contagious foot rot (CFR) remains one of the major economic disease problems in sheep management. It has been estimated that infection can result in a 10% loss in body condition as well as impair wool growth.[1] The annual cost of treatment of this condition in Australia has been estimated at greater than $43 million.

ETIOLOGY

The principal causative agent in sheep foot rot is *Dichelobacter nodosus*, formally *Bacteroides nodosus*. This organism is an obligate anaerobic pathogen of the ovine foot, capable of surviving off the host for no more than 14 days.[2] The organism proliferates best in temperate, humid climates but can be found worldwide. Many cases of foot rot are initiated by a superficial infection of the interdigital area by *Fusobacterium necrophorum*. This organism, like *Dichelobacter*, likes moist temperate climates. It is thought that the inflammation produced by *F. necrophorum* facilitates the attachment and growth of *Dichelobacter*.

PATHOGENESIS AND CLINICAL SIGNS

Differences in the production of proteases by various strains of *D. nodosus* dramatically affect the virulence of this bacterium. The mildest form of foot rot is called foot scald or benign foot rot. This is an inflammatory condition of the interdigital skin causing local erythema and mild, transient lameness which often resolves without treatment. *D. nodosus* strains with low protease production are usually associated with this condition. Increased production of proteases, especially elastase, by *D. nodosus* increases the organism's virulence. The increased protease levels permit the invasion of deeper tissues. Infection starts at the junction of the hoof wall and coronary band and progresses down the lamina of the hoof wall, causing separation and, in many instances, underrunning the sole. Abaxial hoof wall surfaces are usually affected and both claws or more than one foot may be infected. This results in severe lameness. Affected individuals may limp or hop on the infected limb or become so sore that they kneel on the carpi when grazing or become totally recumbent. As a result of their limited mobility, affected sheep show weight loss. Chronically affected individuals may develop malformed hoof walls.

DIAGNOSIS

The clinical examination of lame sheep with the characteristic lesions of CFR in a flock with multiple animals affected is usually sufficient to establish the diagnosis. The anaerobic culturing of fetid exudate from typical lesions can be attempted, but it may be difficult to recover *D. nodosus*, owing to its specialized growth requirements. More commonly, impression smears of exudate from characteristic lesions are examined to find the large, barbell-shaped, slightly curved gram-negative bacteria of *D. nodosus*.

Enzyme-linked immunosorbent assay (ELISA) technology has been developed for use in flocks having CFR.[3, 4] The test can be used to identify infected animals within a flock. It appears to be both sensitive and specific. This test would seem to have its widest application in identifying carrier animals during periods of remission or subclinical infection. This test would not be appropriate for use in flocks using *D. nodosus* vaccines, as there is a titer rise associated with vaccination.

Specific DNA probes have been developed which can identify virulence factors among the strains of *D. nodosus*.[5] This technology is only available as a research tool at this time.

TREATMENT AND CONTROL

F. necrophorum is a normal inhabitant of the environment of sheep and is difficult to avoid; however, *D. nodosus* is an obligate pathogen of sheep's feet and cannot survive for more than 14 days in the environment. Thus a continuing problem with CFR can only occur when sheep carrying *D. nodosus* persist in the flock. The identification and separation of diseased from healthy animals is the first step in limiting the spread of CFR. Thorough

to radical trimming of the affected hoof wall may be necessary to expose infected tissues sufficiently to allow disinfection of the foot via foot bath. Among the most effective foot bath solutions are 10% formalin in water, 10% to 20% copper sulfate in water, and 10% zinc sulfate (w/v) in water. The zinc sulfate solution appears to be at least as efficacious as the other solutions and is less toxic to the environment.

During the initial phase of treatment, affected sheep should be made to stand for 5 to 30 minutes in the foot bath. Subsequent treatment via foot baths should consist of walking through the bath two to three times per week until clinical signs are gone and then weekly as a prophylactic measure.

Antimicrobials have been used successfully in the treatment of CFR in sheep. Antimicrobials commonly used include penicillin, oxytetracycline, tylosin, and erythromycin. In sheep without overgrown or malformed claws and those with milder clinical signs, the injection of oxytetracycline alone has met with good success. Antibiotic dosages in excess of the labeled level may be required to achieve therapeutic concentrations.

There are two vaccines commercially available which are labeled for the prevention of ovine CFR in the United States: one is a *F. necrophorum* bacterin (Volar, Bayer) and the other a *D. nodosus* bacterin (Footvax, Coopers Animal Health). The *D. nodosus* vaccine contains 10 strains which cross-react with 14 of 20 strains found in the United States. Vaccination has been shown to reduce the incidence of CFR in flocks by 45% to 61%, with the most significant reduction in previously infected ewes. Vaccination with *D. nodosus* has shown therapeutic value in reducing the recovery period in clinically affected sheep. This is an oil-adjuvant vaccine and its use is associated with swellings and sterile abscess formation at the injection sites. A two-dose course, 6 weeks to 6 months apart, is required initially, followed by a semiannual or annual booster, depending on the seasonal appearance of the injection in the flock. Boosters should be given several weeks prior to the season in which foot rot is seen in the flock.

A recent study[6] has shown experimentally that single-strain vaccines may be more efficacious than multiple-strain vaccines in providing protection. Vaccines containing multiple serogroups may provide too much antigenic competition to produce high levels of agglutinating antibody compared to monovalent vaccines. Available vaccines used for *Dichelobacter* in the United States and Australia all contain from 9 to 10 strains.

DIFFERENTIAL DIAGNOSIS

Any lameness limited to the foot should be considered in the differential diagnosis of CFR. Among the most common foot lamenesses are toe abscesses and heel abscesses. These tend to affect individuals rather than flocks and more commonly infect a single claw. The causative agent of these conditions is usually *F. necrophorum*.

REFERENCES

1. Stewart DJ: Footrot in sheep. *In* Egerton JR, Young WK, Riffkin GG (eds): Foot Rot and Foot Abscess of Ruminants. Boca Raton, Fla, CRC Press, 1989, pp 5–46.
2. Kimberling CV: Diseases of Feet. *In* Kimberling CV (ed): Jensen and Swift's Diseases of Sheep, ed 3. Philadelphia, Lea & Febiger, 1988, pp 317–324.
3. Whittington RJ, Egerton JR: Application of ELISA to the serological diagnosis of virulent ovine footrot. Vet Microbiol 41(2):147–161, 1994.
4. Whittington RJ, Marshall DJ, Walker RI: ELISA for anti–*D. nodosus* for detection in flocks during subclinical phase. Aust Vet J 67:98–101, 1990.

5. Liu D, Webber J: A polymerase chain reaction assay for improved determination of virulence of *Dichelobacter nodosus*, the specific causative pathogen for ovine footrot. Vet Microbiol 43(2):197–207, 1995.
6. Hunt JD, Jackson DC, Wood PR: Antigenic competition in a multivalent foot rot vaccine. Vaccine 12(5):457–464, 1994.

■ Septic Arthritis

Guy St. Jean, D.M.V., M.S., Diplomate, A.C.V.S.

Septic arthritis is observed secondary to hematogenous infection, traumatic injury, or a septic hoof lesion with local introduction of infectious organisms and iatrogenic inoculation.[1] Infectious arthritis of hematogenous origin is commonly observed in young food-producing animals. The umbilicus is a common site of a septic focus, but septic arthritis may be associated with any systemic infection. Organisms circulating in the blood gain access to the joint. Septic arthritis of hematogenous origin is often polyarticular, with larger joints involved. Traumatic septic arthritis from direct penetration of a foreign body into the joint is commonly associated with mature animals and affects only the damaged joint(s).[2] Organisms associated with septic arthritis are many and varied. Viruses, such as caprine arthritis–encephalitis, mycoplasma, and chlamydia, as well as bacteria, most commonly *Actinomyces pyogenes* and *Escherichia coli*, have been implicated as agents causing septic arthritis.

DIAGNOSIS

A rapid diagnosis of septic arthritis is important because of the progressive destructive nature of the disease on the articular cartilage. The signs associated with septic arthritis include severe lameness, distention of the joint capsule, and heat of the involved joint. Pain on palpation of the joint is often observed. A low-grade fever, depression, and anorexia may be present. In young animals, umbilical cord lesions, pneumonia, and diarrhea may be noted.

Arthrocentesis and synovial fluid evaluation will help to diagnose infectious arthritis. Aseptic techniques must be used in performing arthrocentesis. Results of synovial fluid analysis in cases of infectious arthritis include an increased volume of fluid, a yellow to brown flocculent fluid with a lack of viscosity, protein greater than 2 g/100 mL, and a white blood cell count greater than 30,000 cells per milliliter with 90% or greater being neutrophils. Although a positive bacterial culture confirms the diagnosis, it is often difficult to obtain positive cultures of synovial fluid, even in infected joints. Negative culture may indicate chronic infection with the bacteria isolated in the villous crypts or prior treatment with antibiotics.

Arthroscopy, if not too costly, may assist in the diagnosis of septic arthritis and may help assess joints for prognostication of future soundness.[3] Arthroscopic examination is superior to radiographic examination in diagnosing soft tissue disorders like synovitis and capsulitis and also in evaluating the condition of the articular cartilage.[3] Radiographically demonstrable lesions will seldom be present in acute cases of septic arthritis.[1] Radiographs should be performed to rule out the possibility of traumatic damage to the subchondral bone or osteomyelitis and to establish a baseline for future evaluation. As septic arthritis progresses, radiographic evidence of degenerative joint disease with bone lysis and periosteal proliferation may be noted.[2] Radiographs of advanced cases of septic arthritis may reveal spontaneous ankylosis of a joint.[2]

TREATMENT

Septic arthritis remains a clinical challenge to treat effectively and economically. Treatment of septic arthritis involves eliminating the causative organism and removing the enzymes and proteinaceous material that can damage the articular cartilage. Delay in treatment reduces the prognosis by allowing further periarticular fibrosis and articular damage. Systemic and intra-articular administration of antimicrobial agents is indicated. If intra-articular administration is elected, the dose given into the joint should not exceed the once-a-day dose (based on body weight) that would be given systemically. Treatment should be started before the results of bacteriologic culture are available. Ceftiofur sodium is often used by me as the antibiotic of choice and is administered for 2 weeks beyond return of the joint to clinical normalcy.[4] In cases where the primary source of infection is the umbilicus, surgical resection is indicated.

If antibiotics and synovial aspiration do not bring improvement in 36 hours, joint lavage is indicated. Intermittent joint lavage using two 14-gauge needles introduced into the joint space using aseptic technique with the animal under heavy sedation or light anesthesia may be used in early cases before intra-articular fibrin deposition has occurred. The joint is infused with the lavage solution under pressure to distend the synovial membrane and disrupt adhesions. Large quantities of balanced polyionic fluid are used and allowed to circulate freely through the joint. Periodically blocking the outflow needle helps distend and lavage the entire joint. One to two liters of balanced polyionic solution should be used to lavage a septic joint. An alternative method of joint lavage is arthroscopy. Arthroscopy, if available and economically possible, offers large ingress and egress portals, allowing administration of large volumes of fluid, the ability to identify and remove fibrin clots, and evaluation of articular cartilage.[3] When the inflammatory process becomes chronic, fibrin clots become too large to be removed by anything other than an arthrotomy. The joint is opened and lavaged, fibrin clots are removed, and the abnormal synovial membrane is removed. The open joint must be protected from environmental contamination by a sterile bandage until the joint closes by second intention.

Arthrotomy may be performed for joint debridement, curettage of infected cartilage, and removal of necrotic bone.[2] If indicated, a bone graft and immobilization of the joint may be incorporated in the treatment to produce arthrodesis and a pain-free limb. This procedure may be used successfully in many advanced cases of septic arthritis of the distal and proximal interphalangeal joint.[1] Systemic administration of nonsteroidal anti-inflammatory drugs is indicated to reduce the pain associated with septic arthritis and to encourage early return to normal function. The anti-prostaglandin effect of the nonsteroidal anti-inflammatory drugs can reduce inflammation of the synovium and stop one aspect of the inflammatory process associated with joint sepsis. If possible, the joint affected should be supported with bandages and splints to make the animal more comfortable and avoid flexural deformity. Immobilization should be done only 8 hours/day to avoid reduction in the range of motion of the joint.

REFERENCES

1. DesRochers A, St Jean G: Surgical management of digit disorders in cattle. Vet Clin North Am Food Anim Pract 12:282–285, 1996.
2. DesRochers A, St Jean G, Anderson DE: Use of facilitated ankylosis in the treatment of septic arthritis of the distal interphalangeal joint in cattle. 12 cases (1987–1992). J Am Vet Med Assoc 206:1923–1927, 1995.
3. Gaughan EM: Arthroscopy in food animal practice. Vet Clin North Am Food Anim Pract 12:240–241, 1996.
4. Mills ML, Moore BR, St Jean G, et al: Synovial fluid concentrations, cytologic characteristics and effect on synovism of ceftiofur sodium after intra-articular injection in horses. *In* Proceedings of the 24th Annual Conference of the Veterinary Orthopedic Society, 1997.

■ Stifle Injuries

Dale R. Nelson, D.V.M., M.S.

Most stifle problems can be diagnosed with a thorough physical examination. Satisfactory radiography of the bovine stifle joint is difficult under field conditions. However, when available, radiography is often more valuable for prognostic information aiding in diagnosis. Although clinical signs may appear acute, they may actually be delayed indications of chronic disease, which will affect prognosis and treatment.

With stifle disease, the animal avoids flexing the stifle, keeping the hock and stifle "fixed" when walking. This causes a very abducted stride, which may be confused with a sole abscess involving the lateral claw. Weight is borne on the toe, and the heel does not contact the ground. The fetlock is slightly flexed. Periarticular swelling and joint effusion are evident, especially with acute injuries and infection. Heat in the joint may indicate infection.

Viscosity, turbidity, color change, and clotting can be readily assessed by gross examination of joint fluid.[1] The presence of red blood cells may indicate trauma or synovial membrane involvement.[1] Old hemorrhage may discolor the joint fluid dark yellow, brown, or tan.[1] Increased cell content, especially leukocytes, causes turbidity and flocculence suggesting infection.[1] Normal synovial fluid does not clot because of the absence of fibrinogen.[1] Viscosity is assessed by stringiness of the fluid. Watery synovial fluid indicates infection or possibly recent trauma. Conventional bacterial culturing of septic synovial fluid is usually unrewarding.[2]

Abnormal movement in the stifle can be determined by manipulation of the lower limb or by palpation while the animal is walking. The cranial cruciate ligament may be evaluated with a drawer test on the standing animal.[3] Standing behind the animal and bracing your knees on the back of the hock, the proximal tibia is pulled caudad using both hands on the tibial crest. Generally, a movement of 2 to 3 cm caudally is required to return the tibia to the normal position. To evaluate the collateral ligaments and menisci, a varus/valgus stress test is done.[4] With a finger at the joint space cranial to the medial collateral ligament, the lower leg is abducted and adducted. Widening of the joint space and excessive movement of the meniscus indicate injury. Muscle atrophy, especially within the quadriceps and gluteal muscle groups, develops with stifle lameness. Prolonged lameness (>2 to 3 weeks) in growing animals may cause a varus deformity of the opposite tarsus due to greater weight bearing. This usually disappears in time if the lameness is corrected. As the signs of foot disease are similar to those of stifle lameness, the foot must be carefully examined in all cases of suspected stifle lameness.

PATELLAR LUXATIONS

Clinical signs of upward fixation of the patella in cattle are similar to those seen in ponies.[5] A jerky motion is seen since the limb must be pulled forward more forcefully following extension. Although the anatomy of the femorotibial joint in cattle differs from that of the horse, the limb can become locked in extension and dragged behind the animal.[5] The toes become rounded. Affected cattle seem fractious, but their disposition improves quickly following surgery.[5] Adult Brahman or Brahman-type cattle are more commonly involved.[5] One or both limbs can be affected. Poor conformation, especially "postlegged" cattle with a small quadriceps muscle mass, is an important cause.[5] Hereditary factors may also be important.[6]

A medial patellar desmotomy as performed in the equine is usually successful. Since both limbs may ultimately become involved, surgery should be performed on both stifles.[5]

Lateral luxation of the patella is a congenital problem seen more often in small ruminants and calves. Most cases in calves probably result from atrophy of the quadriceps muscles because of femoral nerve injury during dystocia. The lateral position of the patella hinders support of the stifle. If bilateral, the animal may not stand or may crouch. The patellas should be examined closely in newborns with rear leg lameness. Femoral nerve injury should be recognized because conventional surgical procedures for patellar luxation will not be successful in cases of femoral nerve injury.

FEMORAL NERVE PARALYSIS

Injury to the femoral nerve may occur during dystocia. One study reports on beef calves of exotic breeds that became "hip-locked" in anterior presentation, suffering femoral nerve injuries. Affected calves cannot extend the stifle of the injured leg due to lack of tone in the quadriceps muscle mass. The quadriceps are flaccid the first few days after injury and in 7 to 10 days marked atrophy of these muscles is noticeable. Electromyography may be used to confirm the diagnosis. The prognosis for calves with femoral nerve paralysis is poor to guarded, depending on the degree of nerve injury. If complete disruption of the nerve has not occurred, and if fibrosis does not inhibit reinnervation, quadriceps muscle tone may return within 1 to 6 months.

CRUCIATE LIGAMENT RUPTURE

The cranial cruciate ligament holds the femoral condyles forward on the tibial surface. Cranial cruciate ligament rupture (CCLR) allows the femoral condyles to slide caudad on the tibia, causing marked laxity in the joint. Two scenarios may involve CCLR. Acute signs are often seen in dairy cows after rupture of the ligament from injurious activity such as slipping, struggling to rise, mounting and so forth.[3] However, in older animals, especially bulls, degenerative joint disease (DJD) may be active and the menisci are damaged and disrupted. With laxity in the stifle, the ligament ruptures and only then do the acute signs of CCLR appear.[7, 8] In these animals, radiography, if available, will help establish a prognosis.[9]

CCLR is primarily a disease of adult cattle (>4 years).[9] General signs of stifle disease are present. Laxity of the stifle joint is obvious. Palpation of the stifle while the animal walks reveals excessive movement of the joint which is often accompanied by clicking or knocking sounds. A drawer test will confirm the diagnosis of CCLR.[3]

Prognosis is guarded to poor. DJD is progressive but it may be 6 to 12 months before lameness becomes debilitating. Surgical treatment can benefit some animals. Surgical procedures using fascia or patellar ligament as autogenous replacement of the cruciate ligament or an imbrication procedure of the fascial retinaculum of the stifle have been described.[3, 10, 11] In older animals with suspected chronic DJD preceding CCLR, the prognosis is unfavorable.

MEDIAL COLLATERAL LIGAMENT INJURY

Traumatic injury of the medial collateral ligament (MCL) of the stifle usually stretches the ligament rather than causes rupture. If the meniscus is not involved, recovery usually follows 3 to 4 weeks of stall confinement. However, the medial meniscus may be detached from the joint capsule and the MCL (peripheral detachment of the medial meniscus, PDMM).[4] The mobility of the meniscus and the laxity of the stifle results in disruption of the meniscus and, ultimately, DJD and a poor prognosis.[4] PDMM usually affects younger animals (<2 years).

If present in older animals, PDMM is frequently associated with CCLR. The animal attempts to relieve stress on the medial stifle by placing the foot away from the body. A varus/valgus stress test will cause widening of the joint space and increased movement of the meniscus.[4] The MCL can usually be palpated intact. A detached meniscus can be secured with sutures to the joint capsule and the medial fascia imbricated.[4]

IDIOPATHIC SUPPURATIVE GONITIS

Several reports from the United States, United Kingdom, and Canada have described a suppurative gonitis affecting Holstein or Friesian heifers exclusively.[2, 12, 13] Lameness was acute and ranged from moderate to non–weight bearing in severity. There was joint effusion with the synovial fluid containing large numbers of nucleated cells and a high protein concentration.[2] Gram stain of the fluid did not reveal bacteria, and cultures for bacteria and *Mycoplasma* spp. were negative.[2] An osteolytic lesion on the lateral tibial plateau was commonly seen on radiographs.[2]

Treatment involved joint lavage or arthrotomy, analgesics, and antimicrobials. The prognosis was good, most animals becoming productive herd members, although recovery often required several months. The osteolytic lesions were not accessible by arthroscopy.[2] The cause may be a response to microbial pathogens or microbial antigens.[2] An association with *Brucella abortus* strain 19 vaccination has also been suggested.[12]

REFERENCES

1. Jennings PB: The Practice of Large Animal Surgery. Philadelphia, WB Saunders, 1984, pp 746–751.
2. Madison JB, Tulleners EP, Ducharme NG, et al: Idiopathic gonitis in heifers: 34 cases (1976–1986). J Am Vet Med Assoc 194:273, 1989.
3. Nelson DR: Surgery of the stifle joint in cattle. Compendium Continuing Educ Pract Vet 5:S300, 1983.
4. Nelson DR, Huhn JC, Kneller SK: Surgical repair of peripheral detachment of the medial meniscus in 34 cattle. Vet Rec 127:571, 1990.
5. Baird AN, Angel KL, Moll HD, et al: Upward fixation of the patella in cattle: 38 cases (1984–1990). J Am Vet Med Assoc 202:434, 1993.
6. Gadgil BA, Agarwal SP, Patel UG: A hereditary aspect of luxation of the patella in cattle. Indian Vet J 49:313, 1972.
7. Bartels JE: Femoro-tibial osteoarthrosis in the bull: I. Clinical survey and radiologic interpretation. Am J Vet Radiol Soc 16:151, 1975.
8. Bartels JE: Femoro-tibial osteoarthrosis in the bull: II. A correlation of the radiographic and pathologic findings of the torn meniscus and ruptured cranial cruciate ligament. Am J Vet Radiol Soc 16:159, 1975.
9. Huhn JC, Kneller SK, Nelson DR: Radiographic assessment of cranial cruciate ligament rupture in the dairy cow. Vet Radiol 27:184, 1986.
10. Crawford WH: Intra-articular replacement of bovine cranial cruciate ligaments with an autogenous fascial graft. Vet Surg 19:380, 1990.
11. Moss EW, McCurnin DM, Ferguson TH: Experimental cranial cruciate replacement in cattle using patellar ligament graft. Can Vet J 29:157, 1988.
12. Wyn-Jones G, Baker JR, Johnson PM: A clinical and immunopathological study of *Brucella abortus* strain 19–induced arthritis in cattle. Vet Rec 107:5, 1980.
13. Ducharme NG, Stanton ME, Ducharme GR: Stifle lameness in

cattle at two veterinary teaching hospitals: A retrospective study of forty-two cases. Can Vet J 26:212, 1985.

■ Coxofemoral Luxations

Eric Tulleners, D.V.M.

HISTORY

Coxofemoral luxation is the most common luxation observed in dairy cattle.[1–3] The injury is usually caused by trauma and is almost always unilateral. In newborn calves, coxofemoral luxation may occur as a result of forced extraction. Adult cattle are most commonly affected and often incur the injury in falls; after calving, possibly because of weakness, pelvic ligamentous laxity, and metabolic disturbances such as acetonemia and hypocalcemia; or while being mounted during estrus.[1–3]

LAMENESS EVALUATION

In neonatal calves and immature cattle, a cranial and dorsal coxofemoral luxation is most common. In adult cattle, the direction of luxation is fairly evenly distributed between cranial and dorsal and ventral, with most of the ventral luxations being in a caudal and ventral direction.[1–3]

An animal suffering from a cranial and dorsal luxation is usually ambulatory but is most often not bearing weight on, or is severely lame in the affected limb.[4] The limb is externally rotated (stifle and foot turned outward) and, if bearing weight, the animal's toe touches. When viewed from the rear of the animal, the cranial and dorsal aspect of the affected side of the pelvis is asymmetrical and prominent because of the abnormal position of the greater trochanter. There is a visible and palpable increase in the distance between the greater trochanter and the tuber ischii as compared with the normal side. There is usually minimal soft tissue swelling, and in most instances the limb can be easily flexed. Manipulating the limb does not normally elicit the severe pain, crepitus, and grating characteristic of a fracture; however, the head of the femur has a noticeably abnormal position and range of motion. It is often helpful to examine the animal while it is recumbent, with the affected limb uppermost. An assistant grasps the metatarsus, flexes the limb, and holds it in a moderately abducted position. The assistant then rotates the limb in a circular motion around its longitudinal axis while the examiner presses firmly with the palm of the hand over the greater trochanter to feel the abnormal position and movement of the femoral head and greater trochanter.

Cattle with ventral luxations prefer to remain recumbent and usually rest with the limb in an abnormally abducted position. Cattle with ventral luxations may have serious complicating musculoskeletal injuries such as extensive muscle and ligamentous tearing or, less commonly, fracture of the greater trochanter, and they may be unable to stand. A diagnosis of ventral luxation can be supported by palpating the greater trochanter in an abnormal caudal or cranial and ventral position and by executing the same manipulative tests previously described. The limb can also be abducted to an abnormal extent. The femoral head may be palpable per rectum or per vaginum located cranial to the ilium or pubis in an animal with a cranial and ventral luxation, or in the obturator foramen in an animal with a caudal and ventral luxation.[2, 3]

A definitive diagnosis of coxofemoral luxation can be made by obtaining pelvic radiographs, but this is impractical and unnecessary in most instances. The differential diagnosis of an acute, severe injury localized to the hip region should include fracture of the pelvis or, more commonly, fracture of the capital femoral physis, femoral neck, greater trochanter, or proximal femur. Coxofemoral subluxation, septic arthritis, degenerative joint disease (coxitis), and osteochondrosis should also be considered.

TREATMENT

Most cattle do not thrive with a chronic coxofemoral luxation, so immediate treatment or slaughter is usually indicated. Excisional femoral head and neck arthroplasty is not a viable option for long-term productivity in most cattle.

Nonsurgical closed reduction is most likely to be successful if performed within 12 hours or, at most, 24 hours after injury, making client education and early detection critical. Success with closed reduction has been reported to range from 43% to 75%.[2, 3] To attempt closed reduction, the animal should be restrained in lateral recumbency, with the affected limb uppermost, and heavily sedated with 0.22 mg/kg xylazine given intravenously. Larcombe and Malmo[2] describe their technique as follows:

The position of the cow's pelvis is fixed by a rope passed under the cow's thigh in the inguinal region and tied to a solid object. A second rope is tied to the lower part of the affected limb above the fetlock. Traction is applied using a block and tackle. Initially the direction of pull is in a line which passes through the displaced femoral head and the acetabulum. During traction, the femur is rotated by pushing down on the stifle and lifting the hock. If the femur moves and a sudden "clunk" is felt, the traction is immediately relaxed and the leg examined to see if the dislocation has been reduced. If the greater trochanter of the femur is in its normal anatomic position relative to the pelvic landmarks and the leg can be easily flexed without crepitus, then the replacement has been successful. If not, the process is repeated. If the dislocation is not reduced by this method, the femur is rotated in the opposite direction and if this does not work, prolonged traction is applied so that the head of the femur is pulled away from the pelvis, the leg is rotated as described above and the traction rapidly released. In many cases, the dislocation is reduced as the leg is relaxed. In approximately 30% of cases it is necessary to try different directions of traction before the dislocation is reduced.

In a small number of cases (less than 5%) it is necessary to place a lever under the most proximal part of the femur. This allows the proximal femur to be lifted while the leg is rotated under traction. This assists in reducing the dislocation by lifting the head of the femur over the lip of the acetabulum.[2, p 353]

Jubb and associates[3] delineate the following prognostic factors concerning closed reduction:

Factors demonstrating a statistically significant ($P<0.05$) influence on outcome were: ability to stand with the dislocation (85% vs. 11%), age less than 3 years or more (81% vs. 23%), dislocation in a cranial direction vs. dislocation in a caudal direction (82% vs. 31%), duration of dislocation less than 12 hours vs. duration of dislocation at least 12 hours (56% vs. 8%), occurrence during estrus vs. occurrence when not in estrus (77% vs. 30%), body weight less than 400 kg vs. body weight at least 400 kg (63% vs. 30%).[3, p 356]

Open reduction can be successfully accomplished through a cranial and lateral approach[5] but this requires general anesthesia, assisted traction, and facilities where aseptic surgery can be performed. Open reduction may be successful when closed reduction fails because it allows for hematoma evacuation and for removal of fibrin, tissue fragments, and joint capsule, and the surgeon can be completely confident that the femoral head has been replaced into the acetabulum. In one study involving 22 cattle, 21 (95%) of the luxations could be reduced via a surgical approach.[1] In this study most cattle with cranial and dorsal luxations were ambulatory before surgery, none had concomitant musculoskeletal injuries, and 75% survived long-term. Eighty-three percent of cattle with ventral luxations were unable to stand before surgery, and only 33% survived long-term.

Calves had a better long-term survival rate (75% vs. 50%) and a lower reluxation rate (17% vs. 40%) compared with adults. As with closed reduction, the most common cause of failure was reluxation.

In summary, coxofemoral luxation is a very serious, usually incapacitating orthopedic injury. Treated as an emergency, within 24 hours of injury, closed reduction should be attempted initially. While still associated with a guarded prognosis, open surgical reduction is the treatment of choice for animals with luxations of greater than 24 hours' duration. The prognosis is extremely poor for animals that are weak, recumbent, and unable to rise even momentarily. Most of these animals remain recumbent even with the luxation reduced, or they usually suffer another luxation while struggling to rise.

REFERENCES

1. Tulleners EP, Nunamaker DM, Richardson DW: Coxofemoral luxations in cattle: 22 cases (1980–1985). J Am Vet Med Assoc 191:569–574, 1987.
2. Larcombe MT, Malmo J: Dislocation of the coxo-femoral joint in dairy cows. Aust Vet J 66:351–354, 1989.
3. Jubb TF, Malmo J, Brightling P, et al: Prognostic factors for recovery from coxo-femoral dislocation in cattle. Aust Vet J 66:354–358, 1989.
4. Greenough PR, MacCallum FJ, Weaver DA: Lameness in Cattle. Philadelphia, JB Lippincott, 1972, pp 255–260.
5. Piermattei DL, Greeley RG: An Atlas of Surgical Approaches to the Bones of the Dog and Cat. Philadelphia, WB Saunders, 1979, pp 132–133.

▪ Spondylitis

Bruce L. Hull, D.V.M., M.S.

Spondylitis is inflammation of one or more vertebrae. When applied to the disorder in cattle, the term *spondylitis* is generally synonymous with ankylosing spondylitis, as ankylosis and its sequelae are the causes of the clinical syndrome.

ETIOLOGY

Spondylitis is seen mostly in mature bulls housed in confinement situations. The lesion has also been observed in older cows. Degeneration of the intervertebral disk, allowing excessive intervertebral motion, is probably the initiating cause. This excessive motion in turn stimulates new bone formation around the vertebral bodies. New bone formation is most extensive ventrally but also occurs laterally. The exostosis typically affects the last two or three thoracic and first two or three lumbar vertebrae. However, the entire lumbar spine back to and including the lumbosacral joint may be involved.

CLINICAL SIGNS

Although bridging exostosis may be palpated rectally along the ventral surface of the vertebral bodies, this is not what causes the clinical signs. In fact, palpation of exostosis on the ventral surface of the vertebral bodies could almost be considered a normal finding in an older bull. In one study, 21 of 25 middle-aged dairy bulls showed evidence of vertebral osteophytosis.[1] In some animals, exostosis becomes extensive enough to actually bridge the vertebral bodies and to form a splint along these bodies.

Fracture of this splint of exostosis leads to the clinical signs. Some reports indicate that the splint fractures after a clumsy mount or after a slip. In some cases, the splint may fracture with no apparent predisposing trauma. The clinical signs generally appear suddenly and vary in severity, depending on the extent of the injury. Mild signs include difficulty in rising, reluctance to mount, and a stiff gait. The stiffness of gait may be quite severe, to the point that the animal drags its rear feet. In its most severe form, spondylitis causes a complete posterior paralysis and even absence of spinal reflexes.

Rectal palpation of the exostosis is a helpful diagnostic sign; however, not all cases of spondylitis extend into the posterior lumbar region.

TREATMENT

Treatment, especially in more severely affected animals, is probably hopeless and the destruction of the animal should be considered. Mildly affected animals may respond to stall rest and analgesics; however, the symptoms are very likely to recur, often more severely. As the signs are the result of spinal cord trauma, high doses of prednisolone for an extended period may give some relief to early cases. If used the dose is usually 0.5 mg/lb for 5 to 10 days followed by half this dose for another 5 to 10 days.

REFERENCE

1. Weisbrode SE, Monke DR, Dodaro ST, et al: Osteochondrosis, degenerative joint disease and vertebral osteophytosis in middle-aged bulls. J Am Vet Med Assoc 181:700–705, 1982.

■ Fractures

David E. Anderson, D.V.M., M.S., Diplomate, A.C.V.S.

FRACTURES IN FOOD ANIMALS

Fractures involving the limbs of farm animals are common, mostly found in young stock, and often occur subsequent to trauma during dystocia. The most common fractures diagnosed include metacarpus and metatarsus ($\sim$ 50%), tibia ($\sim$ 12%), radius and ulna ($\sim$ 7%), femur (< 5%), humerus (< 5%), pelvis (< 5%), and phalanges (< 1%).[1] Occasionally, fractures of the axial skeleton (mandible, vertebra, ribs, pelvis) are found. Food animals are considered to be excellent patients for treatment of orthopedic injuries because they spend a majority of time lying down, have a tremendous osteogenic potential, are more resistant to limb breakdown and laminitis, and usually do not resist having appliances on their limbs. The decision to treat a fracture in a food animal is made by considering the cost and success rate of the treatment, the perceived or potential economic or genetic value of the animal, and the location and type of fracture.

EMERGENCY TREATMENT AND FIRST AID

Prior to the decision for treatment, a thorough physical examination should be conducted on all animals suspected of having a fracture. However, the patient first must be made safe from continued trauma. If the animal is recumbent, it should be allowed to remain recumbent until the physical examination and fracture assessment have been conducted. Assessment of

hydration and cardiopulmonary and shock status is of utmost importance. Adequate passive antibody transfer to newborn calves is critical to preoperative preparation and success of the procedure. If colostrum ingestion is unknown, serum immunoglobulin or total protein should be determined. Calves that are hydrated and have a serum protein of less than 5.0 g/dL should be considered to have poor colostral antibody transfer and receive a plasma transfusion before attempting repair.

Temporary stabilization of limb fractures may be performed before moving the animal or attempting to get the animal to stand. As a general rule, fractures below the level of the midradius or midtibia may be temporarily stabilized with splints or casts. Field stabilization of fractures proximal to this level should not be attempted. These efforts often result in the creation of a "fulcrum effect" at the fracture site and also in increased soft tissue trauma, damage to neurovascular structures, or compounding of the fracture. Cattle with these fractures should be carefully loaded into the trailer and allowed time to lie down before beginning transport. External coaptation for temporary stabilization of the fracture may be done by using two splints or a cast. Two boards or pieces of a large polyvinyl chloride (PVC) pipe cut in half, placed 90 degrees to each other (e.g., caudal and lateral aspect of the limb), create a stable external coaptation. A padded bandage is placed on the limb, the splints positioned, and elastic tape applied firmly. The injury should be centered within the coaptation with as much support proximal and distal to the injury as possible. All external coaptation devices should extend to the ground (below the sole). For injuries distal to the carpus or hock, the splints should be placed at the level of the proximal radius or tibia, respectively. For injuries proximal to the carpus or hock and distal to the midradius or midtibia, the lateral splint should extend to the level of the proximal scapula or pelvis, respectively.

PRINCIPLES OF FRACTURE MANAGEMENT

The location of the fracture, the presence of soft tissue and neurovascular trauma, closed or open fracture environment, behavioral nature of the animal, and experience of the veterinarian are important factors in considering what type of treatment is chosen.[2] Fractures of the axial skeleton are often treated by stall rest alone, because external or internal fixation is not required. For fractures involving the appendicular skeleton, the following questions must be answered: Is treatment required? Can the fracture be acceptably reduced closed or is internal reduction required? Can the fracture be adequately immobilized using external coaptation alone, or is use of internal fixation required? What is the cost-benefit analysis?

Walking Block for Bovine Digit

Cattle have two weight-bearing digits for each limb and therefore may stand on one digit during convalescence of the paired digit (e.g., phalangeal fracture). A wooden, rubber, or plastic block (2.5 to 5.0 cm in height and formed to the size and shape of the healthy hoof) can be applied to the sole of the healthy digit. The animal is confined to a stall or small pen for 6 to 10 weeks while fracture healing proceeds and the block is removed. Often, wooden blocks will become worn and removal is not necessary.

Casting

Half-limb casts can be used for immobilization of phalangeal, distal metacarpal, or metatarsal fractures. The cast is placed from a point immediately distal to the carpus or hock extending to the ground and encasing the foot. The dewclaws and the top of the cast are padded, but only stockinette or foam padding (3M Custom Support Foam, 3M Animal Care Products) is placed on the remainder of the limb. Thick padding placed along the limb will quickly become compressed, leaving room for the limb to move within the cast and displacement of the fracture to occur. Full-limb casts are used for fractures occurring at or proximal to the midmetacarpus or metatarsus but distal to the midradius or midtibia. Full-limb casts are placed similarly to half-limb casts, but the prominences of the accessory carpal bone, styloid process of the ulna, calcaneus, and medial and lateral malleolus of the tibia must be padded.

Placement of the cast is facilitated by use of rope restraint, sedation, or anesthesia, as needed. An assistant should help to maintain alignment of the limb during application, being sure to check the position of the limb in the cranial to caudal and lateral to medial planes. Tension on the limb during casting may be obtained by placing wires through holes drilled in the hoof wall and tightening them. The hoof should be positioned in a normal to slightly flexed position. Fiberglas casting tape should be used, but the thickness of the cast is usually based on clinical judgment; casts six to eight layers thick may be used for calves less than 150 kg body weight, but adult cattle may require 12 to 16 layers thickness. Casts used on the hind limbs must be thicker because of stress concentration by the angulation of the hock. Incorporation of metal rods within the cast (two rods placed 90 degrees to each other) may be needed in extremely large patients. Scheduled cast changes at 3-week intervals may be required for rapidly growing calves or for calves that become lame during convalescence. Physeal fractures are usually healed within 4 weeks, but nonphyseal fractures often require 6 weeks to reach clinical union in calves. Fractures in adult cattle often heal within 8 to 10 weeks, but may require 12 to 16 weeks for clinical union to occur. Radiographic union of the fracture (defined as bone union with resolution of the fracture line) is not seen for weeks to months after clinical union (defined as sufficient bridging callus to allow weight bearing without additional support to the limb) has been reached.

Thomas Splint-and-Cast Combination

Use of a Thomas splint-and-cast combination is appropriate for fractures proximal to the midradius and midtibia but distal to the elbow or stifle.[3] The length of the splint should be measured from the normal limb. The fracture is reduced and a cast applied from the foot to the level of the proximal radius or tibia. The splint is placed on the limb, the foot is attached to the base of the splint by drilling holes in the hoof walls and wiring the foot to the splint base, and casting tape is used to attach the cast to the splint frame. The limb cast should be firmly attached to the splint frame to prevent rotation of the limb along the splint during ambulation. The hoop of the splint must be firmly placed into the axilla or groin to allow maximal weight transference, and therefore the hoop must be heavily padded. Cattle should be assisted to stand until they are able to rise on their own. Also, these patients must be checked several times daily to ensure that they have not lain down on top of the splint. Cattle may not be able to rise after lying down on the splint, and severe rumen tympanites may occur if they remain trapped for a prolonged period.

Transfixation Pinning and Casting and External Skeletal Fixation

Transfixation pinning and casting may be applied either as a "hanging-limb pin-cast" or as an external skeletal fixator.[2] Hanging limb pin-cast refers to placement of transfixing, or transcortical, pins through the bone proximal to the injury, followed by application of a full-limb cast. The body weight is transferred to the cast by the pins and transmitted through the cast to the ground. Therefore, the distal limb "hangs" inside the pin-cast. Pin-casts may be used for external skeletal fixation (ESF) by placing transfixation pins proximal and distal to the injury. The advantage of using pin-casts for ESF compared with hanging-limb casts is that the fracture is more stable, the fracture fragments are not able to move within the pin-cast after the swelling within the limb resolves, and the pin-cast may not need to span adjacent joints (in cattle weighing less than 300 kg). Pin selection is made based on the body weight of the animal, the size of the bone involved, and the configuration of the fracture. The diameter of the pin should not exceed 20% to 30% of the diameter of the bone. Defects larger than 30% of the diameter of the bone cause marked loss of the bone's resistance to torsion loading. In general, $\frac{3}{32}$- to $\frac{1}{8}$-in. (2.4 to 3.2 mm) pins are used in calves weighing less than 100 kg, $\frac{1}{8}$- to $\frac{3}{16}$-in. (3.2 to 4.8 mm) pins are used in cattle weighing 100 to 300 kg, $\frac{3}{16}$- to $\frac{1}{4}$-in. (4.8 to 6.4 mm) pins are used in cattle weighing 300 to 600 kg, and $\frac{1}{4}$-in. (6.4 mm) pins are used in cattle weighing more than 600 kg. Pins should be placed in the bone such that they are separated by a minimum of four times the diameter of the pin. This will minimize the risk of the concentration of mechanical forces between the two pins ("stress riser effect"). Before pin insertion, a hole should be predrilled through the bone to accommodate the pin. This hole should not be smaller than 0.5 mm less than the diameter of the pin (e.g., 2.7-mm hole for a 3.2-mm pin). Veterinary orthopedic pins are not designed to be drilled while being inserted. Therefore, significant thermal and mechanical injury occurs in the bone during insertion. Predrilling, using an orthopedic drill bit, will prevent or limit this injury.

For management of open fractures, daily access to the wound is desired. This may be accomplished by leaving a hole in the cast ("window cast") at the site of the injury, but this often gives unsatisfactory access to the wound and is uncomfortable to the patient because the swelling in the limb becomes concentrated at the defect in the cast. Alternatively, metal or acrylic side bars may be used. These side bars must be made large enough to sustain the weight of the patient.

Internal Fixation (Plate, Intramedullary Interlocking Nail)

Internal fixation of fractures has been done in cattle of high perceived economic value. In general, application of bone plates is not recommended for cattle younger than 3 months old. Calves less than 3 months old have thin cortices with limited holding power for bone screws. Recently, intramedullary interlocking nails have become available. These implants may prove to be useful for young cattle, and for management of fractures with historically poor success with bone plating (e.g., humerus fracture). Application of bone plates in cattle is similar to that for horses.

Closed vs. Open Fractures

Overall, closed fractures without damage to the blood supply to the limb have a good to excellent prognosis for healing in cattle. The prognosis is less good for older cattle or cattle of high body weight. Open fractures have a guarded prognosis for healing in cattle. The success rate depends on the severity of soft tissue damage, the bone affected, the age of the patient, the duration and degree of contamination of the wound, and the economic limitations placed on fracture management. Prolonged antibiotic therapy is indicated, and open wound management is preferable to enclosing the wound within a cast. Mature cattle are better able to overcome bone infection associated with open fractures than young calves.

TREATMENT AND PROGNOSIS OF SPECIFIC FRACTURES

Mandible

Mandibular fractures occur during dystocia or direct trauma. Fracture of one mandible may be treated by stall confinement and providing soft feed. Repair of mandible fractures is indicated if the patient has difficulty eating. Bilateral mandibular fractures usually require treatment. Intramedullary pins placed from the rostral to the caudal aspect of the body of the mandible provide adequate stabilization of fractures occurring in the rostral half of the body of the mandible. Fractures occurring rostral to the ramus of the mandible may be treated by application of an external skeletal fixator or a bone plate. Fractures occurring in the ramus of the mandible may be treated by application of a bone plate. Fractures of the mandible have a good to excellent prognosis for healing. The presence of an open wound does not significantly worsen the prognosis.

Vertebrae

Vertebral fractures occur as a result of trauma during handling for vaccination or when mounting for breeding. Vertebral fractures causing paralysis of the limbs have a grave prognosis and euthanasia is indicated. Minimally displaced fractures associated with minor neurologic deficits may be treated by stall confinement. However, progressive neurologic deficits may be seen weeks to months after the injury because of compression of the spinal cord by fibroplasia or callus. Treatment of fracture of the sacrum or caudal vertebrae may be done for cosmesis. Application of a four- or five-hole bone plate allows restoration of normal anatomy. These injuries are often associated with tail paralysis, and the prognosis for return to normal function is guarded.

Pelvis

Fractures of the ilium or sacroiliac junction are the most common pelvic fractures in cattle. These injuries occur because of falls during mounting or on slippery flooring. Fractures of the ilium or sacroiliac junction respond well to stall confinement. Ilium fractures may become open, with bone projecting through the skin. Infection rapidly becomes established and bone sequestration occurs. Surgical removal of the fracture fragment of the ilium is indicated when sepsis or debilitating lameness is present. Internal fixation of ilium fractures is rarely indicated, but may be requested for cosmetic reasons. These fractures may be repaired by application of a bone plate, but reduction of the fracture is often difficult or impossible.

Rib

Rib fractures usually occur during manual extraction for dystocia but may be caused by rough handling in restraint chutes. Treatment of rib fractures is not indicated unless flail chest is present or lung injury is imminent. Owners should be warned that fracture of the first three ribs may cause progressive tracheal collapse weeks to months after injury. Tracheal collapse is caused by compression of the trachea by the forming callus or by the fibrous tissue response to the injury. When this occurs, rib resection is indicated.

Humerus

Nonarticular, minimally displaced fractures of the humerus are best treated by stall confinement. Open reduction and internal fixation of the humerus with bone plates may cause permanent radial nerve paralysis. Use of an intramedullary interlocking nail may allow rigid fixation with minimal risk of radial nerve injury. The prognosis for healing the fracture with stall confinement is good, but the prognosis for return to normal productivity is guarded. Severely displaced or articular fracture of the humerus requires attempted internal fixation, but the prognosis is guarded to poor for return to normal productive use.

Radius and Ulna

Closed fractures of the distal physis of the radius may be treated by a full-limb cast and have a good prognosis for success. Fracture of the midradius and ulna requires use of a Thomas splint-cast, transfixation pinning and casting, or bone plating. The prognosis for healing is good, but significant contralateral limb injury may occur in animals treated by the Thomas splint-cast. Transfixation pinning and casting and bone plating have good to excellent prognoses with minimal risk of permanent injury to the contralateral limb.

Femur

Femoral fractures most often occur in calves during forced extraction for dystocia but occasionally are found in adult cattle after falling during mounting or on slippery flooring. Femoral fractures in mature cattle have a grave prognosis because of body weight and an inability to reduce the fracture. Capital physeal fractures (fracture through the physis of the head of the femur) in mature cattle may be successfully repaired using cross-pins or cannulated screws.[4, 5] Selected femoral fractures may respond to stall rest for 8 to 10 weeks. These cattle require assistance in standing during the first 2 to 4 weeks after the injury. In calves, stack pinning of the femur has a good prognosis for success.[6] Open reduction of the fracture is performed, and two to five intramedullary pins are placed into the femur. If large cortical defects are present, then an external skeletal fixator may be applied in addition to the intramedullary pins. These fractures are usually healed by 6 weeks after surgery. Sepsis is the most common reason for failure of fracture healing.

Tibia

Although fracture of the tibia has been seen as a result of forced extraction during dystocia, tibia fractures are usually caused by trauma. Fracture of the distal physis of the tibia may be treated with a full-limb cast, but these fractures are uncommon. Fractures of the middle portion of the tibia are treated similarly to fractures of the radius and have similar complications.

Metacarpus and Metatarsus III/IV

Fractures involving the metacarpus (MC) or metatarsus (MT) III/IV are the most common fractures to occur in food animals. Closed fracture of the distal physis of the MC or MT may be treated using a half-limb cast. Closed fracture of the middle portion of the MC or MT may be treated with a full-limb cast. Open fractures in mature cattle may be treated by debriding and flushing the wound, applying a full-limb cast, and administering antibiotics for 10 to 14 days. In valuable cattle and young calves, open fractures are best treated by use of an external skeletal fixator and daily wound care until healed. Bone sequestra are often present in open fractures, and healing may not occur until these have been removed. If prolonged sepsis has been present, cancellous bone grafts may facilitate bone union. The optimal sites for harvesting cancellous bone grafts are the wing of the ilium and the proximal tibia. Also, implantation of antibiotic-impregnated bone cement beads will provide prolonged local release of antibiotics.

Phalanges

Closed fractures of the phalanges may be treated by application of a block (see Walking Block for Bovine Digit).

REFERENCES

1. Ferguson JG: Management and repair of bovine fractures. Compendium Continuing Educ Pract Vet 4:S128–135, 1982.
2. Anderson DE, St Jean G: External skeletal fixation in ruminants. Vet Clin North Am Food Anim Pract 12:117–152, 1996.
3. Anderson DE, St Jean G, Vestweber JG, et al: Use of a Thomas splint-cast combination for stabilization of tibial fractures in cattle: 21 cases (1973–1993). Agri Pract 15:16–23, 1994.
4. Wilson DG, Crawford WH, Stone WC, et al: Fixation of femoral capital physeal fractures with 7.0 mm cannulated screws in five bulls. Vet Surg 20:240–244, 1991.
5. Hull BL, Koenig GJ, Monke DR: Treatment of slipped capital femoral epiphysis in cattle: 11 cases (1974–1988). J Am Vet Med Assoc 197:1509–1512, 1990.
6. St Jean G, DeBowes RM, Hull BL, et al: Intramedullary pinning of femoral diaphyseal fractures in neonatal calves: 12 cases (1980–1990). J Am Vet Med Assoc 200:1372–1376, 1992.

■ Tendon Injuries in Cattle

David E. Anderson, D.V.M., M.S., Diplomate, A.C.V.S.

Tendon injuries in cattle can be classified as congenital, developmental, or acquired. Tendon injuries are common in cattle but are frequently overlooked as part of a more severe disease complex. Most congenital and developmental defects occur as tendon contraction. Acquired tendon injury occurs as tendon disruption or tendon sheath infection.

CONTRACTED TENDONS

Contracted tendons may be present at birth or develop in rapidly growing calves. Congenital tendon contracture may be caused by malpositioning of the calf in the uterus or ingestion of toxins by the cow during early gestation (e.g., ingestion of lupine plants between 40 and 70 days' gestation), or be associated with arthrogryposis caused by in utero infection with Akabane virus or bluetongue virus, or by an inherited disorder (arthrogryposis and cleft palate of Charolais cattle, simple autosomal recessive gene).[1, 2] Contracted tendons caused by toxins, viral infection, or inherited disorders are usually severe, associated with arthrogryposis, and have a poor prognosis for correction and survival. Affected calves are usually euthanized. When treatment is attempted, tenotomy of the superficial and deep digital flexor tendons, in addition to transection of the caudal and palmar joint capsules of the carpus and fetlock, respectively, may be required to straighten the limb. If this is done, splinting or casting of the limb for 4 to 8 weeks may be required to allow the flexor tendons to heal. Contracted tendons caused by malpositioning in the uterus of calves usually is seen in large-birth-weight calves with rapid growth rates. For flexor tendon contracture in which the sole of the foot does not come into contact with the ground, physical therapy and splinting or casting are indicated. Casting alone is only indicated for calves in which the limb can be straightened and held in a near-normal conformation. For calves in which the limb cannot be straightened, daily physical therapy in addition to splinting of the limb usually will effect a cure. Constant splinting of the limb for 2 to 4 days followed by a regimen of 12 hours' splinting and 12 hours off, during which forced exercise and physical therapy are done, for 5 to 7 days may be used. Physical therapy is done by forcibly extending the limb to the maximum allowable extent for 20 to 40 cycles over a 10- to 15-minute period done two to three times during the 12 hours that the splint is off. If sufficient improvement is not observed after 7 to 10 days, then tenotomy of the most severely affected flexor tendon should be considered. Once the limb has been corrected to a near-normal conformation, forced exercise is needed to complete rehabilitation. Placement of extended toe splints on the hoofs will increase tension on the flexor tendons during ambulation. Toe splints are easily applied by using hoof acrylic to form an extension onto the hoof wall at the toe. These extensions will usually remain in place for 2 to 3 weeks, at which time the calf should no longer require assistance. Administration of nonsteroidal anti-inflammatory drugs will provide analgesia and increase voluntary exercise. Developmental contracted tendons usually occur in 6- to 10-month-old show calves when they are being fed for maximal growth. Affected calves are usually presented with a complaint of "standing on the toes." These calves have an upright or slightly flexed joint posture at the fetlock, but the dorsal one third of the sole still contacts the ground. Extended toe splints, forced exercise, and limitation of concentrate feeding will usually effect a cure. Application of a half-limb cast after forced extension of the fetlock can be used for 3 to 4 weeks.

TENDON LACERATION AND DISRUPTION

Tendon laceration occurs most commonly in adult, female, dairy breed cattle. These injuries are usually caused by accidents involving farm machinery (72%) and the multiple flexor tendons most often are involved (70%).[3] An open wound is almost always present and the injury most commonly occurs at the proximal or midmetatarsus. The tendons of affected cattle should be immobilized as soon as possible to prevent further injury to the neurovascular structures of the distal limb. The wound should be cleaned and debrided and the tendons inspected. If the laceration involves the flexor tendons of a single digit, treatment may be done using a wooden claw block attached to the sole of the healthy digit. If the flexor tendons of both digits are involved, then external coaptation, with or without tenorrhaphy, is indicated. In one retrospective study, the outcome was not improved by the use of tenorrhaphy.[3] External coaptation is needed for approximately 10 weeks (74 ± 34 days), with an additional 2 weeks of confinement (total convalescence of 88 ±

60 days).[3] The prognosis for return to productivity (87%) and long-term productivity (73%) is good. Long-term complications include persistent lameness (56%) and hyperextension of the digits (19%).

Tendon disruption may occur secondary to sepsis and tendon necrosis. The deep digital flexor tendon is most commonly involved because of avulsion from the third phalanx as an extension of the sole ulcer complex. Treatment is performed by debridement and cleaning of the wound and providing support for the tendon. Tendon repair by fibroplasia will occur if the initiating disease is resolved.

TENOSYNOVITIS

Tenosynovitis most commonly involves the digital flexor tendon sheath, is caused by a laceration or puncture wound, and is septic. Affected cattle do not bear weight or bear minimal weight on the limb. Distention of the flexor tendon sheath is noted by swelling immediately proximal to the dewclaws. Synovial fluid analysis is diagnostic (nucleated cell count [NCC] > 50,000 cells per microliter; total protein > 5.0 g/dL). Surgical debridement and implantation of a drain within the sheath for 5 to 7 days is the treatment of choice.[4] Antibiotics should be administered for 14 to 21 days. The prognosis for return to productivity is good when intensive treatment is initiated early in the process of the disease. If flexor tendon disruption has occurred, the prognosis is poor.

REFERENCES

1. Leipold HW, Hiraga T, Dennis SM: Congenital defects of the bovine musculoskeletal system and joints. Vet Clin North Am Food Anim Pract 9:93–104, 1993.
2. Anderson DE, St-Jean G: Diagnosis and management of tendon disorders in cattle. Vet Clin North Am Food Anim Pract 12:85–116, 1996.
3. Anderson DE, St-Jean G, Morin DE, et al: Traumatic flexor tendon injuries in 27 cattle. Vet Surg 25:320–326, 1996.
4. Anderson DE, Allen D, St-Jean G, et al: Use of a multifenestrated indwelling lavage system for treatment of septic digital tenosynovitis in cattle. Aust Vet J 75:796–799, 1997.

■ Osteomyelitis

Bimbo Welker, D.V.M., M.S.

Septic inflammation of the cortical and medullary components of bone is called osteomyelitis. In food animals it is most commonly a result of either hemotogenous spread of infection or contamination of bone as a sequela to trauma. The clinical signs, treatment, and prognosis of osteomyelitis will depend on the route of infection, the age and immune status of the animal, the virulence and susceptibility of the organism, and the chronicity of the problem.

PATHOPHYSIOLOGY

Osteomyelitis is caused by bacterial infection which originates in or is spread by the blood, or from wounds. Neonates are more commonly affected as a result of immunocompromise due to partial or total failure of passive transfer and the fact that long bone fractures are seen with a higher frequency in younger cattle. The typical sites of infection resulting from hematogenous spread are the joints and the ends of long bones. The architectural arrangement of the vasculature in the metaphyseal and epiphyseal regions creates blood flow patterns more conducive to bacterial colonization. The medullary vessels that course toward the metaphysis of immature long bones terminate in small capillaries that loop back onto themselves and empty into wider-diameter venous sinusoids. This creates a condition of low blood flow and pressure. The result is thought to be conducive to bacterial invasion, proliferation, and cellular infiltration. Occlusion of the vessels and subsequent necrosis of the bone ensues. As the animal ages the vascular patterns change with the nutrient vessels anastomosing with the epiphyseal arteries, thus eliminating the sluggish blood flow phenomenon.

Open fractures, deep wounds, foreign bodies, and soft tissue infections can all lead to the development of secondary osteomyelitis. The sequence of events is similar pathophysiologically, except for the source of the bacteria and the location of the infection.

The organisms most commonly isolated from cases of osteomyelitis resulting from hematogenous spread include *Pasteurella* spp. and *Salmonella* spp. Typical isolates from contaminated wounds include coliforms, *Staphylococcus* spp., *Streptococcus* spp., and *Actinomyces* spp.

The immune status of the animal plays a very important role in the outcome of bacterial invasion. Osteomyelitis is much more likely to occur in immunocompromised individuals. If infection occurs the body may mount a defense that can totally eliminate the infection or at least attenuate it or wall it off. Unchallenged, the infection may progressively destroy surrounding bone, joint, and soft tissue.

CLINICAL SIGNS AND DIAGNOSIS

Osteomyelitis should be a consideration in any calf presented for acute onset of lameness or with a history of trauma. In the initial stages of hematogenous osteomyelitis there may be minimal or no evidence of swelling unless there is concomitant septic osteoarthritis. The temperature and even the white blood cell count may be only mildly elevated or within normal limits. If there is a primary source of infection elsewhere in the body responsible for the bacteremia, then clinical signs associated with that source may predominate. As the infection develops, swelling and pain on deep palpation will become more evident. The temperature will respond accordingly. Unfortunately, by this time the infection has had several days to become established. Because of the anatomy of the vasculature, most of these cases will be found associated with the metaphyseal, physeal, or epiphyseal regions of the bone. If trauma was the predisposing cause, then the location can include any area, and the addition of crepitation on palpation may help in establishing an earlier diagnosis.

Radiographs of the area of pain and swelling may show evidence of osteomyelitis—bone lysis (radiolucency), sclerosis, and possibly sequestra, although sequestra will not become radiographically visible for 5 to 7 days. Therefore, if the radiographs are negative on the initial examination they should be repeated if the problem is not resolving with therapy. As the process fulminates, new bone formation will be evident along with extensive osteolysis, soft tissue swelling, and abscessation.

TREATMENT

The basic principles of treatment of osteomyelitis include debridement, removal of infected and necrotic material, stabilization when indicated, and aggressive antibiotic therapy. Antibiotic therapy should be based on susceptibility patterns when available or on the commonly known infectious organisms. The antibiotic should be broad-spectrum and have good bone-penetrating ability, and attention must be paid to the milk and meat withholding period. Therapy should continue for a minimum of 3 weeks and in many cases longer. The infected site should be surgically debrided and stabilized. Analgesics are of value in controlling the pain associated with the infection and the debridement.

The immunoglobulin status of calves should be evaluated in all cases. If a deficiency is found, appropriate immunoglobulin therapy is necessary.

The prognosis of osteomyelitis is dependent on the severity, duration, and aggressiveness of therapy. Localized cases treated early and aggressively with appropriate therapy should respond well. When the cases go undiagnosed or unrecognized for days before therapy is instituted, a poorer prognosis may be expected.

BIBLIOGRAPHY

Ames NK: Current Veterinary Therapy, ed 2. Philadelphia, WB Saunders, 1986, pp 892–893.
Auer JA: Equine Surgery. Philadelphia, WB Saunders, 1992, pp 932–939.
Greenough PR, Weaver DA: Lameness in Cattle, ed 3. Philadelphia, WB Saunders, 1997, pp 242–244.
Martins RJ, Auer JA, Carter GK: Equine pediatrics: Septic arthritis and osteomyelitis. J Am Vet Med Assoc 188:582–585.

■ Super Foot Rot

Charles Guard, D.V.M. Ph.D.

Treatment-resistant foot rot has been diagnosed as a herd problem on dairies in North America since January 1993; it is characterized as difficult to treat and leads to variable to severe losses within affected herds. Eleven affected farms visited by me were all freestall-housed and ranged in population from 70 to 700 cows. At the onset of the problem, there were typically about 8% of cows affected within the first month. During the ensuing months, foot rot cases became less frequent, and in most herds the problem disappeared after about 6 months.

CLINICAL DESCRIPTION

Reports of dairy cows with foot rot that was difficult to treat were made to me in January 1993. The descriptions were of typical-appearing foot rot that failed to respond to conventional therapy[1, 2]; it was dubbed "super foot rot." The following observations were made of an affected herd of 550 milking cows that used a walk-through foot bath with 5.0% copper sulfate or 0.1% tetracycline daily. Twelve affected cows were restrained on a tilt table and examined. The cows were severely lame. The affected legs were swollen from the region of the dewclaws distally. The claws had no lesions. The skin of the interdigital space was split, and the tissue beneath was necrotic and bloody. A foul odor was present. Seven of the cows had been affected for about 1 week and had evidence of claw separation between the horny and sensitive laminae around the coronary band. The owner reported that nine cows had sloughed one or more claws and had been euthanized. In the more severely affected cows, it was possible to insert four fingers 6 to 8 cm into the interdigital fissure where the necrosis was extensive. The owner reported that about 20 cows had been sold or had died due to foot rot since the outbreak began. Treatments had included parenteral penicillin, ampicillin, and oxytetracycline. Topical treatment was with copper sulfate and ichthammol. None of the treatments had seemed effective.

Transmission from affected to new herds in some instances appears to have followed the introduction of infected cattle. It also seems that the disease may be spread by contaminated hoof-trimming instruments or contaminated trucks and trailers. In these cases the disease usually appears 7 to 10 days after contamination.

DIAGNOSIS

The appearance of cases of super foot rot is identical to that of the more common treatment-responsive foot rot but for which treatment was delayed or inappropriate. Affected cattle become acutely lame with diffuse, symmetrical swelling beginning at the level of the coronary band and progressing proximally. In some cases, there is no obvious fissure in the interdigital skin at first examination. Within 2 days there is extensive interdigital necrosis with a defect in the interdigital tissues. The odor associated with the necrosis is typical of *Fusobacterium necrophorum*. The disease does not seem to be self-limiting; super foot rot in many cows has resulted in recumbency and humane slaughter or euthanasia. In cases of super foot rot, there is often a trail of exudate left on the floor as the cow walks resulting from the rapid liquefaction of affected tissues. Differentiation of super foot rot from nonresistant foot rot is commonly made by failure to respond to conventional treatments with penicillin, amoxicillin, sulfonamides, or tetracyclines. A similar syndrome of treatment-resistant foot rot has been described in the United Kingdom.

Swabs and tissue samples from interdigital lesions were submitted for anaerobic bacteriology study to the New York State Veterinary Diagnostic Laboratory. Under anaerobic conditions *F. necrophorum* and *Bacteroides melaninogenicus* were isolated. These bacteria are considered the primary pathogens in classic interdigital necrobacillosis, or foot rot.[3] However, sensitivity testing of these isolates revealed extensive resistance to commonly used antimicrobials. Testing for sensitivity to sulfonamides was not performed.

TREATMENT

Treatment with erythromycin was tried in four cows with no apparent benefit. Treatments that have been effective are parenteral ceftiofur (Naxcel, Pharmacia & Upjohn) at 1.1 mg/kg s.i.d. or tylosin (Tylan, Elanco Animal Health) at 17 mg/kg s.i.d. and local treatment with a topical poultice of lincomycin and spectinomycin powder (L-S 50, Pharmacia & Upjohn). Following this protocol for 5 to 10 days resulted in some cases that were cured and a reduction to one case in five that went to slaughter. Similar response to treatment has been reported with 5 to 8 days of sulfadimethoxine (Albon Injection 40%, Pfizer Animal Health).

PREVENTION

Adding to the frustration in dealing with this disease has been the apparent failure of preventive foot-bathing programs to alter the incidence of cases. There has been no perceived benefit from daily foot bathing in 5% copper sulfate, 5% or 10% zinc sulfate, 0.1% to 0.4% tetracycline, or 5.0% formalin. One herdsman felt that there were more cases when the tetracycline foot bath was in use. The failure of prevention through foot bathing suggests additional *F. necrophorum* virulence factors or unrecognized environmental effects that promote super foot rot. Cases have only occurred in lactating and dry cows, with a noticeably higher rate in older cows. The hygiene in the barns of affected herds has ranged from exemplary to average.

REFERENCES

1. Berg JN, Loan RW: *Fusobacterium necrophorum* and *Bacteroides melaninogenicus* as etiologic agents of foot rot in cattle. Am J Vet Res 47:1422, 1986.
2. Braun K, Bates D, Shearer JK, et al: Efficacy of amoxicillin trihydrate for the treatment of experimentally induced foot rot in cattle. Am J Vet Res 48:175, 1987.
3. Rebhun WC, Person EG: Clinical management of bovine foot problems. J Am Vet Med Assoc 181:572, 1982.
4. Cook NB, Cutler KL: Treatment and outcome of a severe form of foul-in-the-foot. Vet Rec 136:19, 1995.

▪ Digital Dermatitis

Charles Guard, D.V.M., Ph.D.

A relatively new infectious disease of unknown etiology that causes lameness in cattle has become widespread in most regions of the world where modern dairying is practiced. The condition is called hairy heel warts, strawberry foot, verrucous dermatitis, digital warts, interdigital papillomatosis, and probably most correctly, digital dermatitis. The condition is identical to that described by various authors in Europe and North America and known as mortellaro after one of the Italian writers who described it in 1974.[1] The condition was seen as a few isolated cases in New York in 1979[2] and then it disappeared until the mid-1980s. Within the last 4 years the disease has developed to epidemic proportions in northern Europe and spread throughout the United States.

CLINICAL DESCRIPTION

Digital dermatitis occurs as a herd problem. The spread through the herd will be faster in moist conditions such as in a freestall barn than in a stanchion barn. In the desert, transmission from cow to cow may be extremely slow. The earliest lesion recognizable as digital dermatitis is a reddened circumscribed area typically just above the interdigital cleft on the plantar aspect of the pastern, with erect and elongated hair. This progresses to hair loss and a moist granular surface, the strawberry lesion. These lesions bleed very easily, as when wiped with cotton. The most striking feature of the lesion is the degree of pain expressed by the cow. Hairs at the periphery of the lesion are often erect and matted in exudate to form a rim. As the lesion progresses, focal hypertrophy of the dermis and epidermis leads to raised conical projections appearing much like wet, gray terry cloth. At later stages, papilliform projections of blackened keratin may extend 10 to 15 mm from the surface, the hairy wart stage. In even more advanced lesions, a cauliflower-like tumor will develop with a pedunculated base.

Many cows have simultaneous infection with *Dichelobacter nodosus* leading to significant erosion of the horn of the heels in a hemispheric pattern surrounding the axial space. The hoof may be noticeably overgrown in the heel region from reduced wear caused by altered use of the limb. Interdigital fibromas regardless of cause are commonly infected with digital dermatitis in herds where the disease is endemic. In my experience, after digital dermatitis has been present in a herd for a year or so, most cases of lameness are found in the first-lactation animals even though lesions may be seen on the digits of older cows during routine hoof trimming or other inspections.

Cattle of all breeds are susceptible to digital dermatitis. The disease has so far been seen primarily in dairy cattle with most herds recognizing the problem only in animals of lactating age. Cattle as young as 4 months old are susceptible to developing digital dermatitis. Conditions predisposing to infection are chronically moist digital skin and exposure to the agent(s). Lesions of digital dermatitis have not been recognized proximal to the dewclaws. Some cattle may develop immunity to digital dermatitis; however, some cattle definitely do not become immune and are repeatedly lame during periods of at least 4 years. A currently inexplicable feature of digital dermatitis is the waxing and waning of pain as evidenced by lameness without detectable changes in the causative lesion. This feature makes the evaluation of interventions problematic.

DIAGNOSIS

Diagnosis of the disease is based on the recognition of one of the various stages of digital dermatitis lesions. The skin will have a circumscribed, well-demarcated area of moist, granular to proliferative dermatitis, primarily on the plantar surface of the rear digits. The lesions are extremely painful to slight pressure. Typically, numerous members of a herd are affected. Prevalence can reach 80% of adults in a dairy herd with no control program in place.

After early histologic and ultrastructural studies revealed a lesion similar to that caused by a papilloma virus, Guard and Carmichael[3] and Read et al.[4] used bovine papilloma virus gene probes on tissue specimens from many cases and found no evidence of papilloma virus DNA in any.[4] Dutch researchers observed a spirochete in specially stained samples of lesions in 1981.[5] There were reports in 1992 from California that two distinct spirochetes had been identified in material from cases there.[4] Another laboratory has reported routinely finding in digital dermatitis lesions a gram-negative, spiral-shaped, motile rod which is so far unidentified.[6] Specimens from lesions may be submitted to diagnostic laboratories and examined histologically for the presence of spirochetes with the use of special stains. The initial event in the development of digital dermatitis is a folliculitis with infiltration of inflammatory cells throughout the dermis. Hyperkeratosis develops as capillaries proliferate in the dermis. Spirochetes may be seen throughout the epidermis and at the apex of dermal papillae.

TREATMENT

I had been recommending topical treatment with formaldehyde solutions and routine foot bathing with 5% formalin as a control program with generally good results. No one likes working with formalin and it has been prohibited in some districts for foot bathing by state environmental regulatory officials. A topical tetracycline and gentian violet wound spray has been in routine use in Europe for some time for individual treatment of digital dermatitis lesions. I now recommend topical tetracycline in the form of 5 to 15 mL of injectable oxytetracycline, tetracycline powder, or lincomycin powder applied on a cotton dressing with a flimsy wrap. Since the response is rapid, bandages should be removed in 3 days to prevent other problems developing under the dressing.

For very large proliferative lesions, surgical removal under local anesthesia may be more effective than topical medication for prompt resolution. The numerous recesses in the tissue mass preclude topical applications of antibiotics from reaching all infected regions.

PREVENTION

For many herds, the use of walk-through foot baths with antibiotic solutions have been successful in providing adequate herd level control. Solutions of tetracycline at 0.1% to 0.4% or lincomycin at 0.01% should be used at intervals appropriate to the prevalence and severity of the disease in the herd. In the United States this is an extralabel drug use and must be undertaken with veterinary involvement. The cheapest current source is a poultry water medication that is 70% active ingredient and goes by various names, including "324" (324 g/lb). In addition, another once-weekly foot bath of 5% to 10% copper sulfate or zinc sulfate seems to provide acceptable control of foot rot and interdigital dermatitis.

Some dairymen are making a solution of either tetracycline or lincomycin and spraying the feet of lame cows daily for a few days as an alternative to foot bathing. Florida researchers have recommended spraying all feet of all cows daily for several days at about monthly intervals to control digital dermatitis in drylot dairies.[7]

REFERENCES

1. Cheli R, Mortellaro C: Digital dermatitis in cattle [in Italian]. *In* Proceedings of the Eighth Meeting on Diseases of Cattle, Milan, September 1974, p. 208.
2. Rebhun WC, Payne RM, King JM, et al: Interdigital papillomatosis in dairy cattle. J Am Vet Med Assoc 177:437, 1980.
3. Guard CL, Carmichael LE: Unpublished data, 1989.
4. Read DH, Walker RL, Castro AE: An invasive spirochaete associated with interdigital papillomatosis of dairy cattle. Vet Rec 130:59, 1992.
5. Cornelisse JL, Peterse DL, Toussaint Raven E: A digital disorder in dairy cattle. Dermatitis digitalis? [in Dutch]. Tijdschr Diergeneesk, 106:452, 1981.
6. Leedle JAZ, Gaines JD: Isolation and characterization of a novel, actively motile, spiral-shaped bacterium from a bovine digital papilloma (abstract). Presented at 74th Annual Meeting, Conference of Research Workers in Animal Disease, Chicago 1993, p. 26.
7. Shearer JK, Elliot JB, Injoque RE: Control of digital dermatitis in dairy herds using a topical spray application of oxytetracycline. J Dairy Sci 78 (suppl 1):170, 1995.

Dermatologic Diseases

Consulting Editor

Jimmy L. Howard, D.V.M., M.S., Diplomate, A.B.V.P.

■ Viral Skin Diseases

Danny W. Scott, D.V.M., Diplomate, A.C.V.D.

Cutaneous lesions may be the only feature associated with a viral infection, or they may be part of a more generalized disease. A clinical examination of the skin often provides valuable information that assists the veterinarian in the differential diagnosis of several viral disorders.

An in-depth discussion of all the viral diseases—especially their extracutaneous clinical signs and pathology and their elaborate diagnostic and control schemata—is beyond the scope of this section. The reader is referred to appropriate sections of this text for details.

POXVIRUS INFECTIONS

The Poxviridae are a large family of DNA viruses. The genera include *Orthopoxvirus* (cowpox, vaccinia), *Capripoxvirus* (sheeppox, goatpox, bovine lumpy skin disease), *Suipoxvirus* (swinepox), *Parapoxvirus* (pseudocowpox, bovine papular stomatitis, contagious viral pustular dermatitis), and other unclassified poxviruses (ovine viral ulcerative dermatosis).

Pox lesions in the skin have a typical clinical evolution, beginning as erythematous macules and becoming papular and then vesicular. The vesicular stage is well developed in some pox infections and transient to nonexistent in others. Vesicles evolve into umbilicated pustules with a depressed center and a raised, often erythematous border. This lesion is the so-called pock. The pustules rupture and form a crust. Healed lesions often leave a scar.

Many of the poxviruses of food animals can produce skin lesions in humans: vaccinia, cowpox, goatpox, pseudocowpox, bovine papular stomatitis, and contagious viral pustular dermatitis. The most commonly zoonotic of these are contagious viral pustular dermatitis (orf, contagious ecthyma), pseudocowpox, and bovine papular stomatitis (milker's nodule).

Vaccinia. The orthopoxvirus that causes vaccinia is known to infect cattle and swine, producing syndromes clinically identical to cowpox and swinepox, respectively.

Cowpox. Cowpox is a rare disease of cattle in Europe. Tenderness of the teats is followed by the typical cutaneous sequence of events leading to pocks. The classic thick, red crust, ranging in diameter from 1 to 2 cm, is reported to be pathognomonic. In typical cases of cowpox, lesions are confined to the teats and udder. In severe cases, lesions may be seen on the medial thighs, perineum, vulva, scrotum of bulls, and mouth of nursing calves.

Sheeppox. Sheeppox is the most serious of the pox diseases and occurs in Africa, Asia, and the Middle East. Skin lesions follow a typical pock evolutionary sequence and have a predilec-tion for the eyelids, cheeks, nostrils, ears, neck, axillae, groin, prepuce, vulva, udder, scrotum, and ventral surface of the tail.

Goatpox. Goatpox occurs in Africa, Asia, Europe, and the United States. Skin lesions may or may not follow a typical pock evolutionary sequence and have a predilection for the head, neck, ears, axillae, groin, perineum, and ventral surface of the tail. Some outbreaks are characterized by only muzzle and lip lesions, whereas others involve only the udder, teats, scrotum, prepuce, perineum, and ventral tail.

Bovine Lumpy Skin Disease. Lumpy skin disease is an acute to subacute infectious disease of cattle in Africa. There is a sudden appearance of multiple papules and nodules. The lesions are firm, well circumscribed, and flattened and may be generalized or fairly localized. The neck, chest, back, legs, perineum, udder, and scrotum are commonly affected. Although the lesions can persist for months, they usually proceed to necrosis and disappear within 4 to 12 weeks. A narrow moat forms around the lesions and separates them from normal skin. These so-called sit-fasts then slough, leaving crateriform ulcers that heal by scarring.

Swinepox. Swinepox occurs worldwide and is endemic in areas of intensive swine production. Skin lesions follow the typical gross pock sequence and occur most commonly on the ventrolateral abdomen and thorax and the medial thighs and forelegs.

Pseudocowpox. Pseudocowpox is a common parapoxvirus infection of cattle throughout the world. Typically, the first clinical signs are focal edema, erythema, and pain of affected teats. A small orange papule develops, followed by the formation of a dark-red crust. The edges of the lesions extend peripherally, and the central crust may appear umbilicated. Peripheral extension of the lesion continues, and the central area of the crust begins to desquamate, leaving a slightly raised crust commonly called a ring or horseshoe scab. This type of crust is said to be pathognomonic. Lesions occur on the teats and udder and, occasionally, the medial thighs and perineum.

Bovine Papular Stomatitis. In bovine papular stomatitis, which is found worldwide, initial lesions are erythematous macules, which evolve into papules. These papules then undergo central necrosis and become encrusted and often papillomatous. Lesions occur most commonly on the muzzle, nostrils, and lips and occasionally on the sides, abdomen, hind legs, scrotum, and prepuce. A chronic form of the disease results in a proliferative and necrotizing stomatitis and a generalized, multifocal exudative and necrotizing dermatitis. Bovine papular stomatitis has also been incriminated as a cause of the so-called rat-tail syndrome in cattle.

Contagious Viral Pustular Dermatitis. Contagious viral pustular dermatitis is a cosmopolitan disease (contagious ecthyma, sore mouth, orf) of sheep and goats. Lesions usually occur on the lips, muzzle, nostrils, and eyelids. In severe cases, they may be seen on the genitals, perineum, coronets, interdigital spaces, pasterns, fetlocks, and oral cavity. Skin lesions follow a typical pock progression but are quite proliferative.

Ovine Viral Ulcerative Dermatosis. Ovine viral ulcerative dermatosis occurs throughout the world and is also known as ovine venereal disease and lip and leg ulcer. Granulating ulcers, 1 to 5 cm in diameter, containing pus and adherent crusts, are present in the skin between the upper lips and nostrils, on the cranial and lateral aspect of the feet above the coronets, and interdigitally.

HERPESVIRUS INFECTIONS

Infectious Bovine Rhinotracheitis. Infectious bovine rhinotracheitis occurs worldwide and is caused by bovine herpesvirus 1. Skin lesions include erythema, pustules, necrosis, and ulceration of the muzzle or the vulva or both. Rarely, pustules, crusts, oozing, alopecia, and lichenification may be seen in the perineal and scrotal areas.

Bovine Herpes Mammillitis. Bovine herpes mammillitis occurs worldwide and is caused by bovine herpesvirus 2. Skin lesions may be confined to one teat or involve several and may extend to the udder and perineum. Classically, the disease is sudden in onset, with swollen, tender teats. Vesicles may be seen, but in many cases the epithelium simply sloughs. The severity of the dermatitis varies from lines of erythema, often in circles, which enclose dry skin or papules with occasional ulceration, to annular red to blue plaques, which evolve into shallow 0.5- to 2.0-cm ulcers, to large areas of bluish discoloration, necrosis, slough, ulceration, and serum exudation.

Bovine Pseudolumpy Skin Disease. This skin disorder is also caused by bovine herpesvirus 2 and is found worldwide. Skin lesions are similar in distribution and appearance to those of true lumpy skin disease but are located much more superficially in the skin (slightly raised plaques with a central depression and superficial necrosis).

Bovine Herpes Mammary Pustular Dermatitis. This type of dermatitis, associated with bovine herpesvirus 4, has been reported from the United States. Lesions consist of multiple 1- to 10-mm vesicles and pustules on the lateral and ventral aspects of the udder.

Bovine Malignant Catarrhal Fever. This sporadic, acute, highly fatal systemic disease affects cattle in most parts of the world. Skin lesions include erythema, scaling, necrosis, and ulceration of the muzzle, the face, and, occasionally, the udder, teats, vulva, and scrotum. In addition, purplish discolorations, papules, crusts, thickening, oozing, and necrosis may affect the skin of the perineal, axillary, inguinal, and back regions. Similar dermatologic lesions may occur at the coronet, horn-skin junction, and caudal pastern area and may result in sloughing of hooves or horns.

Pseudorabies. Pseudorabies (Aujeszky's disease, "mad itch") is an acute, rapidly fatal herpesvirus infection that is worldwide in distribution. In ruminants and occasionally in swine, pseudorabies causes an intense, localized, unilateral pruritus with frenzied, violent licking, chewing, rubbing, and kicking at the affected area. Any part of the body may be affected, especially the head, neck, thorax, flanks, and perineum. Severe excoriations are produced.

TOGAVIRUS INFECTIONS

Hog Cholera. Hog cholera is a highly infectious disease of swine caused by a *Pestivirus* that remains a problem in South America, parts of Europe, Asia, and Africa. Early cutaneous lesions consist of erythema and then purplish discoloration of the abdomen, snout, ears, and medial thighs. Areas of necrosis

may develop on the pinnae, tail, and vulva. Chronically diseased swine develop a characteristic purplish blotching of the pinnae and generalized hypotrichosis.

Bovine Virus Diarrhea. Bovine virus diarrhea (mucosal disease) occurs worldwide and is caused by a *Pestivirus*. Skin lesions begin as discrete erosions, which may coalesce and lead to necrosis of the muzzle, lips, and nostrils. Similar lesions may be present on the vulva, prepuce, coronet, and interdigital space. Occasionally, crusts, scales, and alopecia occur on the perineum, medial thighs, and neck.

Ovine Border Disease. Ovine border disease is a congenital infectious disease reported in most parts of the world. It results in an abnormal fleece (hairy shakers, fuzzies) and frequently a darkly pigmented area of fleece on the back of the neck.

PICORNAVIRUS INFECTIONS

Foot-and-Mouth Disease. Foot-and-mouth disease is a highly contagious infectious disease (aphthous fever) of cattle, sheep, goats, and swine. Clinical signs include vesicles and bullae, which rupture to leave painful erosions in the mouth and on the muzzle, nostrils, coronet, interdigital spaces, udder, and teats. Occasionally, hooves may be sloughed.

Vesicular Exanthema. Vesicular exanthema, a calicivirus infection of swine, has not been reported in the United States since 1959. Clinical signs include vesicles and painful erosions on the snout, legs, oral mucosa, coronet, interdigital spaces, and occasionally the udder and teats.

Swine Vesicular Disease. An acute infectious disease, swine vesicular disease occurs in Africa, Asia, and parts of Europe. Vesicles and erosions are seen on the snout, lips, coronet, and occasionally the belly and legs.

MISCELLANEOUS VIRAL INFECTIONS

Vesicular Stomatitis. Vesicular stomatitis is an infectious disease of swine and cattle that is enzootic in North, Central, and South America. Vesicles progress rapidly to painful erosions of the oral cavity, lips, muzzle, feet, and occasionally the prepuce, udder, and teats.

Rinderpest. Rinderpest is an acute, highly contagious systemic disease of ruminants and swine in Africa and Asia. Skin lesions are characterized by erythema, papules, oozing, crusts, and alopecia over the perineum, flanks, medial thighs, neck, scrotum, udder, and teats. Occasionally, a generalized exfoliative dermatitis is seen.

Bluetongue. An insect-borne infectious disease of sheep, goats, and cattle, bluetongue occurs throughout the world. Sheep and goats develop erythema, edema, and occasionally ulceration of the muzzle, lips, and oral mucosa. In addition, some animals develop coronitis with a dark-red to purple band in the skin above the coronet. Cattle develop edema, dryness, cracking, and peeling of the muzzle and lips. Ulceration and crusting may be seen on the udder and teats. The neck, chest, flanks, back, and perineum may become scaly, wrinkled, alopecic, and fissured and may develop areas of moist superficial dermatitis.

African Swine Fever. African swine fever is a peracute, fatal, highly contagious infection of swine in Africa and also Europe. Severely affected swine develop a red to reddish-blue to purplish discoloration of the skin of the snout, ears, belly, legs, sides, and rump.

Bovine Ephemeral Fever. Transmitted by insects, bovine ephemeral fever affects cattle in Africa, Asia, and Australia.

Clinical signs may include widespread subcutaneous emphysema and periarticular edema.

Caprine Viral Dermatitis. This virus infection is an acute highly fatal disease of goats in India. The entire cutaneous surface, including the lips, gums, and tongue, is covered with papules and nodules that become necrotic, then ulcerated.

Swine Parvovirus Vesicular Disease. Outbreaks of parvovirus-related vesicular disease have been reported in swine in the midwestern United States. Lesions consist of vesicles and erosions on the snout and coronet and in the interdigital space and the mouth.

Scrapie. Scrapie is a vertically and horizontally transmissible disease of sheep and goats in many parts of the world. Clinical signs include intermittent, bilaterally symmetrical pruritus, which often begins over the tail head and progresses cranially to involve the flanks, thorax, and occasionally the head and ears. Chronic rubbing and biting lead to alopecia, excoriations, and even hematomas.

BIBLIOGRAPHY

Scott DW: Large Animal Dermatology. Philadelphia, WB Saunders, 1988.

Yeruham I, Abraham A, Insler G, et al: Bovine papular stomatitis in calves with apparent transmission to man. J Vet Med 46:110–113, 1991.

Yeruham I, Abraham A, Nyska A: Clinical and pathological description of a chronic form of bovine papular stomatitis. J Comp Pathol 111:279–286, 1994.

■ Bacterial Skin Diseases

Stephen D. White, D.V.M., Diplomate, A.C.V.D.

Bacterial skin diseases of food animals are among the more devastating diseases in terms of economic loss. Numerous bacteria have been noted to cause skin disease in cattle, sheep, goats, pigs, and llamas; only the more important and common diseases are covered here. For other diseases the reader is encouraged to consult the sources listed in the bibliography.

DERMATOPHILOSIS

Dermatophilosis is a common superficial, pustular, crusting, or ulcerative dermatitis of cattle, sheep, goats, swine, and llamas caused by *Dermatophilus congolensis*.

Etiology and Pathogenesis

D. congolensis is a gram-positive facultative anaerobic actinomycete whose natural habitat is unknown. Attempts to isolate the bacteria from soils have been unsuccessful. *D. congolensis* has been isolated only from the skin of infected animals. The three most common factors in the initiation and development of dermatophilosis are skin damage, moisture, and (theoretically) the presence of asymptomatic, chronically infected carrier animals. Moisture causes the release of the infective, motile, flagellated zoospore form of the organism. Important sources of skin damage include biting flies and arthropods, prickly vegetation, and maceration. The tick *Amblyomma variegatum* has been shown to be associated epidemiologically with dermatophilosis in cattle and sheep. In the latter species, the tick seems to have a systemic effect on the sheep which aggravates the dermatophilosis. The distribution of clinical lesions (e.g., dorsum, distal extremities) often mirrors these environmental insults or sources of moisture (e.g., rain, mud, moist or unclean stalls). Crusts from infected animals are important potential sources of infection and reinfection. Dermatophilosis is a contagious disease. The incubation period averages about 2 weeks but may vary from 1 day to 5 weeks.

Clinical Signs

No age, breed, or sex predilection for dermatophilosis has been noted. Infections may infect a single animal or a majority of the herd.

The primary lesions in dermatophilosis are follicular and nonfollicular papules and pustules. However, these lesions rapidly coalesce and become exudative, which results in groups of hairs becoming matted together, resembling a paintbrush. Close examination shows the proximal portions of these hairs to be embedded in dried exudate. When these paintbrush-like mats are plucked off, areas of purulent or ulcerated skin are revealed. Active lesions contain a thick, creamy, whitish, yellowish, or greenish pus that adheres to the skin surface and to the undersurface of the crusts. Acute active lesions of dermatophilosis are often painful, but the disease is rarely pruritic, except in llamas. The healing or chronic stage of the disease is characterized by dried crusts, scaling, and alopecia, which may resemble dermatophytosis (ringworm).

In goats, the lesions of dermatophilosis are commonly seen on the pinna and tail of kids and the muzzle, dorsal midline, and scrotum of adults. Lesions may be limited to the distal limbs, resembling the strawberry foot rot form of dermatophilosis found in sheep.

In sheep, the most common clinical forms of dermatophilosis are crusts occurring from the coronary bands to the tarsi and carpi with underlying bleeding, fleshy masses of tissue (strawberry foot rot); pyramidal crusts over the topline and flanks (so-called mycotic dermatitis); and crusts on the ears, nose, and face of lambs.

In cattle, dermatophilosis may affect the rump and topline; face and ears (especially in calves [milk scald] and bulls); brisket, axillae, and groin; udder and teats or scrotum and prepuce; distal limbs; and perineum and tail. Animals with over 50% of their body affected often show rapid weight loss and dehydration and die.

Dermatophilosis has been noted in the llama, usually over the dorsum, sides, or distal extremities during warm, rainy weather. Lesions are generally not painful but may be pruritic.

Dermatophilosis is very rare in swine. Affected pigs have a generalized exudative crusting dermatitis. Dual infections with *D. congolensis* and *Staphylococcus hyicus* have been reported. It should be remembered that dermatophilosis is a zoonosis, although human infections are relatively rare.

Diagnosis

The differential diagnosis of dermatophilosis is extensive, including dermatophytosis, staphylococcal folliculitis and furunculosis, viral infections, zinc-responsive dermatosis, and pemphigus foliaceus. In general, cutaneous crusts in food animals should be considered dermatophilosis until proved otherwise. Definitive diagnosis is based on direct smear, skin biopsy, and culture. Direct smears of pus or saline-soaked and minced crust may be stained with new methylene blue, Diff-Quik, or Gram stains. *D. congolensis* appears as fine branching and multiseptate hyphae that divide transversely and longitudinally to form cuboidal packets of coccoid cells arranged in parallel rows within branching filaments (railroad track appearance). In the healing or chronic stages of the disease, direct smears are rarely positive. Skin biopsy usually reveals varying degrees of folliculitis, intradermal pustular dermatitis, and superficial perivascular dermatitis. Intracellular edema with keratinocytes may be striking. The surface crust is characterized by alternating layers of orthokeratosis or parakeratosis and leukocytic debris (palisading crusts). *D. congolensis* is usually seen in the keratinous debris on the surface of the skin and within hair follicles. The organism is best visualized with Giemsa's, Brown and Brenn's, or acid orcein–Giemsa stains. A nodular to diffuse dermatitis resulting from granulomatous inflammation may be noted occasionally. *D. congolensis* grows well in blood agar when incubated in a microaerophilic atmosphere with increased carbon dioxide. However, the culture can be unsatisfactory as a result of rapid overgrowth of secondary invaders and contaminating saprophytes and in the chronic nonexudative stage. In such instances, incubating the crusts for several hours in saline and subsequently culturing this "broth" may be helpful.

Treatment

Recommended topical therapy includes the iodophors, 2.0% to 5.0% lime sulfur, 0.2% copper sulfate, 0.5% zinc sulfate, and 1.0% potassium aluminum sulfate (alum). The first three substances may stain hair and wool. Topical solutions are applied as total body washes, sprays, or dips for 3 to 5 consecutive days and then weekly until healing has occurred. In flocks of sheep where elimination of dermatophilosis is impractical, routine summer and fall protective dips with a 0.5% zinc sulfate or 1.0% potassium aluminum sulfate are reported to be effective.

The most commonly used systemic antibiotics in the treatment of dermatophilosis are penicillin and streptomycin. Various regimens have been recommended; the most common of these for cattle, sheep, goats, and llamas is 5000 IU/kg procaine penicillin G and 5 mg/kg streptomycin daily for 4 to 5 days. In addition, every attempt should be made to remove and dispose of crusts, to keep the animals dry, to give good-quality nutrition, and to control the biting arthropod population. Control of *A. variegatum* is especially important. Studies have shown a decrease in the incidence of dermatophilosis in cattle treated with acaricide.

STAPHYLOCOCCAL INFECTIONS

Most investigators recognize three clinically important coagulase-positive species of staphylococci: *S. aureus*, *S. intermedius*, and *S. hyicus*. The relative percentage of the first two species isolated from lesions may vary among animal species. However, differences in antimicrobial susceptibility patterns between *S. aureus* and *S. intermedius* are probably not significant. *S. hyicus* is usually clinically important only in swine. When possible, bacterial cultures should always be performed in cases of staphylococcal pyoderma. It is my impression that the number of penicillinase-resistant coagulase-positive staphylococci species in food animals is increasing.

Impetigo

Impetigo is defined as a superficial pustular dermatitis that does not involve hair follicles. It occurs in goats, sheep, and cattle. Predisposing factors may include the stress of parturition, moist and filthy environments, showering of lactating cows (to decrease heat stress), and trauma. No age or breed predilection is apparent, but female animals appear to be predisposed to infection. Lesions occur most commonly on the udder, with the base of the teats and the intramammary sulcus most often affected. Occasionally, lesions may spread to the teats, ventral abdomen, medial thighs, perineum, and ventral surface of the tail. Superficial vesicles readily become pustular, rupture and leave erosions, and yield a brown crust. Pruritus and pain are rare, and affected animals usually suffer no systemic disturbance unless staphylococcal mastitis ensues. The differential diagnosis includes dermatophilosis, dermatophytosis, and viral infections. The definitive diagnosis is based on direct smear, skin biopsy, and culture. Skin biopsy reveals subcorneal pustular dermatitis with cocci often visible within the pustules. Therapy with daily topical medicines (chlorhexidine, iodophors) usually results in rapid healing within a few days. Systemic antibiotics are rarely needed but when indicated should be based on results of culture and sensitivity testing. Impetigo may be spread by the milker to other cattle and goats. Affected animals should be milked last, single-service paper towels should be used, and the hands of the milker should be washed after contact with infected animals.

Exudative Epidermitis

Exudative epidermitis is an acute generalized exudative vesicopustular disease of suckling pigs caused by *S. hyicus*. Research suggests that this disease may be caused not by *S. hyicus* infection per se but by some toxins elaborated by the microorganism. In particular a toxin designated *S. hyicus* exfoliative toxin (shET) has been implicated. Because *S. hyicus* can be isolated from the skin, ears, and nostrils of most normal pigs, many authors believe that clinical disease requires some combination of the bacteria and predisposed piglets (skin trauma, inadequate nutrition, other diseases, or stress). The incidence of this disease is not high, but the disease can be a severe problem on individual farms. Exudative epidermitis is most commonly seen in suckling pigs of 1 to 7 weeks of age with no breed or sex predilection. Morbidity varies from 10% to 90% and mortality from 5% to 90% (average 20%). The disease is nonseasonal, and hygiene and management are often good in affected herds. The incubation period is 3 to 4 days.

Clinically, exudative epidermitis may be divided into peracute, acute, and subacute forms. In the peracute form, a dark-brown, greasy exudate appears periocularly, followed by a vesicopustular eruption on the nose, lips, tongue, gums, and coronets. Red-brown macules then appear behind the ears and on the ventral abdomen and medial thighs. The entire body is then covered by erythema, a moist greasy exudate, and thick brown crusts, hence the older term *greasy pig disease*. The feet are frequently affected, with erosions of the coronary band and heel. Conjunctivitis is common, and excessive exudation may result in the adherence of eyelids and blindness. The piglets show progressive depression, anorexia, and polydipsia and usually die within 3 to 5 days. Pruritus, pain, and fever are usually absent.

The acute form follows the general pattern of the peracute form. The skin becomes thicker and wrinkled, and the total body exudate then becomes hardened and cracked, resulting in a furrowed appearance. Death often occurs within 4 to 8 days.

In the subacute form, skin lesions are often confined to the head and ears and are less exudative. The piglets are usually healthy otherwise and recover spontaneously.

The differential diagnosis of exudative epidermitis includes swine parakeratosis, streptococcal pyoderma, biotin deficiency, and viral infections. The definitve diagnosis is based on skin biopsy and culture. Skin biopsy reveals subcorneal vesicular pustular dermatitis. A mild to moderate degree of acantholysis, detachment of the stratum corneum, parakeratosis, hydropic degeneration of the basal cell layer, and degeneration of the hair root sheath may be seen. With special stains, gram-positive cocci may be seen within the vesicles and pustules. *S. hyicus* may be cultured from vesicopustules and consistently from the conjunctiva. Necropsy findings in pigs with exudative epidermitis include dilatation of ureters and renal pelves as a result of ureteral obstruction caused by edema, cellular infiltration, hyperplasia, and mucoid degeneration of ureteral epithelium; serous lymphadenitis; and mild catarrhal gastroenteritis.

The efficacy of any treatment for exudative epidermitis decreases as the duration and severity of the infection increases. Clinical and experimental evidence suggests that vitamin B (especially biotin) supplementation is helpful in therapy and prevention. Antimicrobial susceptibility tests should be performed in cases of exudative epidermitis owing to regional differences in antibiotic resistance. In penicillin-susceptible strains, early treatment with penicillin 5000 IU/kg twice daily, given intramuscularly for 3 to 5 days, may be effective. Tylosin 8 mg/kg, given intramuscularly for 2 to 3 days, has also been reported to be beneficial. An in vitro sensitivity study in Denmark of 100 strains of *S. hyicus* isolated from piglets with exudative epidermitis indicated that novobiocin and trimethoprim-sulfadiazine were the most active compounds against those strains. Topical treatment with a cleansing, degreasing, and antimicrobial agent is also helpful. If conjunctivitis is severe, an antibiotic eye ointment is helpful. Affected piglets should be kept isolated, and exposed piglets should also be treated. Reducing factors predisposing to skin injuries and scrupulous hygiene will often limit an outbreak of exudative epidermitis.

Folliculitis and Furunculosis

Staphylococcal folliculitis (inflammation of the hair follicle) and furunculosis (a folliculitis that has broken through the wall of the hair follicle and now involves the surrounding dermis) are common in goats, sheep, and llamas, and uncommon in cattle and swine. The primary skin lesion of folliculitis is a follicular papule. Pustules may arise from these papules. Erect hairs are frequently noticed over a papule that is more easily felt than seen. These lesions often progressively enlarge and then become encrusted. The chronic healing phase is characterized by progressive flattening of the lesion and a gradually expanding circular area of alopecia and scaling. Hairs at the periphery of these lesions are often easily epilated, thus mimicking dermatophytosis (ringworm). Some lesions progress to furunculosis. This stage is distinguished by varying combinations of nodules, draining tracts, ulcers, and crusts. Scarring and occasionally leukoderma and leukotrichia may follow.

In goats, staphylococcal folliculitis and furunculosis have no age, breed, or sex predilection. Skin lesions are most commonly seen on the face, pinna, udder, ventral abdomen, medial thigh, perineum, and distal limbs. Deeper lesions are often warm and painful. Severe infections, especially with secondary mastitis, may produce pyrexia, anorexia, depression, and septicemia.

Staphylococcal folliculitis and furunculosis are also common in sheep. They may occur as a benign pustular dermatitis (plooks) in otherwise healthy 3- to 4-week-old lambs, especially on the lips and perineum, which spontaneously regresses within 3 weeks. The condition also occurs as a severe facial dermatitis (facial and periorbital eczema, eye scab) in sheep of all ages, but especially in adult ewes just prior to lambing. Pustules, nodules, ulcers, and black scabs develop on the face, pinna, and horn base. This facial form appears to be contagious, and spread through a flock has been attributed to infections of head abrasions while animals are feeding in troughs or fighting.

In llamas, staphylococcal folliculitis usually presents as focal, usually nonpruritic, asymmetrical areas of alopecia causing an exudation. The head or distal extremities are most commonly involved. In a limited number of animals, *S. intermedius* has been the most consistently recovered organism on culture.

Staphylococcal folliculitis and furunculosis are uncommon in cattle. Trauma and poor hygiene are believed to be initiating factors. Lesions are most commonly found on the tail and perineum and less commonly on the scrotum and face. Pruritus and pain are variable.

In swine, staphylococcal folliculitis and furunculosis are also uncommon. No breed or sex predilection is apparent. The condition is most frequently seen in pigs younger than 8 weeks of age, and asymptomatic erythematous pustular dermatitis covers much of the body, especially the hindquarters, abdomen, and chest. The dermatosis usually regresses spontaneously within 3 weeks.

The most important differential diagnosis of staphylococcal folliculitis or furunculosis on the general body surface includes dermatophilosis and dermatophytosis. Definitive diagnosis is based on direct smears, skin biopsy, and culture. Skin biopsy reveals varying degrees of perifolliculitis, folliculitis, and furunculosis, with extensive tissue eosinophilia often accompanying the furunculosis. Bacteria may be visible with special stains.

Therapy of staphylococcal folliculitis or furunculosis varies with severity and stage of the disease. Most cases require topical cleansing, drying, and systemic antibacterial therapy. I recommend daily applications of chlorhexidine for 5 to 7 days and then twice weekly until the infection is resolved. The choice of systemic antibiotics is best made on the basis of culture and sensitivity testing.

Corynebacterium pseudotuberculosis INFECTIONS

Corynebacterium pseudotuberculosis is a gram-positive, pleomorphic short rod. This bacterium requires various predisposing factors to become established as an infection; good management practices may be the most important means of controlling infections. The most common manifestation of *C. pseudotuberculosis* involving the skin in food animals is caseous lymphadenitis of sheep and goats. This is a common disease in these species and is the most frequent cause of abscesses. As a general rule, any abscess associated with a lymph node of a sheep or goat should be assumed to be due to *C. pseudotuberculosis* until proved otherwise. Lesions of caseous lymphadenitis are characterized by abscesses of lymph nodes and nodules and draining tracts in the skin. The purulent discharge is usually thick, creamy or cheesy, and yellowish, greenish, or tan. Confirmation of a tentative diagnosis can readily be made by examination of a Gram-stained smear (gram-positive pleomorphic rods) and confirmed by submitting a sample of pus to a diagnostic laboratory. A closed abscess can be sampled with a syringe and a fine needle. Since the pus is usually very thick, the syringe and needle are sent to the laboratory for flushing and later cultivation of the organism. The skin biopsy specimen shows nodular to diffuse dermatitis associated with tuberculoid granulomatous inflammation. An outer fibrovascular capsule is usually present. It may be possible to identify the organisms with tissue Gram's or Brown and Brenn's stain.

Although *C. pseudotuberculosis* is sensitive to a wide variety of antibiotics in vitro, treatment of caseous lymphadenitis with antibiotics is not very successful in vivo. The most common method of treating superficial abscesses is to wait until they are sufficiently large and "ripe" and simply open them surgically and allow them to drain thoroughly. The skin should be clipped and cleaned at the site, a vertical, bold incision made, and the contents completely expressed. This is followed by careful flushing of the abscess cavity with hydrogen peroxide or chlorhexidine. The cavity may be flushed daily or packed with swabs to ensure complete drainage. Sheep and goats with opened abscesses should be isolated from the herd until the wound has healed completely. During the summer a suitable insect repellent should be applied to open abscesses. The pus from draining abscesses contains large numbers of bacteria that can survive for long periods (months) in the environment. It is desirable to open abscesses and house animals with open abscesses in places not frequented by other animals in the herd. Isolation stalls or a shed where animals are unlikely to become contaminated at a later date is recommended. All pus-contaminated swabs and other material should be removed and disposed of. The clinician should remember that human infection with *C. pseudotuberculosis*, although rare, can occur. Care should be taken to minimize the chances of any human contamination by infected pus.

An alternative to simple abscess drainage is complete removal of the abscess. This may be used in certain selected cases such as in show animals or animals that cannot be isolated. This procedure enables the return of the animal immediately to the flock. The abscesses seldom recur, at least not at that site.

When a large number of animals in the flock are affected, one must rely on general principles of hygiene and preventive medicine. Vaccination programs are controversial.

An outbreak of an ulcerative skin disease with abscesses has been reported in seven herds of dairy cows, all in the San Joaquin Valley in California. *C. pseudotuberculosis* was isolated from the lesions of 19 of 22 affected cows; the isolate was in pure culture in 13 of the 22. Treatment was not extensively reported.

SPIROCHETOSIS

The spirochete *Borrelia suilla* is believed to be a secondary invader of dermatoses of swine, often associated with poor hygiene and skin trauma (abrasions, lacerations, fight wounds, surgical sites). Bilateral ulcerative spirochetosis of the ears is often associated with the trauma of sarcoptic mange or the vice of ear biting. Young pigs, especially 2 to 3 weeks post weaning, are most commonly affected. Although any region of the body may be involved, lesions are most frequently seen on the head, ears, gums, shoulders, side of the body, and scrotum (after castration). The lesions are characterized by initial erythema and edema, which are followed by necrosis and ulceration or swelling and fistulas. A grayish-brown, glutinous pustular discharge is typical. The central area of large swelling often sloughs off. Ear lesions frequently begin bilaterally at the base of the pinnae and extend distally and slough off, leaving a ragged bleeding margin. The major differential diagnosis includes other infectious granulomas and various forms of necrosis (pressure, septicemia). Definitive diagnosis is based on direct smears, biopsy, and culture. Direct smears or dark-field illumination of wet preparations from lesions reveal spirochetes. Skin biopsy reveals varying degrees of necrosis, ulceration and granulation tissue, granulomatous inflammation, and vasculitis. Spirochetes are best visualized histologically with silver stains.

Porcine spirochetosis has been reported to respond to several days of injectable penicillin, 3 to 5 days of oral or injectable sulfonamides, or several days of potassium iodide given orally at a dosage of 1 g/35 kg, up to 3 g total dose. Ulcerative lesions on the pinna are reported to respond rapidly to topical tetracycline. Control measures should include improved sanitation and management.

A spirochete-associated bovine digital dermatitis (papillomatous digital dermatitis) has been described in the United States, Canada, and Europe. Lameness, decreased feed intake, and decreased milk production in dairy cows are common clinical signs. Examination of the hoof reveals exophytic growths involving the bulb of the heel, sometimes extending medially to the axial groove. Lesions are 3 to 4 cm in diameter, grayish with moist, red, ulcerated areas, have thick surface projections, and

are painful and bleed when disturbed. As the lesions progress, there is necrosis and undermining of the horn in the bulb region. Histologic examination shows marked parakeratosis, thick cornified surface projections, papillate epidermal hyperplasia with keratinocytes that are either necrotic or ballooned, and, on silver staining, spirochetes within the outer layers of the epidermis. Treatment with foot baths of 5% formalin or tetracycline (4 g/L or greater), debriding ulcerative lesions, and debulking proliferative lesions has been suggested.

CLOSTRIDIAL INFECTIONS

Clostridial species are ubiquitous anaerobic spore-forming gram-positive rods. They produce a wide variety of toxins and diseases.

Malignant edema (gas gangrene) is an acute wound infection of cattle, sheep, horses, and swine caused by various *Clostridium* spp., including *C. septicum*, *C. sordellii*, and *C. perfringens*. Clinical signs appear within 12 to 48 hours of infection. There is a local lesion at the site of infection consisting of a soft, doughy swelling (pitting edema) with marked local erythema. As the disease progresses, the swelling becomes tense and occasionally hot and painful and the skin becomes dark and taut and eventually sloughs. Emphysema (crepitus) may or may not be present. Lesions may occur anywhere, especially in the inguinal, abdominal, cervical, shoulder, and head areas. A high fever is usually present. Affected animals are weak and depressed, may show muscle tremors and lameness, and usually die within 1 to 2 days.

Blackleg is an acute infectious disease of cattle, sheep, and swine caused by *Clostridium chauvoei*. Clinical signs appear within 12 to 48 hours of infection. The early lesion is a hot painful swelling that progresses to a cold, painless, edematous, and emphysematous swelling. The skin is discolored and becomes dry and cracked. Lesions occur most commonly on an upper limb, the rump, and the neck. Affected animals have a high fever, are depressed and anorectic, and often die within 2 days.

Clostridial swelled head (big head) is an acute wound infection of sheep and goats usually caused by *Clostridium novyi* and less commonly by *Clostridium sordellii*. It is usually seen in rams and bucks at 1 to 2 years of age, especially in the summer and early fall when fighting is common. Lesions begin around the eyes and head and may spread to the neck and consist of subcutaneous edema and fluid exudation. Emphysema is quite rare. Affected animals are pyrectic and toxemic and usually die within 2 to 3 days.

Dermatohistopathologic findings in clostridial infections include diffuse subcutaneous and dermal edema and cellulitis with large numbers of degenerative neutrophils and bacteria. The latter are best visualized with special stains. Septic thrombi may be seen in subcutaneous blood vessels. The clinical signs of these diseases (e.g., swelling followed by necrosis, subcutaneous emphysema) are fairly suggestive of clostridial infection. The organisms may be isolated from lesions; however, owing to the rapid onset of these diseases and rapid death of the animal, any treatment attempted must be administered on an emergency basis. Early surgical drainage and debridement with administration of high levels of penicillin (50,000 IU/kg) or tetracycline (10 to 20 mg/kg) can be tried, but these measures are often futile. In endemic areas, it is recommended that cattle and sheep be vaccinated and that they be excluded from pastures known to be heavily contaminated by these organisms.

ERYSIPELAS

Erysipelas is an infectious disease of swine caused by *Erysipelothrix insidiosa* (*rhusiopathiae*). The organism is a gram-positive pleomorphic facultative anaerobe. Erysipelas is worldwide in distribution and a serious economic problem in swine operations. Erysipelas occurs in acute, subacute, and chronic clinical forms. In the acute form, fever, depression, anorexia, and lameness are accompanied by bluish-purplish discoloration of the skin, especially of the abdomen, ears, and extremities. Pinkish to red macules and papules may also be seen. In the subacute phase, erythematous papules and wheals (urticaria) enlarge and become square, rectangular, or rhomboid (diamond skin disease). These lesions often develop a purplish center and either regress spontaneously or progress to the chronic phase. The chronic phase is characterized by necrosis and sloughing, resulting in dark dry firm areas of skin that peel away. Occasionally the ears, tail, and feet may slough as well. Dermatohistopathologic findings include marked dermal vascular dilation and engorgement in the acute phase and a neutrophilic vasculitis (arteritis) and suppurative hidradenitis in the subacute and chronic phases. The organisms may occasionally be visualized in sections stained with Gram's stain. Penicillin (11,000 IU/kg/day) is the antibiotic of choice for treatment. Pigs at risk may also be protected by penicillin therapy. Vaccinations are recommended to prevent herd outbreaks. Humans are susceptible to infections with *E. insidiosa*. The disorder, termed *erysipeloid*, is an occupational disease of humans, such as veterinarians who come into contact with animals. Lesions are most commonly seen on the hands and fingers and consist of a slowly progressive discrete, violaceous to erythematous, and usually painful cellulitis.

BIBLIOGRAPHY

Anderson ML, Lean IJ, Blanchard PC: *Corynebacterium pseudotuberculosis*–associated skin disease of Holstein cattle in the San Joaquin Valley, California. Bovine Pract 25:73–75, 1990.

Atlee BA, Barbet J: Llama dermatology. *In* Ihrke PJ, Mason IS, White SD (eds): Advances in Veterinary Dermatology, vol 2. Oxford, Pergamon Press, 1992 pp 413–416.

Borgmann IE, Bailey J, Clark EG: Spirochete-associated bovine digital dermatitis. Can Vet J 37:35–37, 1996.

Cameron RDA: Skin Diseases of the Pig. Sydney, University of Sydney Postgraduate Foundation in Veterinary Science, 1984.

Fubini SL, Campbell SG: External lumps on sheep and goats. Vet Clin North Am Large Anim Pract 5:457–476, 1983.

Hadril DJ, Walker AR: Effect of acaricide control of *Amblyomma variegatum* ticks on bovine dermatophilosis on Nevis. Trop Anim Health Prod 26:28–34, 1994.

Lofstedt J: Dermatologic diseases of sheep. Vet Clin North Am Large Anim Pract 5:427–448, 1983.

Oh KS, Lee CS: Pathological studies on exudative epidermitis in experimentally infected pigs. I. Macroscopical and histopathological observations. Korean J Vet Res 34:787–799, 1994.

Rosychuk RAW: Llama dermatology. Vet Clin North Am Food Anim Pract 5:203–215, 1989.

Rosychuk RAW: Llama dermatology. Vet Clin North Am Food Anim Pract 10:228–239, 1994.

Scott DW: Large Animal Dermatology. Philadelphia, WB Saunders, 1988.

Tanabe T, Sato H, Sato H, et al: Correlation between occurrence of exudative epidermitis and exfoliative toxin-producing ability of *Staphylococcus hyicus*. Vet Microbiol 48:1–17, 1996.

Wegener HC, Watts JL, Salmon SA, et al: Antimicrobial susceptibility of *Staphylococcus hyicus* isolated from exudative epidermitis in pigs. J Clin Microbiol 32:793–795, 1994.

Yeruham I, Elad D, Perl S, et al: Contagious impetigo in a dairy cattle herd. Vet Dermatol 7:239–242, 1996.

■ Dermatophytosis (Ringworm)

Susan D. Semrad, V.M.D., Ph.D., Diplomate, A.C.V.I.M.
Karen Moriello, D.V.M., Diplomate, A.C.V.D.

Fungi are ubiquitous in the environment and most are soil organisms or plant pathogens; fewer than 300 species of fungi have been reported to be animal pathogens. Depending upon the pathogenic characteristics of the fungal species, fungal infections may be superficial, subcutaneous, or deep. A *superficial fungal infection*, more commonly known as a dermatophyte infection, occurs when a pathogenic dermatophyte invades keratinized tissues, for example, nails, hair, stratum corneum. Dermatophytosis is the most common fungal skin disease of large animals. *Subcutaneous fungal infections* occur when an opportunistic pathogen is traumatically implanted into the skin; subcutaneous fungal infections occur because of compromised cellular immunity. *Deep fungal infections* are caused by dimorphic fungi. The most common route of infection is via inhalation of infective spores and hematogenous spread to the skin.

ETIOLOGY AND PATHOGENESIS

In food animals, dermatophytosis is caused primarily by species of the genera *Trichophyton* and *Microsporum*; *Epidermophyton* spp. are rarely isolated and may represent human-to-animal transmission. Dermatophytosis is common in cattle and uncommon in small ruminants and swine. The most commonly isolated dermatophytes from food-producing animals include *Trichophyton verrucosum* (cattle, goats, sheep, horses), *Trichophyton mentagrophytes* (cattle, sheep, goats, and rarely swine), *Trichophyton equinum* (horses and cattle in contact with infected horses), *Microsporum nanum* (swine and rarely cattle), and the geophilic fungus *Microsporum gypseum* (cattle, sheep, goats, swine). All of these pathogenic fungi are potential human pathogens.

Susceptible hosts may become exposed, and subsequently infected, via contact with an actively infected host or via contact with a contaminated environment or object (e.g., housing, fencing, feed bunks, blankets, dust, or grooming tools). Fungal spores may also be spread mechanically via vectors such as flies, fleas, and lice. The environment is an overlooked source of infection as fungal spores protected in crusts and hair shafts may remain viable for many months, if not years.

There is a great deal of debate about "reservoirs" of dermatophyte infection. From a practical perspective, there are two major reservoirs of infection—the environment and animal hosts. As mentioned above, the environment is an overlooked source of infection and may actually be a more important reservoir of infection than animal hosts on some farms. Rodents are considered the reservoirs of *T. mentagrophytes*. Small animals may also serve as sources of infection. *Microsporum canis* is the primary pathogen of cats, and dogs can be infected with *T. mentagrophytes*, *T. verrucosum* (rare), *M. canis*, and *M. gypseum*. In addition, many animals may mechanically carry infective spores on their hair coat, also serving as a source of infection. Persons handling infected animals should wear gloves and change clothing before working with uninfected animals.

Dermatophytosis is most common in young, old, or debilitated hosts. Risk factors for infection also include poor nutrition, overcrowding, warmth and humidity leading to maceration of the skin, hot humid climates, concurrent disease, immunosuppression, and lack of exposure to sunlight. With respect to juvenile animals, age and lack of exposure are the most important risk factors; cellular immunity develops after exposure. Crowding of animals during the winter months in temperate climates results in increased incidence of disease. Adult cows may become infected or reinfected after the introduction of infected freshening heifers into a milking herd. When animals are chronically or recurrently infected with dermatophytosis, environmental conditions (unsanitary conditions, high moisture and humidity, or crowding) or immunosuppression (underlying diseases, chronic diseases, or nutritional deficiencies) should be investigated.

Exposure to infective spores does not guarantee an infection. Spores may be mechanically removed from the hair coat or may not be able to establish an infection because of competition from resident flora. Infective spores must reach the epidermis or invade an anagen hair follicle for an infection to occur; moisture enhances the germination of spores. Once spores begin to germinate the infection will continue to spread and progress until it is recognized by the immune system. The clinical signs of infection are directly related to the pathogenesis of infection. Invaded hairs are structurally weakened leading to easy fracturing of hair shafts and subsequent hair loss. Crusting and scaling are the result of an increase in epidermal cell turnover, presumably in response to the presence of the fungal infection. An increase in the epidermal cell turnover time would lead to an increase in exfoliation of epidermal cells and a sloughing of the infective epidermis.

Dermatophytosis is a self-limiting disease and most healthy hosts will recover within 1 to 4 months. Animals mount both a humoral and cellular immune response to infection, but recovery is dependent upon the development of cell-mediated immunity.[1] The duration of immunity to reinfection is unknown, but immunity is "relative." In other words, "immune hosts" can be reinfected upon exposure to a large enough spore challenge.

CLINICAL FEATURES

The incubation period from exposure to clinical disease may range from 1 to 6 weeks; however, clinical symptoms usually begin to develop within 1 to 2 weeks of exposure. The gross appearance of dermatophytosis is quite variable, but characteristically lesions are multifocal, variable in size, alopecic, and scaly. The classic ringworm-like lesion is characterized by an annular area of alopecia, stubbled hairs, and variable amounts of scaling, crusting, and dermatitis. Dermatophyte lesions begin as subtle thickening and scaling of the skin. As the agent invades the hair shaft, hairs fracture and alopecia and scaling become more obvious. The lesion expands circumferentially for about 4 to 8 weeks and then begins to resolve as the animal develops an immune response. The lesion regresses and hair growth resumes after 8 to 16 weeks.

In cattle, clinical lesions of *T. verrucosum* are usually characterized by thick, well-demarcated, tightly adherent, grayish crusts, but may vary from discrete, circular areas of alopecia to severe scaling, crusting, suppuration, and ulceration. Pruritus and pain are variable. In calves, round or oval areas of crusting and alopecia that range from 1 to 5 cm in diameter are typical. Early lesions in calves may appear raised due to serum oozing or secondary pyoderma beneath the crust. Folliculitis and furunculosis are also manifestations of dermatophytosis. Lesions may include papules, nodules, ulcers, and sinuses. There is some evidence that lesion sites of *T. verrucosum* in cattle are sex- and age-dependent. Calves with *T. verrucosum* commonly develop multiple lesions, often around the eye, head, and neck. In adult cows and heifers, the lesions often appear on the neck, trunk, and limbs and less frequently on the face. Lesions may also occur on the udder. The dewlap and intermaxillary space are common sites of lesions in bulls.

In contrast to *T. verrucosum*, infection with *T. mentagrophytes* and *T. equinum* may cause herd outbreaks in cattle characterized by generalized areas of circular alopecia or multifocal and small 0.5- to 2.0-cm lesions with minimal scaling or crusting.

In goats, *T. verrucosum* commonly causes lesions on the face, pinnae, neck, udder, and limbs. The lesions are circular to uneven, to diffuse areas of alopecia, scaling, erythema, and yellowish-gray crusts. Pruritus and pain are rare. In sheep, *T. verrucosum* lesions are most commonly seen on the face, neck, thorax, and back and are characterized by circular areas of alopecia and thick grayish crusts.

In swine, *M. nanum* causes annular areas of red to brown discoloration of the skin and dry, brown to orange crusts, especially behind the ears and on the trunk. Alopecia and pruritus are rare. Lesions in swine need to be differentiated from pityriasis rosea, an inherited, idiopathic disease of young pigs. *M. nanum* causes very inflammatory lesions in humans.

DIAGNOSIS

Dermatophytosis in ruminants needs to be differentiated from bacterial skin infections, primarily *Staphylococcus* spp., dermatophilosis, demodicosis, zinc-responsive dermatoses, and pemphigus foliaceus. Impression smears of the skin are most helpful in differentiating bacterial skin infections from dermatophytosis. Dermatophilosis can be diagnosed via skin biopsy, bacterial culture of the crusts, or more practically by cytologic examination of impression smears made from the skin and underside of a freshly removed crust. Organisms are best visualized under oil immersion. Skin scrapings will rule in or rule out demodicosis. Zinc-responsive dermatoses are more common in goats and sheep than in cattle. Skin biopsy is most helpful in these cases. Pemphigus foliaceus in goats may resemble dermatophytosis in the early course of the disease. Again, skin biopsy is most cost-effective and helpful in making a diagnosis.

In the vast majority of cases, dermatophytosis in food animals is diagnosed based on the history and clinical signs; cost constraints often limit diagnostic testing. There may often be a history of human exposure. When multiple animals are infected and lesions are typical, the diagnosis is not very difficult. Diagnosis may be more difficult when clinical presentations are less typical or when examining a single animal, for example, a pet goat, sheep, or pig.

Dermatophytosis can be diagnosed via fungal culture and microscopic examination of the colony, skin biopsy, or hair microscopy. The last is not very cost-effective with respect to time and is a low-yield test. Artifacts are common and often misleading. Invasion of hair shafts is more readily seen with *M. canis* infections than with most of the infections that occur in large animals. The most cost-effective diagnostic test in large animal dermatology is a skin biopsy. Care should be taken to select early lesions or the most representative lesions available. It is critical not to scrub or prepare the biopsy site. Many of the important skin pathologic changes are present in the superficial crusts attached to hairs. Dermatophytes are usually visible with routine staining (hematoxylin-eosin [H&E]), but special stains such as periodic acid–Schiff (PAS), Gomori's methenamine silver (GMS), or acid orcein–Giemsa (AOG) may be needed in some cases.

Fungal cultures and subsequent microscopic examination of fungal cultures can both confirm the infection and identify the agent. Hairs and crust should be collected from the advancing edge of a new lesion. Prior to collecting the samples, the site should be gently swabbed with alcohol to minimize the growth of contaminants. Suspect infective material is best transported to the laboratory in a sealed container and inoculated onto a fungal culture plate as soon as possible. We prefer Sab-Duets (Bacti-labs, Mountainview, Calif.) because the plates are easy to inoculate and are split; one side of the plate contains dermatophyte test medium (DTM) and the other side contains plain Sabouraud's dextrose agar. DTM can sometimes inhibit the growth of some fungal pathogens. Plates should be inoculated by gently pressing the material onto the surface; avoid embedding the material into the media as dermatophytes are not anaerobic organisms. Plates should be stored medium side up and in a dark area; plates are incubated at room temperature and should be examined daily. Some *Trichophyton* spp. are slow-growing and may need special incubation conditions; all plates should be held for 21 days. A red color change in the DTM is *not* diagnostic for a pathogen, only suggestive. All colonies should be examined microscopically with lactophenol cotton blue stain and colonies identified, if possible. Dermatophytes are pale or buff-colored and are never colored or heavily pigmented.

CLINICAL MANAGEMENT AND TREATMENT

Dermatophytosis is a nonfatal self-limiting disease that will resolve anywhere from 30 to 120 days after infection. Treatment is recommended to speed resolution of the infection, minimize the spread of infection to other animals and humans, and minimize contamination of the environment.

Infected or suspect animals should be isolated from healthy animals and housed in a dry environment with exposure to sunlight. Overcrowding of animals should be avoided. Nutrition should be enhanced. The environment, feed bunks, grooming utensils, and such should be cleaned and disinfects. The most important step in decontamination is an aggressive gross cleaning of the environment and scrubbing of all surfaces with a detergent. Household bleach at a dilution of 1:10 is the most cost-effective disinfectant. Areas should be thoroughly wetted for at least 10 minutes with the bleach dilution and then allowed to dry. Two commercial imidazole disinfectants are available. Enilconazole smoke bombs (Clinafarm SG, Mallinckrodt) and environmental spray (Clinafarm EG, Mallinckrodt) products are available in the United States for disinfecting stables, infected tools and gear, blankets and baskets, and such. Repetition of the treatment depends on the extent of the risk of reinfection.

Topical antifungal agents are the most practical method of treatment of dermatophytosis in food animals. Treatment of the entire animal with topical therapy is recommended as dermatophytes may be present on apparently unaffected areas of the skin and spot therapy may lead to a carrier state. Prior to treatment, crusts and scabs should be removed with a brush. An inexpensive brush (e.g., household scrub brush) that can be destroyed after use is ideal. Topical ointments are best avoided. Recommended topical treatments include lime sulfur 2% to 5% or 1% iodophors applied as a spray or dip once daily for 5 days, then once weekly until clinical cure is observed. Both may be drying and irritating to the skin. Chlorhexidine and captan have been shown to be ineffective against *M. canis* and it is likely they are ineffective against *Trichophyton* spp.

Enilconazole (Imaverol, Janssen Pharmaceutica Animal Health Department, Beerse, Belgium), is very efficacious against dermatophytes in large and small animals. A topical solution is approved for use in Europe and Canada but not yet in the United States.

Whenever a topical antifungal agent is used, remember to (1) treat all in-contact animals (clinically affected or normal), (2) decontaminate the environment and disinfect possible fomites, and (3) dispose of infectious materials (crusts, hair, bedding, and so on) via burning, if feasible. Removal of crusts and scraping lesions with a soft wire brush allows better penetration of local medications. The skin debris removed should be properly disposed of to prevent reinfection and contamination of the environment. Gloves and protective clothing should be worn whenever contacting affected and exposed animals or contaminated materials to reduce the risk of disease transmission to humans.

The efficacy of systemic therapy is unknown; anecdotal reports suggest it is effective. Griseofulvin has most commonly been recommended, although the correct dose and efficacy have not been fully determined. Recommended oral doses range from 7.5 to 60 mg/kg for 7 to 20 days. Feeding low levels of griseofulvin premix in the feed halted the spread of lesions in one study. Intravenous infusion of a 10% to 20% solution of sodium iodide (1 g/14 kg), repeated at 3- to 7-day intervals, has been reported to be efficacious. Iodide may cause abortion in pregnant animals or may induce iodism. Vitamins A and D may be indicated in animals deprived of access to sunlight. Itraconazole 5 to 10 mg/kg orally for 20 days will abort the infection, but this treatment is cost-prohibitive.

PREVENTION

Treatment of all affected and contact animals is necessary to prevent spread of disease. Effective decontamination of the environment can be achieved with enilconazole as a spray or smoke bomb after organic debris has been removed from the area. Provision of good nutrition, dry, well-ventilated housing, and maintenance of general good health are also important in prevention of dermatophytosis.

The use of a fungal vaccine to prevent clinical infection is controversial. A modified live *T. verrucosum* vaccine has been shown to successfully prevent infection with trichophytosis in calves in the former Soviet Union and Scandinavia.[2, 3] Two injections given at 1 and 3 weeks of age were shown to be protective against natural challenge exposure to *T. verrucosum*, but not other dermatophytes. Injection site reactions were common, but systemic reactions were seen in only a few animals. Full protection against infection was also reported in calves receiving a live, freeze-dried vaccine against ringworm, produced by Bioveta, Ivanovice na Hane, Czechoslovakia.[4] Field trials with a crude ribosomal fraction of *T. verrucosum* or a vaccine containing an inactivated strain of *T. verrucosum* showed a reduction in clinical lesions in treated calves and cattle.[5, 6] These vaccines are not available in the United States.

REFERENCES

1. Scott DW: Large Animal Dermatology. Philadelphia, WB Saunders, 1988, pp 168–182.
2. Aamodt O. Vaccination of Norwegian cattle against ringworm. Zentralbl Vet Med B29:451, 1982.
3. Gudding R, Naess B: Vaccination in cattle against ringworm caused by *Trichophyton verrucosum*. Am J Vet Res 47:2415, 1986.
4. Rybnikar A, Chumela J, Vrzal V, et al: Immunity in cattle vaccinated against ringworm. Mycoses 34:443, 1991.
5. Elad D, Segal E: Immunogenicity in calves of a crude ribosomal fraction of *Trichophyton verrucosum*: A field trial. Vaccine 13:83, 1995.
6. Wawrzkiewicz K, Wawrzkiewicz J: An inactivated vaccine against ringworm. Comp Immunol Microbiol Infect Dis 15:31, 1992.

■ Protozoal Skin Diseases

Danny W. Scott, D.V.M., Diplomate, A.C.V.D.

Parasitic protozoa are an important cause of food animal disease in many areas of the world. Some of these protozoal diseases have an associated dermatosis, but the cutaneous disorders are of minimal importance compared with disorders that involve other organ systems. For detailed information on other clinicopathologic, diagnostic, and therapeutic aspects of these diseases, see the appropriate sections of this textbook.

TRYPANOSOMIASIS

Trypanosoma brucei has been reported to cause urticarial plaques over the neck, chest, and flanks of cattle in Africa.

SARCOCYSTOSIS

Affected cattle may lose the tail switch (hence the name *rat-tail syndrome*) and develop alopecia of the pinnae and distal extremities. Sarcocystosis may cause a poor hair coat and patchy alopecia in goats.

BESNOITIOSIS

Besnoitiosis (globidiosis) is reported to affect cattle and goats in Africa, Asia, southern Europe, and South America. In cattle, warm, painful, edematous swellings are present predominantly over the head, ears, distal extremities, and genitalia. These same areas then become alopecic, thickened, and folded (elephantiasis).

In goats, besnoitiosis (dimple) is characterized by thickening, folding, alopecia, fissuring, and oozing of the skin on the legs, ventral thorax and ventral abdomen ("ventrum"), and scrotum. In addition, subcutaneous papules may be present over the hindquarters.

THEILERIASIS

Theileria parva is the cause of East Coast fever in cattle in Africa. The disease may be associated with the development of papules and nodules over the neck and trunk. *Theileria annulata* is a cause of bovine theileriasis in Asia, southern Europe, and northern Africa. Cutaneous lesions may be seen and include wheals or papules that begin on the face, neck, and shoulders and then become generalized. The lesions are firm, and pruritus may be intense.

BIBLIOGRAPHY

Franc M, Gourreau JM, Ferrie J: La besnoitiose bovine. Point Vet 19:445–455, 1987.
Scott DW: Large Animal Dermatology. Philadelphia, WB Saunders, 1988.

■ Flies, Lice, and Grubs

John E. Lloyd, Ph.D.

MUSCOID FLIES OF RANGE CATTLE

The horn fly, *Haematobia irritans*, was introduced into the United States before 1887 and is now common throughout the country. The face fly, *Musca autumnalis*, arrived in the United States around 1950 and has become established in most of the country, but not the Southwest. In semiarid regions of the Midwest the face fly is found in low-lying, moist areas along waterways and is rarely seen on the open prairie. Face flies and horn flies are primarily pests of pasture or range cattle. The face fly is also attracted to horses, and the horn fly may be found on both sheep and horses when they are in close proximity to cattle.

The adult face fly is the same size as the house fly. It has sponging mouthparts and feeds on liquid or liquefied food. The mouthparts of the female face fly also have spines that abrade the surface of eye tissue. The horn fly is approximately one-half the size of the face fly and both sexes of the horn fly have piercing-sucking mouthparts.

The behavior of the adult flies on the host may aid in their identification. Horn flies are with their host constantly, and are located on the back, the belly, and occasionally the base of the horns. During extremely hot, sunny, or rainy weather, the flies congregate on the underside of the belly. The number of flies on an individual animal often reaches the high hundreds in northern climates and the thousands in the South.

The majority of face flies on the host are female. The female face fly is an obligate feeder on body secretions and other fluids, usually probing the eyes and nostrils. It will also feed on open wounds and secretions on other parts of the body. Both males and females feed on plant fluids and fresh cattle dung. Because they come to the host only to feed, a small percentage of the population is present on the host at any given time. On range cattle, the number of face flies is usually considerably lower than the number of horn flies.

Depending on ambient temperatures, horn flies may prefer darker animals, and usually they are more abundant on bulls and older cows. The horn fly has a limited flight range of a few miles, and can migrate to nearby cattle herds. Other than for purposes of migration, the adult female leaves the host only to oviposit. She deposits her eggs on the underside of the edge of a fresh dung pat. The larval horn fly develops through three stages in the dung pat. Pupae are found in the edge of the dung pat or in adjacent soil.

Horn fly larval and pupal development in the field may be quite rapid, for example, 9 to 12 days. Consequently, populations can build up rapidly, and many generations are possible within a season. In cooler climates a single seasonal population peak of adults is usually seen. In regions where summer temperatures are high, however, a midsummer reduction in fly numbers results in a bimodal population curve. In northern climates, horn flies overwinter in the diapausing pupal stage.

Female face flies insert their eggs into fresh cattle droppings which is where all three larval stages develop, requiring a period of 2 to 3 weeks. Following the last larval stage, the white puparium is usually found in soil beneath the pat. Face fly feeding generally occurs during the middle of the day. Face flies remain outdoors, are very mobile, and can fly several miles. Like the horn fly, the number of adult face flies may drop in midsummer in warmer climates. Both male and female face flies overwinter in shelters and can be household pests in the spring when they emerge from hibernation in large numbers.

Horn fly stress may reduce milk yield and weight gains, including weaning weights. Reductions in weight gains as high as ½ lb/day have been reported. Even at relatively low population levels, for example, less than 100 per animal, horn flies will reduce rates of weight gain. In the western United States, the horn fly is an intermediate host and vector of *Stefanofilaria stilsi*, a minute filarial worm that is a parasite of cattle. Infestations by this parasite can lead to secondary infection and an extensive dermatitis along the ventral midline that can spread to other parts of the body.

The face fly is an annoyance to cattle and horses. It affects time of grazing by cattle, but effects on production remain to be demonstrated. The face fly contributes significantly to bovine keratoconjunctivitis. The spines of the female face fly mouthparts physically damage the cornea of the eye, and the fly is most likely a vector of *Moraxella bovis*, the principal agent of infectious bovine keratoconjunctivitis. The face fly is also a vector and intermediate host of mammalian eye worms of the genus *Thelazia*, some of which parasitize horses and cattle.

Treatment

Control of both horn flies and face flies has been considered using dung beetles imported from other parts of the world. Releases of imported dung beetles have been made in the United States, and the beetles have become established in certain areas of the South, apparently to the detriment of horn flies.

Muscoid flies may be effectively controlled through the use of insecticides. One may determine from the insecticide label whether an insecticide is approved for the particular animal and the pest and at what rate of application. Read the insecticide label and observe all instructions, precautions, warnings, and so on, including withdrawal times.

A variety of insecticides and treatment methods are available for control of muscoid flies on range cattle. In general, horn flies are easier to control than are face flies. Care must be taken to be sure the faces are treated for face fly control.

Depending on weather conditions, range cattle may be provided several weeks of relief from fly attack by spray, dip vat, dust, or pour-on treatments with residual insecticides. A few organochlorine insecticides, and a variety of organophosphate and pyrethroid insecticides are available for this purpose. Avermectins can be used for horn fly control up to 28 days, but only in the pour-on formulation. Retreatment of cattle for fly control is necessary, but not more frequently than allowed by the insecticide label.

Frequent applications of fast-acting insecticides (e.g., pyrethrins, the pyrethroids, or some of the organophosphates), repellents, or insecticide-repellent mixtures are effective when cattle are available for frequent handling. These might be applied in a number of ways, including dusts, mist sprays, and pour-ons. Again, when treating for face fly control, pay particular attention to the head and face.

Continuous application of insecticide through the use of self-treatment or sustained release devices is popular for treatment of range cattle because the animals need be handled only once or not at all. Oilers, back rubbers, and dust bags are the most popular of the self-treatment devices.

Oil solutions of insecticides can be applied by means of commercially made oilers or homemade back rubbers. Generally, oilers have reserve tanks that hold insecticide, and they must be recharged less frequently. The back rubber is less expensive but must be tended and recharged more frequently. The homemade back rubber consists of a length of cable, chain, or wire around which burlap is wrapped. The burlap is held in place by additional wire. The back rubber is either suspended between two posts or one end is attached to a post and the other is anchored to the ground. The rubber is positioned approximately 6 in. below the topline so that animals may stand under it to rub. If one end of the rubber is anchored to the ground, animals can rub their flanks and bellies also. The insecticide is mixed in No. 2 diesel fuel or mineral oil and applied at the rate of 1 gal for each 20 linear ft of back rubber. The back rubber must be recharged with sufficient frequency to keep it moist, usually every 1 or 2 weeks.

The dust bag is a simple, self-treatment device developed primarily for horn fly control but it will aid in face fly control also. Dust bags are heavy (usually 10 oz) burlap sacks filled with an approved insecticide dust and suspended approximately 6 in. below backline height. When an animal bumps against the bag a small quantity of dust sifts through the fabric. Ready-made dust bags can be purchased. These often consist of a burlap sack with grommets for hanging and a plastic hood to protect the bag from rain.

Oilers, back rubbers, and dust bags should be placed in outdoor areas where cattle will use them, for example, in loafing areas, near water tanks or mineral licks. Water tanks or mineral licks may be fenced and self-treatment devices installed in a gate so that cattle are forced to use them. To control or aid in the control of face flies, dust bags (and perhaps other devices) can be lowered as cattle become used to them, to the point where the face comes in contact with the bag.

Sustained release devices or formulations include insecticide ear-tags, insecticide feed-throughs (mineral or feed additives, oral larvicides), and sustained or continuous release boluses. The insecticide ear-tag is by far the most popular sustained release device for fly control. These are plastic ear-tags that are formulated with pyrethroid, synergized pyrethroid, organophosphate insecticides, or various combinations. The insecticide slowly migrates to the surface of the tag, comes in contact with the hair coat, and subsequently is spread over the body. All of the tags control nonresistant horn flies and will either control or aid in the control of face flies. Many of the pyrethroid tags are approved for face fly control. Where horn fly resistance to pyrethroids is a concern, an alternative pyrethroid or an organophosphate may provide effective control.

The objective behind the use of the various feed-through and sustained release insecticide formulations is to have the insecticide pass through the bovine digestive tract in sufficient quantity to kill developing fly larvae in the manure pat. Some larvicides currently on the market will control horn flies only, and others have label claims for both horn flies and face flies. One organophosphate insecticide and two insect growth regulators are currently available for this purpose. The insect growth regulators are chemicals that affect the molting process of the larval flies and kill them as they transform from one stage to the next. The products can be administered in a feed supplement, mineral mix, salt block, and so on, or they may be administered via a sustained release bolus. Some of the products that are fed to cattle are purchased ready to use; others must be mixed with supplemental feed or mineral. The boluses, which are administered to the cattle via a balling gun, release active ingredient into feces over an extended period, usually a season.

The larvicide program should be started before the fly season as there will be no effect on adult flies that are already on the cattle. The level of adult fly control may be affected by uneven consumption of larvicidal material fed as a supplement. Also, flies may migrate from neighboring, untreated cattle herds. If adult flies are on the cattle, supplemental fly control measures should be taken.

A number of fly traps have been developed for control of adult flies on range and pasture cattle. Various kinds of traps that are visually attractive to flies may be set near areas where cattle are pastured. Walk-through traps, set in areas where cattle normally pass, remove flies from cattle as they pass through. The flies that are removed from the cattle or are attracted to the traps are then killed by an electric grid, an insecticide-treated surface, or they are entangled and killed in a sticky substance.

LICE INFESTATION (PEDICULOSIS)

Lice are highly specialized ectoparasites that live permanently in the hair coat or plumage of the host. They are flattened, wingless insects with tarsal claws that enable them to grasp individual hairs. Lice tend to be highly host-specific. The species found on cattle, sheep, goats, and swine are usually smaller than 5 mm. Sucking lice are blood feeders, and chewing or biting lice feed on epidermal debris and sebaceous secretions. In temperate areas lice numbers increase, and they are common pests in winter and early spring. In summer they are normally at low levels that escape detection.

Sucking Lice

The sucking lice (suborder Anoplura) are blue to gray in color. They have mouthparts that consist of stylets that are withdrawn into the head capsule when not in use. The head is usually elongated and is always narrower than the thorax. Most of the tarsal claws of sucking lice are large and crablike. The following species of sucking lice are those most commonly encountered in the United States.

Cattle

- *Haematopinus eurysternus* (short-nosed cattle louse)
- *Linognathus vituli* (long-nosed cattle louse)
- *Solenopotes capillatus* (little blue cattle louse)
- *Haematopinus quadripertusus* (cattle tail louse; found only in Gulf States and southern California)

Sheep

- *Linognathus ovillis* (face and body louse)
- *Linognathus pedalis* (sheep foot louse)
- *Linognathus africanus* (African blue louse)

Goats

Linognathus stenopsis (goat-sucking louse)
Linognathus africanus (African blue louse)

Swine

- *Haematopinus suis* (hog louse)

Biting or Chewing Lice

Generally, chewing or biting lice are placed in the suborder Mallophaga, but some authors place them in the suborder Ischnocera. These lice are yellow to red in color. Adults may have distinct dark bands on the abdomen. The chewing lice have mandibular mouthparts that are used for grasping individual hairs as well as for feeding. The head is broad, wider than the thorax. The genus *Damalinia*, which includes the most common species of chewing lice on livestock, is also known as *Bovicola*. The following are the most common species of chewing lice on livestock in the United States. Note that swine are not infested with chewing lice.

Cattle

- *Damalinia (Bovicola) bovis* (cattle-biting louse)

Sheep

- *Damalinia (Bovicola) ovis* (sheep-biting louse)

Goats

- *Damalinia (Bovicola) caprae* (goat-biting louse)
- *Damalinia (Bovicola) limbatus* (Angora goat–biting louse)

- *Damalinia (Bovicola) crassipes* (sometimes called the goat-biting louse)

Lice eggs, also called nits, are cemented to individual hairs close to the skin. There are three nymphal stages or instars of increasing size and an adult stage. Typically, the cycle from egg to adult requires a month.

At most, lice live for a few days off the host. Transfer between animals is primarily through direct contact, and to a lesser extent via fomites. Both chewing and sucking lice may be transferred via attachment to flies (phoresy).

Susceptibility to pediculosis varies considerably between animals. Animals that are sick, or otherwise in poor condition, frequently are heavily infested. In turn, animals that are heavily infested may become more susceptible to disease. Highly susceptible hosts are sometimes referred to as "carriers." These carrier animals are thought to be important in maintaining an infestation in a herd or flock and should probably be culled.

The most obvious effects of lice infestation—excoriation, alopecia, self-wounding—result from pruritus and occur with both chewing and sucking lice infestations. The degree of irritation varies with the animal, and may not necessarily be correlated with the density of lice. Lightly infested animals in a herd may groom and rub as much or more than heavily infested animals. Hairballs in cattle may result from excessive licking. Pelt damage is a direct result of scratching and rubbing, as is damage to structures, fences, and so forth. The signs of pediculosis in livestock may easily be confused with diseases of the skin caused by mites, for example, psoroptic, sarcoptic, chorioptic, and psorergatic mange. Lower weight gains have been attributed to sucking lice. Animals heavily infested with sucking lice may become anemic, and death losses and abortions have been attributed to very heavy infestations of sucking lice.

Most lice species have preferred areas on the host. For some species, these sites change seasonally, and in heavy infestations, most can occur just about anywhere on the body. Lice are usually more noticeable in areas of the body where the hair coat is thinner. The cattle-biting louse is generally most abundant in the topline in the area of the withers. It spreads from the withers to elsewhere on the body, including the poll and tail and dewlap areas. Sucking lice on cattle are heaviest on the head, neck, poll, brisket, inguinal, and axillary regions. The little blue cattle louse is generally restricted to the head. The short-nosed cattle louse is most abundant in the region of the poll and ears or in the scrotal area of bulls in the summer.

Chewing lice on sheep affect the neck, back, and body region of the host. Sucking lice are usually found on the face, lower legs, and flanks. Goat lice seem to be more generally distributed over the host. Both chewing and sucking lice may be found on the neck, ventral and lateral trunk, and inguinal region. Lice are extremely irritating to sheep and goats, and chewing lice are especially damaging to wool production. There is usually much evidence of scratching and biting, and the wool of both sheep and Angora goats may be matted or pulled from the skin. The foot louse, as its name implies, is found on the lower legs and feet and may cause lameness in sheep.

Swine are infested with one species of lice, the hog louse. Found mostly on the ears, in the folds of skin behind the ears, and in the inguinal and axillary regions, this is the largest species of louse that occurs on domestic animals. An infestation by sarcoptic mange of swine may easily be confused with pediculosis and can occur concurrently. Most treatments are directed against both pests.

Treatment

Lice are effectively controlled through the use of insecticides. One may determine from the insecticide label whether an insecticide is approved for the particular animal and the pest. Read the insecticide label and observe all instructions, precautions, warnings, and so on, including withdrawal times. Some of the compounds that are effective against cattle lice may not be used on female dairy animals of breeding age because the withdrawal time for milk has not been established.

In flocks or herds of animals with a history of lice infestation, fall treatment before lice populations increase to damaging levels is advisable. Treatment may also be at time of shearing or other husbandry practice. A variety of insecticides and treatment methods are available. Generally, two applications are recommended, separated by a period of 15 days, in order to kill the lice that were present in the egg stage at the time of the first treatment.

In regions of the country where there is no danger of host-parasite reaction to larvae of cattle grubs in the esophagus or neural canal (see Cattle Grubs), a number of animal systemic insecticides (organophosphates and avermectins) may be used to control lice. Most of the organophosphate systemics may be applied as dips, sprays, or pour-ons, and will control both chewing and sucking cattle lice. Avermectin pour-ons are approved for all cattle lice species, but the injectable, oral paste, and sustained release formulations are labeled only for sucking lice control.

Though the number of systemic insecticides is limited, swine may also be treated with injectable or premix formulations of avermectin or a pour-on formulation of an organophosphate for lice control.

In addition to the animal systemics, pour-ons and whole-body sprays or dips of nonsystemic insecticides, mainly organophosphates, pyrethroids, a few organochlorines, and a formamadine may be applied in the fall to prevent lice buildup. They may also be applied in the winter or spring to control established infestations. More popular for winter and spring treatments, however, are low-volume applications of sprays and pour-ons, which are easier to apply and less stressful to animals when the weather is cold. Treatment of cattle with systemic insecticides at this time of year may not be advisable because of the possibility of an adverse host-parasite reaction. If, however, the cattle were treated earlier for cattle grubs or are otherwise known to be free of grubs, there should be no problem.

If an individual animal or group of animals become reinfested, retreatment is generally recommended for most insecticides as permitted by the label, and if the appropriate withdrawal period is observed. Again, treatment of cattle with systemics at this time of year is not advisable unless they have already been treated with a systemic for cattle grub control.

Because of the tendency for lice-infested cattle to rub, the use of self-treatment devices like back rubbers may aid in control of lice. A variety of insecticides may be used in these devices. It is important to tend to them regularly and ensure that they are charged. Several insecticide ear-tags that provide sustained release of insecticides are now labeled and approved for lice control on cattle. These tags may contain an organophosphate, pyrethroid, or synergized pyrethroid or various combinations of the three as the active ingredients.

CATTLE GRUBS

Two cattle grub species, *Hypoderma lineatum* and *Hypoderma bovis*, are parasites of cattle in the United States. The common cattle grub, *H. lineatum*, is found in most of the continental United States and Canada. The northern cattle grub, *H. bovis*, occurs principally in the northern states and Canada. Densities are greatest in young cattle with no previous exposure to infestation. Occasionally, cattle grubs occur in other hosts, horses for example.

The incidence of *Hypoderma* has decreased considerably in the United States and other parts of the world over the past 30 years, presumably because of the effectiveness and extensive use of animal systemic insecticides for their control.

The adult insects, called "heel flies," are relatively large. The adult of the common cattle grub resembles a honeybee and the northern cattle grub, which is a little larger, somewhat resembles a bumblebee. The adult flies live only 3 to 5 days, and do not feed.

The life cycles of the two species are similar, but in areas of the United States where they are sympatric, events in the life cycle of the common cattle grub generally occur 4 to 6 weeks earlier than those of the northern cattle grub. Depending on local weather conditions, latitude, and altitude, the adults are on the wing seeking a host from early spring through late summer. Ova are attached singly or in rows to individual hairs on the legs and lower body regions. The aggressive egg-laying behavior of the northern cattle grub, which deposits its eggs singly with a flight between each oviposition, is frightening to cattle and produces a running or gadding behavior of the animals under attack. The egg-laying behavior of the common cattle grub, on the other hand, does not normally cause a fright reaction. This species of cattle grub either lands on the host or walks to the host after landing on the ground. The common cattle grub lays eggs in rows on individual hairs. Under optimal temperature conditions eggs hatch in about 3 days and newly emerged larvae penetrate the skin.

Penetration of the skin is via proteolytic enzymes secreted by the larvae and may cause irritation at the site of penetration. Once in the host, first-instar larvae migrate through the body for 4 to 6 months. Movement of the larvae is through connective tissue, through fascial planes between muscles, and along nerve pathways. Eventually the larvae of the common cattle grub move to the submucosal connective tissue of the esophagus and northern cattle grub larvae move to epidural fat of the spinal cord in the region of the thoracic and lumbar vertebrae. Both species may be found in these regions for periods of 2 to 4 months. The presence of larvae produces localized areas of edematous connective and adipose tissue. Yellowish to greenish localized foci or tracks of edematous tissue are attributed to the presence or migration of larvae. In the region of the spinal canal, *H. bovis* larvae have been associated with meningitis, periostitis, osteomyelitis, and with necrosis of connective tissue and epidural fat. Only rarely have nervous disorders been reported.

From the esophagus and the spinal canal, both species, still in the first instar, migrate to subdermal tissue in the mid-dorsal region of the back. They cut breathing holes to the outside and then position their posterior spiracles at the opening. The larvae grow considerably and molt two times within a warble or cyst that is of host origin. The period within the cyst might require up to 2 months. Eventually, fully developed larvae emerge through their breathing holes, drop to the ground, and form puparia. A puparium lasts 15 days to 8 weeks depending on air temperature and humidity, and then adults emerge and seek mates.

Injury to cattle may result from the gadding that occurs in the presence of the adult fly. Effects of the larvae on weight gains and milk production are somewhat equivocal. Considerable damage to hides and carcasses results from breathing holes and jellied tissues in the back at the time of slaughter.

Treatment

Cattle grubs are effectively controlled through the use of insecticides. One may determine from the insecticide label whether an insecticide is approved for the particular site (cattle in this case) and pest. Read the insecticide label and observe all instructions, precautions, warnings, and so on, including withdrawal times. Some of the compounds that are effective against cattle grubs may not be used on female dairy animals of breeding age because the withdrawal time in milk has not been established.

Cattle grubs are most effectively controlled through the use of animal systemic insecticides applied in a variety of ways: high-pressure whole-body spray, dipping vat, pour-on, or injectable. Application of these systemic insecticides in the fall to control cattle grubs will aid in the prevention of damaging cattle lice infestations later in the year. Several organophosphate insecticides are approved for use as a spray, dip, or pour-on. Systemic sprays must be applied at high pressure, 250 to 350 psi, to ensure that the skin is wet and the insecticide is absorbed. Dipping vats are very effective for thorough wetting of the animals, but in some regions of the country disposal of used insecticide is a problem. The pour-on method, which involves the application of relatively low dosages (e.g., a few milliliters to a 0.5 oz/100 lb body weight), is very popular because of ease of application. Various avermectin insecticides may also be applied as pour-on, injectable, or sustained release bolus formulations, and all are effective against both species of cattle grub.

Especially in areas where grub numbers are known to be high, cattle should be treated as soon as possible after the adult heel fly season. If larvae are killed by systemic insecticides, an inflammatory edematous reaction while the larvae are in the tissues of the esophagus or in the spinal canal may lead to adverse host-parasite reactions. Swelling may occlude the lumen of the esophagus in *H. lineatum*–infested cattle resulting in difficulty in swallowing and profuse salivation. Eructation may cease and the animal may become bloated. If *H. bovis* larvae are killed while in the epidural fat of the spinal canal, a transitory irritation of the spinal tissues may result, and mild to severe paraplegia may develop. The host-parasite reaction is generally most severe around 24 hours following treatment though it may occur later. Usually it is over in 48 to 72 hours.

Should a host-parasite reaction occur, anti-inflammatory and antibiotic therapy is indicated. Cattle on a low-energy ration at the time of treatment are less likely to bloat severely. Bloat may be relieved by trocarization. A stomach tube should not be used as the esophagus may be easily traumatized. Atropinization is contraindicated as it reduces rumen motility.

Cutoff dates to avoid treatment while grubs are in the esophagus or spinal canal can be provided by local veterinarians or extension specialists. The local cutoff date may not be appropriate for cattle that have been shipped in from a different geographic location.

Though not a common practice, cattle grubs in the warbles may be controlled by manual extraction or by insecticide treatment, i.e., dressing the backs of cattle with a topical insecticide or treating the animal with a systemic insecticide that is effective against the second and third larval stages. Caution should be taken to avoid the host-parasite reaction if the latter is used.

BIBLIOGRAPHY

Muscoid Flies of Range Cattle

Bruce WG: The history and biology of the horn fly, *Haematobia irritans* (L.) with comments on control. North Carolina Agricultural Experiment Station Technical Bulletin No. 157, 1964.
Byford RL, Craig ME, Crosby BL: A review of ectoparasites and their effect on cattle production. J Anim Sci 70:597–602, 1992.
Drummond RO, Lambert G, Smalley HF Jr, et al: Estimated losses of livestock to pests. *In* Pimentel D (ed): Handbook of Pest Management in Agriculture, vol 1. Boca Raton, Fla, CRC Press, 1981, pp 317–346.

Morgan CE, Thomas GD: Annotated bibliography of the horn fly, *Haematobia irritans* (L.), including references on the buffalo fly, *H. exigua* (de Meijere), and other species belonging to the genus *Haematobia*. US Department of Agriculture miscellaneous publication No. 1278, 1974.
Morgan CE, Thomas GD: Annotated bibliography of the horn fly, *Haematobia irritans* (L.), including references on the buffalo fly, *H. exigua* (de Meijere), and other species belonging to the genus *Haematobia*. US Department of Agriculture miscellaneous publication No. 1278(suppl). 1977.
Teskey HJ: A review of the life history and habits of *Musca autumnalis* DeGeer (Diptera: Muscidae). Can Entomol 92:360–367, 1960.

Lice Infestation (Pediculosis)

Barker SC: Phylogeny and classification, origins, and evolution of host associations of lice. Int J Parasitol 24:1285–1291, 1994.
Crauford-Benson HJ: The cattle lice of Great Britain. Part I. Biology, with a special reference to *Haematopinus eurysternus*. Parasitology 33:331–342, 1941.
Crauford-Benson HJ: The cattle lice of Great Britian. Part II. Lice populations. Parasitology 33:343–358, 1941.
Hopkins GHE: The host-associations of the lice of mammals. Proc Zool Soc London 119:387–604, 1949.
Lancaster JL: Cattle lice. Agricultural Experiment Station, University of Arkansas, Fayetteville, Bull No. 951, 1957.
Matthysse JG: Cattle lice: Their biology and control. Cornell Experiment Station Bull No. 832, 1946.
Meleney WP, Kim KC: A comparative study of cattle-infesting *Haematopinus*, with redescription of *H. quadripertusus* Fahrenholz, 1916 (Anoplura: Haematopinidae). J Parasitol 60:507–522, 1974.
Watson DW, Lloyd JE, Kumar R: Density and distribution of cattle lice (Phthiraptera: Haematopinidae, Linognathidae, Trichodectidae) on six steers. Vet Parasitol 69:283–296, 1997.

Cattle Grubs

Cox DD, Mozier JO, Mullee MT: Posterior paralysis in a calf caused by cattle grubs (*Hypoderma bovis*) after treatment with a systemic insecticide for grub control. J Am Vet Med Assoc 157:1088–1092, 1970.
Panciera RJ, Ewing SA, Johnson EM, et al: Eosinophilic mediastinitis, myositis, pleuritis, and pneumonia of cattle associated with migration of first-instar larvae of *Hypoderma lineatum*. J Vet Diagn Invest 5:226–231, 1993.
Scharff DK, Sharman GAM, Ludwig P: Illness and death in calves induced by treatments with systemic insecticides for the control of cattle grubs. J Am Vet Med Assoc 141:582–587, 1962.
Scholl PJ: Biology and control of cattle grubs. Annu Rev Entomol 39:53–70, 1993.
Wolfe LS: Observations on the histopathological changes caused by the larvae of *Hypoderma bovis* (L.) and *Hypoderma lineatum* (DeVill.) (Diptera: Oestridae) in tissues of cattle. Can J Anim Sci 39:145–159, 1959.

■ Ticks and Mites

Bill C. Clymer, Ph.D., B.C.E.

TICKS THAT COMMONLY INFECT LIVESTOCK

The economic importance[1] of ticks varies based on the geographic region of the United States, time of the year, climatic conditions, and many other factors. Although some species may not cause major losses to the livestock industry, their ability to transmit disease (e.g., Lyme disease) causes ticks to be of primary importance, not only to livestock but also humans. They have been proved to transmit rickettsiae, spirochetes, protozoan blood parasites, and viruses to livestock.[2] Ticks are blood feeders and many species feed on a variety of hosts. In some areas, the blood loss and irritation from tick feeding will greatly decrease the ability of an animal to gain weight or produce milk. Lesions produced by feeding ticks may predispose animals to secondary infections and myiasis. Ticks also cause tremendous losses to wildlife populations. In some of the southeastern states, the loss of the deer fawn crop caused directly and indirectly by ticks has been reported at over 40%. Light to moderate tick populations may cause a substantial loss in tourism income because people shun infested areas.

Ticks, which belong to the class Arachnida, are very similar to mites and differ from insects (Insecta) in the following ways: (1) the head, thorax, and abdomen are all fused into a single body region; (2) antennae are absent; and (3) four pairs of legs are present in the nymphal and adult stages (larvae have only three pairs of legs).[3] There are two types of ticks that attack livestock, the hard ticks (Ixodidae) and the soft ticks (Argasidae). They can be separated by the presence of a dorsal shield or scutum on the hard ticks, which is absent on soft ticks. See Table 1 for general information on the distribution, hosts, and

preferred feeding sites on host animals. Many species of ticks have the ability to live for long periods of time off the host without taking a blood meal. This trait increases the difficulty of control.

Ticks undergo four stages in their development: (1) egg, (2) six-legged larvae, (3) eight-legged nymph, and (4) adult. Their reproduction is sexual. After eggs hatch, the small larvae crawl up onto nearby vegetation and await a suitable host. With the three host ticks, this procedure is repeated again as a nymph and as an adult. Tick mortality is usually very high but most species lay large numbers of eggs. The time spent on the host may be from a few minutes (15 to 30) to several months. When ticks are not on a host, they are usually found on the ground or near the ground in vegetation awaiting an opportunity to parasitize another host. Large numbers of ticks may be found in bedding areas of host animals. Ticks are attracted to their hosts in a variety of ways. Many times the contact may be accidental, but ticks do move toward carbon dioxide, which is released by

Table 1
PARTIAL LIST OF TICKS THAT PARASITIZE LIVESTOCK IN THE UNITED STATES

Tick Species	Generalized Life Cycle	Principal Hosts	Feeding Areas on Domestic Hosts	Distribution
Lone Star tick (Amblyomma americanum)	3-host	Cattle, horses, dogs, and humans, as well as a wide variety of birds and wild mammals	Indiscriminant (all areas of the body subject to attack)	Southern and southeastern United States
Cayenne tick (Amblyomma cajennense)	3-host	Cattle, horses, sheep, goats, and dogs, as well as wild birds and mammals	Indiscriminant	Southern Texas
Gulf Coast tick (Amblyomma maculatum)	3-host	Adults: cattle, sheep, deer, coyotes Immatures: ground-dwelling birds and small mammals	Outer portion of cattle ears	Gulf States north through Oklahoma to southeastern Kansas
Cattle tick (Boophilus annulatus)*	1-host	Cattle, horses, sheep, goats, dogs, deer	Indiscriminant	Southern Texas and Mexico
Tropical cattle tick (Boophilus microplus)*	1-host	Cattle, horses, sheep, goats, dogs, deer	Indiscriminant	Southern Texas and Mexico
Winter tick (Dermacentor albipictus in synonymy with Dermacentor nigrolineatus)	1-host	Horses, mules, cattle, elk, deer, moose	Indiscriminant	Southern, southwestern, and northwestern regions of United States
Rocky Mountain wood tick (Dermacentor andersoni)	3-host	Adults: cattle, horses, dogs, humans, elk, deer, and other wild mammals Immatures: small mammals	Indiscriminant	Rocky Mountains from northern New Mexico to Canada, eastern slopes of the Cascade Range and Sierra Nevada
Pacific Coast tick (Dermacentor occidentalis)	3-host	Adults: cattle, horses, sheep, dogs, humans, deer Immatures: many species of small mammals	Indiscriminant	Oregon and California, western slopes of the Cascade Range and Sierra Nevada
Tropical horse tick (Dermacentor [Anocentor] nitens)	1-host	Equines	Outer ear	Coastal regions of states from southern Texas to Florida and Georgia
American dog tick (Dermacentor variabilis)	3-host	Adults: prefer canines; will feed on humans, cattle, horses Immatures: small rodents	Indiscriminant	Texas to Montana and east to the Atlantic; Pacific seaboard from Washington to California
Black-legged tick (Ixodes scapularus)	3-host	Adults: cattle, horses, sheep, swine, man, deer Immatures: small mammals and birds	Indiscriminant	Eastern, central, and southern United States
Spinose ear tick (Otobius megnini)	Modified 1-host	Immatures: cattle, horses, sheep, cats, dogs, rabbits, elk, mountain sheep	Inner portion of outer ear	Western and southwestern United States

*Ticks suspected of being *B. annulatus* or *B. microplus* should be reported to state animal health agencies and U.S. Department of Agriculture, Animal and Plant Health Inspection Service, veterinary services officials. State and federal regulations require quarantine and eradication procedures for these species.

animals. It is also thought that movement and body heat attract them. Climatic factors play a major role in the severity of tick problems. Some species can overwinter in extremely cold climates, while others can withstand high temperatures and very arid conditions.

There are several types of life cycles, depending on the number of hosts involved. In one-host ticks such as the Texas cattle fever tick (*Boophilus annulatus*), all the parasitic stages beginning with the unfed larvae are passed on a single host. They molt twice on the host and do not leave until they are fully engorged and fertilized, at which time they drop to the ground to molt and lay eggs. Three-host ticks such as the Lone Star tick (*Amblyomma americanum*) generally start their larval stage on a small mammal, drop off, and molt to a nymph, which also attacks a small to medium-sized mammal. The engorged nymph then drops to the ground, molts to an adult, and then searches for a larger animal to complete the cycle. Ground-inhabiting birds and rodents are often preferred hosts for the larval and nymphal stages.

Owing to the rapid and frequent movement of livestock all over the United States, ticks can be easily transported into areas where they are normally not found. This may create some identification problems. Several species of ticks are gradually increasing their "territory." The Gulf Coast tick (*Amblyomma maculatum*) was only found along the Gulf Coast for a number of years, but has spread its territory across Texas, Oklahoma, and into southern Kansas. The spinose ear tick (*Otobius megnini*) has always been considered a semiarid species, but is now found in the more humid areas of the United States.

Ticks can cause large economic losses, as well as the irritation and disease risk. If heavy populations are present, control efforts should be made. Losses to the beef cattle industry have been estimated at over $275 million per year.[1] Both the Environmental Protection Agency and Food and Drug Administration have approved several acaricides for use on livestock for tick control. Because of the life cycle of ticks, several applications per season may be necessary to achieve effective control. Proper identification of the pest species is very important to determine the correct treatment procedure necessary.[4] If suspected as being *B. annulatus* or *Boophilus microplus*, ticks should be sent to the state animal health agencies or the U.S. Department of Agriculture, Animal and Plant Health Inspection Service (USDA, A & PHIS) veterinary services. It is a good practice to have a specimen properly identified if there is some question of its correct identification. Most tick species feed indiscriminately on their host, attaching to various areas of the body, which usually requires whole-body treatment for effective control. Some species are predisposed to feeding in and on the ears of livestock, for example, *A. maculatum*, *O. megnini*, and *Dermacentor nitens*. These species may be effectively controlled with insecticidal ear-tags, tapes, or aerosol spray formulations.

Some species of ticks have developed resistance to some of the acaricides available for control. The list of approved products for use on livestock and pets is constantly changing. Some of the types of products that are currently labeled for tick control include organophosphates and synthetic pyrethroids. The avermectins and milbemycins are also showing some effect on ticks. Safe use of acaricides is mandatory to ensure safety for both applicator and livestock. Before any pesticide is used, read and follow the label. Some breeds of cattle (e.g., Brahman) may show a toxic reaction to some pesticides, and dairy animals are often excluded from the label. Since labeling varies from state to state, consult your state extension service or department of agriculture for a list of currently approved and recommended products. If you have questions about tick identification, send specimens to the National Veterinary Services Laboratory; USDA, A&PHIS; P.O. Box 844, Shipping & Receiving; Ames, Iowa, 50010. Specimens should be placed in 80% ethanol and labeled as to collection date, location, host, and collector.

MITES

Mites, like ticks, belong to the order Acari, class Arachnida. Parasitic mites of domestic animals are usually representatives of three different suborders.[5] The following information lists the suborders and common mites in each one: suborder Mesostigmata—chicken mite (*Dermanyssus gallinae*), northern fowl mite (*Ornithonyssus sylviarum*), and tropical fowl mite (*Ornithonyssus bursa*); suborder Prostigmata—chiggers (*Trombicula* and allies in the family Trombiculidae) and follicle mites (*Demodex* spp.); suborder Astigmata—mange and itch mites (*Sarcoptes*, *Psoroptes*, *Chorioptes*, and *Notoedres*).

Mites differ greatly from one species to another, but, like ticks, the adults have four pairs of legs and many of the mites have the appearance of "small" ticks. The generalized life cycle is very similar to that of ticks except that more than one nymphal stage is usually present. Typically, female mites deposit eggs which hatch into larvae that pass through two or more nymphal stages to eventually mature into adults. The larvae have only three pairs of legs and may be distinguished from later stages by this character. The first nymphal stage (protonymph) has four pairs of legs, one or more plates on the dorsal side, and a single, short sternal plate with three pairs of setae. The second nymphal stage (deutonymph) has four pairs of legs, a single dorsal plate, and a longer sternal plate, extending at least to the fourth pair of coxae, which bears four pairs of setae. The book *Introduction to Veterinary Entomology*, by Bay and Harris,[3] has a very good mite chapter.

Poultry Mites

Poultry mites usually occur on or under the skin or feathers; however, some species may be found in body tissues, feather quills, or nasal and respiratory passages such as the air sac. They live on bits of skin or feather or by piercing the skin or tissue and sucking blood or body fluids. Some species transmit serious and often fatal, disease-producing organisms. Some of the more important species are: Northern fowl mite (*Ornithonyssus sylviarum*), tropical fowl mite (*Ornithonyssus bursa*), chicken mite (*Dermanyssus gallinae*), scaly-leg mite (*Knemidocoptes mutans*), depluming mite (*Knemidocoptes gallinae*), and the turkey chigger (*Neoschoengastia americana*).

Livestock Mites

The four most common species of mites found on domestic livestock in the United States belong to four different genera. They are *Psoroptes*, *Chorioptes*, *Sarcoptes*, and *Demodex*. There still exists in the scientific community a discussion as to whether or not the mites found on the different species of animals (i.e., horses, cattle, swine, sheep) are different species or varieties or strains of the same species. Regardless of their taxonomic classification, their life history, nature of damage, and method of control are similar for all members of the same genus. The *Psoroptes*, *Chorioptes*, and *Sarcoptes* mites are collectively referred to as mange or scab mites, while the *Demodex* mites are referred to as follicle mites. Accurate microscopic diagnosis is important since all three of the mange mites may cause similar damage to the host animal.

The *Psoroptes ovis* (var. *bovis*) mite is small, less than ¹⁄₄₀ in. long, but causes a great deal of irritation to the host animal. It is very detrimental to weight gain, milk production, and feed conversion. Heavily infested animals may experience a 56% decrease in average daily gain.[5] Scabies mites are fairly active on the animal and do not burrow like the sarcoptic or the demodectic mite. Scabies mites are usually spread by animal-to-animal contact, but may also be spread by livestock equipment.

The life cycle of this mite, which lasts 10 to 12 days, is as follows: the eggs hatch in 3 to 5 days, the larval stage takes 2 to 3 days, the nymphal stage (nonsexual form of the adult) lasts 3 to 5 days, and the sexually mature adult is ready to mate and start laying eggs in 1 to 2 days. Each female lays 15 to 24 eggs. Research indicates that mites may survive off the host for up to 10 days.

Initially, scabies infestations may resemble a lice infestation and are often noticed on the withers area first. Small patches of hair will be missing, and the animals will lick and rub those areas. However, scabies is associated with intense pruritus. The constant licking and rubbing that results can lead to severe abscesses, bruises, and cuts. Affected areas enlarge and can quickly (within 24 hours) become lesions that spread over the entire body. In severe infestations, scab formation is so heavy that the hide appears to double in thickness and causes the condition known as elephant hide.

The entire surface of the body is susceptible to infestation. Some animals become almost denuded of hair while others will have severe lesions beneath the hair. This parasite was originally thought to be a "cool season" pest, but I have seen animals with long hair have serious problems during the hotter part of the year. *Psoroptes* spp. cause a quarantinable disease and an accurate diagnosis is very important. Skin scrapings should be taken and checked with a microscope. If identification is uncertain, it should be sent to a diagnostic laboratory for a positive identification.

Animal self-grooming is probably responsible for limiting the number of clinical cases in a group. A limited number of products are currently approved by the federal veterinary services for control of this quarantinable pest. These products need to be used in strict accordance with the label instructions since this mite is one of the dose-limiting parasites for a number of products.

Scabies mites can be very damaging pests but do not normally kill the animal. It has been found that severe scabies infestations have a tremendous effect on the white blood cell count and may over time have a negative effect on the bone marrow. With this lowered immune response, the animal is often predisposed to other stress factors (e.g., respiratory infection) which may result in death.

Sarcoptic mange or itch mites (*Sarcoptes* spp.) are often referred to as barn itch mites and closely resemble the psoroptic mites.[4] One major difference is that the mouthparts of the sarcoptic mites are bluntly rounded whereas the psoroptic mites have slender pointed mouthparts. This mite is also a burrowing mite and is of the most economic importance in large commercial swine operations. They are also the most common type of mange mite found in dairy cattle and horses.

Eggs are laid by fertilized females in the burrows. Females may lay 40 to 50 eggs over a 2 to 4 week period, which hatch within 3 to 5 days. The larvae stay in the old tunnel and may start a new one. The larval stage lasts 4 to 6 days with the nymphal stage lasting only 2 days. Adults may live over 2 months. The burrowing and feeding activity results in severe skin inflammation, accompanied by a serous exudate which hardens into a crust or scab. Lesions may appear anywhere on the body but are more prevalent on the head and neck of swine. In cattle, infested areas are usually found above the scrotum or udder and on the inner surface of the thighs. Secondary bacterial infection is a frequent complication.

Chorioptic mites (*Chorioptes* spp.) are slightly smaller in size than the psoroptic mites. Livestock hosts include cattle, horses,

sheep, and goats and the mites usually spread by direct contact. They are not a burrowing mite but spend their entire life cycle on the host. Chorioptic mites feed on skin debris rather than piercing the skin of the hosts as do the *Psoroptes* and *Sarcoptes* mites. Under laboratory conditions, the complete life cycle requires 21 to 26 days. Infestations normally occur during the winter months, but the disease is milder and typically occurs on the lower hind legs and around the tail. In advanced cases, scabs may become thick and crusted. Infestations normally disappear in the spring. This mite is frequently found on animals in "dairy show strings."

The demodectic or follicular mange mites infect hair follicles and glands of the skin of the hosts. The bodies of the mites are "cigar-shaped" and the legs are short and stubby. The life cycle is not well known, but infestations are more common in cattle, especially dairy breeds. This pest usually is not an economic problem, but it may be hard to control due to the mites being in the hair follicles. Acaricides that are effective for sarcoptic and psoroptic mites will help alleviate the problem.

Research has shown that the avermectin and milbemycin compounds as both pour-ons and injections provide effective mite reduction. Dips and sprays of several different types of compounds are also effective.

REFERENCES

1. Drummond RO, George JE, Kunz SE: Control of Arthropod Pests of Livestock: A Review of Technology. Boca Raton, Fla, CRC Press, 1988, pp 12–14.
2. Teel PD: Ticks. In Williams RE, Hall RD, Broce AD, et al (eds): Livestock Entomology. New York, Wiley, 1985, pp. 129–149.
3. Bay DE, Harris RL: Introduction to Veterinary Entomology. Bryan, Tex, Stonefly, 1988, pp 70–84.
4. Whitlock JH: Diagnosis of Veterinary Parasitisms. Philadelphia, Lea & Febiger, 1960, pp 61–71.
5. Fisher WF, Wright FC: Effects of sheep scab mite on cumulative weight gains in cattle. J Econ Entomol 74:254–257, 1981.

■ Immunologic Skin Diseases

Danny W. Scott, D.V.M., Diplomate, A.C.V.D.

Immunologic skin disorders typically affect only one animal in a group and thus are of minimal concern from an economic or production standpoint. For detailed information on immunologic skin disorders, the reader is referred to the bibliography.

URTICARIA

Urticarial reactions are characterized by localized or generalized wheals, which may or may not be pruritic and which may or may not exhibit serum leakage. The lesions are cold swellings that pit with digital pressure. Characteristically, the wheals are evanescent lesions, with each individual lesion persisting only a few hours. Urticarial lesions may assume bizarre shapes (serpiginous, linear, arciform, papular).

In cattle, urticaria has been reported in association with insect and arthropod stings and bites, infections, systemic medicaments (penicillin, streptomycin, oxytetracycline, chloramphenicol, neomycin, sulfonamides, diethylstilbestrol, carboxymethylcellulose, hydroxypropyl methylcellulose), biologicals (various vaccines and toxoids, especially for leptospirosis, *Brucella abortus* strain 19, foot-and-mouth disease, shipping fever, salmonellosis, rinderpest, and contagious pleuropneumonia), physical trauma (dermatographism), hypodermiasis, feedstuffs (pasture plants, moldy hay or straw, or potato and walnut leaves), inhalants, and plants (stinging nettle). Lesions are most commonly seen on the face, ears, and trunk. Milk allergy is a unique autoallergic disease of cattle, especially Jerseys and Guernseys, which become sensitized to the casein in their own milk. The disorder is believed to be familial and is triggered by circumstances that cause milk retention or unusual engorgement of the udder with milk.

In swine, urticaria has been reported in association with insect and arthropod stings and bites, infections (especially erysipelas), topical applications (especially parasiticides), feedstuffs, systemic medicaments, plants (stinging nettle), and biologicals. Lesions are most commonly seen over the trunk and proximal limbs.

Therapy for urticaria includes elimination and avoidance of known etiologic factors and symptomatic treatment with systemic glucocorticoids (dexamethasone 0.1 mg/kg, intravenously [IV] or intramuscularly [IM], or prednisone or prednisolone 1 mg/kg IV or IM) or nonsteroidal anti-inflammatory agents (aspirin 5 mg/kg; phenylbutazone 2 mg/kg; flunixin meglumine 1 to 2 mg/kg). Antihistamines are rarely beneficial.

ATOPY

Atopy is a genetically determined pruritic dermatitis in which the animal becomes sensitized to inhaled environmental allergens. Atopy has been presumptively diagnosed in Suffolk sheep. These animals had recurrent seasonal (spring, summer, fall) pruritic skin disease. The face, ears, ventral abdomen, and distal limbs were chiefly affected. Secondary lesions, developing over time, included excoriations, alopecia, lichenification, and hyperpigmentation. Intradermal skin testing revealed numerous positive reactions to various plant pollens and molds. Treatment was not initiated in these sheep, although systemic glucocorticoids, systemic antihistamines, or hyposensitization would be therapeutic options.

FOOD HYPERSENSITIVITY

Food hypersensitivity is an extremely rarely reported cause of pruritic skin disease in food animals. Incriminated substances have included wheat, maize, soybeans, rice bran, and clover hay in cattle and pasture plants in swine. Affected animals manifested generalized pruritus with or without papules, plaques, or wheals. Diagnosis would be established by feeding a hypoallergenic diet for 4 weeks (until the symptoms have resolved), then readministering the original diet (whereupon the clinical syndrome is reproduced within 1 to 7 days). Treatment would require avoiding offending foodstuffs.

DRUG ERUPTIONS

Drug eruptions are rarely reported in food animals. Drugs responsible for skin eruptions may be administered orally, topically, or by injection. Any drug may cause an eruption, and there is no specific type of reaction for any one drug. Thus, drug eruption may mimic virtually any dermatosis (e.g., urticaria, vasculitis, vesicobullous dermatitis, erythema multiforme, generalized pruritus, exfoliative dermatitis). The only reliable test for the diagnosis of drug eruption is to withdraw the drug and observe for the disappearance of the eruption in 10 to 14 days.

PEMPHIGUS FOLIACEUS

Pemphigus foliaceus is a rare autoimmune dermatosis of goats. Pustules or vesicles or both are the primary skin lesions but are difficult to find among the secondary lesions of annular erosions with epidermal collarettes, annular crusts, oozing, scaling, and alopecia. Lesions are most prominent on the face, ears, and limbs but may be generalized. Affected goats may or may not have pruritus and may or may not exhibit signs of systemic illness (fever, anorexia, depression, weight loss). Diagnosis is confirmed by skin biopsy (subcorneal pustules or vesicopustules containing numerous acantholytic keratinocytes and neutrophils), bacterial and fungal cultures (negative), and, if available, direct immunofluorescence testing (immunoglobulin with or without complement deposited in the intercellular spaces of the epidermis in primary skin lesions). The disease is chronic and incurable, thus necessitating long-term control with systemic glucocorticoids or injectable gold salts (aurothioglucose).

BOVINE EXFOLIATIVE ERYTHRODERMA

A cow with severe exfoliative erythroderma was studied. Her calves and an unrelated calf that were fed her colostrum developed exfoliative erythroderma. From birth to 4 days of age, the calves developed erythema and vesicles on the muzzle. Between 4 and 50 days of age, the calves developed generalized erythema, scaling, easy epilation, and alopecia. By 4 months of age, the calves had recovered. Skin biopsy specimens revealed intraepidermal pustules containing neutrophils. An immune-mediated disorder associated with colostrum was postulated.

BIBLIOGRAPHY

Bassett H: Bovine exfoliative dermatitis: a new bovine skin disease transferred by colostrum. Irish Vet J 39:106–107, 1985.
Rude TA: Postvaccination type I hypersensitivity in cattle. Agri Pract 11:29–33, 1990.
Scott DW: Large Animal Dermatology. Philadelphia, WB Saunders, 1988.
Scott DW, Campbell SG: A seasonal pruritic dermatitis in sheep resembling atopy. Agri Pract 8(6):46–49, 1987.
Scott DW, Smith MC, Smith CA, et al: Pemphigus foliaceus in a goat. Agri Pract 5(4):38–45, 1984.

■ Environmental Skin Diseases
Danny W. Scott, D.V.M., Diplomate, A.C.V.D.

Environmental disorders are common and often a cause of substantial economic loss in livestock production. In many instances (chemical toxicoses, mycotoxicoses, hepatotoxic plant toxicoses) the dermatologic abnormalities are clinically spectacular and of important diagnostic significance but are of rather trivial overall importance prognostically, therapeutically, and financially compared with abnormalities in other organ systems. For detailed clinicopathologic information on these disorders, the reader is referred to the appropriate sections of this book.

MECHANICAL INJURIES

Intertrigo

Intertrigo is a superficial inflammatory dermatosis that occurs in places where skin is in apposition and is thus subject to the friction of movement, increased local heat, maceration from retained moisture, and irritation from accumulation of debris. When these factors are present to a sufficient degree, dissolution of stratum corneum, exudation, and secondary bacterial infection are inevitable.

Intertrigo is most commonly seen in dairy cattle and dairy goats. Congestion of the udder at parturition is physiologic but may be sufficiently severe to cause edema of the belly, udder, and teats. In most cases, the edema disappears within 2 to 3 days after parturition, but if extensive and persistent it can lead to intertrigo where the skin of the udder contacts the skin of the medial thighs. Erythema is followed by oozing, erosion, crusting, secondary bacterial infection, and, in severe cases, necrosis and a foul odor.

Udder-thigh intertrigo is generally treated with gentle antiseptic soaps (chlorhexidine) and astringent rinses (aluminum acetate) two or three times daily. In severe cases, diuretics (chlorothiazide 0.5 g intravenously [IV] every 12 hours; furosemide 0.5 g IV every 12 hours) and frequent massage are beneficial in reducing udder edema. When the dermatosis is no longer moist and exudative, dusting with powders two or three times daily helps to reduce friction. Healing is usually complete within 4 to 12 weeks.

Hematoma

A hematoma is a circumscribed area of hemorrhage into the tissues. It arises from vascular damage associated with sudden, severe, blunt external trauma (e.g., a fall) or with more prolonged physical trauma (e.g., head shaking because of irritation from ear mites). The lesions are usually acute in onset, subcutaneous, and fluctuant and may or may not be painful.

Hematomas are commonly seen in swine, usually over the shoulders, flanks, and hindquarters, following severe nonpenetrating trauma. Aural hematomas, most frequently seen in lop-eared breeds of swine, are associated with head shaking (from sarcoptic mange, pediculosis, or meal in the ears from overhead feeders) or ear biting. Vulvar hematomas are seen in the postpartum gilt and sow, associated with trauma from faulty farrowing crate doors or large piglets at farrowing. In cattle, hematomas may be seen over the stifle, ischial tuberosity, lateral thorax, point of the shoulder, and middle of the back.

Diagnosis is based on history and physical examination. Needle aspiration and cytologic examination reveal blood. Most hematomas are simply allowed to organize and partially resolve. Occasional herd outbreaks of hematomas, in which 10% of the sows died of massive hemorrhage, have been reported. Increasing the level of vitamin K in the feed corrected the problem.

Gangrene

Gangrene is a clinical term used to describe severe tissue necrosis and sloughing. The necrosis may be moist or dry. The pathologic mechanism of gangrene is an occlusion of either the arterial or venous blood supply. Moist gangrene is produced by impairment of lymphatic and venous drainage plus infection (putrefaction) and is a complication of decubital ulcers associated with bony prominences and pressure points in recumbent animals. Moist gangrene presents as swollen, discolored areas with a foul odor and progressive tissue decomposition. Dry gangrene occurs when the arterial blood supply is occluded, but venous and lymphatic drainage remain intact and infection is absent (mummification).

The causes of gangrene include external pressure (pressure sores, rope galls, constricting bands, and porcine skin necrosis), internal pressure (severe edema), burns (thermal, chemical, friction, radiation, or electrical), frostbite, envenomation (snake bite), vasculitis, ergotism, fescue toxicosis, and various infections (salmonellosis, streptococcosis, spirochetosis, necrobacillosis, erysipelas, malignant catarrhal fever, bovine herpes mammillitis,

bovine lumpy skin disease, and staphylococcal and clostridial infections).

Subcutaneous Emphysema

Subcutaneous emphysema is characterized by free gas in the subcutis. Possible causes include air entering through a cutaneous wound (from an accident or surgery), a lung punctured by the end of a fractured rib, internal penetrating wounds (traumatic reticuloperitonitis), rumen gases migrating from a rumenotomy or rumenal trocarization, extension from pulmonary emphysema, extension from tracheal rupture, gas gangrene infections, and bovine ephemeral fever.

Subcutaneous emphysema is characterized by soft, fluctuant, crepitant subcutaneous swellings. The lesions are usually not painful, and the animals are not acutely ill, except in the case of gas gangrene (clostridial infections).

Diagnosis is based on history and physical examination. Treatment is directed at the underlying cause. Sterile subcutaneous emphysema requires no treatment unless it is extensive and incapacitating, when multiple skin incisions may be necessary.

Black Pox

Black pox is a sporadic condition seen in dairy cattle. It is believed to be a traumatically induced teat disorder caused by poor milking machine techniques. *Staphylococcus aureus* is consistently cultured from the lesions but is presumed to be a secondary invader.

Lesions occur most commonly on the tip of the teat and are characterized by crateriform ulcers with raised edges and a black spot in the pitted center. The affected area may spread to involve the teat sphincter, whereupon mastitis is a possible sequela.

Black pox is usually quite intractable to topical and systemic medicaments. The milking machinery should be carefully analyzed as to pressure and technique.

THERMAL INJURIES

Burns

Burns are occasionally seen in livestock and may be thermal (barn, forest, and brush fires or accidental spillage of hot solutions), electrical (electrocution or lightning strike), frictional (rope burns or abrasions from falling), chemical (improperly used topical medicaments or maliciously used caustic agents), or caused by radiation. The reader is referred to the appropriate section of this book for discussion of the pathophysiology of burns and the management of severely burned animals with extracutaneous complications.

Burns are most commonly seen over the dorsum, face, or teats and udder. Animals with burns over more than 50% of their body usually die. First-degree burns involve the superficial epidermis, are characterized by erythema, edema, and pain, and generally heal without complication. Second-degree burns affect the entire epidermis, are characterized by erythema, edema, pain, and vesicles, and usually re-epithelialize with proper wound care. Third-degree burns include the entire epidermis, dermis, and appendages and are characterized by necrosis, ulceration, anesthesia, and scarring. Fourth-degree burns involve the entire skin, subcutis, and underlying fascia, muscle, and tendon.

In a study of Australian dairy cattle with teat burns (from brush fires), mature cows were more likely to return to normal function than heifers (78% vs. 40%). Major post-burn complications included occlusion of teat orifice, twisted and distorted teats, and mastitis.

Frostbite

Frostbite is more common in neonates; animals that are sick, debilitated, or dehydrated; animals with heavily pigmented skin; and animals having preexisting vascular insufficiency. Also at risk are dairy cattle and goats turned out into cold weather after udders and teats have been washed but inadequately dried off.

Frostbite most commonly affects ears, tails, teats, scrotum, and feet. Mild cases present as erythema, scaling, and alopecia. Severe cases present as necrosis, dry gangrene, and sloughing. The affected skin is usually anesthetic.

Therapy varies with the severity of the frostbite. In mild cases, treatment is usually not needed. In more severe cases, rapid thawing in warm water (41 to 44°C) is indicated as soon as possible after it is known that refreezing can be prevented. Rewarming may be followed by the application of bland, protective ointments or creams. In very severe cases with necrosis and sloughing, symptomatic therapy with topical wet soaks and systemic antibiotics is indicated, and surgical excision is postponed until an obvious boundary between viable and nonviable tissue is present. Once-frozen tissue may be increasingly susceptible to cold injury.

PRIMARY IRRITANT CONTACT DERMATITIS

Primary irritant contact dermatitis is common in livestock and has numerous causes. The dermatologic findings reflect the mode of encounter with the contactant. Primary irritants have one thing in common: they invariably produce dermatitis if they come into direct contact with skin in sufficient concentration for a long enough period. Moisture is an important predisposing factor, since it decreases the effectiveness of normal skin barriers and increases the intimacy of contact between the contactant and the skin surface.

Commonly incriminated causes of primary irritant contact dermatitis include body excretions (feces, urine), wound secretions, caustic substances (acids, alkalis), crude oil, diesel fuel, turpentine, improperly used topical parasiticides (sprays, dips, wipes), irritating plants, wood preservatives, bedding, and a filthy environment.

Because direct contact is required, the face, distal extremities, and ventral abdomen are most commonly affected. The dermatitis varies in severity (depending on the nature of the contactant) from erythema, papules, edema, and scaling, to vesicles, erosions, ulcers, necrosis, and crusts. Pruritus and pain are variable. Severe irritants or self-trauma can result in alopecia, lichenification, and scarring. Leukotrichia and leukoderma can be transient or permanent sequelae.

In most instances, the nature of the contactant can be inferred from the distribution of the dermatitis: muzzle and distal extremities (plants and environmental substances such as sprays, fertilizers, and filth); a single limb (topical medicament); face and dorsum (sprays, dips, wipes); perineum and rear legs (urine, feces); and ventral abdomen (bedding, filth). Salt produces large, irregularly shaped erythematous plaques in contact areas of swine. Pentachlorophenol (a component of waste motor oil, fungicides, wood preservatives) produces severe contact dermatitis in swine. During breeding season, buck goats urinate on their own face, beard, and forelimbs producing urine scald. A dermatitis may be seen on the muzzle, lips, and ear tips of kids and calves fed milk or milk replacer from pans and buckets. "Transit erythema" is a contact dermatitis of swine associated with exposure to lime. A severe contact dermatitis was reported in swine receiving tiamulin orally for the prevention of dysentery. It was hypothesized that the contactant was tiamulin or a metabolite in feces or urine.

Diagnosis is based on history, physical examination, and recovery when the offending contactant is removed. The contact irritant must be identified and eliminated. Residual contactant and other surface debris can be removed with copious amounts of water and gentle cleansing soaps. Moist, oozing dermatoses will benefit from the application of astringent soaks (aluminum acetate, magnesium sulfate). Other measures for treatment of symptoms, depending on the presence and severity of secondary bacterial infection or pruritus, may include topical or systemic antibiotics or glucocorticoids. In most instances, when the irritant is removed, the dermatitis will improve markedly within 7 to 10 days.

PORCINE SKIN NECROSIS

Porcine skin necrosis is becoming increasingly common as more swine are kept under intensive husbandry systems with minimal bedding. Necrotic lesions usually occur bilaterally over bony prominences and other areas easily damaged by environmental contact or fighting. The occurrence of most forms of porcine skin necrosis has been associated with rough concrete flooring, alkaline pH (alkalis and lime-washed pens), and contact dermatitis (formalin and calcium hypochlorite disinfectants, other caustic agents). Porcine ear necrosis is believed to be precipitated by fighting and bite wounds, which may become secondarily infected with *Staphylococcus hyicus* and β-hemolytic streptococci. Severe bacterial infection leads to vasculitis, thrombosis, and necrosis.

Although most forms of porcine skin necrosis are epidemic, mortality is negligible with most forms. In most instances, the initial skin lesion seen in piglets is a reddish-brown macule or patch over a joint or other prominent cutaneous site where contact is made with the ground. The lesions are always bilateral and may be seen within a few hours after birth. The lesions progress through necrosis, erosion, and ulceration, reaching maximum severity in about 7 days. A blackish-brown crust forms over the lesions, which begin to heal after about 3 weeks and are usually healed within 5 weeks of their onset. Lameness and local infections may or may not be seen. The knees are most commonly affected, followed in decreasing order of frequency by the fetlocks, hocks, elbows, coronets, chin, sternum, vulva, stifles, and rump.

Decubital ulcers (pressure sores) occur in sows most commonly over the scapula, hip, mandible, hock, elbow, and carpus. Risk factors include prolonged recumbency during parturition, reduced activity in early lactation, periparturient illness, thin body condition, moist skin, and rough concrete floors.

Teat necrosis is also a herd problem, often being bilateral and affecting the cranial pair of teats most frequently. Tail biting and tail necrosis are often noted. A small abraded area appears on the dorsal or ventral surface of the tail root soon after birth and proceeds to necrose, ulcerate, and encircle the tail root, resulting in sloughing of the entire tail.

Ear necrosis begins as ear biting at the margins of the pinnae. Early lesions may resolve completely or evolve through a vesicular, exudative, and crusted phase (*S. hyicus* infection) and terminate as a scalloping of the ear margins. Sporadically, severe cellulitis develops (β-hemolytic streptococci) and progresses through vasculitis, thrombosis, and severe necrosis and ulceration. This severe form may be accompanied by sloughing of the entire pinna, bacteremia, polyarteritis, and pneumonia.

Diagnosis is based on history and physical examination. In most instances, therapy is of no benefit. Severe cellulitis of the ear is reported to respond to tylosin 100 g/ton of food, ampicillin 10 to 20 mg/kg/day per os, or sodium selenite 0.3 ppm in feed. Prevention is the key. Ensuring proper bedding and freedom from exposure to irritating chemicals is paramount. Gauze pads covered with adhesive tape applied over susceptible anatomic sites as soon as possible after birth will significantly reduce the incidence of skin necrosis in piglets.

OVINE FLEECE ROT

Under natural and experimental conditions, continued wetting of sheep, such that saturation of the skin surface persists, will produce fleece rot. Approximately 1 week of continual skin wetting is sufficient to produce the disorder. The seasonal incidence of fleece rot hence coincides with months of maximum rainfall. Certain sheep show a predisposition to fleece rot, which may be attributed to variations in physical characteristics of the fleece and skin that exist among sheep of different breeds and strains and even among individual sheep. Predisposing factors include increased staple length, less compact fleece, low wax (sebum) content of fleece, and high suint content of fleece. Subsequent to wetting of the skin, a marked proliferation of bacteria, especially *Pseudomonas* spp., produces a superficial exudative dermatitis and fleece discoloration. Considerable economic losses are accrued owing to depreciation of fleece value.

Lesions are most common over the withers and along the back. Initially, the skin in affected areas assumes a deep purple hue. This is followed by the exudation and accumulation of seropurulent material, which causes the characteristic band of matted fleece. The wool in affected areas is saturated and may be easily epilated. Discoloration of the wool by green, blue, brown, orange, or pink bands may occur at any level of the staple. The area of fleece rot emanates putrid odors, which attract gravid blowflies. Affected sheep are otherwise healthy.

Diagnosis is based on history and physical examination. Therapy is not usually undertaken and is usually of no benefit. Chemical drying of the fleece decreases wetness and the incidence of fleece rot. Immunization of sheep with a cell-free vaccine containing high concentrations of soluble antigens from *P. aeruginosa* was reported to reduce the severity of fleece rot. Prevention, through selecting sheep for inherent resistance to fleece rot, would appear to be the most logical approach to dealing with the problem.

CHEMICAL TOXICOSES

A number of chemical toxicoses are known to produce cutaneous abnormalities. In most instances, these skin changes are diagnostically valuable cutaneous markers of important systemic diseases. Details of pathophysiology, diagnosis, and management of these toxicoses are presented elsewhere in this book.

Selenosis

Chronic selenosis may be seen in cattle, sheep, and swine and is suspected to be the cause of alopecia in the flanks and beards of goats. Typically, animals develop sore feet and lameness, which begin in the hind feet and progress to involve all four feet. The coronary band area becomes tender, and transverse cracks and separations appear in the hoof. In severe cases, hooves may become necrotic and slough. The hair coat is rough, and there is progressive loss of especially the long hairs of the tail and fetlock regions.

Molybdenosis

Molybdenosis produces copper deficiency in ruminants. A rough, brittle, faded hair coat and varying degrees of pruritus may be seen. Black hairs often turn red or gray, especially around the eyes, producing a "spectacled" appearance. In sheep, wool loses its crimp, becoming straight and steely. The tensile strength of wool is reduced.

Arsenic Toxicosis

Arsenic toxicosis may produce a dry, dull, rough, easily epilated hair coat, progressing to alopecia and severe seborrheic skin disease. Occasionally, focal areas of skin necrosis and slow-healing ulcers may be seen.

Mercurialism

In cattle, mercurialism may be associated with a generalized loss of body hair and then a loss of the long hairs of the tail and fetlocks.

Chlorinated Naphthalene Toxicosis

The cutaneous changes of chlorinated naphthalene toxicosis in cattle begin over the withers and the sides of the neck and extend cranially, caudally, and ventrally. The skin becomes progressively more hyperkeratotic, scaly, thickened, alopecic, and fissured. Pruritus is absent. Horns may become loose and develop asymmetrical growth.

Thallotoxicosis

In swine, thallotoxicosis may produce generalized alopecia and erythema and necrosis and oozing of the skin around the eyes and mouth.

Polybrominated and Polychlorinated Biphenyl Toxicosis

In cattle, polybrominated biphenyl toxicosis produces hematomas and abscesses over the back, abdominal veins, and rear legs and matting of the coat and alopecia over the lateral thorax, neck, and shoulders. In swine, polychlorinated biphenyl toxicosis produces erythema of the snout and anus.

Iodism

Cutaneous manifestations of iodism include variable degrees of scaling (seborrhea sicca) with or without partial alopecia, which is most prominent over the dorsum, neck, head, and shoulders.

PHOTODERMATITIS

Photodermatitis is ultraviolet light–induced inflammation of the skin. Phototoxicity is a dose-related response of all animals to light exposure (e.g., sunburn). Photosensitivity implies that the skin has been rendered increasingly susceptible to the damaging effects of ultraviolet light. Photoallergy is a reaction to a chemical (systemic or contact) and ultraviolet light in which an immune mechanism can be demonstrated. Photocontact dermatitis occurs when contactants cause photosensitivity or photoallergy. Phytophotodermatitis is caused by contact with certain plants.

Sunburn is a phototoxic reaction caused by excessive exposure to ultraviolet light B in animals that have lightly pigmented, thinly haired skin. Dairy goats that are light-skinned may develop sunburn, especially on the lateral aspects of the udder and teats, when turned outside in summer. The skin becomes erythematous and scaly and if severely burned may exude, necrose, and crust. White pigs may develop sunburn, especially along the back and behind the ears. Severely affected swine may slough their pinnae and tails.

Photosensitization of livestock, particularly sheep, goats, and cattle under range conditions, can be a major obstacle to production. Although photosensitized animals seldom die, resultant weight loss, damaged udders, refusal to allow the young to nurse, and the occurrence of secondary infections and fly strike may lead to severe economic losses. There are three features basic to all types of photosensitization: (1) the presence of a photodynamic agent within the skin, (2) the concomitant exposure to a sufficient amount of ultraviolet light A, and (3) the lack of pigment in skin with a thin hair coat. Photosensitization is classified according to the source of the photodynamic agent: primary (a preformed or metabolically derived photodynamic agent reaches the skin by ingestion, injection, or contact), hepatogenous (elevated blood phylloerythrin levels in association with liver disease), aberrant pigment synthesis (porphyria), and uncertain etiology. The major causes of photosensitization in livestock are listed in Tables 1 and 2.

The dermatologic findings in photosensitization are essentially identical, regardless of the cause. Cutaneous lesions are often restricted to light-skinned, sparsely haired areas, but in severe cases may extend into the surrounding dark-skinned areas as well. The eyelids, lips, face, pinnae, perineum, udder, teats, and coronary bands are commonly involved. There is usually an acute onset of erythema, edema, and variable degrees of pruritus or pain. Vesicles and bullae may be seen, which often progress to oozing, necrosis, and ulceration. In severe cases, the pinnae, eyelids, tail, teats, and feet may slough. In New Zealand, a vesicobullous disease resembling foot-and-mouth disease was seen in swine fed parsnips or celery infected with the fungus *Sclerotinia sclerotiorum.*

MYCOTOXICOSES

Ergotism

Ergotism typically produces lameness of the hind limbs followed by swelling at the coronary bands, which progresses to the fetlocks. The feet become necrotic, cold, and anesthetic, and a distinct line separates viable from dead tissue (usually just above the coronary band). The front feet, pinnae, tail, and teats may be similarly affected and, in severe cases, may slough. Occasionally, large areas of skin (shoulder, lateral thorax, neck, muzzle) may be affected.

Fescue Toxicosis

Fescue toxicosis in cattle produces cutaneous changes similar to those described for ergotism.

Stachybotryotoxicosis

Stachybotryotoxicosis produces focal areas of necrosis and ulceration, especially of mucocutaneous areas, in cattle, sheep, and swine.

Table 1

PRIMARY PHOTOSENSITIZATION AND THAT DUE TO ABERRANT PIGMENT SYNTHESIS AND UNCERTAIN ETIOLOGY IN LIVESTOCK

Source	Photodynamic Agent
Primary	
Plants	
St. Johnswort (*Hypericum perforatum*)	Hypericin
Buckwheat (*Fagopyrum esculentum, Polygonum fagopyrum*)	Fagopyrin, photofagopyrin
Bishop's weed (*Ammi majus*)	Furocoumarins (xanthotoxin, bergapten)
Dutchman's breeches (*Thamnosma texana*)	Furocoumarins
Wild carrot (*Daucus carota*) and spring parsley (*Cymopterus watsonii*)	Furocoumarins
Cooperia pedunculata	Furocoumarins
Parsnips (*Pastinaca sativa*) or celery (*Apium graveolens*)	Furocoumarins
Perennial ryegrass (*Lolium perenne*)	Perloline
Burr trefoil (*Medicago denticulata*)	Aphids
Alfalfa silage	
Chemicals	
Phenothiazine	Phenothiazine sulfoxide
Thiazides	?
Acriflavines	?
Rose bengal	?
Methylene blue	?
Sulfonamides	?
Tetracyclines	?
Aberrant Pigment Synthesis	
Bovine protoporphyria	Protoporphyrin
Bovine erythropoietic porphyria	Uroporphyrin I, coproporphyrin I
Uncertain Etiology	
Clover, alfalfa, lucerne, vetch, oats, field pennycress	?

MISCELLANEOUS PLANT TOXICOSES

Leucaenosis

Leucaenosis in livestock may produce a gradual loss of the long hairs of the tail and fetlock or a sudden, fairly generalized alopecia. Hoof dystrophies and laminitis may be seen.

Hairy Vetch Toxicosis

Hairy vetch toxicosis produces cutaneous lesions in cattle. Early lesions include papules and plaques that ooze a clear to slightly yellowish puslike material that becomes encrusted. Lesions begin on the udder, tail head, and neck and spread to the face, trunk, and limbs. Pruritus is often marked and associated with considerable alopecia. Chronically, the skin becomes thickened, less pliable, and pleated in appearance.

ZOOTOXICOSES

Snake Bite

Snake bites occur most commonly on the nose, head, neck, and legs. The exact site of envenomation is rarely visible.

Table 2
HEPATOGENOUS PHOTOSENSITIZATION IN LIVESTOCK

Source	Hepatotoxin
Plants	
Burning bush, fireweed *(Kochia scoparia)*	?
Kleingrass, dikkor *(Panicum coloratum)*	?
Ngaio tree *(Myoporum spp.)*	Ngaione
Lecheguilla *(Agave lecheguilla)*	Saponins
Caltrops, goat head, geeldikkop *(Tribulus terrestris)*	Saponins
Rape, kale *(Brassica spp.)*	?
Coal-oil brush, spineless horsebrush *(Tetradymia spp.)*	?
Sacahuiste *(Nolina texacana)*	?
Salvation Jane *(Echium lycopsis)*	Pyrrolizidine alkaloids (echiumidine, echimidine)
Lantana *(Lantana camara)*	Triterpene (lantadene A)
Heliotrope *(Heliotropium europaeum)*	Pyrrolizidine alkaloids (lasiocarpine, heliotrine)
Ragworts, groundsels *(Senecio spp.)*	Pyrrolizidine alkaloids (retorsine, jacobine)
Tarweed, fiddle-neck *(Amsinckia spp.)*	Pyrrolizidine alkaloids
Crotalaria, rattleweed *(Crotalaria spp.)*	Pyrrolizidine alkaloids (monocrotaline, fulvine, crispatine)
Millet, panic grass *(Panicum spp.)*	?
Ganskweed *(Lasiospermum bipinnatum)*	?
Vervain *(Lippia rehmanni, Lippia pretoriensis)*	Triterpenes (icterogenin, rehmannic acid)
Bog asphodel *(Narthecium ossifragum)*	Saponins
Alecrim *(Holocalyx glaziovii)*	?
Vuursiektebossie *(Nidorella foetida)*	?
Anthanasia trifurcata	?
Asaemia axillaris	?
Mycotoxicoses	
Pithomyces chartarum (on pasture, esp. rye)	Sporodesmin
Anacystis (Microcystis) spp. (blue-green algae in water)	Alkaloid
Periconia spp. (on Bermuda grass)	?
Phomopsis leptostromiformis (on lupines)	Phomopsin A
Fusarium spp. (on moldy corn)	T-2 toxin (diacetoxyscirpenol)
Aspergillus spp. (on stored feeds)	Aflatoxin
Infection	
Leptospirosis	Leptospires
Liver abscess	Bacterial toxins
Parasitic liver cyst (flukes, hydatids)	Parasites
Rift Valley fever	Virus
Neoplasia	
Lymphosarcoma	Malignant lymphocytes
Hepatic carcinoma	Malignant hepatocytes
Chemicals	
Copper, phosphorus, carbon tetrachloride, phenanthridium	

Shortly after the bite, pronounced swelling obliterates the fang marks. Erythema and edema may progress to necrosis and sloughing. The affected area is usually painful.

Vampire Bats

Vampire bats feed on all regions of the body in cattle, but prefer the front legs, dorsum, hind legs, and withers. Lesions consist of multiple bleeding, crusted ulcers.

Hyalomma Toxicosis

The cutaneous manifestations of *Hyalomma* toxicosis in livestock are characterized by a moist dermatitis that may be confined to the pinnae, face, neck, axillae, or groin but is often generalized. The skin is erythematous, edematous, oozing, and foul-smelling. The hair coat becomes matted and is easily epilated, leaving a raw surface. The skin is painful. Cattle with nonpigmented hooves show distinct erythema of the coronets.

In animals that do not die, the skin becomes dry, scaly, thickened, and alopecic.

DERMATITIS, PYREXIA, AND HEMORRHAGE IN DAIRY COWS

This syndrome has often been associated with the ingestion of diureidoisobutane. Initial cutaneous manifestations include a pruritic papulocrustous dermatitis on the head and neck that spreads to the back, udder, tail head, perineum, and distal extremities. Rubbing, kicking, and licking produce excoriations and alopecia.

BIBLIOGRAPHY

Davies PR, Morrow WEM, Miller DC, et al: Epidemiologic study of decubital ulcers in sows. J Am Vet Med Assoc 208:1058–1062, 1996.
Gevrey J: Les morsures de vipères. Point Vet 25:193–199, 1993.

Harper PAW, Cook RW, Gill PA, et al: Vetch toxicosis in cattle grazing *Vicia Villosa* spp. *dasycarpa* and *V. benghalensis*. Aust Vet J 70:140–144, 1993.

House JK, George LW, Oslund KL, et al: Primary photosensitization related to ingestion of alfalfa silage by cattle. J Am Vet Med Assoc 209:1604–1607, 1996.

Molyneux RJ, Johnson AE, Olsen JD, et al: Toxicity of pyrrolizidine alkaloids from Riddell grounsel (*Senecio riddellii*) to cattle. Am J Vet Res 52:146–151, 1991.

Panciera RJ, Mosier DA, Ritchey JW: Hairy vetch (*Vicia villosa* Roth) poisoning in cattle: Update and experimental induction of disease. J Vet Diagn Invest 4:318–325, 1992.

Piccinini RS, Perocchi AL, Souza JCP, et al: Comportamento do morcego hematofago *Desmodus rotundus* (Chiroptera) relacionado com a taxa de ataque a bovinos em cativeiro. Pesq Vet Bras 5:111–116, 1985.

Scott DW: Environmental skin diseases. *In* Howard JL (ed): Current Veterinary Therapy-Food Animal Practice. Philadelphia, WB Saunders, 1992, pp 901–906.

Scruggs DW, Blue GK: Toxic hepatopathy and photosensitization in cattle fed moldy alfalfa hay. J Am Vet Med Assoc 204:264–266, 1994.

Spickett AM, Burger DB, Crause JC, et al: Sweating sickness: Relative curative effect of hyperimmune serum and a precipitated immunoglobulin suspension and immunoblot identification of proposed immunodominant tick salivary gland proteins. Onderstepoort J Vet Res 58:223–226, 1997.

■ Disorders of Pigmentation and Epidermal Appendages

Danny W. Scott, D.V.M., Diplomate, A.C.V.D.

DISORDERS OF PIGMENTATION

Hyperpigmentation

Hyperpigmentation (melanosis) is frequently encountered as an acquired condition, usually associated with chronic inflammation and irritation. Hyperpigmentation may affect only the skin (melanoderma), only the hair (melanotrichia), or both.

Lentigo is an idiopathic macular melanosis of swine. Annular, well-circumscribed, deeply and evenly pigmented macules are present, especially over the trunk. These lesions may be seen in combination with cutaneous melanoma.

Hypopigmentation

Hypopigmentation (hypomelanosis), amelanosis (achromoderma, achromotrichia), and depigmentation are not synonymous. *Hypopigmentation* refers to a decrease in normal melanin pigmentation. *Amelanosis* indicates a total lack of melanin. *Depigmentation* means a loss of preexisting melanin. *Leukoderma* and *leukotrichia* are clinical terms used to indicate acquired depigmentation of skin and hair, respectively.

Albinism. Albinism is an autosomal recessive disorder of melanin synthesis that affects the skin, hair, and eyes. Affected animals have white skin and hair, pink eyes, and photophobia.

Albinism is rarely diagnosed in food animals and has been most completely studied in Icelandic sheep. In albinism, electron microscopic examination of skin shows that melanocytes are present but melanin synthesis is defective.

Chédiak-Higashi Syndrome. The Chédiak-Higashi syndrome is an autosomal recessive partial oculocutaneous albinism of Hereford cattle. Affected cattle also have photophobia, increased susceptibility to infections, hemorrhagic tendencies, and an average life span of about 1 year.

Light and electron microscopic examinations of skin reveal abnormally large and clumped melanosomes, which are transferred with difficulty to keratinocytes.

Leukoderma. Leukoderma is an acquired depigmentation of the skin that follows various traumatic and inflammatory injuries, such as pressure sores, regressing viral papillomatosis, freezing, and burns (chemical, thermal, radiation). Leukoderma has also been reported to follow contact with phenols and rubber. Many rubbers contain monobenzyl ether of hydroquinone (antioxidant), which inhibits melanogenesis.

Vitiligo. Vitiligo is an idiopathic acquired depigmentation. There are no preceding or concurrent signs of cutaneous inflammation or injury. Vitiligo has been reported in cattle (some cases of which may have a hereditary basis) and in swine with cutaneous melanoma (in which the condition may be immune-mediated).

In cattle, especially Holstein-Friesians, vitiligo begins as a more or less symmetrical development of well-circumscribed, annular areas of depigmentation. The depigmented areas are usually less than 1 cm in diameter (macule) but may occasionally be much larger (patch). Hairs may become depigmented as well. The muzzle, lips, and periocular areas are most commonly affected, but lesions may be seen on many mucocutaneous junctions, the hooves, and even the general body surface. Pruritus and pain are absent, and affected animals are usually healthy otherwise.

The diagnosis of vitiligo is confirmed by a skin biopsy that demonstrates a complete absence of melanin and melanocytes. The depigmentation may wax and wane in intensity but is usually permanent. There is no effective therapy.

Leukotrichia. Leukotrichia is an acquired depigmentation of the hair that follows various traumatic and inflammatory injuries to the skin. Precocious hereditary graying has been reported in Holstein-Friesian cattle in the Netherlands and is called "blau."

Porcine Erythema and Cyanosis

Swine frequently develop noninflammatory erythema or cyanosis of the skin for a number of reasons. Erythema may be seen with dermatosis erythematosa (especially the ventral abdomen, flanks, ears), sunburn (especially the dorsum), transit erythema (especially the ventral abdomen), carbon monoxide poisoning (generalized), viral infections (especially the ears, tail, and extremities with hog cholera and African swine fever), and bacterial infections (especially the ears, tail, and extremities with streptococcosis, erysipelas, and actinobacillosis). Cyanosis may be seen with benign periportal cyanosis (sows at farrowing time, generalized), porcine stress syndrome (blotchy, then coalesced on the dependent side), bacterial infections (especially the ears, tail, and extremities with *Haemophilus parasuis* or *Haemophilus pleuropneumoniae* infections, *Escherichia coli* enteritis, hemagglutinating encephalomyelitis, salmonellosis, pasteurellosis, erysipelas, actinobacillosis), thiamine deficiency, and organophosphate or carbamate poisoning (generalized).

DISORDERS OF EPIDERMAL APPENDAGES

Hypotrichosis

Hypotrichosis means a less than normal amount of hair. The condition may be regional or multifocal but is usually generalized. It has been reported in all food animal species and is usually hereditary.

Curly Coat

Abnormal curliness of the hair coat has been reported as an inherited condition in cattle and swine.

Hypertrichosis

Hypertrichosis means a greater than normal amount of hair. It has been reported as an inherited condition in cattle and swine and with in utero border disease infection in lambs. Hypertrichosis may also be seen focally as a result of local injury or irritation. The hair in these focal areas may become excessive, thicker, stiffer, and darker than normal.

Hair Follicle Dysplasia

Hair follicle dysplasias have been reported in black-and-white and tan-and-white ("buckskin") Holstein cattle. Although the pathogenesis has not been elucidated, it is probable that heredity plays an important role.

Affected animals are born with normal hair coats but begin to lose the hair in the black- or tan-haired areas very early in life. These areas are hypotrichotic, often containing dull, stubbled hairs and a mild degree of scaling on the surface of the skin. The white-haired areas are normal. Affected cattle are otherwise healthy.

Diagnosis is based on skin biopsy, which shows dysplastic hair follicles and hair shafts, and abnormal melanin clumping within hair follicle outer root sheaths, hair shafts, and piliary canals. There is no effective therapy.

Abnormal Shedding

Normal shedding in food animals is basically controlled by photoperiod and, to a lesser extent, environmental temperature. Thus, most animals in temperate regions shed, to one degree or another, in spring and fall. In some animals, especially individual cattle or goats, abnormal spring shedding may result in excessive hair loss. Areas of marked hypotrichosis or alopecia may develop on the face, shoulders, and rump or may be fairly generalized and symmetrical. The skin in affected areas is normal, and the animals are otherwise healthy. The pathogenesis of abnormal shedding is not understood.

Abnormal shedding may be confused with anagen defluxion, telogen defluxion, alopecia areata, or endocrine skin disease. However, affected animals spontaneously and completely recover within 1 to 3 months.

Anagen Defluxion

In anagen defluxion, a circumstance (antimitotic drugs, infectious diseases, endocrine disorders, metabolic diseases) interferes with anagen (the growth phase of hair follicles), resulting in hair follicle and hair shaft abnormalities. Hair loss occurs within days, as the growth phase continues. This is typical of the sudden hair loss that occurs within days of a very high fever, systemic illness, and malnutrition in calves, lambs, and kids. Hair loss is usually symmetrical and widespread.

Diagnosis is based on microscopic examination of affected hairs. Anagen defluxion hairs are characterized by irregularities and dysplastic changes. The diameter of the shaft may be irregularly narrowed and deformed, and breaking often occurs at such structurally weak sites, resulting in ragged points. Anagen defluxion spontaneously resolves when the constitutional stress is relieved.

Telogen Defluxion

In telogen defluxion, a stressful circumstance (high fever, pregnancy, shock, severe illness, surgery, anesthesia) causes the abrupt, premature cessation of growth in anagen hair follicles and the sudden synchrony of many hair follicles in catagen, then telogen (the resting phase of hair follicles). Two to 3 months later, a large number of telogen hairs are shed as a new wave of hair follicle cyclic activity begins. Hair loss is usually symmetrical and widespread.

Diagnosis is based on microscopic examination of affected hairs. Telogen defluxion hairs are characterized by a uniform shaft diameter and a slightly clubbed, nonpigmented root end that lacks root sheaths. Telogen defluxion spontaneously resolves within 1 to 2 months of its appearance.

Alopecia Areata

Alopecia areata is a rare disorder of cattle. There is no apparent age, breed, or sex predilection. The cause and pathogenesis are unknown.

Clinically, alopecia areata is characterized by focal or multifocal, well-circumscribed, annular patches of noninflammatory alopecia. The skin in affected areas appears normal. The face, neck, and trunk are most commonly affected. Pruritus and pain are absent, and affected animals are otherwise healthy. When hair regrows, it may be a lighter color than normal (leukotrichia).

The differential diagnosis includes other causes of annular alopecia: dermatophytosis, dermatophilosis, demodicosis, stephanofilariasis, staphylococcal folliculitis, and sterile eosinophilic folliculitis. All of these are characterized by various gross inflammatory changes: erythema, oozing, crusts, scales, and so forth, which are not seen with alopecia areata. Definitive diagnosis is based on skin biopsy (peribulbar lymphocytic perifolliculitis).

The prognosis appears to vary according to the distribution of lesions. Animals having localized lesions may undergo spontaneous remission within months to 2 years. Animals with widespread lesions may fail to recover. There is no effective therapy.

BIBLIOGRAPHY

Miller WH Jr, Scott DW: Black-hair follicular dysplasia in a Holstein cow. Cornell Vet 80:273–277, 1990.

Ostrowski S, Evans A: Coat-color-linked hair follicle dysplasia in "buckskin" Holstein cows in central California. Agri Pract 10:12–13, 1989.

Paradis M, Fecteau G, Scott DW: Alopecia areata (pelade) in a cow. Can Vet J 29:727–729, 1988.

Scott DW: Large Animal Dermatology. Philadelphia, WB Saunders, 1988, pp 387–398.

Scott DW, Guard CL: Alopecia areata in a cow. Agri Pract 9:16–19, 1988.

■ Neoplastic Skin Diseases

Danny W. Scott, D.V.M., Diplomate, A.C.V.D.

Veterinary oncology has come into its own as a specialty. Detailed information on the various aspects of the pathogenesis, immunology, and pathology of neoplasia is available in other publications and is not presented here. This discussion serves as a clinical overview of the most common cutaneous neoplasms and non-neoplastic tumors in food animals.

In general, the risk of cutaneous neoplasia increases with age. Specific sex predilections for cutaneous neoplasia are evident in female goats (udder papillomatosis, squamous cell carcinoma), female sheep (squamous cell carcinoma), and male swine (scrotal hemangioma). Breed predilections for cutaneous tumors are presented in Table 1.

The skin is one of the most common sites of neoplasia in food animals. The most common cutaneous neoplasms, by animal affected and in approximate descending order of frequency, are papilloma, squamous cell carcinoma, melanoma, and mast cell tumor (cattle); squamous cell carcinoma, papilloma, and melanoma (goats); squamous cell carcinoma and papilloma (sheep); and melanoma, hemangioma, and squamous cell carcinoma (swine).

The key to appropriate management and accurate prognosis of cutaneous neoplasms is *specific diagnosis*. This can be achieved only by biopsy and histologic evaluation. Exfoliative cytology (aspiration and impression smear) is easy and rapid and often gives valuable information on neoplastic cell type and differentiation. However, exfoliative cytology is inferior to, and no substitute for, biopsy and histopathology.

EPITHELIAL NEOPLASMS

Papillomatosis

Papillomatosis (warts, verrucae) is common in cattle, uncommon in goats and sheep, and rare in swine. In most instances, papillomatosis is known to be caused by DNA papovaviruses. In cattle, there are many papovaviruses that tend to have site specificity on the animal. In general, papovaviruses are host-specific infectious agents that are transmitted by direct and indirect (fomite) contact. The incubation period varies from 2 to 6 months. Papillomas have occurred at the sites of ear marking, dehorning, tuberculin testing, liquid nitrogen tatoos and freeze- or heat-branding. Cattle can harbor latent papillomaviruses which can cause skin lesions when the cattle are immunosuppressed with azathioprine or bracken fern.

In cattle, papillomatosis is common and is caused by many different types of DNA papovaviruses. Bovine papovavirus type 1 (BPV-1) causes typical fibropapillomas on the teats and penises of animals younger than 2 years of age. These lesions often spontaneously regress within 1 to 12 months. BPV-2 causes typical fibropapillomas on the head, neck, and dewlap of animals younger than 2 years of age. These lesions are usually multiple, gray, firm, hyperkeratotic, pedunculated, or broad-based, are 1 mm to several centimeters in diameter, and often spontaneously regress within 1 to 12 months. BPV-3 causes so-called atypical warts in cattle of all ages. These lesions are low, flat, circular, and nonpedunculated, have delicate frondlike projections on their surfaces, and may occur anywhere on the body, including the teats. BPV-3–induced papillomas do *not* regress spontaneously. BPV-4 causes papillomas in the gastrointestinal tract. BPV-5 causes so-called rice grain warts on the teats of cattle of all ages. These lesions are small, white, and elongated and do *not* regress spontaneously.

In sheep, papillomatosis is uncommon and has no apparent breed or sex predilection. Two different DNA papovaviruses appear to be involved. Lesions are usually verrucous and multiple and occur most frequently on the hairy skin of the face and legs of adults and the lower forelegs of lambs. Ovine papillomas have the potential of transforming into squamous cell carcinomas in adult animals.

In goats, papillomatosis is uncommon and no age predilection is apparent. Viral etiology is suspected but not proved. Caprine papillomatosis occurs in two clinical forms, and the lesions are usually verrucous. In one form, lesions occur commonly on the face, neck, shoulders, and forelegs and have no apparent sex or breed predilection. These lesions usually regress spontaneously, and transformation into squamous cell carcinoma may occur.

In swine, papillomatosis is rare and no age, breed, or sex predilection is apparent. Viral etiology is suspected but not proved. Lesions may be solitary or multiple and occur on the face, genitalia, and limbs.

The literature on the therapeutic management of papillomatosis is confusing and contradictory. Most of the confusion centers around two major points: (1) the failure to consider the self-limiting nature of many forms of papillomatosis and (2) the relatively recent discovery that there are many types of papovaviruses that produce papillomatosis in food animals. In cattle, papillomatosis caused by BPV-1 and BPV-2 usually regresses spontaneously, as does papillomatosis of sheep and papillomatosis of the head, neck, and forelegs in goats. Spontaneous remission usually occurs within 1 to 12 months, and animals that have persistent lesions should be suspected of having inappropriate immune responses. On the other hand, cattle with papillomatosis caused by BPV-3 or BPV-5, and goats with papillomatosis of the udder have persistent disease, with spontaneous regression occurring rarely.

For lesions that must be removed for aesthetic or health reasons, surgical excision or cryosurgery is effective. It has been anecdotally stated that surgical excision, cryosurgical removal, or crushing of larger lesions may cause other lesions to regress. There is no scientific support for such a statement.

Many topical agents have been tried on individual lesions when surgery was impractical. The most commonly recommended agents include podophyllin (50% podophyllin; 20% podophyllin in 95% ethyl alcohol; 2% podophyllin in 25% salicylic acid) and dimethyl sulfoxide (undiluted medical grade DMSO). These agents are usually applied once daily until remission occurs.

The subject of vaccination (autogenous or commercial) in the treatment and prevention of papillomatosis is very confusing, mostly because experimental and clinical trials were conducted prior to the recognition of the numerous types of papovaviruses involved in papillomatosis. When one allows for the different types of papovaviruses, the following generalizations seem justified. Autogenous vaccines and commercial bovine wart vaccines are ineffective in the treatment of caprine udder papillomatosis and ineffective in the treatment or prevention of bovine papillomatosis caused by BPV-3 and BPV-5. Vaccines containing BPV-1 and BPV-2 are effective in the prevention but not the treat-

Table 1	
BREED PREDILECTIONS FOR CUTANEOUS TUMORS	
Breed	**Tumor**
Shorthorn cattle	Papillomatosis
Saanen goats	Udder papillomatosis
Hereford cattle	Squamous cell carcinoma
Ayrshire cattle	Squamous cell crcinoma
Angora goats	Squamous cell carcinoma, melanoma
Merino sheep	Squamous cell carcinoma, follicular cyst
Berkshire swine	Scrotal hemangioma
Yorkshire swine	Scrotal hemangioma
Angus cattle	Melanoma
Suffolk sheep	Melanoma
Duroc-Jersey swine	Melanoma
Sinclair miniature swine	Melanoma
Nubian goats	Wattle cyst

ment of bovine papillomatosis caused by BPV-1 and BPV-2. Recent studies have shown that immunity following infection and vaccination with papillomaviruses is type-specific.

General therapeutic adjuvants in all cases of papillomatosis, when feasible, include isolation of affected animals from noninfected animals, reduction of cutaneous injuries associated with the environment, and disinfection of the environment (e.g., with formaldehyde or lye).

Uncomplicated papillomatosis is usually of little concern, except in valuable animals destined for competitive shows or overseas sales. Economic losses can occur through hide damage, secondary infection or myiasis, and carcass condemnation. In cattle, it has been stated that animals with papillomatosis affecting over 20% of their bodies have a poor prognosis.

Squamous Cell Carcinoma

Squamous cell carcinomas are common malignant neoplasms of food animals. The cause of squamous cell carcinoma is not clear in all cases, but in most instances it is related to the chronic exposure of poorly pigmented, poorly haired skin to ultraviolet light. In some instances, squamous cell carcinomas may arise from viral papillomas or follicular cysts, or at the sites of liquid nitrogen tatoos or freeze- or heat-branding.

In goats, squamous cell carcinomas occur in adult to aged animals, with does and Angoras being predisposed. The tumors are usually solitary and occur most commonly on the perineum, vulva, and udder of female animals and on the ears of both sexes. The lesions may be ulcerative or proliferative, and metastasis is not uncommon. Caprine squamous cell carcinomas are known to arise from papillomas of the udder, especially in Saanens.

In sheep, squamous cell carcinomas occur in adult to aged animals with ewes and Merinos being predisposed. The lesions may be solitary or multiple and commonly occur on the pinnae, eyelids, muzzle, lips, and perineal region. The lesions may be ulcerative or proliferative, and metastasis may occur. Ovine squamous cell carcinomas are believed to occasionally arise from viral papillomas and follicular cysts, and vulvar squamous cell carcinomas occur most frequently in ewes that have had a radical Mules operation to reduce susceptibility to fly strike.

In cattle, squamous cell carcinomas occur in adult to aged animals with no sex predilection. Breed predilections include poorly pigmented animals, especially Herefords and Ayrshires. The lesions most commonly occur at mucocutaneous junctions, especially periocular and vulvar. Lesions may be ulcerative or proliferative, and metastasis is not uncommon.

In swine, squamous cell carcinomas occur in adult to aged animals with no sex or breed predilection. Lesions may be single or multiple and ulcerative or proliferative and occur especially on the pinnae and trunk. Metastasis may occur.

The therapy of choice is wide surgical excision. Other treatment modalities that may be successful in selected cases include cryosurgery, radiofrequency hyperthermia, and radiation therapy.

MESENCHYMAL NEOPLASMS

Hemangioma

Hemangiomas are benign tumors arising from the endothelial cells of blood vessels. They are uncommon in swine and cattle and rare in sheep and goats. The cause of hemangiomas is unknown.

In swine, hemangiomas occur most commonly in the scrotum of mature Yorkshire and Berkshire boars. The condition may be genetically determined. Lesions are usually multiple, beginning

as tiny purple papules and progressing to hyperkeratotic, hyperpigmented, verrucous papules and plaques. Profuse hemorrhage may occur when lesions are traumatized.

In cattle, hemangiomas are usually solitary (especially head and limbs) in adults and multiple in calves. So-called angiomatosis has been described in mature dairy and beef cattle in the United States and Europe. One or several black to reddish-gray to pink, soft, sessile to pedunculated masses, 0.5 to 2.5 cm in diameter, are most commonly found over the back. These lesions are often initially detected because of recurrent hemorrhage, which can be profuse.

The therapy of choice of hemangiomas is surgical excision.

Mast Cell Tumor

Mast cell tumors are uncommon in cattle and rare in swine. Mast cell tumors may be benign or malignant, and they arise from cutaneous mast cells. The cause of these tumors is unknown.

In cattle, mast cell tumors occur in animals 6 months to 7 years of age, with no breed or sex predilections. Lesions are usually multiple, 1 to 40 cm in diameter, firm to fluctuant, and dermal or subcutaneous in location; they may or may not be ulcerated or alopecic. They can occur anywhere, but especially over the neck and trunk. The majority of bovine mast cell tumors are malignant and metastatic.

In swine, mast cell tumors have been reported in animals 6 to 18 months of age, with no breed or sex predilection. Lesions may be single or multiple, 2 to 20 mm in diameter, firm to fluctuant, dermal to subcutaneous in location, and may occur anywhere on the body. Porcine mast cell tumors may be limited to the skin or may involve internal organs.

The therapy of choice is wide surgical excision when practical. Cryosurgery and radiation therapy are treatment options.

LYMPHORETICULAR NEOPLASIA

Lymphosarcoma

Cutaneous lymphosarcoma is a rare malignancy of cattle, and is extremely rare in sheep, goats, and swine. In cattle, enzootic lymphosarcoma is caused by the bovine leukemia virus, but most cases of bovine cutaneous lymphosarcoma are sporadic and not associated with this retrovirus.

In cattle, cutaneous lymphosarcoma usually occurs in young adult animals, 1 to 4 years of age, with no sex or breed predilection. The lesions are usually multiple, are 1 to 8 cm in diameter, and may occur anywhere on the body, but especially over the neck and trunk. The overlying skin may be normal (urticaria-like) or alopecic, crusted, hyperkeratotic, and ulcerated (ringworm-like). Initially, affected cattle are otherwise healthy. Frequently, the cutaneous lesions spontaneously regress. However, remission is usually followed by relapse and fatal internal involvement.

Effective therapy has not been reported.

MELANOCYTIC NEOPLASMS

Melanomas (malignant) and melanocytomas (benign) are neoplasms arising from melanocytes or melanoblasts. These neoplasms are common in certain breeds of swine, uncommon in cattle and goats, and rare in sheep. The cause of melanomas is unknown. In Sinclair miniature and Duroc-Jersey swine, these neoplasms appear to have a genetic basis.

In cattle, melanomas occur in animals of any age, newborn to aged, with no sex predilection. Dark-haired breeds appear to be predisposed, especially Angus. Lesions may be solitary or multiple and black to gray, are frequently ulcerated, and may occur anywhere on the body, but especially on the head, neck, and distal limbs. About 80% of all melanocytic neoplasms in the skin of cattle are benign (melanocytomas).

In goats, melanomas occur most commonly in adult to aged animals with a predilection for does. Angoras appear to be predisposed to develop these tumors. Lesions may be solitary or multiple and black to gray to brown, are frequently ulcerated, and occur most commonly on the perineum, tail, udder, pinnae, and coronets. Caprine cutaneous melanomas often metastasize.

In sheep, melanomas usually occur in adult to aged animals with no sex predilection. Suffolks appear to be predisposed. Lesions are often multiple and subcutaneous, are black to gray, and tend to occur in pigmented skin. Metastases are frequent.

In swine, melanomas occur in animals of any age, newborn to adult, with no sex predilection. Duroc-Jersey and Sinclair miniature swine are genetically predisposed to develop these tumors. The incidence of melanomas in some swine herds can reach 20%, and littermates may be affected. Lesions may be solitary or multiple and may occur anywhere on the body, especially the trunk. In general, the lesions may be flat, well circumscribed, and evenly pigmented (lentigo or melanocytic nevus stages) or raised, black, and frequently ulcerated (melanoma stage). The smaller, flatter lesions often spontaneously regress, and regression may be associated with the development of vitiligo. Larger, raised lesions often metastasize.

Surgical excision, where feasible, is the only effective therapy.

CYSTS

Cysts are uncommon in goats and sheep and rare in cattle and swine. These cysts are benign, non-neoplastic lesions characterized by an epithelial wall, with keratinous to amorphous contents.

Follicular cysts develop by retention of follicular or glandular products resulting from congenital or acquired loss or obliteration of follicular orifices. The cysts may be solitary or multiple, firm to fluctuant, well circumscribed, smooth, and round, and the overlying skin is often normal in appearance. Cysts that have been traumatized or ruptured can develop foreign body granuloma or secondary infection. Follicular cysts are most commonly seen in adult sheep and may have an inherited basis in Merinos. Lesions occur without apparent sex or site predilection and can cause aesthetic damage, damage to hides and fleece, and increased difficulty in shearing. Secondary squamous cell carcinomas may develop in the cyst walls.

Wattle cysts occur in goats. These cysts are believed to be developmental abnormalities, possibly arising from the branchial cleft. Nubian goats and Nubian crossbreeds are most commonly affected, and the lesions may have a hereditary basis. The cysts are present at the base of the wattle at birth but may not be noticed until the animal is 2 to 3 months of age. They are usually rounded, smooth, soft, and fluctuant, and the overlying skin is normal in appearance.

The treatment of choice for all cysts, when necessary, is surgical excision.

BIBLIOGRAPHY

Campo MS, Jarrett WFH, O'Neil W, et al: Latent papillomavirus infection in cattle. Res Vet Sci 56:151–157, 1994.
Gourreau JM, Scott DW, Cesarini JP: Les tumeurs mélaniques cutanées des bovins. Point Vet 26:785–792, 1995.
Hayward MLR, Baird PJ, Meischke HRC: Filiform viral squamous papillomas on sheep. Vet Rec 132:86–88, 1993.
Jarrett WFH, O'Neil BW, Gaukroger JM, et al: Studies on vaccination against papillomaviruses: A comparison of purified virus, tumour extract, and transformed cells in prophylactic vaccination. Vet Rec 126:449–452, 1990.
Jarrett WFH, O'Neil BW, Gaukroger JM, et al: Studies on vaccination against papillomaviruses: The immunity after infection and vaccination with bovine papillomaviruses of different types. Vet Rec 126:473–475, 1990.
Johnstone AC, Hughes PL, Haines DM: Papillomavirus-induced dermatofibroma in cattle following tuberculin testing. N Z Vet J 42:233–235, 1994.
Miller MA, Weaver AD, Stogsdill PL, et al: Cutaneous melanocytoma in 10 young cattle. Vet Pathol 32:479–484, 1995.
Scott DW, Anderson WI: Bovine cutaneous neoplasms: Literature review and retrospective analysis of 62 cases. Compendium Continuing Educ Pract Vet 14:1405–1418, 1992.
Scott DW, Gourreau JM: Les tumeurs des vaisseaux sanguins cutanés chez les bovins. Point Vet 27:941–946, 1996.
Yeruham I, Perl S, Yakobson B, et al: Skin tumors in cattle following tatooing by liquid nitrogen. Isr J Vet Med 48:38–40, 1993.
Yeruham I, Perl S, Nyska A: Skin tumours in cattle and sheep after freeze- or heat-branding. J Comp Pathol 114:101–106, 1996.

■ Nonparasitic Skin Diseases of Swine

Ralph F. Hall, D.V.M.

Integumentary diseases of swine, in addition to those primary conditions such as swine erysipelas and ectoparasitic diseases, are manifest by a vast array of etiologic agents, including infection by viruses (parvovirus of swine, the vesicular viruses), mycotic agents, bacterial infections, trauma to feet and legs, environmental agents (sunburn, radiant energy from heat lamps), nutritional deficiencies, and conditions of unknown cause such as pityriasis rosea (Table 1, pp 726–727). Many of these conditions have been well reviewed recently.[1, 2]

Zoonotic skin diseases acquired from swine include erysipeloid, *Erysipelothrix rhusiopathiae* being the most common infection. Dermatophytosis from zoophilic species is occasionally though incompletely reported.[3]

REFERENCES

1. Straw B: Diagnosis of skin disease in swine. Compendium Continuing Educ Pract Vet 7:11, 1985.
2. Cowart RP: Integumentary diseases. *In* An Outline of Swine Diseases, a Handbook. Ames, Iowa State University Press, 1995.
3. Merchant S: Zoonotic diseases with cutaneous manifestations in food animals—Part 2. Compendium Continuing Educ Pract Vet 12:11, 1990.

■ Dermatologic Disorders of Sheep

Christopher K. Cebra, V.M.D., M.A., M.S., Diplomate, A.C.V.I.M.

PARASITIC DERMATOSES

Sheep may suffer dermatoses from infestations by five types of ectoparasite: mites, flies, lice, keds, and ticks, as well as from internal infestation with a nematode. The psoroptic and sarcoptic mange mites, keds, ticks, and sucking lice ingest blood or lymph, leading to anemia and general unthriftiness, while harvest mites, chorioptic mange mites, biting lice, and flies feed off surface cells and secretions. All ectoparasites irritate the skin by mechanical trauma or reaction to the parasite's saliva, causing restlessness, interrupted feeding behavior, feet stamping, rubbing against objects, and self-mutilation. Depending on the degree of pruritus, skin lesions consist of mild erythema and scaling or will have progressed to severe ulcerated wounds covered with thick crusts of dried exudates and denuded of hair or wool. The economic importance of ectoparasite infestation can be very high and relates to treatment costs, impaired feed efficiency, decreased wool quality and production, damage to hides, and death losses.

Infestation by the psoroptic mange mite (*Psoroptes ovis*) causes intense pruritus with self-trauma leading to alopecic areas covered with yellow crust and tags of matted wool (sheep scab). The margins of the lesion where active inflammation is occurring are moist. Infestation is usually subclinical during warmer months when the mites retreat to the relatively hairless areas (ear, axilla, and groin) and becomes clinical during the winter when the mites multiply rapidly in the wooled regions of the withers and back. Economic losses due to psoroptic mange can be severe. The mite has been eradicated from the United States, Australia, and New Zealand, but has resisted eradication in several other countries, including the United Kingdom. Local veterinary officials should be contacted if psoroptic mange is suspected.

Sarcoptes scabei, *Demodex ovis*, and *Psororgates* (*Psorobia*) *ovis* live within the skin. *Sarcoptes* is a true burrowing mite which creates long tunnels to lay eggs within the epidermis. The mite spreads slowly across the haired regions, especially the ears, face, and groin of wooled sheep and the whole bodies of haired sheep. Infestation causes such intense pruritus that scratching behavior frequently supersedes eating and weight loss is common. Sarcoptic mange has not been reported in the United States and is a reportable disease. *Demodex* lives within the hair follicles of the face and is rarely of clinical importance in sheep. Although not a burrowing mite, *Psororgates* lives within the superficial layers of the skin. The mite is spread between shorn sheep and rarely seen in young animals. Sheep may show clinical signs and a distribution of lesions similar to psoroptic mange, although they can take years to develop generalized disease. Other sheep appear to become tolerant to the mite and have mild chronic signs. The disease is most common and severe in fine-wooled breeds.

Two mites principally affect the legs of sheep. The ovine subspecies of *Chorioptes bovis* often causes no clinical signs, but mild or severe pruritic dermatitis can occur. Lesions spread from the legs to the face and ventral abdomen in some cases, and fertility may be affected if the scrotum becomes inflamed. Trombiculid or harvest mite (chigger) larvae may infest the legs of sheep during the early fall. The nymph and adult stages do not parasitize mammals. Infestation is most common in sheep with access to unimproved pasture or woods and usually resolves spontaneously as the larvae mature and the ambient temperature drops.

Lice and keds may be found on sheep in all seasons, but are most important in unshorn sheep during the winter. Transmission usually requires direct contact between animals, and is most common when sheep are in confinement, such as winter housing, sale pens, or transporters. The biting louse (*Damalinia* or *Bovicola ovis*) and the sheep ked (*Melophagus ovinus*), a wingless fly, are most abundant on the wooled regions of the neck and back. The sucking louse (*Linognathus ovillus*) is most abundant around the haired areas of the head and limbs. The sucking foot louse (*Linognathus pedalis*) is most abundant on the limbs, but reaches the ventral abdomen with heavy infestations. This louse may cause lameness. *Damalinia* is considered to be more important than sucking lice because it is more active and its feces and inflammatory exudates damage the fleece. Keds are also important due to the staining of the fleece and damage to

the hide (creating "cockles"), but have a much slower rate of multiplication and hence take longer to reach significant numbers. Pruritus is variable with both louse and ked infestations, and is more common with high numbers of parasites. Both of these types of parasite have become more common in North America since the eradication of psoroptic mange led to a relaxation of dipping protocols.

Sheep in areas of the western half of the United States populated by wild cervids are susceptible to infestation by *Eleaophora schneideri* (sorehead). This nematode parasite lives in the large arteries of the neck and head and releases microfilariae which lodge in superficial capillaries. In sheep, this causes intense pruritus with eosinophilic and granulomatous inflammation, principally of the neck but occasionally also of the coronary bands.

Tick infestation is most common during the spring and fall, and heaviest in well-vegetated areas. Unlike lice, mites, or keds, ticks spend only a short period of their life cycle on sheep. They tend to attach to the hairless or haired areas or adjacent wooly areas, but rarely are found deep in the thick wool. Pruritus and alopecia are uncommon. Animal death due to blood loss is rare, except in tropical climates; most losses are due to decreased weight gain, damage to hides, transmission of blood-borne pathogens, and tick paralysis.

Fly bite dermatitis and fly strike are very seasonal, based on the presence of flies. The head fly (*Hydrotaea irritans*) causes wounds around the horn buds of juveniles and head lesions on fighting rams. The fly bite itself is thought to be minor but extremely pruritic, with most of the damage due to self-trauma. Black flies, biting midges, horn flies, and horse flies have much more painful bites and also lead to self-mutilation due to pruritus. Sheep irritated by flies have very interrupted feeding behavior and may even stampede.

The primary blowflies (*Lucilia* or *Phormia* spp.) are attracted to soiled areas of wool and wounds. Previous damage to the skin may be necessary to attract flies. Lesions can occur anywhere on the body in damp climates, but are most common around the tail head, prepuce, or site of a wound or surgical procedure. Merino sheep appear to be especially susceptible due to well-developed perineal skin folds. The flies lay their eggs on the wool, and the maggots migrate to the soiled skin and begin their digestive process. This creates a moist, fetid wound (blowfly strike or cutaneous myiasis) which attracts other flies and allows secondary bacterial invasion and toxemia to occur. The lesion often is obscured by the soiled wool, and the first clinical signs noted are dullness or death. However, blowfly strike appears to be very painful or pruritic, and careful observation will reveal that affected sheep constantly bite at or rub lesions. Parting the fleece over the lesion reveals the maggots and liquefactive necrosis of the skin. Careful inspection of wounds to find the maggots may be necessary because necrosis often follows fascial planes, resulting in deep, honeycombed lesions.

The screwworm flies (*Cochliomyia hominivorax* or *Cochliomyia macellaria* and *Chrysomia bezziana*) or secondary blowflies rarely initiate lesions, but lay eggs within a wound. The wound can be that created by primary blowfly strike or from another source. There is often cohabitation of a wound by several types of fly larvae, but screwworm larvae appear to have a competitive advantage. Screwworm maggots are carnivorous, and invade deep into the living tissue at the edges of the wound. Their digestive process creates large, deep, exudative, foul-smelling lesions. They can also occasionally digest the larvae of other flies. Efforts to eradicate screwworm flies from certain areas, including the United States, through the release of sterilized males have been largely successful, but the long range of the fly and transport of animals with myiasis could lead to reinfestation. Screwworm strike is reportable in many countries.

Table 1
NONPARASITIC SKIN DISEASES OF SWINE

Infectious Skin Diseases

Conditions	Etiology	Predisposing Factors and Age	Lesions	Diagnosis	Treatment and Prevention
Actinobacillosis	*Actinobacillus equuli* or *actinobacillus suis*	Contact with horses in some cases of *A. equuli*; young pigs	Septicemia, multiple hemorrhages on ears and ventral abdomen, necrosis of tail and skin over joints, swollen joints, arthritis, cyanosis of extremities, subcutaneous abscesses, pericarditis, endocarditis, pleural effusion, pneumonia, petechiae in kidneys	Clinical signs, lesions on necropsy, bacterial culture; differentiate from other septicemias, streptococcal and *Corynebacterium* abscesses	Tetracycline, ampicillin, cephalosporins, chloramphenicol, trimethoprim-sulfamethizole, streptomycin
Actinomycosis	*Actinomyces bovis*	Bites and scratches of udder; sows	Extensive granulomas of skin esp. over udder; secondary mastitis; wasting due to visceral infection; most common in sows	Clinical signs, bacterial culture; differentiate from ulcerative granuloma caused by *Borrelia suilla*	Oral KI, streptomycin
Corynebacterial abscesses	*Corynebacterium pyogenes*	Trauma, lacerations, bite wounds, faulty injection technique, castration, tail biting; any age	Abscesses	Bacterial culture; differentiate from streptococcal abscesses	Surgical drainage, antibiotics generally ineffective; no vaccines
Erysipelas	*Erysipelothrix rhusiopathiae*	Contamination of environment by pig feces, surface water, turkey manure, flies; subclinical aflatoxin toxicity, poor nutrition, changes in nutrition, stress, fatigue, temperature changes; not common under 3 mo and over 3 yr	Generalized septicemia; temperature 40–43°C; diamond-shaped skin lesion; anorexia, firm, dry feces; abortion; conjunctivitis; vomition, arthritis, endocarditis	Clinical signs, bacterial culture, serology in chronic cases	Erysipelas antiserum; porcine penicillin 50,000 units/kg; tetracycline, tylosin, vaccination; improve sanitation, remove chronically affected animals
Exudative epidermitis	*Staphylococcus hyicus*	Entry via umbilicus, abrasion on feet and legs, lacerations, vesicular virus lesions, bite wounds, biotin deficiency, agalactia; 5–35 days of age	Marked erythema, greasy skin exudate, erosions of coronary band, brown skin scabs, white precipitate on papillary ducts and renal pelvis	Clinical signs, bacterial culture, slide agglutination with absorbed antisera	Systemic antibiotics; cloxacillin in lanolin base locally, dip in chlorhexidine; improve sanitation, supplement diet with soybean oil, vitamins A, B, D, and E; clip needle teeth; keep surgical instruments clean; tetracycline in feed; control external parasites; no vaccine commercially available
Oral necrobacillosis	*Fusobacterium necrophorum*	Fight wounds, spread by teeth-cutting instruments, poor hygiene; suckling pigs 1–4 wk of age	Necrotic ulcers of cheeks, lips gums, tongue, and legs; listlessness, necrotic odor to lesions	Clinical signs	Curette and swab lesions with hydrogen peroxide or antibiotic spray; sulfadimidine, penicillin, or streptomycin systemically for 3–4 days; remove milk teeth; improve sanitation; sterilize teeth-cutting instruments
Cervical lymphadenitis, jowl abscesses, streptococcal abscesses	β-Hemolytic *Streptococcus* sp. Lancefield group E	Carrier animals, contaminated feed or water, concurrent swinepox and lice infestation; 10–50 wk of age	Enlarged lymph nodes rupture and discharge pus; anorexia, moderate depression, diarrhea, retarded growth	Clinical signs, slaughter inspection, culture; differentiate from *Corynebacterium* abscesses	Surgical drainage; chlortetracycline, sulfamethazine, or tylosin in feed; modified live vaccine; eliminate lice
Ulcerative spirochetosis	*Borrelia suilla*	Poor hygiene; most common in sows	Ulcers on udder up to 30 cm in diameter; secondary mastitis	Clinical signs; examine smears of lesion under dark-field illumination, smears from formalin-fixed tissue stained with silver stain; bacterial culture; differentiate from actinomycosis	Oral KI, penicillin systemically; dust lesions with sulfanilamide, arsenic trioxide, or tartar emetic; intralesional injection of sodium arsenite; tetracycline, tylosin, erythromycin, and spectinomycin orally may be beneficial

Disease	Cause	Epidemiology	Lesions / Clinical signs	Diagnosis	Treatment / Control
Swinepox	Poxvirus	Lice infestation; dry scabs in environment; more common in young animals	Pustular lesions on back and sides, may spread to ventral abdomen; no lesions on mucosal surfaces	Clinical signs, presence of lice, histology and serology	Improve hygiene, control lice
Foot-and-mouth disease	Picornavirus (rhinovirus); not present in United States since 1929	Spread by direct contact, aerosol animal products such as meat, milk, or hides; all ages	Vesicles and erosions on oral mucosa, tongue, snout, lips, gums, pharynx, palate, coronary band, interdigital space, dewclaws, and teats; lameness, anorexia	NOTIFIABLE DISEASE: NOTIFY FEDERAL VETERINARIANS; cannot distinguish clinically from vesicular stomatitis, vesicular exanthema, and swine vesicular disease; identify virus	Eradication policy; prevent import of animals and animal products from enzootic countries; avoid feeding garbage; vaccination in enzootic counties
Swine vesicular disease	Picornavirus (enterovirus); not present in United States	Similar to foot-and-mouth disease	Similar to foot-and-mouth disease; no ruminants affected	NOTIFIABLE DISEASE: NOTIFY FEDERAL VETERINARIANS; identify virus, serology, demonstration of virus antigen	As for foot-and-mouth disease
Vesicular exanthema	Picornavirus (calicivirus); not reported since 1959	As for foot-and-mouth disease	As for foot-and-mouth disease	As for foot-and-mouth disease	As for foot-and-mouth disease
Vesicular stomatitis	Rhabdovirus; two antigenic strains: New Jersey and Indiana	Spread by direct contact and arthropod vectors	Similar to foot-and-mouth disease	Isolation of virus, serum antibody titers	Keep water and soft feed in front of animals at all times; antibiotics for secondary infections
Ringworm	Most cases *Microsporum nanum*, also *Microsporum canis*, *Microsporum gypseum*, *Trichophyton verrucosum*	Persists in environment for up to 12 mo; carrier animals; all ages affected; *M. nanum* adults	Circular lesions coalesce; on most parts of body but not ventral abdomen; some lesions pruritic; thin, dark, crusty scabs	Clinical signs, examination of skin scraping, culture in Sabouraud's dextrose agar; if on ventral midline probably pityriasis rosea	Nystatin locally; griseofulvin in feed; spray with iodine, captan, or salicylic acid
Noninfectious Skin Diseases					
Melanoma	Possibly hereditary	More common in Durocs, young pigs	Single or multiple black nodular cutaneous tumors	Clinical signs, histologic examination	Surgical removal if individual nodule
Feed ingredient deficiency	Several deficiencies reported causing dermatologic lesions	Biotin, inositol, linoleic acid, protein, riboflavin, vitamins A, C, E, K, selenium deficiencies; growing pigs	Various; a scurfy hair coat is often present; long hair with protein deficiency; subcutaneous hemorrhages with vitamin K deficiency	Clinical signs and ration analysis	Correct deficiencies
Zinc deficiency, parakeratosis	Zinc deficiency in ration	Excess calcium, copper, and phytic acid; deficiency in unsaturated fatty acids; Concurrent transmissible gastroenteritis or intestinal clostridial infections; growing pigs	Small circumscribed erythematous areas on ventral abdomen, papules, keratinous crusts; differentiate from sarcoptic mange, exudative epidermitis, pityriasis rosea	Clinical signs, zinc ration < 40 mg/kg, serum zinc and alkaline phosphatase decreased; response	Supplement ration with 200 g/ton zinc carbonate; correct calcium levels
Skin necrosis	Trauma to knees and teats	New concrete farrowing crates, alkaline disinfectants, estrogens in feed in teat necrosis; congenital splayleg; 1–14 days	Reddish-brown areas followed by necrosis on fetlock coronets, elbows, hocks, and teats	Clinical signs	Extra bedding alongside farrowing crate; adhesive bandages or acrylic resin-reinforced plastic skin on anterior teats
Photosensitization	Many plants, phenothiazine, tetracycline, sulfa drugs, chlorothiazide	Grazing pigs; secondary photosensitization if liver disease; all ages	White parts only affected; erythema; edema; pain, serum exudate; lameness, dry, hard, cracked skin, pruritus	Clinical signs, history; differentiate ergotism, sunburn, erysipelas in nursing piglets	Remove from pasture, house in dark area; laxative orally, emollients to skin
Sunburn	Unacclimatized to bright sunlight	Severity depends on length of exposure; all ages	Erythema, edema, and pain	Clinical signs; less severe than photosensitization; no exposure to photodynamic agents	Protect from sun, provide shade
Pityriasis rosea	Unknown, possibly hereditary	1–14 wk	Small papule with brown scab surrounded by reddened zone, spreads centrifugally, lesions coalesce; no loss of hair, most on ventral midline	Clinical signs; negative skin scraping; differentiate from ringworm	None effective; spontaneous cure in 6–8 wk

Diagnosis of Parasitic Dermatoses

Ticks, keds, flies, maggots, and lice may be found on visual inspection of sheep, but mites often require microscopic examination of skin scrape samples. For burrowing mites, deep scrapes must be performed, and because of the intense host response to relatively few mites, multiple scrapes often are necessary to find the parasite. Skin biopsies may be necessary in some cases, and are the only means of visualizing the *Eleaophora* microfilariae. With fly bite dermatosis, the parasite may not be identified, but may be seen swarming around lesions and presumed to be the cause. If the clinical signs are compatible with parasitic dermatoses, appropriate treatment measures should be instituted in spite of negative diagnostic tests.

Adult psoroptic, sarcoptic, and chorioptic mange mites are all of similar size (0.6 to 0.8 mm long) and shape (rounded bodies with two pairs of legs directed craniad and two pairs caudad). *Psoroptes* has long legs with long, jointed pedicles, *Sarcoptes* has short legs with long, unjointed pedicles, and *Chorioptes* has long legs with short unjointed pedicles. *Psororgates* is much smaller (less than 0.2 mm long) and has its eight legs spaced roughly evenly around its body, and trombiculids are about 0.6 mm long, have plumelike filaments at the end of their legs, and are often bright orange. *Demodex* is very small (0.2 mm long), but can be easily recognized by its four anterior pairs of legs and long, cigar-shaped body.

Lice and keds are wingless insects, with three pairs of legs along the thorax followed by a long, bulbous abdomen. Adult lice are 1 to 2 mm long, while keds are up to 7 mm long. Biting lice have broad, flat heads and may have a red hue, while sucking lice have long, narrow, conical heads and are blue. Keds are hairy and have large, leathery abdomens. Lice eggs (nits) and ked larvae often are found cemented to hair or wool fibers.

The adults of fly bite dermatitis often are not captured, and a presumptive diagnosis is made based on season and signs. Adult blowflies are metallic green or blue. Their larvae are pale yellow, segmented, and between 1 and 2 cm long. They have spiracles on their anterior segment and also on a posterior plate, as well as a pair of anterior hooks to grasp flesh. Screwworm larvae have spicules at the anterior end of each segment, while larvae from the other blowflies do not.

Prevention and Treatment of Parasitic Dermatoses

Since ivermectin became available and licensed for use in sheep it has proved to be a convenient, effective preventive and therapeutic treatment for all the parasitic agents of dermatoses in sheep, excepting flies and biting lice. Newer avermectins may prove to be equally efficacious, but have not been licensed or used extensively in sheep. For many infestations, a single oral or subcutaneous (extralabel) dose of ivermectin is effective, while with psoroptic mange or severe sucking louse infestations a second dose may be necessary 1 and 2 weeks later, respectively. Residual killing activity may be maintained for up to 30 days after administration.

The main disadvantages to ivermectin are the cost of the drug and need for individual dosing. Organophosphate, carbamate, pyrethrin, and pyrethroid dips or sprays may also be used, with repeated administration as for ivermectin above. There are a number of these products labeled for use in sheep and the individual manufacturer's directions should be followed. Lime sulfur solutions may be used when residues are a major concern, as with dairy sheep. Full-immersion dipping is greatly superior to spraying, especially for parasites of the wooled regions. Flies may be controlled with topical sprays of similar products (except lime sulfur), with retreatment based on the danger of fly strike and residual effects of the treatment. Pour-on insect growth regulators are also available.

Other treatments may be necessary. Shearing the fleece greatly reduces the load of biting lice and keds, while selectively shearing the fleece from the perineal region ("crutching") decreases susceptibility to fly strike. Avoiding surgical wounds from disbudding, castration, or tail-docking during fly season and performing the Mules operation to remove the skin folds of Merino sheep may also aid in the prevention of fly strike. Once fly strike has occurred, clipping the fleece and cleaning, debriding, and covering wounds are necessary for lesions to heal and prevent further occurrence. Maggots can be killed by the topical application of the same agents used to kill adult flies. Systemic antibiotics and supportive therapy may be necessary to treat secondary infections and toxemia.

In addition to treating all contact animals, environmental treatment may be necessary. Keds and biting lice survive very short periods off the host, especially in extremes of environmental temperature or humidity, but the sucking foot louse and *Chorioptes* may survive up to 3 weeks under favorable conditions. Parasites that can spend entire generations without infesting sheep, such as flies, ticks, and harvest mites, are best controlled by treating the environment with effective products or eliminating their sites of reproduction.

NONPARASITIC DERMATOSES

Nonparasitic dermatoses are less common in sheep than those caused by arthropods, but are often no less damaging economically. In some cases, the skin lesion is the product of a poor environment, while in other cases it is the most visible manifestation of an internal condition. In either case, diagnostic evaluation of sheep with skin lesions is a valuable part of a total flock health strategy.

Affecting Wooled Areas

The two most common nonparasitic skin diseases which cause wool loss are dermatophilosis (lumpy wool, streptotrichosis, or mycotic dermatitis) and *Pseudomonas* infection (fleece rot or green wool). Both are most common during wet periods of the year or when the fleece is otherwise damp. *Dermatophilus congolensis* is a gram-positive, facultative anaerobic actinomycete which grows in branching filaments. The bacterium colonizes moist breaks in the skin leading to a characteristic ulcerative dermatitis covered with hemorrhagic or purulent exudate which dries into thick crusts. Morbidity and mortality are usually low. An environmental reservoir for infection is suspected, but the organism has only been cultured from exudates and crusts; bacteria within crusts can survive for several years.

Two forms of dermatophilosis are recognized in sheep: strawberry foot rot, which affects the coronary band and lower limb, and lumpy wool, which affects the dorsum and flanks. Both forms usually are multifocal, nonpruritic, and surrounded by tags of wool matted with dried exudates. Which form predominates in a given flock probably depends on the factors contributing to dampness and skin breaks on that farm. Light wooled lambs up to 5 months old appear to be the most susceptible, although any sheep with a damp fleece and skin trauma is at risk. Human infections can occur but are rare.

Pseudomonas aeruginosa is a gram-negative, pigment-producing bacillus, the proliferation of which may be stimulated by protein exuded from chronically damp skin. The bacteria release colorful pigments and produce exudative dermatitis with a putrid odor. Although the disease itself causes little morbidity, the colored exudate decreases the value of the fleece and the dermatitis attracts fly strike.

Most cases of crusting, nonpruritic, ulcerative dermatitis in sheep are attributed to dermatophilosis, but the diagnosis can be confirmed by culture, fluorescent antibody testing, or direct smear of exudates or crusts. Dissolving some crust in saline and a stain often helps in visualization of the branching hyphae of *Dermatophilus* with both transverse and longitudinal septa ("railroad tracks"). Bacteriologic techniques can also be used for *Pseudomonas* infections, but diagnosis can usually be made based on history and the finding of green-, brown-, or yellow-stained, malodorous wool.

Specific treatment of *Dermatophilus* and *Pseudomonas* infection is rarely indicated; techniques to dry the fleece and treatments of secondary fly strike are more important. Some radical therapies have been proposed, including the use of chemotherapeutic agents to promote epilation. Vaccination and selection for genetic resistance have both shown promise in preventing fleece rot.

Scrapie can cause wool loss and signs of pruritus similar to a parasitic dermatosis. The nibbling reflex elicited when scratching the back is taken by some to be a pathognomonic sign of scrapie but is not specific to any one cause of pruritus. Abnormal wool growth in neonates can occur due to border disease (hairy shakers), genetic diseases, or iodine or copper deficiency. Copper deficiency also can affect adults, and characteristically causes the wool to have a dilute color and no crimp, while iodine deficiency leads to alopecia and scaly skin. These diseases also affect other organ systems, and are covered elsewhere in this book.

Affecting Haired Areas or Mucous Membranes

While both *Dermatophilus* and *Pseudomonas* are most pathogenic on the wooled areas of sheep, *Staphylococcus* spp. typically affect the face and extremities. The bacteria may just colonize the skin surface (impetigo) or invade the hair shafts (folliculitis). Infection is most common on the face and perineum of month-old lambs, and is usually self-limiting. A similar, mild infection can occur in the inguinal region and on the udder of adults. The characteristic lesion is the pustule (plook) surrounded by erythema and scales. Because affected hairs epilate easily, focal alopecia usually surrounds the lesion. Pruritus appears to be minimal. Occasional persistent or deeper infections occur. Contagious spread of a severe form (eye scab) has been documented in adult sheep which display an ulcerative, pustular dermatitis around the lips, eyes, ears, and horn base. It is assumed that the bacteria spread by direct contact (fighting) or indirect contact between sheep at common water or feed troughs. A previous wound may aid in bacterial colonization.

Contagious ecthyma (orf, sore mouth) is caused by a parapoxvirus and occurs in sheep, goats, various other ruminants, and humans. The basic lesions are papules or vesicles which can rupture to form erosions covered by scabs. The disease usually occurs in periodic outbreaks which coincide with lambing seasons, as young, susceptible lambs are infected by carrier adults. The virus can be recovered from lesions, saliva, and scabs, and transmission is thought to occur through both direct and indirect contact. Lesions develop 4 to 7 days after infection and usually regress spontaneously in 2 to 4 weeks. Infection results in partial immunity which decreases with time. On young animals, lesions are most common on the lips and gums, coronary bands, eyelid margins, and nares. Adults are additionally affected on the udder, which presumably is infected by nursing lambs. Lesions appear to be painful, and decreased nursing behavior by lambs and decreased tolerance of nursing by dams lead

to poor weight gain. Death losses due to contagious ecthyma are rare.

Diagnosis can usually be made by clinical signs, especially in a flock with a history of contagious ecthyma or addition of new animals. A definitive diagnosis can be achieved by isolation of the virus from swabs of lesions or scabs. Fluorescent antibody staining or histopathologic study of tissue biopsy samples has also been used. Epithelial cell proliferation, ballooning of cells, and occasional eosinophilic intracytoplasmic inclusion bodies may be seen microscopically. Treatment of lesions is not usually necessary and may delay healing. There is a dried, modified live virus vaccine used to control morbidity due to contagious ecthyma.

Ulcerative dermatosis is a more severe disease causing lesions with approximately the same distribution as contagious ecthyma. The disease appears to be caused by a virus with some similarities to the contagious ecthyma virus, but affects all ages of sheep without association with the lambing season. Lesions are ulcerative without evidence of epithelial cell proliferation, and often become infected by bacteria. Lameness and decreased feed intake are common, but lesions usually resolve within 6 weeks. There is also a genital form of this disease which affects both sexes during the breeding season, and interferes with copulation. Contagious ecthyma and ulcerative dermatosis should be differentiated from the more severe viral infections which cause mucous membrane ulceration, including sheeppox, bluetongue, rinderpest, and foot-and-mouth disease. These latter viral diseases are usually much more pathogenic and affect multiple organ systems.

Photosensitization can occur due to an inherited metabolic defect, ingestion of primary photosensitizing toxins, or secondary to hepatic damage and decreased metabolism of phylloerythrin (a chlorophyll metabolite). Lesions often involve all areas covered by light hair or shorn wool, because skin covered by heavy fleece or dark hair is protected from light. Erythema, photophobia, and pruritus with self-trauma are seen. A variety of plant and mold toxins have been implicated in secondary photosensitization. These are often different from the toxins commonly associated with liver damage in other species; sheep are reported to be 30 times more resistant to the effects of pyrollizidine alkaloids than horses or cattle, and are hence often used to graze pastures considered unsuitable for large herbivores. A flock history of exposure to a primary or secondary photosensitizing agent, evidence of liver damage, or evidence of disease which follows family lines is helpful in making a diagnosis of photosensitization.

Individual cases or flock outbreaks of multiple, circular, nonpruritic, alopecic lesions on the face, ears, or extremities of sheep may be caused by dermatophytic fungi (ringworm), a papovavirus (warts), or squamous cell carcinoma. All may also affect wooled skin. Ringworm lesions typically are round, slightly raised, and covered with a light-gray scaly crust. On rare occasions, sheep with facial ringworm display signs of intense pruritus similar to those seen with a parasitic dermatosis. Ringworm results from colonization of the skin surface and hair fibers by *Trichophyton* spp. or *Microsporum canis*. Diagnosis of ringworm may be accomplished by microscopic visualization of fungal hyphae or conidia on hair shafts or a skin scrape sample. Placing the sample on a slide in a few drops of a 20% potassium hydroxide solution and heating the slide over a flame for 15 seconds helps digest background material. Growth of fungal colonies on dermatophyte test medium and simultaneous change of the indicator dye color from yellow to red (usually within 7 days) can also be used. Certain dermatophytes require supplemental nutrients or warmer incubation temperatures to produce conidia. Wart lesions range from raised nodules to pedunculated masses of epithelium-wrapped fibrous tissue and have a highly vascular base. Squamous cell carcinoma is more likely to be ulcerated or covered with horny material, and is most common in older Merino sheep. There is currently no recommended treatment for these diseases, although ringworm may be treated as in other species. Ringworm and warts usually regress in 1 to 3 months. Persistent infections often indicate poor immune function and usually do not justify the cost of treatment.

BIBLIOGRAPHY

Kaufmann J: Parasitic Infections of Domestic Animals: A Diagnostic Manual. Boston, Birkhäuser, 1996.
Lofstedt J: Dermatologic diseases of sheep. Vet Clin North Am Food Anim Pract 5:203–215, 1989.
Urquhart GM, Armour J, Duncan JL, et al: Veterinary Parasitology, ed 2. Oxford, Blackwell, 1996.

■ Miscellaneous Skin Diseases

Danny W. Scott, D.V.M., Diplomate, A.C.V.D.

BOVINE STERILE EOSINOPHILIC FOLLICULITIS

Sterile eosinophilic folliculitis is a recently reported, apparently rare disorder of cattle. There are no apparent age, breed, or sex predilections. The cause and pathogenesis are unknown.

The disorder is nonseasonal in occurrence and is characterized by a more-or-less symmetrical papulocrustous eruption. Lesions progress to annular areas of alopecia, crusting, scaling, and plaques. The head, neck, and trunk are commonly affected. Pruritus is usually mild to absent. The lesions are usually not painful, and affected animals are otherwise healthy. Typically, only one animal in a herd is affected.

The differential diagnosis includes other causes of annular, alopecic, crusty lesions: dermatophytosis, dermatophilosis, demodicosis, stephanofilariasis, *Pelodera* dermatitis, and staphylococcal folliculitis. Definitive diagnosis is based on exfoliative cytology (predominantly eosinophils, no intracellular microorganisms), skin biopsy (eosinophilic folliculitis or furunculosis, special stains for microorganisms negative), and negative cultures for bacteria and fungi.

The natural course of the disease is unknown. Although the condition is known to clear with topical or systemic glucocorticoid administration, relapses occur when therapy is stopped.

PORCINE DERMATOSIS ERYTHEMATOSA

Porcine dermatosis erythematosa is a poorly characterized dermatosis. The cause and pathogenesis are unknown, and meaningful clinicopathologic studies have apparently not been conducted.

The dermatosis is reported to be quite common in white pigs and can occur in swine grazing new pasture or in fattening pigs and breeding stock housed entirely indoors. There is striking acute erythema over large areas of the body, including the ears, sides, and abdomen. There is no pruritus or pain, and affected swine are usually otherwise healthy.

Therapy is unnecessary, since complete, spontaneous recovery occurs within a few days.

PANNICULITIS

Panniculitis is inflammation of subcutaneous fat, and is a multifactorial cutaneous reaction pattern. Lesions are subcutaneous, firm to fluctuant, and more or less well circumscribed. The overlying skin and hair coat are initially normal. Lesions may or may not be painful or develop draining tracts. Subcutaneous injections (especially clostridial vaccines) are a well-known cause of panniculitis. Idiopathic sterile granulomatous panniculitis has been described in a yearling steer with multiple lesions on the neck, proximal limbs, axillae, and groin.

DERMATITIS AND NEPHROPATHY IN SWINE

A sporadic dermatitis-nephropathy syndrome has been described in 5-week to 9-month-old swine. Multiple flat or slightly raised red-blue areas, one to several millimeters in diameter, are seen over the thighs, forelimbs, sides of the body, and sometimes the ears. Vasculitis and necrosis are seen in the skin and kidneys. The condition is usually fatal.

SELF-DESTRUCTIVE BEHAVIOR

A possibly genetically based condition was described in Israeli Holstein dairy cattle. Affected cattle would constantly lick their udder and teats at calving, producing either large ulcers between the teats, or ulceration and necrosis of the teats.

EOSINOPHILIC GRANULOMA

Multiple cutaneous nodules were described in 10- to 44-month-old Japanese Friesian cattle. Lesions occurred in the summer and resolved with glucocorticoid and antihistamine therapy. Biopsies revealed eosinophilic granulomas with collagen degeneration.

BOVINE LINEAR KERATOSIS

A possibly genetically based linear keratosis was recognized in a 1-month-old East Flemish × Belgian Blue calf. The lesions consisted of numerous vertically oriented, slightly wavy bands of hyperkeratosis and alopecia on the right thoracic and abdominal walls. The condition was asymptomatic.

BIBLIOGRAPHY

Deprez P, DeCock H, Sustronck B, et al: A case of bovine linear keratosis. Vet Dermatol 6:45–49, 1995.
Rogers GM, King CM: The comparison of injection site reactions caused by two commercial multivalent clostridial vaccines. Agri Pract 17:28–33, 1996.
Scott DW: Large Animal Dermatology. Philadelphia, WB Saunders, 1988.
Scott PR, Pyrah IH, Gough MR, et al: Panniculitis in a yearling steer. Vet Rec 139:262–263, 1996.
van Halderen A, Bakker SK, Wessels JC, et al: Dermatitis/nephropathy syndrome in pigs. J S Afr Vet Assoc 66:108–110, 1995.
Wada Y, Okumura T: Three cases of eosinophilic dermatitis in Holstein-Friesian cattle. J Jpn Vet Med Assoc 46:1018–1021, 1993.
Yeruham I, Markusfield O: Self destructive behaviour in dairy cattle. Vet Rec 138:308, 1996.

▪ External Parasiticides

Larry F. Moore, D.V.M.

External parasiticides are compounds used in the control of insects and arachnids (mites, ticks, and so on). They are more commonly referred to as animal insecticides. External parasiticides are normally used on food-producing animals (1) to treat severe infestations that result in clinical disease, (2) to increase production of meat and other products of animal origin, and (3) to stop or prevent the spread of insect- or arachnid-borne disease.

BOTANICAL AND CHLORINATED HYDROCARBON COMPOUNDS

The first products used for the control of external parasites of food-producing animals were botanicals. Examples are rotenone, nicotine, and natural pyrethrin. These compounds had limited application and usefulness. The first highly effective compounds were the chlorinated hydrocarbons, such as DDT and toxaphene. Their development coincided with the beginning of the modern era of agriculture, at which time there occurred a great increase in agricultural productivity. Humanity was no longer at the mercy of parasitic pests that affected its domesticized plants or animals.

The chlorinated hydrocarbon insecticides, although highly effective, had some serious shortcomings. They were quite persistent, being chemically stable and slow to degrade in the environment. In addition, a stable body residue developed in exposed organisms. With some compounds, an interesting phenomenon developed, termed *biologic magnification*. Biologic magnification, which led to harmful consequences in the environment, began as a residue in the lowest or the first organism in the food chain. An aquatic insect with a residue was eaten by a fish which, in turn, was consumed by a larger fish, which was eaten by a bird. Each succeeding species accumulated a greater body residue than did the organism it consumed. In some cases, this process extended toxic manifestation to the species at the top of the food chain. Even after years of extensive study, these compounds' toxic mode of action was poorly understood, and there were no antidotes. Most chlorinated hydrocarbons have been removed from the market owing to environmental issues with the re-registration process required by the Environmental Protection Agency (EPA).

ORGANOPHOSPHATE COMPOUNDS

The subsequent development of organophosphate compounds gave the agriculturist and the veterinarian effective tools to control pests on plants or animals. These compounds are systemic in action, that is, they are translocated in the body of the plant or animal. Dermal application of a systemic organophosphate compound controls parasites in remote anatomic locations. The most important indicator of the presence of organophosphate compounds is cholinesterase depression. This class of compounds is in general more acutely toxic than are the chlorinated hydrocarbon compounds. Atropine is the most effective antidote for organophosphate parasiticides, but with the bovine an elevated dose is required; thus, the label should be consulted for dosage directions. The oxime compound 2-PAM (2-pyridine aldoxine methchloride), in combination with atropine, is effective for treating intoxication by organophosphate compounds. Organophosphate compounds are rather unstable after application and do not magnify in the environment. They are rapidly metabolized and eliminated from the body. The re-registration process by the EPA has caused elimination of many products because of environmental issues or economics.

PYRETHROIDS

Some of the more recently developed external parasiticide compounds are synthetic pyrethrin or pyrethroid compounds. They are more effective and economical than are the natural pyrethrins. The advent of insecticide ear tags was followed by a wide variety of usages and formulations containing these pyrethroids.

AVERMECTINS

The newest animal parasiticides developed are the avermectins. Avermectins have a broad spectrum of activity against both internal and external parasites. These compounds were isolated from fermentation of the soil organism *Streptomyces avermitilis* and have a neurotoxic action on the parasite.

External parasites controlled by avermectins include grubs, mites, lice, and horn flies with the pour-on formulation. Products for food animals include an injectable ivermectin for cattle and swine, a combination injectable ivermectin and flukicide for cattle, an oral drench for sheep, a pour-on ivermectin for cattle, a sustained-release ivermectin bolus for cattle, and a feed premix for swine.

A doramectin formulation for cattle was recently introduced as an injectable for cattle. Other formulations of doramectin are to be marketed in the future.

PARASITICIDE USE

Modern chemistry has provided the veterinarian with highly effective external parasiticides. It is important that they be used according to label recommendations. Every product should be used solely on the animal species for which it is labeled, and only the label-prescribed dose should be applied for that specific parasitic infestation. The misuse of animal medications has brought unfavorable publicity because of illegal residues in human food. When examining the label, one must pay strict attention to the duration after treatment in which milk must be discarded or animals held from slaughter for food. To adhere to all label recommendations is the professional responsibility of every veterinarian who uses or recommends the use of an animal medication. Veterinarians must resist the thought that a product labeled for the control of a parasite in one species of animal may be used in another species without residue or toxic problems. The product should not be used on a host species for which there is no label recommendation. There could be several reasons for lack of label recommendations, including a lack of residue data, excessive residue of the compound or its metabolites in the host, and insufficient margin between safe and harmful doses. Products vary in safety factors. In any occurrence of toxicity associated with an external parasiticide, there is usually a history of accidental exposure or use contrary to label directions. Veterinarians are often required to make difficult clinical decisions when they encounter a severe infestation that is causing a pathologic condition in host animals that may be complicated by adverse climatic conditions. A product and method of application must be selected that will control the parasite without causing undue stress to the host animal. The products that are available as external parasiticides for use on food animals have all been reviewed and approved by a government agency for ensuring that the product is effective as labeled, is safe to the host species, and will not result in an unacceptable residue.

TREATMENT

Active ingredients have been formulated into a number of products for application by several treatment methods. These include the following approaches.

Pour-on products are formulated in a dilute solution so that they may be poured down the back of the animal. They are easy to use and have become a popular method for treating cattle for grubs (*Hypoderma* spp.). Some of these products are also approved for the control of cattle and swine lice.

The low-volume products such as fenthion are formulated with a higher concentrate of active compound than are the pour-on products. They are also applied to the backs of cattle. They are easy to apply, and their spectrum of activity is similar to that of pour-on products.

Solutions for dip vat use and whole-body spray (applied with a high-pressure sprayer) have similar uses, advantages, and disadvantages. These treatment methods are used effectively for ticks, flies, grubs, lice, and mange control. The dip vat is an effective application method and is used in cattle feedlot operations and tick control programs. Whole-body sprays, although still used, are not as popular as they were in earlier times. The main disadvantage of both treatment methods is their use during severe cold weather. The back rubber is one of the oldest "self-treatment" methods used for applying parasiticides to cattle or swine. There are several types on the market. This application method has several advantages, one of which is ease of application, because infested animals tend to seek out and use a rubber. The disadvantage of the back rubber is that it must be serviced regularly so that proper dispensing of the parasiticide is ensured.

Dust bags have generally the same advantages as the back rubber but are usually more effective because they require less servicing and dispense the parasiticide more consistently when used by cattle. They may be hung where cattle are forced to dust themselves, such as in gateways to pastures, or they may be located where cattle congregate.

The insecticide ear tag containing pyrethroids was widely used in the early 1980s. It proved to be a useful method for horn fly control, especially when continuous control was important. Approved insecticidal ear tags gave season-long control in some areas. The pyrethroid-resistant fly became a problem in the mid 1980s; therefore insecticide ear tags were developed containing organophosphate compounds. In the late 1980s, second-generation pyrethroids (i.e., lambdacyhalothrin and cyfluthrin) were introduced in an ear tag formulation.

Other methods of application, such as mist sprayers, foggers, and treadle sprayers, do not have wide application. They may be of use in special situations.

The introduction of avermectins in injectable formulations represented an alternative to the dip vat and pour-on products. Market figures show wide acceptance because of spectrum or dosage form.

In determining what product or treatment method to use, several considerations need to be made. It is obvious that the treatment of choice should be effective in the control of the parasite, cause no untoward reaction in the host, and be easy to apply and economical to use. These several considerations are the reasons that so many products and methods of application have been developed.

Tables 1 to 4 list common products used for external parasite control on cattle, sheep, goats, and swine. The products are listed by common (generic) name and trade name where possible. These tables are not intended to be an all-inclusive listing of products for the noted indications but are only representative. The current label must be studied thoroughly before the use of any external parasiticide for specific use directions, safety considerations, and proper meat or milk withdrawal periods.

Table 1
SOME COMMON PRODUCTS USED FOR EXTERNAL PARASITE CONTROL ON CATTLE

Product	Company and Address	Marketed Formulation	Pest	Method of Application	Withdrawal Period Before Slaughter (days)	Comments
Amitraz Taktic E.C.	Hoescht Roussel Vet Box 2500 Somerville, NJ 08876-1258	Liquid	Ticks, mites, and lice	Spray	0	Do not treat animals more than 4 times per year
Coumaphos Co-Ral	Bayer Corp. Agriculture Division P.O. Box 390 Shawnee Mission, KS 66201	Wettable powder	Horn flies, lice, ticks, grubs, screwworms, and mites	Spray or dip	0	Treat lactating dairy cattle only at lower dilution
	Bayer Corp.	Flowable	Horn flies, lice, ticks, screwworms, and mites	Spray or dip	0	Treat lactating dairy cattle only at lower dilution
	Bayer Corp.	Liquid emulsifiable livestock insecticide	Horn flies, face flies, lice, ticks, and grubs	Spray or back rubber	0	Treat lactating dairy cattle only at lower dilution
	Bayer Corp.	Liquid livestock insecticide spray	Horn flies, face flies, lice, and ticks	Spray or back rubber	0	Treat lactating dairy cattle only at lower dilution
	Various formulators	Dust (1%)	Horn flies and lice	Dust bag or shaker can	0	Apply no more than 2 oz per animal per day
Dichlorvos, tetrachlorvinphos Ravap E.C.	Boehringer Ingelheim Animal Health 2621 North Belt Highway St. Joseph, MO 64506	Liquid	Horn flies, face flies, lice and ticks	Spray and back rubber	0	Approved for lactating dairy and beef cattle; do not spray more often than every 10 days
Doramectin Dectomax	Pfizer, Inc 812 Springdale Drive Exton, PA 19341-2803	Injectable	Grubs, mites, and sucking lice	Injectable subcutaneously or intramuscularly	35	Do not use in female dairy cattle 20 mo of age or older
Famphur Warbex	Schering-Plough Animal Health Corp. 1095 Morris Ave. Union, NJ 07083	Pour-on	Grubs and lice	Backline treatment	35	Do not treat lactating dairy cattle or within 21 days of freshening; do not treat Brahman bulls
Fenthion Lysoff	Bayer Corp.	Pour-on	Lice and horn flies	Backline treatment	21 Single treatment	Dilute with water before use; do not treat lactating dairy cattle
Spotton	Bayer Corp.	Low-volume pour-on	Grubs and lice	Spot treatment on the backline	45	Do not treat dairy cattle of breeding age
Tiguvon	Bayer Corp.	Pour-on	Grubs and lice	Backline treatment	35 Single treatment	Do not treat lactating dairy cattle
Ivermectin Ivomec	Merial Limited 2100 Ronson Rd. Iselin, NJ 08830-3077	Injectable	Grubs, mites, and sucking lice	Inject subcutaneously	35	Do not use in female dairy cattle of breeding age
Ivomec plus	Merial Limited	Injectable	Grubs, mites, and sucking lice	Inject subcutaneously	49	Do not use in female dairy cattle of breeding age
Ivomec pour-on	Merial Limited	Pour-on	Grubs, mites, sucking and biting lice, and horn flies	Backline treatment	48	Do not use in female dairy cattle of breeding age
Ivomec SR bolus	Merial Limited	Sustained release bolus	Grubs, mites, sucking lice, and ticks	Oral	180	Do not use in female dairy cattle of breeding age
Permethrin Atroban or Expar	Schering-Plough	Liquid	Horn and face flies, mites, ticks, lice, and various other flies	Spray	0	Repeat application as needed but not more often than every 14 days
Atroban or Expar	Schering-Plough	Pour-on	Lice, horn flies, and face flies	Backline treatment	0	Repeat application as needed but not more often than every 14 days

Table continued on following page

Table 1
SOME COMMON PRODUCTS USED FOR EXTERNAL PARASITE CONTROL ON CATTLE *Continued*

Product	Company and Address	Marketed Formulation	Pest	Method of Application	Withdrawal Period Before Slaughter (days)	Comments
Boss	Schering-Plough	Pour-on	Horn flies, lice, and control of horse flies, stable flies, mosquitos, black flies, and ticks	Backline treatment	0	Lactating dairy and beef cattle
Brute	Y-TEX Corp. 1825 Big Horn Ave. Cody, WY 82414	Pour-on	Control of horn flies and lice; aid in control of face flies, stable flies, horse flies, deer flies, house flies, mosquitoes, and black flies	Backline treatment	0	Repeat application as needed but not more often than every 2 wk
Ectiban	Numerous suppliers	Liquid	Horn and face flies, mites, ticks, lice, and various other flies	Spray	0	Repeat application as needed but not more often than every 14 days
GardStar 40% EC	Y-TEX Corp.	Liquid	Horn flies, face flies, stable flies, house flies, horse flies, deer flies, black flies, mosquitoes, eye gnats, mange mites, scabies mites, ticks, and lice	Spray	0	Repeat application as needed
Permectrin II	Numerous suppliers	Liquid	Horn flies, face flies, stable flies, horse flies, lice, ticks, and mites	Spray	0	Re-treat not more than once every 2 wk
Permectrin CDS and CD	Various suppliers	Pour-on	Horn flies, face flies, stable flies, horse flies, lice, ticks, and mites	Backline treatment	0	Re-treat not more often than once every 2 wk
Cyfluthrin CyLence	Bayer Corp.	Pour-on	Horn flies, face flies, biting and sucking lice	Backline treatment	0	Beef and dairy cattle (including lactating) not more often than every 3 wk
Lambdacyhalothrin Saber	Schering-Plough	Pour-on	Horn flies, lice	Backline treatment	0	For use in beef cattle
Phosmet Del-Phos	Schering-Plough	Liquid	Horn flies, lice, Lone Star tick, Gulf Coast ear ticks, sarcoptic mange mites	Spray, back rubber	3	For use in beef cattle
GX118	Starbar/Sandoz Animal Health A division of Sandoz Agro, Inc. 1300 East Toughy Ave. Des Plaines, IL 60018	Liquid	Grubs, lice, horn flies, ticks, and mites	Spray, dip, or pour-on	21	For use on beef cattle only
Lintox HD, Prolate	Starbar	Liquid	Horn flies, lice, and ticks	Spray	3	Do not use on nonlactating cattle within 28 days of freshening
Tetrachlorvinphos Rabon 50 WP	Boehringer Ingelheim Animal Health 2621 North Belt Highway St. Joseph, MO 64506	Wettable powder	Horn flies, lice, and ticks	Spray	0	Do not treat dairy cattle
Rabon 3%	Boehringer Ingelheim	Dust	Horn flies and lice	Dust bag or shaker can	0	Apply no more than 2 oz per animal per day

Table 2
INSECTICIDE EAR TAG AND LARVICIDE PRODUCTS USED FOR EXTERNAL PARASITE CONTROL ON CATTLE

Product	Company and Address	Marketed Formulation	Pest	Method of Application	Withdrawal Period Before Slaughter (Days)	Comments
Pyrethroids						
Cyfluthrin Cutter Gold	Bayer Corp. Agriculture Division P.O. Box 390 Shawnee Mission, KS 66201	Ear-tag	Horn flies, Gulf Coast ticks, spinose ear ticks; and as aid in control of face flies	2 Tags per animal, 1 in each ear	0 Remove tags at the end of the fly season or before slaughter	Approved for lactating dairy cattle
Fenvalerate Ectrin	Boehringer Ingelheim Animal Health 2621 North Belt Highway St. Joseph, MO 64506	Ear-tag	Horn and face flies, Gulf Coast and spinose ear ticks	2 Tags per animal, 1 in each ear	0 Remove tags before slaughter	Approved for lactating dairy cattle
Lambdacyhalothrin Saber	Schering-Plough Animal Health Corp. 1095 Morris Avenue Union, NJ 07083	Ear-tag	Horn flies and face flies	2 Tags per animal, 1 in each ear	Remove tags before slaughter	Do not use in lactating dairy cattle
Permethrins Atroban or Expar	Schering-Plough	Ear-tag	Horn flies, face flies, Gulf Coast and spinose ear ticks	2 Tags per animal, 1 in each ear	0 Remove tags before slaughter	Approved for lactating dairy cattle
GardStar	Y-TEX Corp. 1825 Big Horn Ave. Cody, WY 82414	Ear-tag	Face flies, susceptible horn flies, and Gulf Coast ticks	1 Tag per animal for horn flies; 2 tags for face flies	0 Remove tags before slaughter	Approved for lactating dairy cattle
Zetacypermethrin						
Python ZetaGard	Y-TEX Corp.	Ear-tag	Horn flies, face flies, lice, Gulf Coast ticks, spinose ear ticks, and aid in control of stable flies, black flies, house flies, and small horse flies.	1 Tag for horn flies, 2 tags per animal, 1 in each ear, for control of face flies, ear ticks, and lice	0 Remove tags before slaughter	Approved for lactating dairy cattle
Pyrethroid-organophosphate	Y-TEX Corp.	Ear-tag	Horn and face flies, Gulf Coast and spinose ear ticks	2 Tags per animal, 1 in each ear	0	Approved for lactating dairy cattle
Cypermethrin, chlorpyrifos, and piperonyl butoxide Max-Con						
Lambdacyhalothrin, pirimiphos Double Barrel	Schering-Plough	Ear-tag	Horn flies and face flies	2 Tags per animal, 1 in each ear	0	Do not use in lactating dairy cattle

Table continued on following page

Table 2
INSECTICIDE EAR TAG AND LARVICIDE PRODUCTS USED FOR EXTERNAL PARASITE CONTROL ON CATTLE *Continued*

Product	Company and Address	Marketed Formulation	Pest	Method of Application	Withdrawal Period Before Slaughter (Days)	Comments
Organophosphate **Diazinon**						
Cutter Gold	Bayer Corp.	Ear-tag	Horn flies, Gulf Coast ticks, spinose ear ticks, and as an aid in control of face flies, lice, stable flies, and house flies	1 Tag per animal for horn flies; 2 tags per animal, 1 in each ear, for other labeled pests	0 Remove tags before slaughter	Do not use in lactating dairy cattle
Optimizer	Y-TEX Corp.	Ear-tag	Horn flies, Gulf Coast and spinose ear ticks	2 Tags per animal, 1 in each ear	0	Do not use in lactating dairy cattle
Patriot	Boehringer Ingelheim	Ear-tag	Horn flies, Gulf Coast ticks, spinose ear ticks, and as an aid in control of face flies, lice, stable flies, and house flies	1 Tag per animal for horn flies; 2 tags per animal, 1 in each ear, for other labeled pests	0 Remove tags before slaughter	Do not use in lactating dairy cattle
X-Terminator	Destron-Fearing 490 Villaume Avenue St. Paul, MN 55075	Ear-tag	Horn flies	2 Tags per animal, 1 in each ear	0	Do not use in lactating dairy cattle
Diazinon and chlorpyrifos Warrior and Diaphos Rx	Y-TEX Corp.	Ear-tag	Horn flies, biting lice, sucking lice, Gulf Coast ticks, spinose ear ticks, and aid in control of face flies, stable flies and house flies	1 Tag for 3–4 mo. for control of horn flies	0 Remove tag before slaughter	Do not use in lactating dairy cattle
Fenthion Cutter Blue	Bayer Corp.	Ear-tag	Horn flies and aid in control of face flies	2 Tags per animal, 1 in each ear	0 Remove tags at end of season or before slaughter	Approved for lactating dairy cattle
Pirimiphos Dominator	Schering-Plough	Ear-tag	Horn flies	2 Tags per animal, 1 in each ear	0 Remove tags before slaughter	Do not use in lactating dairy cattle
Larvicide-type Products Diflubenzuron Vigilante	Hoechst Roussel Vet Box 2500 Somerville, NJ 08876-1258	Standard release bolus	Horn flies, face flies, house flies, and stable flies	½–1 bolus	0	Approved for lactating dairy cattle; do not administer to cattle weighing less than 300 lb, and no more than one bolus to any single animal
Tetrachlorvinphos Rabon	Boehringer Ingelheim	Oral larvicide premix	Horn flies, face flies, house flies, and stable flies	Mixed in feed	0	Mix uniformly into cattle feed ration

Table 3
SOME COMMON PRODUCTS USED FOR EXTERNAL PARASITE CONTROL ON SHEEP AND GOATS

Product	Company and Address	Marketed Formulation	Pest	Method of Application	Withdrawal Period Before Slaughter (days)	Comments
Coumaphos	Bayer Corporation Agriculture Division P.O. Box 390 Shawnee Mission, KS 66201	Wettable powder	Lice, ticks, horn flies, screwworms, fleeceworms, and keds; mites in sheep only	Spray or dip	15	Do not treat lactating dairy goats
Diazinon Dryzon	Y-TEX Corp. 1825 Big Horn Ave. Cody, WY 82414	Wettable powder	Sheep keds and lice	Pour-on or spray	14	Do not treat lactating dairy goats or goats intended for slaughter
Fenvalerate Ectrin	Boehringer Ingelheim Animal Health 2621 North Belt Highway St Joseph, MO 64506	Liquid	Lice and keds	Spray or pour-on	2	Repeat at 30-day intervals on sheep and nonlactating goats
Ivermectin Ivomec drench	Merial Limited 2100 Ronson Road Iselin, NJ 08830-3077	Drench	Nasal bots	Oral drench	11	No label direction for goats
Permethrin Atroban or Expar	Schering-Plough Animal Health Corp. 1095 Morris Ave. Union, NJ 07083	Liquid	Keds, lice, ticks, and various flies	Spray	0	Repeat applications as needed but not more often than every 14 days; no label directions for goats
	Schering-Plough	Pour-on	Lice and keds	Pour-on	0	Repeat applications as needed but not more often than every 14 days; labeled for sheep only
Boss pour-on	Schering-Plough	Pour-on	Lice and keds	Pour-on	0	Pour along back; repeat treatment as needed but not more often than every 14 days; labeled for sheep only
Ectiban	Various suppliers	Liquid	Lice and keds	Spray	0	Repeat applications as needed but not more often than every 14 days
GardStar 40% EC	Y-TEX Corp.	Liquid	Horn flies, face flies, stable flies, house flies, horse flies, deer flies, black flies, mosquitoes, eye gnats, mange mites, scabies mites, ticks, lice, and sheep keds	Spray	0	Repeat application as needed
Permectrin II	Numerous suppliers	Liquid	Lice, ticks, and blowflies	Spray	0	No label directions for goats
		Wettable powder	Lice, ticks, and blowflies	Spray	0	No label directions for goats

Table 4
SOME COMMON PRODUCTS USED FOR EXTERNAL PARASITE CONTROL ON SWINE

Product	Company and Address	Marketed Formulation	Pest	Method of Application	Withdrawal Period Before Slaughter (days)	Comments
Coumaphos	Bayer Corp. Agriculture Division P.O. Box 390 Shawnee Mission, KS 66201	Wettable powder	Lice, ticks, horn flies and screwworms	Spray	0	Repeat as necessary
	Bayer Corp.	Liquid emulsifiable livestock insecticide and livestock insecticide spray	Lice	Spray	0	Apply to complete wetting
Amitraz Point-Guard	Hoechst Roussel Vet Box 2500 Somerville, NJ 08876-1258	Pour-on	Mites and lice	Apply to back and in each ear	7	Consult label for control and maintenance program
Taktic E.C.	Hoechst Roussel Vet	Liquid	Mites and lice	Spray	3	Do not treat more than 4 times per year
Fenthion Tiguvon	Bayer Corp.	Ready to use pour-on	Lice	Pour-on	14	Pour uniformly along the animal's back
Fenvalerate Ectrin	Boehringer Ingelheim 2621 North Belt Highway St. Joseph, MO 64506	Liquid	Lice and mites	Spray or pour-on (lice only)	1	Pour uniformly along the animal's back
Ivermectin Ivomec	Merial Limited 2100 Ronson Road Iselin, NJ 08830-3077	Injectable liquid	Lice and mites	Inject subcutaneously	18	Reinfestation is possible from hatching eggs
Premix	Merial Limited	In-feed	Lice and mites	Oral, in feed	5	Formulated for use in swine only
Permethrin Atroban or Expar	Schering-Plough Animal Health Corp. 1095 Morris Ave. Union, NJ 07083	Liquid	Lice and mites	Spray	5	Repeat application as needed, but not more often than every 14 days
Ectiban	Various suppliers	Dust	Lice	Direct application	0	A second treatment in 14 days is recommended
GardStar	Y-TEX Corp. 1825 Big Horn Ave. Cody, WY 82414	Liquid (EC)	Lice and mange mites	Spray or dip	5	For mange, spray pen floors, sides, and bedding; repeat at 14 days
Permectrin II	Various suppliers	Liquid	Lice, ticks, horn flies, and mites	Spray	5	Re-treat after 4–6 wk
	Boehringer Ingelheim Animal Health 2621 North Belt Highway St. Josephs, MO 64506-2002	Wettable powder	Lice, ticks, horn flies, and mites	Spray, paint, or dip	5	Re-treat after 4–6 wk
	Anchor Division Boehringer Ingelheim	Dust	Lice, ticks, horn flies, and mites	Direct application	5	Re-treat after 4–6 wk
Phosmet Prolate	Starbar/Sandoz Animal Health A Division of Sandoz Agro, Inc. 1300 East Toughy Ave. Des Plaines, IL 60018	Liquid	Lice and mites	Spray	1	Repeat in 14 days if needed
Del-Phos	Schering-Plough	Liquid	Lice and sarcoptic mange mites	Spray	1	One treatment is usually effective; second treatment may be applied 14 days after first treatment
Tetrachlorvinphos Rabon	Boehringer Ingelheim	Wettable powder	Lice	Spray	0	Repeat in 2 wk if necessary
		Dust	Lice	Direct application and on bedding	0	Repeat in 2 wk if necessary
		Oral larvicide premix	House flies	Mixed into feed	0	Mix uniformly into daily feed

Index

Note: Page numbers in *italics* refer to illustrations; page numbers followed by t refer to tables.

Q